THE LIBRARY
THE LEARNING AND DEVELOPMENT CENTRE
THE CALDERDALE ROYAL HOSPITAL
HALIFAX HX3 0PW

£195.00

D1423220

# Expert | CONSULT

## Online + Print

### Online access activation instructions

**This Expert Consult** title comes with access to the complete contents online. **Activate your access today** by following these simple instructions:

1. Gently scratch off the surface of the sticker below, using the edge of a coin, to reveal your **activation code**.

2. Visit **www.expertconsultbook.com** and click on the **"Register"** button.

3. **Enter your activation code** along with the other information requested...and begin enjoying your access.

**It's that easy!** For technical assistance, email **online.help@elsevier.com** or **call 800-401-9962** (inside the US) or **+1-314-995-3200** (outside the US).

S8C7MC6

# Urologic Surgical Pathology

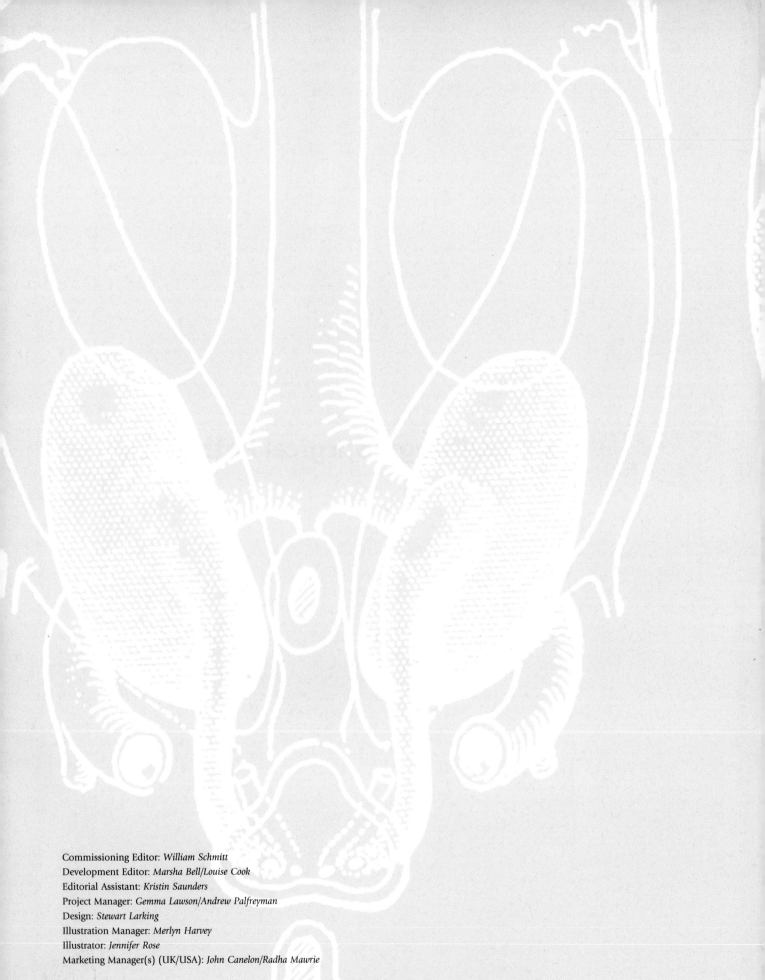

Commissioning Editor: *William Schmitt*
Development Editor: *Marsha Bell/Louise Cook*
Editorial Assistant: *Kristin Saunders*
Project Manager: *Gemma Lawson/Andrew Palfreyman*
Design: *Stewart Larking*
Illustration Manager: *Merlyn Harvey*
Illustrator: *Jennifer Rose*
Marketing Manager(s) (UK/USA): *John Canelon/Radha Mawrie*

Second Edition

# Urologic Surgical Pathology

## David G. Bostwick MD, MBA

Chief Medical Officer
Bostwick Laboratories
Glen Allen, VA, USA

## Liang Cheng MD

Professor of Pathology and Urology
Chief of Genitourinary Pathology Division
Director of Molecular Pathology Laboratory
Department of Pathology and Laboratory Medicine and Clarian Pathology
Laboratory
Indiana University School of Medicine
Indianapolis, IN, USA

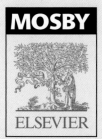

MOSBY

ELSEVIER

## MOSBY
ELSEVIER

is an imprint of Elsevier Inc.

© 2008, Elsevier Inc. All rights reserved.

First published 2008
First edition 1996

No part of this publication may be reproduced or transmitted in any form or by any means, electronic or mechanical, including photocopying, recording, or any information storage and retrieval system, without permission in writing from the publisher. Permissions may be sought directly from Elsevier's Rights Department: phone: (+1) 215 239 3804 (US) or (+44) 1865 843830 (UK); fax: (+44) 1865 853333; e-mail: healthpermissions@elsevier.com. You may also complete your request on-line via the Elsevier website at http://www.elsevier.com/permissions.

ISBN: 978-0-323-01970-5

**British Library Cataloguing in Publication Data**
A catalogue record for this book is available from the British Library

**Library of Congress Cataloging in Publication Data**
A catalog record for this book is available from the Library of Congress

**Notice**
Medical knowledge is constantly changing. Standard safety precautions must be followed, but as new research and clinical experience broaden our knowledge, changes in treatment and drug therapy may become necessary or appropriate. Readers are advised to check the most current product information provided by the manufacturer of each drug to be administered to verify the recommended dose, the method and duration of administration, and contraindications. It is the responsibility of the practitioner, relying on experience and knowledge of the patient, to determine dosages and the best treatment for each individual patient. Neither the Publisher nor the author assume any liability for any injury and/or damage to persons or property arising from this publication.

*The Publisher*

**ELSEVIER** your source for books, journals and multimedia in the health sciences

**www.elsevierhealth.com**

Working together to grow
libraries in developing countries

www.elsevier.com | www.bookaid.org | www.sabre.org

ELSEVIER    BOOK AID International    Sabre Foundation

The publisher's policy is to use **paper manufactured from sustainable forests**

Printed in China
Last digit is the print number: 9 8 7 6 5 4 3 2 1

# Contents

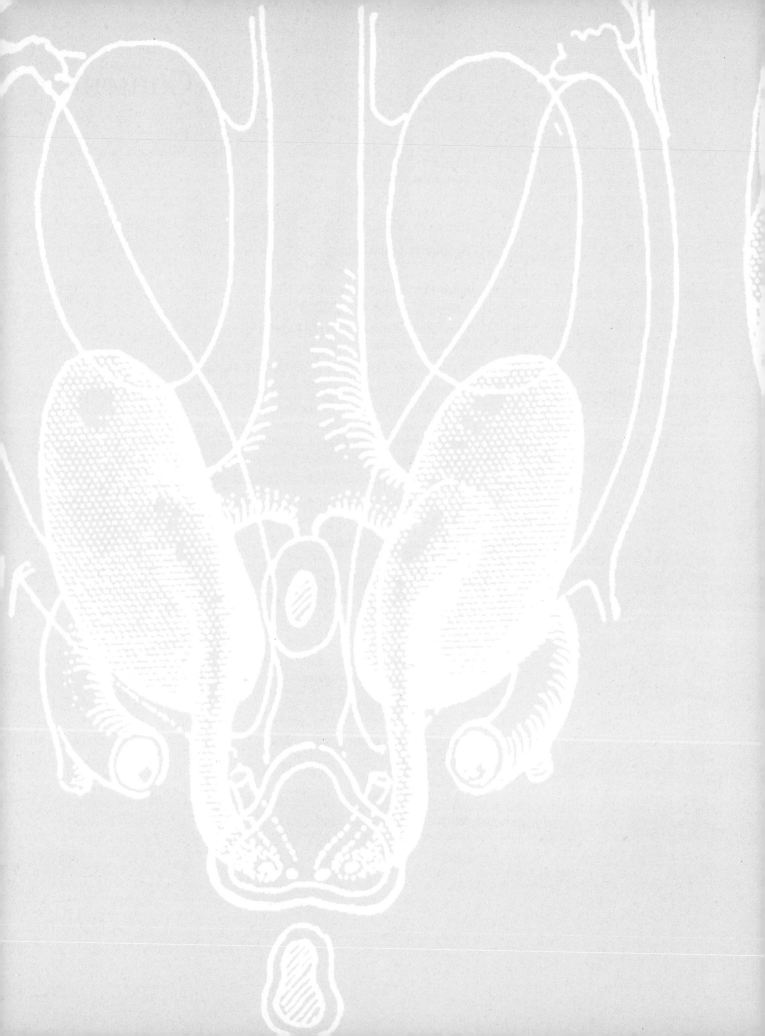

# Preface to Second Edition of Urologic Surgical Pathology

In the 12 years since the publication of the first edition of *Urologic Surgical Pathology*, great strides have been made in our understanding of urologic diseases. Many clinically important new histopathologic entities have been described or more fully defined in virtually every genitourinary organ. Numerous clinically important diagnostic and prognostic markers have entered routine practice, including alpha-methylacyl-CoA racemase, the most widely discussed biomarker in surgical pathology in this century. Genetic testing for the early detection of bladder and prostate cancer and the molecular classification of renal cell carcinomas has become increasingly important. This is an age of enlightenment in urologic surgical pathology, and we have attempted to capture the sense of excitement herein.

Our specialty of surgical pathology continues to evolve. The emergence of personalized medicine has created a paradigm shift in diagnostic and prognostic biomarker analysis. Diagnostic tests are now linked to individualized treatments. The dream of digital imaging is slowly being realized; high resolution images are now routinely captured and transmitted across the internet for multiple purposes. Central pathology review of clinical trial cases has become common practice, and central review protocols will likely be standardized in the near future. The accuracy of predictive outcome models for individual patients continues to be improved. New algorithms, nomograms, neural networks, and other models emerge virtually every month. Further, evidence-based practice with an emphasis on levels of scientific evidence is replacing the "intuitive" practice of medicine, resulting in more consistent outcomes.

Throughout this renaissance in the classification and diagnosis of urologic diseases and in the prediction of individual patient outcome, the histopathologic examination of tissue and cells remains the gold standard. Today's surgical pathologist in any part of the world finds urologic specimens to be an increasingly important part of everyday sign-out. The expectation for excellence in diagnosis remains very high. It is with this understanding that we have produced our second edition.

This book is intended chiefly for use by surgical pathologists in their daily practice. The numerous comments and suggestions from readers of the first edition have been carefully considered and incorporated into the current effort. The text has expanded more than 30%, and the number of full-color illustrations now exceeds 1200. Two new chapters have been added (Urine Cytology and Fine Needle Aspiration of the Kidney) to reflect increasing emphasis on cellular diagnosis in urologic pathology. We have remained true to our purpose of providing a framework for comparison, evaluation, and integration into clinical practice of the evolving urologic diagnosis. The emphasis remains on the practical aspects of diagnostic pathology.

We are exceedingly grateful to our contributing colleagues for sharing their knowledge and experience. We continue to solicit constructive criticism to ensure greater usability in future editions.

David G. Bostwick, MD, MBA
Liang Cheng, MD
March, 2008

# Contributors List

**Urologic Surgical Pathology, 2nd Edition**

**Mahul B. Amin, M.D.**
Professor and Chairman
Department of Pathology and Laboratory Medicine
Cedars-Sinai Medical Center
Los Angeles, CA
USA

**Alberto G. Ayala, M.D.**
Professor of Pathology
Weill Medical College of Cornell University
Deputy Chairman, Department of Pathology
The Methodist Hospital
Ashbel-Smith Professor Emeritus of Pathology
The University of Texas M.D. Anderson Cancer Center
Houston, TX
USA

**Stephen M. Bonsib, M.D.**
Albert G. and Harriet G. Smith Endowed Professor and Chair
Department of Pathology
Louisiana State University Heath Sciences Center
Shreveport, LA
USA

**David G. Bostwick, M.D., MBA**
Chief Medical Officer
Bostwick Laboratories
Glen Allen, VA
USA

**Liang Cheng, M.D.**
Professor of Pathology and Urology
Chief of Genitourinary Pathology Division
Director of Molecular Pathology Laboratory
Department of Pathology and Laboratory Medicine and
Clarian Pathology Laboratory
Indiana University School of Medicine
Indianapolis, IN
USA

**Deloar Hossain, M.D.**
Associate Medical Director
Bostwick Laboratories
Glen Allen, VA
USA

**Janet L. Johnston, B.A., CT (ASCP)**
Director of Advanced Cytodiagnostics
Bostwick Laboratories
Glen Allen, VA
USA

**Kyu-Rae Kim, M.D., Ph.D.**
Professor of Pathology
Asan Medical Center
The University of Ulsan College of Medicine
Seoul
Korea

**Ernest E. Lack, M.D.**
Director of Anatomic Pathology
Washington Hospital Center
Washington, DC
USA

**Antonio Lopez-Beltran, M.D., Ph.D.**
Professor of Anatomic Pathology
Unit of Anatomic Pathology
Department of Surgery
Cordoba University School of Medicine
Cordoba
Spain

**Gregory T. MacLennan, M.D.**
Professor of Pathology, Urology and Oncology
University Hospitals of Cleveland
Institute of Pathology, Case Western Reserve University
Cleveland, OH
USA

**Isabelle Meiers, M.D.**
Chief of Histopathology Department
University Hospital Lewisham
London
UK

**Rodolfo Montironi, M.D.**
Professor of Pathology
Section of Pathological Anatomy
School of Medicine, Polytechnic University of the Marche
Region
United Hospitals
Ancona
Italy

**John F. Morrow, M.D.**
Associate Medical Director
Bostwick Laboratories
Glen Allen, VA
USA

**Manuel Nistal, M.D., Ph.D.**
Head of Service of Pathology, Hospital La Paz
Professor of Histology, Departamento de Morfología
Universidad Autómoma de Madrid
Madrid
Spain

**Ricardo Paniagua, M.D., Ph.D.**
Professor of Cell Biology
Department of Cell Biology and Genetics
University of Alcalá
Madrid
Spain

**Junqi Qian, M.D.**
Director of Molecular Diagnostics
Bostwick Laboratories
Glen Allen, VA
USA

**Andrew A. Renshaw, M.D.**
Staff Pathologist
Department of Pathology
Baptist Hospital of Miami
Miami, FL
USA

**Victor Reuter, M.D.**
Professor of Pathology
Weil Medical College of Cornell University
Attending Pathologist and Vice-Chair
Memorial Sloan-Kettering Cancer Center
New York, NY
USA

**Jae Y. Ro, M.D., Ph.D.**
Professor of Pathology
Director of Surgical Pathology
Department of Pathology
The Methodist Hospital
Weill Medical College of Cornell University
Houston, TX
USA

**Thomas M. Ulbright, M.D.**
Lawrence M. Roth Professor of Pathology
Director of Anatomic Pathology
Department of Pathology and Laboratory Medicine and
Clarian Pathology Laboratory
Indiana University School of Medicine
Indianapolis, IN
USA

**Jacqueline A. Wieneke, M.D.**
Chief, Division of Otorhinolaryngic-Head &
Neck Pathology
Staff Pathologist
Department of Endocrine and Otorhinolaryngic-Head &
Neck Pathology
Armed Forces Institute of Pathology
Washington, DC
USA

**Robert H. Young, M.D.**
Robert E. Scully Professor of Pathology
Harvard Medical School
Pathologist, James Homer Wright Pathology Laboratories
Massachusetts General Hospital
Boston, MA
USA

# CHAPTER 1

# Non-neoplastic diseases of the kidney

Stephen M. Bonsib

*Study with me, then, a few things in the spirit of truth alone so we may establish the manner of Nature's operation. For this essay which I plan, will shed light upon the structure of the kidney. Do not stop to question whether these ideas are new or old, but ask, more properly, whether they harmonize with Nature. I never reached my idea of the structure of the kidney by the aid of books, but by the long and varied use of the microscope. I have gotten the rest by the deductions of reason, slowly, and with an open mind, as is my custom.*[1]

**Marcello Malpighi,**
**1666**

In keeping with the spirit of Marcello Malpighi, this chapter aspires to reveal 'the manner of Nature's operations' as it affects the kidney.[1] However, unlike Malpighi, today's knowledge draws extensively upon the labors, discoveries, and insights of investigators over the last four centuries.

Our knowledge of the normal structure and function of the kidney has been acquired over centuries of scholarly effort. We have come a long way since Aristotle taught that urine was formed by the bladder and that kidneys were present 'not of actual necessity, but as matters of greater finish and perfection.'[1] The foundations of urology were established in the 16th century by Leonardo da Vinci and Vesalius, who provided the first accurate and detailed drawings of the female and male genitourinary tracts (Fig. 1-1).[2,3] Over 300 years passed before William Bowman, in 1842, coupled intravascular dye injection with microscopic examination to demonstrate the structural organization of the nephron and its vascular supply (Fig. 1-2).[4,5] Bowman's observations provided morphologic support for Malpighi's 17th-century speculation of a filtration function for the malpighian body (the glomerulus).[1] Sixty years later, embryologic development of the nephron was demonstrated by Huber in a thin-section serial reconstruction study of embryos (Fig. 1-3). Huber's observations were refined and elegantly illustrated by Brödel in 1907.[6,7] Potter and Osathanondh[8–11] validated the findings in a series of microdissection studies of developing kidneys that were published in the 1960s.

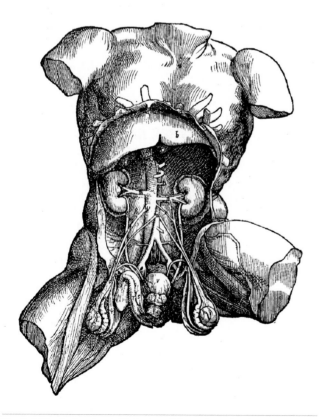

**Fig. 1-1** Vesalius' anatomic illustration of the male genitourinary tract published in 1543. Note that the left kidney is placed lower than the right. (From Murphy LJT. The history of urology, Springfield, MA: Charles C. Thomas, 1972; with permission.)

The ultrastructural features and immunohistochemical profiles of the normal kidney and many diseases were elucidated in the 1970s and 1980s following refinement of the percutaneous biopsy technique and advances in morphologic analysis. Today, we are on the threshold of discovering the genetic basis of many mechanisms that mediate normal and abnormal renal development and physiology.

# Embryologic development and normal structure

This chapter begins with a brief review of the embryology and normal gross and microscopic structure of the kidney. For more in-depth coverage of these topics several excellent resources are available.[12–15]

The development of the urinary and genital tracts is closely related (Fig. 1-4). Both develop from paired longitudinal cords of tissue lateral to the aorta, known as the intermediate mesoderm.[12,13] From the portion caudal to the seventh somite, known as the nephrogenic mesoderm (or nephrogenic cord), three nephronic structures develop in quick succession: the pronephros, the mesonephros, and the metanephros. Although the pronephros and the mesonephros are transient organs, they are crucial for proper development of the urinary and reproductive tracts.

## Pronephros

The first embryologic derivative of the nephrogenic cord is the pronephros, a structure that is functional only in the lowest forms of fish. It arises from the cranial portion of the mesonephric cord during the third week of gestation (1.7 mm stage). Approximately seven pairs of tubules form, only to regress 2 weeks later (Fig. 1-4). The pronephros is important because the pronephric tubules grow caudally and fuse with the next pronephric unit, giving rise to the pronephric duct, now called the mesonephric duct.

## Mesonephros

Cells of the mesonephric duct continue to proliferate caudally (Fig. 1-4) and begin to form the mesonephric kidney during the fourth week of gestation (4 mm). The mesonephros is a highly differentiated structure and is the functional kidney of higher fish and amphibians. Portions of the mesonephric kidney can be easily identified in small embryos (1–3 cm in size) that are occasionally encountered in surgical specimens such as those from ectopic pregnancies (Fig. 1-5).

The mesonephric kidney consists of approximately 40 pairs of nephrons. The cranial nephrons regress sequentially while caudal nephrons form, with 7–15 nephrons being functional at all times (Fig. 1-4). The nephrons are induced in a fashion analogous to that of their metanephric counterparts. A fully developed mesonephric nephron consists of a glomerulus connected to the mesonephric duct by a convoluted proximal tubule (Fig. 1-6A). The glomerulus is vascularized by capillaries that branch from small arterioles originating from the aorta, and its efferent arteriole empties into the posterior cardinal vein. The

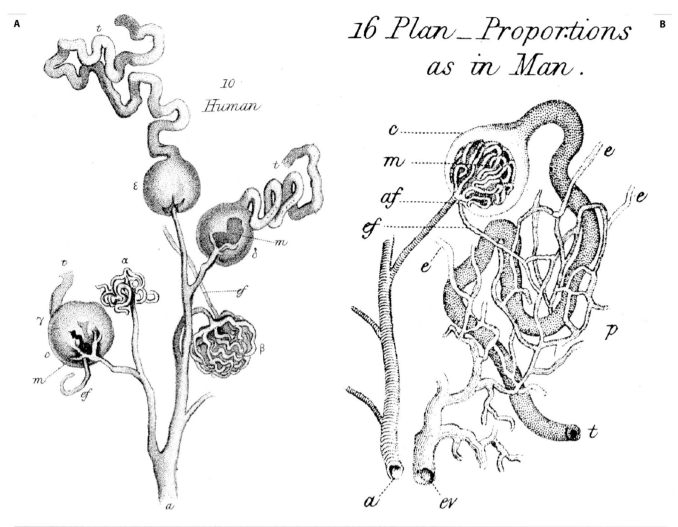

**A**

*t*

*10*
*Human*

*ε*

*t*

*m*

*δ*

*ef*

*τ*

*α*

*γ*

*c*

*m*

*ef*

*β*

*a*

**B**

*16 Plan _ Proportions*
*as in Man .*

*c*

*m*

*af*

*ef*

*e*

*e*

*e*

*p*

*t*

*a*

*ev*

**Fig. 1-2** William Bowman's illustration of the vascular supply to glomeruli and the relationship of the efferent arteriole to the convoluted tubules. (From Bowman W. On the structure and use of the malpighian bodies of the kidney, with observations on the circulation through that gland. Philos Trans Roy Soc Lond Biol 1842; 132: 57; with permission.)

glomerulus appears to filter plasma. Its tubule possesses a brush border and appears capable of nutrient resorption, and concentration and dilution of urine. The mesonephric kidney remains functional until the end of the fourth month of gestation.

## Metanephros

The metanephric kidney is the product of a complex orchestration of embryologic processes. While the collecting system and renal pyramids are forming there is simultaneous induction of thousands of nephrons, and neurovascular and lymphatic components ramify in a carefully organized architecture throughout the cortex and medulla.

While the metanephric kidney is forming, substantial changes also are occurring in the adjacent müllerian and mesonephric ducts (Fig. 1-4) proximal to the origin of the ampullary bud.[12] Following degeneration of mesonephric nephrons in males, the persisting mesonephric duct develops into male genital secretory structures: epididymis, vas deferens, seminal vesicle, and ejaculatory duct. In females,

the müllerian ducts form the fallopian tubes, uterus, and proximal vagina while the mesonephric ducts largely regress, although several embryologic remnant structures persist, including the epoöphoron, paroöphoron, and Gartner's ducts.

Formation of the adult metanephric kidney begins during the fifth and sixth weeks of gestation (4–5 mm), after the mesonephric duct has established communication with the urogenital sinus. A diverticulum, known as the ampullary (or ureteric) bud, forms on its posterior medial aspect (Fig. 1-4), establishing contact with the sacral portion of the nephrogenic mesoderm, the nephrogenic blastema. A complex reciprocal inductive process occurs, resulting in dichotomous ampullary bud branching and nephron induction, eventually culminating in the adult metanephric kidney. The metanephros is therefore a product of two embryonic derivatives: the nephrons are of blastemal origin whereas the ureter, pelvis, calyces, cortical, and medullary collecting ducts are derived from the ampullary bud.

Upon contact with metanephric blastema, the ampullary bud undergoes a rapid sequence of dichotomous branching

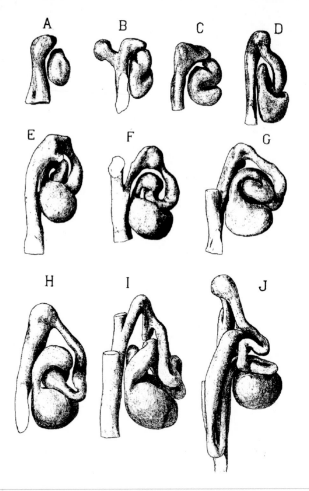

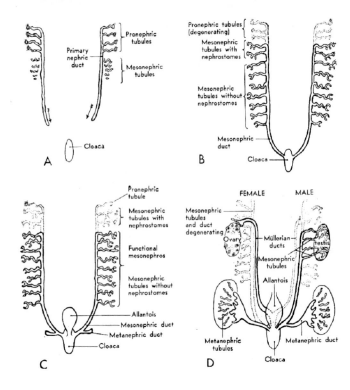

**Fig. 1-4** Diagram illustrating the relationship between reproductive tract and urinary tract development. (From Patton BM. Human embryology. New York: McGraw Hill, 1968; with permission.)

**Fig. 1-3** Wax model serial reconstruction of nephron differentiation by Huber. (From Huber GC. On the development and shape of uriniferous tubules of certain of the higher mammals. Am J Anat 1905; 4: 29; with permission.)

and fusion, forming the renal collecting system by the 14th week.[8] The initial two branches form the renal pelvis, the third to sixth branches form the major and minor calyces, and the sixth to 11th branches form the papillary ducts (Fig. 1-7). Ampullary bud branching is more rapid in the upper and lower poles, resulting in more numerous calyces and papillae in those regions.

While the collecting system is forming, nephron induction has already begun (Fig. 1-5). The kidneys move into the flanks owing to a combination of migration out of the pelvis and rapid caudal growth of the embryo (Fig. 1-8). The kidney also rotates from its original position with the pelvis anterior, to its final position with the pelvis medial.[7] By week 13 or 14, the minor calyces and renal pyramids are well formed and the lobar architecture can be appreciated grossly (Figs 1-9, 1-10). At this time, the cortex contains several generations of nephrons and the lateral portions of adjacent lobes begin to merge to form the columns of Bertin.

By weeks 20–22, the renal lobes are well formed and the kidney is a miniature of the adult kidney (Fig. 1-11). The ampullae (or collecting ducts at this time) cease branching but continue to lengthen.[9,10] As they lengthen, they induce arcades of four to seven nephrons that are connected to the

collecting duct by a connecting tubule (Fig. 1-12). Additional groups of three to seven nephrons then form, each attached directly to a collecting duct without a connecting tubule. Therefore, each cortical collecting duct has 10–14 generations of nephrons attached, with the most recently formed and least mature nephrons located beneath the renal capsule.

## Nephron differentiation

The formation of individual nephrons begins as early as 7 weeks of gestation, resulting in a limited degree of 'renal function' by 9 weeks. In the subcapsular nephrogenic zone of the immature kidney (Fig. 1-13), the sequence of nephron induction can be observed in its various stages of completion. Wax models made by Huber and the drawing by Brödel (Figs 1-3, 1-14) provide a three-dimensional perspective for understanding the cellular events visible in Figure 1-13.

An individual nephron begins to form when the metanephric blastema aggregates adjacent to the ampullary bud to form a hollow vesicle.[9–11] The molecular basis for this event is complex and appears to involve growth factors, adhesion molecules, matrix components, and other regulatory proteins.[16–19] The cells within the vesicle grow differentially, resulting in elongation and the formation of two indentations creating an S-shaped structure with three segments. The upper and middle segments are destined to become the proximal and distal tubules. They form tubular structures and establish communication with each other and

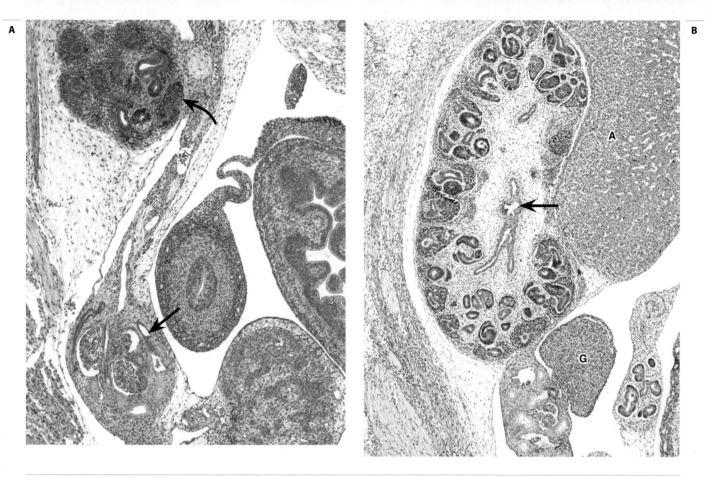

**Fig. 1-5 (A)** An embryo of 7 weeks' gestation showing initial induction of the metanephric kidney (curved arrow) and glomeruli of the mesonephric kidney (arrow). **(B)** Embryo of 12 weeks' gestation, showing a metanephric kidney with a rudimentary collecting system (arrow) and active nephrogenesis. The adrenal gland (A), gonad (G), and mesonephric kidney are also visible.

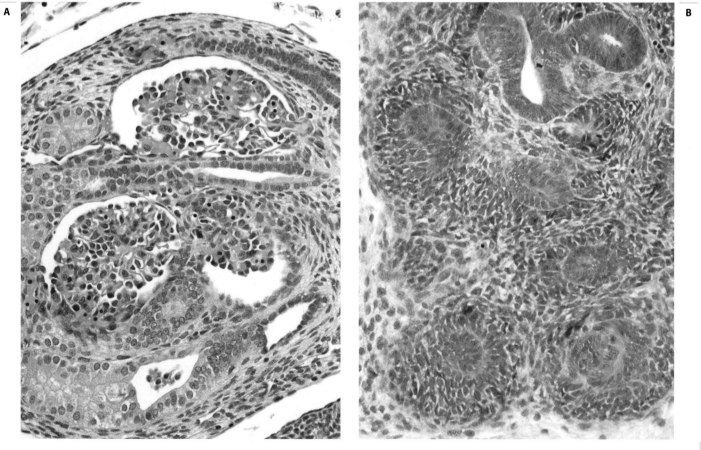

**Fig. 1-6 (A)** A portion of the mesonephric kidney (from Fig. 1-5A) showing well-developed glomeruli and proximal tubules. **(B)** Metanephric kidney (from Fig. 1-5A) beginning to form, showing condensations of cells destined to form glomeruli.

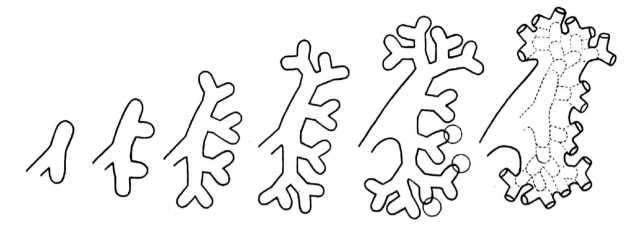

**Fig. 1-7** Development of the renal pelvis. Diagram showing branches of ureteral bud. Circles indicate possible locations of minor calyces at level of third-, fourth-, or fifth-generation branches. Figure at right indicates ureteral bud branches that may dilate to form renal pelvis. (From Osathanondth V, Potter EL. Development of the human kidney as shown by microdissection III. Formation and interrelationship of collecting tubules and nephrons. Arch Pathol 19643; 76: 61; with permission.)

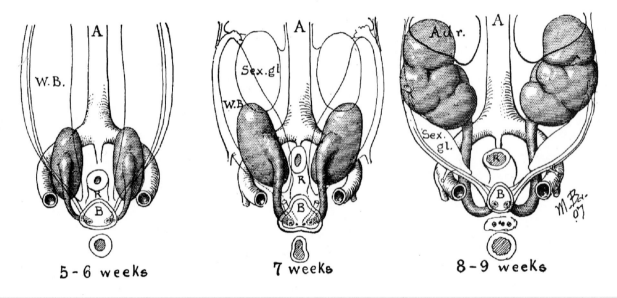

**Fig. 1-8** A 1907 diagram by Max Brödel showing the ascent and medial rotation of the kidney. (From Kelly HA, Burnam CF. Diseases of kidneys, ureters and bladder. New York: Appleton, Century Crofts,1914; with permission.)

the collecting duct. A capillary grows into the lower indentation and branches, and there is broadening and separation of the lower segment into two cell layers, forming a podocyte-invested and vascularized glomerular tuft within Bowman's capsule.

Cells of the upper layer continue to proliferate to form a connecting duct and the distal convoluted tubule, while cells of the middle limb produce the proximal convoluted tubule and the limb of Henle. Finally, the limb of Henle grows down along the collecting duct to form the medullary rays. Nephrogenesis is usually complete by 32–36 weeks' gestation. Maturation occurs beyond this period and continues until adulthood, resulting in renal enlargement that reflects elongation and enlargement of the tubular portions of the nephron.

## Gross anatomy

The kidneys are paired retroperitoneal organs that normally extend from the 12th thoracic vertebra to the third lumbar vertebra. The upper poles are tilted slightly toward the midline, and the right kidney is slightly lower and shorter than the left. The average adult kidney is 11–12 cm long, 5–7 cm wide, 2.5–3 cm thick, and weighs 125–170 g in males and 115–155 g in females.[7,12,15] The combined mass of the kidneys correlates with body surface area. Its volume can increase or decrease by 15–40% with major fluctuations in blood pressure, hydration, or interstitial expansion by edema.

The posterior surfaces are flatter than the anterior and the medial surface is concave, with a 3 cm slit-like space called the hilum. The hilum is the vestibule through which pass the collecting system, nerves, and vessels. In the adult, these structures are invested by fat within the renal sinus.

The subcapsular surface of the renal cortex may be smooth and featureless or may show grooves corresponding to indi-vidual renal lobes (Fig. 1-15). Persistence of distinct fetal lobes is common and is a normal anatomic variant. In some kidneys, three zones are created by two shallow superficial grooves that radiate from the hilum to the lateral border (Fig. 1-16). The three regions are the upper pole, middle zone, and lower pole, and usually reflect regions drained by the three lobar veins.

The normal adult kidney has a minimum of 10–14 lobes, each composed of a central conical medullary pyramid sur-rounded by a cap of cortex (Fig. 1-17). Often, there are six lobes in the upper pole and four lobes each in the middle zone and lower pole. However, there is substantial variability in the number of lobes in the adult kidney and in their visibility when the renal capsule is removed.

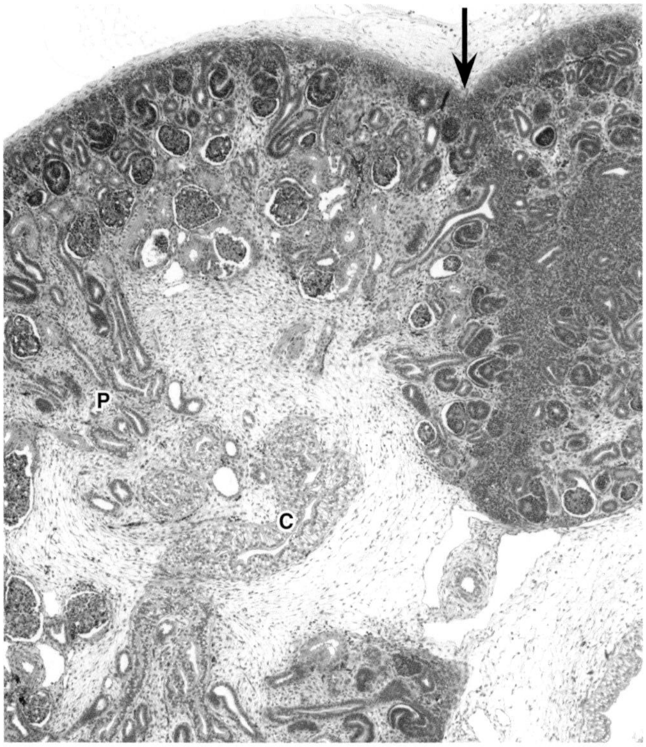

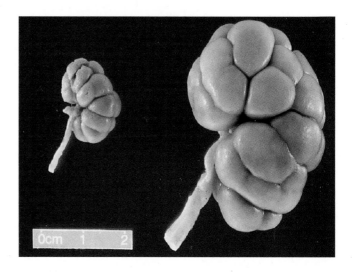

**Fig. 1-11** A 22-week fetal kidney (left) and a 40-week term kidney (right) showing distinct fetal lobes.

**Fig. 1-9** Kidney from a 13-week fetus (compare with Fig. 1-10) showing a renal lobe with a pyramid (P) and the collecting system (C). There is fusion of adjacent lobes forming columns of Bertin (arrow).

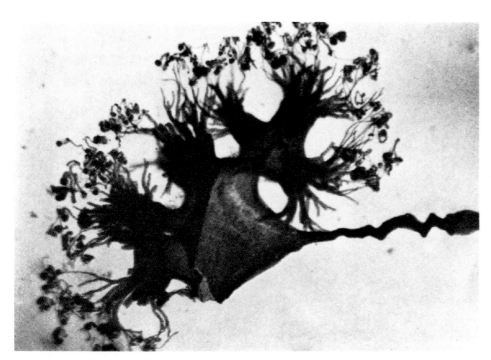

**Fig. 1-10** Microdissected 13-week kidney showing collecting system, renal pyramids, and several generations of glomeruli. Most of the tubules have been removed. (From Osathanondth V, Potter EL. Development of the human kidney as shown by microdissection III. Formation and interrelationship of collecting tubules and nephrons. Arch Pathol 1963; 76: 61; with permission.)

The renal parenchyma consists of cortex and medulla, which are grossly quite distinct (Fig. 1-17). The renal cortex is the nephron-containing parenchyma. It forms a 1.0 cm layer beneath the renal capsule and extends down between the renal pyramids forming the columns of Bertin. The mid-plane of a column of Bertin is the line of fusion of two renal lobes. The medulla consists of renal pyramids and is divided into an outer medulla and the inner medulla or papilla (Fig. 1-17). The outer medulla receives input from nephrons in the overlying cortex and nephrons in the adjacent half of a column of Bertin. The papilla protrudes into a minor calyx. Its tip contains from 20 to 70 openings of the papillary collecting ducts (Bellini's ducts).[14,15]

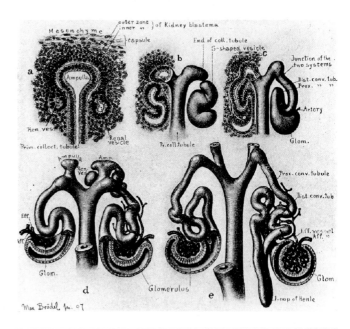

**Fig. 1-14** 1907 illustration by Max Brödel showing the sequence of nephron induction. (From Kelly HA, Burnam CF. Diseases of kidneys, ureters and bladder. New York: Appleton, Century Crofts, 1914; with permission.)

**Fig. 1-12** Kidney showing arrangement of nephrons at birth. **(A)** usual pattern; **(B)** possible variations. (From Osathanondth V, Potter EL. Development of the human kidney as shown by microdissection III. Formation and interrelationship of collecting tubules and nephrons. Arch Pathol 1963; 76: 61; with permission.)

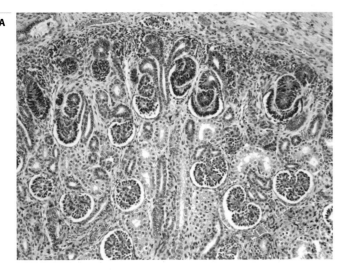

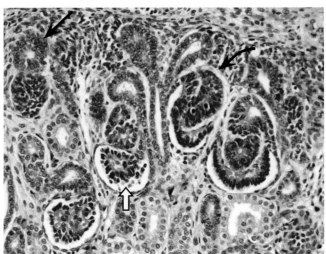

**Fig. 1-13** Nephrogenic zone of a 14-week kidney. Notice ampullary bud and hollow vesicles (arrow), early S-phase (curved arrow), primitive glomerular tuft (open arrow), and increasingly mature glomeruli.

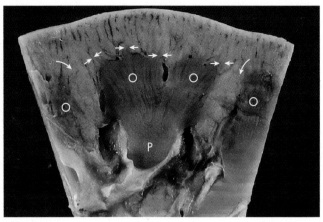

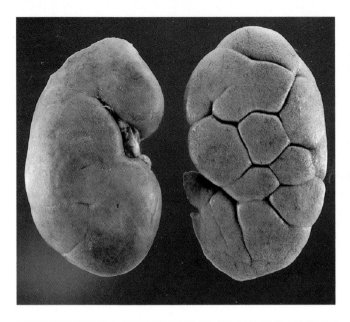

**Fig. 1-17** This renal lobe shows the cortical medullary rays. The columns of Bertin invest the outer medulla (O), while the papilla (P) or inner medulla is nestled within a minor calyx.

**Fig. 1-15** Two adult kidneys with capsules removed showing subtle fetal lobation (left) and prominent fetal lobation (right).

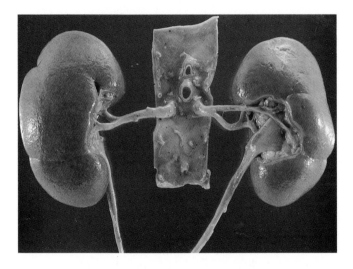

**Fig. 1-16** Kidneys showing two grooves defining the renal poles. In each kidney an anterior and posterior division of the renal artery is visible. The left kidney (right side) is incompletely rotated.

The arterial supply to the kidney follows a general overall blueprint, and knowledge of its details is useful when evaluating lesions in a kidney affected by vascular abnormalities.[20–22] In 1901, Brödel first appreciated the distinctive renovascular segmentation of the kidney.[20] (The nomenclature used here was established by Graves in 1954.[21]) The main renal artery arises from the aorta and divides into an anterior and a posterior division, and five segmental arteries are usually derived from these two divisions (Figs 1-16, 1-18).

The anterior division supplies most of the kidney and often divides into four segmental arteries: the apical, upper, middle, and lower segmental branches. The apical and lower segmental arteries supply the anterior and posterior aspects of the upper and lower poles, respectively (Fig. 1-18). In 20–30% of kidneys, one or both of these arteries arise separately from the aorta, forming supernumerary arteries (also known as aberrant, accessory, or polar arteries). The posterior division becomes the posterior segmental artery. It passes behind the pelvis and supplies the middle two-thirds of the posterior surface. The five segmental arteries and all of their branches are end arteries with no collateral blood flow. Thus, occlusion of a segmental artery or any of its subsequent branches results in infarction of the zone of parenchyma it supplies.[22]

From segmental arteries, the interlobar arteries, arcuate arteries, interlobular arteries, and arterioles are sequentially derived. A segmental artery branches within the renal sinus, giving rise to several interlobar arteries. An interlobar artery enters the parenchyma in a column of Bertin between two renal pyramids (i.e., at the junction of two lobes) and forms a splay of six to eight arcuate arteries. The arcuate arteries course along the corticomedullary junction and terminate at the mid-point of a renal lobe. At perpendicular or slightly oblique angles, the interlobular arteries arise from an arcuate artery and may branch as they pass through the cortex toward the renal capsule. The interlobular arteries course between medullary rays and are encircled by tiers of five to six glomeruli that they supply with afferent arterioles (Fig. 1-19). The glomerular efferent arteriole forms a portal system of capillaries that supplies the adjacent tubules that arise from more than one glomerulus (see Fig. 1-2B).

The renal medulla has a dual blood supply.[23] Its principal supply arises from the efferent arterioles of the juxtamedullary glomeruli that course directly into the medulla, forming the vasa rectae (Fig. 1-20). In addition, as an interlobar artery courses along a minor calyx it gives rise to several spiral arteries that supply arterioles to the papillary tip. These arterioles anastomose freely with arterioles from the opposite side, forming a plexus around the ducts of Bellini.

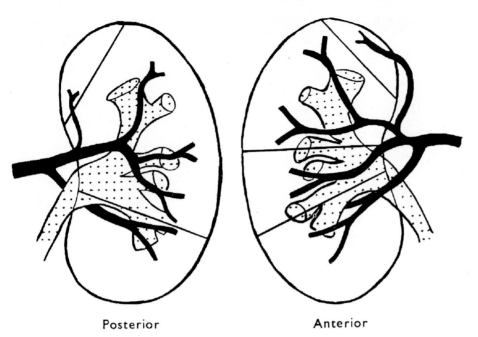

**Fig. 1-18** A diagram of the most common arterial pattern of the kidney showing main renal artery, anterior and posterior divisions, segmental, interlobar, and arcuate arteries. (From Graves FT. The anatomy of the intrarenal arteries and its application to segmental resection of the kidney. Br J Surg 1954; 42: 133; with permission.)

Posterior          Anterior

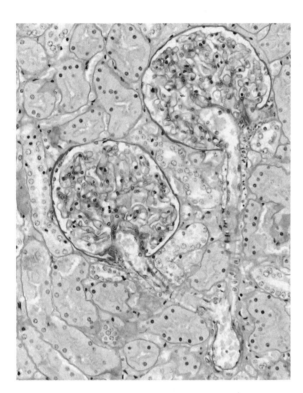

**Fig. 1-19** The interlobular artery supplies arterioles to glomeruli. PAS stain.

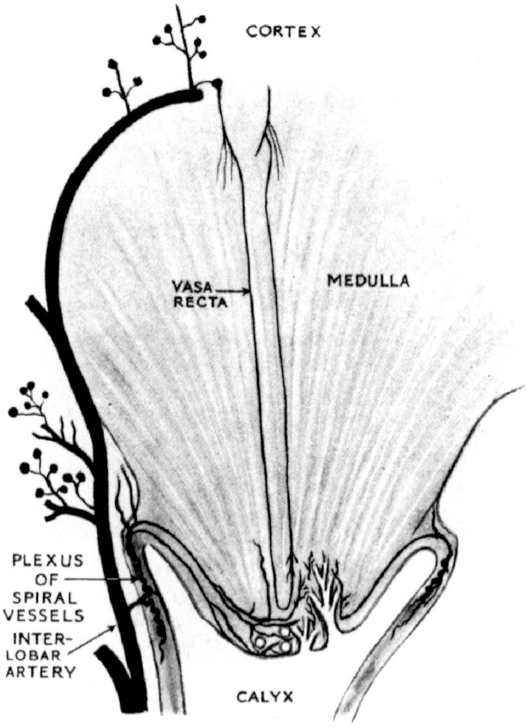

**Fig. 1-20** Diagram of the dual blood supply to the papillae. (From Baker SB. The blood supply to the renal papillae. Br J Urol 1959; 31: 57; with permission.)

The interlobular, arcuate, and interlobar veins parallel the arteries. Unlike the arcuate arteries, the arcuate veins have abundant anastomoses. They combine to form three large lobar veins that drain the three poles of the kidney.[20] These veins lie anterior to the pelvis and unite to form the main renal vein.

The lymphatic drainage is a dual system. The major lymphatic drainage follows the blood vessels from parenchyma to the renal sinus, to the hilum, and terminates in lateral para-aortic lymph nodes. There also is a capsular lymphatic drainage from the superficial cortex that courses into the capsule and then around to the hilum to join the major lymphatic flow.

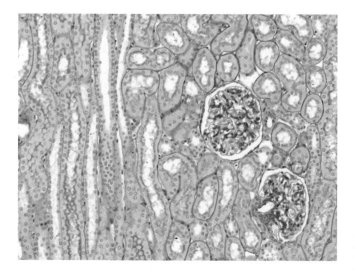

**Fig. 1-21** Renal cortex sectioned perpendicular and parallel to the renal capsule showing medullary rays and the cortical labyrinth. B-PAS stain.

## Microscopic anatomy

The cortex is organized into two regions: the cortical labyrinth and the medullary rays (Fig. 1-21). The labyrinth contains glomeruli, proximal and distal convoluted tubules, connecting tubules, the initial portion of the collecting ducts, as well as interlobular vessels, arterioles, capillaries, and lymphatics. The principal components of the labyrinth are mostly proximal tubules. In the normal cortex the tubules are closely packed, with basement membranes in close contact (Figs 1-19, 1-21). The interstitial space is scant. It contains the peritubular capillary plexus. A medullary ray consists of collecting ducts and the proximal and distal straight tubules that course down into and back up from the medulla. The nephrons that empty into the collecting ducts of a single medullary ray comprise a renal lobule, the functional unit of the kidney.

The medulla is divided into an outer medulla composed of an outer stripe and an inner stripe, and the inner medulla or papilla. Each zone contains specific tubular segments arranged in an elaborate architecture to create the countercurrent concentration system. For further details of the microscopic anatomy of the medulla or for the ultrastructural features of the nephron components, Clapp[14] and Venkatachalam and Kris[15] are two excellent resources.

## Parenchymal maldevelopment and cystic diseases

*The more complicated an organ in its development, the more subject it is to maldevelopment, and in this respect the kidney outranks most other organs.*[13]

*Edith Potter*

Abnormalities of development of the genitourinary tract occur in approximately 10% of the population.[26] Congenital anomalies represent the most common cause of renal failure in children, accounting for over 50% of cases.[19] As captured in the quote by Potter, this is not surprising in light of the complicated organogenesis of this system.[13]

It is difficult to develop a completely satisfactory classification of the diverse array of anomalies that affect the urinary tract (Table 1-1). The ideal schema would account for pathogenesis, morphologic features, and clinical significance. The occurrence of multiple malformations in a single patient and the occurrence of a specific malformation in multiple hereditary and non-hereditary syndromes, coupled with limitations in our understanding of pathogenesis, make classification difficult. Although knowledge of the embryologic development of the kidney provides a tempting basis for explaining departures from the normal renal development, it must be accepted that there is little experimental evidence to defend most conjectures.

Classification of developmental anomalies and cystic diseases based on the underlying genetic defects has been

**Table 1-1** Developmental abnormalities and cystic diseases of the kidney

| |
| --- |
| Abnormalities in form and position |
|     Rotation anomaly |
|     Ectopia |
|     Fusion |
| Abnormalities of mass and number |
| Supernumerary kidney |
| Renal hypoplasia |
|     Simple hypoplasia |
|     Oligomeganephronia |
| Renal agenesis |
|     Unilateral agenesis |
|     Potter's syndrome |
|     Syndromic agenesis |
| Parenchymal maldevelopment and cystic diseases |
| Renal dysplasia |
|     Multicystic and aplastic dysplasia |
|     Segmented dysplasia |
|     Dysplasia associated with lower tract obstruction |
|     Dysplasia associated with hereditary syndromes |
|     Hereditary renal dysplasia and urogenital dysplasia |
| Polycystic kidney disease |
|     Recessive polycystic kidney disease |
|     Dominant polycystic kidney disease |
| Cysts (without dysplasia) in hereditary syndromes |
|     Nephronophthisis |
|     Medullary cystic disease |
|     von Hippel–Lindau disease |
|     Tuberous sclerosis |
|     Glomerulocystic kidney disease |
|     Congenital nephrotic syndrome of the Finnish type |
| Miscellaneous |
|     Renal tubular dysgenesis |
|     Acquired cystic disease |
|     Segmental cystic disease |
|     Medullary sponge kidney |
|     Simple cortical cyst |
|     Pyelocalyceal ectasia and diverticuli |

proposed, and will probably replace current schemes as further information in humans is collected about candidate genes and the dynamic interplay between those genes and their products.[19,24,25] A complicating factor is the polygenetic nature of many disorders in which variable accumulation of multiple minor genetic defects affect susceptibility and influence the nature of each malformation. Evolution in our understanding of the genetic and molecular basis of the broad family of urinary tract malformations will minimize the importance of the simplistic anatomic contribution of urinary tract obstruction popular for so many years by placing it within a larger paradigm of sequential genetic and molecular misadventures that culminate in the malformed kidney and urinary tract.

This section emphasizes diagnostic features and their clinical importance.

## Abnormalities in form and position

It is useful to group abnormalities of form and position because they often occur in combination. For instance, fused kidneys are always ectopic, and most ectopic or fused kidneys are abnormally rotated. Each anomaly may occur in isolation or may represent one component of a more serious complex of malformations affecting other urologic sites or other organ systems. Each may be completely innocent and asymptomatic; however, if urinary tract symptoms develop, they invariably result from impaired urinary drainage that may cause hydronephrosis or pain and may be complicated by infection or nephrolithiasis.

### Rotation anomaly

During ascent of the kidney to a lumbar location, the renal pelvis rotates 90° from an anterior to a medial position (Fig. 1-8). Failure of the pelvis to assume a medial orientation, reverse rotation, or over-rotation to a posterior or even a lateral location, comprise a spectrum of orientation abnormalities known as rotation anomalies.[27] Some degree of malrotation occurs in 1:400–1:1000 individuals.[26] The most common rotation anomaly is non-rotation or incomplete medial rotation resulting in an anterior location of the pelvis and ureter (Figs 1-16, 1-22). This may occur as an isolated abnormality in an otherwise normal kidney. It always accompanies renal ectopia or renal fusion. Ureteropelvic obstruction from a crossing vessel may occasionally result (Fig. 1-22). Excess rotation or reverse rotation with the pelvis posterior or lateral pelvis are very rare.[27]

### Renal ectopia

Failure of the kidney to assume its proper location in the renal fossa is known as renal ectopia.[28–30] There are several varieties named according to location (Table 1-2). Renal ectopia should be distinguished from renal ptosis, in which a normally situated kidney shifts to a lower position. The origin of the renal artery from a normal aortic location identifies a lower-situated kidney as ptotic rather than ectopic. The incidence of ectopia at autopsy ranges from 1:660 to 1:1200.[28,29] Renal ectopia is bilateral in 10% of cases.

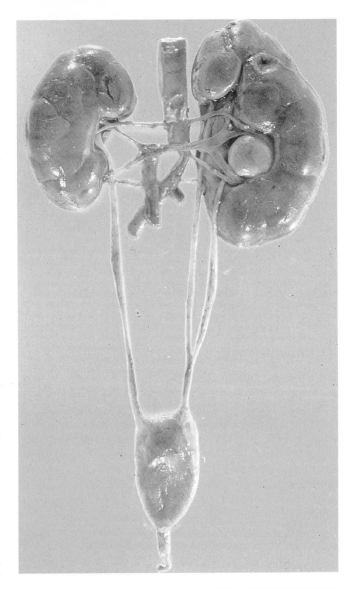

**Fig. 1-22** A duplex left kidney with a bifid ureter and a non-rotated (anterior) lower pelvis. An inferior supernumerary artery and a normal vein cross the ureter, resulting in ureteropelvic junction obstruction.

**Table 1-2** Types of renal ectopia

| |
|---|
| Pelvic – opposite sacrum |
| Iliac – opposite sacral prominence |
| Abdominal – above iliac crest |
| Cephaloid – subdiaphragmatic |
| Thoracic – supradiaphragmatic |
| Crossed – contralateral<br>　With fusion (90%)<br>　Without fusion (10%)<br>　Solitary crossed (rare)<br>　Bilateral crossed (rarest) |

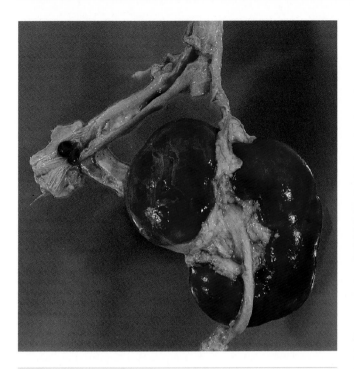

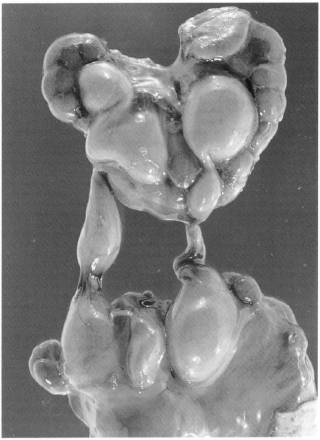

**Fig. 1-23** A hypertrophic pelvic kidney with an anterior ureter in an asymptomatic patient with unilateral agenesis.

**Fig. 1-24** Horseshoe kidney showing hydroureteronephrosis from a neonate with trisomy 18 and multiple congenital anomalies.

The three most common forms of renal ectopia are inferiorly located kidneys.[28,29] The kidney may be non-reniform in shape, its pelvis and ureter are anterior (non-rotated), and the ureter is short and usually placed in the bladder, but may have a high insertion on the pelvis leading to obstruction. The vascular supply is influenced by the final location of the kidney, arising from the aorta, common iliac, internal or external iliac, or inferior mesenteric arteries (Fig. 1-23). The contralateral kidney may be normal, or occasionally absent or even dysplastic. Other anomalies of urologic organs and cardiovascular, skeletal, and gastrointestinal systems are frequent in both males and females.[28,29]

Cephaloid ectopia is usually associated with an omphalocele.[30] The kidney appears to continue its ascent when the abdominal organs herniate into the omphalocele sac. The ureter and pelvis are typically normal. Thoracic ectopia is very rare and usually involves the left kidney.[31] The kidney resides in an extrapleural location in the posterior mediastinum. The diaphragm must be intact to distinguish this from herniation of the kidney (and possibly other abdominal organs) into the thorax secondary to diaphragmatic hernia. The lower lobe of the lung may be hypoplastic, but other anomalies are not present. Thoracic ectopia is usually asymptomatic with a normal ureter and pelvis.

In crossed ectopia the kidney is situated opposite the side of insertion of its ureter in the trigone.[32,33] Four combinations are possible (Table 1-2). In 90% of cases there is also fusion with the other kidney. In crossed fused ectopia the kidneys may assume a variety of shapes and positions, giving rise to six 'types': inferior, superior, lump, sigmoid, disc, and L-shaped.[28] The kidneys function normally and their ureters are normally located within the bladder, but their pelves are non-rotated. Extrarenal anomalies (genital, skeletal, and anorectal) occur in 20–25% of patients.[32,33]

### Horseshoe kidney

Horseshoe kidney is the most common form of renal fusion.[34,35] It is the midline fusion of two distinct renal masses, each with its own ureter and pelvis (Fig. 1-24, 1-25). Horseshoe kidney is relatively common (1:400–2000) with a 2:1 male predominance.[34] The fusion is typically at the lower poles but can vary greatly in the quantity of fused parenchyma. A horseshoe kidney is ectopic and usually situated anterior to the aorta and vena cava. Occasionally the fusion will be posterior to the vena cava or posterior to both the aorta and the vena cava. The ureters and pelves are always anterior. This coupled with commonly encountered high insertion of the ureter on the pelvis can result in obstruction (Fig. 1-24). Approximately 30% of patients will also have other anomalies of the urinary tract, central nervous system, heart, gastrointestinal tract, or skeletal system.[34,35]

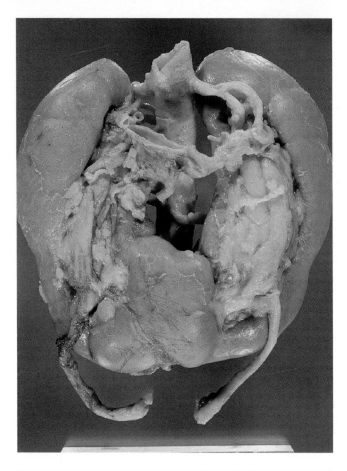

**Fig. 1-25** Horseshoe kidney as an incidental autopsy finding in an adult.

## Abnormalities in mass and number

In contrast to those anomalies listed in the preceding section, the following group of anomalies are much less common and are unrelated abnormalities. Hypoplasia is usually bilateral, whereas supernumerary kidney is usually unilateral and neither is hereditary. The renal parenchyma in each is normally formed. In contrast, renal agenesis can be either unilateral or bilateral and may be hereditary.

### Supernumerary kidney

Supernumerary or duplicated kidney is one of the rarest disorders.[36,37] It has been defined as 'a free accessory organ that is a distinct, encapsulated, large or small parenchymatous mass topographically related to the usual kidney by a loose, cellular attachment at most and often by no attachment whatsoever.'[36] It may be located below (most common), above, or adjacent to the kidney, and is rarely bilateral. It is connected to the lower urinary tract by either a bifid ureter or its own completely separate ureter (Fig. 1-26). In half the reported cases, complications have developed related to obstruction and infection.[36,37]

### Hypoplasia

Hypoplasia refers to a small (<50% of normal) but otherwise normally developed kidney.[22,38] By definition, dysplastic elements are absent. There are two types of hypoplasia: simple

hypoplasia and oligomeganephronia. Previously included in this category was the so-called segmental hypoplasia or Ask–Upmark kidney that is now regarded as an acquired lesion secondary to vesicoureteral reflux.

### Simple hypoplasia

Simple hypoplasia is a rare, usually bilateral, non-hereditary disease in which the small size of the kidney usually reflects a marked reduction in the number of renal lobes.[38,39] Frequently only one to five lobes are present. Occasionally the small size reflects a decrease in the number of cortical glomeruli. Hypertrophic nephrons and dysplastic elements are absent. When bilateral, the small kidneys may eventually fail to provide renal function with body growth and renal insufficiency or renal failure may develop, the severity determined by the degree of hypoplasia.

### Oligomeganephronia

Oligomeganephronia, the most common form of renal hypoplasia, is a bilateral non-hereditary disorder.[40,42] The kidneys are small owing to a reduction in the number of renal lobes and in the number of nephrons within each lobe. Microscopically the nephrons present are tremendously enlarged (Fig. 1-27). Glomerular and tubular volumes have been measured to be 12-times and 17-times normal, respectively.[41]

Children with oligomeganephronia present with a concentration defect that causes polyuria, polydipsia, and salt wasting, resembling patients with juvenile nephronophthisis. Renal insufficiency and proteinuria gradually develop with body growth as progressive glomerular and tubulointerstitial scarring develops. The absence of a family history of renal disease, the presence of proteinuria, and imaging studies revealing symmetrically small non-cystic kidneys, usually permit separation from nephronophthisis.

### Renal agenesis

Absence of the kidney and its corresponding ureter is known as renal agenesis (Table 1-3).[43-48] The corresponding bladder hemitrigone is also absent because it represents the distal continuation of the ureteral smooth muscle (Fig. 1-28).[46] Failure to identify a kidney in a child or an adult does not prove congenital absence of the kidney because small aplastic kidneys identified in newborns have been shown to regress further over time and may become undetectable.[49,50]

### Unilateral renal agenesis

In unilateral agenesis, the contralateral kidney may be hypertrophic up to twice the normal size. The overall renal function may be normal and the condition may be entirely asymptomatic (Fig. 1-23). Several genetic and environmental factors have been associated with an increased risk, such as African-American race, maternal diabetes mellitus and maternal age less than 18 years.[48] In up to 70% of patients, agenesis is associated with additional anomalies most often affecting the genital tracts.[45-52] This presumably reflects a common abnormality affecting the development of both the mesonephric duct and müllerian duct-derived structures. The genital anomalies in females include absence of the ipsilateral fallopian tube, uterine horn, and proximal vagina,

A                                                                                                                                    B

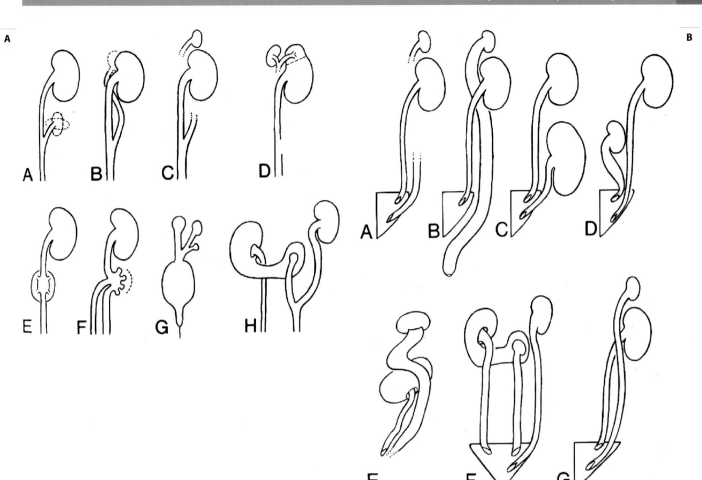

**Fig. 1-26** Morphologic variants of supernumerary kidneys with (**A**) bifid ureters and (**B**) separate ureters. (From N'Guessan G, Stephens FD. Supernumerary kidney. J Urol 1983; 130: 651; with permission.)

**Table 1-3** Classification of renal agenesis

Sporadic forms
    Unilateral
    Bilateral (Potter's syndrome)

Syndromic renal agenesis
    Chromosomal anomalies (trisomies 13 and 18)
    VATER association
    Müllerian aplasia syndrome (MURCS)
    Sirenomelia (caudal regression syndrome)
    Cloacal exstrophy
    Fraser's syndrome
    Williams' syndrome
    Multiple malformation syndromes, NOS
    Hereditary renal adysplasia

**Table 1-4** Oligohydramnios phenotype

Potter facies

Increased interocular distance

Broad flattened nose

Prominent inner canthic folds (sweep downward and lateral)

Receding chin

Large, low-set ears with little cartilage

Positional deformities (flexion of hips and knees, clubbed feet)

Dry skin

Hypoplastic lungs

Small bladder with absent trigone

Placenta – amnion nodosum

or uterine didelphia or vaginal septum.[47–52] In males there may be absence of the ipsilateral epididymis, vas deferens, or seminal vesicle, or a seminal vesicle cyst may be encountered.[45,46] Identification of a patient with a unilateral genital anomaly or renal agenesis should therefore prompt evaluation of the other organ system.

### Potter's syndrome (bilateral renal agenesis)

Bilateral agenesis is a uniformly fatal disorder known as Potter's syndrome.[43] Approximately 40% of affected fetuses are stillborn, and those born alive die of pulmonary failure within 48 hours. Mothers present with severe oligohydramnios because fetal urine normally accounts for most of the amniotic fluid in the second half of gestation. Oligohydramnios impairs pulmonary development, resulting in pulmonary hypoplasia, and produces a variety of distinctive gross features known as the Potter's or oligohydramnios phenotype[44,53,54] (Table 1-4). Figures 1-29 to 1-31 demonstrate some of these characteristic findings.

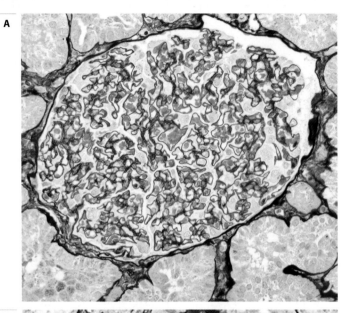

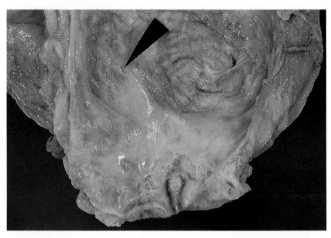

**Fig. 1-28** Bladder showing absent left hemitrigone in an adult with a sporadic form of unilateral renal agenesis. The right hemitrigone is indicated by an arrow.

**Table 1-5** Causes of oligohydramnios

| Common causes |
| --- |
| Potter's syndrome (bilateral renal agenesis) |
| Bilateral renal dysplasia |
| Distal (complete) urinary tract obstruction |
| Uncommon causes |
| Infantile polycystic kidney disease |
| Glomerulocystic kidney disease |
| Renal tubular dysgenesis |
| Chronic amniotic fluid leak |
| In utero acute renal failure |
| Idiopathic |

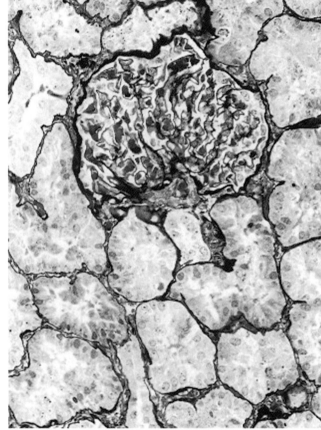

**Fig. 1-27 (A)** Oligomeganephronia in a 22-month-old with an enlarged glomerulus. **(B)** Normal-size glomerulus in a 2-year-old.

Some doctors refer to any fetus born with the oligohydramnios phenotype as having Potter's syndrome, rather than reserving the term for the entity of bilateral renal–ureteral agenesis as initially described. This can be confusing because oligohydramnios has several other causes[55,56] (Table 1-5).

### Syndromic renal agenesis

A large number of syndromes have absence of one (or rarely both) kidney as a component of a constellation of congenital anomalies.[45,52,57–67] This includes chromosomal anomalies, several malformation complexes, and multiple malformation events affecting the gastrointestinal, cardiac, central nervous, or skeletal systems that do not conform to a specific syndrome. Finally, it may also occur in a familial disorder with renal dysplasia (see Hereditary Renal Adysplasia later in this chapter).[64–68] In each disorder, identification of extrarenal components and a detailed family history are essential for proper classification and appropriate genetic counseling. The extrarenal anomalies are responsible for many complications and for the lethal nature of many of the syndromes.

Abnormalities of development and cystic diseases are an often confusing group of anomalies that are important because several forms have hereditary implications. They create confusion because of the inconsistent use of terminology, a failure to understand existing classifications, and the rarity of certain forms.

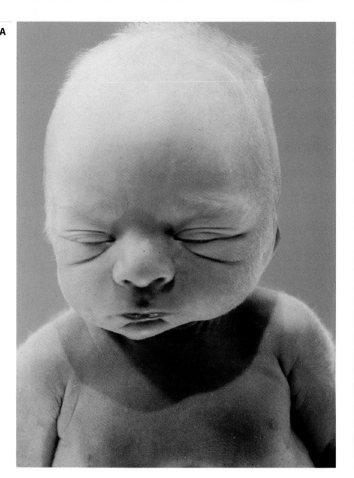
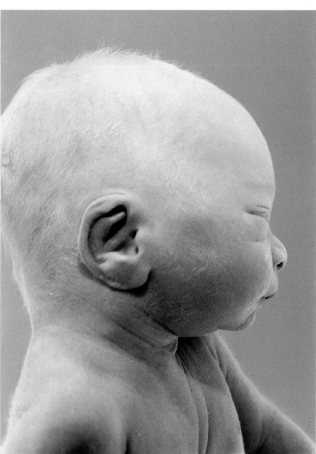

**Fig. 1-29** A fetus born with oligohydramnios showing the characteristic Potter's facies in **(A)** anterior and **(B)** lateral views.

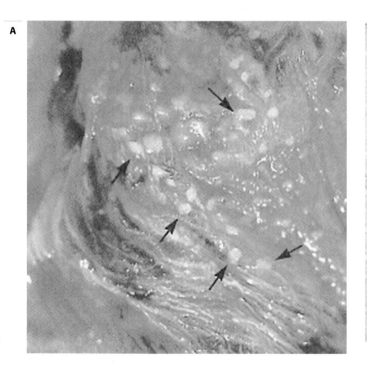
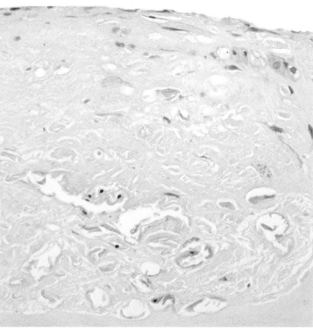

**Fig. 1-30 (A)** Placenta with plaques of amnion nodosum (arrow). **(B)** Plaques of amnion nodosum contain clumps of fetal squames embedded in dense collagen.

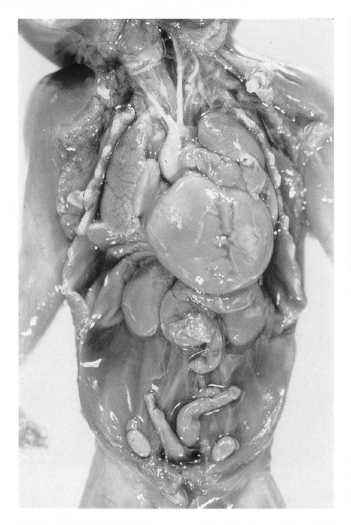

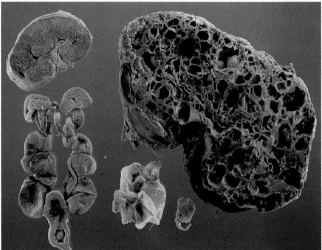

**Fig. 1-32** Autosomal recessive polycystic kidney and autosomal dominant polycystic kidney (upper left and right) and three forms of renal dysplasia: aplastic dysplasia from a 35-year-old, multicystic dysplasia from a neonate, and bilateral dysplasia associated with lower tract obstruction (lower left).

**Table 1-7** Comparison of common cystic diseases

|  | Dysplasia | ARPKD | ADPKD |
|---|---|---|---|
| Incidence | 1 : 1000–2000 | 1 : 50 000 | 1 : 500–1000 |
| Bilateral | +/− | + | + |
| Segmental | +/− | − | − |
| Ureter abnormal | + | − | − |
| Reniform shape | +/− | + | + |
| Uniform cysts | − | + | − |
| Liver abnormal | − | + | + |
| Other malformations | +/− | − | − |

ARPKD, autosomal recessive polycystic kidney disease; ADPKD, autosomal dominant polycystic kidney disease.

**Fig. 1-31** The third consecutive fetus affected with bilateral renal–ureteral agenesis in familial renal adysplasia. The small and large bowel have been removed to reveal adrenal glands but absent kidneys.

**Table 1-6** Potter's classification of cystic disease

| Type I | Autosomal recessive polycystic kidney disease |
|---|---|
| Type IIa | Multicystic renal dysplasia |
| Type IIb | Aplastic renal dysplasia |
| Type III | Autosomal dominant polycystic kidney disease<br>Focal renal dysplasia<br>Dysplasia in hereditary syndromes<br>Autosomal recessive polycystic kidney disease |
| Type IV | Dysplasia associated with lower tract obstruction |

When a cystic kidney is encountered, the initial task is classification. Potter's classification of congenital cystic disease (Table 1-6) first introduced some order into this perplexing field.[13] The classification is based on microdissection of cystic kidneys that localized the cysts to specific segments of the nephron. Unfortunately, this approach did not translate into a clinically useful formulation because hereditary and non-hereditary forms were not separated and dysplasia appeared in three of the four types (Table 1-6). A more

practical formulation separates the two hereditary polycystic kidney diseases (recessive and dominant) from renal dysplasia, and divides dysplasia into sporadic forms and those occurring in hereditary syndromes with multiple malformations.[69–71]

Although there are numerous conditions that can give rise to cystic kidneys, three are of the greatest importance: renal dysplasia, autosomal recessive polycystic kidney disease (ARPKD), and autosomal dominant polycystic kidney disease (ADPKD). Although subtle versions of each occur, most cases encountered are sufficiently distinctive that they can be recognized by gross examination (Fig. 1-32 and Table 1-7).

Both polycystic kidney diseases are hereditary, and in their most severe form result in enormous, bilateral, diffusely cystic kidneys with reniform shapes and normal ureters (Fig. 1-32). Although the kidneys are cystic, there is

**Table 1-8** Multiple malformation syndromes associated with renal dysplasia

Common association
  VATER (VACTERL) association
  MURC syndrome
  Prune-belly syndrome
  Caudal regression syndrome
  Cloacal exstrophy
  Urogenital sinus syndrome
  Urorectal septum syndrome sequence
  Meckel–Gruber syndrome*
  Dandy–Walker syndrome*
  Short rib–polydactyly syndrome*
  Elejalde's syndrome*

Uncommon association
  Trisomy C
  Trisomy 13
  Trisomy 18
  Persistant mesonephric duct syndrome
  Zellweger syndrome*
  Jeune's syndrome*
  Smith–Lemli–Opitz syndrome*
  Beckwith–Wiedemann syndrome*
  Laurence–Moon–Bardet–Biedl syndrome*

*Autosomal recessive inheritance.

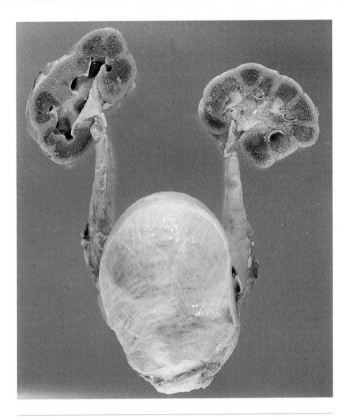

**Fig. 1-33** Megacystis and hydroureteronephrosis without renal dysplasia in a term infant with complete urinary tract obstruction secondary to urethral atresia.

no parenchymal maldevelopment. Each kidney has an associated hepatic lesion, but other visceral malformations are absent. In contrast, dysplastic kidneys are by definition maldeveloped (Fig. 1-32). They are usually not reniform, they vary greatly in size and appearance, and they occur in several patterns: unilateral, bilateral, or confined to the upper pole of a duplex kidney. Approximately 90% of cases have a ureteral abnormality or are associated with distal obstruction, resulting in ureteral stenosis or dilation and megacystis or bladder hypertrophy. Renal dysplasia is most commonly sporadic, but may be familial, part of a multiple malformation complex, or a component of an hereditary malformation syndrome (Table 1-8).

## Renal dysplasia

A dysplastic kidney is a metanephric structure with aberrant nephronic differentiation.[13,69–72] The term *dysplasia* is used in a developmental sense and does not connote any relationship to neoplasia. Dysplastic kidneys should not be confused with hypoplastic kidneys that are small but otherwise normally developed, nor with polycystic kidney diseases that, albeit cystic, do not contain dysplastic elements.

The pathogenesis of renal dysplasia has not been established. There are two major theories that are not mutually exclusive. Dysplasia has traditionally been attributed to 'in utero' urinary tract obstruction, a reasonable concept in light of the common association between obstruction and dysplasia.[70,71] However, normal renal development can occur in the face of complete urinary tract obstruction (Fig. 1-33), and dysplasia resembling the human disease has been very diffi-

cult to produce in experimental animals by early in utero urinary tract obstruction.[73]

The second theory implicates a fundamental defect in inducer tissue (ampullary bud) or responding tissue (blastema).[16,17,74,75] This postulate can also account for the combination of ureteral and renal maldevelopment and can accommodate the occurrence of dysplasia in hereditary syndromes and malformation complexes where diverse genetic, teratogenic, and developmental field defects have been implicated. The identification of specific genetic defects, and progress in unraveling the role of specific genes and their products on the development of the kidneys and the urinary tract, have strengthened this postulate, and represent the key to understanding the molecular basis of malformation events.[19,24,25]

## Multicystic and aplastic dysplasia

Dysplastic kidneys vary tremendously in gross appearance, ranging from large multicystic to small and aplastic (Fig. 1-32). These represent a morphologic continuum and differ only in the extent of cyst formation. When multicystic dysplasia or aplastic dysplasia is bilateral the infant presents with Potter's syndrome and dies of pulmonary hypoplasia. Multicystic kidney is the most common cause of a renal mass in a child and is usually unilateral (Figs 1-34, 1-35).

The histologic appearance of a dysplastic kidney can be quite varied.[13,70–76] Primitive or dysplastic ducts and fetal or immature-appearing cartilage often are present

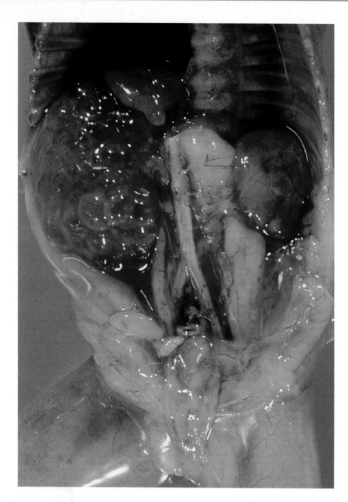

**Fig. 1-34** Unilateral multicystic dysplasia shown in situ.

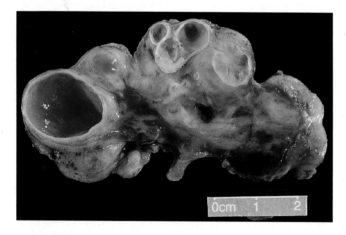

**Fig. 1-35** Transverse section of a multicystic dysplastic kidney.

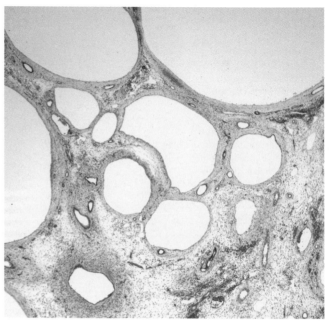

**Fig. 1-36** A dysplastic kidney composed of cysts, dysplastic ducts and primitive tubules.

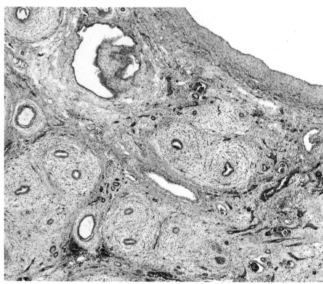

**Fig. 1-37** A dysplastic kidney containing abnormally formed glomeruli and immature tubules.

(Figs 1-36–1-39). Dysplastic ducts are lined with columnar epithelium and surrounded by collars of spindle cells (Fig. 1-36). They are thought to originate from the ampullary buds, whereas the immature cartilage is believed to be derived from blastema.[77] The number of ducts is variable and may be few. Cysts lined by flattened cells, immature tubules, and aberrantly formed glomeruli may predominate, or more normal tubules and well-formed glomeruli may also be present.

Occasionally an infant will present with renal insufficiency and small reniform kidneys with normal ureters and pelves. Simple hypoplasia may be suspected, but biopsy reveals a focal form of dysplasia characterized by an admixture of normal nephrons and aberrantly formed nephrons, usually with microcysts and cartilage or dysplastic ducts. The renal prognosis is bleak,

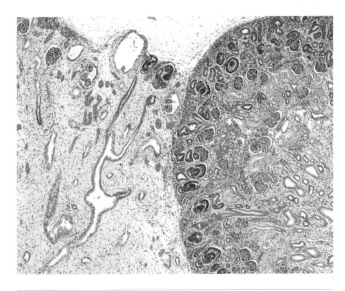

**Fig. 1-38** Aplastic dysplasia showing immature cartilage with a few dysplastic ducts.

**Fig. 1-39** A segmental form of renal dysplasia.

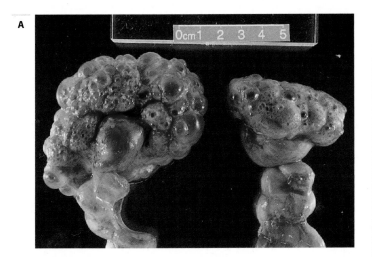

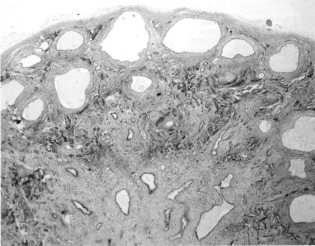

**Fig. 1-40** **(A)** Renal dysplasia associated with urinary tract obstruction. **(B)** Cortical medullary development is present, but few differentiated elements.

and the infant usually develops progressive renal failure as it grows.[78]

## Segmental dysplasia

Segmental dysplasia occurs only in kidneys where the collecting system is duplicated (duplex kidney).[71,79] Usually the duplication is complete with two separate ureters. The upper pole moiety is affected and histologically shows the same range of aberrant nephrogenesis as is encountered in aplastic and multicystic dysplasia (Fig. 1.39). The upper pole ureter is usually ectopic, in a more cranial or caudal location relative to the normally situated lower pole ureter. The incidence of dysplasia increases with the severity of the ectopia.[74]

## Dysplasia associated with lower tract obstruction

Bilateral renal dysplasia can be associated with distal obstruction due to urethral stenosis, posterior urethral valves, or bladder neck obstruction. This form of dysplasia has a distinctive gross appearance. The kidneys are typically reniform, may be large or small, but show distinct corticomedullary differentiation. The bladder is either hypertrophic or greatly dilated, and the ureters are dilated and tortuous (Figs 1-32, 1-40). There may be a severe degree of dysplasia with scant nephronic elements (Fig. 1-40), or only a peripheral zone of dysplastic elements with normal deeper nephrons.

## Dysplasia associated with malformation syndrome

Renal dysplasia may develop in association with numerous multiple malformation syndromes, chromosomal anomalies, and hereditary malformation syndromes[55–68,80–86] (Table 1-8). When multiple malformations are encountered in a pediatric autopsy, it is important to obtain tissue for karyotyping and to meticulously document all anomalies. Consultation with specialists in pediatrics and genetics is advisable to provide the proper classification of the disease so that appropriate family counseling can be provided.

## Hereditary renal adysplasia and urogenital adysplasia

Renal agenesis, aplastic dysplasia, and multicystic dysplasia are the most severe forms of metanephric kidney maldevelopment. When not associated with extrarenal anomalies of a multiple malformation syndrome, they usually are sporadic events with little risk of a subsequently affected sibling. Rarely, however, renal agenesis or renal dysplasia, either unilateral or bilateral (Fig. 1-31), or combined agenesis and dysplasia may be familial (usually autosomal dominant); this is known as hereditary renal adysplasia.[65–68] There may also be concomitant malformation of müllerian structures,

a condition referred to as hereditary urogenital adysplasia.[64] Unfortunately, neither syndrome can be anticipated until a second family member is identified with either agenesis or dysplasia.

## Polycystic kidney diseases

### Autosomal recessive polycystic kidney disease

In autosomal recessive polycystic kidney disease (ARPKD), parents lack the disease and 25% of siblings will be affected.[13,87–93] It is associated with mutations of the *PCKD1* gene, 6p12.[91–93] (Table 1-9) The product of this gene, fibrocystin/polyductin, localizes to the primary cilium and centrosome of renal tubular epithelial cells. Organogenesis in ARPKD appears normal based on microdissection studies of severe neonatal forms.[13] There is ectasia of cortical and medullary collecting ducts that often is accompanied by a liver lesion that in older patients is identical to congenital hepatic fibrosis.

Recessive polycystic kidney disease was originally believed to be an invariably lethal neonatal disorder. Observation of some cases that survived into childhood prompted Blyth and Ockenden[88] to propose a subclassification of the disease into forms: perinatal, neonatal, infantile, and juvenile. These vary in the degree of cyst formation. Although conceptually

**Table 1-9** The genetic basis of hereditary cystic disease

| Cystic disease | Inheritance | Locus | Gene | Gene product |
| --- | --- | --- | --- | --- |
| Polycystic kidney disease | | | | |
| ADPKD 1 | AD | 16p13.3 | *PKD 1* | Polycystin-1 |
| ADPKD 2 | AD | 4q21-23 | *PKD 2* | Polycystin-2 |
| ARPKD | AR | 6p12 | *PKHD1* | Fibrocystin |
| Nephronophthisis | | | | |
| NPHP 1 | AR | 2q12-13 | *NPHP1* | Nephrocystin |
| NPHP 2 | AR | 9q22-31 | *NPHP2* | Inversin |
| NPHP 3 | AR | 3q21-22 | *NPHP3* | Nephrocystin 3 |
| NPHP 4 | AR | | *NPHP4* | Nephrocystin 4 |
| NPHP 5 | AR | | *NPHP5* | Nephrocystin 5 |
| NPHP6/SLSN6 | AR | | *NPHP6* | NPHP6 |
| Medullary cystic disease | | | | |
| MCKD1 | AD | 1q21 | ? | ? |
| MCKD2/FJHN | AD | 16p12 | *UMOD* | Uromodulin |
| Von Hippel–Lindau | AD | 3p25-26 | *VHL* | VHL protein |
| Tuberous sclerosis complex | | | | |
| TSC 1 | AD | 9q34 | *TSC 1* | Hamartin |
| TSC 2 | AD | 16p13.3 | *TSC 2* | Tuberin |
| Glomerulocystic disease | AD | 17q21-3 | *HNF-1B* | HNF-1B protein |
| Finnish type CNS | AR | 19q12-13 | *NPHS 1* | Nephrin |

ADPKD, autosomal dominant polycystic kidney disease; ARPKD, autosomal recessive polycystic kidney disease; NPHP, nephronophthisis; MCKD, medullary cystic kidney disease; FJHN, familial juvenile hyperuricemic nephropathy; TSC, tuberous sclerosis complex; CNS, congenital nephrotic syndrome; AD, autosomal dominant; AR, autosomal recessive.

useful, it is often difficult to place a patient into a given category. The *PKHD1* gene encodes for several isoforms that may account for the clinical spectrum. It appears that as the extent of cyst formation decreases, there is better pulmonary development and a greater likelihood of survival. Unfortunately, with increasing duration of survival there is worsening of the liver disease which in some patients culminates in congenital hepatic fibrosis.[88–91] If one examines the kidneys of children with congenital hepatic fibrosis, two-thirds have some degree of medullary cyst formation and a concentrating defect similar to ARPKD. This has led to the suggestion that ARPKD and congenital hepatic fibrosis may be different manifestations of a single entity.[90]

Most cases of ARPKD result in stillbirth, early neonatal death, or end-stage kidney disease by the age of 20. Affected neonates have massively enlarged and diffusely cystic kidneys that produce abdominal distension and compress thoracic organs (Fig. 1-41). The lungs cannot develop normally and death is from pulmonary hypoplasia. Despite the impressive cyst formation the kidneys may be functional. If they are non-functional, oligohydramnios and a Potter's phenotype may develop.

The cysts extend through the cortex and medulla in a distinctive radiating pattern, imparting a spongy quality (Fig. 1-41). Histologically, the cysts consist of dilated collecting ducts lined with uniform cuboidal cells (Figs 1-42, 1-43). The nephrons between the collecting ducts appear normal.

In the hepatic lesion in patients dying in the neonatal period, the portal bile ducts proliferate and assume a dilated and irregular pattern of anastomosing channels at the periphery of portal triads (Fig. 1-44). There is a marked increase in the size of portal areas with increased fibrous tissue. In older patients, congenital hepatic fibrosis develops, resulting in portal hypertension and hepatosplenomegaly.

In less severely affected kidneys of older children the appearance is variable and the diagnosis may be less obvious. The kidneys are smaller and the cysts fewer. Medullary cysts are always present and tend to be elongated. The cortical cysts are often rounded and variably distributed (Fig. 1-45). The parenchyma adjacent to the cysts eventually develops atrophic changes with tubulointerstitial scarring and glomerulosclerosis. This may create a resemblance to ADPKD. The liver lesion of congenital hepatic fibrosis, therefore, is a useful diagnostic feature. However, a number of diseases

**A**

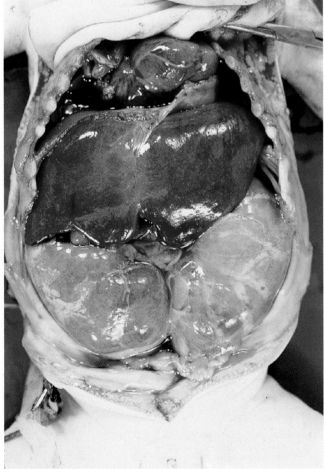

**B**

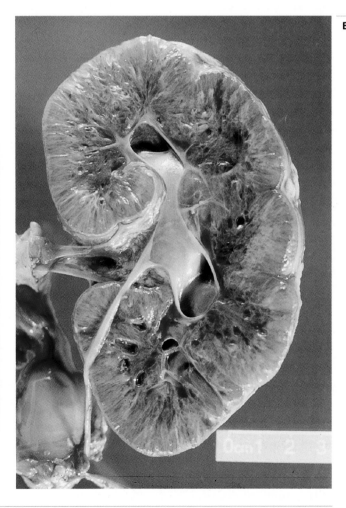

**Fig. 1-41 (A)** Autosomal recessive polycystic kidney disease showing massive kidneys that distend the abdomen, elevate the diaphragm, and compromise the thoracic cavity. **(B)** The bivalved kidney shows a reniform shape and normal collecting system. The cortex and medulla contain diffuse, relatively uniform cysts.

23

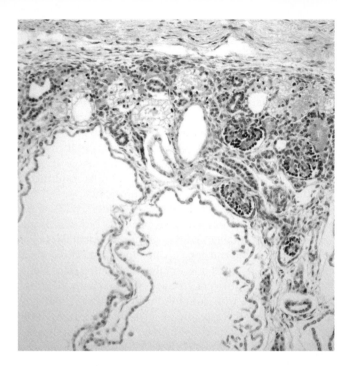

**Fig. 1-42** The cysts in ARPKD are elongated and involve the cortical and medullary collecting ducts.

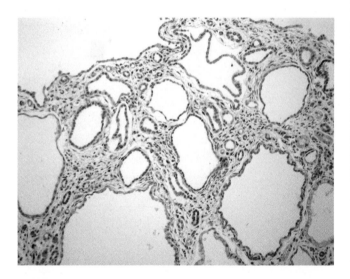

**Fig. 1-43** The cysts in ARPKD are lined with uniform cuboidal epithelium with normal nephron elements in between.

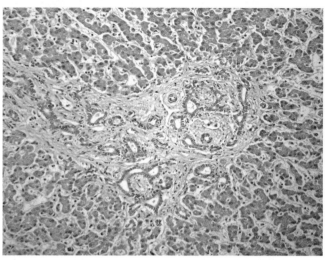

**Fig. 1-44** The liver in perinatal ARPKD disease showing the irregular architecture of portal bile ducts and portal fibrosis.

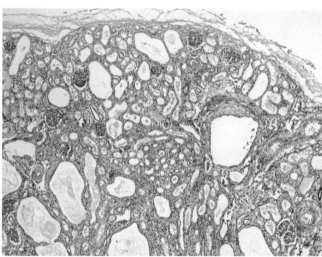

**Fig. 1-45** An infantile form of ARPKD in a 4-year-old showing less prominent collecting duct ectasia. Interstitial fibrosis is developing.

**Table 1-10** Cystic renal disease associated with congenital hepatic fibrosis or biliary dysgenesis

| |
| --- |
| Autosomal recessive polycystic kidney disease |
| Autosomal dominent polycystic kidney disease |
| Nephronophthisis |
| Meckel–Gruber syndrome* |
| Zellweger syndrome* |
| Ivemark's syndrome* |
| Chondrodysplastic syndromes* |
| Trisomy C* |
| Trisomy D* |

*Additional malformations are present.

may be associated with renal cysts and liver disease that require awareness of additional anomalies for proper classification[81] (Table 1-10).

### Adult dominant polycystic kidney disease

Autosomal dominant polycystic kidney disease is the most common cystic renal disease and the most common genetically transmitted disease.[91,94,95] It occurs with an estimated frequency between 1:500 and 1:1000. It is the third to fourth leading cause of end-stage renal disease, and patients comprise 5% to 10% of dialysis patients. Although patients vary greatly in the age of onset of symptoms, most present in their 30s to 50s.[94–97] There is almost 100% penetrance if the individual survives to age 80. Approximately 25% of affected patients lack a family history and presumably represent a new mutation. The disease results from mutations of *PKD1* and *PKD2* that localize to chromosome 16 in 90% of patients and to chromosome 4 in 10%, respectively.[91,94,98,99] The gene product of *PKD1* is polycystin-1, a transmembrane glycoprotein involved in cell signaling (Table 1-9). *PKD2* encodes for polycystin-2, a member of the transient receptor potential channel (TRCP) superfamily of non-selective cation channels.

Patients with ADPKD present with a variety of symptoms, most referable to the urinary tract.[94–97] Chronic flank pain is the most common and correlates with renal weight and cyst size >3 cm. Acute flank pain often reflects hemorrhage into a cyst. Hematuria is the second most common symptom. This may be gross, resulting in clot formation and urinary tract obstruction. Hypertension often develops early in the disease, and activation of the renin–angiotensin system secondary to intrarenal vascular occlusion by expanding cysts has been implicated. Urinary tract infection develops in 50–75% of patients and affects women more often than men. The infection may be confined to the collecting system or a cyst, or may involve the parenchyma. Perinephric extension with abscess is a serious complication with a 60% mortality rate. Urate or calcium oxalate nephrolithiasis develops in 10% of patients, and renal cell carcinoma in 1–5%. Extrarenal complications related to hypertension and berry aneurysms develop in 5–15%. Infection and cardiovascular disease represent the most common causes of death.[96,97]

Early in the disease (Fig. 1-46), the kidney may appear nearly normal with only scattered cysts in the cortex and medulla and normal intervening parenchyma.[100–102] Initially the cysts are small and develop in only about 1% of nephrons. Microdissection studies have shown that they develop

in all segments of the nephron.[102] Scanning electron microscopy and immunohistochemistry of cyst lining cells have confirmed these observations.[103,104]

As the disease progresses, the cysts grow in size and number, resulting in massive renal enlargement (Fig. 1-47). Despite the cystic transformation, the kidneys retain a reniform shape and preserve their collecting systems. The cysts range in size from a few millimeters to several centimeters, and their contents vary from transparent to opaque to hemorrhagic fluid.

Most of the cysts are lined with a single layer of flattened to cuboidal epithelium (Fig. 1-48). Hyperplastic foci or polyp formation (Fig. 1-49) are detectable in some cysts, and renal neoplasms, often of a papillary architecture, may also be present.[105,106] The cyst contents may be proteinaceous or contain red cells or calcific deposits. The intervening parenchyma shows interstitial fibrosis with a lymphoid infiltrate, tubular atrophy, glomerular, and vascular sclerosis.

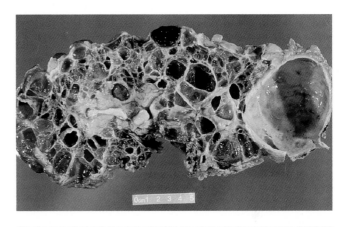

**Fig. 1-47** Transverse section of ADPKD kidney.

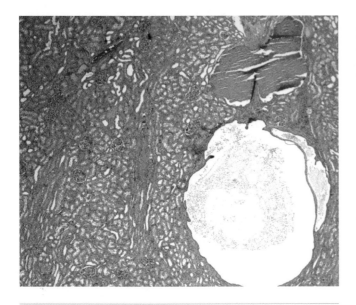

**Fig. 1-46** Infantile onset of ADPKD at age 7 years showing a largely intact cortex and multiple cysts.

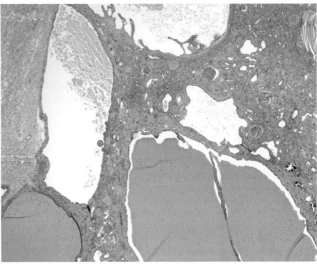

**Fig. 1-48** Advanced ADPKD showing severe interstitial scarring and cysts that contain proteinaceous fluid and calcium oxalate crystals, from an adult in renal failure.

A

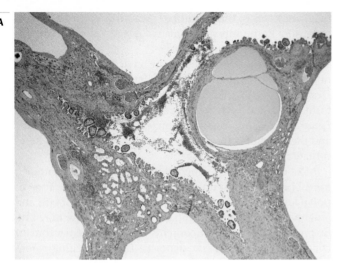

B

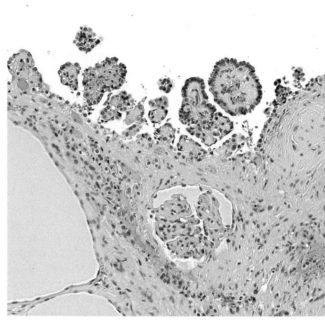

**Fig. 1-49** Papillary tufts lining a cyst in ADPKD.

## Cysts (without dysplasia) in hereditary syndromes

### Nephronophthisis

Nephronophthisis (NPHP) comprises a group of at least six hereditary progressive forms of renal disease.[107–110] All are recessive, present in childhood, and develop into end-stage disease in adolescence. Although fundamentally the diseases are tubulointerstitial, 15% have extrarenal components, retinal dystrophy (Senior–Loken syndrome), oculomotor apraxia (Cogan syndrome), situs inversus (infantile NPHP), and rarely, congenital hepatic fibrosis. Affected individuals present with polyuria and polydipsia due to salt wasting, a concentration defect, anemia disproportionately severe for the level of renal insufficiency, and growth retardation. The genetic loci responsible for all six have been mapped and the protein product of most identified (Table 1-9).[111–114] The encoded proteins are expressed in the primary cilium, centrosome, and cell junctions of renal epithelial cells.

The kidneys in NPHP are usually small. Renal cysts may occur and are confined to the corticomedullary junction. There is a non-specific chronic interstitial nephritis with tubular atrophy, interstitial fibrosis, and periglomerular fibrosis. A prominent lymphoid infiltrate is usually present. As the tubulointerstitial nephritis worsens glomerulosclerosis develops.

### Medullary cystic disease

Medullary cystic disease (MCKD) is autosomal dominant, and, like NPHP, is a progressive tubulointerstitial disease.[112–114] Affected individuals present in the third to fourth decades with polyuria and polydipsia due to salt wasting, a concentration defect, and anemia disproportion-ately severe for the level of renal insufficiency. They progress to end-stage disease in the fourth to seventh decades.

Two forms of MCKD have been identified, MCKD1 and MCKD2. The mutated gene of MCKD2 has been identified and its product is uromodulin (Tamm–Horsfall protein). The gene responsible for MCKD1 has not been identified. Apart from the occurrence of gout and hyperuricemia in MCKD2, these disorders are clinically identical. Currently, there is the suspicion that MCKD2 and familial juvenile hyperuricemic nephropathy may be the same entity.

The kidneys in MCKD may be enlarged if cysts are prominent. Although medullary cysts are common, within a given family not all affected individuals have cysts. The cysts congregate at the corticomedullary junction and range up to 1 cm in size (Fig. 1-50). Cyst formation does not appear to increase as the disease progresses. Microscopically, the appearance is that of a non-specific chronic interstitial nephritis with tubular atrophy, interstitial fibrosis, and periglomerular fibrosis. If cysts are present, they are lined with a flattened to cuboidal epithelium.

### Von Hippel-Lindau disease

Von Hippel–Lindau disease is an uncommon autosomal dominant disorder in which renal and extrarenal cysts and neoplasms develop.[115–118] The syndrome includes retinal, cerebellar, and spinal hemangioblastomas, pheochromocytoma, and epididymal and pancreatic cysts and cystadenomas. In addition, multiple and bilateral renal cysts develop in 75% of patients and renal cell carcinomas, often bilateral and multicentric, in approximately 50% (Fig. 1-51).[117,118] The mutant gene has been localized to the short arm of chromosome 3, 3p25, adjacent to the gene implicated in clear cell renal cell carcinoma (Table 1-9).[118]

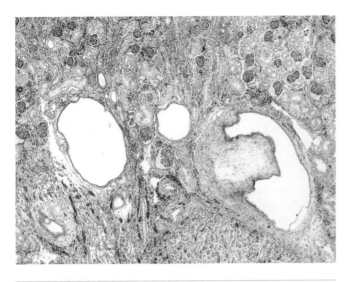

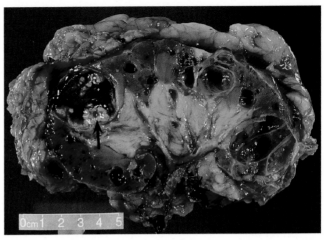

**Fig. 1-51** Nephrectomy in von Hippel–Lindau disease showing multiple cysts. One cyst side contains a mural nodule (arrow) of renal cell carcinoma.

**Fig. 1-50** Medullary cystic disease showing cysts along the outer medulla.

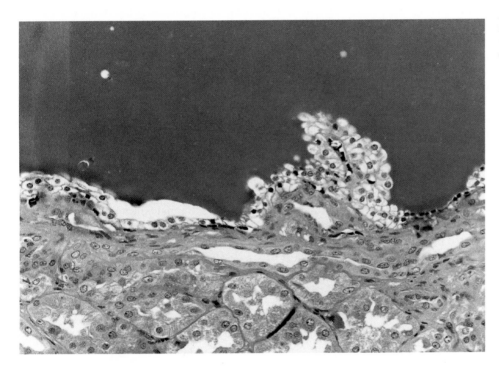

**Fig. 1-52** Cyst (from Fig. 1-51) in von Hippel–Lindau disease lined with clear cells with a papillary tuft.

The renal cysts are lined with glycogen-rich cells similar to those of grade 1 clear cell renal cell carcinoma (Fig. 1-52).[115–118] These range from a benign-appearing lining of one to two cell layers of clear cells to multiple layers of cells. Papillary tufts of mildly atypical cells, solid mural nodules, and cystic masses that are clearly neoplastic in nature also develop. Deoxyribonucleic acid (DNA) analysis has shown aneuploidy in both the cells of cysts and those of solid tumors.[119] This morphologic spectrum represents a challenge in the classification of lesions in biopsy and nephrectomy material. The appropriate morphologic threshold for a malignant diagnosis has yet to be established.

## Tuberous sclerosis

Tuberous sclerosis complex (TSC) is an autosomal dominant disorder characterized by mental retardation, epilepsy, angiofibromas, cardiac rhabdomyomas, renal angiomyolipomas, and renal cysts.[119–123] Two genes have been identified that cause tuberous sclerosis complex, *TSC1* and *TSC2*, mapped to chromosomes 9 and 13, respectively (Table 1-9).[122,123] The latter locus is within a few nucleotides of the *PKD1* locus. Although renal cysts are uncommon and usually not extensive, some individuals – usually children – develop a diffuse cystic renal disease with numerous large cortical and medullary cysts that resemble autosomal dominant polycystic disease, known as the contiguous gene syndrome.[122,123]

The cysts in tuberous sclerosis are distinctive and appear to have diagnostic specificity in the recognition of this disorder.[120,123] The cysts are lined with large eosinophilic cells having large hyperchromatic nuclei. They may form papillary or polypoid masses and may show occasional mitotic activity. Renal cell carcinomas have rarely developed, but this is far less common than in von Hippel–Lindau disease.[121]

## Glomerulocystic kidney disease

Glomerular cysts develop in several forms of pediatric and adult cystic disease (Table 1-11), either as the predominant abnormality or accompanied by renal dysplasia or extrarenal abnormalities of a congenital syndrome.[124–130] Glomerulocystic kidney disease comprises the subgroup in which glomerular cysts constitute the principal abnormality and other abnormalities outside the kidney are absent. In one case report stenosis of the glomerulotubular junction was identified on serial sections and implicated in development of the cystic lesion.[129] There is clinical and genetic heterogeneity within the glomerulocystic kidney disease category (Table 1-11).

Most glomerulocystic kidney diseases are autosomal dominant disorders. Approximately half of all cases will be found to have a family history typical of autosomal dominant polycystic kidney disease. The patient is usually an infant and appears to have early onset of severe autosomal dominant polycystic kidney disease that begins with glomerular cysts as the major finding.[124,126–128] Other kindreds have a strong family history of renal disease that is not consistent with adult polycystic kidney disease and in which biopsies of siblings or parents consistently show only glomerular cysts. Several kindreds have also been found to have small kidneys with reduced or absent renal pyramids, called familial hypoplastic glomerulocystic kidney disease.[130] Mutation in the hepatocyte nuclear factor-1B gene has been identified in these families when this hypoplastic form is associated with early-onset diabetes.[130] Rare sporadic forms have been reported. However, when a family history is absent, the prospect of a new mutation with early onset of a genetic form should always be entertained.

The glomerular cysts in glomerulocystic kidney diseases may be microscopic or sufficiently large to be grossly visible and result in nephromegaly (Fig. 1-53). The cysts may be confined to a subcapsular zone, affect the entire cortex, or be confined to the inner cortex. Tubulointerstitial scarring may also develop or be absent. Once glomerular cysts are recognized, additional morphologic and clinical data are required to resolve the differential possibilities. If extrarenal anomalies are present or if features of renal dysplasia are present, then this is not a primary glomerulocystic kidney disease.

## Congenital nephrotic syndrome of the Finnish type

Congenital nephrotic syndrome of the Finnish type is an autosomal recessive disease caused by two mutations, Fin-major and Fin-minor, in the *NPHS1* gene that encodes for nephrin, a component of the podocyte slit diaphragm (Table 1-9).[131–137] Although rare, it is the most common cause of nephrotic syndrome in the first 3 months of life. It is included in this section because it is also known as 'microcystic disease.' Although most prevalent in Finland, it has been recognized throughout the world.

The affected fetus is born prematurely with a low birthweight and a large placenta. The kidneys may be grossly enlarged due to edema and microcysts resulting from mild ectasia of tubules, especially collecting ducts, and often of Bowman's capsule. Progressive nephrotic syndrome, poor growth, and renal insufficiency develop. As the nephrotic syndrome continues, progressive glomerulosclerosis and tubular atrophy develop and renal failure ensues (Fig. 1-54). Most infants die of infection by 3 years of age unless transplantation is successful.

---

**Table 1-11** Classification of glomerulocystic kidney (From Bernstein J, Landing BH. Genetics of kidney disorders. New York, Alan R. Liss, 1989; with permission)

Glomerulocystic kidney disease
  Autosomal dominant glomerulocystic kidney disease
  Familial hypoplastic glomerulocystic kidney disease
  'Sporadic' glomerulocystic kidney disease

Syndromes with glomerular cysts
  Tuberous sclerosis
  Familial juvenile nephronophthisis with hepatic fibrosis
  Zellweger cerebrorenal–hepatic syndrome
  Trisomy 13 syndrome
  Orofacial–digital syndrome, type I
  Brachymesomelia–renal syndrome
  Short rib–polydactyly syndrome, Majewski type

Dysplastic glomerulocystic kidneys
  Hereditary and syndromal renal dysplasia

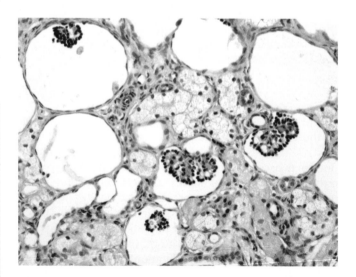

**Fig. 1-53** Glomerulocystic kidney disease showing microcysts principally involving Bowman's capsules.

A

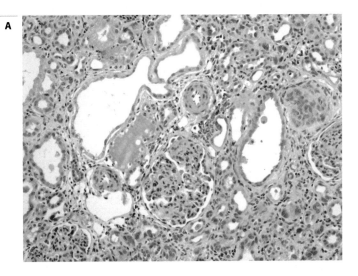

B

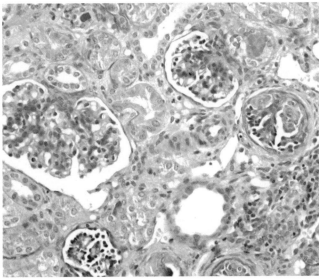

**Fig. 1-54** Congenital nephrotic syndrome of the Finnish type in a 2-year-old at the time of renal transplantation. There is mild ectasia of tubules and Bowman's capsule, glomerular sclerosis, and tubular atrophy.

## Miscellaneous conditions

### Renal tubular dysgenesis

Failure of differentiation of normal-appearing tubules is known as renal tubular dysgenesis.[138-141] It results in neonatal renal failure with the oligohydramnios sequence, a Potter's syndrome phenotype, and may result in death from pulmonary hypoplasia. The kidneys are usually grossly normal, although they may be increased in weight. The glomeruli are close together and appear increased in number. The intervening tubules are small and appear undifferentiated on routine section (Fig. 1-55). Ultrastructurally and with lectin staining, they exhibit features of the distal tubule and collecting duct.

The original reports of renal tubular dysgenesis indicated a hereditary pattern consistent with an autosomal recessive disorder.[138] However, clinical heterogeneity is encountered with this lesion. It has recently been described in monochorionic twins with twin–twin transfusions in which only the donor twin was affected.[139] It has also been reported to be associated with hypocalvaria as a complication of maternal use of angiotensin-converting enzyme inhibitors.[140] Finally, abnormalities in the renin–angiotensin system has been identified that may provide a unifying abnormality.[141]

### Acquired cystic kidney disease

Acquired cystic kidney disease refers to the development of multiple and bilateral renal cysts in patients whose chronic renal failure cannot be attributed to an hereditary cystic disease.[142-148] Although it was identified as long ago as 1847 by Simon,[143] in 1977 Dunnill[144] revived interest in this phenomenon when in an autopsy study of hemodialysis patients he observed not only a high prevalence of renal cysts but also renal tumors in 20% of the patients. One patient died of metastatic renal cell carcinoma. The development of both cysts and tumors appears to be related to the uremic state

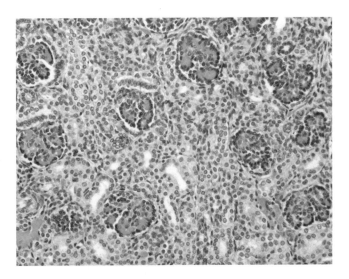

**Fig. 1-55** Congenital renal tubular dysgenesis presenting with oliguric acute renal failure. No normal proximal tubules are present.

because it is independent of the type of dialysis and the cause of original renal disease.[145-148]

Acquired cystic kidney disease is bilateral and asymptomatic in its early stages. Cysts are present in 8% of patients at the time dialysis is initiated, and increase in incidence, number, and size proportional to the duration of dialysis. After 3–5 years of dialysis approximately 50% of patients develop cysts, and by 10 years almost 90% have cysts. The complications of acquired cystic kidney disease include intrarenal and retroperitoneal hemorrhage, cyst infection, and renal cell carcinoma that may account for 3–4% of all deaths.[145-148] Compared to sporadic cases of renal cell carcinoma where the clear type predominates, in acquired cystic kidney disease papillary tumors predominate. Although

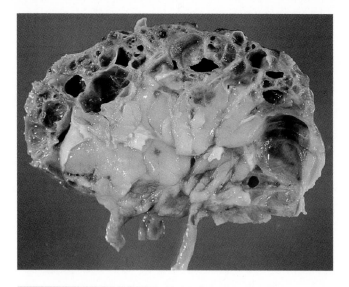

**Fig. 1-56** Acquired cystic disease of the kidney. Although diffusely cystic, the kidney is small and the renal sinus fat is prominent.

improvement in the cystic disease occurs in many patients following a successful transplantation, the influence of transplantation on neoplastic complications remains unclear. As the number of dialysis patients increases and their survivals improve, the occurrence of cystic disease and neoplastic complications can also be expected to increase.

The cysts initially form in the proximal tubules of end-stage kidneys. Most are smaller than 0.5 cm, but cysts 2–3 cm in size can develop. Initially the cysts are cortical, but in advanced cases medullary cysts form and the entire kidney may be replaced by cysts and resemble a smaller version of adult polycystic kidney disease (Fig. 1-56). The cysts are lined with flattened, cuboidal, or columnar epithelium and may contain a proteinaceous to hemorrhagic fluid. Foci of epithelial hyperplasia are common in the cysts and tubules.

### Segmental cystic disease

The literature contains several cases of a unilateral and segmental form of cystic disease that histologically resembles dominant polycystic kidney disease but lacks the progression, extrarenal complications, and familial nature.[149] An early stage of dominant polycystic kidney disease is often entertained because early on one kidney may be more severely affected. Careful imaging of the opposite kidney and inquiry into family history is required.

The differential includes a broad range of other diseases: multiple simple cysts, cystic dysplasia, cystic nephroma, and cystic carcinoma. In multiple simple cysts, the cysts are widely separated and do not congregate in a single region. In segmental forms of dysplasia, ureteral duplication is present. Cystic nephromas are more circumscribed and well demarcated, and cystic carcinomas will show a neoplastic vascular pattern and usually have solid areas. Despite these differences, excision and follow-up may be required to confidently establish the nature of the disease and the hereditary implications.

### Medullary sponge kidney

In medullary sponge kidney there is ectasia of the papillary collecting ducts of one or more renal pyramids.[150,151] Usually bilateral and more common in males, medullary sponge kidney is usually detected radiographically in adults evaluated for nephrolithiasis. The kidneys are not enlarged and renal function is normal, although a concentrating defect may be present in more severely affected patients.

Microscopically, the collecting ducts are dilated and lined with cuboidal or flattened epithelium[150,151] (Fig. 1-57). Intratubular calcifications are common. If stones have obstructed the ducts, localized scarring may be present. Medullary sponge kidney can be distinguished from medullary cystic disease and infantile polycystic kidney disease by the age of the patient and the location of the cysts. In medullary cystic disease the cysts are located at the corticomedullary junction, whereas in the juvenile form of recessive polycystic kidney disease the cysts are in the cortex and medulla and do not congregate at the papillary tips.

### Simple cortical cyst

Simple cortical cysts are the most common cystic renal lesion.[152,153] They are rare before the age of 40, so cysts in a child or young adult, especially if bilateral, can be an important clue to the presence of a cystic renal disease. Simple cysts increase in frequency with advancing age. In older patients they may be multiple and large (Fig. 1-58). They are lined with a flattened layer of cells or lack an epithelial lining. The cyst wall may occasionally calcify, a radiographic finding mimicking infection or malignancy.[122–123]

### Pyelocalyceal ectasia and diverticula

There are several lesions (hydrocalyx, megacalycosis, and calyceal diverticulum) that have in common a cavity lined with urothelium that communicates with the collecting system and is associated with recurrent infections and nephrolithiasis.[154–156] In hydrocalyx there is calyectasis secondary to infundibular stenosis. The stenosis may be congenital or the sequela of inflammation. In contrast, in megacalycosis obstruction is not evident.[154] In both lesions the renal pyramid is flattened or concave, and in cases complicated by infection, parenchymal inflammation and scarring may be present.

In calyceal diverticulum the cavity communicates with a minor calyx via a narrow isthmus[155,156] and no obstruction is present. The upper pole calyx is involved in 54% of cases and parenchymal inflammation and scarring usually are absent unless the case is complicated by infections.

# Vascular diseases

## Hypertension-associated renal disease

Vascular disease, in its various forms (Table 1-12), is the most common cause of renal injury encountered at autopsy owing to the high incidence of atherosclerosis and hypertension (Fig. 1-59).[157–159] A connection between hypertension and renal and cardiovascular diseases has been recognized

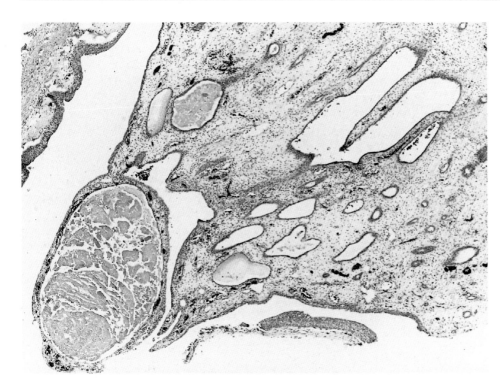

**Fig. 1-57** Medullary sponge kidney showing prominent ectasia and a microlith within a papillary collecting duct.

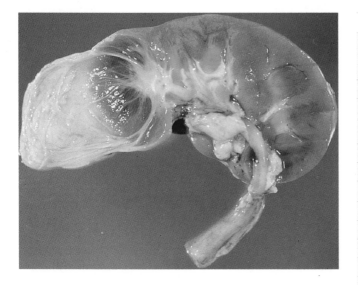

**Fig. 1-58** A large simple cortical cyst found incidentally at autopsy.

**Table 1-12** Classification of vascular diseases of the kidney

| |
| --- |
| Hypertension-associated renal disease |
|    Benign nephrosclerosis |
|    Malignant nephrosclerosis |
| Thrombotic microangiopathy |
| Renal artery stenosis |
|    Atherosclerosis |
|    Fibromuscular dysplasia |
| Renal artery dissection |
| Renal artery aneurysm |
| Arteriovenous malformation and fistula |
| Renal emboli and infarcts |
| Renal cortical necrosis |
| Renal cholesterol microembolism syndrome |
| Renal artery thrombosis |
| Renal vein and renal venous thrombosis |
| Bartter's syndrome |
| Vasculitis |

for over 100 years.[160–162] Hypertension-associated renal disease was first separated from other forms of renal disease in 1914 by Volhard and Fahr, who first recognized the existence of two forms.[163] The most common form, *benign nephrosclerosis*, occurred in elderly individuals who had mild hypertension and little renal impairment. The second form, *malignant nephrosclerosis*, occurred in younger patients with severe hypertension and renal failure. Although most patients with hypertension (90–95%) have idiopathic disease, there are numerous secondary causes that can produce either benign or malignant nephrosclerosis (Table 1-13).

## Benign nephrosclerosis

Benign (or essential) hypertension is an asymptomatic disorder affecting approximately 50 million Americans.[158,159,164] Its pathogenesis is unknown but is probably multifactorial. Genetic factors appear important, but no specific genetic marker has been identified. It is more common in black people. Hypertension usually first appears around age 45–54 years, and if unchecked places the patient at risk for renal insufficiency, congestive heart failure, coronary artery disease, and stroke in later years. Although benign hypertension will

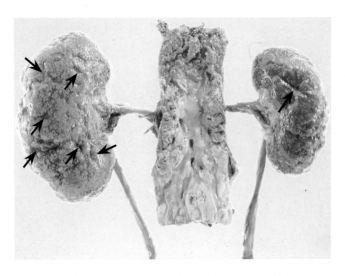

**Fig. 1-59** Complicated atherosclerotic vascular disease showing arterial nephrosclerosis, small atheroembolic infarcts (arrows), and an atrophic right kidney from renal artery stenosis.

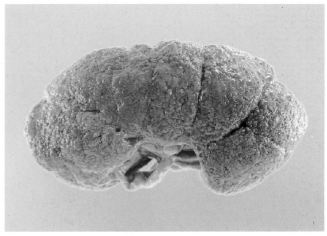

**Fig. 1-60** Granular subcapsular surface of benign hypertension-associated arterial nephrosclerosis.

**Table 1-13** Types and causes of hypertension

| |
| --- |
| Primary |
|    Benign (essential) hypertension |
|    Malignant hypertension |
| Secondary |
|    Renal artery stenosis |
|    Acute glomerulonephritis |
|    Chronic renal diseases |
|    Neoplasms |
|       Renin-producing tumors |
|       Adrenal cortical tumors |
|       Pheochromocytoma |
| Endocrine abnormalities |
|    Thyrotoxicosis |
|    Adrenal cortical hyperplasia |
|    Hyperparathyroidism |
|    Oral contraceptives |
| Neurogenic |
| Miscellaneous vascular |
|    Pre-eclampsia |
|    Thrombotic microangiopathy |
|    Vasculitis |
|    Coarctation of aorta |

not cause renal failure in most patients, it is sufficiently prevalent to account for approximately 15–30% of patients with end-stage renal disease.[158,164]

In benign nephrosclerosis the kidneys are symmetrically reduced in size and weigh between 60 and 100 g (Fig. 1-60). They have granular subcapsular surfaces and thin cortices, the extent of which is influenced by the severity and duration of the hypertension.[159,164] Microscopically, arteries of interlobular size or greater show fibrous intimal thickening with reduplication or fragmentation of the elastic lamina.[157,164,165] Lipid and calcification are not usually present. The grossly visible subcapsular granularity corresponds to shallow subcapsular scars that contain sclerotic glomeruli, atrophic tubules, and thick-walled hyalinized or hyperplastic arterioles (Fig. 1-61).[157,164–167] Similar hyaline arteriolar thickening also occurs in diabetes mellitus and develops to a mild degree in individuals over the age of 60 in the absence of hypertension. Hyaline arteriolar thickening may be encountered in young adults, where it is associated with early-onset coronary artery disease.[168]

## Malignant nephrosclerosis

Malignant nephrosclerosis develops as a consequence of malignant hypertension.[169,170] Malignant hypertension usually arises in a patient with pre-existing benign hypertension, but may develop as a de novo disorder. Patients present with headache, dizziness, and impaired vision. Their diastolic blood pressure exceeds 120–140 mmHg, and retinal hemorrhages and exudates and papilledema are present. Hematuria, proteinuria, and a microangiopathic hemolytic anemia develop. Without treatment, the patient will develop renal failure and may die suddenly from heart failure, myocardial infarct, or cerebral hemorrhage.

The kidney in malignant nephrosclerosis often has petechial subcapsular hemorrhages, or a mottled red and yellow cortex if infarcts are present. Microscopically, a range of lesions is encountered depending on whether the lesions are acute or chronic.

In the acute phase of malignant hypertension an acute thrombotic microangiopathy develops (Fig. 1-62). The glomeruli show capillary loop thrombosis and mesangiolysis, reflecting necrosis of endothelial and mesangial cells, and may develop segmental capillary loop necrosis with crescent formation. The arterioles develop fibrinoid necrosis (necrotizing arteriolitis) and thrombosis, reflecting necrosis of endothelium and medial smooth muscle cells. The intralobular arteries and arcuate arteries show a distinctive

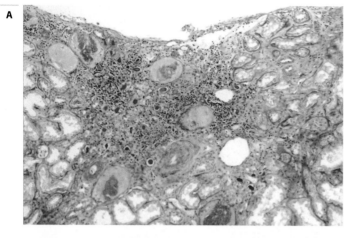

A

**Fig. 1-61 (A)** The shallow subcapsular scars contain sclerotic glomeruli and atrophic tubules and thickened arterioles. PAS stain. **(B)** Glomerular injury in hypertension showing ischemic glomerular basement membrane wrinkling and end-stage ischemic obsolescence. PAS stain. **(C)** Fibrointimal thickening of an artery.

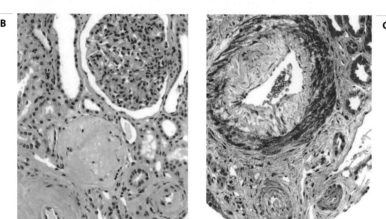

B      C

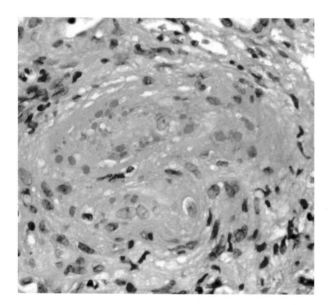

**Fig. 1-62** Necrotizing arteriolitis with thrombosis and extravasated red cells in malignant hypertension.

mucoid or edematous-appearing intimal thickening, and may also contain subendothelial fibrin and fragmented red blood cells.

In more protracted cases chronic or reparative changes are present, either alone or superimposed upon the acute throm-

botic microangiopathy. At this stage, with basement membrane stains such as periodic acid–Schiff (PAS) or a silver stain, the glomeruli may either show ischemic wrinkling and collapse (Fig. 1-63) or an impressive lucent subendothelial expansion and capillary loop basement membrane reduplication. The arterioles and arteries show concentric (onion-skin) myointimal proliferation resulting in severe luminal occlusion (Fig. 1-63).

## Thrombotic microangiopathy

The two classic syndromes dominated by thrombotic microangiopathy are thrombotic thrombocytopenic purpura, described by Moschcowitz[171] in 1925, and hemolytic uremic syndrome described by Gasser et al.[172] in 1955. Thrombotic microangiopathy is a term coined by Symmers[173] in 1952 for the microvascular lesions that develop in thrombotic thrombocytopenic purpura. Since that time, the use of the term has been expanded (Table 1-14) and now includes a group of largely non-inflammatory microvascular thrombotic diseases accompanied by renal disease, hemolytic anemia, and thrombocytopenia.[174–181]

The relationship between the two classic forms of primary thrombotic microangiopathy, thrombotic thrombocytopenic purpura and hemolytic uremic syndrome, remains controversial.[174,180–183] In thrombotic thrombocytopenic purpura the clinical picture is dominated by central nervous

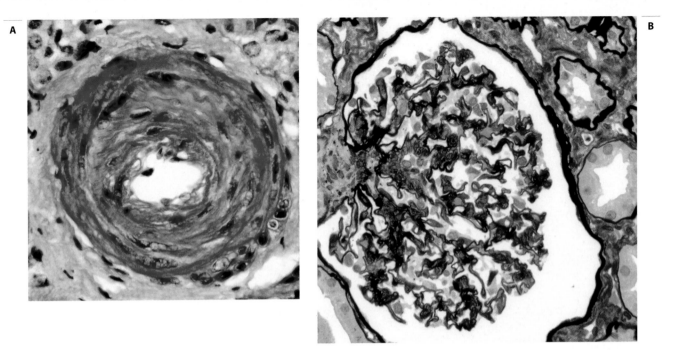

**Fig. 1-63** **(A)** Hyperplastic arteriolitis and **(B)** ischemic capillary loop wrinkling in malignant hypertension. A: PAS stain; B: silver stain.

**Table 1-14** Classification of thrombotic microangiopathy

| |
|---|
| Thrombotic thrombocytopenic purpura |
| Hemolytic uremic syndrome |
| Malignant hypertension |
| Disseminated intravascular coagulation |
| Scleroderma renal crisis |
| Postpartum acute renal failure |
| Irradiation |
| Drugs<br>   Oral contraceptives<br>   Chemotherapeutic agent<br>   Ciclosporin |

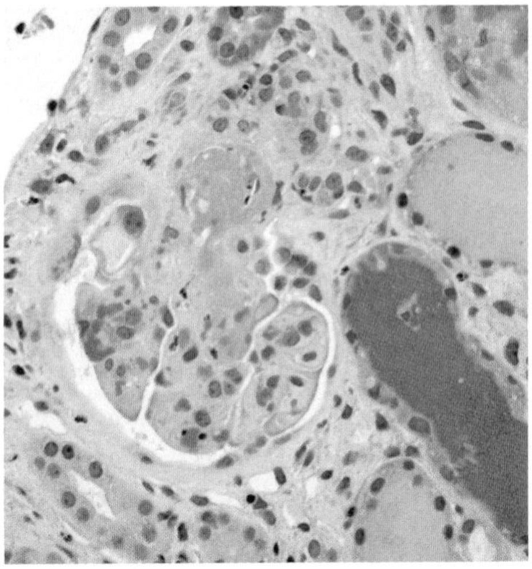

**Fig. 1-64** Hemolytic–uremic syndrome showing arteriolar and glomerular capillary thrombosis.

system involvement and only mild renal disease.[171,174,181] It usually develops in adults and has a fulminant course. If not promptly diagnosed and treated by plasma exchange or plasma infusion it has a high fatality rate.

In contrast, the clinical picture of hemolytic uremic syndrome is dominated by acute renal failure, and patients are usually children.[172,174,183–186] It has an acute, usually gastrointestinal diarrhea prodrome (occasionally upper respiratory infection prodrome) that has been shown to result from infection by verotoxin-producing stains of *Escherichia coli* in 80–90% of cases.[184–186] It is the most common cause of pediatric acute renal failure, but most children recover. Children over the age of 4 and those lacking the diarrhea prodrome have a poorer prognosis.

The histopathologic spectrum of the microvascular lesions in thrombotic microangiopathy is similar regardless of cause and identical to that described for malignant hypertension. Therefore, clinical correlation is required to distinguish thrombotic thrombocytopenic purpura from hemolytic uremic syndrome, or to implicate one of the secondary forms. Unfortunately, even when a secondary form is excluded not all patients are readily classified as either primary thrombotic thrombocytopenic purpura or hemolytic uremic syndrome because an insidious onset can occur with milder forms of both central nervous system and renal disease. Furthermore, acute renal failure and severe hyper-

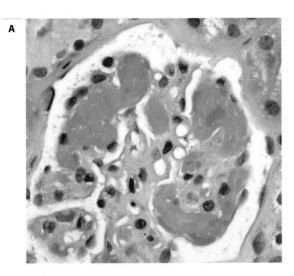
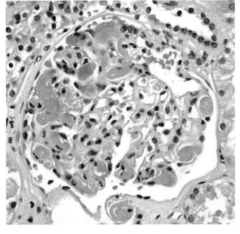

**Fig. 1-65** **(A)** Disseminated intravascular coagulation showing glomerular capillary thrombi. **(B)** Ciclosporin toxicity showing glomeruli capillary loop thrombi in a renal allograft.

tension may both be present, making separation between hemolytic uremic syndrome and primary malignant hypertension difficult if not impossible.

In acute thrombotic microangiopathy, glomeruli, arterioles and arteries may each be affected (Figs 1-64, 1-65). Glomeruli show endothelial cell and often mesangial cell necrosis with capillary loop thrombosis and mesangiolysis. The arterioles show luminal thrombosis and fibrin extravasation beneath the endothelium and into the media. The arteries show severe intimal edema or so-called mucoid intimal thickening, and may also contain fibrin and red cells. Fragmented red cells can be seen in all structures, and cortical infarcts may develop.

In the chronic phase observed in treated patients or in patients with a more insidious onset of the disease, the glomeruli show prominent mesangial expansion, microaneurysms, and reduplication of the capillary loop basement membranes (Fig. 1-66). Arterioles may show hyaline luminal occlusion, or both arterioles and arteries may show hyperplastic concentric myointimal proliferation resulting in severe luminal occlusion.

## Renal artery stenosis

In 1934 Goldblatt et al.[188] established a role for decreased renal perfusion in the generation of systemic hypertension by partially occluding one renal artery of a dog, producing hypertension that was reversed after restoration of blood flow. Hypertension resulting from decreased renal perfusion and relieved by restoration of flow is known as renovascular hypertension. Renal artery stenosis is the most common cause.[189,190] The two major etiologies of renal artery stenosis (Table 1-15) are atherosclerosis (66% of cases) and fibromuscular dysplasia (33% of cases). The remaining causes, although numerous, comprise less than 1% of cases. Renal artery stenosis may result in several complications (Table 1-15).

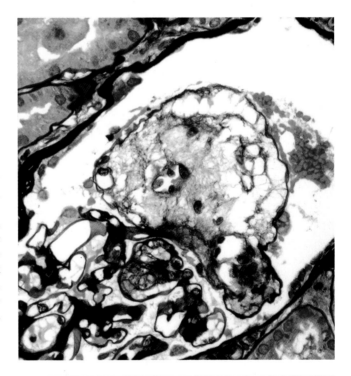

**Fig. 1-66** Chronic therapy-related thrombotic microangiopathy showing basement membrane duplication and severe mesangiolysis in a bone marrow transplant patient. Silver stain.

### Atherosclerosis-related renal artery stenosis

Atherosclerosis is associated with several renal complications (Tables 1-16 and 1-17) and is responsible for 60–70% of cases of renal artery stenosis. There is a male preponderance and patients usually present from age 50 to 70 with significant atherosclerosis of the aorta and other major arteries that influences the management of the disease and its prognosis. Because atherosclerosis develops over many years and is a complication of prolonged essential hypertension, the kidney may exhibit benign nephrosclerosis or may contain remote infarcts from aortic atheroemboli (Fig. 1-59). Bilateral disease occurs in 30% of cases and, if severe, causes ischemic chronic renal failure. Revascularization can improve renal function in some patients; however, because these patients have a long history of hypertension, arterial nephrosclerosis is usually implicated in the renal failure and renal artery stenosis is not recognized.

The renal artery is occluded by eccentrically thickened intima at its aortic ostium or in its proximal portion (Fig. 1-67). Intimal thickening begins when myointimal cells enter the media and synthesize connective tissue components and mucopolysaccharides.[165] Lipid and foam cells accumulate and fibrosis develops. The advanced lesion contains atheromatous material in the form of acingulate cholesterol clefts, foamy macrophages, and calcification. There is irregular duplication of the elastica lamina with sclerosis and atrophy of medial smooth muscle.

## Fibromuscular dysplasia

Fibromuscular dysplasia is the second most common cause of renal artery stenosis in adults and the most common cause in children.[191–193] It consists of a group of lesions (Table 1-18) that, despite histological differences, have a similar clinical presentation, affecting women in their 20s to 40s. The prognosis for fibromuscular dysplasia is much better than for atherosclerosis-associated renal artery stenosis because the patient is younger, the hypertension is of recent onset, and hypertension and atherosclerosis-related diseases in other sites are absent. There are five subtypes (dissection is discussed later in this chapter).

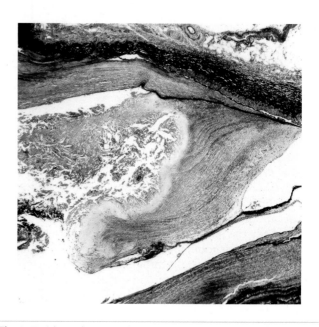

**Fig. 1-67** Atherosclerotic renal artery stenosis with a plaque at the renal artery ostium. Elastic stain.

**Table 1-15** Causes of renal artery stenosis

| |
|---|
| Atherosclerosis |
| Fibromuscular dysplasia |
| Rare other causes |
|    Renal artery dissection |
|    Renal artery aneurysm |
|    Renal artery thrombosis |
|    Renal artery emboli |
|    Arteriovenous malformation |
|    Arteritis |
|    Radiation injury |
|    Transplant artery stenosis |
|    Neurofibromatosis |

**Table 1-16** Renal complications of atherosclerotic vascular disease

| |
|---|
| Renal artery stenosis |
| Atherosclerotic emboli (macroemboli) |
| Cholesterol microembolization |

**Table 1-18** Classification of fibromuscular dysplasia

| |
|---|
| Intimal fibroplasia |
| Medial fibroplasia |
|    Medial hyperplasia |
|    Medial fibroplasia with aneurysms |
|    Perimedial fibroplasia |
| Periarterial fibroplasia |

**Table 1-17** Large vessel renal disease and potential complications

| Primary disorder | Hypertension | Dissection | Aneurysm | Infarct | Rupture |
|---|---|---|---|---|---|
| Renal artery stenosis | + | + | + | + | |
| Renal artery dissection | + | + | + | + | + |
| Renal artery aneurysms | + | + | + | + | + |
| Renal artery thrombosis | + | − | − | + | |
| Renal artery emboli | + | − | − | + | |
| AV malformation fistula | + | − | − | − | + |
| Renal arteritis | + | − | + | + | |
| Renal vein thrombosis | + | − | − | − | |

## Intimal fibroplasias

Intimal fibroplasia is a rare (<1% of cases) form of fibromuscular dysplasia. It produces circumferential intimal thickening in a substantial segment of the renal artery and may also extend into its segmental branches. The thickened intima is composed of fibroblastic tissue (Fig. 1-68). It is distinguished from atherosclerotic intimal thickening by the absence of lipids and calcification and the presence of an intact internal elastic lamina. It is prone to develop thrombosis and dissection.

## Medial hyperplasia

Medial hyperplasia consists of a localized segment of disorganized medial smooth muscle thickening. Radiographically it resembles the intimal form and is also prone to develop thrombosis and dissection. The intima is not thickened and the internal elastic lamina is intact.

## Medial fibroplasia with aneurysms

Medial fibroplasia with aneurysms is the most frequent and distinctive form of fibromuscular dysplasia. It tends to involve the distal main renal artery and its segmental branches and is commonly bilateral. It is characterized by ridges of medial thickening without fibrosis, alternating with areas of extreme medial thinning in which there is close approximation of the internal and external elastic lamina (Figs 1-69, 1-70). These areas of thinning represent the 'aneurysms' and result in a characteristic pattern (string of pearls) on angiogram.

## Perimedial fibroplasia

Perimedial fibroplasia is the second most common form of fibromuscular dysplasia. It is characterized by an irregular pattern of fibrosis that replaces the outer one-half to two-thirds of the media by fibrous tissue (Fig. 1-71). It can lead

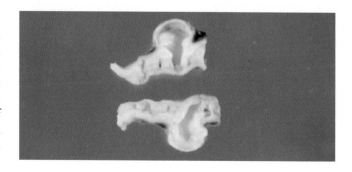

**Fig. 1-69** A segment of the main renal artery showing medial fibroplasia complicated by a saccular aneurysm.

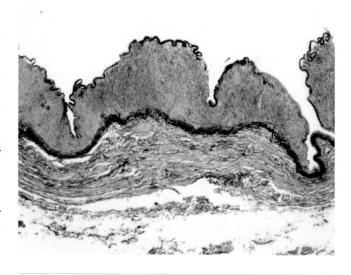

**Fig. 1-70** Medial fibroplasia. Elastic stain.

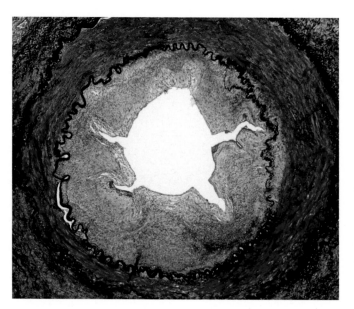

**Fig. 1-68** Intimal fibromuscular dysplasia showing fibroblastic intimal thickening and intact internal elastic lamina. Elastic stain.

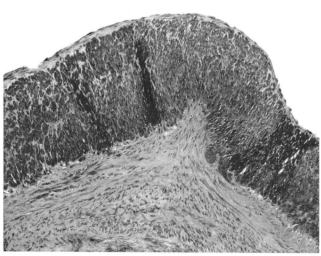

**Fig. 1-71** Perimedial fibroplasia. Trichrome stain.

to severe stenosis and the development of thrombosis and renal infarcts.

### Periarterial fibroplasia

Periarterial fibroplasia is the rarest form of fibromuscular dysplasia. It consists of dense collagenous tissue that forms within the adventitia and restricts arterial expansion during systole. The collagenous tissue can extend into the adjacent fibrofatty tissue, creating a vague similarity to retroperitoneal fibrosis.

### The kidney in renal artery stenosis

In renal artery stenosis of recent onset there is initial enlargement of the juxtaglomerular apparatus resulting from an increase in the number of the extraglomerular mesangial cells, or lacis cells (Fig. 1-72). There is metaplasia of smooth muscle cells of the afferent arteriole to form contractile filament-poor renin-synthesizing cells. Distinctive renin protogranules and mature renin granules can be detected in increased quantities in these cells by the Bowie stain, immunocytochemistry, or electron microscopy.

After several weeks of renal artery stenosis the juxtaglomerular apparatus shrinks, again becoming inconspicuous. At this time the parenchyma supplied by the stenotic artery shows a very distinctive alteration. Grossly there is uniform cortical thinning (Fig. 1-73) resulting from diffuse atrophy of tubules and causing close approximation of glomeruli due to loss of tubular volume (Fig. 1-74). The glomeruli appear slightly contracted but remain viable. If the main renal artery is the site of stenosis then the entire kidney becomes small (40–70 g) and uniformly contracted with a smooth subcapsular surface. If a segmental artery is stenotic, or conversely, if it is free of stenosis whereas the main renal artery is stenotic (Fig. 1-75), then a characteristic line of transition from a thinned cortex to a thicker cortex will be grossly apparent.

### Renal artery dissection

Dissection of the renal artery refers to a disruption of the intima that extends into the media (Figs 1-76, 1-77) with the creation of a false lumen or a double channel, or results in a complete vascular occlusion causing renal infarction.[194–196] Dissection is associated with hypertension, flank pain, and hematuria. The hypertension may not always precede the dissection but is invariably present afterwards. Renal artery dissection has several etiologies[194–196] (Table 1-19).

The most common cause of renal artery dissection is extension from an aortic dissection. Primary renal artery dis-

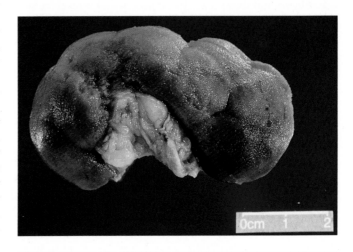

**Fig. 1-73** A small contracted kidney with a smooth surface in chronic renal artery stenosis secondary to fibromuscular dysplasia.

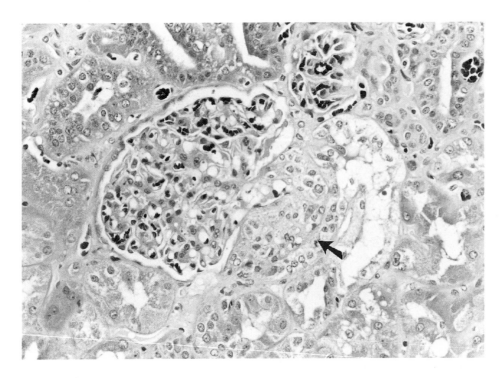

**Fig. 1-72** Acute renal artery stenosis in a renal transplant showing prominent enlargement of the juxtaglomerular apparatus (arrow).

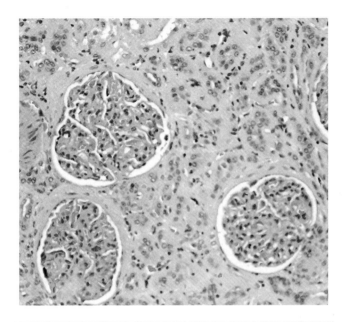

**Fig. 1-74** The thin cortex in chronic renal artery stenosis shows diffuse small atrophic tubules and crowding of non-sclerotic glomeruli.

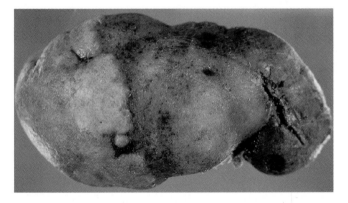

**Fig. 1-75** Chronic renal artery stenosis affecting the middle and lower poles. The upper pole was supplied by a patent supernumerary (polar segmental) artery.

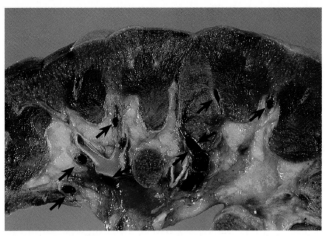

**Fig. 1-76** Extensive renal artery dissection (arrows) following an unsuccessful angioplasty.

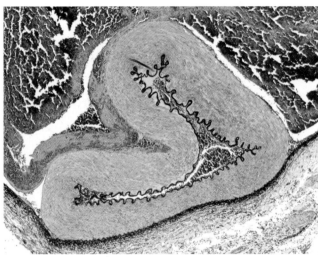

**Fig. 1-77** The dissection (from Fig. 1-76) developed at the interface of the media and adventitia.

section is rarer and in the past was usually a complication of pre-existing fibromuscular dysplasia. Catheter-related causes are increasing with more frequent use of this procedure to correct renal artery stenosis. Dissection due to blunt trauma is rare and usually the consequence of an automobile accident.

## Renal artery aneurysm

Aneurysm of the main renal artery or one of its tributaries is rare, found in 0.01% of autopsies.[196–200] It may be classified as true aneurysm that is congenital or acquired, or false aneurysm that is usually the result of trauma. Most are small and asymptomatic. If a large vessel is involved, renal artery aneurysm may be associated with thrombosis and vascular occlusion leading to infarction or hypertension. Pain is an ominous symptom that usually indicates impending rupture

| Table 1-19 Causes of renal artery dissection |
| --- |
| Extension from aortic dissection |
| Fibromuscular dysplasia |
| Blunt abdominal trauma |
| Catheter injury |
| Spontaneous or idiopathic |

or dissection. The risk of rupture is greatest during pregnancy and parturition and is usually fatal. Three categories of aneurysm have been identified: saccular, fusiform, and intrarenal. Dissecting aneurysm is not included in this list because aneurysmal enlargement is not a feature of renal arterial dissection.

## Saccular aneurysm

Saccular aneurysm develops in the main renal artery at the bifurcation of the anterior and posterior divisions or at a branch point of a segmental artery. Although it is frequently calcified or shows atherosclerotic changes, it is usually regarded as congenital, the atherosclerosis being considered a secondary event. It may be small or enlarge to 4–5 cm. Especially if non-calcified, the large aneurysm is prone to rupture or may erode into an adjacent vein, producing an arteriovenous fistula.

## Fusiform aneurysm

Fusiform aneurysm usually occurs in young patients and represents post-stenotic dilation that develops distal to renal artery stenosis, often secondary to fibromuscular dysplasia. Thrombosis with secondary renal infarction is a serious potential complication.

## Intrarenal aneurysm

Intrarenal aneurysm is usually a false aneurysm.[200] It may result from a wide variety of causes, including trauma (biopsy, surgery), arteritis (polyarteritis nodosa), postinflammatory injury (tuberculosis or transplant rejection), and neurofibromatosis. Rarely, intrarenal aneurysm may be congenital.

## Arteriovenous malformation and fistula

Direct communication between renal arteries and veins may either be congenital or acquired.[201–203] Congenital lesions are referred to as arteriovenous malformations, and acquired lesions are called arteriovenous fistulas. High-output heart failure, hypertension, and hematuria may develop, depending on the size of the shunt and the location of the lesion. The most common type is an acquired fistula (65–75% of cases). It usually has a single point of communication between an artery and a vein,[201] and results from one of several causes, the most common of which is iatrogenic[203] (Table 1-20).

Congenital arteriovenous malformation is rare. Most consist of circoid arteriovenous communications in which there are multiple points of communication between artery and vein. Most are located within the medulla or in the calyceal or pelvic mucosa, and usually cause gross hematuria. Hilar vessels may also be affected. When a single cavernous channel connects an artery with a vein, an abdominal bruit may be heard.

## Renal emboli and infarct

Renal artery emboli invariably cause infarction because of the end-artery organization of the renal blood flow.[18–20] If the infarct is small, it may be clinically and functionally asymptomatic. Larger infarcts cause flank pain, hematuria, and hypertension.[204–211] If bilateral and widespread, renal insufficiency results. Emboli originate either from the heart in patients with valvular disease or atrial fibrillation, or from the aorta.[204–207] Aortic atheroemboli are by far the most frequent (Fig. 1-78). If an infected vegetation is responsible, a more complicated picture develops, with hematogenous pyelonephritis and microabscesses (Fig. 1-79).

Familiarity with the arterial supply to the kidney often enables one, on gross examination, to infer the caliber of vessel occluded by virtue of the size of the infarct and its relationship to the renal lobes (Figs 1-80 and 1-81 and Table 1-21).

The acute infarct shows a sharply demarcated zone of transcortical coagulation necrosis that will also involve the medulla if an arcuate or larger artery is involved (Figs 1-82, 1-83). The margins of the infarct are hemorrhagic and contain many neutrophils and histiocytes. Cholesterol clefts or infected material in the arteries may reveal the source of the embolus (Figs 1-78, 1-79).

Eventually, infarcts become depressed cortical scars (Figs 1-80, 1-81, 1-84). Within them, ghost-like remnants of glomeruli and tubules are present (Fig. 1-84). A PAS stain is helpful in determining whether a scar is an infarct or a more chronic form of injury, because infarcted glomeruli contain condensed masses of capillary loop basement membranes without the collagenous tissue in Bowman's space that forms with other causes of glomerulosclerosis.

## Renal cortical necrosis

Renal cortical necrosis is a serious bilateral ischemic injury that can complicate a variety of extrarenal diseases[212–214] (Table 1-22). Obstetric causes are most frequent. Patients develop acute renal failure, usually associated with anuria and hematuria that may be gross. The condition has a high fatality rate related to extrarenal complications.

The kidneys develop diffuse or patchy sharply demarcated zones of cortical pallor with hyperemic rims that also involve the columns of Bertin. The renal pyramids and a thin subcapsular rim of cortex are spared. There is coagulation

**Table 1-20** Causes of acquired arteriovenous fistula

| Surgical injury |
| --- |
| Needle biopsy |
| Penetrating injury |
| Neoplasia |
| Arterial aneurysm erosion |
| Inflammation |

**Table 1-21** Relationship of infarct size to the arterial supply to the kidney

| Artery | Size of infarct (cm) | Relationship to lobes |
| --- | --- | --- |
| Segmental | 4–5 | Entire lobe and portion of adjacent lobe |
| Interlobar | 2–3 | Columns of Bertin and portion of adjacent lobe |
| Arcuate | 0.5–1.0 | 1/6–1/8 of a lobe, extending to the middle of the lobe |
| Interlobular | 0.1–0.2 | Small portion of a lobe |

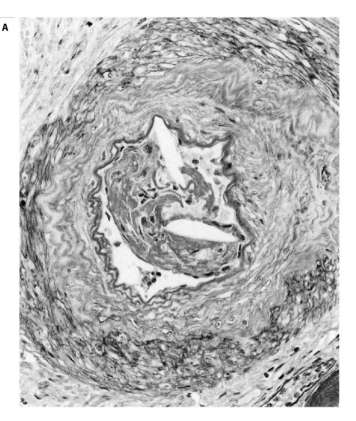

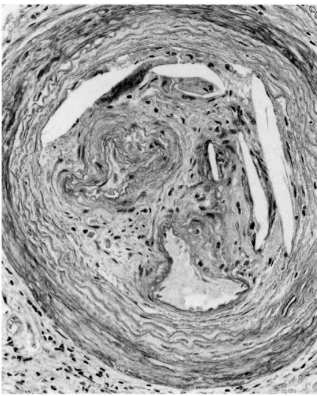

**Fig. 1-78** **(A)** Recent and **(B)** remote atheroemboli showing respectively a fibrin thrombus and recanalization with giant cells.

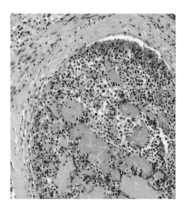

**Fig. 1-79** This thromboembolus from a patient with infective endocarditis contains Gram-positive cocci and has destroyed a portion of the arterial wall.

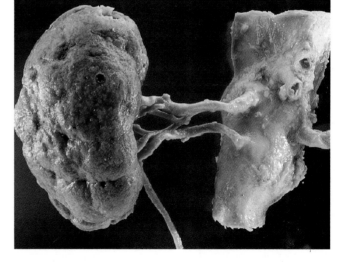

**Fig. 1-80** Multiple depressed scars resulting from arcuate and interlobular atheroembolic infarcts.

necrosis of glomeruli and tubules, usually with widespread thrombosis.

## Renal cholesterol microembolism syndrome

Atherosclerotic vascular disease affects the kidneys in several ways (Fig. 1-85). In 1965 Richards and colleagues[206] distinguished embolic complications of fragments of atherosclerotic plaques that occlude large arteries and result in infarcts, from microemboli of cholesterol crystals. This syndrome usually develops after a vascular procedure such as catheterization or aneurysm surgery, but occasionally arises spontaneously. Emboli shower the microvasculature of multiple organs, including the kidneys, skin, brain, and gastrointestinal tract, producing a systemic disease resembling systemic vasculitis with abdominal pain, acute onset of hypertension, livedo reticularis, and neurologic symptoms. In the initial reports of microembolic disease that appeared in the 1960–1980s, the fatality rate was very high. More recently, patients

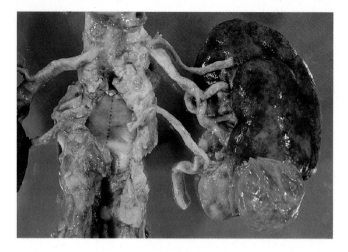

**Fig. 1-81** A remote lower pole infarct and cyst resulting from occlusion of a supernumerary (lower pole segmental) artery during aortic aneurysm repair.

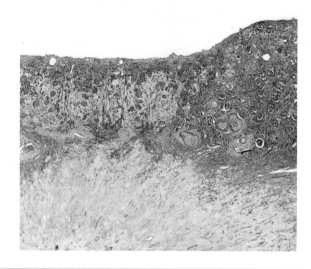

**Fig. 1-84** Remote atheroembolic cortical infarct. PAS stain. Note solid PAS-positive glomeruli and tubules.

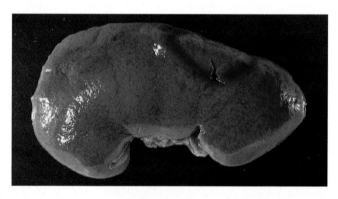

**Fig. 1-82** An acute infarct resulting from an interlobar artery occlusion.

**Table 1-22** Causes of renal cortical necrosis

| |
| --- |
| Obstetric complications |
|   Abruptio placentae |
|   Septic abortion |
|   Intrauterine fetal demise |
| Infections |
|   Sepsis |
|   Peritonitis |
| Burns |
| Gastrointestinal hemorrhage |
| Transfusion reactions |
| Toxins |
| Hemolytic–uremic syndrome |

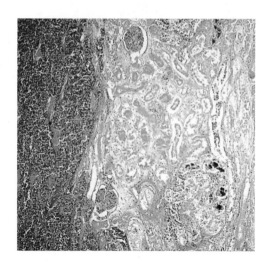

**Fig. 1-83** An acute infarct showing coagulation necrosis with peripheral hemorrhage.

with milder forms have been identified who may completely or partially recover renal function.[206,207,209]

Cholesterol microembolization is associated with several potentially confusing laboratory findings.[208–210,216] Cholesterol microembolization is associated with eosinophilia in 15–80% of cases. In a given patient it may be impressive, with absolute eosinophils counts reported as high as 19 700/mm³. Eosinophiluria is infrequent. Less commonly encountered but potentially more confusing are hypocomplementemia, thrombocytopenia, and proteinuria that may be nephrotic range.

Not every biopsy with a cholesterol crystal should elicit alarm. Asymptomatic cholesterol embolization has been identified at autopsy in 4% of patients with aortic atherosclerotic disease, attesting that cholesterol embolization can be clinically insignificant.[210,215] When multiple emboli are noted on biopsy concern escalates because the percentage of the kidney examined in a single biopsy is minute. Many thousands of emboli may have been delivered to the kidneys for every crystal noted in a biopsy. If the patient presents with impaired renal function and no other cause is identi-

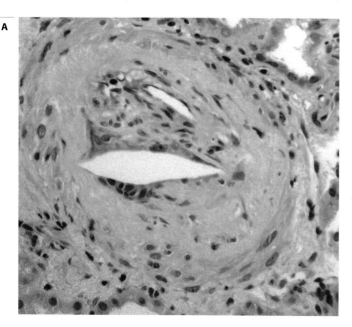 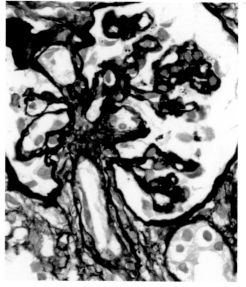

**Fig. 1-85** Renal cholesterol microembolism syndrome with cholesterol emboli **(A)** in an arteriole and **(B)** in the glomerular hilum.

fied, implicating cholesterol embolization as the cause of the renal failure becomes unavoidable. Autopsy studies have demonstrated that fresh or recent cholesterol crystals are intraluminal without a cellular reaction.[210] Within days, macrophages appear, followed by a fibroblastic reaction. Eventually endothelial cell and collagen investment incorporates the crystals into the wall, or provokes further fibroblastic reaction with luminal obliteration. Correlation of the clinical event that may have caused cholesterol embolization with the above features may assist interpretation of finding crystals in a renal biopsy.

## Renal artery thrombosis

Thombosis of the renal artery is an uncommon event that usually follows a traumatic injury either to the artery or to the aorta[204,217] (Table 1-23). Renovascular hypertension and renal infarction are the major complications (see Table 1-17).

## Renal vein and renal venous thrombosis

In the past renal vein thrombosis was believed to cause nephrotic syndrome.[218,219] With the increasing use of renal biopsy and advances in our understanding of the physiologic consequences of nephrotic syndrome, it is now clear that renal vein thrombosis is a complication of the hypercoagulable state that develops in patients with nephrotic syndrome. Patients with renal vein thrombosis present with flank pain or tenderness and hematuria and often have hypertension. Renal failure and pulmonary emboli are serious complications. Although there are no pathognomonic histologic findings, interstitial edema and marginating neutrophils within dilated glomerular capillaries have been described in acute cases. Organizing thrombi are seen in veins at autopsy.[219-221]

**Table 1-23** Causes of renal artery thrombosis

| |
| --- |
| Umbilical artery catheters in neonates |
| Blunt abdominal trauma |
| Intra-aortic balloons in adults |
| Renal transplantation |
| Electrical injury |

Renal venous thrombosis differs from renal vein thrombosis in that smaller intrarenal vessels are affected, such as interlobular and arcuate veins, rather than the main renal vein.[221,222] Infants are usually affected and the condition is associated with serious illnesses such as diarrhea, congenital heart disease, maternal diabetes mellitus, seizures, and birth trauma. Hemorrhagic cortical infarcts may develop if the thrombosis is sufficiently widespread to interfere with collateral blood flow.

## Bartter's syndrome

Bartter's syndrome is characterized by hyperplasia of the juxtaglomerular apparatus, hyperaldosteronism, and hypokalemic alkalosis.[223] Despite the impressive enlargement of the juxtaglomerular apparatus and hyperreninemia, both renal artery stenosis and systemic hypertension are absent. It is most commonly identified in children and in many cases appears to be familial with an autosomal recessive inheritance.

## Vasculitis

Vasculitis comprises a large and heterogeneous group of disorders that have in common inflammatory injury to vascular structures. The first major description of vasculitis dates

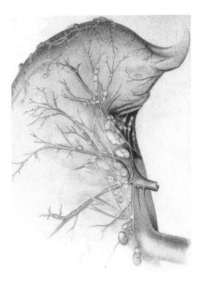

**Fig. 1-86** Nodules along renal arteries in polyarteritis nodosa, from the 1866 description by Küssmaul and Maier. (From Küssmaul A, Maier R. Ueber eine bisher niche beschriebene eigenthumliche arteriener-krankung (periarteritis nodosa), die mit morbus Brightii und rapid fortschreitender ailgemeiner muskellahmung. Dtsch Arch Klin Med 1866; 1: 484; with permission.)

to the 1866 description of periarteritis (polyarteritis) nodosa by Küssmaul and Maier (Fig. 1-86)[224] The seriousness of systemic vasculitis with major visceral involvement was graphically captured in their report. They stated: 'He was one of those patients for whom one could make the prognosis even before making the diagnosis; he gave the impression of being one whose days were numbered.'[224]

A major advance in the diagnosis and management of patients with vasculitis was the discovery of a serologic marker for certain forms of vasculitis, the antineutrophil cytoplasmic antibody.[225–231] Antineutrophil cytoplasmic antibodies (ANCA) are a family of autoantibodies detectable in the serum of patients with the major forms of systemic vasculitis involving the kidney and in idiopathic (immune complex negative or 'pauci-immune') crescentic glomerulo-nephritis (Table 1-24).[227–231] ANCAs have specificity for one of several lysosomal enzymes within neutrophils and mono-cytes. They are detected by indirect immunofluorescence on alcohol-fixed neutrophils. Two principal patterns are detected, a cytoplasmic pattern (C-ANCA) and a perinuclear pattern (P-ANCA). The former is principally due to antipro-teinase 3 specificity, whereas the latter is principally due to antimyeloperoxidase specificity.

Although C-ANCA correlates with Wegener's granuloma-tosis and P-ANCA correlates with polyarteritis and idiopathic crescentic glomerulonephritis, there are sufficient exceptions to make the presence of a positive antineutrophil cytoplas-mic antibody test important, rather than its subtype. Anti-neutrophil cytoplasmic antibody is useful because it simplifies the morphologic and clinical differential (Table 1-24). It can also be used to monitor response to therapy (insensitive due to slow decline in titer with remission) and to distinguish clinical relapse (rising titer) from therapeutic complication (falling titer).

**Table 1-24** Antineutrophil cytoplasmic antibody (ANCA) status in vasculitides

| |
|---|
| **ANCA-positive vasculitis (% positive)** |
| Wegener's granulomatosis (>90) |
| Microscopic polyarteritis (>90) |
| Polyarteritis nodosa (30–50) |
| Idiopathic crescentic vasculitis (>90) |
| Kawasaki disease (50) |
| Churg–Strauss syndrome (50–60) |
| **ANCA-negative vasculitis** |
| Temporal arteritis |
| Takayasu's arteritis |
| Henoch–Schönlein purpura* |
| Connective tissue diseases* |
| Glomerulonephritis |
| Cryoglobulenemia |
| Drug reaction* |
| Infectious arteritis |

*Rare positive cases.

**Table 1-25** Direct immunofluorescence in crescentic glomerulonephritis

| |
|---|
| **Linear immunofluorescence** |
| Goodpasture's syndrome |
| Antiglomerular basement membrane disease |
| **Granular immunofluorescence** |
| Immune complex glomerulonephritis |
| **Negative immunofluorescence** |
| Systemic vasculitis |
| Idiopathic ('pauci-immune') crescentic glomerulonephritis |

The kidney is the most commonly affected organ in sys-temic vasculitis.[232–234] Either necrotizing and crescentic glomerulonephritis (most common) or true arteritis may develop. Crescentic glomerulonephritis is the most common pattern of renal involvement by vasculitis.[232–235] Following necrosis of the glomerular capillary wall a crescent forms.[236] Extravasation of fibrin, protein, and red cells ensues, and epithelial cell proliferation occurs in the area of damage (Fig. 1-87). If healing occurs, a segmental to circumferential scar (fibrous crescent) forms, the size of which varies with the size of the initial necrosis. If the percentage of glomeruli affected by necrosis exceeds 50%, the patient presents with rapidly progressive renal failure. Their urine contains protein, red cells, and often red cell casts.

The process of crescent formation is not specific for vas-culitis: crescents also form in other types of glomerulone-phritis. The process is subclassified by the findings on direct immunofluorescence[235] (Table 1-25). Vasculitis is distinctive because of the absence of appreciable detectable immune reactants by direct immunofluorescence. Most are antineu-trophil cytoplasmic antibody positive.

Necrotizing arteritis and arteriolitis is less common than crescentic glomerulonephritis when vasculitis affects the kidney.[234,235] It is characterized by fibrinoid necrosis of the

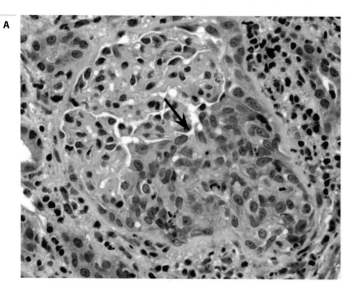

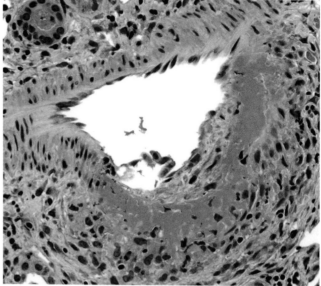

**Fig. 1-87** **(A)** A cellular crescent (arrow) in a patient with classic Wegener's granulomatosis. **(B)** Segmental fibrinoid necrosis of an artery in a patient with polyarteritis nodosa.

vessel wall, karyorrhexis, and a mixed inflammatory cell response rich in neutrophils (Fig. 1-87). The prominent inflammatory component distinguishes vasculitis from acute thrombotic microangiopathy. Although necrotizing arteritis is most common in classic polyarteritis nodosa and Wegener's granulomatosis, it can develop in other forms of vasculitis (see Table 1-24). Serologic data and clinical correlation are crucial to proper classification.[235]

## Tubulointerstitial diseases

Disorders of tubules and interstitium are discussed together because they rarely occur in isolation: any alteration in one affects the other. Tubules make up 90% of the renal cortex, whereas the renal interstitium consists of a slender zone separating the cortical tubules. The renal interstitium contains peritubular capillaries, collagen fibers, and a few interstitial cells (see Figs 1-19 and 1-21). Although normally scant, the interstitium can expand rapidly following an acute tubular or interstitial disease. This is the principal non-neoplastic manner in which gross renal expansion can occur. Conversely, because tubules comprise 90% of the cortical mass, tubular atrophy is responsible for most of the cortical thinning that occurs in any form of chronic renal disease. Interstitial expansion is also the parameter most closely linked to the level of renal insufficiency, even in those diseases that primarily affect vessels or glomeruli.[237–239]

In no other area of renal disease is clinical information more crucial in establishing the etiology of an abnormality than in a tubulointerstitial disease. This is a consequence of the limited spectrum of histologic abnormalities that may result from a large number of different injuries. Because tubulointerstitial alterations correlate with renal dysfunction, most forms of tubulointerstitial disease present with

**Table 1-26** Classification of infection-related tubulointerstitial nephritides

| Acute infection |
| --- |
| Acute pyelonephritis |
| Pyonephrosis |
| Perinephric abscess |
| Emphysematous pyelonephritis |
| Renal papillary necrosis |
| Fungal infections |
| Viral infections |
| **Chronic infection** |
| Chronic pyelonephritis |
| Xanthogranulomatous pyelonephritis |
| Malakoplakia |
| Tuberculosis |

some degree of renal insufficiency. The rate of development of renal insufficiency can be used to formulate a classification of tubulointerstitial diseases. This is useful because it separates entities with the greatest potential for recovery of renal function (acute forms) from those in which some irreversible injury is present (chronic forms). It also is convenient to separate infection-related entities into a third group (Table 1-26) because their etiology is usually more obvious and many forms are interrelated.

Acute tubulointerstitial diseases have a rapid clinical onset and are associated with edema and variable inflammation, and are potentially reversible.[239] The inflammation is usually neutrophilic in infectious etiologies (pyelonephritis) and principally lymphohistiocytic in allergic and autoimmune forms. Chronic tubulointerstitial diseases have a gradual or insidious onset and are associated with irreversible tubular atrophy and interstitial fibrosis. A lymphocytic

**Table 1-27** Complications of acute pyelonephritis

| |
| --- |
| Renal abscess |
| Pyonephrosis |
| Perinephric abscess |
| Emphysematous pyelonephritis |
| Sepsis |

infiltrate is also present, even in forms associated with infection.

## Infection-related tubulointerstitial nephritis

### Acute pyelonephritis

Acute pyelonephritis is a bacterial infection of the kidney.[240] Patients present with fever, leukocytosis, and flank tenderness, and may suffer a variety of complications (Table 1-27). Pyuria and urinary white blood cell casts usually are present. The kidneys may be seeded by organisms via two major pathways: ascending infection and hematogenously.

The most common avenue of infection is ascent from a lower urinary tract infection. *Escherichia coli* is the most frequent organism, followed by other enteric organisms such as *Proteus*, *Klebsiella*, and *Enterobacter*. In most individuals with bacterial cystitis the infection remains localized to the bladder. In susceptible individuals vesicoureteral reflux occurs, permitting colonization of the upper tracts.[240–244] This most often occurs in children with primary vesicoureteral reflux, a congenital (often hereditary) abnormality in the anatomy of the ureterovesical junction.[245] Reflux can also develop in non-refluxing systems if the cystitis is severe, or if there is distal obstruction or a neurogenic bladder.

Even with an upper tract infection, parenchymal infection is not inevitable. The organisms must first gain access to the papillary collecting ducts, a process known as intrarenal reflux.[241–247] The architecture of the renal pyramids influences their susceptibility to intrarenal reflux (see Reflux Nephropathy, later in this chapter). Following initial infection of the pyramids, the infection extends up the medullary rays prior to more generalized cortical spread.

Acute pyelonephritis in surgical and autopsy specimens represents the most severe example. The collecting system is thickened, and yellow-white suppurative foci or overt abscesses are present in both pyramids and cortex (Fig. 1-88). Microscopically, there is mucosal ulceration and an intense neutrophilic response within the tubules and interstitium (Fig. 1-89). Occasionally, in sites of early involvement, bacteria or neutrophils can be seen in the collecting ducts of the cortex and medulla (Fig. 1-90). Glomeruli may be spared initially, but with increasing severity generalized parenchymal destruction occurs that may liquefy, resulting in abscess formation.

Hematogenous pyelonephritis usually complicates prolonged sepsis or infectious endocarditis. The kidneys are usually peppered with abscesses that are more numerous in the cortex than the medulla (Figs 1-91, 1-92). The organisms responsible are more often Gram-positive bacteria or fungi.

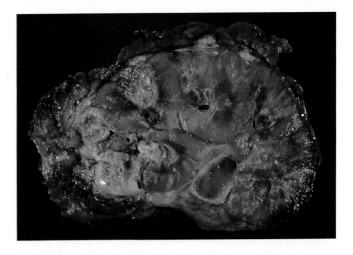

**Fig. 1-88** Ascending acute pyelonephritis complicated by abscess formation most severely affecting the lower pole (left).

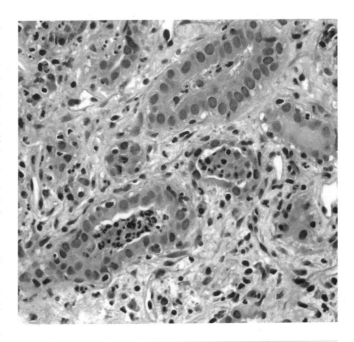

**Fig. 1-89** Acute pyelonephritis showing numerous neutrophils within renal tubules (destined to form urinary white blood cell casts).

### Pyonephrosis

Pyonephrosis is the near total destruction of an obstructed kidney by acute pyelonephritis. The parenchyma is replaced by suppurative inflammation, transforming the kidney into a large abscess. The patient is typically septic. Urine cultures may be negative because of the urinary tract obstruction.

### Perinephric abscess

Perinephric abscess is the accumulation of infectious material and neutrophils within perinephric fat (Fig. 1-93). It usually originates from rupture of a renal abscess or from pyonephrosis, but can develop following a surgical procedure such as renal transplantation or surgery for calculi. Rarely, it may originate from an infected nidus extrinsic to

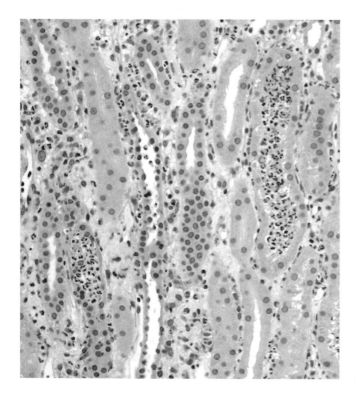

**Fig. 1-90** Ascending acute pyelonephritis with neutrophils in medullary collecting ducts.

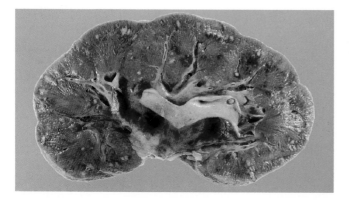

**Fig. 1-91** Hematogenous pyelonephritis showing miliary abscesses in a patient with bacterial sepsis.

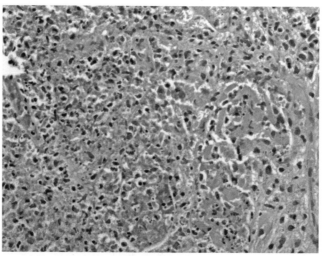

**Fig. 1-92** A cortical microabscess.

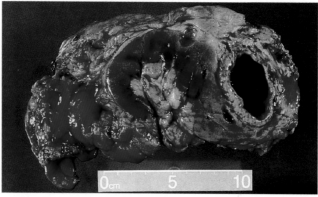

**Fig. 1-93** A perinephric abscess.

the kidney, such as the gastrointestinal tract in diverticulitis and Crohn's disease, or from bone in osteomyelitis.[240,248,249] Either Gram-negative or Gram-positive organisms can be responsible.

### Emphysematous pyelonephritis

Emphysematous pyelonephritis is an uncommon but potentially life-threatening complication of acute suppurative bacterial (rarely fungal) infection of the kidney.[250–253] In emphysematous pyelonephritis gas bubbles develop within the renal parenchyma and may extend into perinephric and even retroperitoneal sites. It should be distinguished from emphysematous pyelitis and ureteritis, which are far less dangerous conditions. Approximately 90% of patients with this infection have diabetes mellitus, and urinary tract

obstruction is present in approximately 40%. Women outnumber men by a ratio of 2:1. *E. coli* is the responsible organism in 68% of cases and *Klebsiella* in 9%, with a mixed infection in 19% of cases. No reported cases have been attributed to *Clostridium* spp.

Grossly the kidney of a patient with emphysematous pyelonephritis shows widespread abscesses with papillary necrosis and cortical infarcts. It may have a cystic appearance due to gas bubbles. Microscopically, the characteristic feature is empty spaces lacking epithelial cell linings and distorting the parenchyma (Fig. 1-94). Adjacent areas show vascular thrombosis, ischemic necrosis, suppurative inflammation, and abscesses.

### Renal papillary necrosis

Necrosis of portions of the renal medulla is known as renal papillary necrosis.[254–259] A number of diseases are associated with papillary necrosis (Table 1-28). When bilateral and diffuse, it presents as an acute devastating illness with renal failure, fever, chills, flank pain, and hematuria. Alternatively, it may be an insidious process that manifests as a urinary concentrating defect or with the gradual devel-

**Table 1-28** Causes of renal papillary necrosis

| Diabetes mellitus |
| --- |
| Urinary tract obstruction |
| Acute pyelonephritis |
| Analgesic abuse |
| Sickle cell disease |
| Hypoxia |
| Dehydration |
| Combination of above=55% |

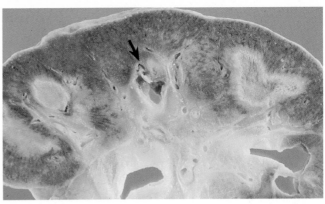

**Fig. 1-95** Renal papillary necrosis in a diabetic patient. The papilla in the center has sloughed (arrow).

**Fig. 1-96** Papillary necrosis showing coagulation necrosis and peripheral inflammation.

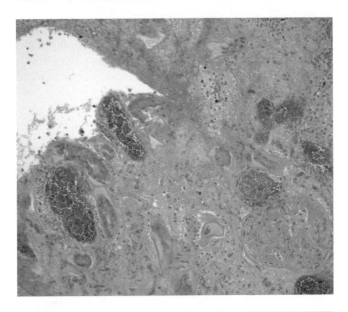

**Fig. 1-94** Emphysematous pyelonephritis showing gas within necrotic parenchyma.

opment of renal failure. Renal papillary necrosis is always the complication of some other disease process, and most patients have more than one risk factor present. In the United States, diabetes is the most prevalent underlying disorder.

Renal papillary necrosis is often included in discussions of pyelonephritis owing to the strong association with infection. However, its pathogenesis is ischemia related to the marginal medullary blood supply. This accounts for its association with disorders that compromise medullary blood flow.

This is usually a disease of adults, although infants can also develop renal papillary necrosis. Although it is often referred to in the pediatric literature as renal medullary necrosis, approximately 25–30% of patients will also develop focal cortical infarcts.[258] Infants with renal papillary necrosis are usually less than 1 month old and have perinatal asphyxia or a severe infantile disease associated with vascular collapse and dehydration, such as gastroenteritis.

In the 1950s and 1960s renal papillary necrosis became a serious problem, particularly in Australia and in Scandinavian countries where analgesic combinations were in widespread use.[260-264] Analgesic nephropathy, as it came to be known, rapidly became the leading cause of chronic renal failure and renal papillary necrosis in those regions (see Analgesic Nephropathy later in this chapter).

In renal papillary necrosis the necrosis usually does not involve the entire medulla. The papillary tip is most vulnerable, whereas the outer medulla is often preserved. A medullary form and a papillary form have been described.[258,259] In the medullary form, the calyceal spiral arteries are patent and peripheral or fornical portions of the pyramid are intact, with the central portions being necrotic (Fig. 1-95). In the papillary form, the necrosis is more extensive and the entire papilla or inner medulla is necrotic (Fig. 1-96). In both forms the necrosis is of a coagulation type, in keeping with its ischemic etiology.

## Fungal infection

Acute fungal tubulointerstitial nephritis is usually encountered in immunocompromised or diabetic patients. Antibiotic therapy and urinary tract instrumentation are other major risk factors.[265-267] As with bacterial infections, the kidney may be seeded either by the ascending or the hematogenous route. *Candida* species and *Torulopsis* are the most common organisms. In patients with acquired immunodeficiency syndrome (AIDS) almost any fungus may be encountered. The kidney shows a mixed neutrophilic and

**Table 1-29** Classification of viral renal diseases

Acute tubulointerstitial nephritis
    Cytomegalovirus
    Adenovirus
    HIV
    Polyoma virus (BK type)

Glomerulonephritis
    Hepatitis B
    Hepatitis C
    HIV
    Rare others:
        Mumps
        Varicella
        Echovirus
        Cytomegalovirus

Arteritis
    Hepatitis B

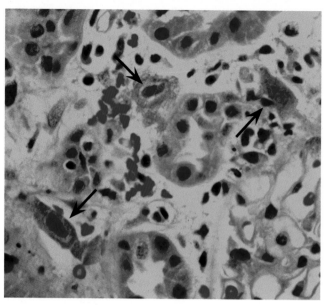

**Fig. 1-98** Cytomegaloviral (arrows) acute interstitial nephritis in an immunocompromised patient.

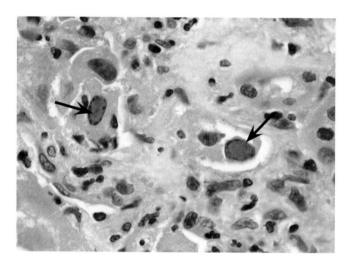

**Fig. 1-97** Polyoma virus in a renal allograft. Several large intranuclear inclusions are present (arrows).

granulomatous response, and fungal elements are usually demonstrable.

## Viral infection

Viruses can produce a variety of renal diseases, including acute tubulointerstitial nephritis, glomerulonephritis (most common), and arteritis (Table 1-29).[268–280] Cytomegalovirus, adenovirus, and polyomavirus can cause a typical acute interstitial nephritis in which viral inclusions are visible within the kidney. Both polyomavirus and adenovirus result in smudgy-appearing intranuclear inclusions within tubular cells (Fig. 1-97).[270,278–280] Cytomegalovirus produces the characteristic large intranuclear inclusions with haloes and eosinophilic cytoplasmic inclusions in tubular cells, podocytes, and endothelial cells (Fig. 1-98).[268,269]

Viral inclusions are not visible in the other viral renal diseases and most produce a glomerulonephritis, often with immune complex deposits.[272–277] Human immunodeficiency virus (HIV) causes a complex renal disease known as HIV nephropathy. This is characterized by a triad of interstitial nephritis with large tubular casts, glomerulonephritis due to focal–segmental glomerulosclerosis, and numerous endothelial reticulotubular inclusions.[274,275] Hantavirus (nephropathica epidemica, hemorrhagic fever with renal syndrome) can produce an uncommon rodent-derived, acute, self-limited influenza-like illness with an acute interstitial nephritis.[276,277]

## Chronic pyelonephritis

Chronic pyelonephritis is a chronic destructive tubulointerstitial disease usually regarded as a sequela of recurrent or persistent episodes of bacterial infection of the kidney. It is responsible for 5–15% of end-stage kidney disease. Usually it is subdivided into reflux nephropathy (or chronic non-obstructive pyelonephritis) and obstructive pyelonephritis.

### Reflux nephropathy (chronic non-obstructive pyelonephritis)

In 1960 Hodson and Edwards[243] established a link between non-obstructive chronic pyelonephritis and vesicoureteral reflux. Appreciation of the nearly ubiquitous association between non-obstructive forms of chronic pyelonephritis and vesicoureteral reflux led Bailey, in 1973, to coin the term 'reflux nephropathy.'[281] Reflux nephropathy appears to be responsible for the majority of pyelonephritic scars.

Vesicoureteral reflux is a congenital disorder in which there is regurgitation of urine from the bladder into a ureter because of inadequate development of its musculature or because the submucosal portion of the ureter is too short.[245–247,282] Often it is a familial disorder and is usually detected after a urinary tract infection at an early age. Although reflux tends to decrease in severity with age as the

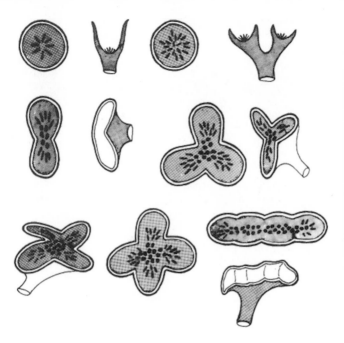

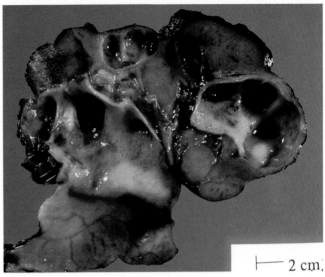

**Fig. 1-100** Reflux nephropathy showing dilated calices with overlying thin cortices separated by intact lobes of cortex.

**Fig. 1-99** Various possible shapes of simple and compound pyramids. (From Hodson CJ. Reflux nephropathy: a personal historical review. AJR Am J Roentgenol 1981; 137: 456; with permission.)

submucosal ureteral segment matures or lengthens, the renal scars are already present, possibly developing at the time of the first infection.[242-244] Scars are usually noted in patients with the most severe degrees of reflux.

Not all patients with urinary tract infections and vesicoureteral reflux develop reflux nephropathy. This observation was explained by Ransley and Risdon,[245] who identified two types of renal pyramid, simple and compound (Fig. 1-99). In simple pyramids Bellini's ducts open through a convex papilla at an oblique angle and close with an increase in intrapelvic pressure. However, compound pyramids that drain multiple lobes have concave surfaces and the orifices of Bellini's ducts fail to close, resulting in reflux. It is believed that reflux nephropathy represents the combined effect of recurrent or persistent vesicoureteral reflux and interrenal reflux that permits infection within the urinary tract to gain access to the renal parenchyma. It also is possible that high pressures in the absence of infection may also result in similar segmental scarring. Compound papillae are usually located in the polar regions of the kidney, the location of most scars in reflux nephropathy.

The kidneys are small and irregularly contracted, usually weighing between 30 and 50 g. Their capsular surfaces show broad depressed scars, usually in polar regions. On cut surfaces there is scalloping and loss of the renal pyramids beneath the cortical scars, resulting in dilated calices (Fig. 1-100). The cortex adjacent to the scars may be unaffected or hypertrophic. The pelvicalyceal system and ureter usually are dilated and their walls thickened.

Microscopically, the cortical scars show chronic interstitial nephritis with a lymphoid interstitial infiltrate (Fig. 1-101). There is extensive tubular atrophy and tubules frequently contain eosinophilic casts (thyroidization). Periglo-

merular fibrosis and global glomerular sclerosis also are typical. The vessels show a striking intimal sclerosis, a finding not present in the adjacent cortex. The uninvolved cortex may appear essentially normal or show a compensatory hypertrophy of nephrons. The collecting system shows chronic pyelitis and ureteritis with lymphoid aggregates or germinal centers in the mucosa.

In some patients hypertension, proteinuria, and progressive renal failure develop. Proteinuria (often in the nephrotic range) is an important finding because it identifies patients at risk for renal failure. The glomerular lesion of focal segmental glomerulosclerosis (Fig. 1-101) is responsible for the proteinuria.[283,284] Unfortunately, correction of the reflux or prevention of recurrent infection does not prevent progression of the glomerular lesion.

### Ask–Upmark kidney

Some patients, mostly children, develop hypertension leading to the identification of vesicoureteral reflux and small kidneys that have one or more circumferential cortical grooves with an underlying dilated calyx.[285,286] These lesions were originally regarded as developmental, leading to the term segmental hypoplasia (or Ask–Upmark kidney). This condition is now regarded as a form of reflux nephropathy, possibly beginning in utero. The cortical scars are distinctive because the glomeruli have disappeared and there is a sharp junction between the uninvolved cortex and the scar, which generally lacks residual inflammation.

### Chronic obstructive pyelonephritis

In chronic obstructive pyelonephritis the kidney is damaged by a combination of pressure-related atrophy and bacterial infection.[287] In advanced cases the kidney is hydronephrotic with diffuse calyceal dilation, blunting or effacement of papillae, and cortical thinning. This uniform alteration is in contrast to the irregular pattern of scarring characteristic

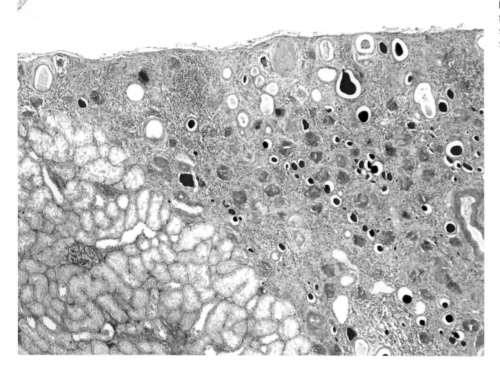

**Fig. 1-101** Reflux nephropathy showing focal chronic interstitial nephritis (right side) with normal cortex on left side. PAS stain.

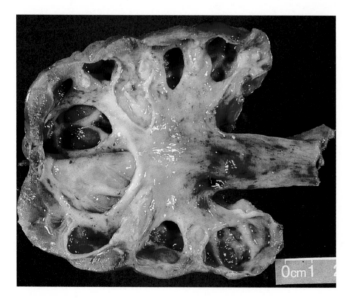

**Fig. 1-102** Chronic obstructive pyelonephritis showing a diffusely attenuated cortex, effaced pyramids, and a dilated collecting system and ureter.

**Table 1-30** Classification of granulomatous diseases of the kidney

| |
|---|
| Xanthogranulomatous pyelonephritis |
| Malakoplakia |
| Mycobacterial infection |
| Fungal infection |
| Parasitic infection |
| Urate nephropathy |
| Sarcoidosis |
| Vasculitis |
| Drug hypersensitivity |

of reflux nephropathy (Fig. 1-102). Microscopically, the picture is that of a diffuse chronic interstitial nephritis with tubular atrophy, interstitial fibrosis, and glomerular sclerosis (Fig. 1-103). Sections including the renal pyramid may show mild blunting of the papillary tip in mild cases, or complete effacement of the pyramid in advanced cases.

## Xanthogranulomatous pyelonephritis

A number of granulomatous diseases may affect the kidney and urinary tract[288-297] (Table 1-30). Most are the result of infections. Xanthogranulomatous pyelonephritis is the inflammatory sequela of chronic suppurative renal infections and usually develops in an obstructed kidney in which portions of the renal parenchyma are transformed into a xanthomatous and suppurative inflammatory mass.[288-291] Although a variety of theories of pathogenesis have been proposed, such as metabolic abnormalities, aberrant immune responses, lower-virulence organisms, or ineffective antimicrobial therapy, the most plausible and simplest mechanism is renal outflow obstruction in the face of a pyogenic infection. This view accommodates the major clinical and pathologic features encountered in the majority of patients. The principal importance of xanthogranulomatous pyelonephritis relates to the difficulty of preoperative diagnosis and its ability clinically, radiographically, and grossly to mimic the destructive growth of a renal neoplasm.

Xanthogranulomatous pyelonephritis begins with suppurative inflammation and edema within the pelvic lamina

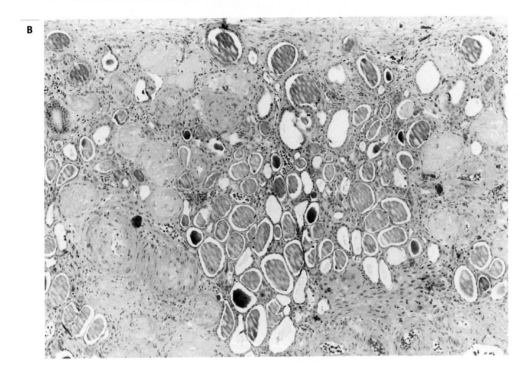

A

B

**Fig. 1-103** End-stage chronic obstructive pyelonephritis showing effaced pyramid, 'thyroidization' of tubules, glomerulosclerosis, and secondary occlusive vascular changes.

propria and adjacent sinus fat, resulting in pelvicalyceal ulceration and fat necrosis. The inflammatory process extends into the medulla, also resulting in necrosis. The cortex, perinephric fat, and even retroperitoneal tissue may eventually be involved. The gross extent of the process has been classified into three 'stages.'[288] In stage I (nephric stage) the process is confined within the renal capsule. In stage II (perinephric stage) the perinephric fat is involved. In stage III (paranephric stage) there is extension outside Gerota's capsule.

Xanthogranulomatous pyelonephritis may involve all or only portions of the renal parenchyma, giving rise to three general patterns: diffuse, segmental, and focal.[289] The diffuse form is most common (Fig. 1-104). It arises in a completely obstructed kidney, usually due to calculi, often of staghorn form (Fig. 1-105). The kidney is non-functional and nephrectomy is the treatment of choice. Preoperative diagnosis is most accurate in this form. The segmental and focal forms are more difficult to diagnose preoperatively and are more likely to be mistaken for neoplasms. They show the same microscopic features as diffuse xanthogranulomatous pyelonephritis, but differ anatomically. Segmental xanthogranulomatous pyelonephritis is polar and is more common in

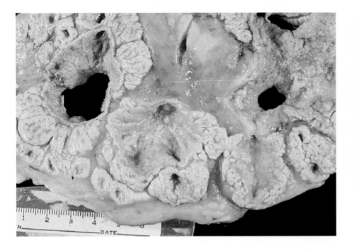

**Fig. 1-104** Xanthogranulomatous pyelonephritis showing xanthomatous nodules centered on pyramids and xanthomatous thickening of the collecting system.

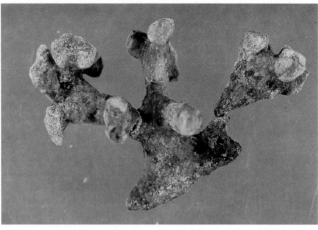

**Fig. 1-105** Staghorn calculus from a patient with xanthogranulomatous pyelonephritis.

A

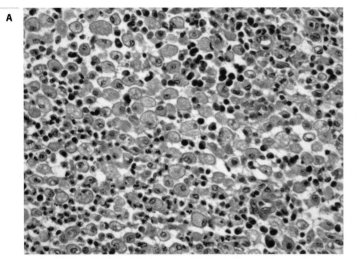

B

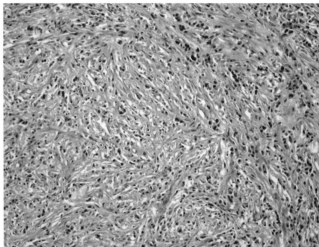

**Fig. 1-106 (A)** The center of a xanthogranulomatous nodule usually contains neutrophils and cell debris, and is surrounded by foamy macrophages. **(B)** The peripheral areas show fibrosis, chronic inflammation, and giant cells.

children. The focal (or tumefactive) form is a cortical variant that lacks communication with the pelvis and is not associated with pyelitis or urinary tract obstruction. These two forms are amenable to partial nephrectomy.

Histologically, xanthogranulomatous nodules show a zonal pattern. There is a central nidus of necrotic debris and neutrophils surrounded by a zone of foamy macrophages (Fig. 1-106). The most peripheral tissue shows a fibroblastic response as the host attempts to confine or organize the inflammatory process.

The presence of the xanthogranulomatous mass, coupled with its histologic cellularity, can elicit concern regarding a neoplasm, particularly if a biopsy or frozen section is examined. The foam cells can resemble clear cell renal carcinoma, and the fibroblastic response can resemble a spindle cell neoplasm. The bubbly microvesicular fat of the foam cells contrasts with the cleared-out cytoplasm char-

acteristic of renal carcinoma. Additional features include a lack of cohesive growth on touch preparations and the absence of cytologic atypia or mitoses. If diagnostic dilemma persists, glycogen stains or demonstration of epithelial markers by immunohistochemistry or electron microscopy can be used.

## Malakoplakia

Malakoplakia is an uncommon chronic granulomatous disease most frequently observed in the urinary tracts of middle-aged women as a complication of recurrent infections.[291,292] Bladder involvement is four to 10 times as common as upper tract involvement, and renal involvement is rare. Diverse extraurinary tract sites also are rarely affected, a situation often associated with a concomitant malignancy. In addition, similar to nephrogenic adenoma, increasing numbers of immunosuppressed patients have been reported to develop urinary tract malakoplakia.

A
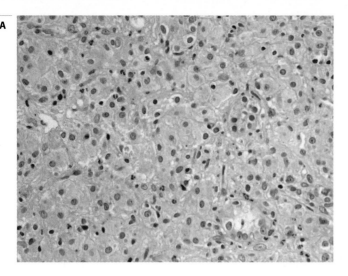

B
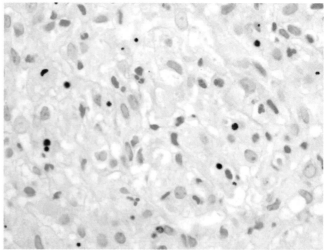

**Fig. 1-107** **(A)** Malakoplakia showing von Hansemann histiocytes. **(B)** Michaelis–Gutmann bodies revealed by von Kossa's stain for calcium.

The typical mucosal lesion of malakoplakia is characterized by a yellow-brown soft (*malakos*) plaque (*plakos*) that often has a central umbilication. The parenchymal lesions consist of similar soft yellow-brown nodules. Microscopically, masses of large eosinophilic histiocytes (von Hansemann histiocytes) are present, many of which contain basophilic inclusions (Michaelis–Gutmann bodies) (Fig. 1-107). PAS stain and special stains for calcium or iron enhance the target-like appearance of these cytoplasmic inclusions and indicate their mineralized nature. They have been shown by a variety of methods to represent incompletely digested bacilli.[292]

### Tuberculosis

The genitourinary tract is the most common extrapulmonary site of tuberculosis infection, which occurs in up to 5% of patients.[293,294] It is principally a disease of the young to middle-aged, with 75% of patients under the age of 50. Most patients will not have radiographic or clinical evidence of pulmonary disease at the time the genitourinary tract involvement is identified.[293]

The renal parenchyma initially becomes infected by hematogenous dissemination, resulting in the bilateral development of small cortical neutrophilic microabscesses that gradually evolve into more typical granuloma and may caseate. Although progressive active disease may occur, in most patients the process is arrested. It may reactivate after a long latency period following a perturbation in the immune system.

Medullary involvement results with reactivation. The organisms appear to favor the thin limbs of Henle, where they proliferate, causing destructive granulomatous lesions that caseate and cavitate (Fig. 1-108). Papillary necrosis follows, with seeding of the collecting system and lower urinary tract. Infection in these sites elicits granulomatous and fibrotic sequelae resulting in contraction of the collection system, ureter, and bladder. The patient thus presents with a concentrating defect, dysuria, and hematuria. Cavitary lesions, calyceal deformity, and ureteral strictures are demonstrable by various imaging studies.

### Acute tubulointerstitial disease

Acute tubulointerstitial disease usually causes a sudden deterioration in renal function and a rise in serum creatinine of 0.5–1.0 mg/dL/day. The urine may contain red cells, but red cell and white cell casts are absent, urinary protein is less than 2 g/day, and the urinary sodium concentration is increased. Many patients also are oliguric (<400 mL urine/day). The rapid evolution of renal failure correlates with the rapid expansion of the interstitial areas by edema. Tubular cell injury and edema, with or without inflammation, are the principal morphologic findings, known respectively as acute tubular necrosis and acute interstitial nephritis.

### Acute tubular necrosis

Acute tubular necrosis is the most common renal parenchymal cause of acute renal failure.[298–301] It is characterized by morphologic evidence of tubular cell injury and is associated with interstitial edema.[299] There is little or no cortical inflammation, although inflammatory cells may accumulate in the vasa recta of the outer medulla.[299] Glomeruli and other vessels are not affected. It usually is divided into ischemic and toxic forms.[298–304] Ischemic injury is more common. Although its etiology usually can be established because it results from decreased renal perfusion secondary to hemorrhage, hypotension, or dehydration, in some patients these are not observed directly but are inferred based on the clinical setting. The etiologies of toxic acute tubular necrosis are more diverse (Table 1-31) and may be difficult to identify because they often develop in the context of therapy for other illnesses or may result from exogenous agents.[302–304] In heavy metal lesions such as those caused by bismuth,

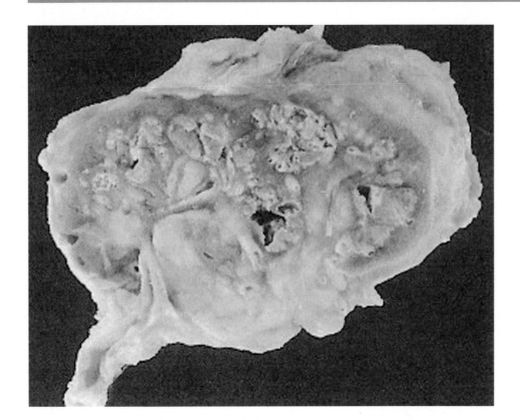

**Fig. 1-108** Renal tuberculosis with caseating granulomas and contracted renal pelvis and ureter.

**Table 1-31** Causes of acute tubular necrosis

Ischemia

Antibiotics
  Aminoglycosides
  Amphotericin B
  Polymixin B
  Rifampicin
  Cephalosporin
  Colistin

Radiographic contrast agents

Non-steroidal anti-inflammatory drugs

Chemotherapeutic agents
  Cis-platinum

Organic solvents
  Carbon tetrachloride
  Ethylene glycol
  Trichloroethylene

Insecticides and herbicides
  Heavy metals
  Mercury
  Bismuth
  Lead
  Cadmium
  Uranium
  Arsenic

Rhabdomyolysis

Hemolysis

Cocaine

Toxins
  Insect stings
  Snake bites
  Mushroom poisoning

cadmium, and lead, proximal tubular intranuclear inclusions are present. Myeloid bodies detectable by electron microscopy are present in lesions caused by aminoglycoside antibiotics, although their presence does not correlate with toxicity.[303] Pigmented casts in distal tubules are present in lesions caused by hemolysis and rhabdomyolysis. Some agents can also produce an acute and a chronic interstitial nephritis.

For acute tubular necrosis to result in acute renal failure it must be diffuse and bilateral. If it is unilateral, or even focal in one kidney, then renal insufficiency will not occur. The size and weight of the kidney are increased as a consequence of interstitial edema. In certain situations with underlying renal atrophy (such as older patients with arterial nephrosclerosis), acute tubular necrosis may result in normal renal size and weight. The cortex usually is pale and may bulge slightly compared to the medulla. The medulla, particularly the outer medulla, is often congested and dark, secondary to dilation of the vasa recta.

In acute tubular necrosis there is interstitial expansion without significant inflammation. If inflammation is present, it consists of a predominantly mononuclear cell infiltrate at the corticomedullary junction or within the vessels in the vasa recta of the outer medulla. The tubules themselves can show two patterns of injury. In the more obvious and severe form there is extensive coagulative necrosis of tubular cells, particularly in the proximal tubules, with loss of nuclei (Fig. 1-109). This form is most common in toxic injuries and at autopsy. In autopsy material this alteration must be distinguished from autolysis. Autolytic tubules may be recognized by the tendency of their epithelium to separate from their tubular basement membranes and from each other, with preservation of their nuclei and intact cell membranes (Fig. 1-109).

The second pattern of acute tubular necrosis is more subtle. It is characterized by attenuation or flattening of the tubular epithelium causing luminal enlargement and widely spaced nuclei (Fig. 1-110). At low magnification this imparts a microcystic appearance to the cortex as a result of single cell necrosis and sloughing. The remaining cells lose their brush border and spread out to cover the basement membrane. There may be short segments of denuded tubular basement membranes. Mitotic figures may be present but are

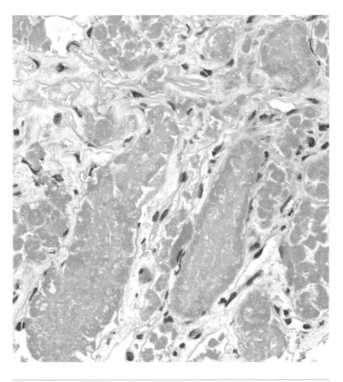

**Fig. 1-109** Acute tubular necrosis at autopsy showing coagulation necrosis.

usually very infrequent. Distal tubules and collecting ducts may contain granular casts of sloughed cells.

## Acute interstitial nephritis

Acute interstitial nephritis is an inflammatory cause of acute renal failure.[302-309] The term *acute* refers to the rapid development of renal failure rather than the character of the infiltrate, which actually consists of lymphocytes, plasma cells, histiocytes, and scattered eosinophils. Acute interstitial nephritis is a hypersensitivity reaction to a variety of stimuli (Table 1-32), and most are cell-mediated reactions.[309,310] However, immune complex formation can occur in connective tissue diseases such as lupus, and rarely in drug reactions.[310] Antitubular basement antibody may also develop in a rare drug reaction, in renal transplant rejection, associated with antiglomerular basement membrane disease (most common), and also as an idiopathic disorder.[310-312] Direct immunofluorescence is required to identify immune complex and antitubular basement membrane-mediated lesions.

Patients often have enlarged, tender kidneys secondary to edema. Morphologically, there is interstitial expansion by edema, resulting in tubular separation.[307-313] There is a variably distributed mixed cell infiltrate that consists principally of lymphocytes and monocytes (Fig. 1-111). Fewer plasma cells and eosinophils may be present, but eosinophils are not required to implicate an allergic reaction. The lymphocytes infiltrate between tubular epithelial cells (tubulitis) that may appear reactive or may show individual cell necrosis. In antibody-mediated cases immune complex deposits may be identified within tubular basement membranes or peritubular capillaries, or a linear tubular basement membrane reaction can be demonstrated if antitubular basement membrane antibody is present. Occasionally a necrotizing vasculitis or granulomas may also develop in allergic reactions.[297,303]

The history and certain laboratory data are required to establish the cause because, except for identifying an infective agent or an antibody-mediated lesion, there are no

**A**

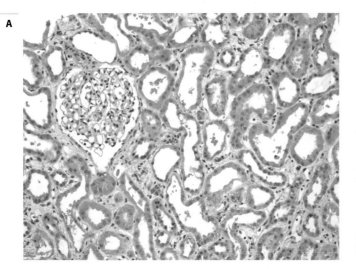

**B**

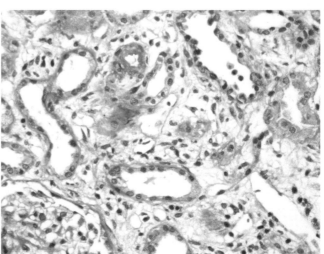

**Fig. 1-110** Mild acute tubular necrosis on renal biopsy showing attenuation of tubular epithelium **(A)** and interstitial edema **(B)**.

**Table 1-32** Causes of acute interstitial nephritis

Drug-associated
　β-Lactam and other antibiotics
　Diuretics
　Non-steroidal anti-inflammatory drugs
　Allopurinol
　Rifampicin
　Cimetidine
　Sulfa drugs
　Phenytoin

Connective tissue diseases
　Systemic lupus erythematosus
　Sjögren's syndrome

Transplant rejection

Sarcoidosis

Acute interstitial nephritis–uveitis syndrome

Antitubular basement membrane disease

Bacterial infections
　Scarlet fever
　Diphtheria
　Typhoid fever
　Brucellosis
　Leptospiral infection
　Rickettsia

Viral infection
　Cytomegalovirus
　Epstein–Barr virus
　Polyomavirus
　HIV
　Hantavirus

**Table 1-33** Exogenous causes of chronic interstitial nephritis

Drugs
　Analgesics
　　Combined analgesics
　　Non-steroidal anti-inflammatory drugs
　Chemotherapeutic agents
　　Cis-platinum
　　Methyl CCMU
　Ciclosporin
　Lithium

Heavy metals
　Lead
　Cadmium

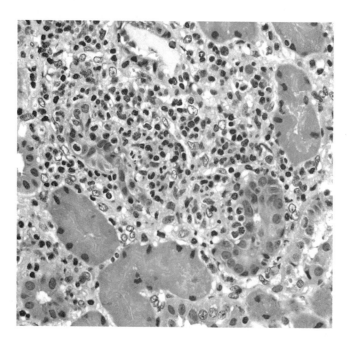

**Fig. 1-111** Allergic acute interstitial nephritis secondary to drug reaction.

morphologic features to discriminate between the various possible causes. Prior to the use of antibiotics, acute interstitial nephritis was usually caused by infections, most often scarlet fever or diphtheria.[307] Today, an allergic drug reaction is clearly the first consideration.[303,308–313] The presence of a rash, fever, eosinophilia, or eosinophiluria can corroborate that impression, but often these are absent. Although the most frequently implicated drugs are listed in Table 1-32, almost any drug can cause an allergic reaction. Frequently, the clinician will attribute it to the drug most recently taken. Proteinuria is usually less than 1 g/day, so the presence of significant proteinuria is very useful because it is most commonly associated with non-steroidal anti-inflammatory drugs (NSAIDs). In patients with a systemic disease that can be associated with acute interstitial nephritis, the underlying disease should be considered the cause.[308,313–316]

## Chronic interstitial nephritis

Chronic interstitial nephritis refers to the gradual development of renal failure due to tubulointerstitial disease. As in acute interstitial nephritis, lymphocytes and histiocytes are the predominant inflammatory cells. However, the histologic picture is dominated by interstitial fibrosis and tubular atrophy (Fig. 1-112). Many of the same agents that cause acute tubular necrosis or acute interstitial nephritis also produce chronic interstitial nephritis (Table 1-33), such as

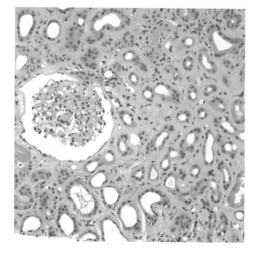

**Fig. 1-112** Idiopathic chronic interstitial nephritis showing interstitial fibrosis, tubular atrophy, and scant inflammation.

heavy metals, drugs, connective tissue diseases, and sarcoidosis.[303,304,317-321] Therefore, in a single patient there may be a combination of acute and chronic features. The lack of a specific cause for the histology requires careful clinical correlation to understand the cause of chronic interstitial nephritis. In some patients no specific cause can be established, and this is called idiopathic chronic interstitial nephritis.

## Drugs and heavy metals

A variety of therapeutic agents and heavy metal exposures can cause the insidious development of chronic interstitial nephritis.[302,303,321-327] The tubulointerstitial scarring is irreversible, but if the toxic injury is recognized and the agent eliminated, some improvement in renal function is often possible. For most agents, no distinctive histologic features develop. However, in lead and cadmium toxicity intranuclear inclusions in tubular cells may be present, and chronic lead toxicity often presents with gout and hypertension. Papillary necrosis is the principal underlying lesion in analgesic nephropathy.

## Analgesic nephropathy

Analgesic nephropathy is characterized by renal papillary necrosis and cortical chronic interstitial nephritis resulting from the prolonged use (10–20 years) of phenacetin-containing compound analgesic preparations.[261-264] This association was first recognized after a marked increase in chronic interstitial nephritis and renal papillary necrosis in several geographic regions in Scandinavia and Australia. Originally the chronic interstitial nephritis was recognized; however, Kincaid-Smith[261] demonstrated that papillary necrosis was the primary injury and the cortical scarring was secondary. Analgesic abuse has been implicated as the cause of 80–90% of renal papillary necrosis in non-diabetic Australians. In addition to chronic renal disease, approximately 34% of patients develop coronary artery disease and other atherosclerotic complications.[264] Furthermore, 8% of patients develop transitional cell carcinoma.

Phenacetin and aspirin combined with caffeine or codeine were the original offending preparations. The substitution of acetaminophen for phenacetin, control over marketing practices, and increased recognition of risk factors have substantially lowered the prevalence of analgesic nephropathy. However, a similar chronic renal disease has now been identified in connection with chronic misuse of NSAIDs.[264]

The renal lesions of analgesic abuse begin in the inner medulla and have been divided into three stages.[261-263] In the first stage there is a yellowish radiating discoloration of the papillary tip. Microscopically, there is necrosis of the loops of Henle and interstitial cells, with thickening and sclerosis of small vessels. In the second stage the process involves the entire inner medulla, with widespread necrosis of collecting ducts, loops of Henle, and vasa recta. Interstitial calcification frequently is present.

During the third stage, cortical changes develop following necrosis of the renal pyramid. The cortex overlying the pyramid becomes thin and atrophic, histologically showing

a non-specific chronic interstitial nephritis with tubular atrophy, interstitial fibrosis, and a lymphoid infiltrate. The columns of Bertin may be spared, producing an alternating pattern of atrophy and thickening of the cortex. The necrotic papillae have often been described as darkly colored, and focally may detach and slough. In contrast to other forms of papillary necrosis, a neutrophilic response is not evident. A distinctive capillary sclerosis affects the small vessels of the papillary tip and the small mucosal vessels of the renal pelvis, ureter, and bladder, characterized by extensive reduplication of the basal lamina best demonstrated by PAS stain.

## Metabolic abnormalities and tubulointerstitial diseases

A variety of metabolic abnormalities may affect the kidney. The four most important involve calcium, uric acid, oxalate, and cystine. Each can exert its effect by parenchymal deposition or by formation of calculi.

### Hypercalcemic nephropathy

Hypercalcemia can result from many systemic diseases (Table 1-34) and has several renal consequences.[328-330] The most common are a decrease in glomerular filtration rate and a decrease in concentrating capacity that may lead to polyuria and, when severe and prolonged, to volume depletion and acute renal failure. Hypercalcemia also can have direct morphologic effects: nephrolithiasis, calcium oxalate crystal formation in tubules, and calcium deposition along cortical tubular basement membranes (Fig. 1-113).

### Nephrolithiasis

Nephrolithiasis is a common abnormality affecting 500 000 Americans each year.[331-333] It is not a single disease, but rather a common endpoint with obstructive complications that may arise in the context of diverse abnormalities of metabolism and renal tubular cell function, or result from urinary tract diseases such as obstruction or bacterial infection. Nephrolithiasis is a dynamic process. In its early stages there is the potential for medical therapy to control or prevent its complications by modifying factors that permit crystallization. There are several types of calculi, which may be pure or heterogeneous in composition (Table 1-35). Each has multiple etiologies and clinical associations.[331-333]

**Table 1-34** Major causes of hypercalcemia

| |
| --- |
| Primary and secondary hyperparathyroidism |
| Vitamin D intoxication |
| Milk alkali syndrome |
| Sarcoidosis |
| Malignant neoplasms |
| Increased bone turnover |
| Idiopathic |

Calcium-containing stones are the most common variety and can have a variable composition, such as calcium oxalate or calcium phosphate (hydroxyapatite, carbonate–apatite, or brushite). Most patients with calcium oxalate-containing stones do not have an abnormality of oxalate metabolism. Hypercalciuria is the most common underlying metabolic abnormality, encountered in 60% of patients.

Struvite stones (infection or triple phosphate stones) are a combination of struvite and carbonate–apatite. They form only in the presence of urea-splitting organisms such as *Proteus*, *Staphylococcus albus*, *Pseudomonas*, and *Klebsiella*.[334] Struvite stones can form very rapidly and create most staghorn calculi (Fig. 1-105).

Not all stones are heavily mineralized. Matrix stones are composed principally of a glycoprotein matrix with focal calcification.[335,336] Matrix stones form large casts of the collecting system and have a soft yellow to tan gross appearance and a laminated structure histologically. They are often associated with urinary tract infection.

Because nephrolithiasis can result from or cause urinary tract obstruction, affected kidneys may show diverse changes such as hydronephrosis, acute or chronic pyelonephritis, or xanthogranulomatous pyelonephritis. Many will also contain small calcified plaques along the papillary tips known as Randall's plaques. In the 1950s Randall[337] noted that 20% of patients with stones had 2–4 mm of submucosal calcified plaques that he felt represented precursor lesions in stone formation.[338] These plaques are derived from interstitial and tubular basement membrane calcification (Fig. 1-114), which in certain patients becomes a nucleation site for stone formation.

## Oxalate-associated renal disease

Oxalic acid is the simplest dicarboxylic acid found in nature.[339] It is a major constituent of many plants and a metabolic byproduct of endogenous and exogenous compounds. The kidneys may be confronted with an excessive oxalate load in several situations (Table 1-36), and this results in oxalosis and calcium oxalate calculi.[339] However, most patients with calcium oxalate stones have none of these disorders but do have abnormalities in calcium metabolism.[330,331]

Primary hyperoxaluria types I and II are autosomal recessive, inborn errors in metabolism that result in excessive

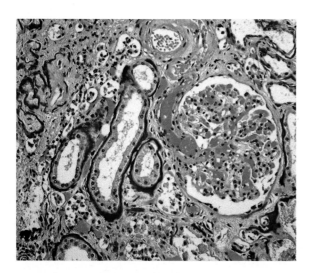

**Fig. 1-113** Nephrocalcinosis showing tubular basement membranes encrusted with calcium.

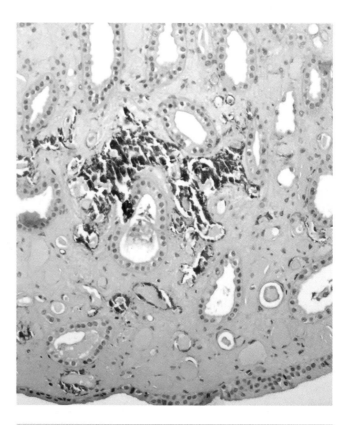

**Fig. 1-114** Randall's plaque in a papillary tip from a patient with nephrolithiasis.

**Table 1-35** Classification of renal calculi

| Calcium phosphate |
| Calcium oxalate |
| Struvite |
| Uric acid |
| Cystine |
| Matrix stone |

**Table 1-36** Causes of hyperoxaluria

| Primary hyperoxaluria, types I and II |
| Secondary hyperoxaluria |
|     Ethylene glycol ingestion |
|     Methoxyflurane anesthesia |
|     Gastrointestinal disease |
|     Pancreatobiliary disease |
|     Chronic renal failure |
|     Idiopathic |

production of oxalate.[339,341,346] Calcium oxalate deposits form in vessels in several extrarenal tissues, such as the heart, brain, eye, and bone marrow. Renal tubular oxalosis and calcium oxalate calculi form and result in renal failure at an early age.

Secondary hyperoxaluria and renal oxalosis may result from ethylene glycol (automobile antifreeze) ingestion or from methoxyflurane anesthesia and cause acute renal failure with renal tubular oxalosis.[339,341,342] In ethylene glycol intoxication glycol is metabolized to oxalate, which precipitates in the distal tubules causing obstruction (Fig. 1-115). There is also a direct toxic effect of glycol on tubular epithelium that contributes to the renal injury. The free fluoride in methoxyflurane appears to stimulate excessive oxalate production by the liver, causing a heavy acute oxalate load to the kidney. In renal tubular oxalosis, calcium oxalate crystals are found within both renal tubular lumina and tubular epithelial cells. The crystals are strongly birefringent under polarized light (Fig. 1-115).

Secondary hyperoxaluria of a more chronic form, leading to stone formation, occurs in patients with small bowel or pancreatobiliary tract disease (enteric oxalosis) and may be a complication of star fruit ingestion.[339,343,347] Unabsorbed lipids bind intraintestinal calcium, leaving insufficient calcium to precipitate the oxalate within the gut, leading to increased oxalate absorption. Finally, it also is common to encounter scattered calcium oxalate crystals in renal tubules at autopsy in patients with chronic renal failure and in the absence of overt renal disease.[344]

## Cystinosis

Cystinosis is an autosomal recessive storage disease characterized by impaired transport of the amino acid cystine across lysosomal membranes, resulting in its excessive accumulation in several organs, including the kidney.[348-353] Three forms are recognized: an infantile nephropathic form, an adolescent form, and an adult form. In the infantile nephropathic form there is initial tubular dysfunction characterized by Fanconi's syndrome that progresses to uremia and death by 9–10 years of age if untreated.[348-351] This is accompanied by growth retardation, photophobia, and hypothyroidism. Its progress can be arrested by treatment with cysteamine, which reduces intracellular cystine levels.[352] The adolescent form is rare and slowly progressive, whereas the adult form causes only ocular disease.

In the early phase of nephropathic cystinosis the kidneys may have enlarged multinucleated podocytes (referred to as polykaryocytosis) and cystine crystals may be visible in macrophages within glomeruli or in interstitial areas.[349-351] With progression of the disease a chronic interstitial nephritis develops, with tubulointerstitial scarring and clusters of crystal-containing macrophages in the interstitium (Fig. 1-116). Because cystine crystals are birefringent and soluble in water, alcohol fixation and polarization provide optimum demonstration and retention of the crystals.

## Uric acid-associated renal disease

Uric acid is the final degradation product of purine metabolism in humans. It is poorly soluble in plasma, and when symptomatic and deposited in tissues it is known as gout. Outside the joints, the kidney is the major site of clinically significant disease caused by hyperuricemia. Three forms of disease occur: acute uric acid nephropathy, uric acid lithiasis, and chronic gouty nephropathy.[354-357]

In acute uric acid nephropathy there is acute renal failure caused by intratubular uric acid crystals. It develops as a complication of rapid tumor lysis in lymphoproliferative and myeloproliferative disorders following the initiation of chemotherapy.[354] The acidity and concentration in the collecting ducts favor uric acid crystal formation. The renal medulla, particularly the papilla, may have grossly visible yellow streaks. Uric acid crystals are very soluble in water and birefringent. Therefore, the histologic demonstration of uric acid crystals requires tissue fixed in absolute alcohol (or the use of touch smears or frozen sections) and viewing under polarized light. Crystals may also form within the collecting system and be detectable in the urine.

A
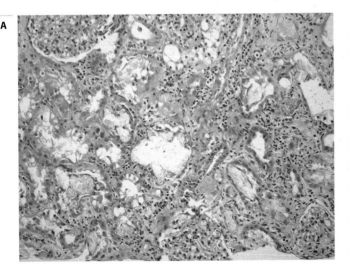

B
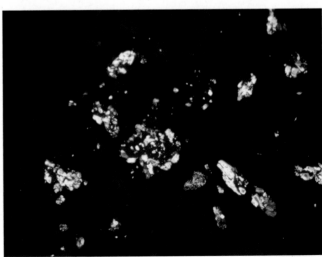

**Fig. 1-115** Calcium oxalate crystals under polarized light in a patient with acute renal failure secondary to ethylene glycol ingestion.

A
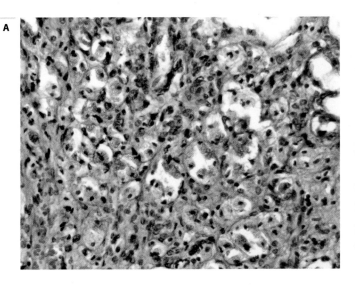

B
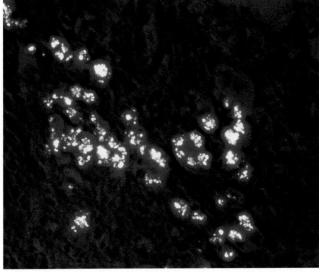

**Fig. 1-116** Infantile nephropathic cystinosis showing cystine crystals in a 6-year-old.

Hydration, alkalization of urine, and pretreatment with allopurinol have greatly reduced the incidence of crystal formation.

Uric acid stones, which may be composed of pure uric acid, are either radiolucent or mixed with calcium oxalate and radio-opaque. They develop in 20% of patients with gout,[354,355] and become more prevalent with the increase in the amount of uric acid excreted. Stone formation can be inhibited by alkalinization of the urine and hydration.

Chronic gouty nephropathy develops in patients with sustained hyperuricemia (Table 1-37). It is characterized by the interstitial deposition of sodium urate. Urate elicits a mononuclear cell and giant cell reaction resulting in the formation of microtophi (Fig. 1-117). These lesions develop mainly within the outer medulla. Small urate granulomas can also be seen in azotemia of other causes, and occasionally in otherwise normal kidneys.[356] In patients with renal failure attributed to chronic gout the cortex shows changes of hypertension-associated arterial nephrosclerosis and chronic interstitial nephritis. Tophi usually are not identified.

It was previously believed that primary gout caused renal failure in a substantial number of gouty patients. This concept has been challenged on the grounds that the gout in many of the patients in older reports was probably secondary, and that the renal disease was actually caused by lead toxicity and underlying diabetes and hyperten\sion.[357-359] It is now known that chronic lead nephropathy causes clinical gout and hypertension and produces the same histologic findings previously regarded as typical of chronic gouty nephropathy.

## Renal transplantation

There are two major considerations in a patient with allograft dysfunction, rejection or drug nephrotoxicity (ciclosporin and FK 506). An allograft biopsy is the only method currently available to distinguish between these possibilities; each manifests a variety of lesions.[260]

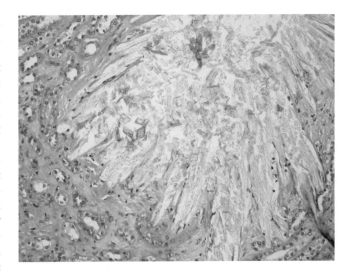

**Fig. 1-117** Medullary urate granuloma.

**Table 1-37** Causes of hyperuricemia and gout

| |
| --- |
| Lymphoproliferative disorders |
| Myeloproliferative disorders |
| Lead (saturnine gout) |
| Diuretics |
| Alcohol |
| Aspirin |
| Endocrine dysfunctions |
| Starvation |
| Hypoxanthine–guanine phosphoribosyltransferase deficiency |
| Phosphoribosylpyrophosphate synthetase increased activity |

**Table 1-38** Renal transplant rejection (abridged version of Banff '97'/ CCTT modification)

| |
| --- |
| Normal/negative |
| Hyperacute rejection |
| Suspicious for acute rejection/borderline acute rejection |
| Type I rejection/acute cellular or interstitial rejection +/− acute transplant glomerulopathy |
| Type II rejection/acute vascular rejection |
| Type III rejection/fibrinoid necrosis |
| Chronic vascular rejection/chronic allograft nephropathy +/− Chronic transplant glomerulopathy |

**Table 1-39** Classification of acute transplant rejection according to pathogenic mechanism

| |
| --- |
| Cellular rejection |
|    Acute interstitial rejection/Banff type I rejection |
|    Acute vascular rejection/Banff type II rejection |
| Antibody-mediated rejection |
|    Hyperacute rejection |
|    Acute antibody-mediated (C4d positive) rejection |
|    Arterial fibrinoid necrosis/Banff type III rejection |

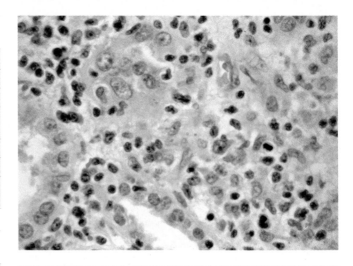

**Fig. 1.118** Acute cellular (type 1) rejection. Edema and a mixed cell infiltrate are present.

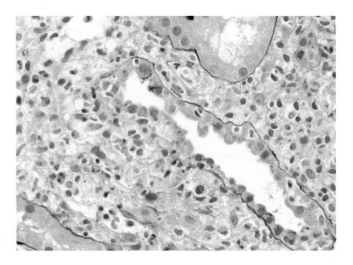

**Fig. 1-119** Acute interstitial (type 1) rejection. Silver stain lights the tubulitis and basement membrane disruption. Jones methenamine silver stain.

The classification of renal transplant rejection has evolved substantially over the last decade, with attempts to establish minimum diagnostic thresholds, provide quantitative parameters for multicenter trials, and to resolve pathogenetically distinct groups that may require different therapies. Multidisciplinary workshops involving pathologists and clinicians convened in Banff, Canada, in 1993 and 1995 led to the Banff Working Formulation.[361] This formulation was later influenced by the results of the NIH-funded Cooperative Clinical Trials of Transplantation (CCTT), leading to a hybrid schema formulated during the 1999 Banff meeting, the Banff '97' Working Formulation (Table 1-38).[362,363] Although quantitative assessment with numerical codes for tubular, interstitial, vascular and glomerular findings is an integral component of the full-blown formulation, this is mostly applicable to biopsy standardization for multicenter studies. Quantitative evaluation is of limited use in the individual patient. More recently, identification of a new form of antibody-mediated rejection, identified by deposition of C4d in peritubular capillaries and arterioles, has prompted reconsideration of the classification, with the proposal of a classification more tightly linked to pathogenic mechanisms (Table 1-39).[364,367]

Acute cellular (interstitial) rejection usually develops in the first few weeks to months following transplantation.[360] A predominance of T lymphocytes with fewer monocytes is observed. Eosinophils and plasma cells are present in modest numbers, but may occasionally be numerous. Acute rejection is classified by the renal compartment affected. Acute cellular rejection, or type I rejection, is most common. Its hallmark is an interstitial infiltrate associated with infiltration of the tubular epithelium by mononuclear cells, known as tubulitis (Fig. 1-118).[360,366] Tubulitis is best recognized with the aid of a basement membrane stain such as PAS or silver stain (Fig. 1-119). Edema and tubular epithelial and tubular basement membrane damage are also present. The minimum inflammatory threshold for acute cellular rejection was established by the CCTT at 5% of the unscarred cortex showing interstitial inflammation with tubulitis, and by Banff '97' at 10%.[362,363]

Acute vascular rejection, or type II, is a more serious form of rejection, less responsive to immunosuppressive treatment.[360,367] It is characterized by endothelial cell enlargement with subendothelial mononuclear cells, known as endovasculitis or endothelialitis (Fig. 1-120). Fibrin may be observed, but is not required for the diagnosis. Endothelial cell necrosis can develop with thrombosis. Glomeruli can also be involved in acute rejection, known as acute transplant glomerulopathy. This is characterized by mononuclear cell accumulation within glomerular capillary loops and mesangium. The hypercellular appearance of glomeruli resembles a proliferative glomerulonephritis that can develop in allografts as a recurrent or 'de novo' condition.[368] If glo-

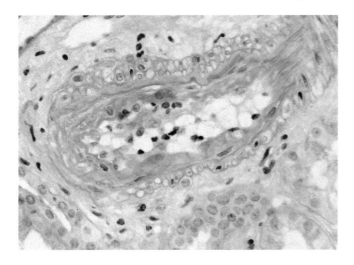

**Fig. 1.120** Acute vascular (type 2) rejection. Enlarged endothelial cells and subendothelial mononuclear cells are present. PAS stain.

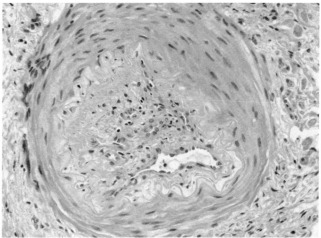

**Fig. 1.121** Chronic vascular rejection. Severe occlusive fibrointimal thickening is present.

merular hypercellularity is associated with changes of type I rejection, or especially type II rejection, a recurrent or 'de novo' glomerulonephritis is unlikely. Immunofluorescence and electron microscopy may be required, however, to exclude the presence of immune deposits in certain cases.

There are also three forms of antibody-mediated rejection. Hyperacute rejection was first recognized, but is extremely rare today.[360,362–364] Hyperacute rejection develops when preformed antibodies in the recipient have specificity for donor-related endothelial antigens, such as blood group ABO antigens, histocompatibility antigens, or other antigens. The antibodies immediately bind to peritubular and glomerular endothelium following vascular anastomosis leading to complement activation. Neutrophils target the endothelium, resulting in cell necrosis and thrombosis. Interstitial hemorrhage and cortical necrosis follow. Direct immunofluorescence demonstrates IgG, complement, and fibrin along capillaries. The surgeon is aware of this catastrophic event shortly after blood flow is established because the graft becomes dark, mottled and edematous, with no urine output. If left in place, the graft becomes necrotic within hours to days.

Acute (C4d-associated) antibody-mediated rejection is the most common form of antibody-mediated rejection.[365,366] Clinically it resembles acute cellular rejection, but is more resistant to immunosuppressive reversal. A cellular infiltrate of type I or II cellular rejection is usually observed. In addition, neutrophils may be located within peritubular capillaries, a feature not typically observed in pure cellular rejections. C4d is detectable in peritubular capillaries and arterioles, regarded as evidence of a pre-existing antibody event. Immunoglobulins are not detected.

The third form of antibody-mediated rejection is arterial fibrinoid necrosis, a very uncommon form of rejection. It referred to as type III rejection, but has also been labeled delayed hyperacute rejection and accelerated acute vascular rejection. It is regarded as antibody-mediated rejection based on serologic studies, although antibody deposition in tissues is not observed.

Chronic rejection is a disease of uncertain and probably multifactorial pathogenesis. Clinically it is characterized by a slowly progressive decline in renal function, beginning at least 2 months after transplantation. The kidney shows tubular atrophy with interstitial fibrosis and glomerulosclerosis.[360] Arteries of all caliber exhibit occlusive fibrointimal thickening similar to hypertensive changes (Fig. 1-121). A modest mononuclear cell infiltrate, foam cells and fibrin can be observed within the intima.

Rendering a specific diagnosis of chronic vascular rejection in a biopsy can be difficult because the larger arteries requisite for the diagnosis may not be sampled. Furthermore, the tubular, interstitial and vascular changes are non-specific, and may be caused by other insults, such as hypertension, donor-related conditions, or nephrotoxic drugs. The term chronic allograft nephropathy has been coined for use in the biopsy setting when chronic changes exist but the diagnostic large arterial changes are not present. Recently, a lesion has been identified by electron microscopy, peritubular capillary basement membrane duplication, that appears quite specific for chronic vascular rejection (Fig. 1-122), although it has been rarely observed in other conditions.[369]

There is also a glomerular form of chronic rejection known as chronic transplant glomerulopathy.[370] The glomerulus shows variable mesangial hypercellularity and sclerosis with capillary loop thickening due to duplication of glomerular basement membranes. These alterations resemble a primary glomerulonephritis, but differ by an absence of immune complex deposits. As patients also have significant proteinuria, immunofluorescence and electron microscopy may be required in selected cases.

# Ciclosporin and FK 506 nephrotoxicity

Ciclosporin and FK 506 have effects on several cell types in the kidney, producing a variety of acute and chronic lesions (Table 1-40).[322,323,371,372] However, the most common mani-

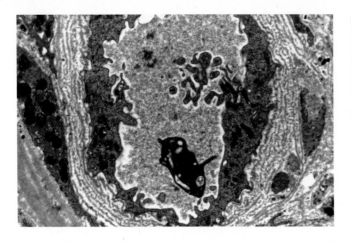

**Fig. 1.122** Chronic vascular rejection. A peritubular capillary has multiple layers of duplicated basement membrane. Electron photomicrograph.

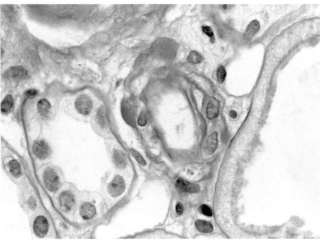

**Fig. 1.123** Ciclosporin-associated hyaline arteriopathy. There are PAS-positive hyalinotic lesions on the outer aspect of this arteriole. PAS stain.

| Table 1-40 Histologic findings with ciclosporin and FK 506 nephrotoxicity |
| --- |
| Normal histology |
| Acute thrombotic microangiopathy |
| Hyaline arteriopathy |
| Tubular isometric vacuolization |
| Interstitial fibrosis |

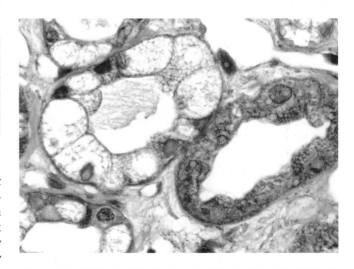

**Fig. 1.124** Ciclosporin-associated isometric tubular epithelial cell vacuolization. Trichrome stain.

festation of nephrotoxicity is an absence of morphologic findings. Renal failure results from arteriolar vasoconstriction and a reversible decrease in the glomerular filtration rate. This form of toxicity is implicated when urinary tract obstruction has been clinically excluded, and the biopsy shows no signs of rejection, acute tubular necrosis, or any lesion described below.

Two nephrotoxic lesions affect the arterioles and glomeruli. An acute thrombotic microangiopathy with glomerular and/or arteriolar thrombi may develop, usually in the initial weeks to months following transplantation (see Fig. 1-65B).[371,372] A second chronic hyaline arteriopathy may develop, in which hyaline deposits replace smooth muscle cells (Fig. 1-123) preferentially along the outer aspect of the arteriole. The external location of hyaline distinguishes this lesion from hypertension and diabetic arteriolar hyalinosis, where the deposits form along the inner aspect of the arteriole.

A distinctive tubular lesion of acute reversible nephrotoxicity is isometric vacuolization. The tubular epithelial cell cytoplasm contains numerous small vacuoles, imparting a foamy appearance, representing dilated smooth endoplasmic reticulum (Fig. 1-124). A second chronic irreversible lesion of nephrotoxicity is interstitial fibrosis with tubular atrophy. It usually appears months to years following transplantation. When ciclosporin was first introduced, however, interstitial fibrosis was observed to develop rapidly when large loading doses were administered in the context of acute tubular necrosis.

## Miscellaneous conditions

### Sarcoidosis

Sarcoidosis is a chronic disease of unknown cause in which multiple organ systems are affected, usually by non-caseating granulomas. Symptomatic renal disease occurs in less than 10% of sarcoidosis patients.[318–320] The most frequent renal abnormalities result from hypercalcemia, which causes a reduction in glomerular filtration rate, a decrease in concentrating ability, renal tubular acidosis, nephrocalcinosis, or results in calcium stones. In addition, a granulomatous acute interstitial nephritis (Fig. 1-125) or chronic interstitial nephritis may develop.

### Amyloidosis and paraprotein-associated tubulointerstitial disease

Patients with multiple myeloma, lymphoma, or leukemia frequently develop renal disease, either from a direct effect

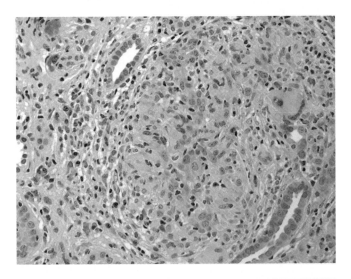

**Fig. 1-125** Sarcoid granuloma in a patient with acute renal failure.

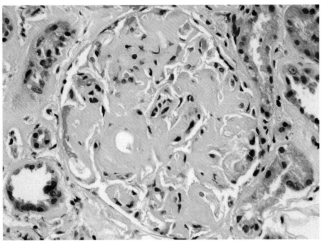

**Fig. 1-126** A glomerulus replaced with homogeneous eosinophilic material characteristic of amyloid.

of the neoplasm or from a therapeutic complication (Table 1-41). Either glomerular or tubulointerstitial lesions may develop and result in proteinuria and renal insufficiency.[373-379] Three light chain- or immunoglobulin-associated diseases may develop: amyloidosis, light-chain cast nephropathy, or light-chain/immunoglobulin deposition disease.

Amyloidosis is a group of diseases that that have in common the tissue deposition of thin (8–11 nm) fibrils rich in β-pleated sheet structure as demonstrated by X-ray diffraction.[373-375] This structure resists proteolysis, leading to perpetuation of the fibrils in tissue. Deposition usually occurs in multiple organs, in diverse combination, although localized deposits (amyloidomas) or organ-isolated forms also occur. Organ-isolated forms may evolve into a systemic process. Renal involvement is usually manifest as nephrotic syndrome with the eventual development of renal failure, although occasional cases of interstitial-limited or vascular-limited disease occur. Cardiomyopathy, enteropathies, neuropathies, ocular involvement, and hepatic involvement are other major clinical presentations. Almost any organ or site may be affected. Although renal disease is a poor prognostic finding, cardiac involvement represents the gravest threat to the patient's survival.

Amyloid can be classified by its clinical syndrome or by its precursor molecule. AL amyloid is the most common type, followed by AA amyloid. The third most common category is familial amyloid. Seven familial forms have been identified: transthyretin, fibrinogen Aa, apolipoprotein AI, apolipoprotein AII, lysozyme, cystatin C, and gelsolin.[377] All are autosomal dominant and most may involve the kidney.

The kidneys in amyloidosis are often stated to be grossly enlarged. However, they may initially be normal in size because early involvement affects the glomeruli that are not appreciably expanded. Conversely, in advanced cases amyloid deposition may result in renal contraction because tubular atrophy accompanies glomerular obliteration, resulting in a decrease in cortical mass. The kidneys may have a

**Table 1-41** Classification of clinical syndromes with amyloid protein

| Clinical syndrome | Amyloid protein | Precursor molecule |
|---|---|---|
| Primary, myeloma-associated | AL | Immunoglobulin light/heavy chain |
| Secondary reactive | AA | Serum AA protein |
| Familial amyloid syndromes | ATTR | Transthyretin |
| | Afib | Fibrinogen Aα cahin |
| | AApol | Apolipoprotein AI |
| | AApoll | Apolipoprotein AII |
| | AGel | Gelsolin |
| | ALys | Lysozyme |
| | ACys | Cystatin C |
| Senile cardiac | ATTR | Transthyretin |
| Familial Mediterranean fever | AA | Serum AA protein |
| Dialysis-associated | Aβ2M | β₂-Microglobulin |

pale or sallow gross appearance, the delineation of cortex and medulla being blurred.

Renal amyloidosis presents in three forms or patterns, defined by the location and appearance of the amyloid fibrils (Table 1-41).[373-375] Amyloid characteristically forms in the glomerulus, initially expanding the mesangium and forming acellular nodules. Later the capillary loops are involved, leading to glomerular obliteration (Fig. 1-126). This form is most common, and is referred to as nodular amyloidosis. Extraglomerular deposition in arterioles and arteries, and deposition in the interstitium of the cortex and medulla occurs in advanced cases. Rarely amyloid deposition is confined to vessels in the kidney and elsewhere, resulting in renovascular hypertension and systemic occlusive vascular disease. This form is known as vascular amyloidosis.

Amyloid deposits have a distinctive homogeneous eosinophilic appearance. A giant cell reaction may be elicited, but usually no tissue reaction is observed. The nodular mesangial deposits resemble nodular diabetic glomerulosclerosis (Kimmelstiel–Wilson lesion) and nodular light-chain deposition disease. Amyloid has affinity for Congo red stain and thioflavin-T stain, permitting identification by light and fluorescent microscopy, respectively (Fig. 1-127). Electron microscopy can resolve equivocal cases by demonstrating the delicate, randomly arrayed fibrils (Fig. 1-128). The methenamine silver stain, a common component of the renal biopsy staining profile, assists in the recognition of amyloid because of its distinctive staining properties. Most deposits of amyloid are silver negative, or stain weakly, in contrast to the two other entities in the differential. Conversely, in some cases of amyloidosis the amyloid fibrils extend through the capillary loop basement membrane in parallel arrays, and have affinity for the silver stain, forming long delicate spike-like arrangements (Fig. 1-129). This is the third form of amyloidosis, known as spicular amyloid. Patients with this form often demonstrate rapid progression of disease.

## Light-chain cast nephropathy (myeloma kidney)

Light-chain cast nephropathy (myeloma kidney) is a disease resulting from the intratubular formation of large eosinophilic (often cracked or fractured) casts composed of a Bence Jones protein and Tamm–Horsfall glycoprotein.[373,376] The

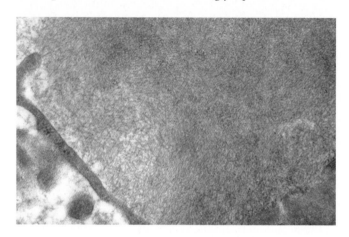

**Fig. 1-128** Electron micrograph showing thin delicate random arrays of fibrils characteristic of amyloid.

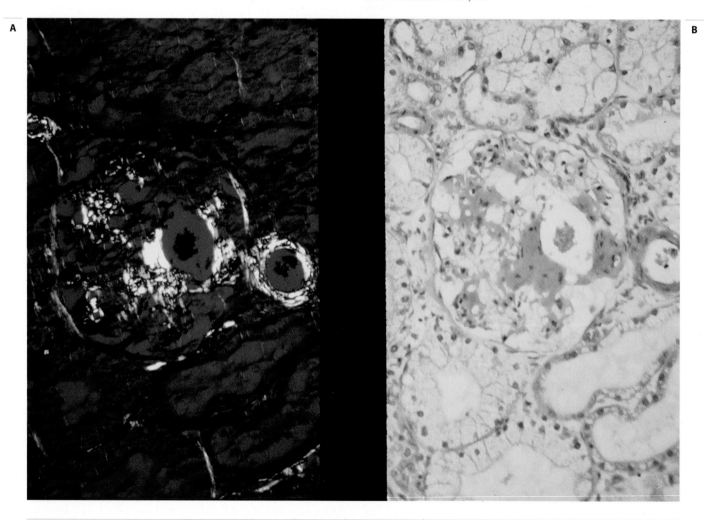

**Fig. 1-127** Congo red stain under bright field and polarization showing the apple green birefringence of amyloid in a glomerulus and its arteriole. Congo red stain.

casts form in the distal tubules and collecting ducts and may extend into the adjacent interstitium. They elicit an inflammatory response that includes neutrophils and histiocytes that may form giant cells (Fig. 1-130).

Immunoglobulin and light-chain deposition disease refers to the deposition of granular paraprotein deposits in glomeruli, tubulointerstitial areas, or both, causing nephrotic syndrome, Fanconi's syndrome, and renal insufficiency (Figs 1-131, 1-132). The glomerular lesion resembles amyloid, but the deposits are granular rather than fibrillar in appearance on electron microscopy.[373,376,378] Similar tubulointerstitial deposits form along the outside of the tubular basement membrane, within the interstitium, and in small vessels. Similar to amyloidosis, systemic involvement also occurs.

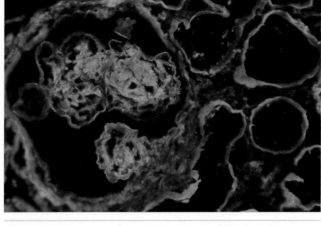

**Fig. 1-131** Direct immunofluorescence showing κ light-chain deposition along tubular and glomerular capillary basement membranes and within the mesangium.

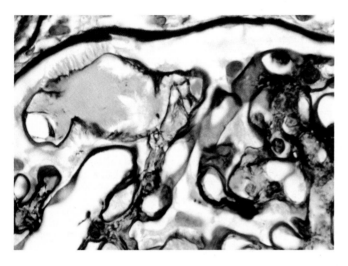

**Fig. 1-129** Spicular amyloid. There is silver-negative amyloid within the capillary loop, and thin spicular silver-positive arrays of amyloid extending perpendicular to the capillary loop basement membrane. Jones methenamine silver stain.

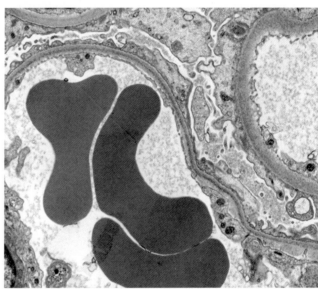

**Fig. 1-132** Granular paraprotein deposits of κ light chains along inner aspect of a capillary loop basement membrane.

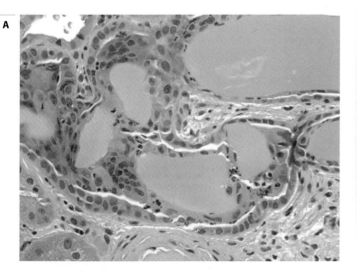

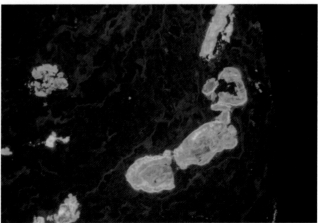

**Fig. 1-130 (A)** Light-chain cast nephropathy causing renal failure. **(B)** Direct immunofluorescence for λ chain within casts.

# REFERENCES

1. Hayman JM Jr. Malpighi's 'Concerning the structure of the kidneys.' A translation and introduction. Ann Med Hist 1925; 7: 242–263.
2. Clark W. The drawings of Leonardo Da Vinci in the collection of Her Majesty the Queen at Windsor Castle. Edinburgh: R & R Clark, 1969.
3. Murphy LJT (ed) The history of urology. Springfield, MA: Charles C. Thomas, 1972.
4. Bowman W. On the structure and use of the malpighian bodies of the kidney, with observations on the circulation through that gland. Philos Trans Roy Soc Lond Biol 1842; 132: 57–80.
5. Fine LG. William Bowman's description of the glomerulus. Am J Nephrol 1985; 5: 433–440.
6. Huber GC. On the development and shape of uriniferous tubules of certain of the higher mammals, Am J Anat 1905; 4: 1–98.
7. Kelly HA, Burnam CF. Diseases of the kidneys, ureters and bladder. New York: Appleton, Century Crofts, 1914.
8. Osathanondh V, Potter EL. Development of the human kidney as shown by microdissection II. Renal pelvis, calyces and papillae. Arch Pathol 1963; 76: 276–289.
9. Osathanondh V, Potter EL. Development of the human kidney as shown by microdissection III. Formation and interrelationship of collecting tubules and nephrons. Arch Pathol 1963; 76: 290–302.
10. Osathanondh V, Potter EL. Development of the human kidney as shown by microdissection IV. Development of tubular portions of nephrons. Arch Pathol 1966; 82: 391–402.
11. Osathanondh V, Potter EL. Development of the human kidney as shown by microdissection V. Development of vascular pattern of glomeruli. Arch Pathol 1966; 82: 403–411.
12. Patten BM. Human embryology. New York: McGraw-Hill, 1968.
13. Potter EL. Normal and abnormal development of the kidney. Chicago: Year Book Medical Publishers, 1972.
14. Clapp WL. Adult kidney. In: Sternberg SS, ed. Histology for the pathologist, 2nd edn. New York: Raven Press, 1997; 839–907.
15. Bonsib SM. Renal anatomy and histology. In: Jennette JC, Olson JL, Schwartz MM, Silva FG, eds. Heptinstall's pathology of the kidney. Baltimore: Lippincott Williams & Wilkins, 2007; Chapter 1.
16. Brenner BM. Determinants of epithelial differentiation during early nephrogenesis. J Am Soc Nephrol 1990; 1: 127–139.
17. Fouser L, Avner ED. Normal and abnormal nephrogenesis. Am J Kidney Dis 1993; 21: 64–70.
18. Kanwar YS, Carone FA, Kumar A, et al. Role of extracellular matrix, growth factors and proto-oncogenes in metanephric development. Kidney Int 1997; 52: 589–606.
19. Pohl M, Bhatnagar V, Mendoza SA, Nigam SK. Towards an etiologic classification of developmental disorders of the kidney and upper urinary tract. Kidney Int 2002; 61: 10–19.
20. Brodel M. The intrinsic blood vessels of the kidney and their significance in nephrotomy. Bull Johns Hopkins Hosp 1901; 12: 10–13.
21. Graves FT. The anatomy of the intrarenal arteries and its application to segmental resection of the kidney. Br J Surg 1954; 42: 132–139.
22. Hodson J. The lobar structure of the kidney. Br J Urol 1972; 44: 246–261.
23. Baker SB. The blood supply to the renal papillae. Br J Urol 1959; 31: 53–59.
24. Ichikawa I, Kuwayama F, Pope JC. Paradigm shift from classic anatomic theories to contemporary cell biological views of CAKUT. Kidney Int 2002; 61: 889–989.
25. Matsell DG. Renal dysplasia: New approaches to an old problem. Am J Kidney Dis 1998; 32: 535–543.
26. Campbell MF. Urology. Philadelphia: WB Saunders, 1986.
27. Weyrauch HM Jr. Anomalies of renal rotation. Surg Gynecol Obstet 1939; 69: 183–199.
28. Thompson GJ, Pace JM. Ectopic kidney: a review of 97 cases. Surg Gynecol Obstet 1939; 69: 935–943.
29. Kelalis PP, Malek RS, Segura JW. Observations on renal ectopia and fusion in children. J Urol 1973; 110: 588–593.
30. Aliotta PJ, Seidel FG, Karp M, et al. Renal malposition in patients with omphalocele. J Urol 1987; 137: 942–944.
31. Malter IJ, Stanley RJ. The intrathoracic kidney; with a review of the literature. J Urol 1972; 107: 538–541.
32. McDonald JH, McClellan DS. Crossed renal ectopia. Am J Surg 1957; 93: 995–1002.
33. Hendren WH, Donahoe PK, Pfister RC. Crossed renal ectopia in children. Urology 1976; 7: 135–144.
34. Boatman DL, Kolln CP, Flocks RN. Congenital anomalies associated with horseshoe kidney. J Urol 1972; 107: 205–207.
35. Zondek LH, Zondek T. Horseshoe kidney and associated congenital malformations. 1964; Urol Int 18: 347–350.
36. Geisinger JF. Supernumerary kidney. J Urol 1936; 38: 331–356.
37. N'Guessan G, Stephens FD. Supernumerary kidney. J Urol 1983; 130: 649–653.
38. Risdon RA, Young LW, Chrispin AR. Renal hypoplasia and dysplasia: a radiological and pathological correlation. Pediatr Radiol 1975; 3: 213–225.
39. Schwartz RD, Stephens RD, Cussen LJ. The pathogenesis of renal dysplasia. I. Quantitation of hypoplasia and dysplasia. Invest Urol 1981; 19: 94–96.
40. Royer P, Habib R, Mathieu H, et al. Bilateral congenital renal hypoplasia with reduction in number and hypertrophy of the nephrons in children. Ann Pediatr 1962; 38: 753–766.
41. Fetterman GH, Habib R. Congenital bilateral oligomeganephronic renal hypoplasia with hypertrophy of nephrons (oligomeganephronie). Am J Clin Pathol 1969; 52: 199–207.
42. Moerman PH, van Damme B, Proesmans W, et al. Oligomeganephronic renal hypoplasia in two siblings. J Pediatr 1984; 105: 75–77.
43. Potter EL. Bilateral absence of ureters and kidneys. A report of 50 cases. Obstet Gynecol 1965; 25: 3–12.
44. Potter EL. Facial characteristics of infants with bilateral renal agenesis. Am J Obstet Gynecol 1946; 51: 885–888.
45. Scott RJ, Goodburn SF. Potter's syndrome in the second semester – prenatal screening and pathological findings in 60 cases of oligohydramnios sequence. Prenat Diagn 1995; 15: 519–525.
46. Rush WH Jr, Currie DP. Hemitrigone in renal agenesis or single ureteral ectopia. Urology 1978; 11: 161–163.
47. Emanuel B, Nachman R, Aronson N, et al. Congenital solitary kidney: a review of 74 cases, J Urol 1974; 111: 394–397.
48. Parikh CR, McCall D, Engelman C, Schrier RW. Congenital renal agenesis: case–control analysis of birth characteristics. Am J Kidney Dis 2002; 39: 689–694.
49. Thompson DP, Lynn HB. Genital anomalies associated with solitary kidney. Mayo Clin Proc 1966; 41: 538–548.
50. Hiraoka M, Tsukahara H, Ohshima Y, et al. Renal aplasia is the predominant cause of congenital solitary kidney. Kidney Int 2002; 61: 1840–1844.
51. Acien P, Ruiz JA, Hernandez JF, et al. Renal agenesis in association with malformation of the female genital tract. Am J Obstet Gynecol 1991; 165: 1368–1370.
52. Duncan PA, Shapiro LR, Stangel JJ, et al. The MURCS association: müllerian duct aplasia, renal aplasia,

and cervicothoracic somite dysplasia. J Pediatr 1979; 95: 399–402.

53. Thomas IT, Smith DW. Oligohydramnios, causes of the nonrenal features of Potter's syndrome, including pulmonary hypoplasia. J Pediatr 1974; 84: 811–814.

54. Salazar H, Kanbour AI, Pardo M. Amnion nodosum. Ultrastructure and histopathogenesis. Arch Pathol 1974; 98: 39–46.

55. Bain AD, Scott JS. Renal agenesis and severe urinary tract dysplasia. Br Med J 1960; 1: 841–846.

56. Curry CJR, Jensen K, Holland J, et al. The Potter sequence: a clinical analysis of 80 cases. Am J Med Genet 1984; 19: 679–702.

57. Escobar LF, Weaver DD, Bixler D, et al. Urorectal septum malformation sequence. Am J Dis Child 1987; 141: 1021–1024.

58. Ingelfinger JR, Newburger JW. Spectrum of renal anomalies in patients with Williams syndrome. J Pediatr 1991; 119: 771–773.

59. Hurwitz RS, Manzoni GAM, Ransley PG, et al. Cloacal exstrophy: a report of 34 cases. J Urol 1987; 138: 1060–1064.

60. Quan L, Smith DW. The VATER association, vertebral defects, and atresia, T-E fistula with esophageal atresia, radial and renal dysplasia: a spectrum of associated defect. J Pediatr 1973; 82: 104–107.

61. Khoury MJ, Cordero JF, Greenberg F, et al. A population based study of the VACTERL association: evidence for its etiologic heterogeneity. Pediatrics 1983; 71: 815–820.

62. Burn J, Marwood RP. Fraser syndrome presenting as bilateral renal agenesis. J Med Genet 1982; 19: 360–361.

63. Rubenstein MA, Bucy JG. Caudal regression syndrome: the urologic implications. J Urol 1975; 114: 934–937.

64. Biedel CW, Pagon RA, Zapata JO. Müllerian anomalies and renal agenesis: autosomal dominant urogenital adysplasia. J Pediatr 1984; 104: 861–864.

65. Buchta RM, Viseskul C, Gilbert EF, et al.: Familial bilateral renal agenesis and hereditary renal adysplasia. Z Kinderheilkd 1973; 115: 111–129.

66. Cain DR, Griggs D, Lackey DA, et al. Familial renal agenesis and total dysplasia. Am J Dis Child 1974; 128: 377–380.

67. Roodhooft AM, Birnholz JC, Holmes LB. Familial nature of congenital absence and severe dysgenesis of both kidneys. N Engl J Med 1984; 310: 1341–1345.

68. Murugasu B, Cole BR, Hawkins EP, et al. Familial renal adysplasia. Am J Kidney Dis 1991; 18: 490–494.

69. Woolf AS, Price KL, Scambler PJ, Winyard PJD. Evolving concepts in human renal dysplasia. J Am Soc Nephrol 2004; 15: 998–1007.

70. Bernstein J: Renal cystic disease: classification and pathogenesis. Congen Anom 1993; 33: 5–13.

71. Woolf AS, Winyard PJ. Advances in the cell biology and genetics of human kidney malformations. J Am Soc Nephrol 1998; 9: 1114–1125.

72. Osathananth V, Potter EL. Pathogenesis of polycystic kidneys. Arch Pathol 1964; 77: 459–465.

73. Berman DJ, Maizals M. The role of urinary obstruction in the genesis of renal dysplasia. J Urol 1982; 128: 1091–1096.

74. Schwartz RD, Stephens FD, Cussen LJ. The pathogenesis of renal dysplasia II. The significance of lateral and medial ectopy of the ureteric orifice. Invest Urol 1981; 19: 97–100.

75. Cussen LJ. Cystic kidneys in children with congenital urethral obstruction. J Urol 1971; 106: 939–941.

76. Ichikawa I, KuwayamaF, Pope IV JC, et al. Paradigm shift from classic anatomic theories to contemporary cell biological views of CAKUT. Kidney Int 2002; 61: 889–989.

77. Maizals M, Simpson SB Jr. Primitive ducts of renal dysplasia induced by culturing ureteral buds denuded of condensed renal blastema. Science 1983; 219: 509–510.

78. Bonsib SM, Koontz P. Renal maldevelopment: A pediatric renal biopsy study. Mod Pathol 1997; 10: 1233–1238.

79. Mackie GG, Stephens FD. Duplex kidneys: a correlation of renal dysplasia with position of the ureteral orifice. J Urol 1975; 114: 274–280.

80. Bernstein J, Brough AJ, McAdams AJ. The renal lesion in syndromes of multiple congenital malformations. Birth Defects 1974; 10: 35–43.

81. Bernstein J. Hepatic and renal involvement in malformation syndromes. Mt Sinai J Med 1986; 53: 421–428.

82. Osler W. Congenital absence of abdominal muscles with distended and hypertrophied urinary bladder. Bull Johns Hopkins Hosp 1901; 12: 331.

83. Manivel JC, Pettinato G, Reinberg Y, et al. Prune belly syndrome: clinicopathological study of 29 cases. Pediatr Pathol 1989; 9: 691–711.

84. Zerres K, Valpel M-C, Weib H. Cystic kidneys. Genetics, pathological anatomy clinical picture and prenatal diagnosis. Hum Genet 1984; 68: 104–135.

85. Kravtzova GI, Lazjuk GI, Lurie IW. The malformations of the urinary system in autosomal disorders. Virchows Arch [A] 1975; 368: 167–178.

86. Duncan PA, Shapiro LR. Interrelationship of the hemifacial microsomia–VATER, VATER and sirenomelia phenotype. Am J Med Genet 1993; 47: 75–84.

87. Capisonda R, Phan V, Traubuci J, et al. Autosomal recessive polycystic kidney disease: outcomes from a single-center experience. Pediatr Nephrol 2003; 18: 119–126.

88. Blyth H, Ockenden BG. Polycystic disease of kidneys and liver presenting in childhood. J Med Genet 1971; 8: 257–284.

89. Lonergan GJ, Rice RR, Suarez ES. Autosomal recessive polycystic kidney disease: radiologic–pathologic correlations. Radiographics 2000; 20: 837–855.

90. Gang DL, Herrin JT. Infantile polycystic disease of the liver and kidneys. Clin Nephrol 1986; 28: 28–36.

91. Igarashi P, Somlo S. Genetics and pathogenesis of polycystic kidney disease. J Am Soc Nephrol 2002; 13: 2384–2398.

92. Wang S, Luo Y, Wilson PD, et al. The autosomal recessive polycystic kidney disease protein is localized to primary cilia, with concentration in the basal body. J Am Soc Nephrol 2004; 15: 592–602.

93. Zerres K, Muecher G, Becker J, et al. Prenatal diagnosis of autosomal recessive polycystic kidney disease (ARPKD): molecular genetics, clinical experience, and fetal morphology. Am J Med Genet 1998; 76: 137–144.

94. Igarashi P, Somlo S. Genetics and pathogenesis of polycystic kidney disease. J Am Soc Nephrol 2002; 13: 2384–2398.

95. Leiske JC, Toback FG. Autosomal dominant polycystic kidney disease. J Am Soc Nephrol 1993; 3: 1442–1450.

96. Fick GM, Johnson, AM, Hammond WS, Gabow PA. Causes of death in autosomal dominant polycystic kidney disease. J Am Soc Nephrol 1995; 5: 2048–2056.

97. Perrone RD. Extrarenal manifestations of ADPKD. Kidney Int 1997; 51: 2022–2036.

98. Grantham JJ. Polycystic kidney disease: from the bedside to the gene and back. Curr Opin Nephrol Hypertens 2001; 10: 533–542.

99. Foggensteiner L, Bevan AP, Thomas R, et al. Cellular distribution of polycystin-2, the protein product of the PKD2 gene. J Am Soc Nephrol 2000; 11: 814–827.

100. Porch P, Noe HN, Stapleton FB. Unilateral presentation of adult type polycystic kidney disease in children. J Urol 1986; 135: 744–746.

101. Shokeir MHK. Expression of 'adult' polycystic renal disease in the fetus and newborn. Clin Genet 1978; 14: 61–72.

102. Baert L. Hereditary polycystic kidney disease (adult form): a microdissection study of two cases at an early stage of the disease. Kidney Int 1978; 13: 519–525.

103. Grantham JJ, Geiser JL, Evan AP. Cyst formation and growth in autosomal dominant polycystic kidney disease. Kidney Int 1987; 31: 1145–1152.

104. Verani RR, Silva FG. Histogenesis of the renal cysts in adult (autosomal dominant) polycystic kidney disease: a

histochemical study. Mod Pathol 1988; 1: 457–463.

105. Bernstein J, Evan AP, Gardner KD Jr. Epithelial hyperplasia in human polycystic kidney diseases. Am J Pathol 1987; 129: 92–101.

106. Gregoiri JR, Torres VE, Holley KE, et al. Renal epithelial hyperplastic and neoplastic proliferation in autosomal dominant polycystic kidney disease. Am J Kidney Dis 1987; 9: 27–38.

107. Saunier S, Salomon R, Antignac C. Nephronophthisis. Curr Opin Genet Dev 2005; 15: 324–331.

108. Waldherr R, Lennert T, Weber H-P, et al. The nephronophthisis complex. A clinicopathologic study in children. Virchows Arch [A] 1982; 394: 235–254.

109. Hildebrandt F, Strahm B, Nothwang H-G, et al. Molecular genetic identification of families with juvenile nephronophthisis type 1: rate of progression to renal failure. Kidney Int 1997; 51: 261–269.

110. Orman H, Fernandez C, Jung M, et al. Identification of a new gene locus for adolescent nephronophthisis, on chromosome 3q22 in a large Venezuelan pedigree. Am J Hum Genet 2000; 66: 118–127.

111. Christodoulou K, Tsingis M, Stavrou C, et al. Chromosome 1 localization of a gene for autosomal dominant medullary cystic kidney disease (ADMCKD). Hum Mol Genet 1988; 7: 905–911.

112. Scolari F, Puzzer D, Amoroso A, et al. Identification of a new locus for medullary cystic disease on chromosome 16p12. Am J Hum Genet 1999. 64: 1655–1666.

113. Wolf MT, Mucha BE, Hennes HC, et al. Medullary cystic disease type 1: mutational analysis in 37 genes on haplotype sharing. Hum Genet 2006; 119: 649–658.

114. Bleyer AJ, Hart TC, Willingham MC, et al. Clinico-pathologic findings in medullary cystic kidney disease type 2. Pediatr Nephrol 2005; 20: 824–827.

115. Lamiell JM, Salazar FG, Hsia YEL. Von Hippel–Lindau disease affecting 43 members of a single kindred. Medicine 1989; 68: 1–29.

116. Solomon O, Schwartz A. Renal pathology in von Hippel–Lindau disease. Hum Pathol 1988; 19: 1072–1079.

117. Chauveau D, Duvic C, Chretien Y, et al. Renal involvement in von Hippel–Lindau disease. Kidney Int 1996; 50: 944–951.

118. Neuman HPH, Zbar B. Renal cysts, renal cancer and von Hippel–Lindau disease. Kidney Int 1997; 51: 16–26.

119. Ibrahim RE, Weinberg DS, Weidner N. Atypical cysts and carcinomas of the kidneys in phacomatoses. Cancer 1989; 63: 148–157.

120. Bernstein J, Robbins TO, Kissane JM. The renal lesions of tuberous sclerosis. Semin Diagn Pathol 1986; 3: 97–105.

121. Ahuja S, Loffler W, Wegener O-H, et al. Tuberous sclerosis with angiomyolipoma and metastasized hypernephroma. Urology 1986; 28: 413–419.

122. Torra R, Badenas C, Darnell A, et al. Facilitated diagnosis of the contiguous gene syndrome: tuberous sclerosis and polycystic kidneys by means of haplotype studies. Am J Kidney Dis 1998; 31: 1038–1043.

123. Martignoni G, Bonetti F, Pea M, et al. Renal disease in adults with TSC2/PKD1 contiguous gene syndrome. Am J Surg Pathol 2002; 26: 198–205.

124. Bernstein J, Landing BH. Glomerulocystic kidney diseases. In: Bartsocas CS, ed. Genetics of kidney disorders. New York: Alan R. Liss, 1989; 27–43.

125. Kaplan BS, Gordon I, Pincott J, et al. Familial hypoplastic glomerulocystic kidney disease: a definite entity with dominant inheritance. Am J Med Genet 1989; 34: 569–573.

126. Romero R, Bonal J, Campo E, et al. Glomerulocystic kidney disease: a single entity? Nephron 1993; 63: 100–103.

127. Bernstein J. Glomerulocystic kidney disease – nosological considerations. Pediatr Nephrol 1993; 7: 464–470.

128. Dedeoglu IO. Spectrum of glomerulocystic kidneys: a case report and review of the literature. Pediatr Pathol Lab Med 1996; 16: 941–949.

129. Hotta O, Sato M, Furuta T, Taguma Y. Pathogenic role of the glomerulo-tubular junction stenosis in glomerulocystic disease. Clin Nephrol 1999; 3: 177–180.

130. Bingham C, Bulman MP, Ellard S, et al. Mutations in the hepatocyte nuclear factor-1B gene are associated with familial hypoplastic glomerulocystic kidney disease. Am J Hum Genet 2001; 68: 219–224.

131. Hallman N, Hjelt L. Congenital nephrotic syndrome. J Pediatr 1959; 55: 152–162.

132. Hallman N, Norio R, Rapola J. Congenital nephrotic syndrome. Nephron 1973; 11: 101–110.

133. Fujinami M, Hane Y, Ito K, et al. Congenital nephrotic syndrome (Finnish type). Acta Pathol Jpn 1985; 35: 517–525.

134. Sibley RK, Mahan J, Mauer SM, et al. A clinicopathologic study of forty-eight infants with nephrotic syndrome. Kidney Int 1985; 27: 544–552.

135. Holtzman LB, St. John PL, Kovari IA, et al. Nephrin localizes to the slit pore of the glomerular epithelial cell. Kidney Int 1999; 56: 1481–1491.

136. Tryggvason K. Unraveling the mechanisms of glomerular ultrafiltration: nephrin, a key component of the slit diaphragm. J Am Soc Nephrol 1999; 10: 2440–2445.

137. Patrakka J, Kestila M, Wartiovaara J, et al. Congenital nephrotic syndrome (NPHS1): features resulting from different mutations in Finnish families. Kidney Int 2000; 58: 972–980.

138. Swinford AE, Bernstein J, Toriello HV, et al. Renal tubular dysgenesis: delayed onset of oligohydrananios. Am J Med Genet 1989; 32: 127–132.

139. Genest DC, Lage JM. Absence of normal appearing proximal tubules in the fetal and neonatal kidney: prevalence and significance. Hum Pathol 1991; 22: 147–153.

140. Pryde PG, Sedman AB, Nugent CE, et al. Angiotensin-converting enzyme inhibitor fetopathy. J Am Soc Nephrol 1993; 3: 1575–1582.

141. Bernstein J, Barajas L. Renal tubular dysgenesis: evidence of abnormality in the renin–angiotensin system. J Am Soc Nephrol 1994; 5: 224–227.

142. Simon J. On subacute inflammation of the kidney. Medico-chir Trans 1847; 30: 141–164.

143. Dunnill MS, Millard PR, Oliver D. Acquired cystic disease of the kidneys: a hazard of long-term intermittent maintenance hemodialysis. J Clin Pathol 1977; 30: 868–877.

144. Grantham JJ. Acquired cystic disease. Kidney Int 1991; 40: 143–152.

145. Bretan PN Jr, Busch MP, Hricak H, et al. Chronic renal failure: a significant risk factor in the development of acquired renal cysts and renal cell carcinoma. Cancer 1986; 57: 1871–1879.

146. Matson MA, Cohen EP. Acquired cystic kidney disease: occurrence, prevalence and renal cancers. Medicine 1990; 69: 217–226.

147. Hughson MD, Schmidt L, Zbar B, et al. Renal cell carcinoma of end-stage renal disease: a histopathologic and molecular genetic study. J Am Soc Nephrol 1996; 7: 2461–2468.

148. Chudek J, Herbers J, Wilhelm M, et al. The genetics of renal tumors in end-stage renal failure differs from those occurring in the general population. J Am Soc Nephrol 1998; 9: 1045–1051.

149. Cho KJ, Thornburg JR, Bernstein J, et al. Localized cystic disease of the kidney: 'angiographic'–pathologic correlation. AJR Am J Roentgenol 1979; 132: 891–895.

150. Pyrah LN. Medullary sponge kidney. J Urol 1966; 90: 274–283.

151. Indridason OS, Thomas L, Berkoben M. Medullary sponge kidney associated with congenital hemihypertrophy. J Am Soc Nephrol 1996; 7: 1123–1130.

152. Dalton D, Neiman H, Grayhack JT. The natural history of simple renal cysts: a preliminary study. J Urol 1986; 135: 905–908.

153. Laucks SP Jr, McLachlan MSF. Aging and simple cysts of the kidney. Br J Radiol 1981; 54: 12–14.

154. Kimche D, Lask D. Megacalycosis. Urology 1978; 19: 478–481.

155. Timmons JW Jr, Malek RS, Hattery RR, et al. Caliceal diverticulum. J Urol 1975; 114: 6–9.

156. Mathieson AJM. Calyceal diverticulum: a case with a discussion and review of the condition. Br J Urol 1953; 25: 147–154.

157. Sommers SC, Relman AS, Smithwick RH. Histologic studies of kidney biopsy specimens from patients with hypertension. Am J Pathol 1958; 34: 685–701.

158. Walker WG. Hypertension-related renal injury: a major contributor to end stage renal disease. Am J Kidney Dis 1993; 22: 164–173.

159. Schwartz GL, Strong CG. Renal parenchymal involvement in essential hypertension, Med Clin North Am 71: 843–858, 1987.

160. Bright R: Tubular view of the morbid appearances in 100 cases connected with albuminous urine: with observations. Guy's Hosp Rep 1836; 1: 380.

161. Johnson GI. On certain points in the anatomy and pathology of Bright's disease. Trans Med Chir Soc 1868; 51: 57–78.

162. Mahomed FA. Some of the clinical aspects of Bright's disease. Guy's Hosp Rep 1879; 24: 363.

163. Volhard F, Fahr T. Die Brightsche Nierenkrankheit: Klinik, pathologie und atlas. Berlin: Julius Springer, 1914.

164. Ono H, Ono Y. Nephrosclerosis and hypertension. Med Clin North Am 1997; 81: 1273–1288.

165. Ratliff NB. Renal vascular disease: pathology of large blood vessel disease. Am J Kidney Dis 1985; 5: A93–A103.

166. Kashgarian M. Pathology of small blood vessel disease in hypertension. Am J Kidney Dis 1985; 5: A104–A110.

167. McManus JFA, Lupton GH Jr. Ischemic obsolescence of renal glomeruli. Lab Invest 1960; 9: 413–434.

168. Tracy RE, Strong JP, Newman III WP, et al. Renovasculopathies of nephrosclerosis in relation to atherosclerosis at ages 25 to 54. Kidney Int 1996; 49: 564–570.

169. MacMahon HE. Malignant nephrosclerosis-a reappraisal. Pathol Annu 1968; 3: 297–334.

170. Ruggenenti P, Remuzi G. Malignant vascular disease of the kidney: nature of the lesions, mediators of disease progression, and the case for bilateral nephrectomy. Am J Kidney Dis 1996; 27: 459–475.

171. Moschcowitz E. An acute febrile pleiochromic anemia with hyaline thrombosis of the terminal arterioles and capillaries. Arch Intern Med 1925; 36: 89–93.

172. Gasser VC, Gautier E, Steek A, et al. Hämolytisch–uramische syndrome: bilaterale Nierenyindennekrosen bei akuten erworbenen hamolytischen anamien. Schweiz Med Wochenschr 1955; 38: 905–909.

173. Symmers WSC. Thrombotic microangiopathic hemolytic anemia (thrombotic microangiopathy). Br Med J 1952; 2: 897–903.

174. Ruggenenti P, Lutz J, Remuzzi G. Pathogenesis and treatment of thrombotic microangiopathy. Kidney Int 1997; 51: S97–S101.

175. Murgo AJ. Thrombotic microangiopathy in cancer patients, including those induced by chemotherapeutic agents. Semin Hematol 1987; 24: 161–177.

176. Churg J, Strauss L. Renal involvement in thrombotic microangiopathy. Semin Nephrol 1985; 5: 46–56.

177. Donohoe JF. Scleroderma and the kidney. Kidney Int 1992; 41: 462–477.

178. Stratta P, Canavese C, Colla L. Microangiopathic hemolytic anemia and postpartum acute renal failure. Nephron 1986; 44: 253–255.

179. Hauglustaine D, van Damme B, et al. Recurrent hemolytic uremic syndrome during oral contraception. Clin Nephrol 1981; 15: 148–153.

180. Remuzzi G, Bertani T. Renal vascular and thrombotic effect of cyclosporine. Am J Kidney Dis 1989; 13: 261–272.

181. Kwaan HC. Clinicopathologic features of thrombotic thrombocytopenic purpura. Semin Hematol 1987; 24: 71–81.

182. Remuzzi G. HUS and TTP: variable expression of a single entity. Kidney Int 1987; 32: 292–308.

183. Kaplan BS, Proesmans W. The hemolytic uremic syndrome of childhood and its variants. Semin Hematol 1987; 24: 148–160.

184. Ashkenazi S. Role of bacterial cytotoxins in hemolytic uremic syndrome and thrombotic thrombocytopenic purpura. Ann Rev Med 1993; 44: 11–18.

185. Richardon SE, Karmali MLA, Becker LE, et al. The histopathology of the hemolytic uremic syndrome associated with verocytotoxin-producing Escherichia coli infections. Hum Pathol 1988; 19: 1102–1108.

186. Kaplan BS, Meyers KE, Schulman SL. The pathogenesis and treatment of hemolytic uremic syndrome. J Am Soc Nephrol 1998; 9: 1126–1133.

187. Cruz DN, Perzella MA, Mahnensmith RL. Bone marrow transplant nephropathy: a case report and review of the literature. J Am Soc Nephrol 1997; 8: 166–173.

188. Goldblatt H, Lynch J, Hanzal RF, et al. Studies in experimental hypertension I. The production of persistent elevation of systolic blood pressure by means of renal ischemia. J Exp Med 1934; 59: 347–357.

189. Wise KL, McCann RL, Dunnick NR, et al. Renovascular hypertension. J Urol 1988; 140: 911–924.

190. Stimpel M, Groth H, Greminger P, et al. The spectrum of renovascular hypertension. Cardiology 1985; 72: 1–9.

191. Harrison EG Jr, McCormack LJ. Pathologic classification of renal arterial disease in renovascular hypertension. Mayo Clin Proc 1971; 46: 161–167.

192. Youngberg SP, Sheps SG, Strong CG. Fibromuscular disease of the renal arteries. Med Clin North Am 1977; 61: 623–641.

193. Ingelfinger JR. Renovascular disease in children. Kidney Int 1993; 43: 493–505.

194. Edwards BS, Stanton AW, Holley KE, et al. Isolated renal artery dissection. Presentation, evaluation, management and pathology. Mayo Clin Proc 1982; 57: 564–571.

195. Rao CW, Blaivas JG. Primary renal artery dissection: a review. J Urol 1977; 118: 716–719.

196. Tynes WV II: Unusual renovascular disorders, Urol Clin North Am 11: 529–542, 1984.

197. Poutasse EF. Renal artery aneurysms. J Urol 1975; 113: 443–449.

198. Altebarmakian VK, Caldamone AA, Dachelet RJ, et al. Renal artery aneurysm. Urology 1979; 13: 257–260.

199. Harrow BR, Sloane JA. Aneurysm of renal artery: report of five cases. J Urol 1956; 81: 35–39.

200. Smith JN, Hinman F Jr. Intrarenal arterial aneurysms. J Urol 1967; 97: 990–996.

201. Maldonado JE, Sheps SG. Renal arteriovenous fistula. Postgrad Med 1966; 40: 263–269.

202. Kopchick JH, Jacobson HA, Bourne NK, et al. Congenital renal arteriovenous malformations. Urology 1981; 17: 13–17.

203. Takaha M, Matsumoto A, Ochi K, et al. Intrarenal arteriovenous malformations. J Urol 1980; 124: 315–318.

204. Hoxie HF, Coggin CB. Renal infarction. Arch Intern Med 1940; 65: 587–594.

205. Thurlbeck WM, Castleman B. Atheromatous emboli to the kidneys after aortic surgery. N Engl J Med 1957; 257: 442–447.

206. Richards AM, Eliot RS, Kanjuh VL, et al. Cholesterol embolism. A multiple-system disease masquerading as polyarteritis nodosa. Am J Cardiol 1965; 15: 696–707.

207. Colt HG, Begg RJ, Saporito J, et al. Cholesterol emboli after cardiac catheterization. Medicine 1988; 67: 389–400.

208. Gasparini M, Hofman R, Stoller M. Renal artery embolism: clinical features and therapeutic options. J Urol 1992; 147: 567–572.

209. Fine MJ, Kapoor W, Falanga V. Cholesterol crystal embolization: a review of 221 cases in the English literature. Angiology 1987; 38: 769–784.

210. Thadhani RI, Camargo CA, Xavier RJ, et al. Atheroembolic renal failure after invasive procedure. Natural history based upon 52 histologically confirmed cases. Medicine 1995; 74: 350–358.

211. Scolari F, Tardanico R, Zani R, et al. Cholesterol crystal embolism: a recognizable cause of renal disease. Am J Kidney Dis 2000; 36: 1089–1109.

212. Wells JD, Margolin ELG, Gall EA. Renal cortical necrosis: clinical and pathologic features in 21 cases. Am J Med 1960; 29: 257–267.

213. Kleinknecht D, Grunfeld JP, Gomez PC, et al. Diagnostic procedures and long term prognosis in bilateral renal cortical necrosis. Kidney Int 1973; 4: 390–400.

214. Grunfeld JP, Ganeval D, Bournerias F. Acute renal failure in pregnancy. Kidney Int 1980; 18: 179–191.

215. Jones DB, Iannaccone PM. Atheromatous emboli in renal biopsies. Am J Pathol 1975; 78: 261–276.

216. Kasinath BS, Corwin HL, Bidoni AK, et al. Eosinophilia in the diagnosis of atheroembolic renal disease. Am J Nephrol 1987; 7: 173–177.

217. Stables DP, Fouche RE, DeVillers JP, et al. Traumatic renal artery occlusion: 21 cases. J Urol 1976; 115: 229–233.

218. Llach F. Hypercoagulability, renal vein thrombosis, and other thrombotic complications of nephrotic syndrome. Kidney Int 1985; 28: 429–439.

219. Rosenmann E, Pollack VE, Pirani CL. Renal vein thrombosis in the adult: a clinical and pathologic study based on renal biopsies. Medicine 1968; 47: 269–335.

220. Llach F, Papper S, Massry SG. The clinical spectrum of renal vein thrombosis: acute and chronic. Am J Med 1980; 69: 819–827.

221. Arneil GC, MacDonald AM, Murphy AV, et al. Renal venous thrombosis. Clin Nephrol 1973; 1: 119–131.

222. Ricci MA, Lloyd DA. Renal venous thrombosis in infants and children. Arch Surg 1990; 125: 1195–1199.

223. Christensen JA, Bader H, Bohle A, et al. The structure of the juxtaglomerular apparatus in Addison's disease, Bartter's syndrome and in Conn's syndrome. Virchows Arch [A] 1976; 370: 103–112.

224. Küssmaul A, Maier R. Ueber eine bisher nicht beschriebene eigenthumliche arterienerkrankung (periarteritis nodosa), die mit morbus Brightii und rapid fortschreitender allgemeiner muskellahmung einherght. Dtsch Arch Klin Med 1866; 1: 484–516.

225. Davies D, Moran ME, Niall JF, et al. Segmental glomerulonephritis with antineutrophil antibody: possible arbovirus aetiology. Br J Med 1982; 285: 606.

226. van der Woude FJ, Rasmussen N, et al. Autoantibodies against neutrophils and monocytes: tool for diagnosis and marker of disease activity in Wegener's granulomatosis. Lancet 1985; 1: 425–429.

227. Jennette JC, Falk RJ. Antineutrophil cytoplasmic autoantibodies and associated diseases: a review. Am J Kidney Dis 1990; 15: 517–529.

228. Goeken JA. Anti-neutrophil cytoplasmic antibody-a useful serological marker for vasculitis. J Clin Immunol 1991; 11: 161–174.

229. Gross WL, Csernok E, Helmchen U. Antineutrophil cytoplasmic autoantibodies, autoantigens, and systemic vasculitis. APMIS 1995; 103: 81–97.

230. Savige J, Davies D, Falk RJ, et al. Antineutrophil cytoplasmic antibodies and associated diseases: a review of the clinical and laboratory features. Kidney Int 2000; 57: 846–862.

231. Savage COS. ANCA-associated renal vasculitis. Kidney Int 2001; 60: 1614–1627.

232. Balow JE. Renal vasculitis. Kidney Int 1985; 27: 954–964.

233. Adu D, Howie AJ, Scott DGI, et al. Polyarteritis and the kidney. QJ Med 1987; 62: 221–237.

234. Churg J, Churg A. Idiopathic and secondary vasculitis: a review. Mod Pathol 1989; 2: 144–160.

235. Couser WG. Rapidly progressive glomerulonephritis: classification, pathogenetic mechanisms and therapy. Am J Kidney Dis 1988; 11: 449–464.

236. Bonsib SM. Glomerular basement membrane necrosis and crescent organization: a scanning electron microscopic study. Kidney Int 1988; 33: 966–974.

237. Bohle A, Gise HV, Mackensen-Haen S, et al. The obliteration of the postglomerular capillaries and its influence upon the function of both glomeruli and tubules. Klin Wochenschr 1981; 59: 1043–1051.

238. Fine LG, Ong ACM, Norman JT. Mechanisms of tubulo-interstitial injury in progressive renal diseases. Eur J Clin Invest 1993; 23: 259–265.

239. Heptinstall RH. Interstitial nephritis. A brief review. Am J Pathol 1976; 83: 214–233.

240. Roberts JA. Pyelonephritis, cortical abscess and perinephric abscess. Urol Clin North Am 1986; 13: 637–645.

241. Funfstuck R, Smith JW, Tschape H, Stein G. Pathogenetic aspects of uncomplicated urinary tract infections: recent advances. Clin Nephrol 1997; 47: 13–18.

242. Hodson CJ. Reflux nephropathy: a personal historical review. AJR Am J Roentgenol 1981; 137: 451–462.

243. Hodson CJ, Edwards O. Chronic pyelonephritis and vesicoureteral reflux. Clin Radiol 1960; 11: 219–231.

244. Arant BS Jr. Vesicoureteral reflux and renal injury. Am J Kidney Dis 1991; 17: 491–511.

245. Ransley PG, Risdon RA. Renal papillary morphology in infants and children. Urol Res 1975; 3: 111–114.

246. Tamminen TE, Kaprio EA. The relation of the shape of papillae and of collecting duct openings to intrarenal reflux. Br J Urol 1977; 49: 345–354.

247. Dillon MJ, Goonaskera CDA. Reflux nephropathy. J Am Soc Nephrol 1998; 9: 2377–2383.

248. Edelstein H, McCabe RE. Perinephric abscess: modern diagnosis and treatment in 47 cases. Medicine 1988; 67: 118–131.

249. Sheinfeld J, Erturk E, Spataro RF, et al. Perinephric abscess: current concepts. J Urol 1987; 137: 191–194.

250. Michaeli J, Mogle P, et al. Emphysematous pyelonephritis. J Urol 1984; 131: 203–208.

251. Klein FA, Smith MJV, Vick CW III, et al. Emphysematous pyelonephritis: diagnosis and management. South Med J 1986; 79: 41–46.

252. Shahatto N, al Awadhi NZ, Ghazali S. Emphysematous pyelonephritis: surgical implications. Br J Urol 1990; 66: 572–574.

253. Shokeir AA, El-Azab M, Mohsen T, El-Diasty T. Emphysematous pyelonephritis: a 15-year experience with 20 cases. Urology 1997; 49: 343–346.

254. Eknoyan G, Qunibi WY, Grissom RT, et al. Renal papillary necrosis: an update. Medicine 1982; 61: 55–73.

255. Harvald B. Renal papillary necrosis. A clinical survey of sixty-six cases. Am J Med 1963; 35: 481–486.

256. Pandya KK, Koshy M, Brown N, et al. Renal papillary necrosis in sickle cell hemoglobinopathies. J Urol 1976; 115: 497–501.

257. Griffin MD, Bergstrlh EJ, Larson TS. Renal papillary necrosis – a sixteen-year clinical experience. J Am Soc Nephrol 1995; 6: 248–256.

258. Davies DJ, Kennedy A, Roberts C. Renal medullary necrosis of infancy and childhood. J Pathol 1969; 99: 125–130.

259. Kozlowski K, Brown RW. Renal medullary necrosis in infants and children. Pediatr Radiol 1978; 7: 85–89.

260. Kincaid-Smith P. Pathogenesis of the renal lesion associated with the abuse of analgesics. Lancet 1967; 1: 859–862.

261. Burry A. Pathology of analgesic nephropathy: an Australian experience. Kidney Int 1978; 13: 34–40.

262. Gloor FJ. Changing concepts in pathogenesis and morphology of analgesic nephropathy as seen in Europe. Kidney Int 1978; 13: 27–33.

263. Nanra RS. Analgesic nephropathy in the 1990s – an Australian experience. Kidney Int 1993; 44: S86–S92.

264. Gault MH, Barrett BJ. Analgesic nephropathy. Am J Kidney Dis 1998; 32: 351–360.

265. Michigan S. Genitourinary fungal infections. J Urol 1976; 116: 390–397.

266. Wise GJ, Silver D. Fungal infections of the genitourinary system. J Urol 1993; 149: 1377–1388.

267. Sinniah R, Churg J, Sobin LH. Renal disease: classification and atlas of infectious and tropical diseases. Chicago: American Society of Clinical Pathologists Press, 1988.

268. Platt JL, Sibley RK, Michael AF. Interstitial nephritis associated with cytomegalovirus infection. Kidney Int 1985; 28: 550–552.

269. Fetterman GH, Sherman FE, Fabrizio NS, et al. Generalized cytomegalic inclusion disease. Arch Pathol 1968; 86: 86–94.

270. Ito M, Hirabayashi N, Uno Y, et al. Necrotizing tubulointerstitial nephritis associated with adenovirus infection. Hum Pathol 1991; 22: 1225–1231.

271. Vas SI. Primary and secondary role of viruses in chronic renal failure. Kidney Int 1991; 401: 52–54.

272. Johnson RJ, Couser WG. Hepatitis B infection and renal disease: clinical, immunopathogenetic and therapeutic considerations. Kidney Int 1990; 37: 663–676.

273. Johnson RJ, Gretch DR, Yamabe H, et al. Membranoproliferative glomerulonephritis associated with hepatitis C virus infection. N Engl J Med 1993; 378: 465–470.

274. D'Agati V, Suh J-I, Carbone L, et al. Pathology of HIV-associated nephropathy: a detailed morphologic and comparative study. Kidney Int 1989; 35: 1358–1370.

275. Cohen AH, Nast CC. HIV-associated nephropathy. A unique combined glomerular, tubular and interstitial lesion. Med Pathol 1988; 1: 87–97.

276. Bruno P, Hassell LH, Brown J, et al. The protean manifestations of hemorrhagic fever with renal syndrome. Ann Intern Med 1990; 113: 385–391.

277. Collan Y, Mihatsch MJ, Lahdevirta J, et al. Nephropathia epidemica: mild variant of hemorrhagic fever with renal syndrome. Kidney Int 1991; 40: S62–S71.

278. Rosen S, Harmon W, Krensky AM, et al. Tubulointerstitial nephritis associated with polyomavirus (BK type) infection. N Engl J Med 1983; 308: 1192–1196.

279. Drachenberg CB, Beskow CO, Cangro CB, et al. Human polyoma virus in renal biopsies: morphological findings and correlation with urine cytology. Hum Pathol 1999; 30: 970–977.

280. Nickeleit V, Hirsch HH, Binet IF, et al. Polyomavirus infection of renal allograft recipients: from latent infection to manifest disease. J Am Soc Nephrol 1999; 10: 1080–1089.

281. Bailey RR. The relationship of vesico-ureteric reflux to urinary tract infection and chronic pyelonephritis–reflux nephropathy. Clin Nephrol 1973; 1: 132–141.

282. Huland H, Buchardt P, Kollerman M, et al. Vesicoureteral reflux in end stage renal disease. J Urol 1979; 121: 10.

283. Torres VE, Velosa JA, Holley KE, et al. The progression of vesicoureteral reflux nephropathy. Ann Intern Med 1980; 92: 766–784.

284. Cotran RS. Glomerulosclerosis in reflux nephropathy. Kidney Int 1982; 21: 528–534.

285. Arant BS Jr, Sotelo-Avila C, Bernstein J. Segmental 'hypoplasia' of the kidney (Ask–Upmark). J Pediatr 1979; 95: 931–939.

286. Shindo S, Bernstein J, Arant BS Jr. Evolution of renal segmental atrophy (Ask–Upmark kidney) in children with vesicoureteral reflux: radiographic and morphologic studies. J Pediatr 1983; 102: 847–854.

287. Klahr S. Obstructive nephropathy. Kidney Int 1998; 54: 286–300.

288. Malek RS, Elder JS. Xanthogranulomatous pyelonephritis: a clinical analysis of 26 cases and of the literature. J Urol 1978; 119: 589.

289. Hartman DS, Davis CJ Jr, Goldman ST, et al. Xanthogranulomatous pyelonephritis: sonographic–pathologic correlation of 16 cases. J Ultrasound Med 1984; 3: 481.

290. Parsons MA, Harris SC, Longstaff AJ, et al. Xanthogranulomatous pyelonephritis: a pathological clinical and aetiologic analysis of 87 cases. Diagn Hist 1983; 6: 203.

291. Esparza AR, McKay DB, Cronan JJ, et al. Renal parenchymal malakoplakia: histologic spectrum and its relationship to megalocytic interstitial nephritis and xanthogranulomatous pyelonephritis. Am J Surg Pathol 1989; 13: 225–236.

292. Dobyan DC, Truong LD, Eknoyan G. Renal malakoplakia revisited. Am J Kidney Dis 1993; 22: 243–252.

293. Narayana AS. Overview of renal tuberculosis. Urology 1982; 19: 231–237.

294. Farer LS, Lowell AM, Meador MP. Extrapulmonary tuberculosis in the United States. Am J Epidemiol 1979; 109: 205–217.

295. Cohen MS. Granulomatous nephritis. Urol Clin North Am 1986; 13: 6477–6659.

296. Casella FJ, Allan M. The kidney in sarcoidosis. J Am Soc Nephrol 1993; 3: 1555–1562.

297. Magil AB. Drug-induced acute interstitial nephritis with granulomas. Hum Pathol 1983; 13: 36–41.

298. Wilke BM, Mailloux LU. Acute renal failure: pathogenesis and prevention. Am J Med 1986; 80: 1129–1135.

299. Solez K, Morel-Maroger L, Sraer JD. The morphology of 'acute tubular necrosis' in man: analysis of 57 renal biopsies and a comparison with the glycerol model. Medicine 1979; 58: 362–376.

300. Beaman M, Turney JH, Rodger RSC, et al. Changing pattern of acute renal failure. QJ Med 1987; 62: 15–23.

301. Leiberthal W. Biology of acute renal failure: therapeutic implications. Kidney Int 1997; 52: 1102–1115.

302. Schreiner GE, Maher FJ. Toxic nephropathy. Am J Med 1965; 38: 409–449.

303. Jao W. Iatrogenic renal disease as revealed by renal biopsy. Semin Diagn Pathol 1988; 5: 63–79.

304. Abuelo JG. Renal failure caused by chemicals, foods, plants, animal venoms and misuse of drugs. An overview. Arch Intern Med 1990; 150: 505–510.

305. Paller MS. Drug-induced nephropathies. Med Clin North Am 1997; 74: 909–917.

306. Cooper K, Bennett WM. Nephrotoxicity of common drugs used in clinical practice. Arch Intern Med 1987; 147: 1213–1218.

307. Councilman WT. Acute interstitial nephritis. J Exp Med 1898; 3: 393–418.

308. Laberke H-C, Bohle A. Acute interstitial nephritis. Correlations between clinical and morphological findings. Clin Nephrol 1980; 14: 263–273.

309. Rossert J. Drug-induced acute interstitial nephritis. Kidney Int 2001; 6: 804–817.

310. McClusky RT. Immunologically mediated tubulointerstitial nephritis. Contemp Issues Nephrol 1983; 10: 121–150.

311. Andres GA, McCluskey RT. Tubular and interstitial renal disease due to immunological mechanisms. Kidney Int 1975; 7: 271–289.

312. Ten RM, Torres VE, Milliner DS, et al. Acute interstitial nephritis: immunologic and clinical aspects. Mayo Clin Proc 1988; 63: 921–930.

313. Sibley RK, Payne W. Morphologic findings in the renal allograft biopsy. Semin Nephrol 1985; 5: 294–306.

314. Dobrin RS, Vernier RL, Fish AJ. Acute eosinophilic interstitial nephritis and renal failure with bone marrow-lymph node granulomas and anterior uveitis. Am J Med 1975; 59: 325–333.

315. Park MH, D'Agati V, Appel GB, et al. Tubulointerstitial disease in lupus nephritis – relationship to immune deposits, interstitial inflammation, glomerular changes, renal function and prognosis. Nephron 1986; 44: 309–319.

316. Winer RL, Cohen AH, Sawhney AS, et al. Sjögren's syndrome with immune complex tubulointerstitial disease. Clin Immunol Immunopathol 1977; 8: 494–503.

317. Yang C-S, Lin C-H, Chang S-H, Hsu H-C. Rapidly progressive fibrosing interstitial nephritis associated with Chinese herbal drugs. Am J Kidney Dis 2000; 35: 313–318.

318. Park MH, D'Agati V, Appel GB, Pirani P. Tubulointerstitial disease in lupus nephritis: relationship to immune deposits, interstitial inflammation, glomerular changes, renal function, prognosis. Nephron 1986; 44: 309–319.

319. Casella FJ, Allon M. The kidney in sarcoidosis. J Am Soc Nephrol 1993; 3: 1555–1562.

320. Brause M, Magnusson K, Degenhardt S, et al. Renal involvement in sarcoid – a

report of 6 cases. Clin Nephrol 2002; 57: 142–148.

321. Gonzalez-Vitale JC, Hayes DM, Cuitovic E, et al. The renal pathology in clinical trials of cis-platinum (II) diamine-dichloride. Cancer 1977; 39: 1362–1371.

322. Farnsworth A, Horvath JS, Hall BM, et al. Renal biopsy morphology in renal transplantation. Am J Surg Pathol 1984; 8: 243–252.

323. Myers BD, Ross J, Newton L, et al. Cyclosporine-associated nephropathy. N Engl J Med 1984; 311: 699–705.

324. Walker RG. Lithium toxicity. Kidney Int 1993; 44: 593–598.

325. Richter GW Kress Y, Cornwall CC. Another look at lead inclusions. Am J Pathol 1968; 53: 189–207.

326. Beaver DL, Burr RE. Bismuth inclusions in the human kidney. Arch Pathol 1963; 76: 89–94.

327. Fowler BA. Mechanisms of kidney cell injury from metals. Environ Health Perspect 1992; 100: 57–73.

328. Benabe JE, Martinez-Maldonado M. Hypercalcemic nephropathy. Arch Intern Med 1978; 138: 777–779.

329. Ibels LS, Alfrey AC, Huffer WE, et al. Calcifications in endstage kidneys. Am J Med 1981; 71: 33–37.

330. Haggitt RC, Pitcock JA. Renal medullary calcifications: a light and electron microscopic study. J Urol 1971; 106: 342–347.

331. Smith LH. Pathogenesis of renal stones. Miner Electrolyte Metab 1987; 13: 21–219.

332. Pac CYC. Etiology and treatment of urolithiasis. Am J Kidney Dis 1991; 18: 624–637.

333. Griffith DP. Struvite stone. Kidney Int 1978; 13: 372–382.

334. Kok DJ, Khan SR. Calcium oxalate nephrolithiasis, a free or fixed particle disease. Kidney Int 1994; 46: 847–852.

335. Williams DI. Matrix calculi. Br J Urol 1963; 35: 411–415.

336. Allen TD, Spence HM. Matrix stones. J Urol 1966; 95: 284–290.

337. Randall A. Papillary pathology as a precursor of primary renal calculus. J Urol 1940; 44: 580–589.

338. Prien EL Sr. The riddle of Randall's plaques. J Urol 1975; 114–500–507.

339. Williams HE. Oxalic acid and the hyperoxaluric syndrome. Kidney Int 1978; 13: 410–417.

340. Scheinam JI. Primary hyperoxaluria: therapeutic strategies for the 90s. Kidney Int 1991; 40: 389–399.

341. Levinsky NG, Robert NJ. Case record 38–1979. N Engl J Med 1979; 301: 650–657.

342. Hollenberg NK, McDonald FD, Cotran R. Irreversible acute oliguric renal failure. A complication of methoxyflurane anesthesia. N Engl J Med 1972; 296: 877–879.

343. Drenik EJ, Stanley TM, Border WA, et al. Renal damage with intestinal bypass. Ann Intern Med 1978; 89: 594–599.

344. Salzer, WR, Keren D. Oxalosis as a complication of chronic renal failure. Kidney Int 1973; 4: 61–66.

345. Aikhunaizi AM, Chan L. Secondary oxalosis: a cause of delayed renal function in the setting of acute renal failure. J Am Soc Nephrol 1996; 11: 2320–2326.

346. Cochat P. Primary hyperoxaluria type 1. Kidney Int 1999; 55: 2533–2547.

347. Chen C-L, Fang H-C, Chou K-J. Acute oxalate nephropathy after ingestion of star fruit. Am J Kidney Dis 1999; 37: 418–422.

348. Foreman JW. Cystinosis. Semin Nephrol 1989; 9: 62–64.

349. Spear GS, Slusser RJ, Schulman JD, et al. Polykaryocytosis of the visceral glomerular epithelium in cystinosis with description of an unusual clinical variant. Johns Hopkins Med J 1971; 129: 83–99.

350. Spear GS, Slusser RJ, Tonsimis AJ, et al. Cystinosis: an ultrastructural and electron-probe study of the kidney with unusual findings. Arch Pathol 1971; 21: 206–221.

351. Bonsib SM, Horvath F Jr. Multinucleated podocytes in a child with nephrotic syndrome and the Fanconi's syndrome: a unique clue to the diagnosis. Am J Kidney Dis 1999; 34: 966–971.

352. Markello TC, Bernardini IM, Gahl WA. Improved renal function in children with cystinosis treated with cysteamine. N Engl J Med 1993; 328: 1157–1162.

353. Town M, Jean G, Cherqui S. A novel gene encoding an integral membrane protein is mutated in nephropathic cystinosis. Nature Genet 1998; 18: 319–324.

354. Boss GR, Seegmiller JE. Hyperuricemia and gout. N Engl J Med 1979; 300: 1459–1468.

355. Talbot JH, Terplan KL. The kidney in gout. Medicine 1960; 39: 405–463.

356. Linnane JW, Burry AF, Emmerson BT. Urate deposits in the renal medulla. Prevalence and association. Nephron 1981; 29: 216–222.

357. Batuman V. Lead nephropathy, gout and hypertension. Am J Med Sci 1993; 305: 241–247.

358. Bennett WM. Lead nephropathy. Kidney Int 1985; 28: 212–220.

359. Beck LH. Requiem for gouty nephropathy. Kidney Int 1986; 30: 280–287.

360. Colvin RB. The renal allograft biopsy. Kidney Int 1996; 50: 1069–1082.

361. Solez K, Axelsen RA, Beneditsson H, et al. International standardization of nomenclature and criteria for the histologic diagnosis of renal allograft rejection: the Banff working classification of kidney transplant pathology. Kidney Int 1993; 44: 411–422.

362. Colvin RB, Cohen AH, Saiontz C, et al. Evaluation of pathologic criteria for acute renal allograft rejection.

Reproducibility, sensitivity, and clinical correlation. J Am Soc Nephrol 1997; 8: 1930–1941.

363. Rascusen LC, Solez K, Colvin, et al. The Banff 97 working formulation of renal allograft pathology. Kidney Int 1999; 55: 713–723.

364. Mauiyyedi S, Crespo M, Pascul M, et al. Cd4 deposition in peritubular capillaries. The morphology and immunophenotype of acute humoral rejection. Transplantation 2000; 69: S402–S408.

365. Mauiyyedi S, Crespo M, Collins AB, et al. Acute humoral rejection in kidney transplantation: II. Morphology, immunopathology, and pathologic classification. J Am Soc Nephrol 2002; 13: 779–787.

366. Bonsib SM, Abul-ezz SR, Ahmad I, et al. Acute rejection-associated tubular basement membrane defects and chronic allograft nephropathy, Kidney Int 58: 2206–2214, 2000.

367. Nicheleit V, Vamvakas EC, Pascual M, et al. The prognostic significance of specific arterial lesions in acute allograft rejection. J Am Soc Nephrol 1998; 9: 1301–1308.

368. Denton MD, Singh AK. Recurrent and de novo glomerulonephritis in the renal allograft. Semin Nephrol 2000; 20: 164–175.

369. Ivanyi B, Fahmy H, Brown H, et al. Peritubular capillaries in chronic renal allograft rejection: A quantitative ultrastructural study. Hum Pathol 2000; 31: 1129–1138.

370. Habib R, Zurowska A, Hinglais N, et al. A specific lesion of the allograft: Allograft nephropathy. Kidney Int 1993; 44: S104–S111.

371. Bergstrand A, Bohman SO, Farnsworth A, et al. Renal histopathology in kidney transplant recipients immunosuppressed with cyclosporine A: Results of an international workshop. Clin Nephrol 1985; 24: 107–119.

372. Zarifian A, Meleg-Smith S, O'Donovoan R, et al. Cyclosporine-associated thrombotic microangiopathy in renal allografts. Kidney Int 1999; 55: 2457–2466.

373. Silva FG, Pirani CL, Mesa-Tejada R, et al. The kidney in plasma cell dyscrasias: a review and a clinicopathologic study of 50 patients. Prog Surg Pathol 1983; 5: 131–176.

374. Gillmore JD, Hawkins PN, Pepys MB. Amyloidosis: A review of recent diagnostic and therapeutic developments. Br J Haematol 1997; 99: 245–256.

375. Gertz MA, Lacy MQ, Dispenzieri A. Immunoglobulin light chain amyloidosis and the kidney. Kidney Int 2002; 61: 1–9.

376. Cohen AH. The kidney in plasma cell dyscrasias: Bence-Jones cast nephropathy and light chain deposition disease. Am J Kidney Dis 1998; 32: 529–532.

377. Benson MD. The hereditary amyloidoses. Best Pract Res Clin Rheum 2003; 17: 909–927.

378. Yazaki M, Liepnieks JJ, Yamashita T, et al. Renal amyloidosis caused by a novel stop-codon mutation in the apolipoprotein A-II gene. Kidney Int 2001; 60: 1658–1665.

379. Sanders PN, Herrera GA, Kirk KA, et al. Spectrum of glomerular and tubulointerstitial renal lesions associated with monotypical immunoglobulin light chain deposition. Lab Invest 1991; 64: 527–537.

THE LIBRARY
THE LEARNING AND DEVELOPMENT CENTRE
THE CALDERDALE ROYAL HOSPITAL
HALIFAX HX3 0PW

# CHAPTER 2

# Neoplasms of the kidney

Gregory T. MacLennan, Liang Cheng

THE LIBRARY
THE LEARNING AND DEVELOPMENT CENTRE
THE CALDERDALE ROYAL HOSPITAL

The first renal neoplasm was reported nearly 200 years ago.[1] Thereafter, it became evident that a variety of different tumors could arise within the kidney. By 1953, according to Dr Lauren Ackerman in his influential textbook, *Surgical Pathology*,[2] the inventory included perirenal lipoma, leiomyoma, liposarcoma, rhabdomyosarcoma, a 'well-circumscribed mucin-producing adenocarcinoma of the cortex,' renal adenoma, Wilms' tumor, and renal adenocarcinoma. Although Ackerman acknowledged that renal adenocarcinoma has 'various patterns . . . granular . . . clear . . . papillary,' it was his opinion that 'it does not appear logical to make subdivisions in nomenclature; better to call it simply an adenocarcinoma of renal tubule origin.' Remarkably, Ackerman's entire description of renal adenocarcinoma was encompassed within 30 lines of text. During the following 50 years the list expanded further, and classification systems became increasingly sophisticated as distinctive morphologic patterns in renal neoplasms were recognized and correlated with clinical findings. Ancillary diagnostic tools, including electron microscopy, immunohistochemistry, cytogenetics and molecular diagnostic techniques, made it possible to detect distinctions between various types of renal neoplasm; some tumors, such as Xp11 translocation carcinoma and synovial sarcoma, are essentially defined by their molecular characteristics. As a consequence of the contributions of numerous investigators over many decades, the most recent World Health Organization classification of renal neoplasms includes almost 50 distinct entities. In this chapter we examine these entities, following a slightly modified version of the outline developed by the World Health Organization.[216]

# RENAL CELL TUMORS

Renal cell neoplasms are tumors that arise in renal tubular epithelium. Papillary adenoma and oncocytoma are considered benign. Multilocular cystic renal cell carcinoma and mucinous tubular and spindle cell carcinoma are indolent neoplasms with very low risk of cancer progression. The remaining renal cell neoplasms are considered malignant.

## Papillary adenoma

Criteria for the definition of papillary adenoma of the kidney were refined over a period of several decades.[3] It was observed in 1938 that renal tumors less than 3 cm in diameter rarely metastasized.[4] A subsequent study in 1950 documented metastases in 65 tumors less than 5 cm in diameter;[5] nonetheless, tumors less than 3 cm were still classified as adenoma. The recognition of oncocytoma as a neoplasm with a benign behavior, regardless of size, only partially resolved the dilemma.[6] In other types of renal epithelial neoplasm it remained impossible to distinguish renal adenoma from adenocarcinoma on the basis of light microscopy, histochemistry, and electron microscopy.[7]

It was proposed that the diagnosis of renal adenoma should be limited to tumors of low histologic grade and less than 1 cm in diameter;[8] this was complicated by the docu-

mentation of metastasis occurring in tumors as small as 9 mm.[9] It became apparent from autopsy studies of small renal cortical tumors that they are quite frequent, being present in 21% of patients overall, and their frequency increases linearly with age, being found in 10% of patients aged 21–40 years, and in 40% of those aged 70–90 years.[10,11] They are also frequently observed in patients undergoing chronic dialysis, occurring in 33% of patients with acquired cystic renal disease.[12] In one autopsy study, only 6% of tumors were larger than 3 mm in diameter, and only 1 of 251 tumors exceeded 10 mm in diameter.[13] Mean size increased from 1.2 to 2.0 mm from age 30 to 60 but did not increase thereafter, meaning that tumors larger than 10 mm demonstrated more proliferative capability than 99.5% of renal cortical epithelial neoplasms.[13] Furthermore, it was observed that certain morphologic types of renal epithelial neoplasm, specifically those with papillary, tubular, and mixed tubulopapillary architecture, were less likely to exhibit malignant behavior. The importance of distinguishing between small papillary and clear cell neoplasms was noted many decades ago, and the importance of this distinction was reinforced by reports of small clear cell renal carcinomas with metastases.

It has been suggested that cytogenetic changes can be used to help define papillary adenoma.[14,15] Whereas papillary renal carcinoma exhibits a wide range of cytogenetic abnormalities, including trisomy of chromosomes 7, 12, 16, 17, and 20 and loss of the Y chromosome, small papillary renal cortical tumors ranging from 2 to 5.5 mm in diameter and of low nuclear grade exhibit only loss of the Y chromosome and a combined trisomy of 7 and 17. Comparative genomic hybridization studies showed genomic changes in four of six papillary renal tumors less than or equal to 5 mm in diameter; all four showed a gain of chromosome 7.[16]

Whereas more than 20% of patients over the age of 20 harbor papillary renal neoplasms less than 5 mm in diameter, and only about 4500 new cases of papillary renal cell carcinoma are diagnosed each year, it seems evident that the growth potential for tumors less than 5 mm in diameter is quite limited.[3] On the other hand, tumors larger than 5 mm have shown growth potential exceeding that of the remaining 90%.

On the basis of the data noted above, it was proposed that papillary adenoma should be defined as a neoplasm having papillary or tubular architecture, low nuclear grade, and a diameter less than or equal to 5 mm.[17-19] It has additionally been suggested that such tumors should lack histologic resemblance to clear cell, chromophobe, or collecting duct renal cell carcinoma.

Papillary adenoma is visible in the renal parenchyma, often just below the renal capsule, as one or more well circumscribed gray-white to tan nodules (Fig. 2-1), varying in shape from conical to roughly spherical. Although most are solitary, in some patients they are multiple and bilateral, and in rare cases innumerable; this latter condition has been termed 'renal adenomatosis.'[20-22] Most have a seamless interface with the adjacent renal parenchyma, but a thin fibrous pseudocapsule is apparent in some. Tumor architecture may be papillary, tubular, or tubulopapillary (Fig. 2-2). In most,

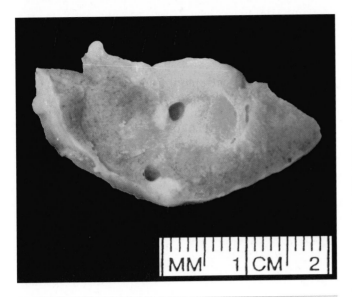

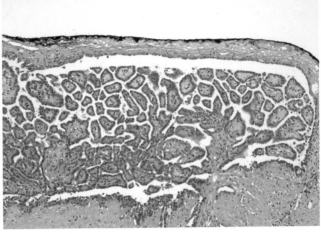

**Fig. 2-3** Papillary adenoma. Higher-power view of lesion in Figure 2.2, showing delicate papillary structures lined by cells with small dark nuclei and scant cytoplasm.

**Fig. 2-1** Papillary adenoma. Circumscribed oval nodule just below the capsule, approximately 3 mm.

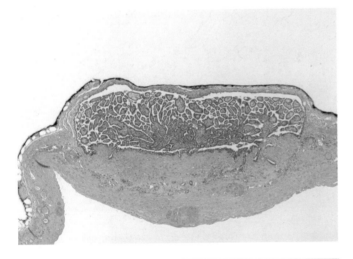

**Fig. 2-2** Papillary adenoma. This was found incidentally in the wall of a benign cyst.

the tumor cells resemble those of type 1 papillary renal cell carcinoma, bearing nuclei that are round to oval and occasionally grooved, with stippled to clumped chromatin and inconspicuous nucleoli, lacking mitotic activity, and accompanied by scant cytoplasm that varies from pale to eosinophilic to basophilic[3,23] (Fig. 2-3). Much less frequently, tumor cells resemble those of type 2 papillary renal cell carcinoma, exhibiting voluminous eosinophilic cytoplasm. Psammoma bodies and foamy macrophages are frequently present.[18]

Immunohistochemically, the majority of cases of papillary adenoma show positive staining for epithelial membrane antigen, low molecular weight cytokeratin, high molecular weight keratin, and peanut agglutinin.[24,25] More than 80% show strong positive immunostaining for α-methylacyl-coenzyme A racemase (AMACR) in a fashion similar to that seen in papillary renal cell carcinoma,[26,27] but

immunoreactivity is typically absent or very limited for glutathione S-transferase (GST-α), a marker overexpressed in most cases of clear cell renal cell carcinoma.[26,28] Both diploid and aneuploid papillary adenoma have been reported.[29]

The relationship between papillary adenoma and papillary renal cell carcinoma has not been fully elucidated. Multifocal papillary adenoma is genetically distinct and arises independently of concurrent papillary renal cell carcinoma, virtually eliminating the likelihood that adenoma represents intrarenal metastasis from a dominant papillary renal carcinoma.[30] Clearly, as noted previously, renal adenoma is far more common than papillary renal cell carcinoma. On the other hand, adenoma is more numerous in kidneys harboring papillary renal cell carcinoma than in kidneys removed for other pathologic entities, particularly clear cell renal cell carcinoma.[26] There is a strong association between the presence of renal adenoma and concomitant papillary renal carcinoma in cases of renal adenomatosis.[20–22,26] Furthermore, the cytogenetic and immunohistochemical staining similarities between adenoma and papillary renal cell carcinoma suggest that the two entities may represent a continuum of one biologic process, particularly in cases of type 1 papillary renal cell carcinoma.[15,26] Evidence for a relationship between papillary adenoma and type 2 papillary renal cell carcinoma and papillary renal neoplasms that arise in the setting of end-stage renal disease is less compelling.[26,31,32]

## Oncocytoma

Following an initial report in 1942 and a few sporadic reports thereafter,[33] interest in this neoplasm was stimulated by a report in 1976 suggesting that renal oncocytoma was relatively common, distinctly separable from renal carcinoma, and benign.[6] For several years, uncertainty concerning its malignant potential persisted;[34] the identification of chromophobe renal cell carcinoma in 1985 helped considerably in resolving this uncertainty.[35]

Renal oncocytoma is believed to arise from the intercalated cells of renal collecting tubules[35,36] and accounts for 5–7% of surgically resected non-urothelial renal neoplasms.[5–7] Patients range in age from 10 to 94 years old (median, 62 years) and the majority are males, with a male:female ratio of 1.7:1 in combined series totalling nearly 400 patients.[2,5–11] Approximately 75% of patients are asymptomatic at the time of diagnosis; their tumor is discovered incidentally during investigation of non-renal complaints. In some patients the diagnosis is prompted by the discovery of a palpable mass; in others, the lesion is identified during investigation of hypertension, hematuria, and/or flank or abdominal pain. Radiologic findings are too nonspecific to discriminate between oncocytoma and renal carcinoma, with the result that oncocytoma generally is managed by surgical excision.[36,37]

Grossly, oncocytoma is typically solid, ranging from 0.3 to 26 cm in greatest dimension, with reported mean size ranging from 4.8 to 8.1 cm. It is commonly mahogany brown and less often tan to pale yellow, and well circumscribed, with varying degrees of encapsulation (Fig. 2-4). An area of central scarring is often present (in up to 33%, particularly in larger tumors); other gross findings may include recent hemorrhage (up to 20%), and rarely, foci of cystic degeneration.[6,38–43] Gross extension of tumor into perirenal fat and rarely into large blood vessels is sometimes evident. Multiplicity is common: up to 13% of oncocytomas are multifocal, and up to 13% are bilateral[40–42,44] (Fig. 2-5). Other benign renal neoplasms are often present, including papillary adenoma and angiomyolipoma, and concurrent renal cell carcinoma has been observed in up to 32% of cases.

Microscopically, oncocytoma is composed predominantly of round to polygonal cells with densely granular eosinophilic cytoplasm, round uniform nuclei with smoothly dispersed chromatin, and a central nucleolus, embedded in a hypocellular hyalinized or myxoid stroma[6,39–41] (Figs 2-6,

2-7). Scattered binucleated cells are often present.[45] A minor component of cells with scant granular cytoplasm, dark hyperchromatic nuclei, and a high nuclear/cytoplasmic ratio may be present (Fig. 2-8). Cells with pronounced nuclear atypia are often present. Mitotic figures are only rarely identified. Tumor architecture may be nested, organoid (classic), tubulocystic, or mixed. In the classic pattern tumor cells form nests, islands, organoid clusters, cords, trabeculae, or confluent solid sheets of cells lacking stroma. The tubulocystic pattern exhibits variably sized luminal structures lined by cells indistinguishable from those of the classic pattern (Fig.

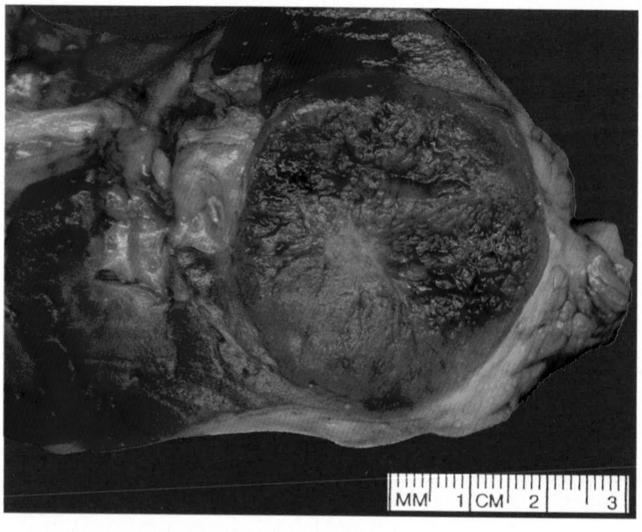

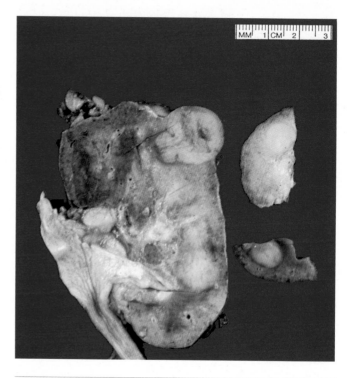

**Fig. 2-5** Renal oncocytoma. Multiple oncocytomas were present in this nephrectomy specimen.

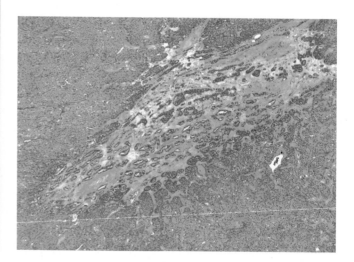

**Fig. 2-6** Renal oncocytoma. Low-power view of an area of scarring demonstrates organoid architecture and the disposition of cell nests in a hyalinized hypocellular stroma.

**Fig. 2-4** Renal oncocytoma. Tumor is circumscribed, mahogany brown and slightly hemorrhagic, with a central stellate scar. (Courtesy of Philip Bomeisl, MD.)

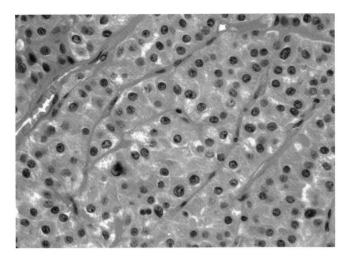

**Fig. 2-7** Renal oncocytoma. Typical oncocytic cells with abundant densely granular eosinophilic cytoplasm, and uniform round nuclei with inconspicuous nucleoli.

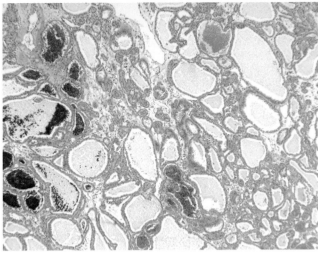

**Fig. 2-9** Renal oncocytoma. This tumor was remarkable by the degree of cystic change that was present; otherwise, it was entirely compatible with oncocytoma.

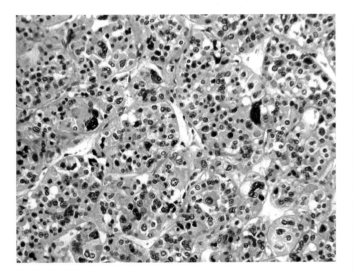

**Fig. 2-8** Renal oncocytoma. Compact nests of cells, some of which show pronounced nuclear pleomorphism and hyperchromasia.

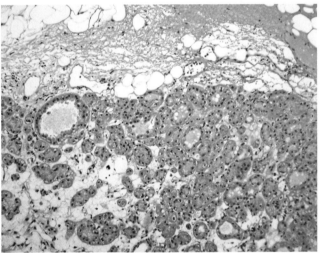

**Fig. 2-10** Renal oncocytoma. This otherwise typical oncocytoma showed areas of extension into perirenal fat.

2-9). The mixed pattern includes both organoid and tubulocystic components. Findings observed in some tumors include focal papillary structures projecting into dilated luminal structures, stromal calcifications, and osseous and myeloid metaplasia.

Certain histologic findings, although of concern, are considered compatible with a diagnosis of oncocytoma, provided their extent is very limited. Rare mitotic figures, hemorrhage, small foci of necrosis, focal nuclear pleomorphism, extension of tumor into perinephric fat or adjacent renal parenchyma, small clusters of cells with clear cytoplasm embedded in hyalinized stroma, minute papillary projections into dilated tubules, and invasion of small, capillary-sized or even venous-type vessels are considered permissible in an otherwise typical oncocytoma[39–41] (Fig. 2-10). Findings that are considered impermissible for a diagnosis of oncocytoma include areas of clear cell or spindle cell car-

cinoma, prominent papillary architecture, macroscopic or conspicuous microscopic necrosis, and significant mitotic activity, including atypical mitotic figures. Accurate assessment of these features necessitates adequate sampling of the tumor; consequently, an accurate diagnosis of an oncocytic renal neoplasm based on needle core biopsy or fine needle aspiration may not always be possible.

Ultrastructurally, tumor cells have basal lamina, rare intercellular or cytoplasmic lumina, and apical short stubby microvilli. The cytoplasm is closely packed with mitochondria showing lamellar or focally stacked cristae. Rare lysosomes and small amounts of lipid are seen, but glycogen is absent. Rare microvesicles similar to those seen abundantly in chromophobe renal cell carcinoma may be noted in a few tumor cells.[46,47] Histochemical staining for Hale's colloidal iron typically is weak and focally distributed in the form of fine dust-like granules, with a tendency to accumulate at the luminal aspect of tubules.[48] Although in many instances the findings are distinctly different from the staining patterns typical of chromophobe renal cell carcinoma, the distinction is not always clear-cut or reliable.[49]

Renal oncocytoma shows frequent positive immunostaining for epithelial membrane antigen (EMA) and pancytokeratin, and negative immunostaining for vimentin, CD10, and renal cell carcinoma marker (RCC Ma).[50] From a practical standpoint, immunohistochemical stains that reliably separate oncocytoma from its chief mimic, the eosinophilic variant of chromophobe renal cell carcinoma, are most desirable. The use of immunostains and other diagnostic techniques in making this distinction is discussed further in the section on chromophobe renal cell carcinoma.

From a molecular perspective, oncocytoma tends to fall into one of three categories: those with no identifiable clonal cytogenetic alterations, those that show losses of a sex chromosome and chromosome 1, and those that exhibit structural rearrangements involving chromosome region 11q12~q13.[51–56] Partial or complete loss of chromosome 14 is another frequently reported abnormality.[57–59]

As noted previously, bilaterality and multifocality are relatively common in oncocytoma. Extreme examples of multifocality, variably termed oncocytosis or oncocytomatosis, often involving both kidneys, have been reported.[60–65] The number of oncocytomas present in such cases may be impossible to determine, and rarely such cases are associated with renal failure.[62,66,67] Typically, at least one dominant tumor is present – usually oncocytoma – and less frequently chromophobe renal cell carcinoma, accompanied by innumerable other oncocytic nodules. Other findings in these cases include diffuse oncocytic change in non-neoplastic tubules, benign oncocytic cortical cysts, and an 'interstitial pattern' characterized by diffuse intermingling of oncocytic tubules and cell clusters with the normal renal interstitium. In some cases 'hybrid tumors' are present, with mixed histologic features of both oncocytoma and chromophobe renal cell carcinoma, raising the intriguing possibility that renal oncocytoma and chromophobe renal cell carcinoma may arise from a common progenitor lesion.

Follow-up of nearly 400 patients with renal oncocytoma reported in several series has disclosed no examples of patient deaths attributable to metastases.[6,38–43] Consequently, renal oncocytoma is considered to be benign.

# Renal cell carcinoma

## Incidence and epidemiology

About 2% of all new cancer cases worldwide originate in the kidney.[68] In the United States, 51 190 new cases and 12 890 deaths from kidney cancer were expected in 2007. About 85% of kidney cancers are of renal cell origin, 12% are urothelial cancer of the renal collecting system, and the remainder are rare malignancies.[69]

Renal cell carcinoma afflicts males approximately twice as often as females, and is most commonly diagnosed in patients in their early 60s.[68] Both the overall incidence of renal cell carcinoma and the incidence of late-stage renal cell carcinoma have gradually increased each year in the United States and Europe over the past 30 years, whereas the incidence of unsuspected renal cell carcinoma diagnosed only at autopsy has diminished.[70,71] The incidence has been increasing more rapidly in females than in males, as well as more rapidly in African-Americans than in white Americans.[72] Age-adjusted incidence rates for black men, white men, black women and white women from 1992 to 2002 were 16.8, 13.8, 8.0, and 6.6/100 000 person-years, respectively.[73] The overall prognosis has improved in the past 40 years, with 5-year relative survival rates approaching 64% by 2002, compared to less than 40% in the early 1960s.[5] There is a 10-fold variation in the international rates of renal cell carcinoma, suggesting that exogenous risk factors, genetic susceptibility, and diagnostic variability may play significant roles in determining the reported incidence of renal cell carcinoma. Rates are highest in several eastern and western European countries, Italy, North America, Australia and New Zealand, and lowest in Asia and Africa.

The risk of developing renal cell carcinoma is two to three times higher in individuals who have a first-degree relative with renal cell carcinoma.[74] Approximately 2–4% of cases of renal cell carcinoma are associated with several distinctive hereditary cancer syndromes that will be discussed under the appropriate headings. The great majority of cases of renal cell carcinoma are considered sporadic, occurring in the absence of apparent genetic predisposition.

Cigarette smoking has consistently been shown to be a causal risk factor for renal cell carcinoma, and has been estimated to account for about 20–30% of such cancers in men and about 10–20% in women.[75] The risk increases with consumption level, and gradually decreases after years of cessation.[76] Obesity is another factor that is consistently linked to an increased risk of renal cell carcinoma. There appears to be a summary relative risk for renal cell carcinoma of 1.07/U increase in body mass index, and excess weight has been estimated to account for more than 40% of cases of renal cell carcinoma in the United States and more than 30% in Europe.[77,78] Although the role of hypertension in the development of renal cell carcinoma is difficult to assess, the bulk of epidemiologic evidence implicates it as a causal risk factor.[73] Long-term renal dialysis exposes patients to a considerably higher average annual incidence of renal cell carcinoma than the general population.[79] The major risk factor in such patients appears to be the presence of acquired cystic kidney disease.[80]

Cumulative evidence has failed to establish a significant relationship between the occurrence of renal cell carcinoma and a number of putative inciting factors, including analgesic use, specific dietary elements, alcohol consumption, hormone-associated variables, and occupational exposures, with the possible exception of arsenic compound exposure, which has been reported to increase the risk of renal cell carcinoma by 30%.[73,81]

## Associations with other disorders

Renal cell carcinoma has been reported in patients with hemihypertrophy, situs inversus totalis, and in a non-

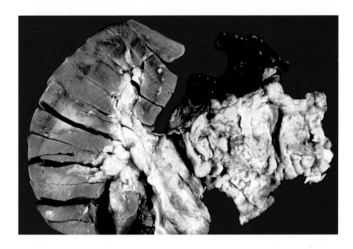

**Fig. 2-11** Extrarenal renal cell carcinoma. A bulky malignancy, histologically a classic clear cell renal cell carcinoma, was found in soft tissues adjacent to an entirely normal kidney.[88]

functioning transplanted kidney, although the nature of the association in these cases is unclear and the occurrences may have been fortuitous.[82–84] Renal cell carcinoma has been reported to occur in teratoma[85] and in supernumerary kidney,[86] and there are several convincing reports of renal cell carcinoma apparently arising outside the confines of the kidney, possibly in ectopic renal tissue[87–89] (Fig. 2-11). Renal cell carcinoma has been linked to cystic kidney disease. Its occurrence in von Hippel–Lindau disease and in end-stage renal disease is quite prevalent, as will be discussed in the sections on clear cell renal cell carcinoma and renal cell carcinoma associated with end-stage renal disease, respectively. More than 40 cases of renal cell carcinoma occurring in patients with tuberous sclerosis have been reported, and it has been speculated that patients with tuberous sclerosis are at increased risk for developing renal cell carcinoma.[90–92] However, meta-analysis of reported cases fails to demonstrate conclusively that the risk of developing renal cell carcinoma is any higher in patients with tuberous sclerosis than in the general population.[93,94] Similarly, although more than 30 patients with autosomal dominant polycystic kidney disease and about half a dozen patients with multicystic dysplastic kidney have reportedly developed renal cell carcinoma, there is no convincing evidence that patients with these conditions have a higher risk of developing renal cell carcinoma than the general population.[93,95,96] However, autosomal dominant polycystic kidney disease does seem to be a risk factor for the development of renal cortical adenoma,[97] and the rare renal cell carcinoma that arises in a setting of autosomal dominant polycystic kidney disease tends to occur in relatively younger patients, to be more frequently bilateral or multifocal, and to have a sarcomatoid component.[69]

## Clinical presentation

Renal cell carcinoma presents clinically in myriad ways, and has been called one of the great masqueraders. Even prior to the availability of today's sophisticated imaging modalities, it was well recognized that urinalysis is an unreliable screen-

ing test for this cancer, and that the classic triad of signs and symptoms of renal cell carcinoma – flank pain, renal mass and gross hematuria – is of little value for early diagnosis as nearly 40% of patients did not have genitourinary symptoms at the time of diagnosis.[98] Currently less than 15% of patients have the 'classic triad.'[99]

In up to one-third of patients the presenting manifestations are paraneoplastic, related to the presence of a neoplasm but not a consequence of either direct tumor extension or metastasis. Some paraneoplastic signs and symptoms in patients with renal cell carcinoma are non-specific and constitutional; others are caused by elaboration of specific proteins by the tumor cells, and in some circumstances the underlying pathogenesis is unknown. Fever, malaise, night sweats, anorexia, nausea, symptoms of neuropathy, muscle tenderness, weight loss and/or fatigue are typical constitutional symptoms that may herald the onset of renal cell carcinoma.[100] Fever occurs in 20–30% of patients, and is the sole presenting complaint in 2%.[101] It is postulated that these constitutional symptoms are mediated by cytokines, including TNF-α and IL-6, that may be elaborated directly by tumor cells or by the immune system in response to the tumor.[99,102,103] Anemia is noted in 20–40% of patients with renal cell carcinoma, thought to be secondary to marrow suppression by inflammatory cytokines associated with the presence of renal cell carcinoma.[104]

Approximately 20% of patients with renal cell carcinoma present with symptoms and signs that are believed to be related to the release of various proteins by tumor cells. Non-metastatic hypercalcemia, affecting between 13% and 20% of patients, has been attributed to a parathyroid hormone-like peptide.[99,105–107] Erythrocytosis has been observed in 1–8% of patients, and is attributed to erythropoietin production by tumor cells.[108,109] The exact relationship between renal cell carcinoma and hypertension is not well established; however, elevated serum renin levels have been found in 37% of patients with renal cell carcinoma, and in some instances hypertension has improved following tumor resection.[104] Other reported associations include gynecomastia secondary to tumoral production of prolactin or gonadotropin,[110,111] galactorrhea related to prolactin production, masculinization of a woman with elevated levels of human chorionic gonadotropin, testosterone and follicle-stimulating hormone, and Cushing's syndrome due to ectopic adrenocorticotrophic hormone (ACTH) production.

The pathogenetic mechanisms underlying a number of paraneoplastic syndromes associated with renal cell carcinoma have not been elucidated. Elevation of erythrocyte sedimentation rate is common in patients with renal cell carcinoma.[112] Non-metastatic hepatic dysfunction (Stauffer's syndrome) is seen in 3–20% of patients with renal cell carcinoma and is characterized by hepatosplenomegaly, coagulopathy, elevation of serum alkaline phosphatase, transaminase, and α$_2$-globulin concentrations; these findings resolve in 66% of patients after nephrectomy, and have been shown to return with tumor recurrence.[99,101] Among non-lymphoid malignancies, renal cell carcinoma is most commonly associated with systemic amyloidosis, a complication observed in 3–5% of patients.[100,113] Other infrequently reported clinical associations related to renal cell carcinoma include leukocytoclastic vasculitis, subacute necrotic myelopathy and myopathy, hyperglycemia, hypertrophic pulmonary osteoarthropathy, symptoms mimicking amyotrophic lateral sclerosis, light-chain nephropathy, and extramembranous glomerulonephritis.[104]

## Radiologic aspects of renal neoplasms

Not long after the development of increasingly sophisticated radiologic imaging tools, it became apparent that the rate of incidental detection of renal cancer had risen; furthermore, the tumor stage was lower in incidentally discovered cancers, and the 5-year survival rate was better than in cases not diagnosed incidentally.[114] In the past three decades the prevalence of incidentally detected renal tumors in some surgical series has risen to as high as 61%.[115] The percentage of small tumors in large series that measure 3 cm or less has risen dramatically, and it is notable that almost all of these are discovered incidentally.[116] Most importantly, it has been demonstrated that incidentally discovered tumors are at significantly lower stage when discovered, fewer of them are of high nuclear grade, and patients with incidentally discovered renal carcinoma have fewer local and distant recurrences and better 5-year cancer-specific survival rates than those in whom the discovery was not incidental.[117,118] The detection of ever smaller tumors has stimulated increased use of minimally invasive and less radical therapeutic procedures, such as partial nephrectomy, laparoscopic resections, radiofrequency ablation, and cryotherapy. Ultrasound is useful for initial imaging, but detects only about two-thirds of renal lesions less than 3 cm in diameter. Computed tomography (CT) is the reference standard for staging and lesion characterization. Magnetic resonance imaging (MRI) is generally used as a problem-solving tool, especially for evaluating small lesions and complex cystic lesions. Increasingly sophisticated enhancements have been developed with all of these technologies, and these have resulted in more accurate characterization of renal tumors.[119] Nonetheless, there are limitations to radiologic accuracy: up to 16% of lesions removable by partial nephrectomy prove to be benign, reinforcing the concept that conservative resection is desirable when technically possible.[120]

## Grading renal cell carcinoma

*Grading is notoriously difficult to perform reproductively and depends heavily on experience and understanding of the criteria of the categories. The latter problem often means it is easier to invent one's own classification than to abide by another's.*

*Donald Skinner MD, 1971[121]*

It is well documented that one of the most important features of renal cell carcinoma for predicting outcome is nuclear grade.[121–139] Several grading systems have been proposed in the past 40 years,[8,121,123,125,138,140,141] but there is no consensus as to which is the most advantageous, as each system appears to have intrinsic advantages and disadvantages. There is a lack of uniformity in the number of grades

**Table 2-1** Fuhrman nuclear grading[123]

| | |
|---|---|
| 1 | Small round uniform nuclei, approximately 10 μm, inconspicuous or absent nucleoli |
| 2 | Nuclei slightly irregular, approximately 15 μm, nucleoli visible at high power (400×) |
| 3 | Nuclei obviously irregular, approximately 20 μm, prominent nucleoli visible at low power (100×) |
| 4 | Similar to grade 3 but with bizarre, often multilobed nuclei and clumped chromatin |

used, and criteria for the cut points between different grades have varied. Definitions of grading criteria are often vague, leading to lack of interobserver consistency. In recognition of some of the inherent problems with existing grading systems, it has been recommended by the Union Intérnationale Contre le Cancer (UICC) and the American Joint Committee on Cancer (AJCC) that an ideal grading system should be based on standardized and reproducible criteria that reflect the heterogeneity of nuclear and nucleolar features within a tumor, and that the criteria should be stratified by histologic subtype. In an ideal grading system, significant outcome differences should be demonstrable between patients with different tumor grades, both univariately and after adjusting for important clinical and pathologic features. The most widely used grading system in North America was proposed by Fuhrman et al.[123] The grading criteria for this system are noted in Table 2-1. Although this system has been used extensively and has withstood the test of time, it has drawn frequent criticism, largely because of its somewhat vague terminology, the limited number of patients studied, the fact that several different histologic tumor subtypes were included in the study, and the fact that deaths were recorded as those due to any cause, rather than being cancer-specific deaths. The independent predictive value of the Fuhrman nuclear grading system has been demonstrated by some investigators.[142,143] Others have found that it is an independent predictor of cancer-specific survival only after grouping grades.[137,144,145] Currently, a number of questions regarding nuclear grading remain unanswered: the definition of adequate tumor sampling; whether sarcomatoid change, even focally, should influence tumor grading; whether interobserver reproducibility can be improved by better definition of grading criteria; whether a three-grade system would be better than a four-grade one; and the question of the degree of practical clinical relevance of any nuclear grading system.[146] The influence of nuclear grading on patient outcome is discussed in several sections to follow and in the section on prognostic factors in renal cell carcinoma.

## Staging renal cell carcinoma

Tumor stage reflects the extent of anatomic spread and involvement of disease and is considered the most important factor in predicting the clinical behavior and outcome of renal cell carcinoma.[147] Staging systems for renal cell carcinoma have been in use for nearly 50 years, and have been continually updated and improved. Since undergoing sim-

**Table 2-2** American Joint Committee ON Cancer TNM Staging of Renal Cell Carcinoma (2002)[150]

| Primary Tumor (T) | |
|---|---|
| TX | Primary tumor cannot be assessed |
| T0 | No evidence of primary tumor |
| T1a | Confined to kidney, 4.0 cm or less |
| T1b | Confined to kidney, more than 4.0 cm but 7.0 cm or less |
| T2 | Confined to kidney, more than 7.0 cm |
| T3a | Tumor invades the perinephric fat or the adrenal gland but not beyond Gerota's fascia |
| T3b | Tumor grossly extends into the renal vein(s) or vena cava below the diaphragm |
| T3c | Tumor grossly extends into the renal vein(s) or vena cava above the diaphragm |
| T4 | Tumor invades beyond Gerota's fascia |

| Regional Lymph Nodes (N) | |
|---|---|
| NX | Regional lymph nodes cannot be assessed |
| N0 | No regional lymph node metastases |
| N1 | Metastasis in a single regional lymph node |
| N1 | Metastasis in more than one regional lymph node |

| Distant Metastases (M) | |
|---|---|
| MX | Distant metastases cannot be assessed |
| M0 | No distant metastases |
| M0 | Distant metastasis |

| Stage groupings | T | N | M |
|---|---|---|---|
| I | T1 | N0 | M0 |
| II | T2 | N0 | M0 |
| III | T1 | N1 | M0 |
| | T2 | N1 | M0 |
| | T3 | N0, N1 | M0 |
| IV | T4 | N0, N1 | M0 |
| | Any T | N2 | M0 |
| | Any T | Any N | M1 |

plifications and refinements in 1992, the Tumor, Nodes, and Metastasis (TNM) staging system has become the predominant staging system for renal cell carcinoma.[148] It was created with several aims in mind: to aid clinicians in planning treatment; to give some indication of prognosis; to assist in evaluating the results of treatment; to facilitate the exchange of information between cancer centers; and to contribute to continuing investigation of human malignancies.[149] The fifth (1997) edition, a collaborative effort of both the UICC and the AJCC, was modified only slightly, subdividing T1 lesions into T1a and T1b, resulting in the current (2002) AJCC version of the system[150] (Table 2-2). Since its inception the TNM system has been shown to be an excellent prognostic factor for patients with renal cell carcinoma.[144,145,148,151–158] The elements of the TNM classification can be reduced to four stage groups: in brief, stage I corresponds to T1 without known lymph node or distant metastases; stage II corre-

sponds to T2 without known lymph node or distant metastases; stage IV corresponds to T4 with any lymph node or distant metastasis status; and stage III includes all other TNM combinations (Table 2-2). The influence of staging on prognosis in renal cell carcinoma is discussed in detail in a later section.

## Clear cell renal cell carcinoma

Clear cell carcinoma accounts for 60–70% of all cases of renal cell carcinoma.[8,159] It is believed to arise in epithelial cells lining the proximal tubule.[160,161] Although patients in all age groups, including children, are at risk for its occurrence, the great majority develop in patients over 40 years of age, and the majority are males with a ratio of approximately 1.5 : 1.[162,163]

More than 90% of cases of clear cell carcinoma have characteristic cytogenetic abnormalities that involve loss of genetic material from the short arm of chromosome 3 (3p) and mutations in the *VHL* gene.[164–170] The VHL gene, which is located at 3p25-26 and functions as a tumor suppressor gene, was identified through studies of patients with von Hippel–Lindau (VHL) disease, and subsequent investigations implied the presence of one or more additional genes near this site.[166,170–172] The VHL gene in clear cell carcinoma is typically found to be inactivated by a combination of allelic deletion and either mutation or, less often, hypermethylation.[173,174] It is suspected that other genes on 3p may act as tumor suppressors and may be involved in the development of clear cell carcinoma, particularly 3p14.2 deletions, possibly resulting in inactivation of the FHIT gene, as well as another tumor suppressor gene at 3p12.[175] A continuous deletion from 3p14.2-p25, including the FHIT and VHL genes, can be identified in up to 96% of cases.[176] Following the initiating event involving the 3p gene, additional genetic alterations occur in clonal tumor cell populations as tumor progression occurs and metastatic capability increases. Consequently, these additional genetic abnormalities, when detectable, are often associated with higher histologic grade, higher pathologic stage, and an adverse prognosis. The genetic abnormalities associated with these effects are loss of 9p, 14q, and loss of heterozygosity on chromosome 10q around the PTEN/MAC locus.[177–180]

There are several familial settings in which clear cell carcinoma may arise, including von Hippel–Lindau disease. This condition affects one in every 36 000 births. It is an autosomal dominant disease associated with the development of retinal angioma, cerebellar and spinal angioma and hemangioblastoma, bilateral multifocal pheochromocytoma, papillary cystadenoma of the epididymis, pancreatic cyst and malignant neuroendocrine tumor, inner ear endolymphatic sac tumor, and renal cyst. In addition, 35–45% of affected patients with VHL develop bilateral multifocal renal cell carcinoma that is always of the clear cell type. An average VHL kidney may harbor as many as 1100 cysts and 600 microscopic clear cell carcinomas.[181] Onset of renal carcinoma in VHL patients is often early: clinically evident renal cancer has been reported in adolescence, and the mean age at diagnosis is 39 years. Historically, without treatment, up

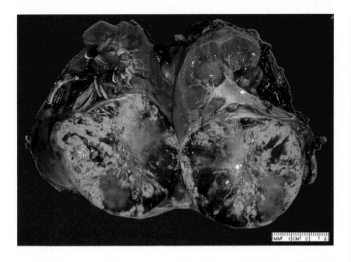

**Fig. 2-12** Renal cell carcinoma. Bosselated well-circumscribed low-grade clear cell carcinoma, bright golden-yellow with extensive hemorrhage and fibrosis. (Courtesy of Carmen Kletecka, MD.)

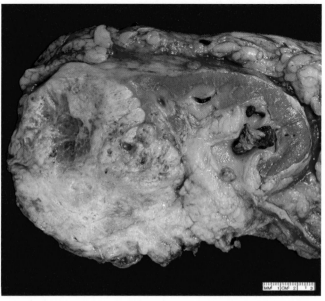

**Fig. 2-13** Renal cell carcinoma. High-grade clear cell carcinoma, not sharply circumscribed, extensively involving renal sinus and perirenal fat as well as Gerota's fascia. (Courtesy of Paul Grabenstetter, MD.)

to 40% of VHL patients died of advanced renal carcinoma. In VHL disease, patients are born with a germline defect in one of the two alleles of the VHL gene, located on chromosome 3p925-26, which functions as a tumor suppressor. Loss of the second allele results in clinical disease expression.[181] Additional heritable settings in which clear cell renal cell carcinoma may develop include families segregating constitutional chromosome 3 translocations,[182] and families with SDHB-associated heritable paraganglioma.[183]

Grossly, clear cell carcinoma ranges in size from a few millimeters to very large, weighing several kilograms; the average size is about 7 cm. It is usually unilateral and unicentric; bilaterality and/or multicentricity are features of hereditary clear cell carcinoma. It commonly forms a bosselated mass that protrudes from the cortical surface (Fig. 2-12). The cut surface is at least in part a characteristic bright golden yellow color, owing to the abundance of cholesterol, phospholipids, and neutral lipids within the tumor cells. The cut surface is typically variegated with areas of gray-white fibrosis and recent or old hemorrhage. It usually has an expansile, pushing growth pattern, and is well demarcated from the adjacent normal kidney by a fibrous pseudocapsule of varying thickness; in some cases it may appear to infiltrate the adjacent renal parenchyma (Fig. 2-13). Areas of cystic change and calcification are commonly found, particularly within areas of necrosis.

Microscopically, clear cell carcinoma displays a variety of architectural patterns: tumor cells are arranged most often in sheets, compact nests, alveolar, acinar and microcystic or even macrocystic structures, separated by an abundance of thin-walled blood vessels (Fig. 2-14). Tubular structures are variable in size. Microcysts contain extravasated red blood cells or eosinophilic fluid. Infrequently, small papillary structures lined by clear cells may be present focally, but account for an insignificant proportion of the overall architecture.

The classic cell of clear cell carcinoma has distinct cell membranes and optically clear cytoplasm due to loss of cytoplasmic lipids and glycogen during histologic process-

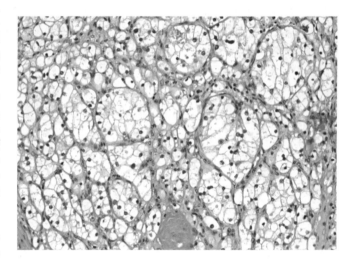

**Fig. 2-14** Renal cell carcinoma. Clear cell carcinoma composed of nests of cells with clear cytoplasm, surrounded by abundant thin-walled blood vessels.

ing. Some cases of clear cell carcinoma display varying numbers of cells with granular eosinophilic cytoplasm; such cells are more often seen in high-grade cancer or near areas of hemorrhage or necrosis. The nuclei of clear cell carcinoma show considerable variation in size, shape, and nucleolar prominence, as discussed in the section on grading, and these features are assessed when assigning a nuclear grade to an individual tumor (Figs 2.15–2.18).

Sarcomatoid differentiation is evident in about 5% of cases[184–188] (Fig. 2-19). The relevance of this finding is discussed in the section on prognosis. Numerous uncommon histologic variations have been described in renal cell carcinoma, including rhabdoid morphology, heterotopic bone

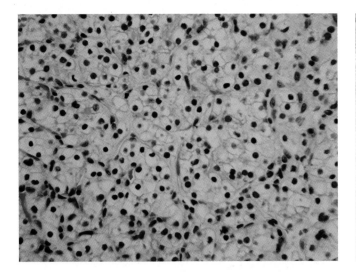

**Fig. 2-15** Renal cell carcinoma. Clear cell carcinoma, Fuhrman grade 1. Nuclei are round and barely larger than red cells; nucleoli are inconspicuous at 400×.

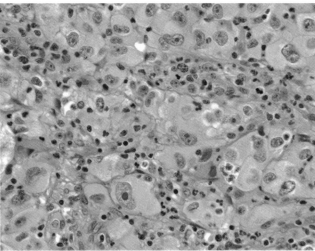

**Fig. 2-17** Renal cell carcinoma. Clear cell carcinoma, Fuhrman grade 3. Nuclei are irregular, at least 20 μm and larger, and have large prominent nucleoli.

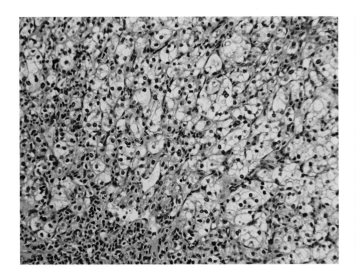

**Fig. 2-16** Renal cell carcinoma. Clear cell carcinoma, Fuhrman grade 2. Nuclei are slightly irregular and about twice as big as red cells; nucleoli are easily visible at 200×.

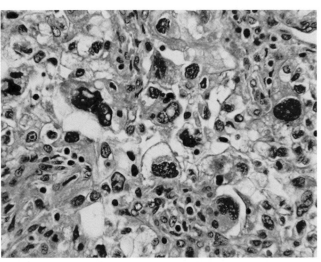

**Fig. 2-18** Renal cell carcinoma. Clear cell carcinoma, Fuhrman grade 4. Nuclei are very large, irregular and multilobed, with clumped chromatin and large prominent nucleoli.

formation, intra- and extracellular hyaline globules, basophilic cytoplasmic inclusions, abundant multinucleated giant cells, sarcoid-like granulomas, myospherulosis, and lymphomatoid features[189–197] (Figs 2-19, 2-20). The significance of these rare findings is unknown.

Immunohistochemically, clear cell carcinoma typically shows positive immunostaining for vimentin, epithelial membrane antigen (EMA), renal cell carcinoma marker (RCC Ma), and CD10. It also tends to show positive immunostaining for low molecular weight cytokeratins (LMWCK) 8, 18, and 9; and keratins AE1/AE3 and Cam 5.2, although the frequency of staining with these markers varies considerably. Immunostaining reactions for CK7, CK20, MUC1, parvalbumin, AMACR, E-cadherin, and CD117 are negative in most cases.[27,50,198–210]

The prognosis for patients with clear cell carcinoma is discussed in the section on prognosis in renal cell carcinoma.

## Multilocular cystic renal cell carcinoma

The first report of a multilocular cystic renal tumor with a component of clear cells appeared in 1928, followed by another in 1957.[211,212] The term 'multilocular cystic renal cell carcinoma' first appeared in print in 1982,[213] and this is the term that has been adopted in the recent WHO classification of renal tumors. By 1991, it had become apparent that multilocular cystic renal neoplasms with very limited components of clear cells should be classified separately from ordinary renal cell carcinoma.[214] Analysis of the cumulative experience with this neoplasm led to the proposal that the term multilocular cystic renal cell carcinoma should be

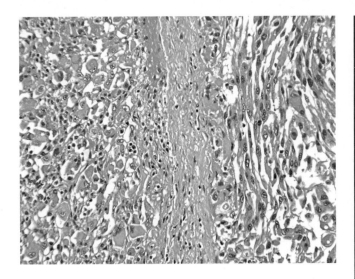

**Fig. 2-19** Renal cell carcinoma. This area of a clear cell carcinoma showed sarcomatoid differentiation on the right and rhabdoid morphology on the left.

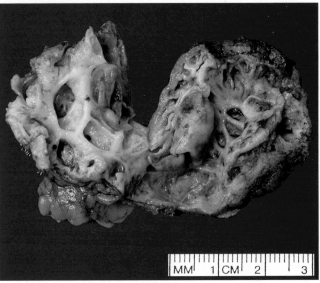

**Fig. 2-21** Multilocular cystic renal cell carcinoma. This small renal neoplasm was composed entirely of variably-sized cysts. (Courtesy of Shams Halat, MD.)

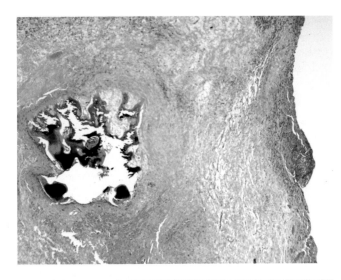

**Fig. 2-20** Renal cell carcinoma. This clear cell carcinoma, a small focus of which is visible on the right, showed heterotopic bone formation on a background of fibrosis and hyalinization.

restricted to renal neoplasms with a fibrous pseudocapsule and composed entirely of cysts and septa with no expansile solid nodules; the septa should contain aggregates of epithelial cells with clear cytoplasm.[215] These criteria define multilocular cystic renal cell carcinoma in the recent WHO classification.[216]

Multilocular cystic renal cell carcinoma is an uncommon tumor of the kidney composed of multiple cysts with clear cells in the septa indistinguishable from grade 1 renal cell carcinoma.[216] It constitutes about 1–5% of all renal cell carcinomas and has a male preponderance with a male:female ratio of 2–3:1.[215,217–220] Age range is 20–76 years; the great majority of patients are in their 50s or 60s, and females tend to present at a younger age than males.

Although most patients are asymptomatic and their tumor is discovered incidentally, a minority have either a palpable mass, gross hematuria, abdominal or back discomfort, or rarely, systemic symptoms. Laboratory findings may include anemia and microhematuria, but most patients have no laboratory abnormalities. Imaging studies usually reveal a complex cystic mass which may have focal calcification.

Grossly, multilocular cystic renal cell carcinoma ranges from 0.5 to 13.0 cm in greatest dimension. It is typically a unilateral and solitary well-circumscribed mass composed entirely of cysts, separated from adjacent renal parenchyma by a fibrous wall; however, it can be multifocal as well as bilateral[220] (Fig. 2-21). The cysts are variable in size and contain clear or hemorrhagic fluid. The septa between cysts are thin. Necrosis is absent, and there are no grossly visible nodules expanding the septa, a feature that differentiates this tumor from extensively cystic conventional clear cell renal cell carcinoma.

Microscopically, the cysts are lined by epithelial cells, usually as a single layer but occasionally multilayered, and occasionally forming minute papillary structures; some cysts lack any lining cells (Fig. 2-22). The lining cells have variable amounts of cytoplasm that may be clear or lightly eosinophilic; however, the cytologic characteristics of the lining epithelial cells do not constitute part of the criteria for defining multilocular cystic renal cell carcinoma, as renal cystic lesions of many types may sometimes be lined by epithelium with clear cells.[215] The septa consist of fibrous tissue. More than 20% of tumors show calcifications within the septa, and metaplastic bone formation is sometimes observed. Within the septa in all cases there are clusters of epithelial cells with clear cytoplasm (Fig. 2-23). These cells resemble the cyst lining cells, usually have small dark nuclei, and do not form expansile nodules (Figs 2-24, 2-25). They are often difficult to distinguish from histiocytes or from lymphocytes with surrounding retraction artifact.[216] Increased vascularity is sometimes associated with septal

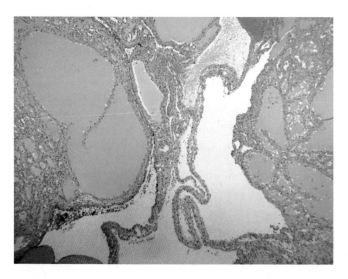

**Fig. 2-22** Multilocular cystic renal cell carcinoma. Tumor consists of cysts separated by delicate septa.

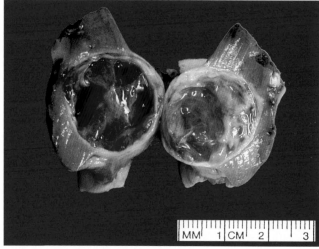

**Fig. 2-24** Extensively cystic clear cell carcinoma. Grossly, the differential in this case included multilocular cystic renal carcinoma; however, mural thickening is evident in the cystic portion on the right, and demonstrated microscopically in Figure 2-25. (Courtesy of Amber Petrolla, MD.)

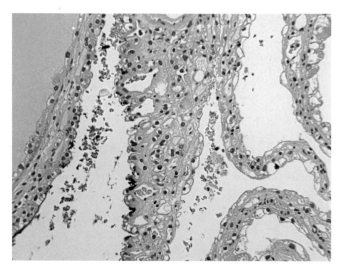

**Fig. 2-23** Multilocular cystic renal cell carcinoma. The delicate septa are lined by clear cells, and clear cells are present within the septa, but are not forming expansile nodules.

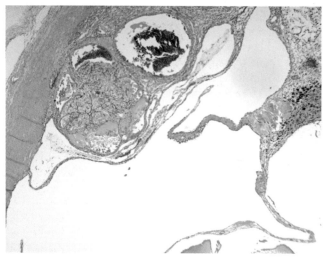

**Fig. 2-25** Extensively cystic clear cell carcinoma. The expansile nodule of clear cell carcinoma weighs against a diagnosis of multilocular cystic renal cell carcinoma.

tumor cell clusters, and this feature may aid in recognizing their presence. In difficult cases the epithelial nature of the tumor cell clusters can be confirmed by their immunoreactivity to antibodies against cytokeratin and epithelial membrane antigen; immunostains for histiocytic markers are negative.[215]

Ploidy studies reveal diploid DNA content in more than 90% of cases.[217] Electron microscopy in one case revealed apical microvilli and other ultrastructural features in the tumor cells that were similar to those seen in conventional clear cell carcinoma of the kidney.[215] Molecular analysis has shown VHL gene mutations in multilocular cystic renal cell carcinoma, supporting its classification as a type of clear cell renal cell carcinoma.[221]

Only rare cases have shown extension beyond the kidney into the perirenal fat.[217,220] This, in conjunction with the fact that the epithelial tumor cells are by definition of low nuclear grade, may explain why there are no reports of recurrence or metastasis of multilocular cystic renal cell carcinoma.[139,215,217–220] The proper diagnosis hinges on strict adherence to the diagnostic criteria for this entity. Surgical resection is indicated to exclude extensively cystic clear cell renal cell carcinoma.

## Papillary renal cell carcinoma

Papillary carcinoma, the second most common type of renal cell carcinoma, accounts for approximately 10–15% of all renal epithelial neoplasms.[139,222,223] It has characteristic cytogenetic, gross and histologic features that distinguish it from other types of renal cell carcinoma.

The great majority of cases occur sporadically, but some develop in members of families with hereditary papillary renal carcinoma (HPRC), an inherited renal cancer characterized by mutations in the *MET* oncogene at 7q31 and by a predisposition to develop multiple bilateral papillary renal tumors.[224–229] It is notable that c-*met* mutations are also detectable in about 13% of patients with papillary renal cell carcinoma who have no family history of renal tumors.[228] In addition, rare cases occur in the setting of a separate autosomal dominant tumor syndrome caused by germline mutations in the fumarate hydratase gene; this syndrome is known as hereditary leiomyomatosis and renal cell cancer (HLRCC).[230] Patients with this syndrome typically develop cutaneous leiomyomas, and females also develop uterine leiomyomas. The syndrome is also characterized by a predisposition to developing papillary renal cell carcinoma, and less frequently, uterine leiomyosarcoma.[230–232]

Overall, papillary renal cell carcinoma is a genetically heterogeneous group of tumors that demonstrate complex numeric chromosomal abnormalities and unique patterns of allelic imbalances that often reveal gains of chromosomes 7, 8, 12q, 16q, 17, and 20q and losses of chromosomes 1p, 4q, 6q, 9p, 11p, 13q, 14q, 18, 21q, X and Y.[233,234] Sporadic cases are most commonly characterized cytogenetically by trisomy or tetrasomy 7, trisomy 17, and loss of chromosome Y.[235] It has been postulated that the progression from papillary adenoma to papillary carcinoma is related to the acquisition of additional abnormalities in chromosomes 12, 16, and 20;[235–237] however, there is no significant difference in the frequency of gains of chromosomes 7, 17, 12, 16, and 20 evident in these two entities.[238] Although genomic deletions of the short arm of chromosome 3 have been regarded as typical for clear cell renal cell carcinoma and rare in papillary renal cell carcinoma,[239] it has been shown that loss of the 3p allele occurs in papillary renal cell carcinoma;[240,241] in fact, the incidence of 3p loss of heterozygosity is similar in papillary, chromophobe and clear cell carcinoma.[175] Deletions of 9p are present in approximately 20% of cases of papillary renal cell carcinoma, and loss of heterozygosity at 9p13 has been linked to short patient survival.[242] Mutations of the p53 gene do not appear to play a role in the pathogenesis of papillary renal cell carcinoma.

The mean age of patients with papillary renal cell carcinoma ranges from 52 to 66 years, and males are affected slightly more than twice as often as females (M:F = 2.4:1).[222,243,244] Patients present with symptoms and signs that are typical of renal cell carcinoma, as previously described; there are no presenting signs and symptoms that are unique to the papillary subtype of renal cell carcinoma. The radiologic findings are non-specific; however, in the era of renal angiography, papillary renal cell carcinoma was found to be much more likely than other subtypes to be avascular or very hypovascular, and was more likely to exhibit radiologically evident mural calcifications. Papillary renal cell carcinoma is also more likely to be multifocal (8% of cases) and necrotic (46%) than other common renal cell carcinoma subtypes,[139] as well as being overrepresented in end-stage renal disease.[245] When multiple papillary tumors are found in patients without a family history of renal tumors, each papillary tumor arises independently: multifocality is not the result of intrarenal metastasis.[30,246] In patients with hereditary papillary renal cancer, it has been estimated that each kidney may harbor as many as 3400 separate microscopic papillary tumors.[225]

Grossly, papillary renal cell carcinoma is typically well circumscribed, and up to 90% of cases are confined to the renal parenchyma.[139] Multifocality may be grossly evident, particularly in cases of hereditary papillary renal cell carcinoma[224,225] (Figs 2-26, 2-27). A thick fibrous pseudocapsule is present in up to two-thirds of cases[243,244,247] (Fig. 2-28). The degree of pseudocapsule formation often parallels the extent

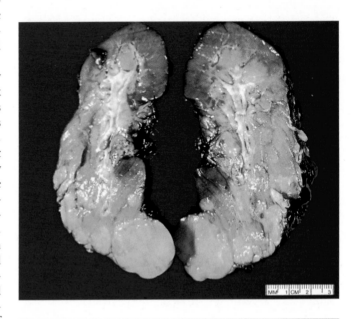

**Fig. 2-26** Papillary renal cell carcinoma. Multiple tumors are evident. There was no family history of renal neoplasms. (Courtesy of Ana DelRio Perez, MD.)

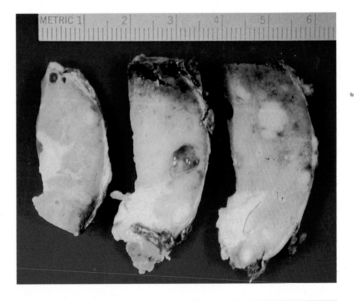

**Fig. 2-27** Papillary renal cell carcinoma. Multiple tumors are evident. This was a well documented case of hereditary papillary renal carcinoma (HPRC).

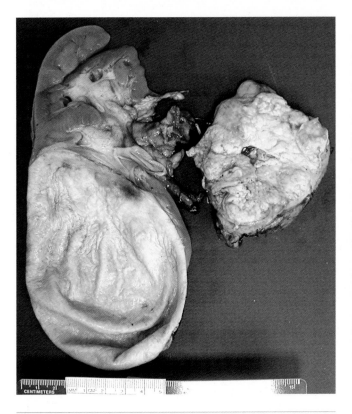

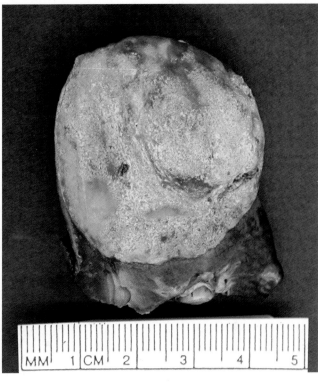

**Fig. 2-28** Papillary renal cell carcinoma. Grossly, this tumor had the appearance of a thick-walled cyst filled with liquefied bloody material; a sarcomatoid papillary renal carcinoma in the wall had already metastasized to form a large hilar mass. (Courtesy of Ed Reineks, MD.)

**Fig. 2-29** Papillary renal cell carcinoma. Tumor is well circumscribed. The yellow color reflects an abundance of stromal macrophages. (Courtesy of Mark Costaldi, MD.)

of hemorrhage and necrosis present in the tumor; the frequency and prominence of these findings varies considerably in reported series, and perhaps reflects the general trend in recent decades towards the detection of tumors incidentally, when they are smaller and more viable. The cut surface varies from light gray-tan to golden yellow to red-brown, depending on the preponderance of macrophages in the stroma and the degree of remote hemorrhage and hemosiderin accumulation (Figs 2-29, 2-30).

Microscopically, papillary renal cell carcinoma is composed of varying proportions of papillary and tubular structures, and in some instances contains cysts with papillary excrescences or with tumor infiltrating the cyst wall.[244] Because papillary structures are also seen in collecting duct carcinoma, and as papillary renal cell carcinoma can exhibit extensive tubule formation and even solid areas, the term 'papillary' is neither specific for nor entirely descriptive of this neoplasm.[23,248–250] Papillae are lined by a single layer of tumor cells that may sometimes appear pseudostratified[23,244] (Fig. 2-31). The stalks of the papillary structures contain fibrovascular cores, and are commonly infiltrated by variable numbers of macrophages; the prevalence of macrophages has no apparent correlation with the extent of accompanying hemorrhage and/or necrosis. The architectural arrangement of the papillary stalks varies. They may form exquisite and readily recognizable papillae; compact and tight packing in some tumors results in a solid appearance; and in some

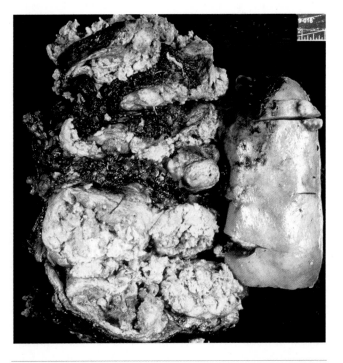

**Fig. 2-30** Papillary renal cell carcinoma. The small renal cortical nodule was a papillary renal cell carcinoma that had metastasized to form a large hilar mass.

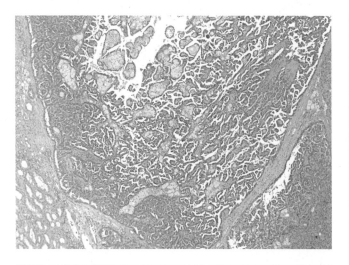

**Fig. 2-31** Papillary renal cell carcinoma. This low-power view demonstrates the papillary architecture. Abundant stromal macrophages are evident.

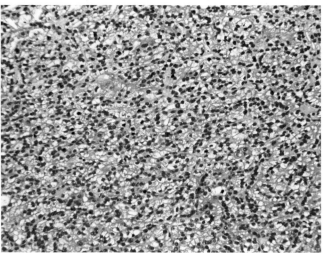

**Fig. 2-32** Papillary renal cell carcinoma. In the solid variant, papillae may not be readily evident.

tumors the papillae are arranged in long parallel arrays, creating a trabecular appearance[243] (Figs 2-32, 2-33).

It has been proposed that papillary renal cell carcinoma can be subclassified into two morphologic variants,[8] which have been designated types 1 and 2.[23,251] Comparative genomic hybridization studies and studies of allelic imbalance by microsatellite analysis show significant molecular differences between the two types.[32,33] Before discussing the differences between the two, it should be noted that both exhibit tumor-associated acute and chronic inflammation, extensive necrosis, evidence of recent hemorrhage, psammoma bodies, cholesterol clefts, foreign body-type giant cells, and areas of dystrophic calcification.[23,251]

Type 1 papillary renal cell carcinoma is composed of papillae covered by a single or double layer of small epithelial cells of low nuclear grade, bearing small round to ovoid nuclei with inconspicuous nucleoli, and possessing minimal pale or clear cytoplasm (Fig. 2-34). Tubular structures in these neoplasms have similar lining cells. The papillae of type 1 tumors are usually thin, delicate, and often short, and frequently show expansion by edema fluid.[23,251] The short complex papillae may impart a glomeruloid appearance. Aggregates of foamy macrophages are commonly noted within the papillary cores or within sheets of tumor cells. Type 1 tumor morphology, as well as being seen in sporadically occurring tumors, is also characteristic of papillary neoplasms that occur in hereditary papillary renal carcinoma (HPRC).[228]

Type 2 papillary renal cell carcinoma tends to be larger than type 1 (mean diameters, 6 cm for type 1, and 9.5 cm for type 2), and are of significantly higher nuclear grade.[23,251] Tumor cells in type 2 cancer exhibit large and spherical nuclei, prominent nucleoli, and varying degrees of nuclear pseudostratification. The cytoplasm is abundant and typically eosinophilic (Fig. 2-35). The fibrovascular cores of the majority of type 2 tumors tend to be dense and fibrous rather than thin and delicate, and edema and glomeruloid bodies are less prevalent than in type 1 tumors. Macrophages, rather

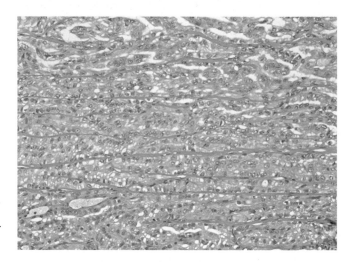

**Fig. 2-33** Papillary renal cell carcinoma. Papillary structures are compactly packed into long parallel arrays.

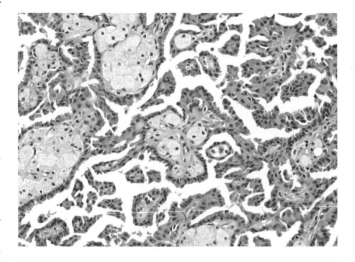

**Fig. 2-34** Papillary renal cell carcinoma. In this type 1 tumor, the papillae are delicate and are lined by cells with small dark nuclei and scant cytoplasm. Abundant stromal macrophages are present.

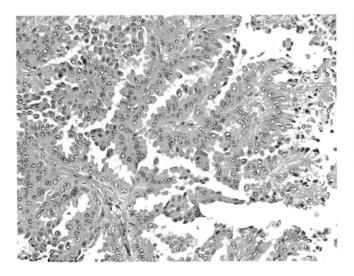

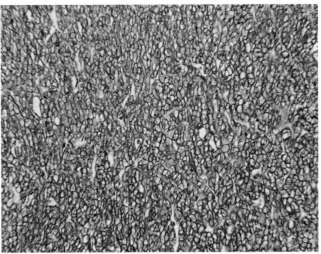

**Fig. 2-35** Papillary renal cell carcinoma. In this type 2 tumor the papillae are thicker and lined by cells with large irregular nuclei and abundant eosinophilic cytoplasm.

**Fig. 2-36** Papillary renal cell carcinoma. Diffuse strongly positive CK7 immunostaining is evident in this solid variant of papillary renal carcinoma.

than populating the papillae, are more likely to be found near areas of necrosis. Type 2 tumors exhibit significantly higher silver-staining nucleolar organizer region (AgNOR) scores and Ki67 indices,[5] and significantly less frequent expression of MUC1, a transmembrane mucin expressed in a variety of normal epithelial cell types and carcinomas.[252] Type 2 tumor morphology, as well as being seen in sporadically occurring cancer, is also characteristic of the papillary neoplasms that occur in hereditary leiomyomatosis and renal cell cancer (HLRCC).[230,231]

The practicality of subtyping papillary renal cell carcinoma is supported by data showing that tumor type is an independent predictor of outcome, with type 1 tumors having significantly better survival than type 2.[251-253] The issue is somewhat complicated by the fact that a clear-cut distinction may be difficult in some cases.[31,254] Specifically, some papillary tumors exhibit nuclear features typical of type 1 but cytoplasmic features typical of type 2,[8,31,254] and some are composed of mixtures of cells of generally low nuclear grade but with substantial variations in cytoplasmic characteristics. Further investigation of these neoplasms is needed to allow optimal correlation of morphology with biologic behavior.

Immunohistochemically, papillary renal cell carcinoma virtually always expresses pancytokeratin, α-methyl-acyl CoA racemase (AMACR), and CD15. The great majority of cases express CD10 and RCC Ma. Type 1 tumors are more likely than type 2 to express CK7 and MUC1; conversely, type 2 tumors are more likely to express E-cadherin and CK20 (Fig. 2-36). There is lack of uniformity in the reporting of CD117 expression in papillary renal cell carcinoma.[23,27,50,204,210,253,255–257] Ultrastructurally, cells of papillary renal cell carcinoma exhibit variably sized luminal microvilli and variable numbers of mitochondria (more in cells with abundant eosinophilic cytoplasm) with lamellar cristae.

They contain little or no glycogen, and do not contain the microvesicles typically observed in chromophobe renal cell carcinoma.[47]

Five-year survival rates for papillary renal cell carcinoma range from 49% to 91%.[139,222,244] Reduced survival has been positively correlated with increasing nuclear grade and stage, vascular invasion, a relative paucity of foam cells, DNA aneuploidy, increased AgNOR score, increased Ki67 index, and the presence of sarcomatoid differentiation.[139,243,247,251,258,259] The presence of tumor necrosis has been identified as a significant adverse finding by some investigators[252] but not by others.[139,243,247,251,259] The relevance of traditional Fuhrman nuclear grading in predicting outcome in papillary renal cell carcinoma has been challenged by data indicating that assessment of nucleolar prominence as a single parameter correlates better with outcome than assessment of multiple nuclear parameters (nuclear size, nuclear shape, and nucleolar prominence) to assign a Fuhrman grade.[123,260] Patients with type 1 cancer have significantly longer survival than those with type 2. Compared to other common types of renal cell carcinoma, the cancer-specific survival rates at 5 years following surgery for a large series of patients with clear cell renal cell carcinoma, papillary renal cell carcinoma and chromophobe renal cell carcinoma were 72%, 91%, and 88%, respectively.[139]

## Chromophobe renal cell carcinoma

Chromophobe cells were first described in chemically induced renal tumors in rats. Chromophobe renal cell carcinoma was first reported in 1985; its name was derived from the morphologic similarity between the predominant tumor cells in the human tumor to those comprising the experimentally produced rat kidney tumor.[261] Subsequently, the eosinophilic variant was described in 1988.[262]

Chromophobe renal cell carcinoma is believed to arise from the intercalated cells of the collecting duct system.[263] Most cases arise sporadically, but some have a hereditary basis, occurring in patients with Birt–Hogg–Dube syndrome, a genetic skin disorder characterized by cutaneous nodules (hair follicle fibrofolliculomas), mainly on the face and neck. Patients with this syndrome are also at risk for the development of pulmonary cysts that predispose to spontaneous pneumothorax and bilateral multifocal renal tumors.[264] Chromophobe renal cell carcinoma comprises approximately 34% of the renal neoplasms that occur in patients with this syndrome; the remainder are oncocytoma (7%), clear cell carcinoma (9%), and hybrid tumors composed of a mixture of oncocytoma and chromophobe carcinoma (50%).

Chromophobe renal cell carcinoma accounts for 4.9% of surgically excised renal epithelial neoplasms. It comprises a higher proportion of renal cancers in the Middle East, for reasons that are inapparent. Patients range in age from 23 to 86 years, and males and females are affected almost equally.[259,265–270] The percentage of cases discovered incidentally in reported series varies considerably, from 19% to 70%; symptomatic patients typically complain of flank pain or gross hematuria, and a mass is palpable only rarely. Some patients note weight loss; paraneoplastic symptoms are generally absent in most patients. Radiologically, there are no features that reliably distinguish chromophobe renal cell carcinoma from other renal epithelial neoplasms, including oncocytoma.

Sporadic chromophobe renal cell carcinoma is typically solitary, with rare exceptions. Tumors are well circumscribed and vary widely in size, from 1.5 to 25 cm in diameter; mean diameters range from 6.9 to 8.5 cm.[259,265–267,269,270] The cut surface is usually solid, homogeneous and light brown or beige; less often the tumor is gray-tan, light pink, or yellow-white (Figs 2-37, 2-38). A minority show hemorrhage and/or necrosis, and these features, when present, are limited in extent. An area of central scarring is infrequently present.

Microscopically, the tumor cells of chromophobe renal cell carcinoma are typically arranged in solid sheets; in some cases, areas of tubulocystic architecture are present.[35] Tumors are intersected randomly by delicate to broad fibrous septa and blood vessels that are predominantly of medium caliber, in contrast to the small sinusoidal vessels that are seen in clear cell carcinoma[271,272] (Fig. 2-39). Two types of tumor cells may be present in varying proportions. One type – the chromophobe cell – is a large polygonal cell with abundant almost transparent and slightly flocculent cytoplasm and prominent, often 'plant-like' cell membranes (Fig. 2-40). The chromophobe cells are frequently found adjacent to vascular channels. Usually they are admixed with a second population of smaller cells with less abundant cytoplasm that is granular and eosinophilic (Fig. 2-41). This combination of cell types characterizes the 'typical' variant of chromophobe renal cell carcinoma.[35] A variant of chromophobe renal cell carcinoma that is virtually entirely composed of intensively

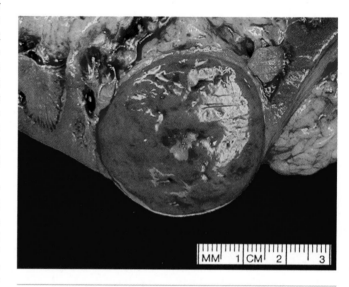

**Fig. 2-38** Chromophobe renal cell carcinoma. This eosinophilic type of chromophobe carcinoma is mahogany and well circumscribed. (Courtesy of Mark Costaldi, MD.)

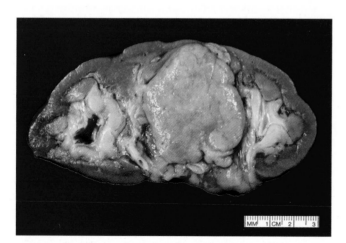

**Fig. 2-37** Chromophobe renal cell carcinoma. This classic type of chromophobe carcinoma is tan and well circumscribed.

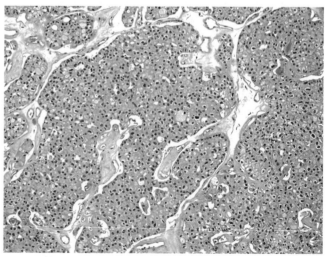

**Fig. 2-39** Chromophobe renal cell carcinoma. Sheets of tumor cells intersected by delicate to broad fibrous septa.

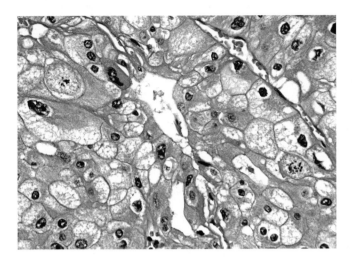

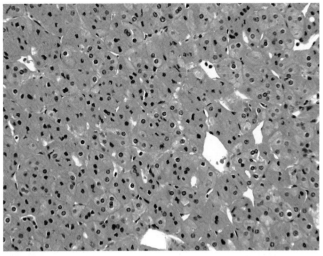

Fig. 2-40 Chromophobe renal cell carcinoma. Numerous chromophobe cells with abundant flocculent cytoplasm and sharply outlined plant-like cell membranes.

Fig. 2-42 Chromophobe renal cell carcinoma. This eosinophilic variant closely mimicked oncocytoma, but showed strong and diffusely positive immunostaining for CK7.

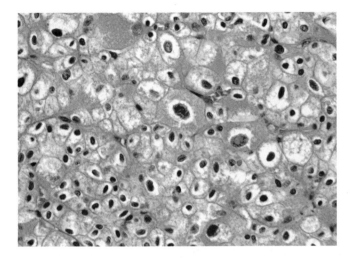

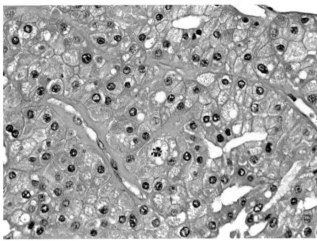

Fig. 2-41 Chromophobe renal cell carcinoma. The tumor cells are smaller, with more densely granular eosinophilic cytoplasm, raisinoid nuclei, and perinuclear haloes.

Fig. 2-43 Chromophobe renal cell carcinoma. This eosinophilic variant closely mimicked oncocytoma, but mitotic figures were readily evident in parts of the tumor.

eosinophilic cells with prominent cell membranes has been designated the eosinophilic variant of this neoplasm[262] (Figs 2-42, 2-43). The nuclei of both cell types are typically hyperchromatic with irregular wrinkled nuclear contours; binucleation is common. Perinuclear halos are frequently present in the more eosinophilic cells, and this feature can be of considerable diagnostic importance. Sarcomatoid transformation, a feature common to other types of renal cell carcinoma, may be found in up to 9% of cases,[185,186,273,274] and in certain geographic locations may be unusually prevalent (Fig. 2-44). Rare cases with osteosarcoma-like differentiation, rhabdoid differentiation, or extensive calcification and ossification have been reported.[200,275,276]

Ultrastructurally, chromophobe cells contain numerous round, ovoid, or elongated microvesicles ranging from 150 to 300 nm in diameter, scanty numbers of small mitochondria with tubulovesicular cristae, and rare glycogen particles.[262,277] The nature and origin of the microvesicles are

unknown: it is postulated that they are derived from mitochondria.[35] Eosinophilic cells have fewer microvesicles and more abundant mitochondria with tubulovesicular or lamellar cristae.[262,275] The relative abundance of microvesicles correlates with the intensity of Hale's colloidal iron staining. A diffuse cytoplasmic staining reaction with Hale's colloidal iron is generally regarded as being supportive of a diagnosis of chromophobe renal cell carcinoma;[35,48] however, since at least 11% of cases of oncocytoma also show diffuse cytoplasmic staining for Hale's colloidal iron, the staining results must be used in conjunction with other findings in finalizing a diagnosis.[49]

The genetic abnormalities that characterize chromophobe renal cell carcinoma have been studied by classic cytogenetic methods, comparative genomic hybridization, single-strand conformational polymorphism, and fluorescence in situ

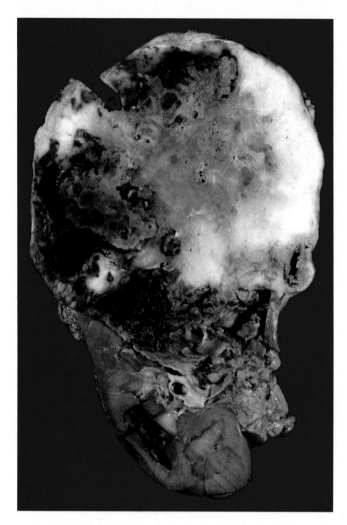

**Fig. 2-44** Chromophobe renal cell carcinoma. Sarcomatoid differentiation was evident in this large chromophobe carcinoma. The patient died of cancer 6 months after surgery.

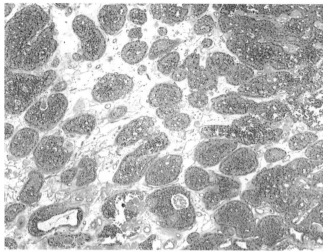

**Fig. 2-45** Chromophobe renal cell carcinoma. The compact tumor cell nests in this chromophobe carcinoma mimic the findings in oncocytoma. Same case as in Figure 2-43.

hybridization analysis.[239,278–293] The abnormalities most consistently observed have been multiple losses of whole chromosomes, most frequently Y, 1, 2, 6, 10, 13, 17, and 21.[262,289] Chromosomal losses result in a hypodiploid DNA index.[267,293,292] Mutation of the p53 tumor suppressor gene has been identified in a minority of chromophobe renal cell carcinomas, but this does not seem to affect prognosis. In contrast to non-sarcomatoid chromophobe renal cell carcinomas, which typically manifest multiple chromosome losses, sarcomatoid chromophobe renal cell carcinomas frequently have multiple gains (polysomy) of chromosomes 1, 2, 6, 10 and 17. However, the capacity to metastasize does not appear to depend on chromosomal gain: distant metastases in cases of metastatic chromophobe renal cell carcinoma show the same genetic patterns, typically monosomy associated with chromosomal loss, found in the primary tumors. Clinical manifestations of the Birt–Hogg–Dube syndrome have been linked to mutations at a locus on chromosome 17p11.2.[294] It has been proposed, based on cytogenetic studies of a case of oncocytosis, that chromophobe renal cell carcinoma may result from loss of additional chromosomes from oncocytoma cells that have already lost chromosomes

X or Y and 1.[65]

Chromophobe renal cell carcinoma virtually always shows positive immunohistochemical staining for pancytokeratin, epithelial membrane antigen (EMA), and parvalbumin, and virtually always shows negative immunostaining for vimentin, CK20, and AMACR.[27,50,198–200,210,295,296]

Distinguishing between oncocytoma and the eosinophilic variant of chromophobe renal cell carcinoma is a significant and relatively frequent problem for surgical pathologists, one that has led to myriad investigations on many levels – histological, histochemical, ultrastructural, immunohistochemical, cytogenetic, and molecular (Fig. 2-45). Frequent binucleation and the presence of 'raisinoid' nuclei with perinuclear haloes, with an appearance mimicking koilocytosis, is characteristic of chromophobe renal cell carcinoma, whereas foci of 'degenerative' nuclear atypia with pleomorphism are seen in 20% of oncocytomas but not in chromophobe renal cell carcinoma.[45] Diffuse colloidal iron staining, although regarded as a classic finding in chromophobe renal cell carcinoma, is also noted in 11% of oncocytomas.[48,49] Similarly, because of an overlap in ultrastructural findings between the two entities, electron microscopy cannot be relied on to make the distinction in all cases.[46,47,277] A large number of immunohistochemical stains have been evaluated and shown to be insufficiently specific as single markers for distinguishing between oncocytoma and chromophobe renal cell carcinoma, including epithelial membrane antigen (EMA), vimentin, parvalbumin, antimitochondrial antibody (113-1), caveolin-1, c-Kit, vinculin, peanut agglutinin antigen (PNA), Ulex europaeus agglutinin (UEA-1), cytokeratin KL1, S100 protein, lysozyme, E-cadherin, MIB-1, cyclin D1, epithelial cell adhesion molecule (EpCam), CK7, and RON proto-oncogene.[49,50,198,199,207,270,271,295,296,298–307] Single markers that show promise but that have not been extensively evaluated include S100A1 protein,[308] ankyrin-repeated protein with a proline-rich region (ARPP),[309] CD63,[310] and MOC31.[311] Several panels of immunohistochemical markers have been proposed for making this distinction: CK7/parvalbumin,[312]

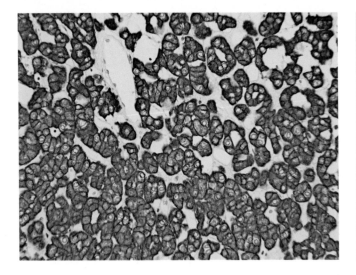

**Fig. 2-46** Chromophobe renal cell carcinoma. Typically, chromophobe carcinoma shows strong and diffusely positive immunostaining for CK7.

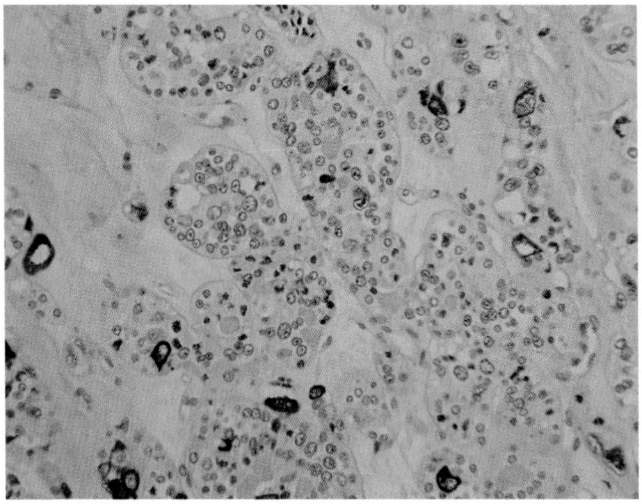

**Fig. 2-47** Oncocytoma. In contrast to the findings in Figure 2-46, this oncocytoma has only scattered cells that show positive immunostaining for CK7.

**Table 2-3** Oncocytoma versus chromophobe renal cell carcinoma[50,312,313]

|  | CK7 | Parvalbumin | PAX2* | CK20 | CD15 | Chromosome loss 2, 6, 10, 17 |
|---|---|---|---|---|---|---|
| Oncocytoma | Neg or focally pos | Pos 47% | Pos | Pos | Pos | No |
| CHRCC | pos | Pos | Neg | Neg | Neg | Yes |

*PAX2: Paired box gene 2.

**Table 2-4** Chromophobe renal cell carcinoma versus clear cell renal carcinoma (CHRCC)/(CCRCC)[50]

|  | CK7 | RCC Ma | CD10 | Vimentin | CD117 | Parvalbumin | E-cadherin |
|---|---|---|---|---|---|---|---|
| CCRCC | Neg | Pos | Pos | Pos | Neg | Neg | Neg |
| CHRCC | Pos | Neg | Neg | Neg | Pos | Pos | Pos |

CK7/c-KIT/PAX2,[313] and CK7/CK20/CD15. Cytokeratin 7 immunostaining is potentially helpful in distinguishing chromophobe renal cell carcinoma (staining pattern strong and diffuse) from oncocytoma (staining pattern focal and patchy) (Figs 2-46, 2-47). It is probable that the ideal single marker or panel of markers is yet to be identified. Genetic analysis allows separation of these entities based on the finding that oncocytomas do not demonstrate combined losses of heterozygosity at chromosomes 1, 2, 6, 10, 13, 17, and 21, characteristic of chromophobe renal cell carcinoma.[314] Furthermore, fluorescence in situ hybridization studies indicate that detection of losses of chromosomes 2, 6, 10, or 17 effectively excludes the diagnosis of oncocytoma and supports the diagnosis of chromophobe renal cell carcinoma[289] (Table 2-3).

Distinguishing chromophobe renal cell carcinoma from clear cell renal cell carcinoma with granular eosinophilic cytoplasm may also be challenging. A number of studies have addressed this problem.[50,198–200,202,206,210,295,315,316] The most common profile for chromophobe renal cell carcinoma is 'CK7++/RCC Ma-/CD10-/vimentin-CD117+/parvalbumin+/E-cadherin+/EMA+/MUC1+/CK20-/AMACR-.' The most prevalent clear cell renal cell carcinoma immunoprofile is CK7-/RCC Ma+/CD10+/vimentin+/CD117-/parvalbumin-/E-cadherin-/EMA+/MUC1+/CK20-/AMACR-/.Consequently, the markers most useful in distinguishing between these entities are CK7, RCC Ma, CD10, vimentin, CD117, parvalbumin, and E-cadherin (Table 2-4).

The prognosis for chromophobe renal cell carcinoma has been shown in a number of large series to be significantly better than for clear cell renal cell carcinoma.[139,259,266] Stage at presentation with chromophobe renal cell carcinoma is significantly lower than with clear cell renal cell carcinoma. Only 4% of patients with chromophobe renal cell carcinoma present with metastases, compared to 27% of patients with clear cell renal cell carcinoma. As noted previously, the cancer-specific survival rates at 5 years following surgery at the Mayo Clinic for a large series of patients with clear cell renal cell carcinoma, papillary renal cell carcinoma and chromophobe renal cell carcinoma were 72%, 91%, and 88%, respectively. The presence of histologic tumor necrosis is significantly associated with death from chromophobe renal cell carcinoma. Sarcomatoid differentiation appears to confer a dismal prognosis: cancer-specific survival at 2 years following surgery for chromophobe renal cell carcinoma with sarcomatoid differentiation was 25%, compared to 96% 2-year survival in patients without sarcomatoid differentiation.[139] Median cancer-specific survival for patients with metastatic chromophobe renal cell carcinoma is 0.6 years, which is not substantially different from the prognosis for patients with other types of metastatic renal cell carcinoma.[139] It appears there is no significant difference in outcome between the typical and the eosinophilic variants of chromophobe renal cell carcinoma.[259]

## Collecting duct carcinoma

The notion that renal carcinoma could originate in collecting duct epithelium was proposed in the late 1970s, and supported by a number of publications over the next 15 years.[248,317–331] This neoplasm arises in the principal cells of the collecting ducts of Bellini. Although it is among the least common types of renal cell carcinoma, accounting for less than 1% of renal malignancies, almost 200 cases have now been reported.

Patients range from 13 to 84 years of age, with a mean age of 55. Collecting duct carcinoma occurs more commonly in males, with a male-to-female ratio of at least 2:1,[332] and even higher (almost 3:1) in the largest reported series.[333] A strong family history of various types of cancer in other family members has been noted in some reports. One case occurred in a horseshoe kidney, and another arose on a background of end-stage renal disease. Up to 25% of cases are discovered incidentally, but the majority of patients present with symptoms, including abdominal or flank pain and hematuria. Less common symptoms include weight loss, fatigue, fever, musculoskeletal pain, anorexia, and gastrointestinal disturbances,[332,334] and rarely the presenting symptoms are those of metastatic cancer.[335] Imaging studies usually disclose the presence of a predominantly solid mass consistent with renal carcinoma.[324,332,336] Urine cytology is positive for malignant cells in a small percentage of cases.[327,333,337] Bone metastases, which may be present at the time of diagnosis, are often osteoblastic.

Small collecting duct carcinomas are usually located centrally, and may be localized to a medullary pyramid. However, because collecting ducts extend from the medulla to the cortex, collecting duct carcinoma can originate anywhere in the parenchyma, and identification of the site of origin may not be possible, particularly in large tumors. Tumors range in size from 1 to 16 cm in greatest dimension.[332,333] The cut surface of collecting duct carcinoma is usually gray-white and firm, and areas of necrosis may be evident (Fig. 2-48). In contrast to other types of renal cell carcinoma, the borders of collecting duct carcinoma are indistinct. Intrarenal metastases may be evident as satellite tumor nodules. Tumor involvement of the adrenal gland, perirenal fat, renal sinus fat, renal pelvis, Gerota's fascia, renal vein and/or regional lymph nodes is grossly evident in the majority of cases.

Microscopically, collecting duct carcinoma shows a complex tubulopapillary architecture which may coexist with solid cord-like areas (Fig. 2-49). Tubules lined by clearly

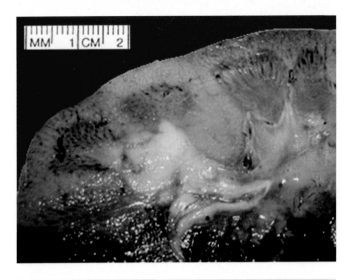

**Fig. 2-48** Collecting duct carcinoma. A gray-white tumor with ill-defined borders occupies a medullary pyramid. (Courtesy of Rodolfo Montironi, MD.)

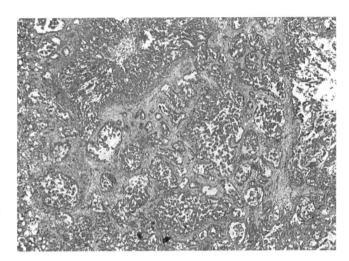

**Fig. 2-49** Collecting duct carcinoma. At low power this tumor demonstrates complex tubulopapillary architecture.

malignant cells are present, singly or arranged to form complex interanastomosing structures. Some tumors have microcysts with intracystic papillary proliferations of high-grade carcinoma (Figs 2-50, 2-51). The borders of the tumor are ill-defined, with extensive infiltration of adjacent parenchyma and often an acute and chronic inflammatory cell infiltrate at the interface between tumor and normal parenchyma (Fig. 2-51). Pronounced stromal desmoplasia is a constant feature (Fig. 2-52). Some tumors show intratubular extension with microscopic subcapsular deposits distant from the main tumor. The epithelium lining native ducts adjacent to or distant from the main tumor mass may show marked cytologic atypia or frank carcinoma in situ. Tumor cells are almost always of high nuclear grade, with nuclear pleomorphism and prominent nucleoli (Fig. 2-53) and varying amounts of eosinophilic cytoplasm. Cells lining luminal structures may display a 'hobnail' appearance, a finding that is not typical of other types of renal cell carci-

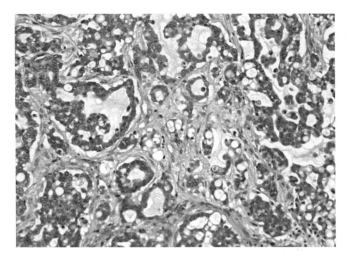

**Fig. 2-50** Collecting duct carcinoma. Tubules and complex interanastomosing structures containing mucin.

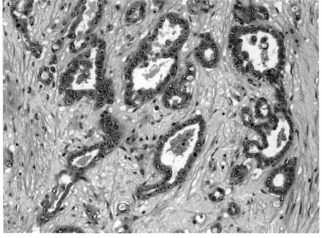

**Fig. 2-53** Collecting duct carcinoma. Neoplastic tubules lined by frankly malignant cells.

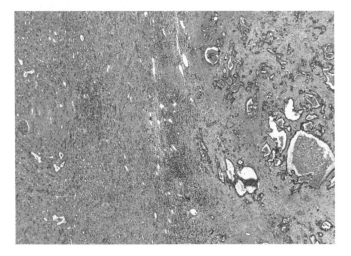

**Fig. 2-51** Collecting duct carcinoma. Pronounced inflammatory reaction at the interface between tumor and normal adjacent parenchyma.

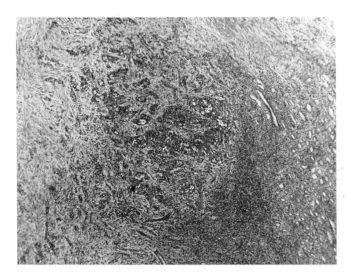

**Fig. 2-52** Collecting duct carcinoma. Marked stromal desmoplasia and intense inflammation at the interface between tumor and normal kidney.

noma. Small vessel invasion is common, and renal vein involvement is evident in about 20% of cases.[332] The incidence of sarcomatoid differentiation varies from 16% to 36%.[186,325,330]

The presence of mucin is often demonstrable by mucicarmine, Alcian blue, or periodic acid–Schiff (PAS) stains, within the tumor cell cytoplasm, at the luminal borders, or extracellularly.[248,320,326] Tumor cells typically show positive immunohistochemical staining for peanut lectin agglutinin, *Ulex europaeus* agglutinin-1 (UEA-1), low molecular weight keratins and pancytokeratin. Positive staining for CK19 and high molecular weight keratin (34βE12) is common. Immunostains for CD15, vimentin, and epithelial membrane antigen show variable results, and immunostains for proximal tubular markers such as villin and CD10 are usually negative. DNA ploidy studies have shown aneuploidy in a high percentage of tumors.[324] There are few descriptions of the ultrastructural features of collecting duct carcinoma. Organelles are abundant; mitochondria comprise up to 30% of cytoplasmic volume. Tumor cells have tight junction complexes, and some show scant microvilli.[320,321]

Cytogenetic findings have been variable. Losses of heterozygosity in 1q (specifically 1q32), 6p, 8p 13q and 21q have been reported, as well as loss of Y.[332,338–340] Loss of heterozygosity in 3p is reported by some investigators,[339,341] but not by others. Amplification of the c-erbB-2 oncogene is evident in about half of collecting duct carcinomas.[342]

Tumor stage is often advanced at the time of presentation, and not surprisingly the prognosis is generally poor. Nearly half of patients have nodal and/or distant metastases at the time of initial diagnosis.[332,333] Approximately two-thirds of patients with collecting duct carcinoma die of cancer within 2 years,[334] and mortality rates as high as 83% have been reported by some investigators. Although a few node-positive patients without distant metastases appear to have had long-term disease-free survival after being given adjuvant therapy, accumulated data suggest that chemotherapy and immunotherapy are of very little benefit in managing collecting duct carcinoma.

# Renal medullary carcinoma

First reported in 1995, renal medullary carcinoma is an uncommon, highly aggressive renal malignancy. It is believed to arise in the terminal collecting ducts and their adjacent papillary epithelium.[343–346] Its occurrence is very strongly associated with sickle cell hemoglobinopathies, so it has been postulated that the above-noted epithelium suffers chronic ischemic damage related to sickling erythrocytes, and that renal medullary carcinoma originates in a setting of chronic regenerative proliferation of this damaged epithelium. The majority of affected patients have been African-Americans with sickle cell trait (HbAS) or hemoglobin SC disease (HbSC), but it has also been reported in a patient with sickle cell disease (HbSS) as well as in white patients without evidence of sickle cell hemoglobinopathies.[343,347]

Almost 100 patients with renal medullary carcinoma have been reported, males ranging from 5 to 40 years of age with a mean age at diagnosis of 19 years, and females ranging from 8 to 39 with a mean age at diagnosis of 22 years. The male:female ratio is 1.9:1, and for reasons that are inapparent, about 75% of tumors occur on the right and 25% occur on the left.[348] The great majority (90%) of patients are African-American; 5% of patients are white and 5% are Hispanic. In reported cases in which sickle cell status was known, 85% had sickle cell trait (HbAS), 9% had hemoglobin SC disease (HbSC), 4% had sickle cell disease (HbSS), and 2% had no evidence of sickle cell hemoglobinopathy.

Abdominal and/or flank pain (52%), gross hematuria (52%) and weight loss (23%) are the most common presenting symptoms;[348] fever, nausea and vomiting are also common, and about 10% of patients have a palpable abdominal mass.[343,346,347,349] Duration of symptoms prior to diagnosis ranges from 2 days to 60 weeks, but the median is relatively short (8 weeks).

Grossly, these tumors typically occupy the renal medulla and are poorly circumscribed, lobulated, firm to rubbery, tan to gray, with varying degrees of hemorrhage and necrosis (Figs 2-54, 2-55). They range in size from 1.8 to 13 cm in greatest dimension, with a mean of 7 cm.[343,350,351] Satellite nodules are commonly present, as is extension into the perinephric and sinus fat. Microscopically, they demonstrate a variety of morphologic patterns (Figs 2-56, 2-57). The most characteristic finding is a reticular or microcystic growth pattern that resembles yolk sac tumor of the testis. Areas that resemble adenoid cystic carcinoma are often noted. Other common patterns include tubule formation and growth in diffuse sheets or solid nodules. Tumor cells are typically pleomorphic, with large nuclei, prominent nucleoli, and varying amounts of eosinophilic cytoplasm. Tumor cells may have a squamoid or rhabdoid appearance, particularly in areas of sheet-like growth. Abundant neutrophils may be noted within the tumor, and there is often an intense inflammatory response at the interface between tumor and the

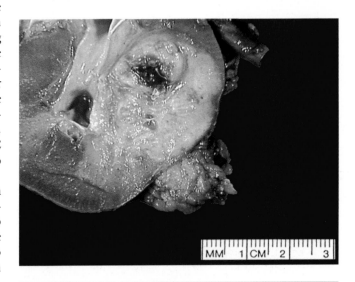

**Fig. 2-55** Renal medullary carcinoma. Nephrectomy specimen from the patient noted in Figure 2-54. Partially necrotic tumor with ill-defined borders, occupying medulla and cortex. (Courtesy of Erica Steele, MD.)

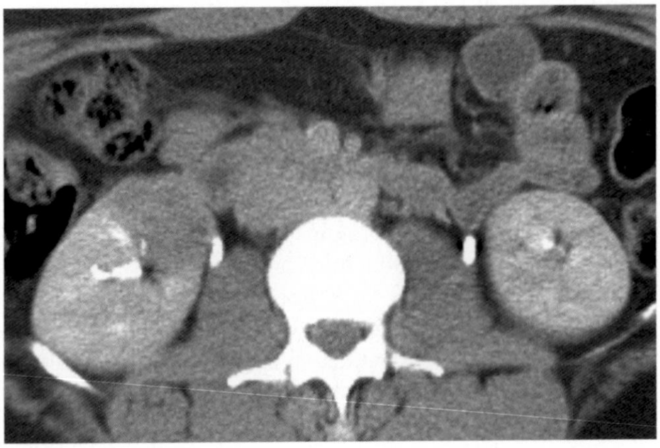

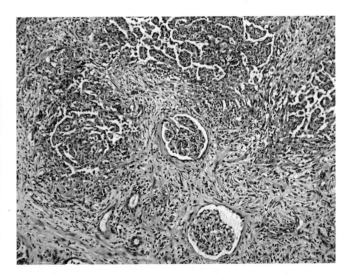

**Fig. 2-54** Renal medullary carcinoma. Ill-defined solid mass evident in left kidney of a 28-year-old African-American woman with sickle cell trait and a 6-month history of intermittent hematuria.

**Fig. 2-56** Renal medullary carcinoma. Tumor freely infiltrates the renal interstitium, showing complex tubulopapillary architecture and desmoplastic host response.

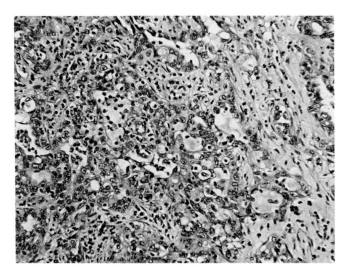

**Fig. 2-57** Renal medullary carcinoma. Malignant tubules containing mucin and a significant infiltrate of neutrophils.

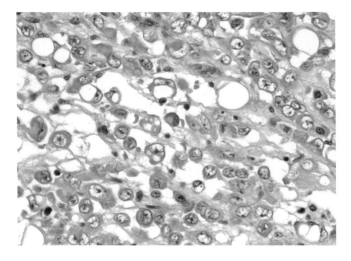

**Fig. 2-58** Renal medullary carcinoma. Some of the tumor cells show rhabdoid morphology. Sickled erythrocytes are readily apparent.

adjacent renal parenchyma (Fig. 2-57). The tumor incites a prominent desmoplastic stromal reaction. Varying degrees of mucin production are evident in the majority of renal medullary carcinomas. In most histologic sections, sickled erythrocytes are identified (Fig. 2-58).

Tumor cells show variable degrees of positive immunostaining for keratin immunostains, carcinoembryonic antigen (CEA), and epithelial membrane antigen (EMA).[343,344,349] Molecular profiling studies indicate that renal medullary carcinoma does not cluster with clear cell or papillary renal cell carcinoma.[346] Renal medullary carcinoma strongly expresses keratin 19 and topoisomerase IIa; the expression of keratin 19 differentiates it from conventional renal cell carcinoma, and the expression of topoisomerase II differentiates it from urothelial carcinoma. A *BCR-ABL* translocation was noted in one case, but although *ABL* gene amplification was noted in another study, an *ABL* translocation was not identified.[348] It

**Table 2-5** Xp11 translocation neoplasms (Modified from Argani P, Ladanyi M. The evolving story of renal translocation carcinomas. Am J Clin Pathol 2006; 126: 332–334)

| Gene fusion | Chromosome translocation | Neoplasm |
| --- | --- | --- |
| ASPL-TFE3 | der(17)t(X;17)(p11.2;q25) | Alveolar soft part sarcoma |
| ASPL-TFE3 | t(X;17)(p11.2;q25) | Renal carcinoma |
| PRCC-TFE3 | t(X;1)(p11.2q21) | Renal carcinoma |
| PSF-TFE3 | t(X;1)(p11.2q34) | Renal carcinoma |
| NonO-TFE3 | inv(X)(p11;q12) | Renal carcinoma |
| CLTC-TFE3 | t(X;17)(p11.2;q23) | Renal carcinoma |

has recently been reported that renal medullary carcinoma and malignant rhabdoid tumor share loss of INI1 expression and may be related entities.[352]

In view of the fact that 95% of patients with renal medullary carcinoma have metastatic cancer at the time of diagnosis or shortly thereafter,[348] it is not surprising that the prognosis for this neoplasm is poor. Common sites of metastasis are the lymph nodes, lung, liver and adrenals. Long-term disease-free survival is rare,[350,351] survival ranging from 2 to 68 weeks, with a mean of 19 weeks. Survival is somewhat longer overall in patients given adjuvant therapy, but is usually limited in duration, and even in cases of prolonged remission, recurrence and death are the usual outcome.[353,354]

## Translocation carcinoma

Renal carcinoma accounts for less than 5% of pediatric renal neoplasms. A number of cytogenetic and molecular discoveries in recent years have disclosed that approximately one-third of renal carcinomas in young patients are in the recently established category of Xp11 translocation carcinomas.[163,233,355–371] In patients aged 18–45 years such tumors are less frequent, accounting for less than 3% of one large series.[372] These cancers are defined by a variety of chromosome translocations, all of which involve a breakpoint at Xp11.2, and all of which result in the fusion of any one of multiple translocation partners with the TFE3 transcription factor gene at this locus[368,373] (Table 2-5). The t(X; 1)(p11.2; q21) translocation, which fuses the *PRCC* and *TFE3* genes, was the first reported Xp11.2 renal cancer. Subsequently, several additional rare translocations were reported, including t(X; 1)(p11.2; p34), which fuses the *PSF* and *TFE3* genes, the inv(X)(p11; q12) which fuses the *NonO (p54^{nrb})* and *TFE3* genes, and the t(X; 17)(p11.2; q23), which fuses the *CLTC* and *TFE3* genes. A more common Xp11.2 translocation carcinoma bears intriguing molecular similarities to alveolar soft part sarcoma, which has been shown to bear an unbalanced translocation, der(17)t(X; 17)(p11.2; q25), which fuses the *TFE3* gene to a novel gene, *ASPL*, on 17q25. It has been demonstrated that renal carcinomas bearing a balanced t(X; 17)(p11.2; q25) translocation share the same *ASPL-TFE3* gene fusion as alveolar soft part sarcoma. Despite this molecular similarity, the two tumors differ in their overall clinical, morphologic, and cytogenetic features.

Although almost all patients with translocation carcinoma are less than 18 years old, this tumor is not restricted to that age group.[356,368,374] Translocation carcinoma occurs with approximately equal frequency in males and females, and it has been observed that at least 15% of these cancers occur in patients who have previously received chemotherapy.[233,373,375] About half of patients present with abdominal or flank pain or hematuria; some tumors are detected as a palpable mass, and some are found incidentally.

PRCC-TFE3 carcinoma bearing the t(X; 1)(p11.2; q21) translocation is typically yellow or gray, ranges in size from 3 to 14 cm in diameter, and has a fibrous pseudocapsule that has varying degrees of calcification in the majority of cases, sometimes substantial enough to impart an egg-shell consistency[374] (Fig. 2-59). It is composed of tumor cells in papillary formations and in nests surrounded by thin-walled capillary vessels (Figs 2-60, 2-61). The tumor cell nests are usually solid, but may be centrally dyscohesive, imparting an alveolar appearance, and some nests have central lumina; fresh blood in these lumina imparts a 'bloody-gland' appearance typical of conventional renal cell carcinoma. The extent of the papillary component is variable: it may be the predominant pattern, or it may account for less than 10% of the tumor. Foam cells are evident in the minority of papillae. Psammoma bodies are often present, and although usually rare and isolated, may be abundant in some tumors. Transitions between areas of nested and papillary architecture are usually sharply demarcated. Tumor cells are uniformly polygonal, with sharply defined borders and abundant cytoplasm that varies from clear and finely granular to distinctly eosinophilic. Proportions of clear and eosinophilic cells vary from tumor to tumor. Nuclei appear rounded at low power, but at high power are wrinkled and irregular; Fuhrman nuclear grade is 2 or 3 in most cases. Areas of necrosis are seen in the majority of cases, but mitotic activity is very limited. Ultrastructurally, all tumors show features typically found in conventional renal cell carcinoma, including fat vacuoles, abundant glycogen, plentiful mitochondria, and microvilli and cell junctions.

ASPL-TFE3 carcinoma associated with the t(X; 17)(p11.2; q25) translocation is usually well circumscribed but

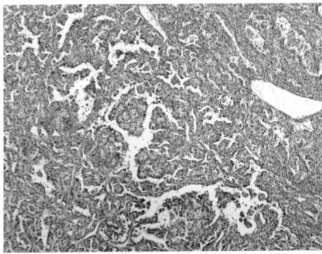

**Fig. 2-60** Translocation carcinoma. PRCC-TFE3 renal carcinoma showing compact nested and papillary architecture at low power.

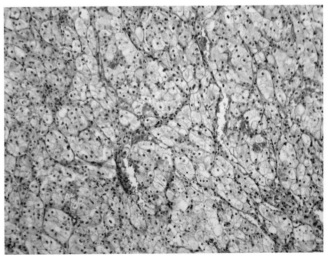

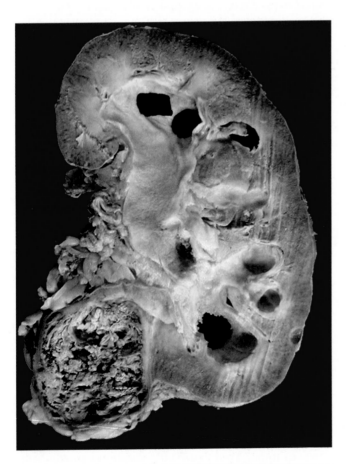

**Fig. 2-59** Translocation carcinoma. Diagnosis was based on tumor morphology and immunoreactivity of tumor cells to antibodies against TFE3. (Courtesy of Rodolfo Montironi, MD.)

**Fig. 2-61** Translocation carcinoma. PRCC-TFE3 renal carcinoma at high power, showing clear to faintly eosinophilic cytoplasm and sharply defined cell borders.

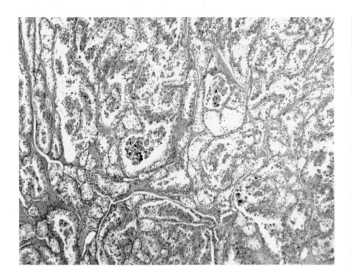

**Fig. 2-62** Translocation carcinoma. ASPL-TFE3 renal carcinoma at low power, showing nested to pseudopapillary architecture and numerous psammomatous calcifications.

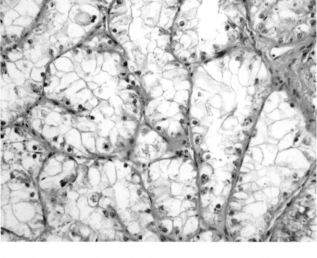

**Fig. 2-63** Translocation carcinoma. ASPL-TFE3 renal carcinoma at higher power showing cells with voluminous clear cytoplasm, and vesicular nuclei with prominent nucleoli.

unencapsulated.[363] It displays nested and pseudopapillary growth patterns and psammomatous calcifications (Figs 2-62, 2-63). Papillary structures lack foam cells and intracytoplasmic hemosiderin.[369] Tumor cells are epithelioid, with well-defined cell borders and voluminous cytoplasm that is predominantly clear but may also be finely granular, eosinophilic, or densely granular. Nuclei have vesicular chromatin and a single prominent nucleolus. Ultrastructurally, tumor cells show a combination of features of alveolar soft part sarcoma (dense granules and rhomboid crystals) and epithelial features (cell junctions, microvilli, and true lumina). The extent and degree of epithelial differentiation is considerably less than in typical renal cell carcinomas.

About 10 cases of an additional rare and distinctive renal carcinoma in this category have been reported, characterized by a t(6,11)(p21; q12) translocation that results in fusion of the 5' portion of the *Alpha* gene with the transcription factor gene *TFEB* at 6p21, and it has been suggested that they be named 't(6; 11) renal carcinomas' or '*Alpha-TFEB* renal carcinomas.'[365,367,376,377] Patients range in age from 9 to 33 years, with a mean age of 17. About half of patients complain of abdominal pain or hematuria, and the rest are asymptomatic. Tumors are solid with focal cyst formation, confined within a pseudocapsule, and range from 2 to 12 cm in greatest dimension (mean diameter 7 cm). They typically display a homogeneous tan-yellow-brown color, without evidence of necrosis. Microscopically, tumors demonstrate a solid, nested pattern of growth, and are composed of two cell populations. The predominant cell type is epithelioid, with well-defined borders, abundant clear, finely granular, or eosinophilic cytoplasm, and rounded or vesicular nuclei that have prominent nucleoli evident at low magnification and mild nuclear membrane irregularities at high power. In all cases there is a second cell population comprising 5–30% of the tumor and consisting of smaller cells with denser chromatin, usually clustered around nodules of hyaline basement membrane material. Mitotic figures are

inapparent. Abortive papillae, psammomatous calcifications, and well-formed tubules are seen in the minority of cases.

Renal carcinoma with Xp11.2-associated translocations typically underexpresses vimentin and epithelial immunohistochemical markers; only about half of these tumors show positive staining for various cytokeratins or EMA, and the staining is often weak and/or focal. Immunostaining for CD10 and the RCC Ma antigen is fairly consistent; however, the most distinctive, sensitive and specific immunohistochemical characteristic of these tumors is nuclear labeling for TFE3 protein, employing an antibody against a segment of the TFE3 gene that is retained in the gene fusions.[378] This marker stains alveolar soft part sarcoma and all Xp11.2 renal carcinomas, but does not stain clear cell or papillary renal cell carcinomas. Rarely, PSF-TFE3 or CLTC-PFE3 carcinomas will show positive immunostaining for melanocytic markers such as HMB-45 or MelanA.[14] In contrast, t(6; 11) renal carcinomas (*Alpha-TFEB* renal carcinomas) are consistently positive for HMB-45 and MelanA, and occasionally focally positive for CD10, but do not stain for epithelial markers, the RCC marker, S100 protein, or TFE3.[376] However, TFE3 is one of four closely related members of the transcription factor family MiT; the other members are Mitf, TFEB, and TFEC.[368] As a result of the *Alpha-TFEB* gene fusion in t(6; 11) renal carcinomas, TFEB protein production is upregulated, an occurrence not observed in any other tumor; consequently, nuclear immunostaining for TFEB is a sensitive and specific diagnostic marker for this tumor.

It is the opinion of some investigators that t(6; 11) renal carcinomas are related to Xp11-translocation carcinoma because they have related molecular pathology, they are morphologically similar, and they have similar immunohistochemical profiles.[368] These investigators have proposed that t(6; 11) renal carcinomas and Xp11-translocation carcinomas should all be classified as members of the 'MiTF/TFE translocation carcinoma family.'[373]

The number of patients with documented follow-up after treatment for the various types of translocation carcinoma is limited.[233,363,369,374] Whereas clinical stage at the time of diagnosis of PRCC-TFE3 carcinoma tends to be fairly evenly distributed, ASPL-TFE3 carcinomas typically present at a high clinical stage. In contrast, as noted above, t(6; 11) renal carcinomas are generally confined within an intact pseudocapsule.[376] Available evidence suggests that ASPL-TFE3 carcinoma is the most aggressive and has the worst prognosis, and that t(6; 11) renal carcinoma is quite indolent; in the largest series of t(6; 11) renal carcinomas, no tumor had recurred or metastasized following surgical excision. The prognosis for PRCC-TFE3 is uncertain, and late recurrence after many years has been documented.[368,374]

## Post-neuroblastoma renal cell carcinoma

Secondary malignant neoplasms develop in approximately 13% of children treated for cancer.[379] In the past 40 years, 21 patients have been diagnosed with renal cell carcinoma following treatment for neuroblastoma during the first 2 years of life.[163,380–392] This is notable, in light of the fact that the occurrence of renal cell carcinoma after treatment for other childhood malignancies is exceptionally uncommon: three renal cell carcinomas have been reported after childhood therapy for Wilms' tumor,[393] and one after treatment for acute promyelocytic leukemia.[394]

Of the 21 reported patients with post-neuroblastoma renal cell carcinoma, 9 were male and 12 were female.[163,391,392] All were diagnosed with neuroblastoma in the first 24 months of life. Fifteen patients were treated with chemotherapy, and 10 had radiation therapy; eight patients had both types of treatment. Remarkably, two patients, both with stage IV-S neuroblastoma, were treated with neither radiation nor chemotherapy; they developed renal cell carcinoma 7 and 8 years, respectively, after being diagnosed with neuroblastoma.[390,391] Renal cell carcinoma developed in the other patients from 2.4 to 34 years after the original diagnosis of neuroblastoma (average 14.5 years), and were between 3 and 36 years old at the time of diagnosis of renal cell carcinoma. In 14 cases with available data, six were asymptomatic at the time of diagnosis of renal cell carcinoma, and eight had a variety of symptoms and physical findings, including abdominal pain in two, back pain in one, fatigue in one, hypertension in two, and abdominal mass in two. Tumors were unilateral in 13 patients, and bilateral (and not infrequently multifocal) in eight.

Detailed pathologic descriptions of post-neuroblastoma renal cell carcinoma are found in only some of the reports.[390,391] Maximum sizes range from 3.5 to 8.0 cm; in multifocal cases, the tumor may be as small as 0.1 cm. Some tumors are confined to the kidney; others are metastatic to lymph nodes or distant sites either at the time of diagnosis or subsequently. Microscopically, the distinctive tumor recognized as post-neuroblastoma renal cell carcinoma is composed of cells arranged in solid sheets or nest and in papillae. Occasional psammoma bodies are present. Tumor cells have sharply defined cell membranes and abundant eosinophilic granular cytoplasm, giving it an 'oncocytoid' appearance. In addition, small foci of cells with abundant reticular cytoplasm are present, with some morphologic resemblance to chromophobe cells. Tumor cell nuclei are medium-sized and irregular, and many bear prominent nucleoli. Only occasional mitotic figures are observed. Some cases clearly have more ominous findings, including high nuclear grade and diffuse parenchymal infiltration with an accompanying desmoplastic reaction; some cases have been described as having a 'pseudosarcomatous' or 'anaplastic' appearance.[380,392]

Ultrastructurally, tumor cells have intercellular junctions, surface microvilli, numerous lysosomal granules, moderate to large numbers of mitochondria, and varying amounts of glycogen.[390] Immunohistochemically, tumor cells typically show positive staining for EMA and keratin Cam 5.2, and patchy staining for vimentin. Immunostaining for cytokeratins 8, 19, and 20 is inconsistent; staining for S100 protein, HMB-45, and cytokeratins 7 and 14 is negative. The cytogenetic features of post-neuroblastoma renal cell carcinoma are not well characterized, but it is clear that none of the known patterns of genetic changes that typify many types of renal cell carcinoma are seen in this neoplasm.

Because of the paucity of cases, and the limited follow-up in many of those cases, it is difficult to draw conclusions concerning prognosis for post-neuroblastoma renal cell carcinoma. The first reported patient had a sarcomatoid component in her tumor and died of widespread metastases shortly after the diagnosis.[380] However, cumulative experience suggests that these neoplasms are minimally aggressive. About half of the patients were free of disease at last follow-up, and even some with known metastases are reported to have stable disease after several years.[380,391,392]

Although it is tempting to speculate that post-neuroblastoma renal cell carcinoma is caused by exposure to chemotherapy and/or radiation therapy in early childhood, some investigators believe that the development of these tumors is more likely due to an underlying genetic relationship or susceptibility, similar to the experience of patients with familial cancer syndromes. This hypothesis is supported by the fact that at least two patients with post-neuroblastoma renal cell carcinoma were never exposed to chemotherapy or radiation therapy, and also by the observation that renal cell carcinoma is a rare second malignancy in children treated for cancer, and the great majority of reported cases have occurred in patients diagnosed with neuroblastoma in early childhood.[390,392,393]

## Mucinous tubular and spindle cell carcinoma

Five examples of this tumor were first reported in 1997 by MacLennan and colleagues under the name of 'low grade collecting duct carcinoma.'[395] Since then, the number of reported cases has risen to about 80. The tumor occurs predominantly in females, with a male:female ratio of 1:4. Patients range in age from 13 to 82 years, with a mean age of 53. Although some tumors are symptomatic, the majority are discovered incidentally. Tumors range in diameter from 2.2 to 12 cm, averaging 6–7 cm. Tumors are sharply circumscribed, gray-white, tan, or yellow, sometimes with minimal hemorrhage and/or necrosis (Fig. 2-64). Microscopically,

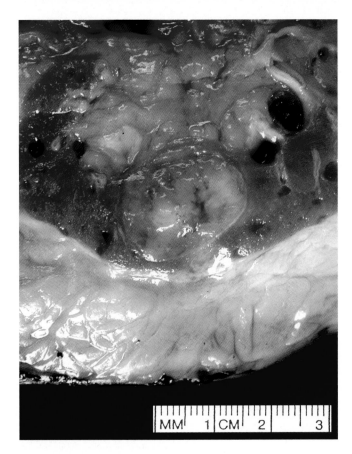

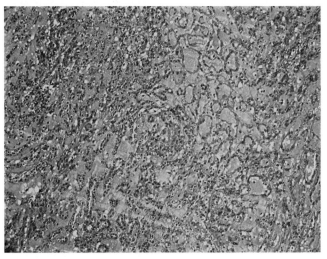

**Fig. 2-65** Mucinous tubular and spindle cell carcinoma. Abundant mucin fills and separates variably sized tubular structures.

**Fig. 2-64** Mucinous tubular and spindle cell carcinoma. Sharply defined gray-white neoplasm with a slightly bulging glistening cut surface. (Courtesy of Christine Kosloski.)

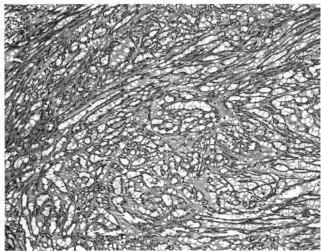

**Fig. 2-66** Mucinous tubular and spindle cell carcinoma. Round and closely packed elongated tubular structures filled and separated by 'bubbly' mucin.

they consist of tightly packed, small elongated tubules separated by abundant basophilic extracellular mucin, sometimes with a 'bubbly' myxoid appearance[395–397] (Figs 2-65, 2-66). Focally, aggregates of spindled cells may be present[398,399] (Fig. 2-67). The mucin stains strongly with Alcian blue at pH 2.5 (Fig. 2-68). Tubules are lined by uniform low cuboidal cells with scant cytoplasm, and round nuclei of low nuclear grade with absent or inconspicuous nucleoli. Mitotic figures are rare. As more experience has been gained with these tumors, it has become apparent that the histologic spectrum may include cases in which the spindle cell component rivals or even exceeds the tubular component, as well as cases with relative paucity of mucinous matrix, aggregates of foamy macrophages, papillations or small components of well formed papillae, focal clear cell change in tubular cells, focal necrosis, oncocytic tubules, numerous small vacuoles, psammomatous calcification, or heterotopic bone formation[400] (Figs 2-69, 2-70).

The exact cell of origin of this neoplasm is not well defined. Accumulated evidence suggests that these tumors originate either from cells of the loop of Henle or from collecting duct epithelium, with more support for the latter site. Tumor cells have a complex and markedly variable immunophenotype, but are typically immunoreactive for EMA, keratin AE1/AE3, CK7, CK19, 34βE12, and AMACR[395–397,399,401] Evidence of neuroendocrine differentiation, with tumor cell immunostaining for neuron-specific enolase, chromogranin, and synaptophysin, has been reported in two cases, supported by ultrastructural findings.[402] It has been pointed out that there is considerable overlap between the immunophenotype of mucinous tubular and spindle cell carcinoma and that of papillary renal carcinoma, warranting caution in the use of immunohistochemistry to distinguish these two entities, and emphasizing the possibility that mucinous tubular and spindle cell carcinoma is simply a variant of papillary renal cell carcinoma.[403,404] Despite morphologic similarities to papillary renal cell carcinoma in some cases, the gains of chromosomes 7 and 17 and loss of Y chromosome that are characteristic of papillary RCC are not seen in mucous tubules and spindle cell carcinoma.[405] Cytogenetic analyses and comparative genomic

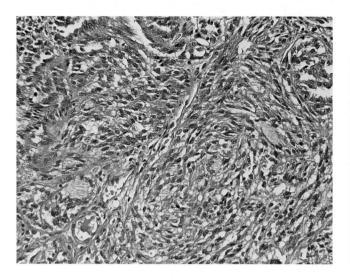

**Fig. 2-67** Mucinous tubular and spindle cell carcinoma. Aggregates of spindled cells are present.

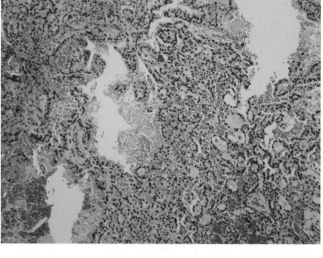

**Fig. 2-69** Mucinous tubular and spindle cell carcinoma. In this example, small papillary structures were focally present.

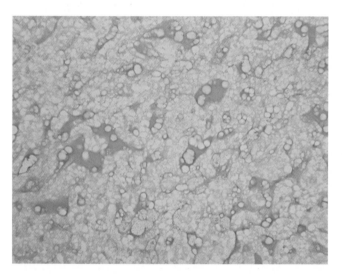

**Fig. 2-68** Mucinous tubular and spindle cell carcinoma. The tumor-associated mucin shows positive staining with Alcian blue.

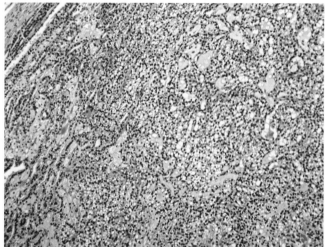

**Fig. 2-70** Mucinous tubular and spindle cell carcinoma. In this variant case, mucin-filled tubules are at the upper right, abundant macrophages at the upper left, and centrally the cells have clear cell morphology.

hybridization studies have revealed multiple genetic alterations that include losses of chromosome 1, 4, 6, 8, 9, 13, 14, 15, 18 and 22.[397,399,406,407]

These tumors are generally of low pathologic stage at the time of excision, and they behave in an indolent fashion: only two patients have experienced metastasis during follow-up as long as 24 years, and no tumor-related deaths have been reported.[395–397,406]

## Renal cell carcinoma, unclassified

This is a diagnostic category for the designation of renal cell carcinomas that do not fit readily into one of the accepted categories.[17,216] It is not possible to specify more stringently the criteria for inclusion in this category. Examples of tumors that are appropriately assigned to this category are tumors that are composites of recognized types, tumors composed of unrecognizable cell types, and renal carcinomas with

entirely sarcomatoid morphology, lacking recognizable epithelial elements.[216] Although the current WHO classification does not recognize tubulocystic carcinoma or the two distinctive types of renal cell carcinomas that arise in a background of end-stage renal disease, it seems probable that these entities will be included in the next version of this classification. Several of these entities are discussed below.

## Tubulocystic carcinoma

Examples of this rare distinctive neoplasm were presented at a meeting of the United States and Canadian Academy of Pathology and described in abstract form in 1994, and several illustrations of the microscopic appearance of these neoplasms were presented in the AFIP *Atlas of Tumor Pathology*, Series III, in 1994.[408,409] Details of the clinical and pathological details of eight examples of this neoplasm were first reported in 1997 by MacLennan and colleagues.[395,410] It was emphasized that although the neoplasm had some features suggestive of collecting duct origin, it was distinctly different from classic collecting duct carcinoma (CDC) in many ways. Because these tumors were clearly composed of tubules and duct-like structures, showed areas of hobnail change, and had immunohistochemical characteristics similar to those of classic CDC (i.e., positivity for 34βE12 and UEA-1), it was hypothesized that they were of collecting duct origin and that they represented the low-grade end of a spectrum of findings in CDC, hence the term 'low-grade collecting duct carcinoma'.[395] Subsequently, the clinical and pathologic features of additional examples of similar tumors were reported, and the name of the lesion was changed to tubulocystic carcinoma.[411] Additional examples of this neoplasm have been reported subsequently.

Tubulocystic carcinoma of the kidney is a well circumscribed tumor that ranges in size from 2 to 17 cm, is often grossly cystic, and lacks hemorrhage or necrosis; some show a 'bubble-wrap' appearance of the cut surface (Fig. 2-71). The microscopic appearance at very low power is reminiscent of a spider web or lace doily (Fig. 2-72). The tumor is composed of tubules and cystic structures of markedly variable size, separated by septa that are commonly delicate and 'spider web-like,' or by fibrotic septa of variable thickness (Fig. 2-73). Tubules are lined by a single layer of low cuboidal epithelial cells with modest to abundant amounts of eosinophilic cytoplasm, commonly with areas of hobnail appearance (Fig. 2-74). Nuclei are round, with evenly dispersed chromatin, and have readily evident nucleoli in some cases. Nuclear grade is 1 or 2 in all instances. No necrosis is present, and mitotic activity is extremely limited.[395,411]

Immunohistochemical studies show expression of proximal convoluted tubule (PCT)-related markers (CD10 (85%), AMACR (77%)) and markers related to distal nephron (parvalbumin (100%), 34βE12 HMWCK (15%) and CK19 (100%)). Ultrastructurally, tumors show abundant microvilli with brush border organization similar to cells of the PCT, but with shorter microvillous height and cytoplasmic interdigitation (similar to intercalated cells of the collecting duct). However, microvesicles normally seen in intercalated cells are not evident. In short, the histogenesis of this tumor

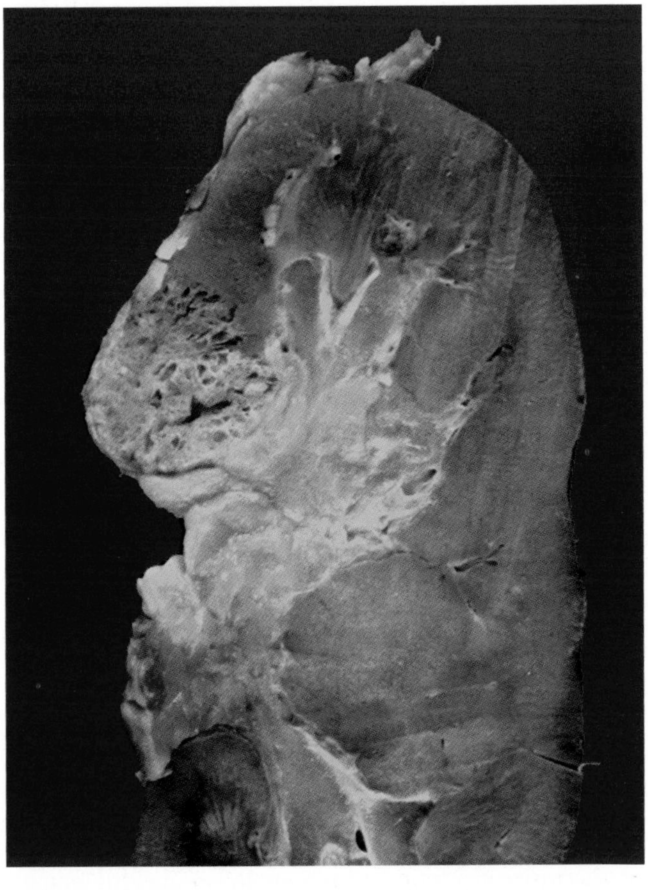

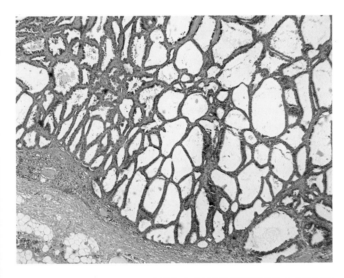

**Fig. 2-72** Low-grade collecting duct carcinoma (tubulocystic carcinoma). The tumor is composed of small cystic spaces separated by delicate septa, with a 'spider-web' or 'lace doily' appearance.

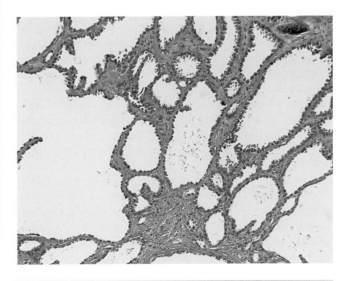

**Fig. 2-73** Low-grade collecting duct carcinoma (tubulocystic carcinoma). Delicate septa lined by eosinophilic cells with a 'hobnail' appearance.

**Fig. 2-71** Low-grade collecting duct carcinoma (tubulocystic carcinoma). The tumor is composed of myriad small cysts. Some examples have a 'bubble-wrap' appearance on sectioning.

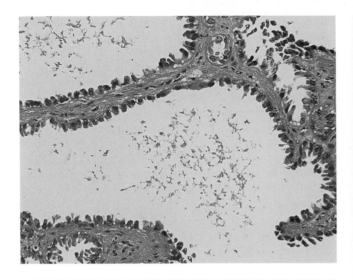

**Fig. 2-74** Low-grade collecting duct carcinoma (tubulocystic carcinoma). At high power the hobnail cells have small dark nuclei; nucleoli are absent or inconspicuous.

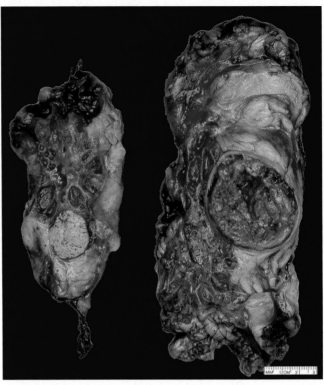

**Fig. 2-75** ESRD-associated renal cell carcinoma. This kidney with acquired cystic renal disease had both types of tumor commonly seen in this setting: the larger tumor on the right is 'acquired cystic disease-associated RCC,' and the smaller yellow tumor on the left is 'clear cell papillary RCC of end-stage kidneys.' (Courtesy of Matthew Kuhn, MD.)

remains unresolved, as ultrastructural and immunohistochemical findings show features characteristic of cells of the PCT and also of intercalated cells of the collecting duct.[412]

Stage and nuclear grade are typically low and biologic activity is indolent, with a potential for metastasis that is less than 10%.[395] Follow-up in 22 patients (median 52.5 months) showed that one patient had bone metastases, and one had both bone and liver metastases and died of cancer.[395,411]

## Acquired cystic disease-associated renal cell carcinoma

Patients with end-stage renal disease (ESRD) are unusually prone to kidney neoplasms, with an incidence of 4.2–5.8%.[413] About half of dialysis patients develop acquired cystic kidney disease (ACKD), a condition that depends on the duration of dialysis (87% incidence after 9 years of dialysis) and is three times more frequent in men than in women, but has no relationship to age, dialysis method, race, or the underlying cause of renal failure.[32] Patients with ACKD are especially prone to the development of carcinoma, with an incidence of 3–7% and a risk 100 times that of the general population.[32,414] Patients with ACKD-associated renal cell carcinoma tend to be relatively young and predominantly male, and their cancers are more frequently multicentric and bilateral, but less aggressive than sporadic renal cell carcinomas. The biological basis for increased renal carcinogenesis in ESRD is undefined. Depressed immunity, excessive free radical production related to inflammation, impaired antioxidant defenses and, more recently, deposition of oxalate crystals, have been postulated. Some tumors are discovered during radiologic evaluation of flank pain or hematuria, whereas others are diagnosed incidentally.

Recent studies have challenged the notion that most ESRD-associated renal cell carcinomas (RCCs) are classic histological types.[32,415] Although approximately 40% are classic clear cell, papillary or chromophobe RCC, the major-

ity may be represented by two newly described subtypes with unique histological and immunohistochemical characteristics. The first and more common of these is designated 'acquired cystic disease-associated RCC,' and the second 'clear cell papillary RCC of end-stage kidneys.' The first type occurs only in kidneys with ACKD, whereas the second occurs in non-cystic end-stage kidneys and in those with ACKD.

Examples of renal neoplasms with abundant intratumoral calcium oxalate deposition, arising in a background of ESRD and ACKD, were first reported in 1998. Grossly, acquired cystic disease-associated RCCs range from 1 to 8 cm, and are often multifocal and bilateral (Fig. 2-75). Such tumors are generally well circumscribed. Foci of hemorrhage and necrosis are common, and some have focally calcified capsules. Many appear to have arisen in cysts. Histologically the tumor architecture demonstrates various combinations of solid sheet-like, papillary, acinar, cribriform and tubulocystic patterns. The tumor cells are typically large with abundant granular eosinophilic cytoplasm, and large round to oval, mildly irregular nuclei with prominent nucleoli.[32,413,416] About 80% of these tumors show abundant intratumoral calcium oxalate crystals within luminal structures and in the stroma (Fig. 2-76). The crystals are not associated with fibrosis, necrosis, increased mitoses or inflammation. Intratumoral calcium oxalate deposition is a feature that appears to be restricted to tumors arising in a background of ACKD. Tumor cells show positive immunostaining for keratin AE1/

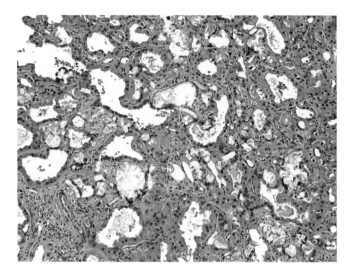

**Fig. 2-76** ESRD-associated renal cell carcinoma. This acquired cystic disease-associated carcinoma exhibits tubulocystic architecture and abundant calcium oxalate crystals.

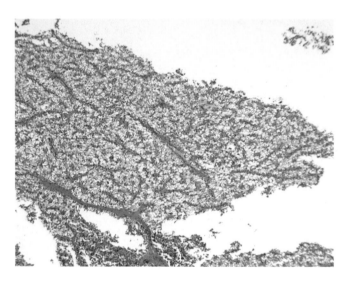

**Fig. 2-77** ESRD-associated renal cell carcinoma. This clear cell papillary RCC of end-stage kidneys shows papillary architecture, but the tumor cells have copious clear cytoplasm.

AE3, CD10, RCC Ma, and often for AMACR.[413,417] Gains in chromosomes 1, 2, 6, and 10 have been documented in a limited number of such cases by fluorescence in situ hybridization studies.

The second tumor type, designated clear cell papillary renal cell carcinoma of end-stage kidneys, occurs with almost equal frequency in ACKD and non-cystic ESRD.[32] Recently, this tumor was also described in patients without ESRD. Grossly, such tumors are typically well circumscribed, often cystic, with a thin fibrous capsule and without hemorrhage or necrosis (Fig. 2-75). Histologically the architecture is predominantly papillary. However, the majority of cells lining the papillary structures exhibit clear cytoplasm and a low nuclear grade (Fig. 2-77). In contrast to the immunostaining profile of typical sporadic papillary RCC, characterized by positive immunostaining for cytokeratin 7 and AMACR, these tumors demonstrate positive immunostaining for cytokeratin 7 but negative immunostaining for racemase.

The prognosis for renal cell carcinoma in ESRD is generally considered more favorable than for non-ESRD cases, possibly because ESRD-associated carcinomas are on the whole biologically less aggressive or because constant medical surveillance of these patients facilitates diagnosis at an early stage. Nonetheless, sarcomatoid morphology, metastasis and death from cancer have been documented in ESRD-associated RCC, and may be more common in acquired cystic disease-associated RCC.[32]

## Purely sarcomatoid renal cell carcinoma

The first evidence that many so-called renal sarcomas included components of renal carcinoma was reported in 1949.[418] Before that time, renal tumors with sarcomatoid morphology were regarded as true sarcomas.[184] Based on observation of morphologic transitions between carcinoma and sarcoma, it was hypothesized in 1968 that the sarcomatous areas resulted from metaplastic transformation of malignant epithelial cells, justifying use of the term sarcomatoid renal carcinoma.[419] It is now recognized that tumor components with sarcomatoid morphology can be seen in clear cell, papillary, chromophobe, collecting duct and renal medullary carcinoma.[274] There is no evidence that renal sarcomatoid carcinoma ever arises de novo. In clear cell carcinoma, it has been shown that the clear cell and sarcomatoid components are derived from the same progenitor cell, indicative of genetic divergence during the clonal evolution of renal cell carcinoma.[420] It seems probable that entirely sarcomatoid renal carcinomas are those in which the sarcomatoid component overgrows and obliterates the carcinoma from which it arose, and consequently such tumors are not regarded as a unique type of renal cell carcinoma[216] (Figs 2.78–2.80).

Approximately 3% of renal carcinomas are purely sarcomatoid and hence unclassified. Compared to purely clear cell carcinoma matched for TNM stage, Fuhrman nuclear grade, and ECOG performance status, purely sarcomatoid renal cell carcinoma is significantly larger, significantly more likely to invade the adrenal gland or other adjacent organs, significantly more likely to metastasize to regional and non-regional lymph nodes and bone, and associated with a significantly lower survival. Almost all patients succumb to cancer, and median survival is short (4.3 months).[421]

## Other rare epithelial neoplasms

The spectrum of renal epithelial neoplasms includes other rarely described tumors, including spiradenocylindroma,[422] and thyroid follicular carcinoma-like carcinoma[402] (Fig. 2-81). The former was a component of a 7 cm solid–cystic renal tumor in a 58-year-old man. The solid component exhibited combined morphologic features of cylindroma and spiradenoma, an overlap well recognized in sporadic skin tumors. The tumor showed cytogenetic features suggestive of isochrome 1(16p), consistent with gene alterations that characterize familial cylindromatosis and sporadic spi-

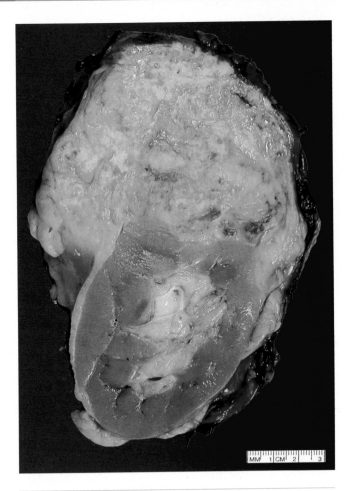

**Fig. 2-78** Purely sarcomatoid renal cell carcinoma. This aggressive tumor extensively infiltrates perirenal fat and extends to the inked Gerota's fascia. (Courtesy of Shams Halat, MD.)

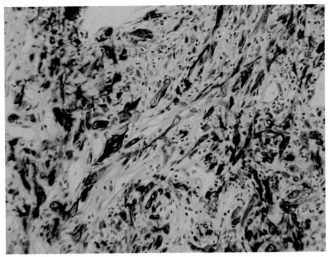

**Fig. 2-80** Purely sarcomatoid renal cell carcinoma. Immunostaining of the tumor illustrated in Figure 2-79 shows diffuse strongly positive staining for keratin Cam 5.2.

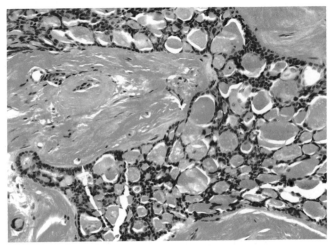

**Fig. 2-81** Thyroid follicular carcinoma-like carcinoma. This unusual renal neoplasm is remarkably reminiscent of a thyroid follicular neoplasm, set in a diffusely hyalinized fibrotic background.

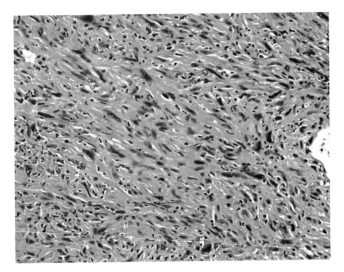

**Fig. 2-79** Purely sarcomatoid renal cell carcinoma. Tumor is composed entirely of spindled and pleomorphic cells. Despite extensive sampling, no epithelial component was found.

radenocylindromas.[422] The patient was well 30 months after surgery. The latter tumor, arising in a 32-year-old woman without demonstrable thyroid disease, measured 11.8 cm and exhibited follicular architecture with inspissated colloid-like material in their lumina, remarkably mimicking follicular thyroid carcinoma. Immunostains for thyroid markers were negative, and cytogenetic findings were dissimilar to those of other recognized renal carcinomas. The patient was well 6 months after surgery. Tumors with similar findings have been reported in abstract form.[423]

## Prognostic factors in renal cell carcinoma

Prognostic factors are features or markers that may be employed to project the course or endpoint of a disease. With regard to renal cell carcinoma, these elements are most often used to predict clinical outcome, but with the advent of novel therapeutic strategies for this type of cancer these elements may also be used in determining a patient's eligibility for entry into a study, for choosing a specific treatment option, and in assessing response to therapy.[424] Prognostic factors can be subdivided into patient-related and tumor-related factors, and each of these categories can be subdivided into one of three categories, depending on the level of evidence or degree of acceptance attributed to them. Category I prognostic factors are regarded as well supported by the literature and/or generally used in clinical management.

In 1997 members of an international workshop on renal cell carcinoma agreed on a number of category I patient-related factors for renal cell carcinoma, all of which are associated with an unfavorable clinical result. These include symptomatic presentation, a poor Eastern Cooperative Oncology Group (ECOG) performance status (performance status of 2–3), elevated erythrocyte sedimentation rate (ESR >30), and anemia (defined as <10 g/dL in females and <12 g/dL in males). Weight loss exceeding 10% of body weight, hypercalcemia, and elevated serum alkaline phosphatase levels are unfavorable findings in patients with metastatic renal cell carcinoma.[107,424–426] More recently, it has been shown that cachexia-like symptoms and signs (weight loss, anorexia and/or malaise, and hypoalbuminemia) are independently predictive of a worse prognosis in patients with stage T1 renal cell carcinoma.[103] Thrombocytosis (platelet count >400 000/mm$^3$) is an independent predictor of poor outcome in patients with metastatic renal cell carcinoma; furthermore, its presence preoperatively in patients with clinically localized renal cell carcinoma is associated with a significantly worse disease-specific outcome than in patients without thrombocytosis.[427,428]

Extensively documented and well-accepted tumor-related prognostic factors include TNM staging parameters (tumor size, local tumor extension, adrenal involvement, large vessel involvement, lymph node involvement, distant metastases), histologic subtype, nuclear grade, sarcomatoid differentiation, and histologic tumor necrosis.[139,429]

Currently, pT1 tumors are subdivided into pT1a and pT1b; pT1a tumors are 4 cm or less, and pT1b tumors are more than 4 cm but not more than 7 cm in size. Regardless of the type of surgical resection, 5-year cancer-specific survival rates for pT1a and pT1b are 97% and 87%, respectively. There is ongoing discussion concerning the optimal pT1 size criteria, with some groups advocating reductions in the upper size limit for pT1 tumors to 5 or 5.5 cm.[430,431] It has also been noted that tumor size is an independent prognostic factor even after accounting for the TNM classification and nuclear grade.[139,145,148,155]

The 5-year cancer-specific survival for pT2 tumors – defined as tumors larger than 7 cm – is 71–74%.[144] Some groups have suggested subcategorizing the pT2 category, providing evidence of worsening outcome at various tumor size cutpoints, specifically 10 cm and 13 cm.[156,432] Future versions of the TNM staging system may be revised to address these issues.

The 5-year cancer-specific survival for stage pT3 ranges from 37% to 67%, possibly reflecting the fact that this is a

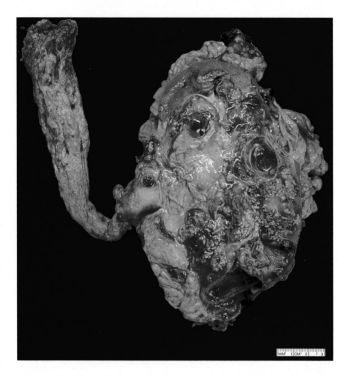

**Fig. 2-82** Stage T3b renal cell carcinoma. High-grade type 2 papillary renal cell carcinoma extending into the renal vein and up the vena cava, ending below the diaphragm.

very broad category that includes varying levels of tumor extension into adjacent structures, specifically perirenal fat, sinus fat, adrenal gland, renal vein and vena cava (Fig. 2-82). Studies reported since the last version of the TNM staging system was published in 2002 indicate that patients whose tumors directly invade the adrenal have a much worse prognosis than those whose tumors only extend into perirenal fat.[433–436] It has been suggested that direct adrenal invasion by tumor should be reclassified as pT4 disease.[434,437,438] Involvement of renal sinus fat appears to portend a worse prognosis than involvement of only perirenal fat.[439,440] Other data suggest that various combinations of the components of the pT3 category, e.g., renal vein or vena cava involvement as well as perirenal fat involvement, result in outcomes worse than predicted by only one of those parameters.[431,441] Patients with tumor thrombi in the renal vein or below the diaphragm (stage pT3B) have been shown to have significantly better outcomes than those whose tumor thrombi extend above the diaphragm (stage pT3c).[442] Future versions of the TNM system may be revised to reflect data from these studies.

Numerous studies have confirmed that outcome is poor in patients with renal cell carcinoma whose lymph nodes are involved by metastatic renal cell carcinoma; the 5-year cancer-specific survival for these patients is reportedly 11–35%.[139,429] The role of lymphadenectomy in treating renal cell carcinoma is unclear.[139] Recent reports indicate that the current pN category may need to be revised, as there appears to be no significant difference in outcome between patients with pN1 disease and those with pN2 disease.[139]

The presence of distant metastases is predictive of a poor outcome in patients with renal cell carcinoma, regardless of histologic type (Figs 2-83, 2-84). Median cancer-specific survival for patients with metastatic clear cell, papillary and chromophobe renal cell carcinoma is 15 months or less for all three tumor types.[139]

It is generally agreed that nuclear grading is important in predicting prognosis in patients with renal cell carcinoma; however, as noted in a previous section, there is a lack of uniform agreement on several crucial issues with respect to grading. As noted, the independent predictive value of the

Fuhrman nuclear grading system has been demonstrated by some investigators.[142,143] The 5- and 10-year cancer-specific survival rates were as follows: for grade 1 tumors, 86–89% and 77–81%, respectively; for grade 2 tumors, 72–79% and 56–68%, respectively; for grade 3 tumors, 50–59% and 30–46%, respectively; and for grade 4 tumors, 28–29% and 19%, respectively. Other investigators have found that the Fuhrman grading system is an independent predictor of cancer-specific survival only after grouping grades.[137,144,145] As noted previously, the relevance of Fuhrman nuclear grading in predicting outcome in papillary renal cell carcinoma has been questioned by investigators who find that assessment of nucleolar prominence as a single parameter correlates better with outcome than assessment of multiple nuclear parameters (nuclear size, nuclear shape, and nucleolar prominence) to assign a Fuhrman grade.[260]

With regard to the influence of histologic subtype on prognosis in renal cell carcinoma, the available data are somewhat conflicting. In one large series, cancer-specific survival rates at 5 years for clear cell, papillary, and chromophobe carcinoma were 68.9%, 87.4%, and 86.7%, respectively. Patients with clear cell carcinoma had a significantly poorer prognosis than patients with chromophobe and papillary carcinoma, even after stratifying for 1997 TNM stage and nuclear grade. The 1997 TNM stage, tumor size, presence of a sarcomatoid component, and nuclear grade were significantly associated with death from all three tumor types.[443] In contrast, in another large study the findings indicated that in multivariate analysis, TNM stage, Fuhrman nuclear grade and ECOG performance status, but not histologic subtype, were valid independent prognostic variables.[143]

Sarcomatoid differentiation was first described in renal cell carcinoma in 1968; it may be found in all of the major renal cell carcinoma subtypes (Fig. 2-85). Sarcomatoid differentiation in renal cell carcinoma is generally associated with a poor prognosis: median survival after diagnosis is less

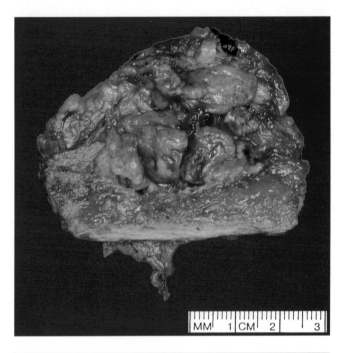

**Fig. 2-83** Metastatic renal cell carcinoma. Resection of this rib metastasis of clear cell renal carcinoma was undertaken because it was symptomatic and was the only demonstrable metastasis. (Courtesy of Shams Halat, MD.)

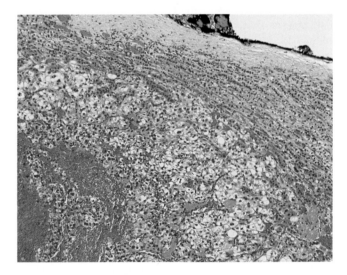

**Fig. 2-84** Metastatic renal cell carcinoma. Clear cell carcinoma involving adrenal in a radical nephrectomy specimen.

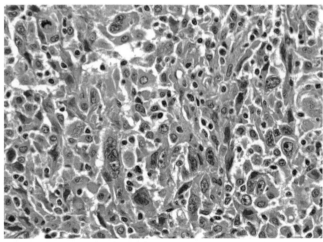

**Fig. 2-85** Sarcomatoid differentiation in renal cell carcinoma. This spindled and pleomorphic area was found in a papillary renal cell carcinoma, but similar findings can occur in clear cell, chromophobe and collecting duct carcinomas.

than 1 year, and the poor prognosis is irrespective of the type of underlying renal cell carcinoma.[184-188] For patients with clear cell, papillary, and chromophobe renal cell carcinoma with sarcomatoid differentiation, cancer-specific survival rates at 2 years are 30%, 40%, and 25%, respectively, in contrast to 84%, 96%, and 96% respectively for patients with non-sarcomatoid clear cell, papillary and chromophobe carcinoma.[139] Sarcomatoid differentiation has been shown in at least one study to provide independent prognostic information for patients with clear cell carcinoma.[259]

Tumor necrosis is frequently associated with aggressiveness. The presence of histologic necrosis has been found by a number of investigators to be independently predictive of poor outcome and survival in clear cell renal cell carcinoma; this does not, however, apply to papillary or chromophobe renal cell carcinoma.[145,259,426]

In recent years, a wide variety of molecular markers have been evaluated as potentially important prognostic markers, including hypoxia-inducible factors (hypoxia-inducible factor, carbonic anhydrase IX, VHL tumor-suppressor protein, vascular endothelial growth factor), regulators of apoptosis (p53, Bcl-2, Smac/DIABLO), regulators of cell cycle (p27, PTEN), and adhesion molecules (EpCam, EphA2). Currently it is unclear how these prognostic markers will be incorporated into future paradigms for assessing prognosis and tailoring specific therapies for renal cell carcinoma.[429]

## Renal cell carcinoma in children

Renal cell carcinoma accounts for less than 0.3% of all tumors and 2.6% of renal neoplasms in patients less than 15 years old,[444] and less than 1% of all resected renal cell carcinomas. Renal cell carcinomas occurring in patients in the first two decades of life are a heterogeneous group of neoplasms that have some striking differences from their adult counterparts.

The median age at presentation is about 10–14 years. There is no striking gender predominance in the pediatric population,[163,445,446] whereas in adults, renal cell carcinoma affects males twice as frequently as females. In contrast to adults, in whom up to 61% of renal cell carcinomas are currently being discovered incidentally,[115] pediatric patients tend to be symptomatic at presentation, in 64–75% of cases, with presenting symptoms and signs including gross hematuria, abdominal or flank pain, fever, weight loss, erythrocytosis, palpable abdominal mass, or combinations thereof.[233,446] Bilaterality is uncommon. von Hippel–Lindau syndrome seems to play little or no role in the occurrence of pediatric renal cell carcinoma.

The morphologic and genetic spectrums of pediatric and adult renal cell carcinomas are substantially different.[163] The most recent WHO classification of renal cell carcinoma includes entities that were not well characterized when the older literature on pediatric renal cell carcinoma appeared;[216] consequently, there are few reports characterizing these neoplasms in the context of current understanding.[163,233] Morphologically, renal cell carcinoma in the pediatric age group is diverse, including (in one series) unclassified carcinoma (24%), papillary carcinoma (22%), translocation

carcinoma (20%), clear cell carcinoma (15%), and rare examples of chromophobe carcinoma, collecting duct carcinoma, post-neuroblastoma carcinoma, and carcinoma combined with nephroblastoma.[163] Another recent series had a higher percentage (54%) of translocation carcinoma.[233] It has been estimated that approximately one-third of pediatric renal cell carcinomas are of translocation type.[368]

A further striking difference between pediatric and adult renal cell carcinomas is that nearly three-quarters of patients who present with lymph node metastases were alive at last follow-up, a survival rate nearly triple that of historical adult controls.[447]

## Metanephric tumors

### Metanephric adenoma

Originally described in the French literature in 1980 as nephrogenic nephroma,[448] and subsequently named metanephric adenoma,[449] examples of this tumor were reported sporadically,[450-452] and eventually most of its clinical and pathologic features were described in two large series published in 1995.[343,453] Its name reflects its morphologic resemblance to the cytologic and architectural features of early metanephric tubular differentiation and to the metanephric hamartomatous element of nephroblastomatosis.[449,453,454] Some investigators have suggested that its occurrence is related to the developing proximal tubule of the fetal kidney or nephrogenic rests, based on morphologic, immunohistochemical and ultrastructural similarities between metanephric adenoma and metanephric tubular epithelium.[453-456] Similarities in patterns of immunohistochemical expression of CD56, CD57, WT1, and CK7 between metanephric adenoma and maturing Wilms' tumor/nephrogenic rests support the premise of a histogenetic relationship between the two entities, and furthermore support the contention of some investigates that metanephric adenoma represents the most hyperdifferentiated, mature form of Wilms' tumor.[456,457] Striking morphologic and immunohistochemical similarities have been observed between metanephric adenoma, Wilms' tumor and nephrogenic rests and two uncommon entities, embryonal hyperplasia of Bowman's capsular epithelium (associated with end-stage renal failure and dialysis) and a morphologically similar entity, metanephric metaplasia of Bowman's capsular epithelium (associated with terminal malignancies with extensive liver metastases), leading some to hypothesize a possible link between these entities.[458,459]

Currently, more than 100 patients with metanephric adenoma have been reported.[460] The majority are female, with a female : male ratio of about 2 : 1.[343,453,456,461] Although most patients are in their fifth or sixth decade, the reported age range for metanephric adenoma is 15 months to 83 years.[343,452,453] In at least half of cases the tumor produces no symptoms and is discovered incidentally. Less frequently a mass is palpable, or patients complain of flank or abdominal pain, intermittent fever, or hematuria. An association with polycythemia has been reported in as many as 12% of cases.

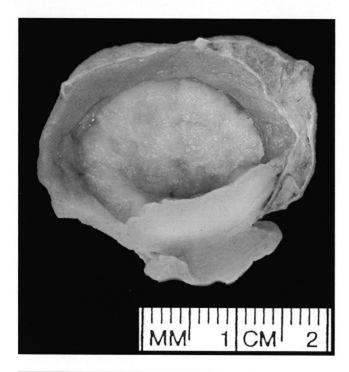

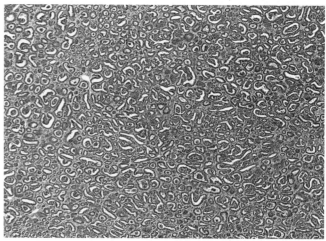

**Fig. 2-87** Metanephric adenoma. The tumor is composed of small embryonal epithelial cells forming densely packed tubules, set in a very limited hyalinized paucicellular stroma. Numerous 'glomeruloid bodies' are present.

**Fig. 2-86** Metanephric adenoma. Light tan, well-circumscribed but unencapsulated renal tumor in a 48-year-old woman. (Courtesy of Mark Costaldi, MD.)

Metanephric adenoma ranges in size from 0.3 to 20 cm in greatest dimension,[343,455] with a mean of 5.5 cm. It is typically unilateral and rarely multifocal. The majority are either unencapsulated or have only a limited and discontinuous pseudocapsule. Tumors are tan to gray to yellow, and soft to firm (Fig. 2-86). Although most are solid, some have areas of hemorrhage, necrosis and cystic degeneration. Calcification within the solid areas or within the walls of cystic structures is common. Infrequently, coexistent renal cell carcinoma is present.[343,462,463]

Microscopically, metanephric adenoma may appear solid at low power, but on closer inspection it is composed of very small acini separated by acellular stroma consisting only of edema fluid or a smoothly hyalinized matrix.(Fig. 2-87). The degree of acinar crowding is variable. Extensive replacement of tumor by hyalinized scar is observed in about one-third of cases. In some, tumor cells are arranged to form nests and tubules. In about half of cases papillary structures are noted, consisting of polypoid fronds or short papillary infoldings within tubular or cystic spaces, producing a glomeruloid appearance. Less commonly, tumor cells form solid aggregates that resemble blastemal nodules of Wilms' tumor, and infrequently microcysts are present, lined by flattened tumor cells similar to those noted elsewhere in the tumor. The great majority of tumors display calcification, either in the form of calcific deposits and foci of dystrophic calcification within areas of stromal hyalinization and scarring, or as psammoma bodies associated with papillary structures.

Tumor cells of metanephric adenoma possess little cytoplasm, which is usually pink or clear (Fig. 2-88). Nuclei are slightly bigger than lymphocytes, irregularly rounded or

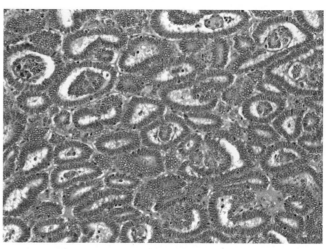

**Fig. 2-88** Metanephric adenoma. At higher power tumor cells are uniform, with evenly dispersed chromatin and scant cytoplasm, lacking nucleoli and mitotic activity.

ovoid, sometimes displaying a central fold. Nuclear chromatin is delicate, nucleoli are absent or inconspicuous, and mitotic figures are rare or entirely absent. Tumor cells are closely spaced and often overlapping. Ultrastructurally, tumor cells show well-developed basal lamina and cell junctions, and short microvilli at the luminal borders. Cytoplasmic organelles are scant.

The differential diagnosis of metanephric adenoma is essentially limited to epithelial-predominant Wilms' tumor (WT) and the solid variant of papillary renal cell carcinoma (PRCC), and the distinction between these entities can be aided by the use of immunohistochemical and cytogenetic studies. Staining profiles for most keratin markers and vimentin are inconsistent.[249,343,453–455,464–466] However, metanephric adenoma typically shows negative immunostaining for epithelial membrane antigen (EMA) and only focal

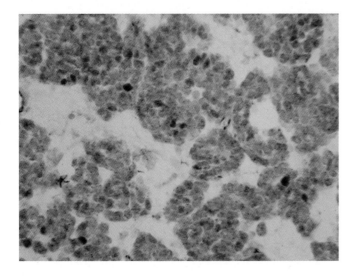

**Fig. 2-89** Metanephric adenoma. Tumor cells show positive immunostaining for WT1.

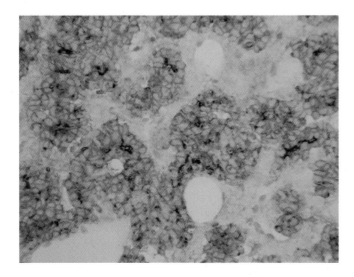

**Fig. 2-90** Metanephric adenoma. Tumor cells show positive immunostaining for CD57.

immunostaining for cytokeratin 7 (CK7). A panel of immunostains including WT1, CD57, α-methylacyl-CoA racemase (AMACR), and CK7 has been shown to be helpful in distinguishing metanephric adenoma from WT and PRCC. Metanephric adenoma is typically immunopositive for WT1 and CD57 and immunonegative for AMACR and CK7, an immunoprofile that is the exact opposite to that of PRCC (Figs 2-89, 2-90). Metanephric adenoma and WT share immunopositivity for WT1 and immunonegativity for racemase and CK7, but are distinguishable by positive staining for CD57 in metanephric adenoma, and negative immunostaining for this marker in Wilms' tumor[456,467] (Table 2-6).

DNA content analysis of metanephric adenoma by flow cytometry yields diploid histograms.[453,465] Although most cytogenetic analyses have revealed normal karyotypes,[453,454,468] exceptions have included a balanced pericentric inversion

**Table 2-6** Metanephric adenoma, Wilms' tumor, solid variant of papillary RCC[457,468]

|  | CK7 | CD57 | AMACR | WT-1 |
|---|---|---|---|---|
| Metanephric adenoma | Neg | Pos | Neg | Pos |
| Wilms' tumor | Neg | Neg | Neg | Pos |
| Papillary RCC, solid | Pos | Neg | Pos | Neg |

involving the short and long arms of chromosome 9 [46,XX,inv (9) (p13q12) c], a commonly described normal constitutional variant not known to be associated with increased risk of neoplasia or other diseases, as well as a case displaying the presence of the dual t(1; 22)(q22; q13) and t(15; 16)(q21; p13) translocations.[460] Abnormalities in chromosome 2 have been reported, specifically partial monosomy 2p,[469] and alterations at 2p13 in 56% of informative cases, providing evidence that metanephric adenoma is a genetic entity distinct from Wilms' tumor and papillary renal neoplasms.[470] Furthermore, the chromosome 11p13 deletion that is characteristic of Wilms' tumor has not been identified in metanephric adenoma.

The possibility of a close histogenetic relationship between metanephric adenoma and papillary renal neoplasms was suggested by reports that demonstrated similar chromosome 7 and 17 gain and loss of sex chromosomes in each;[471] however, these findings have been disputed by other investigators, in whose opinion trisomy of 7 and 17 and loss of Y chromosomes, classic findings in papillary renal neoplasms, are not features of metanephric adenoma.[249,461,466,470,472,473]

Most investigators regard metanephric adenoma as a benign neoplasm. In one case, a nephrectomy specimen that harbored metanephric adenoma also had demonstrable regional lymph node metastases. It has been suggested that in this case the underlying neoplasm was a Wilms' tumor that metastasized and subsequently matured into a metanephric adenoma.[457,474,475] Other cases of metanephric adenomas with putative malignant behavior have been less compelling.[462,463,473]

## Metanephric stromal tumor

Following recognition of a distinctive and unique biphasic renal neoplasm, metanephric adenofibroma,[476] it was recognized that a separate subset of renal neoplasms consisted entirely of stromal elements identical to the stromal component of metanephric adenofibroma. This subset was designated metanephric stromal tumor, reported in an abstract and described more fully in a large series of cases.[477,478] Some investigators have hypothesized that metanephric stromal tumor may arise from intralobar nephrogenic rests that have matured with loss of blastemal elements.[457]

Most patients are children, ranging from a few days old to 15 years, with a mean age of 2 years.[479,480] A single adult patient has been reported.[457] The majority are detected as a palpable abdominal mass, and about 20% have hematuria. Less common manifestations of tumor include hypertension, flank pain, or tumor rupture.[479,481] Some are found incidentally.

Metanephric stromal tumor is typically a tan, lobulated, partially cystic fibrous tumor with a mean diameter of 5 cm. It is often centered in the renal medulla and is usually unifocal, but about one-sixth of cases are multifocal.[479] Mean diameter is 5 cm. It is unencapsulated, and has a scalloped border that on close inspection subtly infiltrates the adjacent normal parenchyma.

Microscopically it is composed of spindled and stellate cells with thin hyperchromatic nuclei and indistinct cytoplasmic extensions[457] (Fig. 2-91). Scattered epithelioid stromal cells may be noted. Metanephric stromal tumor tends to surround native renal tubules and blood vessels, forming concentric 'onion-skin' rings or collarettes around these structures in a myxoid background (Fig. 2-92). Geographic differences in the degree of cellularity versus the

degree of myxoid change produce a vaguely nodular variation in tumor cellularity at low power. In most tumors angiodysplasia is evident within entrapped arterioles, manifested by epithelioid transformation of medial smooth muscle cells and myxoid change. Juxtaglomerular cell hyperplasia within entrapped glomeruli is observed in one-quarter of cases, a feature that may be responsible for hypertension with hyperreninism (Fig. 2-93). Heterologous stromal differentiation results in the presence of glia or cartilage in one-fifth of cases; the association of glial elements with metaplastic embryonal epithelium produces 'glial–epithelial complexes.'

Immunohistochemically, tumor cells of metanephric stromal tumor shows patchy reactivity for CD34, and no immunostaining for cytokeratins, S100 protein, or desmin.[7] Areas with glial differentiation show positive immunostaining for S100 protein and glial fibrillary acidic protein.

Metanephric stromal tumor may be difficult to distinguish from the classic type of congenital mesoblastic nephroma, as both are centered in the renal medulla and both are composed of bland spindled cells. However, congenital mesoblastic nephroma is deeply infiltrative at its interface with adjacent normal parenchyma, whereas metanephric stromal tumor has a scalloped and subtly infiltrative border. In addition, the cellularity of metanephric stromal tumor is much less uniform than that of congenital mesoblastic nephroma, resulting in a vaguely nodular appearance of metanephric stromal tumor at low power, compared to the sharply outlined, linear variations in cellularity seen in congenital mesoblastic nephroma.[457] Cellular or hypodense onion-skin perivascular collarettes, angiodysplasia, juxtaglomerular cell hyperplasia, and heterologous differentiation to glial tissue – features often observed in metanephric stromal tumor – are not seen in congenital mesoblastic nephroma. Cartilaginous differentiation may be seen in either, but is rare in congenital mesoblastic nephroma. Whereas metanephric stromal tumor commonly shows positive immunostaining for CD34, this is uncommon in congenital mesoblastic

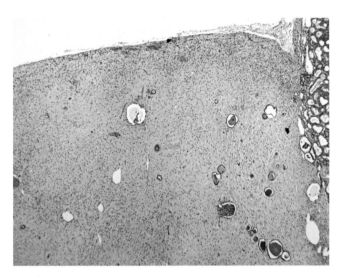

**Fig. 2-91** Metanephric stromal tumor. Spindle cell neoplasm entrapping native renal elements and subtly infiltrative at its interface with the adjacent kidney.

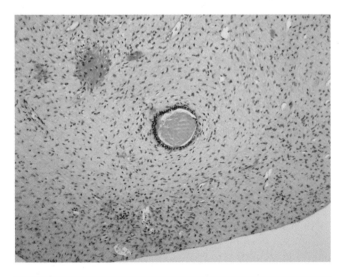

**Fig. 2-92** Metanephric stromal tumor. Spindle cells forming concentric collarettes that encircle a native tubule ('onion-skinning').

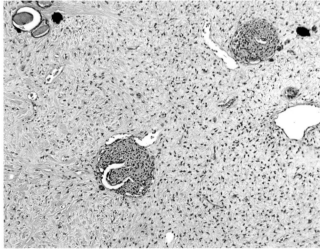

**Fig. 2-93** Metanephric stromal tumor. Entrapped glomerulus demonstrating juxtaglomerular cell hyperplasia.

nephroma. Furthermore, the oldest reported patient with congenital mesoblastic nephroma was 29 months of age, whereas about one-third of patients with metanephric stromal tumor are more than 29 months old.[479-481]

Metanephric stromal tumor may also be difficult to distinguish from spindled clear cell sarcoma of the kidney. The regular branching capillary vascular pattern characteristic of clear cell sarcoma of the kidney is not seen in metanephric stromal tumor; angiodysplasia and heterologous stromal differentiation are absent in clear cell sarcoma of the kidney.[457] Clear cell sarcoma of the kidney shows uniformly negative immunostaining for CD34, in contrast to the findings in metanephric stromal tumor.

Metanephric stromal tumor is considered benign; there are no reports of metastases or of local recurrence.[457]

## Metanephric adenofibroma

This is a rare biphasic renal neoplasm with epithelial and stromal components. It was initially designated nephrogenic adenofibroma,[476] and later renamed metanephric adenofibroma.[482] It was originally described as being composed of a spindled mesenchymal component resembling the classic type of congenital mesoblastic nephroma, admixed with an embryonal epithelial component resembling nephroblastomatosis.[476] It was later recognized that the epithelial component is indistinguishable from metanephric adenoma, and that the stromal component, in addition to being distinct from congenital mesoblastic nephroma, is morphologically identical to metanephric stromal tumor.[457,475,482]

Metanephric adenofibroma is typically a tumor of young people. Patients range in age from 5 months to 36 years (median age 30 months; mean age 72 months), with a male:female ratio of 2:1.[475] Patients with usual histology have a mean age of 10.2 years, and 50% have polycythemia. Patients whose tumors showed increased mitotic activity have a mean age of 30.5 months and have no polycythemia, and patients with composite metanephric adenofibroma/ Wilms' tumor are even younger (mean age 1 year) and also do not have polycythemia. Those with composite metanephric adenofibroma/papillary renal cell carcinoma are the oldest, with a mean age of 13.8 years, and have a low incidence of polycythemia (12.5%).[457]

Metanephric adenofibroma is typically solitary, centered in the renal medulla, and sometimes grossly papillary, occasionally protruding into the renal pelvis.[475] Tumor borders are indistinct. Tumors range in size from 1.8 to 11 cm, with a median size of 3.85 cm. Most are yellow-tan and partially cystic. Areas of hemorrhage and necrosis usually denote the presence of a component of Wilms' tumor.[475,482,483]

Microscopically, there is marked variability in the relative proportions of stromal and epithelial components. All tumors have the same stromal component, indistinguishable from metanephric stromal tumor, but there is variability in the epithelial component. Tumors with usual histology have epithelial components identical to those of metanephric adenoma, and are mitotically inactive. Other tumors have epithelial components identical to those of metanephric adenoma but focally demonstrate increased mitotic activity

(>5 mitoses/20 hpf). In addition, some are composite tumors composed of metanephric adenofibroma and Wilms' tumor, and still others are composite tumors composed of metanephric adenofibroma and papillary renal cell carcinoma composed of well-formed papillae containing stromal macrophages, and lined by cells with vesicular chromatin and abundant eosinophilic cytoplasm.[475] These areas of papillary carcinoma show strong diffuse immunostaining for CK7 and EMA, in contrast to the negative or focal weak staining for these markers shown by the metanephric adenoma-like epithelial components.

The outcome for patients with metanephric adenofibroma has been good, regardless of the nature of the epithelial component. No recurrences have been reported in 21 patients with available follow-up.[457]

## Metanephric adenosarcoma

A single case of this unique lesion has been reported.[484] The patient was a 21-year-old woman who presented with metastatic cancer and rapidly succumbed to it. The cancer originated in one kidney and was a well-demarcated 10 cm solid/cystic tumor, tan-brown, focally hemorrhagic and focally fleshy. The tumor was biphasic, consisting of an epithelial component with morphologic and immunohistochemical features typical for metanephric adenoma, admixed with a malignant spindle cell component. The metastases were morphologically, immunohistochemically and ultrastructurally similar to the spindle cell component of the renal tumor. FISH studies on the metastatic tumor showed disomy for the centromeres of chromosomes 3, 7, 12, and 17. It was concluded that the tumor was part of the spectrum of metanephric neoplasia, currently being the only reported example of a tumor in this category with a benign epithelial component and a malignant stromal component.

# Nephroblastic tumors

## Nephroblastoma (Wilms' tumor)

Reports of malignant mixed renal tumors occurred as early as 1814; however, the first accurate description of nephroblastoma was recorded in 1872.[485,486] After a long period of debate over the derivation of this tumor, Wilms[487] suggested that it was derived from undifferentiated mesoderm, so that the presence of the various morphologic elements of the tumor, such as smooth and striated muscle, bone, and rudimentary renal structures, could be satisfactorily explained by eventual differentiation into myotome, sclerotome, and nephrotome early in fetal life. His theory was generally accepted, and his name has been associated with it ever since.

Nephroblastoma accounts for about 8% of all pediatric cancers[488] and is the most common malignant renal tumor of childhood, comprising about 85% of such tumors.[5] It is the most common genitourinary cancer in children, occurring in approximately 1 in 8000–10 000 children; approximately 400 new cases are seen yearly in the United States.[489-491] Nearly 50% of nephroblastomas are seen in children under 3 years old, 90% occur in children less than 6 years old, and 98% occur in children less than 10 years old.[490,492-494] Nephroblastoma occurs slightly more often in females than in males, particularly when it is bilateral.[495] The risk of its occurrence is lowest among Asians, higher in whites, and highest among blacks.[489,496,497] Although nephroblastoma is considered relatively rare in adolescents and adults, the numbers of reported cases have been sufficient for the development of useful treatment protocols.[498,499]

The vast majority of nephroblastomas arise in the kidney; synchronous or metachronous bilateral involvement occurs in 5–10% of patients.[500,501] Oddly, patients with horseshoe kidneys have a twofold risk of developing nephroblastoma compared to the general population, for reasons that are currently unclear; management of these patients is uniquely challenging.[502-505] In addition, primary tumors that are morphologically indistinguishable from renal nephroblastomas have been reported to arise in a variety of sites, including the chest wall,[506] testis,[507-509] uterus,[510] scrotum,[511] inguinal canal,[512,513] retroperitoneum,[514,515] the sacrococcygeal region,[516,517] and in subcutaneous tissue in the lumbosacral region.[518] It is hypothesized that these extrarenal nephroblastomas arise in ectopic nephrogenic rests, a topic discussed later in this chapter. In support of this concept, ectopic nephrogenic rests have been reported in a number of extrarenal locations, including lumbosacral subcutaneous tissue,[519] adrenal gland,[520] heart,[521] colon,[522] thorax,[523,524] and the inguinal region.[525]

Nephroblastoma is a tumor that attempts to replicate the histology of the developing kidney. It is generally believed to be derived from pluripotential renal precursors that produce undifferentiated blastemal cells, primitive epithelial structures, and stromal components.[526] Despite the fact that 98–99% of cases of nephroblastoma are sporadic and unilateral,[491] nearly 10% of patients manifest clinical and biologic features that suggest an influence of predisposing germline mutations.[527] Congenital anomalies such as aniridia and genitourinary anomalies accompany nephroblastoma in 1% and 3% of cases, respectively, and about 4% of cases are accompanied by somatic overgrowth syndromes. Approximately 2% of nephroblastoma patients have a family history.[491] Furthermore, children with unilateral tumors are typically between 42 and 47 months old, whereas those with bilateral tumors have an average age of 30–33 months. Children with congenital anomalies and those with a family history tend to be diagnosed at an earlier age and tend to have an increased frequency of bilateral tumors.[489,528] These features led to the proposal that nephroblastoma may develop as a consequence of two independent rate-limiting genetic events, specifically, biallelic inactivation of a tumor-suppressor gene.[528] Subsequently, much has been learned in the past 35 years concerning the molecular genetics of nephroblastoma.

The best-characterized genetic change in nephroblastoma (Wilms' tumor) is loss of chromosomal material on the short arm of chromosome 11, the site of two distinct tumor suppressor loci. The Wilms' tumor gene (WT1) locus was initially identified in patients with Wilms' tumor, aniridia, genitourinary malformations, and mental retardation (WAGR) syndrome,[529] who were found to have constitutional deletions of 11p13.[54] The WT1 gene was identified in 1990,[530,531] and was found to encode a transcription factor of the zinc-finger family, which is critical to the survival and subsequent differentiation of renal stem cells.[532,533] The WT1 gene is altered by germline heterozygous deletions in the WAGR syndrome, by germline point mutations in the Denys–Drash syndrome (Wilms' tumor, pseudohermaphroditism, and nephropathy), and by somatic biallelic inactivation in 5–10% of sporadic Wilms' tumors.[530,531,534] Other genetic abnormalities in nephroblastoma include activating mutations in the β-catenin gene (CTNNB1) on chromosome 3p22 (often coinciding with WT1 mutations),[535] and epigenetic dysregulation of IGF2 and H19 at the Beckwith–Wiedemann syndrome locus on chromosome 11p15,[536] abnormalities of 16q,[537] gains or losses of chromosome 12, particularly polysomy for chromosome 12,[538,539] and isochrome 7q, which is uncommon in pediatric nephroblastoma, but perhaps relatively common in adult nephroblastoma.[540] It has recently been discovered that about one-third of nephroblastomas can be shown to have somatic deletions involving the WTX gene on the X chromosome.[526] The WTX gene can be inactivated by a monoallelic 'single-hit' event targeting the single X chromosome in tumors from males and the active X chromosome in tumors from females, in contrast to the typical biallelic inactivation of autosomal tumor-suppressor genes. Despite the successes noted above, the genetic abnormalities responsible for the pathogenesis of the majority of nephroblastomas have not yet been identified.[541]

The most common presenting sign of nephroblastoma is a palpable smooth, non-tender abdominal mass, detected by a parent during bathing or clothing an otherwise healthy child. Microscopic and occasionally gross hematuria is observed in 20–25% of patients, hypertension in 20%, anorexia, fever and weight loss in 10%, and flank pain or hematuria following trauma in 10%.[542,543] Anemia, polycythemia due to erythropoietin production by the tumor, free rupture into the peritoneal cavity, and symptoms related to tumor extension into the great vessels (varicocele, hepatomegaly, ascites, congestive heart failure, or sudden death due to tumor embolism) are rarely reported presentations.[542,543] Although radiologic techniques may not specifically distinguish nephroblastoma from other pediatric renal neoplasms, such imaging modalities are helpful in staging the neoplasm; furthermore, demonstration of bilaterality or multifocality is unusual in pediatric renal tumors other than nephroblastoma.[543,544] A number of presumptive tumor markers have been evaluated, but have been found to be insufficiently specific or consistent to be clinically useful.[545,546]

The great majority of nephroblastomas are solitary and unilateral; however, multifocal tumors in a single kidney are found in 7% of cases, and in 5% of cases, bilateral primary tumors are noted.[501,543,547] (Figs 2-94, 2-95). Grossly, nephroblastomas are usually sharply circumscribed and confined within a fibrous pseudocapsule, with a wide size range, and weighing up to 6 kg. Their color varies from pale gray to tan, and consistency varies from soft to firm, depending on the

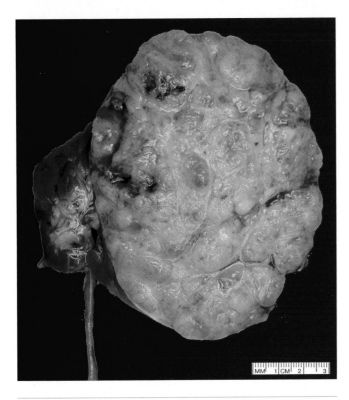

**Fig. 2-94** Wilms' tumor. Well-circumscribed tumor with a bulging cut surface and a thin fibrous pseudocapsule.

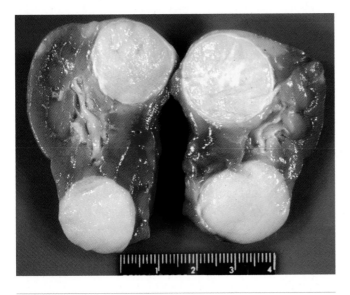

**Fig. 2-95** Wilms' tumor. Multifocal tumors in a single kidney, a finding noted in 7% of cases. (Courtesy of Beverly Dahms, MD.)

content of mature stromal elements.[548,549] Some tumors are extensively cystic; rarely, protrusion of the tumor into the renal pelvis results in a 'botryoid' appearance.[550,551]

Histologically, most nephroblastomas are triphasic, containing elements of blastema, epithelium and stroma in varying proportions; however, biphasic and monophasic nephroblastomas also occur (Fig. 2-96). Each cell or tissue type can exhibit a variable degree of differentiation.

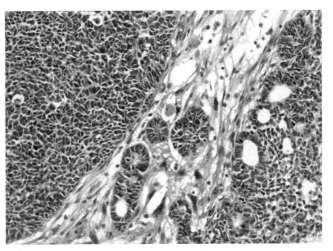

**Fig. 2-96** Wilms' tumor. Three histologic components are typically present: blastema, epithelium forming tubules, and stroma.

Blastema consists of cells that are small, round, densely packed and overlapping, with minimal cytoplasm and little evidence of differentiation. Their nuclei are round or polygonal, relatively uniform in size, with evenly dispersed chromatin and small nucleoli. Abundant mitotic figures are usually present. Blastema exhibits a number of different growth patterns – diffuse, nodular, serpentine, and basaloid – and these are often admixed within a given tumor. The diffuse pattern is characterized by lack of circumscription at the periphery of the tumor, accompanied by extensive invasion of adjacent soft tissues. Nodular and serpentine patterns show sharply defined round or undulating cords or nests of blastemal cells in a myxoid or fibromyxoid stroma, and if a distinctive layer of epithelial cells is arrayed at the periphery of these cell groups, the pattern is designated basaloid.[527,548,549]

The epithelial component, present in most nephroblastomas, is characterized by tubular and occasionally glomeruloid structures that recapitulate the developmental stages of metanephric tubules. The tubules range from primitive rosette-like structures virtually indistinguishable from similar structures seen in neuroblastomas to easily recognizable tubular structures with small lumina. Glomerular structures, reminiscent of those seen in normal kidneys but usually lacking capillaries, are seen in some tumors (Fig. 2-97). An appearance of epithelial maturation may be evident, particularly after therapy; foci of readily recognizable squamous, mucinous, or even ciliated epithelium may be present.[527,548,549]

The stromal component exhibits considerable diversity in its relative abundance and patterns of differentiation. Most often it comprises spindle cells in a myxoid background, resembling embryonal mesenchyme. Skeletal muscle with varying degrees of differentiation is the most commonly observed heterologous stromal component. Other differentiation patterns seen in the stromal component of nephroblastoma include smooth muscle, fibrous tissue, cartilage, bone, adipose tissue, and neuroglia and mature ganglion cells.

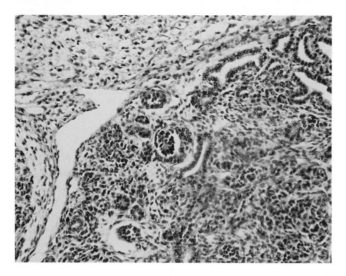

**Fig. 2-97** Wilms' tumor. Blastema, tubules, and a glomerular structure lacking capillaries.

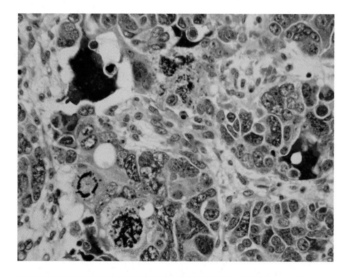

**Fig. 2-98** Wilms' tumor. Nuclear anaplasia: nuclear hyperchromasia and gigantism with multipolar mitotic figures.

In the absence of unfavorable histology most nephroblastomas are highly responsive to chemotherapy. Unfavorable histology is characterized by the presence of nuclear anaplasia, and less commonly by the secondary development of a high-grade sarcoma or carcinoma within a nephroblastoma.[549,552–556] Nuclear anaplasia denotes nuclear hyperchromasia and gigantism with multipolar mitotic figures (Fig. 2-98). It is the cytologic manifestation of extreme polyploidy of tumor cells and is associated with multiple chromosomal rearrangements.[557,558] It can be found in about 5% of nephroblastomas overall; it is rare in tumors from patients less than 2 years old, but its incidence gradually increases to 13% in tumors from patients 5 years of age or older. The definition of anaplasia requires that the nucleus must be hyperchromatic and that all its major dimensions must be at least three times larger than those of neighboring non-anaplastic nuclei.

Each component of the abnormal metaphase of the multipolar polyploid mitotic figures must be as large as, or larger than, a normal metaphase.[548,549]

Anaplasia is significant primarily because its presence portends resistance to chemotherapy and a significantly lower failure-free survival rate.[554,556,559] However, patients with focal anaplasia have outcomes similar to those of patients with favorable histology,[557] whereas an unfavorable outcome is more likely when anaplasia is diffusely distributed throughout the tumor and when present in tumors of advanced stage. Focal anaplasia denotes the presence of one or a few well localized foci of anaplasia within a primary tumor, and criteria for its designation are very restrictive. The diagnosis of focal anaplasia requires reasonable certainty that the entire focus is circumscribed and its periphery has been evaluated, that the anaplastic cells are within renal parenchyma only (not in vascular spaces or in extrarenal sites), and that no 'nuclear unrest' is apparent in non-anaplastic tumor.

Nuclear unrest denotes the presence of disturbing nuclear enlargement, cytologic atypia, and histologic disarray, but without the enlarged multipolar mitotic figures required to meet the criteria for anaplasia. Patients with nuclear unrest are treated adequately by the same protocols used for patients with favorable histology.[560]

Mutations of the p53 gene are known to be associated with anaplasia in nephroblastomas. However, there are inconsistencies between p53 protein overexpression and anaplasia; consequently, p53 expression has not been used as an element in the development of treatment protocols.[549,561–566]

Immunohistochemistry has not been of substantial utility in the pathologic evaluation of nephroblastoma. Nuclear immunostaining for WT1 can be demonstrated in the blastemal and epithelial components of nephroblastoma, but this finding is non-specific, having been demonstrated in other tumors, including desmoplastic small round cell tumor, leukemia, and various carcinomas.[527,549,567,568]

The key determinant of stage is the anatomic extent of tumor invasion. The staging system accepted most widely for staging nephroblastoma is that of the National Wilms' Tumor Study Group (NWTSG-5)[569] (Table 2-7). This takes into account penetration of the renal capsule, involvement of renal sinus vessels, surgical margins, regional lymph nodes, distant metastases, and bilaterality at presentation. Therapy is based on stage, patient age, tumor size, histologic features, and biologic indicators of poor prognosis, such as loss of heterozygosity for specific loci.[549]

Nephroblastomas have limited and usually predictable local and metastatic growth patterns. They extend locally into perirenal soft tissues, renal vein and vena cava (Fig. 2-99). Metastases are most commonly to regional lymph nodes, lungs and liver, and less frequently to the spinal epidural space, central nervous system, and mediastinal lymph nodes following lung metastasis.[570,571] Bone metastasis is quite unusual. Four-year overall survival rates of 96%, 91%, 90%, and 81% are achieved in patients with stage I, II, III, and IV tumors with favorable histology, respectively.[569] Four-year survival rates of 70%, 56%, and 17% are recorded in

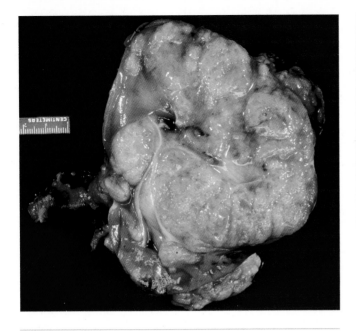

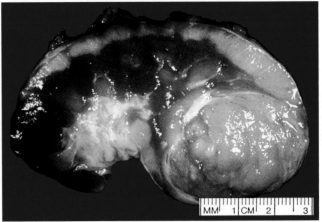

**Fig. 2-100** Nephrogenic rests. Diffuse hyperplastic perilobar nephroblastomatosis: a more or less continuous subcapsular band of nephrogenic rests, associated with a Wilms' tumor, status post preoperative chemotherapy; patient had bilateral Wilms' tumors. (Courtesy of Beverly Dahms, MD.)

**Fig. 2-99** Wilms' tumor. This tumor involved the soft tissues of the renal sinus and extended into the renal vein. (Courtesy of Beverly Dahms, MD.)

**Table 2-7** North American National Wilms' Tumor Study Group Staging System for Renal Tumors[568]

| Stage | Definition |
|-------|-----------|
| I | Tumor limited to the kidney and is resected completely |
| II | Tumor extends beyond kidney and is resected completely<br>Tumor penetrates renal capsule<br>Infiltration into renal sinus vessels<br>Infiltration to adjacent organs or vena cava, but tumor completely resected<br>Biopsy of tumor before removal<br>Tumor spillage focally |
| III | Residual tumor present and confined to the abdomen<br>Resection margins positive for tumor<br>Transected tumor thrombus<br>Inoperable tumor<br>Lymph nodes of abdomen or pelvis involved by tumor<br>Tumor implants on peritoneal surfaces<br>Tumor spillage into peritoneal cavity |
| IV | Hematogenous metastasis or lymph node metastasis outside abdomen and pelvis |
| V | Bilateral renal involvement at diagnosis<br>Tumor in each kidney should be substaged separately |

patients with stage II, III, and IV tumors with unfavorable histology, respectively.[556]

## Nephrogenic rests and nephroblastomatosis

More than one-third of kidneys resected for Wilms' tumor contain putative precursor lesions, which have been designated nephrogenic rests.[572,573] Nephrogenic rests are the result of the abnormal persistence of embryonal cells or their derivatives into postnatal life; they are found in less than 1%

of infants during routine autopsy examination, and are only rarely of intralobar type in this setting.[572-576] There are two distinct categories of nephrogenic rest: perilobar and intralobar.[574,575]

Perilobar nephrogenic rests (PLNR) are strictly confined to the periphery of the renal lobe. They are composed of blastema, embryonal epithelial cells and scant stroma, have an ovoid shape and a subcapsular location, and are sharply demarcated from the adjacent renal parenchyma. Dormant or incipient rests show no features of involution or proliferation. Nephrogenic rests may undergo maturation, sclerosis, involution, obsolescence and eventual disappearance.[574,575] PLNRs that exhibit focal or diffuse overgrowth of blastemal or embryonal epithelial cell types are designated 'hyperplastic rests.' In extreme cases, when one or occasionally both kidneys are involved by a more or less continuous subcapsular band of nephrogenic rests, the condition is designated 'diffuse hyperplastic perilobar nephroblastomatosis'[577] (Figs 2-100, 2-101). The blastema and embryonal epithelium that comprise hyperplastic PLNRs show marked proliferative changes, including abundant mitotic activity and prominent nucleoli. Hyperplastic PLNRs interface directly with adjacent normal renal tissue and lack the pseudocapsule that characterizes nephroblastoma. Furthermore, hyperplastic PLNRs remain subcapsular and tend to be ovoid, in contrast to the spherical expansile growth seen in nephroblastoma. Distinction between the two entities may be virtually impossible on a limited biopsy specimen.

Intralobar nephrogenic rests (ILNRs) can be located anywhere in the renal lobe, and may also be identified in the renal sinus and the walls of the pelvicalyceal system. They are composed of multiple cell types, including abundant immature or mature stroma, and lie between normal nephrons, forming an indistinct interdigitating interface with the adjacent normal tissue (Fig. 2-102). Like PLNRs, ILNRs may be dormant, obsolescent or hyperplastic. Overgrowth in

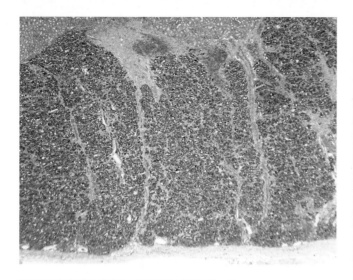

**Fig. 2-101** Nephrogenic rests. Diffuse hyperplastic perilobar nephroblastomatosis, status post preoperative chemotherapy; the patient had bilateral Wilms' tumors.

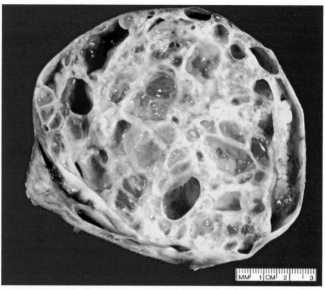

**Fig. 2-103** Cystic partially differentiated nephroblastoma. Tumor is entirely composed of cysts of variable size, and entirely lacks expansile nodules of tumor. (Courtesy of Beverly Dahms, MD.)

## Cystic partially differentiated nephroblastoma

Cystic partially differentiated nephroblastoma is a multilocular cystic Wilms' tumor composed entirely of cysts separated by delicate septa; within the septa are small foci of blastema, primitive or immature epithelium, and immature-appearing stromal cells.[579,580] Virtually all such tumors are identified in children less than 24 months old, and males are affected about twice as often as females.[215] Some of these neoplasms contain no nephroblastomatous elements, and tumors of this sort have been designated 'cystic nephroma,' recognizing that these lesions are distinctly different on many levels from morphologically similar tumors that occur predominantly in adult women.[215]

Cystic partially differentiated nephroblastomas are typically well circumscribed and clearly demarcated from the adjacent normal kidney. They range up to 18 cm in diameter, are entirely composed of cysts of variable size, and entirely lack expansile nodules of tumor[215] (Fig. 2-103).

The cysts are lined by flat, cuboidal or hobnail cells; sometimes no lining epithelium is evident.[580] The septa exhibit variable cellularity and contain blastema, nephroblastomatous epithelial elements in the form of luminal structures resembling tubules and ill-formed papillary structures resembling immature glomeruli, and undifferentiated and differentiated mesenchymal elements, most often in the form of skeletal muscle and myxoid mesenchyme, less often cartilage and fat (Fig. 2-104). Septal elements may form microscopic papillary infoldings within the cysts, or in the papillonodular variant may form grossly evident polyps protruding into cystic spaces.[581]

Complete surgical excision cures cystic partially differentiated nephroblastoma.[581–583] A single reported case of recurrence may have been related to incomplete surgical resection.

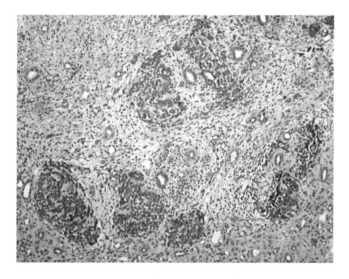

**Fig. 2-102** Nephrogenic rests. Intralobar nephrogenic rests, composed of blastema and immature tubules, forming an indistinct interdigitating interface with the adjacent normal tissue.

ILNRs is usually triphasic, involving stromal prominence, often with heterologous elements.

ILNRs progress to nephroblastoma significantly more often than do PLNRs, and are associated more commonly with WT1 mutations and congenital syndromes. PLNRs rarely progress to malignancy, but there is a strong association between the presence of PLNRs and the development of metachronous bilateral nephroblastoma in children under the age of 12 months.

The treatment of hyperplastic nephroblastomatosis is controversial.[578] Patients with diffuse hyperplastic nephroblastomatosis are commonly treated with chemotherapy, as the risk of development of multiple nephroblastoma as well as anaplastic nephroblastomas is exceptionally high.[549]

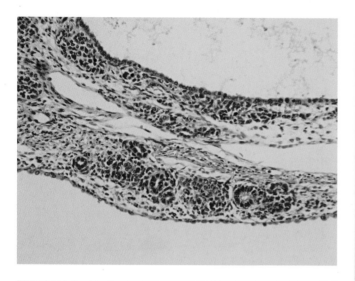

**Fig. 2-104** Cystic partially differentiated nephroblastoma. The delicate septa contain blastema and immature tubules.

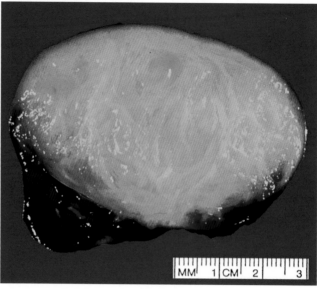

**Fig. 2-105** Congenital mesoblastic nephroma. This example was of the classic type; it has a whorled and myomatous-appearing cut surface. (Courtesy of Beverly Dahms, MD.)

## Mesenchymal tumors occurring mainly in children

### Congenital mesoblastic nephroma

Congenital mesoblastic nephroma was first recognized in 1967.[584] It occurs in approximately 1 in 500 000 infants,[585] accounts for about 4% of malignant renal tumors in children,[541] and has a predilection for very young children. In infants less than 3 months old it is the most common renal neoplasm, and virtually all cases have occurred in children less than 30 months old.[586] It is typically discovered as a palpable abdominal mass. Some are identified in utero by ultrasound, and some cases have been associated with polyhydramnios, hydrops fetalis, and premature delivery.[587–589] Reported tumor-associated biochemical abnormalities include hypercalcemia due to prostaglandin E production by tumor cells,[590] and hyperreninism, probably due to local tumor effects rather than by renin production by tumor cells.[591]

Congenital mesoblastic nephroma is typically unilateral and solitary. It varies in size from 0.8 to 14 cm in greatest dimension, with a mean of 6.2 cm. Most tumors involve the renal sinus.[586,592] There are two variants, designated classic and cellular, with different macroscopic, microscopic and genetic characteristics, and some tumors are composed of mixtures of these elements. Classic congenital mesoblastic nephroma, accounting for about 24% of cases, is typically firm and may exhibit a whorled and myomatous texture; its interface with the adjacent normal kidney is not sharply demarcated (Fig. 2-105). Cellular congenital mesoblastic nephroma, comprising 66% of cases, is more often bulging and soft, with areas of hemorrhage, necrosis, and cystic degeneration, and its interface is the adjacent normal kidney is more sharply delineated[584,586,592–594] (Fig. 2-106).

Microscopically, classic congenital mesoblastic nephroma is composed of bland fibroblastic/myofibroblastic cells

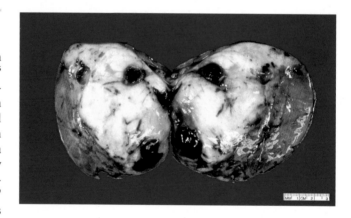

**Fig. 2-106** Congenital mesoblastic nephroma. This cellular mesoblastic nephroma has a bulging cut surface, and areas of hemorrhage and cystic degeneration. (Courtesy of Beverly Dahms, MD.)

arranged in fascicles, with only rare mitotic figures and no necrosis; it is indistinguishable from infantile fibromatosis. It subtly infiltrates adjacent tissues, surrounding islands of native kidney at the interface between tumor and normal renal parenchyma[586,592] (Figs 2-107, 2-108). Long narrow tongues of tumor typically extend into perirenal soft tissue, particularly in the renal hilum.

Cellular congenital mesoblastic nephroma is microscopically indistinguishable from infantile fibrosarcoma.[586,592] It is expansile, with a 'pushing' but unencapsulated border at its interface with normal kidney (Fig. 2-109). It is more densely cellular than the classic variant, and its architecture is more sheet-like than fascicular. It is composed of monomorphic sheets of closely packed small cells with vesicular nuclei and minimal cytoplasm, which may impart a small blue cell appearance (Fig. 2-110). Tumor cells may become

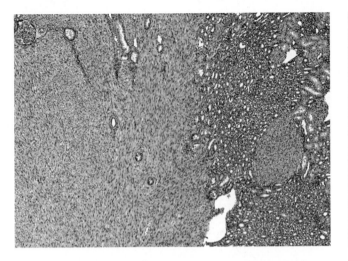

**Fig. 2-107** Congenital mesoblastic nephroma. Classic type of mesoblastic nephroma, composed of bland spindle cells that infiltrate between and around adjacent native renal structures.

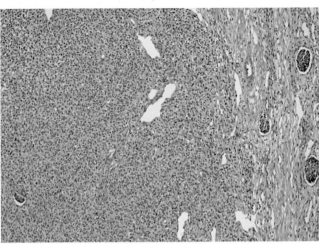

**Fig. 2-109** Congenital mesoblastic nephroma. Cellular type of mesoblastic nephroma, densely cellular, with an expansile pushing border where it meets normal kidney.

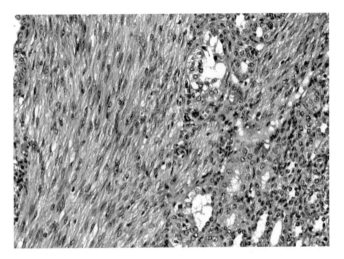

**Fig. 2-108** Congenital mesoblastic nephroma. Classic type of mesoblastic nephroma, composed of spindle cells that lack cytologic atypia or mitotic activity.

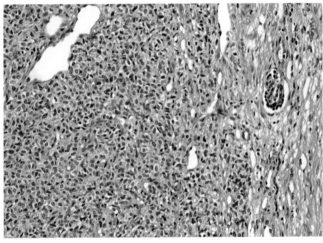

**Fig. 2-110** Congenital mesoblastic nephroma. Cellular type of mesoblastic nephroma, composed of monomorphic sheets of closely packed small cells with vesicular nuclei and minimal cytoplasm.

plump and elongated with slight to moderate nuclear pleomorphism. The presence of tumor cells with prominent nuclei on a background of necrosis may raise concern for rhabdoid tumor. Mitotic figures and necrosis are readily apparent. Mixed congenital mesoblastic nephroma is composed of classic and cellular elements in variable proportions; the classic variant is often seen at the periphery of a centrally expansile nodule of cellular congenital mesoblastic nephroma.

Tumor cells of both variants of congenital mesoblastic nephroma show positive immunostaining for vimentin. They often show positive immunostaining for actin and rarely for desmin. They show no immunostaining for cytokeratins, CD34, Bcl-2, or WT-1, a feature that can help distinguish congenital mesoblastic nephroma from other spindle cell renal tumors in children, specifically primitive undifferentiated stromal Wilms' tumor, clear cell sarcoma of the kidney, and synovial sarcoma.[592,595] Immunostaining for WT-1 is usually positive in primitive undifferentiated stromal Wilms' tumors. Immunostaining for Bcl-2 is positive in synovial sarcomas, primitive undifferentiated stromal Wilms' tumors, and some clear cell sarcomas of the kidney. CD34 outlines the evenly distributed septal capillaries characteristic of clear cell sarcoma of the kidney. It has recently been shown that gene expression profile analysis is a powerful tool for separating these four entities, when used in conjunction with traditional diagnostic tools.[541] Ultrastructurally, tumor cells of congenital mesoblastic nephroma have features of fibroblasts or myofibroblasts.

Classic congenital mesoblastic nephroma is usually diploid, whereas cellular congenital mesoblastic nephroma often shows aneuploidy of chromosomes 11, 8, and 17.[594,596,597] A specific translocation, t(12; 15)(p13; q25), resulting in fusion of the *ETV6* and *NTRK3* genes, characterizes cellular congenital mesoblastic nephroma, but is not found in classic congenital mesoblastic nephroma.[598,599] This translocation and gene fusion is identical to that seen in infantile fibrosarcoma, and is not seen in infantile fibromatosis. It seems appropriate to regard cellular congenital mesoblastic nephroma and infantile fibrosarcomas as a single neoplastic entity, arising in either renal or soft tissue locations.[586,599] It also seems appropriate to draw an analogy between classic congenital mesoblastic nephroma and infantile fibromatosis.[600]

Complete surgical excision is curative in 95% of cases of congenital mesoblastic nephroma.[586,594,600] Recurrences are generally attributed to incomplete resection, and are not related to the variant of tumor.[600] Rarely, tumor-related deaths associated with hematogenous metastases have been reported.[601,602]

## Rhabdoid tumor of kidney

Rhabdoid tumor of the kidney (RTK) was first described in 1978.[552] It accounts for about 2–3% of malignant renal tumors in children.[541,586] Although the component cells resemble rhabdomyoblasts, the tumor does not exhibit muscle differentiation. The cell of origin of RTK is not known. The occurrence is limited to patients less than 5 years old; more than 80% occur in children less than 2 years old, and the median age is 1 year.

In approximately 15% of cases of RTK a brain tumor, most often located in the midline cerebellum, is present simultaneously or becomes apparent a short time later.[603] Most associated brain tumors resemble medulloblastomas, primitive neuroectodermal tumors, or atypical teratoid/rhabdoid tumors,[586,592,604] and have been shown to be second primaries rather than metastases from RTK.[605,606] The molecular hallmark of RTK is biallelic inactivation of the *hSNF5/INI1* tumor-suppressor gene located on the long arm of chromosome 22,[607] a finding that is shared by rhabdoid tumors occurring in the soft tissue, brain, and other tissue sites.

Rhabdoid tumors of the kidney are usually unicentric and unilateral.[592] Most weigh less than 500 g. They are typically bulging, soft, and pale, sometimes with hemorrhage and/or necrosis, and with an ill-defined interface with the adjacent normal kidney[592,603] (Fig. 2-111). Satellite tumor nodules may be evident.[586] Microscopically, RTK is composed of monotonous sheets of loosely cohesive cells with distinct cell borders. The tumor cells are large and polygonal, and characteristically show vesicular nuclei, single cherry-red nucleoli of variable prominence, and juxtanuclear, globular, eosinophilic cytoplasmic inclusions, which are ultrastructurally whorled intermediate filaments. Not all tumor cells contain cytoplasmic inclusions, and cells with such inclusions tend to be clustered rather than diffusely distributed (Figs 2-112, 2-113). Rhabdoid tumors demonstrate aggressive infiltration of adjacent renal parenchyma, and extensive vascular invasion is common.[586,592,608]

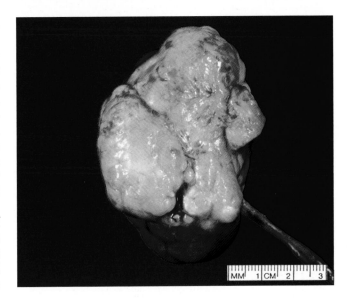

**Fig. 2-111** Rhabdoid tumor of kidney. Tumor is bulging and soft, and pale, with an ill-defined interface with adjacent normal kidney.

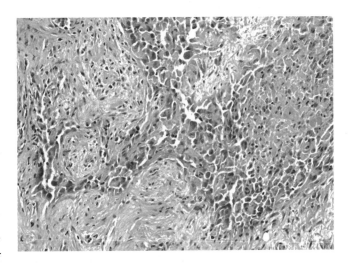

**Fig. 2-112** Rhabdoid tumor of kidney. Sheets of large polygonal loosely cohesive cells with eccentric nuclei; tumor necrosis is evident.

Immunohistochemically, tumor cells of RTK most consistently show positive staining for vimentin, and focal but intense staining for epithelial membrane antigen (EMA). Expression of other markers, including cytokeratin, neuron-specific enolase, S100 protein, CD99, desmin, and Leu 7, is inconsistent. Immunostaining for INI1 is uniformly negative in RTK, but is retained in virtually all tumors that enter into the differential diagnosis. Gene expression profile analysis, used in conjunction with traditional diagnostic tools, has recently been shown to be a powerful tool for separating RTK from Wilms' tumor, clear cell sarcoma of kidney, and cellular mesoblastic nephroma.[541]

Rhabdoid tumor of the kidney is aggressive and lethal. In most cases disease stage is advanced at presentation. To date, no satisfactory treatment for children with RTK has been reported; 5-year survival rates range from 10% to 23%.[586,609]

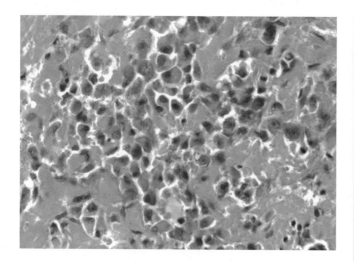

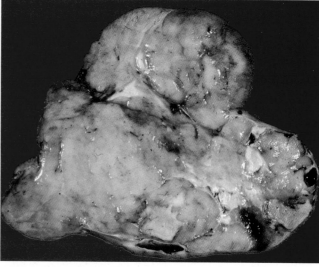

**Fig. 2-113** Rhabdoid tumor of kidney. Tumor cells bear some resemblance to rhabdomyoblasts; they bear juxtanuclear, globular, eosinophilic cytoplasmic inclusions.

**Fig. 2-114** Clear cell sarcoma of kidney. Soft bulging tumor that has almost obliterated the underlying normal kidney. (Courtesy of Beverly Dahms, MD.)

## Clear cell sarcoma of kidney

The existence of a pediatric renal sarcoma with a propensity to metastasize to bone was reported in 1970,[610] and further delineated in 1978 in three separate reports under three different names,[552,611,612] of which 'clear cell sarcoma' eventually became the accepted term for this neoplasm.

Clear cell sarcoma of the kidney (CCSK) comprises approximately 3% of all pediatric renal neoplasms[586] and is seen in patients ranging from 2 months old to 14 years; approximately 50% of patients are in their second or third year of life, and mean age at diagnosis is 3 years.[613] Male patients outnumber females by a ratio of 2:1. CCSK is not familial, is not associated with any known syndrome or with renal dysplasia, and only rarely associated with nephrogenic rests. Recurring findings of translocation t(10; 17) and interstitial deletions of chromosome 14q have been reported, but the significance of these findings is currently unclear.[541,614,615] The cell of origin of CCSK is unknown.

Most CCSK are large unicentric masses that greatly distort or nearly efface the native kidney (Fig. 2-114). Tumors are well circumscribed and sharply demarcated from the adjacent kidney. Apparent origin in the renal medulla is noted in some cases.[478] Tumors range in size from 2.3 to 24 cm in diameter (mean 11.3 cm). Cut surfaces are generally gray-tan, soft, and mucoid, and cysts are noted in most, sometimes representing the dominant gross finding. Hemorrhage and small foci of necrosis are commonly observed, and extension of tumor into the renal vein is present in 5% of cases. Lymph node metastases are present in approximately 30% of patients at the time of diagnosis. Microscopically, tumor cells are separated by regularly spaced fibrovascular septa coursing through the tumor, frequently creating vascular arcades that divide the tumor cells into cords or columns 4–10 cells in width.[478,616] The width of the fibrovascular septa varies considerably, from thin 'chicken-wire' capillaries to capillaries surrounded by sheaths of spindle cells in a collagenous matrix. In classic cases the tumor cells within the

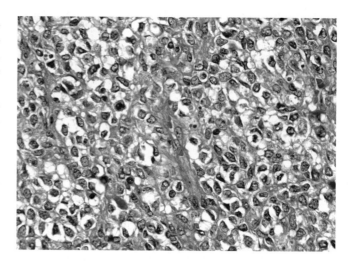

**Fig. 2-115** Clear cell sarcoma of kidney. Tumor cells are plump, ovoid and spindled, with fairly uniform round or oval nuclei, separated by optically clear extracellular mucopolysaccharide matrix material, imparting a clear cell appearance.

cords are plump and ovoid or spindled, with fairly uniform nuclei that are round to oval and often vesicular, with finely dispersed chromatin, inconspicuous nucleoli and infrequent mitotic figures. Tumor cells are separated by optically clear material which consists of extracellular mucopolysaccharide matrix, imparting a clear cell appearance (Fig. 2-115). Tubules and glomeruli are typically entrapped at the periphery of the tumor, and cystic dilation of these tubules may simulate cystic nephroma.

Although about 90% of CCSK exhibit classic microscopic findings, the majority show one of several variant patterns, creating some extraordinarily difficult diagnostic challenges.[6] In the myxoid pattern, cord cells are separated by pools of amphophilic mucinous material. In the sclerosing pattern, osteoid-like material compresses residual cord cells. In the cellular pattern, small nodules of overlapping cord cells may simulate blastemal condensations of Wilms' tumor. The epithelioid patterns, both acinar and trabecular, mimic the tubules of Wilms' tumor and carcinoma, respectively. The palisading pattern simulates the Verocay bodies of schwannoma, the storiform pattern resembles fibrohistiocytic neoplasms, and the purely spindle cell variant is difficult to distinguish from monophasic synovial sarcoma and cellular congenital mesoblastic nephroma. Anaplasia, defined by the same criteria used in Wilms' tumor, is noted in about 3% of cases.[6]

Immunohistochemically, the cord cells of CCSK usually show positive staining for vimentin, and for Bcl-2 in about 50% of cases.[586,595] Immunostains for CD34, S100 protein, desmin, CD99, cytokeratin, and EMA are uniformly negative.[613] CD34 highlights the evenly distributed septal capillaries characteristic of CCSK.[595] Nuclear staining for hSNF5/INI1 is positive, a feature that may assist in separating CCSK from rhabdoid tumor.[617] Furthermore, when used in conjunction with traditional diagnostic tools, gene expression profile analysis has recently been shown to be a powerful tool for distinguishing between CCSK, Wilms' tumor, rhabdoid tumor of kidney, and cellular mesoblastic nephroma.[541]

The overall long-term survival for patients with CCSK is approximately 69%.[478,614] When relapse occurs, it is generally within 4 years of treatment (although later relapses occasionally occur) and is most commonly in bone, followed by lung metastases. The fact that doxorubicin therapy is demonstrably beneficial to patients with CCSK emphasizes the importance of an accurate diagnosis. Remarkably, 98% of stage I patients survive. Survival rates are best for patients between 2 and 4 years old; patients older or younger than this fare worse.[478]

## Ossifying renal tumor of infancy

Ossifying renal tumor of infancy (ORTI) was first described in 1980, and so far only about a dozen cases have been reported.[618–620] ORTI is clinically, radiologically, and morphologically distinct from all other pediatric renal tumors. The majority of patients are males. Patients range in age from 6 days to 17 months old at the time of diagnosis. Most present with gross hematuria,[619,620] or rarely a palpable mass. Radiologic studies disclose upper collecting system abnormalities: dilatation, distortion, filling defects and/or obstructions, associated with punctate calcifications or a calcified mass within the collecting system. The renal contour is not distorted.[619]

At operation, a polypoid neoplasm is noted to be attached to the renal medulla, growing exophytically into the pelvicalyceal system and sometimes reminiscent of a staghorn calculus. In one case, two neoplasms were observed.[619] Although the largest ORTI measured 6.5 cm, most are 2–3 cm in diameter. ORTI is typically firm to hard, sometimes compressing adjacent renal tissue.[619,620] On sectioning, ORTI is usually pink-white or tan-white and solid, rarely with small cysts.

Microscopically, ORTI appears to originate in the papilla of the medullary pyramids. It is composed of proliferating spindle cells admixed with partially calcified osteoid matrix. The precise nature of the spindle cells is unknown. No cases of ORTI have been associated with Wilms' tumor or with WT1/WT2 gene syndromes.

ORTI is regarded as a benign tumor, and conservative surgical excision is recommended whenever possible.[619]

# Mesenchymal tumors occurring mainly in adults

## Leiomyosarcoma

Leiomyosarcoma, a malignant neoplasm demonstrating smooth muscle differentiation, is the most common primary renal sarcoma, accounting for only approximately 0.5% of all primary renal malignancies but comprising 50–60% of primary renal sarcomas.[419,621–624] Slightly more than 100 cases have been reported. Nearly all occur in adults, with a mean age of about 58 years[623] and with no striking gender difference. Renal leiomyosarcoma may arise from the renal parenchyma, renal capsule, main renal vein, or smooth muscle of the renal pelvis, and rarely, in a background of renal angiomyolipoma[622,624–626] (Fig. 2-116). Presenting symptoms may include hematuria, flank pain, fever, or

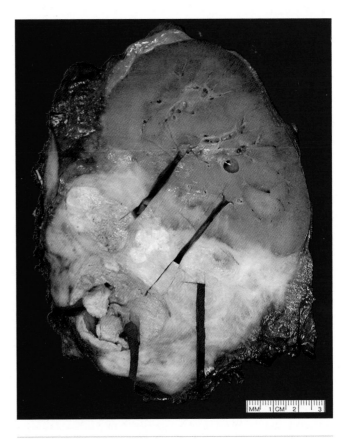

**Fig. 2-116** Leiomyosarcoma of kidney. This tumor arose in a background of renal angiomyolipoma; it diffusely infiltrates normal kidney and surrounding soft tissues, with abundant necrosis. (Courtesy of John Miedler, MD.)

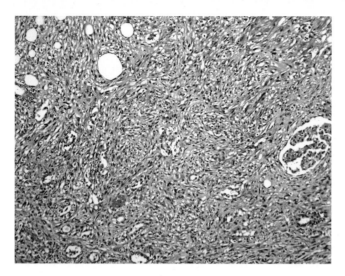

**Fig. 2-117** Leiomyosarcoma of kidney. Same case as shown in Figure 2-116. Spindle cell neoplasm diffusely infiltrating native kidney. Adipose cells of underlying angiomyolipoma visible at upper left.

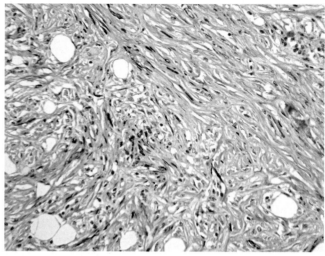

**Fig. 2-118** Leiomyosarcoma of kidney. Same case as shown in Figure 2-116. Spindled tumor cells show positive immunostaining for smooth muscle actin.

symptoms related to metastases; in some patients a mass is palpable.[419,623,627–630]

Tumor size is variable: most are large (up to 23 cm)[622] and solid. Necrosis is seen in up to 90% of cases,[623] and cystic degeneration may be apparent. Tumors are generally well circumscribed and may appear encapsulated.[623,629,630] They are typically gray-white, and soft to firm; some have a whorled cut surface. The microscopic features of renal leiomyosarcoma are similar to those of leiomyosarcoma in other sites, composed of spindled non-tapered eosinophilic cells with blunt-ended nuclei, having a fascicular, plexiform or haphazard architecture (Fig. 2-117). Nuclear pleomorphism is evident in a variable proportion of cases. Mitotic rates are remarkably variable, with a mean of 10.6/10 hpf. Myxoid change – usually focal, but sometimes extensive – is frequently observed. Microscopic vascular invasion is commonly noted.

Immunohistochemically, tumor cells typically show positive staining for smooth muscle actin, desmin, calponin, and h-caldesmon (Fig. 2-118). Most show negative immunostaining for cytokeratins, HMB-45, and S100 protein.[623]

Leiomyosarcomas must be distinguished from sarcomatoid renal cell or urothelial carcinoma, angiomyolipoma, and leiomyoma. The distinction from sarcomatoid carcinoma can be difficult, as both can express smooth muscle actin as well as cytokeratins. Desmin and h-caldesmon are usually positive in leiomyosarcoma and negative in sarcomatoid carcinoma. In the distinction of leiomyoma from leiomyosarcoma, tumors exhibiting necrosis, nuclear pleomorphism, and more than rare mitotic figures are considered malignant. Angiomyolipomas generally express melanocytic markers and α-smooth muscle actin, and are negative for S100 protein and desmin.[623] It should be noted, however, that leiomyosarcoma can arise in a background of angiomyolipoma (Figs 2-117 and 2-118).[631]

The prognosis for renal leiomyosarcoma is generally poor: 3-year survival rate was 20% and median survival period was 18 months in one large series.[622] Most tumors are grade 2 or 3. It is notable that patients with low-grade leiomyosarcomas have a relatively favorable prognosis;[623,630] those with high-grade tumors fare poorly.

## Angiosarcoma

Only 2% of all soft tissue sarcomas are angiosarcomas, and less than 5% of angiosarcomas arise in the genitourinary tract.[632] About two dozen cases of renal angiosarcoma have been reported. Mean patient age is 58 years, with a range of 30–77 years, and the great majority of patients are older white males. There are no known etiologic predisposing factors. In one remarkable instance, two brothers developed renal angiosarcoma.[633]

Patients present with hematuria, weight loss, flank pain, hematuria, or symptoms related to metastatic cancer.[632–636] Tumors vary in size up to 23 cm. They have ill-defined borders, are hemorrhagic, yellow to gray-tan, soft, sometimes necrotic, and locally infiltrative.

Microscopically, renal angiosarcoma is similar to angiosarcoma in other sites, exhibiting vasoformative architecture with channels resembling vascular spaces and sinusoids containing red blood cells, lined by pleomorphic epithelioid cells, as well as areas that are more solid, composed of plump atypical spindle cells with eosinophilic cytoplasm, pleomorphic nuclei, and frequent mitotic figures[632,633,635,636] (Fig. 2-119). Tumor cells show positive immunostaining for factor CD31 and CD34.

The prognosis for renal angiosarcoma is uniformly poor.[632–636] Many patients have metastatic cancer at the time of diagnosis, or develop metastases shortly thereafter. Mean survival time after diagnosis is 7.7 months.

## Malignant fibrous histiocytoma

Primary malignant fibrous histiocytoma of the kidney is rare. Its true incidence is difficult to ascertain. Of 17 renal

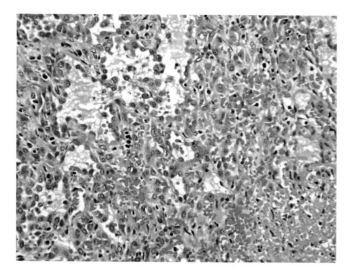

**Fig. 2-119** Renal angiosarcoma. This tumor in a 48-year-old man shows vasoformative architecture with channels resembling vascular spaces and sinusoids containing red blood cells, lined by pleomorphic epithelioid and spindled cells.

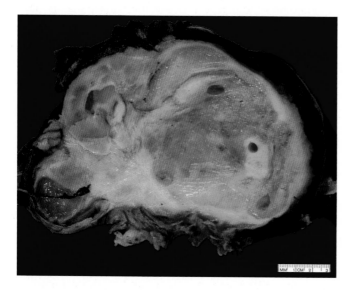

**Fig. 2-120** Malignant fibrous histiocytoma. Tumor invades and largely obliterates native kidney; in this case, the tumor was deemed to have originated in the retroperitoneum and involved the kidney secondarily.

sarcomas in one series, only two were diagnosed as malignant fibrous histiocytoma,[622] and only a few reported cases are well documented.[2-5] It is also difficult to ascertain in some instances whether the kidney was involved primarily or by extension from a retroperitoneal primary (Fig. 2-120).

Patients are middle-aged or older, with equal gender distribution. They present with abdominal or flank pain, weight loss, hematuria, and/or fever, and the majority have palpable tumors.[624,637-640] Tumors vary in size up to 27 cm, and exhibit hemorrhage and necrosis. The majority show a storiform–pleomorphic appearance typical of malignant fibrous histiocytoma in other sites.

Owing to the paucity of well-documented cases the prognosis is difficult to estimate; however, there appear to be few long-term survivors.[622,624,640]

## Hemangiopericytoma

Hemangiopericytoma is a neoplasm believed to be derived from pericytes, contractile cells with processes that wrap around capillaries and aid in autoregulation of blood flow.[641] There are fewer than 30 reported cases of hemangiopericytoma of the kidney, and in at least half of these the tumor involved only the renal capsule or adjacent soft tissues, without renal parenchymal involvement; in one case, tumors involved both kidneys.[642] Patients range in age from 16 to 68 years, with no gender predominance. Presenting symptoms may include flank pain and/or hematuria, and an abdominal mass is often palpable. Some cases are accompanied by paraneoplastic syndromes, including marked hypoglycemia and hypertension.

Tumors range in size from 1.5 to 25 cm in diameter, and are well circumscribed but unencapsulated. Although predominantly solid, tumors often have cysts containing clear, brown or red fluid.[641]

Microscopically, hemangiopericytomas are cellular tumors, composed of sheets of tightly packed round to spindle-shaped cells with elongated nuclei, separated by numerous slit-like and occasionally staghorn-shaped vascular spaces lined by endothelial cells. Tumor cells usually lack hyperchromasia or pleomorphism.[641] Variable numbers of mitotic figures may be present. Tumor cells show positive immunostaining for CD34, and negative immunostaining for CD31, actin, and CD99. The diagnosis of hemangiopericytoma is regarded as one of exclusion; it should be restricted to neoplasms that display a diffuse and consistent hemangiopericytoma pattern throughout the entire tumor. This feature is important, because hemangiopericytoma may be difficult to distinguish from solitary fibrous tumor owing to their common expression of CD34.[643,644]

The prognosis for renal hemangiopericytoma is guarded and difficult to ascertain owing to the paucity of reported cases. There are no pathologic features, such as mitotic rate or tumor size, that are predictive of outcome.[641,642] It has been estimated that approximately 50% of patients with renal hemangiopericytoma die of their disease.

## Osteosarcoma

There are fewer than 20 reported cases of primary renal osteosarcoma.[645-649] Patients are in their fifth to ninth decade of life, and present with abdominal or flank pain, and/or hematuria; there is no gender predilection. In about half of patients an abdominal mass is palpable. Intratumoral calcifications are typically evident radiologically, and may mimic nephrolithiasis.

Tumors may be as large as 28 cm.[648] Most are locally infiltrative high-stage cancers. Tumors are described as friable, brown or gray-pink or gray-white, with hemorrhage, necrosis, and bony hard areas.[645,647,648] Microscopically, the tumors are composed of pleomorphic polygonal to spindled cells with associated fibrous stroma and osteoid formation, as well as osteoclastic giant cells. The osteoid shows lace-like ossification. Abundant mitotic activity is usually noted, and atypical cartilage formation may be focally present.

The overall prognosis for renal osteosarcoma is poor, and most patients die of cancer within a few months of diagnosis;[650–653] long-term survivors are rare.[645]

## Other rare sarcomas

A variety of extremely rare sarcomas apparently originating in the kidney have been reported, including chondrosarcoma,[654] mesenchymal chondrosarcoma,[655] malignant schwannoma,[650,651] malignant mesenchymoma,[652] clear cell sarcoma of soft parts,[653] low-grade fibromyxoid sarcoma of renal capsule,[656] and cystic embryonal sarcoma.[657]

## Angiomyolipoma

The term angiomyolipoma, used to describe the most common mesenchymal tumor of the kidney, has been in use for over 100 years, although it was not popularized in the English literature until 1951.[658] The term accurately describes a mass lesion composed of varying quantities of myoid spindle cells, adipose cells and dysmorphic blood vessels. Although regarded initially as a hamartomatous non-neoplastic overgrowth of native renal tissues, angiomyolipoma has been shown in recent years to be a true neoplasm, as discussed below.

It has long been recognized that angiomyolipoma occurs in patients with tuberous sclerosis as well as those without clinical criteria for this disease.[419,659,660] Tuberous sclerosis is an autosomal dominant tumor-suppressor gene syndrome that affects approximately 1 in 6000 people.[661] It is characterized by seizures, mental retardation, autism, and tumor development in many organ systems, including the brain, retina, heart, kidney, and skin.[662] The tumors in question are cerebral cortical tubers, cardiac rhabdomyomas, renal angiomyolipomas, lymphangioleiomyomas, and facial angiofibromas.[663] Genetic studies of patients with tuberous sclerosis complex have documented that this disease results from mutations in either of two genes: TSC2 on chromosome 16 or TSC1 on chromosome 9;[661,664,665] the clinical findings in either case are indistinguishable. The majority of cases (65%) of TSC are sporadic, caused by a de novo mutational event.[661,666] In recent years, cytogenetic and molecular genetic studies in patients with angiomyolipoma with and without clinical evidence of tuberous sclerosis have provided support for the notion that angiomyolipoma is a neoplasm. Abnormal karyotypes indicative of clonal origin were found in seven of 19 sporadic angiomyolipomas,[667,668] including trisomy 7 and trisomy 8 in two of 10 patients. Angiomyolipomas are frequently observed to show loss of heterozygosity for polymorphic DNA markers of TSC1 and TSC2 genes on 9q34 and 16p13, respectively,[663,669–672] and comparative genomic hybridization studies confirm that a significant proportion of renal angiomyolipomas harbor clonal chromosomal aberrations, particularly genetic imbalances in chromosome 5q.[673] Loss of heterozygosity of the TSC2 gene on 16p13 is the most common clonal abnormality in both TSC-associated and sporadic cases of conventional angiomyolipoma, although the ratio of TSC1 and TSC2 abnormalities in familial cases may be nearly equal. Non-random inactivation of the X chromosome, a finding confirmatory for monoclonality, has frequently been documented in studies of renal angiomyolipoma.[666,670,674–676] One study showed that the adipose tissue and smooth muscle cells of renal angiomyolipoma are both monoclonal but may arise independently from different transformed progenitor cells.

The TSC2 gene on 16p13 functions like a tumor-suppressor gene.[670] Studies of the abnormal molecular mechanisms that underlie the occurrence of renal angiomyolipoma have centered around tuberin, the gene product of the TSC2 gene, and hamartin, the gene product of the TSC1 gene.[662,677] It has been demonstrated that tuberin and hamartin bind directly to form a complex and interact in the process of vesicular trafficking. Inactivating germline mutations in either gene lead to the same phenotypic spectrum, suggesting that both proteins are required for the proper functioning of the tuberin–hamartin complex, and that inactivation of the complex results in the clinical phenotype of TSC. Aberrant vesicular trafficking may be involved in tumorigenesis in TSC, and by extrapolation the same mechanism may account for the development of angiomyolipoma in sporadic cases not associated with TSC.[662,677]

Angiomyolipomas, and an ever-growing number of other neoplasms, are derived from unique cells that have been designated as perivascular epithelioid cells. Evidence for the existence of these unique cells was initially presented in 1991, based on immunohistochemical and ultrastructural investigations of renal and hepatic angiomyolipomas,[678] and confirmed in later studies.[679] The classic perivascular epithelioid cell may be scattered haphazardly within an angiomyolipoma, but is typically clustered around blood vessels; it is large, with abundant clear or acidophilic cytoplasm and a round vacuolated nucleus often exhibiting a nucleolus. Strikingly, it was noted to show immunoreactivity for HMB-45, a marker that had until 1991 been regarded as quite specific for melanocytic tumors. Tumor cells of angiomyolipoma were also noted to contain numerous electron-dense granules, some with transverse striations like those found in melanosomes. Subsequent studies confirmed that tumor cells of pulmonary lymphangiomyomatosis also expressed HMB-45,[680–682] as well as the tumor cells of clear cell 'sugar tumor' of the lung,[683] prompting a proposal of the concept of a family of tumors (PEComas) characterized by the presence of perivascular epithelioid cells. The family has subsequently grown to include a number of unusual visceral, intra-abdominal, soft tissue and bone tumors that have been described under a variety of names.[684–692] The PEComa family has been recognized by the World Health Organization as a group of mesenchymal tumors composed of histologically and immunohistochemically distinctive perivascular epithelioid cells.[693]

In unselected asymptomatic patients the incidence of angiomyolipoma is greater than that of renal cell carcinoma; angiomyolipoma is detectable in up to 0.10% of men and 0.22% of women in such patients.[694] In patients with tuberous sclerosis there is no significant difference in the frequency with which angiomyolipoma is detected in males compared to females.[695] With these data in mind, it is notable that, of patients treated surgically for angiomyolipoma, females outnumber males by a ratio of 4.8 : 1 in those with tuberous sclerosis, and 4.5 : 1 in those without.[696] It seems likely that angiomyolipomas in women more often grow to a size that justifies surgical intervention, perhaps due to hormonal influences, as suggested by the documentation of progesterone receptor immunoreactivity in a subset of surgically excised angiomyolipomas, all of which were removed from female tuberous sclerosis patients less than 50 years old,[697] and by documentation of growth acceleration of angiomyolipoma during pregnancy. In surgical series, the ratio of sporadic angiomyolipomas to those associated with tuberous sclerosis is approximately 4 : 1; however, the relevance of this ratio is questionable, as diagnostic criteria for tuberous sclerosis in some series are unclear, and patients with tuberous sclerosis are more likely to be managed conservatively.[419,696–699]

Angiomyolipoma occurs in patients of all ages. Those undergoing surgical excision of sporadic angiomyolipoma are typically between 45 and 55 years of age, whereas tuberous sclerosis patients having surgical excision of angiomyolipoma are usually 25–35 years old[696] (Fig. 2-121). Patients diagnosed with angiomyolipoma when they are less than 10 years old are likely to have tuberous sclerosis,[695] and a careful search for other lesions of tuberous sclerosis should be conducted in prepubertal patients with angiomyolipoma. Many angiomyolipomas, particularly those less than 4 cm in diameter, produce no symptoms and are found incidentally or during screening in tuberous sclerosis patients.[700] However, more than 80% of angiomyolipomas that exceed 4 cm in diameter are associated with symptoms or signs, which include acute or chronic abdominal or flank pain, hematuria, nausea, vomiting and fever. An abdominal or flank mass is often present, and some patients have associated hypertension. More than half of tumors over 4 cm in diameter are associated with some degree of bleeding, which may be sufficient to result in hypovolemic shock.[698,700] Rupture of angiomyolipoma during pregnancy is a well-recognized complication.[701,702]

Renal angiomyolipoma can be accurately diagnosed in the great majority of cases using ultrasound and/or CT scanning, because of their fat content.[703,704] Exceptions to this include angiomyolipomas that are almost entirely composed of smooth muscle components, and tumors with extensive intratumoral bleeding. Unfortunately, there are rare cases of renal malignancies that contain fat, mimicking angiomyolipoma.[705–709]

Angiomyolipomas may be situated in the renal cortex, medulla, or capsule, and may be solitary or multiple. Most surgically excised specimens are greater than 4 cm in diameter, and can be as large as 30 cm in greatest dimension.[710] Most are smoothly rounded or ovoid, and circumscribed but not encapsulated. They compress and distort the adjacent renal parenchyma but do not infiltrate it. Extension into the perirenal fat is often seen,[703] and rarely angiomyolipomas infiltrate adjacent structures to an extent that makes them unresectable[419] (Fig. 2-122). There are about two dozen reports of angiomyolipomas that extended into the renal vein or vena cava, in one instance even extending as far as the right atrium.[696] Tumors vary from pink-tan or gray to yellow, depending on the relative contents of smooth muscle and fat.

Microscopically, the interface between angiomyolipoma and the adjacent renal parenchyma is sharp, with minimal intermingling of tumor and native renal tubules. Although all angiomyolipomas are composed of smooth muscle, fat, and abnormal blood vessels, the relative proportions of these elements vary from tumor to tumor and even within

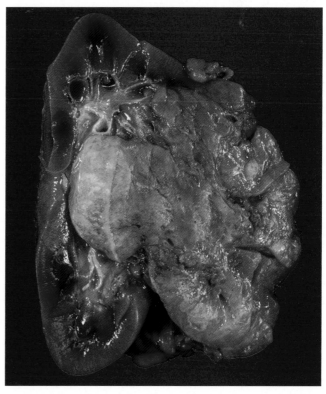

**Fig. 2-122** Renal angiomyolipoma. Bulky lobulated tumor in a 14-year-old girl. (Courtesy of Raymond Redline, MD.)

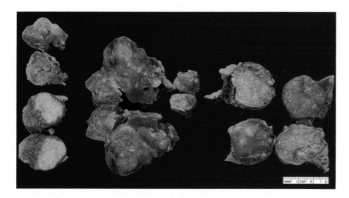

**Fig. 2-121** Renal angiomyolipoma. Multiple tumors resected from a 19-year-old woman with tuberous sclerosis. (Courtesy of Douglas Hartman, MD.)

different regions of the same tumor. Aggregates of thick-walled artery-like blood vessels are admixed with large mature fat cells and smooth muscle cells (Fig. 2-123). The blood vessels typically are devoid of elastica.[711] The smooth muscle cells show some degree of pleomorphism; some are spindled cells resembling normal smooth muscle, and some are rounded epithelioid cells.[696] Although smooth muscle cell nuclei are usually small and regular, lacking mitotic activity, focal areas of marked nuclear atypia may be present, with occasional mitotic figures. The smooth muscle cells typically form a collar around the adventitia of the abnormal blood vessels and may exhibit a perpendicular orientation in relation to it, creating a 'hair on end' appearance[703] (Fig. 2-124). Hemorrhage and areas of necrosis are commonly seen. Intraglomerular microlesions consisting of adipose and smooth muscle cells are observed rarely.[712–714]

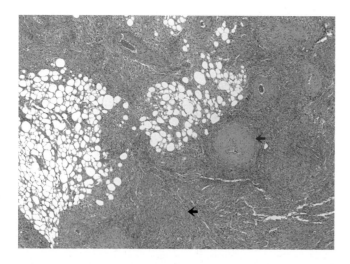

**Fig. 2-123** Renal angiomyolipoma. The tumor is composed of thick-walled artery-like blood vessels, admixed with large mature fat cells and smooth muscle cells.

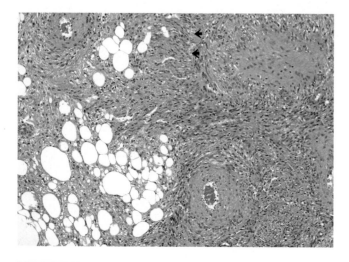

**Fig. 2-124** Renal angiomyolipoma. Arrows indicate the 'hair on end' appearance of smooth muscle cells adjacent to blood vessels.

A recently described variant of angiomyolipoma is characterized by the presence of prominent intratumoral cysts of variable size. Usually there is one large cyst; this may be accompanied by smaller cysts.[715,716] The cysts are lined by cuboidal to hobnail cells. Beneath the epithelium is a compact layer of cellular, müllerian-like stromal tissue with a prominent infiltrate of chronic inflammatory cells. The cysts are generally seen in a background setting of muscle-predominant angiomyolipoma. Prominent curvilinear and branching lymphatic spaces are evident within the smooth muscle, most prominently in the subepithelial myomatous layer. Such tumors may be difficult to distinguish from mixed epithelial and stromal tumor of kidney. The blood vessels seen in mixed epithelial and stromal tumor do not show the dysplastic features seen in angiomyolipoma, such as variable thickness, myxoid change, and disorganization. Furthermore, the smooth muscle cells of mixed epithelial and stromal tumor do not show immunoreactivity to HMB-45 or MelanA, as do the smooth muscle cells of angiomyolipoma. It has been postulated that the epithelial component lining the cysts in these cases represents epithelial differentiation within the angiomyolipoma. This hypothesis deserves further study.

Ultrastructural findings in angiomyolipoma are variable and reflective of the complex morphology of the tumor. Typical smooth muscle cells with abundant glycogen have been observed, as well as smooth muscle cells with intracytoplasmic lipid droplets.[717] Granules containing rhomboid bodies with a crystalline lattice substructure, characteristic of human juxtaglomerular cells, have been identified in epithelioid tumor cells.[718] As noted previously, tumor cells of angiomyolipoma have been noted to contain numerous electron-dense granules, some with transverse striations like those found in melanosomes.[678]

Immunohistochemically, the spindled and epithelioid smooth muscle cells of angiomyolipoma are immunoreactive to antibodies against vimentin, muscle-specific actin, smooth muscle actin, and KIT (CD117).[679,719] About half of tumors show positive immunostaining for desmin, and immunostaining for S100 protein is limited to scattered fat cells and epithelioid cells. Immunostains for cytokeratins and epithelial membrane antigen are consistently negative. The propensity of angiomyolipoma to stain for the melanosome-associated protein HMB-45, as noted previously, has been confirmed by numerous investigators,[679,720–722] and has prompted study of its immunoreactivity to a wide spectrum of melanocytic markers[723–727] (Fig. 2-125). Results of a recent comprehensive study of the utility of melanosome-associated markers in the diagnosis of angiomyolipoma suggest that the combination of HMB-45 and MelanA detects all classic renal angiomyolipomas, and that other markers, such as NK1-C3, tyrosinase, and CD117, are of limited usefulness.

There are more than 40 reported cases of renal angiomyolipoma in which deposits of angiomyolipoma have been observed in regional lymph nodes.[696,728–732] As none of these patients experienced progression of disease, it seems likely that the findings in the lymph nodes represent multicentricity of disease rather than metastasis. Renal angiomyolipoma

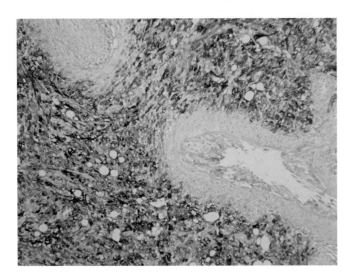

**Fig. 2-125** Renal angiomyolipoma. Tumor cells show positive immunostaining for MelanA.

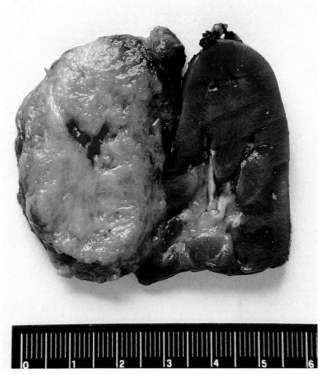

**Fig. 2-126** Renal epithelioid angiomyolipoma. The tumor has a variegated cut surface, whorled in some areas. (Courtesy of of Rodolfo Montironi, MD.)

has also been reported to coexist with angiomyolipomas in the perirenal fat, the opposite kidney, the adrenal, the liver, the lung, and the spleen.[696,733]

Despite the fact that classic angiomyolipoma is regarded as benign, it can be associated with a variety of adverse outcomes. Rupture with massive blood loss can lead to fatal consequences.[696,733] Renal disease, comprising confluent, multiple bilateral angiomyolipomas and renal cysts, causes renal insufficiency in approximately 15% of patients with tuberous sclerosis, and is the second most common cause of death in such patients after central nervous system causes, and the most common cause of death in such patients over the age of 30.[695,696] As noted previously, angiomyolipoma has infrequently been reported to infiltrate local structures to an extent that precludes surgical excision, ultimately causing death.[734,735] Two cases of sarcoma arising in angiomyolipoma have been documented.[631,736] In addition, the epithelioid variant of angiomyolipoma can behave in a clinically malignant fashion, as outlined in the next section. Finally, angiomyolipoma can arise concurrently with renal cell carcinoma, which is most often of clear cell type, and less frequently of chromophobe cell type.[695,737,738]

Studies of large series of patients and observations of the behavior of angiomyolipomas followed radiologically over periods of many years have allowed various management regimens to be proposed.[419,695,698–700,734,739] Currently it is recommended by some that angiomyolipomas larger than 8 cm in diameter should be treated, whether they are causing symptoms or not. Tumors less than 4 cm in diameter can be managed expectantly. Tumors between 4 and 8 cm in diameter have unpredictable behavior and need close monitoring; about half need intervention for bleeding.

## Epithelioid angiomyolipoma

By 1989, pathologists had been well aware of the morphologic features and benign biologic behavior of angiomyolipoma for approximately 100 years.[696] At that point, reports

began to appear of angiomyolipomas that were atypical not only in their morphology, but also in their biologic behavior. In 1989, it was reported that a subset of renal angiomyolipomas exhibited extensive epithelioid smooth muscle components that simulated granular cell renal carcinoma.[740] Two years later, an angiomyolipoma with a predominance of large, hyperchromatic cells that had spindled or bizarre, pleomorphic shapes, accompanied by extensive necrosis and frequent mitotic figures, consistent with high-grade sarcoma, was reported, with demonstrated pulmonary metastases.[736] Subsequently the usefulness of HMB-45 immunostaining in renal angiomyolipoma was demonstrated, and it was increasingly recognized that angiomyolipomas could be composed partly or predominantly of large atypical epithelioid cells and multinucleated giant cells and could be misdiagnosed as renal cell carcinoma.[679,683,741] Since 1996, there have been numerous reports of epithelioid angiomyolipoma characterizing its clinical, radiologic, pathologic and biologic features.[90,91,210,722,742–755]

Males and females are equally affected, and the mean age at diagnosis is 38 years. More than half of reported patients also suffer from tuberous sclerosis. Some tumors are discovered through screening for tuberous sclerosis; in other cases the diagnosis is made through investigation of flank pain, fever, weight loss, palpable abdominal mass, and in one case symptoms of hyperprolactinemia. Because very little fat is present in most epithelioid angiomyolipomas, they mimic carcinoma radiologically. Tumors tend to be large, gray-tan, white, or brown (Fig. 2-126). Hemorrhage is common, and necrosis may be present and sometimes extensive. Gross

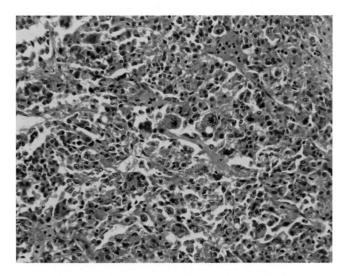

**Fig. 2-127** Renal epithelioid angiomyolipoma. Tumor composed of round to polygonal epithelioid cells with abundant eosinophilid cytoplasm, vesicular nuclei with prominent nucleoli, and abundant mitotic figures.

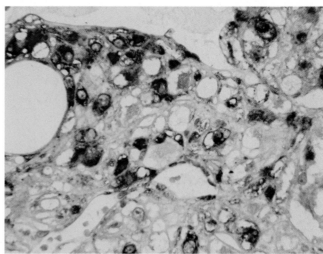

**Fig. 2-128** Renal epithelioid angiomyolipoma. Tumor cells show positive immunostaining for HMB-45.

involvement of perirenal fat, renal veins or vena cava by tumor may be apparent.

Tumors are composed of sheets of round to polygonal epithelioid cells with granular eosinophilic cytoplasm, admixed with variable components of spindle cells. The epithelioid cells show considerable pleomorphism; some have relatively small nuclei, small nucleoli, and limited amounts of cytoplasm; some have large eccentrically placed vesicular nuclei, macronucleoli and copious cytoplasm, and may resemble ganglion cells (Fig. 2-127). In some tumors multinucleated giant cells are present, with multiple peripheral nuclei.[742,743,745,746,749] Tumors show varying degrees of mitotic activity and necrosis. Vascular invasion and extension into perirenal soft tissues may be seen in some cases. Components of classic angiomyolipoma may be apparent.[696,743,746,756] Some tumors are composed partially or predominantly of cells with clear cytoplasm, sometimes with patchy dark-brown melanin pigment.[754,755,757]

Immunohistochemically, epithelioid angiomyolipoma expresses melanocytic markers (HMB-45, HMB-50, microphthalmia transcription factor and Mart-1/MelanA) as well as smooth muscle markers (smooth muscle actin and muscle-specific actin)[210,722,743,746,751] (Fig. 2-128). Cytogenetic studies of epithelioid angiomyolipoma have shown allelic loss of the TS2-containing region on chromosomal arm 16p;[746] the role of TP53 mutation in these tumors is unclear.[752-755]

Malignant behavior has been observed in tumors that have areas of focal classic angiomyolipoma, as well as in tumors entirely composed of epithelioid elements.[91,210,722,743,745,748-750,752,755] Approximately one-third of epithelioid angiomyolipomas have demonstrated metastases to lymph nodes, liver, lung, or spine, and tumors demonstrating necrosis, mitotic activity, nuclear anaplasia and extrarenal extension should be regarded as potentially more aggressive. To date, there have been eight documented deaths from epithelioid angiomyolipoma, and an additional seven cases with documented metastases at the time of reporting.

## Leiomyoma

Leiomyoma is a benign neoplasm with smooth muscle differentiation. It is detectable at autopsy in a surprisingly large number of cases (5%),[10] but larger clinically evident leiomyoma necessitating surgical excision is uncommon; fewer than 40 such cases have been reported.[10,19,626,758-762] Leiomyoma may arise in the renal capsule, cortical vascular smooth muscle, or smooth muscle of the renal pelvis.[19] Most occur in adults, with a median age at presentation of 42 years, although rarely the patient is a child. Two-thirds of patients are female, and 70% are white.[758] Slightly more than half of patients present with pain, either flank or abdominal, and in more than half of patients a mass is palpable. Hematuria is noted in the minority of patients, and with rare exceptions is only microscopic.

Surgically excised renal leiomyoma has an average size of approximately 12 cm;[758] the largest recorded was 57.5 cm in diameter and weighed 37 kg.[763] Renal leiomyoma is typically firm, bulging, and well circumscribed, with a white whorled fibrous or trabeculated cut surface (Fig. 2-129). Calcification or cystic degeneration may be evident, but necrosis is absent. Most are single, but some are multiple.[764]

Microscopically, it is composed of spindled cells usually arranged in small intersecting fascicles, typical of smooth muscle (Fig. 2-130). Nuclear pleomorphism is minimal, and necrosis and mitotic figures are absent, as are adipose cells and abnormal blood vessels.[19,626,762,764] Immunohistochemically, tumor cells show positive immunostaining for desmin, muscle-specific actin, and/or smooth muscle-specific actin, and no immunostaining for cytokeratins.[19,626] Capsular leiomyoma frequently contains populations of cells strongly immunopositive for HMB-45, suggesting an undefined relationship with angiomyolipoma.[19,626]

## Hemangioma

More than 200 cases of renal hemangioma have been reported. Some occur sporadically, and some present in a

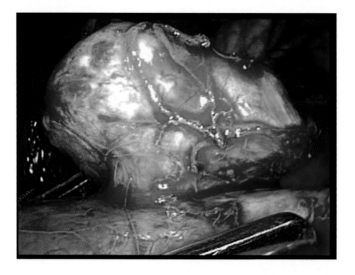

**Fig. 2-129** Renal leiomyoma. The tumor originated in the renal capsule; photo taken during laparoscopic partial nephrectomy. (Courtesy of Lee Ponsky, MD.)

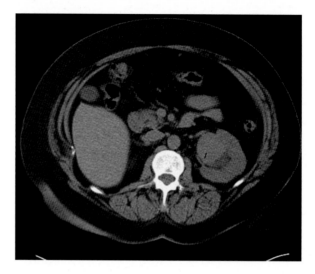

**Fig. 2-131** Renal hilar hemangioma. On CT scan the lesion occupying the hilum of the right kidney was indistinguishable from a malignancy.

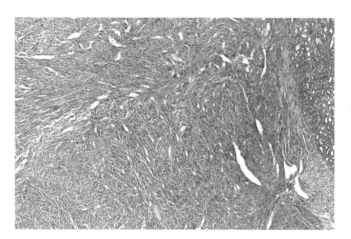

**Fig. 2-130** Renal leiomyoma. Tumor is composed of spindled cells arranged in small intersecting fascicles, typical of smooth muscle.

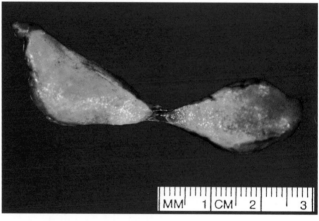

**Fig. 2-132** Renal hilar hemangioma. Same case as shown in Figure 2-131. At surgery, this soft uniformly tan-red lesion was loosely attached to large vessels in the renal hilum, but was not an intrinsic part of the kidney.

background of other vascular disorders, such as Klippel–Trenaunay syndrome, Sturge–Weber syndrome, and systemic angiomatosis. Although the age spectrum of patients with renal hemangioma is broad, ranging from infancy to old age, the majority are young to middle-aged adults. The cardinal manifestation of renal hemangioma is hematuria, but some patients present with abdominal or flank pain, the tumor is discovered incidentally in some, and in small children a palpable mass may draw attention to the lesion.

Most renal hemangiomas are small, 1–2 cm in greatest dimension, but may be as large as 18 cm. They are most often located in the renal pelvis or renal pyramids, but may also be found in the renal cortex, the renal capsule, or within peripelvic blood vessels or soft tissues[764–772] (Fig. 2-131).

Grossly, renal hemangioma may be difficult to visualize, appearing as a small mulberry-like lesion or a small red streak. Larger lesions exhibit varying degrees of circumscription, and often appear red or gray-tan, and spongy (Fig. 2-132).

Microscopically, renal hemangioma is composed of irregular blood-filled vascular spaces lined by a single layer of endothelial cells that lack mitotic activity and nuclear pleomorphism (Fig. 2-133). Both cavernous and capillary hemangiomas have been reported.

## Lymphangioma

Renal lymphangioma, also designated peripyelic–pericalyceal lymphangiectasis, is a rare cystic renal lesion that is regarded as a developmental malformation resulting from failure of developing lymphatic tissue to establish normal communication with the remainder of the lymphatic system.[764,773–775] Fewer than 50 cases have been reported. The

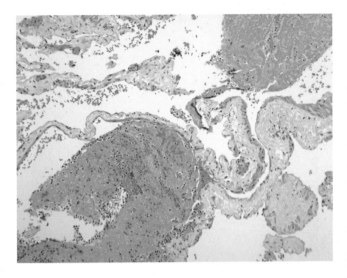

**Fig. 2-133** Renal hilar hemangioma. Cavernous hemangioma/vascular malformation with thick- and thin-walled blood vessels.

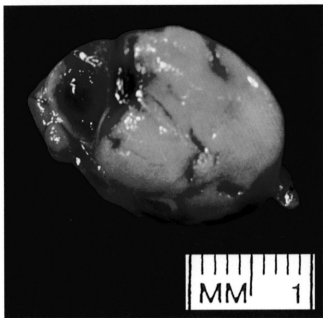

**Fig. 2-134** Juxtaglomerular cell tumor. Small hemorrhagic yellow tumor with bulging cut surface.

great majority of lymphangiomas occur in the head and neck and axillary regions; other sites include the retroperitoneum, mediastinum, mesentery, omentum, colon, and pelvis.[776]

Renal lymphangioma has been reported in neonates, infants, children, and adults.[764,773] Approximately two-thirds occur in adults. The lesion may involve one or both kidneys in localized or diffuse distribution, and rarely may be restricted to the lymphatics of the renal capsule, either unilaterally or bilaterally.[773,777] Some cases manifest as abdominal masses in children,[774,778] some are found incidentally,[776,777,779,780] some present with renin-dependent hypertension, and some present with hematuria and/or pain related to renal obstruction.

Renal lymphangioma is typically a well-encapsulated multicystic mass; the cut surface is composed of innumerable fluid-filled cysts ranging from 0.1 to 2.0 cm, often mimicking polycystic kidney disease or a multilocular renal cyst.

Microscopically, the cysts are lined by flattened endothelial cells, and are separated by a variable amount of stroma that may contain smooth muscle, glomeruli, tubules, lymphoid infiltrates, and blood vessels.[764,778] The nature of the endothelial cells lining the cysts can be ascertained, if necessary, by appropriate immunostains.

Renal lymphangioma is benign. However, once discovered, it is usually excised surgically because the radiologic differential may include cystic renal cell carcinoma in adults, or cystic variant of Wilms' tumor, clear cell sarcoma, or rhabdoid tumor in children.[776,778]

## Juxtaglomerular cell tumor

Juxtaglomerular cell tumor was first described in 1967.[781] It is a renal neoplasm that arises from specialized smooth muscle cells that comprise the vasculature of the juxtaglomerular apparatus. Approximately 70 cases of juxtaglomerular cell tumor have been reported, more often in women than in men (ratio of 1.9:1).[782] Patients range from 6 to 69

years of age, but the majority are in their 20s and 30s, with a mean age of 27 years. Clinical findings often facilitate an accurate preoperative diagnosis. Almost all patients have hypertension that is difficult to control. In the rare instances in which the tumor produces an inactive form of renin, the patient's blood pressure may be normal.[783] Other symptoms reported include pain, headache, polyuria, nocturia, dizziness, and vomiting. Other typical clinical findings include high serum renin levels, elevated serum aldosterone, and hypokalemia.

Grossly, juxtaglomerular cell tumor is usually well circumscribed by a fibrous capsule of variable thickness.[782] It is typically 2–4 cm in diameter, but can be as large as 9 cm.[784] It has a yellow to gray–tan and often hemorrhagic cut surface (Fig. 2-134), and is composed of polygonal to round to elongated, spindle-shaped cells. Cells tend to have slightly eosinophilic cytoplasm and centrally located nuclei. Most cases show some degree of nuclear atypia. Mitotic figures are usually absent. Cell borders may be well defined or ill defined. Cellular arrangement also varies: the cells may be arranged in irregular trabeculae, papilla, organoid patterns, or solid compact sheets.[782,785] The background stroma may be scant, abundant and hyalinized, or edematous, imparting a microcystic appearance. Abundant thin-walled vessels are usually present, and most tumors demonstrate thick-walled vessels, sometimes in clusters, and sometimes branching to an extent that mimics hemangiopericytoma[782,786] (Figs 2-135, 2-136). However, thick-walled blood vessels are not seen in hemangiopericytomas, which also lack the polygonal cells with abundant eosinophilic cytoplasm seen in juxtaglomerular cell tumors.

Because of the varied histological appearance, immuno-histochemical staining of tumors suspected of being

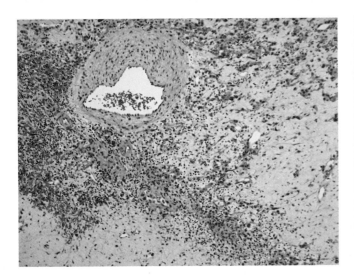

**Fig. 2-135** Juxtaglomerular cell tumor. Round, polygonal, and spindled cells in a myxoid background, with scattered inflammatory infiltrate, and thick-walled blood vessels.

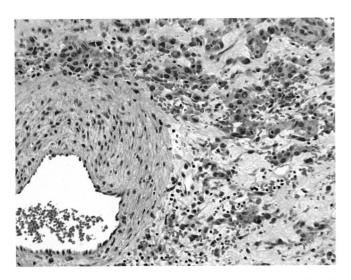

**Fig. 2-136** Juxtaglomerular cell tumor. Higher-power view of findings shown in Figure 2-135.

juxtaglomerular cell tumors can be helpful in confirming the diagnosis and in differentiating them from other renal neoplasms.[782] Juxtaglomerular cell tumor shows positive immunostaining for actin, CD34, and CD117, and negative immunostaining for cytokeratins, desmin, S100 protein, HMB-45, chromogranin, and synaptophysin.[782,786,787] Tumors that may be confused with juxtaglomerular cell tumor include renal cell carcinoma, angiomyolipoma, and glomus tumor. Immunohistochemical staining is helpful in that renal cell carcinomas stain positive for cytokeratins, and angiomyolipoma stains positive for HMB-45; these stains are negative in juxtaglomerular cell tumor. Immunohistochemical staining does not differentiate juxtaglomerular cell tumor from glomus tumor because both arise from smooth muscle cells and stain positive for actin and CD34. However, electron microscopy of juxtaglomerular cell tumor reveals

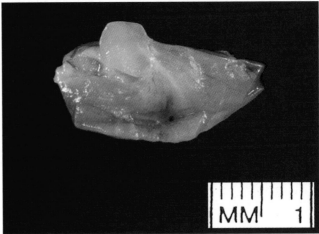

**Fig. 2-137** Renomedullary interstitial cell tumor. Small fibrotic tumor involving the tip of a renal papilla.

both rhomboid-shaped renin protogranules and smooth muscle microfilaments, findings that are unique to this neoplasm, and which account for its characterization as a tumor derived from 'myoendocrine cells.'

Surgical removal of the tumor usually normalizes the patient's blood pressure and relieves other symptoms. These tumors are almost exclusively benign,[781–788] although there has been one documented case of juxtaglomerular cell tumor that metastasized to the lung.[789]

## Renomedullary interstitial cell tumor

Renomedullary interstitial cell tumor is a small benign fibrous lesion in the renal medulla that is found in patients in their teens and older, with a slight female predilection.[10,11] It has been postulated that medullary interstitial cells provide endocrine-like antihypertensive actions, and that renomedullary interstitial cell tumor represents a developmental response to a hypertensive stimulus.[764] This lesion is found incidentally at autopsy, with an incidence of 26–44%, and about 50% are multiple.[10,11,742,764] Most are 0.1–0.5 cm in diameter (Fig. 2-137). Rarely, the lesion is large enough to obstruct renal pelvic outflow and cause pain,[790] and occasionally asymptomatic large lesions are discovered incidentally, requiring surgical excision.

Microscopically, renomedullary interstitial cell tumor is composed of small stellate or polygonal cells set in a background of loose faintly basophilic stroma containing interlacing bundles of delicate fibers[216] (Figs 2-138, 2-139). The stromal matrix at the periphery of the lesion often entraps renal medullary tubules. Amyloid deposits may be observed.[791]

## Schwannoma

Fewer than 20 cases of renal schwannoma have been reported.[792–798] Patients range from 24 to 89 years of age (average 59 years), without apparent gender predilection. The tumor may arise in the renal parenchyma, the renal capsule, or the renal hilar soft tissues. Some are discovered

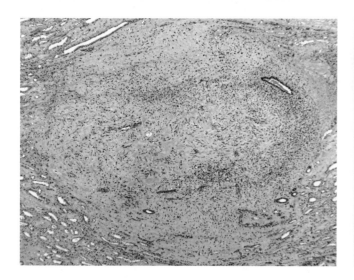

**Fig. 2-138** Renomedullary interstitial cell tumor. Tumor is composed of small stellate cells in a background of loose faintly basophilic stroma containing interlacing bundles of delicate fibers.

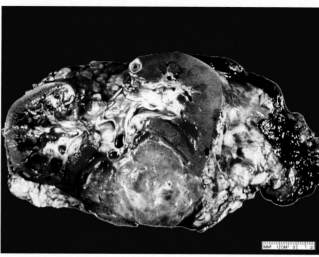

**Fig. 2-140** Renal schwannoma. Well circumscribed tumor in a young female. (Courtesy of Jiaoti Huang, MD.)

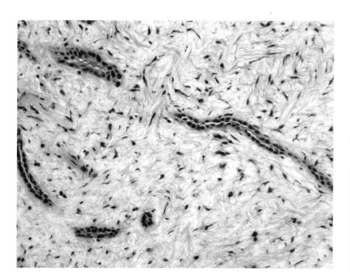

**Fig. 2-139** Renomedullary interstitial cell tumor. Higher-power view of findings described in Figure 2-138.

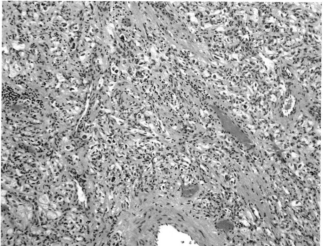

**Fig. 2-141** Renal schwannoma. Although not showing classic findings, this lesion was regarded as most consistent with schwannoma, based primarily on its immunoprofile (the only significant immunostaining was strong and diffuse positivity for S100 protein).

incidentally; in some cases, non-specific symptoms such as malaise, fever, weight loss, or abdominal discomfort are reported, or an abdominal mass is palpable.

Grossly, renal schwannoma ranges from 4 to 16 cm in greatest dimension (mean 9.7 cm). It is typically tan to yellow, well circumscribed, and sometimes multinodular[796,797] (Fig. 2-140).

Microscopically, renal schwannoma is composed of bland uniform spindle cells with wavy nuclei, and is sharply circumscribed with a dense fibrous capsule (Fig. 2-141). Classic schwannoma exhibits variable cellularity, with cellular Antoni A areas alternating with hypocellular Antoni B areas, nuclear palisading, and Verocay body formation.[793–795,797] Cellular schwannoma shows fascicular growth and relatively uniform cellularity, cystic change with macrophage aggregates, and relative paucity of palisading, Verocay bodies and

Antoni A and Antoni B areas. Numerous thick-walled hyalinized blood vessels are present in either type of schwannoma. Mitotic figures and necrosis are absent. Tumor cells show strong and uniformly positive immunostaining for S100 protein, and no immunoreactivity to antibodies against cytokeratin, CD34, CD57, smooth muscle actin, or desmin.

Renal schwannoma is benign.

## Solitary fibrous tumor

Solitary fibrous tumor is a spindle cell neoplasm that was first described in 1931. Although it is most often found in the pleura, it also occurs in a variety of extrapleural sites, including the kidney.[643,799–803] Fewer than two dozen cases of renal solitary fibrous tumor have been reported. It has been postulated that solitary fibrous tumor is a neoplasm of fibroblast/primitive mesenchymal cells with features of multidirectional differentiation.[804] More than half of patients are more than 40 years old (range 28–83 years, average age 52 years), and the male : female ratio is approximately equal.[801,803] Symptoms include flank or abdominal pain and/or hematuria; some patients are asymptomatic, and in others a mass is palpable.[643,799–803]

Renal solitary fibrous tumor ranges in size from 2 to 25 cm, with a mean of 8.75 cm; in one patient bilateral lesions were present.[801,803] It is typically well circumscribed and pseudoencapsulated, lobulated, rubbery, or firm, and has a homogeneous gray or tan-white, whorled cut surface. In most cases necrosis, cyst formation, and hemorrhage are absent. Microscopically, solitary fibrous tumor is composed of a proliferation of spindle cells arranged in a patternless architecture, with areas of alternating hypocellularity and hypercellularity separated from one another by thick bands of hyalinized collagen and branching hemangiopericytoma-like blood vessels (Fig. 2-142). Tumor cells have scant and indistinct cytoplasm, and elongated nuclei with finely dispersed chromatin and only occasional nucleoli. Mitotic activity is limited, and cellular atypia and necrosis are not observed in benign cases.[643,799–803]

Solitary fibrous tumor typically shows strong and diffusely positive immunostaining for CD34, a finding that is considered characteristic and indispensable in making the diagnosis. Seventy percent of solitary fibrous tumors express CD99 and Bcl-2; immunopositivity for epithelial membrane antigen and smooth muscle actin is observed in only about one-quarter of these neoplasms, and immunostaining for S100 protein, cytokeratins, and/or desmin is usually absent or only focal and limited.[800,805]

The differential diagnosis of renal solitary fibrous tumor includes a broad spectrum of epithelial and mesenchymal neoplasms. There are no distinctive ultrastructural findings that aid in the diagnosis of solitary fibrous tumor. The combination of immunopositivity for CD34, Bcl-2, and CD99, and the absence of expression of α-smooth muscle actin, S100 protein, CD31, and c-kit are helpful in distinguishing solitary fibrous tumor from lesions such as monophasic synovial sarcoma, leiomyoma, low-grade leiomyosarcoma, and schwannoma.[800,805]

With a single reported exception, renal solitary fibrous tumor is benign. In one exceptional case, a slowly growing renal lesion in an elderly patient was eventually removed after several years of observation; the tumor was composed of benign-appearing solitary fibrous tumor admixed with a high-grade pleomorphic sarcoma having features that met the criteria for malignancy in solitary fibrous tumors; multiple pulmonary metastases were evident 4 months after surgery.[803]

## Mixed mesenchymal and epithelial tumors

### Cystic nephroma

Cystic nephroma, first described in 1892,[806] is a benign renal neoplasm composed entirely of epithelial-lined cysts separated by septa of variable thickness. The definition of the lesion described as 'cystic nephroma,' and the relationship between cystic nephroma and cystic partially differentiated nephroblastoma, has undergone several revisions in the past six decades.[215,579,582,799,800,807,808] Cystic nephroma and cystic partially differentiated nephroblastoma were distinguished from one another in an early version of the diagnostic criteria by the absence of poorly differentiated tissues and blastemal cells in the septa of cystic nephroma, and the presence of blastemal cells in any amount, with or without other embryonal stromal or epithelial cell types, such as variably differentiated glomeruli, tubules, mesenchyme, striated muscle, cartilage, fibrous tissue or fat, in the septa of cystic partially differentiated nephroblastoma. In a more recent classification the diagnosis of cystic nephroma is restricted to adults; renal neoplasms in children composed entirely of epithelial-lined cysts separated by septa of variable thickness and lacking expansile nodules to alter the rounded contour of the cysts are diagnosed as cystic partially differentiated nephroblastoma, regardless of the presence or absence of blastema or other immature elements in the septa.[215] In support of this classification, several points have been made, based on morphologic observations and analysis of accumulated clinical data from nearly 200 patients in several large series and literature reviews.[582,808–810] Cystic nephroma in adults is seen mainly in females (female : male ratio 8 : 1), is rarely seen before age 30, and does not exhibit nephrogenic rests elsewhere in the kidney or skeletal muscle fibers in the septa. In contrast, cystic partially differentiated nephroblastoma occurs with a slight male preponderance, is rare after the age of 2 years, sometimes exhibits nephrogenic rests elsewhere in the kidney, and commonly shows the presence of skeletal muscle fibers in the septa. In short, it seems probable that the traditional term 'cystic nephroma' embraces

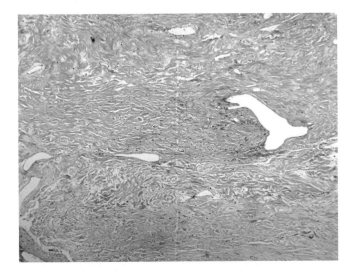

**Fig. 2-142** Solitary fibrous tumor. Patternless architecture, variable cellularity, thick bands of hyalinized collagen and branching hemangiopericytoma-like blood vessels. Grossly the tumor appeared to arise from the renal capsule.

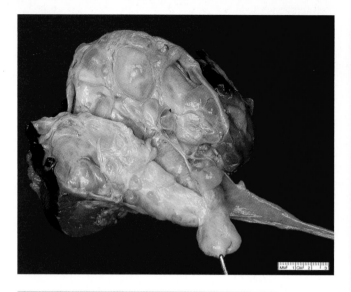

**Fig. 2-143** Cystic nephroma. Tumor extends into renal pelvis. (Courtesy of Carmen Kletecka, MD.)

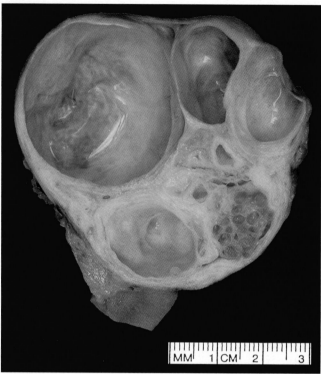

**Fig. 2-144** Cystic nephroma. The tumor is composed of multilocular cysts of variable size. (Courtesy of Mark Costaldi, MD.)

two entirely different lesions, one of which (cystic nephroma) occurs predominantly in adult females and has no relationship to Wilms' tumor, and the other (cystic partially differentiated nephroblastoma) a lesion of young children of both genders, probably representing a mature form of Wilms' tumor.[215]

Cystic nephroma may present as a painless abdominal mass, with flank or abdominal pain, or hematuria.[809,810] Currently, most are discovered incidentally.[811–813] Patients in contemporary series range in age from 22 to 79 years old with a mean age of approximately 55–60 years, and the great majority are female.[811–813] Tumors are well circumscribed, usually unilateral but rarely bilateral,[814] ranging in size from 1.4 to 13 cm, with an average diameter of approximately 6 cm. Most involve the renal cortex, but rarely may be predominantly intrapelvic[815] (Fig. 2-143).

Cystic nephroma is composed of multilocular cysts of varying sizes, filled with serous fluid (Fig. 2-144). The cysts are lined by epithelium that is flattened, cuboidal, or hobnail in appearance. Lining cells with clear cytoplasm are occasionally present. Mitotic figures are absent.[215,811] The septa are thin and correspond to the outlines of the cysts; expansile nodules are absent. The stroma of the septa is composed of spindle cells in a collagenous background (Figs 2-145, 2-146). In some areas stromal cell nuclei are very closely packed, imparting an ovarian stroma-like appearance (Fig. 2-147). In addition, acellular wavy structures somewhat reminiscent of corpora albicantia/corpora fibrosa of the ovary are commonly noted. Small tubular structures resembling renal tubules cut in cross-section may be present in septal stroma, but the septal stroma does not contain aggregates of clear cells, nor does it contain skeletal muscle, fat, smooth muscle, blastema or other immature elements.[215,811–813] The lining epithelium of cysts shows consistent positivity for distal tubule/collecting duct markers (cytokeratin 19 cytokeratin AE1/AE3, epithelial membrane antigen), variable positivity for proximal tubule markers ($\alpha_1$-antitrypsin,

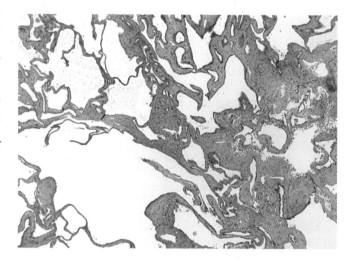

**Fig. 2-145** Cystic nephroma. Variably sized cysts separated by thin septa that correspond to the outlines of the cysts; expansile nodules are absent. Septal stroma is composed of spindle cells in a collagenous background.

lysozyme, CD15, CD10), frequent positivity for CK7, focal positivity for high molecular weight keratin, and negative staining for CK20. The fibrous and ovarian-like stroma both show consistent staining for vimentin and smooth muscle actin, and frequent staining for desmin. However, the fibrous stroma shows no immunostaining for estrogen or progesterone receptors, whereas the ovarian-like stroma shows frequent immunoreactivity for these markers. Stromal cells also

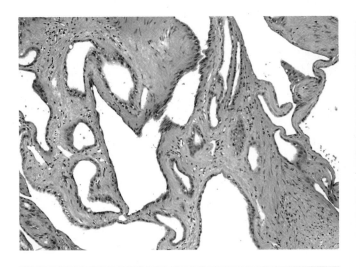

**Fig. 2-146** Cystic nephroma. The lining epithelium is flattened or cuboidal.

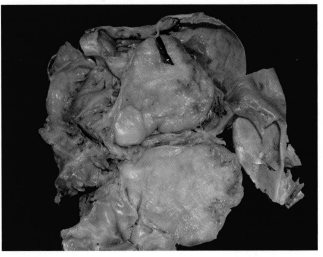

**Fig. 2-148** Cystic nephroma with superimposed sarcoma. A sarcoma has developed, with a solid fleshy cut surface. (Courtesy of John Kunkel, MD.)

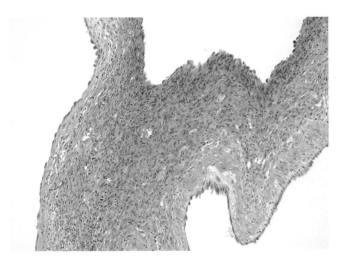

**Fig. 2-147** Cystic nephroma. In some areas stromal cell nuclei are very closely packed, imparting an ovarian stroma-like appearance.

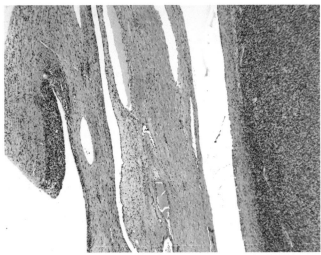

**Fig. 2-149** Cystic nephroma with superimposed sarcoma. On the left is typical cystic nephroma; on the right is a sarcoma.

show no immunoreactivity for HMB-45, WT1, inhibin, or CD117.

Cystic nephroma is regarded as a benign neoplasm, cured by adequate surgical excision. Recurrence has been attributed to incomplete resection.[814] However, there are eight reported instances of sarcoma arising in a background of cystic nephroma in adults, at least three of which have had a fatal outcome[809,816] (Figs 2.148–2.150).

## Mixed epithelial and stromal tumors

Following an initial report in 1973 of the first case of 'congenital mesoblastic nephroma (leiomyomatous hamartoma)' in an adult,[817] there have been numerous single case reports and series of cases of adults with renal neoplasms that are macroscopically solid and cystic, and microscopically biphasic, composed of glands – often cystically dilated – and solid areas of spindle cells with variable growth patterns and cellularity. Such tumors have been assigned a variety of names, including adult mesoblastic nephroma, cystic hamartoma of the renal pelvis, leiomyomatous renal hamartoma, cystic partially differentiated nephroblastoma, adult mature nephroblastoma, multilocular cystic nephroma with ovarian-like stroma, and benign mixed epithelial and stromal tumor.[773,818–832] The term 'mixed epithelial and stromal tumour,' first proposed in 1998, was adopted in the 2004 WHO classification of tumors of the urinary system and male genital organs.

These cases have a number of unifying characteristics. The great majority are female, with a 10 : 1 preponderance and a mean age of 46 years. The majority present with hematuria, flank pain, or symptoms related to urinary infection; however, some tumors are discovered incidentally. Grossly, mixed epithelial and stromal tumor is typically single, unilateral, and well circumscribed, with a mean size of 6 cm

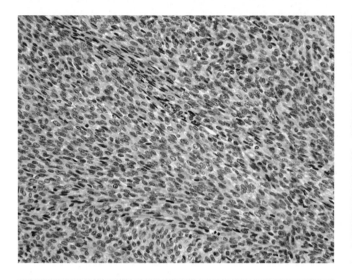

**Fig. 2-150** Cystic nephroma with superimposed sarcoma. Final diagnosis was sarcoma, not otherwise specified, based on inconclusive immunohistochemical and molecular studies.

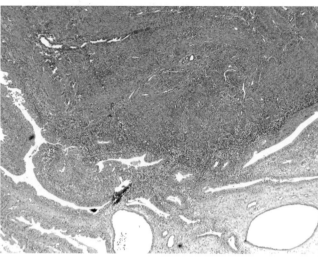

**Fig. 2-152** Mixed epithelial and stromal tumor. Biphasic tumor composed of smooth muscle and fibrous elements admixed with complex epithelial lined structures.

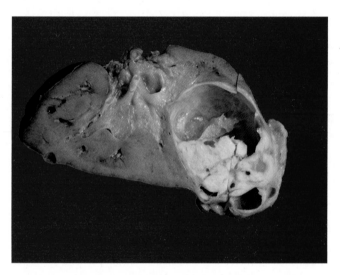

**Fig. 2-151** Mixed epithelial and stromal tumor. Tumor is variably solid and cystic. (Courtesy of Rodolfo Montironi, MD.)

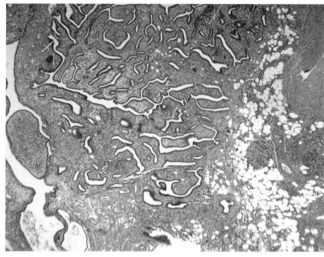

**Fig. 2-153** Mixed epithelial and stromal tumor. Complex branching architecture and broad papillae; stromal component includes fat, smooth muscle, and fibrous tissue.

(range 2–16 cm).[827,830] Some have been noted to protrude into the collecting system.[823] Tumors are variably solid and cystic; the cysts may be clustered or dispersed, and the solid areas may be firm and rubbery, or fleshy (Fig. 2-151).

Microscopically, a smooth muscle capsule of variable thickness is commonly present. Mixed epithelial and stromal tumor is biphasic, with spindle cell and epithelial components, both of which show a wide range of findings (Figs 2-152, 2-153). The spindle cell component typically varies considerably in cellularity, and often shows condensation around cystic areas (Fig. 2-154). It may be hypocellular with extensive collagenization or with myxoid change; it may be cellular and arranged in fascicles resembling smooth muscle or in a woven pattern resembling ovarian stroma; it may be densely cellular and arranged in patterns resembling fibrosarcoma or synovial sarcoma; or it may show alternating zones of hypocellularity and hypercellularity with fibrocytic cells in a keloid-like background resembling solitary fibrous tumor. Fat cells may be present. The epithelial component consists of variably sized glands that may be uniformly dispersed or closely aggregated; in some tumors, tubular structures show complex branching or papillae. Cells lining the glands may be low cuboidal, columnar, or hobnail type, with variable amounts of cytoplasm that may be clear, foamy, eosinophilic or amphophilic. No significant cytologic atypia or mitotic activity is evident within either the spindle cell or the epithelial components.[773,824–830]

Immunohistochemically, the spindle cells show immunoreactivity to antibodies against vimentin and smooth muscle actin, and variable positivity for desmin. They commonly show positive nuclear immunostaining for estrogen

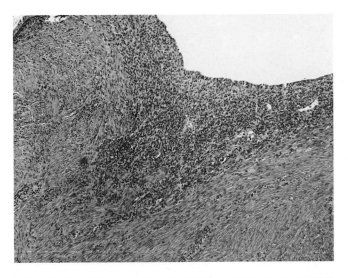

**Fig. 2-154** Mixed epithelial and stromal tumor. Condensation of spindle cell component around cystic areas.

receptors and progesterone receptors in women, a finding that has also been noted in a male patient who had a long history of anti-androgenic therapy for prostate cancer. The epithelial elements show uniformly positive immunostaining for keratin markers; some show positive immunostaining for vimentin, and some demonstrate nuclear positivity for estrogen receptor. Neither component shows immunoreactivity to antibodies against S100 protein, HMB-45, or CD34, antigens that are usually expressed by nerve sheath tumors, angiomyolipomas, and solitary fibrous tumors, respectively. Ultrastructural examination of a limited number of tumors shows features that suggest fibrocytic differentiation in the majority of the spindle cells, with features of myogenic differentiation in a minority of spindle cells. It has been postulated that mixed epithelial and stromal tumor arises from the primary mesenchyme/metanephric blastema, which is capable of both mesenchymal and epithelial differentiation. Alternatively, it may arise from a hormone-sensitive 'periductal fetal mesenchyme' that is postulated to be present around epithelial structures in a number of organs, including kidney, pancreas, and liver.[827]

Mixed epithelial and stromal tumor differs from congenital mesoblastic nephroma by occurring in adults (rather than infants and very young children), by affecting predominantly females (rather than having an equal gender distribution), by having a biphasic composition (rather than a purely mesenchymal composition), and by a demonstrated absence of several cytogenetic alterations that are characteristic of congenital mesoblastic nephroma.[827,829] Only a single report concerning the cytogenetics of mixed epithelial stromal and tumor of the kidney is available, indicating a translocation t(1; 19) detected in a tumor from a young male patient.[832] Mixed epithelial stromal tumor of the kidney differs from adult nephroblastoma by the absence of a component of blastema, and from sarcomatoid renal cell carcinoma by the absence of malignant cytologic characteristics.

The distinction of mixed epithelial and stromal tumor from cystic nephroma is more difficult, and it has been suggested by some investigators that these entities represent a spectrum of the same entity, with a variable ratio of stroma to cyst.[812,813,833,834] It is noted that both entities are rare and occur mainly in adult perimenopausal women. Both occur as a single unilateral well-circumscribed mass composed of mixed solid and cystic areas. Morphologically and immunohistochemically there is extensive overlap between the two lesions, with the exception that the stroma of cystic nephroma is typically nondescript, thin and fibrous, whereas that of mixed epithelial and stromal tumor is dense and ovarian-like. Both are biologically indolent, but both have been associated with rare aggressive behavior. It has been proposed that cystic nephroma may occur in both sexes in the absence of hyperestrinism, and that mixed epithelial and stromal tumor represents a cystic nephroma that has acquired cellular, ovarian-like stroma secondary to hormonal influences.

Although mixed epithelial and stromal tumor was initially considered benign, there have been reports of cases that had clear-cut malignant changes within the stroma,[835,836] as well as reports of cases in which tumors diagnosed as mixed epithelial/stromal demonstrated sarcomatoid morphology, associated with aggressive clinical behavior and an ultimately fatal outcome.[837,838] One case that was reported as mesoblastic nephroma with late recurrence did not have a well-documented epithelial component, and may not have been a mixed epithelial and stromal tumor.[818]

## Synovial sarcoma

Primary renal synovial sarcoma was first reported in 1999[839] after it was recognized that a subset of a heterogeneous group of neoplasms that had been designated 'embryonal sarcoma of the kidney[840] harbored a t(X; 18) chromosome translocation, raising the possibility that it represented the synovial sarcoma-associated t(X; 18)(p11; q11) translocation, which results in fusion of the SYT gene on chromosome 18 to one of the SSX family genes on X (SSX1, SSX2, or SSX4). The clinical, morphologic, immunohistochemical, and molecular features of 23 examples of this tumor have been reported.[841-846] The majority of cases of renal synovial sarcoma demonstrate the SYT-SSX2 gene fusion, a feature that in typical soft tissue synovial sarcoma is commonly associated with monophasic histology.[847]

Renal synovial sarcoma occurs in patients between 20 and 61 years of age, with a slight male preponderance. Tumors are typically large, ranging from 5 to 20 cm in diameter, with a soft or rubbery consistency and variegated cut surfaces. Hemorrhage and necrosis are usually evident, and most exhibit smooth-walled cysts. Extension into large vessels is noted in some cases.[841,842]

Microscopically, renal synovial sarcoma is composed of monomorphic plump spindle cells growing in solid sheets or in short intersecting fascicles that typically infiltrate the adjacent normal renal parenchyma, encircling normal structures (Figs 2-155 and 2-156). Necrosis is present and is often extensive. The spindle cells in most instances are non-pleomorphic, with ovoid nuclei and indistinct cell borders. Recently, however, examples of this tumor with extensive

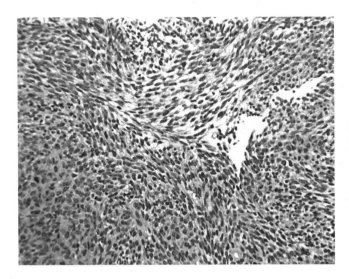

**Fig. 2-155** Synovial sarcoma of kidney. Needle biopsy of an inoperable renal mass in an frail elderly man. Diagnosis confirmed by demonstration of SYT-SSX2 gene fusion.

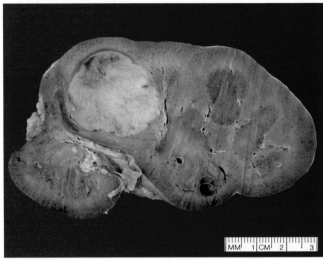

**Fig. 2-157** Carcinoid tumor of kidney. Well circumscribed yellow tumor confined to renal parenchyma. (Courtesy of Rodolfo Montironi, MD.)

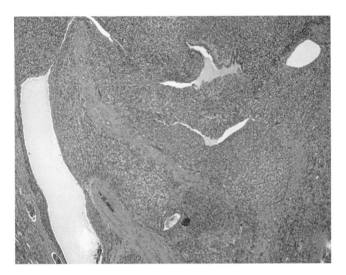

**Fig. 2-156** Synovial sarcoma of kidney. Sheets of monomorphic spindle cells surrounding cysts that are probably trapped and cystically dilated native renal tubules.

rhabdoid cell morphology have been identified, emphasizing that synovial sarcoma needs to be considered part of the differential of mesenchymal kidney tumors with prominent rhabdoid features.[844] Mitotic figures are abundant. Areas of dense cellularity often alternate with hypocellular myxoid, edematous, or sclerotic areas. Cysts of variable size are present, lined by mitotically inactive hobnail epithelium with abundant eosinophilic cytoplasm; the cysts are regarded as entrapped and cystically dilated native renal tubules[841,842] (Fig. 2-156).

Immunohistochemically, tumor cells are consistently immunoreactive to antibodies against vimentin and BCL2, frequently reactive for CD99, and focally reactive for cytokeratins and epithelial membrane antigen. They show no immunoreactivity to antibodies against desmin and muscle-specific actin.[841–844] It has recently been found that

expression of TLE1 is a consistent and prominent feature of synovial sarcoma, whereas its expression was minimal or absent in a wide variety of other spindle cell tumors, including those in the differential diagnosis of synovial sarcoma.[848]

The total number of reported cases of primary renal synovial sarcoma is small, and follow-up data are too limited at present to allow for meaningful comment. In 23 reported cases, six patients are known to have developed local recurrences or distant metastases during follow-up, and an additional three are known to have died of widespread metastatic cancer.[841–846]

## Neuroendocrine tumors

### Renal carcinoid tumor

Primary renal carcinoid tumor, a low-grade malignancy with neuroendocrine differentiation, is uncommon. It is frequently associated with other renal abnormalities, including horseshoe kidney (18%), renal teratoma (14%), and polycystic kidney disease (2%).[849–856] Slightly more than 50 cases have been reported, in patients with an average age of 49 years (range 12–68 years). Almost 30% of cases are discovered incidentally; presenting symptoms in the remainder include abdominal or flank pain, hematuria, constipation, fever, weight loss and testicular pain. Neuroendocrine syndromes occur in about 12% of patients,[857,858] and in 27% a mass is palpable. Renal carcinoid is typically hypovascular or avascular on radiologic studies, and frequently displays intratumoral calcification.[859] Somatostatin receptor scintigraphy can be helpful in pre- and postoperative assessment of disease status.[860]

The tumor ranges in size from 1.5 to 30 cm in greatest dimension, with a mean of 8.4 cm. It is yellow-white to red-tan, and although the majority are solid, about one-third are partially or predominantly cystic (Fig. 2-157). About half are confined to the renal parenchyma, one-third involve

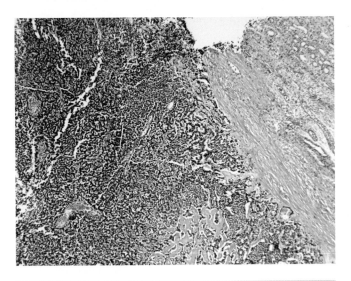

**Fig. 2-158** Carcinoid tumor of kidney. Tumor cells arrayed in ribbons, cords, and solid sheets.

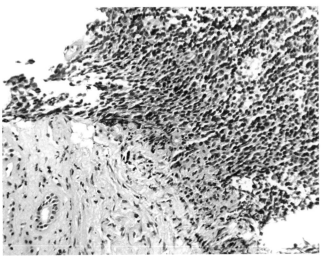

**Fig. 2-159** Small cell carcinoma of kidney. Needle biopsy of an inoperable tumor that was clinically and radiologically primary in the kidney. (Courtesy of Ming Xhou, MD.)

perirenal fat, and renal vein involvement occurs in slightly more than 10% of cases. Histologically, renal carcinoid tumor shows findings typical of carcinoid tumors in other body sites. The majority of tumors have a mixed growth pattern, with cells arranged in a trabecular pattern, solid nests, acinar structures, insular, tubular, or rosette-like structures (Fig. 2-158). Mitotic activity is limited.[853]

The immunoprofile of renal carcinoid is similar to that of carcinoids occurring elsewhere, with positive immunostaining for synaptophysin, chromogranin, neuron-specific enolase, and cytokeratin in a high percentage of cases.[861] It is notable that renal carcinoid often shows positive immunostaining for prostatic acid phosphatase.[862] Cytogenetically, numerical or structural aberrations of chromosomes 3 and 13 have been noted.[863,864] Loss of heterozygosity at the D3F15S2 locus of 3p21 in one case suggested the possibility of a common genetic event in the genesis of renal carcinoid tumor and conventional renal cell carcinoma.

Metastases are present at the time of diagnosis or appear within 7 years of follow-up in 50% of patients. Metastases are more common in patients over 40 years old, and are more often seen in association with tumors that are solid, larger than 4 cm, outside the renal capsule, or that have a mitotic rate higher than 1/10 hpf. The mortality rate is less than 10%, indicating that the disease is relatively indolent, and that resection of positive lymph nodes can be curative.[853]

## Neuroendocrine carcinoma

Fewer than 30 cases of small cell carcinoma of the kidney have been reported, and only 10 of these were composed entirely of small cell carcinoma.[865-870] Some of these 10 cases did not clearly arise from or involve the urothelium of the renal pelvis; in the remainder the exact site of origin was unclear. It is probable that the majority of small cell carcinomas that involve the kidney originate in the urothelium of the renal pelvis or calyces, judging from their reported

locations,[871-875] and from the fact that many are admixed with components of urothelial carcinoma, squamous cell carcinoma, and adenocarcinoma, similar to small cell carcinomas that arise in the urothelium of the urinary bladder.[876]

Patients range in age from 37 to 83 years of age, with a mean of 59 years. Symptoms include hematuria, back or abdominal pain, fatigue and other constitutional symptoms, and non-specific gastrointestinal complaints. The great majority of tumors range between 10 and 18.5 cm in greatest dimension, frequently obliterating large portions of the native kidney.[865,866,868]

Tumors are typically solid, poorly circumscribed, grayyellow, and extensively necrotic and hemorrhagic. Tumor stage at the time of nephrectomy is often advanced, with involvement of perirenal structures, renal vein and regional lymph nodes.[865,866,869] Histologic, immunohistochemical and ultrastructural findings are similar to those of small cell carcinoma in more conventional locations[865,866,868,869] (Fig. 2-159). In one case the following common clonal aberrations were observed: 45,XX, t(X; 10; 18) (p11; p11; q11), -der(18)t(X; 10; 18).[867]

Although some patients have had a favorable outcome,[866,868] the prognosis for most patients with renal small cell carcinoma is poor, possibly because of a propensity for occult metastases at the time of presentation. Median survival is less than 1 year, regardless of the therapeutic regimen employed; survival is prolonged by platinum-based chemotherapy.[874]

## Primitive neuroectodermal tumor

Primitive neuroectodermal tumor and Ewing's sarcoma are viewed as the ends of a common histologic spectrum known as the Ewing family of tumors (EFT).[692] Over 90% of EFT harbor the balanced t(11; 22) (q24; q12)(EWS/FLI-1) translocation; approximately 5% of cases show t(21; 22) (q22;

q12)(EWS/ERG), and less than 1% harbor a variety of rare translocations, all of which involve chromosome 22.[877] Primitive neuroectodermal tumor most commonly arises in the soft tissues of the chest wall, trunk, retroperitoneum, pelvis and extremities, but in recent years more than 50 cases have been reported to arise primarily in the kidney.[675,878–894]

Although the first case of renal PNET was described in 1975,[895] the entity remained largely unrecognized until the early 1990s, at which time it was shown that tumor cells of both Ewing's sarcoma and PNET are immunoreactive for the MIC2 gene product, a finding not shared by classic neuroblastoma or by blastema-predominant nephroblastoma. The specific cytogenetic changes characteristic of EFT, noted above, were also clarified at that time. Since 1994, there have been numerous single case reports as well as small and large series of renal PNET.

Renal PNET arises in patients ranging from 1 month to 72 years of age, with a slight male preponderance and a mean age of 26 years.[892] Most patients are adolescents or young adults; 75% are between 10 and 39 years of age. Patients present with abdominal pain, hematuria, a palpable mass, and sometimes with constitutional symptoms. Tumors are typically large (more than 10 cm in many instances), poorly circumscribed gray-tan to white tumors that extensively obliterate the native renal parenchyma[890] (Fig. 2-160). Hemorrhage, necrosis, and renal vein invasion are common gross findings. Microscopically, PNET consists of sheets of monotonous polygonal cells with high nuclear to cytoplasmic ratios, arranged in a vaguely lobular pattern (Fig. 2-161). Cell overlapping is not prominent. Nuclei are round and hyperchromatic, with dispersed chromatin and absent or inconspicuous nucleoli. Mitotic figures are readily apparent, and may be numerous. In well-preserved specimens cells may show a small amount of clear cytoplasm, corresponding to the presence of intracytoplasmic glycogen. Tumor cells infiltrate adjacent renal parenchyma as broad sheets or

finger-like projections. Pseudorosette formation may be noted (Fig. 2-162).

Immunohistochemically, PNET virtually always shows positive immunostaining for CD99 and for FLI-1 protein, up to 50% of morphologically typical cases show positive immunostaining for pankeratin AE1/3, and 25% show positive immunostaining for CD117.[692] Immunostains for desmin and high molecular weight cytokeratin (34βE12) are negative. PNET is usually not immunoreactive to antibodies against the Wilms' tumor suppressor gene product WT-1,[890] but there are well-documented exceptions to this pattern.[894] It should be noted that neither FLI-1 nor CD99, although highly sensitive for PNET, is entirely specific for PNET. Furthermore, blastema-predominant Wilms' tumor may express cytokeratins. For this reason, it has been suggested that an immunohistochemical panel of antibodies against CD99, FLI-1, and WT-1 should be used to separate renal PNET from

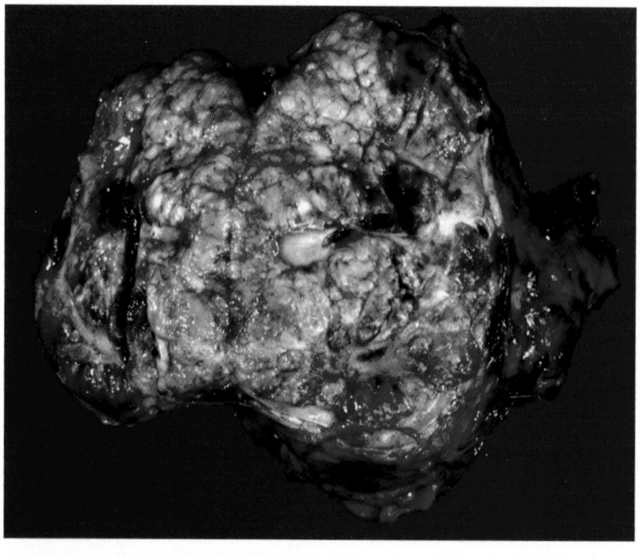

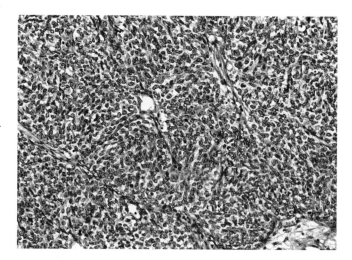

**Fig. 2-161** Primitive neuroectodermal tumor of kidney. Sheets of monotonous polygonal cells with high nuclear to cytoplasmic ratios, arranged in a vaguely lobular pattern. Nuclei are round and hyperchromatic, with dispersed chromatin and absent or inconspicuous nucleoli.

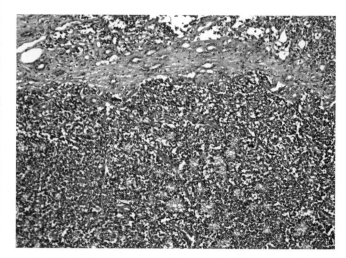

**Fig. 2-162** Primitive neuroectodermal tumor of kidney. An area of rosette formation is demonstrated.

**Fig. 2-160** Primitive neuroectodermal tumor of kidney. Tumor almost entirely obliterates the native kidney. (Courtesy of Beverly Dahms, MD.)

blastema-predominant Wilms' tumor. Although both may express CD99 and cytokeratins, PNET typically expresses FLI-1 and usually does not express WT-1, whereas the opposite is true for Wilms' tumor. It has been pointed out, however, that reliance upon immunohistochemistry as the sole means of ancillary diagnosis in renal PNET can lead to confusing results, and whenever possible the diagnosis should be validated by molecular fusion studies.

The prognosis for renal PNET is guarded. Almost 60% present in advanced stages, with venous tumor thrombi in 33%, and with metastases to lymph nodes (25%), lung (20%) and liver (14%).[892] In a recent analysis of 40 patients with renal PNET, 23 (57%) were free of disease during 5–58 months of follow-up, but 17 (43%) had died of their disease.[892]

## Neuroblastoma

Reports of primary neuroblastoma of the kidney are rare.[878,896,897] By contrast, secondary renal involvement by adrenal or retroperitoneal neuroblastoma is relatively common.[898] Histologic details in the reported cases are limited. The difficulty in distinguishing such lesions from other primary neuroepithelial tumors of the kidney is evidenced by the fact that six neuroblastomas were initially included in an abstract describing a cohort of 101 primary neuroepithelial tumors examined by the National Wilms' Tumor Study Group, but a subsequent publication by the same group concerning 146 primary malignant neuroepithelial tumors of the kidney did not include any examples of primary neuroblastoma.[878,889]

## Paraganglioma

There are fewer than a dozen well-documented cases of renal paraganglioma. Tumors have been detected through evaluation of a palpable abdominal mass, microhematuria, recurrent flank pain, and hypertension. Distinction of intrarenal from capsular lesions is difficult and probably irrelevant, as these tumors are radiologically indeterminate for renal malignancy and are removed on that basis.

The tumors range in size from 1.6 to 18 cm in greatest dimension.[899–905] Some are predominantly solid, with yellow-brown or gray-pink cut surfaces, and others have been predominantly cystic, either unilocular or multilocular, containing hemorrhagic or thick dark-brown fluid. Histologically, most have had the classic 'zellballen' morphology, being composed of organoid clusters of cells surrounded by delicate fibrovascular stroma and sustentacular cells. Some tumors include sheets of large polygonal cells with eccentric nuclei having coarse chromatin and prominent nucleoli. Tumor cells show positive immunostaining for vimentin, neuron-specific enolase, chromogranin, and synaptophysin, and negative or only focally positive staining for cytokeratins. Sustentacular cells show positive immunostaining for S100 protein.

Prognosis for renal paraganglioma is difficult to ascertain, as in most reported cases follow-up has been short. In one remarkable case, lung metastases developed 13 years after the original nephrectomy.[899]

# Hematopoietic and lymphoid tumors

## Lymphoma

Lymphoma involves the genitourinary system more frequently than any other solid organ system.[906] Involvement of the kidneys by lymphoma is not infrequent, and occurs in several patterns, including secondary, primary, post-transplant, and renal intravascular lymphomatosis.[907] Risk factors for renal lymphoma include status post renal transplantation,[908–911] and acquired immunodeficiency syndrome (AIDS).[907,912]

Renal involvement during the course of systemic lymphoma defines secondary renal lymphoma, and is the most common setting for renal lymphoma. Imaging studies at the time of presentation disclose renal involvement in 3–8% of patients with systemic lymphoma, and autopsy evidence of renal involvement has been reported in 34–62% of patients dying of lymphoma.[907,913] When renal involvement is noted at autopsy it is bilateral in 75% of cases. Despite its frequency, the great majority of patients with secondary renal lymphoma do not experience symptoms or clinical findings relative to it.[914]

Primary renal lymphoma accounts for 0.7% of all extranodal lymphomas in North America and 0.1% in Japan.[915] It is defined as lymphoma that presents initially with signs and symptoms related to the kidneys, and is by all diagnostic criteria initially limited to one or both kidneys. It is not rare: it has been reported to account for as many as 3% of surgically excised renal tumors initially regarded clinically as renal carcinoma. Symptoms and signs include flank or abdominal pain or mass, weight loss, fever, malaise, night sweats, hematuria, pyuria, proteinuria, hypertension and azotemia. Nearly all patients tend to fall into one of two clinical scenarios: those with renal masses mimicking renal cell carcinoma,[514,906,907,912–914,916–920] and those who present with acute renal failure associated with massive bilateral renal infiltration by lymphoma.[907,914,915,921–930] In those with renal masses, clinical and radiologic features that suggest renal lymphoma include multifocal and/or bilateral lesions, predominantly perirenal plaques, extrarenal extension of tumor, and very prominent hilar adenopathy, all features that are not typical of other renal neoplasms, including renal cell carcinoma.[907,931] A confounding feature of some lymphomas, however, is tumor extension into the renal vein, and in some cases the vena cava, a radiologic feature typical of renal cell carcinoma.

Post-transplant lymphoproliferative disorder is a nodal or extranodal lymphoid proliferation that follows solid organ or bone marrow transplantation. It is a consequence of therapeutic suppression of T-cell function, which facilitates infection of B lymphocytes by Epstein–Barr virus, resulting in B-cell proliferations that range from benign reactive polyclonal proliferations to monoclonal proliferations (lymphoma).[907] Although the majority of solid-organ transplantation-related lymphoproliferative disorders are of recipient origin,[909] some reported examples of renal lesions have been documented to be of donor origin.[908–911]

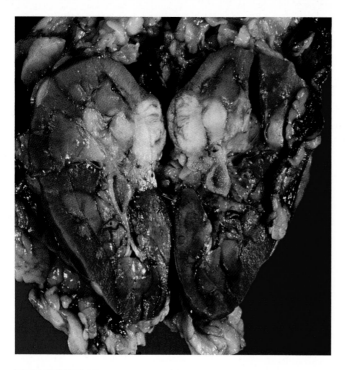

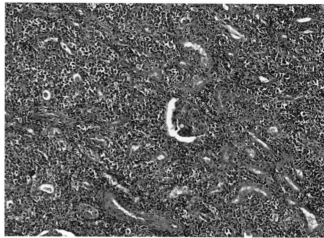

**Fig. 2-164** Renal lymphoma. Sheets of monotonous lymphoma cells infiltrate between native renal tubules and glomeruli.

**Fig. 2-163** Primary renal lymphoma. Nephrectomy performed because of a radiologically indeterminate mass. Lesion was diffuse large B-cell, non-Hodgkin's lymphoma. Complete staging was negative. The patient was in complete remission 18 months post chemotherapy.

Renal intravascular lymphomatosis is a component of angiotropic large cell lymphomas wherein the renal involvement is characterized by extensive infiltration of glomerular and peritubular capillaries by lymphoma cells.[932,933]

Lymphoma in kidneys resected with a presumptive diagnosis of renal carcinoma show single or multiple tumor nodules that are variably described as friable, soft and fleshy, or firm or rock-hard.[912–914,917,918,934] The nodules are typically pale tan, pink, or gray-white, with varying degrees of necrosis and/or hemorrhage (Fig. 2-163). Tumors often obliterate substantial portions of the renal parenchyma, with varying degrees of circumscription. Involvement of perirenal soft tissues and infiltration of the adrenal and/or renal hilar vessels are common findings. Nephrectomy is not usually done in cases presenting with acute renal failure and diffuse bilateral renal enlargement; in these cases the diagnosis is made by percutaneous needle biopsy.[907,914,915,921–930] The kidneys may appear grossly normal in cases of renal intravascular lymphomatosis.[932]

In nephrectomy specimens, lymphoma obliterates the underlying parenchyma except at the interface between tumor and normal kidney, where the lymphoma cells infiltrate in an interstitial pattern, sparing tubules and glomeruli;[914] this interstitial infiltrative pattern is also seen in needle biopsy specimens[921–923,926–928,930] (Fig. 2-164). Virtually all histologic lymphoma subtypes may be encountered. Diffuse large B-cell lymphoma and its variants are the most commonly encountered renal lymphomas.

Renal lymphoma arising in a background of systemic lymphoma has a poor prognosis. The prognosis for primary renal lymphoma is guarded, but there are many reports of complete remission, although reported follow-up periods are often short.[906,912,922–924,929,934] Some patients with renal lymphoma die from complications of therapy.[916,921,926] Detection of extrarenal disease after an initial diagnosis of primary renal lymphoma portends a poor outcome in some instances,[913,916,918,919,925,930] but successful treatment of such relapses, with prolonged remissions, has been reported.[914]

## Leukemia

Myeloid sarcoma is a neoplastic mass formed by proliferating myeloblasts or immature myeloid cells occurring in an extramedullary site. It may arise in a setting of myelodysplastic syndrome, myeloproliferative disorder, or acute myeloid leukemia.[935] Most cases of myeloid sarcoma are identified at autopsy in patients dying of myeloid leukemia, occurring with a frequency of 3–7% of such cases[936] (Fig. 2-165). The frequency of documented renal involvement by myeloid sarcoma in autopsy series varies considerably, but with rare exceptions, in most instances no clinical manifestations of renal involvement are apparent ante mortem.

Rarely, myeloid sarcoma occurs 'de novo' as a forerunner of acute myeloid leukemia in non-leukemic patients.[935,937,938] Patients may have no renal symptoms, or may have flank pain. Renal involvement usually takes the form of diffuse enlargement; in one case the kidney was noted to have an ill-defined green lesion at autopsy, and in another the kidney was diffusely infiltrated by a grayish tumor. Microscopically, renal tissue shows dense interstitial infiltration by immature granulocytic cells. Immunohistochemical stains for anti-lysozyme are usually positive; histochemical stains of biopsy imprints for naphthol ASD-chloroacetate esterase (CAE) may be positive or negative. It has also been suggested that an immunohistochemical panel, including CD20, CD43, CD68, and MPO, can successfully identify the vast majority of myeloid sarcomas in paraffin sections.

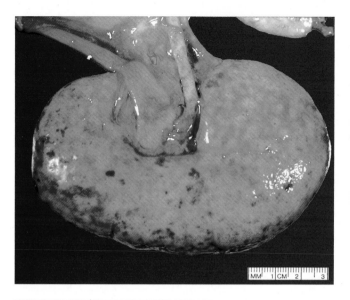

Fig. 2-165 Leukemia involving kidney. Autopsy specimen from a patient recorded as dying from eosinophilic leukemia. Kidney appears swollen, hyperemic, and ecchymotic.

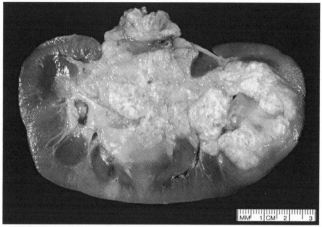

Fig. 2-166 Metastasis to kidney. The patient had had non-small cell carcinoma of lung 4 years previously. The renal lesion was the only clinical lesion, and a renal primary could not be excluded; nephrectomy was carried out and showed squamous cell carcinoma, presumed to be metastatic.

## Plasmacytoma

Fewer than a dozen cases of renal plasmacytoma have been reported.[419,939–944] Some have occurred in patients with a prior history of plasma cell dyscrasia, but most have been diagnosed in kidneys resected with a clinical diagnosis of renal cell carcinoma. The great majority of patients are male; patients range in age from 22 to 64 years of age, although most are in their 50s and 60s. Some are noted to have an abdominal mass, some present with hematuria, and in some cases the renal lesion is found incidentally.

Tumors range in size from 3 to 21 cm in greatest dimension. They are often noted to obliterate large portions of the renal parenchyma and to involve perirenal fat and regional lymph nodes.[939,941,942] Tumors are described as soft or firm and light gray or tan, with small foci of hemorrhage.[940,942,944] Microscopically, tumors are composed of sheets of plasma cells with varying degrees of cytologic atypia and mitotic activity.

Almost all those diagnosed with renal plasmacytoma have a prior, concurrent, or subsequent diagnosis of systemic plasma cell dyscrasia. One remarkable patient underwent nephrectomy and radiation to the renal bed, without further treatment, and lived 16 years symptom free before dying of an acute myocardial infarction.[419]

## Germ cell tumors

There are fewer than a dozen well-documented cases of intrarenal teratoma.[854,855,945–952] In some reports, the precise relationship between the tumor and the renal capsule has been difficult to ascertain, and a large proportion of reported cases may represent Wilms' tumor with teratoid features. Although most have occurred in children less than 7 years old, several have been encountered in adults. Tumors may be single or multiple. Associated anomalies have included renal dysplasia and horseshoe kidney. One case was associated with an ipsilateral malignant neuroepithelial tumor of the adrenal gland,[950] and several had elements of carcinoid tumor. A single case of intrarenal mixed germ cell tumor, composed of yolk sac tumor and teratoma, has been reported.[953] The morphology of reported tumors has been similar to that noted in more conventional sites.

Reported cases of choriocarcinoma metastatic to the kidney are more common than those deemed to have arisen in the kidney.[954,955] Regarding those reported to be renal primaries, it is difficult to exclude the possibility that some originate from spontaneous regression of post-gestational choriocarcinoma, a clinically occult 'burnt-out' testicular primary,[956] or from urothelial carcinoma of the renal pelvis.[957] The morphology of such tumors is indistinguishable from that of their gonadal or uterine counterparts.

## Metastatic tumors

Cancer metastatic to the kidney from other sites is relatively commonly observed at autopsy of patients dying of cancer, occurring in up to 7.2% of cases.[958,959] Occasionally, symptoms related to the renal metastasis are the initial manifestations of disease.[960] The commonest primary sites are the lung, breast, melanoma of skin, opposite kidney, gastrointestinal tract, ovary and testis.[961] In patients with a history of malignancy, renal metastases outnumber renal cell carcinomas by a ratio of about 4:1; a new renal lesion in a patient with advanced incurable cancer is more likely a metastasis than a new primary.[962]

Most metastases are multiple, bilateral, well-defined nodules; some are single and poorly circumscribed (Figs 2-166, 2-167). In some cases metastases are confined to the glomeruli, and rarely this may result in renal insufficiency.[963,964] (Fig. 2-168). It is notable that renal cell carcinoma is the malignant neoplasm most receptive of tumor-to-tumor metastasis; in this circumstance, lung cancer is the tumor most likely to metastasize to renal cell carcinoma.[965]

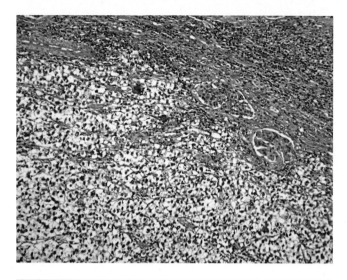

**Fig. 2-167** Metastasis to kidney. Renal neoplasm in a patient with a previous history of seminoma; findings are consistent with metastatic seminoma.

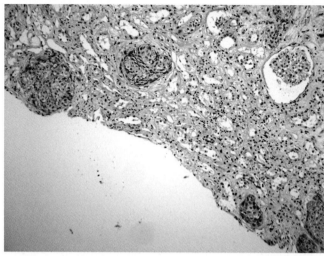

**Fig. 2-168** Metastasis to kidney. The patient was a 68-year-old man who presented with hematuria and renal failure. Clinical diagnosis was acute glomerulonephritis until needle biopsy disclosed the presence of extensive glomerular involvement by metastatic non-small cell lung carcinoma. (Courtesy of Gretta Jacobs, MD.)

# REFERENCES

1. Delahunt B, Eble JN. History of the development of the classification of renal cell neoplasia. Clin Lab Med 2005; 25: 231–246.
2. Ackerman LV. Surgical pathology. Genitourinary tract: kidney. St Louis: Mosby, 1953; 428–451.
3. Delahunt B, Eble JN. Papillary adenoma of the kidney: An evolving concept. J Urol Pathol 1997; 7: 99–112.
4. Bell ET. A classification of renal tumors with observations on the frequencies of various types. J Urol 1938; 39: 238–243.
5. Bell ET. Renal diseases, 2nd edn. Philadelphia: Lea & Febiger, 1950.
6. Klein MJ, Valensi QJ. Proximal tubular adenomas of kidney with so-called oncocytic features. A clinicopathologic study of 13 cases of a rarely reported neoplasm. Cancer 1976; 38: 906–914.
7. Bennington JL. Proceedings: Cancer of the kidney – etiology, epidemiology, and pathology. Cancer 1973; 32: 1017–1029.
8. Thoenes W, Storkel S, Rumpelt HJ. Histopathology and classification of renal cell tumors (adenomas, oncocytomas and carcinomas). The basic cytological and histopathological elements and their use for diagnostics. Pathol Res Pract 1986; 181: 125–143.
9. Talamo TS, Shonnard JW. Small renal adenocarcinoma with metastases. J Urol 1980; 124: 132–134.
10. Xipell JM. The incidence of benign renal nodules (a clinicopathologic study). J Urol 1971; 106: 503–506.
11. Reis M, Faria V, Lindoro J, et al. The small cystic and noncystic noninflammatory renal nodules: a postmortem study. J Urol 1988; 140: 721–724.
12. Hughson MD, Buchwald D, Fox M. Renal neoplasia and acquired cystic kidney disease in patients receiving long-term dialysis. Arch Pathol Lab Med 1986; 110: 592–601.
13. Eble JN, Warfel K. Early human renal cortical epithelial neoplasia. Mod Pathol 1991; 4 33: 139–150.
14. Kovacs G, Emanuel A, Neumann HP, et al. Cytogenetics of renal cell carcinomas associated with von Hippel–Lindau disease. Genes Chromosomes Cancer 1991; 3: 256–262.
15. Kovacs G. Molecular differential pathology of renal cell tumours. Histopathology 1993; 22: 1–8.
16. Presti JC Jr, Moch H, Gelb AB, et al. Initiating genetic events in small renal neoplasms detected by comparative genomic hybridization. J Urol 1998; 160: 1557–1561.
17. Storkel S, Eble JN, Adlakha K, et al. Classification of renal cell carcinoma: Workgroup No. 1. Union Internationale Contre le Cancer (UICC) and the American Joint Committee on Cancer (AJCC). Cancer 1997; 80: 987–989.
18. Grignon DJ, Eble JN. Papillary and metanephric adenomas of the kidney. Semin Diagn Pathol 1998; 15: 41–53.
19. Bonsib SM. Leiomyoma. In: Eble JN, Sauter G, Epstein JI, et al., eds. World Health Organization. Pathology and genetics of tumours of the urinary system and male genital organs. Lyon: IARC Press, 2004, 70.
20. Passega E, Marone C, Pezzoli V, et al. Massive renal adenomatosis: a case exhibiting low-grade malignancy. Hum Pathol 1987; 18: 859–863.
21. Kizaki T, Ugai K, Hirano H, et al. Renal adenomatosis associated with carcinoma of the lower urinary tract: a case report with immunohistochemical study. Pathol Int 1999; 49: 235–240.
22. Kiyoshima K, Oda Y, Nakamura T, et al. Multicentric papillary renal cell carcinoma associated with renal adenomatosis. Pathol Int 2004; 54: 266–272.
23. Delahunt B, Eble JN. Papillary renal cell carcinoma: a clinicopathologic and immunohistochemical study of 105 tumors. Mod Pathol 1997; 10: 537–544.
24. Cohen C, McCue PA, DeRose PB. Immunohistochemistry of renal adenomas and carcinomas. J Urol Pathol 1995; 3: 61–71.
25. Hiasa Y, Kitamura M, Nakaoka S, et al. Antigen immunohistochemistry of renal cell adenomas in autopsy cases: relevance to histogenesis. Oncology 1995; 52: 97–105.
26. Wang KL, Weinrach DM, Luan C, et al. Renal papillary adenoma – a putative precursor of papillary renal cell carcinoma. Hum Pathol 2007; 38: 239–246.
27. Tretiakova MS, Sahoo S, Takahashi M, et al. Expression of alpha-methylacyl-CoA racemase in papillary renal cell carcinoma. Am J Surg Pathol 2004; 28: 69–76.
28. Chuang ST, Chu P, Sugimura J, et al. Overexpression of glutathione

S-transferase alpha in clear cell renal cell carcinoma. Am J Clin Pathol 2005; 123: 421–429.

29. Farnsworth WV, Cohen C, McCue PA, et al. DNA analysis of small renal cortical neoplasms. Comparison with renal carcinomas. J Urol Pathol 1994; 2: 65–79.

30. Jones TD, Eble JN, Wang M, et al. Molecular genetic evidence for the independent origin of multifocal papillary tumors in patients with papillary renal cell carcinomas. Clin Cancer Res 2005; 11: 7226–7233.

31. Yang XJ, Tan MH, Kim HL, et al. A molecular classification of papillary renal cell carcinoma. Cancer Res 2005; 65: 5628–5637.

32. Tickoo SK, dePeralta-Venturina MN, Harik LR, et al. Spectrum of epithelial neoplasms in end-stage renal disease. An experience from 66 tumor-bearing kidneys with emphasis on histologic patterns distinct from those in sporadic adult renal neoplasia. Am J Surg Pathol 30: 2006; 141–153.

33. Zippel L. Zur Kenntnis der Onkocyten. Various archives 1942; 308: 360–382.

34. Lieber MM, Tomera KM, Farrow GM. Renal oncocytoma. J Urol 1981; 125: 481–485.

35. Thoenes W, Storkel S, Rumpelt HJ. Human chromophobe cell renal carcinoma. Virchows Arch B Cell Pathol Mol Pathol 1985; 48: 207–217.

36. Davidson AJ, Hayes WS, Hartman DS, et al. Renal oncocytoma and carcinoma: failure of differentiation with CT. Radiology 1993; 186: 693–696.

37. Gormley TS, Van Every MJ, Moreno AJ. Renal oncocytoma: preoperative diagnosis using technetium 99m sestamibi imaging. Urology 1996; 48: 33–39.

38. Merino MJ, Livolsi VA. Oncocytomas of the kidney. Cancer 1982; 50: 1852–1856.

39. Amin MB, Crotty TB, Tickoo SK, et al. Renal oncocytoma: a reappraisal of morphologic features with clinicopathologic findings in 80 cases. Am J Surg Pathol 1997; 21: 1–12.

40. Perez-Ordonez B, Hamed G, Campbell S, et al. Renal oncocytoma: a clinicopathologic study of 70 cases. Am J Surg Pathol 1997; 21: 871–883.

41. Davis CJ Jr, Sesterhenn IA, Mostofi FK, et al. Renal oncocytoma. Clinicopathological study of 166 patients. J Urogenital Pathol 1991; 1: 41–52.

42. Licht MR, Novick AC, Tubbs RR, et al. Renal oncocytoma: clinical and biological correlates. J Urol 1993; 150: 1380–1383.

43. Choi H, Almagro UA, McManus JT, et al. Renal oncocytoma. A clinicopathologic study. Cancer 1983; 51: 1887–1896.

44. Dechet CB, Bostwick DG, Blute ML, et al. Renal oncocytoma: multifocality, bilateralism, metachronous tumor development and coexistent renal cell carcinoma. J Urol 1999; 162: 40–42.

45. Tickoo SK, Amin MB. Discriminant nuclear features of renal oncocytoma and chromophobe renal cell carcinoma. Analysis of their potential utility in the differential diagnosis. Am J Clin Pathol 1998; 110: 782–787.

46. Tickoo SK, Lee MW, Eble JN, et al. Ultrastructural observations on mitochondria and microvesicles in renal oncocytoma, chromophobe renal cell carcinoma, and eosinophilic variant of conventional (clear cell) renal cell carcinoma. Am J Surg Pathol 2000; 24: 1247–1256.

47. Krishnan B, Truong LD. Renal epithelial neoplasms: the diagnostic implications of electron microscopic study in 55 cases. Hum Pathol 2002; 33: 68–79.

48. Tickoo SK, Amin MB, Zarbo RJ. Colloidal iron staining in renal epithelial neoplasms, including chromophobe renal cell carcinoma: emphasis on technique and patterns of staining. Am J Surg Pathol 1998; 22: 419–424.

49. Cochand-Priollet B, Molinie V, Bougaran J, et al. Renal chromophobe cell carcinoma and oncocytoma. A comparative morphologic, histochemical, and immunohistochemical study of 124 cases. Arch Pathol Lab Med 1997; 121: 1081–1086.

50. Zhou M, Roma A, Magi-Galluzzi C. The usefulness of immunohistochemical markers in the differential diagnosis of renal neoplasms. Clin Lab Med 2005; 25: 247–257.

51. Crotty TB, Lawrence KM, Moertel CA, et al. Cytogenetic analysis of six renal oncocytomas and a chromophobe cell renal carcinoma. Evidence that -Y, -1 may be a characteristic anomaly in renal oncocytomas. Cancer Genet Cytogenet 1992; 61: 61–66.

52. Fuzesi L, Gunawan B, Braun S, et al. Renal oncocytoma with a translocation t(9; 11)(p23; q13). J Urol 1994; 152: 471–472.

53. van den Berg E, Dijkhuizen T, Storkel S, et al. Chromosomal changes in renal oncocytomas. Evidence that t(5; 11)(q35; q13) may characterize a second subgroup of oncocytomas. Cancer Genet Cytogenet 1995; 79: 164–168.

54. Brown JA, Takahashi S, Alcaraz A, et al. Fluorescence in situ hybridization analysis of renal oncocytoma reveals frequent loss of chromosomes Y and 1. J Urol 1996; 156: 31–35.

55. Fuzesi L, Gunawan B, Braun S, et al. Cytogenetic analysis of 11 renal oncocytomas: further evidence of structural rearrangements of 11q13 as a characteristic chromosomal anomaly. Cancer Genet Cytogenet 1998; 107: 1–6.

56. Feder M, Liu Z, Apostolou S, et al. Loss of chromosomes 1 and X in a renal oncocytoma: implications for a possible pseudoautosomal tumor suppressor locus. Cancer Genet Cytogenet 2000; 123: 71–72.

57. Presti JC Jr, Moch H, Reuter VE, et al. Comparative genomic hybridization for genetic analysis of renal oncocytomas. Genes Chromosomes Cancer 1996; 17: 199–204.

58. Lindgren V, Paner GP, Omeroglu A, et al. Cytogenetic analysis of a series of 13 renal oncocytomas. J Urol 2004; 171: 602–604.

59. Fuzesi L, Frank D, Nguyen C, et al. Losses of 1p and chromosome 14 in renal oncocytomas. Cancer Genet Cytogenet 2005; 160: 120–125.

60. Warfel KA, Eble JN. Renal oncocytomatosis. J Urol 1982; 127: 1179–1180.

61. Katz DS, Gharagozloo AM, Peebles TR, et al. Renal oncocytomatosis. Am J Kidney Dis 1996; 27: 579–582.

62. Israeli RS, Wise GJ, Bansal S, et al. Bilateral renal oncocytomatosis in a patient with renal failure. Urology 1995; 46: 873–875.

63. Tickoo SK, Reuter VE, Amin MB, et al. Renal oncocytosis: a morphologic study of fourteen cases. Am J Surg Pathol 1999; 23: 1094–1101.

64. Pavlovich CP, Walther MM, Eyler RA, et al. Renal tumors in the Birt–Hogg–Dube syndrome. Am J Surg Pathol 2002; 26: 1542–1552.

65. Al-Saleem T, Cairns P, Dulaimi EA, et al. The genetics of renal oncocytosis: a possible model for neoplastic progression. Cancer Genet Cytogenet 2004; 152: 23–28.

66. Leroy X, Lemaitre L, De La Taille A, et al. Bilateral renal oncocytosis with renal failure. Arch Pathol Lab Med 2001; 125: 683–685.

67. Farkas LM, Szekely JG, Karatson A. Bilateral, multifocal renal oncocytomatosis with rapid progression leading to renal insufficiency. Nephrol Dial Transplant 1999; 14: 2262–2263.

68. Parkin CM, Whelan SL, Ferlay J, et al. Cancer incidence in five continents. IARC Scientific publications No. 155. Lyon, France: International Agency for Research on Cancer 8, 2002.

69. SEER: Program Public Use Data Tapes 1973–2002, November 2004 Submission. Bethesda: National Cancer Institute, Division of Cancer Control and Population Science, Surveillance Research Program, Cancer Statistics Branch, 2005.

70. Mathew A, Devesa SS, Fraumeni JF Jr, et al. Global increases in kidney cancer incidence, 1973–1992. Eur J Cancer Prev 2002; 11: 171–178.

71. Mindrup SR, Pierre JS, Dahmoush L, et al. The prevalence of renal cell carcinoma diagnosed at autopsy. BJU Int 2005; 95: 31–33.

72. Chow WH, Devesa SS, Warren JL, et al. Rising incidence of renal cell cancer in the United States. JAMA 1999; 281: 1628–1631.

73. Lipworth L, Tarone RE, McLaughlin JK. The epidemiology of renal cell carcinoma. J Urol 2006; 176: 2353–2358.

74. Noordzij MA, Mickisch GH. The genetic make-up of renal cell tumors. Urol Res 2004; 32: 251–254.

75. McLaughlin JK, Lindblad P, Mellemgaard A, et al. International renal-cell cancer study. I. Tobacco use. Int J Cancer 1995; 60: 194–198.

76. Hunt JD, van der Hel OL, McMillan GP, et al. Renal cell carcinoma in relation to cigarette smoking: meta-analysis of 24 studies. Int J Cancer 2005; 114: 101–108.

77. Bergstrom A, Hsieh CC, Lindblad P, et al. Obesity and renal cell cancer – a quantitative review. Br J Cancer 2001; 85: 984–990.

78. Calle EE, Kaaks R. Overweight, obesity and cancer: epidemiological evidence and proposed mechanisms. Natl Rev Cancer 2004; 4: 579–591.

79. Stewart JH, Buccianti G, Agodoa L, et al. Cancers of the kidney and urinary tract in patients on dialysis for end-stage renal disease: analysis of data from the United States, Europe, and Australia and New Zealand. J Am Soc Nephrol 2003; 14: 197–207.

80. Neuzillet Y, Lay F, Luccioni A, et al. De novo renal cell carcinoma of native kidney in renal transplant recipients. Cancer 2005; 103: 251–257.

81. IARC. IARC monographs on the evaluation of carcinogenic risks to humans. Overall evaluations of carcinogenicity: An updating of IARC Monographs volumes 1–41. Lyon, France: IARC Press, 1987.

82. Parker L, Kollin J, Vicario D, et al. Hemihypertrophy as possible sign of renal cell carcinoma. Urology 1992; 40: 286–288.

83. Treiger BF, Khazan R, Goldman SM, et al. Renal cell carcinoma with situs inversus totalis. Urology 1993; 41: 455–457.

84. Kmetec A, Kaplan-Pavlovcic S, Ferluga D. Renal cell carcinoma in nonfunctioning transplanted kidney. Am J Nephrol 2001; 21: 256–258.

85. Carney JA. Wilms' tumor and renal cell carcinoma in retroperitoneal teratoma. Cancer 1975; 35: 1179–1183.

86. Browne MK, Glashan RW. Multiple pathology in a unilateral supernumerary kidney. Br J Surg 1971; 58: 73–76.

87. Marcus PB, Kemp CB. Ectopic renal cell carcinoma: pathologists' problem. Urology 1978; 12: 453–457.

88. Kunkel JF, MacLennan GT, DeOreo GA, et al. Extrarenal renal cell carcinoma. J Urol Pathol 1997; 7: 197–205.

89. Gupta AK, Kamaladevi JC. Extrarenal renal cell carcinoma (a case report). Indian J Pathol Microbiol 1982; 25: 197–205.

90. Al-Saleem T, Wessner LL, Scheithauer BW, et al. Malignant tumors of the kidney, brain, and soft tissues in children and young adults with the tuberous sclerosis complex. Cancer 1998; 83: 2208–2216.

91. Bjornsson J, Short MP, Kwiatkowski DJ, et al. Tuberous sclerosis-associated renal cell carcinoma. Clinical, pathological, and genetic features. Am J Pathol 1996; 149: 1201–1208.

92. Sampson JR, Patel A, Mee AD. Multifocal renal cell carcinoma in sibs from a chromosome 9 linked (TSC1) tuberous sclerosis family. J Med Genet 1995; 32: 848–850.

93. Truong LD, Choi YJ, Shen SS, et al. Renal cystic neoplasms and renal neoplasms associated with cystic renal diseases. Pathogenetic and molecular links. Adv Anat Pathol 2003; 10: 135–159.

94. Tello R, Blickman JG, Buonomo C, et al. Meta analysis of the relationship between tuberous sclerosis complex and renal cell carcinoma. Eur J Radiol 1998; 27: 131–138.

95. Keith DS, Torres VE, King BF, et al. Renal cell carcinoma in autosomal dominant polycystic kidney disease. J Am Soc Nephrol 1994; 4: 1661–1669.

96. Rackley RR, Angermeier KW, Levin H, et al. Renal cell carcinoma arising in a regressed multicystic dysplastic kidney. J Urol 1994; 152: 1543–1545.

97. Gregoire JR, Torres VE, Holley KE, et al. Renal epithelial hyperplastic and neoplastic proliferation in autosomal dominant polycystic kidney disease. Am J Kidney Dis 1987; 9: 27–38.

98. Gibbons RP, Monte JE, Correa RJ, et al. Manifestations of renal cell carcinoma. Urology 1976; 8: 201–206.

99. Palapattu GS, Kristo B, Rajfer J. Paraneoplastic syndromes in urologic malignancy: the many faces of renal cell carcinoma. Rev Urol 2002; 4: 163–170.

100. McDougal WS, Garnick MB. Clinical signs and symptoms of renal cell carcinoma. In: Vogelzand NJ, Shipley WU, Scardino PT, et al., eds. Comprehensive textbook of genitourinary oncology. Baltimore, MD: Williams & Wilkins, 1995; 154–159.

101. Laski ME, Vugrin D. Paraneoplastic syndromes in hypernephroma. Semin Nephrol 1987; 7: 123–130.

102. Tsukamoto T, Kumamoto Y, Miyao N, et al. Interleukin-6 in renal cell carcinoma. J Urol 1992; 148: 78–82.

103. Kim HL, Han KR, Zisman A, et al. Cachexia-like symptoms predict a worse prognosis in localized t1 renal cell carcinoma. J Urol 2004; 171: 1810–1813.

104. Gold PJ, Fefer A, Thompson JA. Paraneoplastic manifestations of renal cell carcinoma. Semin Urol Oncol 1996; 14: 216–222.

105. Strewler GJ, Stern PH, Jacobs JW, et al. Parathyroid hormonelike protein from human renal carcinoma cells. Structural and functional homology with parathyroid hormone. J Clin Invest 1987; 80: 1803–1807.

106. Suva LJ, Winslow GA, Wettenhall RE, et al. A parathyroid hormone-related protein implicated in malignant hypercalcemia: cloning and expression. Science 1987; 237: 893–896.

107. Fahn HJ, Lee YH, Chen MT, et al. The incidence and prognostic significance of humoral hypercalcemia in renal cell carcinoma. J Urol 1991; 145: 248–250.

108. Sufrin G, Mirand EA, Moore RH, et al. Hormones in renal cancer. J Urol 1977; 117: 433–438.

109. Hama Y, Kaji T, Ito K, et al. Erythropoietin-producing renal cell carcinoma arising from autosomal dominant polycystic kidney disease. Br J Radiol 2005; 78: 269–271.

110. Stanisic TH, Donovan J. Prolactin secreting renal cell carcinoma. J Urol 1986; 136: 85–86.

111. Golde DW, Schambelan M, Weintraub BD, et al. Gonadotropin-secreting renal carcinoma. Cancer 1974; 33: 1048–1053.

112. Donmez T, Kale M, Ozyurek Y, et al. Erythrocyte sedimentation rates in patients with renal cell carcinoma. Eur Urol 1992; 21: 51–52.

113. Vanatta PR, Silva FG, Taylor WE, et al. Renal cell carcinoma and systemic amyloidosis: demonstration of AA protein and review of the literature. Hum Pathol 1983; 14: 195–201.

114. Konnak JW, Grossman HB. Renal cell carcinoma as an incidental finding. J Urol 1985; 134: 1094–1096.

115. Jayson M, Sanders H. Increased incidence of serendipitously discovered renal cell carcinoma. Urology 1998; 51: 203–205.

116. Smith SJ, Bosniak MA, Megibow AJ, et al. Renal cell carcinoma: earlier discovery and increased detection. Radiology 1989; 170: 699–703.

117. Tsui KH, Shvarts O, Smith RB, et al. Renal cell carcinoma: prognostic significance of incidentally detected tumors. J Urol 2000; 163: 426–430.

118. Touloupidis S, Papathanasiou A, Kalaitzis C, et al. Renal cell carcinoma: the influence of new diagnostic imaging techniques on the size and stage of tumors diagnosed over the past 26 years. Int Urol Nephrol 2006; 38: 193–197.

119. Coll DM, Smith RC. Update on radiological imaging of renal cell carcinoma. BJU Int 2007; 99: 1217–1222.

120. Kutikov A, Fossett LK, Ramchandani P, et al. Incidence of benign pathologic findings at partial nephrectomy for solitary renal mass presumed to be renal cell carcinoma on preoperative imaging. Urology 2006; 68: 737–740.

121. Skinner DG, Colvin RB, Vermillion CD, et al. Diagnosis and management of renal cell carcinoma. A clinical and pathologic study of 309 cases. Cancer 1971; 28: 1165–1177.

122. Varkarakis MJ, Bhanalaph T, Moore RH, et al. Prognostic criteria of renal cell carcinoma. J Surg Oncol 1974; 6: 97–107.

123. Fuhrman SA, Lasky LC, Limas C. Prognostic significance of morphologic parameters in renal cell carcinoma. Am J Surg Pathol 1982; 6: 655–663.

124. Kloppel G, Knofel WT, Baisch H, et al. Prognosis of renal cell carcinoma related to nuclear grade, DNA content and Robson stage. Eur Urol 1986; 12: 426–431.

125. Delahunt B, Nacey JN. Renal cell carcinoma. II. Histological indicators of prognosis. Pathology 1987; 19: 258–263.

126. Medeiros LJ, Gelb AB, Weiss LM. Renal cell carcinoma. Prognostic significance of morphologic parameters in 121 cases. Cancer 1988; 61: 1639–1651.

127. Storkel S, Thoenes W, Jacobi GH, et al. Prognostic parameters in renal cell carcinoma – a new approach. Eur Urol 1989; 16: 416–422.

128. Grignon DJ, Ayala AG, el-Naggar A, et al. Renal cell carcinoma. A clinicopathologic and DNA flow cytometric analysis of 103 cases. Cancer 1989; 64: 2133–2140.

129. Green LK, Ayala AG, Ro JY, et al. Role of nuclear grading in stage I renal cell carcinoma. Urology 1989; 34: 310–315.

130. Gelb AB, Shibuya RB, Weiss LM, et al. Stage I renal cell carcinoma. A clinicopathologic study of 82 cases. Am J Surg Pathol 1993; 17: 275–286.

131. Takahashi S, Qian J, Brown JA, et al. Potential markers of prostate cancer aggressiveness detected by fluorescence in situ hybridization in needle biopsies. Cancer Res 1994; 54: 3574–3579.

132. Bretheau D, Lechevallier E, de Fromont M, et al. Prognostic value of nuclear grade of renal cell carcinoma. Cancer 1995; 76: 2543–2549.

133. Goldstein NS. The current state of renal cell carcinoma grading. Union Internationale Contre le Cancer (UICC) and the American Joint Committee on Cancer (AJCC). Cancer 1997; 80: 977–980.

134. Delahunt B. Histopathologic prognostic indicators for renal cell carcinoma. Semin Diagn Pathol 1998; 15: 68–76.

135. Usubutun A, Uygur MC, Ayhan A, et al. Comparison of grading systems for estimating the prognosis of renal cell carcinoma. Int Urol Nephrol 1998; 30: 391–397.

136. Onodera Y, Matsuda N, Ohta M, et al. Prognostic significance of tumor grade for renal cell carcinoma. Int J Urol 2000; 7: 4–9.

137. Ficarra V, Righetti R, Martignoni G, et al. Prognostic value of renal cell carcinoma nuclear grading: multivariate analysis of 333 cases. Urol Int 2001; 67: 130–134.

138. Lohse CM, Blute ML, Zincke H, et al. Comparison of standardized and nonstandardized nuclear grade of renal cell carcinoma to predict outcome among 2,042 patients. Am J Clin Pathol 2002; 118: 877–886.

139. Lohse CM, Cheville JC. A review of prognostic pathologic features and algorithms for patients treated surgically for renal cell carcinoma. Clin Lab Med 2005; 25: 433–464.

140. Arner O, Blanck C, von Schreeb T. Renal adenocarcinoma; morphology–grading of malignancy–prognosis. A study of 197 cases. Acta Chir Scand 1965; 346: 1–51.

141. Syrjanen K, Hjelt L. Grading of human renal adenocarcinoma. Scand J Urol Nephrol 1978; 12: 49–55.

142. Ficarra V, Prayer-Galetti T, Novella G, et al. Incidental detection beyond pathological factors as prognostic predictor of renal cell carcinoma. Eur Urol 2003; 43: 663–669.

143. Patard JJ, Leray E, Rioux-Leclercq N, et al. Prognostic value of histologic subtypes in renal cell carcinoma: a multicenter experience. J Clin Oncol 2005; 23: 2763–2771.

144. Tsui KH, Shvarts O, Smith RB, et al. Prognostic indicators for renal cell carcinoma: a multivariate analysis of 643 patients using the revised 1997 TNM staging criteria. J Urol 2000; 163: 1090–1095; quiz 1295.

145. Frank I, Blute ML, Cheville JC, et al. An outcome prediction model for patients with clear cell renal cell carcinoma treated with radical nephrectomy based on tumor stage, size, grade and necrosis: the SSIGN score. J Urol 2002; 168: 2395–2400.

146. True LD. The time for accurate Fuhrman grading of renal cell carcinomas has arrived. Am J Clin Pathol 20021; 18: 827–829.

147. Thrasher JB, Paulson DF. Prognostic factors in renal cancer. Urol Clin North Am 1993; 20: 247–262.

148. Leibovich BC, Blute ML, Cheville JC, et al. Prediction of progression after radical nephrectomy for patients with clear cell renal cell carcinoma: a stratification tool for prospective clinical trials. Cancer 2003; 97: 1663–1671.

149. Gospodarowicz MK, Miller D, Groome PA, et al. The process for continuous improvement of the TNM classification. Cancer 2004; 100: 1–5.

150. Greene FL, Page DL, Fleming ID. AJCC cancer staging manual. New York, Springer; 2002.

151. Javidan J, Stricker HJ, Tamboli P, et al. Prognostic significance of the 1997 TNM classification of renal cell carcinoma. J Urol 1999; 162: 1277–1281.

152. Gettman MT, Blute ML, Spotts B, et al. Pathologic staging of renal cell carcinoma: significance of tumor classification with the 1997 TNM staging system. Cancer 2001; 91: 354–361.

153. Pantuck AJ, Zisman A, Belldegrun AS. The changing natural history of renal cell carcinoma. J Urol 2001; 166: 1611–1623.

154. Gettman MT, Blute ML. Update on pathologic staging of renal cell carcinoma. Urology 2002; 60: 209–217.

155. Frank I, Blute ML, Cheville JC, et al. A multifactorial postoperative surveillance model for patients with surgically treated clear cell renal cell carcinoma. J Urol 2003; 170: 2225–2232.

156. Frank I, Blute ML, Leibovich BC, et al. pT2 classification for renal cell carcinoma. Can its accuracy be improved? J Urol 2005; 173: 380–384.

157. Leibovich BC, Pantuck AJ, Bui MH, et al. Current staging of renal cell carcinoma. Urol Clin North Am 2003; 30: 481–497.

158. Mejean A, Oudard S, Thiounn N. Prognostic factors of renal cell carcinoma. J Urol 2003; 169: 821–827.

159. Reuter VE, Presti JC, Jr. Contemporary approach to the classification of renal epithelial tumors. Semin Oncol 2000; 27: 124–137.

160. Wallace AC, Nairn RC. Renal tubular antigens in kidney tumors. Cancer 1972; 29: 977–981.

161. Yoshida SO, Imam A, Olson CA, et al. Proximal renal tubular surface membrane antigens identified in primary and metastatic renal cell carcinomas. Arch Pathol Lab Med 1986; 110: 825–832.

162. Jemal A, Siegel R, Ward E, et al. Cancer statistics, 2007. CA Cancer J Clin 2007; 57: 43–66.

163. Bruder E, Passera O, Harms D, et al. Morphologic and molecular characterization of renal cell carcinoma in children and young adults. Am J Surg Pathol 2004; 28: 1117–1132.

164. Kovacs G, Szucs S, De Riese W, et al. Specific chromosome aberration in human renal cell carcinoma. Int J Cancer 1987; 40: 171–178.

165. Yoshida MA, Ohyashiki K, Ochi H, et al. Cytogenetic studies of tumor tissue from patients with nonfamilial renal cell carcinoma. Cancer Res 1986; 46: 2139–2147.

166. Anglard P, Tory K, Brauch H, et al. Molecular analysis of genetic changes in the origin and development of renal cell carcinoma. Cancer Res 1991; 51: 1071–1077.

167. Kovacs G, Erlandsson R, Boldog F, et al. Consistent chromosome 3p deletion and loss of heterozygosity in renal cell carcinoma. Proc Natl Acad Sci USA 1988; 85: 1571–1575.

168. Carroll PR, Murty VV, Reuter V, et al. Abnormalities at chromosome region 3p12–14 characterize clear cell renal carcinoma. Cancer Genet Cytogenet 1987; 26: 253–259.

169. Teyssier JR, Ferre D. Chromosomal changes in renal cell carcinoma. No evidence for correlation with clinical stage. Cancer Genet Cytogenet 1990; 45: 197–205.

170. Whaley JM, Naglich J, Gelbert L, et al. Germ-line mutations in the von Hippel–Lindau tumor-suppressor gene are similar to somatic von Hippel–Lindau aberrations in sporadic renal

cell carcinoma. Am J Hum Genet 1994; 55: 1092–102.

171. Goodman MD, Goodman BK, Lubin MB, et al. Cytogenetic characterization of renal cell carcinoma in von Hippel–Lindau syndrome. Cancer 1990; 65: 1150–1154.

172. Latif F, Tory K, Gnarra J, et al. Identification of the von Hippel–Lindau disease tumor suppressor gene. Science 1993; 260: 1317–1320.

173. Gnarra JR, Tory K, Weng Y, et al. Mutations of the VHL tumour suppressor gene in renal carcinoma. Nature Genet 1994; 7: 85–90.

174. Herman JG, Latif F, Weng Y, et al. Silencing of the VHL tumor-suppressor gene by DNA methylation in renal carcinoma. Proc Natl Acad Sci USA 1994; 91: 9700–9704.

175. Velickovic M, Delahunt B, Storkel S, et al. VHL and FHIT locus loss of heterozygosity is common in all renal cancer morphotypes but differs in pattern and prognostic significance. Cancer Res 2001; 61: 4815–4819.

176. Sukosd F, Kuroda N, Beothe T, et al. Deletion of chromosome 3p14.2-p25 involving the VHL and FHIT genes in conventional renal cell carcinoma. Cancer Res 2003; 63: 455–457.

177. Schraml P, Struckmann K, Bednar R, et al. CDKNA2A mutation analysis, protein expression, and deletion mapping of chromosome 9p in conventional clear-cell renal carcinomas: evidence for a second tumor suppressor gene proximal to CDKN2A. Am J Pathol 2001; 158: 593–601.

178. Beroud C, Fournet JC, Jeanpierre C, et al. Correlations of allelic imbalance of chromosome 14 with adverse prognostic parameters in 148 renal cell carcinomas. Genes Chromosomes Cancer 1996; 17: 215–224.

179. Herbers J, Schullerus D, Muller H, et al. Significance of chromosome arm 14q loss in nonpapillary renal cell carcinomas. Genes Chromosomes Cancer 1997; 19: 29–35.

180. Velickovic M, Delahunt B, McIver B, et al. Intragenic PTEN/MMAC1 loss of heterozygosity in conventional (clear-cell) renal cell carcinoma is associated with poor patient prognosis. Mod Pathol 2002 15: 479–485.

181. Linehan WM, Walther MM, Zbar B. The genetic basis of cancer of the kidney. J Urol 2003; 170: 2163–2172.

182. Van EF, Van RC, Bodmer D, et al. Chromosome 3 translocations and the risk to develop renal cell cancer: a Dutch intergroup study. Genent Couns 2003; 14: 149–154.

183. Vanharanta S, Buchta M, McWhinney SR, et al. Early-onset renal cell carcinoma as a novel extraparaganglial component of SDHB-associated heritable paraganglioma. Am J Hum Genet 2004; 74: 153–159.

184. Delahunt B. Sarcomatoid renal carcinoma. the final common dedifferentiation pathway of renal epithelial malignancies. Pathology 2003; 31: 185–190.

185. Cheville JC, Lohse CM, Zincke H, et al. Sarcomatoid renal cell carcinoma: an examination of underlying histologic subtype and an analysis of associations with patient outcome. Am J Surg Pathol 2004; 28: 435–441.

186. de Peralta-Venturina M, Moch H, Amin M, et al. Sarcomatoid differentiation in renal cell carcinoma: a study of 101 cases. Am J Surg Pathol 2001; 25: 275–284.

187. Ro JY, Ayala AG, Sella A, et al. Sarcomatoid renal cell carcinoma: clinicopathologic. A study of 42 cases. Cancer 1987; 59: 516–526.

188. Mian BM, Bhadkamkar N, Slaton JW, et al. Prognostic factors and survival of patients with sarcomatoid renal cell carcinoma. J Urol 2002; 167: 65–70.

189. Haddad FS, Shah IA, Manne RK, et al. Renal cell carcinoma insulated in the renal capsule with calcification and ossification. Urol Int 1993; 51: 97–101.

190. Bonsib SM. Renal cell carcinoma with lymphomatoid. J Urol Pathol 1997; 6: 109–118.

191. Gokden N, Nappi O, Swanson PE, et al. Renal cell carcinoma with rhabdoid features. Am J Surg Pathol 2000; 24: 1329–1338.

192. Fukuoka T, Honda M, Namiki M, et al. Renal cell carcinoma with heterotopic bone formation. Case report and review of the Japanese literature. Urol Int 1987; 42: 458–460.

193. Jagirdar J, Irie T, French SW, et al. Globular Mallory-like bodies in renal cell carcinoma: report of a case and review of cytoplasmic eosinophilic globules. Hum Pathol 1985; 16: 949–952.

194. Datta BN. Hyaline intracytoplasmic globules in renal carcinoma. Arch Pathol Lab Med 1977; 101: 391.

195. Hull MT, Eble JN. Myelinoid lamellated cytoplasmic inclusions in human renal adenocarcinomas: an ultrastructural study. Ultrastruct Pathol 1988; 12: 41–48.

196. Moder KG, Litin SC, Gaffey TA. Renal cell carcinoma associated with sarcoidlike tissue reaction. Mayo Clin Proc 1990; 65: 1498–1501.

197. Chau KY, Pretorius JM, Stewart AW. Myospherulosis in renal cell carcinoma. Arch Pathol Lab Med 2000; 124: 1476–1479.

198. Leroy X, Moukassa D, Copin MC, et al. Utility of cytokeratin 7 for distinguishing chromophobe renal cell carcinoma from renal oncocytoma. Eur Urol 2000; 37: 484–487.

199. Mathers ME, Pollock AM, Marsh C, et al. Cytokeratin 7: a useful adjunct in the diagnosis of chromophobe renal cell carcinoma. Histopathology 2002; 40: 563–567.

200. Wu SL, Kothari P, Wheeler TM, et al. Cytokeratins 7 and 20 immunoreactivity in chromophobe renal cell carcinomas and renal oncocytomas. Mod Pathol 2002; 15: 712–717.

201. McGregor DK, Khurana KK, Cao C, et al. Diagnosing primary and metastatic renal cell carcinoma: the use of the monoclonal antibody 'Renal Cell Carcinoma Marker'. Am J Surg Pathol 2001; 25: 1485–1492.

202. Avery AK, Beckstead J, Renshaw AA, et al. Use of antibodies to RCC and CD10 in the differential diagnosis of renal neoplasms. Am J Surg Pathol 2000; 24: 203–210.

203. Ordonez NG. The diagnostic utility of immunohistochemistry in distinguishing between mesothelioma and renal cell carcinoma: a comparative study. Hum Pathol 2004; 35: 697–710.

204. Kim MK, Kim S. Immunohistochemical profile of common epithelial neoplasms arising in the kidney. Appl Immunohistochem Mol Morphol 2002; 10: 332–338.

205. Langner C, Wegscheider BJ, Ratschek M, et al. Keratin immunohistochemistry in renal cell carcinoma subtypes and renal oncocytomas: a systematic analysis of 233 tumors. Virchows Arch 2004; 444: 127–134.

206. Young AN, Amin MB, Moreno CS, et al. Expression profiling of renal epithelial neoplasms: a method for tumor classification and discovery of diagnostic molecular markers. Am J Pathol 2001; 158: 1639–1651.

207. Petit A, Castillo M, Santos M, et al. KIT expression in chromophobe renal cell carcinoma: comparative immunohistochemical analysis of KIT expression in different renal cell neoplasms. Am J Surg Pathol 2004; 28: 676–678.

208. Miliaras D, Karasavvidou F, Papanikolaou A, et al. KIT expression in fetal, normal adult, and neoplastic renal tissues. J Clin Pathol 2004; 57: 463–466.

209. Langner C, Ratschek M, Rehak P, et al. Expression of MUC1 (EMA) and E-cadherin in renal cell carcinoma: a systematic immunohistochemical analysis of 188 cases. Mod Pathol 2004; 17: 180–188.

210. MacLennan GT, Farrow GM, Bostwick DG. Immunohistochemistry in the evaluation of renal cell carcinoma: a critical appraisal. J Urol Pathol 1997; 6: 195–203.

211. Perlmann S. Uber einen Fall von Lymphangioma cysticum der Niere. Virchows Arch Pathol Ant Physiol Klin Med 1928; 268: 524–535.

212. Robinson GL. Perlmann's tumour of the kidney. Br J Surg 1957; 44: 620–623.

213. Feldberg MA, van Waes PF. Multilocular cystic renal cell carcinoma. Am J Roentgenol 1982; 138: 953–955.

214. Murad T, Komaiko W, Oyasu R, et al. Multilocular cystic renal cell carcinoma. Am J Clin Pathol 1991; 95: 633–637.

215. Eble JN, Bonsib SM. Extensively cystic renal neoplasms: cystic nephroma, cystic partially differentiated nephroblastoma, multilocular cystic renal cell carcinoma, and cystic hamartoma of renal pelvis. Semin Diagn Pathol 1998; 15: 2–20.

216. Eble JN, Sauter G, Epstein JI, et al. World Health Organization: Pathology and genetics of tumours of the urinary system and male genital organs. Lyon, France: IARC Press, 2004.

217. Corica FA, Iczkowski KA, Cheng L, et al. Cystic renal cell carcinoma is cured by resection: a study of 24 cases with long-term followup. J Urol 1999; 161: 408–411.

218. Nassir A, Jollimore J, Gupta R, et al. Multilocular cystic renal cell carcinoma: a series of 12 cases and review of the literature. Urology 2002; 60: 421–427.

219. Imura J, Ichikawa K, Takeda J, et al. Multilocular cystic renal cell carcinoma: a clinicopathological, immuno- and lectin histochemical study of nine cases. Apmis 2004; 112: 183–191.

220. Suzigan S, Lopez-Beltran A, Montironi R, et al. Multilocular cystic renal cell carcinoma: a report of 45 cases of a kidney tumor of low malignant potential. Am J Clin Pathol 2006; 125: 217–222.

221. Grignon DJ, Bismar T, Bianco F, et al. VHL gene mutations in multilocular cystic renal cell carcinoma: evidence in support of its classification as a type of clear cell renal cell carcinoma. Mod Pathol 2004; 17: 154A.

222. Del Vecchio MT, Lazzi S, Bruni A, et al. DNA ploidy pattern in papillary renal cell carcinoma. Correlation with clinicopathological parameters and survival. Pathol Res Pract 1998; 194: 325–333.

223. Mydlo JH, Bard RH. Analysis of papillary renal adenocarcinoma. Urology 1987; 30: 529–554.

224. Zbar B, Tory K, Merino M, et al. Hereditary papillary renal carcinoma. J Urol 1994; 51: 561–566.

225. Ornstein DK, Lubensky IA, Venzon D, et al. Prevalence of microscopic tumors in normal appearing renal parenchyma of patients with hereditary papillary renal cancer. J Urol 2000; 163: 431–433.

226. Fischer J, Palmedo G, von Knobloch R, et al. Duplication and overexpression of the mutant allele of the MET proto-oncogene in multiple hereditary papillary renal cell tumours. Oncogene 1998; 17: 733–739.

227. Zhuang Z, Park WS, Pack S, et al. Trisomy 7-harbouring non-random duplication of the mutant Met allele in hereditary papillary renal carcinomas. Nature Genet 1998; 20: 66–69.

228. Lubensky IA, Schmidt L, Zhuang Z, et al. Hereditary and sporadic papillary renal carcinomas with c-met mutations share a distinct morphological phenotype. Am J Pathol 1999; 155: 517–526.

229. Schmidt L, Junker K, Weirich G, et al. Two North American families with hereditary papillary renal carcinoma and identical novel mutations in the MET proto-oncogene. Cancer Res 1998; 58: 1719–1722.

230. Launonen V, Vierimaa O, Kiuru M, et al. Inherited susceptibility to uterine leiomyomas and renal cell cancer. Proc Natl Acad Sci USA 2001; 98: 3387–3392.

231. Kiuru M, Launonen V, Hietala M, et al. Familial cutaneous leiomyomatosis is a two-hit condition associated with renal cell cancer of characteristic histopathology. Am J Pathol 2001; 159: 825–829.

232. Tomlinson IP, Alam NA, Rowan AJ, et al. Germline mutations in FH predispose to dominantly inherited uterine fibroids, skin leiomyomata and papillary renal cell cancer. Nature Genet 2002; 30: 406–410.

233. Ramphal R, Pappo A, Zielenska M, et al. Pediatric renal cell carcinoma: clinical, pathologic, and molecular abnormalities associated with the members of the mit transcription factor family. Am J Clin Pathol 2006; 126: 349–364.

234. Kattar MM, Grignon DJ, Wallis T, et al. Clinicopathologic and interphase cytogenetic analysis of papillary (chromophilic) renal cell carcinoma. Mod Pathol 1997; 10: 1143–1150.

235. Kovacs G, Fuzesi L, Emanual A, et al. Cytogenetics of papillary renal cell tumors. Genes Chromosomes Cancer 1991; 3: 249–255.

236. Dijkhuizen T, Van den Berg E, Van den Berg A, et al. Chromosomal findings and p53-mutation analysis in chromophilic renal-cell carcinomas. Int J Cancer 1996; 68: 47–50.

237. Henke RP, Erbersdobler A. Numerical chromosomal aberrations in papillary renal cortical tumors: relationship with histopathologic features. Virchows Arch 2002; 440: 604–609.

238. Brunelli M, Eble JN, Zhang S, et al. Gains of chromosomes 5, 7, 12, 16, and 20 and loss of Y occur early in the evolution of papillary renal cell neoplasia: a fluorescent in situ hybridization study. Mod Pathol 2003; 16: 1053–1059.

239. Bugert P, Kovacs G. Molecular differential diagnosis of renal cell carcinomas by microsatellite analysis. Am J Pathol 1996; 149: 2081–2088.

240. Morrissey C, Martinez A, Zatyka M, et al. Epigenetic inactivation of the RASSF1A 3p21.3 tumor suppressor gene in both clear cell and papillary renal cell carcinoma. Cancer Res 2001; 61: 7277–7281.

241. Hughson MD, Dickman K, Bigler SA, et al. Clear-cell and papillary carcinoma of the kidney: an analysis of chromosome 3, 7, and 17 abnormalities by microsatellite amplification, cytogenetics, and fluorescence in situ hybridization.

Cancer Genet Cytogenet 1998; 106: 93–104.

242. Ishikawa I, Kovacs G. High incidence of papillary renal cell tumours in patients on chronic haemodialysis. Histopathology 1993; 22: 135–139.

243. Amin MB, Corless CL, Renshaw AA, et al. Papillary (chromophil) renal cell carcinoma: histomorphologic characteristics and evaluation of conventional pathologic prognostic parameters in 62 cases. Am J Surg Pathol 1997; 21: 621–635.

244. Mancilla-Jimenez R, Stanley RJ, Blath RA. Papillary renal cell carcinoma: a clinical, radiologic, and pathologic study of 34 cases. Cancer 1976; 38: 2469–2480.

245. Schraml P, Muller D, Bednar R, et al. Allelic loss at the D9S171 locus on chromosome 9p13 is associated with progression of papillary renal cell carcinoma. J Pathol 2000; 190: 457–461.

246. Henn W, Zwergel T, Wullich B, et al. Bilateral multicentric papillary renal tumors with heteroclonal origin based on tissue-specific karyotype instability. Cancer 1993; 72: 1315–1318.

247. el-Naggar AK, Ro JY, Ensign LG. Papillary renal cell carcinoma: clinical implication of DNA content analysis. Hum Pathol 1993; 24: 316–321.

248. Fleming S, Lewi HJ. Collecting duct carcinoma of the kidney. Histopathology 10: 1131–1141, 1986.

249. Renshaw AA, Maurici D, Fletcher JA. Cytologic and fluorescence in situ hybridization (FISH) examination of metanephric adenoma. Diagn Cytopathol 1997; 16: 107–111.

250. Renshaw AA, Maurici D, Fletcher JA. Papillary renal cell carcinoma with rare papillae histologically resembling collecting duct carcinoma. J Urol Pathol 1996; 5: 65–73.

251. Delahunt B, Eble JN, McCredie MR, et al. Morphologic typing of papillary renal cell carcinoma: comparison of growth kinetics and patient survival in 66 cases. Hum Pathol 2001; 32: 590–595.

252. Pignot G, Elie C, Conquy S, et al. Survival analysis of 130 patients with papillary renal cell carcinoma: prognostic utility of type 1 and type 2 subclassification. Urology 2007; 69: 230–235.

253. Leroy X, Zini L, Leteurtre E, et al. Morphologic subtyping of papillary renal cell carcinoma: correlation with prognosis and differential expression of MUC1 between the two subtypes. Mod Pathol 2002; 15: 1126–1130.

254. Lefevre M, Couturier J, Sibony M, et al. Adult papillary renal tumor with oncocytic cells: clinicopathologic, immunohistochemical, and cytogenetic features of 10 cases. Am J Surg Pathol 2005; 29: 1576–1581.

255. Renshaw AA, Corless CL. Papillary renal cell carcinoma. Histology and immunohistochemistry. Am J Surg Pathol 1995; 19: 842–849.

256. Gatalica Z, Kovatich A, Miettinen M. Consistent expression of cytokeratin 7 in papillary renal cell carcinoma. J Urol Pathol 1997; 6: 195–203.

257. Pan CC, Chen PC. A distinct expression pattern and point mutation of c-KIT in papillary renal call carcinomas. Mod Pathol 2004; 10: 1440–1441.

258. Lager DJ, Huston BJ, Timmerman TG, et al. Papillary renal tumors. Morphologic, cytochemical, and genotypic features. Cancer 1995; 76: 669–673.

259. Moch H, Gasser T, Amin MB, et al. Prognostic utility of the recently recommended histologic classification and revised TNM staging system of renal cell carcinoma: a Swiss experience with 588 tumors. Cancer 2000; 89: 604–614.

260. Sika-Paotonu D, Bethwaite PB, McCredie MR, et al. Nucleolar grade but not Fuhrman grade is applicable to papillary renal cell carcinoma. Am J Surg Pathol 2006; 30: 1091–1096.

261. Bannasch P, Schacht H, Storch E, Morphogenesis and micromorphology of epithelial tumors of the kidney of nitrosomorpholine intoxicated rats. I. Induction and histology [author's transl]. Z Krebsforsch Klin Onkol Cancer Res Clin Oncol. 1974; 81: 311–331.

262. Thoenes W, Storkel S, Rumpelt HJ, et al. Chromophobe cell renal carcinoma and its variants – a report on 32 cases. J Pathol 1988; 155: 277–287.

263. Storkel S, Steart PV, Drenckhahn D, et al. The human chromophobe cell renal carcinoma: its probable relation to intercalated cells of the collecting duct. Virchows Arch B Cell Pathol Incl Mol Pathol 1989; 56: 237–245.

264. Zbar B, Alvord WG, Glenn G, et al. Risk of renal and colonic neoplasms and spontaneous pneumothorax in the Birt–Hogg–Dube syndrome. Cancer Epidemiol Biomarkers Prev 2002; 11: 393–400.

265. Akhtar M, Kardar H, Linjawi T, et al. Chromophobe cell carcinoma of the kidney. A clinicopathologic study of 21 cases. Am J Surg Pathol 1995; 19: 1245–1256.

266. Amin MB, Tamboli P, Javidan J, et al. Prognostic impact of histologic subtyping of adult renal epithelial neoplasms: an experience of 405 cases. Am J Surg Pathol 2002; 26: 281–291.

267. Crotty TB, Farrow GM, Lieber MM. Chromophobe cell renal carcinoma: clinicopathological features of 50 cases. J Urol 1995; 154: 964–967.

268. Onishi T, Oishi Y, Yanada S, et al. Prognostic implications of histological features in patients with chromophobe cell renal carcinoma. BJU Int 2002; 90: 529–532.

269. Peyromaure M, Misrai V, Thiounn N, et al. Chromophobe renal cell carcinoma: analysis of 61 cases. Cancer 2004; 100: 1406–1410.

270. Taki A, Nakatani Y, Misugi K, et al. Chromophobe renal cell carcinoma: an immunohistochemical study of 21 Japanese cases. Mod Pathol 1999; 12: 310–317.

271. Abrahams NA, MacLennan GT, Khoury JD, et al. Chromophobe renal cell carcinoma: a comparative study of histological, immunohistochemical and ultrastructural features using high throughput tissue microarray. Histopathology 2004; 45: 593–602.

272. Abrahams NA, Tamboli P. Oncocytic renal neoplasms: diagnostic considerations. Clin Lab Med 2005; 25: 317–339.

273. Abrahams NA, Ayala AG, Czerniak B. Chromophobe renal cell carcinoma with sarcomatoid transformation. Ann Diagn Pathol 2003; 7: 296–299.

274. Akhtar M, Tulbah A, Kardar AH, et al. Sarcomatoid renal cell carcinoma: the chromophobe connection. Am J Surg Pathol 1997; 21: 1188–1195.

275. Itoh T, Chikai K, Ota S, et al. Chromophobe renal cell carcinoma with osteosarcoma-like differentiation. Am J Surg Pathol 2002; 26: 1358–1362.

276. Shannon BA, Cohen RJ. Rhabdoid differentiation of chromophobe renal cell carcinoma. Pathology 2003; 35: 228–230.

277. Latham B, Dickersin GR, Oliva E. Subtypes of chromophobe cell renal carcinoma: an ultrastructural and histochemical study of 13 cases. Am J Surg Pathol 1999; 23: 530–535.

278. Kovacs A, Kovacs G. Low chromosome number in chromophobe renal cell carcinomas. Genes Chromosomes Cancer 1992; 4: 267–268.

279. Iqbal MA, Akhtar M, Ali MA. Cytogenetic findings in renal cell carcinoma. Hum Pathol 1996; 27: 949–954.

280. Shuin T, Kondo K, Sakai N, et al. A case of chromophobe renal cell carcinoma associated with low chromosome number and microsatellite instability. Cancer Genet Cytogenet 1996; 86: 69–71.

281. Gunawan B, Bergmann F, Braun S, et al. Polyploidization and losses of chromosomes 1, 2, 6, 10, 13, and 17 in three cases of chromophobe renal cell carcinomas. Cancer Genet Cytogenet 1999; 110: 57–61.

282. Speicher MR, Schoell B, du Manoir S, et al. Specific loss of chromosomes 1, 2, 6, 10, 13, 17, and 21 in chromophobe renal cell carcinomas revealed by comparative genomic hybridization. Am J Pathol 1994; 145: 356–364.

283. Junker K, Weirich G, Amin MB. Genetic subtyping of renal cell carcinoma by comparative genomic hybridization. Rec Res Cancer Res 2004; 162: 169–175.

284. Iqbal MA, Akhtar M, Ulmer C, et al. FISH analysis in chromophobe renal-cell carcinoma. Diagn Cytopathol 2000; 22: 3–6.

285. Moch H, Sauter G, Gasser TC, et al. EGF-r gene copy number changes in renal cell carcinoma detected by fluorescence in situ hybridization. J Pathol 1998; 184: 424–429.

286. Verdorfer I, Hobisch A, Hittmair A, et al. Cytogenetic characterization of 22 human renal cell tumors in relation to a histopathological classification. Cancer Genet Cytogenet 1999; 111: 61–70.

287. Barnabas N, Amin MB, Pindolia K, et al. Mutations in the von Hippel–Lindau (VHL) gene refine differential diagnostic criteria in renal cell carcinoma. J Surg Oncol 2002; 80: 52–60.

288. Sukosd F, Digon B, Fischer J, et al. Allelic loss at 10q23.3 but lack of mutation of PTEN/MMAC1 in chromophobe renal cell carcinoma. Cancer Genet Cytogenet 2001; 128: 161–163.

289. Brunelli M, Eble JN, Zhang S, et al. Eosinophilic and classic chromophobe renal cell carcinomas have similar frequent losses of multiple chromosomes from among chromosomes 1, 2, 6, 10, and 17, and this pattern of genetic abnormality is not present in renal oncocytoma. Mod Pathol 2005; 18: 161–169.

290. Contractor H, Zariwala M, Bugert P, et al. Mutation of the p53 tumour suppressor gene occurs preferentially in the chromophobe type of renal cell tumour. J Pathol 1997; 181: 136–139.

291. Brunelli M, Gobbo S, Cossu-Rocca P, et al. Chromosomal gains in the sarcomatoid transformation of chromophobe renal cell carcinoma. Mod Pathol 2007; 20: 303–309.

292. Akhtar M, Chantziantoniou N. Flow cytometric and quantitative image cell analysis of DNA ploidy in renal chromophobe cell carcinoma. Hum Pathol 1998; 29: 1181–1188.

293. Bonsib SM, Lager DJ. Chromophobe cell carcinoma: analysis of five cases. Am J Surg Pathol 1990; 14: 260–267.

294. Nickerson ML, Warren MB, Toro JR, et al. Mutations in a novel gene lead to kidney tumors, lung wall defects, and benign tumors of the hair follicle in patients with the Birt–Hogg–Dube syndrome. Cancer Cell 2002; 2: 157–164.

295. Khoury JD, Abrahams NA, Levin HS, et al. The utility of epithelial membrane antigen and vimentin in the diagnosis of chromophobe renal cell carcinoma. Ann Diagn Pathol 2002; 6: 154–158.

296. Martignoni G, Pea M, Chilosi M, et al. Parvalbumin is constantly expressed in chromophobe renal carcinoma. Mod Pathol 2001; 14: 760–767.

297. Skinnider BF, Folpe AL, Hennigar RA, et al. Distribution of cytokeratins and vimentin in adult renal neoplasms and normal renal tissue: potential utility of a cytokeratin antibody panel in the differential diagnosis of renal tumors. Am J Surg Pathol 2005; 29: 747–754.

298. Tickoo SK, Amin MB, Linden MD, et al. Antimitochondrial antibody (113–1) in the differential diagnosis of

granular renal cell tumors. Am J Surg Pathol 1997; 21: 922–930.

299. Patton KT, Tretiakova MS, Yao JL, et al. Expression of RON Proto-oncogene in renal oncocytoma and chromophobe renal cell carcinoma. Am J Surg Pathol 2004; 28: 1045–1050.

300. Rampino T, Gregorini M, Soccio G, et al. The Ron proto-oncogene product is a phenotypic marker of renal oncocytoma. Am J Surg Pathol 2003; 27: 779–785.

301. Pan CC, Chen PC, Chiang H. Overexpression of KIT (CD117) in chromophobe renal cell carcinoma and renal oncocytoma. Am J Clin Pathol 2004; 121: 878–883.

302. Garcia E, Li M. Caveolin-1 immunohistochemical analysis in differentiating chromophobe renal cell carcinoma from renal oncocytoma. Am J Clin Pathol 2006; 125: 392–398.

303. Carrion R, Morgan BE, Tannenbaum M, et al. Caveolin expression in adult renal tumors. Urol Oncol 2003; 21: 191–196.

304. Lin BT, Brynes RK, Gelb AB, et al. Cyclin D1 expression in renal carcinomas and oncocytomas: an immunohistochemical study. Mod Pathol 1998; 11: 1075–1081.

305. Tickoo SK, Amin MB, Linden MD, et al. The MIB-1 tumor proliferation index in adult renal epithelial tumors with granular cytoplasm: biologic implications and differential diagnostic potential. Mod Pathol 1998; 11: 1115–1121.

306. Kuroda N, Naruse K, Miyazaki E, et al. Vinculin: its possible use as a marker of normal collecting ducts and renal neoplasms with collecting duct system phenotype. Mod Pathol 2000; 13: 1109–1114.

307. Went P, Dirnhofer S, Salvisberg T, et al. Expression of epithelial cell adhesion molecule (EpCam) in renal epithelial tumors. Am J Surg Pathol 2005; 29: 83–88.

308. Li G, Barthelemy A, Feng G, et al. S100A1: a powerful marker to differentiate chromophobe renal cell carcinoma from renal oncocytoma. Histopathology 2007; 50: 642–647.

309. Shomori K, Nagashima Y, Kuroda N, et al. ARPP protein is selectively expressed in renal oncocytoma, but rarely in renal cell carcinomas. Mod Pathol 2007; 20: 199–207.

310. Mete O, Kilicaslan I, Gulluoglu MG, et al. Can renal oncocytoma be differentiated from its renal mimics? The utility of anti-mitochondrial, caveolin 1, CD63 and cytokeratin 14 antibodies in the differential diagnosis. Virchows Arch 2005; 447: 938–946.

311. Pan CC, Chen PC, Ho DM. The diagnostic utility of MOC31, BerEP4, RCC marker and CD10 in the classification of renal cell carcinoma and renal oncocytoma: an immunohistochemical analysis of 328 cases. Histopathology 2004; 45: 452–459.

312. Adley BP, Papavero V, Sugimura J, et al. Diagnostic value of cytokeratin 7 and parvalbumin in differentiating chromophobe renal cell carcinoma from renal oncocytoma. Anal Quant Cytol Histol 2006; 28: 228–236.

313. Memeo L, Jhang J, Assaad AM, et al. Immunohistochemical analysis for cytokeratin 7, KIT, and PAX2: value in the differential diagnosis of chromophobe cell carcinoma. Am J Clin Pathol 2007; 127: 225–229.

314. Herbers J, Schullerus D, Chudek J, et al. Lack of genetic changes at specific genomic sites separates renal oncocytomas from renal cell carcinomas. J Pathol 1998; 184: 58–62.

315. Wang HY, Mills SE. KIT and RCC are useful in distinguishing chromophobe renal cell carcinoma from the granular variant of clear cell renal cell carcinoma. Am J Surg Pathol 2005; 29: 640–646.

316. Young AN, de Oliveira Salles PG, Lim SD, et al. Beta defensin-1, parvalbumin, and vimentin: a panel of diagnostic immunohistochemical markers for renal tumors derived from gene expression profiling studies using cDNA microarrays. Am J Surg Pathol 2003; 27: 199–205.

317. Cromie WJ, Davis CJ, DeTure FA. Atypical carcinoma of kidney: possibly originating from collecting duct epithelium. Urology 1979; 13: 315–317.

318. O'Brien PK, Bedard YC. A papillary adenocarcinoma of the renal pelvis in a young girl. A light- and electron-microscopic study. Am J Clin Pathol 1980; 73: 427–433.

319. Hai MA, Diaz-Perez R. Atypical carcinoma of kidney originating from collecting duct epithelium. Urology 1982; 19: 89–92.

320. Kennedy SM, Merino MJ, Linehan WM, et al. Collecting duct carcinoma of the kidney. Hum Pathol 1990; 21: 449–456.

321. Rumpelt HJ, Storkel S, Moll R, et al. Bellini duct carcinoma: further evidence for this rare variant of renal cell carcinoma. Histopathology 1991; 18: 115–122.

322. Koikawa Y, Sakamoto N, Naito S, et al. Bellini duct carcinoma of the kidney. Eur Urol 1992; 22: 171–173.

323. Ito F, Horita S, Yanagisawa H, et al. Bellini's duct tumor associated with end stage renal disease: a case diagnosed by lectin immunohistochemistry. Hinyokika Kiyo 1993; 39: 735–738.

324. Dimopoulos MA, Logothetis CJ, Markowitz A, et al. Collecting duct carcinoma of the kidney. Br J Urol 1993; 71: 388–391.

325. Baer SC, Ro JY, Ordonez NG, et al. Sarcomatoid collecting duct carcinoma: a clinicopathologic and immunohistochemical study of five cases. Hum Pathol 1993; 24: 1017–1022.

326. Halenda G, Sees JN, Jr., Belis JA, et al. Atypical renal adenocarcinoma with features suggesting collecting duct origin and mimicking a mucinous adenocarcinoma. Urology 1993; 41: 165–168.

327. Mauri MF, Bonzanini M, Luciani L, et al. Renal collecting duct carcinoma. Report of a case with urinary cytologic findings. Acta Cytol 1994; 38: 755–758.

328. Bielsa O, Arango O, Corominas JM, et al. Collecting duct carcinoma of the kidney. Br J Urol 1994; 74: 127–128.

329. Dodd LG, Madigan SK, Robertson CN, et al. Collecting duct carcinoma occurring in a horseshoe kidney. J Urol Pathol 1995; 3: 51–59.

330. Carter MD, Tha S, McLoughlin MG, et al. Collecting duct carcinoma of the kidney: a case report and review of the literature. J Urol 1992; 147: 1096–1098.

331. Kutta A, Schoenfeld B, Martin W, et al. Multifocal renal cell carcinoma of collecting duct origin. Scand J Urol Nephrol 1993; 27: 531–533.

332. Chao D, Zisman A, Pantuck AJ, et al. Collecting duct renal cell carcinoma: clinical study of a rare tumor. J Urol 2002; 167: 71–74.

333. Tokuda N, Naito S, Matsuzaki O, et al. Collecting duct (Bellini duct) renal cell carcinoma: a nationwide survey in Japan. J Urol 2006; 176: 40–43.

334. Srigley JR, Eble JN. Collecting duct carcinoma of kidney. Semin Diagn Pathol 1998; 15: 54–67.

335. Olivere JW, Cina SJ, Rastogi P, et al. Collecting duct meningeal carcinomatosis. Arch Pathol Lab Med 1999; 123: 638–641.

336. Peyromaure M, Thiounn N, Scotte F, et al. Collecting duct carcinoma of the kidney: a clinicopathological study of 9 cases. J Urol 2003; 170: 1138–1140.

337. Parker R, Reeves HM, Sudarshan S, et al. Abnormal fluorescence in situ hybridization analysis in collecting duct carcinoma. Urology 2005; 66: 1110.

338. Schoenberg M, Cairns P, Brooks JD, et al. Frequent loss of chromosome arms 8p and 13q in collecting duct carcinoma (CDC) of the kidney. Genes Chromosomes Cancer 1995; 12: 76–80.

339. Hadaczek P, Podolski J, Toloczko A, et al. Losses at 3p common deletion sites in subtypes of kidney tumours: histopathological correlations. Virchows Arch 1996; 429: 37–42.

340. Steiner G, Sidransky D. Molecular differential diagnosis of renal carcinoma: from microscopes to microsatellites. Am J Pathol 1996; 149: 1791–1795.

341. Fogt F, Zhuang Z, Linehan WM, et al. Collecting duct carcinomas of the kidney: a comparative loss of heterozygosity study with clear cell renal cell carcinoma. Oncol Rep 1998; 5: 923–926.

342. Selli C, Amorosi A, Vona G, et al. Retrospective evaluation of c-erbB-2 oncogene amplification using competitive PCR in collecting duct carcinoma of the kidney. J Urol 1997; 158: 245–247.

343. Davis CJ Jr, Barton JH, Sesterhenn IA, et al. Metanephric adenoma. Clinicopathological study of fifty patients. Am J Surg Pathol 1995; 19: 1101–1114.

344. Adsay NV, deRoux SJ, Sakr W, et al. Cancer as a marker of genetic medical disease: an unusual case of medullary carcinoma of the kidney. Am J Surg Pathol 1998; 22: 260–264.

345. Dimashkieh H, Choe J, Mutema G. Renal medullary carcinoma: a report of 2 cases and review of the literature. Arch Pathol Lab Med 2003; 127: e135–e138.

346. Yang XJ, Sugimura J, Tretiakova MS, et al. Gene expression profiling of renal medullary carcinoma: potential clinical relevance. Cancer 2004; 100: 976–985.

347. Kalyanpur A, Schwartz DS, Fields JM, et al. Renal medulla carcinoma in a white adolescent. AJR Am J Roentgenol 1997; 169: 1037–1038.

348. Simpson L, He X, Pins M, et al. Renal medullary carcinoma and ABL gene amplification. J Urol 2005; 173: 1883–1888.

349. Mathur SC, Schwartz AM. Pathologic quiz case: a 33-year-old man with an abdominal mass. Arch Pathol Lab Med 2000; 124: 1561–1563.

350. Khan A, Thomas N, Costello B, et al. Renal medullary carcinoma: sonographic, computed tomography, magnetic resonance and angiographic findings. Eur J Radiol 2000; 35: 1–7.

351. Selby DM, Simon C, Foley JP, et al. Renal medullary carcinoma: can early diagnosis lead to long-term survival? J Urol 2000; 163: 1238.

352. Jarzembowski JA, Perry A, Dehner LP. Medullary renal cell carcinoma (MRCC) and malignant rhabdoid tumor (MRT) share loss of INI1 expression and may be related entities. Mod Pathol 2007; 20: 280.

353. Pirich LM, Chou P, Walterhouse DO. Prolonged survival of a patient with sickle cell trait and metastatic renal medullary carcinoma. J Pediatr Hematol Oncol 1999; 21: 67–69.

354. Stahlschmidt J, Cullinane C, Roberts P, et al. Renal medullary carcinoma: prolonged remission with chemotherapy, immunohistochemical characterisation and evidence of bcr/abl rearrangement. Med Pediatr Oncol 1999; 33: 551–557.

355. Tomlinson GE, Nisen PD, Timmons CF, et al. Cytogenetics of a renal cell carcinoma in a 17-month-old child. Evidence for Xp11.2 as a recurring breakpoint. Cancer Genet Cytogenet 1991; 57: 11–17.

356. Meloni AM, Dobbs RM, Pontes JE, et al. Translocation (X; 1) in papillary renal cell carcinoma. A new cytogenetic subtype. Cancer Genet Cytogenet 1993; 65: 1–6.

357. Hernandez-Marti MJ, Orellana-Alonso C, Badia-Garrabou L, et al. Renal adenocarcinoma in an 8-year-old child, with a t(X; 17)(p11.2; q25). Cancer Genet Cytogenet 1995; 83: 82–83.

358. Sidhar SK, Clark J, Gill S, et al. The t(X; 1)(p11.2; q21.2) translocation in papillary renal cell carcinoma fuses a novel gene PRCC to the TFE3 transcription factor gene. Hum Mol Genet 1996; 5: 1333–1338.

359. Weterman MA, Wilbrink M, Geurts van Kessel A. Fusion of the transcription factor TFE3 gene to a novel gene, PRCC, in t(X; 1)(p11; q21)-positive papillary renal cell carcinomas. Proc Natl Acad Sci USA 1996; 93: 15294–15298.

360. Clark J, Lu YJ, Sidhar SK, et al. Fusion of splicing factor genes PSF and NonO (p54nrb) to the TFE3 gene in papillary renal cell carcinoma. Oncogene 1997; 15: 2233–2239.

361. Heimann P, Devalck C, Debusscher C, et al. Alveolar soft-part sarcoma: further evidence by FISH for the involvement of chromosome band 17q25. Genes Chromosomes Cancer 1998; 23: 194–197.

362. Ladanyi M, Lui MY, Antonescu CR, et al. The der(17)t(X; 17)(p11; q25) of human alveolar soft part sarcoma fuses the TFE3 transcription factor gene to ASPL, a novel gene at 17q25. Oncogene 2001; 20: 48–57.

363. Argani P, Antonescu CR, Illei PB, et al. Primary renal neoplasms with the ASPL-TFE3 gene fusion of alveolar soft part sarcoma: a distinctive tumor entity previously included among renal cell carcinomas of children and adolescents. Am J Pathol 2001; 159: 179–192.

364. Heimann P, El Housni H, Ogur G, et al. Fusion of a novel gene, RCC17, to the TFE3 gene in t(X; 17)(p11.2; q25.3)-bearing papillary renal cell carcinomas. Cancer Res 2001; 61: 4130–4135.

365. Argani P, Hawkins A, Griffin CA, et al. A distinctive pediatric renal neoplasm characterized by epithelioid morphology, basement membrane production, focal HMB-45 immunoreactivity, and t(6; 11)(p21.1; q12) chromosome translocation. Am J Pathol 2001; 158: 2089–2096.

366. Argani P, Lui MY, Couturier J, et al. A novel CLTC-TFE3 gene fusion in pediatric renal adenocarcinoma with t(X; 17)(p11.2; q23). Oncogene 2003; 22: 5374–5378.

367. Davis IJ, Hsi BL, Arroyo JD, et al. Cloning of an alpha-TFEB fusion in renal tumors harboring the t(6; 11)(p21; q13) chromosome translocation. Proc Natl Acad Sci USA 2003; 100: 6051–6056.

368. Argani P, Ladanyi M. Translocation carcinomas of the kidney. Clin Lab Med 2005; 25: 363–378.

369. Renshaw AA, Granter SR, Fletcher JA, et al. Renal cell carcinomas in children and young adults: increased incidence of papillary architecture and unique subtypes. Am J Surg Pathol 1999; 23: 795–802.

370. Chian-Garcia CA, Torres-Cabala CA, Eyler RA, et al. Renal cell carcinoma in children and young adults: a clinicopathological and immunohistochemical study of 14 cases. Mod Pathol 2003; 28: 1117–1132.

371. Altinok G, Kattar MM, Mohamed A, et al. Pediatric renal carcinoma associated with Xp11.2 translocations/TFE3 gene fusions and clinicopathologic associations. Pediatr Dev Pathol 2005; 8: 168–180.

372. Cao Y, Paner GP, Perry KT, et al. Renal neoplasms in younger adults: analysis of 112 tumors from a single institution according to the new 2004 World Health Organization classification and 2002 American Joint Committee on Cancer Staging System. Arch Pathol Lab Med 2005; 129: 487–491.

373. Argani P. The evolving story of renal translocation carcinomas. Am J Clin Pathol 2006; 126: 332–334.

374. Argani P, Antonescu CR, Couturier J, et al. PRCC-TFE3 renal carcinomas: morphologic, immunohistochemical, ultrastructural, and molecular analysis of an entity associated with the t(X; 1)(p11.2; q21). Am J Surg Pathol 2002; 26: 1553–1566.

375. Argani P, Lae M, Ballard ET, et al. Translocation carcinomas of the kidney after chemotherapy in childhood. J Clin Oncol 2006; 24: 1529–1534.

376. Argani P, Lae M, Hutchinson B, et al. Renal carcinomas with the t(6; 11)(p21; q12): clinicopathologic features and demonstration of the specific alpha-TFEB gene fusion by immunohistochemistry, RT-PCR, and DNA PCR. Am J Surg Pathol 2005; 29: 230–240.

377. Kuiper RP, Schepens M, Thijssen J, et al. Upregulation of the transcription factor TFEB in t(6; 11)(p21; q13)-positive renal cell carcinomas due to promoter substitution. Hum Mol Genet 2003; 12: 1661–1669.

378. Argani P, Lal P, Hutchinson B, et al. Aberrant nuclear immunoreactivity for TFE3 in neoplasms with TFE3 gene fusions: a sensitive and specific immunohistochemical assay. Am J Surg Pathol 2003; 27: 750–761.

379. Meadows AT, Baum E, Fossati-Bellani F, et al. Second malignant neoplasms in children: an update from the Late Effects Study Group. J Clin Oncol 1985; 3: 532–538.

380. Tefft M, Vawter GF, Mitus A. Second primary neoplasms in children. Am J Roentgenol Radium Ther Nucl Med 1968; 103: 800–822.

381. Li FP, Cassady JR, Jaffe N. Risk of second tumors in survivors of childhood cancer. Cancer 1975; 35: 1230–1235.

382. Fairchild RS, Kyner JL, Hermreck A, et al. Neuroblastoma, pheochromocytoma, and renal cell carcinoma. Occurrence in a single patient. JAMA 1979; 242: 2210–2211.

383. Lack EE, Cassady JR, Sallan SE. Renal cell carcinoma in childhood and adolescence: a clinical and pathological study of 17 cases. J Urol 1985; 133: 822–828.

384. Fenton DS, Taub JW, Amundson GM, et al. Renal cell carcinoma occurring in a child 2 years after chemotherapy for neuroblastoma. AJR Am J Roentgenol 1993; 161: 165–166.

385. Krigman HR, Bentley RC, Strickland DK, et al. Anaplastic renal cell carcinoma following neuroblastoma. Med Pediatr Oncol 1995; 25: 52–59.

386. Donnelly LF, Rencken IO, Shardell K, et al. Renal cell carcinoma after therapy for neuroblastoma. AJR Am J Roentgenol 1996; 167: 915–917.

387. Manion S, Hayani A, Husain A, et al. Partial nephrectomy for pediatric renal cell carcinoma: an unusual case presentation. Urology 1997; 49: 465–468.

388. Vogelzang NJ, Yang X, Goldman S, et al. Radiation induced renal cell cancer: a report of 4 cases and review of the literature. J Urol 1998; 160: 1987–1990.

389. Kato K, Ijiri R, Tanaka Y, et al. Metachronous renal cell carcinoma in a child cured of neuroblastoma. Med Pediatr Oncol 1999; 33: 432–433.

390. Medeiros LJ, Palmedo G, Krigman HR, et al. Oncocytoid renal cell carcinoma after neuroblastoma: a report of four cases of a distinct clinicopathologic entity. Am J Surg Pathol 1999; 23: 772–780.

391. Koyle MA, Hatch DA, Furness PD, 3rd, et al. Long-term urological complications in survivors younger than 15 months of advanced stage abdominal neuroblastoma. J Urol 2001; 166: 1455–1458.

392. Fleitz JM, Wootton-Gorges SL, Wyatt-Ashmead J, et al. Renal cell carcinoma in long-term survivors of advanced stage neuroblastoma in early childhood. Pediatr Radiol 2003; 33: 540–545.

393. Cherullo EE, Ross JH, Kay R, et al. Renal neoplasms in adult survivors of childhood Wilms' tumor. J Urol 2001; 165: 2013–2017.

394. Huang FS, Zwerdling T, Stern LE, et al. Renal cell carcinoma as a secondary malignancy after treatment of acute promyelocytic leukemia. J Pediatr Hematol Oncol 2001; 23: 609–611.

395. MacLennan GT, Farrow GM, Bostwick DG. Low-grade collecting duct carcinoma of the kidney: report of 13 cases of low-grade mucinous tubulocystic renal carcinoma of possible collecting duct origin. Urology 1997; 50: 679–684.

396. Parwani AV, Husain AN, Epstein JI, et al. Low-grade myxoid renal epithelial neoplasms with distal nephron differentiation. Hum Pathol 2001; 32: 506–512.

397. Rakozy C, Schmahl GE, Bogner S, et al. Low-grade tubular-mucinous renal neoplasms: morphologic, immunohistochemical, and genetic features. Mod Pathol 2002; 15: 1162–1171.

398. Srigley JR, Eble JN, Grignon D, et al. Unusual renal cell carcinoma (RCC) with prominent spindle cell change possibly related to the loop of Henle. Mod Pathol 1999; 12: 107.

399. Ferlicot S, Allory Y, Comperat E, et al. Mucinous tubular and spindle cell carcinoma: a report of 15 cases and a review of the literature. Virchows Arch 2005; 447: 978–983.

400. Fine SW, Argani P, DeMarzo AM, et al. Expanding the histologic spectrum of mucinous tubular and spindle cell carcinoma of the kidney. Am J Surg Pathol 2006; 30: 1554–1560.

401. Aubert S, Duchene F, Augusto D, et al. Low-grade tubular myxoid renal tumors: a clinicopathological study of 3 cases. Int J Surg Pathol 2004; 12: 179–183.

402. Jung SJ, Yoon HK, Chung JI, et al. Mucinous tubular and spindle cell carcinoma of the kidney with neuroendocrine differentiation: report of two cases. Am J Clin Pathol 2006; 125: 99–104.

403. Paner GP, Srigley JR, Radhakrishnan A, et al. Immunohistochemical analysis of mucinous tubular and spindle cell carcinoma and papillary renal cell carcinoma of the kidney: significant immunophenotypic overlap warrants diagnostic caution. Am J Surg Pathol 2006; 30: 13–19.

404. Shen SS, Ro JY, Tamboli P, et al. Mucinous tubular and spindle cell carcinoma of kidney is probably a variant of papillary renal cell carcinoma with spindle cell features. Ann Diagn Pathol 2007; 11: 13–21.

405. Cossu-Rocca P, Eble JN, Delahunt B, et al. Renal mucinous tubular and spindle carcinoma lacks the gains of chromosomes 7 and 17 and losses of chromosome Y that are prevalent in papillary renal cell carcinoma. Mod Pathol 2006; 19: 488–493.

406. Srigley JR, Kapusta L, Reuter V, et al. Phenotypic, molecular, and ultrastructural studies of a novel low grade renal epithelial neoplasm possibly related to the loop of Henle. Mod Pathol 2002; 15: 182.

407. Brandal P, Lie AK, Bassarova A, et al. Genomic aberrations in mucinous tubular and spindle cell renal carcinomas. Mod Pathol 2006; 19: 186–194.

408. Hennigar RA, Epstein JI, Farrow GM. Tubular renal cell carcinomas of collecting duct origin. Mod Pathol 1994; 7: 76.

409. Murphy WM, Beckwith JB, Farrow GM. Atlas of tumor pathology, Third Series, Fascicle 11. Tumors of the kidney, bladder, and related urinary structures. Washington, DC: Armed Forces Institute of Pathology, 1994.

410. MacLennan GT, Farrow GM, de Matteis A, et al. Renal cell carcinoma of collecting duct type: a report of 16 cases. Mod Pathol 1996; 9: 77.

411. Amin MB, MacLennan GT, Paraf F, et al. Tubulocystic carcinoma of the kidney: Clinicopathologic analysis of 29 cases of a distinctive rare subtype of renal cell carcinoma (RCC). Mod Pathol 2004; 17: 137A.

412. Radhakrishnan A, MacLennan GT, Hennigar RA, et al. Ultrastructural and immunohistochemical appraisal of tubulocystic carcinoma of the kidney: Histogenetic and diagnostic implications. Mod Pathol 2005; 18: 160A.

413. Sule N, Yakupoglu U, Shen SS, et al. Calcium oxalate deposition in renal cell carcinoma associated with acquired cystic kidney disease: a comprehensive study. Am J Surg Pathol 2005; 29: 443–451.

414. Truong LD, Krishnan B, Cao JT, et al. Renal neoplasm in acquired cystic kidney disease. Am J Kidney Dis 1995; 26: 1–12.

415. Matson MA, Cohen EP. Acquired cystic kidney disease: occurrence, prevalence, and renal cancers. Medicine (Baltimore) 1990; 69: 217–226.

416. Dry SM, Renshaw AA. Extensive calcium oxalate crystal deposition in papillary renal cell carcinoma: report of two cases. Arch Pathol Lab Med 1998; 122: 260–261.

417. Cossu-Rocca P, Eble JN, Zhang S, et al. Acquired cystic disease-associated renal tumors: an immunohistochemical and fluorescence in situ hybridization study. Mod Pathol 2006; 19: 780–787.

418. Griffiths IH, Thackeray AC. Griffiths IH, Thackeray AC. Parenchymal carcinoma of the kidney. Br J Urol 1949; 21: 128–151.

419. Farrow GM, Harrison EG Jr, Utz DC. Sarcomas and sarcomatoid and mixed malignant tumors of the kidney in adults. Cancer 1968; 22: 556–563.

420. Jones TD, Eble JN, Wang M, et al. Clonal divergence and genetic heterogeneity in clear cell renal cell carcinomas with sarcomatoid transformation. Cancer 2005; 104: 1195–1203.

421. Zisman A, Chao DH, Pantuck AJ, et al. Unclassified renal cell carcinoma: clinical features and prognostic impact of a new histological subtype. J Urol 2002; 168: 950–955.

422. Strobel P, Zettl A, Ren Z, et al. Spiradenocylindroma of the kidney: clinical and genetic findings suggesting a role of somatic mutation of the CYLD1 gene in the oncogenesis of an unusual renal neoplasm. Am J Surg Pathol 2002; 26: 119–124.

423. Amin M, Michal M, Radhakrishnan A, et al. Primary thyroid-like follicular carcinoma of the kidney: a histologically distinctive primary renal

epithelial tumor. Mod Pathol 2004; 17: 136–137.

424. Gelb AB. Renal cell carcinoma: current prognostic factors. Union Internationale Contre le Cancer (UICC) and the American Joint Committee on Cancer (AJCC). Cancer 1997; 80: 981–986.

425. Srigley JR, Hutter RV, Gelb AB, et al. Current prognostic factors – renal cell carcinoma. Workgroup No. 4. Union Internationale Contre le Cancer (UICC) and the American Joint Committee on Cancer (AJCC). Cancer 1997; 80: 994–996.

426. Sengupta S, Lohse CM, Cheville JC, et al. The preoperative erythrocyte sedimentation rate is an independent prognostic factor in renal cell carcinoma. Cancer 2006; 106: 304–312.

427. Symbas NP, Townsend MF, El-Galley R, et al. Poor prognosis associated with thrombocytosis in patients with renal cell carcinoma. BJU Int 2000; 86: 203–207.

428. Gogus C, Baltaci S, Filiz E, et al. Significance of thrombocytosis for determining prognosis in patients with localized renal cell carcinoma. Urology 2004; 63: 447–450.

429. Shuch BM, Lam JS, Belldegrun AS, et al. Prognostic factors in renal cell carcinoma. Semin Oncol 2006; 33: 563–575.

430. Cheville JC, Blute ML, Zincke H, et al. Stage pT1 conventional (clear cell) renal cell carcinoma: pathological features associated with cancer specific survival. J Urol 2001; 166: 453–456.

431. Ficarra V, Guille F, Schips L, et al. Proposal for revision of the TNM classification system for renal cell carcinoma. Cancer 2005; 104: 2116–2123.

432. Lam JS, Patard JJ, Goel RH, et al. Can pT2 classification for renal cell carcinoma be improved? An international multicenter experience. J Urol 2006; 175: 240–241.

433. Lam JS, Patard JJ, Leppert JT, et al. Prognostic significance of T3a renal cell carcinoma with adrenal gland involvement: an international multicenter experience. J Urol 2005; 173: 269–270.

434. Thompson RH, Cheville JC, Lohse CM, et al. Reclassification of patients with pT3 and pT4 renal cell carcinoma improves prognostic accuracy. Cancer 2005; 104: 53–60.

435. Thompson RH, Leibovich BC, Cheville JC, et al. Should direct ipsilateral adrenal invasion from renal cell carcinoma be classified as pT3a? J Urol 2005; 173: 918–921.

436. Han KR, Bui MH, Pantuck AJ, et al. TNM T3a renal cell carcinoma: adrenal gland involvement is not the same as renal fat invasion. J Urol 2003; 169: 899–904.

437. Ficarra V, Novara G, Iafrate M, et al. Proposal for reclassification of the TNM staging system in patients with

locally advanced (pT3–4) renal cell carcinoma according to the cancer-related outcome. Eur Urol 2007; 51: 722–729; discussion 729–731.

438. Sandock DS, Seftel AD, Resnick MI. Adrenal metastases from renal cell carcinoma: role of ipsilateral adrenalectomy and definition of stage. Urology 1997; 49: 28–31.

439. Bonsib SM, Gibson D, Mhoon M, et al. Renal sinus involvement in renal cell carcinomas. Am J Surg Pathol 2000; 24: 451–458.

440. Thompson RH, Leibovich BC, Cheville JC, et al. Is renal sinus fat invasion the same as perinephric fat invasion for pT3a renal cell carcinoma? J Urol 2005; 174: 1218–1221.

441. Leibovich BC, Cheville JC, Lohse CM, et al. Cancer specific survival for patients with pT3 renal cell carcinoma – can the 2002 primary tumor classification be improved? J Urol 2005; 173: 716–719.

442. Kim HL, Zisman A, Han KR, et al. Prognostic significance of venous thrombus in renal cell carcinoma. Are renal vein and inferior vena cava involvement different? J Urol 2004; 171: 588–591.

443. Cheville JC, Lohse CM, Zincke H, et al. Comparisons of outcome and prognostic features among histologic subtypes of renal cell carcinoma. Am J Surg Pathol 2003; 27: 612–624.

444. Bernstein L, Linet M, Smith MA, et al. Renal tumors. In: Ries LAG, Smith MA, Gurney JG, eds. Cancer incidence and survival among children and adolescents: United States SEER Program 1975–1995. Bethesda, MD: National Cancer Institute, 1999.

445. Indolfi P, Terenziani M, Casale F, et al. Renal cell carcinoma in children: a clinicopathologic study. J Clin Oncol 2003; 21: 530–535.

446. Cook A, Lorenzo AJ, Salle JL, et al. Pediatric renal cell carcinoma: single institution 25-year case series and initial experience with partial nephrectomy. J Urol 2006; 175: 1456–1460.

447. Geller JI, Dome JS. Local lymph node involvement does not predict poor outcome in pediatric renal cell carcinoma. Cancer 2004; 101: 1575–1583.

448. Pages A, Granier M. Nephronogenic nephroma [author's transl]. Arch Anat Cytol Pathol 1980; 24: 99–103.

449. Mostofi FK, Sesterhenn IA, Davis CJ Jr. Benign tumors of the kidney. Prog Clin Biol Res 1988; 269: 329–346.

450. Nagashima Y, Arai N, Tanaka Y, et al. Two cases of a renal epithelial tumour resembling immature nephron. Virchows Arch A Pathol Anat Histopathol 1991; 418: 77–81.

451. Brisigotti M, Cozzutto C, Fabbretti G, et al. Metanephric adenoma. Histol Histopathol 1992; 7: 689–692.

452. Nonomura A, Mizukami Y, Hasegawa T, et al. Metanephric adenoma of the kidney: an electron microscopic and

immunohistochemical study with quantitative DNA measurement by image analysis. Ultrastruct Pathol 1995; 19: 481–488.

453. Jones EC, Pins M, Dickersin GR, et al. Metanephric adenoma of the kidney. A clinicopathological, immunohistochemical, flow cytometric, cytogenetic, and electron microscopic study of seven cases. Am J Surg Pathol 1995; 19: 615–626.

454. Gatalica Z, Grujic S, Kovatich A, et al. Metanephric adenoma: histology, immunophenotype, cytogenetics, ultrastructure. Mod Pathol 1996; 9: 329–333.

455. Bouzourene H, Blaser A, Francke ML, et al. Metanephric adenoma of the kidney: a rare benign tumour of the kidney. Histopathology 1997; 31: 485–486.

456. Muir TE, Cheville JC, Lager DJ. Metanephric adenoma, nephrogenic rests, and Wilms' tumor: a histologic and immunophenotypic comparison. Am J Surg Pathol 2001; 25: 1290–1296.

457. Argani P. Metanephric neoplasms: the hyperdifferentiated, benign end of the Wilms' tumor spectrum? Clin Lab Med 2005; 25: 379–392.

458. Fischer EG, Carney JA, Anderson SR, et al. An immunophenotypic comparison of metanephric metaplasia of Bowman capsular epithelium with metanephric adenoma, Wilms' tumor, and renal development: a case report and review of the literature. Am J Clin Pathol 2004; 121: 850–856.

459. de Silva K, Tobias V, Kainer G, et al. Metanephric adenoma with embryonal hyperplasia of Bowman's capsular epithelium: Previously unreported association. Pediatr Dev Pathol 2000; 3: 472–478.

460. Lerut E, Roskams T, Joniau S, et al. Metanephric adenoma during pregnancy: clinical presentation, histology, and cytogenetics. Hum Pathol 2006; 37: 1227–1232.

461. Brunelli M, Eble JN, Zhang S, et al. Metanephric adenoma lacks the gains of chromosomes 7 and 17 and loss of Y that are typical of papillary renal cell carcinoma and papillary adenoma. Mod Pathol 2003; 16: 1060–1063.

462. Drut R, Drut RM, Ortolani C. Metastatic metanephric adenoma with foci of papillary carcinoma in a child: a combined histologic, immunohistochemical, and FISH study. Int J Surg Pathol 2001; 9: 241–247.

463. Hes O, Curik R, Malatkova V, et al. Metanephric adenoma and papillary carcinoma with sarcomatoid dedifferentiation of kidney. A case report. Pathol Res Pract 2003; 199: 629–632.

464. Imamoto T, Furuya Y, Ueda T, et al. Metanephric adenoma of the kidney. Int J Urol 1999; 6: 200–202.

465. Birgisson H, Einarsson GV, Steinarsdottir M, et al. Metanephric

adenoma. Scand J Urol Nephrol 1999; 33: 340–343.

466. Tsuji M, Murakami Y, Kanayama H, et al. A case of renal metanephric adenoma: histologic, immunohistochemical and cytogenetic analyses. Int J Urol 1999; 6: 203–207.

467. Olgac S, Hutchinson B, Tickoo SK, et al. Alpha-methylacyl-CoA racemase as a marker in the differential diagnosis of metanephric adenoma. Mod Pathol 2006; 19: 218–224.

468. Granter SR, Fletcher JA, Renshaw AA. Cytologic and cytogenetic analysis of metanephric adenoma of the kidney: a report of two cases. Am J Clin Pathol 1997; 108: 544–549.

469. Stumm M, Koch A, Wieacker PF, et al. Partial monosomy 2p as the single chromosomal anomaly in a case of renal metanephric adenoma. Cancer Genet Cytogenet 1999; 115: 82–85.

470. Pesti T, Sukosd F, Jones EC, et al. Mapping a tumor suppressor gene to chromosome 2p13 in metanephric adenoma by microsatellite allelotyping. Hum Pathol 2001; 32: 101–104.

471. Brown JA, Anderl KL, Borell TJ, et al. Simultaneous chromosome 7 and 17 gain and sex chromosome loss provide evidence that renal metanephric adenoma is related to papillary renal cell carcinoma. J Urol 1997; 158: 370–374.

472. Birgisson H, Einarsson GV. Metanephric adenoma. Scand J Urol Neprol 1999; 33: 340–344.

473. Pins MR, Jones EC, Martul EV, et al. Metanephric adenoma-like tumors of the kidney: report of 3 malignancies with emphasis on discriminating features. Arch Pathol Lab Med 1999; 123: 415–420.

474. Renshaw AA, Freyer DR, Hammers YA. Metastatic metanephric adenoma in a child. Am J Surg Pathol 2000; 24: 570–574.

475. Arroyo MR, Green DM, Perlman EJ, et al. The spectrum of metanephric adenofibroma and related lesions: clinicopathologic study of 25 cases from the National Wilms' Tumor Study Group Pathology Center. Am J Surg Pathol 2001; 25: 433–444.

476. Hennigar RA, Beckwith JB. Nephrogenic adenofibroma. A novel kidney tumor of young people. Am J Surg Pathol 1992; 16: 325–334.

477. Beckwith JB. Metanephric stromal tumor (MST): a new renal neoplasm resembling mesoblastic nephroma (MN) but related to metanephric adenofibroma (MAF). Mod Pathol 1998; 11: 1p.

478. Argani P, Perlman EJ, Breslow NE, et al. Clear cell sarcoma of the kidney: a review of 351 cases from the National Wilms' Tumor Study Group Pathology Center. Am J Surg Pathol 2000; 24: 4–18.

479. Argani P, Beckwith JB. Metanephric stromal tumor: report of 31 cases of a distinctive pediatric renal neoplasm. Am J Surg Pathol 2000; 24: 917–926.

480. Bluebond-Langner R, Pinto PA, Argani P, et al. Adult presentation of metanephric stromal tumor. J Urol 2002; 168: 1482–1483.

481. Palese MA, Ferrer F, Perlman E, et al. Metanephric stromal tumor: a rare benign pediatric renal mass. Urology 2001; 58: 462.

482. Shek TW, Luk IS, Peh WC, et al. Metanephric adenofibroma: report of a case and review of the literature. Am J Surg Pathol 1999; 23: 727–733.

483. Guzman E, Turc-Carel C, Soler C, et al. Nephrogenic adenofibroma in a young child. Pathol Res Pract 2000; 196: 853–856.

484. Picken MM, Curry JL, Lindgren V, et al. Metanephric adenosarcoma in a young adult: morphologic, immunophenotypic, ultrastructural, and fluorescence in situ hybridization analyses: a case report and review of the literature. Am J Surg Pathol 2001; 25: 1451–1457.

485. Klapproth HJ. Wilms' tumor: a report of 45 cases and an analysis of 1351 cases reported in the world literature from 1940 to 1958. J Urol 1959; 81: 633–648.

486. Eberth CJ. Myoma sarcomatodes renum. Arch Path Anat 1872; 55: 518–520.

487. Wilms M. Die Mischgeschwuelste. In: Heft I, ed. Die Mischgeschwuelste der Niere. Leipzig: Verlag Arthur Georgi, 1899; 1–90.

488. Little SE, Hanks SP, King-Underwood L, et al. Frequency and heritability of WT1 mutations in nonsyndromic Wilms' tumor patients: a UK Children's Cancer Study Group Study. J Clin Oncol 2004; 22: 4140–4146.

489. Breslow N, Olshan A, Beckwith JB, et al. Epidemiology of Wilms' tumor. Med Pediatr Oncol 1993; 21: 172–181.

490. Webber BL, Parham DM, Drake LG, et al. Renal tumors in childhood. Pathol Annu 1992; 27: 191–232.

491. Ruteshouser EC, Huff V. Familial Wilms' tumor. Am J Med Genet C Semin Med Genet 2004; 129: 29–34.

492. Crist WM, Kun LE. Common solid tumors of childhood. N Engl J Med 1991; 324: 461–471.

493. Kissane JM, Dehner LP. Renal tumors and tumor-like lesions in pediatric patients. Pediatr Nephrol 1992; 6: 365–382.

494. Breslow N, Beckwith JB, Ciol M, et al. Age distribution of Wilms' tumor: report from the National Wilms' Tumor Study. Cancer Res 1988;48: 1653–1657.

495. Blute ML, Kelalis PP, Offord KP, et al. Bilateral Wilms' tumor. J Urol 1987; 138: 968–973.

496. Stiller CA, Parkin DM. International variations in the incidence of childhood renal tumours. Br J Cancer 1990; 62: 1026–1030.

497. Fukuzawa R, Breslow NE, Morison IM, et al. Epigenetic differences between Wilms' tumours in white and east-Asian children. Lancet 2004; 363: 446–451.

498. Babaian RJ, Skinner DG, Waisman J. Wilms' tumor in the adult patient: diagnosis, management, and review of the world medical literature. Cancer 1980; 45: 1713–1719.

499. Terenziani M, Spreafico F, Collini P, et al. Adult Wilms' tumor: A monoinstitutional experience and a review of the literature. Cancer 2004; 101: 289–293.

500. Paulino AC, Thakkar B, Henderson WG. Metachronous bilateral Wilms' tumor: the importance of time interval to the development of a second tumor. Cancer 1998; 82: 415–420.

501. Shearer P, Parham DM, Fontanesi J, et al. Bilateral Wilms' tumor. Review of outcome, associated abnormalities, and late effects in 36 pediatric patients treated at a single institution. Cancer 1993; 72: 1422–1426.

502. Mesrobian HG, Kelalis PP, Hrabovsky E, et al. Wilms' tumor in horseshoe kidneys: a report from the National Wilms' Tumor Study. J Urol 1985; 133: 1002–1003.

503. Neville H, Ritchey ML, Shamberger RC, et al. The occurrence of Wilms' tumor in horseshoe kidneys: a report from the National Wilms' Tumor Study Group (NWTSG). J Pediatr Surg 2002; 37: 1134–1137.

504. Huang EY, Mascarenhas L, Mahour GH. Wilms' tumor and horseshoe kidneys: a case report and review of the literature. J Pediatr Surg 2004; 39: 207–212.

505. Sawicz-Birkowska K, Apoznanski W, Kantorowicz-Szymik S, et al. Malignant tumours in a horseshoe kidney in children: a diagnostic dilemma. Eur J Pediatr Surg 2005; 15: 48–52.

506. Madanat F, Osborne B, Cangir A, et al. Extrarenal Wilms' tumor. J Pediatr 1978; 93: 439–443.

507. Gillis AJ, Oosterhuis JW, Schipper ME, et al. Origin and biology of a testicular Wilms' tumor. Genes Chromosomes Cancer 1994; 11: 126–135.

508. Michael H, Hull MT, Foster RS, et al. Nephroblastoma-like tumors in patients with testicular germ cell tumors. Am J Surg Pathol 1998; 22: 1107–1114.

509. Emerson RE, Ulbright TM, Zhang S, et al. Nephroblastoma arising in a germ cell tumor of testicular origin. Am J Surg Pathol 2004; 28: 687–692.

510. Muc RS, Grayson W, Grobbelaar JJ. Adult extrarenal Wilms' tumor occurring in the uterus. Arch Pathol Lab Med 2001; 125: 1081–1083.

511. Orlowski JP, Levin HS, Dyment PG. Intrascrotal Wilms' tumor developing in a heterotopic renal anlage of probable mesonephric origin. J Pediatr Surg 1980; 15: 679–682.

512. Luchtrath H, de Leon F, Giesen H, et al. Inguinal nephroblastoma. Virchows Arch A Pathol Anat Histopathol 1984; 405: 113–118.

513. Arkovitz MS, Ginsburg HB, Eidelman J, et al. Primary extrarenal Wilms' tumor in the inguinal canal: case report and review of the literature. J Pediatr Surg 1996; 31: 957–959.

514. Fernandes ET, Kumar M, Douglass EC, et al. Extrarenal Wilms' tumor. J Pediatr Surg 1989; 24: 483–485.

515. Pawel BR, de Chadarevian JP, Smergel EM, et al. Teratoid Wilms' tumor arising as a botryoid growth within a supernumerary ectopic ureteropelvic structure. Arch Pathol Lab Med 1998; 122: 925–928.

516. Abrahams JM, Pawel BR, Duhaime AC, et al. Extrarenal nephroblastic proliferation in spinal dysraphism. A report of 4 cases. Pediatr Neurosurg 1999; 31: 40–44.

517. Martucciello G, Torre M, Belloni E, et al. Currarino syndrome: proposal of a diagnostic and therapeutic protocol. J Pediatr Surg 2004; 39: 1305–1311.

518. Fahner JB, Switzer R, Freyer DR, et al. Extrarenal Wilms' tumor. Unusual presentation in the lumbosacral region. Am J Pediatr Hematol Oncol 1993; 15: 117–119.

519. Horenstein MG, Manci EA, Walker AB, et al. Lumbosacral ectopic nephrogenic rest unassociated with spinal dysraphism. Am J Surg Pathol 2004; 28: 1389–1392.

520. Milliser RV, Greenberg SR, Neiman BH. Heterotopic renal tissue in the human adrenal gland. J Urol 1969; 102: 280–284.

521. Milliser RV, Greenberg SR, Neiman BH. Heterotopic renal tissue in the human heart. J Urol 1972; 108: 21–24.

522. Jain D, Martel M, Reyes-Mugica M, et al. Heterotopic nephrogenic rests in the colon and multiple congenital anomalies: possibly related association. Pediatr Dev Pathol 2002; 5: 587–591.

523. Lozano RH, Rodriguez C. Intrathoracic ectopic kidney: report of a case. J Urol 1975; 114: 601–602.

524. Merimsky E, Firstater M. Ectopic thoracic kidney. Br J Urol 1978; 50: 282.

525. Bennett S, Defoor W, Minevich E. Primary extrarenal nephrogenic rest. J Urol 2002; 168: 1529.

526. Rivera MN, Kim WJ, Wells J, et al. An X chromosome gene, WTX, is commonly inactivated in Wilms' tumor. Science 2007; 315: 642–645.

527. Khoury JD. Nephroblastic neoplasms. Clin Lab Med 2005; 25: 341–361.

528. Knudson AGJ, Strong LC. Mutation and cancer: a model for Wilms' tumor of the kidney. J Natl Cancer Inst 1972; 48: 313–324.

529. Miller R, Fraumeni JF, Manning MD. Association of Wilms' tumor with aniridia, hemihypertrophy and other congenital malformations. N Engl J Med 1964; 270: 922–927.

530. Gessler M, Poustka A, Cavenee W, et al. Homozygous deletion in Wilms' tumours of a zinc-finger gene identified by chromosome jumping. Nature 1990; 343: 774–778.

531. Call KM, Glaser T, Y IC, et al. Isolation and characterization of a zinc finger polypeptide gene at the human chromosome 11 Wilms' tumor locus. Cell 1990; 60: 509–520.

532. Moore AW, McInnes L, Kreidberg J, et al. YAC complementation shows a requirement for Wt1 in the development of epicardium, adrenal gland and throughout nephrogenesis. Development 1999; 126: 1845–1857.

533. Kreidberg JA, Sariola H, Loring JM, et al. WT-1 is required for early kidney development. Cell 1993; 74: 679–691.

534. Rivera MN, Haber DA. Wilms' tumour: connecting tumorigenesis and organ development in the kidney. Natl Rev Cancer 2005; 5: 699–712.

535. Maiti S, Alam R, Amos CI, et al. Frequent association of beta-catenin and WT1 mutations in Wilms' tumors. Cancer Res 2000; 60: 6288–6292.

536. Feinberg AP, Tycko B. The history of cancer epigenetics. Natl Rev Cancer 2004; 4: 143–153.

537. Austruy E, Candon S, Henry I, et al. Characterization of regions of chromosomes 12 and 16 involved in nephroblastoma tumorigenesis. Genes Chromosomes Cancer 1995; 14: 285–294.

538. Slater RM, Mannens MM. Cytogenetics and molecular genetics of Wilms' tumor of childhood. Cancer Genet Cytogenet 1992; 61: 111–121.

539. Soukup S, Gotwals B, Blough R, et al. Wilms' tumor: summary of 54 cytogenetic analyses. Cancer Genet Cytogenet 1997; 97: 169–171.

540. Rubin BP, Pins MR, Nielsen GP, et al. Isochromosome 7q in adult Wilms' tumors: diagnostic and pathogenetic implications. Am J Surg Pathol 2000; 24: 1663–1669.

541. Huang CC, Cutcliffe C, Coffin C, et al. Classification of malignant pediatric renal tumors by gene expression. Pediatr Blood Cancer 2006; 46: 728–738.

542. Grosfeld JL. Risk-based management: current concepts of treating malignant solid tumors of childhood. J Am Coll Surg 1999; 189: 407–425.

543. Wiener JS, Coppes MJ, Ritchey ML. Current concepts in the biology and management of Wilms' tumor. J Urol 1998; 159: 1316–1325.

544. Lowe LH, Isuani BH, Heller RM, et al. Pediatric renal masses: Wilms' tumor and beyond. Radiographics 2000; 20: 1585–1603.

545. Stern M, Longaker MT, Adzick NS, et al. Hyaluronidase levels in urine from Wilms' tumor patients. J Natl Cancer Inst 1991; 83: 1569–1574.

546. Coppes MJ. Serum biological markers and paraneoplastic syndromes in Wilms' tumor. Med Pediatr Oncol 1993; 21: 213–221.

547. Coppes MJ, Arnold M, Beckwith JB, et al. Factors affecting the risk of contralateral Wilms' tumor development: a report from the National Wilms' Tumor Study Group. Cancer 1999; 85: 1616–1625.

548. Eble J, Sauter G, Epstein J. Pathology and genetics of tumours of the urinary system and male genital organs. In: Eble JN, ed. World Health Organization classification of tumours. Lyons, France: IARC Press, 2003.

549. Murphy WM, Grignon DJ, Perlman EJ. Atlas of tumor pathology: Tumors of the kidney, bladder, and related urinary structures (4th series). Washington, DC: Armed Forces Institute of Pathology, 2004.

550. Mahoney JP, Saffos RO. Fetal rhabdomyomatous nephroblastoma with a renal pelvic mass simulating sarcoma botryoides. Am J Surg Pathol 1981; 5: 297–306.

551. Yanai T, Okazaki T, Yamataka A, et al. Botryoid Wilms' tumor: a report of two cases. Pediatr Surg Int 2005; 21: 43–46.

552. Beckwith JB, Palmer NF. Histopathology and prognosis of Wilms' tumors: results from the First National Wilms' Tumor Study. Cancer 1978; 41: 1937–1948.

553. Breslow NE, Churchill G, Nesmith B, et al. Clinicopathologic features and prognosis for Wilms' tumor patients with metastases at diagnosis. Cancer 1986; 58: 2501–2511.

554. Zuppan CW, Beckwith JB, Luckey DW. Anaplasia in unilateral Wilms' tumor: a report from the National Wilms' Tumor Study Pathology Center. Hum Pathol 1988; 19: 1199–1209.

555. Allsbrook WC Jr, Boswell WC Jr, Takahashi H, et al. Recurrent renal cell carcinoma arising in Wilms' tumor. Cancer 1991; 67: 690–695.

556. Green DM, Beckwith JB, Breslow NE, et al. Treatment of children with stages II to IV anaplastic Wilms' tumor: a report from the National Wilms' Tumor Study Group. J Clin Oncol 1994; 12: 2126–2131.

557. Faria P, Beckwith JB, Mishra K, et al. Focal versus diffuse anaplasia in Wilms' tumor – new definitions with prognostic significance: a report from the National Wilms' Tumor Study Group. Am J Surg Pathol 1996; 20: 909–920.

558. Douglass EC, Look AT, Webber B, et al. Hyperdiploidy and chromosomal rearrangements define the anaplastic variant of Wilms' tumor. J Clin Oncol 1986; 4: 975–981.

559. Beckwith JB, Zuppan CE, Browning NG, et al. Histological analysis of aggressiveness and responsiveness in Wilms' tumor. Med Pediatr Oncol 1996; 27: 422–428.

560. Hill DA, Shear TD, Liu T, et al. Clinical and biologic significance of nuclear unrest in Wilms' tumor. Cancer 2003; 97: 2318–2326.

561. Bardeesy N, Falkoff D, Petruzzi MJ, et al. Anaplastic Wilms' tumour, a subtype displaying poor prognosis, harbours p53 gene mutations. Nature Genet 1994; 7: 91–97.

562. Malkin D, Sexsmith E, Yeger H, et al. Mutations of the p53 tumor suppressor gene occur infrequently in Wilms' tumor. Cancer Res 1994; 54: 2077–2079.

563. Takeuchi S, Bartram CR, Ludwig R, et al. Mutations of p53 in Wilms' tumors. Mod Pathol 1995; 8: 483–487.

564. Govender D, Harilal P, Hadley GP, et al. p53 protein expression in nephroblastomas: a predictor of poor prognosis. Br J Cancer 1998; 77: 314–318.

565. Lahoti C, Thorner P, Malkin D, et al. Immunohistochemical detection of p53 in Wilms' tumors correlates with unfavorable outcome. Am J Pathol 1996; 148: 1577–1589.

566. Cheah PL, Looi LM, Chan LL. Immunohistochemical expression of p53 proteins in Wilms' tumour: a possible association with the histological prognostic parameter of anaplasia. Histopathology 1996; 28: 49–54.

567. Barnoud R, Sabourin JC, Pasquier D, et al. Immunohistochemical expression of WT1 by desmoplastic small round cell tumor: a comparative study with other small round cell tumors. Am J Surg Pathol 2000; 24: 830–836.

568. Pritchard-Jones K, Fleming S. Cell types expressing the Wilms' tumour gene (WT1) in Wilms' tumours: implications for tumour histogenesis. Oncogene 1991; 6: 2211–2220.

569. D'Angio GJ, Breslow N, Beckwith JB, et al. Treatment of Wilms' tumor. Results of the Third National Wilms' Tumor Study. Cancer 1989; 64: 349–360.

570. Breslow NE, Takashima JR, Whitton JA, et al. Second malignant neoplasms following treatment for Wilm's tumor: a report from the National Wilms' Tumor Study Group. J Clin Oncol 1995; 13: 1851–1859.

571. Bever CT Jr, Koenigsberger MR, Antunes JL, et al. Epidural metastasis by Wilms' tumor. Am J Dis Child 1981; 135: 644–646.

572. Bove KE, McAdams AJ. The nephroblastomatosis complex and its relationship to Wilms' tumor: a clinicopathologic treatise. Perspect Pediatr Pathol 1976; 3: 185–223.

573. Beckwith JB, Kiviat NB, Bonadio JF. Nephrogenic rests, nephroblastomatosis, and the pathogenesis of Wilms' tumor. Pediatr Pathol 1990; 10: 1–36.

574. Beckwith JB. Precursor lesions of Wilms' tumor: clinical and biological implications. Med Pediatr Oncol 1993; 21: 158–168.

575. Beckwith JB. Nephrogenic rests and the pathogenesis of Wilms' tumor: developmental and clinical considerations. Am J Med Genet 1998; 79: 268–273.

576. Mishra K, Mathur M, Logani KB, et al. Precursor lesions of Wilms' tumor in Indian children: a multiinstitutional study. Cancer 1998; 83: 2228–2232.

577. Barbosa AS, Faria PA, Beckwith JB. Diffuse hyperplastic perilobar nephroblastomatosis (DHLPN): pathology and clinical biology. Lab Invest 1998; 78: 1.

578. Cozzi F, Schiavetti A, Cozzi DA, et al. Conservative management of hyperplastic and multicentric nephroblastomatosis. J Urol 2004; 172: 1066–1070.

579. Brown JM. Cystic partially differentiated nephroblastoma. J Pathol 1975; 115: 175–178.

580. Joshi VV, Banerjee AK, Yadav K, et al. Cystic partially differentiated nephroblastoma: a clinicopathologic entity in the spectrum of infantile renal neoplasia. Cancer 1977; 40: 789–795.

581. Joshi VV, Beckwith JB. Pathologic delineation of the papillonodular type of cystic partially differentiated nephroblastoma. A review of 11 cases. Cancer 1990; 66: 1568–1577.

582. Joshi VV, Beckwith JB. Multilocular cyst of the kidney (cystic nephroma) and cystic, partially differentiated nephroblastoma. Terminology and criteria for diagnosis. Cancer 1989; 64: 466–479.

583. Blakely ML, Shamberger RC, Norkool P, et al. Outcome of children with cystic partially differentiated nephroblastoma treated with or without chemotherapy. J Pediatr Surg 2003; 38: 897–900.

584. Bolande RP, Brough AJ, Izant RJ Jr. Congenital mesoblastic nephroma of infancy. A report of eight cases and their relationship to Wilms' tumor. Pediatrics 1967; 40: 272–278.

585. Tomlinson GE, Argyle JC, Velasco S, et al. Molecular characterization of congenital mesoblastic nephroma and its distinction from Wilms' tumor. Cancer 1992; 70: 2358–2361.

586. Argani P, Ladanyi M. Recent advances in pediatric renal neoplasia. Adv Anat Pathol 2003; 10: 243–60.

587. Angulo JC, Lopez JI, Ereno C, et al. Hydrops fetalis and congenital mesoblastic nephroma. Child Nephrol Urol 1991; 11: 115–116.

588. Favara BE, Johnson W, Ito J. Renal tumors in the neonatal period. Cancer 1968; 22: 845–855.

589. Gray ES. Mesoblastic nephroma and non-immunological hydrops fetalis. Pediatr Pathol 1989; 9: 607–609.

590. Vido L, Carli M, Rizzoni G, et al. Congenital mesoblastic nephroma with hypercalcemia. Pathogenetic role of prostaglandins. Am J Pediatr Hematol Oncol 1986; 8: 149–152.

591. Malone PS, Duffy PG, Ransley PG, et al. Congenital mesoblastic nephroma, renin production, and hypertension. J Pediatr Surg 1989; 24: 599–600.

592. Perlman EJ. Kidney tumors in children. In: Murphy WM, Grignon DJ, Perlman EJ, eds. Atlas of tumor pathology: Tumors of the kidney, bladder, and related urinary structures (4th Series). Washington, DC: Armed Forces Institute of Pathology, 2004; 1–88.

593. Ganick DJ, Gilbert EF, Beckwith JB, et al. Congenital cystic mesoblastic nephroma. Hum Pathol 1981; 12: 1039–1043.

594. Pettinato G, Manivel JC, Wick MR, et al. Classical and cellular (atypical) congenital mesoblastic nephroma: a clinicopathologic, ultrastructural, immunohistochemical, and flow cytometric study. Hum Pathol 1989; 20: 682–690.

595. Shao L, Hill DA, Perlman EJ. Expression of WT-1, Bcl-2, and CD34 by primary renal spindle cell tumors in children. Pediatr Dev Pathol 2004; 7: 577–582.

596. Kovacs G, Szucs S, Maschek H. Two chromosomally different cell populations in a partly cellular congenital mesoblastic nephroma. Arch Pathol Lab Med 1987; 111: 383–385.

597. Schofield DE, Yunis EJ, Fletcher JA. Chromosome aberrations in mesoblastic nephroma. Am J Pathol 1993; 143: 714–724.

598. Knezevich SR, Garnett MJ, Pysher TJ, et al. ETV6-NTRK3 gene fusions and trisomy 11 establish a histogenetic link between mesoblastic nephroma and congenital fibrosarcoma. Cancer Res 1998; 58: 5046–5048.

599. Rubin BP, Chen CJ, Morgan TW, et al. Congenital mesoblastic nephroma t(12; 15) is associated with ETV6-NTRK3 gene fusion: cytogenetic and molecular relationship to congenital (infantile) fibrosarcoma. Am J Pathol 1998; 153: 1451–1458.

600. Argani P, Sorensen PHB. Congenital mesoblastic nephroma. In: Eble JN, Sauter G, Epstein JI, et al., eds. World Health Organization: Pathology and genetics of tumours of the urinary system and male genital organs. Lyon, France: IARC Press, 2004; 60–61.

601. Heidelberger KP, Ritchey ML, Dauser RC, et al. Congenital mesoblastic nephroma metastatic to the brain. Cancer 1993; 72: 2499–2502.

602. Vujanic GM, Delemarre JF, Moeslichan S, et al. Mesoblastic nephroma metastatic to the lungs and heart– another face of this peculiar lesion: case report and review of the literature. Pediatr Pathol 1993; 13: 143–153.

603. Arnholdt H. Pathology and genetics of tumours of the urinary system and male genital organs. In: Eble JN, Sauter G, Epstein JI, et al., eds. World Health Organization: Pathology and genetics of tumours of the urinary system and male genital organs. Lyon, France: IARC Press, 2004; 58–59.

604. Biegel JA, Fogelgren B, Wainwright LM, et al. Germline INI1 mutation in a patient with a central nervous system atypical teratoid tumor and renal rhabdoid tumor. Genes Chromosomes Cancer 2000; 28: 31–37.

605. Fort DW, Tonk VS, Tomlinson GE, et al. Rhabdoid tumor of the kidney with primitive neuroectodermal tumor of the central nervous system: associated tumors with different

histologic, cytogenetic, and molecular findings. Genes Chromosomes Cancer 1994; 11: 146–152.

606. Savla J, Chen TT, Schneider NR, et al. Mutations of the hSNF5/INI1 gene in renal rhabdoid tumors with second primary brain tumors. J Natl Cancer Inst 2000; 92: 648–650.

607. Versteege I, Sevenet N, Lange J, et al. Truncating mutations of hSNF5/INI1 in aggressive paediatric cancer. Nature 1998; 394: 203–206.

608. Weeks DA, Beckwith JB, Mierau GW, et al. Rhabdoid tumor of kidney. A report of 111 cases from the National Wilms' Tumor Study Pathology Center. Am J Surg Pathol 1989; 13: 439–458.

609. Pastore G, Znaor A, Spreafico F, et al. Malignant renal tumours incidence and survival in European children (1978–1997): report from the Automated Childhood Cancer Information System project. Eur J Cancer 2006; 42: 2103–2114.

610. Kidd JM. Exclusion of certain renal neoplasms from the category of Wilms' tumor. Am J Pathol 1970; 58: 16a.

611. Marsden HB, Lawler W, Kumar PM. Bone metastasizing renal tumor of childhood: morphological and clinical features, and differences from Wilms' tumor. Cancer 1978; 42: 1922–1928.

612. Morgan E, Kidd JM. Undifferentiated sarcoma of the kidney: a tumor of childhood with histopathologic and clinical characteristics distinct from Wilms' tumor. Cancer 1978; 42: 1916–1921.

613. Argani P. Clear cell sarcoma. In: Eble JN, Sauter G, Epstein JI, et al., eds. World Health Organization: Pathology and genetics of tumours of the urinary system and male genital organs. Lyon, France: IARC Press, 2004; 56–57.

614. Rakheja D, Weinberg AG, Tomlinson GE, et al. Translocation (10; 17)(q22; p13): a recurring translocation in clear cell sarcoma of kidney. Cancer Genet Cytogenet 2004; 154: 175–179.

615. Brownlee NA, Perkins LA, Stewart W, et al. Recurring translocation (10; 17) and deletion (14q) in clear cell sarcoma of the kidney. Arch Pathol Lab Med 2007; 131: 446–451.

616. Haas JE, Bonadio JF, Beckwith JB. Clear cell sarcoma of the kidney with emphasis on ultrastructural studies. Cancer 1984; 54: 2978–2987.

617. Hoot AC, Russo P, Judkins AR, et al. Immunohistochemical analysis of hSNF5/INI1 distinguishes renal and extra-renal malignant rhabdoid tumors from other pediatric soft tissue tumors. Am J Surg Pathol 2004; 28: 1485–1491.

618. Chatten J, Cromie WJ, Duckett JW. Ossifying tumor of infantile kidney: report of two cases. Cancer 1980; 45: 609–612.

619. Sotelo-Avila C, Beckwith JB, Johnson JE. Ossifying renal tumor of infancy: a clinicopathologic study of nine cases. Pediatr Pathol Lab Med 1995; 15: 745–762.

620. Ito J, Shinohara N, Koyanagi T, et al. Ossifying renal tumor of infancy: the first Japanese case with long-term follow-up. Pathol Int 1998; 48: 151–159.

621. Srinivas V, Sogani PC, Hajdu SI, et al. Sarcomas of the kidney. J Urol 1984; 132: 13–16.

622. Grignon DJ, Ayala AG, Ro JY, et al. Primary sarcomas of the kidney. A clinicopathologic and DNA flow cytometric study of 17 cases. Cancer 1990; 65: 1611–1618.

623. Deyrup AT, Montgomery E, Fisher C. Leiomyosarcoma of the kidney: a clinicopathologic study. Am J Surg Pathol 2004; 28: 178–182.

624. Vogelzang NJ, Fremgen AM, Guinan PD, et al. Primary renal sarcoma in adults. A natural history and management study by the American Cancer Society, Illinois Division. Cancer 1993; 71: 804–810.

625. Brandes SB, Chelsky MJ, Petersen RO, et al. Leiomyosarcoma of the renal vein. J Surg Oncol 1996; 63: 195–200.

626. Bonsib SM. HMB-45 reactivity in renal leiomyomas and leiomyosarcomas. Mod Pathol 1996; 9: 664–669.

627. Ng WD, Chan KW, Chan YT. Primary leiomyosarcoma of renal capsule. J Urol 1985; 133: 834–835.

628. Norton KI, Godine LB, Lempert C. Leiomyosarcoma of the kidney in an HIV-infected child. Pediatr Radiol 1997; 27: 557–558.

629. Krech RH, Loy V, Dieckmann KP, et al. Leiomyosarcoma of the kidney. Immunohistological and ultrastructural findings with special emphasis on the growth fraction. Br J Urol 1989; 63: 132–134.

630. Sharma D, Pradhan S, Aryya NC, et al. Leiomyosarcoma of kidney – a case report with long term result after radiotherapy and chemotherapy. Int Urol Nephrol 2007; 39: 397–400.

631. Lowe BA, Brewer J, Houghton DC, et al. Malignant transformation of angiomyolipoma. J Urol 1992; 147: 1356–1358.

632. Cerilli LA, Huffman HT, Anand A. Primary renal angiosarcoma: a case report with immunohistochemical, ultrastructural, and cytogenetic features and review of the literature. Arch Pathol Lab Med 1998; 122: 929–935.

633. Kern SB, Gott L, Faulkner J, 2nd. Occurrence of primary renal angiosarcoma in brothers. Arch Pathol Lab Med 1995; 119: 75–78.

634. Lee TY, Lawen J, Gupta R. Renal angiosarcoma: a case report and literature review. Can J Urol 2007; 14: 3471–3476.

635. Cason JD, Waisman J, Plaine L. Angiosarcoma of kidney. Urology 1987; 30: 281–283.

636. Pauli JL, Strutton G. Primary renal angiosarcoma. Pathology 2005; 37: 187–189.

637. Lopez JI, Angulo JC, Flores N, et al. Malignant fibrous histiocytoma of the renal capsule and synchronous transitional cell carcinoma of the bladder. Pathol Res Pract 1996; 192: 468–473.

638. Papadopoulos I, Rudolph P. Primary renal malignant fibrous histiocytoma: case report. Urol Int 1999; 63: 136–138.

639. Ptochos A, Karydas G, Iosifidis N, et al. Primary renal malignant fibrous histiocytoma. A case report and review of the literature. Urol Int 1999; 63: 261–264.

640. Tarjan M, Cserni G, Szabo Z. Malignant fibrous histiocytoma of the kidney. Scand J Urol Nephrol 2001; 35: 518–520.

641. Merchant SH, Mittal BV, Desai MS. Haemangiopericytoma of kidney: a report of 2 cases. J Postgrad Med 1998; 44: 78–80.

642. Heppe RK, Donohue RE, Clark JE. Bilateral renal hemangiopericytoma. Urology 1991; 38: 249–253.

643. Magro G, Cavallaro V, Torrisi A, et al. Intrarenal solitary fibrous tumor of the kidney report of a case with emphasis on the differential diagnosis in the wide spectrum of monomorphous spindle cell tumors of the kidney. Pathol Res Pract 2002; 198: 37–43.

644. Suster S, Nascimento AG, Miettinen M, et al. Solitary fibrous tumors of soft tissue. A clinicopathologic and immunohistochemical study of 12 cases. Am J Surg Pathol 1995; 19: 1257–1266.

645. Messen S, Bonkhoff H, Bruch M, et al. Primary renal osteosarcoma. Case report and review of the literature. Urol Int 1995; 55: 158–161.

646. Weingartner K, Gerharz EW, Neumann K, et al. Primary osteosarcoma of the kidney. Case report and review of literature. Eur Urol 1995; 28: 81–84.

647. Watson R, Kanowski P, Ades C. Primary osteogenic sarcoma of the kidney. Aust NZ J Surg 1995; 65: 622–623.

648. Leventis AK, Stathopoulos GP, Boussiotou AC, et al. Primary osteogenic sarcoma of the kidney – a case report and review of the literature. Acta Oncol 1997; 36: 775–777.

649. Ah-Chong AK, Yip AC. Primary osteogenic sarcoma of the kidney presenting as staghorn calculus. Br J Urol 1993; 71: 233–234.

650. Naslund MJ, Dement S, Marshall FF. Malignant renal schwannoma. Urology 1991; 38: 477–479.

651. Romics I, Bach D, Beutler W. Malignant schwannoma of kidney capsule. Urology 1992; 40: 453–455.

652. Quinn CM, Day DW, Waxman J, et al. Malignant mesenchymoma of the kidney. Histopathology 1993; 23: 86–88.

653. Rubin BP, Fletcher JA, Renshaw AA. Clear cell sarcoma of soft parts: report of a case primary in the kidney with cytogenetic confirmation. Am J Surg Pathol 1999; 23: 589–594.

654. Nativ O, Horowitz A, Lindner A, et al. Primary chondrosarcoma of the kidney. J Urol 1985; 134: 120–121.

655. Gomez-Brouchet A, Soulie M, Delisle MB, et al. Mesenchymal chondrosarcoma of the kidney. J Urol 2001; 166: 2305.

656. Silverman JF, Nathan G, Olson PR, et al. Fine-needle aspiration cytology of low-grade fibromyxoid sarcoma of the renal capsule (capsuloma). Diagn Cytopathol 2000; 23: 279–283.

657. Delahunt B, Beckwith JB, Eble JN, et al. Cystic embryonal sarcoma of kidney: a case report. Cancer 1998; 82: 2427–2433.

658. Morgan GS, Straumfjord JV, Hall EJ. Angiomyolipoma of the kidney. J Urol 1951; 65: 525–527.

659. Fischer W. Die nierentumoren bei der tuberosen hirnsklerose. Ziegler Beitr Path Ant Allg Pathol 1911; 50: 235.

660. Moolten SE. Hamartial nature of of the tuberous sclerosis complex and its bearing on the tumor problem: report of a case with tumor anomaly of the kidney and adenoma sebaceum. 1942. Arch Intern Med 1942; 69: 589–623.

661. van Slegtenhorst M, de Hoogt R, Hermans C, et al. Identification of the tuberous sclerosis gene TSC1 on chromosome 9q34. Science 1997; 277: 805–808.

662. Plank TL, Yeung RS, Henske EP. Hamartin, the product of the tuberous sclerosis 1 (TSC1) gene, interacts with tuberin and appears to be localized to cytoplasmic vesicles. Cancer Res 1998; 58: 4766–4770.

663. Smolarek TA, Wessner LL, McCormack FX, et al. Evidence that lymphangiomyomatosis is caused by TSC2 mutations: chromosome 16p13 loss of heterozygosity in angiomyolipomas and lymph nodes from women with lymphangiomyomatosis. Am J Hum Genet 1998; 62: 810–815.

664. Consortium ECTS. Identification and characterization of the tuberous sclerosis gene on chromosome 16. Cell 1993; 75: 1305–1315.

665. Nellist M, Brook-Carter PT, Connor JM, et al. Identification of markers flanking the tuberous sclerosis locus on chromosome 9 (TSC1). J Med Genet 1993; 30: 224–227.

666. Green AJ, Sepp T, Yates JR. Clonality of tuberous sclerosis harmatomas shown by non-random X-chromosome inactivation. Hum Genet 1996; 97: 240–243.

667. de Jong B, Castedo SM, Oosterhuis JW, et al. Trisomy 7 in a case of angiomyolipoma. Cancer Genet Cytogenet 1988; 34: 219–222.

668. Wullich B, Henn W, Siemer S, et al. Clonal chromosome aberrations in three of five sporadic angiomyolipomas of the kidney. Cancer Genet Cytogenet 1997; 96: 42–45.

669. Green AJ, Johnson PH, Yates JR. The tuberous sclerosis gene on chromosome 9q34 acts as a growth suppressor. Hum Mol Genet 1994; 3: 1833–1834.

670. Green AJ, Smith M, Yates JR. Loss of heterozygosity on chromosome 16p13.3 in hamartomas from tuberous sclerosis patients. Nature Genet 1994; 6: 193–196.

671. Henske EP, Neumann HP, Scheithauer BW, et al. Loss of heterozygosity in the tuberous sclerosis (TSC2) region of chromosome band 16p13 occurs in sporadic as well as TSC-associated renal angiomyolipomas. Genes Chromosomes Cancer 1995; 13: 295–298.

672. Carbonara C, Longa L, Grosso E, et al. Apparent preferential loss of heterozygosity at TSC2 over TSC1 chromosomal region in tuberous sclerosis hamartomas. Genes Chromosomes Cancer 1996; 15: 18–25.

673. Kattar MM, Grignon DJ, Eble JN, et al. Chromosomal analysis of renal angiomyolipoma by comparative genomic hybridization: evidence for clonal origin. Hum Pathol 1999; 30: 295–299.

674. Paradis V, Laurendeau I, Vieillefond A, et al. Clonal analysis of renal sporadic angiomyolipomas. Hum Pathol 1998; 29: 1063–1067.

675. Saxena R, Sait S, Mhawech-Fauceglia P. Ewing sarcoma/primitive neuroectodermal tumor of the kidney: a case report. Diagnosed by immunohistochemistry and molecular analysis. Ann Diagn Pathol 2006; 10: 363–366.

676. Cheng L, Gu J, Eble JN, et al. Molecular genetic evidence for different clonal origin of components of human renal angiomyolipomas. Am J Surg Pathol 2001; 25: 1231–1236.

677. Nellist M, van Slegtenhorst MA, Goedbloed M, et al. Characterization of the cytosolic tuberin–hamartin complex. Tuberin is a cytosolic chaperone for hamartin. J Biol Chem 1999; 274: 35647–35652.

678. Weeks DA, Malott RL, Arnesen M, et al. Hepatic angiomyolipoma with striated granules and positivity with melanoma-specific antibody (HMB-45): a report of two cases. Ultrastruct Pathol 1991; 15: 563–571.

679. Ashfaq R, Weinberg AG, Albores-Saavedra J. Renal angiomyolipomas and HMB-45 reactivity. Cancer 1993; 71: 3091–3097.

680. Bonetti F, Pea M, Martignoni G, et al. Cellular heterogeneity in lymphangiomyomatosis of the lung. Hum Pathol 1991; 2: 727–728.

681. Chan JK, Tsang WY, Pau MY, et al. Lymphangiomyomatosis and angiomyolipoma: closely related entities characterized by hamartomatous proliferation of HMB-45-positive smooth muscle. Histopathology 1993; 22: 445–455.

682. Bonetti F, Chiodera PL, Pea M, et al. Transbronchial biopsy in lymphangiomyomatosis of the lung. HMB-45 for diagnosis. Am J Surg Pathol 1993; 17: 1092–1102.

683. Bonetti F, Pea M, Martignoni G, et al. Clear cell ('sugar') tumor of the lung is a lesion strictly related to angiomyolipoma – the concept of a family of lesions characterized by the presence of the perivascular epithelioid cells (PEC). Pathology 1994; 26: 230–236.

684. Martignoni G, Pea M, Bonetti F. Renal epithelioid oxyphilic neoplasms (REON). A pleomorphic monophasic variant of renal angiomyolipoma. Int J Surg Pathol 1995; 2: 539.

685. Zamboni G, Pea M, Martignoni G, et al. Clear cell 'sugar' tumor of the pancreas. A novel member of the family of lesions characterized by the presence of perivascular epithelioid cells. Am J Surg Pathol 1996; 20: 722–730.

686. Folpe AL, Goodman ZD, Ishak KG, et al. Clear cell myomelanocytic tumor of the falciform ligament/ligamentum teres: a novel member of the perivascular epithelioid clear cell family of tumors with a predilection for children and young adults. Am J Surg Pathol 2000; 24: 1239–1246.

687. Vang R, Kempson RL. Perivascular epithelioid cell tumor ('PEComa') of the uterus: a subset of HMB-45-positive epithelioid mesenchymal neoplasms with an uncertain relationship to pure smooth muscle tumors. Am J Surg Pathol 2002; 26: 1–13.

688. Folpe AL, McKenney JK, Li Z, et al. Clear cell myomelanocytic tumor of the thigh: report of a unique case. Am J Surg Pathol 2002; 26: 809–812.

689. Insabato L, De Rosa G, Terracciano LM, et al. Primary monotypic epithelioid angiomyolipoma of bone. Histopathology 2002; 40: 286–290.

690. Govender D, Sabaratnam RM, Essa AS. Clear cell 'sugar' tumor of the breast: another extrapulmonary site and review of the literature. Am J Surg Pathol 2002; 26: 670–675.

691. Bosincu L, Rocca PC, Martignoni G, et al. Perivascular epithelioid cell (PEC) tumors of the uterus: a clinicopathologic study of two cases with aggressive features. Mod Pathol 2005; 18: 1336–1342.

692. Folpe AL, Mentzel T, Lehr HA, et al. Perivascular epithelioid cell neoplasms of soft tissue and gynecologic origin: a clinicopathologic study of 26 cases and review of the literature. Am J Surg Pathol 2005; 29: 1558–1575.

693. Fletcher CDM, Unni KK, Mertens F. Pathology and genetics of tumours of soft tissue and bone, in World Health Organization (WHO) Classification of Tumours. Lyon, IARC Press, 2002.

694. Fujii Y, Ajima J, Oka K, et al. Benign renal tumors detected among healthy adults by abdominal ultrasonography. Eur Urol 1995; 27: 124–127.

695. Cook JA, Oliver K, Mueller RF, et al. A cross sectional study of renal

involvement in tuberous sclerosis. J Med Genet 1996; 33: 480–484.

696. Eble JN. Angiomyolipoma of kidney. Semin Diagn Pathol 1998; 15: 21–40.

697. Henske EP, Ao X, Short MP, et al. Frequent progesterone receptor immunoreactivity in tuberous sclerosis-associated renal angiomyolipomas. Mod Pathol 1998; 11: 665–668.

698. Tong YC, Chieng PU, Tsai TC, et al. Renal angiomyolipoma: report of 24 cases. Br J Urol 1990; 66: 585–589.

699. Kennelly MJ, Grossman HB, Cho KJ. Outcome analysis of 42 cases of renal angiomyolipoma. J Urol 1994; 152: 1988–1991.

700. Oesterling JE, Fishman EK, Goldman SM, et al. The management of renal angiomyolipoma. J Urol 1986; 135: 1121–1124.

701. Yanai H, Sasagawa I, Kubota Y, et al. Spontaneous hemorrhage during pregnancy secondary to renal angiomyolipoma. Urol Int 1996; 56: 188–191.

702. Forsnes EV, Eggleston MK, Burtman M. Placental abruption and spontaneous rupture of renal angiomyolipoma in a pregnant woman with tuberous sclerosis. Obstet Gynecol 1996; 88: 725.

703. Sherman JL, Hartman DS, Friedman AC, et al. Angiomyolipoma: computed tomographic–pathologic correlation of 17 cases. AJR Am J Roentgenol 1981; 137: 1221–1226.

704. Bosniak MA, Megibow AJ, Hulnick DH, et al. CT diagnosis of renal angiomyolipoma: the importance of detecting small amounts of fat. AJR Am J Roentgenol 1988; 151: 497–501.

705. Williams MA, Schropp KP, Noe HN. Fat containing renal mass in childhood: a case report of teratoid Wilms' tumor. J Urol 1994; 151: 1662–1663.

706. Davidson AJ, Davis CJ Jr. Fat in renal adenocarcinoma: never say never. Radiology 1993; 188: 316.

707. Helenon O, Chretien Y, Paraf F, et al. Renal cell carcinoma containing fat: demonstration with CT. Radiology 1993; 188: 429–430.

708. Strotzer M, Lehner KB, Becker K. Detection of fat in a renal cell carcinoma mimicking angiomyolipoma. Radiology 1993; 188: 427–428.

709. Morrison ID, Reznek RH, Webb JA. Case report: renal adenocarcinoma with ultrasonographic appearances suggestive of angiomyolipoma. Clin Radiol 1995; 50: 659–661.

710. Sola JE, Pierre-Jerome F, Sitzmann JV, et al. Multifocal angiomyolipoma in a patient with tuberous sclerosis. Clin Imaging 1996; 20: 99–102.

711. Price EB, Mostofi FK. Symptomatic angiomyolipoma of the kidney. Cancer 1965; 18: 761–774.

712. Nagashima Y, Ohaki Y, Tanaka Y, et al. A case of renal angiomyolipomas associated with multiple and various hamartomatous microlesions. Virchows

713. Kilicaslan I, Gulluoglu MG, Dogan O, et al. Intraglomerular microlesions in renal angiomyolipoma. Hum Pathol 2000; 31: 1325–1328.

714. Martignoni G, Bonetti F, Pea M, et al. Renal disease in adults with TSC2/PKD1 contiguous gene syndrome. Am J Surg Pathol 2002; 26: 198–205.

715. Davis CJ, Barton JH, Sesterhenn IA. Cystic angiomyolipoma of the kidney: a clinicopathologic description of 11 cases. Mod Pathol 2006; 19: 669–674.

716. Fine SW, Reuter VE, Epstein JI, et al. Angiomyolipoma with epithelial cysts (AMLEC): a distinct cystic variant of angiomyolipoma. Am J Surg Pathol 2006; 30: 593–599.

717. Holm-Nielsen P, Sorensen FB. Renal angiomyolipoma: An ultrastructural investigation of three cases with histogenetic considerations. APMIS 1988; 4: 37–47.

718. Yum M, Ganguly A, Donohue JP. Juxtaglomerular cells in renal angiomyolipoma. Ultrastructural observation. Urology 1984; 24: 283–286.

719. Makhlouf HR, Remotti HE, Ishak KG. Expression of KIT (CD117) in angiomyolipoma. Am J Surg Pathol 2002; 26: 493–497.

720. Kaiserling E, Krober S, Xiao JC, et al. Angiomyolipoma of the kidney. Immunoreactivity with HMB-45. Light- and electron-microscopic findings. Histopathology 1994; 25: 41–48.

721. Sturtz CL, Dabbs DJ. Angiomyolipomas: the nature and expression of the HMB-45 antigen. Mod Pathol 1994; 7: 842–845.

722. L'Hostis H, Deminiere C, Ferriere JM, et al. Renal angiomyolipoma: a clinicopathologic, immunohistochemical, and follow-up study of 46 cases. Am J Surg Pathol 1999; 23: 1011–1020.

723. Fetsch PA, Fetsch JF, Marincola FM, et al. Comparison of melanoma antigen recognized by T cells (MART-1) to HMB-45: additional evidence to support a common lineage for angiomyolipoma, lymphangiomyomatosis, and clear cell sugar tumor. Mod Pathol 1998; 11: 699–703.

724. Jungbluth AA, Iversen K, Coplan K, et al. Expression of melanocyte-associated markers gp-100 and Melan-A/MART-1 in angiomyolipomas. An immunohistochemical and rt-PCR analysis. Virchows Arch 1999; 434: 429–435.

725. Zavala-Pompa A, Folpe AL, Jimenez RE, et al. Immunohistochemical study of microphthalmia transcription factor and tyrosinase in angiomyolipoma of the kidney, renal cell carcinoma, and renal and retroperitoneal sarcomas: comparative evaluation with traditional diagnostic markers. Am J Surg Pathol 2001; 25: 65–70.

726. Roma AA, Magi-Galluzzi C, Zhou M. Differential expression of melanocytic markers in myoid, lipomatous, and vascular components of renal angiomyolipomas. Arch Pathol Lab Med 2007; 131: 122–125.

727. Stone CH, Lee MW, Amin MB, et al. Renal angiomyolipoma: further immunophenotypic characterization of an expanding morphologic spectrum. Arch Pathol Lab Med 2001; 125: 751–758.

728. Wilson GC, Lo D. Tuberous sclerosis: a case with pulmonary and lymph node involvement. Med J Aust 1964; 58: 795–796.

729. Ro JY, Ayala AG, el-Naggar A, et al. Angiomyolipoma of kidney with lymph node involvement. DNA flow cytometric analysis. Arch Pathol Lab Med 1990; 114: 65–67.

730. Tallarigo C, Baldassarre R, Bianchi G, et al. Diagnostic and therapeutic problems in multicentric renal angiomyolipoma. J Urol 1992; 148: 1880–1884.

731. Ackerman TE, Levi CS, Lindsay DJ, et al. Angiomyolipoma with lymph node involvement. Can Assoc Radiol J 1994; 45: 52–55.

732. Tawfik O, Austenfeld M, Persons D. Multicentric renal angiomyolipoma associated with pulmonary lymphangioleiomyomatosis: case report, with histologic, immunohistochemical, and DNA content analyses. Urology 1996; 48: 476–480.

733. Abdulla M, Bui HX, del Rosario AD, et al. Renal angiomyolipoma. DNA content and immunohistochemical study of classic and multicentric variants. Arch Pathol Lab Med 1994; 118: 735–739.

734. Farrow GM, Harrison EG, Utz DC, et al. Renal angiomyolipoma. A clinicopathologic study of 32 cases. Cancer 1968; 22: 564–570.

735. Kragel PJ, Toker C. Infiltrating recurrent renal angiomyolipoma with fatal outcome. J Urol 1985; 133: 90–91.

736. Ferry JA, Malt RA, Young RH. Renal angiomyolipoma with sarcomatous transformation and pulmonary metastases. Am J Surg Pathol 1991; 15: 1083–1088.

737. Mai KT, Perkins DG, Robertson S, et al. Composite renal cell carcinoma and angiomyolipoma: a study of the histogenetic relationship of the two lesions. Pathol Int 1999; 49: 1–8.

738. Jimenez RE, Eble JN, Reuter VE, et al. Concurrent angiomyolipoma and renal cell neoplasia: a study of 36 cases. Mod Pathol 2001; 14: 157–163.

739. Steiner MS, Goldman SM, Fishman EK, et al. The natural history of renal angiomyolipoma. J Urol 1993; 150: 1782–1786.

740. Hartwick RWJ, Srigley JR, Shaw P. Uncommon histologic patterns mimicking malignancy in angiomyolipoma. Mod Pathol 1989; 2: 39A.

741. Pea M, Bonetti F, Zamboni G, et al. Melanocyte-marker-HMB-45 is regularly expressed in angiomyolipoma of the kidney. Pathology 1991; 23: 185–188.

742. Mai KT. Giant renomedullary interstitial cell tumor. J Urol 1994; 151: 986–988.

743. Eble JN, Amin MB, Young RH. Epithelioid angiomyolipoma of the kidney: a report of five cases with a prominent and diagnostically confusing epithelioid smooth muscle component. Am J Surg Pathol 1997; 21: 1123–1130.

744. Quek ML, Soni RA, Hsu J, et al. Renal epithelioid angiomyolipoma associated with hyperprolactinemia. Urology 2005; 65: 797.

745. Pea M, Bonetti F, Martignoni G, et al. Apparent renal cell carcinomas in tuberous sclerosis are heterogeneous: the identification of malignant epithelioid angiomyolipoma. Am J Surg Pathol 1998; 22: 180–187.

746. Martignoni G, Pea M, Bonetti F, et al. Carcinoma-like monotypic epithelioid angiomyolipoma in patients without evidence of tuberous sclerosis: a clinicopathologic and genetic study. Am J Surg Pathol 1998; 22: 663–672.

747. Delgado R, de Leon Bojorge B, Albores-Saavedra J. Atypical angiomyolipoma of the kidney: a distinct morphologic variant that is easily confused with a variety of malignant neoplasms. Cancer 1998; 83: 1581–1592.

748. Christiano AP, Yang X, Gerber GS. Malignant transformation of renal angiomyolipoma. J Urol 1999; 161: 1900–1901.

749. Martignoni G, Pea M, Rigaud G, et al. Renal angiomyolipoma with epithelioid sarcomatous transformation and metastases. Demonstration of the same genetic defects in the primary and metastatic lesions. Am J Surg Pathol 2000; 24: 889–894.

750. Cibas ES, Goss GA, Kulke MH, et al. Malignant epithelioid angiomyolipoma ('sarcoma ex angiomyolipoma') of the kidney: a case report and review of the literature. Am J Surg Pathol 2001; 25: 121–126.

751. Stone CH, Lee MW, Amin MB, et al. Renal angiomyolipoma: further immunophenotypic characterization of an expanding morphologic spectrum. Arch Pathol Lab Med 2001; 125: 751–758.

752. Kawaguchi K, Oda Y, Nakanishi K, et al. Malignant transformation of renal angiomyolipoma: a case report. Am J Surg Pathol 2002; 26: 523–529.

753. Ma L, Kowalski D, Javed K, et al. Atypical angiomyolipoma of kidney in a patient with tuberous sclerosis: a case report with p53 gene mutation analysis. Arch Pathol Lab Med 2005; 129: 676–679.

754. Ribalta T, Lloreta J, Munne A, et al. Malignant pigmented clear cell epithelioid tumor of the kidney: clear cell ('sugar') tumor versus malignant melanoma. Hum Pathol 2000; 31: 516–519.

755. Saito K, Fujii Y, Kasahara I, et al. Malignant clear cell 'sugar' tumor of the kidney: clear cell variant of epithelioid angiomyolipoma. J Urol 2002; 168: 2533–2534.

756. Mai KT, Perkins DG, Collins JP. Epithelioid cell variant of renal angiomyolipoma. Histopathology 1996; 28: 277–280.

757. Yu W, Fraser RB, Gaskin DA, et al. C-kit-positive metastatic malignant pigmented clear-cell epithelioid tumor arising from the kidney in a child without tuberous sclerosis. Ann Diagn Pathol 2005; 9: 330–334.

758. Steiner M, Quinlan D, Goldman SM, et al. Leiomyoma of the kidney: presentation of 4 new cases and the role of computerized tomography. J Urol 1990; 143: 994–998.

759. Tawfik OW, Moral LA, Richardson WP, et al. Multicentric bilateral renal cell carcinomas and a vascular leiomyoma in a child. Pediatr Pathol 1993; 13: 289–298.

760. Creager AJ, Maia DM, Funkhouser WK. Epstein–Barr virus-associated renal smooth muscle neoplasm: report of a case with review of the literature. Arch Pathol Lab Med 1998; 122: 277–281.

761. Mohammed AY, Matthew L, Harmse JL, et al. Multiple leiomyoma of the renal capsule. Scand J Urol Nephrol 1999; 33: 138–139.

762. Shum CF, Yip SK, Tan PH. Symptomatic renal leiomyoma: report of two cases. Pathology 2006; 38: 454–456.

763. Clinton-Thomas CL. A giant leiomyoma of the kidney. Br J Surg 1956; 43: 497–501.

764. Tamboli P, Ro JY, Amin MB, et al. Benign tumors and tumor-like lesions of the adult kidney. Part II: Benign mesenchymal and mixed neoplasms, and tumor-like lesions. Adv Anat Pathol 2000; 7: 47–66.

765. Jahn H, Rasmussen L, Nissen HM. Hemangioma of the kidney. Urol Int 1991; 46: 200–202.

766. Zaidi SZ, Mor Y, Scheimberg I, et al. Renal haemangioma presenting as an abdominal mass in a neonate. Br J Urol 1998; 82: 763–764.

767. Hull GW 3rd, Genega EM, Sogani PC. Intravascular capillary hemangioma presenting as a solid renal mass. J Urol 1999; 162: 784–785.

768. Yazaki T, Takahashi S, Ogawa Y, et al. Large renal hemangioma necessitating nephrectomy. Urology 1985; 25: 302–304.

769. Wang T, Palazzo JP, Mitchell D, et al. Renal capsular hemangioma. J Urol 1993; 149: 1122–1123.

770. Gogus C, Kilic S, Ataoglu O, et al. Large cavernous hemangioma of the kidney presenting as a solid renal mass. Int Urol Nephrol 2001; 33: 615–616.

771. Gupta NP, Kumar P, Goel R, et al. Renal sinus hemangioma simulating renal mass: a diagnostic challenge. Int Urol Nephrol 2004; 36: 485–487.

772. Daneshmand S, Huffman JL. Endoscopic management of renal hemangioma. J Urol 2002; 167: 488–489.

773. Bisceglia M, Galliani CA, Senger C, et al. Renal cystic diseases: a review. Adv Anat Pathol 2006; 13: 26–56.

774. Debiec-Rychter M, Kaluzewski B, Saryusz-Wolska H, et al. A case of renal lymphangioma with a karyotype 45,X,-X,i dic(7q). Cancer Genet Cytogenet 1990; 46: 29–33.

775. Leder RA. Genitourinary case of the day. Renal lymphangiomatosis. AJR Am J Roentgenol 1995; 165: 197–198.

776. Honma I, Takagi Y, Shigyo M, et al. Lymphangioma of the kidney. Int J Urol 2002; 9: 178–182.

777. Zapzalka DM, Krishnamurti L, Manivel JC, et al. Lymphangioma of the renal capsule. J Urol 2002; 168: 220.

778. Caduff RF, Schwobel MG, Willi UV, et al. Lymphangioma of the right kidney in an infant boy. Pediatr Pathol Lab Med 1997; 17: 631–637.

779. Anderson C, Knibbs DR, Ludwig ME, et al. Lymphangioma of the kidney: a pathologic entity distinct from solitary multilocular cyst. Hum Pathol 1992; 23: 465–468.

780. Nakai Y, Namba Y, Sugao H. Renal lymphangioma. J Urol 1999; 162: 484–485.

781. Robertson PW, Klidjian A, Harding LK, et al. Hypertension due to a renin-secreting renal tumour. Am J Med 1967; 43: 963–976.

782. Martin SA, Mynderse LA, Lager DJ, et al. Juxtaglomerular cell tumor: a clinicopathologic study of four cases and review of the literature. Am J Clin Pathol 2001; 116: 854–863.

783. Hayami S, Sasagawa I, Suzuki H, et al. Juxtaglomerular cell tumor without hypertension. Scand J Urol Nephrol 1998; 32: 231–233.

784. Kuroda N, Moriki T, Komatsu F, et al. Adult-onset giant juxtaglomerular cell tumor of the kidney. Pathol Int 2000; 50: 249–254.

785. Tetu B, Vaillancourt L, Camilleri JP, et al. Juxtaglomerular cell tumor of the kidney: report of two cases with a papillary pattern. Hum Pathol 1993; 24: 1168–1174.

786. Kodet R, Taylor M, Vachalova H, et al. Juxtaglomerular cell tumor. An immunohistochemical, electron-microscopic, and in situ hybridization study. Am J Surg Pathol 1994; 18: 837–842.

787. Kim HJ, Kim CH, Choi YJ, et al. Juxtaglomerular cell tumor of kidney with CD34 and CD117 immunoreactivity: report of 5 cases. Arch Pathol Lab Med 2006; 130: 707–711.

788. Haab F, Duclos JM, Guyenne T, et al. Renin secreting tumors: diagnosis, conservative surgical approach and long-term results. J Urol 1995; 153: 1781–1784.

789. Duan X, Bruneval P, Hammadeh R, et al. Metastatic juxtaglomerular cell tumor in a 52-year-old man. Am J Surg Pathol 2004; 28: 1098–1102.

790. Glover SD, Buck AC. Renal medullary fibroma: a case report. J Urol 1982; 127: 758–760.

791. Eble JN. Renomedullary interstitial cell tumor. In: Eble JN, Sauter G, Epstein JI, et al., eds. World Health Organization: Pathology and genetics of tumours of the urinary system and male genital organs. Lyon, France: IARC Press, 2004; 74.

792. Somers WJ, Terpenning B, Lowe FC, et al. Renal parenchymal neurilemoma: a rare and unusual kidney tumor. J Urol 1988; 139: 109–110.

793. Ma KF, Tse CH, Tsui MS. Neurilemmoma of kidney – a rare occurrence. Histopathology 1990; 17: 378–380.

794. Ikeda I, Miura T, Kondo I, et al. Neurilemmoma of the kidney. Br J Urol 1996; 78: 469–470.

795. Singer AJ, Anders KH. Neurilemoma of the kidney. Urology 1996; 47: 575–581.

796. Alvarado-Cabrero I. Intrarenal schwannoma. Lyon, France: IARC Press, 2004.

797. Alvarado-Cabrero I, Folpe AL, Srigley JR, et al. Intrarenal schwannoma: a report of four cases including three cellular variants. Mod Pathol 2000; 13: 851–856.

798. Tsurusaki M, Mimura F, Yasui N, et al. Neurilemoma of the renal capsule: MR imaging and pathologic correlation. Eur Radiol 2001; 11: 1834–1837.

799. Gelb AB, Simmons ML, Weidner N. Solitary fibrous tumor involving the renal capsule. Am J Surg Pathol 1996; 20: 1288–1295.

800. Wang J, Arber DA, Frankel K, et al. Large solitary fibrous tumor of the kidney: report of two cases and review of the literature. Am J Surg Pathol 2001; 25: 1194–1199.

801. Znati K, Chbani L, El Fatemi H, et al. Solitary fibrous tumor of the kidney: a case report and review of the literature. Rev Urol 2007; 9: 36–40.

802. Bozkurt SU, Ahiskali R, Kaya H, et al. Solitary fibrous tumor of the kidney. Case report. Apmis 2007; 115: 259–262.

803. Fine SW, McCarthy DM, Chan TY, et al. Malignant solitary fibrous tumor of the kidney: report of a case and comprehensive review of the literature. Arch Pathol Lab Med 2006; 130: 857–861.

804. Hanau CA, Miettinen M. Solitary fibrous tumor: histological and immunohistochemical spectrum of benign and malignant variants presenting at different sites. Hum Pathol 1995; 26: 440–449.

805. Guillou L, Fletcher JA, Fletcher CDM. Extrapleural solitary fibrous tumor and hemangiopericytoma. Lyon, France: IARC Press, 2004.

806. Edmunds W. Cystic adenoma of kidney. Trans Pathol Soc 1892; 432: 89.

807. Boggs LK, Kimmelstiel P. Benign multilocular cystic nephroma: report of two cases of so-called multilocular cyst of the kidney. J Urol 1956; 76: 530–541.

808. Kajani N, Rosenberg BF, Bernstein J. Multilocular cystic nephroma. J Urol Pathol 1993; 1: 33.

809. Madewell JE, Goldman SM, Davis CJ Jr, et al. Multilocular cystic nephroma: a radiographic–pathologic correlation of 58 patients. Radiology 1983; 146: 309–321.

810. Castillo OA, Boyle ET Jr, Kramer SA. Multilocular cysts of kidney. A study of 29 patients and review of literature. Urology 1991; 37: 156–162.

811. Mukhopadhyay S, Valente AL, de la Roza G. Cystic nephroma: a histologic and immunohistochemical study of 10 cases. Arch Pathol Lab Med 2004; 128: 1404–1411.

812. Jevremovic D, Lager DJ, Lewin M. Cystic nephroma (multilocular cyst) and mixed epithelial and stromal tumor of the kidney: a spectrum of the same entity? Ann Diagn Pathol 2006; 10: 77–82.

813. Antic T, Perry KT, Harrison K, et al. Mixed epithelial and stromal tumor of the kidney and cystic nephroma share overlapping features: reappraisal of 15 lesions. Arch Pathol Lab Med 2006; 130: 80–85.

814. Geller RA, Pataki KI, Finegold RA. Bilateral multilocular renal cysts with recurrence. J Urol 1979; 121: 808–810.

815. Kural AR, Obek C, Ozbay G, et al. Multilocular cystic nephroma: an unusual localization. Urology 1998; 52: 897–899.

816. Antonescu C, Bisceglia M, Reuter V, et al. Sarcomatous transformation of cystic nephroma in adults. Mod Pathol 1997; 10: 69A.

817. Block NL, Grabstald HG, Melamed MR. Congenital mesoblastic nephroma (leiomyomatous hamartoma): first adult case. J Urol 1973; 110: 380–383.

818. Levin NP, Damjanov I, Depillis VJ. Mesoblastic nephroma in an adult patient: recurrence 21 years after removal of the primary lesion. Cancer 1982; 49: 573–577.

819. Prats Lopez J, Palou Redorta J, Morote Robles J, et al. Leiomyomatous renal hamartoma in an adult. Eur Urol 1988; 14: 80–82.

820. Trillo AA. Adult variant of congenital mesoblastic nephroma. Arch Pathol Lab Med 1990; 114: 533–535.

821. Van Velden DJJ, Schneider JW, Allen FJ. A case of adult mesoblastic nephroma: ultrastructure and discussion of histogenesis. J Urol 1990; 143: 1216–1219.

822. Durham JR, Bostwick DG, Farrow GM, et al. Mesoblastic nephroma of adulthood. Report of three cases. Am J Surg Pathol 1993; 17: 1029–1038.

823. Pawade J, Soosay GN, Delprado W, et al. Cystic hamartoma of the renal pelvis. Am J Surg Pathol 1993; 17: 1169–1175.

824. Michal M, Syrucek M. Benign mixed epithelial and stromal tumor of the kidney. Pathol Res Pract 1998; 194: 44–48.

825. Truong LD, Williams R, Ngo T, et al. Adult mesoblastic nephroma: expansion of the morphologic spectrum and review of literature. Am J Surg Pathol 1998; 22: 827–839.

826. Michal M, Hes O, Havlicek F. Benign renal angiomyoadenomatous tumor: a previously unreported renal tumor. Ann Diagn Pathol 2000; 4: 311–315.

827. Adsay NV, Eble JN, Srigley JR, et al. Mixed epithelial and stromal tumor of the kidney. Am J Surg Pathol 2000; 24: 958–970.

828. Beiko DT, Nickel JC, Boag AH, et al. Benign mixed epithelial stromal tumor of the kidney of possible mullerian origin. J Urol 2001; 166: 1381–1382.

829. Pierson CR, Schober MS, Wallis T, et al. Mixed epithelial and stromal tumor of the kidney lacks the genetic alterations of cellular congenital mesoblastic nephroma. Hum Pathol 2001; 32: 513–520.

830. Michal M, Hes O, Bisceglia M, et al. Mixed epithelial and stromal tumors of the kidney. A report of 22 cases. Virchows Arch 2004; 445: 359–367.

831. Buritica C, Serrano M, Zuluaga A, et al. Mixed epithelial and stromal tumour of the kidney with luteinised ovarian stroma. J Clin Pathol 2007; 60: 98–100.

832. Comperat E, Couturier J, Peyromaure M, et al. Benign mixed epithelial and stromal tumor of the kidney (MEST) with cytogenetic alteration. Pathol Res Pract 2005; 200: 865–867.

833. Mukhopadhyay S, Valente AL, de la Roza G. Corpora albicantia-like bodies in cystic nephroma: yet another similarity to mixed epithelial stromal tumor of kidney. Int J Surg Pathol 2005; 13: 233.

834. Turbiner J, Amin MB, Humphrey PA, et al. Cystic nephroma and mixed epithelial and stromal tumor of kidney: a detailed clinicopathologic analysis of 34 cases and proposal for renal epithelial and stromal tumor (REST) as a unifying term. Am J Surg Pathol 2007; 31: 489–500.

835. Svec A, Hes O, Michal M, et al. Malignant mixed epithelial and stromal tumor of the kidney. Virchows Arch 2001; 439: 700–702.

836. Bisceglia M, Bacchi CE. Mixed epithelial-stromal tumor of the kidney in adults: two cases from the Arkadi M. Rywlin slide seminars. Adv Anat Pathol 2003; 10: 223–233.

837. Nakagawa T, Kanai Y, Fujimoto H, et al. Malignant mixed epithelial and stromal tumours of the kidney: a report of the first two cases with a fatal clinical outcome. Histopathology 2004; 44: 302–304.

838. Yap YS, Coleman M, Olver I. Aggressive mixed epithelial-stromal tumour of the kidney treated with chemotherapy and radiotherapy. Lancet Oncol 2004; 5: 747–749.

839. Faria PA, Argani P, Epstein JI, et al. Primary synovial sarcoma of the kidney: a molecular reappraisal of a subset of so-called embryonal renal sarcoma. Mod Pathol 1999; 12: 79, 94A.

840. Arnold MM, Beckwith JB, Faria P, et al. Embryonal sarcoma of adult and pediatric kidneys. Mod Pathol 1995; 8: 72A.

841. Argani P, Faria PA, Epstein JI, et al. Primary renal synovial sarcoma: molecular and morphologic delineation of an entity previously included among embryonal sarcomas of the kidney. Am J Surg Pathol 2000; 24: 1087–1096.

842. Kim DH, Sohn JH, Lee MC, et al. Primary synovial sarcoma of the kidney. Am J Surg Pathol 2000; 24: 1097–104.

843. Koyama S, Morimitsu Y, Morokuma F, et al. Primary synovial sarcoma of the kidney: Report of a case confirmed by molecular detection of the SYT-SSX2 fusion transcripts. Pathol Int 2001; 51: 385–391.

844. Jun SY, Choi J, Kang GH, et al. Synovial sarcoma of the kidney with rhabdoid features: report of three cases. Am J Surg Pathol 2004; 28: 634–637.

845. Shannon BA, Murch A, Cohen RJ. Primary renal synovial sarcoma confirmed by cytogenetic analysis: a lesion distinct from sarcomatoid renal cell carcinoma. Arch Pathol Lab Med 2005; 129: 238–240.

846. Perlmutter AE, Saunders SE, Zaslau S, et al. Primary synovial sarcoma of the kidney. Int J Urol 2005; 12: 760–762.

847. Ladanyi M, Antonescu CR, Leung DH, et al. Impact of SYT-SSX fusion type on the clinical behavior of synovial sarcoma: a multi-institutional retrospective study of 243 patients. Cancer Res 2002; 62: 135–140.

848. Terry J, Saito T, Subramanian S, et al. TLE1 as a diagnostic immunohistochemical marker for synovial sarcoma emerging from gene expression profiling studies. Am J Surg Pathol 2007; 31: 240–246.

849. Krishnan B, Truong LD, Saleh G, et al. Horseshoe kidney is associated with an increased relative risk of primary renal carcinoid tumor. J Urol 1997; 157: 2059–2066.

850. Begin LR, Guy L, Jacobson SA, et al. Renal carcinoid and horseshoe kidney: a frequent association of two rare entities – a case report and review of the literature. J Surg Oncol 1998; 68: 113–119.

851. Isobe H, Takashima H, Higashi N, et al. Primary carcinoid tumor in a horseshoe kidney. Int J Urol 2000; 7: 184–188.

852. McVey RJ, Banerjee SS, Eyden BP, et al. Carcinoid tumor originating in a horseshoe kidney. In Vivo 2002; 16: 197–199.

853. Romero FR, Rais-Bahrami S, Permpongkosol S, et al. Primary carcinoid tumors of the kidney. J Urol 2006; 176: 2359–2366.

854. Kurzer E, Leveillee RJ, Morillo G. Rare case of carcinoid tumor arising within teratoma in kidney. Urology 2005; 66: 658.

855. Fetissof F, Benatre A, Dubois MP, et al. Carcinoid tumor occurring in a teratoid malformation of the kidney. An immunohistochemical study. Cancer 1984; 54: 2305–2308.

856. Shibata R, Okita H, Shimoda M, et al. Primary carcinoid tumor in a polycystic kidney. Pathol Int 2003; 53: 317–322.

857. Resnick ME, Unterberger H, McLoughlin PT. Renal carcinoid producing the carcinoid syndrome. Med Times 1966; 94: 895–896.

858. Hamilton I, Reis L, Bilimoria S, et al. A renal lipoma. Br Med J 1980; 281: 1323–1324.

859. Sahin A, Demirbas M, Ozen H, et al. Primary carcinoid of the kidney. Scand J Urol Nephrol 1996; 30: 325–327.

860. McCaffrey JA, Reuter VV, Herr HW, et al. Carcinoid tumor of the kidney. The use of somatostatin receptor scintigraphy in diagnosis and management. Urol Oncol 2000; 5: 108–111.

861. Raslan WF, Ro JY, Ordonez NG, et al. Primary carcinoid of the kidney. Immunohistochemical and ultrastructural studies of five patients. Cancer 1993; 72: 2660–2666.

862. Goldblum JR, Lloyd RV. Primary renal carcinoid. Case report and literature review. Arch Pathol Lab Med 1993; 117: 855–858.

863. van den Berg E, Gouw AS, Oosterhuis JW, et al. Carcinoid in a horseshoe kidney. Morphology, immunohistochemistry, and cytogenetics. Cancer Genet Cytogenet 1995; 845: 95.

864. el-Naggar AK, Troncoso P, Ordonez NG. Primary renal carcinoid tumor with molecular abnormality characteristic of conventional renal cell neoplasms. Diagn Mol Pathol 1995; 4: 48–53.

865. Capella C, Eusebi V, Rosai J. Primary oat cell carcinoma of the kidney. Am J Surg Pathol 1984; 8: 855–861.

866. Tetu B, Ro JY, Ayala AG, et al. Small cell carcinoma of the kidney. A clinicopathologic, immunohistochemical, and ultrastructural study. Cancer 1987; 60: 1809–1814.

867. Chuang CK, Shen YC, Wu JH, et al. Immunobiologic, cytogenetic and drug response features of a newly established cell line (SCRC-1) from renal small cell carcinoma. J Urol 2000; 163: 1016–1021.

868. Gonzalez-Lois C, Madero S, Redondo P, et al. Small cell carcinoma of the kidney: a case report and review of the literature. Arch Pathol Lab Med 2001; 125: 796–798.

869. Akkaya BK, Mustafa U, Esin O, et al. Primary small cell carcinoma of the kidney. Urol Oncol 2003; 21: 11–13.

870. Masuda T, Oikawa H, Yashima A, et al. Renal small cell carcinoma (neuroendocrine carcinoma) without features of transitional cell carcinoma. Pathol Int 1998; 48: 412–415.

871. Essenfeld H, Manivel JC, Benedetto P, et al. Small cell carcinoma of the renal pelvis: a clinicopathological, morphological and immunohistochemical study of 2 cases. J Urol 1990; 144: 344–347.

872. Guillou L, Duvoisin B, Chobaz C, et al. Combined small-cell and transitional cell carcinoma of the renal pelvis. A light microscopic, immunohistochemical, and ultrastructural study of a case with literature review. Arch Pathol Lab Med 1993; 117: 239–243.

873. Kitamura M, Miyanaga T, Hamada M, et al. Small cell carcinoma of the kidney: case report. Int J Urol 1997; 4: 422–424.

874. Majhail NS, Elson P, Bukowski RM. Therapy and outcome of small cell carcinoma of the kidney: report of two cases and a systematic review of the literature. Cancer 2003; 97: 1436–1441.

875. Mirza IA, Shahab N. Small cell cancer of the pleura, kidney, and thymus. . Semin Oncol 2007; 34: 67–69.

876. Cheng L, Pan CX, Yang XJ, et al. Small cell carcinoma of the urinary bladder: a clinicopathologic analysis of 64 patients. Cancer 2004; 101: 957–962.

877. de Alava E, Pardo J. Ewing tumor: tumor biology and clinical applications. Int J Surg Pathol 2001; 9: 7–17.

878. Roloson GJ, Beckwith JB. Primary neuroepithelial tumors of the kidney in children and adults. A report from the NWTS Pathology Center. Mod Pathol 1993; 6: 67A.

879. Mor Y, Nass D, Raviv G, et al. Malignant peripheral primitive neuroectodermal tumor (PNET) of the kidney. Med Pediatr Oncol 1994; 23: 437–440.

880. Chan YF, Llewellyn H. Intrarenal primitive neuroectodermal tumour. Br J Urol 1994; 73: 326–327.

881. Gupta NP, Singh BP, Raina V, et al. Primitive neuroectodermal kidney tumor: 2 case reports and review of the literature. J Urol 1995; 153: 1890–1892.

882. Furman J, Murphy WM, Jelsma PF, et al. Primary primitive neuroectodermal tumor of the kidney. Case report and review of the literature. Am J Clin Pathol 1996; 106: 339–344.

883. Marley EF, Liapis H, Humphrey PA, et al. Primitive neuroectodermal tumor of the kidney – another enigma. A pathologic, immunohistochemical, and molecular diagnostic study. Am J Surg Pathol 1997; 21: 354–359.

884. Sheaff M, McManus A, Scheimberg I, et al. Primitive neuroectodermal tumor of the kidney confirmed by fluorescence in situ hybridization. Am J Surg Pathol 1997; 21: 461–468.

885. Quezado M, Benjamin DR, Tsokos M. EWS/FLI-1 fusion transcripts in three peripheral primitive neuroectodermal tumors of the kidney. Hum Pathol 1997; 28: 767–771.

886. Rodriguez-Galindo C, Marina NM, Fletcher BD, et al. Is primitive neuroectodermal tumor of the kidney a distinct entity? Cancer 1997; 79: 2243–2250.

887. Kuroda M, Urano M, Abe M, et al. Primary primitive neuroectodermal tumor of the kidney. Pathol Int 2000; 50: 967–972.

888. Casella R, Moch H, Rochlitz C, et al. Metastatic primitive neuroectodermal tumor of the kidney in adults. Eur Urol 2001; 39: 613–617.

889. Parham DM, Roloson GJ, Feely M, et al. Primary malignant neuroepithelial tumors of the kidney: a clinicopathologic analysis of 146 adult and pediatric cases from the National Wilms' Tumor Study Group Pathology Center. Am J Surg Pathol 2001; 25: 133–146.

890. Jimenez RE, Folpe AL, Lapham RL, et al. Primary Ewing's sarcoma/primitive neuroectodermal tumor of the kidney: a clinicopathologic and immunohistochemical analysis of 11 cases. Am J Surg Pathol 2002; 26: 320–327.

891. Erkilic S, Ozsarac C, Kocer NE, et al. Primary primitive neuroectodermal tumor of the kidney: a case report. Int Urol Nephrol 2006; 38: 199–202.

892. Ellinger J, Bastian PJ, Hauser S, et al. Primitive neuroectodermal tumor: rare, highly aggressive differential diagnosis in urologic malignancies. Urology 2006; 68: 257–262.

893. Sellaturay SV, Arya M, Cuckow P, et al. Renal primitive neuroectodermal tumor in childhood with intracardiac extension. Urology 2006; 68: 427; e13–e16.

894. Ellison DA, Parham DM, Bridge J, et al. Immunohistochemistry of primary malignant neuroepithelial tumors of the kidney: a potential source of confusion? A study of 30 cases from the National Wilms' Tumor Study Pathology Center. Hum Pathol 2007; 38: 205–211.

895. Kovar H, Dworzak M, Strehl S, et al. Overexpression of the pseudoautosomal gene MIC2 in Ewing's sarcoma and peripheral primitive neuroectodermal tumor. Oncogene 1990; 5: 1067–1070.

896. Shende A, Wind ES, Lanzkowsky P. Intrarenal neuroblastoma mimicking Wilms' tumor. NY State J Med 1979; 79: 93.

897. Gohji K, Nakanishi T, Hara I, et al. Two cases of primary neuroblastoma of the kidney in adults. J Urol 1987; 137: 966–968.

898. Shamberger RC, Smith EI, Joshi VV, et al. The risk of nephrectomy during local control in abdominal neuroblastoma. J Pediatr Surg 1998; 33: 161–164.

899. Lagace R, Tremblay M. Non-chromaffin paraganglioma of the kidney with distant metastases. Can Med Assoc J 1968; 99: 1095–1098.

900. Preger L, Gardner RE, Kawala BO, et al. Intrarenal pheochromocytoma: preoperative angiographic diagnosis. Urology 1976; 8: 194–196.

901. Simon H, Carlson DH, Hanelin J, et al. Intrarenal pheochromocytoma: report of a case. J Urol 1979; 121: 805–807.

902. Dembitzer F, Greenebaum E. Fine needle aspiration of renal paraganglioma: An unusual location for a rare tumor. Mod Pathol 1993; 6: 29A.

903. Rossi G, Oleari G, Botti C, et al. Cystic paraganglioma of the renal capsule. J Urol 2001; 165: 511–512.

904. Rafique M, Bhutta RA, Muzzafar S. Case report: intra-renal paraganglioma masquerading as a renal cyst. Int Urol Nephrol 2003; 35: 475–478.

905. Bezirdjian DR, Tegtmeyer CJ, Leef JL. Intrarenal pheochromocytoma and renal artery stenosis. Urol Radiol 1981; 3: 121–122.

906. Wagner JR, Honig SC, Siroky MB. Non-Hodgkin's lymphoma can mimic renal adenocarcinoma with inferior vena caval involvement. Urology 1993; 42: 720–723; discussion 723–724.

907. Truong LD, Caraway N, Ngo T, et al. Renal lymphoma. The diagnostic and therapeutic roles of fine-needle aspiration. Am J Clin Pathol 2001; 115: 18–31.

908. Wirnsberger GH, Ratschek M, Dimai HP, et al. Post-transplantation lymphoproliferative disorder of the T-cell/B-cell type: an unusual manifestation in a renal allograft. Oncol Rep 1999; 6: 29–32.

909. Cheung AN, Chan AC, Chung LP, et al. Post-transplantation lymphoproliferative disorder of donor origin in a sex-mismatched renal allograft as proven by chromosome in situ hybridization. Mod Pathol 1998; 11: 99–102.

910. Meduri G, Fromentin L, Vieillefond A, et al. Donor-related non-Hodgkin's lymphoma in a renal allograft recipient. Transplant Proc 1991; 23: 2649.

911. Gassel AM, Westphal E, Hansmann ML, et al. Malignant lymphoma of donor origin after renal transplantation: a case report. Hum Pathol 1991; 22: 1291–1293.

912. Tsang K, Kneafsey P, Gill MJ. Primary lymphoma of the kidney in the acquired immunodeficiency syndrome. Arch Pathol Lab Med 1993; 117: 541–543.

913. Salem Y, Pagliaro LC, Manyak MJ. Primary small noncleaved cell lymphoma of kidney. Urology 1993; 42: 331–335.

914. Ferry JA, Harris NL, Papanicolaou N, et al. Lymphoma of the kidney. A report of 11 cases. Am J Surg Pathol 1995; 19: 134–144.

915. Da'as N, Polliack A, Cohen Y, et al. Kidney involvement and renal manifestations in non-Hodgkin's lymphoma and lymphocytic leukemia: a retrospective study in 700 patients. Eur J Haematol 2001; 67: 158–164.

916. Dimopoulos MA, Moulopoulos LA, Costantinides C, et al. Primary renal lymphoma: a clinical and radiological study. J Urol 1996; 155: 1865–1867.

917. Osborne BM, Brenner M, Weitzner S, et al. Malignant lymphoma presenting as a renal mass: four cases. Am J Surg Pathol 1987; 11: 375–382.

918. Kandel LB, McCullough DL, Harrison LH, et al. Primary renal lymphoma. Does it exist? Cancer 1987; 60: 386–391.

919. Uno H, Shima T, Maeda K, et al. Hypercalcemia associated with parathyroid hormone-related protein produced by B-cell type primary malignant lymphoma of the kidney. Ann Hematol 1998; 76: 221–224.

920. Porcaro AB, D'Amico A, Novella G, et al. Primary lymphoma of the kidney. Report of a case and update of the literature. Arch Ital Urol Androl 2002; 74: 44–47.

921. Koolen MI, Schipper P, von Liebergen FJ, et al. Non-Hodgkin lymphoma with unique localization in the kidneys presenting with acute renal failure. Clin Nephrol 1988; 29: 41–46.

922. Dobkin SF, Brem AS, Caldamone AA. Primary renal lymphoma. J Urol 1991; 146: 1588–1590.

923. Sheil O, Redman CW, Pugh C. Renal failure in pregnancy due to primary renal lymphoma. Case report. Br J Obstet Gynaecol 1991; 98: 216–217.

924. van Gelder T, Michiels JJ, Mulder AH, et al. Renal insufficiency due to bilateral primary renal lymphoma. Nephron 1992; 60: 108–110.

925. Brouland JP, Meeus F, Rossert J, et al. Primary bilateral B-cell renal lymphoma: a case report and review of the literature. Am J Kidney Dis 1994; 24: 586–589.

926. Sieniawska M, Bialasik D, Jedrzejowski A, et al. Bilateral primary renal Burkitt lymphoma in a child presenting with acute renal failure. Nephrol Dial Transplant 1997; 12: 1490–1492.

927. Neuhauser TS, Lancaster K, Haws R, et al. Rapidly progressive T cell lymphoma presenting as acute renal failure: case report and review of the literature. Pediatr Pathol Lab Med 1997; 17: 449–460.

928. Chin KC, Perry GJ, Dowling JP, et al. Primary T-cell-rich B-cell lymphoma in the kidney presenting with acute renal failure and a second malignancy. Pathology 1999; 31: 325–327.

929. Abdel Hamid AM, Rogers PB, Sibtain A, et al. Bilateral renal cancer in

children: a difficult, challenging and changing management problem. Clin Oncol 1999; 11: 200–204.

930. Stallone G, Infante B, Manno C, et al. Primary renal lymphoma does exist: case report and review of the literature. J Nephrol 2000; 13: 367–372.

931. Urban BA, Fishman EK. Renal lymphoma: CT patterns with emphasis on helical CT. Radiographics 2000; 20: 197–212.

932. Wick MR, Mills SE, Scheithauer BW, et al. Reassessment of malignant 'angioendotheliomatosis.' Evidence in favor of its reclassification as 'intravascular lymphomatosis.' Am J Surg Pathol 1986; 10: 112–123.

933. Ferry JA, Harris NL, Picker LJ, et al. Intravascular lymphomatosis (malignant angioendotheliomatosis). A B-cell neoplasm expressing surface homing receptors. Mod Pathol 1988; 1: 444–452.

934. Fernandez-Acenero MJ, Galindo M, Bengoechea O, et al. Primary malignant lymphoma of the kidney: case report and literature review. Gen Diagn Pathol 1998; 143: 317–320.

935. Chan YF. Granulocytic sarcoma (chloroma) of the kidney and prostate. Br J Urol 1990; 65: 655–656.

936. Klein B, Falkson G, Simson IW, et al. Granulocytic sarcoma of the kidney in a patient with acute myelomonocytic leukaemia. A case report. S Afr Med J 1986; 70: 696–698.

937. Park HJ, Jeong DH, Song HG, et al. Myeloid sarcoma of both kidneys, the brain, and multiple bones in a nonleukemic child. Yonsei Med J 2003; 44: 740–743.

938. Bagg MD, Wettlaufer JN, Willadsen DS, et al. Granulocytic sarcoma presenting as a diffuse renal mass before hematological manifestations of acute myelogenous leukemia. J Urol 1994; 152: 2092–2093.

939. Catalona WJ, Biles JD 3rd. Therapeutic considerations in renal plasmacytoma. J Urol 1974; 111: 582–583.

940. Morris SA, Vaughan ED Jr, Makoui C. Renal plasmacytoma. Urology 1977; 9: 303–306.

941. Siemers PT, Coel MN. Solitary renal plasmacytoma with palisading tumor vascularity. Radiology 1977; 123: 597–598.

942. Kandel LB, Harrison LH, Woodruff RD, et al. Renal plasmacytoma: a case report and summary of reported cases. J Urol 1984; 132: 1167–1169.

943. Igel TC, Engen DE, Banks PM, et al. Renal plasmacytoma: Mayo Clinic experience and review of the literature. Urology 1991; 37: 385–389.

944. Fan F, Deauna-Limayo D, Brantley Thrasher J, et al. Anaplastic plasmacytoma of the kidney. Histopathology 2005; 47: 432–433.

945. Dehner LP. Intrarenal teratoma occurring in infancy: report of a case with discussion of extragonadal germ cell tumors in infancy. J Pediatr Surg 1973; 8: 369–378.

946. Aubert J, Casamayou J, Denis P, et al. Intrarenal teratoma in a newborn child. Eur Urol 1978; 4: 306–308.

947. Aaronson IA, Sinclair-Smith C. Multiple cystic teratomas of the kidney. Arch Pathol Lab Med 1980; 104: 614.

948. Otani M, Tsujimoto S, Miura M, et al. Intrarenal mature cystic teratoma associated with renal dysplasia: case report and literature review. Pathol Int 2001; 51: 560–564.

949. Mochizuki K, Ohno Y, Tokai Y, et al. Congenital intrarenal teratoma arising from a horseshoe kidney. J Pediatr Surg 2006; 41: 1313–1315.

950. Govender D, Nteene LM, Chetty R, et al. Mature renal teratoma and a synchronous malignant neuroepithelial tumour of the ipsilateral adrenal gland. J Clin Pathol 2001; 54: 253–254.

951. Yoo J, Park S, Lee HJ, et al. Primary carcinoid tumor arising in a mature teratoma of the kidney. A case report and review of the literature. Arch Pathol Lab Med 2002; 126: 979–981.

952. Kojiro M, Ohishi H, Isobe H. Carcinoid tumor occurring in cystic teratoma of the kidney: a case report. Cancer 1976; 38: 1636–1640.

953. Liu YC, Wang JS, Chen CJ, et al. Intrarenal mixed germ cell tumor. J Urol 2000; 164: 2020–2021.

954. Jarrett DD, Pratt-Thomas HR. Metastatic choriocarcinoma appearing as a unilateral renal mass. Arch Pathol Lab Med 1984; 108: 356–357.

955. Ikeda I, Miura T, Kondo I, et al. Metastatic choriocarcinoma of the kidney discovered by refractory hematuria. Hinyokika Kiyo 1996; 42: 447–449.

956. Huang CH, Chen L, Hsieh HH. Choriocarcinoma presenting as a unilateral renal mass and gross hematuria in a male: report of a case. J Formos Med Assoc 1992; 91: 922–925.

957. Vahlensieck W Jr, Riede U, Wimmer B, et al. Beta-human chorionic gonadotropin-positive extragonadal germ cell neoplasia of the renal pelvis. Cancer 1991; 67: 3146–3149.

958. Wagle DG, Moore RH, Murphy GP. Secondary carcinomas of the kidney. J Urol 1975; 114: 30–32.

959. Bracken RB, Chica G, Johnson DE, et al. Secondary renal neoplasms: an autopsy study. South Med J 1979; 72: 806–807.

960. Payne RA. Metastatic renal tumours. Br J Surg 1960; 48: 310–315.

961. Peterson RO. Metastatic neoplasms. In: Urologic pathology. Philadelphia: JB Lippincott, 1986; 134–136.

962. Choyke PL, White EM, Zeman RK, et al. Renal metastases: clinicopathologic and radiologic correlation. Radiology 1987; 162: 359–363.

963. Belghiti D, Hirbec G, Bernaudin JF, et al. Intraglomerular metastases. Report of two cases. Cancer 1984; 54: 2309–2312.

964. Naryshkin S, Tomaszewski JE. Acute renal failure secondary to carcinomatous lymphatic metastases to kidneys. J Urol 1991; 146: 1610–1612.

965. Sella A, Ro JY. Renal cell cancer: best recipient of tumor-to-tumor metastasis. Urology 1987; 30: 35–38.

# CHAPTER 3

# Renal pelvis and ureter

Stephen M. Bonsib, Liang Cheng

The renal pelvis and ureter are muscular conduits lined by urothelium that function to propel urine from the renal calyceal system to the urinary bladder. They are both affected by developmental, reactive, and neoplastic disorders. The developmental disorders are a group of closely related entities that include abnormalities in ureteral number and location, and of the structure and function of pelvic and ureteral muscularis propria. The mucosa is the site of the major reactive and neoplastic disorders.

## Development

The ureter and renal pelvis develop from the ampullary bud, which arises from the distal mesonephric duct during the fourth week of development.[1] Contact of the ampullary bud with metanephric blastema induces nephrogenesis. During the months that follow, the ampullary bud elongates and branches dichotomously in parallel with the development of the nephrons to create the adult metanephric kidney with its renal pelvis and ureter.[1] As the ureter elongates, there is a period of luminal obliteration followed in the fifth week by recanalization. Recanalization begins in the middle of the ureter and extends proximally and distally with the ureteropelvic and ureterovesical junctions the last segments to recanalize.[2]

The mesonephric duct distal to the ampullary bud (the common nephric duct) is incorporated into the developing urogenital sinus, and the ureteral orifice migrates to the trigone of the urinary bladder.[1] The common nephric duct forms the trigone and contributes to the prostatic urethra in the male. Concomitant development of the male and female reproductive tracts from the mesonephric (wolffian) and müllerian ducts respectively, and division of the cloaca into bladder and hindgut, occur nearby as the ureter and kidney develop. Thus multiple malformations in these areas often occur together.

## Anatomy

The lumen of the renal pelvis and ureter is lined by urothelium (also called transitional epithelium), which rests on a basement membrane over a lamina propria composed of highly vascular loose connective tissue (Fig. 3-1A). The urothelium is composed of three to five layers of cells in the pelvis and four to seven layers of cells in the ureter (Fig. 3-1B).[3] The pelvis and ureter have a continuous muscular wall that originates in the fornices of the minor calyces as small interlacing fascicles of smooth muscle cells.[4–7] These take on a spiral architecture in the pelvis and ureter, a structure necessary for effective peristalsis.[4,6] The muscularis propria is not divided into distinct layers. Near the bladder the ureter acquires an external sheath from the detrusor muscle, and the muscle fascicles become oriented longitudinally.[5,8] The longitudinal fibers continue through the wall of the bladder and into the submucosa, where they spread about the ureteral orifice to contribute to the trigone muscle. Ultimately they terminate near the bladder neck in the female and at the verumontanum in the male.

Peristalsis is initiated by 'pacemaker' cells in the renal pelvic muscle near the calyces. These generate electrical impulses that propagate from cell to cell through gap junctions.[9,10] Effective peristalsis requires both continuity of gap junctions and an appropriate quantity and organization of muscle fascicles.[3] As will be discussed later in this chapter, disruption of this pattern, even focally, may cause ureteral incompetence or functional obstruction.

## Congenital malformations

Genitourinary tract malformations occur in 10% of the population and are the most common group of congenital anomalies.[11] Some, such as bifid ureter, are clinically insig-

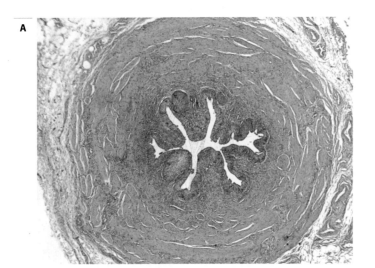
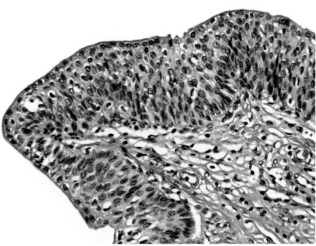

**Fig. 3-1** Adult ureter. **(A)** Cross-section showing adventitia, muscularis propria, and irregular contour of relaxed mucosa. **(B)** The mucosa consists of a few layers of urothelial cells overlying loose connective tissue. No muscularis mucosae is visible.

**Table 3-1** Common associations between ureteral anomalies

|  | Bifid/duplex | Ectopia | Reflux | Obstruction of ureteropelvic junction | Ureterocele | Dysplasia |
|---|---|---|---|---|---|---|
| Bifid/duplex |  | + | + | + | + | + |
| Ectopia | + |  | + | + | + | + |
| Reflux | + | + |  | + | + | + |
| Obstruction of ureteropelvic junction | + | + | + |  | + | + |
| Ureterocele | + | + | + | + |  | + |
| Diverticulum | – | + | + | – | – | + |
| Primary megaureter | – | – | – | – | – | + |

**Table 3-2** Ureteral muscle findings in ureteral anomalies

|  | Muscle normal | Muscle deficient | Muscle dysplastic | Longitudinal fiber predominance | Circular fiber predominance | Sheath thick |
|---|---|---|---|---|---|---|
| Refluxing megaureter | + | + | + | – | – | – |
| Obstruction of ureteropelvic junction | + | + | + | + | – | – |
| Primary megaureter | – | – | + | – | + | + |
| Ureterocele | + | + | + | – | – | – |
| Paraureteral diverticulum | + | + | + | – | – | – |

nificant.[12] Others are associated with ureteral incompetence or obstruction, carrying the risk of renal damage, or are associated with renal dysplasia.[1] Some are components of multiple malformation syndromes (e.g., VATER association or prune belly syndrome), are associated with chromosomal abnormalities (e.g., trisomy syndromes), or have a familial association.[13–20] The various congenital malformations of the ureters frequently occur together (Table 3-1).

Patients with ureteropelvic anomalies usually present with symptoms of ureteral or pelvic distention, such as flank pain or mass, or with complications such as infection, calculi, or renal insufficiency.[1,20] Ultrasound imaging permits the demonstration of ureteropelvic malformations both in utero and in neonates. Most such lesions encountered in surgical pathology consist of intrinsic structural defects of the muscularis, usually involving the ends of the ureters, the last segments to recanalize during embryogenesis. These malformations are congenital and developmental in origin, but patients may present at any age, from newborn to adulthood. Surgical therapy usually consists of excision of the abnormal segment to preserve renal function. The surgical pathologist should define the anatomic basis of the functional deficit, which usually consists of a distinct but localized defect in the quantity or organization of smooth muscle (Table 3-2). Recognition of these lesions requires an appreciation of the normal muscle pattern, and their histologic demonstration requires well-oriented sections in which the pattern of the muscle fascicles is highlighted by a trichrome stain. For most lesions longitudinal orientation of the specimen best shows the deviation from the normal muscle pattern. Primary megaureter (see below) is an exception in which cross-sections display the predominance of circular fibers and thickening of the periureteral sheath.

# Abnormalities in number or location of ureters

Ureteral agenesis, ureteral duplication, and ureteral ectopia are a group of related malformations resulting from defective formation of the ampullary bud.[1] Isolated failure of ampullary bud formation causes ureteral agenesis with absence of the ipsilateral hemitrigone and kidney[1] (see Fig. 1-28). Another cause of agenesis of the ureter and kidney is wolffian duct failure. Wolffian duct failure can be recognized because of its associated genital tract malformations (e.g., absent testis or unicornuate uterus).[1,11] Unilateral agenesis of the kidney and ureter is associated with additional urologic malformations in 20–40% of patients.[21] Bilateral renal agenesis (Potter's syndrome) (see Fig. 1-34) is lethal because of its associated pulmonary hypoplasia.

Bifid ureter and duplex ureter, the most common (0.8% of all autopsies) ureteral anomalies, result from premature branching of the ampullary bud or the development of two separate ampullary buds.[1,22] Premature branching results in two separate renal pelves and proximal ureters that join to form a single ureter at some point above the bladder[12] (Fig. 3-2). Duplex ureters (Fig. 3-3) have two separate ureteral orifices in the bladder.[22,23] The ureter from the lower pole usually has its orifice normally situated on the trigone or displaced laterally. The orifice of the ureter from the upper pole can be normally placed, but displacement toward the bladder neck or to an extravesical location is more typical.[23] Ureteral ectopia results from an abnormally high or low origin of the ampullary bud from the mesonephric duct. Eighty percent of ureteral orifice ectopia is associated with the ureter from the upper pole of a duplicated system.[22,23] The ectopic ureteral orifice may be intravesical (lateral or caudal to the normal site), or extravesical in the urethra,

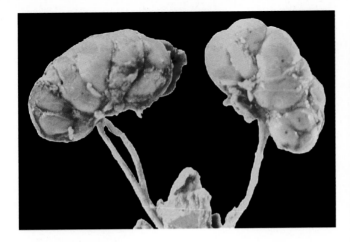

**Fig. 3-2** Bifid ureter joining to form a single ureter above the bladder.

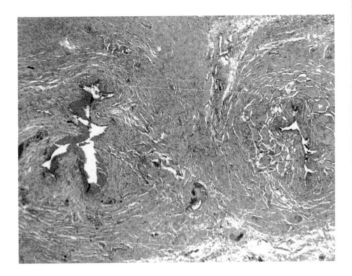

**Fig. 3-3** Duplex ureter near point of confluence.

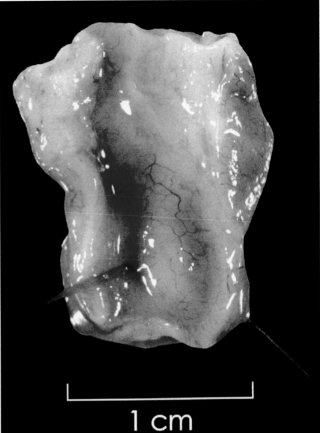

**Fig. 3-4** Longitudinal section showing mucosal aspect of distal ureter in reflux. Note the thin wall.

vestibule, or genitalia. Symptoms are influenced by the patient's gender and the site of the ureteral orifice, and may consist of urethral dribbling, vaginal 'discharge,' epididymo-orchitis, or pyelonephritis if reflux or obstruction are present.[11] The greater the degree of ectopia in a lateral or extravesical location, the more likely it is that the corresponding renal unit will be dysplastic.[23] The surgical pathology specimen thus may include a segmental or complete nephrectomy for dysplasia or pyelonephritis, or a distal ureter excised for reflux, obstruction, or ureterocele.

## Refluxing megaureter

Reflux from the bladder into the ureter is the most common ureteral problem requiring surgical intervention. Patients usually present in early childhood with urinary tract infections and often already have renal scars (reflux nephropathy).[24,25] Reflux may be unilateral or bilateral, and in about one-third of cases the patients' siblings have similar urologic abnormalities.[19] Vesicoureteral reflux is caused by incompetence of the ureterovesical junction. There is a 5 : 1 preponderance of females over males, possibly resulting from the additional mechanical support provided to the bladder by the prostate and seminal vesicles.

The affected ureters have abnormally short submucosal segments or deficiency of longitudinal fibers in the intramural segment, or both.[1,20,25] Abnormally short submucosal segments are apparent to the urologist but difficult to demonstrate histologically. Deficiency of longitudinal fibers can be demonstrated in longitudinal sections of the intramural segment and may appear to the urologist as an abnormally thin and translucent segment of distal ureter (Fig. 3-4). Excision of the defective distal ureteral segment and reimplantation of the ureter is usually effective.[24]

## Ureteropelvic junction obstruction

Ureteropelvic junction obstruction is the most common cause of ureteral obstruction and may present at any age. In childhood it is frequently bilateral (16%), associated with other urologic malformations (15–20%), and predominantly on the left side and in boys.[16,26] In adulthood, ureteropelvic junction obstruction is most often unilateral and in women.[26] The two most common causes are defects in the muscularis (75%), and renal non-rotation associated with polar vessels (6–24%).[27–29]

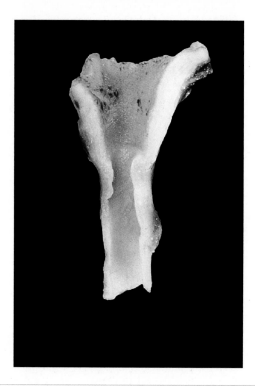

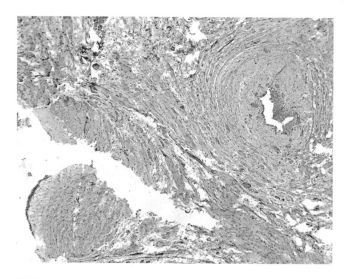

**Fig. 3-6** Ureteropelvic junction obstruction.

**Fig. 3-5** Funnel-shaped zone of ureteropelvic junction obstruction.

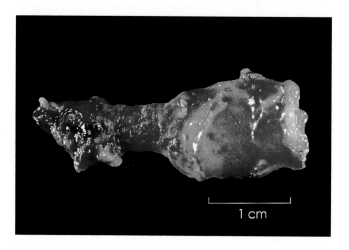

**Fig. 3-7** Primary megaureter with abrupt dilation at superior end.

The obstructed ureteropelvic junction is characteristically funnel shaped (Fig. 3-5). It may have a grossly visible area of thin muscle, a valve-like intraluminal protrusion of edematous mucosa or muscularis, or may be stenotic. The histologic appearance of ureteropelvic junction obstruction is varied. There may be segmental smooth muscle attenuation, often with a preponderance of longitudinal fibers, diffuse lack of fascicular organization of pelvic muscles (i.e., dysplastic; see Ureteral dysplasia, later in this chapter), segmental absence of smooth muscle, or a stenotic lumen with normal muscle (Fig. 3-6).[27,28] 'Valves' or 'pleats' have also been described, which probably result from herniation at a site of muscle abnormality.[29]

Renal polar blood vessels are common anatomic variants of the renal vasculature that usually do not obstruct the ureter because of its medial origin at the renal hilum.[30] In congenitally non-rotated kidneys the pelvis is anterior and polar vessels may cause significant ureteral obstruction[30] (see Fig. 1-22).

## Primary megaureter

Primary megaureter is a non-refluxing, non-obstructive form of ureteral dilation.[20] Its gross appearance is distinctive (Fig. 3-7). The ureters are narrow and straight immediately above the bladder, and above that segment they are fusiform and markedly dilated. This fusiform dilation differs from the tortuous appearance of ureteral dilation secondary to reflux or obstruction. In 80% of these patients there is functional obstruction at the level of the narrow segment, and this must be excised.[31,32] Seen in cross-section, the narrow segment shows either a preponderance of circular fibers, hypoplasia

and fibrosis of the smooth muscle, or thickening of the periureteral sheath (Fig. 3-8).[20] The only abnormality of the dilated segment is hypertrophy of the smooth muscle. In the other 20% of cases of primary megaureter, the narrow segment of ureter has normal muscle and the dilated ureter above it has an almost complete absence of muscle.[32] Such ureters have been called dysplastic ureters (see Ureteral dysplasia, later in this chapter) and are commonly associated with a dysplastic kidney.[33,34]

## Ureterocele

Ureterocele is congenital dilation of the distal ureter within the bladder (Fig. 3-9). Ureterocele balloons into the bladder and occasionally protrudes into the urethra.[35–37] Most ureteroceles occur in the upper pole ureter of a duplicated system. In this situation the ureter usually passes dorsal to the lower pole ureter.[35] Its dilated portion may undermine and distort the trigone, often resulting in obstruction or

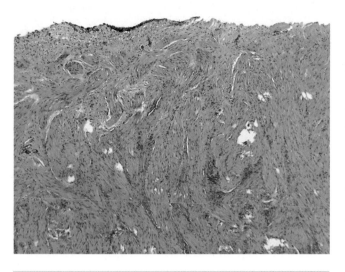

**Fig. 3-8** Primary megaureter segment showing smooth muscle hyperplasia.

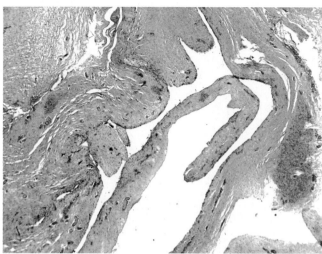

**Fig. 3-10** Ureterocele showing thinning or lacking of muscle in its wall.

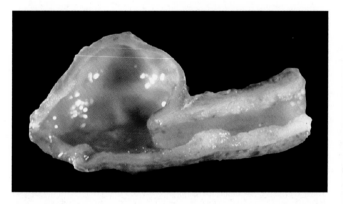

**Fig. 3-9** Ureterocele of upper pole ureter. Orifice was near bladder neck.

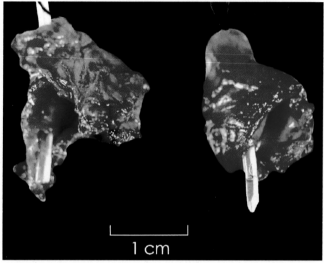

1 cm

**Fig. 3-11** Bilateral paraureteral diverticula. Probes indicate ureteral orifices at the mouth of each diverticulum.

reflux of the normally situated lower pole ureter, or, if the ureterocele is large, the contralateral ureter as well.[35] Uretero-cele rarely affects a single ureter.

Microscopically, the muscle of the wall of the ureterocele varies from hypertrophic to atrophic or absent[36] (Fig. 3-10). Consistent with the usual ectopic location of the ureteral orifice associated with duplex kidneys, 70% of cases have segmental dysplasia of the upper pole of the kidney.[37]

## Paraureteral diverticulum

Herniation of the urinary bladder involving the distal ureter is called paraureteral diverticulum. It is usually congenital and detected in childhood, but may result from urethral or bladder neck obstruction at any age.[38,39] Vesicoureteral reflux is commonly associated with paraureteral diverticulum. The location of the ureteral orifice within the diverticulum cor-relates with the risk of renal dysplasia[38] (Fig. 3-11). When the ureter opens into the dome of the diverticulum (a form of lateral ectopia) rather than near its orifice, the likelihood of renal dysplasia is great. There are few histologic studies of diverticula, but deficient ureteral muscle and sheath devel-opment have been reported.[38]

## Ureteral dysplasia

Ureteral dysplasia refers to ureters composed of infrequent small muscle cells lacking organization and failing to form fascicles.[27] Takunaka[32] showed that these small muscle cells possess thin actin filaments but lack the thick myosin filaments essential for normal muscle contractility. An alternative term, ureteral maldevelopment, was introduced by Hanna in 1979 for this condition. Recognition of dys-plastic ureters is important because of their association with ipsilateral renal dysplasia in 56–70% of cases.[27,28]

Dysplastic ureters are variable in appearance, some appearing atretic (see Fig. 1-40A) whereas others are dilated (Fig. 3-12) as well as anomalous in location. Recognition of their dysplastic nature is not possible with the naked eye, because ureters with normal muscle fascicle formation can have a similar appearance.

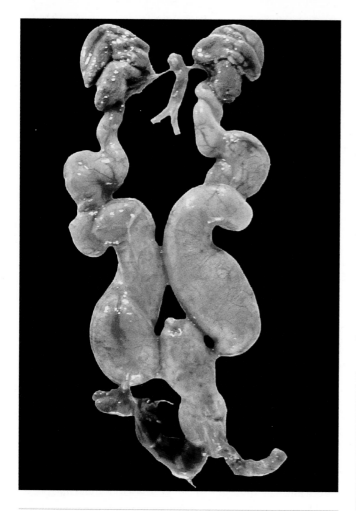

Fig. 3-12 Dysplastic megaureter associated with bilateral renal dysplasia.

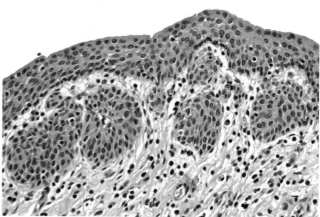

Fig. 3-13 von Brunn's nests of the ureter.

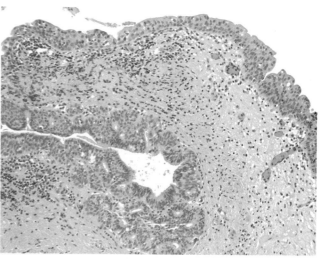

Fig. 3-14 Ureteritis glandularis.

# Non-neoplastic proliferative, metaplastic, and inflammatory lesions

## Hyperplasia, von Brunn's nests, ureteropyelitis cystica et glandularis

The most common non-neoplastic urothelial proliferative lesions are simple hyperplasia, von Brunn's nests, and ureteropyelitis cystica et glandularis.[40,41] Simple hyperplasia is an increase in the number of layers of urothelial cells without cytologic atypia. It commonly accompanies inflammation and neoplasia. Von Brunn's nests are small nests of normal urothelial cells within the lamina propria (Fig. 3-13). They are most common in the trigone of the bladder, but are also found in 10% of normal ureters at autopsy.[41] When von Brunn's nests have central lumina lined by urothelium or columnar cells they are referred to as ureteritis or pyelitis cystica and ureteritis or pyelitis glandularis (Fig. 3-14), respectively. These changes are common in patients with stone disease.[42] Although usually microscopic in size, ureteritis and pyelitis cystica may rarely produce grossly visible fluid-filled cysts that elevate the urothelium[41,43,44] (Fig. 3-15).

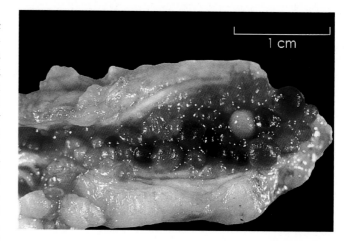

Fig. 3-15 Ureteritis cystica with cobblestone appearance of vesicles protruding into the ureteral lumen.

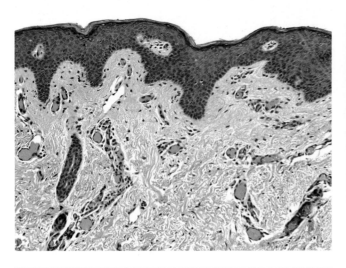

**Fig. 3-16** Keratinizing squamous metaplasia of the ureter.

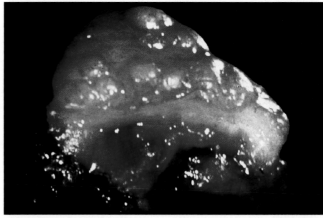

**Fig. 3-17** Malakoplakia of the ureter with yellow mucosal plaques. (Courtesy of Robert H. Young, MD.)

Von Brunn's nests and ureteropyelitis cystica are generally regarded as normal features of the urothelial mucosa. However, they may also be reactive lesions and have arisen following experimental mucosal injury.[45] In that situation they develop within 24–48 hours and persist for months following removal of the inflammatory stimulus.

## Squamous and glandular metaplasia

Squamous metaplasia is the most common form of urothelial metaplasia.[41,43,46–48] It may be non-keratinizing or show keratinization (Fig. 3-16) with or without atypia. When squamous metaplasia is encountered in the renal pelvis and ureter, it is often keratinizing. The keratin may be so copious that squames are seen in the urine or collect in the pelvis, forming a mass.[46] This sequence has prompted the use of terms such as leukoplakia and cholesteatoma when either keratinization or keratin accumulation, respectively, is marked.[46] Keratinizing squamous metaplasia is usually the result of chronic irritation. Conditions such as chronic infection, indwelling catheters, and calculi are present in 60–70% of patients.[44] Keratinizing squamous metaplasia of the urothelial mucosa is associated with an increased risk of squamous cell and urothelial carcinoma.[49,50]

Mucinous (glandular, enteric, intestinal, colonic) metaplasia indicates the presence of colonic-type mucinous epithelium, often containing enterochromaffin cells, in place of urothelium.[45,51–54] In the bladder these alterations may range from numerous minute foci to involvement of the entire mucosa, usually observed in bladder exstrophy.[52] Intestinal metaplasia of the renal pelvis and ureter is rare, and most cases have been associated with adenocarcinoma.[45,53]

## Nephrogenic adenoma

Nephrogenic adenoma is rare in the ureter[55–58] and much more common in the urinary bladder, often appearing as an exophytic lesion which cystoscopically may mimic urothelial carcinoma. Microscopically, it is a benign papillary and tubular proliferation lined by cuboidal or hobnail epithelium.[59,60] Nephrogenic adenoma is discussed in detail in Chapter 4.

## Reactive atypia

Reactive atypia may affect the urothelium and mimic urothelial carcinoma in situ. Thiotepa and mitomycin-C, intravesical chemotherapeutic agents used to treat non-invasive urothelial cancer, are most often implicated.[61,62] However, similar alterations can be produced by irradiation and catheterization. The resultant striking cytologic atypia characteristically affects superficial cells, which, although enlarged, have low nuclear cytoplasmic ratios, nuclear or cytoplasmic vacuoles, and smudged chromatin.[61,62] The mixture of normal urothelial cells with occasional large atypical cells is distinctive. Reactive atypia is characteristically encountered in the bladder, but may also be encountered in the ureteral mucosa in patients with vesicoureteral reflux.[62]

## Malakoplakia

Malakoplakia is an uncommon chronic granulomatous disease originally described by Michaelis and Gutmann[63] in 1902 and elaborated upon by von Hansemann[64] in 1903. Malakoplakia is most frequently observed in the urinary tract of middle-aged women as a complication of recurrent infections.[65–68] Bladder involvement is four to 10 times more common than involvement of the renal pelvis and ureter.[69–71]

The typical lesion of malakoplakia is a yellow-brown soft ('malakos') plaque ('plakos') (Fig. 3-17) that often has a central umbilication. Microscopically, masses of large eosinophilic histiocytes (von Hansemann histiocytes) are present, many of which contain basophilic inclusions (Michaelis–Gutmann bodies). Periodic acid–Schiff (PAS) staining and special stains for calcium and iron enhance the targetoid appearance of these cytoplasmic inclusions and indicate their mineralized nature. Malakoplakia is discussed in detail in Chapter 4.

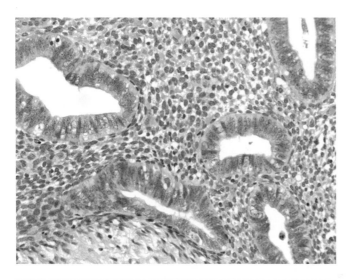

**Fig. 3-18** Endometriosis of the ureter.

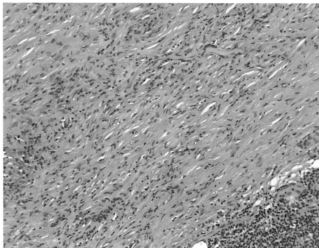

**Fig. 3-19** Retroperitoneal fibrosis.

## Endometriosis

Endometriosis is defined by the presence of endometrial tissue outside the confines of the uterine cavity. It affects approximately 10–20% of premenopausal women,[72] but only 1–2% of cases involve the urinary tract. Ureter endometriosis is even rarer.[73–76] Antonelli[77] reported the largest series of ureteral endometriosis (19 cases), of which four (21%) had coexisting bladder endometriosis. The presenting symptoms include flank pain, gross hematuria, dysuria, uremia, and pelvic mass.[72] Approximately 50% of cases are asymptomatic. The lesion is similar to those appearing in other organ sites, and consists of benign endometriotic glands and stroma (Fig. 3-18). It may also present as a polypoid lesion.[78] Malignant transformation of ureteral endometriosis is rare.[79–81]

## Retroperitoneal fibrosis

Retroperitoneal fibrosis is a proliferative process of inflammation and fibrosis of middle and old age.[82–87] Retroperitoneal structures may be encased, with the ureters frequently exhibiting medial deviation on intravenous pyelography. Retroperitoneal fibrosis may be primary and idiopathic, although a variety of secondary causes have been identified, including iatrogenic (drugs, surgery, irradiation), inflammatory (vasculitis, aneurysms, diverticulitis, inflammatory bowel disease), and neoplastic (sclerosing lymphoma and urothelial carcinoma) disorders.[82–87] Regardless of the etiology, the typical histology is a prominent mixed inflammatory cell infiltrate with fibroplasia and edema (Fig. 3-19). The major challenge is to identify those secondary causes that may merit different therapy.

## Neoplasms

Neoplasms of the ureter and pelvis represent 20–25% of upper tract tumors in adults, and renal cell carcinomas comprise most of the remainder.[88–92] Ureteral and pelvic neoplasms occur with approximately equal frequency, but collectively are only 1/10th as common as their bladder counterparts.[93,94] Ninety-five percent are epithelial and 80% are malignant, with urothelial carcinoma accounting for 90% of these.[88] In a recent series from the University of Texas MD Anderson Cancer Center, primary non-urothelial carcinomas represented 1.9% of all patients with upper urinary tract tumors.[95]

## Benign epithelial neoplasms

### Inverted papilloma

Inverted papilloma is a benign urothelial tumor that occurs less commonly in the renal pelvis and ureter than in the urinary bladder.[96–98] It is almost twice as common in the ureter as in the renal pelvis.[99] Men predominate, and the mean age of presentation is about 65 years.[99] In the upper tract it is found incidentally by intravenous pyelography,[96] or may cause hematuria.[100,101] Inverted papilloma may be multiple and associated with urothelial carcinoma at other sites.[102] Grossly, it may form a mass, mimicking carcinoma (Fig. 3-20). The tumor consists of trabeculae of histologically typical urothelium, which often forms small glandular structures lined by metaplastic mucinous epithelium.[103] The histologic features of these tumors are discussed in more detail in Chapter 5. Rarely, urothelial carcinoma may arise within an inverted papilloma of the ureter.[104,105]

### Urothelial papilloma

Urothelial papilloma is rare. It is usually a small (several millimeters or less), delicate papillary structure most often found incidentally and only rarely biopsied. The latter has been attributed to the tendency for urologists to fulgurate this small, clinically innocent-appearing lesion. Microscopically, papilloma consists of thin delicate fibrovascular fronds invested by epithelium of normal thickness that lacks atypia. By definition, there is no extension into the lamina propria.

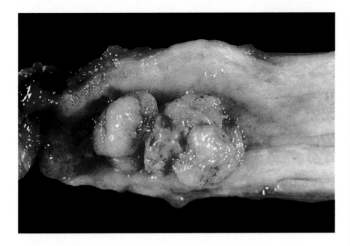

**Fig. 3-20** Inverted papilloma of the ureter.

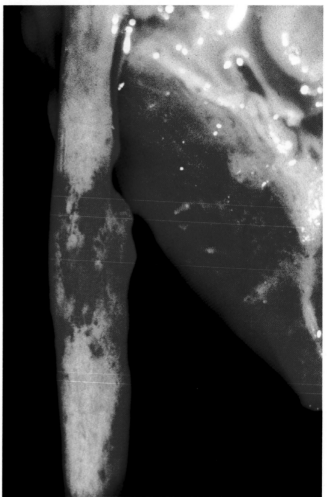

**Fig. 3-21** Red patches of urothelial carcinoma in situ of the ureter. (Courtesy of Robert H. Young, MD.)

## Malignant neoplasms

### Urothelial dysplasia and carcinoma in situ

In keeping with the concept of the urothelium of the renal pelvis, ureter, and bladder as a single anatomic unit affected by similar neoplastic influences, the same relationships between dysplasia and cancer shown for bladder cancer have also been established in the upper tract. The mucosa adjacent to invasive pelvic and ureteral tumors is abnormal (dysplasia or carcinoma in situ) in 95% of specimens. The severity of the mucosal dysplasia correlates with the grade of the adjacent carcinoma and identifies patients at risk for metachronous tumors of other sites.[106-109] Furthermore, ureteral or pelvic muscle invasion occurs in 86–90% of cases of flat urothelial carcinoma but only 30–36% of cases of papillary urothelial carcinoma.[107,108] Grossly, the mucosa appears erythematous (Fig. 3-21) or normal. The histologic criteria are identical to those described in Chapter 5 (Fig. 3-22). An excellent prognosis has been documented for patients with carcinoma in situ of the upper urinary tract who were treated with radical nephroureterectomy[110] or BCG.[111-113]

### Urothelial carcinoma

Urothelial carcinoma of the upper tract is epidemiologically similar to that of the bladder.[89-92] The right and left sides are affected about equally, and approximately 2–4% of cases are bilateral. Tumors of the renal pelvis and calyces are approximately twice as common as tumors of the ureters.[114] There is a male preponderance[114,115] and it is most common in older individuals. Hematuria is the principal symptom, but flank pain also is frequent.[89,109] Cigarette smoking,[116,117] industrial carcinogens[118] and chronic irritation (stones and infection)[119] are risk factors. Phenacetin abuse[120-122] is the most important etiologic factor in some populations, accounting for nearly one-quarter of renal pelvic tumors and more than 10% of ureteral tumors. Balkan nephropathy and exposure to thorium-containing radiologic contrast material[123,124] are risk factors for upper tract carcinoma, but not for urinary bladder tumors. Genetic factors play a role in the carcinogenesis of upper urinary tract urothelial carcinoma.

The risk is significantly increased in patients with a family history of hereditary non-polyposis colon cancer.[125] A high incidence of microsatellite instability (21%) was initially reported in sporadic tumors of the upper urinary tract;[126] others have reported a much lower incidence (7%) of microsatellite instability.[127] Patients with microsatellite-unstable tumor have more familial cases of colorectal cancer.[128] Cytogenetic studies showed that genetic changes in upper tract urothelial carcinoma are similar to those of its counterparts in the urinary bladder.[89]

Multifocality is a significant problem for patients with upper tract tumors.[114,129,130] There is no survival difference between patients with unilateral or synchronous bilateral upper urinary tract cancers,[131] but patients with bilateral subsequent (metachronous) upper tract tumors have a shorter survival.[132] Nearly 50% of patients with upper tract tumors may later develop urothelial carcinoma of the bladder.[89,133] In contrast, the incidence of upper urinary tract tumor is low (0.7–4%) among patients with primary bladder cancer.[89] Patients with multiple bladder tumors are at high risk of developing upper urinary tract cancers.[134] The location of bladder tumors is also an important risk factor: patients with

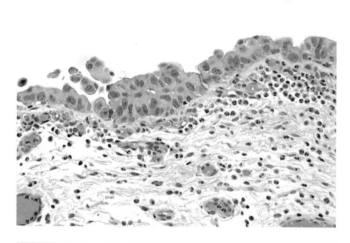

**Fig. 3-22** Urothelial carcinoma in situ of the ureter.

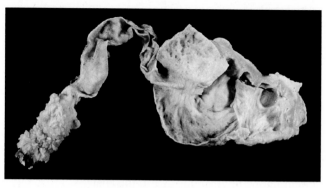

**Fig. 3-24** Papillary urothelial carcinoma of the ureter causing hydronephrosis.

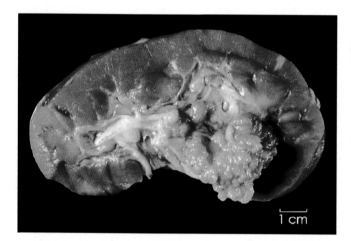

1 cm

**Fig. 3-23** Papillary urothelial carcinoma of the renal pelvis.

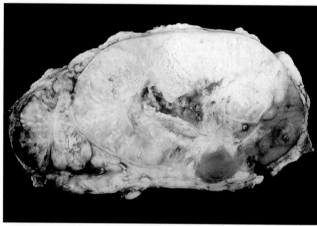

**Fig. 3-25** Infiltrative urothelial carcinoma of the pelvis, replacing most of the kidney.

bladder tumor in the trigone are at approximately six times higher risk for a synchronous tumor in the upper urinary tract.[135] Stage Ta bladder cancer patients with two or more recurrences are also at high risk of developing an upper urinary tract tumor.[136] Some studies suggest that patients with a history of bladder urothelial carcinoma have a worse prognosis than those without.[137]

In the ureter the most common location of tumor is the distal segment.[138] Owing to the high rate of recurrence (more than 15%) in the ureter distal to the resected tumor, nephro-ureterectomy with resection of a cuff of urinary bladder is the operation of choice.[108] Fluorescence in situ hybridization (FISH) analysis of abnormalities of chromosomes 3, 7, 9, and 17 offers greater sensitivity than cytology for the detection of upper urinary tract urothelial carcinoma while maintaining a similar specificity.[139]

### Gross pathology

The gross appearance of the tumors is similar to that seen in the bladder (Fig. 3-23), except that large papillary tumors frequently fill the ureters and cause obstruction, resulting in hydronephrosis (Fig. 3-24). Large tumors of the pelvis may extensively invade the renal parenchyma in an ill-defined infiltrative manner (Fig. 3-25), even extending into the para-cortical fat with a scirrhous response. In some such tumors little evidence remains of a mucosal origin in the pelvis, and extensive histologic sampling is necessary to demonstrate it. Gross fat extension or invasion into renal parenchyma should be documented along with other pertinent prognostic factors, such as tumor size.[140,141]

### Grading and staging

Grade and stage are the most important prognostic factors in urothelial carcinoma of the upper tract,[89,93,142,143] but the multiplicity of tumors also has an effect.[129,134] In one study, approximately 75% of cases were low grade and low stage.[144] Recent studies suggest that upper urinary tract urothelial carcinoma tends to have higher grade and stage than its urinary bladder counterpart.[145] The grading scheme is identical to that applied in the bladder (see detailed discussion in Chapter 5). Both 1973[146] and 1998 ISUP/2004 WHO grading systems[147] have been used in recent years.[148,149] Both have been effective in predicting prognosis, although the 1973 WHO grading system is more widely used and established.[142,145,150–163]

The American Joint Committee on Cancer (AJCC) TNM staging system has been used extensively and is shown in Box 3-1.[164] Muscle invasion is a critical point in the progression of these tumors, and survival is markedly reduced when it is present.[159,165–168] Recent studies suggests that ureteral tumors tend to have a worse prognosis than renal pelvic tumors,[142,158,169] which contrasts with previous data from other groups that showed either no difference[128,162] or a better prognosis for ureteral tumors.[157,170] Thus these tumors should not be lumped together in the analysis.

## Microscopic pathology

The histopathology of urothelial carcinoma of the renal pelvis and ureter (Figs 3-26–30) has the same spectrum as urothelial carcinoma of the urinary bladder,[91,92] including squamous and glandular[171] differentiation and the sarcomatoid (Fig. 3-30),[172–179] lymphoepithelioma-like,[180–186] plasmacytoid,[180] micropapillary,[180,187–189] inverted,[190] microcystic,[191] and small cell[192–195] variants. A complete discussion of the microscopic pathology of urothelial carcinoma appears in Chapter 5. Rare variants, including those with trophoblastic differentiation and osteoclast-type giant cells,[196–198] have

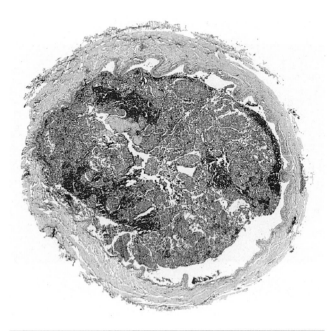

**Fig. 3-26** Papillary urothelial carcinoma filling the lumen of the ureter.

---

### Box 3-1

### The 2002 AJCC TNM Staging of Carcinoma of the Renal Pelvis and Ureter

- Ta  Noninvasive papillary carcinoma
- Tis  Carcinoma in situ
- T1  Invasion of subepithelial connective tissue
- T2  Invasion of muscularis propria
- T3  Invasion of peripelvic fat or renal parenchyma (renal pelvic tumors only)
  Invasion of periureteric fat (ureteral tumors only)
- T4  Invasion of adjacent organs or through kidney into perirenal fat
  Invasion of periureteric fat (ureteral tumors only)
- N0  No regional lymph node metastasis
- N1  Metastasis to a single lymph node less than or equal to 2 cm in maximum diameter
- N2  Metastasis to a single lymph node between 2 cm and 5 cm in maximum diameter or metastasis to multiple lymph nodes none larger than 5 cm in maximum diameter
- N3  Metastasis to a lymph node larger than 5 cm in maximum diameter
- M0  No distant metastasis
- M1  Distant metastasis

---

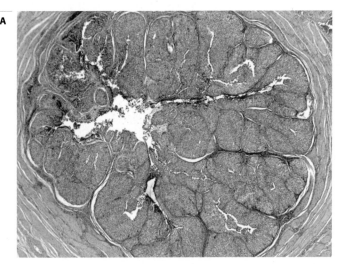

A

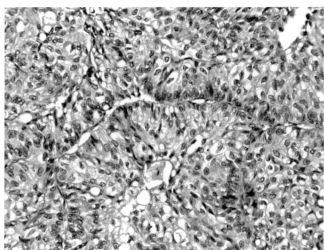

B

**Fig. 3-27** Non-invasive papillary urothelial carcinoma, low-grade or grade 2 **(A, B)**.

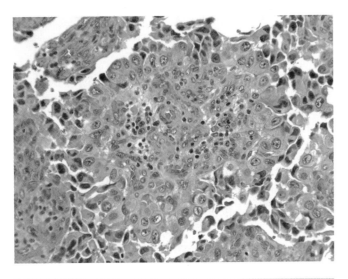

**Fig. 3-28** Non-invasive papillary urothelial carcinoma, high-grade or grade 3.

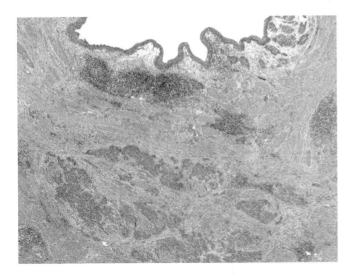

**Fig. 3-29** Invasive urothelial carcinoma involving the muscularis propria wall.

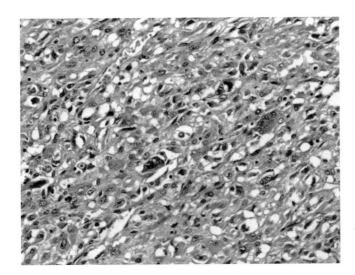

**Fig. 3-30** Sarcomatoid urothelial carcinoma of the ureter.

been reported. When the sarcomatoid elements obscure the clearly carcinomatous elements, immunohistochemical studies[172,174,179,199] or ultrastructural examination[171] may be of diagnostic help.

Mapping studies have shown that virtually all cases of urothelial carcinoma of the renal pelvis and ureter are associated with changes ranging from hyperplasia to carcinoma in situ in the mucosa elsewhere in the specimen.[200] Thickening of basement membranes around capillaries in the lamina propria of the renal pelvis and ureter has been found to be a histologic marker for analgesic abuse, and is termed capillarosclerosis.[120]

In addition to grade and stage, tumor necrosis[201] and vascular invasion[159] have recently been identified as independent prognostic factors for upper urinary tract urothelial carcinoma.

## Squamous cell carcinoma

Approximately 10% of renal pelvic tumors are squamous cell carcinomas,[202] and the percentage of cases of ureteral carcinoma is even smaller. Calculi, horseshoe kidney, and chronic infection are risk factors for squamous cell carcinoma.[50,95] The relationship with squamous metaplasia is more controversial, with some studies of squamous cell carcinoma reporting a strong association[203,204] whereas some studies of squamous metaplasia have reported little association.[46] The disagreement may be the result of the rarity of squamous cell carcinoma of the upper urinary tract. Epstein–Barr virus infection is not associated with the development of upper urinary tract squamous cell carcinoma.[205] The most common presenting symptoms are flank pain and gross hematuria.

Most squamous cell carcinomas of the renal pelvis and ureters are high stage;[152] extensive infiltration of the renal parenchyma is common (Fig. 3-31) and survival for 5 years is rare.[204,206] The histopathology of this tumor is similar to that of squamous cell carcinoma in the urinary bladder. It should be distinguished from metastatic squamous cell carcinoma, which is usually straightforward when clinical and

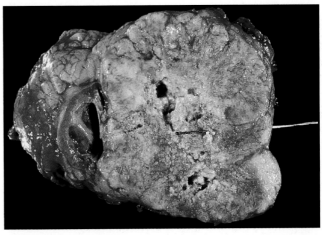

**Fig. 3-31** Squamous cell carcinoma of the renal pelvis. The probe indicates the course of the ureter.

pathological features are considered. An exceptional case of adenosquamous carcinoma of the renal pelvis without urothelial carcinoma was described in association with staghorn calculi.[207]

## Adenocarcinoma

Primary adenocarcinoma of the upper tract is rare and the reports consist of single cases or small series of cases (Fig. 3-32).[95,208–221] Most occur in adults, but rare pediatric cases have been described.[222] Calculi, chronic inflammation, and infection appear to be predisposing conditions. Most patients present with advanced cancer, similar to those with squamous cell carcinoma, and have a poor prognosis. Intestinal metaplasia and villous adenoma[45,51,223,224] may be a precursor lesion, and non-invasive carcinoma is sometimes found in the adjacent mucosa. Variants of adenocarcinoma have been described, and the prognostic significance of subclassification is uncertain. The prognosis is generally poor.[95] Papillary architecture and a resemblance to mucinous adenocarcinoma of the colon (Fig. 3-33) are common. One tumor had

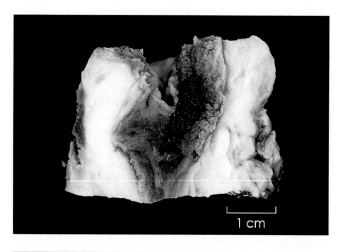

**Fig. 3-32** Mucinous adenocarcinoma of the renal pelvis.

hepatoid areas and contained bile pigment.[218] the formation of collagen spherules has been described.[225]

## Metastases

Neoplastic involvement of the ureters may occur by direct local extension or metastasis.[226–231] Contiguous ureteral involvement is more frequent and is usually caused by carcinoma of the cervix, prostate, or bladder.[226] Metastatic involvement is less common, and breast and colon are the most common sites of primaries.[227,232] Ureteral involvement is rarely the initial manifestation of the neoplasm.

When distant metastasis occurs, the lung is the most common site in patients with urothelial carcinoma of the upper urinary tract.

## Mesenchymal neoplasms

Mesenchymal neoplasms are uncommon in the ureter and pelvis. Fibroepithelial polyps are the most common, followed by benign and malignant smooth muscle tumors. A variety of additional tumors have been reported as single cases, including hemangioma, neurofibroma, and malignant schwannoma.

### Fibroepithelial polyp

Fibroepithelial polyp is more common in the ureters and renal pelvis than in the bladder. It is an uncommon benign mesenchymal tumor of the renal pelvis[233] and ureter.[234] Approximately 70% of patients are male.[235] Fibroepithelial polyp occurs at all ages, from infancy to old age (the mean is approximately 40 years),[236–246] and is the most common benign polypoid lesion of the ureters in children.[237] Colicky flank pain and hematuria are the most common symptoms. The etiology is uncertain.[247]

Grossly, fibroepithelial polyp consists of single or multiple slender, smooth-surfaced vermiform polyps that usually arise from a common base. The ureteropelvic junction is a common site and the polyp may cause obstruction at that narrow point. Rarely, fibroepithelial polyp is bilateral. Microscopically, the polyp is covered by normal urothelium,

A

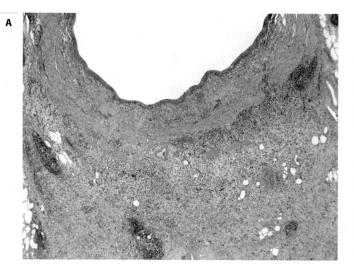
B

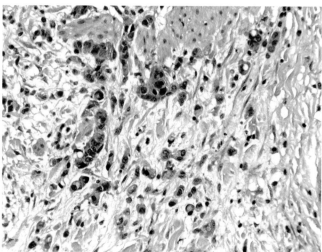

**Fig. 3-33** Mucinous adenocarcinoma of the ureter infiltrating the lamina propria **(A and B).** The tumor cells display signet-ring features.

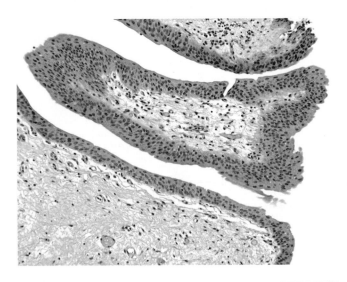

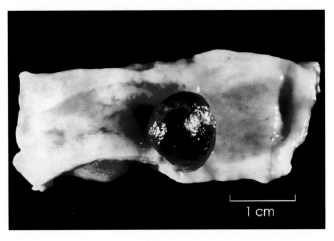

**Fig. 3-36** Hemangioma of the ureter. (Courtesy of Robert H. Young, MD.)

**Fig. 3-34** Fibroepithelial polyp consisting of a fibrovascular core with scattered inflammatory cells and a covering of normal urothelium.

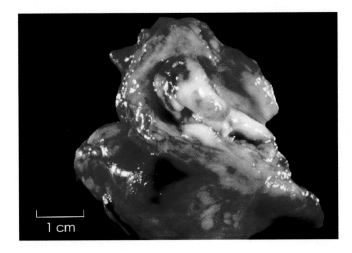

**Fig. 3-35** Leiomyosarcoma of ureter. (Courtesy of Robert H. Young, MD.)

which may be focally eroded. The core of the polyp is composed of a loose edematous and vascular stroma with few inflammatory cells (Fig. 3-34).

### Leiomyoma and leiomyosarcoma

Smooth muscle tumors of the ureter and pelvis are much rarer than those of the kidney, and the frequency of benign[248-256] and malignant tumors is approximately

equal.[257-261] Patients present with hematuria, pain, or mass findings indistinguishable from the presentation of urothelial neoplasms. Grossly, small tumors may form polypoid masses (Fig. 3-35), whereas larger tumors are often infiltrative. Histologically, they resemble their counterparts elsewhere.

### Hemangioma

Hemangioma of the ureter and renal pelvis is an uncommon polypoid tumor (Fig. 3-36) consisting of hypervascular fibrous stroma covered by normal urothelium.[262-266] Occurring in children and adults, this lesion may be multiple and frequently causes obstruction.

### Other tumors

Other sarcomas, such as osteogenic sarcoma,[267] Ewing's sarcoma,[268] liposarcoma,[269] rhabdomyosarcoma,[270] and malignant schwannoma[271] are extremely rare. Malignant melanoma may arise in the mucosa of the renal pelvis.[272] Carcinosarcoma, which combines squamous or urothelial carcinoma with heterologous sarcoma such as osteogenic sarcoma, chondrosarcoma, or rhabdomyosarcoma, is extremely rare.[273,274] Choriocarcinomatous differentiation may be seen in coexisting urothelial carcionoma.[275-277] A pure choriocarcinoma of the renal pelvis has been reported.[278] Inflammatory pseudotumor involving the ureter is rare (see detailed discussion in Chapter 5).[279-281] Obstruction caused by secondary infiltration by malignant lymphoma occurs in approximately 16% of cases of disseminated lymphoma.[282]

## REFERENCES

1. Mackie GG. Abnormalities of the ureteral bud. Urol Clin North Am 1978; 5: 161–174.

2. Ruano-Gil D, Coca-Payeras A, Tejedo-Mateu A. Obstruction and normal recanalization of the ureter in the human embryo. Its relation to congenital ureteric obstruction. Eur Urol 1975; 1: 287–293.

3. Holstein AF, Sandmann J, Bressel M, et al. Reinvestigation of the transitional epithelium (urothelium) of the human ureter. Ann Anat 1994; 176: 109–117.

4. Matsuno T, Tokunaka S, Koyanagi T. Muscular development in the urinary tract. J Urol 1984; 132: 148–152.

5. Itatani H, Koide T, Okuyama A, et al. Development of the ureterovesical

junction in human fetus: in consideration of the vesicoureteral reflux. Invest Urol 1977; 15: 232–238.

6. Itatani H, Koide T, Okuyama A, et al. Development of the calyceal system in the human fetus. Invest Urol 1979; 16: 388–394.

7. Shnorhavorian M, Anderson KR. Anatomic and physiologic

considerations in ureteroscopy. Urol Clin North Am 2004; 31: 15–20.

8. Elbadawi A. Anatomy and function of the ureteral sheath. J Urol 1972; 107: 224–229.

9. Notley RG. Electron microscopy of the upper ureter and the pelvi-ureteric junction. Br J Urol 1968; 40: 37–52.

10. Rizzo M, Faussone Pellegrini MS, Arbi Riccardi R, et al. Ultrastructure of the urinary tract muscle coat in man. Calices, renal pelvis, pelvi-ureteric junction and ureter. Eur Urol 1981; 7: 171–177.

11. Vaughan ED Jr, Middleton GW. Pertinent genitourinary embryology: review for practicing urologists. Urology 1975; 6: 139–149.

12. Lenaghan D. Bifid ureters in children: an anatomical, physiological and clinical study. J Urol 1962; 87: 808–817.

13. Barry JE, Auldist AW. The Vater association: one end of a spectrum of anomalies. Am J Dis Child 1974; 128: 769–771.

14. Straub E, Spranger J. Etiology and pathogenesis of the prune belly syndrome. Kidney Int 1981; 20: 695–699.

15. Egli F, Stalder G. Malformations of kidney and urinary tract in common chromosomal aberrations. I. Clinical studies. Humangenetik 1973; 18: 1–15.

16. Atwell JD, Cook PL, Howell CJ, et al. Familial incidence of bifid and double ureters. Arch Dis Child 1974; 49: 390–393.

17. Atwell JD. Familial pelviureteric junction hydronephrosis and its association with a duplex pelvicaliceal system and vesicoureteric reflux. A family study. Br J Urol 1985; 57: 365–369.

18. Roodhooft AM, Birnholz JC, Holmes LB. Familial nature of congenital absence and severe dysgenesis of both kidneys. N Engl J Med 1984; 310: 1341–1345.

19. Jerkins GR, Noe HN. Familial vesicoureteral reflux: a prospective study. J Urol 1982; 128: 774–778.

20. Belman AB. Megaureter. Classification, etiology, and management. Urol Clin North Am 1974; 1: 497–513.

21. Emanuel B, Nachman R, Aronson N, et al. Congenital solitary kidney: a review of 74 cases. J Urol 1974; 111: 394–397.

22. Caldamone AA. Duplication anomalies of the upper tract in infants and children. Urol Clin North Am 1985; 12: 75–91.

23. Mackie GG, Stephens FD. Duplex kidneys: a correlation of renal dysplasia with position of the ureteral orifice. J Urol 1975; 114: 274–280.

24. Hawtrey CE, Culp DA, Loening S, et al. Ureterovesical reflux in an adolescent and adult population. J Urol 1983; 130: 1067–1069.

25. Tanagho EA, Guthrie TH, Lyon RP. The intravesical ureter in primary reflux. J Urol 1969; 101: 824–832.

26. Johnston JH, Evans JP, Glassberg KI, et al. Pelvic hydronephrosis in children: a review of 219 personal cases. J 1977; Urol 117: 97–101.

27. Foote JW, Blennerhassett JB, Wiglesworth FW, et al. Observations on the ureteropelvic junction. J Urol 1970; 104: 252–257.

28. Hanna MK, Jeffs RD, Sturgess JM, et al. Ureteral structure and ultrastructure. Part II. Congenital ureteropelvic junction obstruction and primary obstructive megaureter. J Urol 1976; 116: 725–730.

29. Maizels M, Stephens FD. Valves of the ureter as a cause of primary obstruction of the ureter: anatomic, embryologic and clinical aspects. J Urol 1980; 123: 742–747.

30. Stephens FD. Ureterovascular hydronephrosis and the 'aberrant' renal vessels. J Urol 1982; 128: 984–987.

31. Tanagho EA, Smith DR, Guthrie TH. Pathophysiology of functional ureteral obstruction. J Urol 1970; 104: 73–88.

32. Tokunaka S, Koyanagi T. Morphologic study of primary non-reflux megaureters with particular emphasis on the role of ureteral sheath and ureteral dysplasia. J Urol 1982; 128: 399–402.

33. Tokunaka S, Gotoh T, Koyanagi T, et al. Muscle dysplasia in megaureters. J Urol 1984; 131: 383–390.

34. Hanna MK. Ureteral structure and ultrastructure. Part V. The dysplastic ureter. J Urol 1979; 122: 796–798.

35. Tanagho EA. Anatomy and management of ureteroceles. J Urol 1972; 107: 729–736.

36. Tokunaka S, Gotoh T, Koyanagi T, et al. Morphological study of the ureterocele: a possible clue to its embryogenesis as evidenced by a locally arrested myogenesis. J Urol 1981; 126: 726–729.

37. Mandell J, Colodny AH, Lebowitz R, et al. Ureteroceles in infants and children. J Urol 1980; 123: 921–926.

38. Tokunaka S, Koyanagi T, Matsuno T, et al. Paraureteral diverticula: clinical experience with 17 cases with associated renal dysmorphism. J Urol 1980; 124: 791–796.

39. Wickramasinghe SF, Stephens FD. Paraureteral diverticula. Associated renal morphology and embryogenesis. Invest Urol 1977; 14: 381–385.

40. Mostofi FK. Potentialities of bladder epithelium. J Urol 1954; 71: 705–714.

41. Wiener DP, Koss LG, Sablay B, et al. The prevalence and significance of Brunn's nests, cystitis cystica and squamous metaplasia in normal bladders. J Urol 1979; 122: 317–321.

42. Ozdamar AS, Ozkurkcugil C, Gultekin Y, et al. Should we get routine urothelial biopsies in every stone surgery? Int Urol Nephrol 1997; 29: 415–420.

43. Morse HD. The etiology and pathology of pyelitis cystica, ureteritis cystica and cystitis. Am J Pathol 1928; 4: 33–49.

44. Askari A, Herrera HH. Pyeloureteritis cystica. Urology 1980; 16: 398–399.

45. Bullock PS, Thoni DE, Murphy WM. The significance of colonic mucosa (intestinal metaplasia) involving the urinary tract. Cancer 1987; 59: 2086–2090.

46. Hertle L, Androulakakis P. Keratinizing desquamative squamous metaplasia of the upper urinary tract: leukoplakia–cholesteatoma. J Urol 1982; 127: 631–635.

47. Reece RW, Koontz WW Jr. Leukoplakia of the urinary tract: a review. J Urol 1975; 114: 165–171.

48. Harada H, Seki T, Togashi M, et al. Squamous metaplasia mimicking papillary carcinoma in the upper urinary tract. Hokkaido Igaku Zasshi 2004; 79: 15–17.

49. Kinn AC. Squamous cell carcinoma of the renal pelvis. Scand J Urol Nephrol 1979; 14: 77–80.

50. Li MK, Cheung WL. Squamous cell carcinoma of the renal pelvis. J Urol 1987; 138: 269–271.

51. Gordon A. Intestinal metaplasia of the urinary tract epithelium. J Pathol Bacteriol 1963; 85: 441–444.

52. Ward AM. Glandular neoplasia within the urinary tract. The aetiology of adenocarcinoma of the urothelium with a review of the literature. I. Introduction: the origin of glandular epithelium in the renal pelvis, ureter and bladder. Virchows Arch A Pathol Anat 1971; 352: 296–311.

53. Krag DO, Alcott DL. Glandular metaplasia of the renal pelvis: report of a case. Am J Clin Pathol 1957; 27: 672–680.

54. Sung MT, Lopez-Beltran A, Eble JN, et al. Divergent pathway of intestinal metaplasia and cystitis glandularis of the urinary bladder. Mod Pathol 2006; 19: 1395–1401.

55. Gokaslan ST, Krueger JE, Albores-Saavedra J. Symptomatic nephrogenic metaplasia of ureter: a morphologic and immunohistochemical study of four cases. Mod Pathol 2002; 15: 765–770.

56. Wong-You-Cheong JJ, Woodward PJ, Manning MA, et al. From the archives of the AFIP: Inflammatory and non-neoplastic bladder masses: radiologic-pathologic correlation. Radiographics 2006; 26: 1847–1868.

57. Bozkurt SU, Erbarut I, Yazici C, et al. Nephrogenic adenoma of the ureter: Case report. Int Urol Nephrol 2007; 39: 65–69.

58. Cheng L, Cheville JC, Sebo TJ, et al. Atypical nephrogenic metaplasia of the urinary tract: a precursor lesion? Cancer 2000; 88: 853–861.

59. Satodate R, Koike H, Sasou S, et al. Nephrogenic adenoma of the ureter. J Urol 1984; 131: 332–334.

60. Lugo M, Petersen RO, Elfenbein IB, et al. Nephrogenic metaplasia of the ureter. Am J Clin Pathol 1983; 80: 92–97.

61. Murphy WM, Soloway MS, Finebaum PJ. Pathological changes associated with topical chemotherapy for superficial bladder cancer. J Urol 1981; 126: 461–464.

62. Mukamel E, Glanz I, Nissenkorn I, et al. Unanticipated vesicoureteral reflux: a possible sequela of long-term thiotepa instillations to the bladder. J Urol 1982; 127: 245–246.

63. Michaelis L, Gutmann C. Ueber Einschlusse in Blasentumoren. Zeitschr Klin Med 1902; 47: 208–215.

64. Von Hansemann D. Uber Malakoplakie der Harnblase. Virchows Arch Pathol Anat Physiol Klin Med 1903; 173: 302–308.

65. Asiyanbola B, Camuto P, Mansourian V. Malakoplakia occurring in association with colon carcinoma. J Gastrointest Surg 2006; 10: 657–661.

66. Teahan SJ, O'Malley KJ, Little DM, et al. Malacoplakia of transplant ureter resulting in anuric renal failure. J Urol 1999; 162: 1375–1376.

67. Baumgartner BR, Alagappian R. Malakoplakia of the ureter and bladder. Urol Radiol 1990; 12: 157–1579.

68. Long JP Jr, Althausen AF. Malacoplakia: a 25-year experience with a review of the literature. J Urol 1989; 141: 1328–1331.

69. Stanton MJ, Maxted W. Malacoplakia: a study of the literature and current concepts of pathogenesis, diagnosis and treatment. J Urol 1981; 125: 139–146.

70. McClure J. Malakoplakia. J Pathol 1983; 140: 275–330.

71. McClure J. Malakoplakia of the urinary tract. Br J Urol 1982; 54: 181–185.

72. Comiter CV. Endometriosis of the urinary tract. Urol Clin North Am 2002; 29: 625–635.

73. Generao SE, Keene KD, Das S. Endoscopic diagnosis and management of ureteral endometriosis. J Endourol 2005; 19: 1177–1179.

74. Strang A, Lisson SW, Petrou SP. Ureteral endometriosis and coexistent urethral leiomyoma in a postmenopausal woman. Int Braz J Urol 2004; 30: 496–498.

75. Tanuma Y. Ureteral endometriosis: a case report and a review of the Japanese literature. Hinyokika Kiyo 2001; 47: 573–577.

76. Dominici A, Agostini S, Sarti E, et al. Ureteral endometriosis: an unusual case of a pelvic mass arising in the ureter and involving the rectum and uterine cervix. Arch Ital Urol Androl 2004; 76: 91–93.

77. Antonelli A, Simeone C, Zani D, et al. Clinical aspects and surgical treatment of urinary tract endometriosis: our experience with 31 cases. Eur Urol 2006; 49: 1093–1098.

78. Parker RL, Dadmanesh F, Young RH, et al. Polypoid endometriosis: a clinicopathologic analysis of 24 cases and a review of the literature. Am J Surg Pathol 2004; 28: 285–297.

79. Salerno MG, Masciullo V, Naldini A, et al. Endometrioid adenocarcinoma with squamous differentiation arising from ureteral endometriosis in a patient with no history of gonadal endometriosis. Gynecol Oncol 2005; 99: 749–752.

80. Jimenez RE, Tiguert R, Hurley P, et al. Unilateral hydronephrosis resulting from intraluminal obstruction of the ureter by adenosquamous endometrioid carcinoma arising from disseminated endometriosis. Urology 2000; 56: 331.

81. Stern RC, Dash R, Bentley RC, et al. Malignancy in endometriosis: frequency and comparison of ovarian and extraovarian types. Int J Gynecol Pathol 2001; 20: 133–139.

82. Mitchinson MJ. The pathology of idiopathic retroperitoneal fibrosis. J Clin Pathol 1970; 23: 681–689.

83. Lepor H, Walsh PC. Idiopathic retroperitoneal fibrosis. J Urol 1979; 122: 1–6.

84. Mitchinson MJ. Retroperitoneal fibrosis revisited. Arch Pathol Lab Med 1986; 110: 784–786.

85. Barbalias GA, Liatsikos EN. Idiopathic retroperitoneal fibrosis revisited. Int Urol Nephrol 1999; 31: 423–429.

86. ILie CP, Pemberton RJ, Tolley DA. Idiopathic retroperitoneal fibrosis: the case for non-surgical treatment. Br J Urol Int 2006; 98: 137–140.

87. Wong C, Sibai H, Bernard C, et al. Localized idiopathic retroperitoneal fibrosis mimicking primary obstructive megaureter in a child. J Urol 2000; 163: 1913–1914.

88. Bennington JL, Beckwith JB. Atlas of tumor pathology, second series, fascicle 12, tumors of the kidney, renal pelvis, and ureter. Armed Forces Institute of Pathology, 1975.

89. Kirkali Z, Tuzel E. Transitional cell carcinoma of the ureter and renal pelvis. Crit Rev Oncol Hematol 2003; 47: 155–169.

90. Kvist E, Lauritzen AF, Bredesen J, et al. A comparative study of transitional cell tumors of the bladder and upper urinary tract. Cancer 1988; 61: 2109–2112.

91. Genega EM, Porter CR. Urothelial neoplasms of the kidney and ureter. An epidemiologic, pathologic, and clinical review. Am J Clin Pathol 2002; 117: S36–48.

92. Melamed MR, Reuter VE. Pathology and staging of urothelial tumors of the kidney and ureter. Urol Clin North Am 1993; 20: 333–347.

93. Booth CM, Cameron KM, Pugh RC. Urothelial carcinoma of the kidney and ureter. Br J Urol 1980; 52: 430–435.

94. McCarron JP, Mills C, Vaughn ED Jr. Tumors of the renal pelvis and ureter: current concepts and management. Semin Urol 1983; 1: 75–81.

95. Busby JE, Brown GA, Tamboli P, et al. Upper urinary tract tumors with non-transitional histology: a single-center experience. Urology 2006; 67: 518–523.

96. Naito S, Minoda M, Hirata H. Inverted papilloma of ureter. Urology 1983; 22: 290–291.

97. Lausten GS, Anagnostaki L, Thomsen OF. Inverted papilloma of the upper urinary tract. Eur Urol 1984; 10: 67–70.

98. Sung MT, Maclennan GT, Lopez-Beltran A, et al. Natural history of urothelial inverted papilloma. Cancer 2006; 107: 2622–2627.

99. Kyriakos M, Royce RK. Multiple simultaneous inverted papillomas of the upper urinary tract. A case report with a review of ureteral and renal pelvic inverted papillomas. Cancer 1989; 63: 368–380.

100. Embon OM, Saghi N, Bechar L. Inverted papilloma of ureter. Eur Urol 1984; 10: 139–140.

101. Arrufat JM, Vera-Roman JM, Casas V, et al. [Inverted papilloma of the ureter]. Actas Urol Esp 1983; 7: 225–228.

102. Palvio DH. Inverted papillomas of the urinary tract. A case of multiple, recurring inverted papillomas of the renal pelvis, ureter and bladder associated with malignant change. Scand J Urol Nephrol 1985; 19: 299–302.

103. Kunze E, Schauer A, Schmitt M. Histology and histogenesis of two different types of inverted urothelial papillomas. Cancer 1983; 51: 348–358.

104. Kimura G, Tsuboi N, Nakajima H, et al. Inverted papilloma of the ureter with malignant transformation: a case report and review of the literature. The importance of the recognition of the inverted papillary tumor of the ureter. Urol Int 1987; 42: 30–36.

105. Grainger R, Gikas PW, Grossman HB. Urothelial carcinoma occurring within an inverted papilloma of the ureter. J Urol 1990; 143: 802–804.

106. McCarron JP Jr, Chasko SB, Gray GF Jr. Systematic mapping of nephroureterectomy specimens removed for urothelial cancer: pathological findings and clinical correlations. J Urol 1982; 128: 243–246.

107. Heney NM, Nocks BN, Daly JJ, et al. Prognostic factors in carcinoma of the ureter. J Urol 1981; 125: 632–636.

108. Nocks BN, Heney NM, Daly JJ, et al. Transitional cell carcinoma of renal pelvis. Urology 1982; 19: 472–477.

109. Nielsen K, Ostri P. Primary tumors of the renal pelvis: evaluation of clinical and pathological features in a consecutive series of 10 years. J Urol 1988; 140: 19–21.

110. Yuasa T, Tsuchiya N, Narita S, et al. Radical nephroureterectomy as initial treatment for carcinoma in situ of upper urinary tract. Urology 2006; 68: 972–975.

111. Nishino Y, Yamamoto N, Komeda H, et al. Bacillus Calmette–Guérin instillation treatment for carcinoma in

situ of the upper urinary tract. Br J Urol Int 2000; 85: 799–801.

112. Kojima Y, Tozawa K, Kawai N, et al. Long-term outcome of upper urinary tract carcinoma in situ: effectiveness of nephroureterectomy versus bacillus Calmette–Guérin therapy. Int J Urol 2006; 13: 340–344.

113. Thalmann GN, Markwalder R, Walter B, et al. Long-term experience with bacillus Calmette– Guérin therapy of upper urinary tract transitional cell carcinoma in patients not eligible for surgery. J Urol 2002; 168: 1381–1385.

114. Mazeman E. Tumours of the upper urinary tract calyces, renal pelvis and ureter. Eur Urol 1976; 2: 120–126.

115. Guinan P, Vogelzang NJ, Randazzo R, et al. Renal pelvic cancer: a review of 611 patients treated in Illinois 1975– 1985. Cancer Incidence and End Results Committee. Urology 1992; 40: 393–399.

116. McLaughlin JK, Blot WJ, Mandel JS, et al. Etiology of cancer of the renal pelvis. J Natl Cancer Inst 1983; 71: 287–291.

117. McLaughlin JK, Silverman DT, Hsing AW, et al. Cigarette smoking and cancers of the renal pelvis and ureter. Cancer Res 1992; 52: 254–257.

118. Schmauz R, Cole P. Epidemiology of cancer of the renal pelvis and ureter. J Natl Cancer Inst 1974; 52: 1431–1434.

119. Chow WH, Lindblad P, Gridley G, et al. Risk of urinary tract cancers following kidney or ureter stones. J Natl Cancer Inst 1997; 89: 1453–1457.

120. Palvio DH, Andersen JC, Falk E. Transitional cell tumors of the renal pelvis and ureter associated with capillarosclerosis indicating analgesic abuse. Cancer 1987; 59: 972–976.

121. Steffens J, Nagel R. Tumours of the renal pelvis and ureter. Observations in 170 patients. Br J Urol 1988; 61: 277–283.

122. Lomax-Smith J, Seymour AE. Unsuspected analgesic nephropathy in transitional cell carcinoma of the upper tract: a morphological study. Histopathology 1980; 4: 255–269.

123. Christensen P, Madsen MR, Jensen OM. Latency of thorotrast-induced renal tumours. Survey of the literature and a case report. Scand J Urol Nephrol 1983; 17: 127–130.

124. Verhaak RL, Harmsen AE, van Unnik AJ. On the frequency of tumor induction in a thorotrast kidney. Cancer 1974; 34: 2061–2068.

125. Watson P, Lynch HT. Extracolonic cancer in hereditary non-polyposis colorectal cancer. Cancer 1993; 71: 677–685.

126. Hartmann A, Zanardo L, Bocker-Edmonston T, et al. Frequent microsatellite instability in sporadic tumors of the upper urinary tract. Cancer Res 2002; 62: 6796–6802.

127. Mongiat-Artus P, Miquel C, Van der Aa M, et al. Microsatellite instability and mutation analysis of candidate genes in urothelial cell carcinomas of upper urinary tract. Oncogene 2006; 25: 2113–2118.

128. Blaszyk H, Wang L, Dietmaier W, et al. Upper tract urothelial carcinoma: a clinicopathologic study including microsatellite instability analysis. Mod Pathol 2002; 15: 790–797.

129. Corrado F, Ferri C, Mannini D, et al. Transitional cell carcinoma of the upper urinary tract: evaluation of prognostic factors by histopathology and flow cytometric analysis. J Urol 1991; 145: 1159–1163.

130. Kang CH, Yu TJ, Hsieh HH, et al. The development of bladder tumors and contralateral upper urinary tract tumors after primary transitional cell carcinoma of the upper urinary tract. Cancer 2003; 98: 1620–1626.

131. Holmang S, Johansson SL. Synchronous bilateral ureteral and renal pelvic carcinomas: incidence, etiology, treatment and outcome. Cancer 2004; 101: 741–747.

132. Holmang S, Johansson SL. Bilateral metachronous ureteral and renal pelvic carcinomas: incidence, clinical presentation, histopathology, treatment and outcome. J Urol 2006; 175: 69–73.

133. Bonsib SM. Pathology of the renal pelvis and ureter. In: Eble JN, ed. Tumors and tumor-like conditions of the kidneys and ureters. New York: Churchill Livingstone, 1990; 177–205.

134. Millan-Rodriguez F, Chechile-Toniolo G, Salvador-Bayarri J, et al. Upper urinary tract tumors after primary superficial bladder tumors: prognostic factors and risk groups. J Urol 2000; 164: 1183–1187.

135. Palou J, Rodriguez-Rubio F, Huguet J, et al. Multivariate analysis of clinical parameters of synchronous primary superficial bladder cancer and upper urinary tract tumor. J Urol 2005; 174: 859–861.

136. Canales BK, Anderson JK, Premoli J, et al. Risk factors for upper tract recurrence in patients undergoing long-term surveillance for stage Ta bladder cancer. J Urol 2006; 175: 74–77.

137. Mullerad M, Russo P, Golijanin D, et al. Bladder cancer as a prognostic factor for upper tract transitional cell carcinoma. J Urol 2004; 172: 2177–2181.

138. Anderstrom C, Johansson SL, Pettersson S, et al. Carcinoma of the ureter: a clinicopathologic study of 49 cases. J Urol 1989; 142: 280–283.

139. Marin-Aguilera M, Mengual L, Ribal MJ, et al. Utility of fluorescence in situ hybridization as a non-invasive technique in the diagnosis of upper urinary tract urothelial carcinoma. Eur Urol 2007; 51: 409–415.

140. Amin MB, Srigley JR, Grignon DJ, et al. Updated protocol for the examination of specimens from patients with carcinoma of the urinary bladder, ureter, and renal pelvis. Arch Pathol Lab Med 2003; 127: 1263–1279.

141. Lopez Beltran A, Bassi P, Pavone-Macaluso M, et al. Handling and pathology reporting of specimens with carcinoma of the urinary bladder, ureter, and renal pelvis. Eur Urol 2004; 45: 257–266.

142. Ozsahin M, Zouhair A, Villa S, et al. Prognostic factors in urothelial renal pelvis and ureter tumours: a multicentre Rare Cancer Network study. Eur J Cancer 1999; 35: 738–743.

143. Akaza H, Koiso K, Niijima T. Clinical evaluation of urothelial tumors of the renal pelvis and ureter based on a new classification system. Cancer 1987; 59: 1369–1375.

144. Blute ML, Tsushima K, Farrow GM, et al. Transitional cell carcinoma of the renal pelvis: nuclear deoxyribonucleic acid ploidy studied by flow cytometry. J Urol 1988; 140: 944–949.

145. Stewart GD, Bariol SV, Grigor KM, et al. A comparison of the pathology of transitional cell carcinoma of the bladder and upper urinary tract. BJU Int 2005; 95: 791–793.

146. Mostofi FK, Sobin LH, Torloni H. Histological typing of urinary bladder tumours. Geneva: World Health Organization, 1973.

147. Eble JN, Sauter G, Epstein JI, et al. World Health Organization classification of tumours: pathology and genetics of tumours of the urinary system and male genital organs. Lyon, IARC Press, 2004.

148. Maclennan GT, Kirkali Z, Cheng L. Histologic grading of noninvasive papillary urothelial neoplasms. Eur Urol 2006; 51: 889–897.

149. Jones TD, Cheng L. Papillary urothelial neoplasm of low malignant potential: evolving terminology and concepts. J Urol 2006; 175: 1995–2003.

150. Reitelman C, Sawczuk IS, Olsson CA, et al. Prognostic variables in patients with transitional cell carcinoma of the renal pelvis and proximal ureter. J Urol 1987; 138: 1144–1145.

151. Vahlensieck W Jr, Sommerkamp H. Therapy and prognosis of carcinoma of the renal pelvis. Eur Urol 1989; 16: 286–290.

152. Strobel SL, Jasper WS, Gogate SA, et al. Primary carcinoma of the renal pelvis and ureter. Evaluation of clinical and pathologic features. Arch Pathol Lab Med 1984; 108: 697–700.

153. Murphy DM, Zincke H, Furlow WL. Primary grade 1 transitional cell carcinoma of the renal pelvis and ureter. J Urol 1980; 123: 629–631.

154. Huben RP, Mounzer AM, Murphy GP. Tumor grade and stage as prognostic variables in upper tract urothelial tumors. Cancer 1988; 62: 2016–2020.

155. Guarnizo E, Pavlovich CP, Seiba M, et al. Ureteroscopic biopsy of upper tract urothelial carcinoma: improved diagnostic accuracy and histopathological considerations using a multi-biopsy approach. J Urol 2000; 163: 52–55.

156. Genega EM, Kapali M, Torres-Quinones M, et al. Impact of the 1998 World Health Organization/International

Society of Urological Pathology classification system for urothelial neoplasms of the kidney. Mod Pathol 2005; 18: 11–18.

157. Suh RS, Faerber GJ, Wolf JS, Jr.: Predictive factors for applicability and success with endoscopic treatment of upper tract urothelial carcinoma. J Urol 2003; 170: 2209–2216.

158. Akdogan B, Dogan HS, Eskicorapci SY, et al. Prognostic significance of bladder tumor history and tumor location in upper tract transitional cell carcinoma. J Urol 2006; 176: 48–52.

159. Langner C, Hutterer G, Chromecki T, et al. pT classification, grade, and vascular invasion as prognostic indicators in urothelial carcinoma of the upper urinary tract. Mod Pathol 2006; 19: 272–279.

160. Bariol SV, Stewart GD, McNeill SA, et al. Oncological control following laparoscopic nephroureterectomy: 7-year outcome. J Urol 2004; 172: 1805–1808.

161. Goel MC, Mahendra V, Roberts JG. Percutaneous management of renal pelvic urothelial tumors: long-term followup. J Urol 2003; 169: 925–930.

162. Keeley FX Jr, Bibbo M, Bagley DH. Ureteroscopic treatment and surveillance of upper urinary tract transitional cell carcinoma. J Urol 1997; 157: 1560–1565.

163. Wolf JS Jr, Dash A, Hollenbeck BK, et al. Intermediate followup of hand assisted laparoscopic nephroureterectomy for urothelial carcinoma: factors associated with outcomes. J Urol 2005; 173: 1102–1107.

164. Greene FL, Page DL, Flemming ID, et al. American Joint Committee on Cancer Staging Manual, 6th edn. New York: Springer-Verlag, 2002.

165. Hall MC, Womack S, Sagalowsky AI, et al. Prognostic factors, recurrence, and survival in transitional cell carcinoma of the upper urinary tract: a 30-year experience in 252 patients. Urology 1998; 52: 594–601.

166. Olgac S, Mazumdar M, Dalbagni G, et al. Urothelial carcinoma of the renal pelvis: a clinicopathologic study of 130 cases. Am J Surg Pathol 2004; 28: 1545–1552.

167. Morioka M, Jo Y, Furukawa Y, et al. Prognostic factors for survival and bladder recurrence in transitional cell carcinoma of the upper urinary tract. Int J Urol 2001; 8: 366–373.

168. Batata MA, Whitmore WF, Hilaris BS, et al. Primary carcinoma of the ureter: a prognostic study. Cancer 1975; 35: 1626–1632.

169. Park S, Hong B, Kim CS, et al. The impact of tumor location on prognosis of transitional cell carcinoma of the upper urinary tract. J Urol 2004; 171: 621–625.

170. Iborra I, Solsona E, Casanova J, et al. Conservative elective treatment of upper urinary tract tumors: a multivariate analysis of prognostic factors for recurrence and progression. J Urol 2003; 169: 82–85.

171. Tajima Y, Aizawa M. Unusual renal pelvic tumor containing transitional cell carcinoma, adenocarcinoma and sarcomatoid elements (so-called sarcomatoid carcinoma of the renal pelvis). A case report and review of the literature. Acta Pathol Jpn 1988; 38: 805–814.

172. Piscioli F, Bondi A, Scappini P, et al. 'True' sarcomatoid carcinoma of the renal pelvis. First case report with immunocytochemical study. Eur Urol 1984; 10: 350–355.

173. Rao SS, Rao NN, Venkataratnam G. Carcinosarcoma of renal pelvis in a child. A case report. Indian J Pathol Microbiol 1986; 29: 313–316.

174. Wick MR, Perrone TL, Burke BA. Sarcomatoid transitional cell carcinomas of the renal pelvis. An ultrastructural and immunohistochemical study. Arch Pathol Lab Med 1985; 109: 55–58.

175. Darko A, Das K, Bhalla RS, et al. Carcinosarcoma of the ureter: report of a case with unusual histology and review of the literature. Int J Urol 2006; 13: 1528–1531.

176. Lee G, Rankin A, Williamson M, et al. Case report: sarcomatoid carcinoma arising from the ureter: a rare case and a treatment dilemma. Int Urol Nephrol 2004; 36: 153–154.

177. Perimenis P, Athanasopoulos A, Geragthy J, et al. Carcinosarcoma of the ureter: a rare, pleomorphic, aggressive malignancy. Int Urol Nephrol 2003; 35: 491–493.

178. Johnin K, Kadowaki T, Kushima M, et al. Primary heterologous carcinosarcoma of the ureter with necrotic malignant polyps. Report of a case and review of the literature. Urol Int 2003; 70: 232–235.

179. Vermeulen P, Hoekx L, Colpaert C, et al. Biphasic sarcomatoid carcinoma (carcinosarcoma) of the renal pelvis with heterologous chondrogenic differentiation. Virchows Arch 2000; 437: 194–197.

180. Perez-Montiel D, Wakely PE, Hes O, et al. High-grade urothelial carcinoma of the renal pelvis: clinicopathologic study of 108 cases with emphasis on unusual morphologic variants. Mod Pathol 2006; 19: 494–503.

181. Leroy X, Zerimech F, Zini L, et al. MUC1 expression is correlated with nuclear grade and tumor progression in pT1 renal clear cell carcinoma. Am J Clin Pathol 2002; 118: 47–51.

182. Terai A, Terada N, Ichioka K, et al. Lymphoepithelioma-like carcinoma of the ureter. Urology 2005; 66: 1109.

183. Roig JM, Amerigo J, Velasco FJ, et al. Lymphoepithelioma-like carcinoma of ureter. Histopathology 2001; 39: 106–107.

184. Cohen RJ, Stanley JC, Dawkins HJ. Lymphoepithelioma-like carcinoma of the renal pelvis. Pathology 1999; 31: 434–435.

185. Ng KF, Chen TC, Chang PL. Lymphoepithelioma-like carcinoma of the ureter. J Urol 1999; 161: 1277–1278.

186. Chalik YN, Wieczorek R, Grasso M. Lymphoepithelioma-like carcinoma of the ureter. J Urol 1998; 159: 503–504.

187. Vang R, Abrams J. A micropapillary variant of transitional cell carcinoma arising in the ureter. Arch Pathol Lab Med 2000; 124: 1347–1348.

188. Holmang S, Thomsen J, Johansson SL. Micropapillary carcinoma of the renal pelvis and ureter. J Urol 2006; 175: 463–467.

189. Perez-Montiel D, Hes O, Michal M, et al. Micropapillary urothelial carcinoma of the upper urinary tract: Clinicopathologic study of five cases. Am J Clin Pathol 2006; 126: 86–92.

190. Kawachi Y, Ishi K. Inverted transitional cell carcinoma of the ureter. Int J Urol 1996; 3: 313–315.

191. Leroy X, Leteurtre E, De La Taille A, et al. Microcystic transitional cell carcinoma: a report of 2 cases arising in the renal pelvis. Arch Pathol Lab Med 2002; 126: 859–861.

192. Essenfeld H, Manivel JC, Benedetto P, et al. Small cell carcinoma of the renal pelvis: a clinicopathological, morphological and immunohistochemical study of 2 cases. J Urol 1990; 144: 344–347.

193. Chang CY, Reddy K, Chorneyko K, et al. Primary small cell carcinoma of the ureter. Can J Urol 2005; 12: 2603–2606.

194. Kim TS, Seong DH, Ro JY. Small cell carcinoma of the ureter with squamous cell and transitional cell carcinomatous components associated with ureteral stone. J Korean Med Sci 2001; 16: 796–800.

195. Tsutsumi M, Kamiya M, Sakamoto M, et al. A ureteral small cell carcinoma mixed with malignant mesodermal and ectodermal elements: a clinicopathological, morphological and immunohistochemical study. Jpn J Clin Oncol 1993; 23: 325–329.

196. Tarry WF, Morabito RA, Belis JA. Carcinosarcoma of the renal pelvis with extension into the renal vein and inferior vena cava. J Urol 1982; 128: 582–585.

197. Kenney RM, Prat J, Tabernero M. Giant-cell tumor-like proliferation associated with a papillary transitional cell carcinoma of the renal pelvis. Am J Surg Pathol 1984; 8: 139–144.

198. Baydar D, Amin MB, Epstein JI. Osteoclast-rich undifferentiated carcinomas of the urinary tract. Mod Pathol 2006; 19: 161–171.

199. Emerson RE, Cheng L. Immunohistochemical markers in the evaluation of tumors of the urinary bladder: a review. Anal Quant Cytol Histol 2005; 27: 301–316.

200. Mahadevia PS, Karwa GL, Koss LG. Mapping of urothelium in carcinomas of the renal pelvis and ureter. A report

of nine cases. Cancer 1983; 51: 890–897.

201. Langner C, Hutterer G, Chromecki T, et al. Tumor necrosis as prognostic indicator in transitional cell carcinoma of the upper urinary tract. J Urol 2006; 176: 9104.

202. Utz DC, Mc DJ. Squamous cell carcinoma of the kidney. J Urol 1957; 78: 540–552.

203. Vyas MC, Joshi KR, Mathur DR, et al. Primary squamous cell carcinoma of the renal pelvis. A report of four cases with review of literature. Indian J Pathol Microbiol 1982; 25: 151–155.

204. Blacher EJ, Johnson DE, Abdul-Karim FW, et al. Squamous cell carcinoma of renal pelvis. Urology 1985 5: 124–126.

205. Ng KF, Chuang CK, Chang PL, et al. Absence of Epstein–Barr virus infection in squamous cell carcinoma of upper urinary tract and urinary bladder. Urology 2006; 68: 775–777.

206. Mizusawa H, Komiyama I, Ueno Y, et al. Squamous cell carcinoma in the renal pelvis of a horseshoe kidney. Int J Urol 2004; 11: 782–784.

207. Howat AJ, Scott E, Mackie DB, et al. Adenosquamous carcinoma of the renal pelvis. Am J Clin Pathol 1983; 79: 731–733.

208. Kim YI, Yoon DH, Lee SW, et al. Multicentric papillary adenocarcinoma of the renal pelvis and ureter. Report of a case with ultrastructural study. Cancer 1988; 62: 2402–2407.

209. Martinez Garcia R, Boronat Tormo F, Dominguez Hinarejos C. Adenocarcinoma de pelvis renal. Actas Urol Esp 1989l 13: 470–472.

210. Onishi T, Franco OE, Shibahara T, et al. Papillary adenocarcinoma of the renal pelvis and ureter producing carcinoembryonic antigen, carbohydrate antigen 19–9 and carbohydrate antigen 125. Int J Urol 2005; 12: 214–216.

211. Yilmaz Y, Dilek H, Odabas O, et al. Primary non-mucinous, non-papillary adenocarcinoma of the ureter. Int Urol Nephrol 1998; 30: 259–262.

212. Terris MK, Anderson RU. Mucinous adenocarcinoma of the renal pelvis in natives of India. Urol Int 1997; 58: 121–123.

213. Iwaki H, Wakabayashi Y, Kushima R, et al. Primary adenocarcinoma of the ureter producing carbohydrate antigen 19-9. J Urol 1996; 156: 1437.

214. Rao DS, Krigman HR, Walther PJ. Enteric type adenocarcinoma of the upper tract urothelium associated with ectopic ureter and renal dysplasia: an oncological rationale for complete extirpation of this aberrant developmental anomaly. J Urol 1996; 156: 1272–1274.

215. Delahunt B, Nacey JN, Meffan PJ, et al. Signet ring cell adenocarcinoma of the ureter. Br J Urol 1991; 68: 555–556.

216. Takezawa Y, Saruki K, Jinbo S, et al. A case of adenocarcinoma of the renal pelvis. Hinyokika Kiyo 1990; 36: 841–845.

217. Stein A, Sova Y, Lurie M, et al. Adenocarcinoma of the renal pelvis. Report of two cases, one with simultaneous transitional cell carcinoma of the bladder. Urol Int 1988; 43: 299–301.

218. Ishikura H, Ishiguro T, Enatsu C, et al. Hepatoid adenocarcinoma of the renal pelvis producing alpha-fetoprotein of hepatic type and bile pigment. Cancer 1991; 67: 3051–3056.

219. Brawer MK, Waisman J. Papillary adenocarcinoma of ureter. Urology 1982; 19: 205–209.

220. Shintaku M, Megumi Y, Maekura S. Adenocarcinoma of the renal pelvis with vimentin-positive intracytoplasmic inclusions. Pathol Int 2000; 50: 48–51.

221. Spires SE, Banks ER, Cibull ML, et al. Adenocarcinoma of renal pelvis. Arch Pathol Lab Med 1993; 117: 1156–1160.

222. Moncino MD, Friedman HS, Kurtzberg J, et al. Papillary adenocarcinoma of the renal pelvis in a child: case report and brief review of the literature. Med Pediatr Oncol 1990; 18: 81–86.

223. Fernando Val-Bernal J, Torio B, Mayorga M, et al. Concurrent tubulovillous adenoma and transitional cell carcinoma associated with diffuse gastric and intestinal metaplasia of the defunctioned ureter. Pathol Res Pract 2001; 197: 507–513.

224. Cheng L, Montironi R, Bostwick D. Villous adenoma of the urinary tract: a report of 23 cases, including 8 with coexistent adenocarcinoma. Am J Surg Pathol 1999; 23: 764–771.

225. Hes O, Curik R, Mainer K, et al. Urothelial signet-ring cell carcinoma of the renal pelvis with collagenous spherulosis: a case report. Int J Surg Pathol 2005; 13: 375–378.

226. Richie JP, Withers G, Ehrlich RM. Ureteral obstruction secondary to metastatic tumors. Surg Gynecol Obstet 1979; 148: 355–357.

227. Cohen WM, Freed SZ, Hasson J. Metastatic cancer to the ureter: a review of the literature and case presentations. J Urol 1974; 112: 188–189.

228. DiPietro M, Zeman RK, Keohane M, et al. Oat cell carcinoma metastatic to ureter. Urology 1983; 22: 419–420.

229. Katsuno G, Kagawa S, Kokudo Y, et al. Ureteral metastasis from appendiceal cancer: report of a case. Surg Today 2005; 35: 168–171.

230. Esrig D, Kanellos AW, Freeman JA, et al. Metastatic renal cell carcinoma to the contralateral ureter. Urology 1994; 44: 278–281.

231. Zorn KC, Orvieto MA, Mikhail AA, et al. Solitary ureteral metastases of renal cell carcinoma. Urology 2006; 68: 428; e5–7.

232. Hudolin T, Nola N, Milas I, et al. Ureteral metastasis of occult breast cancer. Breast 2004; 13: 530–532.

233. Wolgel CD, Parris AC, Mitty HA, et al. Fibroepithelial polyp of renal pelvis. Urology 1982; 19: 436–439.

234. Goldman SM, Bohlman ME, Gatewood OM. Neoplasms of the renal collecting system. Semin Roentgenol 1987; 22: 284–291.

235. Williams PR, Feggetter J, Miller RA, et al. The diagnosis and management of benign fibrous ureteric polyps. Br J Urol 1980; 52: 253–256.

236. Bartone FF, Johansson SL, Markin RJ, et al. Bilateral fibroepithelial polyps of ureter in a child. Urology 1990; 35: 519–522.

237. Macksood MJ, Roth DR, Chang CH, et al. Benign fibroepithelial polyps as a cause of intermittent ureteropelvic junction obstruction in a child: a case report and review of the literature. J Urol 1985; 134: 951–952.

238. Van Poppel H, Nuttin B, Oyen R, et al. Fibroepithelial polyps of the ureter. Etiology, diagnosis, treatment and pathology. Eur Urol 1986; 12: 174–179.

239. Carey RI, Bird VG. Endoscopic management of 10 separate fibroepithelial polyps arising in a single ureter. Urology 2006; 67: 413–415.

240. Lam JS, Bingham JB, Gupta M. Endoscopic treatment of fibroepithelial polyps of the renal pelvis and ureter. Urology 2003; 62: 810–813.

241. Kiel H, Ullrich T, Roessler W, et al. Benign ureteral tumors. Four case reports and a review of the literature. Urol Int 1999; 63: 201–205.

242. Zervas A, Rassidakis G, Nakopoulou L, et al. Transitional cell carcinoma arising from a fibroepithelial ureteral polyp in a patient with duplicated upper urinary tract. J Urol 1997; 157: 2252–2253.

243. Cooper CS, Hawtrey CE. Fibroepithelial polyp of the ureter. Urology 1997; 50: 280–281.

244. Karaca I, Sencan A, Mir E, et al. Ureteral fibroepithelial polyps in children. Pediatr Surg Int 1997; 12: 603–604.

245. Faerber GJ, Ahmed MM, Marcovich R, et al. Contemporary diagnosis and treatment of fibroepithelial ureteral polyp. J Endourol 1997; 11: 349–351.

246. Sharma NK, Stephenson RN, Tolley DA. Endoscopic management of fibroepithelial polyps in the ureter. Br J Urol 1996; 78: 131–132.

247. Stuppler SA, Kandzari SJ. Fibroepithelial polyps of ureter. A benign ureteral tumor. Urology 1975; 5: 553–558.

248. Zaitoon MM. Leiomyoma of ureter. Urology 1986; 28: 50–51.

249. Fitko R, Gallagher L, Gonzalez-Crussi F, et al. Urothelial leiomyomatous hamartoma of the kidney. Am J Clin Pathol 1991; 95: 481–483.

250. Ikota H, Tanimoto A, Komatsu H, et al. Ureteral leiomyoma causing hydronephrosis in type 1 multiple

endocrine neoplasia. Pathol Int 2004; 54: 457–459.

251. Yashi M, Hashimoto S, Muraishi O, et al. Leiomyoma of the ureter. Urol Int 2000; 64: 40–42.

252. Zaitoon MM. Leiomyoma of ureter. Urology 1986; 28: 50–51.

253. Ogata S, Mizoguchi H, Arita M, et al. A case of hemangiomyoma of the ureter in a child. Eur Urol 1985; 11: 355–356.

254. Mondschein LJ, Sutton AP, Rothfeld SH. Leiomyoma of the ureter in a child: the first reported case. J Urol 1976; 116: 516–518.

255. Sekar N, Nagrani B, Yadav RV. Ureterocele with leiomyoma of ureter. Br J Urol 1980; 52: 400.

256. Kao VC, Graff PW, Rappaport H. Leiomyoma of the ureter. A histologically problematic rare tumor confirmed by immunohistochemical studies. Cancer 1969; 24: 535–542.

257. Gislason T, Arnarson OO. Primary ureteral leiomyosarcoma. Scand J Urol Nephrol 1984; 18: 253–254.

258. Tolia BM, Hajdu SI, Whitmore WF Jr. Leiomyosarcoma of the renal pelvis. J Urol 1973; 109: 974–976.

259. Rushton HG, Sens MA, Garvin AJ, et al. Primary leiomyosarcoma of the ureter: a case report with electron microscopy. J Urol 1983; 129: 1045–1046.

260. Griffin JH, Waters WB. Primary leiomyosarcoma of the ureter. J Surg Oncol 1996; 62: 148–152.

261. Nakajima F, Terahata S, Hatano T, et al. Primary leiomyosarcoma of the ureter. Urol Int 1994; 53: 166–168.

262. Uhlir K. Hemangioma of the ureter. J Urol 1973; 110: 647–649.

263. Jansen TT, van deWeyer FP, deVries HR. Angiomatous ureteral polyp. Urology 1982; 20: 426–427.

264. Ogata N, Yonekawa Y. Paramedian supracerebellar approach to the upper brain stem and peduncular lesions. Neurosurgery 1997; 40: 101–105.

265. Maestroni U, Dinale F, Frattini A, et al. Ureteral hemangioma: a clinical case report. Acta Biomed 2005; 76: 115–117.

266. Coulier B, Lefebvre Y, Petein M. Renal pelvis haemangioma demonstrated by MSCT urography with ureteral compression and 3D reconstruction. JBR-BTR 2005; 88: 187–189.

267. Eble JN, Young RH, Storkel S. Primary osteosarcoma of the kidney: a report of three cases. J Urogenital Pathol 1991; 1: 83–88.

268. Charny CK, Glick RD, Genega EM, et al. Ewing's sarcoma/primitive neuroectodermal tumor of the ureter: a case report and review of the literature. J Pediatr Surg 2000; 35: 1356–1358.

269. Raj GV, Madden JF, Anderson EE. Liposarcoma presenting as an intraluminal ureteral mass. Urology 2003; 61: 1035.

270. Townsend MF 3rd, Gal AA, Thoms WW, et al. Ureteral rhabdomyosarcoma. Urology 1999; 54: 561.

271. Fein RL, Hamm FC. Malignant schwannoma of the renal pelvis: a review of the literature and a case report. J Urol 1965; 94: 356–361.

272. Frasier BL, Wachs BH, Watson LR, et al. Malignant melanoma of the renal pelvis presenting as a primary tumor. J Urol 1988; 140: 812–814.

273. Chen KT, Workman RD, Flam MS, et al. Carcinosarcoma of renal pelvis. Urology 1983; 22: 429–431.

274. Yano S, Arita M, Ueno F, et al. Carcinosarcoma of the ureter. Eur Urol 1984; 10: 71.

275. Deodhare S, Leung CS, Bullock M. Choriocarcinoma associated with transitional cell carcinoma in-situ of the ureter. Histopathology 1996; 28: 363–365.

276. Grammatico D, Grignon DJ, Eberwein P, et al. Transitional cell carcinoma of the renal pelvis with choriocarcinomatous differentiation. Immunohistochemical and immunoelectron microscopic assessment of human chorionic gonadotropin production by transitional cell carcinoma of the urinary bladder. Cancer 1993; 71: 1835–1841.

277. Zettl A, Konrad MA, Polzin S, et al. Urothelial carcinoma of the renal pelvis with choriocarcinomatous features: genetic evidence of clonal evolution. Hum Pathol 2002; 33: 1234–1237.

278. Vahlensieck W, Jr., Riede U, Wimmer B, et al. Beta-human chorionic gonadotropin-positive extragonadal germ cell neoplasia of the renal pelvis. Cancer 1991; 67: 3146–3149.

279. Harper L, Michel JL, Riviere JP, et al. Inflammatory pseudotumor of the ureter. J Pediatr Surg 2005; 40: 597–599.

280. Nozawa M, Namba Y, Nishimura K, et al. Inflammatory pseudotumor of the ureter. J Urol 1997; 157: 945.

281. Bramwit M, Kalina P, Rustia-Villa M. Inflammatory pseudotumor of the choroid plexus. AJNR Am J Neuroradiol 1997; 18: 1307–1309.

282. Scharifker D, Chalasani A. Ureteral involvement by malignant lymphoma. Ten years' experience. Arch Pathol Lab Med 1978; 102: 541–542.

THE LIBRARY
THE LEARNING AND DEVELOPMENT CENTRE
THE CALDERDALE ROYAL HOSPITAL
HALIFAX HX3 0PW

# CHAPTER 4

# Fine needle aspiration of the kidney

Andrew A. Renshaw

Fine needle aspiration (FNA) of the kidney is a useful technique for diagnosing a specific subset of renal lesions, and several reviews are available.[1-3] However, most renal lesions are *not* suitable for FNA. The vast majority are either benign cysts (based on their radiographic appearance) that can be left alone or are sufficiently worrisome that resection is indicated, regardless of the results of FNA. It is estimated that less than 10% of all renal masses are candidates for FNA.[4]

FNA of renal lesions is often helpful in the appropriate clinical setting. Although most lesions have a characteristic appearance that allows diagnosis on cytologic material, there are several important pitfalls one must be aware of in order to avoid making mistakes with these specimens.

## Background to renal fine needle aspiration

### Indications for renal fine needle aspiration

There are several indications for FNA. First, it can provide a diagnosis in a patient who is not a candidate for resection. This includes patients who are unresectable because a primary tumor is high stage, patients with presumptive metastatic disease, or patients who are not medically able to undergo resection. In addition, many urologists will follow and do not resect benign lesions such as oncocytomas, and this is a relatively common indication for FNA. Second, FNA has traditionally been used to evaluate patients with radiographically indeterminate lesions, usually cysts. However, the utility of the technique in this setting is quite limited – see the section on Non-neoplastic cysts. Finally, although the ultimate decision to perform partial rather than total nephrectomy is a surgical one, the results of FNA can be useful in triaging these patients. An increasing number of patients are potential candidates for partial nephrectomy, partly because of the availability of higher-resolution imaging techniques. These include patients with small lesions, young patients, and those at risk for multiple and bilateral lesions, such as patients with von Hippel–Lindau syndrome.[5] In the majority of these patients FNA can provide a specific or differential diagnosis.

### Specimen collection and preparation

All renal aspirations are image guided and are performed by radiologists or, rarely, surgeons at the time of operation. Most are fixed in alcohol and stained with Papanicolaou or hematoxylin and eosin stains. Cell blocks can be particularly helpful for identifying papillae and other architectural features, and many lesions are best diagnosed with immunohistochemical support (e.g., angiomyolipoma). Core needle biopsy is useful in specific settings, such as the diagnosis of oncocytoma.

### Complications

Complications of renal FNA are uncommon; they include hemorrhage, pneumothorax, infection, arteriovenous fistula, and urinoma. Death and needle track seeding by carcinoma are extraordinarily rare in the modern era with the use of smaller (less than 18 gauge) needles.

## Accuracy

The accuracy of renal FNA in the literature ranges from 64% to 94%.[6-20] Some tumors are difficult to aspirate, and between 9% and 37% of aspirates are inadequate. Repeat aspiration remains non-diagnostic in over 40% of these cases.[8,10,12,16-20] There are no defined criteria for adequacy, but an FNA is considered adequate when a specific or differential diagnosis can be made. The authors' personal experience with approximately 500 cases reveals that about 10–15% of these specimens simply do not have adequate material for diagnosis, but in the remainder it is extremely rare for the resection specimen to not correlate with the cytologic diagnosis, though this may be a differential rather than specific diagnosis.

Importantly, in the 1998 College of American Pathologists Non-Gynecologic Cytology Program,[21] renal FNA had the highest false positive rate (30.4%) of any organ system, and the second highest false negative rate (13.9%). Many of these errors relate to misinterpreting normal elements as tumor.[22] It appears that many cytologists simply are not familiar with the known pitfalls in these specimens.

## Normal elements

Normal elements, including glomeruli, proximal tubular cells, and distal tubular cells, can resemble and may be misinterpreted as tumor cells.[22] As a general rule, though, normal elements are relatively scant, whereas most tumor aspirates are highly cellular. Therefore, it is prudent to diagnose sparsely cellular aspirates as suspicious rather than positive for malignant cells.

### Glomeruli

Glomeruli (Fig. 4-1) are highly cellular globular structures that may mimic the papillae of papillary renal cell carcinoma, especially at low magnification. In contrast to papillary renal cell carcinoma, however, the endothelial cells lining the capillary loops can be seen at the extreme edge of many glomeruli. In renal cell carcinoma, cancer cells may be at the edge of a large cluster, but the cytoplasm of the cell almost always extends even more peripherally than the nucleus, and the nucleus is rounder than that of an endothelial cell.

### Proximal tubular cells

Proximal tubular cells (Fig. 4-2) consist of single cells with round bland nuclei, small but easily seen nucleoli, and abundant granular cytoplasm. These normal cells have to be ripped from their tubules, and as a result the cell membrane is usually torn and the granules often appear to be spilling out of the cells. These cells are similar if not identical to those seen in oncocytoma and some cases of papillary and chromophobe renal cell carcinoma. However, FNAs of tumors are more cellular, papillary tumors have papillae, and chromophobe cancer cells are often binucleate, with some variation in cell and nuclear size and

**A**

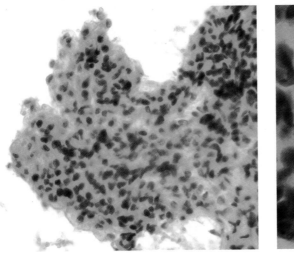

**B**

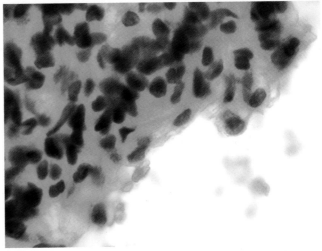

**Fig. 4-1 (A)** Glomeruli appear as rounded masses that superficially resemble papillae. **(B)** On high magnification the capillary loops and flattened endothelial cells are visible at the periphery. H&E, 200× (A); 1000× (B).

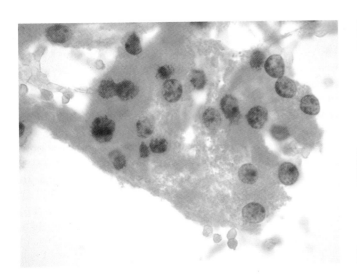

**Fig. 4-2** Proximal tubular cells. The cells have abundant granular cytoplasm and disrupted membranes. H&E, 1000×.

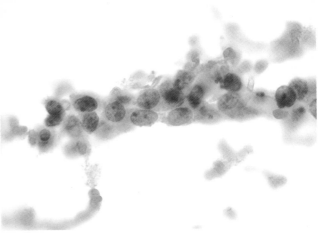

**Fig. 4-3** Distal tubular cells. The cells have scant clear cytoplasm and round nuclei with small nucleoli. H&E, 1000×.

shape, and well-defined cell borders as these cells are loosely cohesive.

## Distal tubular cells

Distal tubular cells (Fig. 4-3) are small, single or cohesive cells appearing as sheets of about 20 cells, with scant clear to slightly granular cytoplasm and small round nuclei that may contain small nucleoli. The cell membrane is intact, but may be difficult to appreciate because the cytoplasm is scant. What little cytoplasm is present is clear or minimally granular, but not vacuolated.[23] These cells are identical to those seen in low-grade clear cell or papillary renal cell carcinoma. However, aspirates of tumors should be more cellular, often have intracytoplasmic hemosiderin, and papillary renal cell carcinoma may form papillae and spherules.

## Benign lesions

### Oncocytoma

Oncocytoma comprises 3–5% of all renal tumors and is benign, although metastases have been reported.[24–29] Current criteria emphasize both cytologic and architectural features. The cells have abundant uniformly granular cytoplasm, small but distinct nucleoli which focally may reach Fuhrman grade 2 or rarely 3 in size, and have a distinctive architecture consisting of small nests and tubules without broad trabeculae that are typically seen in chromophobe renal cell carcinoma.[30] The classic gross description of oncocytoma is mahogany brown with a central stellate scar, but a more accurate description is a well-circumscribed mass that is

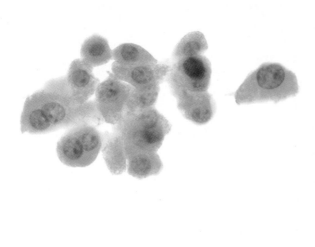

**Fig. 4-4** Oncocytoma. The cells are single, small, and uniform with abundant granular cytoplasm and round nuclei with small nucleoli. H&E, 1000×.

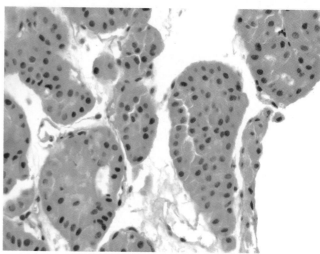

**Fig. 4-5** Oncocytoma on core biopsy. The architecture of small nests is very helpful in confirming the diagnosis. H&E, 200×.

exactly the same color as the adjacent cortex, which is mahogany brown if the kidney is removed without draining the blood first, and more pale gray or tan if the kidney has been drained before resection.

The cells of oncocytoma are easily dissociated and aspirates are typically highly cellular.[31–35] There are numerous single cells and loosely cohesive small clusters up to about 10 cells, with abundant eosinophilic granular cytoplasm, well-defined cell membranes, frequent binucleation, and round nuclei with small but distinct nucleoli (Fig. 4-4). Although atypia may be present in oncocytoma, it is 'endocrine' atypia, and consists of nuclei with marked size variation and relatively dark chromatin without prominent nucleoli. This is in marked contrast to the prominent nucleoli and fine chromatin of most renal cell carcinomas. Hyaline globules have been reported in oncocytoma,[36] but they are not specific.[37]

The differential diagnosis includes normal proximal tubules, clear cell renal cell carcinoma, chromophobe renal cell carcinoma, papillary renal cell carcinoma, and hepatocytes. The cells of proximal tubules are identical, but aspirates are scant and the cell membranes are rarely intact. Although clear cell renal cell carcinoma is always listed in the differential diagnosis of oncocytoma, in practice it is rarely a diagnostic challenge. The aspirates of clear cell renal cell carcinoma are more cohesive, have fewer single cells, have more nuclear atypia, and less uniformly granular cytoplasm. Although some clear cell tumors may have abundant granular cytoplasm, most of these are high grade. Chromophobe renal cell carcinoma may be extremely difficult to distinguish from oncocytoma, but usually has less uniformly granular cytoplasm and often more nuclear outline irregularity. Chromophobe tumors show diffuse cytoplasmic positivity with Hale's colloidal iron staining, which is diagnostic. However, oncocytoma usually displays focal to moderate membranous staining that can be misleading. Rare low-grade papillary tumors may have cells that are

identical to those seen in oncocytoma, but the papillary architecture is diagnostic. As in clear cell tumors, most papillary tumors with granular cytoplasm are higher grade. Rarely, inadvertent sampling of the liver can superficially resemble oncocytoma, as hepatocytes have abundant granular cytoplasm. However, hepatocytes are usually aspirated in groups as well as singly, may have bile, and have more variation in the size of cells and their nuclei.

It is currently controversial whether oncocytoma should be diagnosed on fine needle aspiration alone. There is no specific immunohistochemical marker for oncocytoma. In addition, individual cells in both clear cell and papillary tumors can be identical to those seen in oncocytoma, and large areas of chromophobe renal cell carcinoma can strongly resemble oncocytoma even on resection. Finally, hybrid tumors that have features of both chromophobe renal cell carcinoma and oncocytoma have been described, both sporadically and in association with Birt–Hogg–Dube syndrome.[38] In such cases it may be best to diagnose these lesions as oncocytic neoplasms, list the differential diagnosis, and suggest that, if clinically indicated, partial nephrectomy should be considered. If a definite diagnosis is desired, core needle biopsy may be preferred (Fig. 4-5) in which the nested architecture of oncocytoma can be distinguished from that of chromophobe renal cell carcinoma. At present, the diagnosis of oncocytoma on aspirate material alone is a diagnosis of exclusion. Although it is true that the more cells in an aspirate that resemble oncocytoma the more likely it is that the aspirate is truly oncocytoma and not one of its many mimics, the cellularity necessary to make this diagnosis reliably is not known.

## Cortical adenoma

Renal cortical adenoma is histologically, immunohistochemically, and cytogenetically indistinguishable from low-grade papillary renal cell carcinoma except by size.[39,40] Renal adenoma is defined as a small lesion always less than 0.5 cm in diameter, and usually less than 0.2 cm.[41] As a result, these lesions are too small to be reliably aspirated, and the diagnosis of renal cortical adenoma is inappropriate in FNA specimens.

## Angiomyolipoma

Angiomyolipoma is a benign tumor that can rarely metastasize. It occurs in two distinct clinical settings:[42-44] approximately half of the cases occur in young adults with tuberous sclerosis and are usually multiple and bilateral; the other half occur in young and middle-aged women without any known clinical syndrome, and are usually solitary. This tumor may bleed profusely, and when greater than 5 cm in diameter is often resected to prevent this. Angiomyolipoma is composed of three elements: blood vessels, mature fat, and atypical smooth muscle cells that are reactive for HMB45.

FNA of typical angiomyolipoma with abundant adipose tissue is easy to diagnose,[45-55] but this tumor is rarely aspirated because it can be diagnosed by identifying the fat radiographically. Most FNAs are obtained from masses with little adipose tissue. In general, the vessels are too large to be aspirated, although rarely large intact vessels are identified (Fig. 4-6). As a result, the predominant cell in most aspirates is the atypical smooth muscle cell, and this can be very challenging to diagnose. The aspirates are generally paucicellular and at low magnification consist of relatively large groups of elongated and round cells that resemble abnormal stroma (Fig. 4-7). The cells are cohesive, and single cells are rare. Unlike the cellular groups of renal cell carcinoma, these groups are less dense and have more cytoplasm. At higher magnification, the cells consist predominantly of atypical smooth muscle cells that may be elongated (Fig. 4-8), round (Fig. 4-9), benign-appearing, or markedly atypical. The cytoplasm is often stringy rather than granular or vacuolated, but this may be difficult to appreciate (Fig. 4-10). Infrequently,

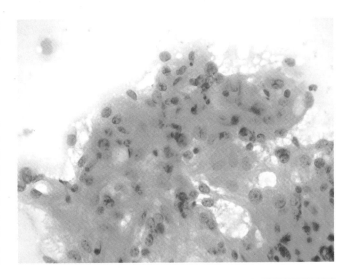

**Fig. 4-7** Angiomyolipoma. On low magnification there are cohesive clusters of cells with abundant cytoplasm. H&E, 200×.

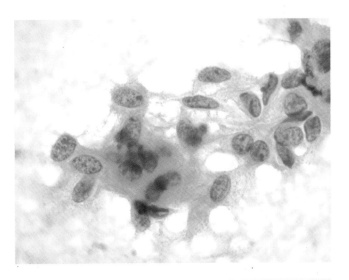

**Fig. 4-8** Angiomyolipoma. Some cells are elongated. H&E, 1000×.

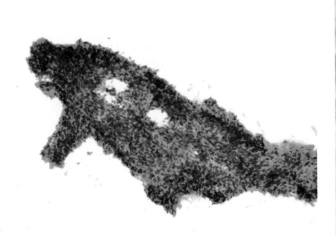

**Fig. 4-6** Angiomyolipoma. Rarely, a large vessel is aspirated. H&E, 200×.

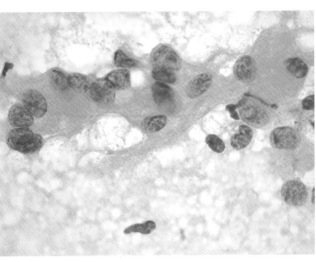

**Fig. 4-9** Angiomyolipoma. Some cells are round. H&E, 1000×.

large clear vacuoles are also present, perhaps representing fat. The atypia consists of markedly enlarged dark hyperchromatic round nuclei (Fig. 4-11). In contrast to the atypia seen in most cases of clear cell rare cell carcinoma, the chromatin is usually much darker, nucleoli are absent, and the atypia is present in rare cells rather than in the majority. However, the atypia in some cases of angiomyolipoma is both marked and varied, and virtually any pattern may be seen in such cases. Immunoreactivity for HMB45 is helpful, and is employed whenever the diagnosis of a renal aspirate is not clear.

Several lesions may mimic angiomyolipoma on FNA. When atypical smooth muscle cells appear round, they resemble clear cell renal cell carcinoma.[12,47,56] Often, the

nuclei will have more granular and dark chromatin and lack prominent nucleoli typical of clear cell renal cell carcinoma. In addition, the quality of the cytoplasm is different, consisting of stringy material with rare large clear vacuoles, rather than the mixture of clear and granular material. Staining with EMA, keratin, and HMB45 is advisable with any pleomorphic round cell aspirate. When the cells are elongated, the major differential diagnosis is sarcoma[57] or sarcomatoid renal cell carcinoma. Immunohistochemistry is the best way to distinguish these lesions.

## Metanephric adenoma

Metanephric adenoma[58–61] is another benign lesion in which metastases have been reported.[62] It typically occurs in women in the fifth decade, and is composed of tubules and papillae that form 'glomeruloid bodies' lined by uniformly benign-appearing cells with occasional psammoma bodies. The tumor is EMA negative and has a normal karyotype, helpful features in distinguishing it from renal cell carcinoma.

Cytologically,[63] metanephric adenoma consist of small short papillae and loose sheets of cells and individual cells pulled out of the papillae with scant cytoplasm, round nuclei, fine even chromatin, and rare small nucleoli. The chromatin resembles that seen in papillary carcinoma of the thyroid.

The differential diagnosis includes Wilms' tumor, low-grade papillary renal cell carcinoma, and metastases. It may not be possible to distinguish metanephric adenoma from Wilms' tumor, although the latter may have larger cells with more hyperchromasia and mitotic figures.[59] Low-grade papillary renal cell carcinoma also has similar features, but has more cytoplasm and is EMA positive.[39,59] Both metanephric adenoma and metastases often have a high nuclear to cytoplasmic (N/C) ratio, but metastases are often EMA positive

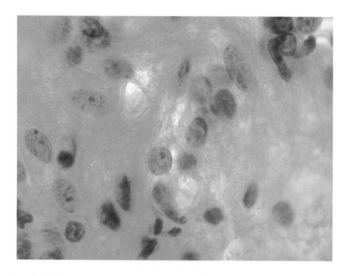

**Fig. 4-10** Angiomyolipoma. The cytoplasm has a stringy appearance. H&E, 1000×.

A

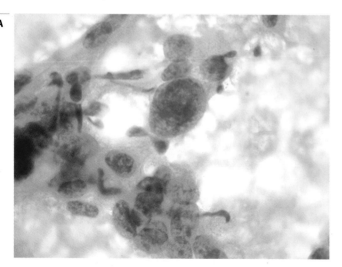

B

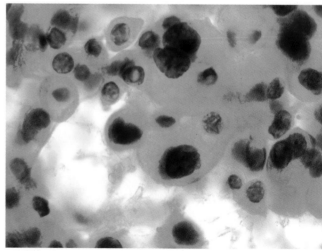

**Fig. 4-11** Angiomyolipoma. The atypia consists most often of single markedly enlarged round nuclei with dark hyperchromatic chromatin and no nucleoli. H&E, 1000×.

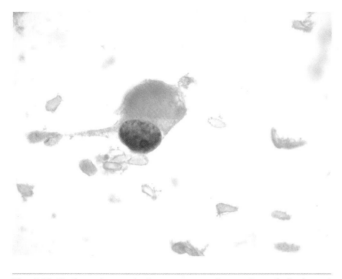

**Fig. 4-12** Cystic nephroma. Aspirates may contain round or spindle-shaped cells with minimal or marked atypia, and may not be distinguishable from renal cell carcinoma. Most aspirates, however, are scant. H&E, 1000×.

and should never be diagnosed in the absence of a clinical history.

## Cystic nephroma

Cystic nephroma is a benign tumor that can mimic renal cell carcinoma and typically presents as an isolated mass.[44] It is composed of stroma and small cysts sometimes lined by atypical epithelium. Importantly, although cystic, this lesion often appears solid radiographically. FNAs are *usually* misdiagnosed as either renal cell carcinoma, angiomyolipoma, or sarcoma[11,64,65] because they contain markedly atypical round cells or, less commonly, spindle cells. The round cells are typically single and contain clear to vacuolated cytoplasm, nuclear membrane irregularity, and prominent nucleoli[66,67] (Fig. 4-12). The spindle cells are large, pleomorphic, and admixed with cells having intracytoplasmic vacuoles simulating fat.[68] Without a cell block or a core biopsy to demonstrate the characteristic arrangement of cysts and cellular stroma, most aspirates consisting of scant atypical round cells with clear cytoplasm cannot be reliably distinguished from clear cell renal cell carcinoma. Nevertheless, these specimens are almost always hypocellular and consist of single cells without large groups. Diagnosing scant specimens as suspicious rather than positive is the best way to avoid a misdiagnosis.

## Xanthogranulomatous pyelonephritis

Xanthogranulomatous pyelonephritis[10] is a reactive process that may present as a mass mimicking renal cell carcinoma. The mass is composed of histiocytes and multinucleated giant cells. The histiocytes may be grouped and resemble clear cell renal cell carcinoma, but are distinguishable by having dirtier cytoplasm, smaller microvesicles in the cytoplasm, an absence of nuclear atypia, and, most often, bean-shaped nuclei rather than the round nuclei typical of renal

cell carcinoma. In addition, histiocytes are positive for CD68 and negative for keratin and EMA.

## Non-neoplastic cysts

Renal cysts are common. Half of men over the age of 50 years have at least one cyst,[69,70] and up to 85% of all renal masses are cysts. The majority are benign, acquired, and solitary, but 1–4% of kidneys with cysts have coexistent renal cell carcinoma which may or may not involve the cyst.[71–77] The renal cell carcinoma is usually either clear cell or papillary type.[44] Although cystic carcinoma is malignant,[78] the prognosis of cystic renal cell carcinoma is generally excellent.[79,80]

Aspirates of cystic renal masses have relatively low sensitivity. In patients with cystic renal cell carcinoma, FNA is more likely to yield a false negative diagnosis than a true positive result.

Cystic lesions are classified based on the radiographic appearance using the four-category Bosniak system.[81–86] Most lesions are category 1 and benign, and receive no further evaluation. Category 4 lesions are highly suspicious for renal cell carcinoma and should be resected directly without the need for additional studies. Category 2 and 3 lesions are indeterminate and problematic. Between 5% and 57% of indeterminate lesions are malignant, and these are often selected for FNA.

It is difficult to determine the exact sensitivity of FNA for Bosniak category 2 and 3 lesions, for several reasons. First, most of the cytology literature on FNA of cystic lesions predates CT and MR imaging,[8,70,74,75,87–90] and certainly includes a high preponderance of both category 1 and category 4 lesions. In general, 9–37% of FNAs of *all* renal cell carcinomas, most of which are solid, are non-diagnostic.[6,8,11,12,91–93] Second, most renal cell carcinomas interpreted as negative on FNA have a cystic component.[93] Third, most radiographically suspicious cysts prove to be renal cell carcinoma.[6,11,12] Finally, in the largest series describing the FNA features of cystic renal cell carcinoma to date (11 cases), only two cases had atypical cells on cytologic examination, and repeat aspirates in these two patients were both negative.[94]

From the cumulative data, we estimate that the sensitivity of renal FNA of Bosniak category 2 and 3 lesions is approximately 10–20%. Obviously, in those patients in which a positive or suspicious diagnosis can be rendered, renal FNA is of value, but this represents a minority of patients. Most patients with Bosniak category 2 and 3 lesions have a negative aspirate. As the risk of malignancy is 5–57% prior to the FNA, a negative result does not change the patient's risk.

How should these aspirates be interpreted? Most often one sees proteinaceous debris and macrophages. These should be signed out as negative, but with a comment stating either that renal cell carcinoma cannot be ruled out or that clinical correlation is necessary to ensure the sample is representative of the underlying lesion. Occasionally, a few small epithelial cells are identified with little or no atypia. Most of these are single cells or very small groups of cells. Again, these can be signed out as negative, with the above comment. In some cases, rare epithelial cells will show either nuclear or cytoplasmic atypia. Nuclear atypia consists of nuclear enlargement with or without prominent nucleoli or nuclear outline irregularity. Cytoplasmic atypia consists of clearing of the cytoplasm, a finding that is distinctly uncommon in normal renal epithelial cells but which may be observed in 'atypical cyst lining cells.' In either case the optimal diagnosis is suspicious for malignancy, knowing that many cases will prove to be reactive cyst lining cells, but that some may be cystic renal cell carcinoma. Unless the case is very cellular, it is prudent not to render a definitive diagnosis.

## Acquired cystic disease and adult polycystic disease

Patients with acquired cystic disease secondary to renal failure often develop multiple cysts, and 9% develop renal cell carcinoma that is often multifocal and papillary.[95–98] Similarly, patients with adult polycystic kidney disease are also at increased risk of renal cell carcinoma that is likewise often multifocal and papillary. In both settings, patients routinely develop papillary hyperplasia[99] within the cysts, and distinction between hyperplasia and carcinoma is not possible on FNA. In contrast to most non-neoplastic cysts, larger groups of cells rather than single cells may be aspirated. Fortunately, the underlying disease is almost always known in these patients, and therefore it is probably best to avoid cyst FNA. However, when presented with an aspirate from a patient with either disease, high cellularity is the strongest diagnostic clue for malignancy.

## Other benign lesions

A variety of unusual benign lesions may be diagnosed by FNA. Abscesses, pyelonephritis,[4,89] and infarcts[100] have been reportedly misdiagnosed as renal cell carcinoma. Each of these lesions may have markedly atypical cells, but the cellularity is scant and thus they should not be diagnosed as posi-tive for malignancy. Other lesions that have been described on FNA include Liesegang rings,[101] malakoplakia,[102] aspergil-losis,[103] actinomycosis,[104] and retroperitoneal fibrosis.[105]

## Malignant lesions

### Renal cell carcinoma

The most common malignant tumor of the kidney is renal cell carcinoma. These tumors are most commonly graded using the 4-tiered Fuhrman system,[106] and there is good cytologic and histologic correlation for this grading scheme.[107,108] Renal cell carcinoma is classified histologically according to the most recent consensus classification system,[41] and histologic subtyping performed on aspiration material correlates well with subtype on resection.[93,109] The cytologic features of each subtype are sufficiently distinct that an accurate diagnosis can often be made by FNA.

#### Conventional clear cell renal cell carcinoma

Clear cell renal cell carcinoma comprises 75% of all renal cell carcinomas. Genetic analysis shows frequent deletions of chromosome 3p, the site of the von Hippel–Lindau gene.[110–113]

The cytology of these tumors can be divided into three overlapping patterns, depending on grade and whether the cells are easily spread out on the slide. The first pattern, the classic pattern, is usually seen with high-grade tumors, and consists of a highly cellular aspirate with large groups of cells and isolated cells containing abundant cytoplasm, a low N/C ratio, and centrally located round to slightly irregular nuclei with prominent nucleoli[8,23,114,115] (Fig. 4-13). The nuclei may be eccentric, sometimes to the point of appearing to be partially extruded. The cytoplasm is translucent and vacuolated, often with peripheral vacuoles. This combina-tion of eccentric round nuclei with central cytoplasm mimics the cytology of plasma cells, and these cells have been

A
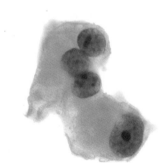

B
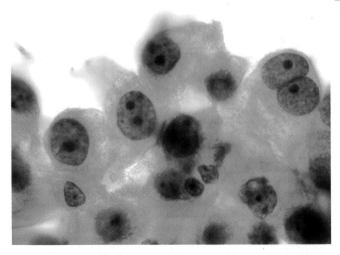

**Fig. 4-13** Clear cell renal cell carcinoma, classic cytology, high-grade tumor. Tumor cells have abundant clear to granular cytoplasm, large round nuclei which are eccentrically located, and prominent nucleoli. H&E, 1000x.

described as plasmacytoid. High-grade tumors have more isolated cells and less vacuolization. Occasionally clear cell tumors – usually high-grade ones – have neutrophils within the cytoplasm, a finding that is relatively specific for the clear cell subtype.

The second cytologic pattern of clear cell carcinoma is seen in low-grade tumors. In this setting, the cells are arranged in small sheets with a bland appearance that resembles normal distal tubular cells (Fig. 4-14). The best way to distinguish these cells from normal cells is by the increased cellularity, although some low-grade cancers are difficult to aspirate. Occasionally, a scant amount of hemosiderin is also present, and this can be quite helpful.[116] However, low-grade clear cell carcinoma is usually difficult to diagnose on direct smears, in contrast to cell block material.

The third cytologic pattern of clear cell carcinoma is observed in both low- and high-grade tumors. In this pattern, the tumor cells are difficult to aspirate as the neoplastic cells are tightly adherent to the fibrous stroma. The aspirate consists of chunks of highly cellular fibrous tissue, and one must go to high magnification and diligently screen the edge of the tissue to identify the neoplastic cells (Fig. 4-15). The tumor cells are best identified by the clear cytoplasm and location lining the fibrous stroma. Similar to the second pattern, direct smears of such cases are extremely difficult to interpret, in contrast with the cell blocks. In some cases an EMA stain may be helpful in distinguishing tumor cells from macrophages.

The differential diagnosis includes benign tubular cells, macrophages, adrenal cortical cells, hepatocytes, cystic

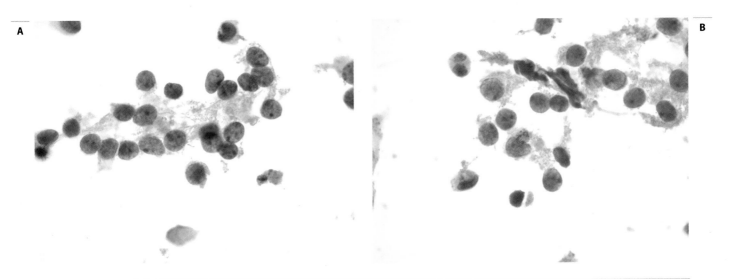

**Fig. 4-14** Clear cell renal cell carcinoma, low-grade. **(A)** The cells are small with scant cytoplasm and minimal atypia, resembling distal tubular cells. **(B)** Some clear cell tumors have a scant amount of hemosiderin in a perinuclear location which is quite characteristic. However, intracytoplasmic hemosiderin is much more common in papillary tumors. Cellularity may be the best clue that this is malignant. H&E, 200× **(A)** 1000× **(B)**.

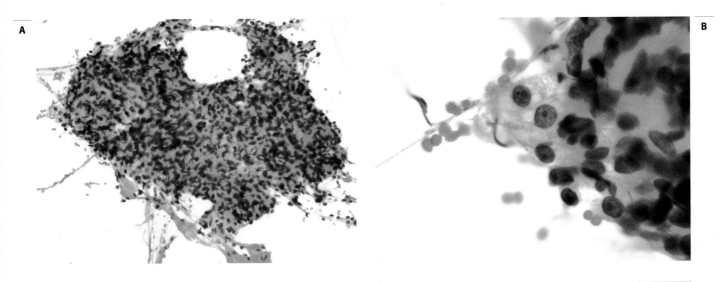

**Fig. 4-15** Clear cell renal cell carcinoma. **(A)** The cells are tightly cohesive, appearing as cellular chunks of tissue. **(B)** In such cases, diligent screening around the edge of the cluster can reveal identifiable neoplastic cells. H&E, 200× **(A)** 1000× **(B)**.

nephroma, cystic renal disease, and other types of renal cell carcinoma. Aspirates of tubular cells are typically scant and rarely contain large groups. The cells do not have vacuolated cytoplasm or contain hemosiderin. Macrophages rarely produce large groups of cells, do not have an extruded nucleus, are more uniformly microvacuolated, have dirty cytoplasm, contain kidney bean-shaped rather than round nuclei, and lack atypia. Adrenal cortical cells are more uniform, have smaller vacuoles, and often have stripped cytoplasm, so that one typically sees bare nuclei in a background of proteinaceous debris (Fig. 4-16). Hepatocytes are more uniformly granular, may contain bile, and have round nuclei of various sizes that are almost always centrally located (Fig. 4-17). Cystic nephroma may have individual cells that are virtually identical to clear cell renal cell carcinoma, and may be markedly atypical. In general, however, these aspirates are paucicellular and should be diagnosed as suspicious rather than positive. Cystic renal disease, including acquired cystic disease and adult polycystic renal disease, can also have cells that are virtually identical to those seen in clear cell renal cell carcinoma, but the cellularity is usually low.

## Papillary renal cell carcinoma

Papillary renal cell carcinoma is defined histologically as a tumor with at least 50% true papillae (although in some cases these are closely packed and may appear solid[39]), and comprises between 7% and 15% of cases of renal cell carcinoma.[39,117,118] This cancer commonly has trisomies of chromosomes 7, 16, and 17,[40,119,120] is associated with renal cortical adenoma,[121] and is often multifocal.[121] Large tumors may be cystic and necrotic, and may appear cystic radiologically. Low-grade/low-stage papillary renal cell carcinoma has an excellent prognosis,[117,118,120] whereas the prognosis for high-grade/high-stage carcinoma is poor.[120,122] Immunohistochemically these tumors are immunoreactive for EMA, low molecular weight keratin, and CK7,[39,123] and negative for high molecular weight keratin 34BE12.

Like clear cell carcinoma, papillary cancer has several overlapping cytologic patterns. The most common is seen in low-grade cancers.[124–127] This tumor can only be recognized by its architectural appearance, as it lacks atypia and the cells are cytologically identical to those of distal tubules with scant clear cytoplasm. Architecturally, papillae are often recognized at low power, but more commonly one sees spherules, tubules, or rosettes that lack fibrovascular cores[128] (Fig. 4-18). The majority have clear cytoplasm, but rare cases contain abundant granular cytoplasm (Fig. 4-19). Cytologically, the cells are identical to those seen in oncocytoma, but the papillary architecture is diagnostic. More commonly, tumors with abundant granular cytoplasm are higher grade and have relatively prominent nucleoli (Fig. 4-20). Some of these tumors have true papillae with fibrovascular cores distended with macrophages, a feature that is best appreciated in cell blocks. The cells have more granular cytoplasm and resemble proximal tubular cells more than distal tubular cells. There is abundant intracytoplasmic hemosiderin, much more than that rarely seen in clear cell carcinoma, and this is strongly suggestive of papillary cancer. Psammoma bodies are helpful when present, but are uncommon. High-grade papillary carcinoma may be mistaken for high-grade clear cell carcinoma owing to the typical presence of large round nuclei, prominent nucleoli, and relatively abundant granular cytoplasm.

The differential diagnosis includes distal tubular cells, proximal tubular cells, oncocytoma, other types of renal cell carcinoma, and cystic renal disease. Low-grade cancer can be distinguished from distal tubular cells by increased cellularity and distinctive architecture, including papillae, spherules, and rosettes. Rare low-grade tumors are cytologically identical to oncocytoma, but the papillary architecture is diagnostic. Most papillary cancers with abundant granular cytoplasm are high grade, and nuclear size and prominent nucleoli are the most useful discriminating features. However, distinguishing high-grade papillary cancer and clear cell renal cell carcinoma in FNA samples can be extremely difficult.[93] Fortunately, this distinction is not usually clinically significant.

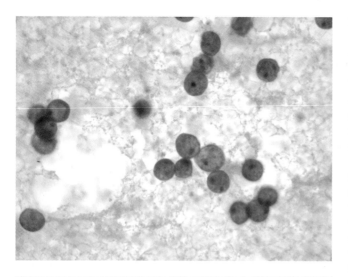

**Fig. 4-16** Adrenal cortical cells consist of bare round nuclei in a background of granular debris representing stripped cytoplasm. H&E, 1000×.

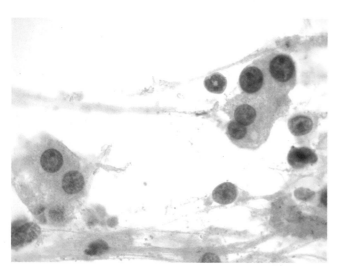

**Fig. 4-17** Hepatocytes are remarkably common in renal aspirates. H&E, 1000×.

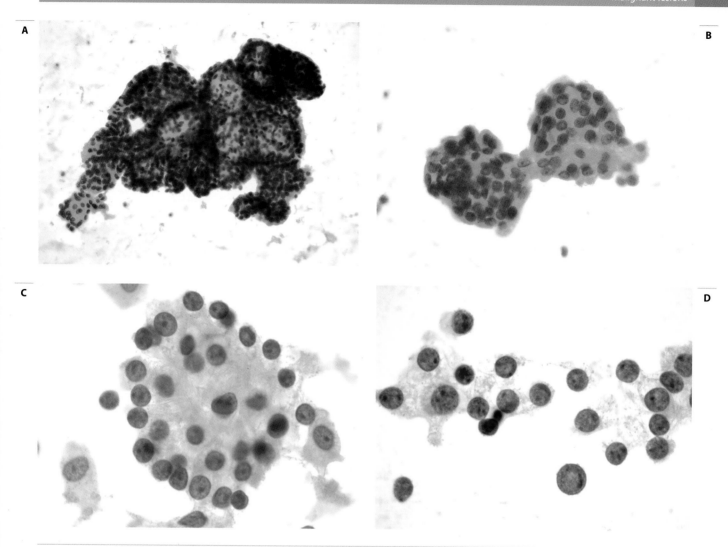

**Fig. 4-18** Papillary renal cell carcinoma, low-grade. Classic features include **(A)** papillae, **(B)** spherules, and **(C)** rosettes. **(D)** Atypia is minimal. H&E, 200× (A,B,C) 1000× (D).

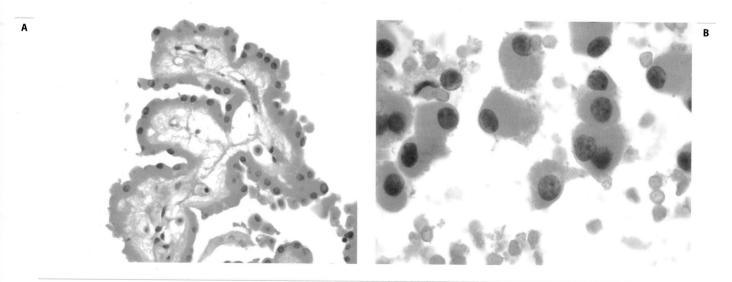

**Fig. 4-19** Papillary renal cell carcinoma, low-grade, with granular cytoplasm. Such tumors are rare. **(A)** The papillae are diagnostic. If only individual cells are seen **(B)**, the tumor cannot be distinguished from oncocytoma H&E, 400× (A) 1000× (B).

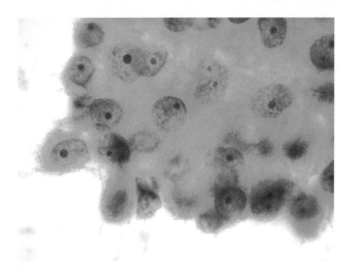

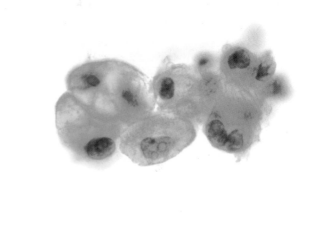

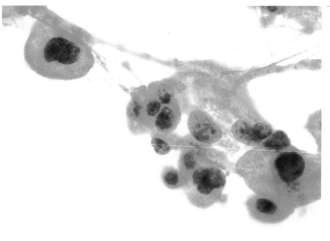

**Fig. 4-20** Papillary renal cell carcinoma. Tumors with abundant granular cytoplasm are typically higher grade, like this one. H&E, 1000×.

**Fig. 4-21** Chromophobe renal cell carcinoma. **(A)** Typical and **(B)** eosinophilic variants. The cells have a 'koilocytic' appearance. H&E, 1000×.

Cystic renal disease, including acquired cystic disease and adult polycystic renal disease, can also have cells that are virtually identical to those seen in papillary renal cell carcinoma, but the cellularity is scant.

### Chromophobe renal cell carcinoma

Chromophobe renal cell carcinoma comprises 3–5% of all renal cell carcinomas,[129-131] is associated with numerous specific chromosomal deletions,[132-134] and unless large or multifocal has an excellent prognosis.[130,135-137]

Most aspirates of chromophobe carcinoma are very cellular, consisting of groups and isolated cells that are generally less cohesive than other clear cell tumors[138-140] (Fig. 4-21). To many cytologists, the cells of chromophobe renal cell carcinoma have a 'koilocytic' appearance as a result of cytoplasmic and nuclear features reminiscent of koilocytes in cervical smears. These features include large cells with prominent cell membranes and abundant fluffy granular cytoplasm. Binucleation is common. Some nuclei are round and bland, but the majority in chromophobe carcinoma have markedly irregular outlines, dark hyperchromatic chromatin, and a marked size variation. Prominent nucleoli are uncommon. These nuclear features are distinctly different from those of most other renal cell carcinomas.

The eosinophilic variant of chromophobe carcinoma has more granular cytoplasm, whereas typical variants have more clear cytoplasm. The cytoplasm stains diffusely positive with Hale's colloidal iron stain.

The differential diagnosis depends upon whether the tumor is typical or eosinophilic variant. Typical chromophobe carcinoma resembles clear cell carcinoma, and the eosinophilic variant resembles oncocytoma. Unlike clear cell tumors, chromophobe cancer has more variation in cell and nuclear size, darker chromatin without nucleoli, and more irregular nuclear outlines. In contrast to oncocytoma, the eosinophilic variant of chromophobe carcinoma has more nuclear size variation and outline irregularity, but some

cases may be impossible to distinguish by cytology alone (Fig. 4-22). Diffuse cytoplasmic staining with Hale's colloidal iron is diagnostic of chromophobe renal cell carcinoma, but oncocytoma may have significant cell membrane staining.

### Sarcomatoid renal cell carcinoma

Sarcomatoid carcinoma comprises about 3% of renal cell carcinomas, is high grade, and has a poor prognosis. Many of these tumors are unresectable at presentation, and are thus potential candidates for FNA.[141,142] Nevertheless, more tumors are being identified at a lower stage and these patients may have a better prognosis. The tumors by definition have foci of high-grade spindle cells[114,143] and may also have a round cell component. If this is lacking, then the tumor should be keratin or EMA positive.

Both the cytologic and the differential diagnoses are strongly dependent upon sampling. Most aspirates are highly cellular and easily diagnosed as high-grade carcinoma. For the diagnosis of sarcomatoid carcinoma a spindle cell component should be identified, although this is often less spindled on cytology than it is in histology. If only the spindle cell area is sampled, sarcoma and angiomyolipoma should be excluded. If only the epithelioid area is sampled, clear cell renal cell carcinoma must be considered.

## Collecting duct renal cell carcinoma

This is a rare tumor[144–154] that is poorly defined,[155] characterized by a medullary location, tubulopapillary histology, high-grade cytology, and prominent desmoplasia. It may be confused with other tumors, especially renal medullary carcinoma[156] and papillary renal cell carcinoma.[149–151,157,158] Characteristically, this tumor is reactive for high molecular weight cytokeratin 34BE12.[146,152] A low-grade variant has been reported,[159] but the cytologic features have not yet been described.

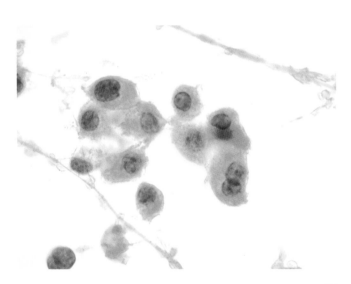

**Fig. 4-22** Chromophobe renal cell carcinoma. Areas like this may be difficult to distinguish from oncocytoma. H&E, 1000×.

Although there are numerous case reports of the cytology of collecting duct carcinoma, given the uncertainty of the diagnostic criteria it is not clear whether the histologic diagnosis in many of these cases is correct. Nevertheless, the features most commonly described include large hyperchromatic nuclei and scant cytoplasm which resemble metastasis.[160–164] The differential includes metastatic disease, urothelial carcinoma, and renal cell carcinoma, NOS.

## Other malignant lesions

### Metastases

Metastases are present in up to 7.2% of all cancer patients at autopsy,[165] but most are clinically silent. It is extremely uncommon for metastases to the kidney to present as the initial manifestation of malignancy, and 'metastases' without a known primary often represent unusual primary tumors[166] (see below). The lung is the most common site of origin for metastases to the kidney, although they may arise from any site (Fig. 4-23).

Cytologically,[6,8,93,167,168] metastases present with scant cytoplasm, a high N/C ratio, irregular nuclear outlines, and hyperchromatic chromatin. These features are unusual for most renal cell carcinomas. One study suggested that the presence of a heterogeneous cell population, small cytoplasmic vacuoles, hemosiderin deposits, and a low N/C ratio were the best features to distinguish metastasis from renal cell carcinoma.[169]

Depending on the site of origin, many metastases are positive for mucicarmine, CEA, and TTF-1, and most are negative for CD10 and RCC antigen,[170] and this combination of stains can be used to rule out a renal cell carcinoma. The differential with typical variants of renal cell carcinoma is usually not difficult, although metastatic thyroid carcinoma, which can present a very long time after the initial resection, may strongly resemble renal cell carcinoma.[171] Distinguishing metastases from urothelial carcinoma can be challenging (see below).

**A**
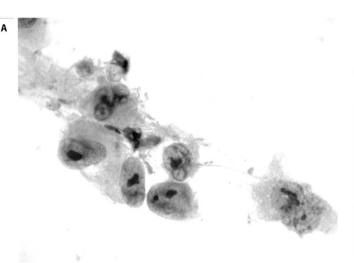
**B**
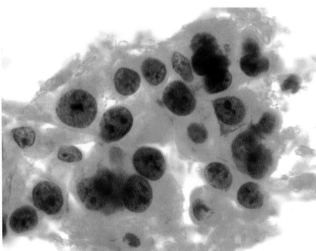

**Fig. 4-23** Metastases. Most metastases have relatively high N/C ratios and granular chromatin. These two examples from **(A)** lung and **(B)** melanoma could easily be confused with primary renal cell carcinoma. History and immunohistochemical findings are essential. H&E, 1000×.

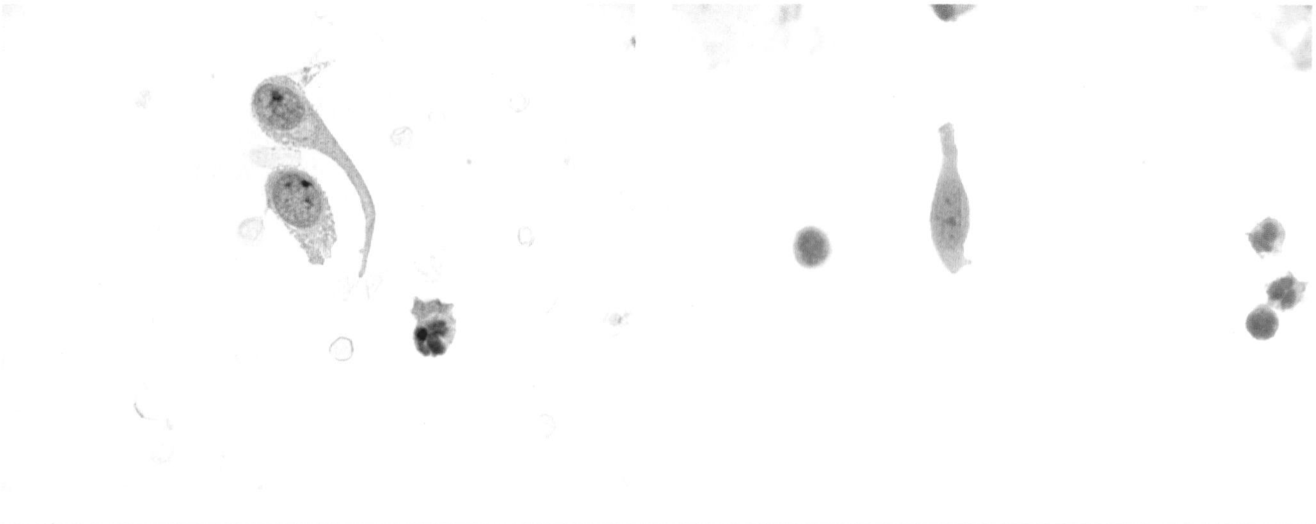

A                                                                                                                                    B

**Fig. 4-24** Urothelial carcinoma. These cercariform cells have long flat tails that are characteristic of urothelial carcinoma. H&E, 1000×.

Metastases rarely present in the kidney without a known primary site, so one should be cautious about diagnosing metastasis without a prior history. When one sees a lesion that looks like a metastasis in the absence of a clinical history, one should first consider urothelial carcinoma and then a variety of rare primary renal tumors, including collecting duct carcinoma, mucin-positive carcinoma,[172] small cell carcinoma,[173] and lymphoma,[174] all of which may not be distinguishable from metastases on cytologic material alone.

### Urothelial carcinoma

Urothelial carcinoma that arises in the renal pelvis is treated differently (nephroureterectomy) from renal cell carcinoma (nephrectomy), so it is clinically important to make this distinction. Cytologically, low- and high-grade urothelial tumors have different appearances.[6–8,175] Low-grade carcinoma is characteristically composed of sheets and papillae of cells with moderate amounts of opaque cytoplasm without vacuolization, containing large hyperchromatic nuclei with granular chromatin. In some cases, cells have long cytoplasmic tails that are narrow in the middle, wider at the ends, and flattened (Fig. 4-24). These cells, termed cercariform cells,[176–178] are characteristic of urothelial carcinoma, and when present in large numbers can be helpful in distinguishing this tumor from those of other sites.

Typically, high-grade urothelial carcinoma consists of isolated cells and small clusters with scant cytoplasm that may contain vacuoles, a high N/C ratio, dense hyperchromatic chromatin, and irregular nuclei (Fig. 4-25). Cercariform cells may also be present, and such cases are usually easy to distinguish from renal cell carcinoma. In difficult cases immunohistochemical studies may be helpful, as urothelial carcinoma is usually positive for keratin 34BE12, CK20, CEA, and mucicarmine, whereas renal cell carcinoma is negative. Separation of urothelial carcinoma and metastases can be very difficult, but it is useful to collectively consider the

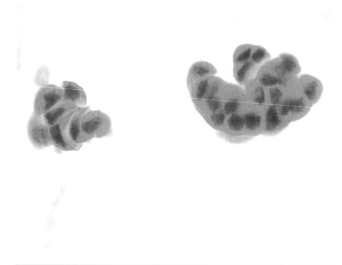

**Fig. 4-25** Urothelial carcinoma, high grade. The hyperchromatic markedly angulated nuclei are easily distinguished from renal cell carcinoma, although metastasis may be difficult to exclude. H&E, 1000×.

clinical history, immunohistochemical results for CK20 and TTF-1 (to exclude lung tumors especially), and the presence of cercariform cells.

### Rare malignant tumors

The cytologic features of a variety of unusual malignant tumors have been described, including mucinous tubular and spindle cell renal cell carcinoma,[179] low-grade myxoid renal epithelial neoplasm,[180] clear cell sarcoma,[181,182] rhabdoid tumor,[183] translocation-associated renal tumor,[184] primitive neuroectodermal tumor,[185,186] synovial sarcoma,[187] mesoblastic nephroma in an adult,[188] low-grade fibromyxoid sarcoma,[189] acute leukemia,[190] renal lymphoma,[191] renal medullary carcinoma,[192] Wilms' tumor in adults,[193] and neuroblastoma.[194]

# Future trends

## Fine needle aspiration in pediatric patients

Renal FNA is a useful technique for selected renal masses. Until recently, FNA was not commonly used in children because, by definition, aspiration of Wilms' tumor, the most common renal tumor in this age group, upstaged the patient, but this has recently been changed. Whether this will encourage the use of FNA in this patient population is unclear. FNA in pediatric patients can be challenging, however, because the cytologic appearance of some tumors, including clear cell sarcoma, can be very difficult.

## Renal mass ablation

Over the past decade radiologists have used a variety of methods, including chemicals, heat, and radiofrequency, to destroy renal masses in situ without resection. The procedure has been shown to be safe, and follow-up in these patients is currently being accrued. Renal FNA with immediate assessment has been shown to be an accurate method of following these treatments.[195]

## REFERENCES

1. Renshaw AA, Granter SR, Cibas ES. Fine needle aspiration of the adult kidney. Cancer Cytopathol 1997; 81: 71–88.

2. Renshaw A. Aspiration cytology. A pattern recognition approach. Philadelphia: Elsevier Saunders, 2005.

3. Renshaw AA. Kidney and adrenal gland. In: Cibas ES, Ducatman BS, eds. Cytology. Diagnostic principles and clinical correlates, 2nd edn. Edinburgh: WB Saunders, 2003; 383–404.

4. Kelley CM, Cohen MB, Raab SS. Utility of fine-needle aspiration biopsy in solid renal masses. Diagn Cytopathol 1996; 14: 14–19.

5. Renshaw AA, Corless CL. Papillary renal cell carcinoma: gross features and histologic correlates. J Urol Pathol 1997; 7: 9–19.

6. Helm CW, Burwood RJ, Harrison NW, Melcher DH. Aspiration cytology of solid renal tumors. J Urol 1983; 55: 249–253.

7. Juul N, Torp-Pedersen S, Gronvall S, et al. Ultrasonically guided fine needle aspiration biopsy of renal masses. J Urol 1985; 133: 579–581.

8. Murphy WM, Zambroni BR, Emerson LD, et al. Aspiration biopsy of the kidney. Cancer 1985; 56: 200–205.

9. Dekmezian RH, Charnsangavej C, Rava P, Katz RL. Fine needle aspiration of kidney tumors in 105 patients: a cytologic and histologic correlation. Acta Cytol 1985; 29: 931.

10. Nguyen GK. Percutaneous fine-needle aspiration biopsy cytology of the kidney and adrenal. Pathol Annu 1987; 22: 163–191.

11. Pilotti S, Rilke F, Alasio L, Garbagnati F. The role of fine needle aspiration in the assessment of renal masses. Acta Cytol 1988; 32: 1–10.

12. Cristallini EG, Paganelli C, Bolis GB. Role of fine-needle aspiration biopsy in the assessment of renal masses. Diagn Cytopathol 1991; 7: 32–35.

13. Truong LD, Todd TD, Dhurandhar B, Ramzy I. Fine-needle aspiration of renal masses in adults: analysis of results and diagnostic problems in 108 cases. Diagn Cytopathol 1999; 20: 339–349.

14. Zardawi IM. Renal fine needle aspiration cytology. Acta Cytol 1999; 43: 184–190.

15. Sengupta S, Zincke H, Blute ML. The accuracy of 250 fine needle biopsies of renal tumors. J Urol 2005; 174: 44–46.

16. Wunderlich H, Hindermann W, Mustafa AMA, et al. The accuracy of 250 fine needle biopsies of renal tumors. J Urol 2005; 174: 44–46.

17. Neuzillet Y, Lechevallier E, Andre M, et al. Accuracy and clinical role of fine needle percutaneous biopsy with computerized tomography guidance of small (less than 4.0 cm) renal masses. J Urol 2004; 171: 1802–1805.

18. Brierly RD, Thomas PJ, Harrison NW, et al. Evaluation of fine-needle aspiration cytology for renal masses. BJU Int 2000; 85: 14–18.

19. Lechevallier E, Andre M, Barriol D, et al. Fine-needle percutaneous biopsy of renal masses with helical CT guidance. Cancer 2000; 216: 506–510.

20. Johnson PT, Nazarian LN, Feld RI, et al. Sonographically guided renal mass biopsy: indications and efficacy. J Ultrasound Med 2001; 20: 749–753.

21. College of American Pathologists. Interlaboratory Comparison Program in Non-Gynecologic Cytopathology, 1999.

22. Young NA, Mody DR, Davey DD. Misinterpretation of normal cellular elements in fine-needle aspiration biopsy specimens: observations from the College of American Pathologists Interlaboratory Comparison Program in Non-gynecologic Cytopathology. Arch Pathol Lab Med 2002; 126: 670–675.

23. Linsk JA, Franzen S. Aspiration cytology of metastatic hypernephroma. Acta Cytol 1984; 28: 250–260.

24. Klein M, Valensi Q. Proximal tubular adenomas of kidney with so called oncocytic features. Cancer 1976; 38: 906–914.

25. Lieber M, Tomera K, Farrow G. Renal oncocytoma. J Urol 1981; 125: 481–485.

26. Merino M, LiVolsi V. Oncocytomas of the kidney. Cancer 1982; 50: 1852–1856.

27. Choi H, Almagro U, McManus J, et al. Renal oncocytoma. A clinicopathologic study. Cancer 1983; 51: 1887–1896.

28. Alanen KA, Ekfors TO, Lipasti JA, Nurmi MJ. Renal oncocytoma: the incidence of 18 surgical and 12 autopsy cases. Histopathology 1984; 8: 731–737.

29. Lieber MM. Renal oncocytoma: prognosis and treatment. Eur Urol 1990; 18: 17–21.

30. Amin MB, Crotty TB, Tickoo SK, Farrow GM. Renal oncocytoma: a reappraisal of morphologic features with clinicopathologic findings in 80 cases. Am J Surg Pathol 1997; 21: 1–12.

31. Rodriguez CA, Buskop A, Johnson J, et al. Renal oncocytoma. Acta Cytol 1980; 24: 355–359.

32. Nguyen GK, Amy RW, Tsang S. Fine needle aspiration biopsy cytology of renal oncocytoma. Acta Cytol 1985; 29: 33–36.

33. Alanen KA, Tyrkko JES, Nurmi MJ. Aspiration biopsy cytology of renal oncocytoma. Acta Cytol 1985; 29: 859–862.

34. Cochand-Priollet B, Rothschild E, Chagnon S, et al. Renal oncocytoma diagnosed by fine-needle aspiration cytology. Br J Urol 1988; 61: 534–544.

35. Liu J, Fanning CV. Can renal oncocytomas be distinguished from renal cell carcinoma on fine-needle aspiration specimens? A study of conventional smears in conjunction with ancillary studies. Cancer 2001; 93: 390–397.

36. Deshpande A, Munshi M. Renal oncocytoma with hyaline globules: cytologic diagnosis by guided fine needle aspiration, a case report. Indian J Pathol Microbiol 2005; 48: 230–235.

37. Nayar R, Bourtsos E, DeFrias DV. Hyaline globules in renal cell carcinoma and hepatocellular carcinoma. A clue or a diagnostic pitfall on fine-needle aspiration. Am J Clin Pathol 2000; 114: 576–582.

38. Adley BP, Schafernak KT, Yeldandi AV, et al. Cytologic and histologic findings in multiple renal hybrid oncocytic tumors in a patient with Birt–Hogg–Dube syndrome: a case report. Acta Cytol 2006; 50: 584–588.

39. Renshaw AA, Corless CL. Papillary renal cell carcinoma: histology and immunohistochemistry. Am J Surg Pathol 1995; 19: 842–849.

40. Corless CL, Aburatani H, Fletcher JA, et al. Papillary renal cell carcinoma: quantitation of chromosome 7 and 17 by FISH, analysis of chromosome 3p for LOH, and DNA ploidy. Diagn Mol Pathol 1996; 5: 53–64.

41. Storkel S, Eble JN, Adlakha K, et al. Classification of renal cell carcinoma: Workgroup No. 1. Union Internationale Contre le Cancer (UICC) and the American Joint Committee on Cancer (AJCC). Cancer 1997; 80: 987–989.

42. Farrow GM, Harrison EG, Utz DC, Jones DR. Renal angiomyolipoma: a clinicopathologic study of 32 cases. Cancer 1968; 22: 564–570.

43. Blute ML, Malek RS, Segura JW. Angiomyolipoma: clinical metamorphosis and concepts for management. J Urol 1988; 139: 20–24.

44. Murphy WM, Beckwith JB, Farrow GM. Tumors of the kidney, bladder, and related urinary structures, 3rd edn. In: Rosai J, ed. Atlas of tumor pathology; Vol. 11.Washington, DC: Armed Forces Institute of Pathology, 1994; 193–288.

45. Nguyen GK. Aspiration biopsy cytology of renal angiomyolipoma. Acta Cytol 1984; 28: 261–264.

46. Glenthoj A, Partoft S. Ultrasound-guided percutaneous aspiration of renal angiomyolipoma. Acta Cytol 1984; 28: 265–268.

47. Taavitsainen M, Krogeris L, Rannikko S. Aspiration biopsy of renal angiomyolipoma. Acta Radiol 1989; 30: 381–382.

48. Sant GR, Ayers DK, Bankoff MS, et al. Fine needle aspiration biopsy in the diagnosis of renal angiomyolipoma. J Urol 1990; 143: 999–1001.

49. Pancholi V, Munjal K, Jain M, et al. Pre-operative diagnosis of a renal angiomyolipoma with fine needle aspiration cytology: a report of 3 cases. Acta Cytol 2006; 50: 466–468.

50. Crapanzano JP. Fine-needle aspiration of renal angiomyolipoma: cytological findings and diagnostic pitfalls in a series of five cases. Diagn Cytopathol 2005; 32: 53–57.

51. Gupta RK, Nowitz M, Wakefield SJ. Fine needle aspiration cytology of renal angiomyolipoma: report of a case with immunocytochemical and electron microscopic findings. Diagn Cytopathol 1998; 18: 297–300.

52. Sangawa A, Shintaku M, Nishmura M. Nuclear pseudoinclusions in angiomyolipoma of the kidney. A case report. Acta Cytol 1998; 42: 425–429.

53. Mojica WD, Jovanoska S, Bernacki EG. Epithelioid angiomyolipoma: appearance on fine-needle aspiration report of a case. Diagn Cytopathol 2000; 23: 192–195.

54. Cibas ES, Goss GA, Kulke MH, et al. Malignant epithelioid angiomyolipoma ('sarcoma ex angiomylipoma') of the kidney: a case report and review of the literature. Am J Surg Pathol 2001; 25: 121–126.

55. Mai KT, Yazdi HM, Perkins DG, Thijssen A. Fine needle aspiration biopsy of epithelioid angiomyolipoma. A case report. Acta Cytol 2001; 45: 233–236.

56. Miranda MC, Saigo PE. Fine needle aspiration biopsies of primary renal neoplasms. [Abstract] Acta Cytol 1996; 40: 1026.

57. Wadih GE, Raab SS, Silverman JF. Fine needle aspiration cytology of renal and retroperitoneal angiomyolipoma. Acta Cytol 1995; 39: 945–950.

58. Jones EC, Pins M, Dickersin GR, Young RH. Metanephric adenoma of the kidney. Am J Surg Pathol 1995; 19: 615–626.

59. Davis CJ, Barton JH, Sesterhenn IA, Mostofi FK. Metanephric adenoma. Clinicopathological study of fifty patients. Am J Surg Pathol 1995; 19: 1101–1114.

60. Gatalica Z, Grujic S, Kovatich A, Petersen RO. Metanephric adenoma: histology, immunophenotype, cytogenetics, ultrastructure. Mod Pathol 1996; 9: 329–333.

61. Strong JW, Ro JY. Metanephric adenoma of the kidney: a newly characterized entity. Adv Anat Pathol 1996; 3: 172–178.

62. Renshaw AA, Freyer DR, Hammers YA. Metastatic metanephric adenoma in a child. Am J Surg Pathol 2000; 24: 570–574.

63. Renshaw AA, Maurici D, Fletcher JA. Cytologic and fluoresence in situ hybridization (FISH) examination of metanephric adenoma. Diagn Cytopathol 1997; 16: 107–111.

64. Taxy JB, Marshall FF. Multilocular renal cysts in adults. Arch Pathol Lab Med 1983; 107: 633–637.

65. Sherman ME, Silverman JML, Balogh K, Tan SS. Multilocular renal cyst. Arch Pathol Lab Med 1987; 111: 732–736.

66. Clark SP, Kung ITM, Tang SK. Fine-needle aspiration of cystic nephroma (multilocular cyst of the kidney). Diagn Cytopathol 1992; 8: 349–351.

67. Hughes JH, Niemann TH, Thomas PA. Multicystic nephroma: report of a case with fine-needle aspiration findings. Diagn Cytopathol 1996; 14: 60–63.

68. Morgan C, Greenberg ML. Multilocular renal cyst: a diagnostic pitfall on fine-needle aspiration cytology. Diagn Cytopathol 1995; 13: 66–70.

69. de Kernion JB, Belldegrun A. Renal tumors. In: Walsh PC, Retik AB, Stamey TA, Vaughan ED, eds. Campbell's urology. Vol. 2. Philadelphia: WB Saunders, 1992; 1055–1067.

70. Lang EK. Renal cyst puncture studies. Urol Clin North Am 1987; 14: 91–102.

71. Gibson TE. Inter-relationship of renal cysts and tumors: report of three cases. J Urol 1954; 71: 241–252.

72. Emmett JL, Levine SR, Woolner LB. Co-existence of renal cyst and tumour: incidence in 1,007 cases. Br J Urol 1963; 35: 403–410.

73. Levine SR, Emmett JL, Woolner LB. Cyst and tumor occurring in the same kidney. J Urol 1964; 91: 8–9.

74. Khorsand D. Carcinoma within solitary renal cysts. J Urol 1965; 93: 440–444.

75. Lang EK. Coexistence of cyst and tumor in the same kidney. Diagn Radiol 1971; 101: 7–16.

76. Navari RM, Ploth DW, Tatum RK. Renal adenocarcinoma associated with multiple simple cysts. JAMA 1981; 246: 1808–1809.

77. Ljunberg B, Holmberg G, Sjodin JG, et al. Renal cell carcinoma in a renal cyst: a case report and review of the literature. J Urol 1990; 143: 797–799.

78. Brunn E, Nielsen K. Solitary cyst and clear cell adenocarcinoma of the kidney: report of 2 cases and review of the literature. J Urol 1986; 136: 449–451.

79. Corica FA, Iczkowski KA, Cheng L, et al. Cystic renal cell carcinoma is cured by resection: a study of 24 cases with long-term follow-up. J Urol 1999; 161: 408–411.

80. Suzigan S, Lopez-Beltran A, Montironi R, et al. Multilocular cystic renal cell carcinoma: a report of 45 cases of a kidney tumor of low malignant potential. Am J Clin Pathol 2006; 125: 217–222.

81. Pollack HM, Banner MP, Arger PH, et al. The accuracy of gray-scale renal ultrasonography in differentiating cystic neoplasms from benign cysts. Radiology 1982; 143: 741–745.

82. Bosniak MA. Difficulties in classifying cystic lesions of the kidney. Urol Radiol 1991; 13: 91–93.

83. Bosniak MA. The small (<3.0 cm) renal parenchymal tumor: detection diagnosis and controversies. Radiology 1991; 179: 307–317.

84. Aronson S, Frazier HA, Baluch JD, et al. Cystic renal masses: usefulness of the Bosniak classification. Urol Radiol 1991; 13: 83–90.

85. Bosniak MA. Problems in the radiologic diagnosis of renal parenchymal tumors. Urol Clin North Am 1993; 20: 217–230.

86. Aubert S, Zini L, Delomez J, et al. Cystic renal cell carcinoma in adults: is preoperative recognition of multilocular cystic renal cell carcinoma possible? J Urol 2005; 174: 2115–2119.

87. Plowden KM, Erozan YS, Frost JK. Cellular atypias associated with benign lesions of the kidney as seen in fine needle aspirates. [Abstract] Acta Cytol 1984; 28: 648–649.

88. Ambrose SS, Lewis EL, Obrien DP, et al. Unsuspected renal tumors

associated with renal cysts. J Urol 1977; 117: 704–707.

89. Koss LG. Diagnostic cytology of the urinary tract. Philadelphia: Lippincott-Raven, 1995.

90. Todd TD, Dhurandar B, Mody D, et al. Fine-needle aspiration of cystic lesions of the kidney. Morphologic spectrum and diagnostic problems in 41 cases. Am J Clin Pathol 1999; 111: 317–328.

91. Lang EK. Roentgenographic assessment of asymptomatic renal lesions. Radiology 1973; 109: 257–269.

92. Nosher JL, Amorosa JK, Leiman S, Plafker J. Fine needle aspiration of the kidney and adrenal gland. J Urol 1982; 128: 895–899.

93. Renshaw AA, Lee KR, Madge R, Granter SR. Accuracy of fine needle aspiration in distinguishing subtypes of renal cell carcinoma. Acta Cytol 1997; 41: 987–994.

94. Kleist H, Jonsson O, Lundstam S, et al. Quantitative lipid analysis in the differential diagnosis of cystic renal lesions. Br J Urol 1982; 54: 441–445.

95. Dunnill M, Millard P, Oliver D. Acquired cystic disease of the kidneys: a hazard of long-term intermittent maintenance haemodialysis. J Clin Pathol 1977; 30: 868–877.

96. Hughson M, Hennigar G, McManus J. Atypical cysts, acquired renal cystic disease, and renal cell tumors in end stage dialysis kidneys. Lab Invest 1980; 42: 475–480.

97. Bretan PN, Busch MP, Hricak H, Williams RD. Chronic renal failure: a significant risk factor in the development of acquired renal cysts and renal cell carcinoma. Cancer 1986; 57: 1871–1879.

98. Williams JC, Merguerian PA, Schned AR, Morrison PM. Acquired renal cystic disease and renal cell carcinoma in an allograft kidney. J Urol 1995; 153: 395–396.

99. Gregoire J, Torres V, Holley K, Farrow G. Renal epithelial hyperplastic and neoplastic proliferation in autosomal dominant polycystic kidney disease. Am J Kidney Dis 1987; 9: 27–38.

100. Silverman JF, Gurley AM, Harris JP, et al. Fine needle aspiration cytology of renal infarcts. Acta Cytol 1991; 35: 736–741.

101. Raso DS, Greene WB, Finley JL, Silverman JF. Morphology and pathogenesis of Liesegang rings in cyst aspirates: report of two cases with ancillary findings. Diagn Cytopathol 1998; 19: 116–119.

102. Kapasi H, Robertson S, Futter N. Diagnosis of renal malakoplakia by fine needle aspiration cytology: a case report. Acta Cytol 1998; 42: 1419–1423.

103. de Medeiros CR, Dantas da Cunha A, Pasquini R, Arns de Cunha C. Primary renal aspergillosis: extremely uncommon presentation in patients trated with bone marrow transplantation. Bone Marrow Transplant 1999; 24: 113–114.

104. Hyldgaard-Jensen J, Sandstrom HR, Pedersen JF. Ultrasound diagnosis and guided biopsy in renal actinomycosis. Br J Radiol 1999; 72: 510–512.

105. Dash RC, Liu K, Sheafor DH, Dodd LG. Fine-needle aspiration findings in idiopathic retroperitoneal fibrosis. Diagn Cytopathol 1999; 21: 22–26.

106. Fuhrman S, Lasky L, Limas C. Prognostic significance of morphologic parameters in renal cell carcinoma. Am J Surg Pathol 1982; 6: 655–663.

107. Nurmi M, Tyrkko J, Puntala P, et al. Reliability of aspiration biopsy cytology in the grading of renal adenocarcinoma. Scand J Urol Nephrol 1984; 18: 151–156.

108. Cajulis RS, Katz RL, Dekmezian R, et al. Fine needle aspiration biopsy of renal cell carcinoma. Acta Cytol 1993; 37: 367–372.

109. Mai KT, Alhalouly T, Lamba M, et al. Distribution of subtypes of metastatic renal-cell carcinoma: correlating findings of fine-needle aspiration biopsy and surgical pathology. Diagn Cytopathol 2003; 28: 66–70.

110. Gnarra JR, Tory K, Weng Y, et al. Mutations of the VHL tumour suppressor gene in renal carcinoma. Nature Genet 1994; 7: 85–90.

111. Foster K, Prowse A, van den Berg A, et al. Somatic mutations of the von Hippel–Lindau disease tumour suppressor gene in non-familial clear cell renal carcinoma. Hum Mol Genet 1994; 3: 2069–2173.

112. Whaley JM, Naglich J, Gelbert L, et al. Germ-line mutations in the von Hippel–Lindau tumor suppressor gene are similar to somatic von Hippel–Lindau aberrations in sporadic renal cell carcinoma. Am J Hum Genet 1994; 55: 1092–1102.

113. Shuin T, Kondo K, Torigoe S, et al. Frequent somatic mutations and loss of heterozygosity of the von Hippel–Lindau tumor suppressor gene in primary human renal cell carcinoma. Cancer Res 1994; 54: 2852–2855.

114. Hidvegi D, DeMay RM, Nunez-Alonso C, Nieman H. Percutaneous transperitoneal aspiration of renal adenocarcinoma guided by ultrasound. Acta Cytol 1979; 23: 467–470.

115. Nguyen GK. Fine needle aspiration biopsy cytology of metastatic renal cell carcinoma. Acta Cytol 1988; 32: 409–414.

116. Renshaw AA, Fletcher JA. Trisomy 3 in renal cell carcinoma. Mod Pathol 1997; 10: 481–484.

117. Mancilla-Jimenez R, Stanley R, Blath R. Papillary renal cell carcinoma. A clinical, radiologic, and pathologic study of 34 cases. Cancer 1976; 38: 2469–2480.

118. Mydlo J, Bard R. Analysis of papillary renal adenocarcinoma. Urology 1987; 30: 529–534.

119. Kovacs G. Molecular differential pathology of renal cell tumours. Histopathology 1993; 22: 1–8.

120. Lager DJ, Huston BJ, Timmerman TG, Bonsib SM. Papillary renal tumors. Cancer 1995; 76: 669–673.

121. Kovacs G, Kovacs A. Parenchymal abnormalities associated with papillary renal cell tumors: A morphologic study. J Urol Pathol 1993; 1: 301–312.

122. Amin MB, Corless CL, Renshaw AA, et al. Papillary (chromophil) renal cell carcinoma: histomorphologic characteristics and evaluation of conventional pathologic prognostic parameters in 62 cases. Am J Surg Pathol 1997; 21: 621–635.

123. Gatalica Z, Kovatich A, Miettinen M. Consistent expression of cytokeratin 7 in papillary renal cell carcinoma. J Urol Pathol 1995; 3: 205–211.

124. Flint A, Cookingham C. Cytologic diagnosis of the papillary variant of renal-cell carcinoma. Acta Cytol 1987; 31: 325–329.

125. Weaver MG, Al-Kaisi N, Abdul-Karim FW. Fine needle aspiration cytology of a renal cell adenocarcinoma with massive intracellular hemosiderin accumulation. Diagn Cytopathol 1991; 7: 147–149.

126. Dekmezian R, Sneige N, Shabb N. Papillary renal-cell carcinoma: fine-needle aspiration of 15 cases. Diagn Cytopathol 1991; 7: 198–203.

127. Wang S, Filipowicz EA, Schnadig VJ. Abundant intracytoplasmic hemosiderin in both histiocytes and neoplastic cells: a diagnostic pitfall in fine-needle aspiration of cystic papillary renal cell carcinoma. Diagn Cytopathol 2001; 24: 82–85.

128. Weir M, Pitman MB. The vascular pattern of renal cell carcinomas on fine needle aspiration biopsy: an aid in the distinction from hepatocellular carcinoma. [Abstract] Acta Cytol 1996; 40: 1081.

129. Thoenes W, Storkel S, Rumpelt H. Human chromophobe cell renal carcinoma. Virchows Archiv B Cell Pathol 1985; 48: 207–217.

130. Thoenes W, Storkel S, Rumpelt H, et al. Chromophobe cell renal carcinoma and its variants – a report on 32 cases. J Pathol 1988; 155: 277–287.

131. Bonsib S, Lager D. Chromophobe cell carcinoma: analysis of five cases. Am J Surg Pathol 1990; 14: 260–267.

132. Kovacs G, Soudah B, Hoene E. Binucleated cells in a human renal cell carcinoma with 34 chromosomes. Cancer Genet Cytogenet 1988; 31: 211–215.

133. Kovacs A, Kovacs G. Low chromosome number in chromophobe renal cell carcinoma. Genes, Chromosomes Cancer 1992; 4: 267–268.

134. Speicher M, Schoell B, du Manoir S, et al. Specific loss of chromosomes 1, 2, 6, 10, 13, 17, and 21 in chromophobe renal cell carcinomas revealed by comparative genomic hybridization. Am J Pathol 1994; 145: 356–364.

135. Crotty TB, Farrow GM, Lieber MM. Chromophobe cell renal carcinoma:

clinicopathologic features of 50 cases. J Urol 1995; 154: 964–967.

136. Akhtar M, Kardar H, Linjawi T, et al. Chromophobe cell carcinoma of the kidney. A clinicopathologic study of 21 cases. Am J Surg Pathol 1995; 19: 1245–1256.

137. Renshaw AA, Henske EP, Loughlin KR, et al. Aggressive variants of chromophobe renal cell carcinoma. Cancer 1996; 78: 1756–1761.

138. Renshaw AA, Granter SR. Fine needle aspiration of chromophobe renal cell carcinoma. Acta Cytol 1996; 40: 867–872.

139. Akhtar M, Ali MA. Aspiration cytology of chromophobe cell carcinoma of the kidney. Diagn Cytopathol 1995; 13: 287–294.

140. Wiatrowska BA, Zakowski MF. Fine-needle aspiration biopsy of chromophobe renal cell carcinoma and oncocytoma. Cancer Cytopathol 1999; 87: 161–167.

141. Ro JY, Ayala AG, Sella A, et al. Sarcomatoid renal cell carcinoma: clinicopathologic. A study of 42 cases. Cancer 1987; 59: 516–526.

142. Bonsib SM, Fischer J, Plattner S, Fallon B. Sarcomatoid renal tumors. Cancer 1987; 59: 527–532.

143. Auger M, Katz RL, Sella A, et al. Fine-needle aspiration cytology of sarcomatoid renal cell carcinoma: a morphologic and immunocytochemical study of 15 cases. Diagn Cytopathol 1993; 9: 46–51.

144. Cromie LJ, Davis CJ, DeTure FA. Atypical carcinoma of kidney. Urology 1979; 13: 315–317.

145. Rumpelt HJ, Storkel S, Moll R, et al. Bellini duct carcinoma: further evidence for this rare variant of renal cell carcinoma. Histopathology 1991; 18: 115–122.

146. Kennedy S, Merino M, Linehan W, et al. Collecting duct carcinoma of the kidney. Hum Pathol 1990; 21: 449–456.

147. Fleming S, Lewi H. Collecting duct carcinoma of the kidney. Histopathology 1986; 10: 1131–1141.

148. Becht E, Muller SC, Storkel S, Alken P. Distal nephron carcinoma: a rare kidney tumor. Eur Urol 1988; 14: 253–254.

149. Fuzesi L, Cober M, Mittermayer C. Collecting duct carcinoma: cytogenetic characterization. Histopathology 1992; 21: 155–160.

150. Kotkaya Y, Sakamoto N, Saito S, et al. Bellini duct carcinoma of the kidney. Eur Urol 1992; 22: 171–173.

151. Carter MD, Tha S, McLoughlin MG, Owen DA. Collecting duct carcinoma of the kidney: a case report and review of the literature. J Urol 1992; 147: 1096–1098.

152. Baer SC, Ro JY, Ordonez NG, et al. Sarcomatoid collecting duct carcinoma: A clinicopathologic and immunohistochemical study of five cases. Hum Pathol 1993; 24: 1017–1022.

153. Mauri MF, Bonzanini M, Luciani L, Palma PD. Renal collecting duct carcinoma. Report of a case with urinary cytologic findings. Acta Cytol 1994; 38: 755–758.

154. Zaman SS, Sack MJ, Ramchandani P, et al. Cytopathology of retrograde renal pelvis brush specimens: collecting duct carcinoma and low-intermediate grade transitional cell carcinoma. Diagn Cytopathol 1996; 15: 312–321.

155. Eble JN. Renal medullary carcinoma: a distinct entity emerges from the confusion of 'collecting duct carcinoma.' Adv Anat Pathol 1996; 3: 233–238.

156. Davis CJ, Mostofi FK, Sesterhenn IA. Renal medullary carcinoma. The seventh sickle cell nephropathy. Am J Surg Pathol 1995; 19: 1–11.

157. Renshaw AA, Maurici D, Fletcher JA. Papillary renal cell carcinoma with rare papillae histologically resembling collecting duct carcinoma. J Urol Pathol 1996; 5: 65–74.

158. Gregori-Romero MA, Morell-Quadreny L, Llombart-Bosch A. Cytogenetic analysis of three primary Bellini duct carcinomas. Genes Chromosomes Cancer 1996; 15: 170–172.

159. Farah R, Ben-Izhak O, Munichor M, Cohen H. Low-grade renal collecting duct carcinoma: a case report with histochemical, immunohistochemical, and ultrastructural study. Ann Diagn Pathol 2005; 9: 46–48.

160. Layfield LJ. Fine-needle aspiration biopsy of renal collecting duct carcinoma. Diagn Cytopathol 1994; 11: 74–78.

161. Caraway NP, Wojcik EM, Katz RL, et al. Cytologic findings of collecting duct carcinoma of the kidney. Diagn Cytopathol 1995; 13: 304–309.

162. Bejar J, Szvalb S, Maly B, et al. Collecting duct carcinoma of the kidney: a cytological study and case report. Diagn Cytopathol 1996; 15: 136–138.

163. Sironi M, Delpiano C, Claren R, Spinelli M. New cytological findings on fine-needle aspiration of renal collecting duct carcinoma. Diagn Cytopathol 2003; 29: 239–240.

164. Sarode VR, Islam S, Wooten D, et al. Fine needle aspiration cytology of collecting duct carcinoma of the kidney: report of a case with distinctive features and differential diagnosis. Acta Cytol 2004; 48: 843–848.

165. Bracken RB, Chica G, Johnson DE. Secondary renal neoplasms, an autopsy study. South Med J 1979; 72: 806–807.

166. Gattuso P, Ramzy I, Truong LD, et al. Utilization of fine-needle aspiration in the diagnosis of metastatic tumors to the kidney. Diagn Cytopathol 1999; 21: 35–38.

167. Giashuddin S, Cangiarella J, Elgert P, Levine PH. Metastases to the kidney: eleven cases diagnosed by aspiration biopsy with histologic correlation. Diagn Cytopathol 2005; 32: 325–329.

168. Khurana KK, Powers CN. Basaloid squamous carcinoma metastatic to renal-cell carcinoma: fine needle aspiration cytology of tumor-to-tumor metastasis. Diagn Cytopathol 1997; 17: 379–382.

169. Tabatabai ZL, Staerkel GA. Distinguishing primary and metastatic conventional renal cell carcinoma from other malignant neoplasms in fine-needle aspiration biopsy specimens. Arch Pathol Lab Med 2005; 129: 1017–1021.

170. Simsir A, Chhieng D, Wei XJ, et al. Utility of CD10 and RCCma in the diagnosis of metastatic conventional renal-cell adenocarcinoma by fine-needle aspiration biopsy. Diagn Cytopathol 2005; 33: 3–7.

171. Renshaw AA. Basophilic tumors of the kidney. J Urol Pathol 1998; 8: 85–101.

172. Grignon DJ, Ro JY, Ayala AG. Primary mucin-secreting adenocarcinoma of the kidney. Arch Pathol Lab Med 1988; 112: 847–849.

173. Capella C, Eusebi V, Rosai J. Primary oat cell carcinoma of the kidney. Am J Surg Pathol 1984; 8: 855–861.

174. Ferry JA, Harris NL, Papanicolaou N, Young RH. Lymphoma of the kidney. Am J Surg Pathol 1995; 19: 134–144.

175. Santamaria M, Jauregui I, Urtasun F, Bertol A. Fine needle aspiration biopsy in urothelial carcinoma of the renal pelvis. Acta Cytol 1995; 39: 443–448.

176. Powers CN, Elbadawi A. 'Cercariform' cells: a clue to the cytodiagnosis of transitional cell origin in metastatic neoplasms? Diagn Cytopathol 1995; 13: 15–21.

177. Renshaw AA, Madge R. Cercariform cells for helping distinguish transitional cell carcinoma from non-small cell lung carcinoma in fine needle aspirates. Acta Cytol 1997; 41: 999–1007.

178. Friedman HD, Nsoulis IS, Krauss DJ, et al. Transitional cell carcinoma arising in a pyelocalyceal cyst. An unusual cystic renal lesion with cytologic and imaging findings. Virchows Arch 1999; 434: 459–462.

179. Ortega JA, Solano JG, Perez-Guillermo M. Cytologic aspect of mucinous tubular and spindle-cell renal carcinoma in fine-needle aspirates. Diagn Cytopathol 2006; 34: 660–662.

180. Sun W, McGregor DK, Ordonez NG, et al. Fine needle aspiration cytology of a low grade myxoid renal epithelial neoplasm: a case report. Acta Cytol 2005; 49: 525–529.

181. Iyer VK, Agarwala S, Verma K. Fine-needle aspiration cytology of clear-cell carcinoma of the kidney: study of eight cases. Diagn Cytopathol 2005; 33: 83–89.

182. Krishnamurthy S, Bharadqaj R. Fine needle aspiration cytology of clear cell carcinoma of the kidney. A case report. Acta Cytol 1998; 42: 1444–1446.

183. Barroca HM, Costa MJ, Carvalho JL. Cytologic profile of rhabdoid tumor of

the kidney. A report of 3 cases. Acta Cytol 2003; 47: 1055–1058.

184. Gupta K, Nijhawan R. Renal-cell carcinoma in a three-year-old child. [Letter] Diagn Cytopathol 2004; 30: 369–370.

185. Maly B, Maly A, Reinhartz T, Sherman Y. Primitive neuroectodermal tumor of the kidney. Report of a case initially diagnosed by fine needle aspiration cytology. Acta Cytol 2004; 48: 264–268.

186. Premalata CS, Gayathri Davi M, Diswas S, et al. Primitive neuroectodermal tumor of the kidney. A report of two cases diagnosed by fine needle aspiration cytology. Acta Cytol 2003; 47: 475–479.

187. Vesoulis Z, Rahmeh T, Nelson R, et al. Fine needle aspiration biopsy of primary renal synovial sarcoma. A case report. Acta Cytol 2003; 47: 668–672.

188. Kumar N, Jain S. Aspiration cytology of mesoblastic nephroma in an adult: diagnostic dilemma. Diagn Cytopathol 2000; 23: 124–126.

189. Silverman JF, Nathan G, Olson PR, et al. Fine-needle aspiration cytology of low-grade fibromyxoid sarcoma of the renal capsule. Diagn Cytopatyol 2000; 23: 279–283.

190. Das DK, Shome DK, Garg A, et al. Pediatric acute leukemia presenting as bilateral renal enlargement. Report of a case with fine needle aspiration cytologic features suggestive of megakaryocytic differentiation. Acta Cytol 2000; 44: 819–823.

191. Truong LD, Caraway N, Ngo T, et al. Renal lymphoma. The diagnostic and therapeutic roles of fine-needle aspiration. Am J Clin Pathol 2001; 115: 18–31.

192. Qi J, Shen PU, Rezuke WN, et al. Fine needle aspiration cytology diagnosis of renal medullary carcinoma: a case report. Acta Cytol 2001; 45: 735–739.

193. Li P, Perle MA, Scholes JV, Yang GC. Wilms' tumor in adults: aspiration cytology and cytogenetics. Diagn Cytopathol 2002; 26: 99–103.

194. Serrano R, Rodriguez-Peralto JL, De Orbe GG, et al. Intrarenal neuroblastoma diagnosed by fine-needle aspiration: a report of two cases. Diagn Cytopathol 2002; 27: 294–297.

195. Moreland WS, Zagoria RJ, Geisinger KR. Use of fine needle aspiration biopsy in radiofrequency ablation. Acta Cytol 2002; 46: 819–822.

# CHAPTER 5

# Non-neoplastic disorders of the urinary bladder

Robert H. Young

# Embryology and anatomy

## Embryology

The common excretory ducts (the dilated segments of the mesonephric ducts distal to the ureteral buds) become absorbed into the urogenital sinus after the fourth week of gestation. Their epithelium merges toward the midline and forms a triangular patch that will become the trigone of the urinary bladder. The ends of the developing ureters implant there. The anterior abdominal wall closes with the caudal migration of the cloacal membrane, and during this process mesenchyme is induced to form the anterior wall of the bladder. During the seventh week of gestation the urorectal septum of the cloaca fuses with the proctodeum, separating the rectum from the parts of the urogenital sinus that will form the dome and posterior wall of the bladder. Thus, most of the bladder is derived from the rostral part of the urogenital sinus.

In early embryogenesis the allantois projects outward from the yolk sac into the body stalk, which later forms the umbilical cord. The allantois originates from the part of the yolk sac that gives rise to the cloaca. As the urinary bladder forms, the allantois remains connected to its apex. The urachus (from the Greek o′ o′υραχυζ, plural urachi) is the intra-abdominal structure that connects the apex of the bladder to the umbilicus and contains the allantois. The urachus grows with the embryo to maintain its bridge between the dome of the bladder and the body stalk. By the sixth month of gestation, the urachus has become a cord-like structure little more than 1 mm in diameter between the umbilicus and the dome of the bladder. At birth, the dome of the bladder is near the umbilicus, the urachus is 2–3 mm long, the adjacent umbilical arteries are 5–7 mm in diameter, and the umbilical vein is 10 mm in diameter. Superiorly, the urachus usually divides into three bands of fibrous tissue. The middle band passes through the abdominal wall into the umbilical cord, where it disperses into fine strands. The other two bands attach to the adventitia of the umbilical arteries.

## Gross anatomy

The bladder is located within the pelvis minor, beneath the peritoneum. When it fills, it expands into the abdomen and may reach the level of the umbilicus. In children younger than 6 years the empty bladder is partially in the abdomen. Between age 6 and puberty, the bladder descends to its adult position. At the bladder neck, the bladder is fixed in place by the pubovesical ligaments in the female and the puboprostatic ligaments in the male. The rest of the bladder is loosely contained by the pelvic fat and fibrous tissue and is free to expand as the need arises. The empty bladder has roughly the shape of an inverted pyramid. The superior surface, the dome, is covered by peritoneum. The most anterior and superior point, the apex, is the usual point of insertion of the median umbilical ligament and the urachus. The posterior surface faces posteriorly and inferiorly, forming the base of the bladder. Between it and the rectum are the uterine

cervix and the superior end of the vagina in females and the lower vasa deferentia and seminal vesicles in the male. On either side, the lateral surfaces are in contact with the fascia of the levator ani muscles.

The trigone lies at the base of the bladder and borders the posterior side of the bladder neck.[1] At the lateral points of the trigone, the ureters empty into the bladder cavity through the ureteral orifices.[2] The muscle of the trigone is derived from the detrusor muscle of the bladder and the muscle of the ureters.[3] Within the wall of the bladder, the ureters are surrounded by sheaths of muscle and fibrous tissue known as Waldeyer's sheath.[4] The ureters pass obliquely through the wall of the bladder in such a way that when the bladder fills, the pressure compresses and closes the ureters, preventing reflux.[5,6] The region where the walls of the bladder converge and connect with the urethra is the neck of the bladder.[7] In this area, muscle fibers from the detrusor muscle, the muscle of the trigone, and the muscle of the urethra merge.[3] The internal sphincter is in the bladder neck and consists principally of fibers from the detrusor muscle.[8]

The urachus lies in the space of Retzius anterior to the peritoneum and surrounded anteriorly and posteriorly by the umbilicovesical fascia. On either side of it lie the umbilical arteries, which are enveloped in the umbilicovesical fascia. Caudally, the layers of the umbilicovesical fascia spread over the dome of the bladder. This space is pyramidal and separated from the peritoneum and other structures by fascial planes. After birth, the apex of the bladder descends and draws the urachus with it, bringing along the obliterated umbilical arteries. Within the umbilical fascial tunnel, the adventitia of the umbilical arteries is teased out into fibrous strands referred to as the plexus of Luschka.

Hammond et al.[9] recognized four anatomic variants of the urachus (Fig. 5-1). Type I consists of a well-formed urachus that extends from the bladder to the umbilicus, distinct from the umbilical arteries. In type II, the urachus is joined with one of the umbilical arteries and these continue jointly to the umbilicus. In type III, the urachus and both umbilical arteries join and continue to the umbilicus as the ligamentum commune. Type IV consists of a short tubular urachus that terminates before fusing with either of the umbilical arteries. Hammond et al.[9] found urachi of type I in almost 33% of adults, type II in 20%, type III in 20%, and type IV in 25%. Blichert-Toft et al.[10] found a different distribution of the types in a study of 81 specimens: 9% type I, 12% type II, 25% type 3, and 54% type IV. In adults, the urachus outside the bladder wall is usually 5–5.5 cm long and at its junction with the bladder is 4–8 mm broad, tapering to approximately 2 mm at the umbilical end. Pathologically and clinically, it is convenient to divide the urachus into supravesical, intramural, and intramucosal segments (Fig. 5-2).

The urinary bladder is supplied by two pairs of vessels, the superior and inferior vesical arteries, branches from the internal iliac arteries.[11,12] The lymphatics of the anterior and posterior bladder walls drain through the internal and middle chains of the external iliac lymph nodes, and those of the trigone drain to both the external iliac nodes and the hypogastric nodes.[13]

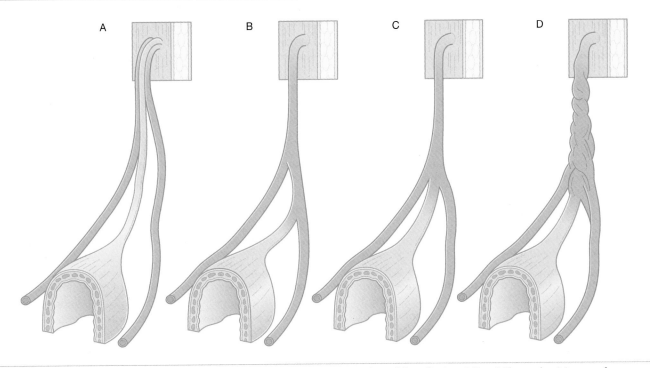

**Fig. 5-1** The four common variants of urachal anatomy. Type I. The urachus extends to the umbilicus (fetal type). Type II. The urachus joins one of the umbilical arteries. Type III. The urachus and umbilical arteries merge and continue to the umbilicus. Type IV. The urachus and umbilical arteries form a complex of fine strands, the plexus of Luschka.

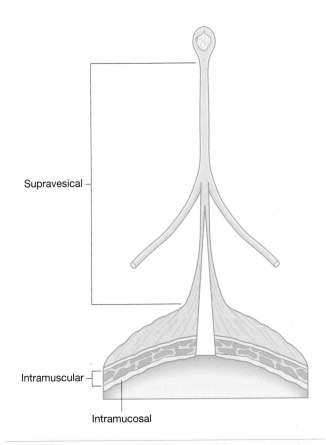

**Fig. 5-2** The urachus is composed of intramucosal, intramuscular, and supravesical segments.

## Histology

The bladder is lined by a specialized epithelium variously referred to as *urothelium* for its adaptation to the urinary environment or *transitional cells* after the anal transition zone, a vestige of the cloaca, or because of its morphology, which early microscopists perceived as transitional between squamous and glandular. The designation *urothelium* is preferred here for its reflection of the function of these cells. The urothelial lining of the human urinary tract is composed of three to six layers of cells. The apparent number of layers varies with the degree of distention or stretching at the time of fixation. There are two subtypes of urothelial cell: the umbrella cells, which cover the surface and are in direct contact with urine, and the underlying cells, which comprise the other layers.

The umbrella cells are the largest cells of the urothelium (Fig. 5-3) and have eosinophilic cytoplasm, which may contain small amounts of mucin. Their nuclei are large and often somewhat irregular, with condensed hyperchromatic chromatin and inconspicuous nucleoli. Ultrastructurally, umbrella cells have asymmetrical cell membranes with a thick outer layer,[14] an irregular angular surface resulting from insertion of stiff segments of membrane, and a variety of intercellular connections.[15] These specializations enable the umbrella cells to cope with the rigors of the urinary environment and maintain the blood–urine barrier as the bladder expands and contracts.[14]

The urothelial cells of the other layers are smaller and more uniform than the umbrella cells,[16] with pale cytoplasm. The nuclei are central, predominantly oval, and, in the deeper layers, oriented perpendicular to the basement membrane.[17] Often there is a noticeable nuclear groove. The chromatin is very fine and evenly dispersed, and nucleoli are small and inconspicuous. Mitotic figures are uncommon and DNA replication studies reveal that the urothelium is renewed approximately once a year. The basal layer of urothelium rests on a basement membrane. Beneath the basement membrane is the lamina propria, a zone of loose connective tissue that contains delicate vessels and thin, delicate bundles of smooth muscle fibers referred to as the muscularis mucosae (Fig. 5-4). The muscularis mucosae of the bladder is variable, ranging from an essentially complete layer analogous to that seen in the colon to a sparse and incomplete array of smooth muscle fibers.[18–22] The connective tissue beneath the muscularis mucosae contains an arcade of larger vessels. Beneath this is the muscularis propria, composed of large bundles of muscle fibers with a scant amount of loose connective tissue. The arrangement of muscle bundles varies in pattern and thickness at different locations in the bladder. Distinct layers, analogous to those of the bowel, are seen only in the area of the internal sphincter. In the bladder neck and superior urethral regions, the muscle bundles are more uniform and densely packed than elsewhere.

Histologically, urachal remnants typically consist of a central lumen lined by epithelium and surrounded by a narrow zone of dense connective tissue, then bundles of smooth muscle fibers, and finally a connective tissue adventitia (Fig. 5-5).[23] Such tubular remnants are present in about 33% of adults.[24] Schubert et al.[24] classified intramural urachal remnants into three groups, ranging from simple tubular structures to more complex canals (Figs 5-6, 5-7). The mucosal segment of the urachus may consist of a papilla, a small opening flush with the surface, a wide diverticular opening, or may be absent (Fig. 5-8, Fig. 5-9). Hammond et al.[9] found a mucosal opening in 10% of specimens. Blichert-Toft et al.[10] found that the epithelial component was present in more than 50% of supravesical segments of the type I variant but was often absent or limited to the segment immediately above the bladder in type IV. Urothelium is the most common lining, present in more than 66% of intra-

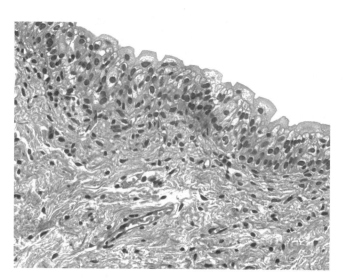

**Fig. 5-3** Umbrella cells have voluminous cytoplasm and large nuclei with inconspicuous nucleoli.

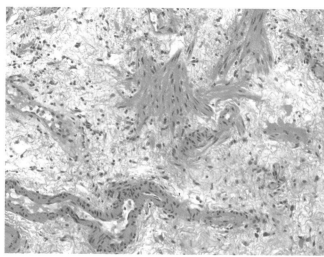

**Fig. 5-4** Smooth muscle in lamina propria is arranged in small irregular bundles.

**Fig. 5-5** The structure of the urachus in cross-section.

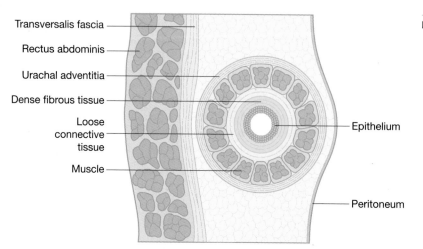

Transversalis fascia

Rectus abdominis

Urachal adventitia

Dense fibrous tissue

Loose connective tissue

Muscle

Epithelium

Peritoneum

mural remnants.[24] The remaining intramural remnants are lined by columnar cells that occasionally may be mucus-secreting.[25]

## Epithelial abnormalities

### von Brunn's nests

Well-circumscribed nests of urothelial cells in the lamina propria, von Brunn's nests,[27–31] arise by a process of budding from the overlying epithelium or by migration[32] and may or may not be attached to the epithelium. Autopsy studies reveal von Brunn's nests in 85–95% of bladders, more commonly in the trigone than elsewhere.[28,30,31,33] Previously, some considered these nests to be related to inflammation or a precursor of carcinoma but neither view is currently accepted. Today they are viewed as normal features of the bladder mucosa.

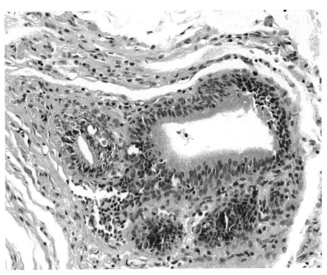

**Fig. 5-7** A complex of urachal channels with focal dilation in the supravesical segment.

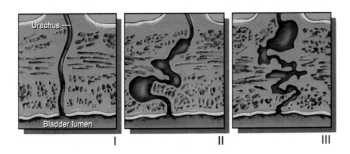

**Fig. 5-6** Variation in the course and structure of the urachus. Type I is a simple canal with a smooth course. Type II has saccular dilations. Type III is more complex with dilations, outpouchings, and an irregular course.

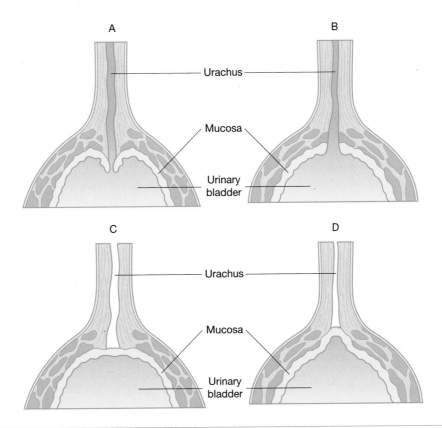

**Fig. 5-8** The intramucosal urachus varies from a lumen terminating in a papilla (**A**), a patent lumen smoothly continuous with bladder mucosa (**B**), smooth bladder mucosa closing the urachal lumen (**C**), to dimpled bladder mucosa covering the urachal lumen (**D**).

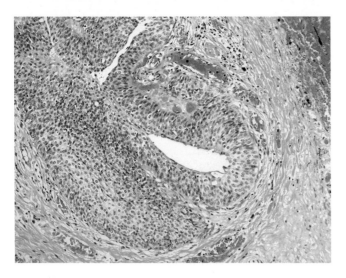

**Fig. 5-9** Type A intramucosal urachus ending in a papilla.

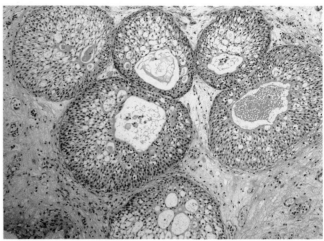

**Fig. 5-11** Cystitis glandularis of the typical type. The lining cells are columnar, goblet cells are not present, and mucus is absent or inconspicuous.

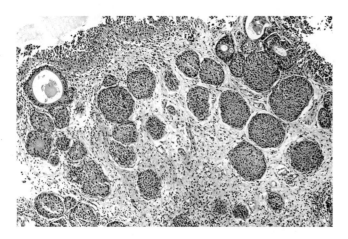

**Fig. 5-10** von Brunn's nests at the mucosal surface and deeper in the lamina propria. Note the smooth round contours of the nests.

Histologically, von Brunn's nests are rounded, well-circumscribed groups of urothelial cells in the lamina propria, usually close to the urothelium but occasionally appreciably deep (Fig. 5-10). Central lumina are often present within florid von Brunn's nests, sometimes with cystic dilatation. Their regular shape and orderly spatial arrangement contrast with the features of rare carcinomas with a nested pattern that are occasionally confused with von Brunn's nests (see Figure 6-30 in Chapter 6). In contrast, small, crowded nests with variable spacing and an infiltrative base characterize the nested variant of urothelial carcinoma.[34] The nuclei of the cells in von Brunn's nests lack significant atypia. Reactive and metaplastic changes in the surface urothelium may also occur in von Brunn's nests. Urothelial carcinoma in situ may extend into von Brunn's nests and should not be mistaken for invasion of the lamina propria. When von Brunn's nests are numerous, closely packed, and

hyperplastic, the distinction from inverted papilloma may be difficult and arbitrary.

Rarely florid epithelial proliferations may occurr in cases of von Brunn's nests, similar to those seen in the setting of radiation or chemotherapy (see Discussion below).

## Cystitis glandularis and cystitis cystica

The term cystitis glandularis refers to a lesion that evolves from and merges imperceptibly with von Brunn's nests.[35–42] Cystitis glandularis is so common that it may be considered a normal feature of the vesical mucosa. Autopsy studies reveal its presence in up to 71% of bladders, most commonly in the trigone.[33] Most foci of cystitis glandularis are microscopic. However, it occasionally forms irregular, rounded, or nodular elevations of the mucosa.[43] Exceptionally, it forms larger polypoid lesions that may be mistaken for a neoplasm prior to microscopic examination.[44–47] Microscopically, cystitis glandularis is composed of glands in the lamina propria which are lined by cuboidal to columnar cells surrounded by one or more layers of urothelial cells (Fig. 5-11). Similar epithelium may also be present on the mucosal surface. The glands of cystitis glandularis may be dilated. Although the lining cells are sometimes characterized as mucinous, they usually do not appear overtly mucinous in sections stained with hematoxylin and eosin,[35] and mucin stains are often negative or weakly positive. Less frequently, the lining cells are tall and columnar with obvious mucin production. In such cases, goblet cells are often present and the glands closely resemble colonic glands. Rarely, Paneth cells and argentaffin-, argyrophil-, or chromogranin A-positive cells are present.[37,42,48–50] The distinction between non-mucinous and mucinous cystitis glandularis has been recognized for many years but is not always made. The more common form can be referred to as the typical type of cystitis glandularis and the second form as the intestinal type.[35] Molecular and immunohistochemical evidence of divergent pathways of histogenesis for these two metaplastic processes has been reported.[50,51] Although the two may coexist, one may predominate or be present exclusively.

Cystitis glandularis of the intestinal type may be extensive, affecting both the lamina propria and the mucosa.[35,47,49,52] Biopsies from such areas closely resemble colonic mucosa, with tubular glands and numerous goblet cells (Fig. 5-12 A and B). The mucin produced by these cells is of the colonic type.[53,54] In some cases, the cells also stain immunohistochemically with antibodies to prostate-specific antigen and prostatic acid phosphatase.[55,56] Rarely, colonic epithelium may be present in the bladder as a developmental abnormality.[57]

Diffuse cystitis glandularis of the intestinal type is termed intestinal metaplasia and usually occurs in chronically irritated bladders, such as those of paraplegics or in patients with stones or long-term catheterization (Fig. 5-13). Unlike focal cystitis glandularis of the intestinal type, persistent extensive or diffuse intestinal metaplasia is associated with an increased risk of bladder carcinoma.[42,48,58,59] It is only the intestinal type of cystitis glandularis that is associated with adenocarcinoma.[60–67]

Cystitis glandularis usually poses no diagnostic problem, but occasional cases are difficult to distinguish from adenocarcinoma.[60,68] This is particularly true of the intestinal type, especially when mucin extravasates into the stroma. An irregular haphazard arrangement of glands in the deeper lamina propria and cytologic atypia should raise the suspicion of adenocarcinoma.

Cystitis cystica consists of von Brunn's nests in which the central cells have degenerated to form small cystic cavities.[13,30,69–71] Albeit somewhat less common than von Brunn's nests and cystitis glandularis, cystitis cystica is present in up to 60% of bladders.[31] It is most common in adults, but also occurs in children. At cystoscopy, its cystic nature is usually apparent.[71] Grossly, the lesions appear as translucent, submucosal cysts that are pearly-white to yellow-brown (Fig. 5-14).[43] Most are less than 5 mm in diameter, but rare examples measuring a few centimeters in diameter[70] have been reported. The cysts contain clear yellow fluid. Microscopically, the cysts are lined by urothelium or cuboidal epithelium (Fig. 5-15) and filled by eosinophilic fluid in which a few inflammatory cells are often present.

## Squamous metaplasia

Metaplastic squamous epithelium is common in patients with severe chronic cystitis,[72–77] such as non-functioning bladders[78,79] or schistosomiasis.[80] It is about four times more common in women than men. Squamous metaplasia may occur anywhere in the bladder, but is most frequent on the anterior wall. Areas of metaplasia often are white or gray-white (Fig. 5-16), and may blend into the surrounding mucosa[72] or be sharply demarcated.[74] Abundantly keratinizing lesions may have a bulky irregular appearance similar to carcinoma.[81,82] Histologically, the lesions show squamous epithelium of variable thickness, often covered by a layer of keratin (Fig. 5-17). In most cases there is no nuclear atypia, but changes as severe as those of carcinoma in situ are occa-

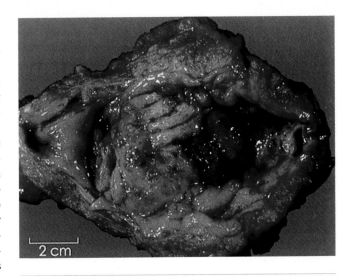

**Fig. 5-13** Extensive cystitis glandularis, intestinal type (intestinal metaplasia). Large and small foci of glistening red mucosa mimic a bladder tumor.

A

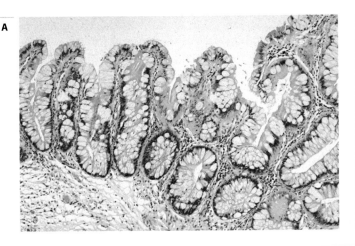

B

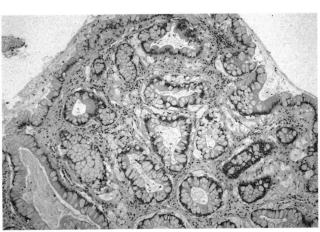

**Fig. 5-12 (A)** Cystitis glandularis, intestinal type. There are spaced tubular glands lined by goblet cells. The surface epithelium is also mucinous. **(B)** Cystitis glandularis, intestinal type. The glands closely resemble colonic glands.

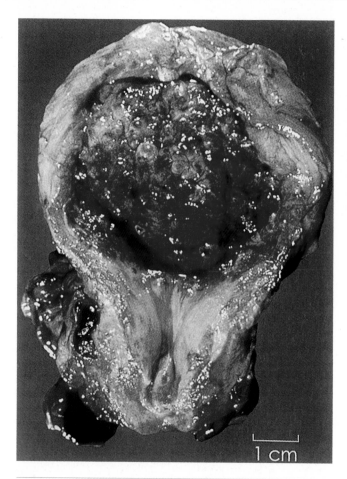

**Fig. 5-14** Cystitis cystica appears as thin-walled domed mucosal cysts or blebs.

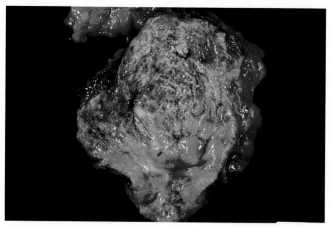

**Fig. 5-16** Keratinizing squamous metaplasia is gray with flecks of light-colored keratin.

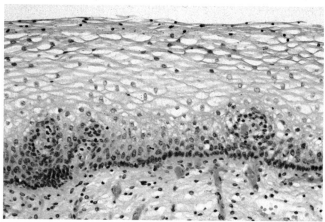

**Fig. 5-17** Squamous metaplasia replacing the urothelium.

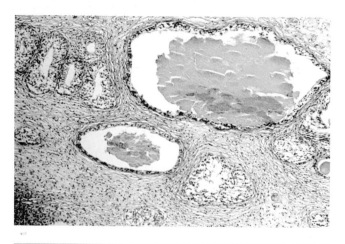

**Fig. 5-15** Cystitis cystica. The cysts are lined by urothelium, and the lumen contains proteinaceous fluid.

sionally seen (Fig. 5-18) and should raise the possibility of invasive carcinoma elsewhere in the specimen or in nearby mucosa.

Keratinizing squamous metaplasia (leukoplakia) appears to be a significant risk factor for the development of carcinoma of the urinary mucosa.[83–85] A Mayo Clinic study of 78 patients with keratinizing squamous metaplasia found that 22% had synchronous carcinoma and another 20% later developed carcinoma (the mean interval was 11 years).[86] Similar findings were reported with a longer duration of follow-up by Khan et al.[87] Most were squamous cell carcinoma. Where schistosomiasis is endemic, squamous metaplasia commonly precedes squamous cell carcinoma.[88,89]

Non-keratinizing glycogenated squamous epithelium, resembling vaginal epithelium (Fig. 5-19), is present in the trigone and bladder neck in up to 86% of women of reproductive age and in almost 75% of postmenopausal women.[90–95] This normal finding should not be diagnosed as squamous metaplasia. Cystoscopically, these areas are pale gray-white with irregular borders, often with a surrounding zone of erythema. The clinical association of this cystoscopic finding with symptoms of urgency and frequency has been called pseudomembranous trigonitis. This type of squamous epithelium is very rare in men, but has been reported in patients receiving estrogen therapy for adenocarcinoma of the prostate.[92,96]

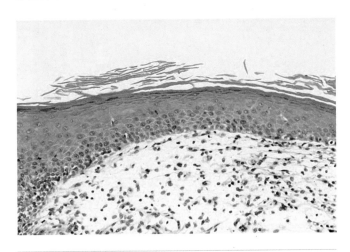

**Fig. 5-18** Keratinizing squamous metaplasia with parakeratosis.

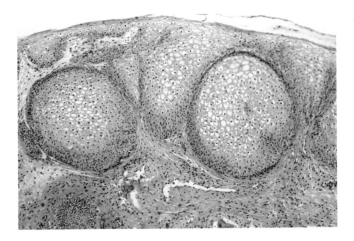

**Fig. 5-19** Non-keratinizing glycogenated squamous epithelium.

## Nephrogenic adenoma

First described as a hamartoma in 1949 by Davis,[97] the name nephrogenic adenoma was given a year later by Friedman and Kuhlenbeck[98] in a report of eight cases. They chose this name because in its most common form the tumor is composed of small tubules resembling renal tubules.[99–105] The terms nephrogenic metaplasia[106,107] and adenomatous metaplasia[102] are preferred by some. More than 75% of reported cases have involved the bladder, but lesions in the urethra, ureter, and rarely the renal pelvis have also been reported.[103] Recent evidence in renal transplant patients suggests that nephrogenic adenoma is derived from tubular renal cells and is not a metaplastic proliferation of the urothelium as that long been thought.[108] Molecular evidence rarely suggests that clear cell adenocarcinoma of the bladder may rarely arise from nephrogenic adenoma.[109]

Approximately 90% of patients with nephrogenic adenoma are adults, and there is a male preponderance of 2:1. In children, it is more common in girls than in boys.[110,111]

Nephrogenic adenoma is frequently found following genitourinary surgery (61% of cases) or associated with calculi (14%), trauma (9%), and cystitis.[103] Renal transplant recipients make up about 8% of patients.[103,112] Complaints of hematuria, dysuria, and frequency are common, but the association with other lesions makes it difficult to categorically attribute any of these symptoms to the nephrogenic adenoma.

Approximately 56% are papillary, 34% sessile, and 10% polypoid. It is rare on the anterior wall of the bladder,[103] but nearly evenly distributed over the rest of the mucosa. About two-thirds are smaller than 1 cm in diameter, most being incidentally discovered microscopic lesions. Approximately 25% are from 1 to 4 cm in diameter and only 10% are larger. In less than 20% of cases there are multiple lesions, which rarely include diffuse involvement of the bladder.

Microscopically, nephrogenic adenoma displays tubular, cystic, polypoid, papillary, and diffuse patterns.[113] The most common architecture is tubular (present in 96% of cases). The tubules are typically small round structures lined by cuboidal epithelium (Fig. 5-20), but occasionally are elongated and solid. Sometimes they are surrounded by a prominent basement membrane. Cystic dilatation of the tubules is common (present in 72% of cases) (Fig. 5-21) and may predominate. Tubules and cysts often contain eosinophilic or basophilic secretions, which may react with mucicarmine (present in 25% of cases). Polypoid and papillary structures (Fig. 5-22) are present in 65% of cases. Edematous polyps are more common than delicate papillae, which are present in only 10% of cases. Focal solid growth (Fig. 5-23) is uncommon.

Most tubules, cysts, and papillae have cuboidal to low columnar epithelium with scant cytoplasm, but epithelium with abundant clear cytoplasm is seen in up to 40% of cases. Hobnail cells (Fig. 5-20B) focally line the tubules and cysts in 70% of cases, rarely they predominte.[113] Larger cysts may be lined by flat epithelium cells. Glycogen is present in some cells in 10–15% of cases.[114] The nuclei are regular and round, and atypia is rare,[113,115] usually appearing degenerative. Mitotic figures are absent or rare. Nephrogenic adenoma is often associated with chronic cystitis, which may obscure it. Rarely, it is associated with stromal calcification,[99,116] squamous metaplasia, or cystitis glandularis.

Nephrogenic adenoma has a number of features that may cause confusion with bladder carcinoma. Tiny mucin-filled tubules apparently lined by a single cell with a compressed nucleus may resemble signet ring cells. The irregular disposition of the tubules may simulate invasive adenocarcinoma, especially when they are among the fibers of the muscularis mucosae. Hobnail cells may bring to mind clear cell adenocarcinoma, which shares architectural features of tubular, cystic, and papillary structures with nephrogenic adenoma (see Chapter 6). Clinical and pathologic features that help to distinguish nephrogenic adenoma from clear cell adenocarcinoma are shown in Table 5-1.

In a few cases of nephrogenic adenoma, papillae are the predominant feature (Fig. 5-24); cytologic atypia may be

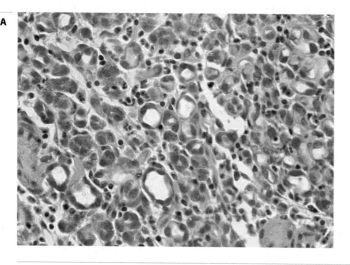
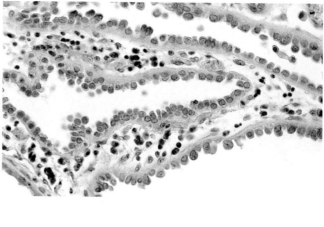

**Fig. 5-20** (**A**) Tubules of nephrogenic adenoma lined by cuboidal epithelium resembling renal medullary tubules. (**B**) Tubules of nephrogenic adenoma lined by hobnail cells.

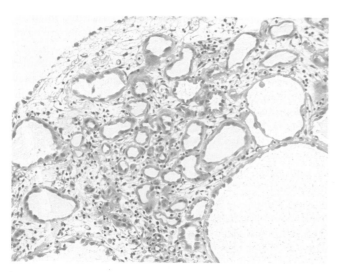

**Fig. 5-21** Cystic dilation of tubules in nephrogenic adenoma.

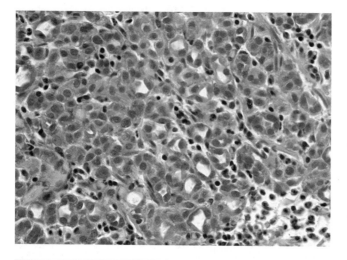

**Fig. 5-23** The diffuse or solid pattern of nephrogenic adenoma. The cells have abundant eosinophilic cytoplasm.

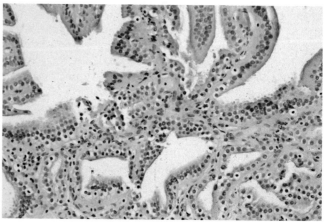

**Fig. 5-22** Papillary nephrogenic adenoma. The papillae are covered by a single layer of cuboidal cells.

**Fig. 5-24** Nephrogenic adenoma with predominance of the papillary component.

present (Figs 5-25 and 5-26) and may cause confusion with other papillary lesions, such as urothelial carcinoma and papillary cystitis. Recognition of the cuboidal epithelium covering the papillae of nephrogenic adenoma differentiates it from these lesions, which are covered by urothelium.

Nephrogenic adenoma may be confused with prostate adenocarcinoma owing to immunoreactivity for racemase (P504S) reactivity, and negative reactivity for basal cell-specific cytokeratin (34βE12) and p63.[117] However, negative reactivity for prostate-specific antigen (PSA) and prostatic acid phosphatase (PAP) differentiates nephrogenic adenoma from prostate adenocarcinoma.[118–120] Immunohistochemical staining for nuclear transcription factor for renal development (PAX2) is useful for differentiating nephrogenic adenoma from prostate adenocarcinoma, benign urothelium, and papillary urothelial carcinoma.[121]

## Papillary hyperplasia

The urothelial mucosa overlying inflammatory or neoplastic processes may occasionally have a papillary appearance on microscopic examination. In some cases, discovery of the bladder lesion precedes identification of the underlying condition, and in these cases the bladder lesion is referred to as a herald lesion.[122] The term papillary hyperplasia is used when papillae are not seen grossly or at cystoscopy.[43] Most often, the underlying lesion originates in the prostate, female genital tract, or colon.[122,123] When associated with prostatic disease, the papillary lesions are found in the trigone in the midline; those associated with uterine disease are found in the midline above the trigone. When associated with intestinal disease, the bladder lesions are often on the left and posterior. Non-specific papillary hyperplasia should be distinguished from the papillary hyperplasia that is seen as the earliest manifestation of papillary carcinoma.

**Table 5-1** Features distinguishing nephrogenic adenoma from clear cell adenocarcinoma

| Feature | Nephrogenic adenoma | Clear cell adenocarcinoma |
| --- | --- | --- |
| Gender predominance | Male | Female |
| Age | 33% < 30 years | All > 43 years |
| Associated genitourinary conditions | Very common | Absent |
| Size | Usually small | Often large |
| Solid growth pattern | Rare | Common |
| Clear cells | Uncommon | Common |
| Glycogen in cytoplasm | Rare | Common and abundant |
| Nuclear atypia and mitotic figures | Rare | Common |

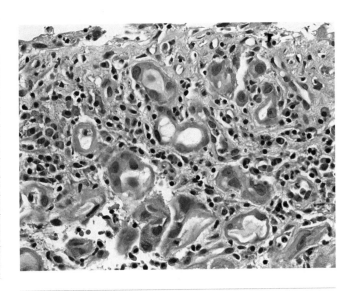

**Fig. 5-25** Cytologic atypia in nephrogenic adenoma.

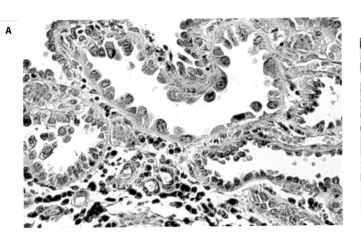

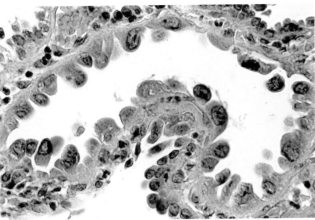

**Fig. 5-26** Cytologic atypia in nephrogenic adenoma (**A** and **B**).

# Inflammation and infection

## Non-specific cystitis

### Polypoid and papillary cystitis

Polypoid and papillary cystitis result from inflammation and edema in the lamina propria, leading to papillary and polypoid mucosal lesions.[124–128] The term papillary cystitis is used for finger-like papillae (Figs 5-27 and 5-28) lined by reactive urothelium, and polypoid cystitis for broad-based edematous lesions (Figs 5-29 and 5-30). The latter are more common. Chronic inflammation in the lamina propria and dilated blood vessels are prominent and diagnostically helpful features of both papillary and polypoid cystitis. Depending on the degree of edema of the lamina propria, there is a continuous morphological spectrum from papillary cystitis to polypoid cystitis to bullous cystitis (Fig. 5-30).

In papillary and polypoid cystitis the lesion is taller than it is wide, whereas in bullous cystitis the opposite applies. There may be associated metaplastic changes in the epithelium covering or adjacent to the lesion.

In the clinical settings of indwelling catheter and vesical fistula, the surgical pathologist should be alert to the possibility that an exophytic bladder lesion may be inflammatory.[129] Polypoid cystitis is present in up to 80% of patients with indwelling catheters.[127] Although most lesions are microscopic in size, polypoid or bullous lesions up to 5 mm in diameter (mostly in the dome or on the posterior wall) are found in about 33% of cases. Prolonged catheterization may induce widespread polypoid and bullous cystitis. Most lesions disappear within 6 months of removal of the irritant.[126]

Vesical fistulae, whether resulting from intestinal diverticulitis,[130] Crohn's disease, colorectal cancer (Fig. 5-31),[130]

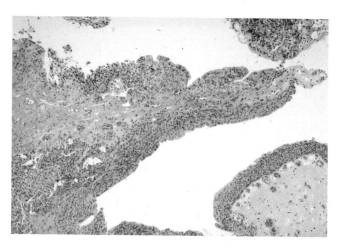

**Fig. 5-27** Papillary cystitis with finger-like fronds covered by a few layers of urothelium.

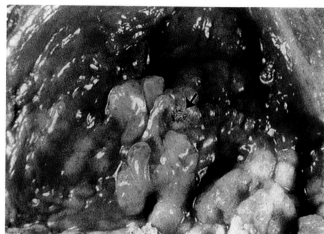

**Fig. 5-29** Polypoid cystitis. Arrow shows biopsy site. (Courtesy of Dr M. El-Bolkainy.)

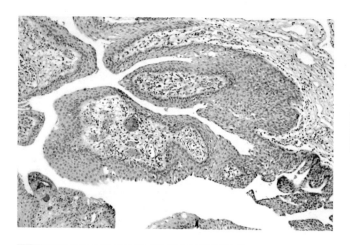

**Fig. 5-28** Papillary cystitis.

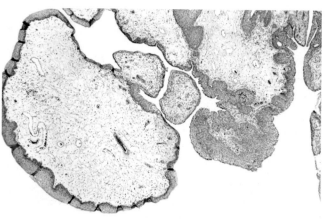

**Fig. 5-30** Polypoid cystitis.

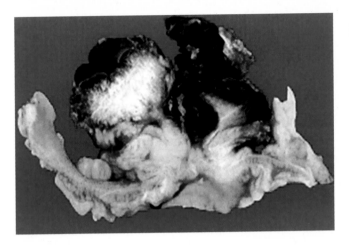

Fig. 5-31 Colovesical fistula secondary to adenocarcinoma of colon. The dimpled outlet in the bladder mucosa (above) connects with the colon (below).

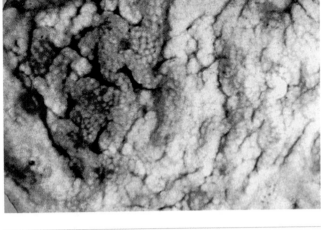

Fig. 5-32 Follicular cystitis. The lymphoid aggregates are visible as small domed lesions on the mucosal surface.

or appendicitis, are often associated with polypoid cystitis, and, less commonly, with papillary cystitis.[131–136] Fistulae between the urinary bladder and the alimentary tract are about three times more common in men than in women.[132,137] Pneumaturia and fecaluria are typical symptoms.[132] In about 50% of cases indications of extravesical disease are initially absent, making the diagnosis more difficult. Patients may present with frequency, urgency, and dysuria. Cystoscopically, the appearance often suggests bladder carcinoma.[126]

Papillary and polypoid cystitis must be distinguished from papillary urothelial carcinoma. Grossly and microscopically, the fronds of polypoid cystitis are much broader than those of most papillary carcinomas. The delicate papillae of papillary cystitis more closely resemble those of carcinoma. Branching is much less prominent in papillary cystitis than in papillary carcinoma. In papillary cystitis the epithelium may be hyperplastic, but usually not to the degree seen in carcinoma. Umbrella cells are more often present in papillary cystitis than in carcinoma.

## Follicular cystitis

Follicular cystitis occurs in up to 40% of patients with bladder cancer[138] and 35% of those with urinary tract infection.[139] Grossly, the mucosa is erythematous with pink, white, or gray nodules (Fig. 5-32).[140–143] Microscopically, the nodules consist of lymphoid follicles in the lamina propria, usually with germinal centers (Fig. 5-33). Malignant lymphoma is the most important differential diagnostic consideration, particularly in biopsies. The criteria used to distinguish lymphoma from chronic inflammation at other sites apply here.

## Giant cell cystitis

Atypical mesenchymal cells with enlarged, hyperchromatic, or multiple nuclei are frequently seen in the lamina propria of the bladder. Wells[144] found them in 33% of cases of cystitis at autopsy and coined the term giant cell cystitis. Such cells are common in bladder biopsies, including those without other evidence of cystitis. Histologically, the cells

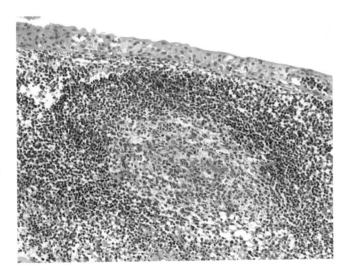

Fig. 5-33 Follicular cystitis. The lamina propria contains a lymphoid follicle.

often have bipolar or multipolar tapering eosinophilic cytoplasmic processes (Fig. 5-34). The nuclei are often irregular in size and shape, and hyperchromatic. Mitotic figures are absent or rare. If present in large numbers, these cells may bring to mind pseudoneoplastic lesions such as postoperative spindle cell nodule and neoplasms such as sarcomatoid urothelial carcinoma or sarcoma. Similar cells may be seen in the lamina propria after radiation therapy and anticancer chemotherapy.[145–148]

## Hemorrhagic cystitis

Cystitis with a predominantly hemorrhagic clinical presentation (Fig. 5-35) may be caused by chemical toxins, radiation, viral infection, or may be idiopathic. Chemical causes include

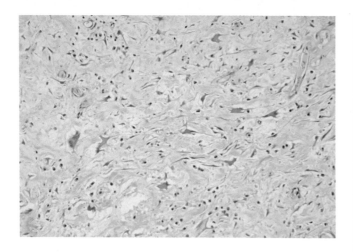

**Fig. 5-34** Giant cell cystitis. The lamina propria contains large stromal cells, some with elongated cytoplasmic processes and some that are multinucleated.

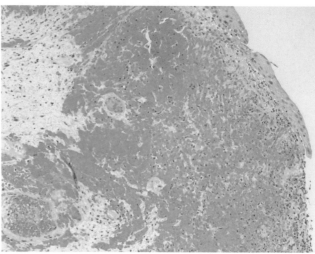

**Fig. 5-36** Hemorrhagic cystitis.

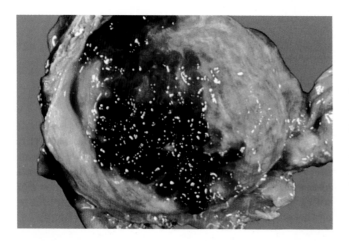

**Fig. 5-35** Hemorrhagic cystitis. (Courtesy of Dr I. Damjanov.)

drugs (such as cyclophosphamide, busulfan, and thiotepa), derivatives of aniline and toluidine (such as dyes and insecticides), and a host of other compounds.[149,150] Radiation and chemotherapy for cancer account for most cases.

Since its introduction in the late 1950s, cyclophosphamide has been recognized as a potent bladder toxin associated with hemorrhagic cystitis.[147,151,152] Hemorrhage may be severe,[153] and early experience reported mortality of nearly 4%.[152] Hemorrhage usually begins during or shortly after treatment. Within 4 hours the mucosa is edematous and congested (Fig. 5-36) and the epithelium shows changes similar to those seen in the irradiated bladder, including nuclear pleomorphism and variable cell size. As the bladder heals, the urothelium becomes hyperplastic and may form papillae. High doses of cyclophosphamide and repeated exposure may lead to irreversible fibrosis and a small contracted bladder.[145] Epithelial and mesenchymal neoplasms have arisen in the bladder following cyclophosphamide therapy.[154–156]

## Special types of cystitis

### Interstitial cystitis

Interstitial cystitis has also been referred to as Hunner's ulcer, but that term is used less frequently today as it has been recognized that ulcers are not always present. The term interstitial cystitis was introduced by Skene[157] in 1887, and Nitze[158] described most of the characteristic features prior to the work by Hunner in 1914.[159] Interstitial cystitis poses diagnostic problems for both pathologists and urologists. The pathologic features are not specific, and the pathologist must correlate them with the clinical and cystoscopic features.

At least 90% of patients with interstitial cystitis are women, and it is seen most often in middle and old age.[160–165] Patients complain of marked frequency, urgency, and pain when the bladder becomes full and when it is emptied.[166] The urine is sterile. Cystoscopy may reveal small foci of hemorrhage (glomerulations), hemorrhagic spots that ooze blood, and linear cracks in the mucosa.[166,167] Occasionally, there are ulcers with radiating scars. Ulcers and scars are more frequent in older patients with long-standing cystitis.[168] In advanced cases the wall of the bladder becomes fibrotic and contracted, resulting in very low bladder capacity (Fig. 5-37). Interstitial cystitis most often affects the dome and posterior and lateral walls.

Biopsy specimens from patients with interstitial cystitis have a variety of appearances. When present, ulcers are often wedge-shaped, and the urothelium is either absent or mixed with a surface exudate of fibrin, erythrocytes, and inflammatory cells (Fig. 5-38). The ulcers usually extend deep into the lamina propria, which is edematous and congested. The muscularis propria may also be edematous or fibrotic. Generally, there is a dense infiltrate of lymphocytes and plasma cells. When ulcers are not present, the changes are less striking. Small mucosal ruptures, edema of the lamina propria, and foci of hemorrhage in the lamina propria are usually

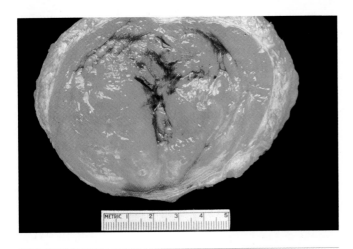

**Fig. 5-37** Chronic interstitial cystitis. The mucosa is punctuated by depressed scars, and the wall is thick and rigid.

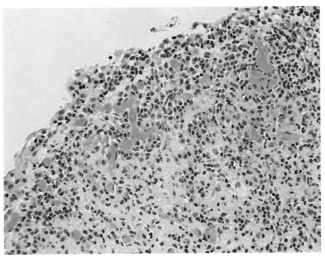

**Fig. 5-39** In eosinophilic cystitis the lamina propria contains sheets of eosinophils.

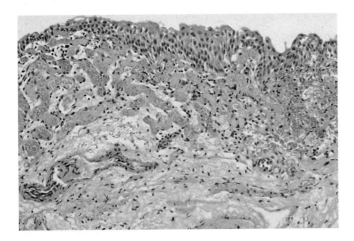

**Fig. 5-38** The lamina propria is prominently vasular in interstitial cystitis.

present and correspond to the glomerulations seen at cystoscopy.

Mast cells are often seen in the mucosa, lamina propria, and muscularis propria in interstitial cystitis. Their significance has been debated for the last four decades. Simmons and Bunce[169] first described an increase in mast cells in interstitial cystitis in 1958. Kastrup et al.[170] concluded that more than 20 mast cells/mm² in the muscularis propria was strongly suggestive of interstitial cystitis, and Larsen et al.[171] found that 28 mast cells/mm² was the upper limit for normal bladders. Johansson and Fall[168] found an average of 164 mast cells/mm² in the lamina propria of patients with ulcers, 93/mm² in those without, and 88/mm² in a control group. The difficulty of counting mast cells and the lack of consensus on what is 'normal' are evident. Conditions of tissue fixation also affect the count. Thus, the histologic features of interstitial cystitis are not pathognomonic.

The extensive mucosal denudation that often occurs with carcinoma in situ may result in an appearance of ulceration, inflammation, and vascular congestion closely resembling that seen in interstitial cystitis. When urothelium is absent or scant in a biopsy, multiple sections should be obtained to look for foci of atypical cells. When other conditions are excluded, often the pathologist can only report that the pathologic findings are consistent with interstitial cystitis.

## Eosinophilic cystitis

Bladder inflammation with a striking infiltrate of eosinophils occurs in two settings: in association with allergic diseases, or without allergic association but usually in association with transurethral resection or invasive urothelial carcinoma.[172] In some cases there is no associated condition.[173] Eosinophilic cystitis associated with allergic disease is rare, and most cases have involved patients with asthma or eosinophilic gastroenteritis.[174,175] Very rarely, eosinophilic cystitis is associated with parasitic infection.[176,177] Patients range in age from newborn to elderly, and more than 33% are children. The ratio of females to males is 2:1. The usual symptoms are dysuria, frequency, and hematuria. At cystoscopy there often are polypoid lesions resembling those of polypoid cystitis, and in children sarcoma botryoides may come to mind. Nodular and sessile lesions and ulcers also are seen. Occasionally, the lesions mimic carcinoma.[178,179] Histologically, the lamina propria is edematous, containing a mixed inflammatory infiltrate in which eosinophils are prominent (Fig. 5-39). Occasionally, edema causes ureteral obstruction and upper tract complications, but most patients respond to non-specific medical treatment, including antihistamines, non-steroidal anti-inflammatory agents, and steroids. However, the disease tends to be persistent or recurrent,[173] so long-term follow-up is recommended.[180]

Patients with no history of allergy are typically older men with various urologic diseases, such as prostatic hyperplasia and carcinoma of the bladder.[181] Many patients give a history of transurethral resection or biopsy, and eosinophilic cystitis may be a reaction to bladder injury. Inflammation with prominent eosinophils is also commonly seen at the periphery of invasive carcinoma in cystectomy specimens.

## Postsurgical necrobiotic granulomas

After transurethral surgery using diathermic cautery the bladder may contain necrotizing palisading granulomas.[182-184] Similar lesions have been reported subsequent to laser surgery.[185] Postsurgical granulomas are found in approximately 10% of cases, and the frequency increases with the number of operations. Typically, these granulomas have elongate linear or serpiginous outlines. Their centers contain acellular, finely granular eosinophilic material in which flecks of brown debris are often present (Fig. 5-40 A, B). Around the necrotic areas is a band of histiocytes arranged radially like the stakes of a palisade fence. Epithelioid histiocytes and foreign body giant cells also are commonly present. Surrounding this layer is a layer of dense chronic inflammation in which eosinophils may be numerous. Eventually the granulomas are replaced by fibrous scars, sometimes with dystrophic calcification.

## Bacillus Calmette–Guérin granulomas

Since 1976, urothelial carcinoma in situ has been treated with intravesical instillation of the mycobacterium bacillus Calmette–Guérin.[186] This therapy often produces remission, but is not usually curative[187,188] A profound inflammatory reaction ensues after instillation,[189] with the result that the urothelium is lost and the lamina propria develops dense chronic inflammatory infiltrates, among which are interspersed small granulomas composed of epithelioid histiocytes and multinucleated giant cells (Fig. 5-41).[190-194] These granulomas are usually round or ovoid lesions in the superficial lamina propria and lack necrosis. Acid-fast stains only rarely demonstrate organisms. Granulomatous inflammatory changes may also be seen in urine cytology specimens.[195,196] Rarely, nephrogenic adenoma may arise following therapy with bacillus Calmette–Guérin.[197]

## Other non-infectious granulomas

Following herniorrhaphy, suture granuloma may produce an inflammatory mass in or near the bladder.[198-204] Usually the herniorrhaphy wound has been infected. Because of the long interval between herniorrhaphy and bladder symptoms (up to 11 years), the clinical diagnosis is often of bladder neoplasm. Microscopic examination shows a predominantly inflammatory process with foreign body giant cells and fibrosis around fragments of suture.

Rarely, diffuse infiltrates of histiocytes without the features specific for malakoplakia may form nodules in the bladder, and this has been termed xanthogranulomatous cystitis.[205] Collections of foamy histiocytes may also be found in the lamina propria in patients with disorders of lipid metabolism and have been called xanthoma of the bladder.[206] Granulomatous inflammation of the bladder has also been reported in association with granulomatous disease of childhood,[207] rheumatoid arthritis,[208] and fistulae of Crohn's disease.[209] Sarcoidosis rarely affects the bladder.[210]

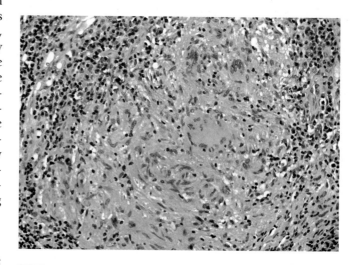

**Fig. 5-41** Granuloma of bacillus Calmette–Guérin.

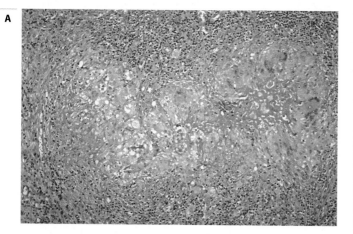

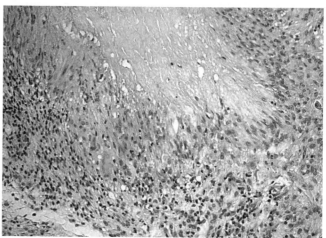

**Fig. 5-40** (**A**) Postoperative granuloma with amorphous debris. (**B**) Postoperative granuloma with strands of coagulated tissue in the center and a palisade of histiocytes surrounding the necrotic material.

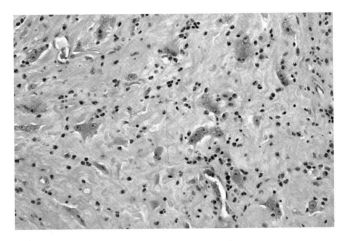

**Fig. 5-42** Radiation cystitis with atypical stromal cells.

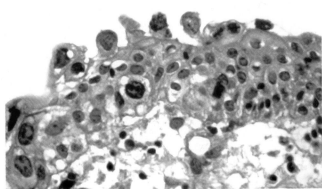

**Fig. 5-44** Epithelial atypia and sloughing associated with intravesical thiotepa.

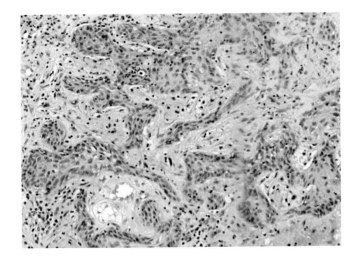

**Fig. 5-43** Florid epithelial proliferation after radiation therapy.

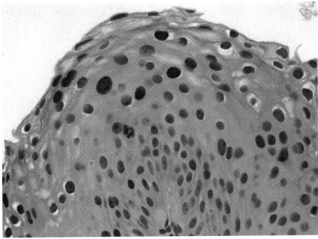

**Fig. 5-45** Epithelial atypia associated with intravenous cyclophosphamide.

## Radiation cystitis

Radiation frequently induces a variety of abnormalities in the bladder.[211-213] Three to 6 weeks after treatment there is acute cystitis, with loss of the urothelium and congestion and edema in the lamina propria.[214] The remaining urothelial cells show varying degrees of nuclear atypicality. Features of radiation injury in the urothelium include vacuoles in the cytoplasm and nuclei, karyorrhexis, and a normal nuclear/cytoplasmic ratio. In the stroma, marked edema and telangiectasis are common. Blood vessels also undergo hyalinization and thrombosis. The lamina propria usually contains atypical spindle cells similar to those of giant cell cystitis (Fig. 5-42). Later, ulcers and fibrosis and contraction of the bladder wall and stricture of the ureters may occur.[214,215]

Florid epithelial proliferations[211-215] that can simulate carcinoma have been seen (Fig 5-43). Attention to the reactive nature of the background is crucial to avoid a misdiagnosis of carcinoma.

## Reaction to chemotherapy

Urothelial carcinoma in situ is commonly treated with intravesical topical chemotherapy. The most frequently used agents are the alkylating agents triethylenethiophosphoramide (thiotepa) and mitomycin C. These drugs induce denudation of the bladder mucosa in 37% of biopsies.[148] The remaining epithelium often shows nuclear changes such as pleomorphism and hyperchromasia, which may be mistaken for residual carcinoma in situ (Figs 5-44, 5-45).[216]

Pseudocarcinomatous lesions similar to those seen in radiation cystitis have been seen in patients who have been treated with chemotherapy.[211]

## Infectious cystitis

### Bacterial cystitis

Bacterial infection is the most common cause of cystitis and is usually caused by coliform organisms such as *Escherichia coli*, *Klebsiella pneumoniae*, and *Streptococcus faecalis*. Less commonly, *Proteus vulgaris*, *Pseudomonas pyocyanea*, *Neisseria gonorrhoeae*, *Salmonella typhi*, and diphtheroids are implicated. A predisposition to bacterial cystitis is associated with structural factors, including exstrophy, urethral malforma-

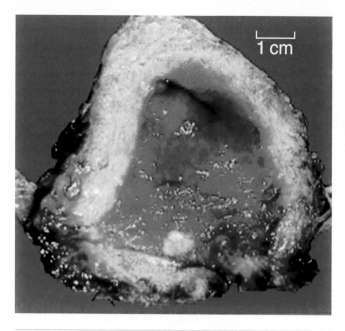

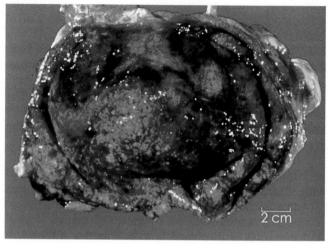

**Fig. 5-47** Gangrenous cystitis from a patient with *Klebsiella* sepsis. The mucosa is diffusely necrotic.

**Fig. 5-46** Bladder of a spinal cord injury patient with chronic and acute cystitis.

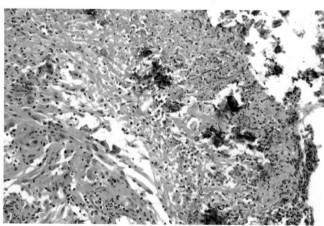

**Fig. 5-48** Encrusted cystitis with deposits of calcium salts.

tions, fistulae with other pelvic organs, diverticula, calculi, and foreign bodies. Urinary stasis and alkalinity also promote infection. Systemic illnesses such as diabetes mellitus, chronic renal disease, and immunosuppression are predisposing conditions. Most pathogens gain access to the bladder by ascending the urethra. Mycobacteria are an exception and usually descend from the upper tract in the urine.

Early in bacterial infection the appearance of the mucosa ranges from moderately erythematous to deeply hemorrhagic; these changes may be diffuse or focal. In addition to the classic symptoms of dysuria, urgency, and frequency, hematuria may result from leakage of erythrocytes through the mucosa. Later, a gray fibrinous membrane may cover the mucosal surface. With progression, a thin purulent exudate may adhere to the surface, creating a suppurative or exudative cystitis. Edema may thicken the vesical wall, and in chronic infections fibrosis may thicken and stiffen the wall, and the mucosa may be ulcerated (Fig. 5-46).

Microscopically, the urothelium may be hyperplastic or metaplastic. Ulceration may be extensive, and the surface of the ulcer may be covered by a fibrinous exudate, in which neutrophils are mixed with bacterial colonies. Early in the infection edema is often the predominant finding. Initially leukocytes are not numerous, but as the infection progresses they become prominent in the lamina propria. In severe cases suppuration is followed by abscess formation, which may involve the entire thickness of the bladder wall. When the inflammatory reaction is less intense and more indolent, the process may be characterized as subacute. In such cases the mucosa is usually denuded, the lamina propria is edematous, and eosinophils may be prominent.

In chronic cystitis the mucosa may be ulcerated and the urothelium thin or hyperplastic. The urothelium may display reactive atypia. Granulation tissue may replace parts of the lamina propria and muscularis propria, eventually becoming densely fibrotic.

## Gangrene

Gangrene is a dangerous complication of vesical infection and may arise as a consequence of circulatory compromise, debilitating systemic illness (such as uncontrolled diabetes mellitus or carcinoma), vascular insufficiency, or instillation of corrosive chemicals.[217-220] Gangrene usually begins in the mucosa and the necrotic tissue is sloughed to expose deeper structures (Fig. 5-47). Occasionally, the muscularis propria is deeply penetrated, and gangrene extends to the serosa. Deposition of mineral salts from the urine may give the sloughed material a gritty texture.

### Encrusted cystitis

When urea-splitting bacteria alkalinize the urine and inorganic salts are deposited in a damaged mucosa (Fig. 5-48), the term encrusted cystitis is applied.[221-227] Encrusted cystitis is most common in women and may occur in association with conditions in which inflammation or trauma damages the mucosa. In recent years, an increasing number of cases of encrusted cystitis have been diagnosed, especially in immunosuppressed patients such as renal transplant recipients. Numerous species of bacteria have been demonstrated in this infection, but *Corynebacterium* group D2 (*Corynebac-*

*terium urealyticum*) is currently isolated in most cases.[228–230] Urine culture in selective media and prolonged incubation are necessary to isolate *Corynebacterium urealyticum*.[231] Patients complain of long-standing dysuria, frequency, and sometimes hematuria. The urine contains gritty material, blood, mucus, and pus. When the salts are rich in calcium, the deposits may be visible on radiographs.[227,232] Cystoscopically, the lesions are usually multiple and have a gritty appearance. Rarely, the entire mucosa is involved. Histologically, the lesions are covered with a shaggy coat of fibrin mixed with calcified necrotic debris and inflammatory cells. The underlying tissue may be quite inflamed early in the course of the disease, but later inflammatory cells become scant and the lamina propria becomes fibrotic. Mineral salts may also be deposited on the surface of urothelial carcinoma, particularly in areas of necrosis or fulguration.[232] Treatment is based on adapted antibiotic therapy, acidification of urine, and excision of calcified plaques. The consequences of treatment failure are serious and can result in graft nephrectomy in kidney transplant recipients.[230]

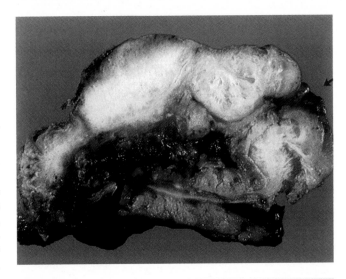

**Fig. 5-49** Urachal abscess. Arrow indicates outlet of urachus in the bladder mucosa.

### Emphysematous cystitis

In some cases of cystitis gas-filled blebs are seen on cystoscopy or at gross examination, a condition termed emphysematous cystitis.[233–242] Emphysematous cystitis is more common in women than men. Approximately half the patients are diabetic, usually having bacterial infections with *E. coli* or *Aerobacter aerogenes*.[243] Less frequently, the infection is fungal.[238,242] Other predisposing conditions include cystoscopy, trauma, fistula, and urinary stasis. The blebs range from 0.5 to 3 mm in diameter and may be present throughout the mucosa. Histologically, the blebs are cavities lined by flattened cells and surrounded by thin septa in the lamina propria. Occasionally they extend into the muscularis propria.

## Xanthogranulomatous cystitis

Xanthogranulomatous inflammation is associated with malignant neoplasms in the bladder, as it is in the kidney and extraurinary sites, as well as with benign neoplasms and nonneoplastic conditions such as urachal diverticula or infections. Less than one dozen cases are reported.[205,206,244–252]

## Urachal abscess

Most bacterial infections of the urachus are associated with a urachal malformation or cyst.[253–255] Many of these develop into abscesses (Fig. 5-49) that may drain into the bladder or through the umbilicus. Rupture through the peritoneum can cause severe peritonitis, a serious complication. When the abscess is large and associated with much inflammation and fibrosis in surrounding tissues, it may be difficult or impossible to determine precisely the nature of the underlying urachal abnormality. The combination of antibiotic therapy with surgical excision of the urachal malformation and abscess is usually curative.[256] On rare occasions, urachal abscess may be caused by tuberculous, echinococcal, or actinomycotic infections.[23]

## Malakoplakia

First described in 1902 and 1903 by Michaelis and Gutmann[257] and by von Hansemann,[258] malakoplakia occurs most frequently in the urinary bladder, where it is visible as yellow-white soft raised plaques on the mucosal surface.[259] It was this appearance, combined with a reluctance to speculate on the pathogenesis of the disorder, that prompted von Hansemann to combine the Greek roots for plaque (*plakos*) and soft (*malakos*) to coin the term malakoplakia.[260] Urinary tract malakoplakia primarily affects women (more than 75% of cases) and has a peak incidence in the fifth decade.[260] It occasionally occurs in children.[261] Malakoplakia is an uncommon granulomatous process that results from impairment of the capacity of mononuclear cells to kill phagocytosed bacteria.[262,263] It is usually associated with infection by coliform organisms. Most patients present with the usual symptoms of urinary tract infection, including hematuria. *E. coli* is most frequently cultured from the urine but *Proteus vulgaris*, *Aerobacter aerogenes*, *K. pneumoniae*, and α-hemolytic streptococci have also been isolated. Despite this, bacteria have rarely been identified within the lesions of malakoplakia without the use of transmission electron microscopy.[264,265]

Grossly, the lesions are usually multiple, soft yellow or yellow-brown plaques (Fig. 5-50). Often there is a central dimple and a rim of congestion about the plaque. Lesions larger than 2 cm are unusual. In some cases the lesions are nodular, but rarely large and polypoid.

Microscopically, there is an accumulation of histiocytes with granular eosinophilic cytoplasm (von Hansemann histiocytes) in the superficial lamina propria beneath the urothelium, which is usually intact (Fig. 5-51). The histiocytes contain the characteristic intracytoplasmic inclusions known as Michaelis–Gutmann bodies. These are typically spherical, 5–8 μm, concentrically laminated bodies with a bull's-eye appearance (Fig. 5-52). Often they are basophilic, but also may be pale and difficult to see. They always contain calcium and sometimes iron salts, so the von Kossa (Fig. 5-53) and Perl's Prussian blue stains highlight them. They also react with the periodic acid–Schiff stain, but so does the cytoplasm of the von Hansemann histiocytes (Fig. 5-54), so this

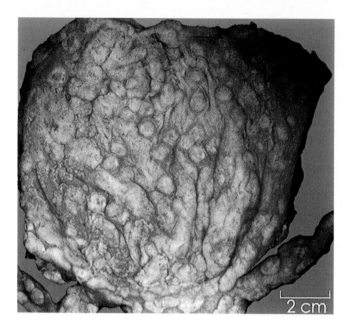

**Fig. 5-50** Malakoplakia of the bladder and ureters.

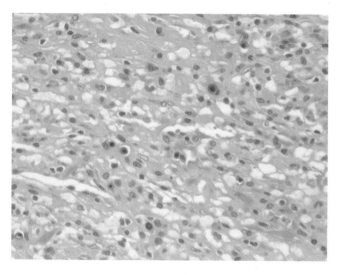

**Fig. 5-51** Malakoplakia.

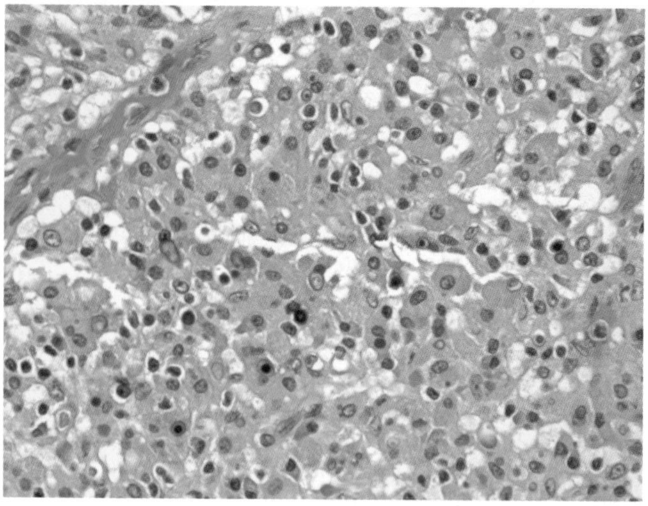

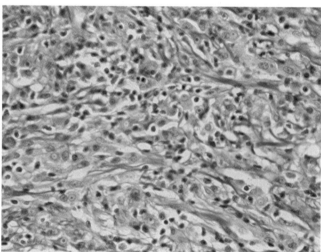

**Fig. 5-52** Malakoplakia. Note von Hausemann cells in the lamina propria.

**Fig. 5-53** Malakoplakia. The von Kossa stain for calcium highlights the Michaelis–Gutmann bodies.

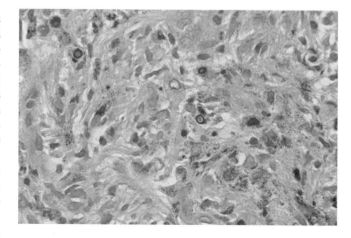

**Fig. 5-54** Malakoplakia. The von Hansemann histiocytes react with the periodic acid–Schiff stain.

technique is less helpful than staining for calcium. Early in the disease, Michaelis–Gutmann bodies may be scant and very difficult to appreciate in sections stained with hematoxylin and eosin. Thus, when there is an infiltrate of histiocytes in the bladder, a section should be stained for calcium to find inapparent Michaelis–Gutmann bodies. These bodies are required for the diagnosis, so it is possible that there is an early prediagnostic phase of the disease in which there is insufficient calcification to make them detectable. In some cases there is abundant granulation tissue, extensive fibrosis, or a dense infiltrate of acute and chronic inflammatory cells that may obscure the von Hansemann histiocytes and Michaelis–Gutmann bodies. Late in the disease, there may be extensive fibrosis and few Michaelis–Gutmann bodies.

Ultrastructural and immunohistochemical studies have shown that the cytoplasm of von Hansemann histiocytes contains many phagolysosomes in which there are frag-

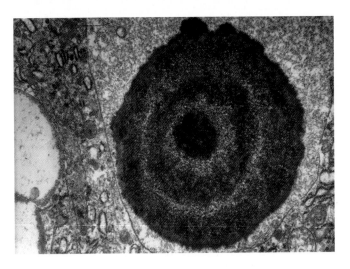

**Fig. 5-55** Ultrastructural appearance of a Michaelis–Gutmann body.

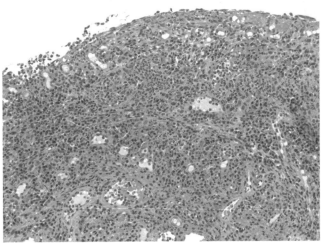

**Fig. 5-56** Candidal cystitis. Fungus is present in the inflammatory exudate and debris.

ments of bacterial cell walls.[266] It appears that Michaelis–Gutmann bodies form when the phagolysosomes fuse and calcium is transported across the phagolysosomal membranes, forming hydroxyapatite crystals with phosphate from the bacterial cell walls. The bodies enlarge over time, producing the typical laminated structure. Ultrastructurally, Michaelis–Gutmann bodies range from 5 to 10 μm in diameter (Fig. 5-55).[267] At the center is a dense crystalline core surrounded by a homogeneous zone that is not crystalline but rather granular or composed of myelin figures.

### Tuberculous cystitis

Tuberculous cystitis is almost always caused by *Mycobacterium tuberculosis*;[268,269] *Mycobacterium bovis* accounts for only about 3% of cases.[270] Tuberculous cystitis is almost always secondary to renal tuberculosis, from which organisms in infected urine implant in the bladder. In one study 66% of patients with surgically treated renal tuberculosis had vesical tuberculosis.[271] Some cases in men appear to be secondary to genital infection, in which case spread of the infection is directly along the mucosa. Frequency, urgency, hematuria, and dysuria are common symptoms.

Early in the infection the lesions are in the region of the ureteral orifices and consist of marked mucosal congestion, sometimes with edema. These lesions may progress to form 1–3 mm tubercles or may ulcerate and become covered by friable necrotic material. Initially the tubercles are sharply circumscribed, firm, and solid. As they enlarge they coalesce and ulcerate.

The tuberculous granuloma in which central caseous necrosis is surrounded by multinucleated giant cells, plasma cells, and lymphocytes is the characteristic histological lesion. Acid-fast or auramine–rhodamine-stained sections will usually disclose mycobacteria.

Chronic tuberculous cystitis may result in a small, scarred, low-capacity bladder. The ureteral orifices may be distorted and obstructed, causing hydronephrosis and hydroureter. Rarely, the infection penetrates the wall of the bladder causing peritonitis or a fistula.

### Fungal and actinomycotic cystitis

Fungal cystitis is uncommon and most often is caused by *Candida albicans*.[272–274] Infection may ascend the urethra or may be hematogenous. Ascending infection is usually limited to the trigone. Most candidal cystitis occurs in debilitated patients or those on antibiotic therapy. Many are diabetic and most are women. Nocturia, constant pain, and marked frequency are typical symptoms. The urine is usually turbid and bloody.

The lesions are typically slightly raised, sharply demarcated white plaques with irregular shapes. Occasionally, a fungus ball may form in the lumen of the bladder. Microscopically, there is ulceration and inflammation of the lamina propria. The typical hyphae and budding yeast forms may be seen in routine sections (Fig. 5-56) or with periodic acid–Schiff or Gomori's methenamine silver stains.

Rare cases of fungal cystitis caused by *Aspergillus* species[275] and other fungi have been reported.[273]

Vesical actinomycosis is rare in the general population but complicates actinomycosis of the ovary or fallopian tube in about 10% of cases.[276] Symptoms are non-specific. Microscopically, the bladder wall is focally or diffusely thickened and there is often continuity with the lesions in adjacent organs. The infection may form a mass simulating a neoplasm. The mucosa may be edematous or ulcerated and, if the infection is transmural, a fistula may form. Microscopically, there is abundant granulation tissue within which are small abscesses containing colonies of *Actinomyces* (sulfur granules).

### Viral cystitis

#### Human papillomavirus

A few dozen cases of condyloma acuminatum of the bladder have been reported.[277–285] There is a female to male preponderance of approximately 2 : 1. Patients range in age from early adult to old age, but most have been younger than 50 years. Most patients, many of whom are immunocompromised, have had condylomata of the urethra, vulva, vagina, anus, or perineum, but some have had condylomata only in the bladder. In some immunocompromised patients the lesions have been particularly difficult to eradicate and may rarely progress to invasive disease.[286,287]

Cystoscopy usually shows a solitary lesion in the bladder neck or trigone. These appear papillary, and the clinical differential diagnosis includes papillary carcinoma and other papillary lesions of the vesical mucosa. Alternatively, the mucosa may have prominent folds and scattered white flecks (Fig. 5-57).[279]

Microscopically, the lesions show the characteristic features of condylomata, including koilocytotic cells with abundant clear cytoplasm (Fig. 5-58) and wrinkled hyperchromatic nuclei. These features distinguish the lesions from the rare squamous papilloma and papillary squamous cell carcinoma of the bladder.

### Other viruses

Adenovirus is recognized as an important cause of hemorrhagic cystitis, especially in children.[288] Otherwise healthy children may be affected, as well as children after bone marrow transplantation. Adenovirus types 11 and 21 are most frequently identified.[289-293] Papovavirus also causes hemorrhagic cystitis in children and adults.[294] Herpes simplex

type 2 has caused hemorrhagic cystitis in a few patients,[295] and herpes zoster has also caused cystitis.[296] Cytomegalovirus also is sometimes seen in the bladder, particularly in immunosuppressed patients.[297]

## Schistosomiasis

Schistosomiasis is the fourth most prevalent disease in the world and the leading cause of hematuria.[298] In humans, the trematode *Schistosoma hematobium* commonly resides in the paravesical veins and causes urinary schistosomiasis, which also is known as bilharziasis.[299] The adult forms of these flat worms are dioecious, living as pairs in veins, with the male surrounding the female. Estimates of adults' life spans vary from 2 to 20 years, and each pair is capable of producing up to 200 eggs per day. In endemic areas children have the highest incidence of infection, but it is adults who suffer the severe effects of chronic infection.

Schistosomiasis has various clinical manifestations, but the underlying process begins with the deposition of eggs in small veins and venules. Subsequently, the eggs may pass into the lumina of hollow organs, such as the bladder, or become trapped in the walls of viscera, where they produce a granulomatous response and may be destroyed or calcified. Alternatively, they may enter the circulation from the small veins and embolize other sites. For unknown reasons, the predominant site for oviposition by *S. hematobium* is the venous systems of the lower urinary tract. *S. hematobium* deposits eggs in clusters, causing a patchy distribution of lesions.[300] The eggs are not acid-fast in histologic sections, whereas those of other common human schistosomes, *S. mansoni, S. intercalatum,* and *S. japonicum,* are acid-fast. *S. mattheei,* which usually infects animals but may cause urinary schistosomiasis in humans, also is not acid-fast. In humans, the eggs of *S. hematobium* are intermediate in size between those of *S. mansoni* and *S. japonicum.*

Schistosomiasis may be categorized as active or inactive. The active form is characterized by the presence of active pairs of flatworms depositing eggs, which elicit a strong granulomatous response (Fig. 5-59). Polypoid inflammatory

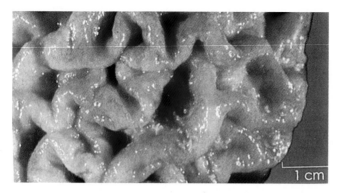

**Fig. 5-57** Condyloma of the bladder with prominent folds.

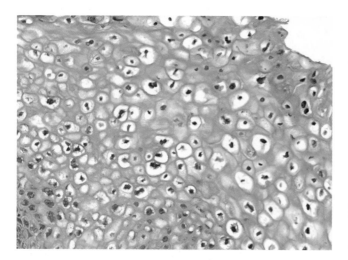

**Fig. 5-58** Koilocytes in the condyloma of the bladder.

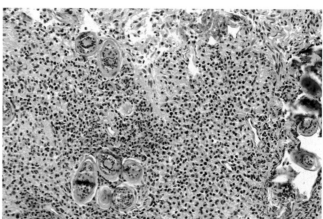

**Fig. 5-59** Schistosomiasis, active form with numerous ova.

masses may obstruct the ureters or the bladder outlet.[300] The number of ova in the urine correlates with the burden of eggs in the bladder wall, and the active stage is most readily diagnosed by examination of the urine. The inactive form occurs after the worms have died and there are no viable eggs in urine or tissue. However, eggs remain in the tissue, and high concentrations of calcified eggs may be detected radiographically. Evaluation of the quantity of ova in tissue requires special digestion techniques.[301-304] In the inactive phase, the patient is not infectious.

The principal non-neoplastic manifestations of schistosomiasis in the bladder are polyps and ulcers. In most cases, the trigone and ureteral orifices are the sites of the lesions,[241] which may lead to bladder neck obstruction.[305] The deposits of ova are heaviest in the submucosa.[80] During active disease, heavy burdens of eggs produce multiple large inflammatory polyps, which may obstruct the ureteral orifices and may bleed sufficiently to cause anemia or clot retention.[306-308] Obstruction may lead to stone formation in the kidneys, ureters, and bladder.[309,310] In inactive schistosomiasis the polyps are fibrocalcific. In a small percentage of cases the polyps are composed of hyperplastic epithelium that appears more villous than polypoid. The inflammation in the bladder also gives rise to polypoid cystitis, biopsy specimens of which may not contain any eggs. In the early active stage, ulcers rarely form when a necrotic polyp detaches. Ulcers are more common in the chronic stage, when large numbers of eggs (more than 250 000/g of bladder tissue) are present. These constantly painful ulcers are often in the posterior bladder wall of young adults and have stellate or ovoid contours.[311] Metaplastic changes, including keratinizing squamous metaplasia and intestinal metaplasia, are also common.[298] The bladder mucosa may also contain raised granules known as bilharzial tubercles.[312] These may calcify to form the classic sandy patches. Neoplastic complications of schistosomiasis are discussed in Chapter 6.

## Calculi

Bladder stones are most common in men with bladder outlet obstruction (Fig. 5-60) and in children in underdeveloped countries. Most are free in the bladder, but occasionally calculi form about a suture after surgery. The symptoms are similar to those of bladder outlet obstruction, including hesitancy, frequency, and nocturia. Other symptoms include hematuria, dysuria, and suprapubic pain radiating down the penis. Radiography or cystoscopy is usually diagnostic of bladder calculus. Because bladder stones may be composed of radiolucent uric acid, cystoscopy is the most definitive diagnostic procedure.

Bladder calculi were common in children in Europe before 1800 and remain relatively common in some parts of Asia and the Middle East. Most patients are boys younger than 10 years, and the stones are composed of calcium oxalate and ammonium acid urate. Patients usually do not have renal stones. A diet low in protein and minerals, along with low fluid intake, seem to be factors that promote stone formation in these children. In North America and Europe, only 2–3% of patients with bladder calculi are children.

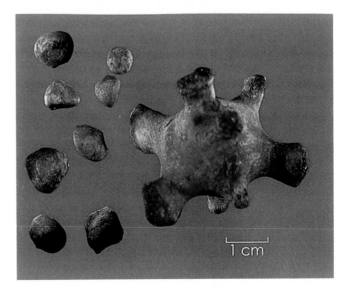

**Fig. 5-60** Bladder calculi from a man with obstructive prostatic hyperplasia.

Most of these also have renal or ureteral calculi, and their stones are composed of calcium oxalate, calcium phosphate, or a mixture of the two. Although most of these children have bacterial infections, the causative organisms do not often produce urease. Children with a history of multiple urologic procedures are more likely to have struvite stones and infections with *Proteus* species.

## Polyps and other mass lesions

### Ectopic prostate

Polyps composed of prostatic epithelium resembling those more commonly seen in the prostatic urethra rarely occur in the bladder.[313-316] Reported cases have occurred in men from 20 to 67 years old, and hematuria has been the most consistent symptom. About two-thirds of the lesions arise in the trigone and the architecture varies from papillary to polypoid. The stroma contains prostatic glands and the surface is covered by columnar epithelium or urothelium. Immunohistochemistry confirms the prostatic character of the glands and columnar cells. Prostatic hyperplasia may also expand into the bladder lumen as a polypoid mass.[317-319]

### Other polyps

Fibroepithelial polyps of the bladder are rare and resemble their more common counterpart in the ureter.[320-322] They are distinguished from polypoid cystitis by being solitary, with a more fibrous core and a paucity of inflammatory cells. Rare cases of collagen polyps resulting from the accumulation of injected collagen in the bladder to control stress incontinence have been reported.[323]

### Hamartoma

Hamartoma of the bladder is a rare (fewer than a dozen reported cases) polypoid mass (Fig. 5-61) composed of

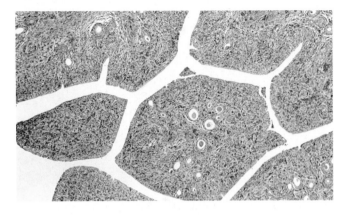

**Fig. 5-61** Bladder hamartoma consisting of polypoid fronds of cellular stroma containing small tubular structures lined by epithelium.

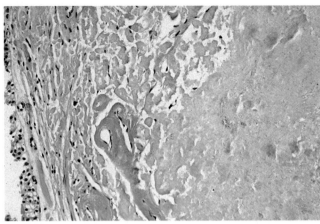

**Fig. 5-62** Amyloid fills the lamina propria in this biopsy specimen.

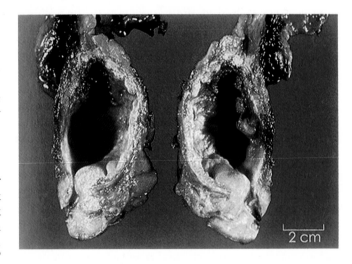

**Fig. 5-63** Postoperative spindle cell nodule in bladder neck.

epithelial elements resembling von Brunn's nests, cystitis glandularis, or cystitis cystica distributed irregularly in a stroma that may be muscular, fibrous, or edematous.[324-328] Occasional cases have intestinal metaplasia of the glands, small tubules resembling renal tubules, or markedly cellular stroma.

## Amyloidosis

More than 100 cases of primary amyloidosis of the bladder have been reported.[329-338] The lesions appear throughout adulthood and are equally common in both sexes. In most cases the deposits are limited to the bladder, but in some cases the ureters and urethra have also been involved. Hematuria is almost always the presenting symptom.[339] On cystoscopy the lesions range from sessile and ulcerated to nodular or polypoid, and often are mistaken for carcinoma.[105] In about 25% of cases there are multiple lesions. In the Mayo Clinic series of 31 cases of primary amyloidosis of the bladder, 24 patients had immunoglobulin light chain, and three had transthyretin-related amyloid. Although local recurrences were common, none of the patients developed systemic amyloidosis.[340] Histologically, the amyloid deposits are predominantly in the lamina propria and muscularis propria (Fig. 5-62). Vascular involvement is less prominent. A foreign body giant cell reaction may be present adjacent to the deposits, and rarely the deposits become calcified.

Secondary involvement of the bladder is rare in systemic amyloidosis.[341] Reported cases are associated with rheumatoid arthritis, Crohn's disease, ankylosing spondylitis, myeloma, and familial Mediterranean fever. Hematuria is universal and often very severe.[339,341] Although primary localized amyloidosis often presents with hematuria, it is generally much less severe than that associated with secondary amyloidosis. On cystoscopy there is diffuse erythema, sometimes with petechiae or necrosis. Histologically the amyloid is mainly in the blood vessels; occasionally there are lesser deposits in the lamina propria.

## Postoperative spindle cell nodule

The term postoperative spindle cell nodule was coined by Proppe et al.[342] in 1984 for a proliferative spindle cell lesion occurring in the lower urinary tract and female genital tract within 120 days of surgery at the site where the lesions arise. Subsequently, others have reported identical lesions.[343,344] At cystoscopy, the bladder lesions are nodular (Fig. 5-63) and described as a 'heaped up tumor' and a 'friable vegetant mass.' The possibility of confusion with malignancy is heightened by the microscopic examination that shows interlacing fascicles (Fig. 5-64) of mitotically active spindle cells (Fig. 5-65) resembling leiomyosarcoma or some other spindle cell sarcoma. Other histologic features include delicate vasculature, scattered inflammatory cells, small foci of hemorrhage, edema, and focal myxoid change. Although there may be many mitotic figures, the nuclei usually show little pleomorphism or hyperchromasia.

The original and subsequent reports have shown that postoperative spindle cell nodules are benign reactive proliferations that resolve spontaneously or with medical therapy and

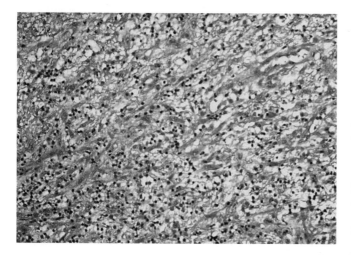

**Fig. 5-64** Postoperative spindle cell nodule composed of cellular bundles of spindle cells.

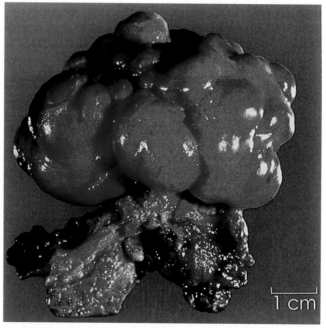

**Fig. 5-66** Pseudosarcomatous fibromyxoid tumor. A polypoid mass projects into the bladder lumen.

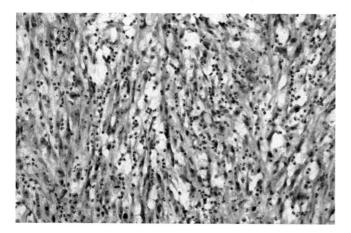

**Fig. 5-65** Postoperative spindle cell nodule with mitotic figure.

must be distinguished from sarcoma. Well-differentiated leiomyosarcoma is the most important consideration in this differential diagnosis. This distinction may be very difficult because both postoperative spindle cell nodule and well-differentiated leiomyosarcoma have similarly bland nuclei, may infiltrate the muscularis propria, and have similar numbers of mitotic figures. The prominent array of delicate blood vessels seen in many postoperative spindle cell nodules is not a common feature of leiomyosarcoma. Myxoid change may be seen in both and is not helpful unless extensive, a finding more common in leiomyosarcoma. The clinical history of recent surgery at the site powerfully suggests postoperative spindle cell nodule. In these cases, follow-up with cystoscopy and additional biopsies is warranted.

## Pseudosarcomatous fibromyxoid tumor (inflammatory pseudotumor)

Patients without a history of recent surgery may also have benign proliferative spindle cell lesions that mimic sarcoma.[345] A variety of terms have been applied to these, but pseudosar-

comatous fibromyxoid tumor is emerging as the preferred term.[346–352] Most patients range in age from 20 to 50 years and there appears to be a slight preponderance of women. Gross hematuria is the most common presenting symptom.

Grossly, the lesions have ranged from a pedunculated mass protruding into the bladder cavity (Fig. 5-66) to small nodules or ulcers in the mucosa. Usually, the lesions are solitary, 2–5 cm polyps with broad bases. Some lesions are sessile and deeply infiltrate the muscularis propria (Fig. 5-67). The cut surface may be gelatinous or mucoid.

Histologically, pseudosarcomatous fibromyxoid tumor is typically composed of spindle cells arranged in a widely spaced haphazard pattern in a myxoid matrix containing a prominent network of small blood vessels (Fig. 5-68).[351] A second pattern that is sometimes seen is more cellular, with spindle cells arranged in fascicles with variable amounts of collagen between them (Fig. 5-69). In both patterns the spindle cells are similar, with long bipolar eosinophilic or amphophilic cytoplasmic processes. In the myxoid pattern stellate and polygonal cells are also present. The nuclei are large and occasionally multiple. In most cases there are fewer than two mitotic figures per 10 high-power fields, but occasional cases have more.[351] The myxoid pattern (Fig. 5-70) usually contains a sparse inflammatory infiltrate, whereas in the second pattern lymphocytes and plasma cells may be prominent. An example of the second pattern has been reported as a plasma cell granuloma.[354] Eosinophils are common in both patterns. Infiltration of the muscularis propria is common, and the process may extend into perivesical fat. ALK-1 staining is often positive in these tumours (Fig 5-71).

The main differential diagnostic consideration for pseudosarcomatous fibromyxoid tumor is malignancy, particularly myxoid sarcomatoid carcinoma and other sarcomas, includ-

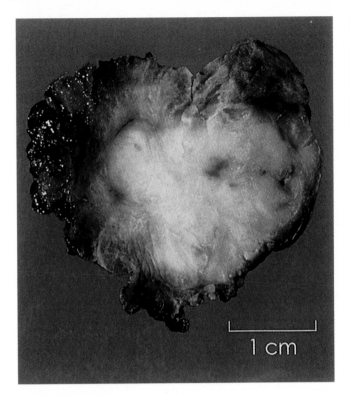

**Fig. 5-67** Pseudosarcomatous fibromyxoid tumor. The cut surface shows involvement of the full thickness of the bladder wall.

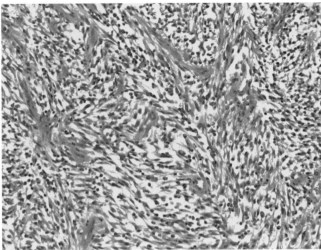

**Fig. 5-69** Pseudosarcomatous fibromyxoid tumor composed of fascicles of spindle cells.

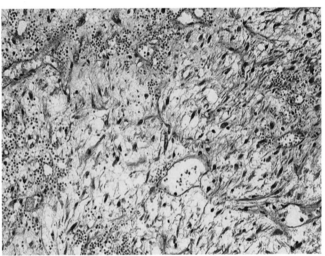

**Fig. 5-70** Pseudosarcomatous fibromyxoid tumor with myxoid areas.

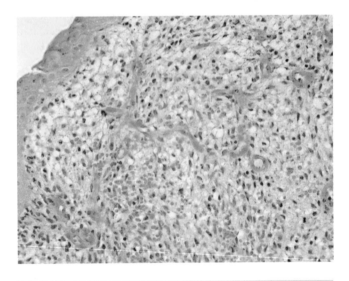

**Fig. 5-68** Pseudosarcomatous fibromyxoid tumor showing delicate blood vessels in a background of spindle cells.

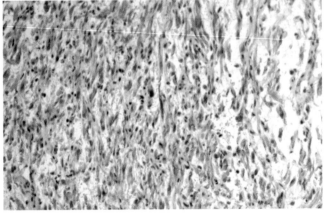

**Fig. 5-71** ALK-1 staining.

ing myxoid leiomyosarcoma. Inflammation and vascularity are more prominent in pseudosarcomatous fibromyxoid tumor than in leiomyosarcoma, and the cellularity is more variable, although a destructively infiltrative margin favors leiomyosarcoma. Pseudosarcomatous fibromyxoid tumor also may invade the muscularis propria. The most reliable criteria to separate sarcoma and pseudosarcomatous fibromyxoid tumor are nuclear atypia and the presence of necrosis at the tumor–detrusor muscle interface in muscle-invasive cases.[353] Sarcoma also shows less prominent microvascula-

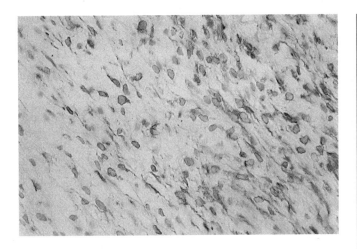

**Fig. 5-72** Cytokeratin immunoreactivity in pseudosarcomatous fibromyxoid tumor.

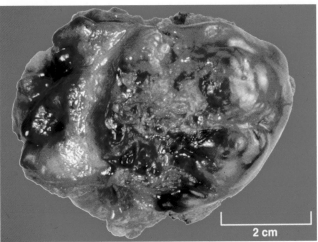

**Fig. 5-73** Endometriosis. A hemorrhagic ill-defined mass projects in the bladder lumen.

ture, less variable cellularity, consistently less than one mitotic figure per 10 high-power fields, and predominant acute inflammation without plasma cells.[353] Immunohistochemical evidence of smooth muscle actin, desmin and other muscle-specific differentiation favors leiomyosarcoma, but this is not absolutely reliable. Immunohistochemically, the spindle cells of pseudosarcomatous fibromyxoid tumor are strongly positive for vimentin, variable for smooth muscle actin, and focally for cytokeratin[355,356] (Fig. 5-72). Fluorescence in situ hybridization (FISH), with translocation of the anaplastic lymphoma kinase (ALK) gene, or immunohistochemical staining for cytoplasmic ALK protein is present in 40–89% of pseudosarcomatous fibromyxoid tumors.[355,357,358]

## Müllerian lesions

### Endometriosis

The bladder is the most common site of urinary tract involvement in endometriosis,[359-364] but only about 1% of women with endometriosis have bladder involvement.[365] As many as 50% of these patients have a history of pelvic surgery, and approximately 12% lack evidence of endometriosis at any other site. The average age is approximately 35 years. Frequency, dysuria, and hematuria are the most common symptoms, but more than 50% of patients have no vesical symptoms. Endometriosis of the muscularis propria may give symptoms similar to those of interstitial cystitis.[366] There is a palpable suprapubic mass in almost 50% of cases, and this may undergo catamenial enlargement. Rarely, endometriosis has been reported in postmenopausal women treated with estrogen[367-369] and in men treated with estrogen for prostate cancer.[370-372] At cystoscopy the lesions usually appear as congested, edematous mucosal elevations overlying blue, blue-black, or red-brown cysts. Grossly, a hemorrhagic ill-defined mass may project into the bladder lumen (Fig. 5-73). The overlying urothelium may be intact or eroded. If the lesions are limited to the muscularis propria (Fig. 5-74) or serosa, the mucosa may be normal. Fibrosis

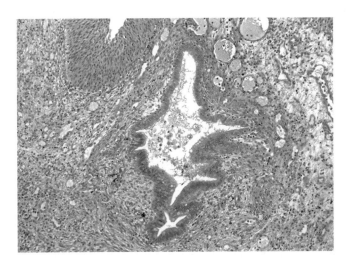

**Fig. 5-74** Endometriosis. Endometrioid glands surrounded by endometrial stroma.

and hyperplastic muscle around the lesions may thicken the bladder wall. Microscopically, the lesions resemble endometriosis as seen elsewhere. In some cases not all of the glands are surrounded by endometrial stroma, and in some foci stroma is absent.[360] A case of malignant transformation of endometriosis of bladder has been reported.[373]

### Endocervicosis

Endocervicosis of the bladder is less common than endometriosis.[374,375] Patients typically present in their fourth and fifth decades with symptoms such as suprapubic pain, dysuria, frequency, or hematuria, and may have catamenial exacerbation of symptoms. They often have a history of cesarean section. Most lesions are in the muscularis propria, but the mucosa (Fig. 5-75A) and adventitia also may be involved. In endocervicosis there is a haphazard proliferation of irregularly shaped mucinous glands in the bladder

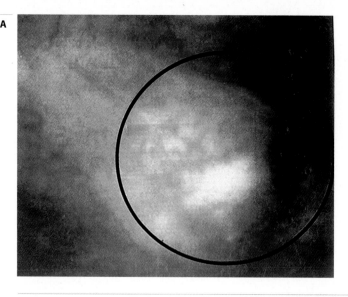

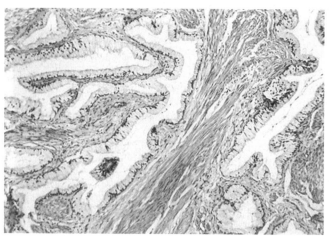

**Fig. 5-75** Endocervicosis. (**A**) Cystoscopy shows vesical endocervicosis as a submucosal nodule. (**B**) Glands lined by benign columnar epithelium are present in the muscularis propria.

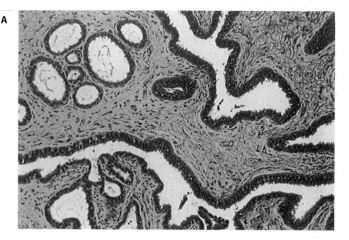

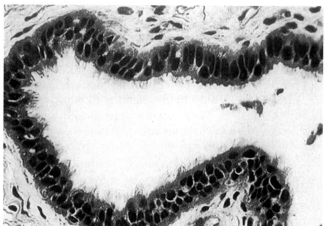

**Fig. 5-76** Endosalpingiosis. (**A**) Glands, some of them branching, are lined by tubal-type epithelium. (**B**) Higher magnification demonstrates cilia on the surfaces of the epithelial cells.

wall (Fig. 5-75B). The epithelium lining the glands consists of a single layer of columnar cells with abundant pale cytoplasm that reacts with periodic acid–Schiff and mucicarmine stains. Ciliated cells often are interspersed among the mucinous cells. When the glands are dilated, the epithelium is cuboidal or flattened. The glandular lumina usually contain mucus. Ruptured glands with extravasated mucus and a stromal reaction may be seen. The most common of the benign müllerian glandular lesions in women, endosalpingiosis, is, enigmatically, the one least often seen in the bladder. Indeed, it has only recently been described.[376] Vesical endosalpingiosis consists of numerous tubal-type glands (Fig. 5-76A) lined at least focally by ciliated cells (Fig. 5-76B). The müllerian epithelium may replace the urothelium of the mucosa and cover polypoid intraluminal projections (Fig. 5-77). In some

cases a mixture of several different types of müllerian epithelium is present and the term müllerianosis may be appropriate.[376]

## Müllerian cyst

In men, müllerian duct cysts usually lie between the bladder and rectum and may involve the posterior wall of the bladder.[377,378] Patients usually present with irritative bladder symptoms and clinical evaluation reveals a midline supraprostatic mass. Grossly, the cyst is unilocular or multilocular and filled with clear or hemorrhagic fluid. Microscopically, the cyst lining is often lost throughout much of its area, but a layer of müllerian epithelium can usually be found at least focally. In contrast to seminal vesicle cysts, spermatozoa are absent from müllerian duct cysts.

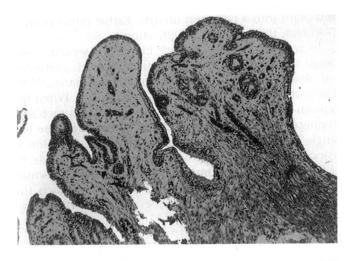

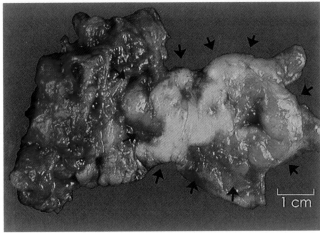

**Fig. 5-77** Müllerianosis. Polyps lined by müllerian epithelium protrude into the bladder lumen. Epithelia of endocervical, endometrial, and tubal types were present in this case.

**Fig. 5-78** Exstrophy of the bladder. The mucosa (arrows) shows congestion, edema, and fibrosis.

Müllerian sinus lined by mucus-secreting epithelium connecting the posterolateral wall of the bladder with the broad ligament is a rare lesion.[379]

# Malformations

## Agenesis

Agenesis of the bladder is rare,[380] and only a few dozen cases have been recorded, almost all of them in girls.[381–385] Agenesis results from failure of separation of the ureters from the wolffian ducts. In this situation, the ureters enter the müllerian tract or posterior urethra. Alternatively, the urorectal septum fails to form, and the cloaca remains. Usually there is ureteral obstruction with megaureter and hydronephrosis. When development of the distal ureters fails, the trigone of the bladder does not develop. Vesical agenesis is strongly associated with sirenomelia, a syndrome characterized by fusion of the lower extremities and other anomalies. Most such cases have no ureters, lending support to the concept that vesical agenesis is related to failure of ureteral development.

## Exstrophy

Exstrophy (incomplete closure) of the bladder and its associated malformations has long been recognized, and the 1855 description and review by Duncan[386] can hardly be improved upon today. Exstrophy is more common than agenesis and occurs in approximately 1 of 10 000–40 000 live births.[387] Although there is little risk (1%) to siblings of patients with exstrophy,[388] among offspring of parents with exstrophy the rate is 1 in 70 live births.[389] Exstrophy occurs in two variants: bladder exstrophy and cloacal exstrophy. The latter is much less common than the former (1 in 200 000 live births).[390]

Exstrophy results from perforation of an abnormally developed cloacal membrane. In normal development, the ingrowth of mesenchyme between the ectodermal and endodermal layers of the cloacal membrane permits fusion of the midline structures below the umbilicus and closure of the abdominal wall. Downward growth of the urorectal septum divides the cloaca into the bladder anteriorly and the rectum posteriorly. The urorectal septum joins the cloacal membrane in the perineum before perforating it to produce the anal and urogenital openings. Before perforation, the genital tubercles migrate medially and fuse in the midline. Defective development of the cloacal membrane with premature perforation results in a variety of abnormalities, including superior vesical fissure, bladder exstrophy, and cloacal exstrophy.[391]

Bladder exstrophy is five to seven times more common in boys than in girls.[392] It is often accompanied by other malformations, such as epispadias, intestinal malformations, and defects of spinal closure. Genital malformations are the rule, with epispadias in 86% of boys and unfused labia in 71% of girls.[393] Epispadias is so often associated with exstrophy that the two are sometimes called the exstrophy–epispadias complex.[389] Spina bifida is present in 18% of cases.[393]

Bladder exstrophy is a true malformation rather than an arrest of development.[394] In exstrophy, the urinary tract is open to the body wall from the urethral meatus to the umbilicus.[391] The mucosa of the bladder and urethra is fused to the adjacent skin, and the urethra and bladder are foreshortened. The ureters end in a widened trigone and are prone to reflux after surgical closure. The pubic symphysis is widely open (3–10 cm).[391] The rectus muscles are widely separated, and umbilical and inguinal hernias are common. At birth, the exstrophic bladder mucosa is usually smooth and has a normal appearance. This condition is short-lived, and trauma and infection quickly produce ulcers and inflammation (Fig. 5-78). The anus is often anteriorly displaced, and there may be rectal prolapse. In girls, the müllerian system shows variable duplication and failure of closure.[395] In boys, the penis is short, with a dorsal chordee. Incomplete variants of this constellation of anatomical lesions are rare.[396]

Histologically, the mucosa often shows acute and chronic inflammation with ulceration and metaplastic changes at the time of surgical closure.[397] Squamous and intestinal metaplasia is absent or slight at birth, and become extensive and profound with time.[398] After closure, the mucosa often remains inflamed and squamous metaplasia is common, although changes such as cystitis cystica and glandularis diminish.[397]

Without surgery, more than 66% of patients with bladder exstrophy die by age 20.[392] Early surgical intervention, with or without urinary diversion, is successful in many cases, allowing preservation of renal function, urinary continence, and eliminating urinary infections in more than 50% of patients.[399,400] The chronic inflammation and metaplasia of untreated exstrophy predispose the patient to carcinoma, particularly adenocarcinoma.[392] Surgical reconstruction prevents this, and exstrophy-associated carcinoma has become rare.[401]

Cloacal exstrophy is a complex malformation that also is known as exstrophia splanchnia, which conveys the extensiveness of the defects.[402] Typically, the lower abdominal wall consists of a large area of exposed mucosa, above which is usually an omphalocele. At the center of the area of mucosa is a patch of intestinal mucosa with one to four orifices. The most superior orifice connects to the ileum, and the lowest connects to a short segment of colon that ends blindly. The other orifices are appendices. The anus is imperforate. Lateral to the intestinal mucosa is exstrophic bladder mucosa containing the ureteral orifices and occasionally the vasa deferentia and vagina. Patches of bladder mucosa may join above or below the intestinal mucosa, or may encircle it. The testes are undescended and the external genitalia are absent or malformed. Double penis is common in boys.[403] The pubic symphysis is diastatic and vertebral abnormalities are common. Abnormalities of other organ systems are rare. Cloacal exstrophy was invariably fatal four decades ago, but modern surgical techniques have greatly improved patient outcome, and survival is now almost 50%.[390]

## Duplication and septation of the bladder

The complete form of duplication is very rare and consists of two fully formed urinary bladders with complete mucosal and muscular elements.[404,405] Each unit receives the ureter from its side and drains into a duplicate urethra.[406] In the great majority of cases this anomaly is accompanied by either diphallus or duplication of the uterus and vagina. In almost 50% of cases the hindgut is duplicated, and the lumbar vertebrae may also be duplicated.[407]

In partial duplication, the bladder is divided either sagittally or coronally by a complete wall, and each side is connected to the ureter from the kidney on its side.[404,405,408] Partial duplication differs from complete duplication in that the two units usually communicate and drain into a common urethra. Partial duplication is even rarer than complete duplication.

In septation of the urinary bladder, a septum composed of mucosa with or without muscularis partitions the bladder

in either the sagittal or the coronal plane.[404,408] The partition may be complete or incomplete. When the septum is in the sagittal plane, the ureter from each side connects with its respective chamber. Because there is a single bladder neck and urethra, complete septation is associated with dysplasia and obstruction of one side.[409] If the partition is incomplete, drainage may be normal. Hourglass bladder is an allied condition in which the bladder narrows near its middle, giving it the shape of an hourglass.[410,411]

## Urachal cysts and persistence

Completely patent urachus is a dramatic lesion in which urine flows from the umbilicus or stump of the umbilical cord. This abnormality is uncommon, with fewer than 300 reported cases.[182,412] The ratio of males to females is approximately 2:1. Most patients with patent urachus have no other developmental abnormality, although Lattimer[413] found that 50% of patients with prune-belly syndrome (congenital deficiency of the abdominal musculature) had patent urachus. In most cases patent urachus does not appear to result from increased intravesical pressure. Schreck and Campbell[414] found that only two of eight children with patent urachus had urinary outlet obstruction. Embryologically, the sequence of development indicates that the urachus is normally already closed before the development of other structures can lead to increased pressure, which might keep it open. The concept that increased pressure later in development might lead to the reopening of the urachus after normal closure was refuted by Begg's[26] anatomical studies.

Incompletely patent urachus is classified by Vaughan[415] as umbilicourachal sinus, vesicourachal sinus or diverticulum, and the blind variant in which the urachus is closed at both ends but remains open centrally (Fig. 5-79). Later, Hinman[416] added alternating urachal sinus to the classification to account for individuals without a history of umbilical urinary drainage in whom urachal infections drained both into the bladder and from the umbilicus. Alternating urachal sinus should be distinguished from completely patent urachus, in which the lumen is patent from bladder to umbilicus at birth. Hinman concluded that, in patients with alternating urachal sinus, the lumen is a potential space in which accumulating epithelial cellular debris becomes a focus for infection. Rarely, stones form within urachal malformations. These may be urinary in origin, similar in composition to other urinary calculi, or may be of different origin, in which case they are usually small and yellow-brown or brown.

Urachal cysts are found at any point in the urachus (Fig. 5-80) and range from small lesions found incidentally (Fig. 5-81, 5-82) to immense masses containing as much as 50 L of fluid.[417] Small cysts are usually lined by urothelium or cuboidal epithelium (Fig. 5-83), but columnar epithelium may be present. The lining of large cysts is usually flattened.

## Diverticulum

Diverticulum of the bladder (Fig. 5-84) is a common clinical problem that infrequently requires surgical treatment. The etiology of bladder diverticulum is generally attributed to

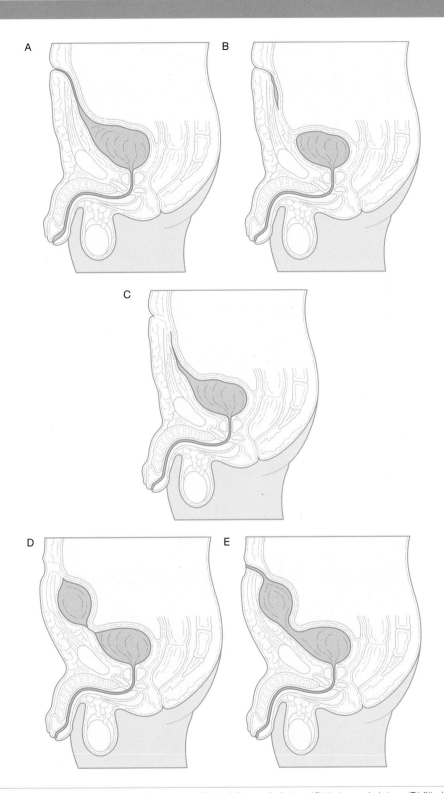

**Fig. 5-79** Types of persistent or patent urachus. (**A**) Complete patency. (**B**) Umbilicourachal sinus. (**C**) Vesicourachal sinus. (**D**) Blindly patent urachus. (**E**) Alternating urachal sinus.

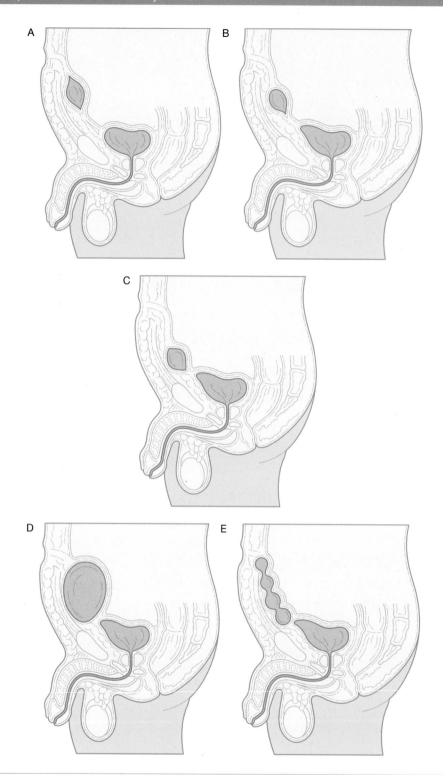

**Fig. 5-80** Classification of urachal cysts. (**A**) Juxtaumbilical. (**B**) Intermediate. (**C**) Juxtavesical. (**D**) Giant cyst. (**E**) Multiple cysts.

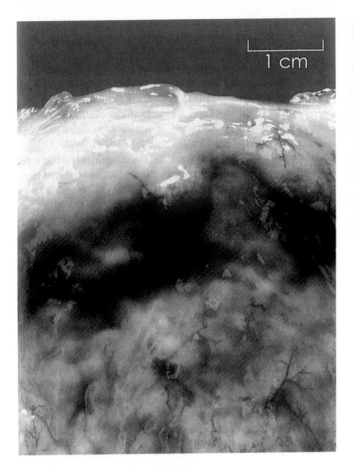

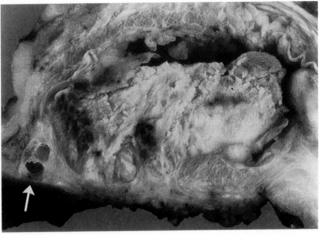

**Fig. 5-82** Urachal cyst. An incidental finding in a radical cystoprostatectomy specimen.

**Fig. 5-81** Small urachal cyst found as a submucosal nodule in the bladder dome.

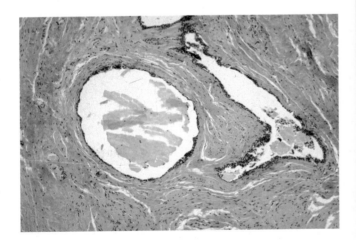

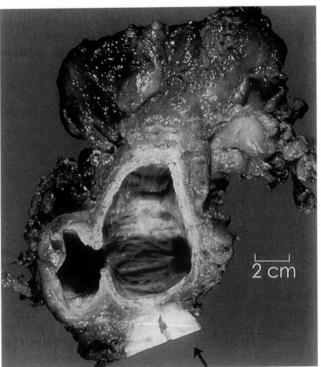

**Fig. 5-83** Multilocular urachal cyst lined by cuboidal and atrophic epithelium.

**Fig. 5-84** Bladder diverticulum (arrow indicates hyperplastic prostate).

increased luminal pressure,[418] although some lesions in children are attributable to localized deficiency of the muscularis propria[419-423] and others to syndromes such as Ehlers–Danlos.[424] Diverticula are common in children with Menkes' syndrome (kinky hair syndrome).[425] They are found in patients of all ages,[426] but most often in men older than 50 years[418] with outflow obstruction caused by prostatic hyperplasia, suggesting that they are caused by increased pressure.[427] Diverticula are most common in the vicinity of the ureteral orifices. At this site, diverticula can cause ureteral obstruction or reflux and predispose the patient to infection. Although most diverticula are small and asymptomatic, large ones may rival or exceed the volume of the bladder[418]

and be associated with infection and stone formation. Less than 10% of diverticula develop neoplasms, most of which are urothelial carcinoma.[428-431]

The excised specimen usually includes a small orifice connecting the bladder and the diverticulum.[427] The passage between the two consists of a narrow intramural neck in the inner layer of the muscularis propria, and the wall of the diverticulum may contain attenuated muscle fibers from the outer layer in patients without a history of chronic inflammation. In patients with a history of chronic inflammation the muscle fibers often are absent, having been replaced by fibrous tissue.[432] Squamous metaplasia also is seen in association with chronic inflammation.[432]

# REFERENCES

1. Tanagho EA, Smith DR, Meyers FH. The trigone: anatomical and physiological considerations. 2. In relation to the bladder neck. J Urol 1968; 100: 633–639.

2. Tanagho EA, Meyers FH, Smith DR. The trigone: anatomical and physiological considerations. I. In relation to the ureterovesical junction. J Urol 1968; 100: 623–632.

3. Woodburne RT. Anatomy of the bladder and bladder outlet. J Urol 1968; 100: 474–487.

4. Elbadawi A. Anatomy and function of the ureteral sheath. J Urol 1972; 107: 224–229.

5. Gosling J. The structure of the bladder and urethra in relation to function. Urol Clin North Am 1979; 6: 31–38.

6. Tanagho EA, Pugh RC. The anatomy and function of the ureterovesical junction. Br J Urol 1963; 35: 151–165.

7. Tanagho EA, Smith DR. The anatomy and function of the bladder neck. Br J Urol 1966; 38: 54–71.

8. Hutch JA, Rambo OS Jr. A study of the anatomy of the prostate, prostatic urethra and the urinary sphincter system. J Urol 1970; 104: 443–452.

9. Hammond G, Yglesias L, Davis JK. The urachus, its anatomy and associated fasciae. Anat Rec 1941; 80: 271–278.

10. Blichert-Toft M, Koch F, Nielsen OV. Anatomic variants of the urachus related to clinical appearance and surgical treatment of urachal lesions. Surg Gynecol Obstet 1973; 37: 51–54.

11. Shehata R. The arterial supply of the urinary bladder. Acta Anat (Basel) 1976; 96: 128–134.

12. Braithwaite JL. The arterial supply of the male urinary bladder. Br J Urol 1952; 24: 64–71.

13. Parker AE. The lymph collectors from the urinary bladder and their connections with the main posterior lymph channels of the abdomen. Anat Rec 1936; 65: 443–460.

14. Koss LG. The asymmetric unit membranes of the epithelium of the urinary bladder of the rat. An electron microscopic study of a mechanism of epithelial maturation and function. Lab Invest 1969; 21: 154–168.

15. Battifora H, Eisenstein R, McDonald JH. The human urinary bladder mucosa. An electron microscopic study. Invest Urol 1964; 1: 354–361.

16. Newman J, Antonakopoulos GN. The fine structure of the human fetal urinary bladder. Development and maturation. A light, transmission and scanning electron microscopic study. J Anat 1989; 166: 135–150.

17. Alroy J, Gould VE. Epithelial-stromal interface in normal and neoplastic human bladder epithelium. Ultrastruct Pathol 1980; 1: 201–210.

18. Ro JY, Ayala AG, el-Naggar A. Muscularis mucosa of urinary bladder. Importance for staging and treatment. Am J Surg Pathol 1987; 11: 668–673.

19. Keep JC, Piehl M, Miller A, et al. Invasive carcinomas of the urinary bladder. Evaluation of tunica muscularis mucosae involvement. Am J Clin Pathol 1989; 91: 575–579.

20. Younes M, Sussman J, True LD. The usefulness of the level of the muscularis mucosae in the staging of invasive transitional cell carcinoma of the urinary bladder. Cancer 1990; 66: 543–548.

21. Weaver MG, Abdul-Karim FW. The prevalence and character of the muscularis mucosae of the human urinary bladder. Histopathology 1990; 17: 563–566.

22. Hasui Y, Osada Y, Kitada S, et al. Significance of invasion to the muscularis mucosae on the progression of superficial bladder cancer. Urology 1994; 43: 782–786.

23. Eble JN. Abnormalities of the urachus. New York: Churchill Livingstone, 1989.

24. Schubert GE, Pavkovic MB, Bethke-Bedurftig BA. Tubular urachal remnants in adult bladders. J Urol 1982; 127: 40–42.

25. Tyler DE. Epithelium of intestinal type in the normal urachus. A new theory of vesical embryology. J Urol 1964; 92: 505–507.

26. Begg RC. The urachus: its anatomy, histology and development. J Anat 1930; 64: 170–183.

27. von Brunn A. Ueber drusenshnliche Bildungen in der Schleimhaut des Nierenbeckens, des Ureters und der Harnblase beim Menschen. Arch Mikrosc Anat 1893; 41: 242–302.

28. Morse HD. The etiology and pathology of pyelitis cystica, ureteritis cystica and cystitis cystica. Am J Pathol 1928; 4: 33–49.

29. Patch FS, Rhea LJ. The genesis and development of von Brunn's nests and their relation to cystitis cystica, cystitis glandularis and primary adenocarcinoma of the bladder. Can Med Assoc J 1935; 33: 597–606.

30. Andersen JA, Hansen BF. The incidence of cell nests, cystitis cystica and cystitis glandularis in the lower urinary tract revealed by autopsies. J Urol 1972; 108: 421–424.

31. Wiener DP, Koss LG, Sablay B, et al. The prevalence and significance of Brunn's nests, cystitis cystica and squamous metaplasia in normal bladders. J Urol 1979; 122: 317–321.

32. Goldstein AM, Fauer RB, Chinn M, et al. New concepts on formation of Brunn's nests and cysts in urinary tract mucosa. Urology 1978; 11: 513–517.

33. Ito N, Hirose M, Shirai T, et al. Lesions of the urinary bladder epithelium in 125 autopsy cases. Acta Pathol Jpn 1981; 31: 545–557.

34. Volmar KE, Chan TY, De Marzo AM, et al. Florid von Brunn nests mimicking urothelial carcinoma: a morphologic and immunohistochemical comparison to the nested variant of urothelial carcinoma. Am J Surg Pathol 2003; 27: 1243–1252.

35. Emmet JL, McDonald JR. Proliferation of the glands of urinary bladder simulating malignant neoplasm. J Urol 1942; 48: 257–267.

36. Lowry EC, Hamm FC, Beard DE. Extensive glandular proliferation of the urinary bladder resembling malignant neoplasm. J Urol 1944; 52: 133–138.

37. Foot NC. Glandular metaplasia of the epithelium of the urinary tract. South Med J 1944; 37: 137–142.

38. Sauer HR, Blick MS. Cystitis glandularis: a consideration of symptoms, diagnosis and clinical course of the disease. J Urol 1948; 61: 446–458.

39. Lane TJD. An uncommon bladder condition simulating carcinoma. Glandular proliferation in the epithelium of the urinary tract, with special reference to cystitis cystica and cystitis glandularis. Br J Urol 1948; 20: 175–179.

40. Kittredge WE, Brannan W. Cystitis glandularis. J Urol 1959; 81: 419–430.

41. Gingell JC, Burn JI. Cystitis glandularis – case report. Br J Urol 1970; 42: 446–449.

42. Ward AM. Glandular neoplasia within the urinary tract. The aetiology of adenocarcinoma of the urothelium with a review of the literature. I. Introduction: the origin of glandular epithelium in the renal pelvis, ureter and bladder. Virchows Arch A Pathol Pathol Anat 1971; 352: 296–311.

43. Striling WC. Chronic proliferative lesions of the urinary tract. J Urol 1941; 45: 342–360.

44. Dann RH, Arger PH, Enterline HT. Benign proliferation processes presenting as mass lesions in the urinary bladder. Am J Roentgenol Radium Ther Nucl Med 1972; 116: 822–829.

45. Imray TJ, Kaplan P. Lower urinary tract infections and calculi in the adult. Semin Roentgenol 1983; 18: 276–287.

46. Davies G, Castro JE. Cystitis glandularis. Urology 1977; 10: 128–129.

47. Edelman L. Muciparous glands in the mucosa of the urinary bladder, report of two cases. J Urol 1928; 20: 211–224.

48. Young RH, Parkhurst EC. Mucinous adenocarcinoma of bladder. Case associated with extensive intestinal metaplasia of urothelium in patient with non-functioning bladder for twelve years. Urology 1984; 24: 192–195.

49. Bullock PS, Thoni DE, Murphy WM. The significance of colonic mucosa (intestinal metaplasia) involving the urinary tract. Cancer 1987; 59: 2086–2090.

50. Bollito ER, Pacchioni D, Lopez-Beltran A, et al. Immunohistochemical study of neuroendocrine differentiation in primary glandular lesions and tumors of the urinary bladder. Anal Quant Cytol Histol 2005; 27: 218–224.

51. Sung MT, Lopez-Beltran A, Eble JN, et al. Divergent pathway of intestinal metaplasia and cystitis glandularis of the urinary bladder. Mod Pathol 2006; 19: 1395–1401.

52. Gordon A. Intestinal metaplasia of the urinary tract epithelium. J Pathol Bacteriol 1963; 85: 441–444.

53. Wells M, Anderson K. Mucin histochemistry of cystitis glandularis and primary adenocarcinoma of the urinary bladder. Arch Pathol Lab Med 1985; 109: 59–61.

54. Hasegawa R, Fukushima S, Hirose M, et al. Histochemical demonstration of colonic type mucin in glandular metaplasia and adenocarcinoma of the human urinary bladder. Acta Pathol Jpn 1987; 37: 1097–1103.

55. Nowels K, Kent E, Rinsho K, et al. Prostate specific antigen and acid phosphatase-reactive cells in cystitis cystica and glandularis. Arch Pathol Lab Med 1988; 112: 734–737.

56. Golz R, Schubert GE. Prostatic specific antigen. immunoreactivity in urachal remnants. J Urol 1989; 141: 1480–1482.

57. Hasegawa R, Fukushima S, Furukawa F, et al. Aberrant colonic epithelium in the bladder. report of a case. J Urol 1986; 136: 901–902.

58. Elem B, Alam SZ. Total intestinal metaplasia with focal adenocarcinoma in a *Schistosoma*-infested defunctioned urinary bladder. Br J Urol 1984; 56: 331–333.

59. Eble JN, Young RH. Benign and low-grade papillary lesions of the urinary bladder: a review of the papilloma–papillary carcinoma controversy, and a report of five typical papillomas. Semin Diagn Pathol 1989; 6: 351–371.

60. Bell TE, Wendel RG. Cystitis glandularis: benign or malignant? J Urol 1968; 100: 462–465.

61. Parker C. Cystitis cystica and glandularis: a study of 40 cases. Proc Roy Soc Med 1970; 63: 239–242.

62. Shaw JL, Gislason GJ, Imbriglia JE. Transition of cystitis glandularis to primary adenocarcinoma of the bladder. J Urol 1958; 79: 815–822.

63. Lin JI, Yong HS, Tseng CH, et al. Diffuse cystitis glandularis associated with adenocarcinomatous change. Urology 1980; 15: 411–415.

64. Kittredge WE, Collett AJ, Morgan C Jr. Adenocarcinoma of the bladder associated with cystitis glandularis. A case report. J Urol 1964; 91: 145–150.

65. Salm R. Neoplasia of the bladder and cystitis cystica. Br J Urol 1967; 39: 67–72.

66. Susmano D, Rubenstein AB, Dakin AR, et al. Cystitis glandularis and adenocarcinoma of the bladder. J Urol 1971; 105: 671–674.

67. Edwards PD, Hurm RA, Jaeschke WH. Conversion of cystitis glandularis to adenocarcinoma. J Urol 1972; 108: 568–570.

68. Talbert ML, Young RH. Carcinomas of the urinary bladder with deceptively benign-appearing foci. A report of three cases. Am J Surg Pathol 1989; 13: 374–381.

68b. Young RH, Bostwick DG. Florid cystitis glandularis of intestinal type with mucin extravasation: a mimic of adenocarcinoma. Am J Surg Pathol 1996; 20: 1462–1468.

69. Kretschmer HL. The pathology and cystoscopy of cystitis cystica. Surg Gynecol Obstet 1908; 7: 274–279.

70. Warrick WD. Cystitis cystica. Bacteriological studies in a series of 18 cases. J Urol 1941; 45: 835–843.

71. Kaplan GW, King LR. Cystitis cystica in childhood. J Urol 1970; 103: 657–659.

72. Thomson GJ, Stein JJ. Leukoplakia of the urinary bladder. a report of 34 clinical cases. J Urol 1940; 44: 639–649.

73. Rabson SM. Leukoplakia and carcinoma of the urinary bladder, report of a case and review of the literature. J Urol 1936; 35: 321–341.

74. O'Flynn JD, Mullaney J. Leukoplakia of the bladder. A report on 20 cases, including 2 cases progressing to squamous cell carcinoma. Br J Urol 1967; 39: 461–471.

75. Scholl AJ. Squamous cell changes and infection in the urinary tract. J Urol 1940; 44: 759–767.

76. Reece RW, Koontz WW Jr. Leukoplakia of the urinary tract: a review. J Urol 1975; 114: 165–171.

77. Widran J, Sanchez R, Gruhn J. Squamous metaplasia of the bladder: a study of 450 patients. J Urol 1974; 112: 479–482.

78. Polsky MS, Weber CH Jr, Williams JE 3rd, et al. Chronically infected and postdiversionary bladders: cytologic and histopathologic study. Urology 1976; 7: 531–535.

79. Kaufman JM, Fam B, Jacobs SC, et al. Bladder cancer and squamous metaplasia in spinal cord injury patients. J Urol 1977; 118: 967–971.

80. Zahran MM, Kamel M, Mooro H, et al. Bilharziasis of urinary bladder and ureter. comparative histopathologic study. Urology 1976; 8: 73–79.

81. Witherington R. Leukoplakia of the bladder: an 8-year follow-up. J Urol 1974; 112: 600–602.

82. Thomas SD, Sanders PW 3rd, Sanders PW Jr. Cholesteatoma of the bladder. J Urol 1974; 112: 598–599.

83. Connery DB. Leukoplakia of the urinary bladder and its association with carcinoma. J Urol 1953; 69: 121–127.

84. O'Flynn JD, Mullaney J. Vesical leukoplakia progressing to carcinoma. Br J Urol 1974; 46: 31–37.

85. DeKock ML, Anderson CK, Clark PB. Vesical leukoplakia progressing to squamous cell carcinoma in women. Br J Urol 1981; 53: 316–317.

86. Benson RC Jr, Swanson SK, Farrow GM. Relationship of leukoplakia to urothelial malignancy. J Urol 1984; 131: 507–511.

87. Khan MS, Thornhill JA, Gaffney E, et al. Keratinising squamous metaplasia of the bladder: natural history and rationalization of management based on review of 54 years experience. Eur Urol 2002; 42: 469–474.

88. El-Bolkainy MN, Mokhtar NM, Ghoniem MA, et al. The impact of schistosomiasis on the pathology of

bladder carcinoma. Cancer 1981; 48: 2643–2648.

89. Khafagy MM, el-Bolkainy MN, Mansour MA. Carcinoma of the bilharzial urinary bladder. A study of the associated mucosal lesions in 86 cases. Cancer 1972; 30: 150–159.

90. Cifuentes L. Epithelium of vaginal type in the female trigone: the clinical problem of trigonitis. J Urol 1947; 57: 1021–1037.

91. Packham DA. The epithelial lining of the female trigone and urethra. Br J Urol 1971; 43: 201–205.

92. Tyler DE. Stratified squamous epithelium in the vesical trigone and urethra. findings correlated with the menstrual cycle and age. Am J Anat 1962; 111: 319–335.

93. Long ED, Shepherd RT. The incidence and significance of vaginal metaplasia of the bladder trigone in adult women. Br J Urol 1983; 55: 189–194.

94. Ney C, Ehrlich JC. Squamous epithelium in the trigone of the human female urinary bladder, with a note on cystoscopic observations during estrogen therapy. J Urol 1955; 73: 809–819.

95. Stephenson TJ, Henry L, Harris SC, et al. Pseudomembranous trigonitis of the bladder. hormonal aetiology. J Clin Pathol 1989; 42: 922–926.

96. Henry L, Fox M. Histological findings in pseudomembranous trigonitis. J Clin Pathol 1971; 24: 605–608.

97. Davis TA. Hamartoma of the urinary bladder. Northwest Med 1949; 48: 182–185.

98. Friedman NB, Kuhlenbeck H. Adenomatoid tumors of the bladder reproducing renal structures (nephrogenic adenomas). J Urol 1950; 64: 657–670.

99. O'Shea PA, Callaghan JF, Lawlor JB, et al. 'Nephrogenic adenoma': an unusual metaplastic change of urothelium. J Urol 1981; 125: 249–252.

100. Navarre RJ Jr, Loening SA, Platz C, et al. Nephrogenic adenoma: a report of 9 cases and review of the literature. J Urol 1982; 127: 775–779.

101. Devine P, Ucci AA, Krain H, et al. Nephrogenic adenoma and embryonic kidney tubules share PNA receptor sites. Am J Clin Pathol 1984; 81: 728–732.

102. Ford TF, Watson GM, Cameron KM. Adenomatous metaplasia (nephrogenic adenoma) of urothelium. An analysis of 70 cases. Br J Urol 1985; 57: 427–433.

103. Young RH, Scully RE. Nephrogenic adenoma. A report of 15 cases, review of the literature, and comparison with clear cell adenocarcinoma of the urinary tract. Am J Surg Pathol 1986; 10: 268–275.

104. Sorensen FB, Jacobsen F, Nielsen JB, et al. Nephroid metaplasia of the urinary tract. A survey of the literature, with the contribution of 5 new immunohistochemically studied cases,

including one case examined by electron microscopy. Acta Pathol Microbiol Immunol Scand [A] 1987; 95: 67–81.

105. Young RH. Pseudoneoplastic lesions of the urinary bladder. Pathol Annu 1988; 23: 67–104.

105b. Cheng L, Cheville JC, Sebo TJ, et al. Atypical nephrogenic metaplasia of the urinary tract: a precursor lesion? Cancer 2000; 88: 853–861.

105c. Hansel DE, Nadasdy T, Epstein JI. Fibromyxoid nephrogenic adenoma: a newly recognized variant mimicking mucinous adenocarcinoma. Am J Surg Pathol 2007; 31: 1231–1237.

106. Lugo M, Petersen RO, Elfenbein IB, et al. Nephrogenic metaplasia of the ureter. Am J Clin Pathol 1983; 80: 92–97.

107. Billerey C, Khamlu K, Regin JP, et al. La métaplasie nephrogenique de la muqueuse urothéliale, a propos de onze observations. Ann Urol 1983; 17: 340–346.

108. Mazal PR, Schaufler R, Altenhuber-Muller R, et al. Derivation of nephrogenic adenomas from renal tubular cells in kidney-transplant recipients. N Engl J Med 2002; 347: 653–659.

109. Hartmann A, Junker K, Dietmaier W, et al. Molecular evidence for progression of nephrogenic metaplasia of the urinary bladder to clear cell adenocarcinoma. Hum Pathol 2006; 37: 117–120.

110. de Jong EA, Scholtmeijer RJ. Nephrogenic adenoma of the bladder in children. Eur Urol 1984; 10: 187–190.

111. Kay R, Lattanzi C. Nephrogenic adenoma in children. J Urol 1985; 133: 99–101.

112. Gonzalez JA, Watts JC, Alderson TP. Nephrogenic adenoma of the bladder: report of 10 cases. J Urol 1988; 139: 45–47.

113. Oliva E, Young RH. Nephrogenic adenoma of the urinary tract. a review of the microscopic appearance of 80 cases with emphasis on unusual features. Mod Pathol 1995; 8: 722–730.

114. Alsanjari N, Lynch MJ, Fisher C, et al. Vesical clear cell adenocarcinoma. V. Nephrogenic adenoma: a diagnostic problem. Histopathology 1995; 27: 43–49.

115. McIntire TL, Soloway MS, Murphy WM. Nephrogenic adenoma. Urology 1987; 29: 237–241.

116. Patel PS, Wilbur AC. Nephrogenic adenoma presenting as a calcified mass. AJR Am J Roentgenol 1988; 150: 1071–1072.

117. Gupta A, Wang HL, Policarpio-Nicolas ML, et al. Expression of alpha-methylacyl-coenzyme A racemase in nephrogenic adenoma. Am J Surg Pathol 2004; 28: 1224–1229.

118. Malpica A, Ro JY, Troncoso P, et al. Nephrogenic adenoma of the prostatic urethra involving the prostate gland: a

clinicopathologic and immunohistochemical study of eight cases. Hum Pathol 1994; 25: 390–395.

119. Skinnider BF, Oliva E, Young RH, et al. Expression of alpha-methylacyl-CoA racemase (P504S) in nephrogenic adenoma: a significant immunohistochemical pitfall compounding the differential diagnosis with prostatic adenocarcinoma. Am J Surg Pathol 2004; 28: 701–705.

120. Xiao GQ, Burstein DE, Miller LK, et al. Nephrogenic adenoma: immunohistochemical evaluation for its etiology and differentiation from prostatic adenocarcinoma. Arch Pathol Lab Med 2006; 130: 805–810.

121. Tong GX, Melamed J, Mansukhani M, et al. PAX2: a reliable marker for nephrogenic adenoma. Mod Pathol 2006; 19: 356–363.

122. Melicow MM, Uson AC. The 'herald' lesion of the bladder. a lesion which portends the approach of cancer or inflammation from outside the bladder. J Urol 1961; 85: 543–551.

123. Melicow MM, Uson AC, Stams U. Herald lesion of urinary bladder. A non-specific but significant pathologic process. Urology 1974; 3: 140–147.

124. Mostofi FK. Potentialities of bladder epithelium. J Urol 1954; 71: 705–714.

125. Buck EG. Polypoid cystitis mimicking transitional cell carcinoma. J Urol 1984; 131: 963.

126. Ekelund P, Johansson S. Polypoid cystitis. a catheter associated lesion of the human bladder. Acta Pathol Microbiol Scand [A] 1979; 87A: 179–184.

127. Ekelund P, Anderstrom C, Johansson SL, et al. The reversibility of catheter-associated polypoid cystitis. J Urol 1983; 130: 456–459.

128. Young RH. Papillary and polypoid cystitis. A report of eight cases. Am J Surg Pathol 1988; 12: 542–546.

129. Milles G. Catheter-induced hemorrhagic pseudopolyps of the urinary bladder. JAMA 1965; 193: 968–969.

130. Slade N, Gaches C. Vesico-intestinal fistulae. Br J Surg 1972; 59: 593–597.

131. Goldstein MJ, Bragg D, Sherlock P. Granulomatous bowel disease presenting as a bladder tumor. Report of a case. Am J Dig Dis 1971; 16: 337–341.

132. Pugh JI. On the pathology and behaviour of acquired non-traumatic vesico-intestinal fistula. Br J Surg 1964; 51: 644–657.

133. Joffe N. Roentgenologic abnormalities of the urinary bladder secondary to Crohn's disease. AJR Am J Roentgenol 1976; 127: 297–302.

134. Lazarus JA, Marks MS. Vesico-intestinal fistula: actual and incipient. Early diagnosis and treatment. Am J Surg 1943; 59: 526–535.

135. Demos TC, Moncada R. Inflammatory gastrointestinal disease presenting as

genitourinary disease. Urology 1979; 13: 115–121.

136. Gray FW, Newman HR. Granuloma of the bladder associated with regional enteritis: case report. J Urol 1957; 78: 393–397.

137. Carson CC, Malek RS, Remine WH. Urologic aspects of vesicoenteric fistulas. J Urol 1978; 119: 744–746.

138. Sarma KP. On the nature of cystitis follicularis. J Urol 1970; 104: 709–714.

139. Marsh FP, Banerjee R, Panchamia P. The relationship between urinary infection, cystoscopic appearance, and pathology of the bladder in man. J Clin Pathol 1974; 27: 297–307.

140. Hinman F, Cordonnier J. Cystitis follicularis. J Urol 1935; 34: 302–308.

141. Stirling WC. Cystitis follicularis, with a discussion of the other proliferative lesions of the bladder and report of four cases. JAMA 1939; 112: 1326–1331.

142. Alexander S. Some observations respecting the pathology and pathological anatomy of the nodular cystitis. J Cutan Genitourin Dis 1893; 11: 245–262.

143. Kretschmer HL. On the occurrence of lymphoid tissue in the urinary organs. J Urol 1952; 68: 252–260.

144. Wells HG. Giant cells in cystitis. Arch Pathol Lab Med 1938; 26: 32–43.

145. Johnson WW, Meadows DC. Urinary-bladder fibrosis and telangiectasia associated with long-term cyclophosphamide therapy. N Engl J Med 1971; 284: 290–294.

146. Beyer-Boon ME, de Voogt HJ, Schaberg A. The effects of cyclophosphamide treatment on the epithelium and stroma of the urinary bladder. Eur J Cancer 1978; 14: 1029–1035.

147. Millard RJ. Busulfan-induced hemorrhagic cystitis. Urology 1981; 18: 143–144.

148. Murphy WM, Soloway MS, Finebaum PJ. Pathological changes associated with topical chemotherapy for superficial bladder cancer. J Urol 1981; 126: 461–464.

149. deVries CR, Freiha FS. Hemorrhagic cystitis: a review. J Urol 1990; 143: 1–9.

150. Treible DP, Skinner D, Kasimain D, et al. Intractable bladder hemorrhage requiring cystectomy after use of intravesical thiotepa. Urology 1987; 30: 568–570.

151. Rubin JS, Rubin RT. Cyclophosphamide hemorrhagic cystitis. J Urol 1966; 96: 313–316.

152. Lawrence HJ, Simone J, Aur RJ. Cyclophosphamide-induced hemorrhagic cystitis in children with leukemia. Cancer 1975; 36: 1572–1576.

153. Stillwell TJ, Benson RC Jr. Cyclophosphamide-induced hemorrhagic cystitis. A review of 100 patients. Cancer 1988; 61: 451–457.

154. Rowland RG, Eble JN. Bladder leiomyosarcoma and pelvic fibroblastic

tumor following cyclophosphamide therapy. J Urol 1983; 130: 344–346.

155. Pedersen-Bjergaard J, Ersboll J, Hansen VL, et al. Carcinoma of the urinary bladder after treatment with cyclophosphamide for non-Hodgkin's lymphoma. N Engl J Med 1988; 318: 1028–1032.

156. Fairchild WV, Spence CR, Solomon HD, et al. The incidence of bladder cancer after cyclophosphamide therapy. J Urol 1979; 122: 163–164.

157. Skene AJC. Treatise on diseases of the bladder and the urethra in women. William and Wood, 1887.

158. Nitze M. Lehrbuch der kystoscopie, 2nd edn. Berlin, 1907.

159. Hunner GL. A rare type of bladder ulcer in women. report of cases. Trans South Surg Gynecol 1914; 27: 247–292.

160. Kretschmer HL. Elusive ulcer of the bladder. J Urol 1939; 42: 385–395.

161. Higgins CC. Hunner ulcer of the bladder (review of 100 cases). Ann Intern Med 1941; 15: 708–715.

162. Hand JR. Interstitial cystitis: report of 223 cases (204 women and 19 men). J Urol 1949; 61: 291–310.

163. Burford EH, Burford CE. Hunner ulcer of the bladder. a report of 187 cases. J Urol 1958; 79: 952–955.

164. DeJuana CP, Everett JC Jr. Interstitial cystitis. experience and review of recent literature. Urology 1977; 10: 325–329.

165. Koziol DE, Saah AJ, Odaka N, et al. A comparison of risk factors for human immunodeficiency virus and hepatitis B virus infections in homosexual men. Ann Epidemiol 1993; 3: 434–441.

166. Messing EM, Stamey TA. Interstitial cystitis. early diagnosis, pathology, and treatment. Urology 1978; 12: 381–392.

167. Meares EM Jr. Interstitial cystitis – 1987. Urology 1987; 29: 46–48.

168. Johansson SL, Fall M. Clinical features and spectrum of light microscopic changes in interstitial cystitis. J Urol 1990; 143: 1118–1124.

169. Simmons JL, Bunce PL. On the use of an antihistamine in the treatment of interstitial cystitis. Am Surg 1958; 24: 664–667.

170. Kastrup J, Hald T, Larsen S, et al. Histamine content and mast cell count of detrusor muscle in patients with interstitial cystitis and other types of chronic cystitis. Br J Urol 1983; 55: 495–500.

171. Larsen S, Thompson SA, Hald T, et al. Mast cells in interstitial cystitis. Br J Urol 1982; 54: 283–286.

172. Hellstrom HR, Davis BK, Shonnard JW. Eosinophilic cystitis. A study of 16 cases. Am J Clin Pathol 1979; 72: 777–784.

173. Castillo J Jr, Cartagena R, Montes M. Eosinophilic cystitis: a therapeutic challenge. Urology 1988; 32: 535–537.

174. Rubin L, Pincus MB. Eosinophilic cystitis: the relationship of allergy in the urinary tract to eosinophilic cystitis and the pathophysiology of

eosinophilia. J Urol 1974; 112: 457–460.

175. Gregg JA, Utz DC. Eosinophilic cystitis associated with eosinophilic gastroenteritis. Mayo Clin Proc 1974; 49: 185–187.

176. Perlmutter AD, Edlow JB, Kevy SV. Toxocara antibodies in eosinophilic cystitis. J Pediatr 1968; 73: 340–344.

177. Oh SJ, Chi JG, Lee SE. Eosinophilic cystitis caused by vesical sparganosis: a case report. J Urol 1993; 149: 581–583.

178. Thijssen A, Gerridzen RG. Eosinophilic cystitis presenting as invasive bladder cancer: comments on pathogenesis and management. J Urol 1990; 144: 977–979.

179. Hansen MV, Kristensen PB. Eosinophilic cystitis simulating invasive bladder carcinoma. Scand J Urol Nephrol 1993; 27: 275–277.

180. Teegavarapu PS, Sahai A, Chandra A, et al. Eosinophilic cystitis and its management. Int J Clin Pract 2005; 59: 356–360.

181. Lowe D, Jorizzo J, Hutt MS. Tumour-associated eosinophilia: a review. J Clin Pathol 1981; 34: 1343–1348.

182. Eble JN, Banks ER. Post-surgical necrobiotic granulomas of urinary bladder. Urology 1990; 35: 454–457.

183. Spagnolo DV, Waring PM. Bladder granulomata after bladder surgery. Am J Clin Pathol 1986; 86: 430–437.

184. Sorensen FB, Marcussen N. Iatrogenic granulomas of the prostate and the urinary bladder. Pathol Res Pract 1987; 182: 822–830.

185. Washida H, Watanabe H, Noguchi Y, et al. Tissue effects in the bladder wall after contact Nd:YAG laser irradiation for bladder tumor. World J Urol 1992; 10: 115–119.

186. Witjes JA, van der Meijden AP, Debruyne FM. Use of intravesical bacillus Calmette–Guérin in the treatment of superficial transitional cell carcinoma of the bladder: an overview. Urol Int 1990; 45: 129–136.

187. Harland SJ, Charig CR, Highman W, et al. Outcome in carcinoma in situ of bladder treated with intravesical bacille Calmette–Guérin. Br J Urol 1992; 70: 271–275.

188. Akaza H, Hinotsu S, Aso Y, et al. Bacillus Calmette–Guérin treatment of existing papillary bladder cancer and carcinoma in situ of the bladder. Four-year results. The Bladder Cancer BCG Study Group. Cancer 1995; 75: 552–559.

189. Patard JJ, Chopin DK, Boccon-Gibod L. Mechanisms of action of bacillus Calmette–Guérin in the treatment of superficial bladder cancer. World J Urol 1993; 11: 165–168.

190. Adolphs HD, Schwabe HW, Helpap B, et al. Cytomorphological and histological studies on the urothelium during and after chemoimmune prophylaxis. Urol Res 1984; 12: 129–133.

191. Lage JM, Bauer WC, Kelley DR, et al. Histological parameters and pitfalls in the interpretation of bladder biopsies in bacillus Calmette–Guérin treatment of superficial bladder cancer. J Urol 1986; 135: 916–919.

192. Shapiro A, Lijovetzky G, Pode D. Changes of the mucosal architecture and the urine cytology during BCG treatment. World J Urol 1988; 6: 61–64.

193. Pagano F, Bassi P, Milani C, et al. Pathologic and structural changes in the bladder after BCG intravesical therapy in men. Prog Clin Biol Res 1989; 310: 81–91.

194. Rigatti P, Colombo R, Montorsi F, et al. Local bacillus Calmette–Guérin therapy for superficial bladder cancer: clinical, histological and ultrastructural patterns. Scand J Urol Nephrol 1990; 24: 191–198.

195. Badalament RA, Gay H, Cibas ES, et al. Monitoring intravesical bacillus Calmette–Guérin treatment of superficial bladder carcinoma by postoperative urinary cytology. J Urol 1987; 138: 763–765.

196. Betz SA, See WA, Cohen MB. Granulomatous inflammation in bladder wash specimens after intravesical bacillus Calmette–Guérin therapy for transitional cell carcinoma of the bladder. Am J Clin Pathol 1993; 99: 244–248.

197. Stilmant MM, Siroky MB. Nephrogenic adenoma associated with intravesical bacillus Calmette–Guérin treatment. a report of 2 cases. J Urol 1986; 135: 359–361.

198. Brandt WE. Unusual complications of hernia repairs: large symptomatic granulomas. Am J Surg 1956; 92: 640–643.

199. Stearns DB, Gordon SK. Granuloma of the bladder following inguinal herniorrhaphy: report of case with gross hematuria. Br Med Q 1959; 10: 52–53.

200. Daniel WJ, Aarons BJ, Hamilton NT, et al. Paravesical granuloma presenting as a late complication of herniorrhaphy. Aust NZ J Surg 1973; 43: 38–40.

201. Helms CA, Clark RE. Post-herniorrhaphy suture granuloma simulating a bladder neoplasm. Radiology 1977; 124: 56.

202. Pearl GS, Someren A. Suture granuloma simulating bladder neoplasm. Urology 1980; 15: 304–306.

203. Katz PG, Crawford JP, Hackler RH. Infected suture granuloma simulating mass of urachal origin: case report. J Urol 1986; 135: 782–783.

204. Flood HD, Beard RC. Post-herniorrhaphy paravesical granuloma. Br J Urol 1988; 61: 266–268.

205. Walther M, Glenn JF, Vellios F. Xanthogranulomatous cystitis. J Urol 1985; 134: 745–746.

206. Nishimura K, Nozawa M, Hara T, et al. Xanthoma of the bladder. J Urol 1995; 153: 1912–1913.

207. Cyr WL, Johnson H, Balfour J. Granulomatous cystitis as a manifestation of chronic granulomatous disease of childhood. J Urol 1973; 110: 357–359.

208. Berman HH, Wilets AJ. Rheumatoid pseudotumor of urinary bladder simulating carcinoma. Urology 1977; 9: 83–85.

209. Greenstein AJ, Janowitz HD, Sachar DB. The extra-intestinal complications of Crohn's disease and ulcerative colitis. a study of 700 patients. Medicine (Baltimore) 1976; 55: 401–412.

210. Tammela T, Kallioinen M, Kontturi M, et al. Sarcoidosis of the bladder: a case report and literature review. J Urol 1989; 141: 608–609.

211. Gowing NFC. III. Pathological changes in the bladder following irradiation, a contribution to a symposium on 'Treatment of carcinoma of the bladder' at the British Institute of Radiology on January 14. Br J Radiol 1960; 33: 484–487.

211b. Chan TY, Epstein JI. Radiation or chemotherapy cystitis with "pseudocarcinomatous" features. Am J Surg Pathol 2004; 28: 909–913.

211c. Lane Z, Epstein JI. Pseudocarcinomatous epithelial hyperplasia in the bladder unassociated with prior irradiation or chemotherapy. Am J Surg Pathol 2008; 32: 92–97.

212. Fajardo LF, Berthrong M. Radiation injury in surgical pathology. Part I. Am J Surg Pathol 1978; 2: 159–199.

213. Baker PM, Young RH. Radiation-induced pseudocarcinomatous proliferations of the urinary bladder: a report of 4 cases. Hum Pathol 2000; 31: 678–683.

214. Warren S. Effects of radiation on tissues. VII. Effects of radiation on the urinary system, the kidneys and ureters. Arch Pathol 1942; 34: 1079–1084.

215. Suresh UR, Smith VJ, Lupton EW, et al. Radiation disease of the urinary tract: histological features of 18 cases. J Clin Pathol 1993; 46: 228–231.

216. Murphy WM, Soloway MS, Lin CJ. Morphologic effects of thio-TEPA on mammalian urothelium. Changes in abnormal cells. Acta Cytol 1978; 22: 550–554.

217. Stirling WC, Hopkins GA. Gangrene of the bladder, review of two hundred seven cases; report of two personal cases. J Urol 1934; 31: 517–525.

218. Cristol DS, Greene LF. Gangrenous cystitis, etiologic classification and treatment. Surgery 1945; 18: 343–346.

219. Maggio AJ Jr, Lupu A. Gangrene of bladder. Urology 1981; 18: 390–391.

220. Devitt AT, Sethia KK. Gangrenous cystitis: case report and review of the literature. J Urol 1993; 149: 1544–1545.

221. Hager BH, Magath TB. The etiology of incrusted cystitis with alkaline urine. JAMA 1925; 85: 1352–1355.

222. Hager BH. Clinical data on alkaline incrusted cystitis. J Urol 1926; 16: 447–457.

223. Letcher HG, Matheson NM. Encrustation of bladder as a result of alkaline cystitis. Br J Surg 1935; 23: 716–720.

224. Randall A, Campbell EW. Alkaline incrusted cystitis. J Urol 1937; 37: 284–299.

225. Jameson RM. The treatment of phosphatic encrusted cystitis (alkaline cystitis) with nalidixic acid. Br J Urol 1966; 38: 89–92.

226. Jameson RM. Phosphatic encrusted cystitis. Br J Clin Pract 1967; 21: 463–465.

227. Harrison RB, Stier FM, Cochrane JA. Alkaline encrusting cystitis. AJR Am J Roentgenol 1978; 130: 575–577.

228. Meria P, Desgrippes A, Arfi C, et al. Encrusted cystitis and pyelitis. J Urol 1998; 160: 3–9.

229. Giannakopoulos S, Alivizatos G, Deliveliotis C, et al. Encrusted cystitis and pyelitis. Eur Urol 2001; 39: 446–448.

230. Meria P, Margaryan M, Haddad E, et al. Encrusted cystitis and pyelitis in children: an unusual condition with potentially severe consequences. Urology 2004; 64: 569–573.

231. Zapardiel J, Nieto E, Soriano F. Evaluation of a new selective medium for the isolation of Corynebacterium urealyticum. J Med Microbiol 1998; 47: 79–83.

232. Pollack HM, Banner MP, Martinez LO, et al. Diagnostic considerations in urinary bladder wall calcification. AJR Am J Roentgenol 1981; 136: 791–797.

233. Mills RG. Cystitis emphysematosa, I. Report of cases in men. J Urol 1930; 23: 289–306.

234. Mills RG. Cystitis emphysematosa, II. Report of a series of cases in women. JAMA 1930; 94: 321–332.

235. Redewill FH. Cystitis cystica emphysematosa. Urol Cutan Rev 1934; 38: 537–543.

236. Levin HA. Gas cysts of urinary bladder. J Urol 1938; 39: 45–52.

237. Bailey H. Cystitis emphysematosa: 19 cases with intraluminal and interstitial collections of gas. Am J Roentgenol Radium Ther Nucl Med 1961; 86: 850–862.

238. Singh CR, Lytle WF Jr. Cystitis emphysematosa caused by Candida albicans. J Urol 1983; 130: 1171–1173.

239. Rocca JM, McClure J. Cystitis emphysematosa. Br J Urol 1985; 57: 585.

240. Hawtrey CE, Williams JJ, Schmidt JD. Cystitis emphysematosa. Urology 1974; 3: 612–614.

241. Maliwan N. Emphysematous cystitis associated with Clostridium perfringens bacteremia. J Urol 1979; 121: 819–820.

242. Bartkowski DP, Lanesky JR. Emphysematous prostatitis and cystitis secondary to Candida albicans. J Urol 1988; 139: 1063–1065.

243. Quint HJ, Drach GW, Rappaport WD, et al. Emphysematous cystitis: a review of the spectrum of disease. J Urol 1992; 147: 134–137.

244. Fornari A, Dambros M, Teloken C, et al. A case of xanthogranulomatous cystitis. Int Urogynecol J 2007; [e-pub ahead of print]

245. Goel R, Kadam G, Devra A, et al. Xanthogranulomatous cystitis. Int Urol Nephrol 2007; 39: 477–478.

246. Hayashi N, Wada T, Kiyota H, et al. Xanthogranulomatous cystitis. Int J Urol 2003; 10: 498–500.

247. Izquierdo Garcia FM, Garcia Diez FS, Miguelez Simon A, et al. [Xanthogranulomatous cystitis: report of a case]. Arch Esp Urol 2001; 54: 263–265.

248. Tai HL, Chen CC, Yeh KT. Xanthogranulomatous cystitis associated with anaerobic bacterial infection. J Urol 1999; 162: 795–796.

249. Bates AW, Fegan AW, Baithun SI. Xanthogranulomatous cystitis associated with malignant neoplasms of the bladder. Histopathology 1998; 33: 212–215.

250. Chung MK, Seol MY, Cho WY, et al. Xanthogranulomatous cystitis associated with suture material. J Urol 1998; 159: 981–982.

251. Garcia AA, Florentine BD, Simons AJ, et al. Xanthogranulomatous cystitis as a cause of elevated carcinoembryonic antigen mimicking recurrent colorectal cancer. Report of a case. Dis Colon Rectum 1996; 39: 1051–1054.

252. Tan LB, Chiang CP, Huang CH, et al. Xanthogranulomatous cystitis. a case report and review of the literature. Int Urol Nephrol 1994; 26: 413–417.

253. Brodie N. Infected urachal cysts. Am J Surg 1945; 69: 243–248.

254. MacMillan RW, Schullinger JN, Santulli TV. Pyourachus: an unusual surgical problem. J Pediatr Surg 1973; 8: 387–389.

255. Hinman F Jr. Surgical disorders of the bladder and umbilicus of urachal origin. Surg Gynecol Obstet 1961; 113: 605–614.

256. Newman BM, Karp MP, Jewett TC, et al. Advances in the management of infected urachal cysts. J Pediatr Surg 1986; 21: 1051–1054.

257. Michaelis L, Gutmann C. Ueber Einschlusse in Blasentumoren. Zeitschr Klin Med 1902; 47: 208–215.

258. von Hansemann D. Uber Malakoplakie der Harnblase. Virchows Arch Pathol Anat Physiol Klin Med 1903; 173: 302–308.

259. Damjanov I, Katz SM. Malakoplakia. Pathol Annu 1981; 16: 103–126.

260. McClure J. Malakoplakia. J Pathol 1983; 140: 275–330.

261. Sinclair-Smith C, Kahn LB, Cywes S. Malacoplakia in childhood. Case report with ultrastructural observations and review of the literature. Arch Pathol 1975; 99: 198–203.

262. Lou TY, Teplitz C. Malakoplakia: pathogenesis and ultrastructural morphogenesis. A problem of altered macrophage (phagolysosomal) response. Hum Pathol 1974; 5: 191–207.

263. Abdou NI, NaPombejara C, Sagawa A, et al. Malakoplakia: evidence for monocyte lysosomal abnormality correctable by cholinergic agonist in vitro and in vivo. N Engl J Med 1977; 297: 1413–1419.

264. McClurg FV, D'Agostino AN, Martin JH, et al. Ultrastructural demonstration of intracellular bacteria in three cases of malakoplakia of the bladder. Am J Clin Pathol 1973; 60: 780–788.

265. Qualman SJ, Gupta PK, Mendelsohn G. Intracellular Escherichia coli in urinary malakoplakia: a reservoir of infection and its therapeutic implications. Am J Clin Pathol 1984; 81: 35–42.

266. Stevens S, McClure J. The histochemical features of the Michaelis–Gutmann body and a consideration of the pathophysiological mechanisms of its formation. J Pathol 1982; 137: 119–127.

267. McClure J, Cameron CH, Garrett R. The ultrastructural features of malakoplakia. J Pathol 1981; 134: 13–25.

268. Auerbach O. The pathology of urogenital tuberculosis. New Int Clin 1940; 3: 21–61.

269. Christensen WI. Genitourinary tuberculosis. review of 102 cases. Medicine (Baltimore) 1974; 53: 377–390.

270. Stoller JK. Late recurrence of Mycobacterium bovis genitourinary tuberculosis: case report and review of literature. J Urol 1985; 134: 565–566.

271. Lazarus JA. Prevention and treatment of delayed wound healing and ulcerative cystitis following surgery for tuberculosis of the urinary tract. J Urol 1946; 55: 160–163.

272. Michigan S. Genitourinary fungal infections. J Urol 1976; 116: 390–397.

273. Wise GJ, Silver DA. Fungal infections of the genitourinary system. J Urol 1993; 149: 1377–1388.

274. Rohner TJ Jr, Tuliszewski RM. Fungal cystitis: awareness, diagnosis and treatment. J Urol 1980; 124: 142–144.

275. Sakamoto S, Ogata J, Sakazaki Y, et al. Fungus ball formation of Aspergillus in the bladder: an unusual case report. Eur Urol 1978; 4: 388–389.

276. McClure J, Young RH. Infectious disease of the urinary bladder, including malakoplakia. New York: Churchill Livingstone, 1989.

277. Kleiman H, Lancaster Y. Condyloma acuminata of the bladder. J Urol 1962; 88: 52–55.

278. Pompeius R, Ekroth R. A successfully treated case of condyloma acuminatum of the urethra and urinary bladder. Eur Urol 1976; 2: 298–299.

279. Keating MA, Young RH, Carr CP, et al. Condyloma acuminatum of the bladder and ureter: case report and review of the literature. J Urol 1985; 133: 465–467.

280. van Poppel H, Stessens R, de Vos R, et al. Isolated condyloma acuminatum of the bladder in a patient with multiple sclerosis: etiological and pathological considerations. J Urol 1986; 136: 1071–1073.

281. Walther M, O'Brien DP 3rd, Birch HW. Condylomata acuminata and verrucous carcinoma of the bladder: case report and literature review. J Urol 1986; 135: 362–365.

282. Del Mistro A, Koss LG, Braunstein J, et al. Condylomata acuminata of the urinary bladder. Natural history, viral typing, and DNA content. Am J Surg Pathol 1988; 12: 205–215.

283. Shirai T, Yamamoto K, Adachi T, et al. Condyloma acuminatum of the bladder in two autopsy cases. Acta Pathol Jpn 1988; 38: 399–405.

284. Jimenez Lasanta JA, Mariscal A, Tenesa M, et al. Condyloma acuminatum of the bladder in a patient with AIDS: radiological findings. J Clin Ultrasound 1997; 25: 338–340.

285. Chrisofos M, Skolarikos A, Lazaris A, et al. HPV 16/18-associated condyloma acuminatum of the urinary bladder: first international report and review of literature. Int J STD AIDS 2004; 15: 836–838.

286. Barber NJ, Kane TP, Conroy B, et al. Condyloma acuminatum-like lesion of the urinary bladder progressing to invasive spindle cell carcinoma. Scand J Urol Nephrol 2003; 37: 512–514.

287. Lewin F, Cardoso AP, Simardi LH, et al. Verrucous carcinoma of the bladder with koilocytosis unassociated with vesical schistosomiasis. Sao Paulo Med J 2004; 122: 64–66.

288. Mufson MA, Belshe RB. A review of adenoviruses in the etiology of acute hemorrhagic cystitis. J Urol 1976; 115: 191–194.

289. Numazaki Y, Shigeta S, Kumasaka T, et al. Acute hemorrhagic cystitis in children. Isolation of adenovirus type II. N Engl J Med 1968; 278: 700–704.

290. Hanash KA, Pool TL. Interstitial and hemorrhagic cystitis: viral, bacterial and fungal studies. J Urol 1970; 104: 705–706.

291. Shindo K, Kitayama T, Ura T, et al. Acute hemorrhagic cystitis caused by adenovirus type 11 after renal transplantation. Urol Int 1986; 41: 152–155.

292. Mufson MA, Belshe RB, Horrigan TJ, et al. Cause of acute hemorrhagic cystitis in children. Am J Dis Child 1973; 126: 605–609.

293. Ambinder RF, Burns W, Forman M, et al. Hemorrhagic cystitis associated with adenovirus infection in bone marrow transplantation. Arch Intern Med 1986; 146: 1400–1401.

294. Apperley JF, Rice SJ, Bishop JA, et al. Late-onset hemorrhagic cystitis associated with urinary excretion of polyomaviruses after bone marrow

transplantation. Transplantation 1987; 43: 108–112.

295. DeHertogh DA, Brettman LR. Hemorrhagic cystitis due to herpes simplex virus as a marker of disseminated herpes infection. Am J Med 1988; 84: 632–635.

296. Richmond W. The genito-urinary manifestations of herpes zoster. Three case reports and a review of the literature. Br J Urol 1974; 46: 193–200.

297. Wong TW, Warner NE. Cytomegalic inclusion disease in adults. Report of 14 cases with review of literature. Arch Pathol 1962; 74: 403–422.

298. Smith JH, Christie JD. The pathobiology of Schistosoma haematobium infection in humans. Hum Pathol 1986; 17: 333–345.

299. Bilharz T. Distomum Haematobium und sein Verhaltniss zu gewissen pathologischen Veranderungen der menschlichen Harnorgane. Wiener Med Wschr 1856; 6: 49–52.

300. Von Lichtenberg F, Erickson DG, Sadun EH. Comparative histopathology of schistosome granulomas in the hamster. Am J Pathol 1973; 72: 149–178.

301. Kamel IA, Cheever AW, Elwi AM, et al. Schistosoma mansoni and S. haematobium infections in Egypt. I. Evaluation of techniques for recovery of worms and eggs at necropsy. Am J Trop Med Hyg 1977; 26: 696–701.

302. Cheever AW, Kamel IA, Elwi AM, et al. Schistosoma mansoni and S. haematobium infections in Egypt. II. Quantitative parasitological findings at necropsy. Am J Trop Med Hyg 1977; 26: 702–716.

303. Christie JD, Crouse D, Pineda J, et al. Patterns of Schistosoma haematobium egg distribution in the human lower urinary tract. I. Noncancerous lower urinary tracts. Am J Trop Med Hyg 1986; 35: 743–751.

304. Gelfand M, Ross CM, Blair DM, et al. Schistosomiasis of the male pelvic organs. Severity of infection as determined by digestion of tissue and histologic methods in 300 cadavers. Am J Trop Med Hyg 1970; 19: 779–784.

305. Fam A, Le Golvan PC. Bilharzial bladder-neck obstruction. Br J Urol 1960; 32: 165–177.

306. Smith JH, Kelada AS, Khalil A, et al. Surgical pathology of schistosomal obstructive uropathy: a clinicopathologic correlation. Am J Trop Med Hyg 1977; 26: 96–103.

307. Smith JH, Torky H, Kelada AS, et al. Schistosomal polyposis of the urinary bladder. Am J Trop Med Hyg 1977; 26: 85–88.

308. el-Badawi AA. Bilharzial polypi of the urinary bladder. Br J Urol 1966; 38: 24–35.

309. Ibrahim A. The relationship between urinary bilharziasis and urolithiasis in the Sudan. Br J Urol 1978; 50: 294–297.

310. Cutajar CL. The role of schistosomiasis in urolithiasis. Br J Urol 1983; 55: 349–352.

311. Smith JH, Kelada AS, Khalil A. Schistosomal ulceration of the urinary bladder. Am J Trop Med Hyg 1977; 26: 89–95.

312. Makar N. Cystoscopic appearance of bilharziosis of the bladder. Br J Urol 1932; 4: 209–216.

313. Gutierrez J, Nesbit RM. Ectopic prostatic tissue in bladder. J Urol 1967; 98: 474–478.

314. Rubin J, Khanna OP, Damjanov I. Adenomatous polyp of the bladder. a rare cause of hematuria in young men. J Urol 1981; 126: 549–550.

315. Klein HZ, Rosenberg ML. Ectopic prostatic tissue in bladder trigone. Distinctive cause of hematuria. Urology 1984; 23: 81–82.

316. Remick DG Jr, Kumar NB. Benign polyps with prostatic-type epithelium of the urethra and the urinary bladder. A suggestion of histogenesis based on histologic and immunohistochemical studies. Am J Surg Pathol 1984; 8: 833–839.

317. Bernstein RG, Siegelman SS, Tein AB, et al. Huge filling defect in the bladder caused by intravesical enlargement of the prostate. Radiology 1969; 92: 1447–1452.

318. Korsower JM, Reeder MM. Filling defect in the urinary bladder. JAMA 1975; 231: 408–409.

319. Faber RB, Kirchner FK Jr, Braren V. Benign prostatic hyperplasia presenting as a massive bladder filling defect in a young man. J Urol 1977; 118: 347–348.

320. Musselman P, Kay R. The spectrum of urinary tract fibroepithelial polyps in children. J Urol 1986; 136: 476–477.

321. Ganem EJ, Ainsworth LB. Benign neoplasms of the urinary bladder in children: review of the literature and report of a case. J Urol 1955; 73: 1032–1038.

322. Young RH. Fibroepithelial polyp of the bladder with atypical stromal cells. Arch Pathol Lab Med 1986; 110: 241–242.

323. Smith VC, Boone TB, Truong LD. Collagen polyp of the urinary tract: a report of two cases. Mod Pathol 1999; 12: 1090–1093.

324. Borski AA. Hamartoma of the bladder. J Urol 1970; 104: 718–719.

325. Keating MA, Young RH, Lillehei CW, et al. Hamartoma of the bladder in a 4-year-old girl with hamartomatous polyps of the gastrointestinal tract. J Urol 1987; 138: 366–369.

326. Duvenage GF, Dreyer L, Reif S, et al. Bladder hamartoma. Br J Urol 1997; 79: 133–134.

327. Brancatelli G, Midiri M, Sparacia G, et al. Hamartoma of the urinary bladder: case report and review of the literature. Eur Radiol 1999; 9: 42–44.

328. Ota T, Kawai K, Hattori K, et al. Hamartoma of the urinary bladder. Int J Urol 1999; 6: 211–214.

329. Kinzel RC, Harrison EG Jr, Utz DC. Primary localized amyloidosis of the bladder. J Urol 1961; 85: 785–795.

330. Tripathi VN, Desautels RE. Primary amyloidosis of the urogenital system: a study of 16 cases and brief review. J Urol 1969; 102: 96–101.

331. Malek RS, Greene LF, Farrow GM. Amyloidosis of the urinary bladder. Br J Urol 1971; 43: 189–200.

332. Akhtar M, Valencia M, Thomas AM. Solitary primary amyloidosis of urinary bladder. Light and electron microscopic study. Urology 1978; 12: 721–724.

333. Nakajima K, Hisazumi H, Okasyo A, et al. Primary localized amyloidosis of bladder. Urology 1980; 15: 302–303.

334. Caldamone AA, Elbadawi A, Moshtagi A, et al. Primary localized amyloidosis of urinary bladder. Urology 1980; 15: 174–180.

335. Khan SM, Birch PJ, Bass PS, et al. Localized amyloidosis of the lower genitourinary tract: a clinicopathological and immunohistochemical study of nine cases. Histopathology 1992; 21: 143–147.

336. Ehara H, Deguchi T, Yanagihara M, et al. Primary localized amyloidosis of the bladder: an immunohistochemical study of a case. J Urol 1992; 147: 458–460.

337. Grainger R, O'Riordan B, Cullen A, et al. Primary amyloidosis of lower urinary tract. Urology 1988; 31: 14–16.

338. Akram CM, Al-Marhoon MS, Mathew J, et al. Primary localized AA type amyloidosis of urinary bladder: case report of rare cause of episodic painless hematuria. Urology 2006; 68: 1343, e15–17.

339. Missen GA, Tribe CR. Catastrophic haemorrhage from the bladder due to unrecognised secondary amyloidosis. Br J Urol 1970; 42: 43–49.

340. Tirzaman O, Wahner-Roedler DL, Malek RS, et al. Primary localized amyloidosis of the urinary bladder: a case series of 31 patients. Mayo Clin Proc 2000; 75: 1264–1268.

341. Nurmi MJ, Ekfors TO, Puntala PV. Secondary amyloidosis of the bladder: a cause of massive hematuria. J Urol 1987; 138: 44–45.

342. Proppe KH, Scully RE, Rosai J. Postoperative spindle cell nodules of genitourinary tract resembling sarcomas. A report of eight cases. Am J Surg Pathol 1984; 8: 101–108.

343. Huang WL, Ro JY, Grignon DJ, et al. Postoperative spindle cell nodule of the prostate and bladder. J Urol 1990; 143: 824–826.

344. Vekemans K, Vanneste A, Van Oyen P, et al. Postoperative spindle cell nodule of bladder. Urology 1990; 35: 342–344.

344b. Wick MR, Brown BA, Young RH, et al. Spindle-cell proliferations of the urinary tract. An immunohistochemical study. Am J Surg Pathol 1988; 12: 379–389.

345. Roth JA. Reactive pseudosarcomatous response in urinary bladder. Urology 1980; 16: 635–637.

346. Nochomovitz LE, Orenstein JM. Inflammatory pseudotumor of the urinary bladder – possible relationship to nodular fasciitis. Two case reports, cytologic observations, and ultrastructural observations. Am J Surg Pathol 1985; 9: 366–373.

347. Ro JY, Ayala AG, Ordonez NG, et al. Pseudosarcomatous fibromyxoid tumor of the urinary bladder. Am J Clin Pathol 1986; 86: 583–590.

348. Young RH, Scully RE. Pseudosarcomatous lesions of the urinary bladder, prostate gland, and urethra. A report of three cases and review of the literature. Arch Pathol Lab Med 1987; 111: 354–358.

349. Stark GL, Feddersen R, Lowe BA, et al. Inflammatory pseudotumor (pseudosarcoma) of the bladder. J Urol 1989; 141: 610–612.

350. Dietrick DD, Kabalin JN, Daniels GF Jr, et al. Inflammatory pseudotumor of the bladder. J Urol 1992; 148: 141–144.

351. Jones EC, Clement PB, Young RH. Inflammatory pseudotumor of the urinary bladder. A clinicopathological, immunohistochemical, ultrastructural, and flow cytometric study of 13 cases. Am J Surg Pathol 1993; 17: 264–274.

352. August CZ, Khazoum SG, Mutchnik DL. Inflammatory pseudotumor of the bladder: a case report with DNA content analysis. J Urol Pathol 1993; 1: 211–217.

352b. Albores-Saavedra J, Manivel JC, Essenfeld H, et al. Pseudosarcomatous myofibroblastic proliferations in the urinary bladder of children. Cancer 1990; 66: 1234–1241.

353. Iczkowski KA, Shanks JH, Gadaleanu V, et al. Inflammatory pseudotumor and sarcoma of urinary bladder: differential diagnosis and outcome in thirty-eight spindle cell neoplasms. Mod Pathol 2001; 14: 1043–1051.

353b. Jones EC, Young RH. Myxoid and sclerosing sarcomatoid transitional cell carcinoma of the urinary bladder: a clinicopathologic and immunohistochemical study of 25 cases. Mod Pathol 1997; 10: 908–916.

354. Jufe R, Molinolo AA, Fefer SA, et al. Plasma cell granuloma of the bladder: a case report. J Urol 1984; 131: 1175–1176.

355. Harik LR, Merino C, Coindre JM, et al. Pseudosarcomatous myofibroblastic proliferations of the bladder: a clinicopathologic study of 42 cases. Am J Surg Pathol 2006; 30: 787–794.

356. Sonobe H, Okada Y, Sudo S, et al. Inflammatory pseudotumor of the urinary bladder with aberrant expression of cytokeratin. Report of a case with cytologic, immunocytochemical and cytogenetic findings. Acta Cytol 1999; 43: 257–262.

357. Freeman A, Geddes N, Munson P, et al. Anaplastic lymphoma kinase (ALK 1) staining and molecular analysis in inflammatory myofibroblastic tumours of the bladder: a preliminary clinicopathological study of nine cases and review of the literature. Mod Pathol 2004; 17: 765–771.

358. Hirsch MS, Dal Cin P, Fletcher CD. ALK expression in pseudosarcomatous myofibroblastic proliferations of the genitourinary tract. Histopathology 2006; 48: 569–578.

358b. Cessna MH, Zhou H, Sanger WG, et al. Expression of ALK1 and p80 in inflammatory myofibroblastic tumor and its mesenchymal mimics: a study of 135 cases. Mod Pathol 2002; 15: 931–938.

359. Lichtenheld FR, McCauley RT, Staples PP. Endometriosis involving the urinary tract. A collective review. Obstet Gynecol 1961; 17: 762–768.

360. O'Conor VJ, Greenhill JP. Endometriosis of the bladder and ureter. Surg Gynecol Obstet 1945; 80: 113–119.

361. Beecham CT, McCrea LE. Endometriosis of the urinary tract. Urol Surv 1957; 7: 2–24.

362. Arap Neto W, Lopes RN, Cury M, et al. Vesical endometriosis. Urology 1984; 24: 271–274.

363. Aldridge KW, Burns JR, Singh B. Vesical endometriosis: a review and 2 case reports. J Urol 1985; 134: 539–541.

364. Stanley KE Jr, Utz DC, Dockerty MB. Clinically significant endometriosis of the urinary tract. Surg Gynecol Obstet 1965; 120: 491–498.

365. Abeshouse BS, Abeshouse G. Endometriosis of the urinary tract: a review of the literature and a report of four cases of vesical endometriosis. J Int Coll Surg 1960; 34: 43–63.

366. Sircus SI, Sant GR, Ucci AA Jr. Bladder detrusor endometriosis mimicking interstitial cystitis. Urology 1988; 32: 339–342.

367. Stewart WW, Ireland GW. Vesical endometriosis in a postmenopausal woman: a case report. J Urol 1977; 118: 480–481.

368. Skor AB, Warren MM, Mueller EO Jr. Endometriosis of bladder. Urology 1977; 9: 689–692.

369. Vorstman B, Lynne C, Politano VA. Postmenopausal vesical endometriosis. Urology 1983; 22: 540–542.

370. Pinkert TC, Catlow CE, Straus R. Endometriosis of the urinary bladder in a man with prostatic carcinoma. Cancer 1979; 43: 1562–1567.

371. Oliker AJ, Harris AE. Endometriosis of the bladder in a male patient. J Urol 1971; 106: 858–859.

372. Schrodt GR, Alcorn MO, Ibanez J. Endometriosis of the male urinary system: a case report. J Urol 1980; 124: 722–723.

373. Balat O, Kudelka AP, Edwards CL, et al. Malignant transformation in endometriosis of the urinary bladder: case report of clear cell adenocarcinoma. Eur J Gynaecol Oncol 1996; 17: 13–16.

374. Clement PB, Young RH. Endocervicosis of the urinary bladder. A report of six cases of a benign mullerian lesion that may mimic adenocarcinoma. Am J Surg Pathol 1992; 16: 533–542.

375. Parivar F, Bolton DM, Stoller ML. Endocervicosis of the bladder. J Urol 1995; 153: 1218–1219.

376. Young RH, Clement PB. Mullerianosis of the urinary bladder. Mod Pathol 1996; 9: 731–737.

377. Ritchey ML, Benson RC Jr., Kramer SA, et al. Management of mullerian duct remnants in the male patient. J Urol 1988; 140: 795–799.

378. Feldeman T, Schellhammer PF, Devine CJ Jr, et al. Mullerian duct cysts: conservative management. Urology 1987; 29: 31–34.

379. Steele AA, Byrne AJ. Paramesonephric (mullerian) sinus of urinary bladder. Am J Surg Pathol 1982; 6: 173–176.

380. Glenn JF. Agenesis of the bladder. JAMA 1959; 169: 2016–2018.

381. Graham SD. Agenesis of bladder. J Urol 1972; 107: 660–661.

382. Vakili VF. Agenesis of the bladder: a case report. J Urol 1973; 109: 510–511.

383. Metoki R, Orikasa S, Ohta S, et al. A case of bladder agenesis. J Urol 1986; 136: 662–664.

384. Krull CL, Heyns CF, de Klerk DP. Agenesis of the bladder and urethra: a case report. J Urol 1988; 140: 793–794.

385. Palmer JM, Russi MF. Persistent urogenital sinus with absence of the bladder and urethra. J Urol 1969; 102: 590–594.

386. Duncan A. An attempt towards a systematic account of the appearances connected with that malconformation of the urinary organs in which the ureters, instead of terminating in a perfect bladder, open externally on the surface of the abdomen. Edin Med Surg J 1855; 1805–82: 43–60.

387. Rickham PP. Incidence and treatment of ectopia vesicae. Clin Med (Northfield IL) 1961; 8: 1971–1972.

388. Ives E, Coffey R, Carter CO. A family study of bladder exstrophy. J Med Genet 1980; 17: 139–141.

389. Shapiro E, Lepor H, Jeffs RD. The inheritance of the exstrophy-epispadias complex. J Urol 1984; 132: 308–310.

390. Hurwitz RS, Manzoni GA, Ransley PG, et al. Cloacal exstrophy: a report of 34 cases. J Urol 1987; 138: 1060–1064.

391. Jeffs RD. Exstrophy and cloacal exstrophy. Urol Clin North Am 1978; 5: 127–140.

392. Mc IJ, Worley G Jr. Adenocarcinoma arising in exstrophy of the bladder: report of two cases and review of the literature. J Urol 1955; 73: 820–829.

393. Engel RM, Wilkinson HA. Bladder exstrophy. J Urol 1970; 104: 699–704.

394. Marshall VF, Muecke EC. Functional closure of typical exstrophy of the bladder. J Urol 1970; 104: 205–212.

395. Blakeley CR, Mills WG. The obstetric and gynaecological complications of bladder exstrophy and epispadias. Br J Obstet Gynaecol 1981; 88: 167–173.

396. Hamdy MH, el-Kholi NA, el-Zayat S. Incomplete exstrophy of the bladder. Br J Urol 1988; 62: 484–485.

397. Rudin L, Tannenbaum M, Lattimer JK. Histologic analysis of the exstrophied bladder after anatomical closure. J Urol 1972; 108: 802–807.

398. Culp DA. The histology of the exstrophied bladder. J Urol 1964; 91: 538–548.

399. Mesrobian HG, Kelalis PP, Kramer SA. Long-term followup of 103 patients with bladder exstrophy. J Urol 1988; 139: 719–722.

400. Oesterling JE, Jeffs RD. The importance of a successful initial bladder closure in the surgical management of classical bladder exstrophy: analysis of 144 patients treated at the Johns Hopkins Hospital between 1975 and 1985. J Urol 1987; 137: 258–262.

401. Nielsen K, Nielsen KK. Adenocarcinoma in exstrophy of the bladder – the last case in Scandinavia? A case report and review of literature. J Urol 1983; 130: 1180–1182.

402. Spencer R. Exstrophia splanchnica (exstrophy of the cloaca). Surgery 1965; 57: 751–766.

403. Johnston JH. The genital aspects of exstrophy. J Urol 1975; 113: 701–705.

404. Senger FI, Santare VJ. Congenital multilocular bladder: a case report. Trans Am Assoc Genitourin Surg 1951; 43: 114–119.

405. Abrahamson J. Double bladder and related anomalies: clinical and embryological aspects and a case report. Br J Urol 1961; 33: 195–214.

406. Satter EJ, Mossman HW. A case report of a double bladder and double urethra in the female child. J Urol 1958; 79: 274–278.

407. Ravitch MM, Scott WW. Duplication of the entire colon, bladder, and urethra. Surgery 1953; 34: 843–858.

408. Burns E, Cummins H, Hyman J. Incomplete reduplication of the bladder with congenital solitary kidney: report of a case. J Urol 1947; 57: 257–269.

409. Tacciuoli M, Laurenti C, Racheli T. Double bladder with complete sagittal septum: diagnosis and treatment. Br J Urol 1975; 47: 645–649.

410. Ockerblad NF, Carlson HE. Congenital hourglass bladder. Surgery 1940; 8: 665–671.

411. Uhlir K. Rare malformations of the bladder. J Urol 1968; 99: 53–58.

412. Sterling JA, Goldsmith R. Lesions of urachus which appear in the adult. Ann Surg 1953; 137: 120–128.

413. Lattimer JK. Congenital deficiency of the abdominal musculature and associated genitourinary anomalies. a report of 22 cases. J Urol 1958; 79: 343–352.

414. Schreck WR, Campbell WA 3rd. The relation of bladder outlet obstruction to urinary–umbilical fistula. J Urol 1972; 108: 641–643.

415. Vaughan GT. Patent urachus, review of cases reported. Operation on a case complicated with stones in the kidneys. A note on tumors and cysts of the urachus. Trans Am Surg Assoc 1905; 23: 273–294.

416. Hinman F Jr. Urologic aspects of the alternating urachal sinus. Am J Surg 1961; 102: 339–343.

417. Cullen TS. Embryology, anatomy, and diseases of the umbilicus together with diseases of the urachus. Philadelphia: WB Saunders, 1916.

418. Fox M, Power RF, Bruce AW. Diverticulum of the bladder – presentation and evaluation of treatment of 115 cases. Br J Urol 1962; 34: 286–298.

419. Barrett DM, Malek RS, Kelalis PP. Observations on vesical diverticulum in childhood. J Urol 1976; 116: 234–236.

420. Kretschmer HL. Diverticula of the urinary bladder, a clinical study of 236 cases. Surg Gynecol Obstet 1940; 71: 491–503.

421. Hernanz-Schulman M, Lebowitz RL. The elusiveness and importance of bladder diverticula in children. Pediatr Radiol 1985; 15: 399–402.

422. Livne PM, Gonzales ET Jr. Congenital bladder diverticula causing ureteral obstruction. Urology 1985; 25: 273–276.

423. Verghese M, Belman AB. Urinary retention secondary to congenital bladder diverticula in infants. J Urol 1984; 132: 1186–1188.

424. Breivik N, Refsum S Jr, Oppedal BR, et al. Ehlers–Danlos syndrome and diverticula of the bladder. Z Kinderchir 1985; 40: 243–246.

425. Harcke HT Jr, Capitanio MA, Grover WD, et al. Bladder diverticula and Menkes' syndrome. Radiology 1977; 124: 459–461.

426. Schiff M Jr, Lytton B. Congenital diverticulum of the bladder. J Urol 1970; 104: 111–115.

427. Miller A. The aetiology and treatment of diverticulum of the bladder. Br J Urol 1958; 30: 43–56.

428. Abeshouse BS, Goldstein AE. Primary carcinoma in a diverticulum of the bladder, a report of four cases and review of the literature. J Urol 1943; 49: 534–557.

429. Knappenberger ST, Uson AC, Melicow MM. Primary neoplasms occurring in vesical diverticula: a report of 18 cases. J Urol 1960; 83: 153–159.

430. Faysal MH, Freiha FS. Primary neoplasm in vesical diverticula. A report of 12 cases. Br J Urol 1981; 53: 141–143.

431. Montague DK, Boltuch RL. Primary neoplasms in vesical diverticula: report of 10 cases. J Urol 1976; 116: 41–42.

432. Peterson LJ, Paulson DF, Glenn JF. The histopathology of vesical diverticula. J Urol 1973; 110: 62–64.

# CHAPTER 6

# Neoplasms of the urinary bladder

Liang Cheng, Antonio Lopez-Beltran, Gregory T. MacLennan, Rodolfo Montironi, David G. Bostwick

Carcinoma of the urinary bladder is the fourth most common malignancy in men, accounting for an estimated 67 160 new cases and 13 750 deaths from cancer in the United States in 2007.[1] Bladder cancer is morphologically heterogeneous: more than 90% of cases are urothelial (transitional cell) carcinoma, whereas primary squamous cell carcinoma, adenocarcinoma, small cell carcinoma, and other tumors are less common. The classification system for urinary bladder neoplasia used in this chapter has been modified according to the most recent World Health Organization (WHO) classification of tumors of the urinary system.[2]

## Benign urothelial (transitional cell) neoplasms

### Urothelial papilloma and diffuse papillomatosis

Urothelial papilloma is a benign exophytic urothelial neoplasm that typically occurs in patients less than 50 years of age.[3] The male:female ratio is 2:1. The most common symptom is hematuria.[3] Most tumors are located near the ureteric orifices. Urothelial papilloma may recur, but recurrent papilloma does not progress.[3,4]

The diagnostic criteria for urothelial papilloma in the 2004 WHO classification[2] are identical to those defined in the 1973 classification.[5] Using the restrictive diagnostic criteria recommended by the WHO, urothelial papilloma represents less than 1% of papillary urothelial neoplasms.[3,6–9] Urothelial papilloma is composed of a delicate fibrovascular core covered by cytologically and architecturally normal urothelium with no more than seven layers of cells (Fig. 6-1). The superficial cells are often prominent and may have vacuolization of the cytoplasm, eosinophilic syncytial morphology, apocrine-like morphology, or demonstrate mucinous metaplasia.[7,9] Mitotic figures are absent to rare and, if present, are located in the basal cell layer. The stroma may show edema and/or inflammatory cells. Rare cases show dilated lymphatics within the fibrovascular fronds. Occasionally,

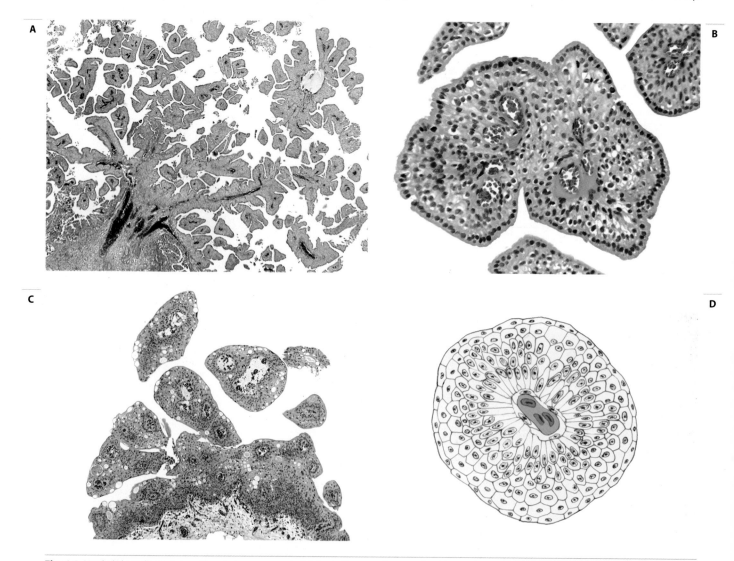

**Fig. 6-1** Urothelial papilloma is a papillary lesion composed of delicate fibrovascular cores lined by cytologically and architecturally normal urothelium less than seven cell layers thick. (**A**) Low-power view of urothelial papilloma. (**B**) High-power view of the same tumor as in A. (**C**). Another example of urothelial papilloma. (**D**) Schematic diagram of urothelial papilloma. (From Cheng L, Darson M, Cheville JC, et al. Urothelial papilloma of the bladder: clinical and biological implications. Cancer 1999; 86: 2098–2101, with permission.)

foamy histiocytes accumulate within the fibrovascular stalks. Secondary budding of small fronds from larger simple primary papillary fronds is commonly observed.

Papilloma is a diploid tumor with a low proliferation rate, undetectable or very limited p53 accumulation, and frequent fibroblast growth factor receptor 3 (FGFR3) mutation (75% of cases).[10] Cytokeratin 20 expression is limited to the superficial (umbrella) cells.[9,11]

The designation diffuse papillomatosis is applicable when the mucosa is extensively involved by multiple small delicate papillary processes, creating a velvety cystoscopic appearance.[7,9,12] These papillary structures are covered by normal urothelium having no cytological atypia (Fig. 6-2). The malignant potential of this lesion is uncertain.

## Inverted papilloma

Inverted papilloma is usually found in men in the sixth or seventh decade of life.[13–17] The male : female ratio is 7 : 1.[13] Hematuria and obstructive symptoms are the most common symptoms at presentation. The majority of inverted papillomas develop in the region of the trigone and bladder neck (Fig. 6-3). Some cases may be multifocal.[13,18] The

incidence of multiplicity ranges from 1.3% to 4.4%.[13,15] A significant number of patients have a history of smoking, suggesting a possible link between tobacco use and inverted papilloma.[13]

Histologically, inverted papilloma shows an inverted growth pattern, usually composed of anastomosing islands and trabeculae of histologically and cytologically normal urothelial cells invaginating from the surface urothelium into the subjacent lamina propria but not into the muscularis propria (Fig. 6-4). Although the term 'inverted papilloma' was initially introduced in 1963 by Potts and Hirst to describe this architecturally distinctive urothelial neoplasm,[19] in 1927 the Viennese urologist Paschkis had previously reported four morphologically identical urothelial tumors under the name of adenomatoid polyp.[20] Kunze et al.[14] proposed the subdivision of inverted papilloma into two morphologically distinct variants, trabecular and glandular. By their criteria, the trabecular variant is composed of anastomosing cords and trabeculae of urothelial cells invaginating the lamina propria at various angles. These invaginating structures demonstrate mature urothelium centrally, with darker and palisading basal cells peripherally, usually surrounded by fibrotic stroma without marked inflammation. The glandular variant is composed of nests of urothelium with either pseudoglandular spaces lined by mature urothelium, or even true glandular elements, containing mucicarminophilic secretions and mucus-secreting cells. The glandular variant, as proposed by these investigators, has considerable morphologic overlap with florid cystitis glandularis, and is not widely accepted as a diagnostic entity.

Within the spectrum of findings in inverted papilloma, vacuolization and foamy xanthomatous cytoplasmic changes may be seen. These 'clear cells' may be concentrated in distinct regions of the tumor, but more frequently are diffusely intermingled with usual inverted papilloma cells. Foci of non-keratinizing squamous metaplasia and neuroendocrine differentiation have been reported.[18] Mitotic figures are either absent or rare. Some cases may demonstrate focal minor cytologic atypia that is probably degenerative in nature and has no clinical significance. Inverted papilloma may coexist with carcinoma, and it is most important to differentiate inverted papilloma from urothelial carcinoma with an inverted growth pattern. Such distinction may be difficult, especially in limited biopsy specimens, or when

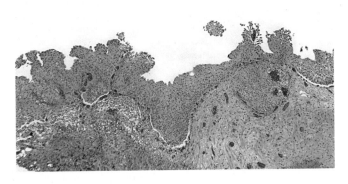

**Fig. 6-2** Diffuse papillomatosis. Multiple papillary excrescences are present in the mucosa. Cytologically, the lining cells are normal.

**Fig. 6-3** Distribution of inverted papillomas in the urinary tract. (From Sung MT, MacLennan GT, Lopez-Beltran A, et al. Natural history of urothelial inverted papilloma. Cancer 2006; 107: 2622–262, with permission.)

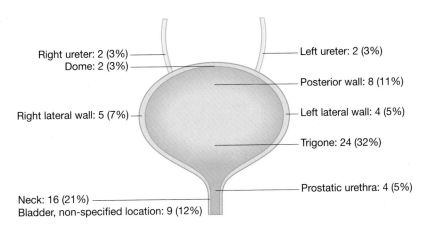

Right ureter: 2 (3%)
Dome: 2 (3%)
Left ureter: 2 (3%)
Posterior wall: 8 (11%)
Right lateral wall: 5 (7%)
Left lateral wall: 4 (5%)
Trigone: 24 (32%)
Prostatic urethra: 4 (5%)
Neck: 16 (21%)
Bladder, non-specified location: 9 (12%)

**A**

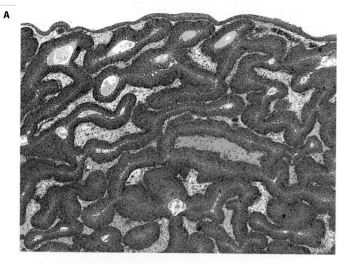

**B**

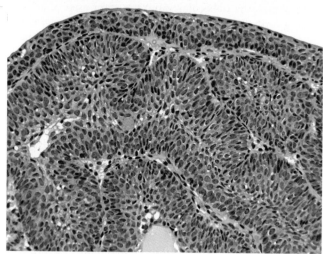

**Fig. 6-4.** Inverted urothelial papilloma. (**A**) The low magnification demonstrates a distinct downward growth pattern of a typical inverted papilloma composed of intact surface lining urothelium and underlying thin anastomosing trabeculae of urothelium in the lamina propria. (**B**) At higher magnification, the trabeculae are lined by uniform urothelial cells without cytologic atypia.

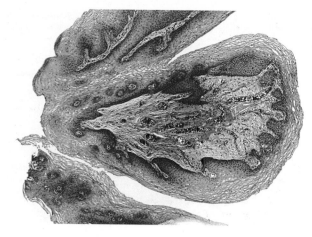

**Fig. 6-5** Squamous cell papilloma of the urinary bladder. (From Cheng L, Leibovich BC, Cheville JC, et al. Squamous papilloma of the urinary tract is unrelated to condyloma acuminata. Cancer 2000; 88: 1679–1686, with permission.)

interpretation is confounded by crush artifact.[21] Inverted papilloma usually exhibits orderly maturation of invaginated trabeculae and cords, composed of spindling and peripherally palisading cells. In contrast, urothelial carcinoma with inverted growth pattern often has thick and irregular tumor columns with transition to more solid nests. Additionally, the presence of an exophytic papillary component and unequivocal tumor invasion into the lamina propria or muscularis propria justify a diagnosis of inverted urothelial carcinoma. Marked cytological atypia, including nuclear pleomorphism, nucleolar prominence, and abundant mitotic activity, further support a diagnosis of malignancy.[21]

Several investigators have voiced concern regarding the malignant potential of inverted papilloma based on the subsequent development of urothelial carcinoma, but the great majority of patients with this complication have a history of a prior or concurrent urothelial carcinoma.[17,22–24] In a large series of 75 patients all but one had an uneventful course without either tumor recurrence or progression to urothelial malignancy during a mean follow-up of 68 months.[13] Consequently, transurethral resection of inverted papilloma is adequate treatment, and surveillance protocols as rigorous as those employed in the management of urothelial carcinoma seem unnecessary for this benign entity.

It has been well documented by the finding of non-random inactivation of X chromosomes that inverted papilloma is a clonal neoplasm that arises from a single progenitor cell.[25] Sung et al.[26–31] studied the status of loss of heterozygosity (LOH) in inverted papilloma using microsatellite markers which are commonly altered in urothelial carcinoma. The incidence of loss of heterozygosity in inverted papilloma is low (8–10%) and contrasts with the high frequency of loss of heterozygosity (29–80%) in urothelial carcinoma and papillary urothelial neoplasm of low malignant potential.[26,27,29,30,32,33] The low frequency of allelic loss in inverted papilloma is similar to that of normal urothelium.[34] The markedly reduced frequency of loss of heterozygosity in inverted papilloma compared to that of urothelial carcinoma suggests that inverted papilloma does not harbor the key genetic abnormalities that predispose to the development of urothelial carcinoma, and may indicate that these entities arise through separate and distinct pathogenetic mechanisms.

## Squamous papilloma

Squamous papilloma is a rare benign neoplasm that may represent the squamous counterpart of urothelial papilloma.[35] It is unrelated to human papillomavirus infection. It usually occurs in elderly women and follows a benign clinical course.[35] Histologically, it is composed of papillary cores with overlying benign squamous epithelium (Fig. 6-5). These tumors are diploid with undetectable or very limited nuclear p53 accumulation. Some demonstrate immunohistochemical expression of epidermal growth factor receptor (EGFR) protein.[36]

# Flat intraepithelial lesions

The classification of non-papillary (flat) intraepithelial lesions and conditions of the urothelium has evolved over the years and was recently redefined at the International Consultation on the Diagnosis of Non-Invasive Urothelial Neoplasms held in Ancona, Italy, in 2001 (Table 6-1).[37] This classification includes epithelial abnormalities (reactive urothelial atypia and flat urothelial hyperplasia), presumed preneoplastic lesions and conditions (keratinizing squamous and glandular metaplasia, and malignancy-associated cellular changes) as well as preneoplastic (dysplasia) and neoplastic non-invasive (carcinoma in situ) lesions.[37,38] Each of these lesions is defined with strict morphological criteria in order to provide more accurate information to urologists for managing patients.

Great advances have been made in the molecular genetic and biomarker characterization of bladder cancer in recent years.[10,28,31,33,39–51] Malignancy-associated cellular change (MACC) is a recently introduced concept, encompassing urothelial abnormalities in bladders harboring neoplasia that are not evident by routine light microscopy but are demonstrable by chromatin analysis or genetic studies.[37,52–54] The clinical relevance of malignancy-associated cellular changes remains to be established, but these parameters may be important in evaluating the status of residual urothelium after surgical bladder tumor resections.[48,53] Recent studies have shown that 50% of the histologically normal urothelium adjacent to superficial urothelial carcinoma harbors genetic anomalies on chromosome 9, similar to the anomalies found in the coexisting carcinoma. In addition, non-diploid nuclear DNA histograms occur in 4–54% of histologically normal urothelium adjacent to bladder tumors.[52] These genetic alterations suggest a neoplastic potential for flat urothelial lesions, regardless of whether cytologic atypia is present or not.

## Flat urothelial hyperplasia (simple hyperplasia)

Normal urothelium is a multilayered epithelium composed of basal, intermediate and superficial cells (Fig. 6-6A). The number of cell layers (usually fewer than seven) may vary because of tangential sectioning.[38] Urothelial hyperplasia is characterized by markedly thickened mucosa with an increase in the number of cell layers, usually to 10 or more (Fig. 6-6B). However, it is not necessary to count the number of cell layers for the diagnosis (Table 6-2). The cells in urothelial hyperplasia show no significant cytologic abnormalities, although slight nuclear enlargement may be focally present. Morphologic evidence of maturation from base to surface is generally evident. Urothelial compression artifact or tangential sectioning of mucosa with pseudopapillary growth (lacking a true vascular core) may resemble flat urothelial hyperplasia.

Flat urothelial hyperplasia has been observed in association with a variety of conditions, including inflammatory disorders, urolithiasis, papillary urothelial hyperplasia, dysplasia, carcinoma in situ, and low-grade papillary tumors.[37] When seen as an isolated phenomenon, there is no evidence to suggest that primary urothelial hyperplasia has a premalig-

**Table 6-1** Classification of flat urothelial lesions of the urinary bladder based on the Ancona International Consultation

| |
|---|
| Flat urothelial hyperplasia |
| Reactive urothelial atypia |
| Presumed preneoplastic lesions and conditions |
|     Keratinizing squamous metaplasia |
|     Intestinal metaplasia |
|     Malignancy associated cellular changes |
| Preneoplastic lesions |
|     Dysplasia |
| Neoplastic non-invasive lesion |
|     Urothelial carcinoma in situ |

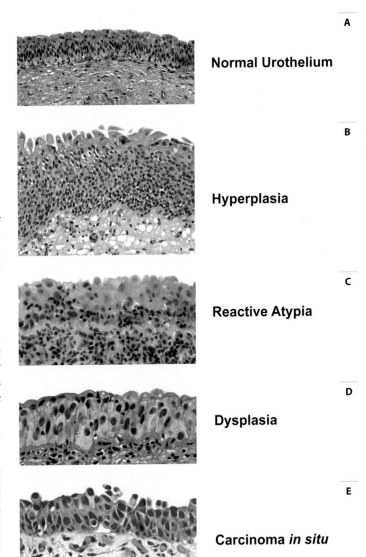

**Normal Urothelium** A

**Hyperplasia** B

**Reactive Atypia** C

**Dysplasia** D

**Carcinoma *in situ*** E

**Fig. 6-6** Flat intraepithelial lesions. (**A**) Normal urothelium. (**B**) Urothelial (simple) hyperplasia. (**C**) Reactive atypia. (**D**) Urothelial dysplasia. (**E**) Urothelial carcinoma in situ (CIS).

**Table 6-2** Comparison of flat intraepithelial lesions

| | Reactive atypia | Hyperplasia | Dysplasia | Carcinoma in situ |
|---|---|---|---|---|
| Cell layers | Variable | >7 cells | Variable | Variable |
| Polarization | Slightly abnormal | Normal | Slightly abnormal | Abnormal |
| Cytoplasm | Vacuolated | Homogeneous | Homogeneous | Homogeneous |
| N:C ratio | Normal or slightly increased | Normal or slightly increased | Slightly increased | Increased |
| Nuclei | | | | |
|   Anisonucleosis | Normal | Normal | Mild | Moderate to severe |
|   Borders | Regular/smooth | Regular/smooth | Notches/creases | Pleomorphic |
|   Chromatin | Fine/dusty | Fine | Slight hyperchromasia | Coarse/hyperchromatic |
|   Chromatin distribution | Even | Even | Even | Uneven |
|   Nucleoli | Large | Small/absent | Small/absent | Large/prominent |
| Mitotic figures | Variable | Absent | Rare | Often |
| Denudation | Variable | No | No | Variable |
| Cytokeratin 20 | Surface | Surface | Variable | Variable |
| Stromal microvascular proliferation | Variable | Variable | Less prominent | Often prominent |

nant potential. However, molecular analyses have shown that this lesion may be clonally related to the papillary tumors in bladder cancer patients.[55,56] Flat urothelial hyperplasia has been considered by some authors to be the source of papillary neoplasia, usually associated with low-grade tumors.[57]

## Urothelial reactive atypia

Urothelial abnormalities whose architectural and cytologic changes are of lesser degree than those of dysplasia have often been termed atypia.[37] The term atypia is, by its very nature, non-specific. The intra- and interobserver variation in recognition and interpretation of 'urothelial atypia' is substantial. Nevertheless, the term 'atypia' is still in use at many institutions. Two similar categories of atypia have been recently recognized, namely reactive atypia and atypia of unknown significance.[58] Both are placed among the 'benign' urothelial abnormalities.[37]

### Reactive atypia

Reactive atypia is characterized by mild nuclear abnormalities occurring in acutely or chronically inflamed urothelium. In most cases there is a history of cystitis, instrumentation, infection, stones, or previous therapy.[38] The epithelium may or may not be thickened in reactive atypia. The cells are often larger than normal, with more abundant cytoplasm than normal urothelial cells (Fig. 6-6C). These features occasionally impart a squamoid appearance. Nuclei are uniformly enlarged, vesicular, and may have prominent, usually centrally located nucleoli. Mitotic figures may be frequent but always occur in the lower epithelial layers. Inflammatory cells occupying the lamina propria and infiltrating into the urothelium are invariably present. CD44 and p53 immunohistochemical stains may be particularly useful from a differential diagnosis perspective (see urothelial dysplasia below).

### Atypia of unknown significance

The term 'atypia of unknown significance' was introduced by the International Society of Urological Pathology (ISUP) Consensus Group to describe lesions in which the pathologist was uncertain whether the changes were reactive or preneoplastic.[58] Atypia of unknown significance is characterized by nuclear changes similar to those seen in reactive atypia. However, the degree of nuclear pleomorphism and hyperchromasia is greater than in reactive atypia, and dysplasia cannot be definitely ruled out. Inflammation in the lamina propria with urothelial infiltration is often present. However, the cellular changes seem to be disproportionate to the degree of inflammation. Atypia of unknown significance is often seen in patients with a previous diagnosis of urothelial neoplasia. Progression to urothelial carcinoma has not been documented.[38] There is currently no evidence supporting a premalignant nature of such lesions. The clinical outcome of patients with atypia of unknown significance is identical to that of patients with reactive atypia.[38] The utility of creating this diagnostic category has been questioned, and the use of the designation 'atypia of unknown significance' is discouraged.

## Urothelial dysplasia (low-grade intraurothelial neoplasia)

Urothelial dysplasia is defined as abnormal urothelium with cytologic and architectural changes that do not meet all the criteria for an unequivocal diagnosis of urothelial carcinoma in situ (Figs 6-6D, 6-7, and 6-8).[37,38,59] The overall appearance is that of the urothelium in low-grade papillary urothelial carcinoma. The cytologic abnormalities in urothelial dysplasia, characterized by cellular crowding, loss of orderly maturation, and loss of cellular polarity, are not present in the full thickness of the urothelium (Figs 6-6D, 6-7 and 6-8). Occasionally there may be an increased number of cell

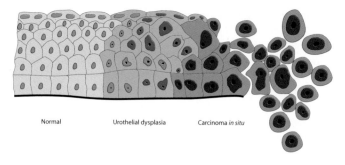

Normal          Urothelial dysplasia          Carcinoma *in situ*

**Fig. 6-7** Morphologic continuum from normal urothelium through dysplasia to carcinoma in situ, and invasion. The dysplastic urothelium shows loss of orderly maturation and cellular polarity. The progression from dysplasia to carcinoma in situ is characterized by increasing nuclear : cytoplasmic ratio, nuclear hyperchromasia, nuclear and nucleolar enlargement. The superficial umbrella cell layer is often absent in urothelial carcinoma in situ, but its loss is not a prerequisite for the diagnosis. Urothelial carcinoma in situ often progresses to invasive cancer.

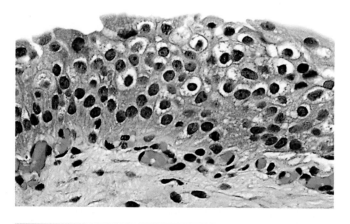

**Fig. 6-8** Urothelial dysplasia. Dysplastic urothelium shows variability in nuclear size and shape, increase in N/C ratio, and loss of cellular polarity. Cytoplasmic clearing is common. The superficial umbrella cell layer is intact. The degree of cytologic atypia is insufficient for an unequivocal diagnosis of carcinoma in situ.

layers. The superficial umbrella cells are usually present. Most cellular abnormalities in dysplasia are restricted to the basal and intermediate cell layers. Individual dysplastic cells show enlarged nuclei and nucleoli with irregular contours and coarsening of the chromatin. Multiple nucleoli and nuclear overlapping may be seen. The cells often show cytoplasmic clearing. Mitotic figures, when present, are generally basally located. The transition from normal to abnormal urothelium is subtle. Non-dysplastic urothelial cells are often dispersed among the dysplastic cells.

The diagnosis of urothelial dysplasia can be made in cases in which the urothelium demonstrates significant cytologic atypia that cannot be attributed to inflammation or a reparative process, and yet lacks the full complement of cytologic abnormalities that characterize carcinoma in situ. Nuclear and architectural features are the primary criteria for distinguishing dysplasia from reactive atypia and urothelial carcinoma in situ. Aberrant cytokeratin 20 expression in urothelial cells plus overexpression of p53 and Ki-67 are indicators of dysplastic change in urothelial mucosa.[60,61] Molecular markers may be helpful in the differential diagnosis. Cytokeratin 20 immunostaining is limited to the superficial cell layers in normal urothelium; in contrast, cytokeratin 20 immunostaining is usually present in the superficial and intermediate cell layers of dysplastic urothelium.[60,62] CD44 may be of particular value in the distinction between urothelial dysplasia and reactive atypia.[61,63] Positive CD44 immunostaining is observed only in the basal cells in normal urothelium, and is either absent entirely or present only in scattered cells in urothelial dysplasia, whereas full-thickness positive membranous CD44 staining is typical of reactive urothelium.[63] Dysplastic cells show increased p53 expression, whereas p53 nuclear accumulation is predominantly undetectable or only weakly evident in the basal and parabasal cells in reactive urothelium. Alterations of p53 and allelic losses, particularly in chromosome 9, may occur in dysplasia.[56]

It has proved difficult to create a standardized nomenclature for intraurothelial cytologic abnormalities. Consequently, grading of urothelial dysplasia is not currently recommended. The use of the term 'atypia' as a synonym for urothelial dysplasia is discouraged. Intraurothelial cytologic abnormalities that cannot be attributed to a reactive or reparative process and yet lack sufficient abnormalities to be diagnosed as carcinoma in situ should be diagnosed as urothelial dysplasia without qualifiers.

## Primary dysplasia

Primary dysplasia occurs in the absence of other urothelial tumors. Its prevalence in the general population is unknown owing to the lack of large-scale screening studies. In an autopsy series of 313 patients without gross lesions, urothelial dysplasia was present in 6.8% of males and 5.7% of females.[64] Only a few studies provide clinical information on patients with primary dysplasia.[38,59,65,66] These patients are predominantly middle-aged men with irritative symptoms with or without hematuria. The lesion has a predilection for posterior wall location.[59] Dysplasia is not cystoscopically visible, although occasionally the urothelium may appear raised and irregular or mildly erythematous. It is estimated that de novo (primary) dysplasia progresses to bladder neoplasia in 14–19% of cases.[38,59,65,66] Using modern criteria for urothelial dysplasia, Cheng et al.[59] found a 19% progression rate in 36 patients with isolated urothelial dysplasia during a mean follow-up of 8.2 years. A similar progression rate (15%) was found in a different cohort of patients.[38]

## Secondary dysplasia

Secondary dysplasia is seen in patients with a history of bladder neoplasia. The incidence of dysplasia in patients with established bladder neoplasia varies from 22% to 86% and approaches 100% in patients with invasive carcinoma.[37,67–72] As many as 24% of random biopsies from patients with stage Ta and T1 carcinoma show epithelial abnormalities that include dysplasia and carcinoma in situ.[73] The presence of urothelial dysplasia indicates urothelial instability and is a harbinger of recurrence and progression.[52,72,74–80] The recurrence rate was 73% in patients with superficial neoplasia and concomitant dysplasia compared to 43% in those without coexisting dysplasia.[73] Of the 30% of patients with superficial urothelial carcinoma who developed muscle invasive cancer within 5 years after the initial diagnosis, most had dysplasia or carcinoma in situ adjacent to the primary tumor.[74] Of the patients with dysplasia elsewhere in the bladder mucosa, 36% eventually developed muscle-invasive tumors, whereas only 7% patients with normal urothelium in adjacent biopsies subsequently developed muscle invasive cancer.

## Urothelial carcinoma in situ (high-grade intraurothelial neoplasia)

Urothelial carcinoma in situ is a flat, non-invasive lesion in which the urothelium is entirely composed of cytologically malignant cells. Melamed et al.[81] first described the natural history of urothelial carcinoma in situ and found that nine of 25 patients (36%) developed invasive carcinoma within 5 years after the initial diagnosis. In Cheng's study of 138 patients with urothelial carcinoma in situ in the absence of invasive cancer, the patient's age at diagnosis ranged from 32 to 90 years (mean, 66 years).[82] The male:female ratio in patients with carcinoma in situ is approximately 7:1. Clinical presentations include gross and microscopic hematuria, irritative symptoms (dysuria, pain, frequency), nocturia, and sterile pyuria. Approximately 25% of patients are asymptomatic. Carcinoma in situ usually is multifocal, with a predilection for the trigone, lateral wall, and dome of the bladder. Cystoscopically, it may appear as erythematous velvety or granular patches, although it may also be visually undetectable. Erythematous changes are often apparent at gross examination (Fig. 6-9).

De novo or isolated carcinoma in situ (often referred to as primary carcinoma in situ ) accounts for 1–3% of bladder neoplasms.[9,37,82–84] The clinical presentation often closely mimics that of interstitial cystitis. Urothelial carcinoma in situ is very often multifocal. Mapping studies of cystectomy

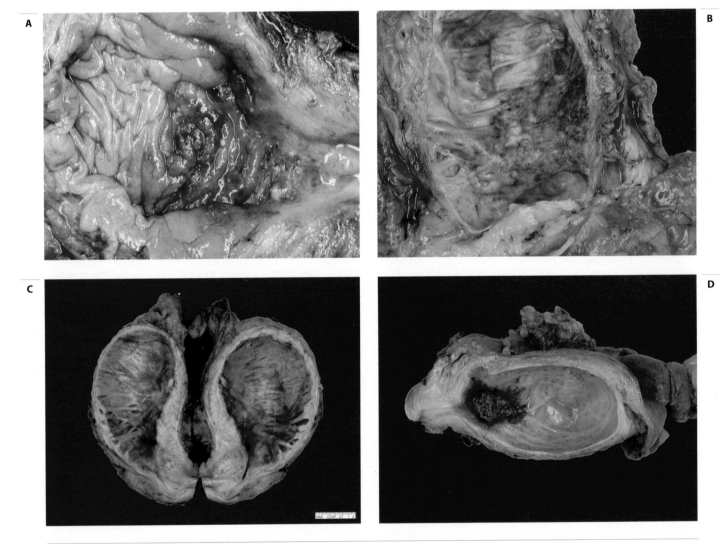

**Fig. 6-9 (A–D)** Gross appearance of urothelial carcinoma in situ. Erythematous changes are common.

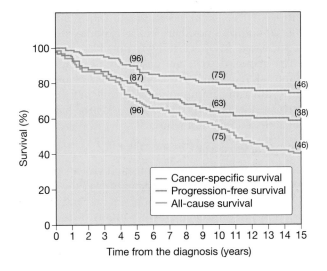

**Fig. 6-10** Kaplan–Meier survival curves for 138 patients with primary urothelial carcinoma in situ of the bladder. No patients had invasive urothelial carcinoma at the time of diagnosis. The numbers in parentheses represent the number of patients under observation at 5, 10, and 15 years. Progression was defined as development of invasive carcinoma, distant metastasis, or death from bladder cancer. (From Cheng L, Cheville JC, Neumann RM, et al. Survival of patients with carcinoma in situ of the urinary bladder. Cancer 1999; 85: 2469–2474, with permission.)

specimens show extensive carcinoma in situ, with involvement of the prostatic urethra and of the ureter in as many as 67% and 57% of cases, respectively.[85–91] Urothelial carcinoma in situ has a high likelihood of progressing to invasive carcinoma if left untreated.[82] The mean interval between a diagnosis of carcinoma in situ and the detection of cancer progression is 5 years. The actuarial progression-free survival, cancer-specific survival, and all-cause survival rates are respectively 63%, 79%, and 55% at 10 years, and 59%, 74%, and 40%, respectively, at 15 years (Fig. 6-10)[82] Factors predictive of progression include multifocality, coexistent bladder neoplasia, DNA aneuploidy, prostatic urethral involvement, and recurrence after treatment.[9,37,40,54,82,92,93]

Urothelial carcinoma in situ is often associated with invasive carcinoma elsewhere in the bladder (referred as secondary carcinoma in situ). The frequency of carcinoma in situ increases with the grade and stage of the associated urothelial neoplasm. Patients with coexisting invasive urothelial carcinoma have higher risk of cancer progression and cancer-specific death than do patients with primary carcinoma in situ.[37]

## Microscopic pathology

Urothelial carcinoma in situ is characterized by flat, disordered proliferation of urothelial cells with marked cytologic abnormalities (Fig. 6-11). The morphological diagnosis of

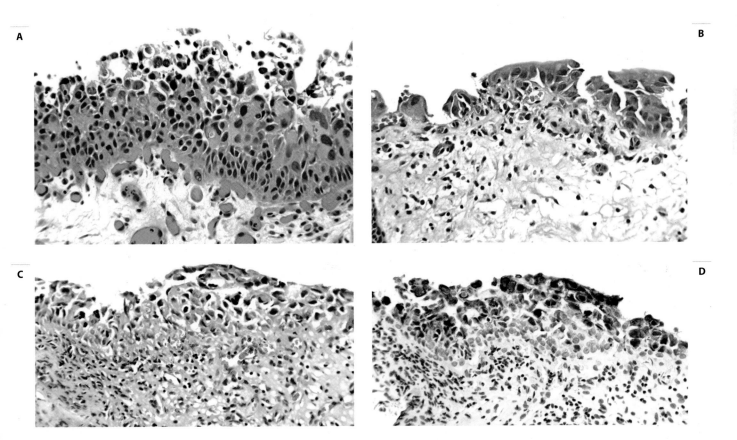

**Fig. 6-11** Urothelial carcinoma in situ displaying disordered proliferation of malignant urothelial cells that demonstrate a high nuclear:cytoplasmic ratio, nuclear pleomorphism, irregular nuclear contours, coarsely granular chromatin, and prominent nucleoli. (**A–C**) There is loss of cellular polarity and cell cohesion in urothelial carcinoma in situ. Vascular proliferation is often prominent in the underlying stroma. Full-thickness involvement is not required for the diagnosis of urothelial carcinoma in situ. Superficial umbrella cell layer may still be present. (**D**) Aberrant expression of cytokeratin 20 is observed.

carcinoma in situ requires severe cytological atypia (anaplasia).[9,37,82] Full-thickness change, which may range from one cell layer to the thickness of hyperplasia (more than seven cells), is not required. Superficial (umbrella) cells may or may not be present. Marked disorganization of cells is characteristic, with loss of cellular polarity and reduced cellular cohesiveness. The tumor cells tend to be large and pleomorphic, with moderate to abundant cytoplasm. Nevertheless, the cells of carcinoma in situ are sometimes small with a high nucleus to cytoplasmic ratio. The chromatin tends to be coarse and clumped. Nucleoli may be multiple, and are large and prominent in at least some of the cells. Mitotic figures, which are often atypical, are seen in the uppermost layers of the urothelium.

The adjacent mucosa often contains lesser degrees of cytologic abnormality. Tissue edema, vascular ectasia and proliferation of small capillaries are frequently observed in the lamina propria (Fig. 6-11).

An immunohistochemical panel consisting of cytokeratin 20, CD44, p53, and Ki-67 may be helpful in the differential diagnosis.[37,60,61,94-98] Carcinoma in situ shows intense cytokeratin 20 and p53 positivity in the majority of malignant cells. Increased Ki-67 labeling is noted in carcinoma in situ. The neoplastic cells are uniformly negative for CD44 immunostaining.[94] In contrast, cytokeratin 20 staining shows patchy cytoplasmic immunoreactivity only in the superficial umbrella cell layer, and CD44 stains only the basal cells in the adjacent normal urothelium.

## Histological variants

A number of morphologic variants and growth patterns of carcinoma in situ have been recognized over the years (Figs 6-12–6-14; Table 6-3). Although it is not necessary to mention these specific growth patterns or morphologic variants in the surgical pathology report, awareness of the histologic diversity of carcinoma in situ may aid in the diagnosis of this therapeutically and biologically important lesion.[37,99] These lesions may be associated with microinvasion, sometimes clinically unsuspected and histologically subtle.

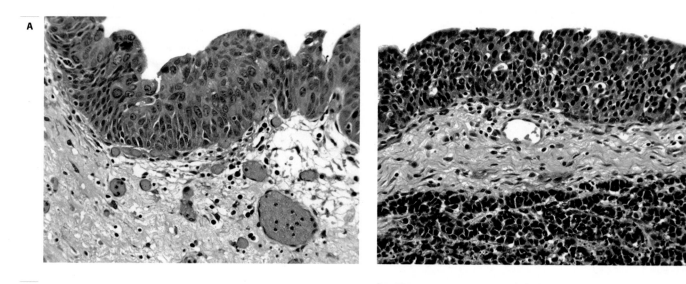

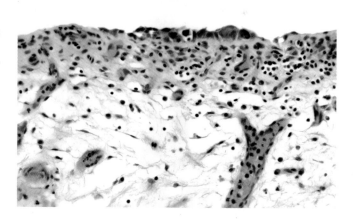

**Fig. 6-12** Histologic variants of urothelial carcinoma in situ (CIS). (**A**) Large cell CIS. (**B**) Small cell CIS. Small cell carcinoma is present in the lamina propria. (**C**) 'Clinging' CIS. (**D**) Denuding CIS. The urothelium is partially denuded; residual CIS cells are present in the remainder of the urothelium.

## Large cell carcinoma in situ

Large cell carcinoma in situ constitutes the most common morphologic form of this entity. Cytologic findings include nuclear pleomorphism, variably abundant cytoplasm, and anaplastic nuclear features (Fig. 6-12A). In rare cases, large cell carcinoma in situ may have minor nuclear pleomorphism but still exhibits architectural disarray.

**Table 6-3** Morphologic patterns of urothelial carcionoma in situ (CIS)

- Large cell CIS
- Small cell CIS
- Denuding and 'clinging pattern' CIS
- Pagetoid and undermining (lepedic) CIS
- CIS with squamous or glandular differentiation
- CIS with microinvasion (CISmic)

## Small cell carcinoma in situ

The small cell pattern refers to the size of the cells and may or may not coexist with small cell carcinoma (Fig. 6-12B), which is unrelated to neuroendocrine differentiation of carcinoma in situ. In such cases the pleomorphism is usually minimal, the cytoplasm is scant and nuclei are enlarged and hyperchromatic, with coarse unevenly distributed chromatin. The scattered prominent nucleoli are distorted and angulated. Recognition of the small cell pattern of carcinoma in situ is important to avoid misdiagnosis of basal cell hyperplasia, which has been observed in patients treated with bacille Calmette–Guérin (BCG). These show a small cell pattern but lack nuclear atypia or loss of polarity.

## Denuding and 'clinging pattern' carcinoma in situ

In some cases the neoplastic urothelial cells are strikingly dyscohesive and undergo extensive exfoliation, with the result that biopsies may show only a few residual carcinoma cells on the surface ('clinging carcinoma in situ') or no rec-

A
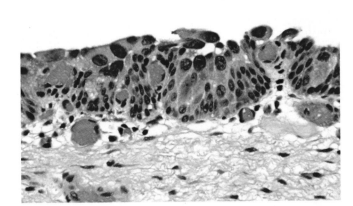

B
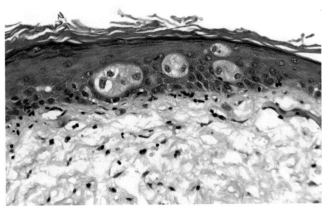

C
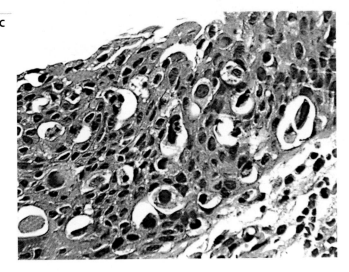

D
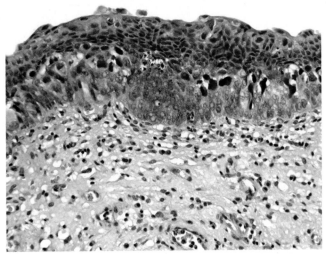

**Fig. 6-13** Pagetoid and lepidic urothelial carcinoma in situ. (**A–C**) Pagetoid spread of urothelial carcinoma in situ. Clusters and isolated single neoplastic cells (**B** and **C**) are present in the urothelium. (**D**) Urothelial carcinoma in situ may also display an undermining or lepidic growth pattern.

ognizable epithelial cells on the surface, a condition referred to as 'denuding cystitis' (Fig. 6-12C, D).[100] In the clinging pattern of carcinoma in situ there is a patchy, usually single layer of atypical cells. In mucosal biopsies entirely lacking surface epithelium, carcinoma in situ may be present only in von Brunn's nests. A careful search for carcinoma in situ in deeper sections or in other submitted biopsy fragments is important, and a recommendation for evaluation of urine cytology for carcinoma cells is warranted.

## Pagetoid and undermining (lepidic) carcinoma in situ

Another pattern of carcinoma in situ, also referred to as cancerization of the urothelium, shows either pagetoid spread (clusters or isolated single cells) or undermining or

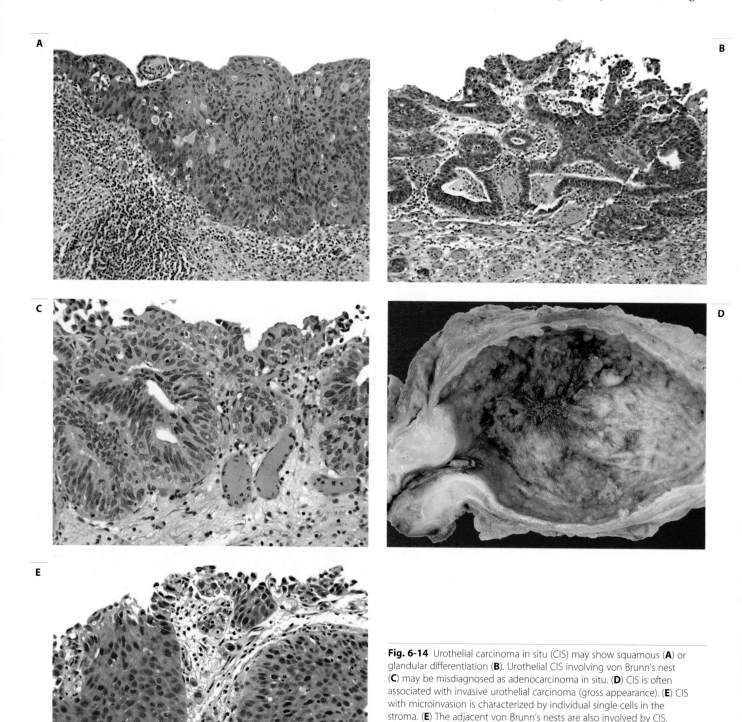

**Fig. 6-14** Urothelial carcinoma in situ (CIS) may show squamous (**A**) or glandular differentiation (**B**). Urothelial CIS involving von Brunn's nest (**C**) may be misdiagnosed as adenocarcinoma in situ. (**D**) CIS is often associated with invasive urothelial carcinoma (gross appearance). (**E**) CIS with microinvasion is characterized by individual single cells in the stroma. (**E**) The adjacent von Brunn's nests are also involved by CIS.

overriding of the normal urothelium (lepidic growth) (Fig. 6-13). Carcinoma in situ exhibiting pagetoid growth is characterized by large single cells or small clusters of cells within otherwise normal urothelium of the ureter, urethra, prostatic ducts, or areas of squamous metaplasia. Individual cells showing pagetoid spread have enlarged nuclei with coarse chromatin; frequently the cytoplasm is clear.

Pagetoid growth patterns can be found in up to 15% of carcinoma in situ cases.[37] Most patients are male and their ages range from 31 years to 78 years (mean, 64 years). Pagetoid carcinoma in situ is usually a focal lesion and is easily overlooked; it occurs in a clinical and histological setting of conventional carcinoma in situ with coexisting invasive urothelial carcinoma, and such patients essentially have the same progression and survival rates as those without pagetoid changes. In cases with extensive urothelial denudation, pagetoid carcinoma in situ may be focally present in adjacent otherwise normal-looking urothelium, thus alerting the surgical pathologist to search for additional carcinoma in situ elsewhere in the bladder.

Because primary extramammary Paget's disease of the external genitalia and of the anal canal may extend to the bladder, and conversely, some cases of pagetoid carcinoma in situ of the bladder may extend to the urethra, ureter, and external genitalia, differentiating between these two entities represents an important diagnostic and therapeutic challenge. A panel of immunostains, including cytokeratin 7, cytokeratin 20, and thrombomodulin, may assist in differentiating pagetoid urothelial carcinoma in situ from extramammary Paget's disease, which is known to be cytokeratin 7 positive and cytokeratin 20 negative.[37]

### Carcinoma in situ with squamous or glandular differentiation

Rare cases of carcinoma in situ may exhibit squamous differentiation characterized by intercellular bridges. Carcinoma in situ with squamous features is most often observed in association with urothelial carcinoma showing extensive squamous differentiation elsewhere in the bladder (Fig. 6-14A). A much less frequently encountered pattern is carcinoma in situ with morphological and immunohistochemical evidence of glandular differentiation (Fig. 6-14B). Some authors refer to this as adenocarcinoma in situ; such lesions may show papillary, cribriform, or flat morphology. Carcinoma in situ involving von Brunn's nests (Fig. 6-14C), cystitis glandularis, or cystitis cystica may be difficult to distinguish from adenocarcinoma in situ in the absence of concurrent invasive adenocarcinoma.

### Carcinoma in situ with microinvasion

Carcinoma in situ with microinvasion was initially defined by Farrow et al.[101] as invasion into the lamina propria to a depth of 5 mm or less from the basement membrane (Fig. 6-14D, E). A recent consensus conference suggested that cases with more than 20 cells measured from the stromal–epithelial interface should be classified as fully invasive.[37] Microinvasion appears as direct extension in cords (tentacular), single cells, or single cells and clusters of cells (Fig. 6-14E). The clusters of cells may have retraction artifact that

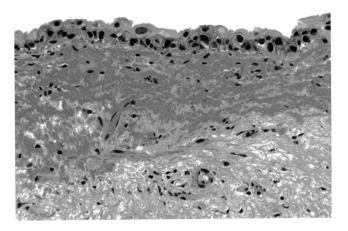

**Fig. 6-15** Cyclophosphamide (cytoxan)-induced changes include urothelial atypia and hemorrhagic cystitis.

mimics vascular invasion. Stromal response may be present, but in most cases is absent. In cases with a prominent stromal inflammatory response the invasive neoplastic cells may be interspersed among lymphocytes, making them inconspicuous. In these circumstances, immunohistochemical staining with antibodies against cytokeratins (such as AE1/AE3) exposes the invading cells.[102]

## Therapy-induced changes

Antineoplastic agents used in the bladder or systemically, such as thiotepa (triethylenethiophosphoramide), mitomycin C, cyclophosphamide, BCG, and radiation therapy produce urothelial changes that can mimic cancer histologically (see also chapter 5). Pathologists must be aware of the diagnostic pitfalls and exercise caution when evaluating urothelial atypia following treatment with chemotherapy or irradiation.[37,103–105] In most cases, knowledge of the prior treatment is crucial to correctly diagnosing the epithelial and stromal changes present (Fig. 6-15). If the distinction between treatment-induced atypia and dysplasia/carcinoma in situ is uncertain, a conservative approach with repeat cystoscopy and biopsy is indicated, preferably after the inflammation has subsided.

Cyclophosphamide therapy may induce stromal fibrosis, vascular intimal thickening, mural fibrin deposition in vessels, and vascular ectasia.[104] It also induces epithelial necrosis followed by rapid atypical regeneration. The metabolic effects of cyclophosphamide, including arrest of cell and nuclear division, produce bi- and multinucleated cells, often with large bizarre nuclei resembling radiation injury changes that can be mistaken for malignancy. Cyclophosphamide may also induce reactivation of polyomavirus infection, causing marked nuclear atypia in the surface urothelium. In rare cases, polyomavirus infection (BK virus) infection mimics flat intraepithelial lesions in immunocompromised patients.

In BCG-treated bladders it is important to bear in mind that residual carcinoma in situ might only be present in von Brunn's nests. Loss of intercellular cohesion in carcinoma in situ may result in the so-called 'denuding cystitis' or in residual neoplastic cells loosely attached to the surface ('clinging' pattern). Also important are the reactive changes associated with BCG therapy, which include both acute and chronic inflammation. There may also be a pattern of reactive epithelial atypia and granulomatous reaction deep in the bladder wall.[104,105]

Mitomycin C and thiotepa, when used as topical chemotherapeutic agents in the bladder, produce identical histologic changes. These include exfoliation, epithelial denudation, multinucleation, cytoplasmic vacuolization, and the appearance of bizarre, non-malignant nuclei in the superficial layer of the urothelium. A marked necroinflammatory process follows the administration of topical mitomycin C. There is a histiocytic response extending deep into the bladder wall. Mitomycin C may also initiate eosinophilic cystitis, a useful clue for the surgical pathologist when evaluating small bladder biopsies in this setting. These agents are not metabolic inhibitors of DNA replication and so do not produce full-thickness urothelial atypia, as is seen after cyclophosphamide therapy.

Radiation therapy produces a variety of bladder lesions associated with a progression of pathologic findings. The earliest change, usually seen after 3–6 weeks, consists of acute cystitis with desquamation of urothelial cells and hyperemia with edema of the lamina propria. The urothelium shows varying degrees of atypia, including cytoplasmic and nuclear vacuolization, karyorrhexis, stromal hyalinization, thrombosis of blood vessels, and mesenchymal cell atypia similar to that seen in giant cell cystitis.[104] Enlarged nuclei may have large nucleoli, but degenerative nuclear features are usually present. Surface ulceration with fibrin deposition, or a reactive, tumor-like epithelial proliferation associated with fibrosis of the lamina propria and/or muscularis propria, arteriolar mural thickening and hyalinization, and atypical and sometimes multinucleated stromal cells, are features seen in late cases of radiation cystitis, usually becoming evident months or years after radiation therapy. An important long-term effect of radiotherapy is the development of de novo radiation-induced bladder cancer, which is usually a urothelial carcinoma; occasionally it is a squamous cell neoplasm. Rare examples of sarcomatoid carcinoma (or carcinosarcoma) and sarcoma of the urinary bladder have been reported.[37,104–108]

Several inflammatory conditions of the urinary bladder, some of them related to treatment, may cause urothelial atypia, leading to overdiagnosis of dysplasia and carcinoma-in-situ. In addition, the damaged mucosa may become ulcerated, with adjacent atypical regenerating urothelium showing pseudoepitheliomatous hyperplasia. This change is more common after ulceration related to radiation therapy.[37,105,109]

# Urothelial (transitional cell) carcinoma

## General features

### Epidemiology and risk factors

Bladder cancer is the seventh most common cancer worldwide, accounting for approximately 336 000 new cases each year.[2,93,110,111] There are significant variations in incidence, morbidity, and mortality rates of bladder cancer in different countries and ethnicity groups. African-American men have a much lower incidence of bladder cancer, but their mortality rates are similar to those of white Caucasians.[93,111–113] Bladder cancer occurs two to five times more frequently in men than in women. This has been attributed to different smoking and occupational exposures between men and women.[93,111–113]

Several risk factors have been linked to bladder cancer. Exogenous factors, such as tobacco smoking, occupational risk, and lifestyle exposure to carcinogens, play an important role. Smokers have two to four times the risk of urothelial cancer as the general population, and heavy smokers have five times the risk.[113] Nevertheless, the specific urothelial carcinogens associated with smoking are still unknown. It is estimated that 20 years of smoking are needed for the development of bladder cancer, and the probability of this event is directly correlated with the lifetime number of cigarettes consumed. The relative risk of active smokers developing bladder cancer compared to never-smokers is 3:1, and for previous smokers it is 1.9:1. Although the exact mechanism by which tobacco causes bladder cancer is not known, many known carcinogens in cigarette smoke, such as acrolein, 4-amino-biphenyl, arylamine, and oxygen free radicals, have been implicated. Furthermore, increased duration of smoking, intensity of tobacco consumption, and degree of inhalation significantly contribute to cancer development. The beneficial effects of smoking cessation, on the other hand, include an almost immediate decline in the risk of bladder cancer. Continued smokers have a worse recurrence-free survival than those who quit at the time of diagnosis.[93,114]

Occupational exposure to aniline dyes and aromatic amines such as 2-naphthylamine and benzidine are the second most prevalent risk factor for bladder cancer. Benzidine, the most carcinogenic aromatic amine, is used in dye production and as a hardener in the rubber industry.[114] The degree of carcinogenesis due to occupational exposure varies with the degree of industrialization, but in heavily industrialized nations occupational exposure may account for up to one-quarter of all urothelial cancers. The latency period between exposure and tumor development is usually prolonged.[93] Occupational bladder cancer has also been observed in gas workers, painters, and hairdressers. Nutrition may also play a role. Vitamin A supplementation apparently reduces the risk of bladder cancer, whereas ingestion of fried foods and fat increases the risk. A high fluid intake reduced the risk of bladder cancer in one study, but this remains controversial. Epidemiologic studies in Taiwan and Chile have shown an increased risk for urothelial cancer in people whose drinking water has a high content of arsenic. Other water contaminants with putative toxic effects on urothelium are also actively being investigated.[93]

Additional factors implicated in the development and progression of bladder cancer include analgesic use; urinary tract infections, whether bacterial, parasitic, fungal, or viral; urinary lithiasis; pelvic radiation; and chemotherapeutic agents such as cyclophosphamide.[115] Although caffeine ingestion has been implicated as a risk factor for bladder cancer, risk estimates for this association decrease after controlling for concomitant tobacco use. Similarly, saccharin containing artificial sweeteners induce bladder neoplasia in rats, but human epidemiological studies have failed to establish this relationship in humans. There is a relationship between the parasite bilharzia (schistosomiasis) and squamous cell cancer in the bladder, more frequently seen in the Middle East, where the waterborne flatworms are endemic.[93]

## Signs and symptoms

The majority of bladder cancer patients present with hematuria. Approximately 20% of patients being evaluated for gross hematuria will subsequently be diagnosed with bladder cancer. Similarly, of patients presenting with microscopic hematuria, up to 10% will be diagnosed with bladder cancer. A significant proportion of patients also have irritative voiding symptoms, including urgency, frequency and dysuria: their symptoms are mistakenly attributed to urinary tract infection.

The initial evaluation and management for patients with suspected bladder cancer involves cystoscopic evaluation of the bladder and prostatic urethra for mucosal lesions. Small lesions and flat lesions worrisome for carcinoma in situ can be sampled with cold-cup biopsy forceps, and larger suspicious lesions are resected transurethrally as completely as possible. Transurethral resections and biopsies should include muscularis propria if possible.[116]

## Field cancerization and tumor multicentricity

The development of multifocal tumors, either synchronous or metachronous, in the same patient is a common characteristic of urothelial malignancy (Fig. 6-16).[91,117-119] Multiple coexisting tumors have often arisen before clinical symptoms are apparent. The separate tumors may or may not share a similar histology. Two theories have been proposed to explain the frequency of urothelial tumor multifocality. The monoclonal theory suggests that the multiple tumors arise from a single transformed cell which proliferates and spreads throughout the urothelium, either by intraluminal implantation or by intraepithelial migration. The second

theory, the field-effect theory, explains tumor multifocality as a development secondary to field cancerization effect. Chemical carcinogens cause independent transforming genetic alterations at different sites in the urothelial lining, leading to multiple genetically unrelated tumors.

The issue of a monoclonal versus an oligoclonal origin for multifocal urothelial carcinomas is clinically important for understanding patterns of early tumor development when planning treatment and surgical strategies.[30,31,40,42,43,48,59,93,120] The cause of multifocality also influences test design for the genetic detection of recurrent or residual tumor cells in post-treatment urine samples. There is currently no consensus concerning which theory is most important in the development of multifocal urothelial carcinoma. Many studies have suggested a monoclonal origin for multifocal urothelial carcinoma,[121-132] but others have shown an independent origin for some multicentric urothelial tumors using similar methods.[55,56,123,126,130,131,133-137] A recent study suggests that both field-cancerization and monoclonal tumor spread may coexist in the same patient.[31] Molecular evidence has been found to support an oligoclonal origin for multifocal urothelial carcinomas in the majority of cases, consistent with the field-cancerization theory for multicentric urothelial carcinogenesis. This finding is clinically important, as an understanding of early tumor development and spread must be considered in the development of appropriate treatment and surgical strategies, and when molecular diagnostic techniques are used in the detection of recurrent or residual disease.

Field cancerization, which is an important cause of multicentric squamous cell carcinomas of the head and neck, postulates that multifocal urothelial carcinomas arise in the same way.[48] In the field cancerization process simultaneous or sequential tumors result from numerous independent mutational events at different sites in the urothelial tract. These independent transformations are a consequence of external cancer-causing influences. In support of the field effect theory is the frequent finding of genetic instability in normal-appearing bladder mucosa in patients with bladder cancer in the adjacent urothelium.[34,138] Premalignant changes, such as dysplasia or carcinoma in situ, often are found in urothelial mucosa away from an invasive bladder cancer. Many genetic comparisons and mapping of atypia in cystectomy specimens have emphasized the role of oligoclonality and field cancerization in the development of multifocal urothelial tumors, especially in early-stage disease. As the monoclonal and oligoclonal theories to explain urothelial tumor multifocality are not mutually exclusive, various theories have been proposed to combine the two mechanisms. It has been suggested that oligoclonality is more common in early lesions, with progression to higher stages leading to the overgrowth of one clone and pseudomonoclonality.[131,139] Thus, early or preneoplastic lesions may arise independently, with a specific clone undergoing malignant transformation, which subsequently spreads through the urothelium by either intraluminal or intraepithelial dissemination. Whereas tumor multifocality seems to be an oligoclonal phenomenon in the majority of cases, in some cases there is undeniable support for the monoclonal hypothesis.[31]

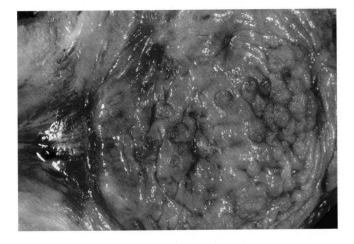

**Fig. 6-16** Gross appearance of multifocal urothelial carcinoma. The papillary architecture of these tumors is apparent.

# Histologic grading

## 1973 World Health Organization (WHO) Classification

Histologic grading is one of the most important prognostic factors in bladder cancer. The first widely accepted grading system for papillary urothelial neoplasms was the WHO (1973) classification system, which divided urothelial tumors into four categories: papilloma, grade 1 carcinoma, grade 2, and grade 3.[5] Histologic grading is based on the degree of cellular anaplasia, with grade 1 tumors having the least degree of anaplasia compatible with a diagnosis of malignancy; grade 3 tumors have the most severe degree of anaplasia, and grade 2 have an intermediate degree of cellular anaplasia (Fig. 6-17). Anaplasia is further defined by the authors of the WHO (1973) classification as increased cellularity, nuclear crowding, disturbed cellular polarity, failure of differentiation from the base to the surface, nuclear pleomorphism, irregular cell size, variations in nuclear shape and chromatin pattern, displaced or abnormal mitotic figures, and giant cells.[5]

The WHO 1973 histologic grading of bladder cancer is one of most successful grading systems among all organ sites and has been validated since its introduction three decades ago.[140-143] It has been accepted by pathologists, urologists, oncologists, and cancer registrars in the United States and elsewhere. An enormous amount of data has been accumulated using this system in studies of the morphologic properties, clinical behavior, treatment, and follow-up of urothelial tumors. Because of its relative simplicity and its well-documented powerful predictive value, it has been well accepted by urologists and used globally in making clinical decisions for management of patients with urothelial cancer for several decades.[140,141]

## Grade 1 urothelial carcinoma

Grade 1 papillary carcinoma consists of an orderly arrangement of normal urothelial cells lining delicate papillae with minimal architectural abnormality and minimal nuclear atypia. Nuclear grooves are usually present. There may be some complexity and fusion of the papillae, but this is usually not prominent. The urothelium is often thickened to more than seven cell layers. The urothelium displays normal maturation and cohesiveness, with an intact superficial cell layer. The nuclei tend to be uniform in shape and spacing, although there may be some enlargement and elongation. The chromatin texture is finely granular, without significant nucleolar enlargement. Mitotic figures are rare or absent, and basally located. Grade 1 tumor should be distinguished from urothelial papilloma which is a benign lesion (Table 6-4).

Grade 1 carcinoma appears to have a predilection for the ureteric orifices. In one study, 69% of grade 1 urothelial carcinomas were centered near a ureteric orifice, but the remainder were seen in all other portions of the bladder. Patients with grade 1 carcinoma are at increased risk of local recurrence, progression, and death from bladder cancer. Significant levels of morbidity and mortality are associated with grade 1 urothelial carcinoma of the bladder if patients are followed for a sufficient interval.[144-157] With 20 years of

**Table 6-4** Diagnostic features of urothelial papilloma and grade 1 non-invasive papillary urothelial carcinoma

| | Papilloma | Grade 1 tumor |
|---|---|---|
| Age | Younger (usually <50 years) | Older (usually >50 years) |
| Sex (Male:female) | 2:1 | 3:1 |
| Size | Small, usually <2 cm | Larger |
| Microscopic findings | | |
| Well-formed papillae | Present | Present |
| Thickness of urothelium | ≤7 layers | usually >7 layers |
| Superficial umbrella cells | Present | Usually present |
| Cytologic atypia | Minimal or absent | Mild |
| Nuclear enlargement | Rare or none | Slight to moderate |
| Nuclear hyperchromasia | Rare or none | Slight |
| Chromatin | Finely granular | Slightly coarse or granular |
| Nucleoli | Absent | May be present |
| Mitotic figures | None | Rare, basally located |
| Stromal invasion | Absent | Uncommon |

follow-up, Holmang et al.[146] found that 14% of patients with non-invasive grade 1 urothelial carcinoma (pTa G1) died of bladder cancer. In a recent review of 152 patients with stage Ta grade 1 urothelial carcinoma, Leblanc et al.[148] found that 83 patients (55%) had tumor recurrence, including 37% with cancer progression. Patients who remained tumor-free for 1 year still had a 43% chance of late recurrence. In Greene's[158] study of 100 patients with grade 1 cancer, 10 (10%) died of bladder cancer after more than 15 years; of 73 patients who had recurrences, 22% were of higher grade than the original tumor. The mean interval from diagnosis to the development of invasive cancer was 8 years. Jordan et al.[156] studied 91 patients with grade 1 papillary urothelial tumors and found that 40% of them had recurrence. Twenty percent of patients with recurrences developed high-grade (grade 3) cancer, and four patients (4%) died of bladder cancer. Long-term follow-up is recommended for patients with grade 1 papillary urothelial carcinoma.

## Grade 2 urothelial carcinoma

Grade 2 carcinoma represents a broad group of tumors encompassing a spectrum of cytologic atypia and some variability in the relative proportions of cells with atypical features. Grade 2 carcinomas retain some of the orderly architectural appearance and maturation of grade 1 carcinoma, but display at least focal moderate variation in orderliness. Cytologic abnormalities are invariably present in grade 2 carcinoma, with moderate nuclear crowding, moderate loss of cell polarity, moderate nuclear hyperchromasia, moderate anisonucleosis, and mild nucleolar enlargement. Mitotic figures are usually limited to the lower

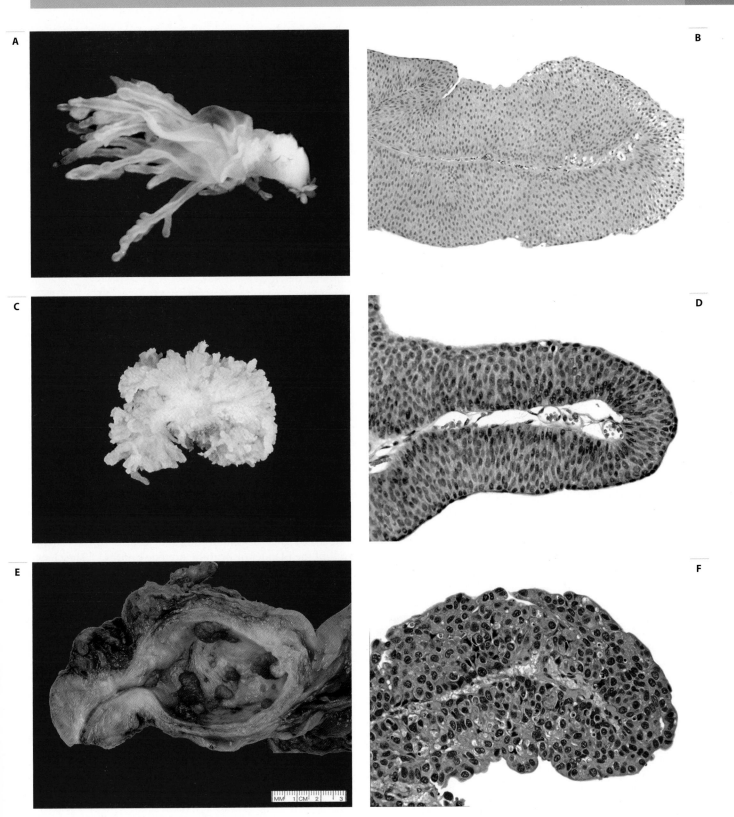

**Fig. 6-17** Gross and microscopic appearance of non-invasive urothelial carcinoma. Grading using the 1973 WHO classification scheme is recommended. (**A, B**) Grade 1 urothelial carcinoma. (**C, D**) Grade 2 urothelial carcinoma. (**E, F**) Grade 3 urothelial carcinoma.

half of the urothelium, but this is an inconstant feature. Superficial cells are usually present, and the urothelial cells are predominantly cohesive, although there may be variations in cohesion. Some tumors may be extremely orderly, reminiscent of grade 1 carcinoma, with only a small focus of obvious disorder or irregularity. These are considered grade 2 cancer, recognizing that tumor grade is based on the highest level of abnormality present.

The prognosis for patients with grade 2 urothelial carcinoma is significantly worse than for those with lower-grade papillary cancer. The recurrence risk for patients with non-invasive grade 2 cancer is 45–67%.[8,9,159] Invasion occurs in up to 20%, and cancer-specific death is expected in 13–20% following surgical treatment.[8,9,159] Patients with grade 2 cancer and invasion of the lamina propria are at even greater risk, with recurrences in 67–80% of cases, the development of muscle-invasive cancer in 21–49%, and cancer-specific death in 17–51% of those treated surgically.[8,9,159] Some authors consider both nuclear pleomorphism and mitotic count as criteria for subdividing grade 2 urothelial cancer (grade 2A and 2B), and they have been successful in identifying groups of cancers with different outcomes.[142,160–163] However, subclassification of grade 2 urothelial carcinoma is not recommended because of significant interobserver variability.

## Grade 3 urothelial carcinoma

Grade 3 carcinoma displays the most extreme nuclear abnormality of any papillary urothelial cancer, similar to changes observed in urothelial carcinoma in situ. The obvious urothelial disorder and loss of polarity are present at scanning magnification. The superficial cell layer is partially or completely absent, accompanied by prominent cellular dyscohesion. There is obvious loss of normal architecture and cell polarity, and frequent atypical mitotic figures. Cellular anaplasia, characteristic of grade 3 carcinoma, is defined as increased cellularity, nuclear crowding, random cellular polarity, absence of normal mucosal differentiation, nuclear pleomorphism, irregularity in cell size, variation in nuclear shape, capricious chromatin pattern, increased frequency of mitotic figures and occasional neoplastic giant cells.[5]

The recurrence risk for patients with non-invasive grade 3 cancer is 65–85%, with invasion occurring in 20–52% and cancer-specific death in up to 35% following surgical treatment.[8,164] Of surgically treated patients with grade 3 cancer and lamina propria invasion, 46–71% develop recurrences, 24–48% develop muscle-invasive cancer, and 25–71% suffer cancer-specific death, emphasizing a need for aggressive treatment of these patients.[9,159,165]

## 1998 International Society of Urological Pathology (ISUP)/2004 World Health Organization (WHO) Classification

The first widely accepted grading system for papillary urothelial neoplasms was the WHO 1973 classification system.[5] In 1998, a revised system of classifying non-invasive papillary urothelial neoplasms of the urinary bladder was proposed[166] and was subsequently formally adopted by the World Health Organization. In 2004, a classification system

for non-invasive papillary urothelial neoplasms, identical to the 1998 WHO/ISUP classification system, was adopted in *Pathology and Genetics of Tumours of the Urinary System and Male Genital Organs*, one of a series of WHO 'Blue Books' for the classification of tumors.[2] This new system separates non-invasive papillary urothelial neoplasms into four categories, designated papilloma, papillary urothelial neoplasm of low malignant potential (PUNLMP), low-grade carcinoma, and high-grade carcinoma. The recommendations in this book reflect the views of a Working Group of urologic pathologists assembled at an Editorial and Consensus Conference held in Lyon, France, in December 2002, and their subsequently reported findings and recommendations were stated to be a work in progress.[2]

### Papillary urothelial neoplasm of low malignant potential (PUNLMP)

PUNLMP is a low-grade urothelial tumor with a papillary architecture and a purported low incidence of recurrence and progression.[140,141,143,165,167–169] This lesion is histologically defined by the WHO (2004) classification system as a papillary urothelial tumor which resembles the exophytic urothelial papilloma, but with increased cellular proliferation exceeding the thickness of normal urothelium. All such tumors would have been considered grade 1 urothelial carcinomas by the WHO 1973 grading system (Fig. 6-18A). Cytologic atypia is minimal or absent, and architectural abnormalities are minimal with preserved polarity. Mitotic figures are infrequent and usually limited to the basal layer. Clinically, these tumors show a male preponderance (3:1) and occur at a mean age of 65 years.[170] They are most commonly identified during investigation of gross or microscopic hematuria. Cystoscopically, the lesions are typically 1–2 cm in greatest dimension, and located on the lateral wall of the bladder or near the ureteric orifices.[170] They have been described as having a 'seaweed in the ocean' appearance.

Several studies have shown that the WHO (2004) classification can differentiate non-invasive papillary urothelial tumors into prognostic groups.[165] When applied to transurethral resection of bladder tumor specimens, this classification system predicted the pathologic stage in the corresponding cystectomy.[170] However, the published recurrence and progression rates are conflicting, and some studies have shown the prognostic value of the WHO (2004) system to be limited.[140,141,171–173] In a series of 112 patients diagnosed with PUNLMP having up to 35 years of follow-up (median, more than 12 years), tumor recurrence was observed in 29%. Seventy-five percent of patients with tumor recurrence had a higher tumor grade (i.e., low-grade or high-grade urothelial carcinoma according to the WHO (2004) classification). The overall disease progression rate in these patients with PUNLMP was 4%.[170] With a median follow-up of 56 months, the WHO (1973) grade 1 tumors had a progression rate of 11%, whereas the WHO (2004) PUNLMP tumors had a progression rate of 8%.[174] The tumor recurrence rate following PUNLMP resection was reported to be 35% in the study by Holmang et al. and 47% in the study by Pich et al.[173,175] These authors concluded that PUNLMP and

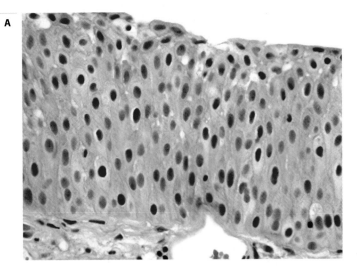

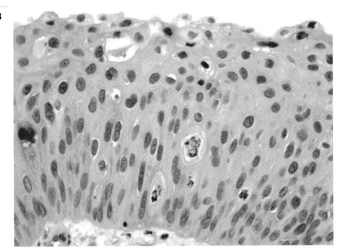

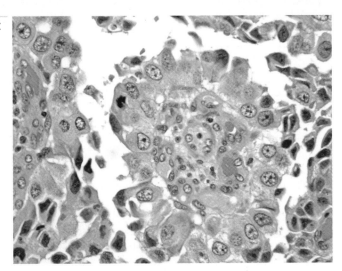

**Fig. 6-18** Histologic grading of urothelial tumors using the 2004 WHO grading system. (**A**) Papillary urothelial neoplasm of low malignant potential (PUNLMP), formerly 1973 WHO grade 1 urothelial carcinoma. (**B**) Low-grade urothelial carcinoma, formerly 1973 WHO grade 2 urothelial carcinoma. (**C**) High-grade urothelial carcinoma; formerly 1973 WHO grade 3 urothelial carcinoma.

low-grade carcinoma have similar risks of progression. Taken together, these data indicate that patients with PUNLMP do not have a benign neoplasm, but instead have a significant risk of tumor recurrence and disease progresssion. PUNLMP is not substantially different from non-invasive Ta grade 1 carcinoma as defined by 1973 WHO criteria; long-term clinical follow-up is recommended for these patients.[140,141]

Despite the provision of detailed histologic criteria for the diagnostic categories in the 2004 WHO system, no improvement in intra- and interobserver variability compared to the 1973 WHO system has been documented.[140,141,176–179] In fact, Mikuz et al.[180] demonstrated that interobserver agreement was higher using the 1973 WHO classification than when using either the 2004 WHO or 1999 WHO/ISUP systems. In a study by Yorokoglu and colleagues[178] the intra- and interobserver reproducibilities of both the 2004 WHO and the 1973 WHO systems were evaluated by assigning six urologic pathologists to the task of independently reviewing 30 slides of non-invasive papillary urothelial tumors in a study set. They found no statistical difference between the reproducibility achieved with either system; the new system failed to improve reproducibility.[178] There was agreement for PUNLMP in only 48% of cases, and reproducibility was lower for low-grade tumors in both the 2004 WHO and the 1973 WHO systems.[178] Murphy et al.[177] recorded a 50% discrepancy rate among pathologists attempting to distinguish between PUNLMP and low-grade papillary urothelial carcinoma after a period of structured pathologist education.

### Low-grade urothelial carcinoma

A low-grade papillary urothelial carcinoma shows fronds with recognizable variation in architecture and cytology.[2,165] The tumor shows slender papillae with frequent branching and variation in nuclear polarity; nuclei show enlargement and irregularity; chromatin is vesicular, and nucleoli are often present (Fig. 6-18B) Mitotic figures may occur at any level in low-grade papillary urothelial carcinoma. The majority of cases would have been considered as grade 2 in the WHO (1973) classification scheme. Altered expression of cytokeratin 20, CD44, p53 and p63 is frequent. Some tumors are diploid, but aneuploidy is the rule. FGFR3 mutations are seen with about the same frequency as in PUNLMP.[2,165] The male:female ratio is 2.9:1 and the mean age is 70 years (range, 28–90 years). Most patients present with hematuria and have a single tumor in the posterior or lateral bladder wall. However, 22% of patients with low-grade papillary urothelial carcinoma have two or more tumors. Tumor recurrence, stage progression and tumor-related mortality are 50%, 10% and 5%, respectively. In some series stage progression may be as high as 13%.[165]

### High-grade urothelial carcinoma

In high-grade papillary urothelial carcinoma the cells lining papillary fronds show an obviously disordered arrangement with cytologic atypia (Fig. 6-18C). All tumors classified as grade 3 in the 1973 WHO scheme, as well as some assigned grade 2 in that classification, would be considered high-grade carcinoma in the 2004 WHO classification. The papillae are frequently fused. Both architectural and cytologic abnormality are recognizable at scanning power.[165] The nuclei are pleomorphic with prominent nucleoli and altered polarity. Mitotic figures are frequent. The thickness of the urothelium varies considerably. Carcinoma in situ is frequently evident in the adjacent mucosa. Changes in cytokeratin 20, p53 and p63 expression, as well as aneuploidy, are more frequent than in low-grade lesions. Molecular alterations in these tumors include overexpression of p53, HER2 or EGFR, and loss of p21Waf1 or p27kip1 as seen with invasive cancers. Genetically, high-grade non-invasive lesions (pTa G3) resemble invasive tumors.[2,165] A comparative genomic hybridization-based study showed deletions at 2q, 5q, 10q, and 18q as well as gains at 5p and 20q.[181] Hematuria is common and the endoscopic appearance varies from papillary to nodular or solid. There may be single or multiple tumors. Stage progression and death due to disease are observed in as many as 65% of patients.[2]

## Other recent proposals for bladder cancer grading and tumor heterogeneity

### The Ancona 2001 refinement of the 1973 WHO classification

In an effort to improve understanding and to standardize use of the 1973 WHO classification, an expanded and refined contemporary description of the scheme was presented in 2001. This proposal is known as the Ancona refinement of the 1973 WHO grading system.[5,9,159] This effort was inspired by discussions during the International Consensus Meeting on Bladder Cancer held in Ancona, Italy, 2001. It was proposed that urothelial tumors be divided into two main groups based on growth pattern: flat and papillary. Flat tumors form a morphologic continuum whose classification includes reactive changes, dysplasia, and carcinoma in situ (see previous discussion). Papillary tumors include papilloma, grade 1 papillary carcinoma, grade 2 papillary carcinoma, and grade 3 papillary carcinoma. The diagnostic criteria for each of these categories were refined and optimized for reproducibility.[9,159] The use of terms that had been recently introduced for new urothelial neoplasia grading schemes, including 'low malignant potential' and 'atypia of uncertain clinical significance,' was discouraged. Grading of bladder cancer should be based on the highest level of abnormality noted. No formal recommendation has so far been made regarding the amount or extent of a higher grade needed for upgrading, but the Ancona refinement requires at least one high-power field.[9,159]

### The 1999 WHO grading proposal

The publication of the 1999 WHO blue book introduced a new grading scheme.[182] This new classification retained the three-tiered numbering system (grade 1, grade 2, and grade 3 carcinoma), but tumors formerly classified as 1973 WHO grade 1 were subdivided into PUNLMP and grade 1 tumors. In the 1999 WHO classification, which differed from the 1998 WHO/ISUP and 1973 WHO classifications, papillary tumors of the urinary bladder were subclassified as papilloma, papillary urothelial neoplasm of low malignant potential, grade 1, grade 2, and grade 3 papillary urothelial carcinoma. The definition of papilloma remains the same in

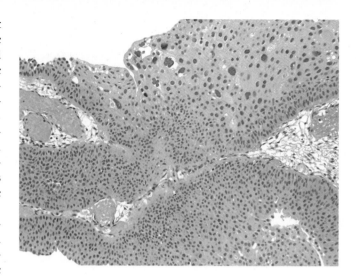

**Fig. 6-19** Cancer heterogeneity of Ta urothelial carcionoma. The same tumor may have areas with different histologic grades.

all new grading systems, and is defined as a papillary tumor with a delicate fibrovascular stroma lined by cytologically and architecturally normal urothelium without increased cellularity or mitotic figures.[3]

## Tumor heterogeneity

Papillary urothelial neoplasms encompass a spectrum of morphologic findings, including tumors that behave aggressively and tumors that are biologically benign. Attempting to differentiate biologic behavior based solely on subtle histopathological criteria is fraught with difficulties and perils, especially considering the significant interobserver variability that has been documented in numerous studies with all classification schemes.[177–180] The WHO (2004)/ISUP system provides clearly defined histologic criteria for each of its diagnostic categories; however, urothelial neoplasms frequently demonstrate features of more than one grade (Fig. 6-19). The grading of papillary urothelial tumors is typically based on the worst grade present. However, cancer heterogeneity could have a significant impact on patient outcome. Cheng et al.[183] examined 164 patients with stage Ta urothelial tumors and found that approximately one-third had morphologic heterogeneity consistent with more than one histologic grade. They graded both the primary and secondary patterns of tumor growth by the WHO (2004)/ISUP criteria, with PUNLMP, low-grade carcinoma, and high-grade carcinoma patterns receiving scores of 1, 2, and 3, respectively. Each tumor was then evaluated by a combined scoring system on a scale of 2–6. With a median follow-up of 9.2 years, the prognosis of patients with a combined score of 6 (the entire tumor consisting of high-grade carcinoma) is considerably worse than for those with a combined score of 5 (a tumor consisting of low- and high-grade carcinoma) (26% 10-year progression-free survival versus 68% 10-year progression free survival, p = 0.02).[183] The significant survival difference (42%) between score 5 and score 6 groups may suffice to warrant different management strategies in appropriate settings. Subsequent studies have also suggested that combined scoring systems may be useful in the grading of bladder tumors.[184] Grading should take cancer heterogeneity into consideration, as prognostic accuracy was increased when the combined primary and secondary grades were applied.[183]

Neither the WHO (2004)/ISUP system nor the WHO 1973 systems take tumor heterogeneity into account; however, the WHO 1973 system does allow a greater amount of diagnostic flexibility in that tumors are frequently classified as grade 1–2 or grade 2–3. This added flexibility may actually give a more accurate representation of the tumor histology than attempting to force a lesion into a single diagnostic category. It appears that prognostic accuracy is improved when heterogeneity is considered.[183] Future investigations will be needed to fully address the impact of tumor heterogeneity on clinical outcome.

## Staging of invasive bladder cancer

### General features of invasive urothelial carcinoma

At gross examination most tumors present as a single, solid, polypoid mass with or without ulceration, and may also appear sessile and extensively infiltrate the bladder wall (Fig. 6-20). Histologically, the neoplastic cells invade the bladder wall as nests, cords, trabeculae, small clusters, or single cells that are often separated by a desmoplastic stroma. The tumor sometimes grows in a more diffuse, sheet-like pattern, but even in these cases focal nests and clusters are generally present. The cells show moderate to abundant amphophilic or eosinophilic cytoplasm and large hyperchromatic nuclei. In larger nests, palisading of nuclei may be seen at the edges of the nests. The nuclei are typically pleomorphic and have irregular contours with angular profiles. Nuclear grooves may be identified in some cells. Nucleoli are highly variable in number and appearance. Some cells contain single or

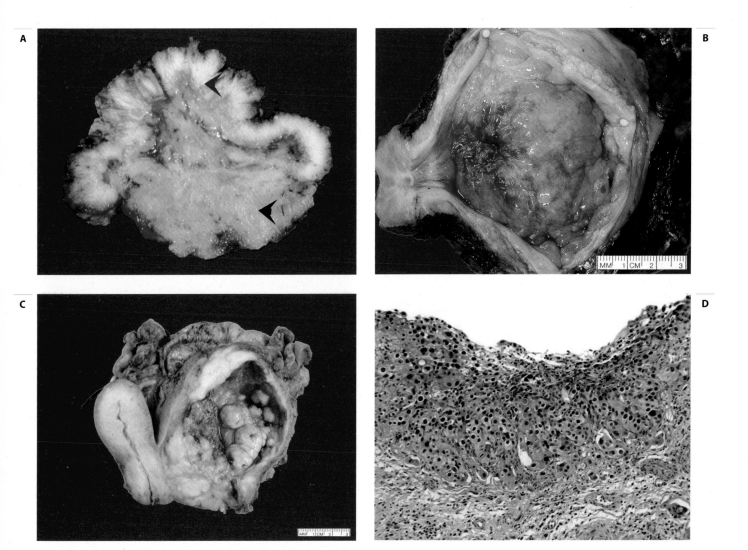

**Fig. 6-20** Urothelial carcinoma of the bladder. (**A**) Tumor is invasive into the lamina propria (blue arrow) but does not involve muscularis propria (black arrow). (**B**) Urothelial carcinoma often coexists with urothelial carcinoma in situ, which was present in the areas of widespread mucosal erythema. (**C**) Invasion into an adjacent organ (uterine cervix) is evident grossly. (**D**) The mucosal surface of invasive cancer is often denuded or ulcerated, with a ragged appearance.

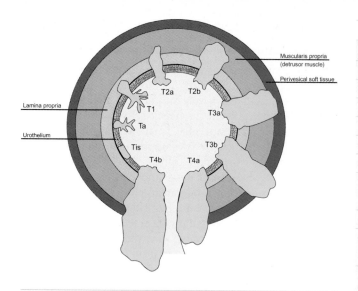

**Fig. 6-21** Schematic diagram of staging of bladder carcinoma according to the 2002 TNM (tumor, lymph node, and metastasis) staging system.

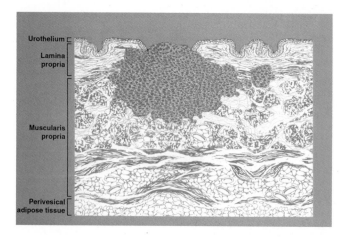

**Fig. 6-22** The bladder is organized into the urothelium, lamina propria, muscularis propria, and perivesical adipose tissue. Adipose tissue can be present in the lamina propria or muscularis propria layer. Current staging system for bladder cancer is based on the depth of invasion. A tumor invading into muscular propria (detrusor muscle) is illustrated. (From Cheng L, Neumann RM, Scherer BG, et al. Tumor size predicts the survival of patients with pathological stage T2 bladder carcinoma: a critical evaluation of the depth of muscle invasion. Cancer 1999; 85: 2638–2647, with permission.)

**Table 6-5** TNM classification of bladder cancer (2002 revision)

| *Primary tumor* | | |
|---|---|---|
| TX | Primary tumor can not be assessed | |
| T0 | No evidence of primary tumor | |
| Ta | Non-invasive papillary carcinoma | |
| Tis | Carcinoma in situ | |
| T1 | Tumor invades subepithelial connective tissue (lamina propria) | |
| T2 | Tumor invades musclularis propria | |
| | T2a | Tumor invades superficial muscle (inner half) |
| | T2b | Tumor invades deep muscle (outer half) |
| T3 | Tumor invades perivesical tissue | |
| | T3a | Microscopically |
| | T3b | Macroscopically (extra-vesical mass) |
| T4 | Tumor invades any of the following: prostate, uterus, vagina, pelvic wall, and abdominal wall | |
| | T4a | Tumor invades prostate or uterus or vagina |
| | T4b | Tumor invades pelvic wall or abdominal wall |

The suffix 'm' should be added to the appropriate T category to indicate multiple tumors. The suffix 'is' may be added to any T to indicate the presence of associated carcinoma in situ

| *Regional Lymph Nodes (N)* | |
|---|---|
| NX | Regional Lymph nodes cannot be assessed |
| N0 | No regional lymph node metastasis |
| N1 | Metastases in a single lymph node, 2 cm or less in greatest dimension |
| N2 | Metastases in a single lymph node, more than 2 cm but not more than 5 cm in greatest dimension, or multiple lymph nodes, none more than 5 cm in greatest dimension |
| N3 | Metastasis in a lymph node more than 5 cm in greatest dimension |

| *Distant Metastasis (M)* | |
|---|---|
| MX | Distant metastasis cannot be assessed |
| M0 | No distant metastasis |
| M1 | Distant metastasis |

multiple small nucleoli, and others have large eosinophilic nucleoli. Foci of marked pleomorphism may be seen, with bizarre and multinuclear tumor cells present. Mitotic figures are common, including many abnormal forms. Invasive tumors are most commonly high grade, usually showing marked anaplasia with focal giant cell formation.

Pathologic stage is most critical for assessing patient prognosis. The 2002 TNM (tumor, lymph node, and metastasis) staging information should be provided in the pathology report (Figs 6-21 and 6-22; Table 6-5).

### Stage pT1 tumor

Infiltrating urothelial carcinoma is defined by the WHO as a urothelial tumor that invades beyond the basement membrane.[185] The 2002 TNM staging system defines pT1 tumors of the bladder as those invading the lamina propria but not the muscularis propria.[186] Recognition of lamina propria invasion by urothelial carcinoma is one of the most challenging fields in surgical pathology, and the pathologist should follow strict criteria in its assessment (Table 6-6, Fig. 6-23).[102,187]

*Histologic grade* Although invasion is not necessarily an unexpected finding in low-grade tumors, it is much more commonly encountered in high-grade lesions, reaching 70–96% in some series (Fig. 6-23A).[102] In addition, in transurethral resection specimens histologic grade has been correlated with pathologic stage at cystectomy.[188]

*Stromal–epithelial interface* Tangentially sectioned, densely packed non-invasive papillary tumors exhibit a stromal–epithelial interface that is smooth and regular. In instances of true invasion, one is likely to see variably sized and irregularly shaped nests or individual tumor cells insinuating

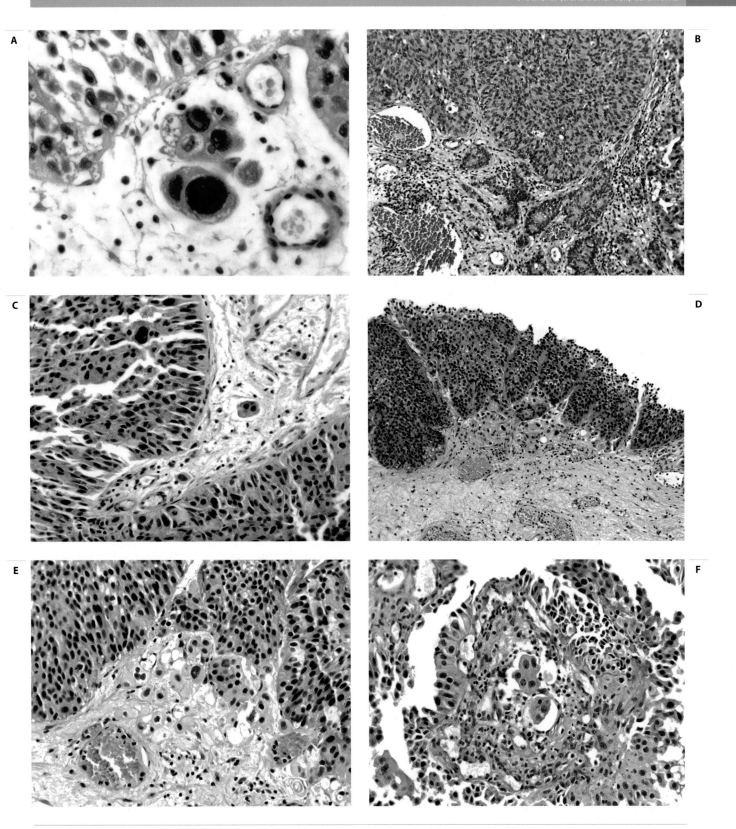

**Fig. 6-23** Histologic features useful for the diagnosis of stromal invasion. (**A**) Histologic grade. (**B**) Irregular contour of invading fronts. (**C**) Single individual cells. (**D, E**) Paradoxical differentiation. Invading tumor cells may have more eosinophilic cytoplasm than overlying non-invading tumor cells. (**F**) Retraction artifact is most useful in the diagnosis of stalk invasion in the papillae.

through the stroma. When the specimen includes tangential sections through non-invasive tumor, or when urothelial carcinoma involves von Brunn's nests, the basement membrane preserves a regular contour, whereas in cases of true invasion it is frequently absent or disrupted. The smoothness of the epithelial–stromal interface may be assessed on H&E stains. In some cases, however, additional findings may be helpful; for example, there is a parallel array of thin-walled vessels that evenly line the basement membrane of non-invasive nests. These are absent in patients with invasive tumors.

*Invading epithelium* The invasive front of the neoplasm may show one of several features. Most commonly, tumors invade the underlying stroma as single cells or irregularly shaped nests of tumor cells (Fig. 6-23B, C). Sometimes tentacular or finger-like extensions can be seen arising from the base of the papillary tumor. Frequently, the invading nests appear cytologically different from cells at the base of

the non-invasive component. Invasive tumor cells often have more abundant cytoplasm and a higher degree of nuclear pleomorphism. In some cases, particularly in microinvasive disease, the invasive tumor cells may acquire abundant eosinophilic cytoplasm. At low- to medium-power magnification these microinvasive cells seem to be more differentiated than the overlying non-invasive disease, a feature known as paradoxical differentiation (Fig. 6-23D, E).

*Stromal response* The stromal response to invading carcinoma is not always uniformly present in invasive urothelial carcinoma, and the diagnosis of invasion may rely on identification of the typical characteristics of the invading epithelium. The stromal reaction in the lamina propria associated with invasive tumor may be inflammatory, myxoid, or fibrous (Fig. 6-24A–E). Assessment of differences in stromal growth pattern provides an important diagnostic clue.[189] Although the majority of bladder tumors with unquestionable lamina propria invasion exhibit some sort of stromal reaction, microinvasive disease usually does not, making its identification even more difficult. In some cases, retraction artifact around superficially invasive individual tumor cells may mimic angiolymphatic invasion. Often this finding is focal, and may itself be one of the early signs of invasion into the lamina propria.

Lamina propria invasion may elicit a brisk inflammatory response. Numerous inflammatory cells in the lamina propria often obscure the interface between epithelium and stroma (Fig. 6-24F, G). This makes small nest or single cell invasion difficult to recognize. Cytokeratin immunostaining is useful in difficult cases (Fig. 6-24H).

Invasive urothelial carcinoma may have a cellular stroma with spindled fibroblasts and variable collagenization, or a hypocellular stroma with a myxoid background. Rarely, the tumor induces an exuberant proliferation of fibroblasts, which may display alarming cellular atypia similar to giant cell cystitis. This feature, although a helpful clue to invasion, should not be mistaken for the spindle cell component of sarcomatoid urothelial carcinoma. Immunostains for cyto-

**Table 6-6** Histologic features that are useful for the diagnosis of stromal invasion

| |
|---|
| Histologic grade: |
|    Invasive cells are usually higher nuclear grade |
| Invading epithelium |
|    Irregularly shaped nests |
|    Single cell infiltration |
|    Irregular or absent basement membrane |
|    Tentacular finger-like projections |
|    Paradoxical differentiation |
| Angiolymphatic invasion |
| Stromal response |
|    Desmoplasia or fibrotic stroma |
|    Retraction artifact |
|    Inflammation |
|    Myxoid stroma |
|    Pseudosarcomatous stroma |

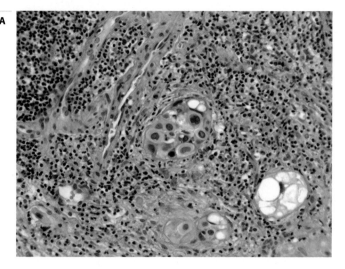

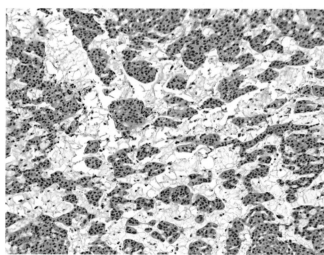

**Fig. 6-24** Diagnosis of stage T1 bladder cancer. The stroma associated with invasive cancer may be (**A**) inflammatory, (**B**) myxoid or (continued on next page).

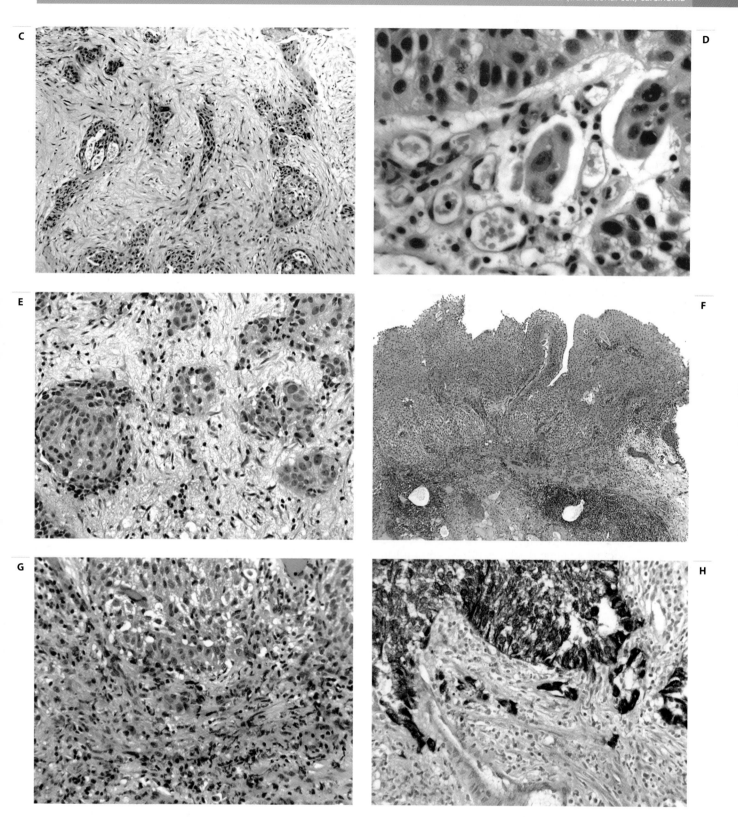

**Fig. 6-24, Cont'd** (**C**) fibrous. (**D**) Retraction artifact around superficially invasive individual tumor cells may mimic angiolymphatic invasion. (**E**) Hypocelluar stroma with myxoid background. (**F, G**) Invasive tumor may also show variable and often brisk inflammation at the tumour-stromal interface. (**H**) Immunostaining with anti-cytokeratin antibodies (AE1/3) is useful for identification of individual tumor cells.

**Table 6-7** Pitfalls in the diagnosis of stage pT1 urothelial carcinoma

- Tangential sectioning and poor orientation
- Obscuring inflammation
- Thermal injury
- Urothelial carcinoma in situ involving von Brunn's nests
- Muscle invasion indeterminate for type of muscle (muscularis propria versus muscularis mucosae)
- Variants of urothelial carcinoma with deceptively bland cytology
- Pseudoinvasive nests of benign proliferative lesions

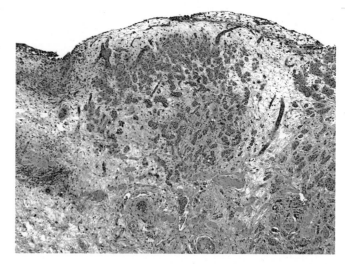

A

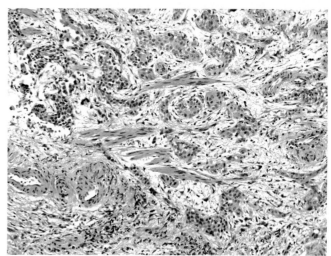

B

**Fig. 6-25** Muscularis mucosae is not uniformly present in the lamina propria. Substaging of pT1 cancer based on muscularis mucosae invasion (**A** and **B**) is not recommended.

keratin are helpful in difficult cases, although some myofibroblasts may also be positive for keratin.[190] The proliferating stroma is usually non-expansile, being limited to areas around the neoplasm, and is composed of cells which have a degenerate or smudged appearance.

*Diagnostic pitfalls* Transurethral resection specimens are excised in a piecemeal fashion. Submitted tissue fragments are of variable shape and size and difficult, if not impossible, to orientate properly (Table 6-7). Furthermore, owing to their complex architecture, papillary tumors are inevitably tangentially sectioned in multiple planes, resulting in the presence of isolated nests of non-invasive tumor cells within connective tissue. Smooth, round, and regular contours favor tangential sectioning, whereas irregular, jagged nests with a haphazard arrangement favor stromal invasion. Papillary tumors may show variable and often brisk inflammation at the tumor–stromal interface. This may obscure isolated cells or small nests of invasive tumor. Diagnosis of invasion in some of these cases can be facilitated by immunohistochemical study with anti-cytokeratin antibodies. Thermal injury or cautery artifact produces severely distorted morphology, rendering accurate diagnosis of invasion difficult. Tumor cells involving von Brunn's nests may also mimic lamina propria invasion. This is especially problematic when von Brunn's nests are prominent, or when they have been distorted by inflammatory or cautery artifact.

*Substaging of pT1 tumors* The recurrence and progression rates for pT1 tumors are highly variable.[102,191] There is a need for an accurate, easy-to-use, reproducible substaging system to stratify pT1 patients into different prognostic groups. Several studies have explored the utility of evaluating the spatial relationship of invasive tumor to the muscularis mucosae for subclassification of pT1 tumors.[102,192–198]

The muscularis mucosae consists of thin, wavy fascicles of smooth muscle frequently associated with large, thin-walled blood vessels. Muscularis mucosae can be identified in 15–83% of biopsy specimens,[102,192–197,199–204] but 6% of radical resection specimens do not have discernable muscularis mucosae.[203] Thus, the 'large' vessels have been used as a surrogate marker of muscularis mucosae in all published studies that have proposed T1 substaging based on muscularis mucosae invasion (Fig. 6-25). For example, Angulo et al.[192] were able to identify muscularis mucosa in 39% of their cases, and used the blood vessel landmark in another 26%. Thus, in 35% of their cases, substaging could not be performed because neither muscularis mucosae nor large

vessels could be found. Platz et al.[196] identified muscularis mucosae in only 33% of their cases and found no significant prognostic value in substaging pT1 cancer using the level of muscularis mucosae invasion. These problems have raised concerns about the practicality and validity of substaging pT1 disease based on assessment of muscularis mucosae invasion, and currently this practice is not universally advocated.[166] Nonetheless, when possible, pathologists should provide an assessment of the depth of lamina propria invasion or the extent of disease.

Recently, Cheng et al. proposed a system for substaging pT1 tumors based on ocular micrometer measurement of tumor invasion into the subepithelial connective tissue[187,199,200] (Fig. 6-26). Using an ocular micrometer to measure the depth of invasion from the mucosal basement membrane, they found a significant correlation between depth of invasion in the transurethral resection specimens and final pathologic stage at cystectomy.[187,205] A depth of invasion of 1.5 mm predicted advanced-stage disease at cystectomy with a sensitivity of 81%, a specificity of 83%, and positive and negative predictive values of 95% and 56%, respectively. They further applied the same criteria to a group of 83 consecutive patients diagnosed with pT1 bladder cancer. With a depth of tumor invasion greater than 1.5 mm they found a 5-year progression-free survival of 67%. With a depth of invasion less than 1.5 mm, the 5-year survival rate was 93%.[199]

Substaging of pT1 bladder tumors may also be facilitated by cytokeratin immunohistochemistry, especially in difficult cases where specimen orientation and tissue artifacts hinder accurate assessment.[102,189,206,207]

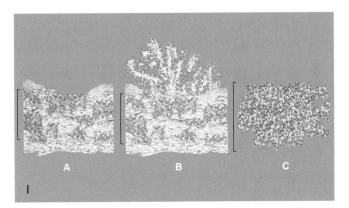

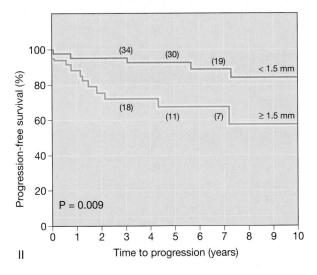

**Fig. 6-26** Substaging of pT1 bladder cancer based on the depth of invasion. The depth of stromal invasion in transurethral resection or biopsy specimens is measured from the basement membrane of the bladder mucosa to the deepest invasive cancer cells using ocular micrometer (IA-B). When tissue fragments contained cancer without intervening stroma or the specimens were not oriented, the depth of invasion was measured from the shortest distance to avoid overestimation of the depth of invasion (IC). Cancer progression-free survival according to the level of depth of invasion (1.5 mm) in the transurethral resection specimens (II). Number in parentheses represents the number of patients under observation at 3, 5, and 7 years. Progression was defined as the development of muscle-invasive or more advanced stage carcinoma, distant metastasis, or death from bladder cancer. (From Cheng L, Weaver AL, Neumann RM, et al. Substaging of T1 bladder carcinoma based on the depth of invasion as measured by micrometer: a new proposal. Cancer 1999; 86: 1035–1043 and Cheng L, Neumann RM, Weaver AL, et al. Predicting cancer progression in patients with stage T1 bladder carcinoma. J Clin Oncol 1999; 17: 3182–3187, with permission.)

### Stage pT2 tumor

The 2002 TNM staging system subclassifies pT2 tumor into two categories: cancer invading less than half of the depth of muscularis propria (pT2a), and cancer invading more than half of the depth of muscularis propria (Fig. 6-27A,B).[186] The clinical utility of substaging of pT2 tumors has been questioned.[200]

The subdivision of the T2 category is based on work by Jewett and Strong in 1952.[208] In a study of 18 patients with muscle-invasive carcinoma (five T2a cases and 13 T2b cases), they found that 80% of this small series of patients with stage T2a bladder carcinoma survived, whereas only 8% of those with stage T2b survived. Data that have accumulated in the 46 years since this original publication do not support the subdivision of T2 by depth of muscularis propria invasion.[209–238] Jewett,[239] in 1978, stated that 'it seems probable that our arbitrary dividing line drawn 30 years ago at the halfway level to separate B1 from B2 tumors was too superficial.'

Cheng et al.[200] found that tumor size, rather the depth of invasion, was predictive of distant metastasis-free and cancer-specific survival in patients with muscularis propria invasion. Ten-year distant metastasis-free and cancer-specific survival rates were respectively 100% and 94% for patients with cancers <3 cm, and 68% and 73%, respectively, for patients with cancer = 3 cm.[200] Jimenez et al.[240] have recently introduced a morphologic classification of invasive bladder tumors distinguishing three patterns of growth (nodular, trabecular, and infiltrative). Tumors with an infiltrative growth pattern are associated with a worse prognosis than those displaying a non-infiltrative (nodular or trabecular) growth pattern.

### Stage pT3 tumor

Stage pT3 bladder carcinoma is defined as tumor invading into perivesical soft tissue (Fig. 6-27C, D). The subdivision of pT3 tumors into T3a (tumors with microscopic extravesical tumor extension) and pT3b (tumors with gross extravesical extension) is also controversial. Quek et al.[241] examined 236 patients with pT3 tumors. With a median follow-up of 8.9 years, no difference in recurrence or survival was found between patients with pT3a and those with pT3b tumors. Lymph node and surgical margin status were the only factors that significantly affected patient prognosis in this study.

### Stage pT4 tumor

Stage pT4 bladder cancer is defined as tumor invading into adjacent organs, including the uterus (Fig. 6-27 E, F), vagina, prostate (Fig. 6-27G, H), pelvic wall or abdominal wall. The designation of prostatic invasion by bladder carcinoma as stage pT4 cancer has been debated. Esrig et al.[242] studied 143 bladder cancers with prostatic involvement, dividing them into two groups: group I penetrated the full thickness of the bladder wall to involve the prostate, and group II involved the prostate by extension from the prostatic urethra. Five-year overall survivals were 21% and 55% for group I and group II patients, respectively. Among group II patients, the presence of prostatic stromal invasion was associated with a worse prognosis than for patients in whom urothelial cancer was confined to the urethral mucosa only.[242] Similarly, Pagano et al.[243] found that 5-year survival was only 7%

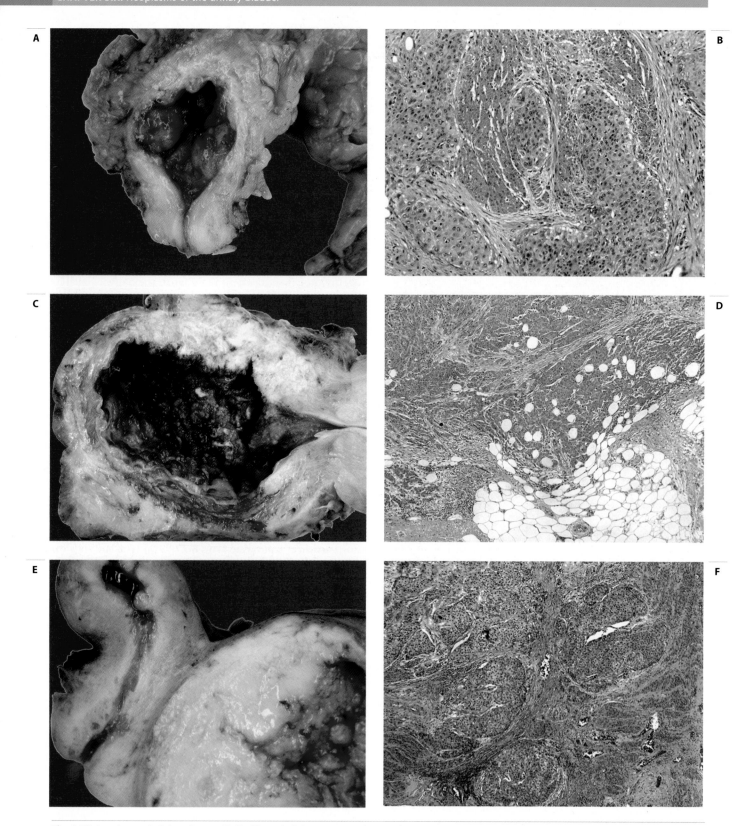

**Fig. 6-27** Invasive urothelial carcinoma. (**A, B**) pT2 urothelial carcinoma with muscularis propria invasion. (**C, D**) pT3 urothelial carcinoma with invasion into perivesicular adipose tissue. Extensive urothelial carcinoma in situ is also present (**C**). (**E, F**) pT4 cancer with invasion into adjacent uterine wall.

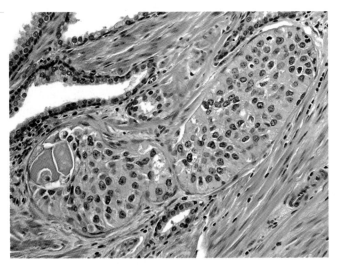

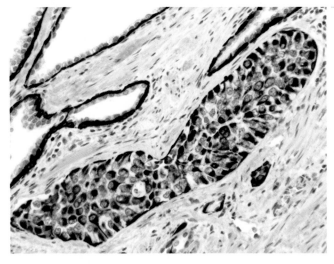

**Fig. 6-27, Cont'd** (**G**) Another pT4 cancer with invasion into the prostate. Immunostaining for high molecular weight cytokeratin highlights tumor cells.

among group I patients, compared to 46% among group II patients. In group II, all patients with only urethral mucosal involvement were alive and free of disease at 5 years, compared to 40–50% survival among patients with prostatic stromal invasion. In a detailed mapping study of 214 radical cystoprostatectomy specimens, Shen et al.[244] found the presence of prostatic involvement and levels of involvement to be significant prognostic factors in patients with bladder cancer. About 26% of the invasive bladder cancers in the prostate resulted from direct prostatic infiltration from the primary tumor in the bladder, and in the remaining 72% of cases the prostate was infiltrated by urothelial carcinoma arising in the prostatic urethra.[244]

## Histologic variants

Urothelial carcinoma has a propensity for divergent differentiation.[185] Virtually the whole spectrum of bladder cancer variants described below may be seen in variable proportions in otherwise typical urothelial carcinoma (Fig. 6-28). The clinical outcome of some variants differs from that of typical urothelial carcinoma. Therefore, recognition of these variants is important (Tables 6-8 and 6-9).

### Urothelial carcinoma with mixed differentiation

About 20% of urothelial carcinomas contain areas of squamous or glandular differentiation (Fig. 6-29). Squamous differentiation, defined by the presence of intercellular bridges or keratinization, occurs in 21% of urothelial carcinomas of the bladder (Fig. 6-29A, B).[245–247] Its frequency increases with grade and stage. Detailed histologic maps of urothelial carcinoma with squamous differentiation have shown wide variations in the proportion of the squamous component. Some cases have urothelial carcinoma in situ as the only urothelial component. Cases with areas of squamous differentiation may have a less favorable response to therapy than pure urothelial carcinoma.[246–249] Of 91 patients with metastatic carcinoma, 83% with mixed adenocarcinoma and 46% with mixed squamous cell carcinoma

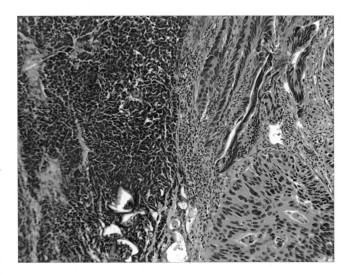

**Fig. 6-28** Urothelial carcinoma shows divergent differentiation with small cell carcinoma (left) and adenocarcinoma component (top right).

experienced disease progression despite intense chemotherapy, whereas in <30% of patients with pure urothelial histology the carcinoma progressed.[250] Low-grade urothelial carcinoma with focal squamous differentiation has a higher recurrence rate than pure low-grade urothelial carcinoma. Tumors with any identifiable urothelial element are classified as urothelial carcinoma with squamous differentiation, and an estimate of the percentage of squamous component should be provided. Cytokeratin 14, L1 antigen and caveolin-1 have been reported as immunohistochemical markers of squamous differentiation in urothelial carcinoma.[251,252]

Glandular differentiation is less common than squamous differentiation and may be present in about 6% of urothelial carcinomas of the bladder (Fig. 6-29C, D).[245,246,251] Glandular differentiation is defined by the presence of true glandular spaces within the tumor. These may be tubular or enteric glands with mucin secretion. A colloid–mucinous pattern

**Table 6-8** Histologic variants of urothelial carcinoma

| |
|---|
| Urothelial carcinoma with mixed differentiation (specify type and percentage)<br>  With squamous cell differentiation<br>  With glandular differentiation<br>  Other |
| Urothelial carcinoma, nested variant |
| Urothelial carcinoma with inverted growth |
| Urothelial carcinoma, micropapillary variant |
| Urothelial carcinoma, microcystic variant |
| Lymphoepithelioma-like urothelial carcinoma |
| Lymphoma-like/plasmacytoid-like urothelial carcinoma |
| Urothelial carcinoma, clear cell (glycogen-rich) variant |
| Urothelial carcinoma, lipoid-cell variant |
| Urothelial carcinoma with syncytiotrophoblastic giant cells |
| Urothelial carcinoma with rhabdoid features |
| Sarcomatoid carcinoma |
| Small cell carcinoma |
| Large cell undifferentiated carcinoma |
| Giant cell carcinoma |
| Urothelial carcinoma with unusual stromal reactions<br>  Pseudosarcomatous stroma<br>  Stromal osseous or cartilaginous metaplasia<br>  Osteoclast-type giant cells<br>  Prominent lymphoid infiltrate |

characterized by nests of cells 'floating' in extracellular mucin, occasionally with signet ring cells, may be present. Cytoplasmic mucin-containing cells are present in 14–63% of typical urothelial carcinomas and are not considered to represent glandular differentiation. The diagnosis of adenocarcinoma is reserved for pure tumors. A tumor with mixed glandular and urothelial differentiation is classified as urothelial carcinoma with glandular differentiation, and an estimate of the percentage of glandular component should be provided.

The expression of MUC5AC-apomucin may be useful as an immunohistochemical marker of glandular differentiation in urothelial tumors.[253,254] When adenocarcinoma is present in association with urothelial carcinoma, even focally, it portends a poor prognosis. Glandular differentiation is an important finding and usually dictates more aggressive therapy (see later in this chapter).

## Urothelial carcinoma, nested variant

The nested variant of urothelial carcinoma is an aggressive neoplasm with fewer than 50 reported cases.[251] There is a marked male preponderance, and 70% of patients die 4–40 months after diagnosis in spite of therapy.[255,256] This rare pattern of urothelial carcinoma was first described as a tumor with a 'deceptively benign' appearance that closely resembles von Brunn's nests infiltrating the lamina propria (Fig. 6-30).[255–258] A variable proportion of infiltrating cell nests may

**Table 6-9** Diverse morphologic manifestations and pitfalls in the diagnosis of urothelial carcinoma variants

| Variants of urothelial carcinoma | Main Differential diagnosis |
|---|---|
| Urothelial carcinoma with squamous and/or glandular differentiation | Squamous cell carcinoma, adenocarcinoma |
| Urothelial carcinoma, nested variant | von Brunn's nest hyperplasia, cystitis glandularis, nephrogenic adenoma, paraganglioma, carcinoid, prostatic adenocarcinoma |
| Urothelial carcinoma, inverted variant | Inverted papilloma |
| Urothelial carcinoma, micropapillary variant | Adenocarcinoma, metastasis from other sites including serous carcinoma of the ovary |
| Urothelial carcinoma, microcystic variant | Cystitis cystica and cystitis glandularis, nephrogenic adenoma, adenocarcinoma |
| Lymphoepithelioma-like (urothelial) carcinoma | Urothelial carcinoma with prominent lymphoid infiltrate, lymphoma (MALTOMA type), chronic cystitis |
| Urothelial carcinoma, plasmacytoid variant | Plasmacytoma, melanoma |
| Urothelial carcinoma, clear cell (glycogen-rich) variant | Clear cell carcinomas from kidney and other sites, clear cell adenocarcinoma |
| Urothelial carcinoma, lipoid cell variant | Carcinosarcoma/sarcomatoid carcinoma with heterologous elements (liposarcoma), signet ring cell adenocarcinoma |
| Urothelial carcinoma with syncytiotrophoblastic giant cells | Choriocarcinoma, sarcomatoid carcinoma |
| Large cell undifferentiated carcinoma | Metastasis from other sites (lung) |
| Urothelial carcinoma with rhabdoid feature | Plasmacytoma, melanoma, inflammatory myofibroblastic tumor, metastasis from other sites |
| Urothelial carcinoma with peudosarcomatous stroma | Sarcomatoid carcinoma |
| Urothelial carcinoma with stromal osseous or cartilaginous metaplasia | Sarcomatoid carcinoma with heterologous elements |
| Urothelial carcinoma with osteoclast-type giant cells | Reactive granulomatous lesion, giant cell carcinoma |
| Urothelial carcinoma with prominent lymphoid infiltrate | Lymphoma, lymphoepithelioma-like carcinoma |
| Rare urothelial carcinomas with discohesive, acinar differentiation or endometrioid-like morphologies | Lobular carcinoma of breast, endometrial carcinoma, prostatic adenocarcioma |

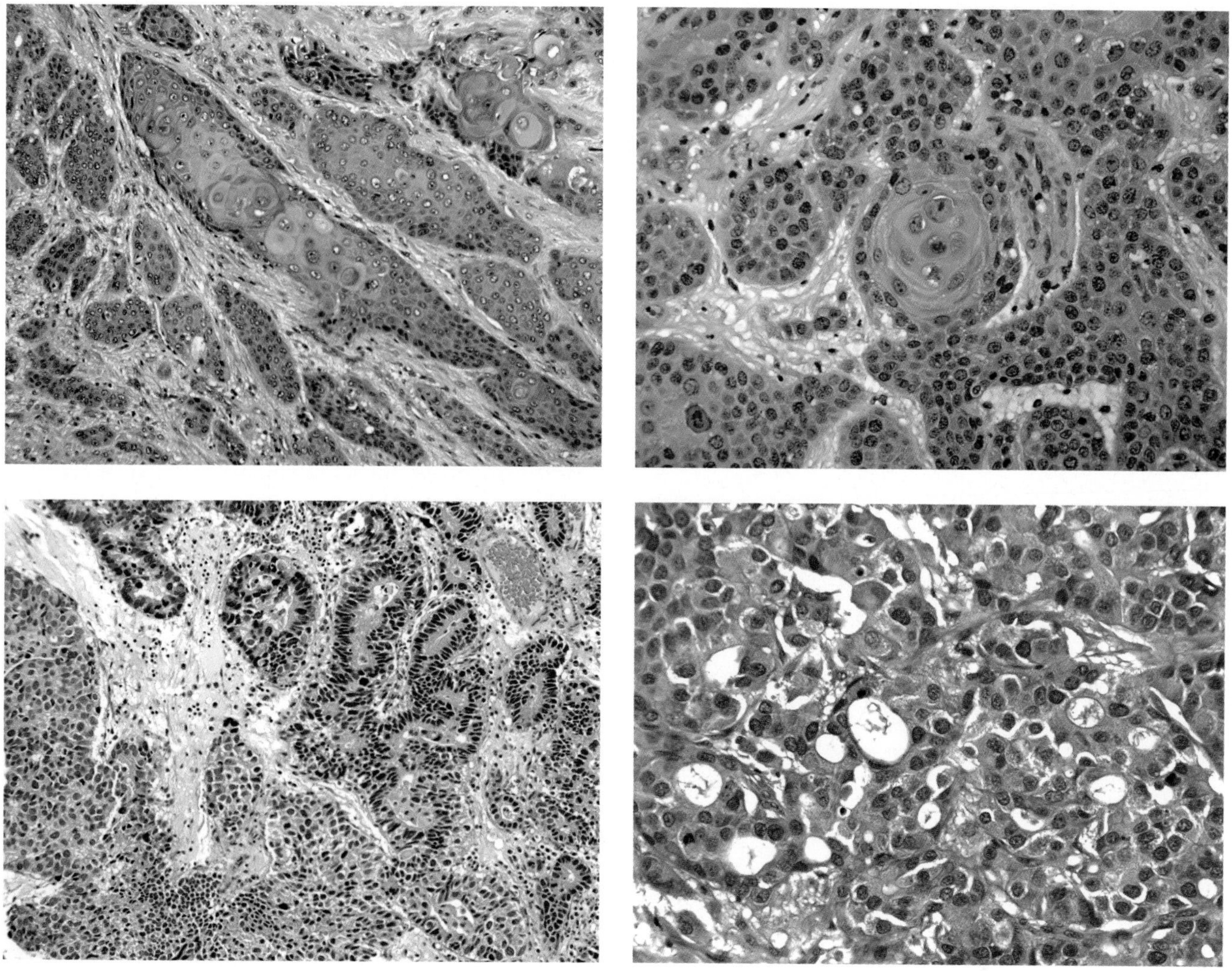

**Fig. 6-29** Urothelial carcinoma with mixed differentiation. (**A, B**) Squamous differentiation. (**C, D**) Glandular differentiation. (**D**) Mucin secretion is noted in the luminal space of glandular differentiation.

exhibit small tubular lumina (Table 6-10). Nuclei generally show little or no atypia, but invariably the tumor contains foci of unequivocal cancer with cells exhibiting enlarged nucleoli and coarse nuclear chromatin. Anaplastic features are often more apparent in the deeper aspects of the cancer.[259] The differential diagnosis of the nested variant of urothelial carcinoma includes prominent von Brunn's nests, cystitis cystica, cystitis glandularis, inverted papilloma, nephrogenic metaplasia, carcinoid tumor, paraganglionic tissue, and paraganglioma.[251,255,259]

The immunohistochemical features of the nested variant of urothelial carcinoma are similar to those of aggressive urothelial carcinomas of the usual type, with frequent loss of p27 and a high MIB-1 labeling index.[260] In the differential diagnosis between florid von Brunn's nests and the nested variant of urothelial carcinoma, CK20 immunohistochemical evaluation does not appear to be useful, but significantly greater MIB-1 expression and p53 expression are seen in nested variant urothelial carcinoma compared to florid von Brunn's nests, with MIB-1 expression in >7% of lesional cells

and p53 expression in >3% of lesional cells seen only in carcinoma.[261]

## Urothelial carcinoma, inverted variant

This variant also has been referred as urothelial carcinoma with endophytic (inverted papilloma-like) growth, or inverted urothelial carcinoma (Fig. 6-31). The potential for misinterpretation of urothelial carcinoma with inverted growth as benign inverted papilloma is high.[21,262–265] The inverted variant of urothelial carcinoma demonstrates significant nuclear pleomorphism, architectural abnormality, and increased mitotic activity. In most cases the surface of the neoplasm shows similar abnormalities and is readily recognized as typical urothelial carcinoma. An exophytic papillary or invasive component is often associated with the inverted element.[21,263] However, in cases of inverted papilloma fragmented during transurethral resection, a pseudo-exophytic pattern may result. Large papillary tumors with prominent endophytic growth may appear to 'invade' the

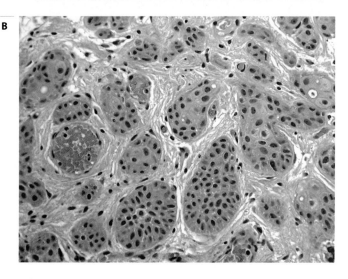

**A**

**B**

**Fig. 6-30** Urothelial carcinoma, nested variant. (**A**) Tumor invades into the lamina propria. (**B**) The cells are relatively uniform without significant cytologic atypia. The key differential diagnostic consideration is von Brunn's nest hyperplasia.

lamina propria with a pushing border. Unless this pattern is accompanied by true destructive stromal invasion the likelihood of metastasis is minimal, because the basement membrane is not truly breached. A recent proposal suggests grading these tumors following the same criteria as for usual urothelial carcinoma.[21,251]

Inverted papillomas of the urinary bladder and urothelial carcinomas with an inverted growth pattern may be distinguished using a combination of morphologic, immunohistochemical, and molecular genetic assessments (Table 6-11).[21] Whereas inverted papillomas usually do not demonstrate immunoreactivity for Ki-67, p53, or cytokeratin 20, urothelial carcinomas with inverted growth pattern frequently express one or more of these biomarkers. Similarly, inverted papillomas do not show the molecular features of urothelial carcinoma on UroVysion FISH analysis, whereas inverted-pattern urothelial carcinomas often demonstrated genetic alterations that are commonly seen in bladder cancer.[21]

## Urothelial carcinoma, micropapillary variant

Micropapillary carcinoma is a distinct variant of urothelial carcinoma that resembles papillary serous carcinoma of the ovary (Fig. 6-32). Approximately 60 cases have been reported in the literature.[251,266] There is a male preponderance and the patient age ranges from the fifth to the ninth decade, with a mean age of 66 years.[267,268] The most common presenting symptom is hematuria. The first description of micropapillary carcinoma included 18 patients whose ages ranged from 47 to 81 years (mean, 67) with a male:female ratio of 5:1. Seven patients died of carcinoma.[251,269] In 80% of reported cases micropapillary carcinoma is accompanied by noninvasive papillary or invasive urothelial carcinoma. The presence of a micropapillary component at the surface in bladder biopsy specimens is an unfavorable prognostic feature. In such cases deeper biopsies may prove useful, as muscle invasion is a significant concern.[251,268] Micropapillary carcinoma is composed of infiltrating slender delicate filiform processes or small tight papillary tumor cell clusters lying within lacunae that resemble lymphovascular spaces; no lining endothelial cells are demonstrable by immunohistochemistry in these small lacunar spaces, however.[269,270] Twenty-five

**Table 6-10** Key features in the differential diagnosis of the nested variant of urothelial carcinoma

| | Lumen formation | Marked cytologic atypia in deeper portion | Infiltrative base | Muscle invasion | Immunohistochemistry |
|---|---|---|---|---|---|
| Nested variant | Present, variable | Present, frequent | Present, frequent | Present, frequent | Low p27$^{kip1}$, high proliferation |
| Florid von Brunn nests | Present, variable | Absent | Absent | Absent | Variable |
| Nephrogenic metaplasia | Present | Absent | Present, frequent | Present, rare | Variable |
| Cystitis cystica, cystitis glandularis | Present | Absent | Absent | Absent | Variable |
| Paraganglionic tissue and paraganglioma | Absent, associated prominent vascular network | Absent | Absent | Present | Neuroendocrine markers positive |

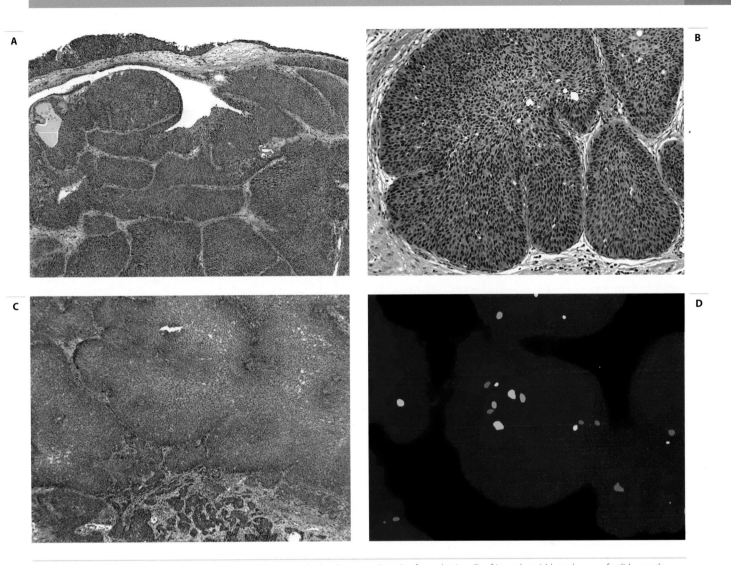

**Fig. 6-31** Urothelial carcinoma, inverted variant. (**A, B**)There are thick columns and cords of neoplastic cells of irregular width and areas of solid growth. (**C**) Stromal invasion is obvious. (**D**) Multicolor interphase fluorescence in situ hybridization (FISH) using the UroVysion probes is useful in difficult cases. The cancer cell showed four copies of chromosome 3 (red), and two copies each of chromosomes 7 (green), 17 (aqua) and p16 gene (gold).

**Table 6-11** Differences between urothelial carcinoma with inverted growth and inverted papilloma

| Characteristics | Urothelial carcinoma, inverted growth | Inverted papilloma |
| --- | --- | --- |
| Surface | Variable, usually exophytic papillary lesion present | Smooth, dome shaped, usually intact cytologically unremarkable surface urothelium |
| Growth pattern | Endophytic, thick trabeculae, circumscription variable | Endophytic, sharply delineated, anastomosing cords and trabeculae |
| Cytologic features | Cytologic atypia is invariably present, mitotic figures often present, less maturation or palisading | Orderly polarized cells, some spindling and palisading at periphery, absence of necrosis and diffuse severe cytologic atypia. Mitotic figures absent or rare. |
| Biologic potential | Recurrences and progression may occur | Benign, no recurrences when completely resected** |
| Immunohistochemistry | Variable with grade; usually high p53 accumulation or Ki67-MIB1 counts | Low p53 accumulation and Ki-67-MIB1 counts. |
| UroVision FISH | Positive | Negative |

*Rare recurrences related to incomplete surgical excision.

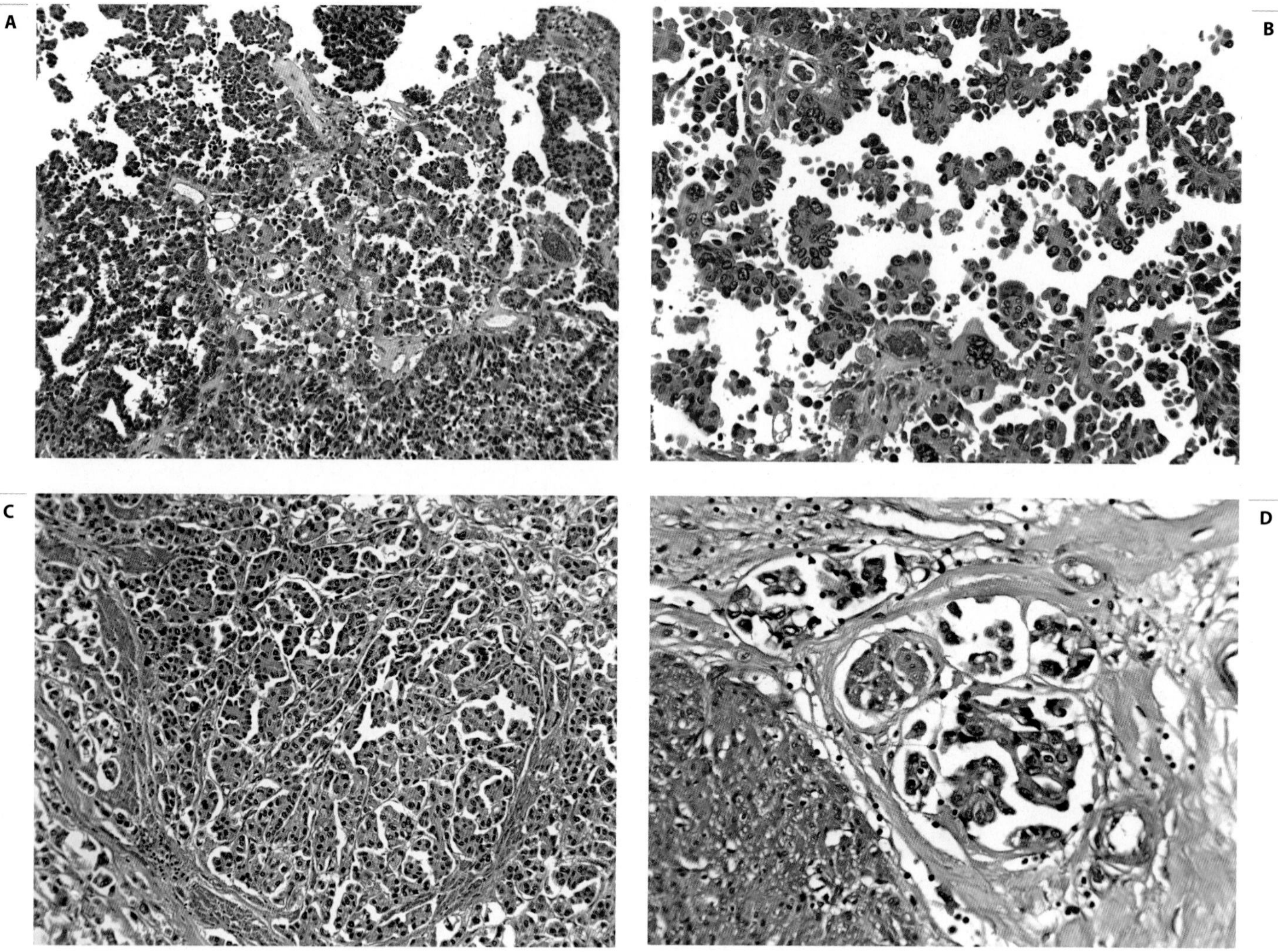

**Fig. 6-32** Urothelial carcinoma, micropapillary variant. (**A**, **B**) Surface component resembling papillary serous carcinoma of the ovary. (**C**) Tumor extends into muscularis propria. (**D**) Infiltrating tumor may form tight clusters of micropapillary aggregates within lacunae.

percent of cases show glandular differentiation, and some authors consider it a variant of adenocarcinoma. Psammoma bodies are infrequent. True vascular and lymphatic invasion is commonly demonstrable, and most cases show invasion of the muscularis propria or deeper. Metastases are common at the time of initial diagnosis.[268] The main differential consideration is metastatic serous micropapillary ovarian carcinoma in women, or mesothelioma in either gender.

The expression of keratins by tumor cells of micropapillary carcinoma is similar to that of typical urothelial carcinoma, but micropapillary carcinomas are much more likely to express CA-125, suggesting that the micropapillary phenotype is a form of glandular differentiation.[271] Micropapillary carcinoma also shows positive immunostaining for EMA, cytokeratins 7 and 20, and Leu M-1 (CD-15). MUC1 expression is seen in the stroma-facing aspect of the tumor cell groups, indicating a reversal of the normal cell orientation in these tumors.[272]

## Urothelial carcinoma, microcystic variant

The microcystic variant of invasive urothelial carcinoma is characterized by microcysts, macrocysts, or tubular structures with cysts ranging from microscopic up to 2 cm in diameter (Fig. 6-33). [273,274] The cysts and tubules may be empty, may contain necrotic debris, or may be filled with mucin demonstrable by periodic acid–Schiff staining after diastase predigestion. This variant of urothelial carcinoma may be confused with benign proliferations such as florid polypoid cystitis cystica and glandularis and nephrogenic metaplasia.[274] This pattern should be separated from the nested variant of urothelial carcinoma with tubular differentiation.[251]

## Lymphoepithelioma-like (urothelial) carcinoma

Carcinoma that histologically resembles lymphoepithelioma of the nasopharynx has been described in the urinary bladder, with fewer than 40 cases reported.[251,273,275–278] It is more

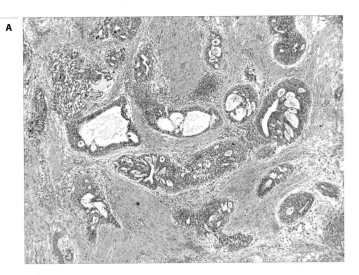

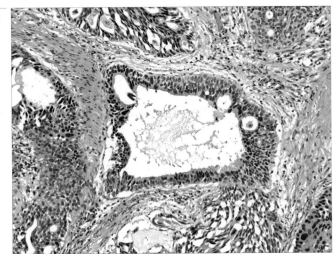

**Fig. 6-33** (**A, B**) Urothelial carcinoma, microcystic variant.

common in men than in women (3:1 ratio) and tends to occur in late adulthood (range 52–81 years; mean, 69 years). Most patients present with hematuria. The tumor is solitary and usually involves the dome, posterior wall, or trigone, often with a sessile growth pattern. Histologically, it may be pure or mixed with typical urothelial carcinoma, the latter being focal and inconspicuous in some instances. Glandular and squamous differentiation may be seen. The epithelial component is composed of nests, sheets, and cords of undifferentiated cells with large pleomorphic nuclei and prominent nucleoli (Fig. 6-34). [251,277] The cytoplasmic borders are poorly defined, imparting a syncytial appearance. The background consists of a prominent lymphoid stroma that includes T and B lymphocytes, plasma cells, histiocytes, and occasional neutrophils or eosinophils. Epstein–Barr virus infection has not been identified in lymphoepithelioma-like carcinoma of the bladder. [279,280] Immunohistochemistry reveals cytokeratin immunoreactivity (keratins AE1/3 and 7) in the malignant cells, confirming their epithelial nature. [251] The epithelial cells are rarely positive for cytokeratin 20. [275] The major differential diagnostic considerations are poorly differentiated urothelial carcinoma with lymphoid

inflammatory response, poorly differentiated squamous cell carcinoma, and lymphoma. Lymphoepithelioma-like bladder carcinoma has been found to be responsive to chemotherapy if the tumor is encountered in its pure form. Although most reported cases occurring in the urinary bladder are associated with a relatively favorable prognosis when pure or predominant, when lymphoepithelioma-like carcinoma is only focally present in an otherwise typical urothelial carcinoma, the prognosis is the same as that for patients with conventional urothelial carcinoma of the same grade and stage.

### Lymphoma-like/plasmacytoma-like urothelial carcinoma

Zukerberg et al. [281] described bladder carcinoma in two patients that diffusely permeated the bladder wall and was composed of cells with a monotonous appearance mimicking lymphoma. The tumor cells were medium sized, with eosinophilic cytoplasm and eccentric nuclei producing a plasmacytoid appearance (Fig. 6-35). [277,282] The epithelial nature of the malignancy was confirmed by immunohistochemistry. [283] Differential diagnostic considerations include lymphoma (plasmacytoid type) and multiple myeloma. Identification of an epithelial component confirms the diagnosis. In a series report of six cases the male:female ratio was 2:1 and the age range was 54–73 years. All cases stained positively for cytokeratin cocktail, and cytokeratins 7 and 20. All were negative for leukocyte common antigen. Five of six patients died of disease (mean survival, 23 months). [273]

### Urothelial carcinoma, clear cell (glycogen-rich) variant

Up to two-thirds of urothelial carcinomas have foci of clear cell change resulting from abundant glycogen. [251,284,285] The glycogen-rich clear cell 'variant' of urothelial carcinoma, recently described, appears to represent the extreme end of the morphologic spectrum. It consists predominantly or exclusively of cells with abundant clear cytoplasm (Fig. 6-36). Tumor cells show positive immunostaining for cytokeratin 7. [286] Recognition of this pattern avoids confusion with clear cell adenocarcinoma of the bladder and metastatic clear cell carcinoma from the kidney or prostate. Cytoplasmic clearing as a result of thermal artifact in transurethral resections should not be mistaken for this variant of bladder cancer. [284,285]

### Urothelial carcinoma, lipoid cell variant

Lipoid cell variant is a rare neoplasm defined as an urothelial carcinoma that exhibits transition to a cell type resembling signet-ring lipoblasts (Fig. 6-37). It is currently considered an ill-defined urothelial tumor variant, and whether it should be classified as carcinosarcoma remains to be established. [251] Gross hematuria was the initial symptom in seven reported cases. [251,287] All patients were elderly men (63–94 years, mean 74 years). On microscopic examination the extent of the lipoid cell pattern varied from 10% to 30% of the tumor, with associated micropapillary ($n = 1$), plasmocytoid ($n = 2$), and grade 3/3 conventional urothelial carcinoma ($n = 4$) predominating. The immunohistochemical results showed

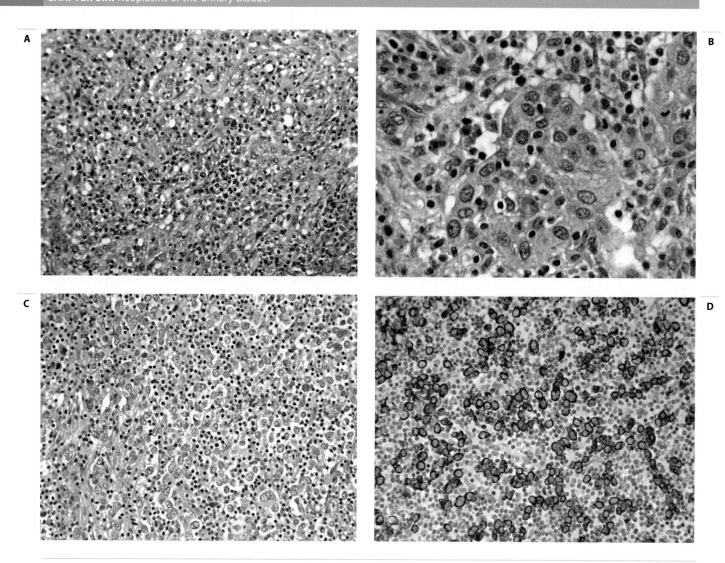

**Fig. 6-34** Lymphoepithelioma-like (urothelial) carcinoma. (**A–C**) Infiltrating tumor shows typical syncytial arrangement of the cells in an inflammatory background with abundant eosinophils. (**D**) The tumor cells display strong immunoreactivity to antibodies again keratin AE1/AE3.

an epithelial phenotype of the lipoid cell component characterized by diffuse staining with cytokeratins AE1/AE3. The reported cases were pathologic stage T2 ($n = 2$), T3a ($n = 1$), T3b ($n = 3$), and T4 ($n = 1$). At follow-up, one patient had died of cancer and two were alive with disease at 58, 14, and 55 months, respectively. Two patients had no evidence of disease at 11 and 29 months of follow-up, and two additional patients had died of other causes at 10 and 15 months, respectively.[251] In another recently reported series four of five patients died of bladder cancer during a mean follow-up of 27 months.[288]

### Urothelial carcinoma with syncytiotrophoblastic giant cells

Syncytiotrophoblastic giant cells are present in up to 28% of urothelial carcinomas, producing substantial amounts of immunoreactive β-human chorionic gonadotropin (hCG) indicative of syncytiotrophoblastic differentiation (Fig. 6-38).[251,289,290] The number of hCG-immunoreactive

cells was associated with cancer grade.[291,292] Secretion of hCG into the serum may be associated with a poor response to radiation therapy.[290,293,294] The most important differential diagnostic consideration is choriocarcinoma. hCG expression in poorly differentiated urothelial carcinoma without overt syncytiotrophoblastic differentiation probably represents a metaplastic phenomenon.[295] It seems likely that previously reported 'primary choriocarcinomas of the bladder' represent urothelial carcinoma with syncytiotrophoblasts.[273,289,293]

### Sarcomatoid urothelial carcinoma

The term sarcomatoid variant of urothelial carcinoma should be used for any biphasic malignant neoplasm that exhibits morphologic or immunohistochemical evidence of both epithelial and mesenchymal differentiation. The presence or absence of heterologous elements should be acknowledged in the report[273,296] (discussed later in the section on Sarcomatoid carcinoma).

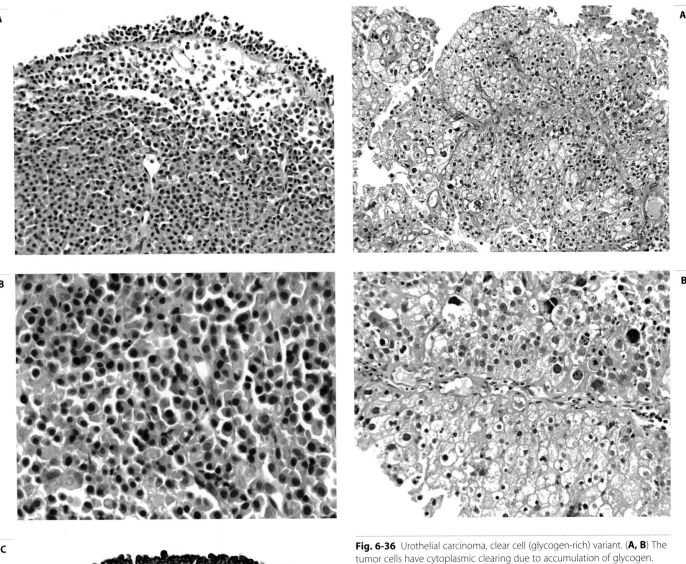

**Fig. 6-36** Urothelial carcinoma, clear cell (glycogen-rich) variant. (**A, B**) The tumor cells have cytoplasmic clearing due to accumulation of glycogen.

## Small cell carcinoma

Small cell carcinoma is a malignant neoplasm derived from the urothelium which mimics its pulmonary counterpart (discussed later in the section on Neuroendocrine tumor). It often coexists with conventional urothelial carcinoma.[297]

## Large cell undifferentiated carcinoma

Large cell undifferentiated carcinoma consists of large cell tumors that cannot be otherwise classified (Fig. 6-39A). The tumor cells are characerized by large nuclei, prominent nucleoli, abundant eosinophilic cytoplasm, and usually well-defined cell borders. They are rare in the urinary tract, aggressive, and of high stage at presentation. One reported case had elevated serum α-fetoprotein levels and α-fetoprotein expression by immunohistochemistry in tumor cells that otherwise showed no morphologically recognizable differentiation.[251] On rare occasions high-grade urothelial carcinoma may contain epithelial tumor giant cells resembling giant cell carcinoma of the lung. The giant cells show immunoreactivity to antibodies against keratins AE1/

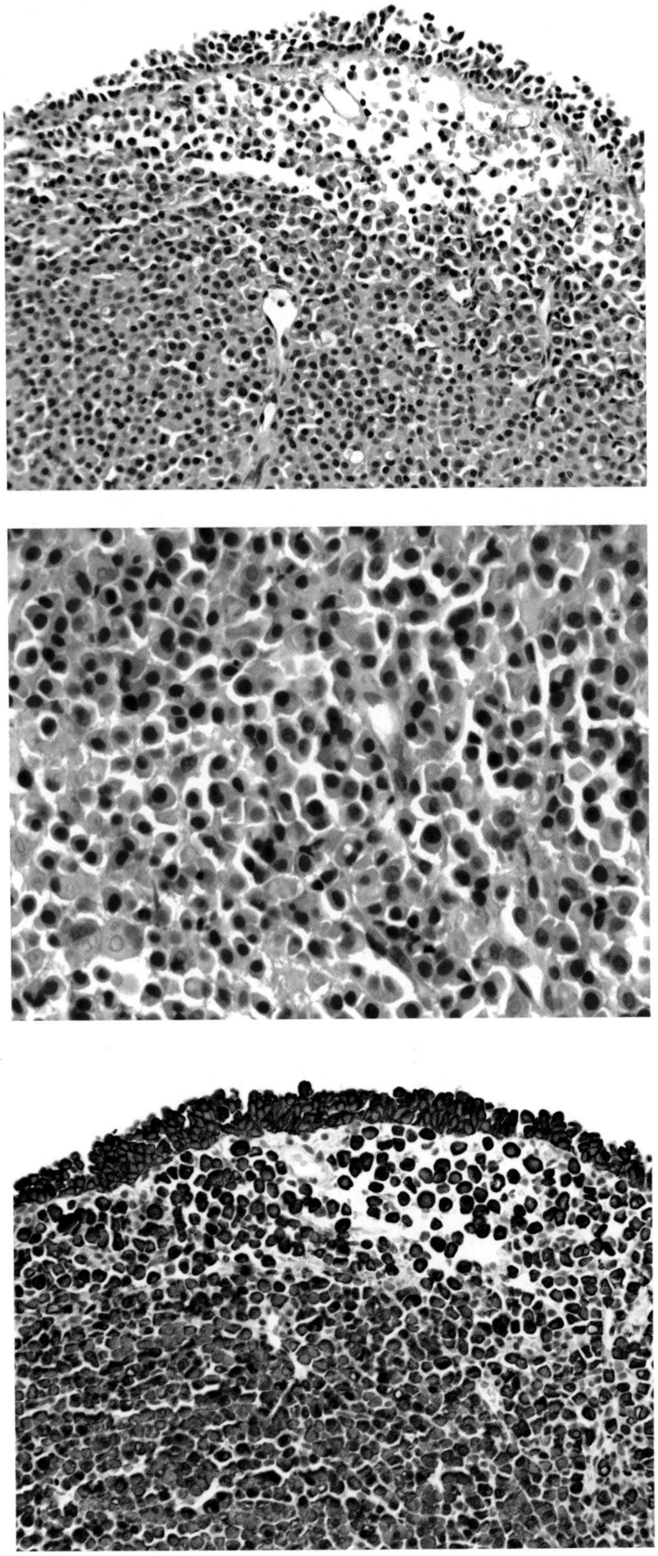

**Fig. 6-35** Urothelial carcinoma, plasmacytoid variant. (**A, B**) The tumor cells have an eccentric nucleus and eosinophilic cytoplasm reminiscent of plasma cells. (**C**) Cytokeratin stain is strongly positive in tumor cells.

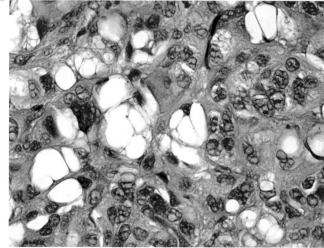

**A**

**B**

**C**

**Fig. 6-37** (**A–B**) Urothelial carcinoma, lipoid variant. (**C**) The tumor cells have a lipoblast-like appearance.

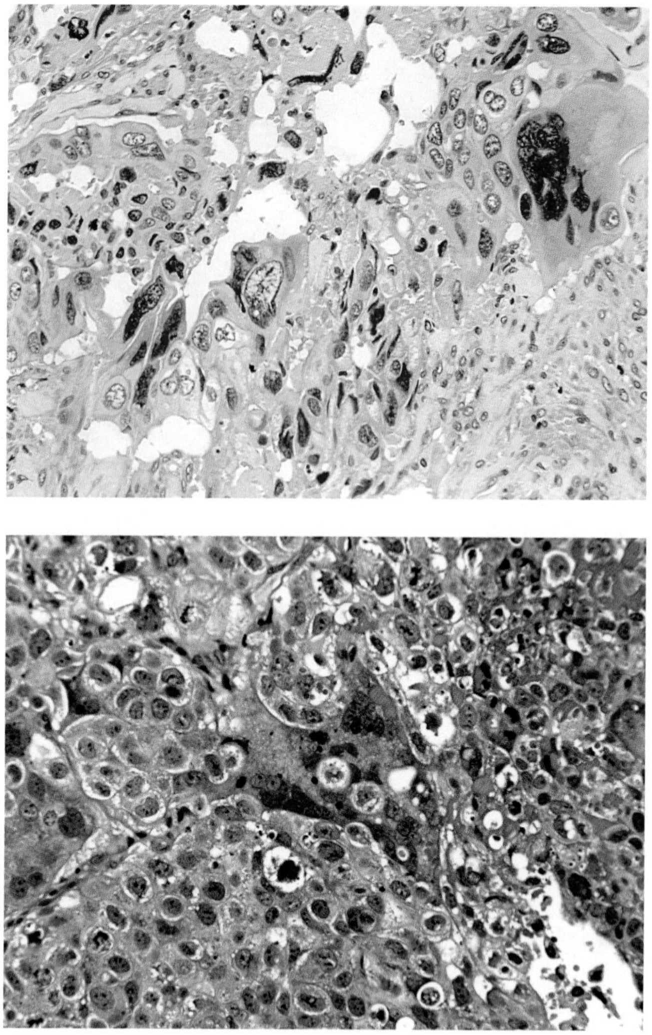

**A**

**B**

**Fig. 6-38** (**A–B**) Urothelial carcinoma with syncytiotrophoblastic giant cells.

AE3 and Cam5.2, and sometimes vimentin.[251,298] We consider (cytokeratin-positive) giant cell carcinoma of the urinary bladder (Fig. 6-39B) to be part of a morphologic spectrum of large cell undifferentiated carcinoma. Malignant giant cells in urothelial carcinoma, when present in great numbers, portend a poor prognosis, similar to that of giant cell carcinoma of the lung or prostate.

The differential diagnosis includes sarcomatoid carcinoma with giant cells, giant cell carcinoma metastatic from other organs to the bladder, and osteoclast-like giant cell tumor of the urinary bladder.[273,299] Giant cells may also be associated with trophoblastic differentiation in some cases, and osteoclast-type giant cells are found in some invasive high-grade urothelial carcinomas.[300] These should not be confused with large cell undifferentiated carcinoma.

## Urothelial carcinoma with rhabdoid features

A variety of tumors with rhabdoid differentiation have been described in the literature, but very few cases have been described in the urinary tract.[301–304] Parwani et al.[305] recently

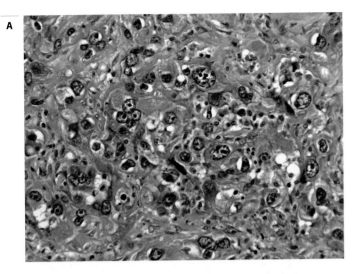

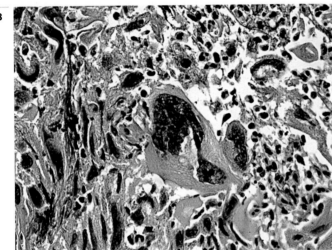

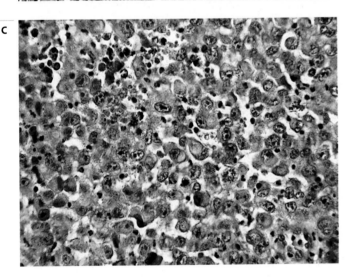

**Fig. 6-39** (**A**) Large cell undifferentiated carcinoma. (**B**) Numerous giant cells may be seen in large cell undifferentiated carcinoma. (**C**) Urothelial carcinoma with rhabdoid features.

reported six cases of urothelial carcinoma with rhabdoid features. Four tumors were located in the bladder and two were in the renal pelvis. In all cases the rhabdoid component was admixed with other components, including conventional urothelial carcinoma, sarcomatoid carcinoma, and/or small cell carcinoma. Rhabdoid cells have abundant eosinophilic cytoplasm, vesicular nuclei, and prominent nucleoli (Fig. 6-39C). They show positive immunostaining for cytokeratin markers (epithelial membrane antigen, CAM5.2, and AE1/3). These tumors are highly aggressive: 50% of patients die of bladder cancer shortly after the diagnosis.[305]

## Urothelial carcinoma with prominent stromal reaction

Infiltrating urothelial carcinoma may be associated with a variety of stromal reactions. There may be a pseudosarcomatous stroma (Fig. 6-40A), which rarely displays sufficient cellularity, cytologic atypia, spindle cell proliferation, or a myxoid appearance to raise serious concern about sarcomatoid carcinoma.[306–308] The stromal cells in these circumstances are invariably cytokeratin negative or only focally positive. Tumor-associated osseous (Fig. 6-40B) or chondroid metaplasia is present in some cases of urothelial carcinoma and its metastases. This stromal reaction may be difficult to differentiate from osteosarcoma or chondrosarcoma.[309–311] The metaplastic bone or cartilage is histologically benign. Zukerberg et al.[312] described the presence of osteoclast-like giant cells in two cases of invasive high-grade urothelial carcinoma. The giant cells had abundant eosinophilic cytoplasm and numerous small, round, regular nuclei (Fig. 6-40C). These giant cells displayed immunoreactivity for vimentin and CD68 but not for epithelial markers.[299] The presence of osteoclast-like giant cells does not appear to influence prognosis.[251] An inflammatory cell response in the stroma adjacent to invasive tumors is relatively common.[313] This response usually takes the form of a lymphocytic infiltrate with a variable admixture of plasma cells (Fig. 6-40D).[314] Generally this cellular reaction is mild to moderate, but occasionally it may be intense. Sometimes a neutrophilic response is observed, with or without extensive eosinophilic infiltration. There is evidence suggesting that carcinomas occurring in the absence of a cellular immune response are likely to behave more aggressively.[314] In a recent study, intense inflammation in bladder carcinoma was indicative of a good prognosis.[315] Exclusion of lymphoepithelioma-like carcinoma of the urinary bladder is important when there is extensive inflammation in the stroma.[251,273]

## Other uncommon morphologic variations in bladder cancer

Baldwin et al.[316] described 10 cases of urothelial carcinoma with a strikingly dyscohesive growth pattern and morphological features mimicking infiltrating lobular carcinoma of the breast and diffuse carcinoma of the stomach. Eight of the patients were male and two were female. The mean age

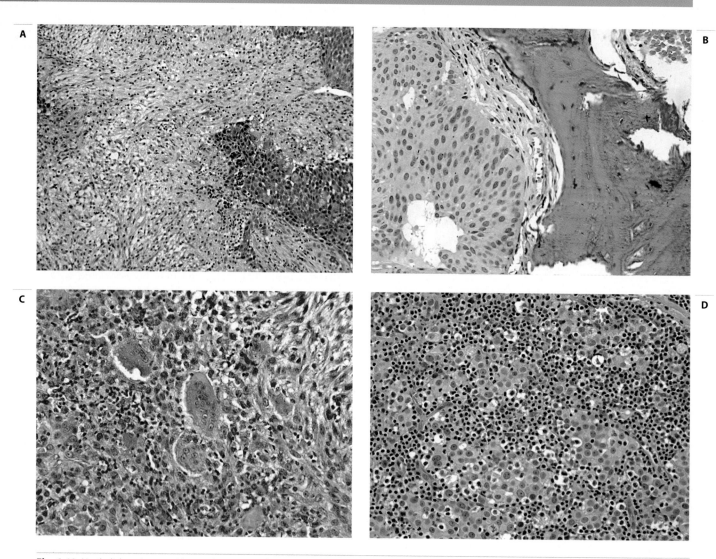

**Fig. 6-40** Urothelial carcinoma with prominent stromal reaction (**A**) Pseudosarcomatous stroma. (**B**) Osteoid formation. (**C**) Osteoclast-type giant cells. (**D**) Lymphoid-rich stroma.

was 67 years at presentation (range, 52–77 years). All the cases showed areas where the tumor was composed of uniform cells with a dyscohesive single-cell, diffusely infiltrative growth pattern (Fig. 6-41). In some areas the tumor cells were arranged in linear single-cell files (Indian-file pattern) and in other areas there were solid sheets of dyscohesive cells. In all cases there were tumor cells showing prominent intracytoplasmic vacuoles.[316] Four cases also showed typical transitional cell carcinoma or carcinoma in situ. The tumor cells expressed cytokeratin 20 but not estrogen receptor, and some were negative for E-cadherin. It is important to recognize this pattern so as to avoid a misdiagnosis of metastatic lobular breast carcinoma, especially in small biopsies.[316] In every case, clinicopathologic correlation is mandatory. Patients with breast or stomach carcinoma metastatic to the bladder almost invariably have a history of the prior malignancy.

Urothelial carcinoma with acinar/tubular type differentiation is uncommon (Fig. 6-42).[317] Gleason pattern 3 prostate

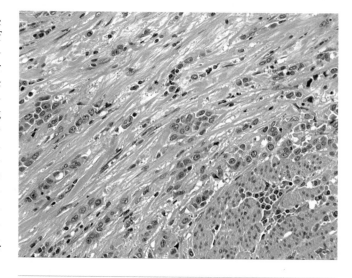

**Fig. 6-41** Urothelial carcinoma with dyscohesive growth pattern, mimicking lobular carcinoma of the breast.

cancer is the main differential consideration in cases of urothelial carcinoma with acinar/tubular type differentiation. Immunohistochemistry for prostate-specific antigens and cytokeratin 20 is helpful in difficult cases.[251]

## Specimen handling and reporting

Appropriate assessment and reporting of pathological findings in cases of urothelial malignancy assist the urologist with management of the patient (Table 6-12).[318,319] The most common bladder specimens are endoscopic biopsies and transurethral resections of the bladder (TURB), both of which contain subepithelial tissue of varying depth.[318] Other specimens include cystectomy (partial or total), cystoprostatectomy, pelvic exenteration (en bloc resection), and diverticular resections. Surgical excision of urachal adenocarcinoma usually includes the bladder dome, urachus, and umbilicus.

A bladder biopsy can provide information that helps to assess risk factors for recurrence, progression, and response to treatment. Small non-invasive papillary neoplasms are often excised by biopsy using cold cup forceps, diathermy forceps, or a small diathermy loop.[318] To avoid tissue distortion, these specimens should be transferred to fixative with minimal handling. Larger neoplasms are often sampled by transurethral resection using a diathermy loop that produces strips of tissue 6 mm in diameter and of variable length. Additional resection of the bladder base after a previous transurethral resection may provide additional information for assessment of tumor staging. Hyperemic or velvety areas of urothelium are typically sampled to exclude carcinoma in situ; random biopsies are commonly taken from macroscopically normal urothelium distant from the tumor site to determine the extent of involvement.[320,321] Some urologists also submit biopsy specimens of the urethra, particularly in patients with high-grade papillary urothelial carcinoma or carcinoma in situ.

The pathology report should include clinically relevant historical information as well as clinically useful macroscopic and microscopic information. Reporting of bladder cancer should include information related to (1) specimen type, (2) tumor site and size, (3) histologic type, (4) associated epithelial lesions, (5) histologic grade, (6) tumor configuration, (7) adequacy of material for determining T category, (8) pathologic staging, and (9) additional pathologic findings.

Muscularis mucosae is often present in the lamina propria, and consists of thin, wavy fascicles of smooth muscle, frequently associated with large-caliber blood vessels (Fig. 6-25).[189,192,322] Muscularis mucosae invasion (pT1) should not be mistaken for muscularis propria invasion (pT2), and it is unacceptable to simply state in the pathology report that smooth muscle invasion is present.[192] The presence or absence of muscularis propria (detrusor muscle) should also be mentioned in the pathology report as an indication of the adequacy of resection.[102,323,324]

An additional feature of importance in bladder tumor evaluation is the presence of blood vessel or lymphatic

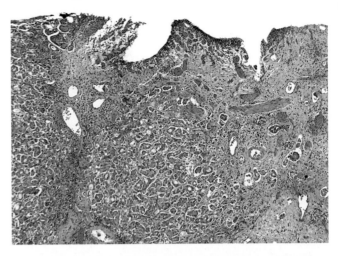

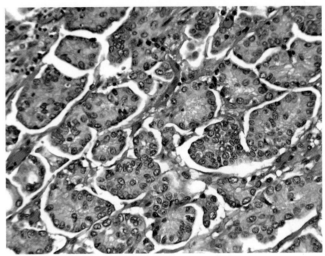

**Fig. 6-42** Urothelial carcinoma with acinar/tubular type differentiation. (**A, B**) The acini are lined by cuboidal cells with abundant eosinophilic cytoplasm. The tumor may mimic prostatic adenocarcinoma.

channel invasion (Fig. 6-43). [325–327] Identifying vascular or lymphatic invasion is sometimes difficult, as lymphovascular spaces may easily be confused with artifactual clefting around nests of invasive carcinoma. In suspicious cases blood vessels can be highlighted by immunohistochemical staining for CD31 or CD34. The presence of vascular or lymphatic invasion, and whether immunohistochemical stains assisted in identifying this finding, should be included in the report.

The presence of associated urothelial carcinoma in situ should also be reported in cases of bladder carcinoma, as patients with associated carcinoma in situ are at much higher risk of tumor recurrence and disease progression.

Tumor involving the resection margin in partial or complete cystectomy specimens is assumed to correspond to residual tumor in the patient. Positive margins should be

**Table 6-12** Parameters for handling and reporting bladder specimens with cancer

| I. | General information |
|---|---|
| | – Pertinent clinical information: name, medical record number, age, sex, ethnicity, referring physician, and relevant clinical history |
| II. | Gross description |
| | – Fresh or fixed specimen |
| | – Nature of the specimens: biopsy, chips (TURB), partial cystectomy, radical cystectomy, cystoprostatectomy, 'en bloc' resection. |
| | – Total weight of resected tissue fragments (TURB); three dimensional measurements of recognizable anatomic structures and tumors or other recognizable lesions |
| | – Site of involvement, gross fat extension |
| III. | Diagnostic and prognostic information |
| | – Histologic type |
| | – Histologic grade: use WHO grading schemes (WHO 1973, WHO 2004, or both) |
| | – Extent of tumor in bladder (degree of invasion)<br>    No invasion<br>    Invasion of the suburothelial connective tissue, muscularis propria, perivesical soft tissue |
| | – Presence or absence of lymphatic/vascular invasion |
| | – Presence or absence of dysplasia and carcinoma in situ |
| | – Presence or absence of tumor multifocality |
| | – Extent of tumor in organs attached to the bladder<br>    Prostate: direct extension to the prostate, involvement of prostatic urethra, involvement of prostatic ducts with or without stromal involvement<br>    Ureter, renal pelvis, and urethra: Report any dysplastic/neoplastic change of the mucosa, and report any invasion into adjacent suburothelial connective tissue or muscularis propria<br>    Seminal vesicles: report spread of carcinoma in these organs either through epithelium or by direct extension of an infiltrative tumor<br>    Vagina/uterus: report direct extension or metastasis to either organ |
| | – Surgical margins<br>    Ureteral margin<br>    Urethral margins<br>    Perivesical soft tissue margin |

classified as macroscopic or microscopic according to the findings at the specimen inked surfaces.[328] The resection margin status should be carefully specified. In particular, statements about deep soft tissue margins should specify whether peritoneal surfaces are involved by tumor. In cases of urachal adenocarcinoma in which partial cystectomy with excision of the urachal tract and umbilicus is performed, the margins of the urachal tract, i.e., the soft tissue surrounding the urachus and the skin around the umbilical margin, should be specified.

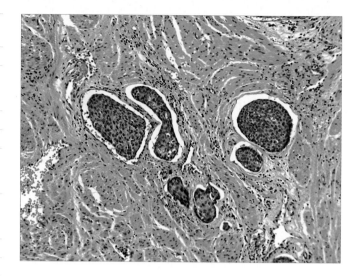

**Fig. 6-43** Lymphovascular invasion of an invasive urothelial carcinoma.

# Glandular neoplasms

## Villous adenoma

Villous adenoma is an uncommon benign glandular epithelial neoplasm with exophytic growth that is often associated with urachal adenocarcinoma (Fig. 6-44).[329,330] Patients often present with hematuria and/or irritative symptoms. Mucusuria may be present in rare cases. There is no apparent gender preponderance. The tumor usually occurs in elderly patients (mean age, 65 years; range, 23–94 years) with a predilection for the urachus, dome, and trigone of the urinary bladder. Its cystoscopic appearance is that of an exophytic tumor. Histologically, villous adenoma of the bladder is identical to villous adenoma of the colon, with columnar mucin-filled goblet cells lining delicate fibrovascular stalks (Fig. 6-45). Nuclear findings include pseudostratification, crowding, occasional prominent nucleoli and hyperchromasia, as in the colon. Villous adenomas of the bladder show positive immunostaining for cytokeratin 20 (100% of cases), cytokeratin 7 (56%), and carcinoembryonic antigen (89%). Acid mucin is demonstrable in 78% of cases with Alcian blue periodic acid–Schiff staining.[329] Patients with an isolated villous adenoma have an excellent prognosis, but progression to adenocarcinoma appears to occur in 21–33% of cases.

The differential diagnosis includes adenocarcinoma of bladder.[329] Villous adenomas of the bladder may coexist with in situ and invasive adenocarcinoma. On limited sampling there may be only changes of villous adenoma. Therefore, the entire specimen should be processed to exclude invasive disease.

## Adenocarcinoma

Adenocarcinoma is defined as a malignant neoplasm derived from the urothelium showing histologically pure glandular phenotype. It accounts for 0.5–2% of all malignant bladder

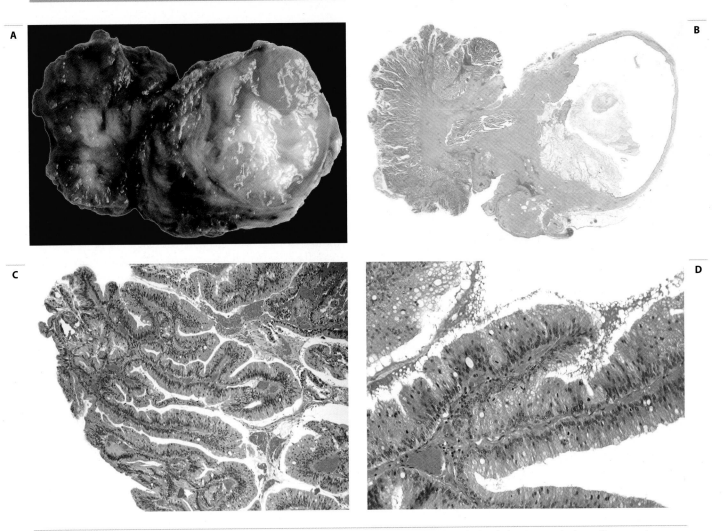

**Fig. 6-44** Villous adenoma. (**A, B**) Tumor located in the dome of the bladder, originating from the urachus, and showing exophytic papillary growth. (**C, D**) The tumor has long papillary fronds lined by intestinal-type columnar epithelium with scattered goblet cells.

tumors. Adenocarcinoma of the urinary bladder occurs more commonly in males than in females, with a peak incidence in the sixth decade of life.[331] Patients typically present with hematuria. Two major categories have been recognized: those arising in the bladder proper, and those arising from urachal remnants. Approximately one-third arise in the urachus (Fig. 6-46).[332] Recent molecular evidence suggest that intestinal metaplasia is a putative precursor for adenocarcinoma.[333]

Adenocarcinoma of the bladder may show different histologic growth patterns (Fig. 6-46): enteric (colonic) type, adenocarcinoma not otherwise specified (NOS), mucinous (colloid) type, signet ring cell type, clear cell type, hepatoid type, and mixed forms (Table 6-13). The enteric type closely resembles adenocarcinoma of the colon.[331] The NOS type consists of adenocarcinoma with a non-specific glandular growth pattern. Tumors that show abundant mucin and tumor cell clusters apparently floating in mucin are classified as mucinous (colloid) type. The signet ring cell variant may be diffuse or mixed, and may have a monocytoid or plasma-

cytoid phenotype. Pure signet ring cell carcinoma carries the worst prognosis of the different histologic types of adenocarcinoma. It is not uncommon to find a mixture of these growth patterns. The grading system for adenocarcinoma of the bladder is based on the degree of glandular differentiation and nuclear pleomorphism, categorized as well, moderately, or poorly differentiated.

The reported immunohistochemical profile of bladder adenocarcinoma is variable, but generally resembles that of colonic adenocarcinoma (Table 6-14).[61,94] Cytokeratin 7 positivity is variable, but cytokeratin 20 is positive in most bladder adenocarcinomas.[331] The 'intestinal marker' CDX2, a nuclear transcription factor, may be misleading in this situation because primary bladder adenocarcinomas are virtually always also CDX2 positive.[334] It is notable that CDX2 positivity has been observed in 2% of urothelial carcinomas in a tissue microarray study; consequently, CDX2 immunostaining cannot be used to exclude a urothelial primary in cases of metastatic carcinoma of uncertain origin.[335] Areas of intestinal metaplasia in the bladder also routinely stain posi-

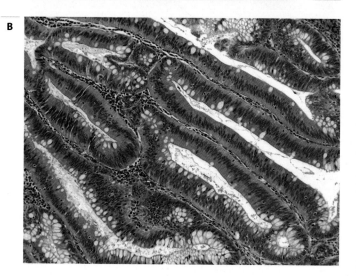

**Fig. 6-45** Villous adenoma of the urinary bladder. (**A**) The microscopic appearance of the tumor is identical to that of its colonic counterparts. (**B**) The epithelial cells display nuclear stratification, nuclear crowding, nuclear hyperchromasia, and occasional prominent nucleoli.

tive for CDX2.[61,336] Villin, an actin-binding protein found in epithelial cells with a brush border, is positive in colon adenocarcinoma and bladder adenocarcinomas of enteric type, but not in urothelial carcinomas with glandular differentiation.[337] Nuclear β-catenin staining is seen in 81% of colorectal carcinomas involving the bladder, whereas staining restricted to the cytoplasm is typical of primary bladder adenocarcinoma.[338]

## Clear cell adenocarcinoma

Clear cell (mesonephric) adenocarcinoma is a rare variant of urinary bladder carcinoma that morphologically resembles its counterpart in the female genital tract. Patients are typically females who present with hematuria or dysuria. Occasionally clear cell adenocarcinoma has been associated with endometriosis or müllerianosis; occurrence in a bladder diverticulum has been reported. Tumors are typically exophytic, nodular, or sessile in appearance (Fig. 6-47). Clear cell adenocarcinomas may infiltrate the bladder wall and metastasize to lymph nodes and distant organs in a pattern similar to other types of bladder cancer.

Clear cell adenocarcinoma exhibits a distinctive histologic appearance with a variety of architectural patterns, forming tubulocystic or papillary structures or growing in diffuse solid sheets. The tubules vary in size and may contain either basophilic or eosinophilic secretions. The papillae are generally small and their fibrovascular cores may be extensively hyalinized. The tumor cells range from flat to cuboidal to

**Table 6-13** Histologic variants of adenocarcinomas of the urinary bladder

| Adenocarcinoma, not otherwise specified (NOS) |
| Enteric (colonic type) |
| Signet ring cell |
| Mucinous clear cell (including colloid) |
| Hepatoid |
| Mixed |
| Urachal |

**Table 6-14** Typical staining patterns of primary and secondary adenocarcinomas of the bladder

|  | 34βE12 | CK7 | CK20 | CEA | PSA | PSAP | CDX2 | Villin | CA-125 | Vimentin |
|---|---|---|---|---|---|---|---|---|---|---|
| Primary bladder adenocarcinoma | + | +/− | +/− | + | − | +/− | + | +/− | +/− | − |
| Prostatic adenocarcinoma | − | − | +/− | +/− | + | + | − | − | − | − |
| Seminal vesicle adenocarcinoma |  | + | − |  |  |  |  |  | + |  |
| Renal cell carcinoma | − | − | − | − | − | − | − | − | − | + |
| Colorectal adenocarcinoma | − | − | + | + | − | − | + | + | +/− | − |
| Endometrial adenocarcinoma |  | + | − | − |  |  | +/− |  | + | + |

34βE12, cytokeratin 34βE12; CK7, cytokeratin 7; CK20, cytokeratin 20; CEA, carcinoembryonic antigen; PSA, prostate-specific antigen; PSAP, prostate-specific acid phosphatase; +, usually positive; +/−, variable staining; −, usually negative.

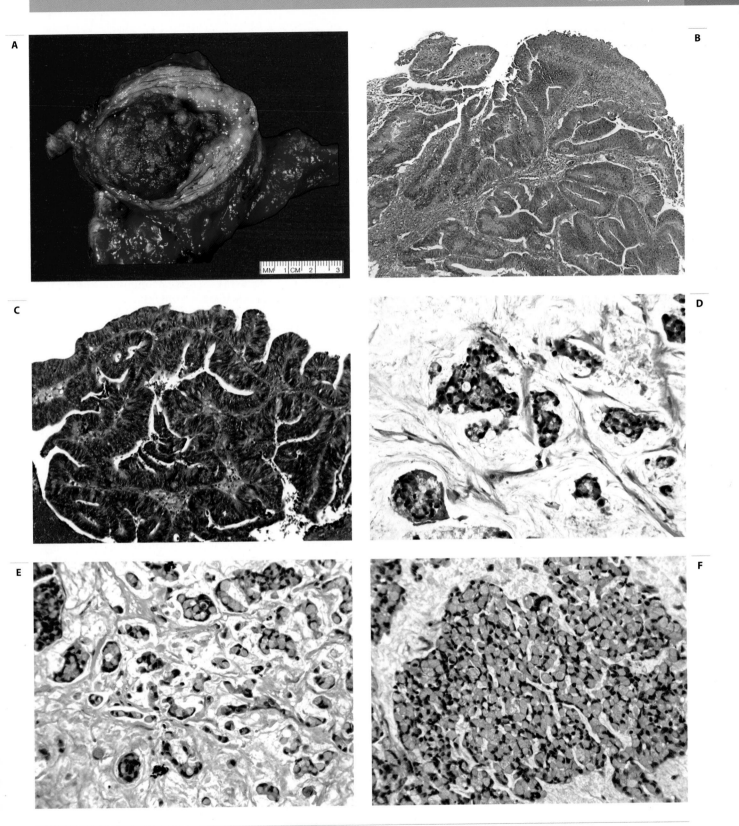

**Fig. 6-46** Adenocarcinoma. (**A**) Gross appearance. (**B**) Adenocarcinoma, NOS (not otherwise specified). (**C**) Enteric type, resembling typical colonic adenocarcinoma. (**D**) Colloid (mucinous) type. Malignant cells float in a pool of mucin. (**E, F**) Signet-ring cell type. (**F**) Mucin pool formation is common.

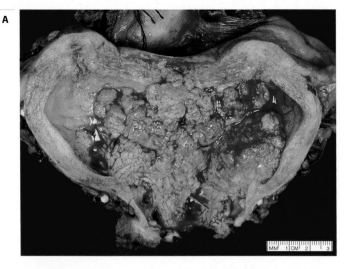

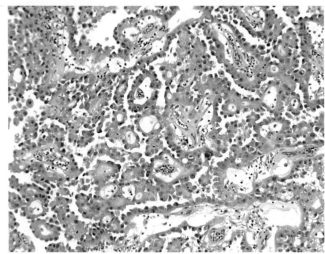

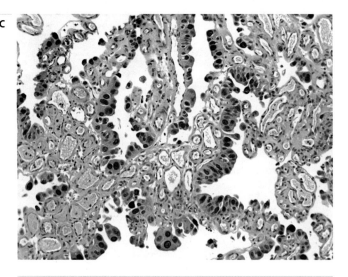

**Fig. 6-47** Clear cell adenocarcinoma. (**A**) Gross appearance at cystectomy. (**B**) The tumor may display various growth patterns similar to clear cell adenocarcinoma of the ovary. (**C**) The tubules are lined by columnar cells with a 'hobnail' appearance.

columnar, and may have either clear or eosinophilic cytoplasm. The cytoplasm often contains glycogen. Hobnail cells are frequently seen. Cytologic atypia is usually moderate to severe, and high mitotic counts are frequently observed. In some cases clear cell adenocarcinoma is associated with urothelial carcinoma, and rarely with adenocarcinoma not otherwise specified (NOS).

Tumor cells are positive for CA-125, suggestive of a müllerian origin, but CA-125 staining may also be seen in urothelial carcinoma and carcinoma from a variety of other sites, so this finding does not prove a müllerian origin.[284,339] These tumors are typically positive for cytokeratin 7 with variable cytokeratin 20 staining.[284] Stains for prostate-specific antigen (PSA) and prostate-specific acid phosphatase (PSAP) are negative.[339] The main differential diagnostic consideration for clear cell carcinoma is nephrogenic metaplasia (Table 6-15).[340] Several immunohistochemical stains have been evaluated for utility in making this distinction, but only p53 and MIB-1 appear useful, with at most focal p53 staining and MIB-1 counts of less than 14 per 200 cells in nephrogenic adenoma and strong p53 staining and MIB-1 counts of more than 32 per 200 cells in clear cell adenocarcinoma.[341] However, p53 nuclear accumulation (up to 20%), increased MIB-1 labeling index (up to 5%), and aneuploid DNA patterns have been observed in atypical nephrogenic metaplasia.[340] All cases of atypical nephrogenic metaplasia display positive immunoreactivity for high-molecular-weight cytokeratin (34βE12), cytokeratin 7, and EMA.[340] In contrast to atypical nephrogenic metaplasia, clear cell carcinomas will typically display greater cytologic atypia, a significant mitotic rate, and necrosis.[341] Clear cell adenocarcinoma of the urinary bladder is positive for both cytokeratin 7 and cytokeratin 20.[342] Positive α-methylacyl-CoA racemase (P504S) (AMACR) immunoreactivity for both clear cell adenocarcinoma and nephrogenic adenoma has been noted.[342,343] CD10 is focally positive in clear cell adenocarcinoma.[342]

The other differential diagnostic considerations include clear cell variant of urothelial carcinoma, metastatic clear cell renal carcinoma, cervical or vaginal clear cell adenocarcinoma, and in males, prostatic adenocarcinoma secondarily involving the bladder. In addition to the immunostaining characteristics noted previously, clear cell adenocarcinoma may show positive staining for carcinoembryonic antigen and Leu-M1, but is negative for estrogen and progesterone receptors, and these stains may be helpful in the differential diagnosis.

## Hepatoid adenocarcinoma

Primary hepatoid adenocarcinoma of the bladder is extremely rare, with only three well-illustrated case reports.[344] The pathological diagnosis is based on a combination of histological features resembling hepatocellular carcinoma and positive immunostaining for α-fetoprotein. The tumor occurs in elderly men and is biologically aggressive. Lymph node metastases are common.[344] The histogenesis is uncertain. Tumors are composed of polygonal cells with abundant granular eosinophilic cytoplasm, vesicular nuclei, and prom-

**Table 6-15** Differential Diagnosis of atypical nephrogenic metaplasia and clear cell adenocarcinoma[340,342]

| Characteristics | Nephrogenic adenoma | Clear Cell Adenocarcinoma |
|---|---|---|
| Sex | Male predominance (male-to-female ratio, 3:1) | Female predominance (male to female ratio, 1:2) |
| Mean Age (years) | 62 | 58 |
| Clinical presentation | Hematuria and voiding symptoms | Hematuria and voiding symptoms |
| Biological behavior | Benign | Aggressive |
| Location | No apparent predilection | Predilection for the urethra |
| Size | Small | Large |
| Microscopic findings | | |
| Necrosis | Absent | Often present (53%) |
| Mitotic figures | Absent or inconspicuous | Easily identifiable |
| Stromal edema | Common | Uncommon |
| Luminal mucin | Common | Common |
| Clear cell change | May be seen | Common |
| Hobnail cells | Common | Common |
| Infiltrative growth | Usually absent | Present |
| Psammoma bodies | Absent | May be seen |
| Inflammation | Invariably present | May be present |
| Cytologic atypia | | |
| Nuclear enlargement | Present | Present |
| Nuclear hyperchromasia | Present | Present |
| Prominent nucleoli | Present | Present |
| Nuclear pleomorphism | Minimal | Present |
| Immunostaining | | |
| PSA | Negative | Negative |
| 34βE12 | Positive | Positive (occasionally negative) |
| Cytokeratin 7 | Positive | Positive |
| Cytokeratin 20 | Negative | Positive |
| EMA | Positive | Positive |
| AMACR(P504S) | Often positive | Often positive |
| MIB Labeling index | <5% | Often >15% |
| P53 | Occasional positive | Positive |
| DNA ploidy | Aneuploid pattern may be seen | Unknown |

#PSA, prostate-specific antigen; 34βE12, high molecular weight cytokeratin; EMA, Epithelial membrane antigen; AMACR, α-methylacyl CoA racemase.

*Nuclear pleomorphism is more pronounced in clear cell adenocarcinoma.

inent nucleoli arranged in nests and trabecular structures; the overall appearance is reminiscent of hepatocellular carcinoma (Fig. 6-48). Occasionally, hyaline globules and bile production are seen. Immunoreactivity for α-fetoprotein (AFP), low molecular weight cytokeratin (CAM 5.2), α₁-antitrypsin (AAT), albumin, hepatocyte paraffin-1(HepPar-1), epithelial membrane antigen (EMA), and a striking canalicular pattern with polyclonal anti-carcinoembryonic antigen (CEA) staining all indicate hepatocellular differentiation.[344] The hepatic nature of the cells was further confirmed by the demonstration of albumin gene mRNA by non-isotopic in situ hybridization.[344]

## Urachal adenocarcinoma

Urachal adenocarcinoma is far less common than non-urachal adenocarcinoma of the bladder. Urachal adenocarcinomas arise from the urachus, the fibrous remnant of the embryonic allantoic stalk connecting the umbilicus to the bladder (Fig. 6-49). Urachal remnants are reported to occur most frequently in the bladder dome or posterior wall. Most cases of urachal adenocarcinoma occur in the fifth and sixth decades of life, which is about 10 years younger than those patients with non-urachal bladder adenocarcinoma. This tumor occurs slightly more often in men than in women.[345] Presenting signs and symptoms may include a suprapubic mass, mucusuria, or irritative symptoms [345]

Urachal carcinoma usually involves the muscular wall of the bladder dome, and it may or may not destroy the overlying mucosa (Fig. 6-49). The mass may be relatively small and discrete, but in some cases it forms a large mass invading the retropubic space of Retzius and may extend as far as the anterior abdominal wall. Mucinous lesions tend to calcify, and these calcifications on plain X-rays of the abdomen may be the initial clinical manifestation.[345] The mucosa of the urinary bladder remains intact in early stages of the disease,

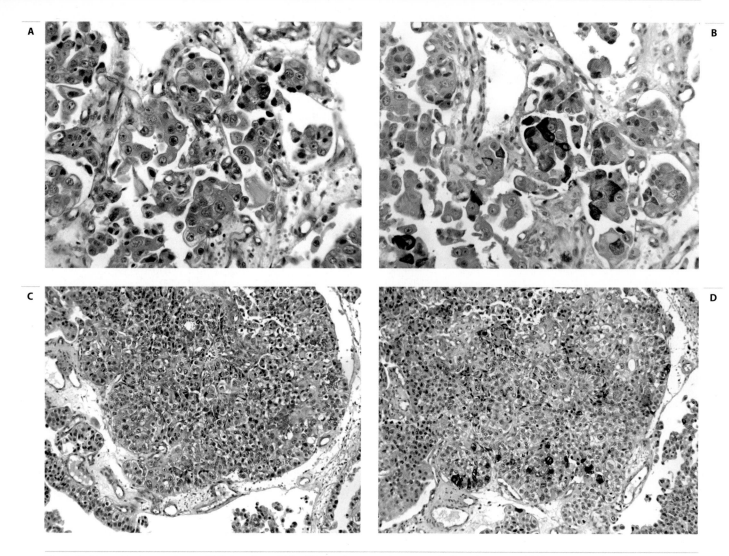

**Fig. 6-48** Hepatoid adenocarcinoma. (**A**) Trabecular and (**C**) solid growth patterns. Immunostains for α-fetoprotein (AFP) are positive (**B** and **D**).

but it eventually becomes ulcerated as the tumor extends towards the bladder cavity. The cut surface of this tumor exhibits a glistening, light-tan appearance, reflecting its mucinous contents. A specific staging system for this neoplasm has been proposed. Histologically, urachal adenocarcinomas are subdivided into mucinous, enteric, not otherwise specified, signet ring-cell, and mixed types; these subtypes are similar to those of adenocarcinoma of the urinary bladder (Fig. 6-49).

Specific criteria to classify a tumor as urachal in origin were initially established by Wheeler and Hill in 1954[346] and consisted of the following: (1) tumor in the dome of the bladder, (2) absence of cystitis cystica and cystitis glandularis, (3) invasion of muscle or deeper structures and either intact or ulcerated epithelium, (4) presence of urachal remnants, (5) presence of a suprapubic mass, (6) a sharp demarcation between the tumor and the normal surface epithelium, and (7) tumor growth in the bladder wall, extending into the space of Retzius. These rather restrictive criteria were modified by Johnson et al.,[346a] who proposed the following

criteria: (1) tumor in the bladder dome, (2) a sharp demarcation between the tumor and the surface epithelium, and (3) exclusion of primary adenocarcinoma located elsewhere that has spread secondarily to the bladder. According to Johnson's criteria, urachal adenocarcinoma may be associated with areas of cystitis cystica and cystitis glandularis in the adjacent or distant bladder mucosa, provided that they show no dysplastic intestinal metaplasia (adenomatous change). Although urachal adenocarcinoma may arise from villous adenoma of the urachus, intestinal metaplasia of the urachal epithelium is believed to be the factor predisposing to malignant transformation at this site.

Whenever urachal adenocarcinoma or primary adenocarcinoma of the bladder is considered, direct extension or metastasis from colorectal carcinoma must be excluded. Management of urachal adenocarcinoma consists of partial or radical cystectomy, including resection of the umbilicus. Recurrences are common, however, especially when a partial cystectomy is done. It is important to distinguish between urachal and non-urachal adenocarcinomas for treatment

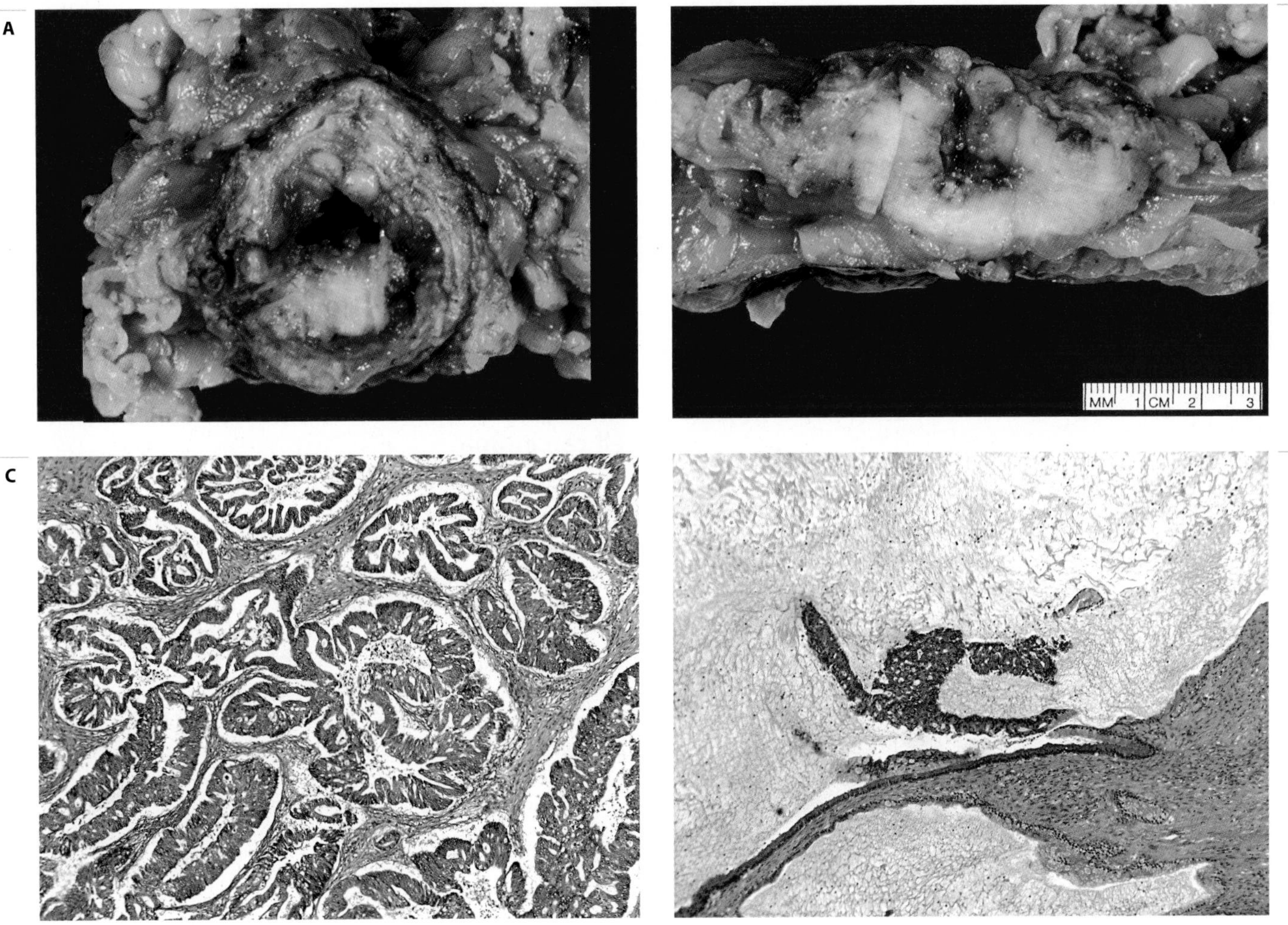

**Fig. 6-49** Urachal adenocarcinoma. (**A, B**) Gross appearance. (**C**) Usual type. (**D**) Colloid type.

purposes. Resection of urachal adenocarcinoma must include removal of the entire urachal remnant.

Non-urachal bladder adenocarcinomas show positive immunostaining with carcinoembryonic antigen in 67% of cases and Leu-M1 (CD15) in 73% of cases, whereas urachal adenocarcinomas consistently stain with both.[61,332]

## Squamous cell neoplasms

### Squamous cell carcinoma in situ

Only a few reports on squamous cell carcinoma in situ (CIS) of the bladder are available. Histologically, it is identical to squamous cell carcinoma in situ found in other organ sites (Fig. 6-50). This finding is often associated with subsequent or concurrent invasive urothelial carcinoma with squamous differentiation. In a recent report of 11 patients, one had no evidence of disease at 8 months, one had residual squamous cell carcinoma in situ at 10 months, one had high-grade urothelial carcinoma (not otherwise specified) at rebiopsy after 6 months, three were noted to have invasive squamous cell carcinoma at intervals of 2, 3, and 4 months, respec-

tively, and one was found to have invasive urothelial carcinoma with squamous features in the cystectomy specimen at 12 months.[36] Wide-range human papillomavirus DNA signal was detected in one case. Enhanced expression of EGFR in these bladder squamous lesions suggests a possible therapeutic target in cases that are difficult to manage clinically.[36]

### Squamous cell carcinoma

Squamous cell carcinoma is defined as a malignant neoplasm derived from the urothelium that shows a pure squamous cell phenotype (Fig. 6-51).[347-349] When urothelial elements (including urothelial carcinoma in situ) are present the tumor should be classified as urothelial carcinoma with squamous differentiation. Risk factors associated with the development of squamous cell carcinoma include tobacco smoking, chronic non-specific urinary tract infections, and schistosomiasis.[350-356] Keratinizing squamous metaplasia may be present in the adjacent epithelium in cases of squamous cell carcinoma of the bladder, and frequently displays the full spectrum of dysplastic lesions and/or carcinoma in situ.[347] Invasive squamous cell carcinoma of the bladder

**A**

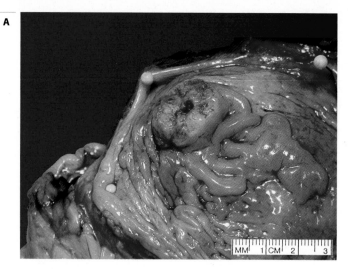

**B**

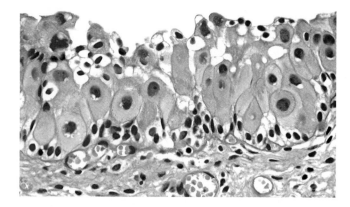

**C**

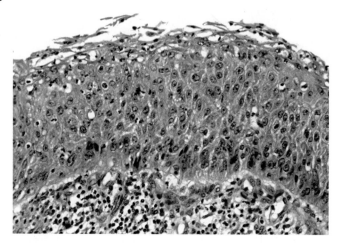

**Fig. 6-50** Invasive squamous cell carcinoma. (**A**) Gross appearance of nodular elevated invasive squamous cell carcinoma, surrounded by extensive areas of dysplastic squamous epithelium. (**B**) Cytologic atypia in squamous cell dysplasia is less severe than squamous cell carcinoma in situ (**C**).

displays a range of differentiation, from well differentiated to poorly differentiated, with a histologic spectrum that can vary from well-defined islands of squamous cells with keratinization, prominent intercellular bridges, and minimal nuclear pleomorphism, to tumors exhibiting marked nuclear pleomorphism and only focal evidence of squamous differentiation. Histologic grading is based on the amount of keratinization and the degree of nuclear pleomorphism using a three-tiered system (grades 1, 2, and 3).[348,357] Several morphologic variants of squamous cell carcinoma, including verrucous, basaloid, and clear cell pattern, have been recognized.

## Schistosoma-associated squamous cell carcinoma

Schistosomiasis is known to be associated with squamous cell carcinoma of the bladder (Fig. 6-52A, B). Tumors arising in this setting are typically large, often filling the bladder lumen, and frequently polypoid or solid with visible necrosis and keratin debris; others are ulcerated infiltrating tumors. Histologically, the presence of keratinizing squamous metaplasia in the adjacent flat epithelium is relatively constant and may be associated with dysplasia or carcinoma in situ. The prevalence of associated squamous metaplasia in cases of squamous cell carcinoma of the bladder ranges from 17% to 60%, and is widely variable according to the geographic location of the patient population. Like non-schistosoma-associated squamous cell carcinoma, these tumors range from well to poorly differentiated, but most commonly are well differentiated with prominent keratinization and intercellular bridge formation with minimal nuclear pleomorphism. Pathologic stage and lymph node status are significant prognostic and predictive factors, and pathologic grade according to the degree of keratinization and the degree of nuclear pleomorphism is also considered an important prognostic indicator. Radical surgical excision is currently the most widely used treatment option; neoadjuvant radiation has been reported to improve survival in aggressive tumors.

## Verrucous squamous cell carcinoma

Verrucous carcinoma is an uncommon variant of squamous cell carcinoma that accounts for 3–5% of squamous bladder cancers. It occurs most often in patients with schistosomiasis, but has also been reported in patients from non-endemic areas.[35] Grossly this tumor appears as a 'warty' mass; histologically, it shows epithelial acanthosis and papillomatosis, minimal nuclear and architectural atypia, and rounded, pushing deep borders (Fig. 6-52C, D; Table 6-16). Cases of squamous carcinoma with verrucous features but which also have an infiltrative component have been described; it is recommended by the WHO (2004)[2] not to diagnose such cases as verrucous carcinoma, but as regular squamous cell carcinoma. Verrucous carcinoma in the bladder is associated with minimal risk of progression whether associated with schistosomiasis or not. No link to human papilloma virus infection has been established.[35]

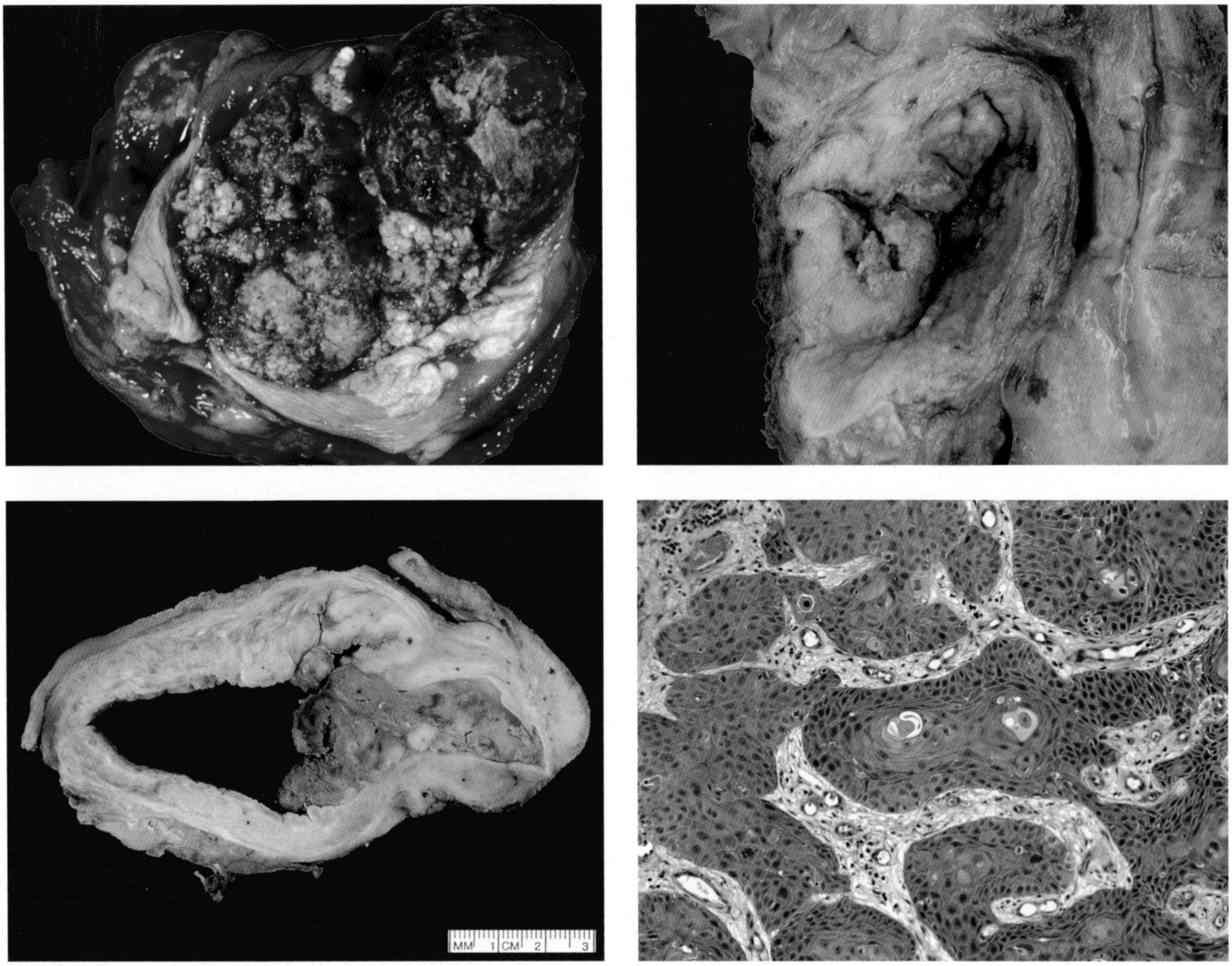

**Fig. 6-51** Squamous cell carcinoma of the urinary bladder. (**A–C**) Tumors are often bulky and exophytic. (**D**) Keratin pearl formation is typical of squamous cell carcinoma.

## Basaloid squamous cell carcinoma

Basaloid squamous cell carcinoma has been recently recognized in the urinary bladder, with one reported case.[358] The patient had a long-standing history of recurrent urinary tract infections. Grossly, it was a sessile multilobulated tan-brown mass involving the posterior wall of the bladder. Architecturally, the tumor was characterized by small nests of basaloid cells with minimal cytoplasm arranged with peripheral palisading (Fig. 6-52E, F). Cytologically, the tumor cells had a high nuclear/cytoplasmic ratio with dense hyperchromatic nuclei. Focally there was central necrosis of the larger nests and a pseudoglandular arrangement of the small nests. The tumor stroma was desmoplastic. Mitotic figures and apoptotic bodies were frequent. The reported case also had microscopic foci of urothelial cell carcinoma with squamous differentiation. Squamous metaplasia was present elsewhere in the bladder in addition to dysplasia and squamous cell carcinoma in situ. The experience with basaloid squamous

cell carcinoma in other organs suggests that these may have a more aggressive course than usual squamous carcinoma. This tumor is probably best categorized as urothelial carcinoma with squamous cell differentiation (basaloid type).

## Neural and neuroendocrine tumors

### Small cell carcinoma

#### Epidemiology and clinical features

Small cell carcinoma is a malignant neuroendocrine neoplasm of the urothelium which histologically mimics its pulmonary counterpart.[297] It is an extremely rare malignancy that accounts for less than 1% of urinary bladder cancers.[297,359-374] The demographic and clinical features of small cell carcinoma of the urinary bladder are similar to those of conventional urothelial carcinoma. The majority of patients are male, and most are in the sixth to seventh decade

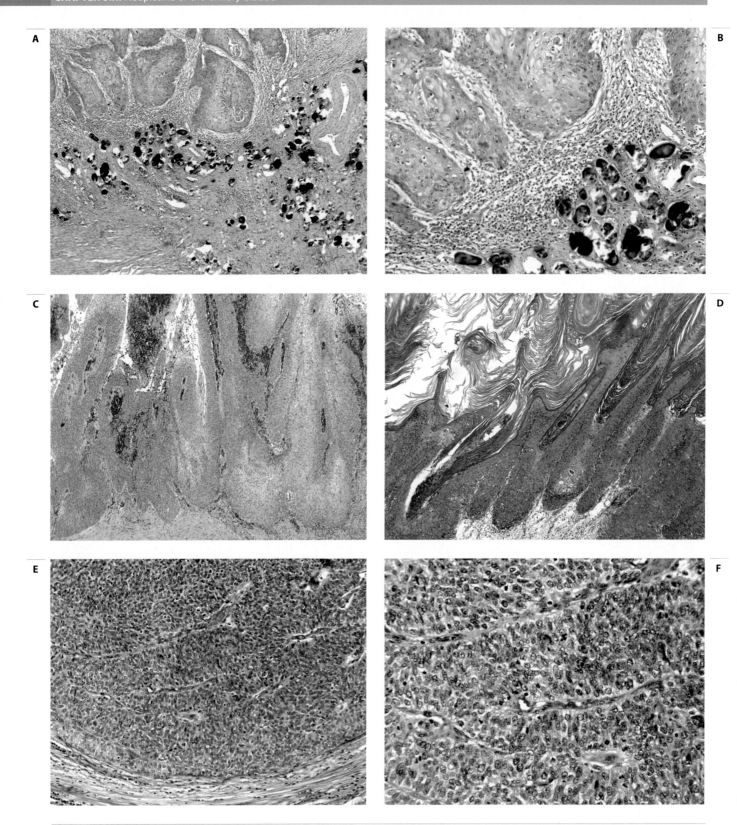

**Fig. 6-52** Variants of squamous cell carcinoma. (**A, B**) Schistosoma-associated squamous cell carcinoma. Numerous schistomal eggs are seen. (**C, D**) Verrucous squamous cell carcinoma. The tumor forms broad endophytic fronds of squamous epithelium with pushing growth pattern at its base. (**E, F**) Basaloid squamous cell carcinoma. The tumor is characterized by nests and trabeculae of basaloid cells with minimal cytoplasm.

**Table 6-16** Differential Diagnosis of Squamous Papilloma, Condyloma Acuminatum, and Verrucous suqamous cell Carcinoma of the Urinary Bladder[35]

| | Squamous papilloma | Condyloma acuminatum | Verrucous squamous cell carcinoma |
|---|---|---|---|
| Age (years) | 62 (range, 32–82). | 40 (range, 17–76) | 66 (range, 43–83) |
| Sex (Male:female) | 1:6 | 1:1.6 | 1.2:1 |
| Clinical history | Non-specific | External genitalia condyloma or history of immunosuppression | Non-specific |
| Clinical presentation | Irritative symptoms | Irritative symptoms | Irritative symptoms |
| Biological behavior | Rarely recurs | Aggressive | Aggressive |
| Location | No predilection | No predilection | No predilection |
| Extent | Small, solitary | Multiple, extensive | Diffuse, extensive |
| Histologic changes | | | |
|   Architecture | Papillary | Papillary | Expansive and endophytic |
|   Pushing margin | Absent | Absent | Present |
|   Cytologic atypia | Usually not seen or mild | Usually not seen or mild | May be present |
|   Stromal invasion | Absent | Absent | Present |
| P53 alteration | –/+ | + | + |
| Human papilloma virus detection | – | + | – |
| DNA ploidy | Diploid | Aneuploid | Aneuploid |

+: usually positive, +/–: variable staining, –: usually negative.

of life. The mean age at the time of diagnosis is 66 years, ranging from 36 to 85 years, with a male preponderance (male:female ratio 3:1).[297] Most patients have a history of cigarette smoking. There is no link between small cell carcinoma of the urinary bladder and human papilloma virus infection.[375] Clinical presentations include site-specific and systemic symptoms. Site-specific symptoms are similar to those of urothelial carcinoma. Clinical presentations include hematuria, irritative symptoms such as dysuria, nocturia, frequency, urinary obstructive symptoms, or localized abdominal/pelvic pain.[297] Systemic symptoms are non-specific and include anorexia and weight loss. Occasionally, patients have paraneoplastic syndromes with hypercalcemia, hypophosphatemia, or ectopic secretion of adrenocortico-tropic hormone (ACTH).[359,366,376,377]

### Staging, treatment, and outcome

The majority of patients have advanced stage disease when first diagnosed, typically with muscularis propria invasion or extravesical extension. A significant proportion of patients also present initially with metastatic cancer, including metastases to regional lymph nodes, bone, liver, and/or lung.[297] Therefore, careful and accurate pathologic and clinical staging is necessary in order to guide further therapy. The overall prognosis is poor, with a median survival time of 1–2 years, although a few patients have survived for longer (Fig. 6-53).[297] In Cheng's[297] report of 64 cases the cancer-specific survival rate at 5 years was 16%, consistent with the 14% rate reported by Choong et al. from the Mayo Clinic.[366] The overall median survival was 1.7 years.[366] Cytotoxic chemotherapy plays a major therapeutic role in the treatment of

limited- and advanced-stage small cell carcinoma of the urinary bladder. Chemotherapy is usually combined with other therapeutic modalities such as radiation or surgical resection. Because of the rarity of small cell carcinoma of the urinary bladder it is difficult to conduct clinical trials, and so treatment will continue to mirror that of small cell lung cancer. Improvement in survival may depend on the identification of new molecular markers for early diagnosis and for the development of novel targeted therapies.[28,372,378–381]

### Histogenesis and genetics

Several hypotheses have been proposed to explain the histogenesis of small cell carcinoma of the urinary bladder. The stem cell theory is that small cell carcinoma originates from multipotential, undifferentiated stem cells. This is supported by the observation that small cell carcinoma frequently coexists with other histologic types of bladder carcinoma.[364,369,382] Another theory is that small cell carcinoma originates from neuroendocrine cells in normal or metaplastic urothelium. It is speculated that Kultschitzky-type neuroendocrine stem cells may exist within the urothelium and may give rise to neuroendocrine tumors.[383,384] Others have suggested that small cell carcinoma of the bladder may be derived from a poorly defined population of submucosal cells of neural crest origin, the same cells from which paragangliomas and neurofibromas arise in the urinary bladder.[385,386] Recent molecular data indicate that both urothelial and small cell carcinoma originate from the same stem cell in the urothelium.[28]

**A**

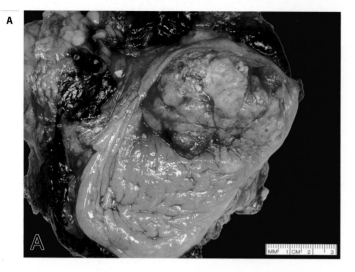

**B**

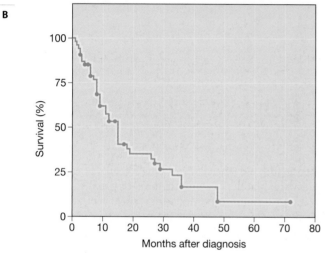

**Fig. 6-53** Small cell carcinoma of the urinary bladder. (**A**) The gross appearance of small cell carcinoma is not different from that of typical urothelial carcinoma. (**B**) Kaplan–Meier survival curve for patients with small cell carcinoma of the urinary baldder. The prognosis is extremely poor. (From Cheng L, Pan CX, Yang XJ, et al. Small cell carcinoma of the urinary bladder: a clinicopathological analysis of 64 patients. Cancer 2004; 101: 957–962, with permission.)

At the molecular level, small cell carcinoma of the urinary bladder demonstrates chromosomal aberrations that are commonly seen in small cell lung cancer.[371,372,379] Loss of 4q, 5q, 10q and 13q is common in small cell carcinoma of the urinary bladder.[387] Cheng et al.,[28] in a large series of small cell carcinoma of the urinary bladder, identified allelic loss at 3p25–26, 9p21, 9q32–33, and 17p13, and non-random inactivation of the X chromosome. Homozygous deletion of p16[388] and gain or high level of amplification at 1p22–32, 3q26.3, 8q24, 12q14–21, and 5q, 6p, 8q and 20q, chromosomes 1–3, 5–7, 9, 11 and 18 have also been found.[387,389] Some of these regions contain oncogenes. For example, 8q24 includes the oncogene c-MYC, which is found to be highly amplified in small cell carcinoma of the urinary bladder.

Small cell carcinoma of the urinary bladder also shares some of the aberrant signaling pathways seen in small cell lung cancer. For instance, an autocrine loop through the c-kit/stem cell factor (SCF) pathway has been frequently identified.[390,391] It is well known that c-kit, a transmembrane receptor tyrosine kinase involved in many physiological and pathological processes, including hematopoiesis and carcinogenesis, is a target of the tyrosine kinase inhibitor imatinib. c-Kit expression can be detected in up to 40% of small cell carcinomas of the urinary bladder.[372]

## Pathology

Most tumors appear as a single large, solid, polypoid mass (Fig. 6-53A), but may also appear sessile and ulcerated, and extensively infiltrate the bladder wall. The lateral walls and dome of the bladder are the most frequent topographies, but rare cases may arise in a bladder diverticulum.[379–381] Histologically, small cell carcinoma of the urinary bladder consists of sheets or nests of small or intermediate-sized cells with nuclear molding, scant cytoplasm, inconspicuous nucleoli and evenly dispersed finely stippled chromatin (Fig. 6-54A–D). Mitotic figures are readily evident and may be frequent.[297] There may be extensive nuclear disruption, which can make diagnosis difficult in biopsy specimens. Punctate or geographical necrosis is common, and DNA encrustation of blood vessel walls (Azzopardi phenomenon) may be noted.[364,368] Occasionally, tumor rosettes are present. Vascular invasion is invariably present.[297,392] In the great majority of cases extensive tumor infiltration of detrusor muscle is evident.

Coexisting non-small cell carcinoma components, in the form of carcinoma in situ, conventional urothelial carcinoma, adenocarcinoma, squamous cell carcinoma, or sarcomatoid carcinoma, are present in 12–61% of cases.[297] In a largest series reported by Cheng et al.,[379] 20 cases (32%) were pure small cell carcinoma, and 44 cases (68%) consisted of small cell carcinoma admixed with other histological types (urothelial carcinoma in 35 cases, adenocarcinoma in four, sarcomatoid urothelial carcinoma in two, and both adenocarcinoma and urothelial carcinoma in three). In another series only 12% of cases were pure small cell carcinoma, whereas a mixture of small cell and urothelial carcinoma was noted in 36 cases (70%), a mixture of small cell carcinoma and adenocarcinoma was present in four (8%), and a mixture of small cell carcinoma and squamous cell carcinoma in five (10%).[360]

Ultrastructurally, tumor cell nuclei are irregular with coarse chromatin. Cytoplasm is scant, with sparse organelles including polyribosomes, short segments of rough endoplasmic reticulum, mitochondria and occasional Golgi complexes. A finding of diagnostic importance is the presence of membrane-limited, rounded dense core granules ranging from 150 to 250 nm in diameter, which have been observed in almost all cases examined.[364,368] Tonofilaments and dendrite-like processes are also present in the some of the cases.

## Immunohistochemistry

The immunohistochemical profile of small cell carcinoma of the urinary bladder has been extensively investigated.[61,360,364,365,372,380,381,393,394] It typically exhibits both epi-

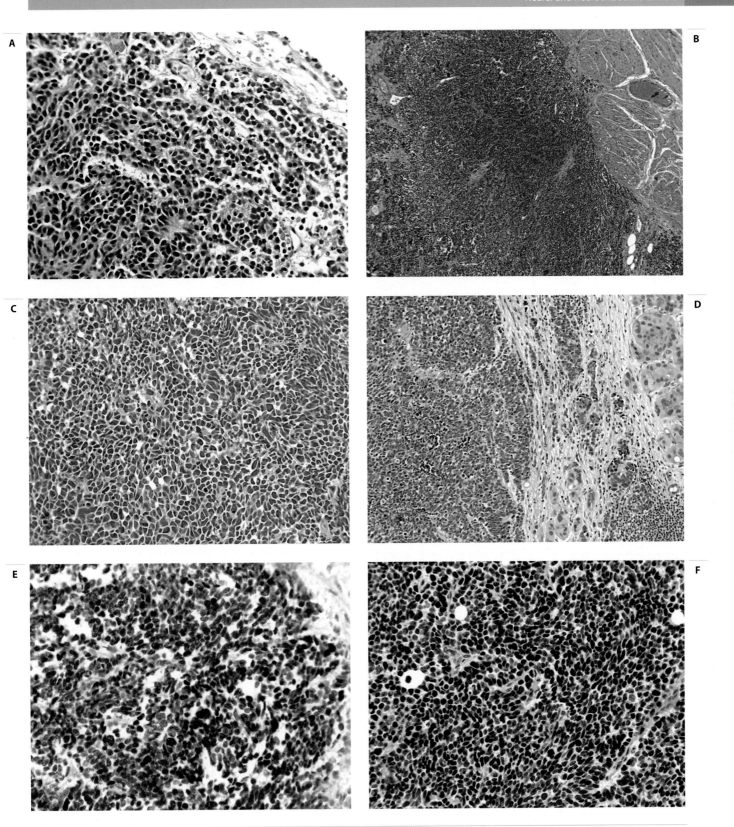

**Fig. 6-54** Small cell carcinoma of the urinary bladder. (**A, C**) Tumors are composed of sheets and cords of small cells with scant cytoplasm and hyperchromatic nuclei with nuclear crowding and overlapping. These tumor typically present with high-stage with invasion into muscularis propria, as evident in (**B**). (**D**) Coexisting urothelial carcinoma component is often present. (**E**) Immunostain for p53 is diffusely positive. (**F**) These tumors often show positive immunostaining for thyroid transcription factor-1 (TTF-1).

thelial and neuroendocrine differentiation. However, the diagnosis of small cell carcinoma can be made on the typical morphologic features alone, even if neuroendocrine differentiation cannot be demonstrated. Markers that have been helpful in confirming neuroendocrine differentiation in small cell carcinoma include neuron-specific enolase, chromogranin, synaptophysin, Leu 7, protein gene product 9.5 (PGP9.5), serotonin, vasoactive intestinal peptide, and others. Neuroendocrine differentiation has been demonstrated in 30–100% of cases of small cell carcinoma by various markers in different studies. Chromogranin A appears to be a relatively insensitive marker, demonstrable immunohistochemically in only a third of cases.

Positive immunostaining for cytokeratin 7 has been observed in about 60% of cases.[364,365,367,394,395] Cytokeratin 20 and uroplakin III immunostains are negative in small cell carcinoma of the urinary bladder.[374,394,396,397] Strong and focally intense cytoplasmic dot-like CAM5.2 reactivity is reported in about two-thirds of cases studied.[360,393] Positive immunostaining for cytokeratin 34βE12 has been observed in 40% of cases,[374] and positive EMA immunostaining in about 78% of cases.[364,365] p53 is overexpressed in 52% of cases (Fig. 6-54E).[381] Reported frequencies of Ki67 expression have varied from 15% to 80%.[374,396]

CD44v6 may be useful in distinguishing poorly differentiated urothelial carcinoma from small cell carcinoma. CD44, a member of a family of transmembrane glycoproteins, mediates cell–cell and cell–matrix adhesion, the latter by serving as a receptor for hyaluronate binding. CD44v6 splice variant is an isoform conferring metastatic potential and has been correlated with aggressive behavior in some cancers. CD44v6 immunoreactivity is demonstrable in 60% of cases of urothelial carcinoma, compared to only 7% positivity in small cell carcinoma.[398,399]

Thyroid transcription factor 1 (TTF-1) is a nuclear transcriptional factor protein expressed in thyroid and lung epithelium. TTF-1 is considered to be a reliable marker for distinguishing primary adenocarcinomas of the lung from adenocarcinomas of extrapulmonary origin, and for distinguishing pulmonary small cell carcinoma from Merkel cell carcinoma. Jones et al.[394] showed that approximately 40% of cases of small cell carcinoma of the urinary bladder had positive TTF-1 staining (Fig. 6-54F). Therefore, TTF-1 immunostaining cannot reliably distinguish between a lung or a urinary bladder primary in cases of metastatic small cell carcinoma of uncertain primary location.

### Differential diagnosis

The main differential diagnoses include metastasis of small cell carcinoma from another site, lymphoma, lymphoepithelioma-like carcinoma, plasmacytoid carcinoma, and poorly differentiated urothelial carcinoma.[297] Immunohistochemical studies can be quite helpful in distinguishing these entities in difficult cases. Small cell carcinoma can occasionally mimic malignant lymphoma when the tumor cells of small cell carcinoma appear to grow in a dyscohesive pattern, a finding that may result from artifacts produced by fixation and specimen processing. Lymphoma shows positive immu-

nostaining for leukocyte common antigen (LCA), and negative immunostaining for keratin and neuroendocrine markers that are typically positive in small cell carcinoma. Plasmacytoid carcinoma, poorly differentiated urothelial carcinoma, and squamous cell carcinoma do not express neuroendocrine markers such as synaptophysin or chromogranin, unlike small cell carcinoma. Large cell neuroendocrine carcinoma is characterized morphologically by large tumor cells with low nuclear/cytoplasmic ratios, coarse chromatin and frequent nucleoli, and high mitotic activity with areas of necrosis; confirmation of its true nature requires positive immunostaining with appropriate neuroendocrine markers.

Small cell carcinoma metastatic to the urinary bladder can only be distinguished from a bladder primary by knowledge of the clinical setting.[394] The identification of co-existing urothelial carcinoma or in-situ component supports the bladder primary.

## Large cell neuroendocrine carcinoma

Large cell neuroendocrine carcinoma is a poorly differentiated and high-grade neuroendocrine tumor (Fig. 6-55), morphologically identical to its counterpart in the lung. Primary large cell neuroendocrine carcinomas of the urinary bladder are rare, and experience with them is limited to a few anecdotal case reports.[400–403] The age at diagnosis ranges from 32 to 82 years. These tumors are either pure or can be associated with other components, such as typical urothelial carcinoma, squamous cell carcinoma, adenocarcinoma or sarcomatoid carcinoma. Immunohistochemically, the tumor cells frequently show immunoreactivity to chromogranin A, CD56, neuron-specific enolase, and synaptophysin. In addition to neuroendocrine markers, the tumor cells typically show positive immunostaining for cytokeratins CAM 5.2 and AE1/AE3 and epithelial membrane antigen (EMA), and may show focal positivity for vimentin. In situ hybridization for the detection of Epstein–Barr virus in one reported case was negative. These tumors are aggressive and tend to metastasize systemically despite aggressive adjuvant therapy. Metastasis from a lung primary should be considered before diagnosing a primary bladder large cell neuroendocrine carcinoma.

## Carcinoid

Carcinoid is a potentially malignant neuroendocrine neoplasm derived from the urothelium. Fewer than two dozen cases of carcinoid tumor of the urinary bladder have been reported, usually occurring in elderly patients (range 29–75 years of age), with a slight male preponderance. Hematuria is common, but irritative voiding symptoms may be the first symptom. Association with carcinoid syndrome has not been reported. Most tumors are submucosal, with a predilection for the trigone, and range in size from 0.3 to 3 cm. Carcinoid tumors are often polypoid at cystoscopy. Coexistence of carcinoid with other urothelial neoplasia, such as inverted papilloma and adenocarcinoma, has been reported.

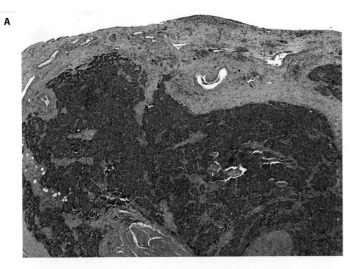

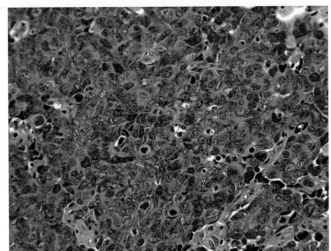

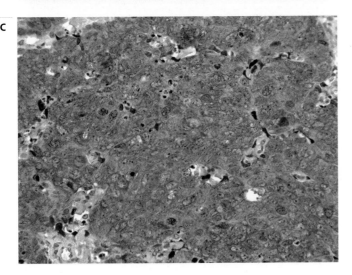

**Fig. 6-55** Large cell neuroendocrine carcinoma. (**A**) The tumor is highly aggressive, with invasion into muscularis propria. (**B**) Tumor forms solid sheets composed of cells with large hyperchromatic nuclei and amphophilic cytoplasm. (**C**) Immunostain for synaptophysin is positive.

Carcinoid tumors of the bladder are histologically similar to their counterparts in other organ sites. The tumor cells have abundant amphophilic cytoplasm and are arranged in an insular, acinar, trabecular, or pseudoglandular pattern with a delicate vascular stroma. An organoid growth pattern, resembling paraganglioma, is sometimes seen. Tumor cell nuclei have finely stippled chromatin and inconspicuous nucleoli. Mitotic figures are infrequent, and tumor necrosis is absent. Tumor cells show immunoreactivity for neuro-endocrine markers (neuron-specific enolase, chromogranin, serotonin, and synaptophysin) and cytokeratin (AE1/AE3). Differential diagnostic considerations include paraganglioma, nested variant of urothelial carcinoma and metastatic prostate carcinoma. About 25% of patients have or develop regional lymph node or distant metastases, but the majority are cured by excision.

## Paraganglioma (pheochromocytoma)

### Clinical features

Primary paraganglioma of the bladder occurs infrequently. The largest series, which included 16 patients followed for a mean of 6.3 years, was reported by Cheng et al.[385] Females are more likely to develop bladder paraganglioma: the male : female ratio is 1 : 3. The tumor tends to occur in young patients (mean, 45 years) and symptoms are present in over 80% of cases. Presenting symptoms include hematuria, hypertension which may be exacerbated during voiding, and other symptoms of catecholamine excess.[404–424] At cystoscopic examination, small (<3 cm), dome-shaped nodules covered by normal mucosa are found in the trigone, dome, or lateral wall of the bladder (Fig. 6-56).

In contrast to extra-adrenal paragangliomas at other sites, of which approximately 10% exhibit malignant behavior, the frequency of malignancy in bladder paragangliomas is about 20%.[385] No reliable histologic criteria exist to distinguish malignant from benign neoplasms.[409,412,423,425–427] The findings of nuclear pleomorphism, mitotic figures, and necrosis are not reliable predictors of clinical outcome in patients with paraganglioma of the urinary bladder.[408,412] Malignancy in these tumors can only be confirmed by the occurrence of regional or distant metastases. No metastases or tumor recurrences have been observed in patients whose tumors were confined within the bladder wall.[385]

### Histogenesis

The origin of paraganglioma of the bladder is uncertain. It is thought to arise from embryonic rests of chromaffin cells in the sympathetic plexus of the detrusor muscle.[385] It is postulated that small nests of paraganglionic tissue may persist along the aortic axis and in the pelvic regions, and that these may migrate into the urinary bladder wall during fetal development.[428–431] In an autopsy study of 409 patients, Honma[432] identified paraganglia of the urinary bladder in 52% of the cases examined and found that paraganglia were present throughout different layers of the bladder wall, with a predilection for the anterior and posterior walls. The

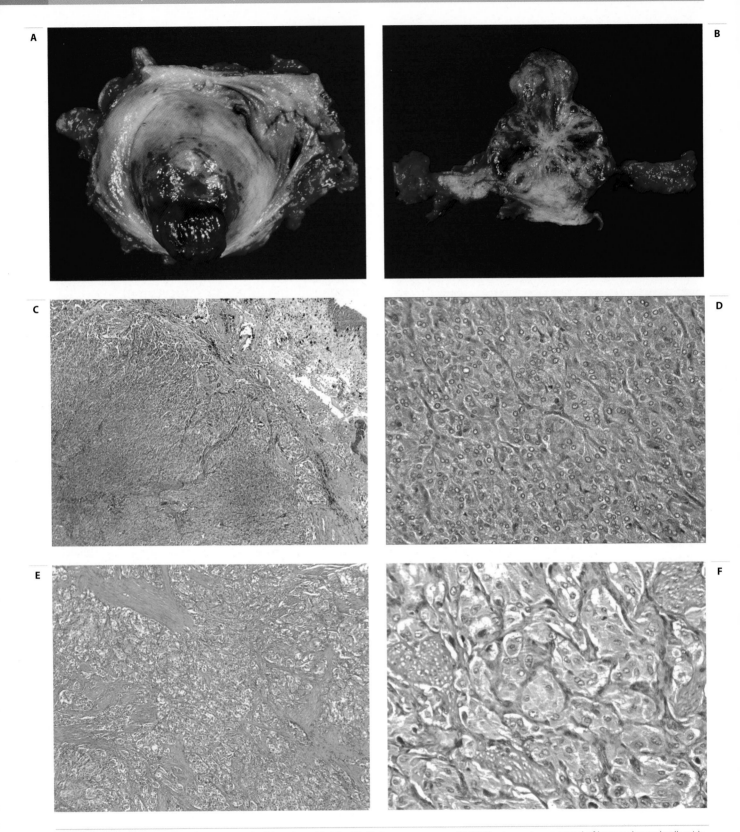

**Fig. 6-56** Paraganglioma (pheochromocytoma) of the urinary bladder. (**A, B**) Gross appearance. (**C, D**) The tumor is composed of large polygonal cells with eosinophilic granular cytoplasm and central vesicular nuclei. (**E**) Tumor invades into the muscularis propria. (**F**) A Zellballen growth pattern is characteristic of paraganglioma (**A** and **B** from Cheng L, Leibovich B, Cheville J, et al. Paraganglion of the urinary bladder: can biologic potential be predicted? Cancer 2000; 88: 844–852, with permission.)

trigone of the bladder was the least common location of paraganglia.[432] In Cheng's study[385] the majority of tumors (94%) involved the muscularis propria of the bladder wall, with a predilection for the posterior and lateral walls. A significant number of patients (37%) also had extravesical extension or pelvic involvement. These findings support the hypothesis that paraganglioma of the bladder originates from paraganglionic cells that migrated into the bladder wall.[428] The high prevalence of paraganglionic cells within the muscular wall (63% of all paraganglia of the bladder)[432] is consistent with the frequent occurrence of paraganglioma in this location.

## Genetics

Genomic analyses have identified germline mutations responsible for sporadic as well as familial paraganglioma syndromes.[433–440] The susceptibility genes include SDHB, SDHC, and SDHD. Succinate dehydrogenase (SDH), which consists of four polypeptides [SDHA, SDHB(1p36), SDHC(1q21), and SDHD(11q23)], is the major mitochondrial enzyme linking the aerobic respiratory chain and the Krebs cycle, which oxidizes succinate to fumarate.[433,435] The SDH genes are tumor suppressor genes, the inactivation of which is involved in the hypoxia–angiogenic pathway activating the transcription factor hypoxia-inducible factor (HIF).[433] Nonsense and missense mutations, insertions, and small and large deletions have been reported in the SDH genes of patients with pheochromocytoma or paraganglioma. These mutations are generally seen in younger patients. SDHD mutations have been identified in patients with pheochromocytoma or functional paraganglioma. Patients with these mutations usually have a paternal family history of disease due to maternal imprinting. SDHB gene mutations are usually associated with abdominal paragangliomas and are often identified in patients with no family history of the disease. The SDHB gene mutation is associated with a high risk of malignancy.[433]

HIF dysregulation is also linked to inactivation of the VHL tumor suppressor gene (3p25–26), which is seen in von Hippel–Lindau disease. Pheochromocytomas or paragangliomas may be seen in this disease.[441] Other autosomally dominant diseases associated with pheochromocytomas/paragangliomas include multiple endocrine neoplasia type 2 (due to mutation of the RET proto-oncogene) and neurofibromatosis type 1 (due to a mutation in NF-1, a tumor suppressor gene). Genetic aberrations at other loci (2q and 16p) have also been recently found to be associated with familial pheochromocytoma.[442] Similarly, Lemeta et al.[443] found abnormalities in tumor suppressor genes located at 6q23–24 which may play a role in the tumorigenesis of pheochromocytomas.

## Pathology

Histologically, bladder paraganglioma is similar to its counterparts in other body sites; most are covered by normal urothelium (Fig. 6-56).[385] The tumor consists of round or polygonal epithelioid cells with abundant eosinophilic or granular cytoplasm. Tumor cell nuclei are centrally located, and are vesicular with finely granular chromatin. The cells are arranged in discrete nests (zellballen), with intervening vascular septa. Sustentacular cells may be present. Mitotic figures, necrosis, and vascular invasion are usually absent.[385]

## Immunohistochemistry

Paraganglioma typically demonstrates immunoreactivity with neuroendocrine markers such as chromogranin, synaptophysin, and neuron-specific enolase.[385] The sustentacular cells exhibit immunostaining for S100 protein. Tumor cells are often immunoreactive for vimentin, but usually show no immunoreactivity for cytokeratins 7, 20, or pancytokeratin AE1/AE3.[433]

## Differential diagnosis

The differential diagnosis for this tumor includes granular cell tumor, nested variant of urothelial carcinoma, metastatic large cell neuroendocrine carcinoma, and malignant melanoma.[255,256,258,385,444,445] Granular cell tumor has abundant eosinophilic granular cytoplasm, shows strongly positive immunostaining for S100 protein, and lacks the zellballen growth pattern, the fine vascular stroma, chromogranin immunoreactivity, and sustentacular cell S100 protein immunostaining.[446–450] The nested variant of urothelial carcinoma also lacks a fine vascular network and is immunohistochemically negative for S100 protein and chromogranin. Metastatic large cell neuroendocrine carcinoma is characterized by necrosis, abundant mitotic activity, and cellular anaplasia. Although it is immunoreactive for neuroendocrine markers similar to paraganglioma, it is also immunoreactive for cytokeratin and negative for sustentacular cell S100 protein immunoreactivity. History is important in differentiating paraganglioma from metastatic carcinoid. Carcinoid tumor is negative for sustentacular cell S100 protein immunoreactivity. Malignant melanoma must be considered in the differential diagnosis, as paraganglioma may contain melanin pigment.

## Neurofibroma

Neurofibroma of the urinary bladder is rare, occurring mostly in the setting of NF-1 rather than as isolated lesions.[386] Classically, neurofibromas of the urinary bladder occur in young patients, with a slight male preponderance. The average age at diagnosis is 17 years. Presenting symptoms include hematuria, irritative symptoms, and a pelvic mass. Neurofibroma is a benign, probably neoplastic tumor of various nerve sheath cells, including Schwann cells, perineurium-like cells, fibroblasts, and intermediate-type cells.[451] The histologic findings are the same as in neurofibromas of other organs: tumors are composed of a hypocellular proliferation of spindle cells, loosely arranged into fascicles with scattered 'shredded carrot' bundles of collagen (Fig. 6-57). Individual cells have wavy, bland nuclei. In a recent series by Cheng et al.,[386] three of four bladder neurofibromas were transmural with both diffuse and plexiform growth patterns. Another case had only diffuse pattern with submucosal involvement and subepithelial pseudo-meissnerian corpuscles on biopsy. Areas of diffuse involvement were hypocellular with small

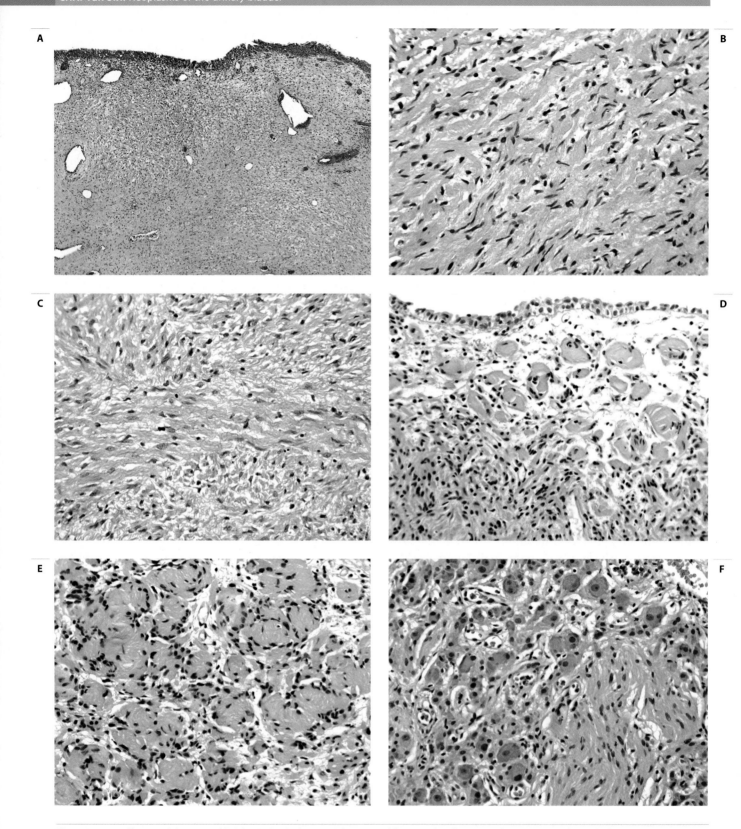

**Fig. 6-57** Neurofibroma of the urinary bladder. (**A, B, C**) The tumor shows a proliferation of uniform neurofibroma cells. (**D, E**) Superficial band-like subepithelial pseudo-meissnerian corpuscles are prominent. (**F**) Ganglion cells may be involved by neurofibroma.

to medium-sized spindle cells having ovoid to elongated nuclei in a collagenized matrix. A few mast cells were present. Immunohistochemical staining was reactive in all cases for S100 protein as well as type IV collagen.[386] Three were positive for neurofilament protein in axons. A recent report indicates that bladder neurofibromas do not express ALK-1 protein. The differential diagnosis of bladder neurofibroma includes other spindle cell tumors, such as leiomyoma, postoperative spindle cell nodule, inflammatory pseudotumor, low-grade leiomyosarcoma, other nerve sheet tumors, and rarely rhabdomyosarcoma.[386]

## Schwannoma

Schwannoma of the urinary bladder is derived from Schwann cells in nerve sheaths. It occurs in both men and women, and is often associated with von Recklinghausen's disease.[452] The age at presentation ranges from the fourth to the sixth decade.[452,453] The presenting symptoms include bladder pressure, suprapubic pain, back pain, urgency, and frequency. No recurrences have been reported during follow-up periods of 1–3 years after surgical resection.[452,453]

Grossly, the tumor appears as a circumscribed mass, often arising from the lateral wall, beneath a normal mucosa. It may or may not extend into the perivesical fat. Histologically, schwannoma consists of spindle cells with uniform round to oval nuclei arranged in a palisading or organoid pattern. There is no nuclear pleomorphism and mitotic figures are infrequent.[452,453] Tumor cells show positive immunostaining for S100 protein, neuron-specific enolase, and vimentin. Immunostains for myoglobin, Factor VIII, keratins, actin (HHF-35), and desmin are negative.[452,453]

## Primitive neuroectodermal tumor

Primary primitive neuroectodermal tumor (PNET) of the bladder is an extremely rare and aggressive neoplasm.[454] Morphologically it is a small round blue cell tumor that are often associated with extensive areas of necrosis (Fig. 6-58). Tumor cells show strong expression of CD99, vimentin, and CD117 (c-kit), and focal reactivity to cytokeratin and S100 protein. Ultrastructural study reveals sparse neurosecretory granules.[454] Molecular genetic analysis supports the diagnosis of PNET by showing the EWS/FLI-1 fusion transcript type 2 by RT-PCR and EWS gene rearrangement by FISH. A patient treated with imatinib following systemic chemotherapy and radical surgery remains alive after 4 years follow-up.[454]

## Malignant peripheral nerve sheath tumor (MPNST)

Malignant peripheral nerve sheath tumor is rare in the urinary bladder. Only a few cases have been documented, predominantly in patients less than 40 years old.[455] Some have arisen in the setting of NF-1, possibly originating in neurofibromas of autonomic nerve plexuses in the bladder wall. MPNST is typically a highly malignant and rapidly growing tumor. Patients present with hematuria, and a suprapubic mass is sometimes noted.[456] The lesion has been

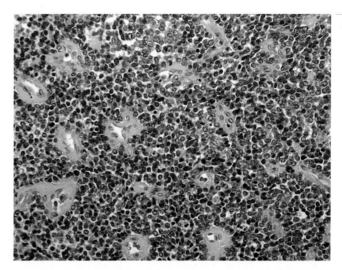

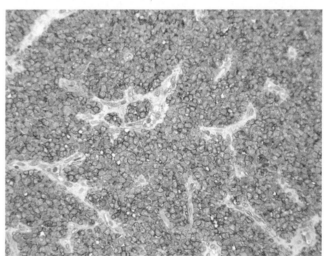

**Fig. 6-58** Primitive neuroectodermal tumor (PNET) of the urinary bladder. (**A**) The tumor is highly cellular and consists of small round blue cells in sheets surrounded by fibrovascular stroma. Pseudorosette formation is apparent. (**B**) The tumor is immunoreactive for CD99.

seen arising from the trigone, as well as from the lateral and posterior walls of the bladder. It may form multiple large nodules with surface ulceration and areas of necrosis. The tumor may infiltrate the entire thickness of the bladder wall, involving perivesical soft tissues or pelvic peritoneum. Distant metastases may be present at diagnosis. Prognosis is generally poor, with local recurrence or distant metastases often evident within 2 months of initial surgical resection.

Histologically, MPNST is a poorly differentiated tumor that grows in sheets and nodules consisting of interlacing fascicles of malignant spindle cells.[455] The tumor cells are pleomorphic, with variable amounts of eosinophilic cytoplasm.[456] Most have a single nucleus, but multinucleated tumor cells may be present. Nuclei are round to oval with prominent irregular eosinophilic nucleoli, or elongated and tapered with marked atypia. Mitotic activity may be moderate. An extensive infiltrate of acute and chronic inflammatory cells, including eosinophils, may be present. An epithelioid variant, as well as a variant with rhabdomyoblastic differentiation (malignant triton tumor), has been described.[456]

Immunohistochemical stains can help with the identification of this tumor, which typically shows positive immunostaining for S100 protein and vimentin, and focally positive staining for neuron-specific enolase (NSE). It does not usually stain for epithelial membrane antigen (EMA), cytokeratin AE1/AE3, muscle-specific actin, desmin, myoglobin, cytokeratin, chromogranin, or neurofilament.[455,456] In one case, rhabdomyoblastic differentiation with focal immunostaining for myoglobin was identified in a tumor that arose in an infant with NF-1.[457]

The differential diagnosis of this tumor includes epithelioid sarcoma, undifferentiated carcinoma, melanoma, epithelioid angiosarcoma, rhabdoid tumor, carcinosarcoma, and epithelioid leiomyosarcoma. Immunoreactivity to HMB45 or MelanA, or strong diffuse S100 protein immunoreactivity would favor melanoma. Carcinosarcoma would show evidence of epithelial differentiation with immuno-reactivity for cytokeratins and EMA. Unlike epithelioid sarcoma, tumor cells of MPNST are immunoreactive for S100 protein, focally immunoreactive for NSE, and not immunoreactive for EMA or cytokeratins. Immunohistochemistry can also be used to help rule out endothelial, muscular and neuroendocrine differentiation as well as anaplastic lymphoma.

# Sarcomatoid carcinoma

## Definition and terminology

The term sarcomatoid carcinoma applies when a malignant neoplasm exhibits morphologic or immunohistochemical evidence of both epithelial and mesenchymal differentiation. Heterologous elements may be present and should be acknowledged in the pathology report.[306] There is considerable confusion and disagreement in the literature regarding nomenclature and histogenesis of these tumors. We postulate that sarcomatoid carcinoma is a common final pathway of all forms of epithelial bladder tumor, a hypothesis supported by molecular data[46] and morphologic evidence (Fig. 6-59). Sarcomatoid transformation has been observed in various epithelial tumors of the urinary bladder, including conventional urothelial carcinoma, small cell carcinoma, adenocarcinoma, squamous cell carcinoma, and large cell neuroendocrine carcinoma.

Various terms have been used for these neoplasms, including carcinosarcoma, sarcomatoid carcinoma, pseudosarcomatous transitional cell carcinoma, malignant mesodermal mixed tumor, spindle cell carcinoma, giant cell carcinoma, and malignant teratoma. In some reports, both carcinosarcoma and sarcomatoid carcinoma are included under the term 'sarcomatoid carcinoma.' In others they are regarded as separate entities. There is an emerging consensus that the most appropriate term for all of these neoplasms is sarcomatoid carcinoma.[46,458] We prefer to use this term for the majority of cases in which there is a spindle cell component with positive vimentin staining. Some may use the term carcinosarcoma for cases with identifiable heterologous elements on hematoxylin and eosin-stained sections or positive

staining for markers of specific mesenchymal differentiation. Both diagnostic categories appear to be variations of the same neoplastic transformation process and have the same clinical features and prognosis.

## Clinical features

Sarcomatoid carcinoma represents approximately 0.3% of bladder carcinomas. The most frequent presenting symptoms are hematuria, dysuria, nocturia, acute urinary retention, and lower abdominal pain. The mean patient age is 66 years (range 50–77 years).[106,459–461] In some patients there is a history of carcinoma treated by radiation, or exposure to cyclophosphamide therapy.[459,460] The presence of specific types of differentiation of the spindle cell component does not influence the prognosis, but sarcomatoid carcinoma is usually high grade, biologically aggressive, and associated with a poor prognosis.[106,461] Pathological stage is the best predictor of survival in sarcomatoid carcinoma.

## Histogenesis and genetics

A recent analysis of 30 sarcomatoid urothelial carcinomas for X-chromosome inactivation status as well as loss of heterozygosity (LOH) has shed light on the pathogenesis of this tumor.[46] The results of this study found identical patterns of allelic loss in the carcinomatous and in the sarcomatous components, identified at four of six polymorphic microsatellite markers where genetic alterations occur frequently in urothelial carcinomas, including D8S261 (86%), D9S177 (75%), IFNA (57%), and D11S569 (78%) loci.[46] Furthermore, discordant allelic loss of microsatellite markers was also found at the various sites as the bladder tumors underwent malignant progression, leading to genetic divergence of high-grade anaplastic malignancies following the initial neoplastic transformation. Additionally, the study found the same pattern of non-random X-chromosome inactivation in both carcinomatous and sarcomatous components in five of eight female patients.[46] The identical X-chromosome inactivation and significant concordance of LOH support the contention that both carcinomatous and sarcomatous components arise from a monoclonal primordial cell. Clonal divergence may occur during tumor progression and lead to differentiation into mesenchymal as well as epithelial phenotypes.[46]

## Pathology

The gross appearance is characteristically 'sarcoma-like,' with a dull gray fleshy cut surface and infiltrative margins. The tumors are often polypoid and tend to form large intraluminal masses (Fig. 6-60). Microscopically, sarcomatoid carcinoma is composed of a urothelial, glandular or small cell epithelial component showing variable degrees of differentiation (Fig. 6-61).[306] Carcinoma in situ is present in 30% of cases and is occasionally the only apparent epithelial component. A small subset of sarcomatoid carcinomas may have a prominent myxoid stroma. The mesenchymal component most frequently observed is an undifferentiated high-grade spindle cell neoplasm. The most common heterologous element is osteosarcoma, followed by chondrosarcoma, rhabdomyosarcoma, leiomyosarcoma, liposarcoma, angiosarcoma, or multiple types of mesenchymal differentiation.

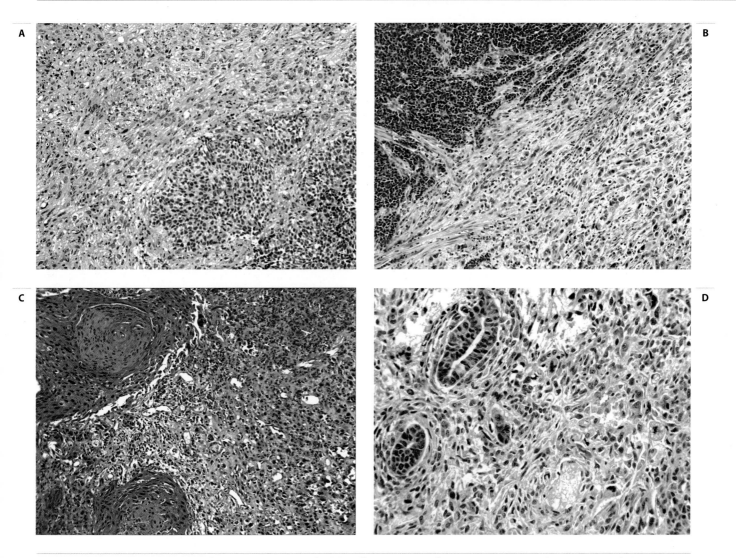

**Fig. 6-59** Sarcomatoid carcinoma is the final common pathway of cellular differentiation. Transformation into sarcomatoid component can be seen in typical urothelial carcinoma (**A**), small cell carcinoma (**B**), squamous cell carcinoma (**C**), and adenocarcinoma (**D**).

### Differential diagnosis and immunohistochemistry

Sarcomatoid carcinoma is characterized by strong staining with keratins (AE1/AE3, CAM5.2) and/or epithelial membrane antigen, with coexpression of vimentin in the majority of cases (Fig. 6-62; Tables 6-17 and 6-18).[61,106,459,461–466] In contrast to smooth muscle neoplasms, actin and desmin are typically negative. However, sarcomatoid carcinomas with heterologous differentiation may rarely be encountered, and in this situation expression of other mesenchymal markers such as actin, desmin, and S100 protein may be observed.[467,468]

Sarcomatoid carcinoma of the urinary bladder is usually biphasic, composed of both epithelial and mesenchymal elements. In cases exclusively composed of spindle cells, the main differential diagnostic consideration is sarcoma, particularly leiomyosarcoma. In view of the rarity of primary bladder sarcoma, any malignant spindle cell tumor in the urinary bladder in an adult should be considered sarcomatoid carcinoma until proven otherwise. Cytokeratin immunostaining may be helpful in this setting.

One should also bear in mind that focal cytokeratin immunoreactivity may be seen in smooth muscle tumors and pseudosarcomatous myofibroblastic proliferations. Smooth muscle tumors are additionally immunoreactive for desmin and vimentin, even when they express cytokeratin antigens.[306,458]

Sarcomatoid carcinoma with prominent myxoid and sclerosing stroma may be mistaken for pseudosarcomatous myofibroblastic tumor, postoperative spindle cell nodule, or urothelial carcinoma with pseudosarcomatous stroma.[464–466] The presence of slit-like vessels and the absence of mitotic figures and significant cytologic atypia favor the diagnosis of a benign lesion.

## Soft tissue tumors

Pure sarcomas of the urinary bladder are all rare and have been described only in small series and isolated case reports.[469,470] Myofibroblastic proliferations, including pseu-

**Table 6-17** Immunohistochemistry of spindle cell lesions of the bladder

| | Sarcomatoid Carcinoma | IMT | LMS | Leiomyoma | MFH | Neurofibroma | PSCN | RMS |
|---|---|---|---|---|---|---|---|---|
| **ALK-1** | | pos | | | | rare pos | neg | |
| **α-1-Antichymotrypsin** | | | | | pos | | | |
| **CD68** | | | | | pos | | | |
| **Cytokeratin** | pos | pos/neg | neg/pos | | neg/pos | neg | neg/pos | neg/pos |
| **Desmin** | peg/pos | pos/neg | pos | pos | neg/pos | | pos/neg | pos |
| **EMA** | pos | pos/neg | neg | | | neg | neg | neg |
| **h-Caldesmon** | | | pos | pos | neg | | | neg |
| **Muscle-specific actin** | pos/neg | pos | pos | pos | neg/pos | | pos | pos |
| **MYOD1** | | | neg | | neg | | | pos |
| **Myogenin** | | | neg | | neg | | | pos |
| **Myoglobin** | | neg | | | | | | pos/neg |
| **NSE** | | | | | | | | neg/pos |
| **Smooth muscle actin** | neg/pos | pos | pos | pos | neg/pos | | pos/neg | neg/pos |
| **S-100 protein** | | neg | neg | | neg | pos | | neg |
| **Vimentin** | pos/neg | pos | pos | pos | pos | | pos | pos |
| **CD31** | | | | | neg | | | |
| **CD34** | | | neg/pos | | neg | | | neg |

ALK = anaplastic lymphoma kinase; IMT = inflammatory myofibroblastic tumor; PSCN = postoperative spindle cell nodule; LMS = leiomyosarcoma; MFH = malignant fibrous histiocytoma; RMS = rhabdomyosarcoma; EMA = epithelial membrane antigen; NSE = neuron-specific enolase; Pos: positive, Neg: negative; Neg/Pos: variable staining.

**Table 6-18** Differential features of selected soft tissue tumors of the urinary bladder

| | Cytologic atypia | Mitotic figures | Atypical mitotic figures | Tumor necrosis | Inflammation | Invasion of muscle | Other features |
|---|---|---|---|---|---|---|---|
| **Sarcomatoid Carcinoma** | present | present | present | present | Often present | may be present | Concomitant carcinoma |
| **IMT** | minimal | few | absent | surface only | often prominent | may be present | Delicate capillaries |
| **Leiomyoma** | minimal | rare | absent | absent | absent | absent | Well circumscribed |
| **Leiomyosarcoma** | present | present | present | present | Sparse | present | Uniform appearance |
| **MFH** | present | present | present | present | present | present | Multinucleated cells |
| **Neurofibroma** | varies | absent | absent | absent | Sparse | absent | Strands of collagen |
| **PSCN** | minimal | variable | absent | absent | present | absent | Delicate capillaries |
| **RMS** | present | present | present | varies | absent | may be present | Cambium layer in Embryonal RMS, Alveolar appearance |
| **Angiosarcoma** | present | present | present | may be present | present | may be present | Anastomosing vessels |

ALK = anaplastic lymphoma kinase; IMT = inflammatory myofibroblastic tumor; MFH = malignant fibrous histiocytoma; PSCN = postoperative spindle cell nodule; RMS = rhabdomyosarcoma.

dosarcomatous myofibroblastic tumor and postoperative spindle cell nodule, still invoke a degree of uncertainty for classification and differential diagnosis. Other rare benign lesions of the bladder include leiomyoma, hemangioma, and neurofibroma. Other examples are rarely described.[469–471] Differentiation of benign from malignant lesions is critical to avoid overly aggressive therapy. Malignant mesenchymal tumors of the urinary bladder include leiomyosarcoma, rhabdomyosarcoma, angiosarcoma and malignant fibrous histiocytoma (undifferentiated sarcoma).

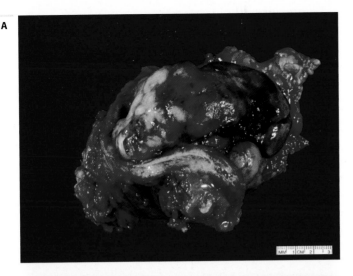

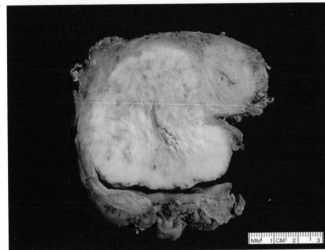

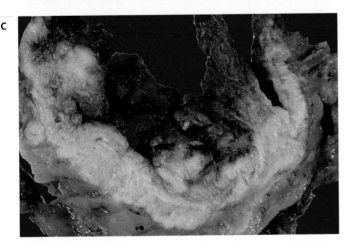

**Fig. 6-60** Sarcomatoid carcinoma. (**A, B**) The tumor may form a large nodular mass protruding into the lumen of the bladder. (**C**) Cross-section shows diffusely infiltrative growth.

Recognizing these spindle cell lesions and differentiating them from sarcomatoid carcinoma is important, as these two diagnostic categories have differing therapeutic as well as prognostic implications.[469,470,472]

## Myofibroblastic proliferations and benign soft tissue tumors

### Inflammatory myofibroblastic tumor (IMT)

Inflammatory myofibroblastic tumor (IMT) of the bladder is a controversial entity and has had many designations, including inflammatory pseudotumor, inflammatory pseudosarcomatous fibromyxoid tumor, nodular fasciitis, pseudosarcomatous myofibroblastic proliferation, and fibromyxoid pseudotumor.[464,473–496] It was initially described as a lesion showing spindle cells in a myxoid stroma with scattered chronic inflammatory cells.[497] The most frequent presenting symptom is hematuria; other symptoms include irritative and/or obstructive voiding symptoms, abdominal pain, or the discovery of a mass lesion. Rarely, constitutional symptoms including fever and weight loss have been reported, possibly due to the release of cytokines. Grossly, the lesion is either a polypoid mass or a submucosal nodule. The tumor may or may not cause surface ulceration and the cut surface is often pale, firm, and glistening. Histologically, there is a proliferation of spindle cells with elongated eosinophilic cytoplasmic processes in a loose edematous or myxoid background (Figs 6-63 and 6-64; Tables 6-17 and 6-18). The nuclei may be large, with occasional atypia.[478,495,498] Single, prominent nucleoli may be present. Occasional mitotic figures are seen, none of which is atypical. The mitotic rates vary from 0 to 20 mitoses per 10 hpf (high-power fields).[488,493,494] Inflammation, usually chronic and consisting of a lymphoplasmacytic infiltrate, is invariably seen. Some lesions have infiltrates of eosinophils or neutrophils, which may be focally prominent. Extravasated red blood cells may be present. Three histologic patterns have been recognized,[476,488] the most common of which is the 'nodular fasciitis-like' pattern with myxoid, vascular, and inflammatory areas. A second pattern, designated 'fibrous histiocytoma-like,' has a more compact spindle cell proliferation and scattered lymphocytes, plasma cells, or eosinophils. The third pattern, designated 'scar or desmoid-like,' has dense collagen with fewer spindled and inflammatory cells (Fig. 6-64). Infiltration into the muscularis propria or even perivesical involvement may be seen. Typically, the lesion occurs in young patients (9–42 years) with a female preponderance. The tumor size ranges from 1.5 to 13 cm. Follow-up data have revealed no evidence of metastases, but the lesion may recur after surgery.[478,495,496]

There is some lack of consistency in the reported immunoprofile, with the result that the utility of immunostaining in separating this lesion from other spindle cell lesions of the bladder is limited. Immunoreactivity for actin and vimentin is usually present but may be focal.[464–466] P53 staining is weak or absent in inflammatory myofibroblastic tumor and postoperative spindle cell nodule, but strongly and diffusely positive in rhabdomyosarcoma, leiomyosarcoma and sarcomatoid carcinoma.[479,492] Pancytokeratin reac-

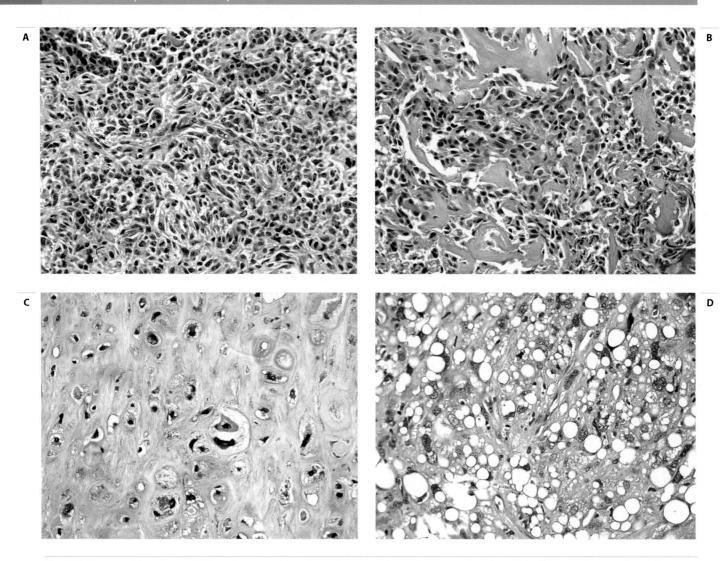

**Fig. 6-61** Sarcomatoid carcinoma. (**A**) Typical sarcomatoid carcinoma is composed of malignant spindle cells with significant cytologic atypia and frequent mitotic figures. (**B–D**) Heterologous differentiation, including (**B**) osteosarcoma, (**C**) chondrosarcoma, and (**D**) liposarcoma, may be seen.

tivity, which may be patchy, is seen in many cases of inflammatory myofibroblastic tumor. Nevertheless, cytokeratin may be seen in other non-epithelial tumors, such as leiomyosarcoma.[493,494] Actin immunoreactivity may not help differentiate benign from malignant tumors, as α-smooth muscle actin (SMA) is positive in 43% of sarcomas, 63% of inflammatory myofibroblastic tumors, and an intermediate percentage of postoperative spindle cell nodule. Rhabdomyosarcoma rarely expresses SMA, but leiomyosarcoma often does. Iczkowski et al.[478,495] found that three of 11 inflammatory myofibroblastic tumors, two of three postoperative spindle cell nodules, and none of eight sarcomas were reactive for desmin, but this marker may be present in leiomyosarcomas at other sites. Inflammatory myofibroblastic tumor shows variable staining for EMA. Inflammatory myofibroblastic tumor is negative for myoglobin, whereas rhabdomyosarcoma is usually positive for skeletal muscle markers such as myogenin or MyoD1. Strong coexpression of SMA and cytokeratin is characteristic of vesical myofibro-

blasts, and thus should characterize inflammatory myofibroblastic tumor.[489]

The main differential diagnoses include postoperative spindle cell nodule, embryonal rhabdomyosarcoma, and leiomyosarcoma.[464–466,478,479,492,495,496] Postoperative spindle cell nodule is reportedly more likely to have eosinophils.[493,494] Inflammatory myofibroblastic tumor may be confused with myxoid leiomyosarcoma, as both may have a myxoid stroma. Morphologically, leiomyosarcoma is more uniform in its cellularity and exhibits more cytologic atypia. Inflammatory myofibroblastic tumor, on the other hand, has a more prominent network of small blood vessels and a more extensive inflammatory infiltrate. Inflammatory myofibroblastic tumor may have necrosis at the site of surface ulceration and may infiltrate into the detrusor muscle, but it typically does not exhibit deep necrosis as may be seen in a sarcoma. However, in a recent series by Harik et al.,[474] 32% of inflammatory myofibroblastic tumor cases showed necrosis in the deep bladder wall, two of which were extensively necrotic.[499–501]

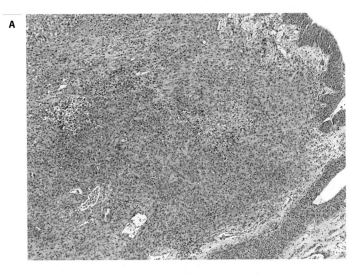

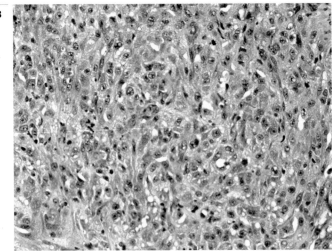

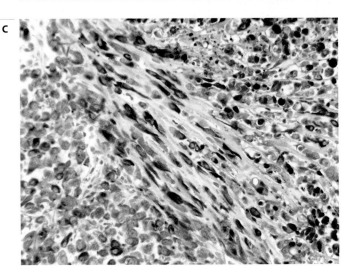

**Fig. 6-62** Sarcomatoid carcinoma. (**A, B**) Inflammatory cells are invariably present in sarcomatoid carcinoma. Sarcomatoid urothelial carcinoma should be distinguished from other benign and malignant spindle cell tumor. (**C**) Strong and diffuse immunoreactivity for cytokeratin AE1/3 confirms the epithelial nature of the tumor.

Recently, positive cytoplasmic immunostaining for anaplastic lymphoma kinase (ALK-1) has been identified in 89% of inflammatory myofibroblastic tumors in the bladder.[479,492,498] The ALK-1 staining was confirmed by fluorescence in situ hybridization to mRNA from a fusion gene resulting from translocation of the ALK gene on chromosome 2p23 to the clathrin heavy-chain region on chromosome 17q23.[498,499] It has been suggested that ALK-negative cases are less likely to recur. Neither ALK-1 staining nor translocation of the ALK-1 gene has been identified in any case of bladder leiomyosarcoma or rhabdomyosarcoma. However, spindle cell lesions in sites other than the urinary bladder may display ALK-1 expression, which has been reported in 40% of inflammatory myofibroblastic tumors, 19% of rhabdomyosarcomas, and 10% of leiomyosarcomas at other sites.[464-466,496,499-501]

It has been proposed by Harik et al.[474] that inflammatory myofibroblastic tumor occurring in the adult bladder and postoperative spindle cell nodule should be combined into a diagnostic category designated 'pseudosarcomatous myofibroblastic proliferations.' These investigators have furthermore suggested that there is enough evidence to distinguish 'pseudosarcomatous myofibroblastic proliferations' of the bladder from inflammatory myofibroblastic tumor of childhood. The latter is often associated with systemic findings, such as fever, weight loss and laboratory abnormalities, including anemia, thrombocytosis and polyclonal hypergammaglobulinemia. Further experience with these lesions may help to validate this approach.

## Postoperative spindle cell nodule (PSCN)

Postoperative spindle cell nodule (PSCN) may be seen in both genders months after surgical instrumentation or resection.[474,479,491,492,502,503] It is characterized by nodules up to 4 cm in size occurring in the lower genital tract and lower urinary tract.[502] Patients range in age from 29 to 79 years, and typically present with hematuria and/or obstructive voiding symptoms. Some PSCN are found incidentally by CT scan or at cystoscopy.[478,495] Microscopically the tumors are uniform, composed of intersecting fascicles of plump spindle cells with delicate vessels, focal hyalinization, and moderate collagen deposition (Fig. 6-65). The spindle cells have abundant, tapering, eosinophilic cytoplasm. The nuclei vary only slightly in size and there is no cytologic atypia. There are numerous mitotic figures, ranging from 1 to 25 per 10 hpf, none of which is abnormal.[464-466,496] All lesions have ulceration with acute inflammatory cells in the ulcer bed, as well as scattered chronic inflammatory cells in deeper areas. The tumor has infiltrating margins with smooth muscle destruction. Moderate edema and small foci of hemorrhage may be identified. No recurrences or metastases have been reported, but bladder wall eosinophilia may be prominent following resection of the lesion.[502] The proliferating cells are immunoreactive for cytokeratin AE1/AE3, CAM5.2 and vimentin in some cases, similar to the findings in IMT. Some cases exhibit only immunoreactivity for vimentin.[496]

The differential diagnoses for PSCN include sarcomatoid carcinoma, myxoid leiomyosarcoma, rhabdomyosarcoma,

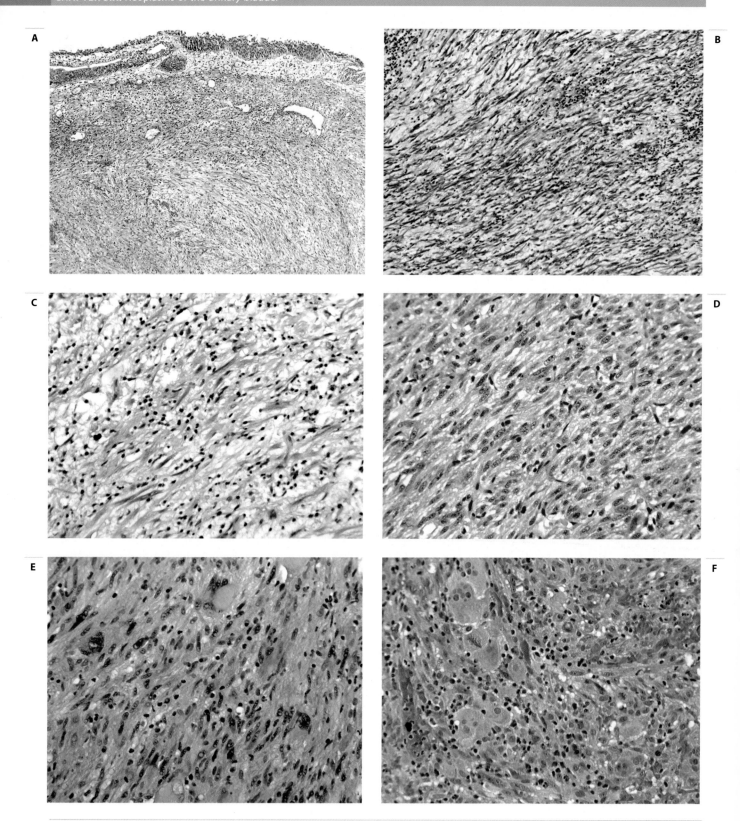

**Fig. 6-63** Inflammatory myofibroblastic tumor. (**A–C**) The tumor is composed of spindle cells in an edematous stroma. Scattered acute and chronic inflammatory cells are typically seen in this lesion. (**D, E**) The lesion may appear hypercellular. (**E, F**) Multinucleated giant cells and mitotic figures may be present.

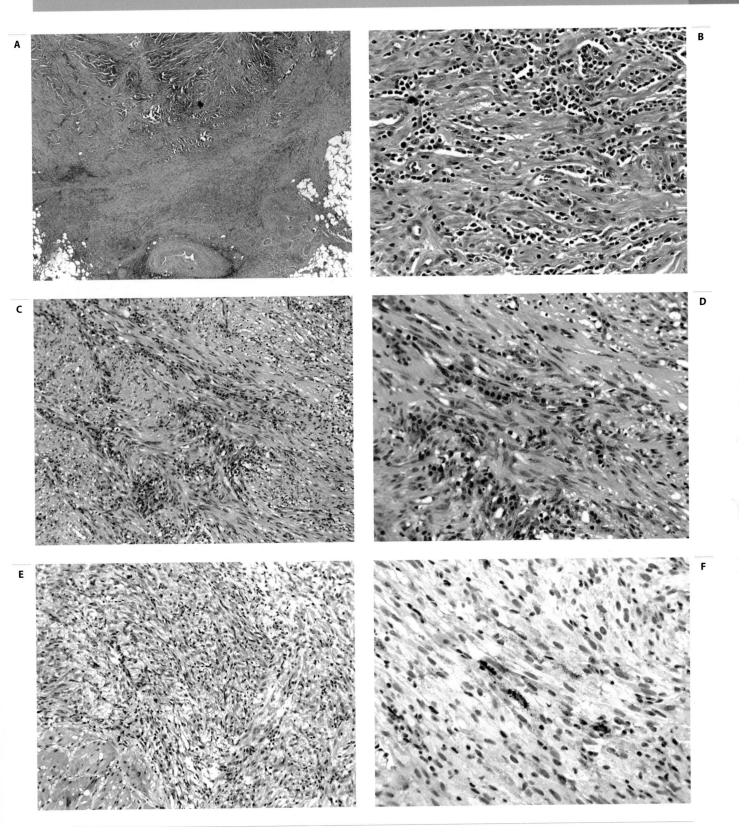

**Fig. 6-64** Inflammatory myofibroblastic tumor. (**A–D**) End stage of sclerotic/fibrotic variant. Inflammatory background is almost always present. (**E**) The lesion may extend into muscle. (**F**) Immunostaining for ALK is useful in confirming the diagnosis.

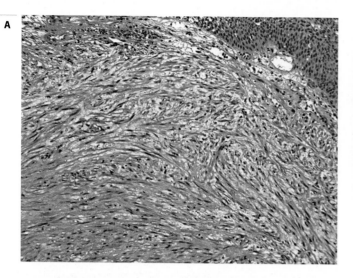

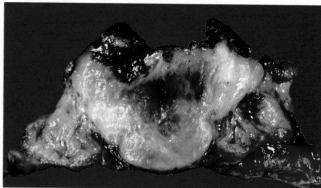

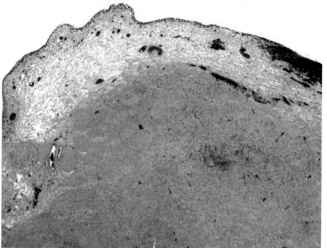

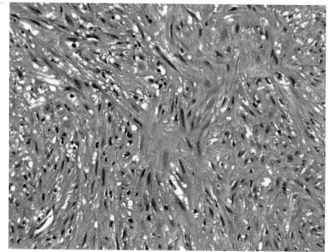

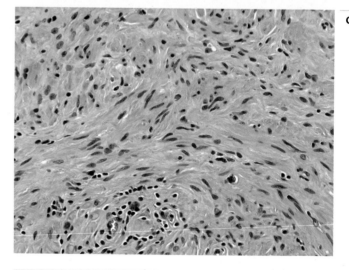

**Fig. 6-65** Postoperative spindle cell nodule. Inflammatory cells are invariably present.

and malignant fibrous histiocytoma (see Inflammatory myofibroblastic tumor for discussion).[488,498] Findings that are helpful in distinguishing PSCN from sarcoma include the lack of necrosis or myxoid degeneration, lack of nuclear atypia, and predominance of chronic over acute inflammation.[479,492] P53 immunostaining may be helpful in distinguishing these lesions, being noted only rarely in PSCN, but showing strong and diffuse staining in malignant lesions.

## Leiomyoma

Although rare, leiomyoma is the most common benign neoplasm of the bladder.[471,472,504,505] A recent review by Goluboff et al.[471] of 37 cases reported that 59% occurred in the third to the sixth decades, with an average patient age of 44 years. Leiomyoma of the bladder is more common in women, with a male:female ratio of 1:3. About 19% of patients are asymptomatic; others present with obstructive voiding symptoms (49%), irritative symptoms (38%), hematuria (11%), or flank pain (13%). Leiomyomas are

**Fig. 6-66** Leiomyoma of the urinary bladder. (**A**) The tumor is well circumscribed with central hemorrhagic areas. (**B, C**) The tumor is composed of intersecting fascicles of benign smooth muscle cells with eosinophilic cytoplasm and cigar-shaped blunt ended nuclei.

most often endovesical, followed by extravesical, or intramural.[471] Grossly, the tumors are small, well-circumscribed white nodules without necrosis, and measure 1.6–5.8 cm (Fig. 6-66). Microscopically, leiomyoma consists of intersecting fascicles of smooth muscle cells with moderate to abundant eosinophilic cytoplasm.[505] Cellularity is usually limited, and myxoid change is absent in most cases. The nuclei are oval to cigar-shaped, centrally located, and blunt-ended, and lack significant nuclear atypia, mitotic activity and necrosis. Examples of angioleiomyoma have been reported. Leiomyoma is immunoreactive for smooth muscle actin (SMA), actin, desmin, and vimentin. Some may express CD34, but most are negative for cytokeratin and S100 protein. Excision is usually curative.

## Hemangioma

Cheng et al.[506] reported the findings in 19 patients with bladder hemangioma. In this series the mean age at diagnosis was 58 years, whereas in previous reports hemangiomas occurred in all age groups but predominantly in patients less than 30 years old. The male : female ratio is 3 : 1.[506] The usual presenting symptom is gross hematuria, but other complaints may include irritative voiding symptoms and abdominal pain. Endoscopically, a sessile, blue, raised mass may be seen. The lesion is usually small (median 0.7 cm). Hemangiomas are most often found on the posterior and lateral walls of the bladder. The histologic findings in bladder hemangioma are the same as those noted in other sites. Cavernous hemangioma is the most common type reported in the bladder, but capillary or arteriovenous types may infrequently be seen (Fig. 6-67). Effective conservative treatment consists of biopsy with or without fulguration. After such treatment, none of the 19 patients reported by Cheng et al. developed recurrence (mean follow-up of 6.9 years).[506] The differential diagnosis for bladder hemangioma includes angiosarcoma and Kaposi's sarcoma, both of which exhibit more cytologic atypia. Exuberant granulation tissue contains prominent inflammation, which is not a feature of hemangioma. Multiple hemangiomas may be associated with syndromes predisposing to their development, including Klippel–Trenaunay–Weber and Sturge–Weber syndromes.[506]

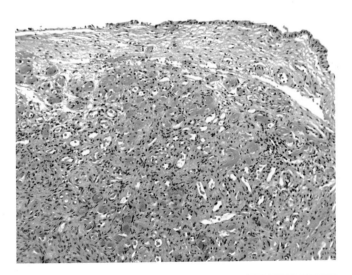

**Fig. 6-67** Hemangioma of the urinary bladder, capillary type.

## Granular cell tumor

This tumor is rarely seen in the urinary bladder but reported cases have occurred in adult patients 23–70 years of age.[446-450,507] There is no gender predilection.[449] The tumors are usually solitary, well circumscribed, and vary in size up to 12 cm. Histologically, the cells have abundant granular eosinophilic cytoplasm and vesicular nuclei. S100 protein is invariably expressed in the tumor cells. A congenital granular cell tumor of the gingiva with systemic involvement including the urinary bladder has been reported. To date, only one malignant granular cell tumor of the bladder has been described.[507]

## Solitary fibrous tumor

Solitary fibrous tumor of the urinary bladder has recently been recognized.[508] It occurs in older patients who present with pain or hematuria. Two of the seven reported cases were incidental findings. The tumor is typically a polypoid submucosal mass. Histopathologic features include spindle cells arranged haphazardly in a variably collagenous stroma. Dilated vessels reminiscent of hemangiopericytoma are present.[509] All solitary fibrous tumors of the bladder have had a benign course, although the number of cases is small and in several cases follow-up has been short. The proliferating cells typically show CD34 immunoreactivity.

## Perivascular epithelioid cell tumor (PEComa)

Perivascular epithelioid cell tumor (PEComa) is a rare mesenchymal neoplasm with indolent biological behavior.[510-512] All cases involving the urinary bladder have occurred in patients less than 50 years old.[510-512] One of the characteristic histologic features of this tumor is the delicate vascular stroma between the tumor cell nests. Clear to eosinophilic, epithelioid and spindled cells are arranged in fascicles or packets (Fig. 6-68). Mitotic figures are inconspicuous. Immunohistochemically the cells are positive for HMB-45 and smooth muscle actin, but negative for S100 protein, MelanA, desmin, and pancytokeratin.

Clear cell myomelanocytic tumor, another member of the PEComa family, has also been reported in the urinary bladder. The single reported case arose from the muscularis propria in a 33-year-old woman. [511]

## Malignant soft tissue tumors

### Leiomyosarcoma

Leiomyosarcoma is the most common malignant mesenchymal tumor of the urinary bladder in adults.[469,470,505,513-515] It is rare, but has been reported in patients ranging from 15 to 75 years of age; most are in the sixth to eighth decades of life. There is a male preponderance. Some leiomyosarcomas develop a number of years after the administration of cyclophosphamide. Acrolein, a degradation product of cyclophosphamide, is thought to be the causative agent.[513,515] Patients present with gross hematuria, obstructive voiding symptoms, dysuria, or an abdominal mass. Most often the

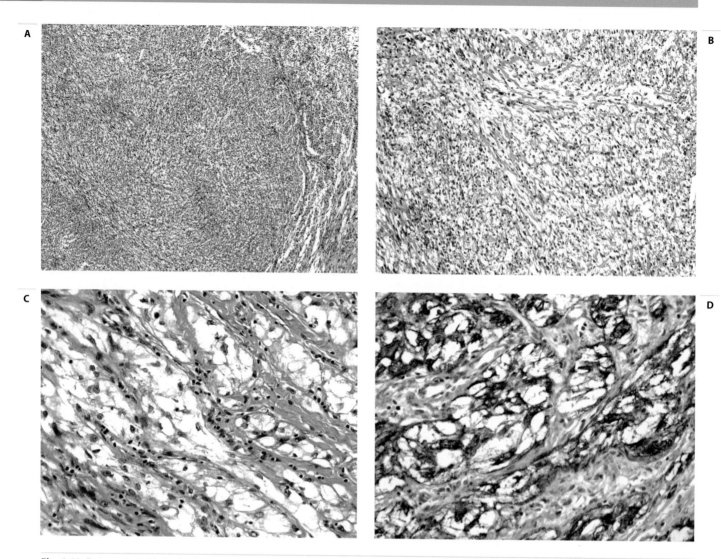

**Fig. 6-68** Perivascular epithelioid cell tumor (PEComa) of the urinary bladder. (**A–C**) PEComa of the urinary bladder consists of a proliferation of epithelioid cells with fascicular arrangement of cells. (**D**) Cells have abundant clear cytoplasm and are HMB45 immunoreactive.

tumor is located in the dome of the bladder, and less frequently in the lateral walls. Grossly, the tumor is large, unencapsulated, often polypoid with surface ulceration, and exhibits invasive growth involving all layers of the bladder (Fig. 6-69). The cut surface is usually firm or fleshy with a fibrous or myxoid appearance. Some are hemorrhagic, with varying degrees of necrosis. Histologically, interlacing bundles and fascicles of elongated, eosinophilic cytoplasmic processes and spindled to elongate hyperchromatic nuclei are common. High-grade lesions have significant nuclear pleomorphism with hyperchromasia and irregular nuclear membranes. Pleomorphic, vesicular nuclei with macronucleoli and frequent bizarre mitotic figures, interspersed with some multinucleated giant cells, characterize high-grade lesions. The pleomorphism of high-grade leiomyosarcoma is usually identifiable at low power, along with tumor cell necrosis, increased mitotic activity, and infiltration of the muscularis propria. Grading influences prognosis and is based on the degree of cytologic atypia and mitotic activity. Low-grade leiomyosarcoma has <5 mitoses per hpf, mild to

moderate cytologic atypia, minimal necrosis and an infiltrative margin.[515] High-grade leiomyosarcoma has >5 mitoses per hpf, moderate to marked cytologic atypia, and may show abundant necrosis.

Several morphologic variants, including myxoid and epithelioid types, have been described. Myxoid leiomyosarcoma may contain moderate numbers of thin-walled blood vessels, and epithelioid leiomyosarcoma has rounded tumor cells, which occasionally exhibit clear and vacuolated cytoplasm.

Immunohistochemically, leiomyosarcomas usually stain positively for vimentin, with variable staining for SMA (43–100%), and desmin (0–60%) (Tables 6-17 and 6-18). Infrequently, they show positive immunostaining with epithelial markers, including cytokeratins (CAM5.2, AE1/AE3) (10%) and epithelial membrane antigen (5%). ALK-1 immunostain is usually negative.

Leiomyosarcoma must be differentiated from several other tumors, including leiomyoma, sarcomatoid carcinoma, rhabdomyosarcoma, postoperative spindle cell tumor, and pseudosarcomatous myofibroblastic prolif-

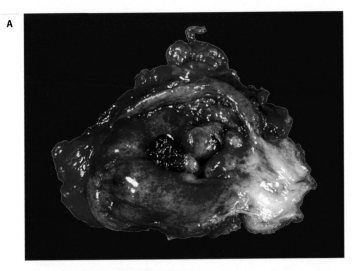

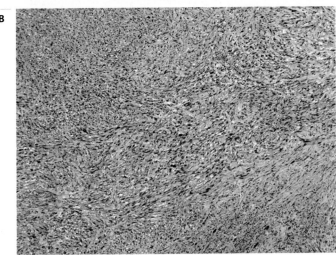

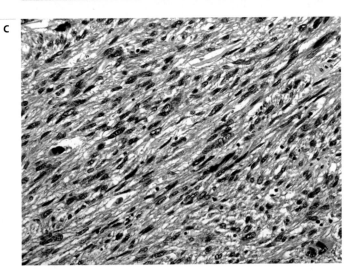

**Fig. 6-69** Leiomyosarcoma of the urinary bladder. (**A**) The tumor is bulky, polypoid, hemorrhagic and necrotic. (**B, C**) It is composed of interwoven fascicles of spindle cells with nuclear pleomorphism, hyperchromasia and atypical mitotic figures.

erations. (Tables 6-17 and 6-18) Sarcomatoid carcinoma can be recognized if one is aware of a history of a high-grade urothelial carcinoma or of concurrent urothelial in situ or invasive carcinoma. Therefore, extensive tissue sampling is recommended before rendering a diagnosis of leiomyosarcoma in the bladder. Sarcomatoid carcinoma is typically immunopositive for low molecular weight cytokeratin and EMA and usually immunonegative for myogenous markers such as desmin and SMA, although in rare cases with muscle differentiation these markers may be diffusely positive.[515] Although leiomyosarcomas may show cytokeratin immunoreactivity, the staining is usually focal and weak. Another differential consideration, rhabdomyosarcoma, may have a myxoid appearance, but this tumor is extremely rare in adults. Features of rhabdomyosarcoma include the presence of cross-striations and/or a cambium layer, as well as positive staining for myogenin.

## Rhabdomyosarcoma

Rhabdomyosarcoma is infrequently seen in the urinary bladder, and the great majority occur during childhood and adolescence.[451,489,516–522] Only a few cases of bladder rhabdomyosarcoma in adults have been reported.[517] Rhabdomyosarcoma is the most frequent malignant tumor of the bladder in children. There is a slight male preponderance. Children with NF-1 have an increased prevalence of rhabdomyosarcoma with a predominance of bladder or prostate primaries. Although the prognosis in adults is generally poor, significant advances in the treatment of childhood rhabdomyosarcoma have been made, resulting in improved survival with preservation of bladder function. Patients with rhabdomyosarcoma classically present with hematuria; some have obstructive voiding symptoms, and in some cases an abdominal mass is evident.[523] The most frequent site of involvement is adjacent to the trigone, a feature that essentially precludes the option of partial cystectomy.

Several histologic variants of rhabdomyosarcoma are seen in the bladder, with the embryonal type, including the botryoid subtype, being the most common.[516] Grossly, rhabdomyosarcoma, including the sarcoma botryoides variant, appears as a polypoid gelatinous and lobulated mass protruding into bladder lumen with variable hemorrhage and necrosis. The shiny, lobulated, grape-like appearance of the most common type of bladder sarcoma in children is the source of the name *sarcoma botryoides*. Most tumors have a superficial covering epithelium. The botryoid subtype of embryonal RMS demonstrates a 'cambium' or condensed layer of small round rhabdomyoblasts under the intact epithelium (Fig. 6-70). The main tumor mass in botryoid rhabdomyosarcoma may be a paucicellular myxoid tumor. These hypocellular areas may be admixed with more cellular areas, especially where the tumor infiltrates deeply into the muscle wall. Histologically, well-differentiated tumor cells (rhabdomyoblasts) have hyperchromatic small nuclei. The cells are small and elongated with frequent cross-striations.[516] Less differentiated rhabdomyoblasts have medium-sized or large, irregularly shaped hyperchromatic nuclei with a small rim of cytoplasm and a high mitotic rate. Often atypical mitotic

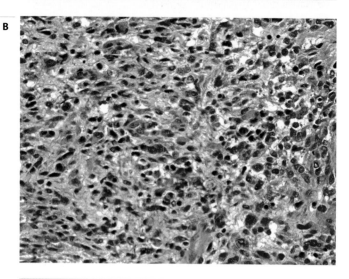

**Fig. 6-70** Rhabdomyosarcoma of the urinary bladder. (**A**) Intact urothelium with underlying cambium layer of malignant cell is seen. (**B**) The tumor is composed of a mixture of small round to spindle-shaped cells, strap cells, and rhabdomyoblasts with abundant eosinophilic cytoplasm.

figures and bizarre cells are seen.[517] A rare variant reported to occur in the bladder is alveolar rhabdomyosarcoma. This has closely packed alveolar spaces separated by thin fibrovascular septa lined by a single layer of cuboidal hyperchromatic tumor cells. The polygonal cells lining the fibrovascular septa have a hobnail appearance, with nuclei projecting away from the basement membrane. Tumor cells floating in the alveolar spaces have been described. The solid type of alveolar rhabdomyosarcoma grows in confluent sheets, but the cells are similar to those of the classic pattern.[516] Mixed alveolar and embryonal types occur, and their biologic behavior is similar to that of pure alveolar RMS. The botryoid subtype, which tends not to infiltrate deeply into the muscle, are associated with an overall excellent prognosis. Deeply infiltrating embryonal RMS and alveolar RMS, on the other hand, often portend a poor prognosis even with modern multimodality therapy. Immunohistochemical stains of rhabdomyosarcoma usually show positivity for desmin, MyoD1 or myogenin. Also, muscle-specific actin,

myoglobin, and myosin may be positive. Rhabdomyoblasts may stain for NSE and infrequently for cytokeratin. The alveolar variant has been reported to stain focally with S100. The differential diagnosis of bladder rhabdomyosarcoma includes pseudosarcomatous myofibroblastic tumor, leiomyosarcoma, neurofibroma, and sarcomatoid carcinoma. These tumors can often be distinguished on morphologic grounds.[517] Immunohistochemistry often points towards skeletal muscle differentiation.

## Angiosarcoma

Angiosarcoma of the bladder, which arises from blood vessel endothelium, is exceedingly rare and carries a very poor prognosis.[524–528] Seventy percent of patients die within 2 years of diagnosis. Angiosarcoma can arise in any part of the bladder, and the age at presentation ranges from 38 to 85 years.[524] There is a male preponderance. The development of angiosarcoma has been linked to certain environmental exposures, including vinyl chloride, arsenic, and therapeutic irradiation. All cases have presented with hematuria. Other reported symptoms include flank or groin pain and dysuria. The disease has often extended locally beyond the bladder or metastasized at time of presentation. Frequent sites of metastasis are the lung and liver.[524] Histologically, angiosarcoma of the bladder is composed of anastomosing vascular channels lined by atypical endothelial cells (Fig. 6-71). The endothelial cells are often pleomorphic with large hyperchromatic nuclei, prominent nucleoli and abundant mitotic figures. The vascular lining cells may protrude into the lumen, imparting a hobnail appearance. There may be no intervening stroma. The vascular channels range in size from small capillaries to sinusoidal spaces. A solid growth pattern of monomorphic epithelioid cells with vesicular chromatin and moderate eosinophilic cytoplasm arranged in sheets and nests has been described. Infiltration into the deep muscle layer may be present with either vascular or solid growth patterns. Immunohistochemically, angiosarcoma stains positively for vimentin, CD31, and CD34. The only reported epithelioid angiosarcoma of the bladder was negative for cytokeratins. The differential diagnosis for angiosarcoma of the bladder is hemangioma, which is usually small and lacks cytologic atypia, anastomosing channels, and solid areas. Kaposi's sarcoma may be seen in the urinary bladder, especially in immunocompromised patients. The differential also includes high-grade urothelial carcinoma.[524]

## Malignant fibrous histiocytoma

Primary malignant fibrous histiocytoma (MFH) of the bladder is rare.[2,472,529] It occurs most commonly in men from 45 to 79 years of age, with gross hematuria at the time of presentation. The tumor is often large at presentation and involves all layers of the bladder wall (Fig. 6-72). The overlying urothelium may be either normal or ulcerated. Four morphologic variants are recognized: myxoid, inflammatory, storiform–fascicular, and pleomorphic. Histologically, these tumors are composed of spindled or polygonal cells with variably sized oval to round nuclei. The nuclei have coarse chromatin and prominent nucleoli. Mitotic activity is

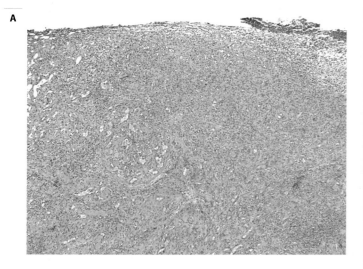

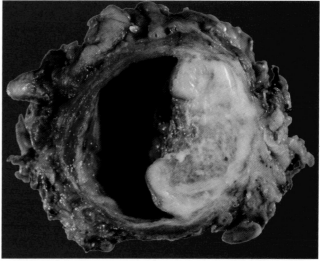

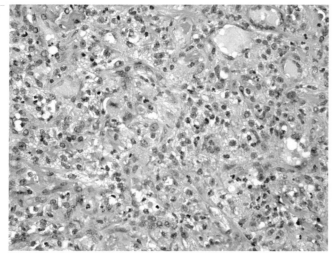

**Fig. 6-71** Angiosarcoma of the urinary bladder. (**A**) The surface epithelium is partially denuded. (**B**) The tumor is composed of anastomosing vascular channels lined by malignant endothelial cells.

**Fig. 6-72** Malignant fibrous histiocytoma of the urinary bladder. (**A**) The tumor is fleshy and necrotic, partially filling the lumen. (**B**) Spindled and pleomorphic cells with nuclear hyperchromasia, admixed with occasional giant cells, are arranged in a storiform and fascicular pattern.

usually moderate to high. Multinucleated giant cells are scattered throughout. Inflammatory-type malignant fibrous histiocytoma is characterized by an abundance of inflammatory cells, especially neutrophils infiltrating between fascicles of tumor cells.

Immunohistochemical stains can help differentiate malignant fibrous histiocytoma from other spindle cell neoplasms in the bladder. Typically, malignant fibrous histiocytoma is non-reactive for cytokeratin. It is often reactive for vimentin and $\alpha_1$-antichymotrypsin, and focally reactive for CD68. Some tumors have stained strongly for NSE and S100 protein.

Several tumors enter into the differential diagnosis of malignant fibrous histiocytoma. Sarcomatoid carcinoma of the bladder may have a similar appearance, but an epithelial component immunoreactive to cytokeratin and EMA is usually identifiable in sarcomatoid carcinoma. Differentiating malignant fibrous histiocytoma from pseudosarcomatous myofibroblastic tumor or postoperative spindle cell

nodule may be difficult. Mixed acute and chronic inflammatory cells and a history of a surgical procedure favor postoperative spindle cell nodule. Malignant fibrous histiocytoma of the bladder is a highly aggressive tumor with a high local recurrence rate and frequent metastases. Treatment usually is surgical with postoperative chemotherapy and radiation, but no therapy has yet been successful at prolonging survival.

## Osteosarcoma

Defined as a malignant tumor showing osteoid production, osteosarcoma of the urinary bladder occurs in males 60–65 years of age.[530–533] Some have a history of radiation therapy for urothelial carcinoma. Most osteosarcomas arise in the trigone region. Hematuria, dysuria, urinary frequency, and recurrent urinary tract infections are the most common presenting symptoms. Osteosarcoma of the urinary bladder presents as a solitary, large, polypoid, gritty, often deeply invasive, variably hemorrhagic mass. Histologically, tumors are composed of cytologically malignant cells surrounding variably calcified, woven bone lamellae. Foci of chondrosarcomatous differentiation or spindle cell areas may also be observed. The cytologic atypia differentiates osteosarcoma from stromal osseous metaplasia occurring in some urothelial carcinomas. By definition, a recognizable malignant epithelial component is diagnostic of sarcomatoid carcinoma even when osteoid is present. Urothelial sarcomatoid carcinoma is the most important differential diagnostic consideration for osteosarcoma of the bladder. Osteosarcoma of the urinary tract is an aggressive tumor associated with a poor prognosis. The majority of patients have advanced stage at presentation and die of disease within 6 months, often with lung metastases. The stage of the disease at time of diagnosis is the best predictor of survival.

## Other rare soft tissue tumors arising in the bladder

Other malignant mesenchymal neoplasms such as malignant peripheral nerve sheath tumor, liposarcoma, chondrosarcoma, hemangiopericytoma, and Kaposi's sarcoma may rarely involve the bladder.[469,470] The diagnosis requires that bladder involvement by direct extension from another site be excluded. In the case of primary chondrosarcoma of the bladder, sarcomatoid carcinoma must be excluded. A rare case of osteoclast-like giant cell tumor of the urinary bladder has been reported in a 73-year-old woman who had recurrence (Fig. 6-73).[298] The tumor is morphologically identical to those seen at osseous sites. Immunostaining for cytokeratin is negative. A single case report on alveolar soft part sarcoma arising in the bladder has been reported;[534] the tumor showed strong nuclear immunoreactivity for TFE3.

## Malignant melanoma

Malignant melanoma may occur in the urinary bladder as a primary tumor or as a metastasis. Primary melanoma in the bladder has been reported in fewer than 20 patients,[535,536] all adults, with men and women being equally affected. Gross hematuria is the most frequent presenting symptom but some patients with bladder melanoma have presented with symptomatic metastases. Metastatic melanoma is much more common than primary melanoma in the bladder. The generally accepted criteria for determining that melanoma is primary in the bladder are lack of a cutaneous lesion history, failure to find a regressed melanoma of the skin with a Woods' lamp examination, failure to find a different visceral primary, and pattern of spread consistent with bladder primary. Almost all of the tumors have appeared darkly pigmented at cystoscopy and on gross pathologic examination (Fig. 6-74). Their sizes range from <1 cm to 8 cm. Histologically the tumors show classic features of malignant melanoma: pleomorphic nuclei, spindle and polygonal cytoplasmic contours, and intracytoplasmic melanin

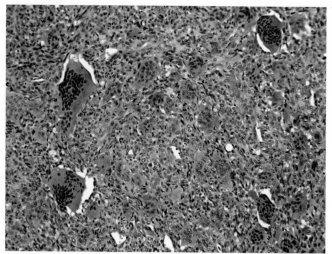

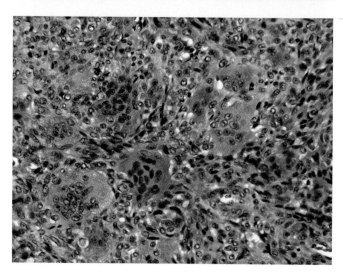

**Fig. 6-73** Osteoclast-like giant cell tumor of the urinary bladder. (**A, B**) Numerous osteoclast-like giants cells are seen. This rare tumor histologically resembles its counterpart in the bone and should not be confused with giant cell carcinoma (which falls into in the morphologic spectrum of large cell undifferentiated carcinoma). Immunohistochemical stains for cytokeratin were negative (not shown).

pigment. Pigment production is variable and may be absent. One example of clear cell melanoma has been reported. A few of the tumors are associated with melanosis of the vesical epithelium. One malignant melanoma arose in a bladder diverticulum.

Immunohistochemical procedures have shown positive reactions with antibodies to S100 protein and with HMB-45 or MelanA. Two-thirds of the patients have died of metastatic melanoma within 3 years of diagnosis. Follow-up of those alive at the time of other reports has been less than 2 years.

## Germ cell tumors

A number of germ cell neoplasms may arise rarely in the bladder, including dermoid cyst, teratoma,

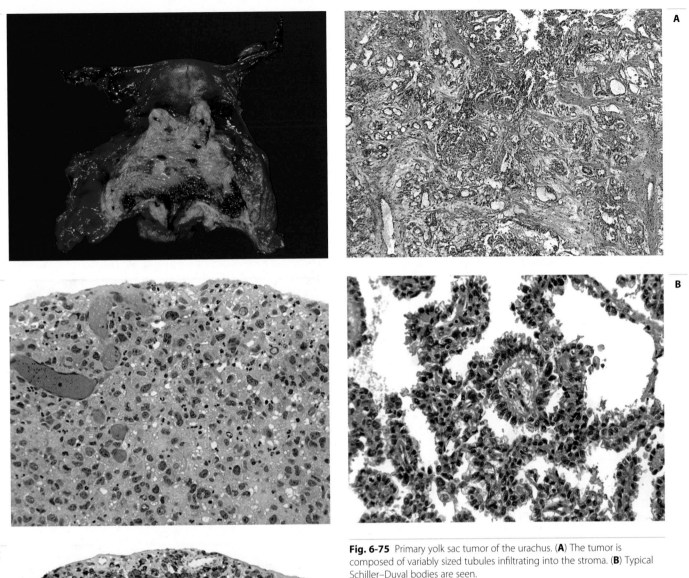

**Fig. 6-75** Primary yolk sac tumor of the urachus. (**A**) The tumor is composed of variably sized tubules infiltrating into the stroma. (**B**) Typical Schiller–Duval bodies are seen.

**Fig. 6-74** Malignant melanoma involving the bladder neck. (**A**) The mucosa displays jet-black pigmentation. (**B**) The tumor cells have abundant eosinophilic cytoplasm and prominent nucleoli. (**C**) HMB-45 immunostaining is strongly and diffusely positive.

seminoma, choriocarcinoma, and yolk sac tumor (Fig. 6-75).[290,291,294,295,529,537–547] Rare cases of teratoma arising in the bladder have been described in both adults and children. Dermoid cyst typically occurs in women between 30 and 49 years of age who present with non-specific bladder symptoms. Typical histologic features include calcifications and structures consistent with hair and/or teeth.

Pure choriocarcinoma of the bladder in the absence of recognizable papillary or solid urothelial carcinoma is rare and is associated with an aggressive clinical course. Diagnostic features include syncytiotrophoblastic giant cells and cytotrophoblast cells that display human chorionic gonadotropin (HCG) immunoreactivity. Choriocarcinoma should not be confused with urothelial carcinoma with syncytiotrophoblastic giant cells (see previous discussion). One reported case had isochromosome 12 by fluorescence in situ hybridization.[548] Patients usually have symptoms typical of other bladder cancers, including hematuria, dysuria, and frequency. Some male patients may have gynecomastia. Increased urinary levels of HCG may be present.

## Hematologic malignancies

Malignant lymphoma may occur in the urinary bladder as a primary lesion or as part of a systemic disease.[549-555] Lymphomas constitute less than 1% of bladder neoplasms. Secondary involvement of the bladder is common (12–20%) in advanced-stage systemic lymphoma. Bladder lymphomas may form solitary (70%) or multiple (20%) masses at cystoscopy. Occasionally (10%) there may be diffuse thickening of the bladder wall. Ulceration is rare (<20%) in primary but common in secondary lesions. Frankly hemorrhagic changes of the mucosa have been observed. The etiology of bladder lymphoma remains unclear. Schistosomiasis is associated with a T-cell lymphoma of the bladder. Papillary uro-

thelial tumors may present simultaneously with bladder lymphoma, either primary or secondary. Primary marginal zone B-cell lymphoma of mucosa-associated lymphoid tissue (MALT lymphoma) of the bladder has an excellent prognosis after therapy (Fig. 6-76).[555] Lymphoepithelial lesions may be seen and should not be confused with lymphoepithelioma-like carcinoma or lymphoid-rich variant urothelial carcinoma. Other types of primary bladder lymphoma, such as Burkitt's lymphoma, T-cell lymphoma, Hodgkin's lymphoma, and plasmacytoma are very rare. Among secondary bladder lymphomas, diffuse large B-cell lymphoma is the single most frequent histological subtype, followed by follicular, small cell, low-grade MALT, mantle cell, Burkitt's and Hodgkin's lymphomas. Involvement of the urinary bladder by acute myeloid leukemia (granulocytic sarcoma or myeloid sarcoma) is rare, and relevant clinical data and a high index of suspicion are critical to avoid misdiagnosis (Fig. 6-77).[556–558]

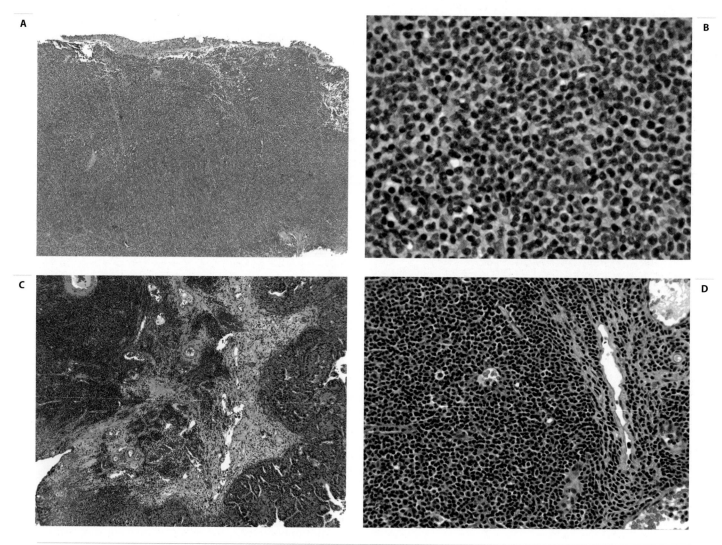

**Fig. 6-76** Lymphoma involving the urinary bladder. (**A, B**) Primary marginal zone B-cell lymphoma of mucosa-associated lymphoid tissue (MALT lymphoma). The surface epithelium is largely intact. The tumor is composed of diffuse sheets of small to medium sized lymphoid cells with pale cytoplasm. (**C, D**) A case of co-existing small lymphocytic lymphoma and transitional cell (urothelial) carcinoma

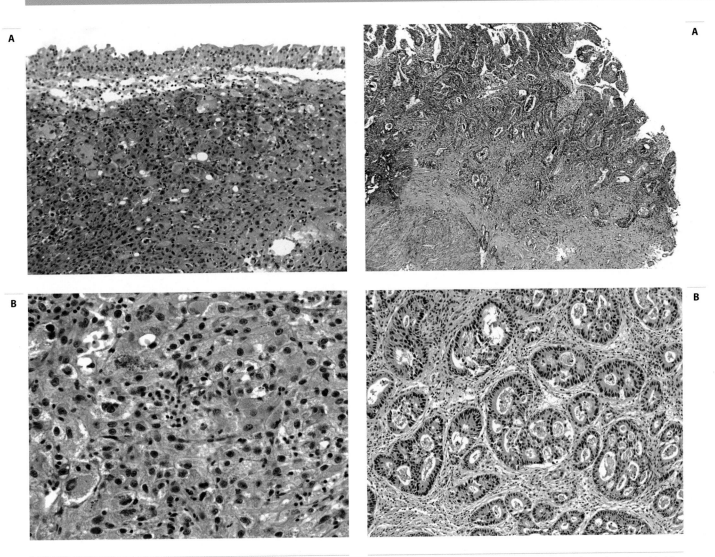

**Fig. 6-77** Granulocytic sarcoma. The bladder is involved by acute myeloid leukemia. Tumor is composed of immature myeloid cells including promyelocytes and myeloblasrs.

**Fig. 6-78** Metastatic colonic adenocarcinoma involving the urinary bladder.

## Metastatic tumors and secondary extension

The urinary bladder is secondarily involved by a wide spectrum of malignancies. The most common primary sites and their relative frequencies include the colon (Fig. 6-78) (21%), prostate (Fig. 6-79), (19%), rectum (12%), and cervix (11%).[559] Most tumors from these sites involve the bladder by direct extension. The most common distant sites of origin of tumors metastatic to the bladder and their relative frequencies are the stomach (4.3%), skin (3.9%), lung (2.8%), and breast (2.5%). Secondary tumor deposits are almost always solitary (96.7%), and 54% of these are located in the bladder neck or trigone. Over half of secondary tumors are adenocarcinomas. In terms of differential diagnosis, few secondary tumors have distinctive histological features, making it difficult to make the appropriate diagnosis. Hence knowledge of the history and clinical setting is particularly important in these cases. Immunohistochemistry is useful for distinguishing primary tumors of the urinary bladder from metastases or direct extension from other sites.[61,560]

### Metastatic urothelial carcinoma

When urothelial carcinoma presents at other sites, recognition of urothelial origin may be difficult, particularly as squamous and glandular differentiation are common in high-grade urothelial carcinoma (Fig. 6-80). Differential cytokeratin expression may be of value in the confirmation of metastatic urothelial carcinoma.[561–564] Expression of the combination of thrombomodulin, high molecular weight cytokeratin (34βE12), and cytokeratin 20 is strongly suggestive of urothelial origin in the setting of metastatic carcinoma of unknown primary, whereas the expression of two

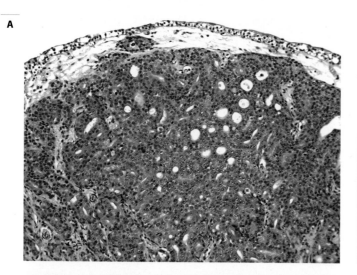

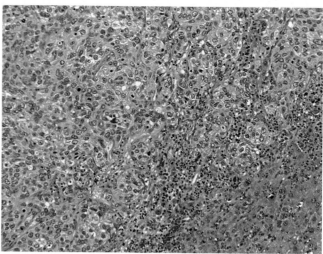

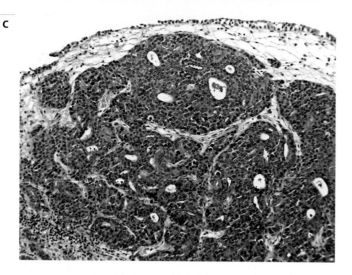

**Fig. 6-79** (**A, B**) Prostatic adenocarcinoma (ductal type) involving the urinary bladder. The urothelium is intact. (**C**) Tumor cells show positive immunostaining for PSA.

**Fig. 6-80** Metastatic urothelial carcinoma involving the liver.

of these three is still suggestive, albeit more weakly.[565] Expression of uroplakin III is highly specific for tumors of urothelial origin[565–568] Ovarian Brenner tumors, which histologically resemble urothelial neoplasms, may stain with uroplakin III and may therefore be included as a possible alternative primary site for uroplakin III-positive metastatic carcinomas in female patients.[566,568] Some immunophenotypic differences between Brenner tumors and urothelial carcinomas of the bladder do exist. Urothelial carcinomas are frequently positive for thrombomodulin and cytokeratin 20, whereas Brenner tumors typically do not stain with these antibodies.[569] Ovarian transitional cell carcinomas rarely (6%) express uroplakin III and typically have a uroplakin III–/cytokeratin 20–/WT1+ phenotype, in contrast to the uroplakin III+ phenotype observed in 82% of Brenner tumors.[568] In fact, the differences in staining with uroplakin III and other markers suggests that Brenner tumors are the only true urothelial neoplasms of the ovary, with ovarian transitional cell carcinomas representing a pattern of poorly differentiated adenocarcinoma.[570]

# REFERENCES

1. Jemal A, Siegel R, Ward E, et al. Cancer statistics, 2007. CA Cancer J Clin 2007; 57: 43–66.

2. Eble JN, Sauter G, Epstein JI, et al. World Health Organization Classification of Tumours: Pathology and genetics of tumours of the urinary system and male genital organs. Lyon, France: IARC Press, 2004.

3. Cheng L, Darson M, Cheville JC, et al. Urothelial papilloma of the bladder: clinical and biologic implications. Cancer 1999; 86: 2098–2101.

4. McKenney JK, Amin MB, Young RH. Urothelial (transitional cell) papilloma of the urinary bladder: a clinicopathologic study of 26 cases. Mod Pathol 2003; 16: 623–629.

5. Mostofi FK, Sobin LH, Torloni H. Histological typing of urinary bladder tumours. Geneva: World Health Organization, 1973.

6. Bergkvist A, Ljungqvist A, Moberger G. Classification of bladder tumours based on the cellular pattern. A preliminary report of a clinical-pathological study of 300 cases with a minimum follow-up of eight years. Acta Chir Scand 1965; 130: 371–378.

7. Eble JN, Young RH. Benign and low-grade papillary lesions of the urinary bladder: A review of the papilloma-papillary carcinoma controversy, and a report of five typical papillomas. Semin Diagn Pathol 1989; 6: 351–371.

8. Bostwick DG. Natural history of early bladder cancer. J Cell Biochem 1992; 161: 31–38.

9. Bostwick DG, Ramnani DM, Cheng L. Diagnosis and grading of bladder cancer and associated lesions. Urol Clin North Am 1999; 26: 493–507.

10. van Rhijn BW, Montironi R, Zwarthoff EC, et al. Frequent FGFR3 mutations in urothelial papilloma. J Pathol 2002; 198: 245–251.

11. Harnden P, Mahmood N, Southgate J. Expression of cytokeratin 20 redefines urothelial papillomas of the bladder. Lancet 1999; 353: 974–977.

12. Mostofi FK. Pathological aspects and spread of carcinoma of the bladder. JAMA 1968; 206: 1764–1769.

13. Sung MT, MacLennan GT, Lopez-Beltran A, et al. Natural history of urothelial inverted papilloma. Cancer 2006; 107: 2622–2627.

14. Kunze E, Schauer A, Schmitt M. Histology and histogenesis of two different types of inverted urothelial papillomas. Cancer 1983; 51: 348–358.

15. Cheng CW, Chan LW, Chan CK, et al. Is surveillance necessary for inverted papilloma in the urinary bladder and urethra? Aust NZ J Surg 2005; 75: 213–217.

16. Witjes JA, van Balken MR, van de Kaa CA. The prognostic value of a primary inverted papilloma of the urinary tract. J Urol 1997; 158: 1500–1505.

17. Cheville JC, Wu K, Sebo TJ, et al. Inverted urothelial papilloma: is ploidy, MIB-1 proliferative activity, or p53 protein accumulation predictive of urothelial carcinoma? Cancer 2000; 88: 632–636.

18. Goertchen R, Seidenschnur A, Stosiek P. Clinical pathology of inverted papillomas of the urinary bladder. A complex morphologic and catamnestic study. Pathologe 1994; 15: 279–285.

19. Potts IF, Hirst E. Inverted papilloma of the bladder. J Urol 1963; 90: 175–179.

20. Paschkis R. Über adenoma der harnblase. Ztschr Urol Chir 1927; 21: 315–325.

21. Jones TD, Zhang S, Lopez-Beltran A, et al. Urothelial carcinoma with an inverted growth pattern can be distinguished from inverted papilloma by fluorescence in-situ hybridization, immunohistochemistry, and morphologic analysis. Am J Surg Pathol 2007; 31: 1861–1867.

22. Asano K, Miki J, Maeda S, et al. Clinical studies on inverted papilloma of the urinary tract: report of 48 cases and review of the literature. J Urol 2003; 170: 1209–1212.

23. Cameron KM, Lupton CH. Inverted papilloma of the lower urinary tract. Br J Urol 1976; 48: 567–577.

24. Mattelaer J, Leonard A, Goddeeris P, et al. Inverted papilloma of bladder: clinical significance. Urology 1988; 32: 192–197.

25. Sung MT, Eble JN, Wang M, et al. Inverted papilloma of the urinary bladder: a molecular genetic appraisal. Mod Pathol 2006; 19: 1289–1294.

26. Baud E, Catilina P, Boiteux J-P, et al. Human bladder cancers and normal bladder mucosa present the same hot spot of heterozygous chromosome-9 deletion. Int J Cancer 1998; 77: 821–824.

27. Keen AJ, Knowles MA. Definition of two regions of deletion on chromosome 9 in carcinoma of the bladder. Oncogene 1994; 9: 2083–2088.

28. Cheng L, Jones TD, McCarthy RP, et al. Molecular genetic evidence for a common clonal origin of urinary bladder small cell carcinoma and coexisting urothelial carcinoma. Am J Pathol 2005; 166: 1533–1539.

29. Louhelainen J, Wijkstrom H, Hemminki K. Multiple regions with allelic loss at chromosome 3 in superficial multifocal bladder tumors. Int J Oncol 2001; 18: 203–210.

30. Paterson RF, Ulbright TM, MacLennan GT, et al. Molecular genetic alterations in the laser-capture-microdissected stroma adjacent to bladder carcinoma. Cancer 2003; 98: 1830–1836.

31. Jones TD, Wang M, Eble JN, et al. Molecular evidence supporting field effect in urothelial carcinogenesis. Clin Cancer Res 2005; 11: 6512–6519.

32. Primdahl H, von der Masse H, Christensen M, et al. Allelic deletions of cell growth regulators during progression of bladder cancer. Cancer Res 2000; 60: 6623–6629.

33. Cheng L, MacLennan GT, Zhang S, et al. Laser capture microdissection analysis reveals frequent allelic losses in papillary urothelial neoplasm of low malignant potential of the urinary bladder. Cancer 2004; 101: 183–188.

34. Junker K, Boerner D, Schulze W, et al. Analysis of genetic alterations in normal bladder urothelium. Urology 2003; 62: 1134–1138.

35. Cheng L, Leibovich BC, Cheville JC, et al. Squamous papilloma of the urinary tract is unrelated to condyloma acuminata. Cancer 2000; 88: 1679–1686.

36. Guo CC, Fine SW, Epstein JI. Non-invasive squamous lesions in the urinary bladder: a clinicopathologic analysis of 29 cases. Am J Surg Pathol 2006; 30: 883–891.

37. Lopez-Beltran A, Cheng L, Andersson L, et al. Preneoplastic non-papillary lesions and conditions of the urinary bladder: an update based on the Ancona International Consultation. Virchows Arch 2002; 440: 3–11.

38. Cheng L, Cheville JC, Neumann RM, et al. Flat intraepithelial lesions of the urinary bladder. Cancer 2000; 88: 625–631.

39. Lopez-Beltran A, Requena MJ, Luque RJ, et al. Cyclin D3 expression in primary Ta/T1 bladder cancer. J Pathol 2006; 209: 106–113.

40. Droller MJ. Bladder cancer: State-of-the-art care. CA Cancer J Clin 1998; 48: 269–284.

41. Cheng L, Bostwick DG, Li G, et al. Conserved genetic findings in metastatic bladder cancer. A possible utility of allelic loss of chromosomes 9p21 and 17p13 in diagnosis. Arch Pathol Lab Med 2001; 125: 1197–1199.

42. Cheng L, Gu J, Ulbright TM, et al. Precise microdissection of human bladder carcinomas reveals divergent tumor subclones in the same tumor. Cancer 2002; 94: 104–110.

43. Jones TD, Carr MD, Eble JN, et al. Clonal origin of lymph node metastases in bladder carcinoma. Cancer 2005; 104: 1901–1910.

44. van Rhijn BW, van der Kwast TH, Vis AN, et al. FGFR3 and P53 characterize alternative genetic pathways in the pathogenesis of urothelial cell carcinoma. Cancer Res 2004; 64: 1911–1914.

45. van Rhijn BW, Lurkin I, Radvanyi F, et al. The fibroblast growth factor receptor 3 (FGFR3) mutation is a strong indicator of superficial bladder cancer with low recurrence rate. Cancer Res 2001; 61: 1265–1268.

46. Sung MT, Wang M, MacLennan G, et al. Histogenesis of sarcomatoid urothelial carcinoma of the urinary bladder: evidence for a common clonal origin with divergent differentiation. J Pathol 2007; 211: 420–430.

47. Muto S, Horie S, Takahashi S, et al. Genetic and epigenetic alterations in normal bladder epithelium in patients with metachronous bladder cancer. Cancer Res 2000; 60: 4021–4025.

48. Davidson DD, Cheng L. Field cancerization in the urothelium of the bladder. Anal Quant Cytol Histol 2006; 28: 337–338.

49. Knowles MA, Currie GA. Genetic alterations in bladder cancer. Lancet 1993; 342: 1184.

50. Knowles MA. The genetics of transitional cell carcinoma: progress and potential clinical application. BJU Int 1999; 84: 412–427.

51. Knowles MA, Habuchi T, Kennedy W, et al. Mutation spectrum of the 9q34 tuberous sclerosis gene TSC1 in transitional cell carcinoma of the bladder. Cancer Res 2003; 63: 7652–7656.

52. Kiemeney L, Witjes J, Heibroek R, et al. Dysplasia in normal-looking urothelium increases the risk of tumour progression in primary superficial bladder cancer. Eur J Cancer 1994; 30A: 1621–1625.

53. Montironi R, Scarpelli M, Mazzucchelli R, et al. Subvisual changes in chromatin organization state are detected by karyometry in the histologically normal urothelium in patients with synchronous papillary carcinoma. Hum Pathol 2003; 34: 893–901.

54. Mazzucchelli R, Barbisan F, Stramazzotti D, et al. Chromosomal abnormalities in macroscopically normal urothelium in patients with bladder pT1 and pT2a urothelial carcinoma: a fluorescence in situ hybridization study and correlation with histologic features. Anal Quant Cytol Histol 2005; 27: 143–151.

55. Hartmann A, Moser K, Kriegmair M, et al. Frequent genetic alterations in simple urothelial hyperplasias of the bladder in patients with papillary urothelial carcinoma. Am J Pathol 1999; 154: 721–727.

56. Hartmann A, Schlake G, Zaak D, et al. Occurrence of chromosome 9 and p53 alterations in multifocal dysplasia and carcinoma in situ of human urinary bladder. Cancer Res 2002; 62: 809–818.

57. Chow N, Cairns P, Eisenberger CF, et al. Papillary urothelial hyperplasia is a clonal precursor to papillary transitional cell bladder cancer. Int J Cancer 2000; 89: 514–518.

58. Epstein JL, Amin MB, Reuter VR, et al. The Bladder Consensus Conference Committee. The World Health Organization/International Society of Urologic Pathology consensus classification of urothelial (transitional cell) neoplasms of the urinary bladder. Am J Surg Pathol 1998; 22: 1435–1438.

59. Cheng L, Cheville JC, Neumann RM, et al. Natural history of urothelial dysplasia of the bladder. Am J Surg Pathol 1999; 23: 443–447.

60. Harnden P, Eardley I, Joyce AD, et al. Cytokeratin 20 as an objective marker of urothelial dysplasia. Br J Urol 1996; 78: 870–875.

61. Emerson RE, Cheng L. Immunohistochemical markers in the evaluation of tumors of the urinary bladder: a review. Anal Quant Cytol Histol 2005; 27: 301–316.

62. Mallofre C, Castillo M, Morente V, et al. Immunohistochemical expression of CK20, p53, and Ki-67 as objective markers of urothelial dysplasia. Mod Pathol 2003; 16: 187–191.

63. McKenney JK, Desai S, Cohen C, et al. Discriminatory immunohistochemical staining of urothelial carcinoma in situ and non-neoplastic urothelium: an analysis of cytokeratin 20, p53, and CD44 antigens. Am J Surg Pathol 2001; 25: 1074–1078.

64. Shirai T, Fukushima S, Hirose M, et al. Epithelial lesions of the urinary bladder in 313 autopsy cases. Jpn J Cancer Res 1987; 78: 1073–1080.

65. Zuk R, Rogers H, Martin J, et al. Clinicopathological importance of primary dsyplasia of bladder. J Clin Pathol 1988; 41: 1277–1280.

66. Baithun S, Rogers H, Martin J, et al. Primary dysplasia of bladder. Lancet 1988; 1: 483.

67. Cooper P, Waisman J, Johnston W, et al. Severe atypia of transitional epithelium and carcinoma of the urinary bladder. Cancer 1973; 31: 1055–1060.

68. Eisenberg R, Roth R, Schweinsberg M. Bladder tumors and associated proliferative mucosal lesions. J Urol 1960; 84: 544–550.

69. Harewood LM. The significance of urothelial dysplasia as diagnosed by cup biopsies. Aust NZ J Surg 1986; 56: 199–203.

70. Kakizoe T, Matumoto K, Nishio Y, et al. Significance of carcinoma in situ and dysplasia association with bladder cancer. J Urol 1985; 133: 395–398.

71. Schade RO, Swinney J. Pre-cancerous changes in bladder epithelium. Lancet 1968; 2: 943–946.

72. Wolf H, Hojgaard K. Urothelial dysplasia in random mucosal biopsies from patients with bladder tumors. Scand J Urol Nephrol 1980; 14: 37–41.

73. Smith G, Elton RA, Beynon LL, et al. Prognostic significance of biopsy results of normal-looking mucosa in cases of superficial bladder cancer. Br J Urol 1983; 55: 665–669.

74. Althausen A, Prout G, Daly J. Non-invasive papillary carcinoma of the bladder associated with carcinoma in situ. J Urol 1976; 116: 575–580.

75. Gibbons R, Mandler J, Harmann W. The significance of epithelial atypia seen in non-invasive transitional cell papillary tumors of the bladder. J Urol 1969; 102: 195–199.

76. Murphy WM, Nagy GK, Rao MK, et al. 'Normal' urothelium in patients with bladder cancer: a preliminary report from the National Bladder Cancer Collaborative Group A. Cancer 1979; 44: 1050–1058.

77. Murphy WM, Soloway MS. Developing carcinoma (dysplasia) of the urinary bladder. Pathol Annu 1982; 17: 197–217.

78. Murphy WM, Soloway MS. Urothelial dysplasia. J Urol 1982; 127: 849–854.

79. Wolf H, Hojgaard K. Urothelial dysplasia concomitant with bladder tumours as a determinant factor for future new occurrences. Lancet 1983; 134–136.

80. Wolf H, Olsen P, Hojgaard K. Urothelial dysplasia concomitant with bladder tumours: a determinant for future new occurrences in patients treated by full-course radiotherapy. Lancet 1985; 1: 1005–1008.

81. Melamed M, Voutsa N, Grabstald H. Natural history and clinical behavior of in situ carcinoma of the human urinary bladder. Cancer 1964; 17: 1533–1545.

82. Cheng L, Cheville JC, Neumann RM, et al. Survival of patients with carcinoma in situ of the urinary bladder. Cancer 1999; 85: 2469–2474.

83. Farrow G. Pathology of carcinoma in situ of the urinary bladder and related lesions. J Cell Biochem 1992; 161: 39–43.

84. Orozco R, Martin A, Murphy W. Carcinoma in situ of the urinary bladder: Clues to host involvement in human carcinogenesis. Cancer 1994; 74: 115–122.

85. Batista J, Palou J, Iglesias J, et al. Significance of urethral carcinoma in situ in specimens of cystectomy. Eur Urol 1994; 25: 313–315.

86. Khan AU, Farrow GM, Zincke H, et al. Primary carcinoma in situ of the ureter and renal pelvis. J Urol 1979; 121: 681–683.

87. Mahadevia PS, Koss LG, Tar IJ. Prostatic involvement in bladder cancer. Prostate mapping in 20 cystoprostatectomy specimens. Cancer 1986; 58: 2096–2102.

88. Farrow G, Utz D, Rife C. Morphological and clinical observations of patients with early bladder cancer treated with total cystectomy. Cancer Res 1976; 36: 2495–2501.

89. Farrow GM, Utz D, Rife C, et al. Clinical observations on sixty-nine cases of in situ carcinoma of the urinary bladder. Cancer Res 1977; 37: 2794–2798.

90. Farrow GM, Barlebo H, Enjoji M, et al. Transitional cell carcinoma in situ. Prog Clin Biol Res 1986; 221: 85–96.

91. Koss LG, Tiamson EM, Robbins MA. Mapping cancerous and precancerous bladder changes. A study of the

urothelium in ten surgically removed bladders. JAMA 1974; 227: 281–286.

92. Lamm DL. Carcinoma in situ. Urol Clin North Am 1992; 19: 499–508.

93. Kirkali Z, Chan T, Manoharan M, et al. Bladder cancer: epidemiology, staging and grading, and diagnosis. Urology 2005; 66: 4–34.

94. McKenney JK, Amin MB. The role of immunohistochemistry in the diagnosis of urinary bladder neoplasms. Semin Diagn Pathol 2005; 22: 69–87.

95. Desai S, Lim SD, Jimenez RE, et al. Relationship of cytokeratin 20 and CD44 protein expression with WHO/ ISUP grade in pTa and pT1 papillary urothelial neoplasia. Mod Pathol 2000; 13: 1315–1323.

96. Soini Y, Turpeenniemi HT, Kamel D, et al. p53 immunohistochemistry in transitional cell carcinoma and dysplasia of the urinary bladder correlates with disease progression. Br J Cancer 1993; 68: 1029–1035.

97. Schmitz-Drager BJ, van Roeyen CR, Grimm MO, et al. P53 accumulation in precursor lesions and early stages of bladder cancer. World J Urol 1994; 12: 79–83.

98. Wagner U, Sauter G, Moch H, et al. Patterns of p53, erbB-2, and EGF-r expression in premalignant lesions of the urinary bladder. Hum Pathol 1995; 26: 970–978.

99. McKenney JK, Gomez JA, Desai S, et al. Morphologic expressions of urothelial carcinoma in situ: a detailed evaluation of its histologic patterns with emphasis on carcinoma in situ with microinvasion. Am J Surg Pathol 2001; 25: 356–362.

100. Owens CL, Epstein JI. Significance of denuded urothelium in papillary urothelial lesions. Am J Surg Pathol 2007; 31: 298–303.

101. Farrow GM, Utz DC. Observation on microinvasive transitional cell carcinoma of the urinary bladder. Clin Oncol 1982; 1: 609–615.

102. Lopez-Beltran A, Cheng L. Stage pT1 bladder carcinoma: diagnostic criteria, pitfalls and prognostic significance. Pathology 2003; 35: 484–491.

103. Lopez-Beltran A, Luque RJ, Mazzuchelli R, et al. Changes produced in the urothelium by traditional and newer therapeutic procedures for bladder cancer. J Clin Pathol 2002; 55: 641–647.

104. Lopez-Beltran A. Bladder treatment. Immunotherapy and chemotherapy. Urol Clin North Am 1999; 26: 535–554.

105. Lopez-Beltran A. Urothelial changes induced by therapeutic procedures for bladder cancer. Anal Quant Cytol Histol 2006; 28: 339.

106. Lopez-Beltran A, Pacelli A, Rothenberg HJ, et al. Carcinosarcoma and sarcomatoid carcinoma of the bladder: clinicopathological study of 41 cases. J Urol 1998; 159: 1497–1503.

107. Pazzaglia S, Chen XR, Aamodt CB, et al. In vitro radiation-induced neoplastic progression of low-grade uroepithelial tumors. Radiat Res 1994; 138: 86–92.

108. Kanno J, Sakamoto A, Washizuka M, et al. Malignant mixed mesodermal tumor of bladder occurring after radiotherapy for cervical cancer: report of a case. J Urol 1985; 133: 854–856.

109. Chan TY, Epstein JI. Radiation or chemotherapy cystitis with 'pseudocarcinomatous' features. Am J Surg Pathol 2004; 28: 909–913.

110. Ferlay J, Bray F, Pisani P, et al. GLOBOCAN 2000: Cancer incidence, mortality and prevalence worldwide. Lyon, France: IARC Press, 2001.

111. Cohen SM, Shirai T, Steineck G. Epidemiology and etiology of premalignant and malignant urothelial changes. Scand J Urol Nephrol 2000; 205: 105–115.

112. Hartge P, Harvey EB, Linehan WM, et al. Unexplained excess risk of bladder cancer in men. 1: J Natl Cancer Inst 1990; 82: 1636–1640.

113. Zeegers MP, Kellen E, Buntinx F, et al. The association between smoking, beverage consumption, diet and bladder cancer: a systematic literature review. World J Urol 2004; 21: 392–401.

114. Droller MJ. Bladder cancer. J Urol 1997; 157: 1266–1267.

115. Escudero AL, Luque RJ, Quintero A, et al. Association of human herpesvirus type 6 DNA with human bladder cancer. Cancer Lett 2005; 230: 20–24.

116. Esrig D, Freeman JA, Stein JP, et al. Early cystectomy for clinical stage T1 transitional cell carcinoma of the bladder. Semin Urol Oncol 1997; 15: 154–160.

117. Weinstein RS. Origin and dissemination of human urinary bladder carcinoma. Semin Oncol 1979; 6: 149–156.

118. Lutzeyer W, Rubben H, Dahm H. Prognostic parameters in superficial bladder cancer: an analysis of 315 cases. J Urol 1982; 127: 250–252.

119. Kiemeney LA, Witjes JA, Heijbroek RP, et al. Predictability of recurrent and progressive disease in individual patients with primary superficial bladder cancer. J Urol 1993; 150: 60–64.

120. Cheng L, MacLennan GT, Pan CX, et al. Allelic loss of the active X chromosome during bladder carcinogenesis. Arch Pathol Lab Med 2004; 128: 187–190.

121. Sidransky EA, Frost P, von Eschenbach A, et al. Clonal origin of bladder cancer. N Engl J Med 1992; 326: 737–740.

122. Habuchi T, Takahashi R, Yamada H, et al. Metachronous multifocal development of urothelial cancers by intraluminal seeding. Lancet 1993; 342: 1087–1088.

123. Miyao N, Tsai YC, Lerner SP, et al. Role of chromosome 9 in human bladder cancer. Cancer Res 1993; 53: 4066–4070.

124. Xu X, Stower MJ, Reid IN, et al. Molecular screening of multifocal transitional cell carcinoma of the bladder using p53 mutations as biomarkers. Clin Cancer Res 1996; 2: 1795–1800.

125. Chern HD, Becich MJ, Persad RA, et al. Clonal analysis of human recurrent superficial bladder cancer by immunohistochemistry of P53 and retinoblastoma proteins. J Urol 1996; 156: 1846–1849.

126. Takahashi T, Kakehi Y, Mitsumori K, et al. Distinct microsatellite alterations in upper urinary tract tumors and subsequent bladder tumors. J Urol 2001; 165: 672–677.

127. Takahashi T, Habuchi T, Kakehi Y, et al. Clonal and chronological genetic analysis of multifocal cancers of the bladder and upper urinary tract. Cancer Res 1998; 58: 5835–5841.

128. Li M, Cannizzaro LA. Identical clonal origin of synchronous and metachronous low-grade, non-invasive papillary transitional cell carcinomas of the urinary tract. Hum Pathol 1999; 30: 1197–1200.

129. Fadl-Elmula I, Gorunova L, Mandahl N, et al. Cytogenetic monoclonality in multifocal uroepithelial carcinomas: evidence of intraluminal tumour seeding. Br J Cancer 1999; 81: 6–12.

130. Hartmann A, Rosner U, Schlake G, et al. Clonality and genetic divergence in multifocal low-grade superficial urothelial carcinoma as determined by chromosome 9 and p53 deletion analysis. Lab Invest 2000; 80: 709–718.

131. Hafner C, Knuechel R, Zanardo L, et al. Evidence for oligoclonality and tumor spread by intraluminal seeding in multifocal urothelial carcinomas of the upper and lower urinary tract. Oncogene 2001; 20: 4910–4915.

132. Simon R, Eltze E, Schafer KL, et al. Cytogenetic analysis of multifocal bladder cancer supports a monoclonal origin and intraepithelial spread of tumor cells. Cancer Res 2001; 61: 355–362.

133. Goto K, Konomoto T, Hayashi K, et al. p53 mutations in multiple urothelial carcinomas: a molecular analysis of the development of multiple carcinomas. Mod Pathol 1997; 10: 428–437.

134. Spruck CH 3rd, Ohneseit PF, Gonzalez-Zulueta M, et al. Two molecular pathways to transitional cell carcinoma of the bladder. Cancer Res 1994; 54: 784–788.

135. Petersen I, Ohgaki H, Ludeke BI, et al. p53 mutations in phenacetin-associated human urothelial carcinomas. Carcinogenesis 1993; 14: 2119–2122.

136. Yoshimura I, Kudoh J, Saito S, et al. p53 gene mutation in recurrent superficial bladder cancer. J Urol 1995; 153: 1711–1715.

341

137. Stoehr R, Hartmann A, Hiendlmeyer E, et al. Oligoclonality of early lesions of the urothelium as determined by microdissection-supported genetic analysis. Pathobiology 2000; 68: 165–172.

138. Cianciulli AM, Leonardo C, Guadagni F, et al. Genetic instability in superficial bladder cancer and adjacent mucosa: an interphase cytogenetic study. Hum Pathol 2003; 34: 214–221.

139. Hafner C, Knuechel R, Stoehr R, et al. Clonality of multifocal urothelial carcinomas: 10 years of molecular genetic studies. Int J Cancer 2002; 101: 1–6.

140. MacLennan GT, Kirkali Z, Cheng L. Histologic grading of non-invasive papillary urothelial neoplasms. Eur Urol 2007; 51: 889–898.

141. Jones TD, Cheng L. Papillary urothelial neoplasm of low malignant potential: evolving terminology and concepts. J Urol 2006; 175: 1995–2003.

142. Cheng L, Bostwick DG. World Health Organization and International Society of Urological Pathology classification and two-number grading system of bladder tumors: reply. Cancer 2000; 88: 1513–1516.

143. Montironi R, Lopez-Beltran A, Mazzucchelli R, et al. Classification and grading of the non-invasive neoplasms: recent advances and controversies. J Clin Pathol 2003; 56: 91–95.

144. Malmstrom PU, Bush C, Norlen BJ. Recurrence, progression, and survival in bladder cancer. A retrospective analysis of 232 patients with greater than or equal to 5-year follow-up. Scand J Urol Nephrol 1987; 21: 185–195.

145. Prout GJBB, Griffin PP, Friedell GH. Treated history of non-invasive grade 1 transitional cell carcinoma. The National Bladder Cancer Group. J Urol 1992; 148: 1413–1419.

146. Holmang S, Hedelin H, Anderstrom C, et al. The relationship among multiple recurrences, progression and prognosis of patients with stages Ta and T1 transitional cell cancer of the bladder followed for at least 20 years. J Urol 1995; 153: 1823–1827.

147. England HR, Paris AMI, Blandy JP. The correlation of T1 bladder tumour history with prognosis and follow-up requirements. Br J Urol 1981; 53: 593–597.

148. Leblanc B, Duclos AJ, Benard F, et al. Long-term followup of initial Ta grade 1 transitional cell carcinoma of the bladder. J Urol 1999; 162: 1946–1960.

149. Pocock RD, Ponder BAJ, O'Sullivan JP, et al. Prognostic factors in non-infiltrating carcinoma of the bladder: A preliminary report. Br J Urol 1982; 54: 711–715.

150. Gilbert HA, Logan JL, Kagan AR, et al. The natural history of papillary transitional cell carcinoma of the bladder and its treatment in any unselected population on the basis of

151. Heney NM, Ahmed S, Flanagan MJ, et al. Superficial bladder cancer: progression and recurrence. J Urol 1983; 130: 1083–1086.

152. Fitzpatrick JM, West AB, Butler MR, et al. Superficial bladder tumors (stage pTa, grades 1 and 2): The importance of recurrence pattern following initial resection. J Urol 1986; 135: 920–922.

153. Prout G, Bassil B, Griffin P. The treated histories of patients with Ta grade 1 transitional-cell carcinoma of the bladder. Arch Surg 1986; 121: 1463–1468.

154. Hemstreet GP 3rd, Rollins S, Jones P, et al. Identification of a high risk subgroup of grade 1 transitional cell carcinoma using image analysis based deoxyribonucleic acid ploidy analysis of tumor tissue. J Urol 1991; 146: 1525–1529.

155. Mufti GR, Virdi JS, Singh M. 'Solitary' Ta-T1 G1 bladder tumour – history and long-term prognosis. Eur Urol 1990; 18: 101–106.

156. Jordan AM, Weingarten J, Murphy WM. Transitional cell neoplasms of the urinary bladder. Can biologic potential be predicted from histologic grading? Cancer 1987; 60: 2766–2774.

157. Fitzpatrick JM. Superficial bladder carcinoma. World J Urol 1993; 11: 142–147.

158. Greene L, Hanash K, Farrow G. Benign papilloma or papillary carcinoma of the bladder. J Urol 1973; 110: 205–207.

159. Bostwick DG, Mikuz G. Urothelial papillary (exophytic) neoplasms. Virchows Arch 2002; 441: 109–116.

160. Pauwels RPE, Schapers RFM, Smeets AWGB, et al. Grading in superficial bladder cancer: morphological criteria. Br J Urol 1988; 61: 129–134.

161. Schapers RF, Pauwels RP, Wijnen JT, et al. A simplified grading method of transitional cell carcinoma of the urinary bladder: reproducibility, clinical significance and comparison with other prognostic parameters. Br J Urol 1994; 73: 625–631.

162. Carbin B, Ekman P, Gustafson H, et al. Grading of human urothelial carcinoma based on nuclear atypia and mitotic frequency. I. Histological description. J Urol 1991; 145: 968–971.

163. Lipponen PK, Eskelinen MJ, Kiviranta J, et al. Prognosis of transitional cell bladder cancer: a multivariate prognostic score for improved prediction. J Urol 1991; 146: 1535–1540.

164. Bostwick DG, Lopez-Beltran A. Bladder biopsy interpretation. Washington DC: United Pathologists Press, 1999.

165. Lopez-Beltran A, Montironi R. Non-invasive urothelial neoplasms: according to the most recent WHO classification. Eur Urol 2004; 46: 170–176.

166. Epstein JI, Amin MB, Reuter VR, et al. The World Health Organization/International Society of Urological Pathology consensus classification of urothelial (transitional cell) neoplasms of the urinary bladder. Bladder Consensus Conference Committee. Am J Surg Pathol 1998; 22: 1435–1448.

167. Alsheikh A, Mohamedali Z, Jones E, et al. Comparison of the WHO/ISUP classification and cytokeratin 20 expression in predicting the behavior of low-grade papillary urothelial tumors. World/Health Organization/Internattional Society of Urologic Pathology. Mod Pathol 2001; 14: 267–272.

168. Alvarez KJ, Lopez-Beltran A, Anglada CF, et al. Clinico-pathologic differences between bladder neoplasm with low malignant potential and low-grade carcinoma. Actas Urol Esp 2001; 25: 645–650.

169. Montironi R, Lopez-Beltran A. The 2004 WHO Classification of Bladder Tumors: a summary and commentary. Int J Surg Pathol 2005; 13: 143–153.

170. Cheng L, Neumann RM, Bostwick DG. Papillary urothelial neoplasms of low malignant potential. Clinical and biologic implications. Cancer 1999; 86: 2102–2108.

171. Fujii Y, Kawakami S, Koga F, et al. Long-term outcome of bladder papillary urothelial neoplasms of low malignant potential. BJU Int 2003; 92: 559–562.

172. Oosterhuis JSR, Janssen-Heijnen ML, Pauwels RP, et al. Histological grading of papillary urothelial carcinoma of the bladder: prognostic value of the 1998 WHO/ISUP classification system and comparison with conventional grading systems. J Clin Pathol 2002; 55: 900–905.

173. Pich A, Chiusa L, Formiconi A, et al. Biologic differences between non-invasive papillary urothelial neoplasms of low malignant potential and low-grade (grade 1) papillary carcinomas of the bladder. Am J Surg Pathol 2001; 25: 1528–1533.

174. Samaratunga H, Makarov DV, Epstein JN. Comparison of WHO/IUP and WHO classification of non-invasive papillary urothelial neoplasms for risk of progression. Urology 2002; 15: 315–319.

175. Holmang S, Andius P, Hedelin H, et al. Stage progression in Ta papillary urothelial tumors: relationship to grade, immunohistochemical expression of tumor markers, mitotic frequency and DNA ploidy. J Urol 2001; 165: 1124–1130.

176. Park YW, Shim SI, Lee QW, et al. ISUP/WHO classification of urothelial neoplasms of urinary bladder. Mod Pathol 2006; 9: 86A.

177. Murphy WM, Takezawa K, Maruniak NA. Interobserver discrepancy using the 1998 World Health Organization/International Society of Urologic Pathology classification of urothelial

neoplasms: practical choices for patient care. J Urol 2003; 168: 968–972.

178. Yorukoglu K, Tuna B, Dikicioglu E, et al. Reproducibility of the 1998 World Health Organization/International Society of Urologic Pathology classification of papillary urothelial neoplasms of the urinary bladder. Virchows Arch 2003; 443: 734–740.

179. Bol MG, Baak JP, Buhr-Wildhagen S, et al. Reproducibility and prognostic variability of grade and lamina propria invasion in stages Ta, T1 urothelial carcinoma of the bladder. J Urol 2003; 169: 1291–1294.

180. Mikuz G. The reliability and reproducibility of the different classifications of bladder cancer. In: Hauptmann S, Dietel M, Sorbrinho-Sinoes M (eds) Surgical pathology update 2001. Berlin: ABW-Wissenschaftsverlag, 2001; 114–115.

181. Habuchi T, Ogawa O, Kakehi Y, et al. Accumulated allelic losses in the development of invasive urothelial cancer. Int J Cancer 1993; 53: 5093–5095.

182. Mostofi FK, Davis CJ, Sesterhenn IA. WHO histologic typing of urinary bladder tumors. Berlin: Springer, 1999.

183. Cheng L, Neumann RM, Nehra A, et al. Cancer heterogeneity and its biologic implications in the grading of urothelial carcinoma. Cancer 2000; 88: 1663–1670.

184. Bircan S, Candir O, Serel TA. Comparison of WHO 1973, WHO/ ISUP 1998, WHO 1999 grade and combined scoring systems in evaluation of bladder carcinoma. Urol Int 2004; 73: 201–208.

185. Lopez-Beltran A, Sauter G, Gasser T, et al. Urothelial tumors: Infiltrating urothelial carcinoma. In: Eble JN, Epstein JI, Sesterhenn I, eds. World Health Organization Classification of Tumors. Pathology and gentics of tumors of the urinary system and male genital organs. Lyon, France: IARC Press, 2004.

186. Greene FL, Page DL, Flemming ID, et al. American Joint Committee on Cancer Staging Manual, 6th edn. New York: Springer-Verlag, 2002.

187. Cheng L, Weaver AL, Neumann RM, et al. Substaging of T1 bladder carcinoma based on the depth of invasion as measured by micrometer. A new proposal. Cancer 1999; 86: 1035–1043.

188. Cheng L, Neumann RM, Weaver AL, et al. Grading and staging of bladder carcinoma in transurethral resection specimens. Correlation with 105 matched cystectomy specimens. Am J Clin Pathol 2000; 113: 275–279.

189. Jimenez RE, Keany TE, Hardy HT, et al. pT1 Urothelial carcinoma of the bladder: Criteria for diagnosis, pitfalls, and clinical implications. Adv Anat Pathol 2000; 7: 13–25.

190. Tamas EF, Epstein JI. Detection of residual tumor cells in bladder biopsy specimens: pitfalls in the interpretation of cytokeratin stains. Am J Surg Pathol 2007; 31: 390–397.

191. Nieder AM, Brausi M, Lamm D, et al. Management of stage T1 tumors of the bladder: International Consensus Panel. Urology 2005; 66: 108–125.

192. Angulo JC, Lopez JI, Grignon DJ, et al. Muscularis mucosa differentiates two populations with different prognosis in stage T1 bladder cancer. Urology 1995; 45: 47–53.

193. Hasui Y, Osada Y, Kitada S, et al. Significance of invasion to the muscularis mucosae on the progression of superficial bladder cancer. Urology 1994; 43: 782–786.

194. Hermann GG, Horn T, Steven K. The influence of the level of lamina propria invasion and the prevalence of p53 nuclear accumulation on survival in stage T1 transitional cell bladder cancer. J Urol 1998; 159: 91–94.

195. Holmang S, Hedelin H, Anderstrom C, et al. The importance of the depth of invasion in stage T1 bladder carcinoma: a prospective cohort study. J Urol 1997; 157: 800–804.

196. Platz CE, Cohen MB, Jones MP, et al. Is microstaging of early invasive cancer of the urinary bladder possible or useful? Mod Pathol 1996; 11: 1035–1039.

197. Younes M, Sussman J, True LD. The usefulness of the level of the muscularis mucosae in the staging of invasive transitional cell carcinoma of the urinary bladder. Cancer 1990; 66: 543–548.

198. Sozen S, Akbal C, Sokmensuer C, et al. Microstaging of pT1 transitional cell carcinoma of the bladder: does it really differentiate two populations with different prognoses? Urol Int 2002; 69: 200–206.

199. Cheng L, Neumann RM, Weaver AL, et al. Predicting cancer progression in patients with stage T1 bladder carcinoma. J Clin Oncol 1999; 17: 3182–3187.

200. Cheng L, Neumann RM, Scherer BG, et al. Tumor size predicts the survival of patients with pathologic stage T2 bladder carcinoma: A critical evaluation of the depth of muscle invasion. Cancer 1999; 85: 2638–2647.

201. Dixon JS, Gosling JA. Histology and fine structure of the muscularis mucosae of the human urinary bladder. J Anat 1983; 136: 265–271.

202. Keep JC, Piehl M, Miller E, et al. Invasive carcinomas of the urinary bladder. Evaluation of tunica muscularis mucosae involvement. Am J Clin Pathol 1989; 91: 575–579.

203. Ro JY, Ayala AG, el-Naggar A. Muscularis mucosa of urinary bladder. Importance for staging and treatment. Am J Surg Pathol 1987; 11: 668–673.

204. Engel P, Anagnostaki L, Braendstrup O. The muscularis mucosae of the human urinary bladder. Scand J Urol Nephrol 1992; 26: 249–252.

205. Cheng L, Weaver AL, Bostwick DG. Predicting extravesical extension of bladder carcinoma: a novel method based on micrometer measurement of the depth of invasion in transurethral resection specimens. Urology 2000; 55: 668–672.

206. Mhawech P, Iselin C, Pelte MF. Value of immunohistochemistry in staging T1 urothelial bladder carcinoma. Eur Urol 2002; 42: 459–463.

207. Humphrey PA. Urinary bladder pathology 2004: an update. Ann Diagn Pathol 2004; 8: 380–389.

208. Jewett HJ. Carcinoma of the bladder: Influence of depth of infiltration on the 5-year results following complete extirpation of the primary growth. J Urol 1952; 67: 672–680.

209. Bayraktar Z GG, Ihsan AT, Sevin G.: Staging error in the bladder tumor: The correlation between stage of TUR and cystectomy. Int J Urol Nephrol 2002; 33: 627–629.

210. Herr HW. Staging invasive bladder tumors. J Surg Oncol 1992; 51: 217–220.

211. Herr HW. A proposed simplified staging system of invasive bladder tumors. Urol Int 1993; 50: 17–20.

212. Hall RR, Prout GR. Staging of bladder cancer: Is the tumor, node, metastasis system adequate? Semin Oncol 1990; 17: 517–523.

213. Skinner DG. Current state of classification and staging of bladder cancer. Cancer Res 1977; 37: 2838–2842.

214. Skinner DG. Current perspectives in the management of high grade invasive bladder cancer. Cancer 1980; 45: 1866–1874.

215. Cummings KB, Barone JG, Ward WS. Diagnosis and staging of bladder cancer. Urol Clin North Am 1992; 19: 455–465.

216. Bowles WT, Cordonnier JJ. Total cystectomy for carcinoma of the bladder. J Urol 1963; 90: 731–735.

217. Cox CE, Cass AS, Boyce WH. Bladder cancer: A 26-year review. Trans Am Assoc Genitourin Surg 1968; 60: 22–30.

218. Boileau MA, Johnson DE, Chan RC, et al. Bladder carcinoma. Results with preoperative radiation therapy and radical cystectomy. Urology 1980; 16: 569.

219. Beahrs JR, Fleming TR, Zincke H. Risk of local urethral recurrence after radical cystectomy for bladder cancer. J Urol 1984; 131: 264–266.

220. Bredael JJ, Croker BP, Glenn JF. The curability of invasive bladder cancer treated by radical cystectomy. Eur Urol 1980; 6: 206–210.

221. Cordonnier JJ. Simple cystectomy in the management of bladder carcinoma. Arch Surg 1974; 108: 190–191.

222. Mathur VK, Krahn HP, Ramsey EW. Total cystectomy for bladder cancer. J Urol 1981; 125: 784–786.

223. Pollack A, Zagars GK, Cole CJ, et al. The relationship of local control to distant metastasis in muscle invasive bladder cancer. J Urol 1995; 154: 2059–2064.

224. Pomerance A. Pathology and prognosis following total cystectomy for

carcinoma of bladder. Br J Urol 1972; 44: 451–458.

225. Prout GRJ. The surgical management of bladder carcinoma. Urol Clin North Am 1976; 3: 149–175.

226. Richie JP, Skinner DG, Kaufman JJ. Radical cystectomy for carcinoma of the bladder: 16 years of experience. J Urol 1975; 113: 186–189.

227. Richie JP, Skinner DG, Kaufman JJ. Carcinoma of the bladder: treatment by radical cystectomy. J Surg Res 18: 271–5, 1975.

228. Roehrborn CG, Sagalowsky AI, Peters PC. Long-term patient survival after cystectomy for regional metastastic transitional cell carcinoma of the bladder. J Urol 1991; 146: 36–39.

229. Skinner DG. Management of invasive bladder cancer: a meticulous pelvic node dissection can make a difference. J Urol 1982; 128: 34–36.

230. Sorensen BL, Ohlsen AS, Barlebo H. Carcinoma of the urinary bladder. Clinical staging and histologic grading in relation to survival. Scand J Urol Nephrol 1969; 3: 189–192.

231. Utz DC, Schmitz SE, Fugelso PD, et al. A clinicopathologic evaluation of partial cystectomy for carcinoma of the urinary bladder. Cancer 1975; 32: 1075–1077.

232. Whitemore WFJ. Management of invasive bladder neoplasms. Semin Urol 1983; 1: 34–41.

233. Wishnow KI, Levinson AK, Johnson DE, et al. Stage B (P 2/3A/N0) transitional cell carcinoma of bladder highly curable by radical cystectomy. Urology 1992; 39: 12–16.

234. Pearse HD, Reed RR, Hodges CV. Radical cystectomy for bladder cancer. J Urol 1978; 119: 216–218.

235. Montie JE, Straffon RA, Stewart BH. Radical cystectomy without radiation therapy for carcinoma of the bladder. J Urol 1984; 131: 477–482.

236. Pagano F, Bassi P, Galetti TP, et al. Results of contemporary radical cystectomy for invasive bladder cancer: A clinicopathological study with an emphasis on the inadequacy of the tumor, nodes and metastases classification. J Urol 1991; 145: 45–50.

237. Yu RJ, Stein JP, Cai J, et al. Superficial (pT2a) and deep (pT2b) muscle invasion in pathological staging of bladder cancer following radical cystectomy. J Urol 2006; 176: 493–498; discussion 498–499.

238. Girgin C, Sezer A, Delibas M, et al. Impact of the level of muscle invasion in organ-confined bladder cancer. Urol Int 2007; 78: 145–149.

239. Jewett HJ. Comments on the staging of invasive bladder cancer: two B's or not to B's: That is the question. [Editorial] J Urol 1978; 119: 39.

240. Jimenez RE, Gheiler E, Oskanian P, et al. Grading the invasive component of urothelial carcinoma of the bladder and its relationship with progression-free survival. Am J Surg Pathol 2000; 24: 980–987.

241. Quek ML, Stein JP, Clark PE, et al. Microscopic and gross extravesical extension in pathological staging of bladder cancer. J Urol 2004; 171: 640–645.

242. Esrig D, Freeman JA, Elmajian DA, et al. Transitional cell carcinoma involving the prostate with a proposed staging classification for stromal invasion. J Urol 1996; 156: 1071–1076.

243. Pagano F, Bassi P, Ferrante GL, et al. Is stage pT4a (D1) reliable in assessing transitional cell carcinoma involvement of the prostate in patients with a concurrent bladder cancer? A necessary distinction for contiguous or noncontiguous involvement. J Urol 1996; 155: 244–247.

244. Shen SS, Lerner SP, Muezzinoglu B, et al. Prostatic involvement by transitional cell carcinoma in patients with bladder cancer and its prognostic significance. Hum Pathol 2006; 37: 726–734.

245. Lopez-Beltran A, Requena MJ, Alvarez-Kindelan J, et al. Squamous differentiation in primary urothelial carcinoma of the urinary tract as seen by MAC387 immunohistochemistry. J Clin Pathol 2007; 60: 332–335.

246. Lopez-Beltran A, Martin J, Garcia J, et al. Squamous and glandular differentiation in urothelial bladder carcinomas. Histopathology, histochemistry and immunohistochemical expression of carcinoembryonic antigen. Histol Histopathol 1988; 3: 63–68.

247. Akdas A, Turkeri L. The impact of squamous metaplasia in transitional cell carcinoma of the bladder. Int Urol Nephrol 1991; 23: 333–336.

248. Gonzalez-Campora R, Davalos-Casanova G, Beato-Moreno A, et al. BCL-2, TP53 and BAX protein expression in superficial urothelial bladder carcinoma. Cancer Lett 2007; 250: 292–299.

249. Wasco MJ, Daignault S, Zhang Y, et al. Urothelial carcinoma with divergent histologic differentiation (mixed histologic features) predicts the presence of locally advanced bladder cancer when detected at transurethral resection. Urology 2007; 70: 69–74.

250. Ro JY, Staerkel GA, Ayala AG. Cytologic and histologic features of superficial bladder cancer. Urol Clin North Am 1992; 19: 435–453.

251. Lopez-Beltran A, Cheng L. Histologic variants of urothelial carcinoma: differential diagnosis and clinical implications. Hum Pathol 2006; 37: 1371–1388.

252. Fong A, Garcia E, Gwynn L, et al. Expression of caveolin-1 and caveolin-2 in urothelial carcinoma of the urinary bladder correlates with tumor grade and squamous differentiation. Am J Clin Pathol 2003; 120: 93–100.

253. Kunze E, Francksen B, Schulz H. Expression of MUC5AC apomucin in transitional cell carcinomas of the urinary bladder and its possible role in the development of mucus-secreting adenocarcinomas. Virchows Arch 2001; 439: 609–615.

254. Kunze E. Histogenesis of nonurothelial carcinomas in the human and rat urinary bladder. Exp Toxicol Pathol 1998; 50: 341–355.

255. Drew PA, Furman J, Civantos F, et al. The nested variant of transitional cell carcinoma: an aggressive neoplasm with innocuous histology. Mod Pathol 1996; 9: 989–994.

256. Talbert ML, Young RH. Carcinomas of the urinary bladder with deceptively benign-appearing foci. A report of three cases. Am J Surg Pathol 1989; 13: 374–381.

257. Young RH, Oliva E. Transitional cell carcinomas of the urinary bladder that may be underdiagnosed. A report of four invasive cases exemplifying the homology between neoplastic and non-neoplastic transitional cell lesions. Am J Surg Pathol 1996; 20: 1448–1454.

258. Murphy WM, Deanna DG. The nested variant of transitional cell carcinoma: a neoplasm resembling proliferation of Brunn's nests. Mod Pathol 1992; 5: 240–243.

259. Holmang S, Johansson SL. The nested variant of transitional cell carcinoma – a rare neoplasm with poor prognosis. Scand J Urol Nephrol 2001; 35: 102–105.

260. Lin O, Cardillo M, Dalbagni G, et al. Nested variant of urothelial carcinoma: a clinicopathologic and immunohistochemical study of 12 cases. Mod Pathol 2003; 16: 1289–1298.

261. Volmar KE, Chan TY, De Marzo AM, et al. Florid von Brunn nests mimicking urothelial carcinoma: a morphologic and immunohistochemical comparison to the nested variant of urothelial carcinoma. Am J Surg Pathol 2003; 27: 1243–1252.

262. Amin MB, Gomez JA, Young RH. Urothelial transitional cell carcinoma with endophytic growth patterns: a discussion of patterns of invasion and problems associated with assessment of invasion in 18 cases. Am J Surg Pathol 1997; 21: 1057–1068.

263. Terai A, Tamaki M, Hayashida H, et al. Bulky transitional cell carcinoma of bladder with inverted proliferation. Int J Urol 1996; 3: 316–319.

264. Sudo T, Irie A, Ishii D, et al. Histopathologic and biologic characteristics of a transitional cell carcinoma with inverted papilloma-like endophytic growth pattern. Urology 2003; 61: 837.

265. Kawachi Y, Ishi K. Inverted transitional cell carcinoma of the ureter. Int J Urol 1996; 3: 313–315.

266. Amin MB, Ro JY, el-Sharkawy T, et al. Micropapillary variant of transitional cell carcinoma of the urinary bladder. Histologic pattern resembling ovarian

papillary serous carcinoma. Am J Surg Pathol 1994; 18: 1224–1232.

267. Dominici A, Nesi G, Mondaini N, et al. Skin involvement from micropapillary bladder carcinoma as the first clinical manifestation of metastatic disease. Urol Int 2001; 67: 173–174.

268. Hong SP, Park SW, Lee SJ, et al. Bile duct wall metastasis from micropapillary variant transitional cell carcinoma of the urinary bladder mimicking primary hilar cholangiocarcinoma. Gastrointest Endosc 2002; 56: 756–760.

269. Johansson SL, Borghede G, Holmang S. Micropapillary bladder carcinoma: a clinicopathological study of 20 cases. J Urol 1999; 161: 1798–1802.

270. Maranchie JK, Bouyounes BT, Zhang PL, et al. Clinical and pathological characteristics of micropapillary transitional cell carcinoma: a highly aggressive variant. J Urol 2000; 163: 748–751.

271. Samaratunga H, Khoo K. Micropapillary variant of urothelial carcinoma of the urinary bladder; a clinicopathological and immunohistochemical study. Histopathology 2004; 45: 55–64.

272. Nassar H, Pansare V, Zhang H, et al. Pathogenesis of invasive micropapillary carcinoma: role of MUC1 glycoprotein. Mod Pathol 2004; 19: 1045–1050.

273. Eble JN, Young RH. Carcinoma of the urinary bladder: a review of its diverse morphology. Semin Diagn Pathol 1997; 14: 98–108.

274. Leroy X, Leteurtre E, De La Taille A, et al. Microcystic transitional cell carcinoma: a report of 2 cases arising in the renal pelvis. Arch Pathol Lab Med 2002; 126: 859–861.

275. Holmang S, Borghede G, Johansson SL. Bladder carcinoma with lymphoepithelioma-like differentiation: a report of 9 cases. J Urol 1998; 159: 779–782.

276. Amin MB, Ro JY, Lee KM, et al. Lymphoepithelioma-like carcinoma of the urinary bladder. Am J Surg Pathol 1994; 18: 466–473.

277. Dinney CP, Ro JY, Babaian RJ, et al. Lymphoepithelioma of the bladder: a clinicopathological study of 3 cases. J Urol 1993; 149: 840–841.

278. Tamas EF, Nielsen ME, Schoenberg MP, et al. Lymphoepithelioma-like carcinoma of the urinary tract: a clinicopathological study of 30 pure and mixed cases. Mod Pathol 2007; 20: 828–834.

279. Cohen RJ, Stanley JC, Dawkins HJ. Lymphoepithelioma-like carcinoma of the renal pelvis. Pathology 1999; 31: 434–435.

280. Gulley ML, Amin MB, Nicholls JM, et al. Epstein–Barr virus is detected in undifferentiated nasopharyngeal carcinoma but not in lymphoepithelioma-like carcinoma of the urinary bladder. Hum Pathol 1995; 26: 1207–1214.

281. Zukerberg LR, Harris NL, Young RH. Carcinomas of the urinary bladder simulating malignant lymphoma. A report of five cases. Am J Surg Pathol 1991; 15: 569–576.

282. Sahin AA, Myhre M, Ro JY, et al. Plasmacytoid transitional cell carcinoma. Report of a case with initial presentation mimicking multiple myeloma. Acta Cytol 1991; 35: 277–280.

283. Tamboli P, Amin MB, Mohsin SK, et al. Plasmacytoid variant of non-papillary urothelial carcinoma. [Abstract] Mod Pathol 2000; 13: 107A.

284. Oliva E, Amin MB, Jimenez R, et al. Clear cell carcinoma of the urinary bladder: a report and comparison of four tumors of müllerian origin and nine of probable urothelial origin with discussion of histogenesis and diagnostic problems. Am J Surg Pathol 2002; 26: 190–197.

285. Braslis KG, Jones A, Murphy D. Clear-cell transitional cell carcinoma. Aust NZ J Surg 1997; 67: 906–908.

286. Kotliar SN, Wood CG, Schaeffer AJ, et al. Transitional cell carcinoma exhibiting clear cell features. A differential diagnosis for clear cell adenocarcinoma of the urinary tract. Arch Pathol Lab Med 1995; 119: 79–81.

287. Lopez-Beltran A, Luque RJ, Oliveira PS, et al. Urothelial carcinoma of the bladder, lipid cell variant (UCBLCV). Immunohistochemical and clinico-pathologic findings in seven cases. [Abstract] Mod Pathol 2002; 15: 171A.

288. Leroy X, Gonzalez S, Zini L, et al. Lipoid-cell variant of urothelial carcinoma: a clinicopathologic and immunohistochemical study of five cases. Am J Surg Pathol 2007; 31: 770–773.

289. Bastacky S, Dhir R, Nangia AK, et al. Choriocarcinomatous differentiation in a high-grade urothelial carcinoma of the urinary bladder: case report and literature review. J Urol Pathol 1997; 6: 223–234.

290. Campo E, Algaba F, Palacin A, et al. Placental proteins in high-grade urothelial neoplasms. An immunohistochemical study of human chorionic gonadotropin, human placental lactogen, and pregnancy-specific beta-1-glycoprotein. Cancer 1989; 63: 2497–2504.

291. Yamase HT, Wurzel RS, Nieh PT, et al. Immunohistochemical demonstration of human chorionic gonadotropin in tumors of the urinary bladder. Ann Clin Lab Sci 1985; 15: 414–417.

292. Oyasu R, Nan L, Smith P, et al. Human chorionic gonadotropin beta-subunit synthesis by undifferentiated urothelial carcinoma with syncytiotrophoblastic differentiation. Arch Pathol Lab Med 1994; 118: 715–717.

293. Fowler AL, Hall E, Rees G. Choriocarcinoma arising in transitional cell carcinoma of the bladder. Br J Urol 1992; 70: 333–334.

294. Martin JE, Jenkins BJ, Zuk RJ, et al. Human chorionic gonadotrophin expression and histological findings as predictors of response to radiotherapy in carcinoma of the bladder. Virchows Arch A Pathol Anat Histopathol 1989; 414: 273–277.

295. Grammatico D, Grignon DJ, Eberwein P, et al. Transitional cell carcinoma of the renal pelvis with choriocarcinomatous differentiation. Immunohistochemical and immunoelectron microscopic assessment of human chorionic gonadotropin production by transitional cell carcinoma of the urinary bladder. Cancer 1993; 71: 1835–1841.

296. Omeroglu A, Paner GP, Wojcik EM, et al. A carcinosarcoma/sarcomatoid carcinoma arising in a urinary bladder diverticulum. Arch Pathol Lab Med 2002; 126: 853–855.

297. Cheng L, Pan CX, Yang XJ, et al. Small cell carcinoma of the urinary bladder: a clinicopathologic analysis of 64 patients. Cancer 2004; 101: 957–962.

298. O'Connor RC, Hollowell CM, Laven BA, et al. Recurrent giant cell carcinoma of the bladder. J Urol 2002; 167: 1784.

299. Amir G, Rosenmann E. Osteoclast-like giant cell tumour of the urinary bladder. Histopathology 1990; 17: 413–418.

300. Baydar D, Amin MB, Epstein JI. Osteoclast-rich undifferentiated carcinomas of the urinary tract. Mod Pathol 2006; 19: 161–171.

301. Kumar S, Kumar D, Cowan DF. Transitional cell carcinoma with rhabdoid features. Am J Surg Pathol 1992; 16: 515–521.

302. Harris M, Eyden BP, Joglekar VM. Rhabdoid tumour of the bladder: a histological, ultrastructural and immunohistochemical study. Histopathology 1987; 11: 1083–1092.

303. Inagaki T, Nagata M, Kaneko M, et al. Carcinosarcoma with rhabdoid features of the urinary bladder in a 2-year-old girl: possible histogenesis of stem cell origin. Pathol Int 2000; 50: 973–978.

304. Duvdevani M, Nass D, Neumann Y, et al. Pure rhabdoid tumor of the bladder. J Urol 2001; 166: 2337.

305. Parwani AV, Herawi M, Volmar K, et al. Urothelial carcinoma with rhabdoid features: report of 6 cases. Hum Pathol 2006; 37: 168–172.

306. Bannach G, Grignon D, Shum D. Sarcomatoid transitional cell carcinoma vs pseudosarcomatous stromal reaction in bladder carcinoma: an immunohistochemical study. J Urol Pathol 1993; 1: 105–113.

307. Kobayashi R, Hirayama Y, Kobayashi E, et al. A germline insertion in the tuberous sclerosis (Tsc2) gene gives rise to the Eker rat model of dominantly inherited cancer. Nature Genet 1995; 9: 70–74.

308. Mahadevia PS, Alexander JE, Rojas-Corona R, et al. Pseudosarcomatous

stromal reaction in primary and metastatic urothelial carcinoma. A source of diagnostic difficulty. Am J Surg Pathol 1989; 13: 782–790.

309. Eble JN, Young RH. Stromal osseous metaplasia in carcinoma of the bladder. J Urol 1991; 145: 823–825.

310. Kinouchi T, Hanafusa T, Kuroda M, et al. Ossified cystic metastasis of bladder tumor to abdominal wound after partial cystectomy. J Urol 1995; 153: 1049–1050.

311. Lamm K. Chondroid and osseous metaplasia in carcinoma of the bladder. J Urol Pathol 1995; 3: 255–262.

312. Zukerberg LR, Armin AR, Pisharodi L, et al. Transitional cell carcinoma of the urinary bladder with osteoclast-type giant cells: a report of two cases and review of the literature. Histopathology 1990; 17: 407–411.

313. Lipponen PK, Eskelinen MJ, Jauhiainen K, et al. Tumour infiltrating lymphocytes as an independent prognostic factor in transitional cell bladder cancer. Eur J Cancer 1992; 29A: 69–75.

314. Flamm J. Tumor-associated tissue inflammatory reaction and eosinophilia in primary superficial bladder cancer. Urology 1992; 40: 180–185.

315. Offersen BV, Knap MM, Marcussen N, et al. Intense inflammation in bladder carcinoma is associated with angiogenesis and indicates good prognosis. Br J Cancer 2002; 87: 1422–1430.

316. Baldwin L, Lee AH, Al-Talib RK, et al. Transitional cell carcinoma of the bladder mimicking lobular carcinoma of the breast: a discohesive variant of urothelial carcinoma. Histopathology 2005; 46: 50–56.

317. Huang Q, Chu PG, Lau SK, et al. Urothelial carcinoma of the urinary bladder with a component of acinar/tubular type differentiation simulating prostatic adenocarcinoma. Hum Pathol 2004; 35: 769–773.

318. Lopez-Beltran A, Bassi P, Pavone-Macaluso M, et al. Handling and pathology reporting of specimens with carcinoma of the urinary bladder, ureter, and renal pelvis. Eur Urol 2004; 45: 257–266.

319. Amin MB, Srigley JR, Grignon DJ, et al. Updated protocol for the examination of specimens from patients with carcinoma of the urinary bladder, ureter, and renal pelvis. Arch Pathol Lab Med 2003; 127: 1263–1279.

320. May F, Treiber U, Hartung R, et al. Significance of random bladder biopsies in superficial bladder cancer. Eur Urol 2003; 44: 47–50.

321. Pagano F, A G, Milani C, et al. Prognosis of bladder cancer I. Risk factors in superficial transitional cell carcinoma. Eur Urol 1987; 13: 145–149.

322. Dalbagni G, Herr HW, Reuter VE. Impact of a second transurethral resection on the staging of T1 bladder cancer. Urology 2002; 60: 822–824.

323. Reuter VE. The pathology of bladder cancer. Urology 2006; 67: 11–17; discussion 17–18.

324. Reuter VE. Bladder. Risk and prognostic factors – a pathologist's perspective. Urol Clin North Am 1999; 26: 481–492.

325. Leissner J, Koeppen C, Wolf HK. Prognostic significance of vascular and perineural invasion in urothelial bladder cancer treated with radical cystectomy. J Urol 2003; 169: 955–960.

326. Lotan Y, Gupta A, Shariat SF, et al. Lymphovascular invasion is independently associated with overall survival, cause-specific survival, and local and distant recurrence in patients with negative lymph nodes at radical cystectomy. J Clin Oncol 2005; 23: 6533–6539.

327. Quek ML, Stein JP, Nichols PW, et al. Prognostic significance of lymphovascular invasion of bladder cancer treated with radical cystectomy. J Urol 2005; 174: 103–106.

328. Algaba F, Arce Y, Lopez-Beltran A, et al. Intraoperative frozen section diagnosis in urological oncology. Eur Urol 2005; 47: 129–136.

329. Cheng L, Montironi R, Bostwick DG. Villous adenoma of the urinary tract: a report of 23 cases, including 8 with coexistent adenocarcinoma. Am J Surg Pathol 1999; 23: 764–771.

330. Seibel JL, Prasad S, Weiss RE, et al. Villous adenoma of the urinary tract: a lesion frequently associated with malignancy. Hum Pathol 2002; 33: 236–241.

331. Bollito ER, Pacchioni D, Lopez-Beltran A, et al. Immunohistochemical study of neuroendocrine differentiation in primary glandular lesions and tumors of the urinary bladder. Anal Quant Cytol Histol 2005; 27: 218–224.

332. Grignon D, Ro J, Ayala A, et al. Primary adenocarcinoma of the urinary bladder: a clinicopathologic analysis of 72 cases. Cancer 1990; 67: 2165–2172.

333. Morton MJ, Zhang S, Lopez-Beltran S, et al. Telomere shortening and chromosomal abnormalities in intestinal metaplasia of the urinary bladder. Clin Cancer Res 2007; 13: 6232–6236.

334. Werling RW, Yaziji H, Bacchi CE, et al. CDX2, a highly sensitive and specific marker of adenocarcinomas of intestinal origin: and immunohistochemical survey fo 476 primary and metastatic carcinomas. Am J Surg Pathol 2003; 27: 303–310.

335. Kaimaktchiev V, Terracciano L, Tornillo L, et al. The homeobox intestinal differentiation factor CDX2 is selectively expressed in gastrointestinal adenocarcinomas. Mod Pathol 2004; 17: 1392–1399.

336. Sung MT, Lopez-Beltran A, Eble JN, et al. Divergent pathway of intestinal metaplasia and cystitis glandularis of the urinary bladder. Mod Pathol 2006; 19: 1395–1401.

337. Tamboli P, Mohsin SK, Hailemariam S, et al. Colonic adenocarcinoma metastatic to the urinary tract versus primary tumors of the urinary tract with glandular differentiation: a report of 7 cases and investigation using a limited immunohistochemical panel. Arch Pathol Lab Med 2002; 126: 1057–1063.

338. Wang HL, Lu DW, Yerian LM, et al. Immunohistochemical distinction between primary adenocarcinoma of the bladder and secondary colorectal adenocarcinoma. Am J Surg Pathol 2001; 25: 1380–1387.

339. Drew P, Murphy WM, Civantos F, et al. The histogenesis of clear cell adenocarcinoma of the lower urinary tract: case series and review of the literature. Hum Pathol 1996; 27: 248–252.

340. Cheng L, Cheville JC, Sebo TJ, et al. Atypical nephrogenic metaplasia of the urinary tract: a precursor lesion? Cancer 2000; 88: 853–861.

341. Gilcrease MZ, Delgado R, Vuitch F, et al. Clear cell adenocarcinoma and nephrogenic adenoma of the urethra and urinary bladder: a histopathologic and immunohistochemical comparison. Hum Pathol 1998; 29: 1451–1456.

342. Sung MT, Zhang S, MacLennan GT, et al. Histogenesis of clear cell adenocarcinoma in the urinary tract: Evidence of urothelial origin by histology, immunohistochemistry and fluorescence in situ hybridization analysis. Clin Cancer Res 2008; 14: 1947–1955.

343. Gupta A, Wang HL, Policarpio-Nicolas ML, et al. Expression of alpha-methylacyl-coenzyme A racemase in nephrogenic adenoma. Am J Surg Pathol 2004; 28: 1224–1229.

344. Lopez-Beltran A, Luque RJ, Quintero A, et al. Hepatoid adenocarcinoma of the urinary bladder. Virchows Arch 2003; 442: 381–387.

345. Lopez-Beltran A, Nogales F, Donne CH, et al. Adenocarcinoma of the urachus showing extensive calcification and stromal osseous metaplasia. Urol Int 1994; 53: 110–113.

346. Wheeler JD, Hill WT. Adenocarcinoma involving the urinary bladder. Cancer 1954; 7: 119–135.

346a. Johnson DE, Hodge GB, Abdul-Karim FW, et al. Urachal carcinoma. Urology 1985; 26: 218–221.

347. Bessette PL, Abell MR, Herwig KR. A clinicopathologic study of squamous cell carcinoma of the bladder. J Urol 1974; 112: 66–67.

348. Faysal MH. Squamous cell carcinoma of the bladder. J Urol 1981; 126: 598–599.

349. Lagwinski N, Thomas A, Stephenson AJ, et al. Squamous cell carcinoma of the bladder: A clinicopathologic analysis of 45 cases. Am J Surg Pathol 2007; 31: 1777–1787.

350. Brennan P, Bogillot O, Cordier S, et al. Cigarette smoking and bladder cancer in men: a pooled analysis of 11 case-control studies. Int J Cancer 2000; 86: 289–294.

351. Fortuny J, Kogevinas M, Chang-Claude J, et al. Tobacco, occupation and non-transitional-cell carcinoma of the bladder: an international case–control study. Int J Cancer 1999; 80: 44–46.

352. Cheever AW. Schistosomiasis and neoplasia. J Natl Cancer Inst 1978; 61: 13–18.

353. IARC: IARC Monographs on the evaluation of carcinogenic risks to humans. Schistosomes, liver flukes, and Helicobacter pylori. Lyon, France: IARC Press, 1994.

354. IARC. IARC Monographs on the evaluation of carcinogenic risks to humans. Tobacco smoke and involuntary smoking. Lyon, France: IARC Press, 2004.

355. Kao J, Upton M, Zhang P, et al. Individual prostate biopsy core embedding facilitates maximal tissue representation. J Urol 2002; 168: 496–499.

356. Mostafa MH, Helmi S, Badawi AF, et al. Nitrate, nitrite and volatile N-nitroso compounds in the urine of Schistosoma haematobium and Schistosoma mansoni infected patients. Carcinogenesis 1994; 15: 619–625.

357. Newman DM, Brown JR, Jay AC, et al. Squamous cell carcinoma of the bladder. J Urol 1968; 100: 470–473.

358. Vakar-López F, Abrams J. Basaloid squamous cell carcinoma occurring in the urinary bladder. Arch Pathol Lab Med 2000; 124: 455–459.

359. Cramer SF, Aikawa M, Cebelin M. Neurosecretory granules in small cell invasive carcinoma of the urinary bladder. Cancer 1981; 47: 724–730.

360. Abrahams NA, Moran C, Reyes AO, et al. Small cell carcinoma of the bladder: a contemporary clinicopathological study of 51 cases. Histopathology 2005; 46: 57–63.

361. Angulo JC, Lopez JI, Sanchez-Chapado M, et al. Small cell carcinoma of the urinary bladder: a report of two cases with complete remission and a comprehensive literature review with emphasis on therapeutic decisions. J Urol Pathol 1996; 5: 1–19.

362. Bastus R, Caballero JM, Gonzalez G, et al. Small cell carcinoma of the urinary bladder treated with chemotherapy and radiotherapy: results in five cases. Eur Urol 1999; 35: 323–326.

363. Holmang S, Borghede G, Johansson SL. Primary small cell carcinoma of the bladder: a report of 25 cases. J Urol 1995; 153: 1820–1822.

364. Blomjous CE, Vos W, De Voogt HJ, et al. Small cell carcinoma of the urinary bladder. A clinicopathologic, morphometric, immunohistochemical, and ultrastructural study of 18 cases. Cancer 1989; 64: 1347–1357.

365. Blomjous CE, Vos W, Schipper NW, et al. Morphometric and flow cytometric analysis of small cell undifferentiated carcinoma of the bladder. J Clin Pathol 1989; 42: 1032–1039.

366. Choong NW, Quevedo JF, Kaur JS. Small cell carcinoma of the urinary bladder. The Mayo Clinic experience. Cancer 2005; 103: 1172–1178.

367. Grignon DJ, Ro JY, Ayala AG, et al. Small cell carcinoma of the urinary bladder. A clinicopathologic analysis of 22 cases. Cancer 1992; 69: 527–536.

368. Mills SE, Wolfe JTD, Weiss MA, et al. Small cell undifferentiated carcinoma of the urinary bladder. A light-microscopic, immunocytochemical, and ultrastructural study of 12 cases. Am J Surg Pathol 1987; 11: 606–617.

369. Kim CK, Lin JI, Tseng CH. Small cell carcinoma of urinary bladder. Ultrastructural study. Urology 1984; 24: 384–386.

370. Lohrisch C, Murray N, Pickles T, et al. Small cell carcinoma of the bladder: long term outcome with integrated chemoradiation. Cancer 1999; 86: 2346–2352.

371. Pan CX, Zhang H, Lara PNJ, et al. Small-cell carcinoma of the urinary bladder. Diagnosis and management. Expert Rev Anticancer Ther 2006; 6: 1707–1713.

372. Pan CX, Yang XJ, Lopez-Beltran A, et al. c-Kit expression in small cell carcinoma of the urinary bladder: prognostic and therapeutic implications. Mod Pathol 2005; 18: 320–323.

373. Alijo Serrano F, Sánchez-Mora N, Angel Arranz J, et al. Large cell and small cell neuroendocrine bladder carcinoma: immunohistochemical and outcome study in a single institution. Am J Clin Pathol 2007; 128: 733–739.

374. Soriano P, Navarro S, Gil M, et al. Small-cell carcinoma of the urinary bladder. A clinico-pathological study of ten cases. Virchows Arch 2004; 445: 292–297.

375. Wang HL, Lu DW. Detection of human papillomavirus DNA and expression of p16, Rb, and p53 proteins in small cell carcinomas of the uterine cervix. Am J Surg Pathol 2004; 28: 901–908.

376. Reyes CV, Soneru I. Small cell carcinoma of the urinary bladder with hypercalcemia. Cancer 1985; 56: 2530–2533.

377. Partanen S, Asikainen U. Oat cell carcinoma of the urinary bladder with ectopic adrenocorticotropic hormone production. Hum Pathol 1985; 16: 313–315.

378. Abbosh PH, Wang M, Eble JN, et al. Hypermethylation of tumor suppressor gene CpG islands in small cell carcinoma of the urinary bladder. Mod Pathol 2008; 21: 355–362.

379. Wang X, MacLennan GT, Lopez-Beltran A, et al. Small cell carcinoma of the urinary bladder: Histogenesis, genetics, diagnosis, biomarkers, treatment, and prognosis. Appl Immunohistochem Mol Morphol 2007; 15: 8–18.

380. Wang X, Zhang S, MacLennan GT, et al. Epidermal growth factor receptor protein expression and gene amplification in small cell carcinoma of the urinary bladder. Clin Cancer Res 2007; 13: 953–957.

381. Wang X, Jones TD, MacLennan GT, et al. P53 expression in small cell carcinoma of the urinary bladder: biological and prognostic implications. Anticancer Res 2005; 25: 2001–2004.

382. Podesta AH, True LD. Small cell carcinoma of the bladder. Report of five cases with immunohistochemistry and review of the literature with evaluation of prognosis according to stage. Cancer 1989; 64: 710–714.

383. Martignoni G, Eble JN. Carcinoid tumors of the urinary bladder. Immunohistochemical study of 2 cases and review of the literature. Arch Pathol Lab Med 2003; 127: e22–e24.

384. Oesterling JE, Brendler CB, Burgers JK, et al. Advanced small cell carcinoma of the bladder. Successful treatment with combined radical cystoprostatectomy and adjuvant methotrexate, vinblastine, doxorubicin, and cisplatin chemotherapy. Cancer 1990; 65: 1928–1936.

385. Cheng L, Leibovich B, Cheville J, et al. Paraganglioma of the urinary bladder: can biologic potential be predicted? Cancer 2000; 88: 844–852.

386. Cheng L, Scheithauer BW, Leibovich BC, et al. Neurofibroma of the urinary bladder. Cancer 1999; 86: 505–513.

387. Terracciano L, Richter J, Tornillo L, et al. Chromosomal imbalances in small cell carcinomas of the urinary bladder. J Pathol 1999; 189: 230–235.

388. Leonard C, Huret JL, and Groupe Française de Cytogénétique Oncologique. From cytogenetics to cytogenomics of bladder cancers. Bull Cancer 2002; 89: 166–173.

389. Atkin NB, Baker MC, Wilson GD. Chromosome abnormalities and p53 expression in a small cell carcinoma of the bladder. Cancer Genet Cytogenet 1995; 79: 111–114.

390. Rohr UP, Rehfeld N, Pflugfelder L, et al. Expression of the tyrosine kinase c-kit is an independent prognostic factor in patients with small cell lung cancer. Int J Cancer 2004; 111: 259–263.

391. Tamborini E, Bonadiman L, Negri T, et al. Detection of overexpressed and phosphorylated wild-type kit receptor in surgical specimens of small cell lung cancer. Clin Cancer Res 2004; 10: 8214–8219.

392. Ali SZ, Reuter VE, Zakowski MF. Small cell neuroendocrine carcinoma of the urinary bladder. A clinicopathologic study with emphasis on cytologic features. Cancer 1997; 79: 356–361.

393. Trias I, Algaba F, Condom E, et al. Small cell carcinoma of the urinary bladder. Presentation of 23 cases and review of 134 published cases. Eur Urol 2001; 39: 85–90.

394. Jones TD, Kernek KM, Yang XJ, et al. Thyroid transcription factor 1 expression in small cell carcinoma of the urinary bladder: an immunohistochemical profile of 44 cases. Hum Pathol 2005; 36: 718–723.

395. Lopez JI, Angulo JC, Flores N, et al. Small cell carcinoma of the urinary bladder. A clinicopathological study of six cases. Br J Urol 1994; 73: 43–49.

396. Helpap B. Morphology and therapeutic strategies for neuroendocrine tumors of the genitourinary tract. Cancer 2002; 95: 1415–1420.

397. Ordonez NG. Value of thyroid transcription factor-1 immunostaining in distinguishing small cell lung carcinomas from other small cell carcinomas. Am J Surg Pathol 2000; 24: 1217–1223.

398. Iczkowski KA, Shanks JH, Allsbrook WC, et al. Small cell carcinoma of urinary bladder is differentiated from urothelial carcinoma by chromogranin expression, absence of CD44 variant 6 expression, a unique pattern of cytokeratin expression, and more intense gamma-enolase expression. Histopathology 1999; 35: 150–156.

399. Iczkowski KA, Shanks JH, Bostwick DG. Loss of CD44 variant 6 expression differentiates small cell carcinoma of urinary bladder from urothelial (transitional cell) carcinoma. Histopathology 1998; 32: 322–327.

400. Lee KH, Ryu SB, Lee MC, et al. Primary large cell neuroendocrine carcinoma of the urinary bladder. Pathol Int 2006; 56: 688–693.

401. Dundr P, Pesl M, Povysil C, et al. Large cell neuroendocrine carcinoma of the urinary bladder with lymphoepithelioma-like features. Pathol Res Pract 2003; 199: 559–563.

402. Evans AJ, Al-Maghrabi J, Tsihlias J, et al. Primary large cell neuroendocrine carcinoma of the urinary bladder. Arch Pathol Lab Med 2002; 126: 1229–1232.

403. Hailemariam S, Gaspert A, Komminoth P, et al. Primary, pure, large-cell neuroendocrine carcinoma of the urinary bladder. Mod Pathol 1998; 11: 1016–1020.

404. Yoffa D, Withycombe J. Bladder-pheochromocytoma metastases. Lancet 1967; 2: 422.

405. Pugh R, Gresham G, Mullaney J. Phaeochromocytoma of the urinary bladder. J Pathol Bacteriol 1960; 79: 89–107.

406. Poirer H, Robinson JO. Pheochromocytoma of the urinary bladder: a male patient. Br J Urol 1962; 34: 88–92.

407. Glucksman MA, Persinger CP. Malignant non-chromaffin paraganglioma of the bladder. J Urol 1963; 89: 822–825.

408. Grignon DJ, Ro JY, Mackay B, et al. Paraganglioma of the urinary bladder: immunohistochemical, ultrastructural, and DNA flow cytometric studies. Hum Pathol 1991; 22: 1162–1169.

409. Leestma JE, Price EB Jr. Paraganglioma of the urinary bladder. Cancer 1971; 28: 1063–1073.

410. Das S, Lowe P. Malignant pheochromocytoma of the bladder. J Urol 1980; 123: 282–284.

411. Das S, Bulusu NV, Lowe P. Primary vesical pheochromocytoma. Urology 1983; 21: 20–25.

412. Davaris P, Petraki K, Arvanitis D, et al. Urinary bladder paraganglioma (UBP). Pathol Res Pract 1986; 181: 101–106.

413. Javaheri P, Raafat J. Malignant phaeochromocytoma of the urinary bladder – report of two cases. Br J Urol 1975; 47: 401–404.

414. Higgins P, Tresidder G. Malignant phaeochromocytoma of the urinary bladder. Br J Urol 1980; 52: 230.

415. Moloney G, Cowdell R, Lewis C. Malignant phaeochromocytoma of the bladder. Br J Urol 1966; 38: 461–470.

416. Shimbo S, Nakano Y. A case of malignant pheochromocytoma producing parathyroid hormone-like substance. Calif Tissue Res 1974; 15: 155.

417. Asbury W, Hatcher P, Gould H, et al. Bladder pheochromocytoma with ring calcification. Abdom Imag 1996; 21: 275–277.

418. Deklerk DP, Catalona WJ, Nime FA, et al. Malignant pheochromocytoma of the bladder: the late development of renal cell carcinoma. J Urol 1975; 113: 864–868.

419. Campbell DR, Mason W, Manchester J. Angiography in pheochromocytomas. J Can Assoc Radiol 1974; 25: 214–223.

420. Lumb B, Gresham G. Phaeochromocytoma of the urinary bladder. Lancet 1958; 1: 81–82.

421. Meyer J, Sane S, Drake R. Malignant paraganglioma (pheochromocytoma) of the urinary bladder: report of a case and review of the literature. Pediatrics 1979; 63: 879–885.

422. Scott W, Eversole S. Pheochromocytoma of the urinary bladder. J Urol 1960; 83: 656–664.

423. Piedrola G, Lopez E, Rueda M, et al. Malignant pheochromocytoma of the bladder: current controversies. Eur Urol 1997; 31: 122–125.

424. Zhou M, Epstein JI, Young RH. Paraganglioma of the urinary bladder: a lesion that may be misdiagnosed as urothelial carcinoma in transurethral resection specimens. Am J Surg Pathol 2004; 28: 94–100.

425. Medeiros L, Wolf B, Balogh K, et al. Adrenal pheochromocytoma: a clinicopathologic review of 60 cases. Hum Pathol 1985; 16: 580–589.

426. Albores-Saavedra J, Maldonado ME, Ibarra J, et al. Pheochromocytoma of the urinary bladder. Cancer 1969; 23: 1110–1118.

427. Jurascheck F, Egloff H, Buemi A, et al. Paraganglioma of urinary bladder. Urology 1983; 22: 659–663.

428. Zimmerman I, Biron R, MacMahon H. Pheochromocytoma of the urinary bladder. N Engl J Med 1953; 249: 25–26.

429. Dixon J, Gosling J, Canning D, et al. An immunohistochemical study of human postnatal paraganglia associated with the urinary bladder. J Anat 1992; 181: 431–436.

430. Fletcher T, Bradley W. Neuroanatomy of the bladder–urethra. J Urol 1978; 119: 153–160.

431. Rode J, Bentley A, Parkinson C. Paraganglial cells of urinary bladder and prostate: potential diagnostic problem. J Clin Pathol 1990; 43: 13–16.

432. Honma K. Paraganglia of the urinary bladder. An autopsy study. Zentralbl Pathol 1994; 139: 465–469.

433. Gimenez-Roqueplo AP. New advances in the genetics of pheochromocytoma and paraganglioma syndromes. Ann NY Acad Sci 2006; 1073: 112–121.

434. Bayley JP, van Minderhout I, Weiss MM, et al. Mutation analysis of SDHB and SDHC: novel germline mutations in sporadic head and neck paraganglioma and familial paraganglioma and/or pheochromocytoma. BMC Med Genet 2006; 7: 1.

435. Mannelli M, Simi L, Ercolino T, et al. SDH mutations in patients affected by paraganglioma syndromes: a personal experience. Ann NY Acad Sci 2006; 1073: 183–189.

436. Braun S, Riemann K, Kupka S, et al. Active succinate dehydrogenase (SDH) and lack of SDHD mutations in sporadic paragangliomas. Anticancer Res 2005; 25: 2809–2814.

437. Koch CA, Vortmeyer AO, Zhuang Z, et al. New insights into the genetics of familial chromaffin cell tumors. Ann NY Acad Sci 2002; 970: 11–28.

438. Amar L, Bertherat J, Baudin E, et al. Genetic testing in pheochromocytoma or functional paraganglioma. J Clin Oncol 2005; 23: 8812–8818.

439. Cascon A, Montero-Conde C, Ruiz-Llorente S, et al. Gross SDHB deletions in patients with paraganglioma detected by multiplex PCR. a possible hot spot? Genes Chromosomes Cancer 2006; 45: 213–219.

440. Astuti D, Hart-Holden N, Latif F, et al. Genetic analysis of mitochondrial complex II subunits SDHD, SDHB and SDHC in paraganglioma and phaeochromocytoma susceptibility. Clin Endocrinol (Oxford) 2003; 59: 728–733.

441. Pollard PJ, El-Bahrawy M, Poulsom R, et al. Expression of HIF-1alpha, HIF-2alpha (EPAS1), and their target genes in paraganglioma and pheochromocytoma with VHL and SDH mutations. J Clin Endocrinol Metab 2006; 91: 4593–4598.

442. Dahia PL. Evolving concepts in pheochromocytoma and paraganglioma. Curr Opin Oncol 2006; 18: 1–8.

443. Lemeta S, Salmenkivi K, Pylkkanen L, et al. Frequent loss of heterozygosity at

6q in pheochromocytoma. Hum Pathol 2006; 37: 749–754.

444. Moyana TN, Kontozoglou T. Urinary bladder paragangliomas. An immunohistochemical study. Arch Pathol Lab Med 1988; 112: 70–72.

445. Moran CA, Albores-Saavedra J, Wenig BM, et al. Pigmented extraadrenal paraganlioma: a clinicopathologic and immunohistochemical study of five cases. Cancer 1997; 79: 398–402.

446. Mouradian J, Coleman J, McGovern J, et al. Granular cell tumor (myoblastoma) of the bladder. J Urol 1974; 112: 343–345.

447. Mizutani S, Okuda N, Sonoda T. Granular cell myoblastoma of the bladder: report of an additional case. J Urol 1973; 110: 403–405.

448. Seery WH. Granular cell myoblastoma of the bladder: report of a case. J Urol 1968; 100: 735–737.

449. Fletcher MS, Aker M, Hill JT, et al. Granular cell myoblastoma of the bladder. Br J Urol 1985; 57: 109–110.

450. Christ M, Ozzello L. Myogenous origin of a granular cell tumor of the urinary bladder. Am J Clin Pathol 1971; 56: 736–749.

451. Sung L, Anderson JR, Arndt C, et al. Neurofibromatosis in children with rhabdomyosarcoma. A report from the Intergroup Rhabdomyosarcoma Study IV. J Pediatr 2004; 144: 666–668.

452. Geol H, Kim DW, Kim TH, et al. Laparoscopic partial cystectomy for schwannoma of urinary bladder: case report. J Endourol 2005; 19: 303–306.

453. Cummings JM, Wehry MA, Parra RO, et al. Schwannoma of the urinary bladder: a case report. Int J Urol 1998; 5: 496–497.

454. Lopez-Beltran A, Perez-Seoane C, Montironi R, et al. Primary primitive neuroectodermal tumour of the urinary bladder: a clinico-pathological study emphasising immunohistochemical, ultrastructural and molecular analyses. J Clin Pathol 2006; 59: 775–778.

455. Rober PE, Smith JB, Sakr W, et al. Malignant peripheral nerve sheath tumor (malignant schwannoma) of urinary bladder in von Recklinghausen neurofibromatosis. Urology 1991; 38: 473–476.

456. Eltoum IA, Moore RJ 3rd, Cook W, et al. Epithelioid variant of malignant peripheral nerve sheath tumor (malignant schwannoma) of the urinary bladder. Ann Diagn Pathol 1999; 3: 304–308.

457. Daimaru Y, Hashimoto H, Enjoji M. Malignant 'triton' tumors: a clinicopathologic and immunohistochemical study of nine cases. Hum Pathol 1984; 15: 768–778.

458. Ikegami H, Iwasaki H, Ohjimi Y, et al. Sarcomatoid carcinoma of the urinary bladder: a clinicopathologic and immunohistochemical analysis of 14 patients. Hum Pathol 2000; 31: 332–340.

459. Torenbeek R, Blomjous CE, de Bruin PC, et al. Sarcomatoid carcinoma of the urinary bladder. Clinicopathologic analysis of 18 cases with immunohistochemical and electron microscopic findings. Am J Surg Pathol 1994; 18: 241–249.

460. Torenbeek R, Hermsen MA, Meijer GA, et al. Analysis by comparative genomic hybridization of epithelial and spindle cell components in sarcomatoid carcinoma and carcinosarcoma: histogenetic aspects. J Pathol 1999; 189: 338–343.

461. Lopez-Beltran A, Escudero AL, Cavazzana AO, et al. Sarcomatoid transitional cell carcinoma of the renal pelvis. A report of five cases with clinical, pathological, immunohistochemical and DNA ploidy analysis. Pathol Res Pract 1996; 192: 1218–1224.

462. Serio G, Zampatti C, Ceppi M. Spindle and giant cell carcinoma of the urinary bladder: a clinicopathological light microscopic and immunohistochemical study. Br J Urol 1995; 75: 167–172.

463. Lahoti C, Schinella R, Rangwala AF, et al. Carcinosarcoma of urinary bladder: report of 5 cases with immunohistologic study. Urology 1994; 43: 389–393.

464. Jones EC, Clement PB, Young RH. Inflammatory pseudotumor of the urinary bladder: a clinicopathological, immunohistochemical, ultrastructural, and flow cytometric study of 13 cases. Am J Surg Pathol 1993; 17: 264–274.

465. Jones E, Young R. Nonneoplastic and neoplastic spindle cell proliferations and mixed tumors of the urinary bladder. J Urol Pathol 1994; 2: 105–134.

466. Jones EC, Young RH. Myxoid and sclerosing sarcomatoid transitional cell carcinoma of the urinary bladder: a clinicopathologic and immunohistochemical study of 25 cases. Mod Pathol 1997; 10: 908–916.

467. Perret L, Chaubert P, Hessler D, et al. Primary heterologous carcinosarcoma (metaplastic carcinoma) of the urinary bladder. a clinicopathologic, immunohistochemical, and ultrastructural analysis of eight cases and a review of the literature. Cancer 1998; 82: 1535–1549.

468. Ogishima T, Kawachi Y, Saito A, et al. Sarcomatoid carcinoma and carcinosarcoma of the urinary bladder. Int J Urol 2002; 9: 354–358.

469. Lott S, Lopez-Beltran A, MacLennan GT, et al. Soft tissue tumors of the urinary bladder. Part I: Myofibroblastic proliferationas, benign neoplasms, and tumors of uncertain malignant potential. Hum Pathol 2007; 38: 963–977.

470. Lott S, Lopez-Beltran A, Montironi R, et al. Soft tissue tumors of the urinary bladder. Part II: Malignant neoplasms. Hum Pathol 2007; 38: 8807–823.

471. Goluboff ET, O'Toole K, Sawczuk IS. Leiomyoma of bladder: report of case

and review of literature. Urology 1994; 43: 238–241.

472. Kunze E, Theuring F, Kruger G. Primary mesenchymal tumors of the urinary bladder. A histological and immunohistochemical study of 30 cases. Pathol Res Pract 1994; 190: 311–332.

473. Lundgren L, Aldenborg F, Angervall L, et al. Pseudomalignant spindle cell proliferations of the urinary bladder. Hum Pathol 1994; 25: 181–191.

474. Harik LR, Merino C, Coindre JM, et al. Pseudosarcomatous myofibroblastic proliferations of the bladder: a clinicopathologic study of 42 cases. Am J Surg Pathol 2006; 30: 787–794.

475. Sty JR, Wells RG, Hardie RC. Inflammatory pseudotumor of the bladder. Wis Med J 1995; 94: 297–297.

476. Lamovec J, Zidar A, Trsinar B, et al. Sclerosing inflammatory pseudotumor of the urinary bladder in a child. Am J Surg Pathol 1992; 16: 1233–1238.

477. Roy A, Pramanik RN, Biswas S, et al. Pseudosarcomatous myofibroblastic proliferation in urinary bladder. J Ind Med Assoc 1993; 91: 18–19.

478. Hojo H, Newton WA Jr, Hamoudi AB, et al. Pseudosarcomatous myofibroblastic tumor of the urinary bladder in children: a study of 11 cases with review of the literature. An Intergroup Rhabdomyosarcoma Study. Am J Surg Pathol 1995; 19: 1224–1236.

479. Hughes DF, Biggart JD, Hayes D. Pseudosarcomatous lesions of the urinary bladder. Histopathology 1991; 18: 67–71.

480. Albores-Saavedra J, Manivel JC, Essenfeld H, et al. Pseudosarcomatous myofibroblastic proliferations in the urinary bladder of children. Cancer 1990; 66: 1234–1241.

481. Ro JY, el-Naggar AK, Amin MB, et al. Inflammatory pseudotumor of the urinary bladder. Am J Surg Pathol 1993; 17: 1193–1194.

482. Wick MR, Brown BA, Young RH, et al. Spindle-cell proliferations of the urinary tract. An immunohistochemical study. Am J Surg Pathol 1988; 12: 379–389.

483. Lopez-Beltran A, Lopez-Ruiz J, Vicioso L. Inflammatory pseudotumor of the urinary bladder. A clinicopathological analysis of two cases. Urol Int 1995; 55: 173–176.

484. Young RH. Spindle cell lesions of the urinary bladder. Histol Histopathol 1990; 5: 505–512.

485. Kapusta LR, Weiss MA, Ramsay J, et al. Inflammatory myofibroblastic tumors of the kidney: a clinicopathologic and immunohistochemical study of 12 cases. Am J Surg Pathol 2003; 27: 658–666.

486. Dietrick DD, Kabalin JN, Daniels GF Jr, et al. Inflammatory pseudotumor of the bladder. J Urol 1992; 148: 141–144.

487. N'Dow J, Brown PA, McClinton S, et al. Inflammatory pseudotumour

of the urinary bladder. Br J Urol 1993; 72: 379–380.

488. Coffin CM, Watterson J, Priest JR, et al. Extrapulmonary inflammatory myofibroblastic tumor (inflammatory pseudotumor). A clinicopathologic and immunohistochemical study of 84 cases. Am J Surg Pathol 1995; 19: 859–872.

489. McKenney JK. An approach to the classification of spindle cell proliferations in the urinary bladder. Adv Anat Pathol 2005; 12: 312–323.

490. Stark GL, Feddersen R, Lowe BA, et al. Inflammatory pseudotumor (pseudosarcoma) of the bladder. J Urol 1989; 141: 610–612.

491. Angulo JC, Lopez JI, Flores N. Pseudosarcomatous myofibroblastic proliferation of the bladder: report of 2 cases and literature review. J Urol 1994; 151: 1008–1012.

492. Iczkowski KA, Shanks JH, Gadaleanu V, et al. Inflammatory pseudotumor and sarcoma of urinary bladder: differential diagnosis and outcome in thirty-eight spindle cell neoplasms. Mod Pathol 2001; 14: 1043–1051.

493. Debiec-Rychter M, Marynen P, Hagemeijer A, et al. ALK-ATIC fusion in urinary bladder inflammatory myofibroblastic tumor. Genes Chromosomes Cancer 2003; 38: 187–190.

494. Dehner LP. Inflammatory myofibroblastic tumor: the continued definition of one type of so-called inflammatory pseudotumor. Am J Surg Pathol 2004; 28: 1652–1654.

495. Hirsch MS, Dal Cin P, Fletcher CD. ALK expression in pseudosarcomatous myofibroblastic proliferations of the genitourinary tract. Histopathology 2006; 48: 569–578.

496. Montgomery EA, Shuster DD, Burkart AL, et al. Inflammatory myofibroblastic tumors of the urinary tract: a clinicopathologic study of 46 cases, including a malignant example inflammatory fibrosarcoma and a subset associated with high-grade urothelial carcinoma. Am J Surg Pathol 2006; 30: 1502–1512.

497. Roth JA. Reactive pseudosarcomatous response in urinary bladder. Urology 1980; 16: 635–637.

498. Freeman A, Geddes N, Munson P, et al. Anaplastic lymphoma kinase (ALK 1) staining and molecular analysis in inflammatory myofibroblastic tumours of the bladder: a preliminary clinicopathological study of nine cases and review of the literature. Mod Pathol 2004; 17: 765–771.

499. Bridge JA, Kanamori M, Ma Z, et al. Fusion of the ALK gene to the clathrin heavy chain gene, CLTC, in inflammatory myofibroblastic tumor. Am J Pathol 2001; 159: 411–415.

500. Cessna MH, Zhou H, Sanger WG, et al. Expression of ALK1 and p80 in inflammatory myofibroblastic tumor and its mesenchymal mimics: a study

of 135 cases. Mod Pathol 2002; 15: 931–938.

501. Chan JK, Cheuk W, Shimizu M. Anaplastic lymphoma kinase expression in inflammatory pseudotumors. Am J Surg Pathol 2001; 25: 761–768.

502. Proppe KH, Scully RE, Rosai J. Postoperative spindle cell nodules of genitourinary tract resembling sarcomas. A report of eight cases. Am J Surg Pathol 1984; 8: 101–108.

503. Mottet-Auselo N, Marsollier C, Chapuis H, et al. Postoperative pseudosarcomatous nodule: report of one case and review of the literature. Eur Urol 1994; 25: 262–264.

504. Chen M, Lipson SA, Hricak H. MR imaging evaluation of benign mesenchymal tumors of the urinary bladder. AJR Am J Roentgenol 1997; 168: 399–403.

505. Martin SA, Sears DL, Sebo TJ, et al. Smooth muscle neoplasms of the urinary bladder: a clinicopathologic comparison of leiomyoma and leiomyosarcoma. Am J Surg Pathol 2002; 26: 292–300.

506. Cheng L, Nascimento AG, Neumann RM, et al. Hemangioma of the urinary bladder. Cancer 1999; 86: 498–504.

507. Kontani K, Okaneya T, Takezaki T. Recurrent granular cell tumour of the bladder in a patient with von Recklinghausen's disease. BJU Int 1999; 84: 871–872.

508. Westra WH, Grenko RT, Epstein J. Solitary fibrous tumor of the lower urogenital tract: a report of five cases involving the seminal vesicles, urinary bladder, and prostate. Hum Pathol 2000; 31: 63–68.

509. Prout MN, Davis HL Jr. Hemangiopericytoma of the bladder after polyvinyl alcohol exposure. Cancer 1977; 39: 1328–1330.

510. Parfitt JR, Bella AJ, Wehrli BM, et al. Primary PEComa of the bladder treated with primary excision and adjuvant interferon-alpha immunotherapy: a case report. BMC Urol 2006; 6: 20.

511. Pan C-C, Yu I-T, Yang A-H, et al. Clear cell myomelanocytic tumor of the urinary bladder. Am J Surg Pathol 2003; 27: 689–692.

512. Kalyanasundaram K, Parameswaran A, Mani R. Perivascular epithelioid tumor of urinary bladder and vagina. Ann Diagn Pathol 2005; 9: 275–278.

513. Pedersen-Bjergaard J, Jonsson V, Pedersen M, et al. Leiomyosarcoma of the urinary bladder after cyclophosphamide. J Clin Oncol 1995; 13: 532–533.

514. Tanguay C, Harvey I, Houde M, et al. Leiomyosarcoma of urinary bladder following cyclophosphamide therapy: report of two cases. Mod Pathol 2003; 16: 512–514.

515. Mills SE, Bova GS, Wick MR, et al. Leiomyosarcoma of the urinary bladder. A clinicopathologic and immunohistochemical study of 15

cases. Am J Surg Pathol 1989; 13: 480–489.

516. Lambert I, Debiec-Rychter M, Dubin M, et al. Solid alveolar rhabdomyosarcoma originating from the urinary bladder in an adult. Diagnostic value of molecular genetics. Histopathology 2004; 44: 508–510.

517. Leuschner I, Harms D, Mattke A, et al. Rhabdomyosarcoma of the urinary bladder and vagina: a clinicopathologic study with emphasis on recurrent disease: a report from the Kiel Pediatric Tumor Registry and the German CWS Study. Am J Surg Pathol 2001; 25: 856–864.

518. Arndt C, Rodeberg D, Breitfeld PP, et al. Does bladder preservation (as a surgical principle) lead to retaining bladder function in bladder/prostate rhabdomyosarcoma? Results from Intergroup Rhabdomyosarcoma Study IV. J Urol 2004; 171: 2396–2403.

519. Lauro S, Lalle M, Scucchi L, et al. Rhabdomyosarcoma of the urinary bladder in an elderly patient. Anticancer Res 1995; 15: 627–629.

520. Aydoganli L, Tarhan F, Atan A, et al. Rhabdomyosarcoma of the urinary bladder in an adult. Int Urol Nephrol 1993; 25: 159–161.

521. Hays DM. Bladder/prostate rhabdomyosarcoma: results of the multi-institutional trials of the Intergroup Rhabdomyosarcoma Study. Semin Surg Oncol 1993; 9: 520–523.

522. Hays DM, Raney RB, Wharam MD, et al. Children with vesical rhabdomyosarcoma (RMS) treated by partial cystectomy with neoadjuvant or adjuvant chemotherapy, with or without radiotherapy. A report from the Intergroup Rhabdomyosarcoma Study (IRS) Committee. J Pediatr Hematol Oncol 1995; 17: 46–52.

523. Qualman SJ, Coffin CM, Newton WA, et al. Intergroup Rhabdomyosarcoma Study: update for pathologists. Pediatr Dev Pathol 1998; 1: 550–561.

524. Engel JD, Kuzel TM, Moceanu MC, et al. Angiosarcoma of the bladder: a review. Urology 1998; 52: 778–784.

525. Schindler S, De Frias DV, Yu GH. Primary angiosarcoma of the bladder: cytomorphology and differential diagnosis. Cytopathology 1999; 10: 137–143.

526. Stroup RM, Chang YC. Angiosarcoma of the bladder: a case report. J Urol 1987; 137: 984–985.

527. Ravi R. Primary angiosarcoma of the urinary bladder. Arch Esp Urol 1993; 46: 351–353.

528. Morgan MA, Moutos DM, Pippitt CH Jr, et al. Vaginal and bladder angiosarcoma after therapeutic irradiation. South Med J 1989; 82: 1434–1436.

529. Egawa S, Uchida T, Koshiba K, et al. Malignant fibrous histiocytoma of the bladder with focal rhabdoid tumor differentiation. J Urol 1994; 151: 154–156.

530. Kato T, Kubota Y, Saitou M, et al. Osteosarcoma of the bladder successfully treated with partial cystectomy. J Urol 2000; 163: 548–549.

531. Berenson RJ, Flynn S, Freiha FS, et al. Primary osteogenic sarcoma of the bladder. Case report and review of the literature. Cancer 1986; 57: 350–355.

532. Ghalayini IF, Bani-Hani IH, Almasri NM. Osteosarcoma of the urinary bladder occurring simultaneously with prostate and bowel carcinomas: report of a case and review of the literature. Arch Pathol Lab Med 2001; 125: 793–795.

533. Young RH, Rosenberg AE. Osteosarcoma of the urinary bladder. Report of a case and review of the literature. Cancer 1987; 59: 174–178.

534. Amin MB, Patel RM, Oliveira P, et al. Alveolar soft-part sarcoma of the urinary bladder with urethral recurrence: a unique case with emphasis on differential diagnoses and diagnostic utility of an immunohistochemical panel including TFE3. Am J Surg Pathol 2006; 30: 1322–1325.

535. Kernek KM, Koch MO, Daggy JK, et al. The presence of benign prostatic glandular tissue at surgical margins does not predict PSA recurrence. J Clin Pathol 2005; 58: 725–728.

536. Tajima Y, Aizawa M. Unusual renal pelvic tumor containing transitional cell carcinoma, adenocarcinoma and sarcomatoid elements (so-called sarcomatoid carcinoma of the renal pelvis). A case report and review of the literature. Acta Pathol Jpn 1988; 38: 805–814.

537. Huang HY, Ko SF, Chuang JH, et al. Primary yolk sac tumor of the urachus. Arch Pathol Lab Med 2002; 126: 1106–1109.

538. Melicow M. Tumors of the urinary bladder: A clinico-pathological analysis of over 2500 specimens and biopsies. J Urol 1955; 74: 498–521.

539. Young RH, Eble JN. Unusual forms of carcinoma of the urinary bladder. Hum Pathol 1991; 22: 948–965.

540. Yokoyama S, Hayashida Y, Nagahama J, et al. Primary and metaplastic choriocarcinoma of the bladder. A report of two cases. Acta Cytol 1992; 36: 176–182.

541. Cho JH, Yu E, Kim KH, et al. Primary choriocarcinoma of the urinary bladder – a case report. J Korean Med Sci 1992; 7: 369–372.

542. Shah VM, Newman J, Crocker J, et al. Ectopic beta-human chorionic gonadotropin production by bladder urothelial neoplasia. Arch Pathol Lab Med 1986; 110: 107–111.

543. Seidal T, Breborowicz J, Malmstrom P. Immunoreactivity to human chorionic gonadotropin in urothelial carcinoma: correlation with tumor grade, stage, and progression. J Urol Pathol 1993; 1: 397–410.

544. Taylor G, Jordan M, Churchill B, et al. Yolk sac tumor of the bladder. J Urol 1983; 129: 591–594.

545. Jacobs MA, Bavendam T, Leach GE. Bladder leiomyoma. Urology 1989; 34: 56–57.

546. Mintz E. Pedunculated neurofibroma of the bladder. J Urol 1940; 43: 268–274.

547. Bolkier M, Ginesin Y, Lichtig C, et al. Lymphangioma of bladder. J Urol 1983; 129: 1049–1050.

548. Hanna NH, Ulbright TM, Einhorn LH. Primary choriocarcinoma of the bladder with the detection of isochromosome 12p. J Urol 2002; 167: 1781.

549. Weaver MG, Abdul-Karim FW. The prevalence and character of the muscularis mucosae of the human urinary bladder. Histopathology 1990; 17: 563–566.

550. Kurtman C, Andrieu MN, Baltaci S, et al. Conformal radiotherapy in primary non-Hodgkin's lymphoma of the male urethra. Int Urol Nephrol 2001; 33: 537–539.

551. Mearini E, Zucchi A, Costantini E, et al. Primary Burkitt's lymphoma of bladder in a patient with AIDS. J Urol 2002; 167: 1397–1398.

552. Krober SM, Aepinus C, Ruck P, et al. Extranodal marginal zone B cell lymphoma of MALT type involving the mucosa of both the urinary bladder and stomach. J Clin Pathol 2002; 55: 554–557.

553. Lemos N, Melo CR, Soares IC, et al. Plasmacytoma of the urethra treated by excisional biopsy. Scand J Urol Nephrol 2000; 34: 75–76.

554. Ohsawa M, Aozasa K, Horiuchi K, et al. Malignant lymphoma of bladder. Report of three cases and review of the literature. Cancer 1993; 72: 1969–1974.

555. Kempton CL, Kurtin PJ, Inwards DJ, et al. Malignant lymphoma of the bladder: evidence from 36 cases that low-grade lymphoma of the MALT-type is the most common primary bladder lymphoma. Am J Surg Pathol 1997; 21: 1324–1333.

556. Al-Quran SZ, Olivares A, Lin P, et al. Myeloid sarcoma of the urinary bladder and epididymis as a primary manifestation of acute myeloid leukemia with inv(16). Arch Pathol Lab Med 2006; 130: 862–866.

557. Hasegeli UA, Altundag K, Saglam A, et al. Granulocytic sarcoma of the urinary bladder. Am J Hematol 2004; 75: 262–263.

558. Aki H, Baslar Z, Uygun N, et al. Primary granulocytic sarcoma of the urinary bladder: case report and review of the literature. Urology 2002; 60: 345.

559. Bates AW, Baithun SI. The significance of secondary neoplasms of the urinary and male genital tract. Virchows Arch 2002; 440: 640–647.

560. Chuang AY, Demarzo AM, Veltri RW, et al. Immunohistochemical differentiation of high-grade prostate carcinoma from urothelial carcinoma. Am J Surg Pathol 2007; 31: 1246–1255.

561. Chu P, Wu E, Weiss LM. Cytokeratin 7 and cytokeratin 20 expression in epithelial neoplasms: a survey of 435 cases. Mod Pathol 2000; 13: 962–972.

562. Wang NP, Zee S, Zarbo RJ, et al. Coordinate expression of cytokeratins 7 and 20 defines unique subsets of carcinomas. App Immunohistochem 1995; 3: 99–107.

563. Moll R, Lowe A, Laufer J, et al. Cytokeratin 20 in human carcinomas: a new histodiagnostic marker detected by monoclonal antibodies. Am J Pathol 1992; 140: 427–447.

564. Jiang J, Ulbright TM, Younger C, et al. Cytokeratin 7 and cytokeratin 20 in primary urinary bladder carcinoma and matched lymph node metastasis. Arch Pathol Lab Med 2001; 125: 921–923.

565. Parker DC, Folpe AL, Bell J, et al. Potential utility of uroplakin III, thrombomodulin, high molecular weight cytokeratin, and cytokeratin 20 in noninvasive, invasive, and metastatic urothelial (transitional cell) carcinomas. Am J Surg Pathol 2003; 27: 1–10.

566. Kaufmann O, Volmerig J, Dietel M. Uroplakin III is a highly specific and moderately sensitive immunohistochemical marker for primary and metastatic urothelial carcinomas. Am J Clin Pathol 2000; 113: 683–687.

567. Moll R, Wu XR, Lin JH, et al. Uroplakins, specific membrane proteins of urothelial umbrella cells, as histological markers of metastatic transitional cell carcinomas. Am J Pathol 1995; 147: 1383–1397.

568. Logani S, Oliva E, Amin MB, et al. Immunoprofile of ovarian tumors with putative transitional cell (urothelial) differentiation using novel urothelial markers: histogenetic and diagnostic implications. Am J Surg Pathol 2003; 27: 1434–1441.

569. Ordonez NG. Transitional cell carcinomas of the ovary and bladder are immunophenotypically different. Histopathology 2000; 36: 433–438.

570. Riedel I, Czernobilsky B, Lifschitz-Mercer B, et al. Brenner tumors but not transitional cell carcinomas of the ovary show urothelial differentiation: immunohistochemical staining of urothelial markers, including cytokeratins and uroplakins. Virchows Arch 2001; 438: 181–191.

# CHAPTER 7

# Urine cytology

John F. Morrow, Janet Johnston, David G. Bostwick

This chapter discusses the spectrum of cytologic abnormalities in voided urine samples and washings in order to allow comparison with the biopsy findings described in Chapters 5 and 6. The clinically significant and common problem of hematuria is also addressed from the perspective of the cytopathologist.

## Utility of urine cytology

### Indications

Cytologic examination of urinary sediment is valuable in the diagnosis of a wide variety of benign and malignant diseases of the bladder, urethra, ureter, and kidney.[1-4] This chapter focuses mainly on diagnostic cytology of the urothelium, with special emphasis on bladder diseases. Urine cytology has important limitations: for example, despite recent improvements it is not highly reliable for the identification of low-grade papillary tumors.[5,6] However, cytology yields good to excellent results in the identification of carcinoma in situ and high-grade urothelial carcinoma.[5,7] The principal indications for the use of cytology in disorders of the urinary tract include:

- Diagnosis of carcinoma in situ, urothelial dysplasia, and high-grade carcinoma.
- Follow-up of patients with urothelial tumor, regardless of grade.
- Monitoring of patients with urothelial tumor undergoing or following treatment.[2,8-12]
- Evaluation of hematuria, including separation of kidney (upper-tract disease) and non-kidney (lower-tract) causes.

The major diagnostic categories are presented in Table 7-1.

### Types of cytology specimen

The sources of urologic cytology specimens include voided or randomly voided urine, catheterized urine, bladder washing (barbotage), brushing,[13,14] ureter and renal pelvis brushing and washing,[14] and neobladder urine from an ileal conduit or colonic pouch. A recent prospective study showed that spontaneously voided specimens were superior to post-cytometrogram and bladder irrigation specimens (adequacy 97%, 94%, and 12%, respectively).[15] Collection method was significantly associated with specimen adequacy and cell count.[15]

### Normal components of urinary sediment

Urothelial cells are the most variably sized cells in urinary sediment. They vary from 20 μm in diameter to the typical 'umbrella' cell whose size may approach 100 μm. These cells are often multinucleate with reactive nuclei. Urothelial cells typically have round to oval nuclei with abundant homogeneous, predominantly basophilic cytoplasm. Cells from the basal urothelium are smaller, round, and display well-defined thickened cytoplasmic membranes. Chromocenters

**Table 7-1** Cytologic diagnostic categories in urinary sediment

| Non-Tumor-Associated Cytology* |
| --- |
| Normal cells/negative for malignant cells |
| Inflammatory changes<br>    Specific type<br>    Non-specific |

| Tumor-Associated Cytology |
| --- |
| Rare single cells and clusters of mildly to moderately atypical urothelial cells; this may represent a reactive process, but neoplasm should be considered; clinical correlation is indicated |
| Rare highly atypical urothelial cells, favor neoplasm; a reactive process cannot be excluded; repeat study and/or further investigation may be of value |
| Severely atypical urothelial cells highly suspicious for neoplasm; clinical correlation is recommended |
| Malignant cells present most suggestive of urothelial carcinoma |
| Malignant cells present/specify: squamous cell carcinoma, adenocarcinoma, prostatic adenocarcinoma, renal cell carcinoma, other |
| Malignant cells present, not otherwise specified |

*In addition, evaluation of urinary sediment in patients with hematuria allows separation of kidney (upper-tract disease) and non-kidney (lower-tract) causes.

and multiple eosinophilic micronucleoli may be prominent, especially in cases with accompanying inflammation.

Fragments of urothelial cells are commonly found in catheterized specimens as well as bladder washes; however, it is abnormal to see urothelial fragments in spontaneously voided urine, and their presence may be associated with papilloma or low-grade urothelial cancer. Occasionally, a large urothelial fragment displays cytoplasmic vacuoles containing neutrophils. Multinucleation, nuclear enlargement, and hyperchromasia can be found in inflammatory processes within the lower urinary tract.

### Superficial (umbrella) cells

Regardless of the type of sample and the collection technique used, superficial urothelial cells are a common component of the urinary sediment. These cells have one or more nuclei that are large, measuring up to 30 μm in diameter, comparable to superficial squamous cells (Fig. 7-1).[2] Binucleate cells are common. Such cells are often larger than the mononucleate superficial cells, and their nuclei are somewhat smaller. Large multinucleate superficial cells are by far the most striking component of the urinary sediment (excluding contaminating squamous epithelial cells), particularly in washings or brushings of the bladder or ureter. Multinucleate superficial cells are particularly large, and may be mistaken for giant cells. A common error in diagnosis is misinterpretation of large superficial cells as macrophages or tumor cells. The DNA content of superficial cells may be twice that of other urothelial cells (tetraploid nuclei).[16,17]

The chromatinic rim of the nucleus is thick and sharply demarcated. The chromatin is finely granular, often with a 'salt and pepper' appearance, and may contain one or more promi-

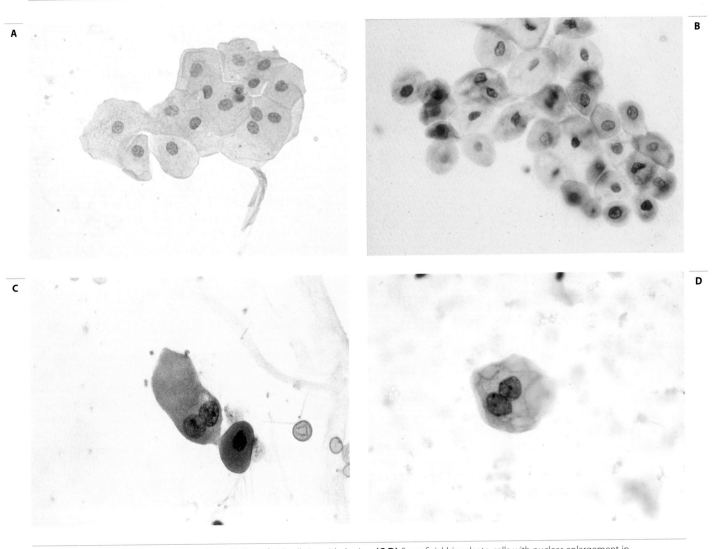

**Fig. 7-1** Normal superficial (umbrella) cells. **(A,B)** Superficial cells in voided urine. **(C,D)** Superficial binucleate cells with nuclear enlargement in catheterization specimens.

nent chromocenters. The structure of the nucleus is better preserved in bladder washings than in voided urine. In women, there may be a sex chromatin body attached to the nuclear membrane. The cytoplasm of these cells is usually eosinophilic, often finely granular, and sometimes vacuolated.

## Cells originating from the deeper layers of the urothelium

Epithelial cells smaller than the superficial cells that are derived from the deeper layers of the urothelium often exfoliate in clusters, particularly if the specimen was obtained with an instrument. Single small urothelial cells are observed in voided urine, usually in the presence of inflammation and destruction of the superficial cell layer. Clusters of urothelial cells may be tightly packed and assume spherical 'papillary' configurations with sharp borders. Such clusters are often misinterpreted as low-grade papillary carcinoma.[18,19] When the deep cells are removed by an instrument, they often

appear in loose clusters. These cells are polygonal or elongated, sometimes columnar, and almost always display cytoplasmic extensions in contact with other cells. The amount of basophilic cytoplasm in such cells depends on the layer of origin, and is more abundant in cells derived from superficial layers. Single cells resemble parabasal squamous cells in both size and configuration. They are often spherical or round, particularly in voided urine, but may also show cytoplasmic extensions.[2] The nuclei of the smaller urothelial cells are approximately the same size, measuring about 5 μm in diameter. They are usually finely granular and benign appearing, containing one or rarely two small chromocenters. In voided urine, the nuclei may be pale or opaque and occasionally somewhat darker.

## Mucus-containing epithelial cells

Occasionally, urine cytology specimens contain mucus-secreting columnar epithelial cells with peripheral nuclei

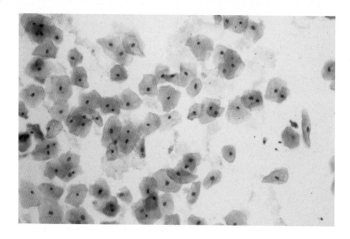

**Fig. 7-2** Squamous cells in the urine.

and distended clear cytoplasm. These cells may be ciliated. Such cells derive from cystitis cystica or cystitis glandularis.

## Squamous cells

Squamous cells of varying size and degrees of maturation are common in urinary sediment, particularly in voided specimens (Fig. 7-2). Such cells are more abundant in females than in males.[2] In women, these cells originate in the squamous epithelium and in the trigone of the urinary bladder, and may be glycogenated. Voided urinary sediment may also contain squamous cells derived from the vulva, vagina, or uterine cervix. In men, the origin of the squamous cells is the terminal portion of the urethra, or, in rare cases, a vaginal type of squamous metaplasia. Among the benign squamous cells there may be superficial cells, intermediate cells, and smaller parabasal cells. Navicular cells are intermediate squamous cells with a large cytoplasmic glycogen content and peripheral nuclei; these cells stain yellow with Papanicolaou stain. Such cells may be observed during pregnancy, early menopause, and sometimes in women or men receiving hormonal therapy (androgen deprivation therapy for prostate cancer). In women, the population of squamous cells in the urinary sediment may be used to determine the level of estrogenic activity (the so-called urocytogram). Squamous cells may also be anucleate and fully keratinized. The presence of such 'ghost' cells may be of diagnostic significance, representing leukoplakia or squamous cell carcinoma of the bladder.[1]

## Renal epithelial cells

Collecting duct cells derived from the renal tubules are commonly seen in the urine sediment (<1 per HPF) in a concentrated cell preparation from normal individuals. They are small, cuboidal in appearance with a polygonal shape and single, slightly eccentric nucleus. In patients with medical conditions such as diabetes, hypertension and kidney related diseases, their numbers can be markedly increased and accompany renal casts of many varieties as well as fragments from the proximal and distal collecting ducts. Renal epithelial fragments are indicative of renal ischemia or com-

promised perfusion of the tubules. Three distinct types of renal epithelial cells that can be identified and quantified in the urine sediment and include convoluted tubular cells of proximal and distal types, and collecting duct cells. Necrotic cells of these types may also be identified by their characteristic size, shape and texture of their cytoplasm.

## Convoluted tubular cells

Cells from the convoluted tubular epithelium are the largest cells in the nephron, present at the entrance to Bowman's capsule and extending to the beginning of the loop of Henle. These cells are rarely seen in normal individuals, but are shed in large numbers in cases of renal toxicity and renal ischemia caused by a wide variety of drugs, heavy metals, immunosuppressants, and other toxins.

Proximal tubular cells in urine are easily identified by their large size (20–60 μm in diameter) irregular, elongated, or cigar-like appearance, and coarsely granular basophilic cytoplasm (Fig. 7-3A). Cytoplasmic borders are indistinct and may be ragged or torn. Ultrastructurally the granular cytoplasm contains large numbers of mitochondria. Nuclei are slightly larger than erythrocytes and may occasionally be multinucleate. Interestingly, proximal and distal tubular cells appear singly, never in fragments or clusters. These cells are often mistaken for granular casts in unstained brightfield microscopy. Proximal and distal renal tubular cells slough from their basement membranes and can be found in urine as intact preserved cells, or as 'ghost' or necrotic forms that retain their size and cytoplasmic characteristics (Fig. 7-3B).

## Collecting duct cells

Renal tubular cells lining the proximal and distal collecting ducts are small (12–18 μm in diameter), and each contains a single slightly eccentric nucleus with coarse and evenly distributed chromatin. There may be an occasional nucleolus, as these cells may be reactive, with prominent nucleoli, but they are never multinucleate. The cytoplasm is polygonal to columnar, finely granular and uniformly basophilic, with distinct borders (Fig. 7-3C). Vacuolization may occasionally be seen, especially in reactive states. The cells may phagocytose cast-like material, crystals, and pigments.

Collecting duct cells may be seen in very low numbers in the urine of normal individuals, but are significant when found with renal casts and/or as fragments. An abnormal number (more than one per high power field) may be found in a wide variety of clinical conditions, including shock, trauma, burn, and exposure to toxins; in addition, an increased number of cells in renal transplant patients heralds clinical rejection by up to 48 hours.

Renal epithelial cell fragments in urine indicate a severe form of renal tubular injury (ischemic necrosis), and are exclusively from the collecting duct. This reflects loss of blood flow (ischemic injury) to the renal tubules and subsequent sloughing of entire segments or portions of the renal tubules with regeneration of lost epithelium, a process similar to repair in cervical smears. There are five types of fragments, and these are classified according to morphology: (1) spindle fragments; (2) fragments attached to or surrounding cast

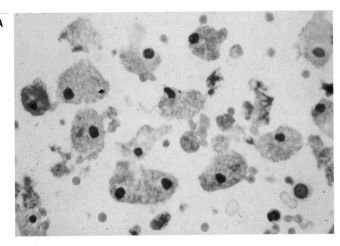

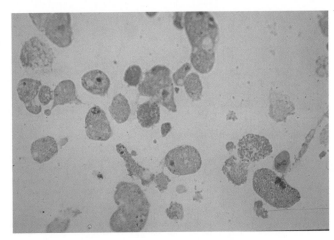

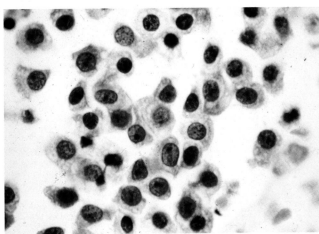

**Fig. 7-3** Proximal and distal convoluted tubular cells from the nephron **(A).** Necrotic proximal and distal convoluted tubular cells **(B).** Collecting duct cells **(C).**

material; (3) pavement or 'en-face' fragments; (4) fragments with reactive cellular or non-cellular inclusions (cast-like, crystal or pigmented (bile) inclusions); and (5) cylindrical, tube-like fragments.

## Other benign cells

Occasionally, cells of prostatic and seminal vesicle origin may be present in the urinary sediment. Such cells accompany spermatozoa and are common after prostatic massage.[21,22]

Macrophages are often observed in inflammatory reactions of the urinary tract. The cells may be mononucleate or multinucleate, and contain fine cytoplasmic vacuoles, sometimes with phagocytic debris. Normal urinary sediment contains very few lymphocytes or neutrophils. The presence of large numbers of such cells may precede clinical evidence of inflammation. Erythrocytes are a frequent component of the urinary sediment, particularly in patients with clinical evidence of hematuria (see below).[1]

## Non-cellular components of urinary sediment

Polygonal transparent crystalline precipitates of urates are common in voided urine. Their presence results from changes in the acidity of urine after collection, but has no diagnostic significance. Crystals derived from true uric acid are rare. Other crystals are very rarely of diagnostic value.[23] Voided urine and occasional specimens obtained by instrumentation may contain contaminants.

## Renal casts in urine sediment

Renal casts are observed in urinary sediment from patients with glomerular and renal parenchymal diseases. Casts are composed of Tamm–Horsfall protein and originate in the distal tubules and collecting ducts. In normal individuals, hyaline and rare granular casts may occasionally appear owing to dehydration, fever, exercise, and other factors; these casts are considered physiologic. Conversely, non-physiologic casts made of abnormal urinary protein and those that contain cells of various types are easily identified. The types of cell contained within the cast matrix, the width of the casts, and the number of casts is indicative of the severity of the underlying disease. The presence of abnormal amounts of protein, blood, leukocytes, nitrites, and bilirubin correlates with the type of cast.

## Urolithiasis (stone formation)

About one in 15 people in the industrialized world develops kidney stones, and all age groups and both genders are affected, with an apparent genetic predisposition.

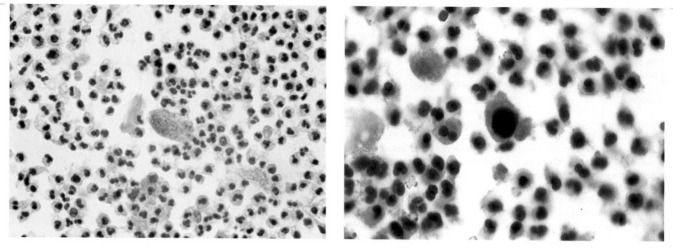

**Fig. 7-4** Acute cystitis **(A)**, consisting of marked inflammation, degenerate urothelial cells **(B)**, and scattered superficial cells.

Urinary tract calculi are composed of waste products, and hematuria commonly occurs during the earliest stages. Calculi form as the result of increased excretion of solutes (calcium oxalate, calcium phosphate, magnesium ammonium phosphate, struvite or triple phosphate, uric acid, cystine), abnormal urinary pH, stasis, dehydration, and/or urinary concentration. Once a stone grows to a significant size the patient may experience symptoms that range from a dull ache to severe pain, often equated with the pain of childbirth or abdominal surgery without the benefit of anesthesia. Stones originate as microscopic grains of mineral debris, enlarging to the size of gravel and later to a large stone.

Stones may occur anywhere along the urinary tract, and many patients pass them spontaneously. Large calculi require surgical intervention or shock wave extracorporeal lithotripsy to create passable fragments.

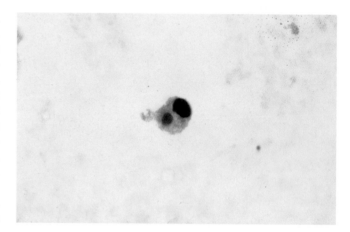

**Fig. 7-5** Degenerate urothelial cells with cytoplasmic inclusions.

## Diagnostic criteria

### Inflammatory processes

#### Bacteria

A wide variety of bacteria may affect the epithelium of the urinary tract. Most are coliforms and other Gram-negative rods. Cystitis may be acute or chronic. Acute cystitis is usually associated with symptoms that rarely require confirmatory tissue biopsy or cytologic examination. In those cases in which the urine is studied, the sediment may contain numerous exfoliated urothelial cells, necrotic material, and inflammatory cells, with a predominance of neutrophils (Fig. 7-4). Marked necrosis and inflammation may also occur in the presence of necrotic tumors, particularly high-grade urothelial carcinoma and squamous cell carcinoma.

The urinary sediment in chronic cystitis usually contains a background of chronic inflammation with macrophages and erythrocytes.[1] Urothelial cells may be abundant and poorly preserved, occasionally forming small clusters. The cytoplasm in these cells tends to be granular and vacuolated; when the cells are degenerate, the cytoplasm contains spheri-

cal eosinophilic inclusions of no significance (Fig. 7-5). These may have slight nuclear enlargement and hyperchromasia, but the contours of the nuclei are usually regular and the chromatin texture is finely granular without the coarse granularity of urothelial cancer cells. There may be necrosis of urothelial cells, with nuclear pyknosis and marked cytoplasmic vacuolization. In ulcerative cystitis, large sheets of urothelial cells may be observed.

Interstitial cystitis, a form of chronic cystitis associated with chronic inflammation, displays non-specific cytologic changes.[2] Eosinophilic cystitis has a preponderance of eosinophils, a pattern that may be seen in patients with allergic disorders, previous biopsies, or following mitomycin C treatment.[24]

Tuberculous cystitis may be observed in patients with AIDS and those receiving treatment for urothelial carcinoma with BCG (Bacille Calmette–Guérin). In such patients, the urine or bladder wash shows inflammatory cells, and rarely contains fragments of tubercles consisting of clusters of elongated carrot-shaped epithelioid cells, sometimes accompanied by multinucleated Langerhans'-type giant cells and reactive atypia of urothelial cells.[25–27] The sediment or bladder biopsy occasionally contains 'decoy' cells with glassy hyperchromatic nuclei.[25] Similar findings may occur in patients with tuberculosis of the bladder.

## Fungi

Fungi occasionally affect the lower urinary tract, particularly the urinary bladder, and *Candida albicans* is the most common, usually seen in pregnant women, diabetics, and those with impaired immunity, such as patients with AIDS, those undergoing chemotherapy for cancer, and bone marrow transplant recipients. In urinary sediment the fungi may appear as yeast forms, with small oval bodies, or pseudohyphae, having oblong branching non-encapsulated filaments (Fig. 7-6). Other fungi are uncommon, including *Blastomyces dermatitidis*, *Aspergillus*, and *Mucormyces*. A fungus of the species *Alternaria* is a common laboratory contaminant.[2]

## Viruses

Several important viruses cause significant morphologic changes in the urothelial cells, many of which may be confused with malignancy. The dominant feature of viral infection is the formation of nuclear and cytoplasmic inclusions (Table 7-2).

Herpes simplex is an obligate intracellular virus, and florid infection with permissive replication of the virus causes abnormalities in urothelial cells that are readily recognized. In the early stages of viral replication, the nuclei of infected cells appear hazy, with a ground-glass appearance. Multinucleation is commonly observed in such cells. Multiple nuclei are often densely packed, with nuclear molding and tightly fitting contoured nuclei. In later stages of infection, the viral particles concentrate in the center of the nuclei, forming bright eosinophilic inclusions with a narrow clear zone or halo at the periphery. Infected cells may contain single or multiple nuclei.[2,23]

Cytomegalovirus is usually seen in newborn infants with impaired immunity and is common in adults with AIDS. The characteristic changes are readily recognized in the urinary sediment, including large cells with large basophilic nuclear inclusions surrounded by a large peripheral clear zone (Fig. 7-7). There is a distinct outer band of condensed nuclear chromatin.

Polyomavirus infection is widespread, according to serologic studies of adults. The occult virus can become activated and recognized in voided urinary sediment. One form of polyomavirus, the BK virus, plays a major role in urine cytology because it produces cell abnormalities that may be readily confused with cancer; these cells are also known as 'decoy cells' (Fig. 7-8).[28] In permissive infections, the BK virus produces large, homogeneous, basophilic nuclear inclusions that occupy almost the entire volume of the nuclei.[29,30] Occa-

**Table 7-2** Characteristic cytologic changes associated with specific types of virus

**CMV**
Enlarged cells
High nucleus: cytoplasmic (N/C) ratio
Basophilic intranuclear inclusion with 'owl's-eye' appearance; occasionally small, dark intracytoplasmic inclusions

**Herpes virus**
Enlarged, multinucleated cells with 'ground-glass' chromatin
High N/C ratio
Opaque, structureless chromatin
Eosinophilic intranuclear inclusion

**Polyomavirus**
Enlarged cells
High N/C ratio
Opaque, structureless chromatin, chromatinic membrane is common
Nuclei stain with a magenta hue
Intranuclear inclusion fills almost the entire nuclear area

**Papillomavirus**
Perinuclear clear cytoplasmic zones (koilocytosis)
Nuclear enlargement and homogeneous hyperchromasia

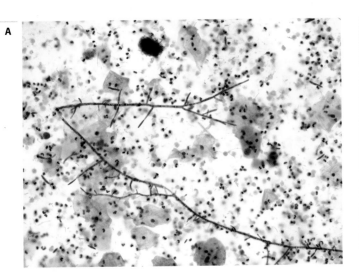

A

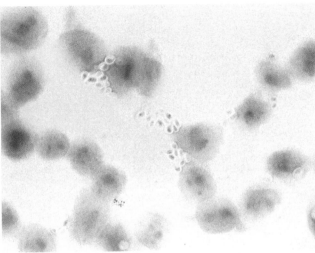

B

**Fig. 7-6** *Candida albicans* in the urinary sediment. **(A)** Distinctive branching fungal hyphae are abundant in this urine specimen. **(B)** Note the small oval budding spores that stand in contrast to the urothelial cells.

sionally, a narrow rim of clearing separates the inclusion from the chromatinic rim. The infected cells are often enlarged and usually contain a single nucleus, but binucleation and occasional large multinucleated cells may be seen.[31] The cytologic picture in some cases may be quite dramatic and has led to misdiagnoses of carcinoma.[32] Another rare form of polyomavirus infection of the urine is caused by the JC virus, which is associated with progressive multifocal leukoencephalopathy.

More than 70 types of human papillomavirus have been identified, and types 6 and 11 are associated with condyloma acuminatum. Condyloma may also appear in the urethra, and invariably induces koilocytosis. Urothelial carcinoma exhibits a low incidence of human papillomavirus types 16 and 18 infection.[33]

### Trematodes and other parasites

The most important of these is *Schistosoma haematobium* (bilharzia). There are two important cytologic manifestations of infection with *Schistosoma haematobium*: recognition of the ova, and the malignant tumors that may be associated with it.[24] The ova are elongated structures with a thick transparent capsule and a sword-shaped protrusion known as the terminal spine located at the narrow end of the ovum. Fresh or calcified ova may be readily recognized in the urinary sedi-

ment. The embryonal form of the parasite, known as miracidium, is released in human stool and urine, retaining the shape of the ovum with its terminal spine.

Other common intestinal parasites that affect the bladder include *Ascaris lumbricoides*, *Enterobius vermicularis*, and agents of filariasis.

## Reactive cytologic changes

Numerous reactive and atypical changes involving the urothelium may be mistaken for malignancy (Tables 7-3, 7-4).

### Lithiasis

About 40% of patients with calculi have abnormal cytologic findings in voided urine.[18] These patients have numerous large, smooth-bordered clusters of benign urothelial cells with an abundance of superficial cells (Fig. 7-9). These changes may overlap with the spectrum of findings with low-grade urothelial carcinoma, but the cells tend to cluster, with fewer single cells.[18] Calculi are abrasive to the mucosa when present in the renal pelvis, ureter, or urinary bladder, and the resultant cytologic specimens closely resemble the effects of instrumentation. Significant atypia of urothelial cells due to lithiasis is uncommon.[2] Nonetheless, lithiasis remains a major diagnostic pitfall in urinary cytology interpretation.

### Drug effects

Intravesically administered agents and drugs, including BCG (see Bacteria, above), mitomycin C, and thiotepa are commonly used for treatment of primary and recurrent bladder

**Table 7-3** Differential diagnosis of urothelial atypia found in urinary sediment

| Urinary tract conditions |
|---|
| Urethral catheterization |
| Urinary calculi |
| Chronic cystitis and cystitis glandularis |
| Cellular changes due to radiation therapy and chemotherapy |
| Atypical and/or hyperplastic urothelium |
| Papillary urothelial tumor of low malignant potential and low-grade urothelial carcinoma |

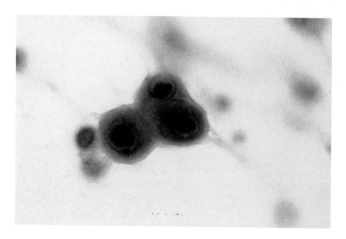

**Fig. 7-7** CMV infection; characteristic 'owls eye' intranuclear inclusion.

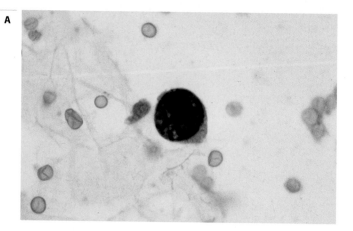

A

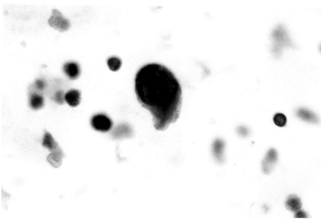

B

**Fig. 7-8** Decoy cells in polyomavirus infection. **(A, B)** These may be mistaken for malignant cells.

**Table 7-4** Cellular features of reactive urothelial atypia versus urothelial neoplasia

|  | Atypia | CIS | Grade 1 carcinoma | Grades 2 and 3 carcinoma |
|---|---|---|---|---|
| **Cells** | | | | |
| Arrangement | Papillary aggregates | Numerous single cells | Papillary and loose clusters | Isolated and loose clusters |
| Size | Increased | Increased | Increased, uniform | Increased, pleomorphic |
| Number | Variable | Variable | Often numerous | Variable |
| Cytoplasm | Variable | Variable maturation | Homogeneous | Variable |
| Nucleus/cytoplasmic ratio | Normal/increased | Increased | Increased | Increased |
| **Nuclei** | | | | |
| Position | Non-eccentric | Non-eccentric | Eccentric | Eccentric |
| Size | Enlarged | Enlarged | Enlarged | Variable |
| Morphology | Uniform within aggregates | Aggregates, cannibalism | Variable within aggregates | Variable |
| Borders | Smooth/slightly irregular | Marked membrane irregularity | Irregular (notches, creases) | Irregular |
| Chromatin | Dusty-peripheral concentration | Increased chromatin coarsely, granular, evenly distributed | Fine, even | Coarse, uneven |
| Nucleoli | Often large | Rare nucleoli | Small/absent | Variable |
| **Background** | Variable | Clean | Clean | Dirty, tumor diathesis |

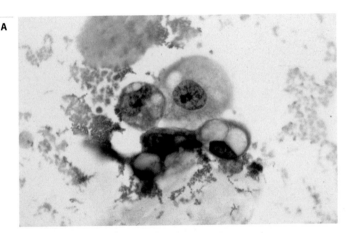

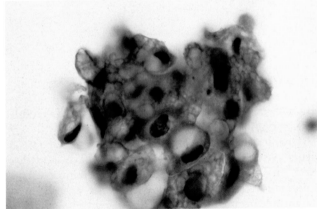

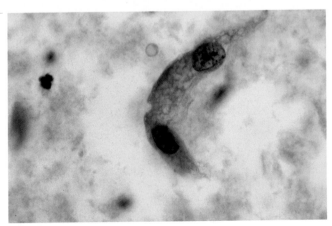

**Fig. 7-9** Renal lithiasis, with findings that may be mistaken for malignancy. **(A)** Cluster of benign urothelial cells. **(B)** Tissue fragment resembling the effects of instrumentation. **(C)** Superficial cells with mild nuclear atypia.

A

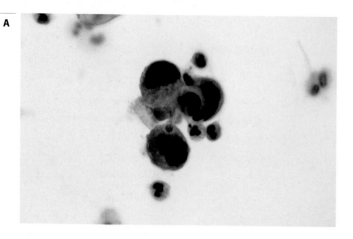

B

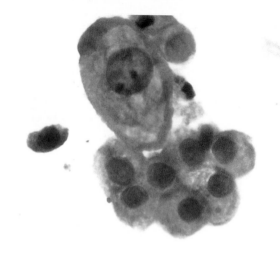

C

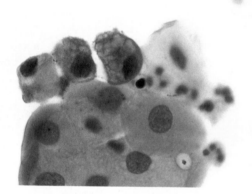

**Fig. 7-10** Mitomycin C changes in the urine mimicking malignancy.

tumors (Figs 7-10, 7-11). They may induce cell enlargement, cytoplasmic vacuolization, and other reactive changes. Intravesical chemotherapy can contribute to false-positive results in urine cytology.[6]

Systemically administered drugs, such as the alkylating agents cyclophosphamide and busulfan, have a marked effect on the urothelium, inducing significant cytologic abnormalities (Fig. 7-12). These drugs may cause changes that include bizarre urothelial cells with marked nuclear and nucleolar enlargement, mimicking poorly differentiated carcinoma.[2,34,35] Large doses of cyclophosphamide have been shown to induce urothelial carcinoma, leiomyosarcoma, and carcinosarcoma.[36,37]

### Effects of radiation therapy

Radiation therapy typically induces marked cell enlargement, with bizarre cell shapes and vacuolated nuclei and cytoplasm (Fig. 7-13). These findings may persist for years after treatment.[2]

## Urine cytology in renal transplant recipients

The epithelial cells of collecting tubules are well preserved in patients following renal transplantation. The cells that appear in urine specimens have scant vacuolated cytoplasm

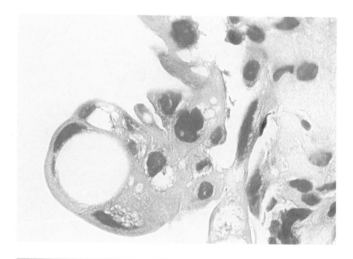

**Fig. 7-11** Thiotepa-induced changes, including urothelial detachment with nuclear atypia and cytoplasmic vacuolization.

with spherical and somewhat opaque nuclei. A feature of impending rejection is the presence in the urine of numerous T lymphocytes and increasing numbers of collecting duct cells of renal origin. The erythrocytes have a thick outer border and a clear center suggestive of a renal origin. In rejection, tissue fragments may be present, including necrotic renal tubules and casts.[20]

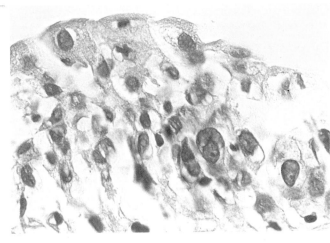

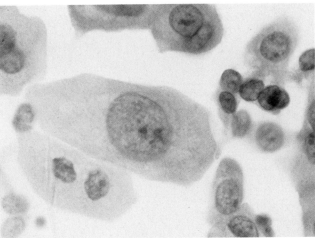

**Fig. 7-12** Cyclophosphamide changes. Atypical urothelial cells with large hyperchromatic nuclei **(B, C)** that may be mistaken for malignant cells. **(A)** Tissue section, urine cytology.

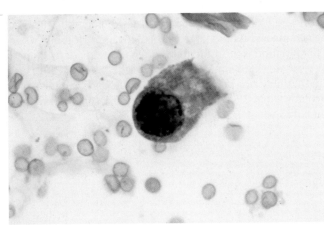

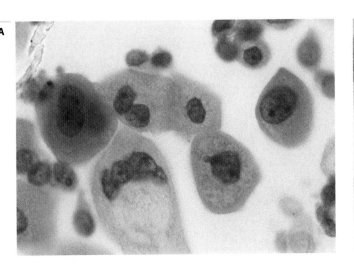

**Fig. 7-13** Radiation changes. Note bizarre enlarged urothelial cells with numerous vacuolations **(A, B)**.

## Other benign conditions

Partial or complete keratinization of the squamous epithelium, referred to clinically as leukoplakia, often replaces the urothelium, resulting in a cystoscopic gray-white appearance of the mucosa. In the urinary sediment, anucleated keratin-ized cell – so-called ghost cells – may be present. When such cells are identified, further investigation should be undertaken to exclude the possibility of squamous cell carcinoma.[1,2] Cystitis glandularis may shed ciliated mucus-containing epithelial cells that contain peripheral nuclei and clear cytoplasm. Such cells may be mistaken for adenocarcinoma. Large numbers of macrophages may be present in urine samples from patients with malakoplakia, but the release of such inflammatory cells usually occurs after biopsy and is detected in the urine stream. The spherical, intracytoplasmic, eosinophilic, or calcified Michaelis–Guttmann bodies in the cytoplasm of the macrophages are usually readily identified.

## Benign tumors and tumor-like processes

There are no cell changes that are characteristic of inverted papilloma or nephrogenic adenoma, and cytologic findings from these processes may be difficult to interpret.[38]

Condyloma acuminatum of the urinary bladder is uncommon, and may be associated with condyloma of the urethra or external genitalia. Koilocytosis is characterized by squamous cells with large hyperchromatic nuclei and perinuclear clear zones or haloes. These changes result from infection by human papillomavirus types 6 and 11. The presence of koilocytes in voided urinary sediment in males often indicates a lesion in the bladder or urethra. In women, such cells may also indicate contamination from the lower genital tract. Occasionally, koilocytes may mimic squamous cell carcinoma. Endometrial-type glandular cells in urinary sediment have been reported in women with endometriosis.[39]

## Cytologic diagnosis of urothelial tumors

### Dysplasia

In cases of dysplasia, the only cytologic finding is the presence of atypical urothelial cells (Fig. 7-14).[40] It is difficult, if not impossible, to recognize specific cell changes that correspond to low- to intermediate-grade dysplasia.[2] We consider high-grade (severe) dysplasia and carcinoma in situ to be synonymous (see below).

### Carcinoma in situ

Urothelial carcinoma in situ (CIS) is characterized by the presence of malignant cells that are often uniform in size and which may be small or large (Fig. 7-15) (Table 7-5).[7,35] The background of the smears is often clean, free of necrotic debris, and lacks inflammation. Occasionally, the cells may be heterogeneous and large, particularly after biopsies. When inflammation is prominent it is often prudent not to attempt to separate CIS from invasive carcinoma. Microinvasive carcinoma may not be recognizable in cytologic samples, particularly when CIS is present. CIS may persist after intravesical therapy such as BCG (Fig. 7-16).

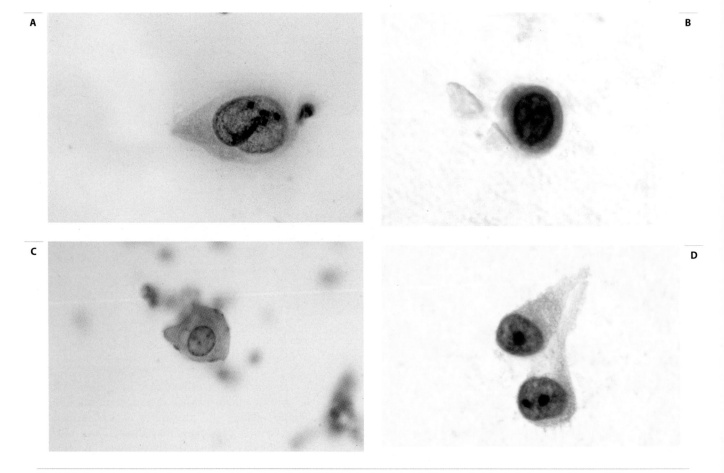

**Fig. 7-14** Atypical urothelial cells consistent with dysplasia **(A–D)**. Multiple biopsies of the bladder revealed dysplasia, but no evidence of CIS.

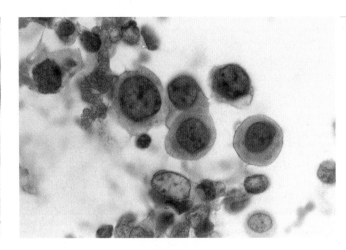

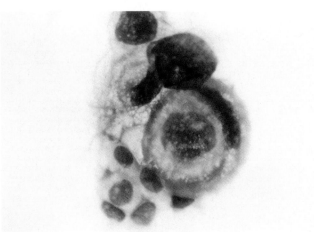

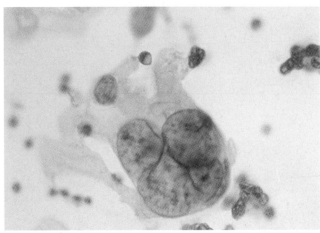

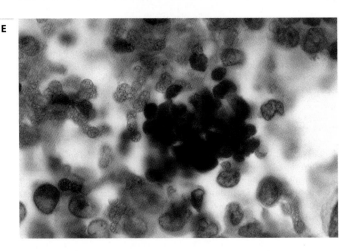

**Fig. 7-15** **(A)** CIS (right) in association with atypical cells of dysplasia (left); **(B, C)** Cluster of cells of CIS. **(D)** Multinucleated cell of CIS. **(E)** Small cell variant of CIS.

## Papilloma, WHO grade 1 carcinoma, papillary neoplasm of low malignant potential, and low-grade papillary carcinoma

It may be difficult cytologically to separate WHO grade 1 urothelial carcinoma (papillary urothelial neoplasm of low malignant potential) from papilloma.[41,42] The urothelial cell clusters are often arranged in a papillary configuration, and are difficult to distinguish from those shed from the normal benign urothelium after palpation, instrumentation, or irritation by calculi or inflammation Fig 7-17.[18,19] In voided

urine, spontaneously shed complex clusters of morphologically benign urothelial cells may be suggestive of a papillary tumor, provided that trauma can be excluded clinically. Diagnostic features of WHO grade 1 carcinoma (papillary neoplasm of low malignant potential) include the presence of tumor fragments with connective tissue stalks or central capillary vessels (Table 7-5).[43] Numerous attempts to define the precise microscopic features of tumor fragments that separate benign urothelial cell clusters from WHO grade 1 carcinoma have met with limited success.[44] Some authors claim that low- to intermediate-grade papillary urothelial

**Table 7-5** Criteria for cytologic grading of urothelial cancer (Modified from Shenoy MA, Colby TV, Schumann GB. Reliability of urinary cytodiagnosis in urothelial neoplasms. Cancer 1985; 56: 2041–2045)

| Morphologic features | CIS | Grade 1 carcinoma (papillary neoplasm of low malignant potential) | Grade 2 carcinoma (low grade urothelial carcinoma) | Grade 3 carcinoma (high grade urothelial carcinoma) |
|---|---|---|---|---|
| Background | Clean | Clean | Clean | Dirty, tumor diathesis |
| Cellular arrangement | Numerous single cells, rare fragments | Large fragments of urothelium | Large fragments of urothelium and single cells | Large fragments and numerous single cells |
| Nuclear features | Syncytia,* cannibalism | Slightly enlarged | Nuclear crowding and overlap | Syncytia*, cannibalism |
| Nuclear membrane | Marked membrane irregularity | Minimal membrane irregularity | Moderate membrane irregularity | Marked membrane irregularity |
| Chromatin | Increased chromatin, coarsely granular, evenly distributed | Finely granular, vesicular | Coarse, unevenly distributed | Increased chromatin, coarsely granular, unevenly distributed |
| Nucleolus | Rare nucleoli | Occasional micronucleoli | Variable micronucleoli | Macronucleoli |
| Cytoplasmic features | Variable maturation | Cell maturation present | Moderate degree of maturation | Maturation absent, squamoid and/or glandular features |

*Loss of cell borders.

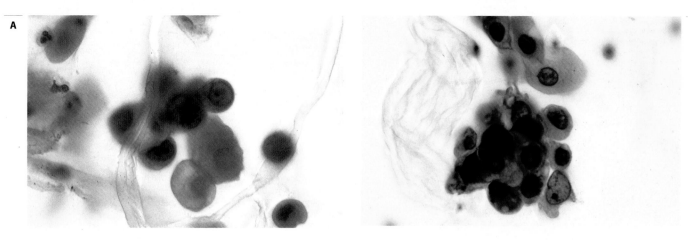

**Fig. 7-16** CIS resistant to BCG therapy, with clusters of hyperchromatic neoplastic cells. **(A, B)**

tumors shed recognizable cells in the urinary sediment:[45] characteristic features include increased nuclear/cytoplasmic ratio, enlarged and eccentric nuclei, and inconspicuous nucleoli, features present in 70% of such tumors.[46] Others report correct cytologic diagnosis in 33% of cases.[44]

Differentiation of WHO grade 1 carcinoma (papillary urothelial neoplasm of low malignant potential) from instrumentation artifacts is based on the presence of cell clusters with ragged borders, unlike the smooth borders lined by densely stained cytoplasm at the edge of benign cell clusters.[19] Grade 1 carcinoma can be identified with 45% sensitivity and 98% specificity based on the cytologic criteria of increased nuclear/cytoplasmic ratio, irregular nuclear borders, and cytoplasmic homogeneity.[47] Overall observer accuracy was 76%, with a sensitivity of 82% for a definitive negative diagnosis and a specificity for a definitive positive

diagnosis of 96%.[48] In another study, the sensitivity of 90% and specificity of 65% for grade 1 carcinoma was based on the absence of inflammation, the presence of single and overlapping groups of cells with high nuclear/cytoplasmic ratio, hypochromasia, nuclear grooves and notches, and small nucleoli.[6] A third study showed 26% sensitivity and 95% specificity for grade I urothelial carcinoma,[5] and another showed 37% sensitivity (suspicious or malignant diagnoses) and 94% specificity; 48% of these cytology specimens were classified as atypical.[49] WHO grade I carcinoma is a major source of false-negative results in urine cytology.[6]

Ancillary techniques that may be valuable for separating benign and neoplastic urothelial cells include fluorescence in situ hybridization,[50–53] immunocytochemical tests,[54–57] and DNA ploidy analysis.[45] Digital image analysis is superior to bladder wash cytology for predicting tumor recurrence.[58]

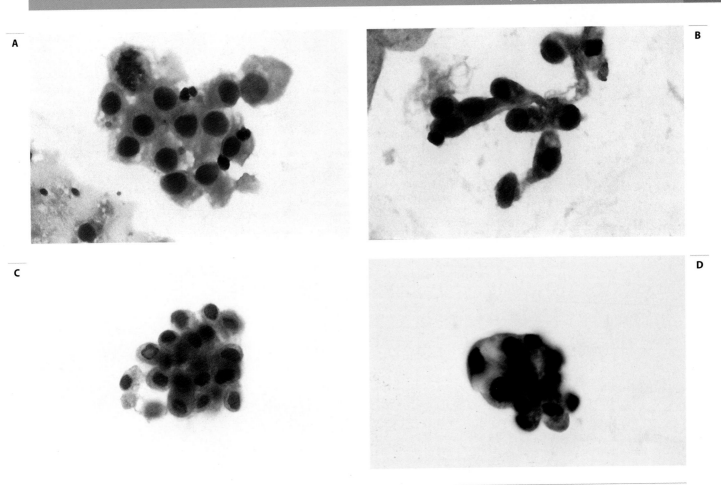

**Fig. 7-17** Examples of grade 1 (of 3) papillary urothelial carcinoma. In each case, the diagnosis was confirmed by biopsy **(A–D)**.

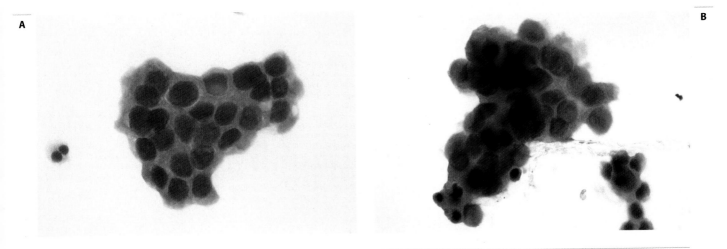

**Fig. 7-18** Examples of grade 2 (of 3) papillary urothelial carcinoma. In each case, the diagnosis was confirmed by biopsy **(A–H)**.

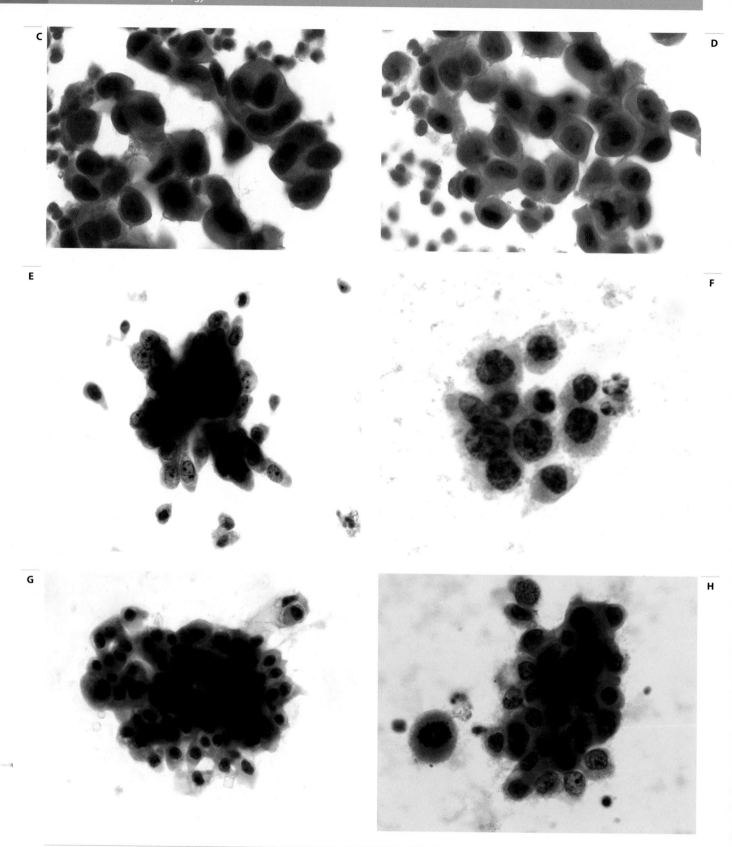

**Fig. 7-18** *Continued*

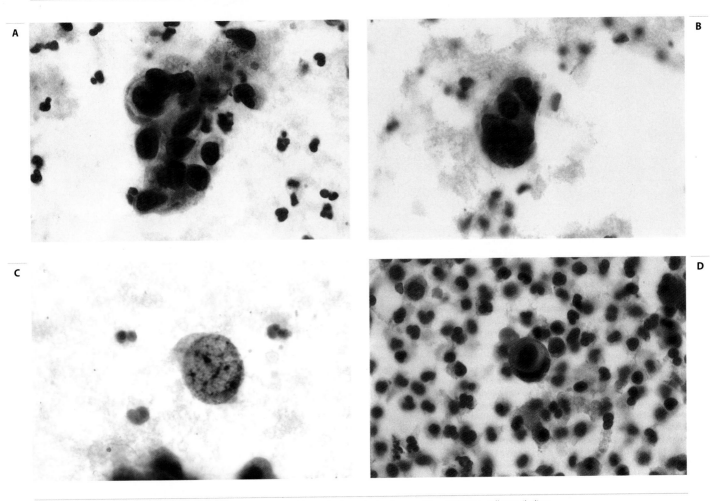

**Fig. 7-19 (A-C)** Grade 3 (of 3) papillary urothelial carcinoma with marked cytologic abnormalities. **(D)** Note cell cannibalism.

## WHO grade 2 (low-grade) and grade 3 (high-grade) urothelial carcinoma

It may be difficult to separate grade 2 and grade 3 urothelial carcinoma from urothelial carcinoma in situ (CIS) (Table 7-5). Unlike benign urothelial cells, these cells have substantial nuclear and cytoplasmic abnormalities (Fig. 7-19). The principal value of urine cytology is the diagnosis and monitoring of high-grade tumors that may not be evident cystoscopically, including CIS and occult invasive carcinoma.[7,59]

In voided urine, low-grade and high-grade urothelial carcinoma cells vary in size and shape and may be small or large. The nuclei are enlarged, with coarsely granular chromatin, hyperchromasia, abnormal nuclear contours, and prominent nucleoli. Multinucleate cancer cells and mitotic figures are often readily identified.[60]

In bladder washings, urothelial carcinoma may demonstrate a lower degree of nuclear hyperchromasia, perhaps resulting in more prominent large nucleoli. The cells may be poorly preserved, particularly when there is inflammation or necrosis, and a variety of changes may be present, including frayed or vacuolated cytoplasm, non-specific eosinophilic cytoplasmic inclusions, and pyknotic nuclei. In some high-

grade papillary tumors, the dominant cytologic finding may be the presence of isolated cancer cells, either singly or in groups of two or three.

Grade 2 carcinoma may present cytologic diagnostic challenges,[2,49,59,61] as it is often similar cytologically to grade 1 carcinoma.[49,61] Fortunately, in most cases atypical urothelial cells are observed, and these alert the clinician to the need for cystoscopic examination. For high-grade urothelial carcinoma, digital image analysis and bladder wash cytology are equally predictive.[58]

## Correlation of urine cytology and biopsy findings (diagnostic accuracy)

The diagnostic accuracy of urine cytology is high in patients who are symptomatic or being followed after diagnosis and treatment for bladder cancer. The reported results vary considerably. In general, all reports of series of bladder tumors indicate that papilloma and papillary urothelial neoplasms of low malignant potential cannot be reliably diagnosed by urine cytology despite the inclusion of several key cytologic findings. Reported sensitivity of urine cytology for grade 1

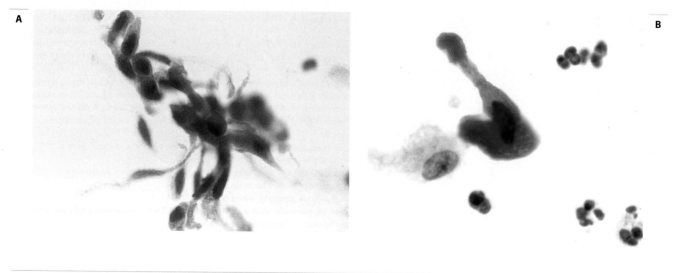

**Fig. 7-20** High-grade squamous cell carcinoma in urine **(A, B)**.

urothelial carcinoma varies from 26% to 90%.[5,6] The sensitivity increases to 80% for grade 2, and to 95% for grade 3. Urothelial carcinoma in situ can be diagnosed as suspicious or positive in virtually all instances. The overall sensitivity of urine cytology for primary carcinoma of the bladder ranges from 45% to 97%. In a recent report, urine cytology predicted 82% of all recurrent tumors in the bladder.[62] Two major drawbacks of urinary cytology are the high rate of false-positive results in patients on intravesical chemotherapy, and the high rate of false-negative results in those with grade 1 carcinoma.

Urine cytology after BCG therapy had a sensitivity of 56% and a specificity of 56% for cancer recurrence; when combined with cystoscopy, the results were 88% and 82%, respectively, obviating the need for routine biopsy in many patients.[63] Urine cytology after radical cystectomy is an early indicator of cancer recurrence, preceding radiographic failure by a mean of 2.1 years.[64] Ureteral margin involvement at cystectomy was a significant predictor of failure.

Immunohistochemical expression of HER-2/neu and high molecular weight cytokeratin in cells from voided urine predicted those patients at high risk for bladder cancer recurrence with a minimum of 3 years' follow-up.[65] HER-2/neu was expressed in 7% of cases without recurrence, compared to 85% of those with recurrence; results for high molecular weight cytokeratin were 43% versus 64%, respectively.

## Other types of carcinoma

### Squamous cell carcinoma

Invasive squamous cell carcinoma is common in Africa and the Middle East, particularly in patients infected with *Schistosoma haematobium*, but is relatively uncommon in developed countries, accounting for no more than 3% of bladder tumors.[24] Squamous cell carcinoma has been observed with increasing frequency in long-term survivors with severe spinal cord injury and neurogenic bladder.

Squamous cell carcinoma may display varying degrees of differentiation (Fig. 7-20). In well-differentiated invasive cell carcinoma, the cytologic findings in voided urine are somewhat characteristic. The presence of markedly keratinized cells with thick, yellow or orange cytoplasm and large, irregular, often dark pyknotic nuclei is useful. Squamous pearls, characterized by cell aggregates concentrically arranged around a core of keratin, may be observed.[2] The background of the smear often shows evidence of marked necrosis, and ghost cells may be present. A mixture of cancer cells is observed in the urine of patients with poorly differentiated squamous cell carcinoma, including sharply demarcated cells with eosinophilic cytoplasm and large nuclei.[1,2] Most cases are aneuploid.[66]

### Adenocarcinoma

In colonic-type adenocarcinoma of the bladder, the urinary sediment contains columnar cancer cells with large, hyperchromatic nuclei and large nucleoli, sometimes in clusters. In poorly differentiated mucus-producing carcinoma, the cancer cells are small, spherical or cuboidal in shape, and contain large hyperchromatic nuclei, often with prominent nucleoli. The cytoplasm is usually basophilic, often scant, and sometimes poorly preserved. When there are large cytoplasmic vacuoles containing mucus, the nuclei may be pushed to the periphery of the cell, a feature diagnostic of signet-ring cell carcinoma.

In clear cell adenocarcinoma, the cancer cells are large, with abundant finely vacuolated or granular cytoplasm, open vesicular nuclei, and prominent nucleoli. Such cells usually form around papillary clusters.[1] Most cases are DNA aneuploid.[67]

### Small cell undifferentiated carcinoma (oat cell carcinoma)

In small cell carcinoma, the cancer cells are small – about four times the size of lymphocytes – and contain compact, often pyknotic nuclei, and scant basophilic cytoplasm.[68] Nucleoli are not visible. The presence of small clusters of tightly packed tumor cells with nuclear molding may be diagnostically useful.[2] The presence of cell clusters without prominent nucleoli is helpful in differentiating these cells from malignant lymphoma. In lymphoma, the cells do not cluster and usually contain small nucleoli. The demonstration of neuroendocrine differentiation in small cell carcinoma may require immunohistochemical or ultrastructural studies.

## Mixed carcinoma

Urothelial cancer may contain foci with more than one histologic type, including squamous cell carcinoma, adenocarcinoma, and small cell carcinoma. The cytologic findings in such tumors rarely permit the diagnosis of mixed carcinoma. Usually, one cytologic pattern is dominant, although rarely a mixed population of cancer cells may be observed.

## Other malignant tumors

Rare cases of carcinoid (low-grade neuroendocrine carcinoma) have been diagnosed by urine cytology.[69] Other rare cancers that may be diagnosed by cytology include sarcoma, carcinoma, primary and secondary lymphoma,[70] and choriocarcinoma. In many cases, urine cytology may not be diagnostic.

## Major diagnostic pitfalls

Most errors in urine cytology are overdiagnoses of benign cellular changes as malignant (Table 7-6). Knowledge of these changes is fundamental to the practice of cytology. Below is a summary of some of the most vexing problems, which are also described and illustrated elsewhere in this chapter and the rest of this book.

## Trauma or instrumentation

The normal urothelium tends to exfoliate in the form of round or oval tissue fragments that are commonly designated papillary clusters. Vigorous palpation, catheterization, or any form of instrumentation may result in the formation of such clusters which, when present in large numbers, may be misinterpreted as papillary carcinoma,[19] Another important source of error is the presence of numerous superficial urothelial cells that may be mistaken for cancer cells because of their variable nuclear features.[35]

**Table 7-6** Major diagnostic pitfalls in lower urinary tract cytology

| |
|---|
| Overdiagnosis of normal and degenerated urothelium as malignant |
| Overdiagnosis of human polyomavirus infection as malignant |
| Overdiagnosis of effects of cyclophosphamide as malignant |
| Underdiagnosis of grade 1 or grade 2 urothelial carcinoma (papillary urothelial neoplasia of low malignant potential or low-grade urothelial carcinoma) as benign |

## Cell preservation

Cells in voided urinary sediment, particularly in the first morning voiding, are often poorly preserved, compounding the diagnostic difficulty. The diagnosis of cancer in voided urine should be avoided unless the findings are unequivocal.[2]

## Human polyomavirus

Polyomavirus (BK virus) infection forms large intranuclear inclusions that may mimic cancer cell nuclei. However, the inclusions are homogeneous and lack the coarse granularity of chromatin seen in cancer.[2,31] This is an important source of diagnostic errors that can contribute to costly and lengthy patient investigations.

## Lithiasis

Calculi anywhere in the lower urinary tract may act as abrasive instruments, dislodging epithelial fragments that may be quite large and display papillary appearances mimicking low-grade papillary carcinoma.[18] The presence of numerous superficial cells may also create diagnostic difficulty due to nuclear abnormalities.[2,6,35]

## Drugs and other therapeutic procedures

Urothelial cell changes may result from a wide variety of inciting agents, including chemotherapeutic agents, radiotherapy, and other interventions. Intravesical chemotherapy is responsible for a high rate of false-positive results.[6] A further source of diagnostic difficulty may be synchronous infection with polyomavirus in patients who are immunocompromised.[2] It should be remembered that urothelial carcinoma or sarcoma may develop in patients receiving cyclophosphamide for the treatment of malignant lymphoma.[36,37]

## Special aspects of anatomic sites other than the urinary bladder

It is rare for a primary cancer of the urethra not to be associated with a bladder tumor. The most common are squamous cell carcinoma, adenocarcinoma, and urothelial carcinoma, although all are rare. Other rare cancers include malignant melanoma and clear cell adenocarcinoma.

A common cytologic examination of the urethra occurs after cystectomy for bladder cancer. Often these examinations may reveal carcinoma in situ or early invasive carcinoma.[7]

Urine cytology is usually diagnostic in urothelial carcinoma of the renal pelvis and ureter, particularly when the cancers are high grade. In low-grade urothelial malignancies, the same diagnostic problems are encountered as in the bladder.[71]

Urine cytology is unsatisfactory for detection of renal cell carcinoma. When malignant cells are present, they are large with clear or vacuolated cytoplasm and distinct nucleoli.

Prostatic adenocarcinoma may yield cells in voided urine spontaneously or after prostatic massage, particularly if the carcinoma is high grade. The cancer cells in the urinary sediment are usually small, often spherical, and columnar. Small cell clusters may be observed. The cytoplasm is usually basophilic with open vesicular nuclei and prominent nucleoli. This procedure is not considered useful for the early detection of prostatic carcinoma.

## Secondary tumors

Numerous metastatic malignant tumors may be observed in the urinary sediment. The most common arise from adjacent or contiguous organs, including the uterine cervix and endometrium or ovary in women, the prostate in men, and the colon in both sexes; urine cytology may then show squamous cell carcinoma or adenocarcinoma. Clinicopathologic correlation is usually required for diagnosis. Rare cases of lymphoma, leukemia, and melanoma may be diagnosed from urine samples.

## Ancillary studies

### Flow cytometry

Voided urine is generally not adequate for flow cytometry, and the cell samples must be obtained by vigorous flushing of the bladder through a soft rubbery catheter five to ten times with saline solution, or during cystoscopy by lavage. Subpopulations of bladder epithelial cells can be identified by interactive digital image analysis. The diagnosis of cancer is strongly suspected in cases with an aneuploid stemline or 16% or more of measured cells with hyperdiploid DNA (>2 x DNA content). A specimen is less likely to be malignant if no aneuploid stemline is detected and fewer than 11% of the cells are hyperdiploid. If 11–15.9% of the cells measured are hyperdiploid and no aneuploid stemline is detected, the samples are considered suspicious. Recurrent cancer can be detected by using combined urine cytology and image analysis.[72,73]

### Digital image analysis

Digital image analysis was superior to flow cytometry for DNA ploidy analysis, with sensitivities of 91% and 71%, respectively.[50] Further, image analysis was superior to cytologic examination for prediction of tumor recurrence after normal findings at cystoscopic examination, and was equivalent to cytology for the detection of high-grade lesions.[58]

### Blood group antigens and other tumor markers detected by immunohistochemistry

Deletion of A, B, and H blood group antigens is associated with biochemical and structural changes of glycoprotein and glycolipid components of the cell surface during neoplastic transformation. Blood group reactivity is reduced in high-grade and aggressive tumors. Carcinoembryonic antigen has been used in the evaluation of exfoliated urothelial cancer cells. The proliferation marker Ki67 and reactivity to the URO series of monoclonal antibodies may also be useful but are not routinely employed.[56]

## Fluorescence in situ hybridization (FISH)

Multitarget fluorescence in situ hybridization (FISH) containing probes to chromosomes 3, 7, 17, and the 9p21 band has high sensitivity and specificity for detecting urothelial carcinoma,[52,53] and is useful for investigating numeric abnormalities in bladder cancer[50–53,74,75] (Fig. 7-21). FISH revealed abnormalities of chromosomes 8 and 12 in 83% of bladder tumors of all grades.[50] It had greater sensitivity than cytology for detecting upper urinary tract urothelial carcinoma (77% vs 36%, respectively) while maintaining similar specificity (95% vs 100%, respectively).[76]

About 27% of patients under surveillance for recurrent bladder cancer with no immediate clinical evidence of recurrence have positive multitarget FISH, and about 65% of these anticipatory positive patients develop recurrent cancer within 29 months.[77]

## The problem of hematuria

Hematuria is the most common symptom of urinary tract disease, present in about 21% of the US population, including 2% of children.[78] It is defined as excretion of three or more red blood cells per high-power field (hpf) in freshly voided centrifuged urine, preferably documented on up to three separate occasions.[79] Normally, up to 3% of adults excrete small numbers of red blood cells (up to two red cells per hpf, or the equivalent of 1000 red cells/mL), so it is important in such cases to avoid overdiagnosis. Hematuria

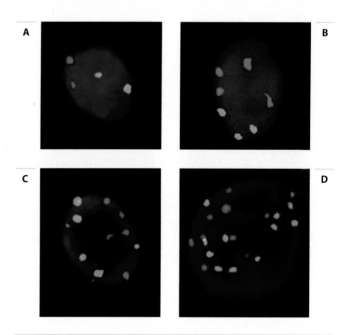

**Fig. 7-21** Fluorescence in situ hybridization (FISH) in voided urine cytology. **(A)** Normal urothelium showing two copies of chromosome 3 (red) and two of chromosome 7 (green) by fluorescence in-situ hybridization (FISH). **(B)** Aneusomic urothelial cell showing four copies of chromosome 3 (red) and three copies of chromosome 7 (green) by FISH. **(C)** Aneusomic urothelial cell showing six copies of chromosome 3 (red) and five of chromosome 7 (green) by FISH. **(D)** Urothelial carcinoma cell showing gains of chromosome 3 (red) and 7 (green) by FISH.

may be occult (not visible with the naked eye, usually discovered incidentally during laboratory studies accompanying routine physical examination), gross (usually obvious to the patient), or associated with blood clots, often presenting as an abnormal color ranging from pink to bright or dark red. As little as 1 mL of blood per liter creates a noticeable change in the color of urine.

Hematuria may be asymptomatic or symptomatic and transient or persistent, and is often associated with other findings such as proteinuria, hypertension, edema or other physical findings. A through history and physical examination should always be performed with attention to family history.

Hematuria may occur anywhere along the urinary tract. There are many causes, including anatomic abnormalities, calculi, medications, vigorous exercise, foreign bodies, trauma, hemoglobinopathies and coagulopathies, glomerulonephritis, and malignancy (Tables 7-7, 7-8).[80] It is critical that the source of persistent hematuria be identified, according to the Best Practice Policy of the American Urologic Association.[79] There is no 'safe' level of hematuria, and the patient should undergo urologic workup, including urinalysis, urine culture, cystoscopy, imaging studies, urine chemistry and serum panels, and urine cytology.

## Routine laboratory investigation of hematuria

Routine urinalysis combines macroscopic reagent strip (dipstick) testing with microscopic examination of the sediment to detect chemical and structural disorders of the urinary tract. Dipstick examination has about 90% sensitivity to detect three or more red blood cells or the equivalent amount of free hemoglobin or myoglobin.[81] The degree of hematuria bears no relation to the seriousness of the underlying disease, so hematuria should be considered a symptom of serious disease until proven otherwise.[82]

The dipstick test and confirmatory tests for protein, glucose, and bilirubin are standardized and easy to perform, but there is a great deal of inconsistency in the performance of the microscopic examination. Procedures are not standardized, and variables include the amount of urine examined, the method of processing, the method of evaluation and reporting, and the technical ability of the individual performing the examination. Unfortunately, most abnormal urinalyses are not pursued clinically, except perhaps to obtain repeat urinalysis, often with progression of treatable disease that could be prevented.[83]

Microscopic examination is often performed only if the dipstick test is abnormal, but this approach should be discouraged. Exclusive reliance on the dipstick test significantly reduces the sensitivity of urinalysis for the detection of serious and treatable disease; the combination of dipstick and microscopic examination greatly improves the detection of urinary tract disease, and is recommended.

## Pathogenesis of hematuria

Red cells in the urine result from trauma or a spontaneous response to a multitude of causes or conditions throughout the urinary tract. This process, known as diapedesis, is caused by the oozing of red or white blood cells through blood

**Table 7-7** Site-specific causes of hematuria

| Lower urinary tract bleeding | Upper urinary tract (renal) bleeding |
| --- | --- |
| Tumors (urethra, bladder, prostate, ureters, renal pelvis) | **Primary glomerulopathies** |
| Obstructive uropathy | IGA nephrology |
| Benign prostatic hyperplasia | Postinfectious glomerulonephritis |
| Lithiasis (stones) | Membranoproliferative glomerulonephritis |
| Infections (cystitis, prostatitis, schistosomiasis, tuberculosis, condyloma acuminatum) | Focal glomerular sclerosis |
| Systemic bleeding disorders or coagulopathy | **Secondary glomerulopathy** |
| Trauma | Lupus nephritis |
| Radiation therapy | Henloch–Schönlein syndrome |
| Instrumentation | Vasculitis (polyarteritis nordosa) |
| Vigorous exercise | Wegner's granulomatosis |
| Menstrual contamination | Hemolytic–uremic syndrome |
| Endometriosis | Essential mixed cryoglobulinema |
| | Interstitial nephritis |
| | **Familial conditions** |
| | Hereditary nephritis (Alport's syndrome) |
| | Renal tumors (renal cell carcinoma) |
| | Vascular disorders (malignant hypertension) |
| | Sickle cell trait or disease |
| | Metabolic disorders (hypercalciuria) |
| | Polycystic kidney |
| | **Infections** |
| | Pyelonephritis (acute or chronic) |
| | Tuberculosis |
| | Cytomegalovirus |
| | BK polyomavirus |
| | **Nephrolithiasis** |
| | **Increased light chain immunoglobulins (multiple myeloma)** |
| | **Diabetes** |
| | **Amyloid** |

vessel walls. The vessels are usually preserved, except with glomerular hematuria, in which there is damage to the endothelial cells and glomerular basement membranes.

## Dysmorphic red blood cells indicate glomerular disease

Red cells of glomerular origin are referred to as 'dysmorphic' (abnormal and misshapen), whereas red cells leaking though vessels in the renal tubules and in the lower urinary tract are

**Table 7-8** Etiologic classification of causes of hematuria by ingestion and pigments

| Drugs and medications | Pigments | Other |
|---|---|---|
| **Antibiotics** | | **Diuretics** |
| Penicillin | Rhabdomyosis (myoglobin) | Thiazides |
| Cephalosporin | Hemoglobin (transfusion reaction) | Furosemide |
| Rifampin | Heme pigment (hemolysis) | Triamferene |
| Erythromycin | | Chlorthalidone |
| Sulfonamides | | **Other:** |
| Aminoglycosides | | Radiocontrast agents |
| Tetracycline | | Cis-platinum |
| **NSAIDS** | | Heavy metals (gold, cadmium, mercury) |
| Acetaminophen | | Organic solvents |
| Acetylsalicylic acid | | |
| Naproxen | | |
| Ibuprofen | | |
| Indomethacin | | |
| Phenylbutazone | | |
| Tolmetin | | |
| Mefenamic acid | | |
| Fenoprofen | | |
| **Other drugs** | | |
| Captopril | | |
| Cimetidine | | |
| Phenobarbital | | |
| Dilantin | | |
| Interferon | | |
| Lithium | | |

'isomorphic' (normal size and shape, smooth cell membranes, and uniform hemoglobin content)[23,84] (Fig. 7-22). There are two defining features of dysmorphic red blood cells: each 'target' cell should have a clear and distinct central inclusion of heme pigment surrounded by a clear zone, as well as one or several abnormal outpouchings ('blebs') of the red cell membrane.

Most investigators agree that the presence of even one dysmorphic red blood cell in urine is clinically significant, but some debate on this point persists. The presence of dysmorphic red blood cells accompanied by even a small amount of protein is especially significant, indicating a glomerular source of bleeding.

## Optimal cytodiagnostic urinalysis for evaluation of hematuria

Optimal cytodiagnostic urinalysis refers to the comprehensive quantitative evaluation of urinary sediment.[23,84] This method incorporates advances in routine urinalysis, including the dipstick test and confirmatory tests such as the SSA test for protein, the Ictotest for bilirubin, and the Clinitest tablet test for glucose. In addition, enhanced cytopreparation improves cell recovery to maximize microscopic visualization and quantitative assessment. Diagnostic findings are correlated with serum findings as well as with quantatitive urine chemistries including albumin, microalbumin, B-2 immunoglobulin and creatinine, providing the clinician with the full spectrum of chemical and morphologic abnormalities that are present, together with recommendation for additional testing and possible treatment.

There are six components of optimal cytodiagnostic urinalysis:

- Patient history
- Physical examination of the urine sample, including color, character, and specific gravity
- Chemical examination, consisting of multiparameter reagent dipstick testing and confirmatory chemical tests
- Microscopic urinary sediment examination using standardized sediment recovery and high-contrast transparent Papanicolaou stain
- Quantitative microscopic examination of the sediment entities and 10 specific morphologic categories: background, cellularity, epithelial fragments, inclusion-bearing cells, red blood cells, neutrophils, eosinophils, lymphocytes, renal tubular cells, and casts
- Diagnostic interpretation, with appropriate recommendations, including possible confirmatory testing and clinical follow-up.

Optimal cytodiagnostic urinalysis is an improvement over routine unstained sediment examination because this method:

- Improves visualization of urinary sediment entities
- Provides additional information on the nature of urinary tract disorders
- Allows early cost-effective triaging of patients to an appropriate specialist (e.g. urologist, nephrologist)
- Provides a non-invasive method for monitoring patients
- Optimizes clinicopathologic correlation of results
- Standardizes results reporting
- Is adaptable to various laboratory sizes and settings
- Requires a minimum of equipment and space
- Is adaptable to automation
- Provides a permanent record of urinary sediment findings for review and quality control.

The clinical utility of optimal cytodiagnostic urinalysis is its ability to detect various types of mononuclear cells, viral and non-viral inclusions, and pre-cancerous and cancerous cells. It is valuable in differential diagnosis and the monitoring of renal tubular injury for conditions such as acute tubular necrosis (ATN), tubulointerstitial inflammation (nephritis), acute renal allograft rejection, and primary and secondary renal lesions. It can also help to discriminate inflammatory,

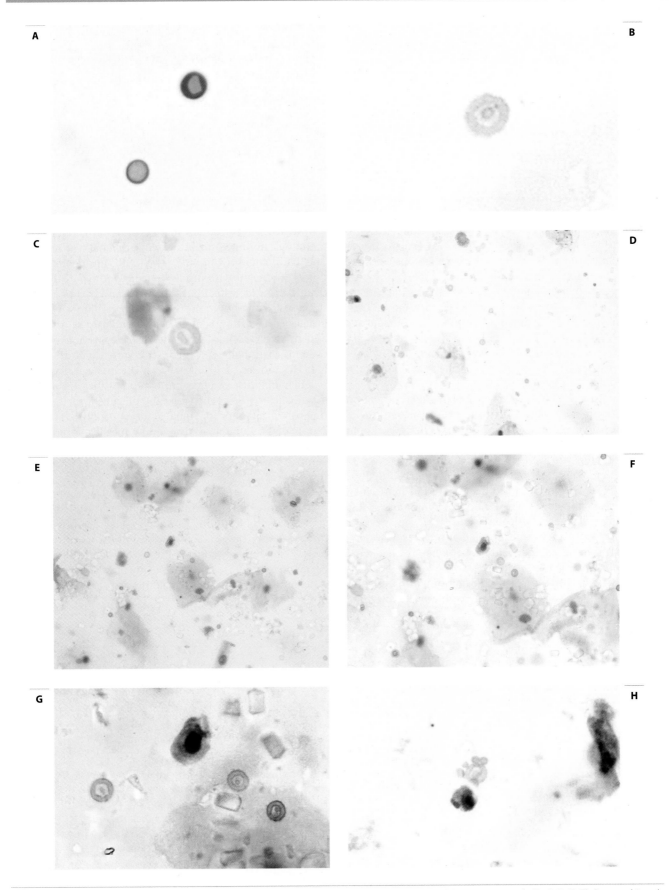

**Fig. 7-22 (A)** Isomorphic red blood cells. Note the smooth membranes and uniform amount of hemoglobin. Compare with **(B, C, D, E, F)**: Dysmorphic red blood cells, 'target cell type.' Note the central inclusion of heme pigment. **(G, H)** Dysmorphic red blood cells with prominent 'blebs' or protrusions of red cell membranes.

**Table 7-9** Correlation of optimal cytodiagnostic urinalysis with renal biopsy

| Lesion location | Sensitivity | Specificity | Accuracy | Positive predictive value | Negative predictive value |
|---|---|---|---|---|---|
| Glomerular | 0.95 | 0.85 | 0.91 | 0.90 | 0.92 |
| Tubular | 0.80 | 0.89 | 0.88 | 0.57 | 0.96 |
| Interstitial | 0.78 | 0.87 | 0.82 | 0.88 | 0.76 |
| Tubulointerstitial (combined) | 0.91 | 0.91 | 0.91 | 0.95 | 0.83 |
| Vascular | 0.50 | 0.74 | 0.64 | 0.58 | 0.67 |

infectious, degenerative or neoplastic conditions of the kidney and the lower urinary tract; evaluate and monitor immunosuppressed patients; screen patients with nephrotoxic or carcinogenic exposure; often explain inconclusive results; and prevent unnecessary renal biopsy in some cases.

There is a high level of intra- and interobserver agreement in determining the origin of renal cells (glomerular, tubular, interstitial, or vascular cells) by optimal cytodiagnostic urinalysis.[23,84] Similarly, the correlation is high with biopsy findings: 89% correlation of native kidneys and 77% of transplant kidneys. Sensitivity and specificity for glomerular lesions alone in native and transplant kidneys was 91%, and 85%, respectively. Severity scores showed good correlation between optimal cytodiagnostic urinalysis results and renal biopsy in native and transplanted kidneys (Table 7-9), and correlated well with increased creatinine concentration. In cases with biopsy-proven glomerular lesions, more severe changes were found by optimal cytodiagnostic urinalysis when the biopsy showed a proliferative lesion than when only normal glomeruli were found by light microscopy. Optimal cytodiagnostic urinalysis has an advantage over renal biopsy in that it can be repeated as often as necessary, and thus allows the progression or regression of a renal lesion to be observed over time.[23,84]

The accuracy of optimal cytodiagnostic urinalysis for determining the origin and etiology of blood in the urine was studied in 100 consecutive patients with occult hematuria.[1] For the sake of the study, only cancer and lithiasis were considered positive. A total of 13% of patients had pathologic findings, including two with renal cell carcinoma, one with angiomyolipoma, two with urothelial bladder cancer, and eight with urinary calculi; optimal cytodiagnostic urinalysis identified both bladder cancers, seven of eight urinary calculi, but none of the renal tumors (probably because a renal tumor must be of significant size and stage and in direct contact with the distal collecting system in order to shed malignant cells). The presence of dysmorphic red cells and red blood casts was strongly suggestive of renal parenchymal disease. The authors found that optimal cytodiagnostic urinalysis increased the diagnostic yield and distinguished bladder or renal causes of microhematuria. Automated cellular analysis had low specificity for discriminating glomerular from non-glomerular causes of hematuria compared with microscopic sediment analysis (42% vs 93%, respectively).[85]

Emerging methods for quantitative measurement of marker proteins (e.g., albumin, transferrin, IgG, $\alpha_1$-microglobulin, retinol-binding protein, $\alpha_2$-macroglobulin, Bence Jones proteins) have challenged the dominant role of microscopy. Renal biopsy abnormalities were identified in all cases by marker protein excretion, but in only 41% of cases by cellular urinary sediments.[86] Future studies should determine the reproducibility of these results.

## REFERENCES

1. Fracchia JA, Motta J, Miller LS, et al. Evaluation of asymptomatic microhematuria. Urology 1995; 46: 484–489.
2. Koss LG. Errors and pitfalls in cytology of the lower urinary tract. Monogr Pathol 1997; 39: 60–74.
3. Ooms EC, Veldhuizen RW. Cytological criteria and diagnostic terminology in urinary cytology. Cytopathology 1993; 4: 51–54.
4. Potts SA, Thomas PA, Cohen MB, Raab SS. Diagnostic accuracy and key cytologic features of high-grade transitional cell carcinoma in the upper urinary tract. Mod Pathol 1997; 10: 657–662.
5. Bastacky S, Ibrahim S, Wilczynski SP, Murphy WM. The accuracy of urinary cytology in daily practice. Cancer 1999; 87: 118–128.
6. Maier U, Simak R, Neuhold N. The clinical value of urinary cytology: 12 years of experience with 615 patients. J Clin Pathol 1995; 48: 314–317.
7. Gamarra MC, Zein T. Cytologic spectrum of bladder cancer. Urology 1984; 23: 23–26.
8. Badalament RA, Gay H, Cibas ES, et al. Monitoring endoscopic treatment of superficial bladder carcinoma by postoperative urinary cytology. J Urol 1987; 138: 760–762.
9. Berlac PA, Holm HH. Bladder tumor control by abdominal ultrasound and urine cytology. J Urol 1992; 147: 1510–1512.
10. Chow NH, Tzai TS, Cheng HL, et al. Urinary cytodiagnosis: can it have a different prognostic implication than a diagnostic test? Urol Int 1994; 53: 18–23.
11. Koss LG, Deitch D, Ramanathan R, Sherman AB. Diagnostic value of cytology of voided urine. Acta Cytol 1985; 29: 810–816.
12. Schwalb DM, Herr HW, Fair WR. The management of clinically unconfirmed positive urinary cytology. J Urol 1993; 150: 1751–1756.
13. Matzkin H, Moinuddin SM, Soloway MS. Value of urine cytology versus bladder washing in bladder cancer. Urology 1992; 39: 201–203.
14. Bian Y, Ehya H, Bagley DH. Cytologic diagnosis of upper urinary tract neoplasms by ureteroscopic sampling. Acta Cytol 1995; 39: 733–740.

15. Hundley AF, Maygarden S, Wu JM, et al. Adequacy of urine cytology specimens: an assessment of collection techniques. Int Urogynecol J 2007; 18: 977–1001.

16. Amberson JB, Laino JP. Image cytometric deoxyribonucleic acid analysis of urine specimens as an adjunct to visual cytology in the detection of urothelial cell carcinoma. J Urol 1993; 149: 42–45.

17. Kline MJ, Wilkinson EJ, Askeland R, et al. DNA tetraploidy in Feulgen-stained bladder washings assessed by image cytometry. Anal Quant Cytol Histol 1995; 17: 129–134.

18. Highman W, Wilson E. Urine cytology in patients with calculi. J Clin Pathol 1982; 35: 350–356.

19. Kannan V, Bose S. Low grade transitional cell carcinoma and instrument artifact. A challenge in urinary cytology. Acta Cytol 1993; 37: 899–902.

20. Roberti I, Reisman L, Burrows L, Lieberman KV. Urine cytology and urine flow cytometry in renal transplantation – a prospective double blind study. Transplantation 1995; 59: 495–500.

21. Rupp M, O'Hara B, McCullough L, et al. Prostatic carcinoma cells in urine specimens. Cytopathology 1994; 5: 164–170.

22. Gutmann EJ. Seminal vesicle cell in a spontaneously voided urine. Diagn Cytopathol 2006; 34: 824–825.

23. Marcussen N, Schumann J, Campbell P, Kjellstrand C. Cytodiagnostic urinalysis is very useful in the differential diagnosis of acute renal failure and can predict the severity. Renal Fail 1995; 17: 721–729.

24. Eltoum IA, Suliaman SM, Ismail BM, et al. Evaluation of eosinophiluria in the diagnosis of Schistosomiasis hematobium: a field-based study. Am J Trop Med Hyg 1992; 46: 732–736.

25. Bhan R, Pisharodi LR, Gudlaugsson E, Bedrossian C. Cytological, histological, and clinical correlations in intravesical Bacillus Calmette–Guérin immunotherapy. Ann Diagn Pathol 1998; 2: 55–60.

26. Betz SA, See WA, Cohen MB. Granulomatous inflammation in bladder wash specimens after intravesical bacillus Calmette–Guérin therapy for transitional cell carcinoma of the bladder. Am J Clin Pathol 1993; 99: 244–248.

27. Schwalb MD, Herr HW, Sogani PC, et al. Positive urinary cytology following a complete response to intravesical bacillus Calmette–Guérin therapy: pattern of recurrence. J Urol 1994; 152: 382–387.

28. Crabbe JG. 'Comet' or 'decoy' cells found in urinary sediment smears. Acta Cytol 1971; 15: 303–305.

29. Maghrabi M, Marwan D, Osoba AO. BK virus infection in a renal transplant Saudi child. Saudi Med J 2007; 28: 121–124.

30. Burgos D, Lopez V, Cabello M, et al. Polyomavirus BK nephropathy: the effect of an early diagnosis on renal function or graft loss. Transplant Proc 2006; 38: 2409–2411.

31. Koss LG, Sherman AB, Eppich E. Image analysis and DNA content of urothelial cells infected with human polyomavirus. Anal Quant Cytol 1984; 6: 89–94.

32. Seftel AD, Matthews LA, Smith MC, Willis J. Polyomavirus mimicking high grade transitional cell carcinoma. J Urol 1996; 156: 1764.

33. Lopez-Beltran A, Escudero AL, Carrasco-Aznar JC, Vicioso-Recio L. Human papillomavirus infection and transitional cell carcinoma of the bladder. Immunohistochemistry and in situ hybridization. Pathol Res Pract 1996; 192: 154–159.

34. Forni AM, Koss LG, Geller W. Cytological study of the effect of cyclophosphamide on the epithelium of the urinary bladder in man. Cancer 1964; 17: 1348–1355.

35. Murphy WM. Current status of urinary cytology in the evaluation of bladder neoplasms. Hum Pathol 1990; 21: 886–896.

36. Travis LB, Curtis RE, Boice JD Jr, Fraumeni JF Jr. Bladder cancer after chemotherapy for non-Hodgkin's lymphoma. N Engl J Med 1989; 321: 544–545.

37. Wall RL, Clausen KP. Carcinoma of the urinary bladder in patients receiving cyclophosphamide. N Engl J Med 1975; 293: 271–273.

38. Stilmant M, Murphy JL, Merriam JC. Cytology of nephrogenic adenoma of the urinary bladder. A report of four cases. Acta Cytol 1986; 30: 35–40.

39. Schneider V, Smith MJ, Frable WJ. Urinary cytology in endometriosis of the bladder. Acta Cytol 1980; 24: 30–33.

40. Murphy WM, Soloway MS. Urothelial dysplasia. J Urol 1982; 127: 849–854.

41. Wolinska WH, Melamed MR, Klein FA. Cytology of bladder papilloma. Acta Cytol 1985; 29: 817–822.

42. Renshaw AA, Nappi D, Weinberg DS. Cytology of grade 1 papillary transitional cell carcinoma. A comparison of cytologic, architectural and morphometric criteria in cystoscopically obtained urine. Acta Cytol 1996; 40: 676–682.

43. Green LK, Meistrich H. Dramatically increased specificity and sensitivity in detecting low grade papillary TCC via a combination of cytospin and cell blocking techniques [Abstract]. Mod Pathol 1995; 8: 40A.

44. Wiener HG, Vooijs GP, van't Hof-Grootenboer B. Accuracy of urinary cytology in the diagnosis of primary and recurrent bladder cancer. Acta Cytol 1993; 37: 163–169.

45. Sack MJ, Artymyshyn RL, Tomaszewski JE, Gupta PK. Diagnostic value of bladder wash cytology, with special reference to low grade urothelial neoplasms. Acta Cytol 1995; 39: 187–194.

46. Murphy WM, Soloway MS, Jukkola AF, et al. Urinary cytology and bladder cancer. The cellular features of transitional cell neoplasms. Cancer 1984; 53: 1555–1565.

47. Raab SS, Lenel JC, Cohen MB. Low grade transitional cell carcinoma of the bladder. Cytologic diagnosis by key features as identified by logistic regression analysis. Cancer 1994; 74: 1621–1626.

48. Raab SS, Slagel DD, Jensen CS, et al. Low-grade transitional cell carcinoma of the urinary bladder: application of select cytologic criteria to improve diagnostic accuracy [corrected]. Mod Pathol 1996; 9: 225–232.

49. Whisnant RE, Bastacky SI, Ohori NP. Cytologic diagnosis of low-grade papillary urothelial neoplasms (low malignant potential and low-grade carcinoma) in the context of the 1998 WHO/ISUP classification. Diagn Cytopathol 2003; 28: 186–190.

50. Cajulis RS, Haines GK 3rd, Frias-Hidvegi D, et al. Cytology, flow cytometry, image analysis, and interphase cytogenetics by fluorescence in situ hybridization in the diagnosis of transitional cell carcinoma in bladder washes: a comparative study. Diagn Cytopathol 1995; 13: 214–223; discussion 224.

51. Halling KC, King W, Sokolova IA, et al. A comparison of cytology and fluorescence in situ hybridization for the detection of urothelial carcinoma. J Urol 2000; 164: 1768–1775.

52. Skacel M, Fahmy M, Brainard JA, et al. Multitarget fluorescence in situ hybridization assay detects transitional cell carcinoma in the majority of patients with bladder cancer and atypical or negative urine cytology. J Urol 2003; 169: 2101–2105.

53. Bubendorf L, Grilli B, Sauter G, et al. Multiprobe FISH for enhanced detection of bladder cancer in voided urine specimens and bladder washings. Am J Clin Pathol 2001; 116: 79–86.

54. Olsson H, Zackrisson B. ImmunoCyt a useful method in the follow-up protocol for patients with urinary bladder carcinoma. Scand J Urol Nephrol 2001; 35: 280–282.

55. Fradet Y, Lockhard C. Performance characteristics of a new monoclonal antibody test for bladder cancer: ImmunoCyt trade mark. Can J Urol 1997; 4: 400–405.

56. Panosian KJM, Lopez-Beltran A, Croghan G. An immunohistochemical evaluation of urinary bladder cytology utilizing monoclonal antibodies. World J Urol 1989; 7: 73–79.

57. Lodde M, Mian C, Negri G, et al. Role of uCyt+ in the detection and surveillance of urothelial carcinoma. Urology 2003; 61: 243–247.

58. van der Poel HG, Boon ME, van Stratum P, et al. Conventional bladder wash cytology performed by four experts versus quantitative image analysis. Mod Pathol 1997; 10: 976–982.

59. Rife CC, Farrow GM, Utz DC. Urine cytology of transitional cell neoplasms. Urol Clin North Am 1979; 6: 599–612.

60. Shenoy UA, Colby TV, Schumann GB. Reliability of urinary cytodiagnosis in urothelial neoplasms. Cancer 1985; 56: 2041–2045.

61. Curry JL, Wojcik EM. The effects of the current World Health Organization/ International Society of Urologic Pathologists bladder neoplasm classification system on urine cytology results. Cancer 2002; 96: 140–145.

62. Loh CS, Spedding AV, Ashworth MT, et al. The value of exfoliative urine cytology in combination with flexible cystoscopy in the diagnosis of recurrent transitional cell carcinoma of the urinary bladder. Br J Urol 1996; 77: 655–658.

63. Guy L, Savareux L, Molinie V, et al. Should bladder biopsies be performed routinely after bacillus Calmette– Guérin treatment for high-risk superficial transitional cell cancer of the bladder? Eur Urol 2006; 50: 516– 520; discussion 520.

64. Raj GV, Bochner BH, Serio AM, et al. Natural history of positive urinary cytology after radical cystectomy. J Urol 2006; 176: 2000–20005; discussion 20005.

65. Raica M, Zylis D, Cimpean AM. Cytokeratin 20, 34betaE12 and overexpression of HER-2/neu in urine cytology as predictors of recurrences in superficial urothelial carcinoma. Rom J Morphol Embryol 2005; 46: 11–15.

66. Shaaban AA, Tribukait B, el-Bedeiwy AF, Ghoneim MA. Characterization of squamous cell bladder tumors by flow cytometric deoxyribonucleic acid analysis: a report of 100 cases. J Urol 1990; 144: 879–883.

67. Tribukait B. Clinical DNA flow cytometry. Med Oncol Tumor Pharmacother 1984; 1: 211–218.

68. Rollins S, Schumann GB. Primary urinary cytodiagnosis of a bladder small-cell carcinoma. Diagn Cytopathol 1991; 7: 79–82.

69. Rudrick B, Nguyen GK, Lakey WH. Carcinoid tumor of the renal pelvis: report of a case with positive urine cytology. Diagn Cytopathol 1995; 12: 360–363.

70. Tanaka T, Yoshimi N, Sawada K, et al. Ki-1-positive large cell anaplastic lymphoma diagnosed by urinary cytology. A case report. Acta Cytol 1993; 37: 520–524.

71. Gourlay W, Chan V, Gilks CB. Screening for urothelial malignancies by cytologic analysis and flow cytometry in a community urologic practice: a prospective study. Mod Pathol 1995; 8: 394–397.

72. Mora LB, Nicosia SV, Pow-Sang JM, et al. Ancillary techniques in the follow-up of transitional cell carcinoma: a comparison of cytology, histology and deoxyribonucleic acid image analysis cytometry in 91 patients. J Urol 1996; 156: 49–54; discussion 55.

73. de la Roza GL, Hopkovitz A, Caraway NP, et al. DNA image analysis of urinary cytology: prediction of recurrent transitional cell carcinoma. Mod Pathol 1996; 9: 571–578.

74. Arentsen HC, de la Rosette JJ, de Reijke TM, Langbein S. Fluorescence in situ hybridization: a multitarget approach in diagnosis and management of urothelial cancer. Expert Rev Mol Diagn 2007; 7: 11–19.

75. Stroganova AM, Khachaturian AV. [Fluorescence in situ hybridization in diagnosis of urinary bladder cancer]. Arkh Patol 2006; 68: 43–46.

76. Marin-Aguilera M, Mengual L, Ribal MJ, et al. Utility of fluorescence in situ hybridization as a non-invasive technique in the diagnosis of upper urinary tract urothelial carcinoma. Eur Urol 2007; 51: 409–415.

77. Yoder BJ, Skacel M, Hedgepeth R, et al. Reflex UroVysion testing of bladder cancer surveillance patients with equivocal or negative urine cytology: a prospective study with focus on the natural history of anticipatory positive findings. Am J Clin Pathol 2007; 127: 295–301.

78. Sprinack JP. Hematuria. In: Resnick MJ, Caldimore AA, Spirnack JP, eds. Decision making in urology. Philadelphia: BC Decker, 1985; 4–32.

79. Grossfeld GD, Wolf JS, Litwin MS. Asymptomatic microscopic hematuria in adults: Summary of the AUA Best Practice Policy Recommendations. Am Fam Phys 2001; 63: 440–444.

80. Neiberger RE. The ABCs of evaluating children with hematuria. Am Fam Phys 1994; 49: 176–181.

81. Sutton JM. Evaluation of hematuria in adults. JAMA 1990; 129: 2475–2480.

82. Thaller TR, Wang LP. Evaluation of asymptomatic microscopic hematuria in adults. Am Fam Phys 1999; 60: 366–370.

83. Ritchie CD, Bevan TA. Importance of occult haematuria found at screening. Br Med J 1986; 292: 681–683.

84. Marcussen N, Schumann JL, Schumann GB. Analysis of cytodiagnostic urinalysis findings in 77 patients with concurrent renal biopsies. Am J Kidney Dis 1992; 20: 618–628.

85. Scharnhorst V, Gerlag PG, Nanlohy Manuhutu ML, van der Graaf F. Urine flow cytometry and detection of glomerular hematuria. Clin Chem Lab Med 2006; 44: 1330–1334.

86. Ottiger C, Savoca R, Yurtsever H, Huber AR. Increased sensitivity in detecting renal impairments by quantitative measurement of marker protein excretion compared to detection of pathological particles in urine sediment analysis. Clin Chem Lab Med 2006; 44: 1347–1354.

CHAPTER **8**

# Non-neoplastic diseases of the prostate

David G. Bostwick, Junqi Qian, Deloar Hossain

## Embryology and fetal–prepubertal history

The prostate is derived from the urogenital sinus.[1,2] During the first 10 weeks of gestation, testosterone from the embryonic testes stimulates ingrowth of epithelial buds into urogenital sinus mesenchyme through a feedback loop.[2] The mesenchyme induces the urogenital sinus epithelium to undergo ductal morphogenesis and differentiation, which in turn signals the urogenital mesenchyme to differentiate into smooth muscle cells surrounding the epithelial ducts.[2–4] At the same time, the seminal vesicles, epididymis, vas deferens, and ejaculatory ducts develop from wolffian (mesonephric) ducts stimulated by fetal testosterone. At 31–36 weeks of gestation, the basic structure of the prostate is fully formed. In the fetal prostate, prostatic acini consist of tight aggregates of immature basal cells, often with squamous metaplasia of ducts and the urethra (Fig. 8-1).

After birth, the size of the prostate remains stable until 10–12 years of age, but duct formation and solid epithelial outgrowth continue.[5–8] During puberty there is a marked androgen-driven increase in gland size. By age 20, the mean prostate weighs about 20 g and remains stable for up to 30 years.[2,6,7]

Maldevelopment of the prostate is rare, and includes aplasia, hypoplasia, cystic change, and mesonephric remnants. Aplasia and hypoplasia are associated with androgen deficiency. Cystic change is uncommon and may be congenital or acquired, including utricular and müllerian duct cyst,[9–11] ejaculatory duct cyst,[12–14] vas deferens cyst, and seminal vesicle cyst, and rarely produces clinical symptoms.[14–16] Cysts may be also associated with infertility due to ejaculatory duct obstruction.[17,18] Mesonephric remnants in the prostate are an unusual mimic of adenocarcinoma[19–23] that consists of a proliferation of benign acini arranged in lobules or showing infiltrative growth between smooth muscle bundles without stromal desmoplasia (see below).[23]

## Anatomy and histology of the prostate

### Prostatic urethra and verumontanum

The urethra serves as a reference landmark for the study of prostate anatomy (Figs 8-2, 8-3).[24] There is a single 35° bend in the center of the prostatic urethra, creating proximal and distal segments of nearly equal length. The verumontanum bulges from the posterior wall at the urethral bend and tapers distally to form the crista urethralis. Most prostatic ducts and the ejaculatory ducts empty into the urethra in the mid and distal prostatic urethra, whereas the small periurethral glands of Littré have minute openings throughout the length of the urethra. Immediately proximal to the verumontanum is the utricle, a small 0.5 cm long epithelium-lined cul de sac. Recent studies revealed that the utricle is derived from the urogenital sinus, in contrast to the previous belief that it is a müllerian remnant.[11,25]

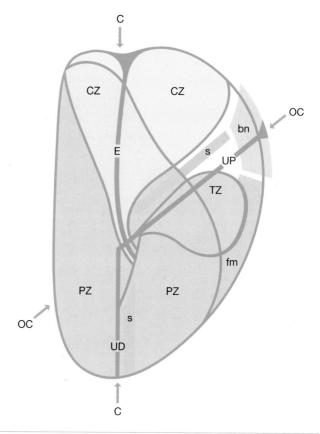

**Fig. 8-2** Sagittal diagram of the distal prostatic urethral segment (UD), proximal urethral segment (UP), and ejaculatory ducts (E), showing their relationships to a sagittal section of the anteromedial non-glandular tissues (bladder neck (bn), anterior fibromuscular stroma (fm), preprostatic sphincter (s), and distal striated sphincter (s)). These structures are shown in relation to a three-dimensional representation of the glandular prostate (central zone (CZ), peripheral zone (PZ), and transition zone (TZ)). The coronal plane (C) and the oblique coronal plane (OC) are indicated by arrows. (Reprinted with permission from McNeal JE, Bostwick DG. Anatomy of the prostate: implications for disease. In: Bostwick DG, ed. Pathology of the prostate. New York: Churchill Livingstone, 1990; 2.)

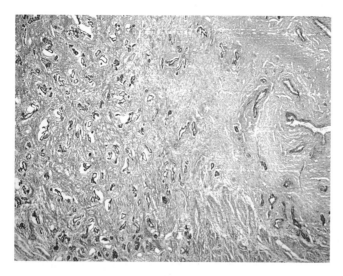

**Fig. 8-1** Fetal prostate at 35 weeks with immature epithelial elements.

A circumferential sleeve of muscle surrounds the entire urethra. This muscular layer includes a proximal preprostatic smooth muscle sphincter that prevents retrograde ejaculation and a distal sphincter of striated and smooth muscle at the apex that is important in control of micturition.

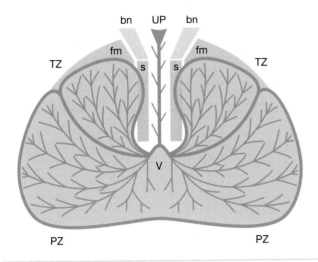

**Fig. 8-3** Oblique coronal section diagram of the prostate showing location of the peripheral zone (PZ) and transition zone (TZ) in relation to the proximal urethral segment (UP), verumontanum (V), preprostatic sphincter (s), bladder neck (bn), and periurethral region with periurethral glands. The branching pattern of the prostatic ducts is indicated; medial transition zone ducts penetrate into the sphincter. (Reprinted with permission from McNeal JE, Bostwick DG. Anatomy of the prostate: implications for disease. In: Bostwick DG, ed. Pathology of the prostate. New York: Churchill Livingstone, 1990; 2.)

## Zonal anatomy of the prostate

The prostate is composed of three zones: the peripheral zone, central zone, and transition zone (Table 8-1).[2,3,26,27] The peripheral zone contains about 70% of the volume of the prostate and is the most common site of prostatic intraepithelial neoplasia (PIN) and carcinoma. Peripheral zone acini are simple, round to oval, and set in a loose stroma of smooth muscle and collagen (Fig. 8-4). Digital rectal examination often includes a description of the left and right 'lobes' based on palpation of the median furrow in the midline that divides the peripheral zone into left and right halves.[2,3,26,27]

The central zone is a cone-shaped area that includes the entire base of the prostate and encompasses the ejaculatory ducts; it comprises about 25% of the volume of the prostate. Central zone acini are large and complex, with intraluminal ridges, papillary infoldings, and occasional epithelial arches and cribriform glands mimicking PIN (Fig. 8-5).[2,28] The ratio of epithelium to stroma is higher in the central zone than the rest of the prostate, and the stroma is composed of compact interlacing smooth muscle bundles.[2,26]

The transition zone contains the smallest volume of the normal prostate – about 5% – but often enlarges together with the anterior fibromuscular stroma to a massive size owing to benign prostatic hyperplasia and dwarfs the remainder of the prostate. Transition zone glands tend to be simple, small, and round, similar to those in the peripheral zone but are embedded in a compact stroma that forms a distinctive boundary with the loose stroma of the peripheral zone (Fig. 8-6).[2,29] The central and peripheral zones are often referred to together as the outer prostate or 'non-transition

**Table 8-1** Zonal anatomy of the human prostate: histological features

|  | Central zone | Transition zone | Peripheral zone |
|---|---|---|---|
| Volume of normal prostate (%) | 25 | 5 | 70 |
| ***Anatomic landmarks*** | | | |
| Intraprostatic relationships | Ejaculatory ducts | Surrounds proximal prostatic urethra | Distal prostatic urethra |
| Adjacent structures | Seminal vesicles | Bladder neck | Rectum |
| Urethral orifices of ducts | Verumontanum adjacent to ejaculatory ducts | Posterolateral wall of proximal prostatic urethra at its distal end | Posterolateral wall of distal prostatic urethra |
| ***Distinctive histologic features*** | | | |
| Epithelium | Complex large polygonal acini with intraluminal ridges | Simple small round acini | Simple small round acini |
| Stroma | Compact | Compact | Loose |
| ***Biochemical differences*** | | | |
| Production of pepsinogen II | Yes | No | No |
| Production of tissue plasminogen activator | Yes | No | No |
| ***Lectin binding patterns*** | | | |
| LCA, Con-A, WGA, PNA-N, RCA-1 | Yes | No | Yes |
| UEA-1, S-WGA, PNA | Yes | No | No |
| DBA, SBA, BS-1 | No | No | No |
| ***Proposed embryonic origin*** | Wolffian duct | Urogenital sinus | Urogenital sinus |

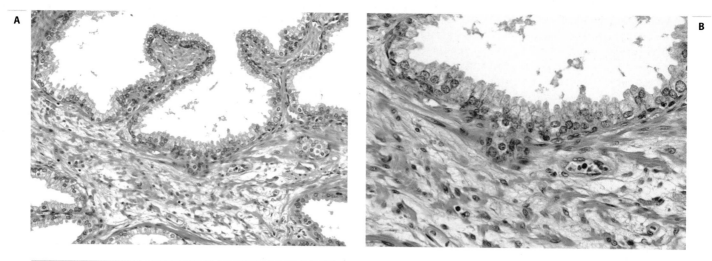

**Fig. 8-4** **(A)** Normal peripheral zone, consisting of simple acini and a loose stroma of smooth muscle and collagen. **(B)** The epithelium is columnar, with small round basal nuclei and an inconspicuous flattened basal cell layer.

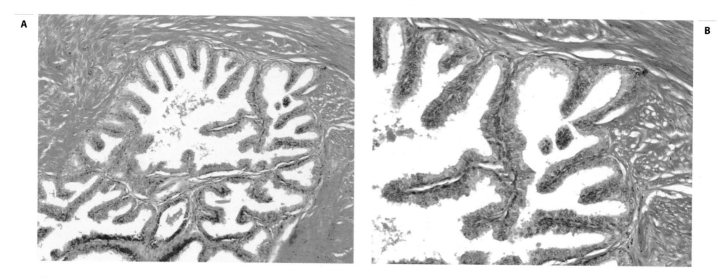

**Fig. 8-5** **(A)** Normal central zone consisting of large acini with complex intraluminal ridges, papillary infoldings, and epithelial arches set in a stroma of compact smooth muscle. **(B)** The epithelium varies from cuboidal to columnar.

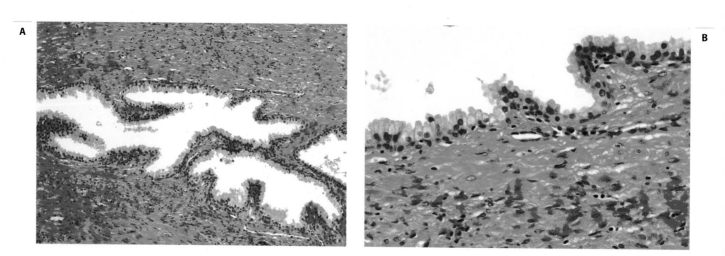

**Fig. 8-6** **(A)** Normal transition zone, consisting of simple acini and a compact stroma. **(B)** The epithelium is cuboidal or low columnar with apical cytoplasmic blebs.

zone,' whereas the transition zone and anterior fibromuscular stroma are often referred to as the inner prostate.[26]

Gene expression differs between the peripheral zone and the transition zone,[30,31] and stromal–epithelial interactions might be responsible for the distinct zonal localization of diseases.

## Normal epithelium of the prostate

The epithelium of the prostate is composed of three principal cell types according to light microscopy: secretory cells, basal cells, and neuroendocrine cells. An additional type, intermediate cells, can only be convincingly demonstrated by the unique immunophenotype (keratin phenotype intermediate between basal and luminal cells that coexpress high levels of keratin 5 and keratin 18 (K5/18) and hepatocyte growth factor receptor c-MET).

The secretory luminal cells are cuboidal to columnar, with small round nuclei, punctuate or inconspicuous nucleoli, finely granular chromatin, and pale to clear cytoplasm; they account for the bulk (73%) of epithelial volume.[2,6,32] Despite having the lowest proliferative activity, the terminally differentiated secretory cells produce prostate-specific antigen (PSA),[1] prostatic acid phosphatase (PAP), androgen receptors, acidic mucin, and other secretory products. They also express high levels of keratins 8 and 18 but lack keratins 5 and 14 and lack p63.

The basal cells of the prostate form a flattened attenuated layer of inconspicuous elongate cells at the periphery of the glands surmounting the basement membrane (Fig. 8-7).[33–35] These cells possess the highest proliferative activity of the prostatic epithelium, albeit low, and are thought to act as stem or 'reserve' cells that repopulate the secretory cell layer.[33–37] Basal cells apparently retain the ability to undergo metaplasia, including squamous differentiation in the setting of infarction and myoepithelial differentiation in sclerosing adenosis. Epidermal growth factor receptors have been identified in basal cells but not in secretory cells, suggesting that these cells play a role in growth regulation.[38,39] Basal cells are

selectively labeled with antibodies to high molecular weight keratins such as clone 34β-E12 (keratin 903), a property that is exploited immunohistochemically in separating benign acinar processes such as atrophy (which retains a basal cell layer) from adenocarcinoma (which lacks a basal cell layer) (Fig. 8-7). The nuclear protein p63 is another diagnostically useful basal cell marker, consistently decorating nuclei.[40] Basal cell cocktail (the combination of 34β-E12 and p63) increases the sensitivity of the basal cell detection and reduces staining variability compared to either stain alone.[41–43] Basal cells also express high levels of keratins 5 and 14, as well as p63, in contrast to secretory and intermediate cells. Basal cells contain little or no PSA, PAP, androgen receptors, keratins 8 or 18, or mucin. The normal prostatic epithelium frequently displays foci of basal cell proliferation that are too small to warrant the diagnosis of basal cell hyperplasia. Prostatic basal cells do not possess myoepithelial differentiation, unlike basal cells in the breast, salivary glands, pancreas, and other sites, probably because the massive smooth muscle stroma of the prostate propels secretions downstream without the need for assistance from basal cells.

Neuroendocrine cells are the least common cell type of the prostatic epithelium and are usually not identified in routine hematoxylin and eosin-stained sections, except for rare cells with large eosinophilic granules.[44,45] Although their function is unknown, neuroendocrine cells probably have an endocrine–paracrine regulatory role in growth and development, similar to neuroendocrine cells in other organs, and contain numerous neuropeptides that modulate cell growth and proliferation.[46–48] Androgen deprivation therapy does not appear to influence the number or distribution of neuroendocrine cells in the normal or neoplastic prostate.[49] These cells coexpress PSA[49] and androgen receptors, suggesting a common cell of origin for epithelial cells and neuroendocrine cells in the prostate. Neuroendocrine cells are in greatest number near the verumontanum, suggesting a role in luminal constriction and dilatation. Serotonin and chromogranin are the best immunohistochemical markers of neuroendocrine cells in formalin-fixed sections of the pros-

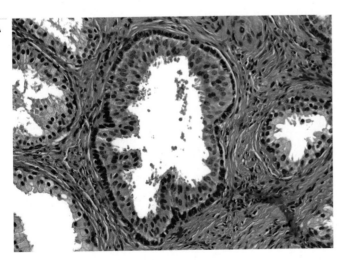
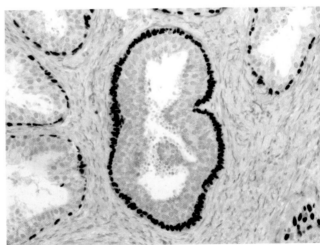

A

B

**Fig. 8-7** **(A)** Normal prostatic acinus with prominent basal cell layer due to nuclear crowding and hyperchromasia. The basal cell layer is usually inconspicuous. **(B)** Immunostains for high molecular weight keratin and p63 demonstrate a continous circumferential layer of basal cells.

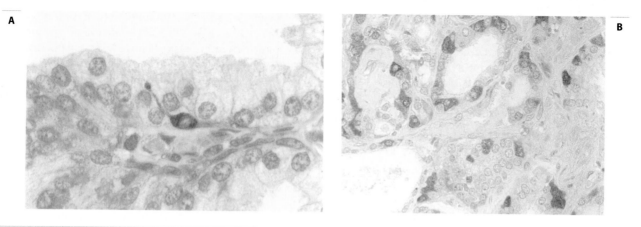

**Fig. 8-8** Neuroendocrine cells. **(A)** When present in normal prostatic epithelium, they are infrequent and variable in shape. **(B)** The cells in prostatic adenocarcinoma display dark cytoplasmic reaction product which fills the cytoplasm of scattered cells, obscuring the nuclei. (Immunohistochemical stains for serotonin **(A)** and chromogranin **(B)**).

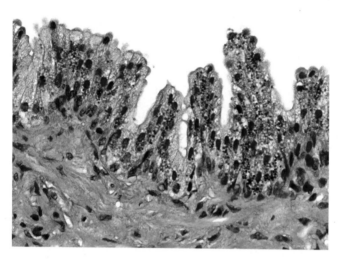

**Fig. 8-9** Melanin-like pigment in benign prostatic epithelium.

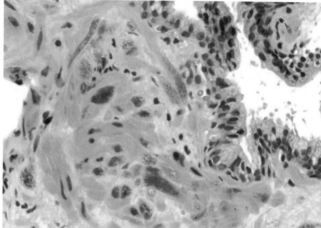

**Fig. 8-10** Melanin-like pigment in prostatic stroma (melanosis).

tate (Fig. 8-8).[44,46,47,50] African-American men have comparatively low prostatic neuroendocrine cell expression compared to other ethnic groups, and this may play a role in their increased risk of cancer.[51]

## Pigment

Pigment is occasionally observed in the cytoplasm of the secretory epithelium, including lipofuscin and melanin.[52,53] Lipofuscin granules are golden-brown, gray-brown, or blue by H&E staining (Fig. 8-9), positive for Fontana–Masson, periodic acid–Schiff with diastase, Congo red, Luxol fast blue, and oil-red O, and exhibit autofluorescence. Similar pigment may also be found in seminal vesicle and ejaculatory duct epithelium, high-grade PIN, and adenocarcinoma. Special attention should be paid to avoid misinterpretation of pigmented acini adjacent to carcinoma as evidence of seminal vesicle invasion on needle biopsy. This pigment represents 'wear and tear' or 'old age' pigment, resulting from endogenous cellular byproducts of the prostate epithelium.[26] It is present in all zones of the prostate, and is randomly distributed. Less commonly, melanin-like (Fontana–Masson

positive) pigment is found in scattered foci in the normal and hyperplastic prostatic epithelium and stroma (Fig. 8-10) (see Melanosis, below).[54]

## Luminal products

The intraluminal contents of benign prostatic acini include mucin, degenerating epithelium, crystalloids, proteinaceous debris, corpora amylacea, calculi, and spermatozoa.[55–57]

Mucin is not usually present in benign acini. Histochemical staining demonstrates neutral mucins (periodic acid–Schiff with diastase), whereas neoplastic acini often demonstrate neutral and acidic mucins (Alcian blue, pH 2.5 positive).[58–62] However, acid mucin is not specific for prostate cancer as other benign conditions also express it, including mucinous metaplasia, sclerosing adenosis, atypical adenomatous hyperplasia, and high-grade PIN. MUC1 (EMA), MUC2, MUC4, MUC5AC and MUC6 are not found in benign prostatic epithelium,[63] although conflicting results have been found with MUC1[64,65] and MUC4.[66] Positive staining for MUC6 in seminal vesicular epithelium may be useful for excluding prostatic origin.[67]

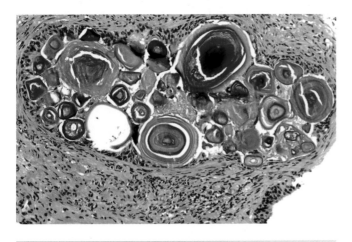

**Fig. 8-11** Corpora amylacea fill benign prostatic acini.

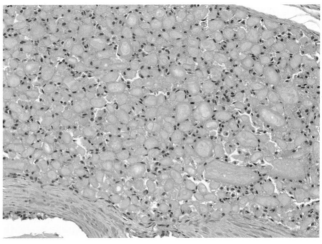

**Fig. 8-13** Corpora amylacea mimicking signet ring-cell carcinoma.

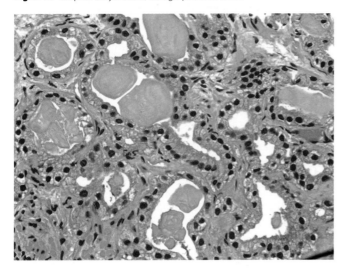

**Fig. 8-12** Corpora amylacea in prostatic adenocarcinoma.

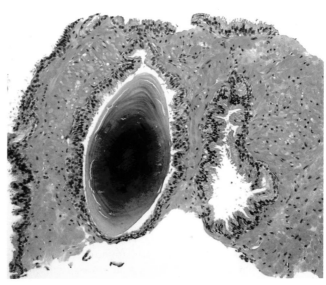

**Fig. 8-14** Prostatic calculus in dilated acinus.

Corpora amylacea are luminal secretions present in up to 78% of benign prostatic acini[57,68–70] but are only rarely observed in adenocarcinoma (0.4% of needle biopsies with cancer) (Figs 8-11, 8-12).[57] They vary in size and shape, but most are round (Fig. 8-13). Color ranges from pink-purple to orange, and the presence of concentric laminations is variable. Corpora amylacea are thought to be related to epithelial cell desquamation and degeneration. Ultrastructurally, they are composed of bundles of fibrils and occasional interspersed electron-dense areas.[68–70] Biochemical analysis and X-ray diffraction reveal that their main constituent is sulfated glycosaminoglycans.[55,71]

Proteinaceous secretions are a frequent non-specific finding in benign and neoplastic acini (overall 8% incidence in one study, with 100% incidence in men over 70 years of age),[72] and are considered the precursor of corpora amylacea and calculi.[73] In an animal model, luminal secretions increased significantly in the presence of inflammation.[74]

Calculi (microcalcifications), present in 31–100% of prostates, are typically found in central, large prostatic ducts (Fig. 8-14).[75] They are often observed in association with inflammation, benign prostatic hyperplasia (BPH), and basal cell hyperplasia.[56,76] Whereas luminal microcalcifica-

tions are commonly observed in breast cancer, prostatic calculi are rarely seen in malignant acini. Interestingly, stromal microcalcifications are observed in about 3% of needle biopsies, invariably in association with chronic inflammation.[77] Calcific deposits of Monckeberg's medial calcinosis are occasionally observed in arteries and large arterioles in the periprostatic tissue.

Calcification was more prevalent in autopsy prostates from African-Americans in Washington, DC than from Africans from West Africa, perhaps reflecting different diets of the two population groups.[78] There was a positive association between prostatic calcification and age.

Intraprostatic spermatozoa can be identified with Berg's stain, and are present in 26% of prostates at radical prostatectomy, including the peripheral zone (72%), central zone (22%), and transition zone (6%).[79] They are frequently associated with inflammation and atrophy, including post-atrophic hyperplasia (PAH).

## Rectal tissue in needle biopsies

Rectal tissue is often seen in needle biopsies of the prostate and when distorted may be misinterpreted as carcinoma.[80] Immunoreactivity for racemase and negative staining for basal cell-specific antikeratin 34B-E12 further confounds the diagnostic difficulty, although the combination of PSA and PAP should provide accurate differentiation in all cases. Useful histologic clues to identify rectal mucosa include the presence of detached tissue with an epithelium containing goblet cells, a lamina propria and muscularis propria, and abundant inflammatory cells.

## Capsule

The capsule of the prostate consists of an inner layer of smooth muscle and an outer covering of collagen, with marked variability in the relative amounts in different areas (Fig. 8-15). At the apex, the acinar elements become sparse, and the capsule becomes ill-defined, composed of a mixture of fibrous connective tissue, smooth muscle, and striated muscle. As a result, the prostatic capsule cannot be regarded as a well-defined anatomic structure with constant features.[81] In biopsy and surgical specimens, the capsule at the apex and bladder base is difficult to identify; consequently, it is often not possible to determine the presence of extraprostatic extension of cancer at these sites.

Along the lateral aspect of the prostate, the lateral pelvic fascia and the prostatic capsule are separated by adipose tissue in 52% of cases, whereas in the remainder they are adherent.[82] Denonvilliers' fascia and the prostatic capsule are tightly adherent posteriorly in 97% of cases. A smooth transition from the capsule to the anterior fibromuscular stroma is invariably present, but the capsule is only recognizable anteriorly in 11% of cases. In 85% of cases the lateral pelvic fascia connects and fuses with the anterior fibromuscular stroma and covers the outermost regions of the lateral and anterior surfaces.[82]

Abundant adipose tissue is present around most of the prostate, and is a reliable marker of extraprostatic tissue in biopsies. In a series of radical prostatectomies, periprostatic adipose tissue was present on 48% of all prostatic surfaces examined.[83]

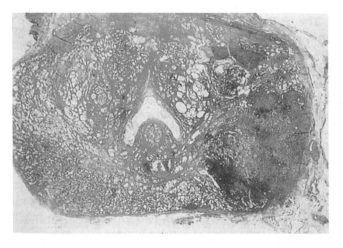

**Fig. 8-15** Whole-mount prostate showing the capsule and neurovascular bundles (bottom right). Contrast with the contralateral region (bottom left), where the bundle has been spared and left within the patient.

The distribution varied among the different surfaces of the prostate, with the anterior, posterior, right, and left surfaces showing respectively 44%, 36%, 59%, and 57% adipose tissue. Nerve-sparing prostatectomy resulted in slightly less adipose tissue (46%) than non-nerve-sparing procedures (54%).

Intraprostatic fat is very rarely observed and, when present, consists of a small microscopic focus of a few adipocytes.[84,85] Sung and colleagues[86] examined 313 consecutive totally embedded radical prostatectomies and found no evidence of intraprostatic fat in any case. For practical purposes, identification of fat in biopsies is considered sampling of extraprostatic tissue.[85]

Small (15–20 μm) eosinophilic hyaline bodies, referred to as stromal hyaline bodies, are sometimes observed within the muscular wall of the seminal vesicles, vas deferens, and prostate.[87–89] These round to oval structures result from degeneration of smooth muscle fibers, and transition forms can be seen. Stromal hyaline bodies stain with Masson's trichrome and PAS, but not with phosphotungstic acid hematoxylin method (PTAH), methyl green pyronine, Feulgen, Alcian blue at pH 2.5, or Congo red.

## Nerve and blood supply

The nerve supply of the prostate is furnished by paired neurovascular bundles that run along the posterolateral edge of the prostate from apex to base. Surgical sparing of these structures during radical prostatectomy may preserve sexual potency.[90] Autonomic ganglia are clustered near the neurovascular bundles, sending out small nerve trunks that arborize over the surface of the prostate, penetrating through the capsule and branching to form an extensive network of nerve twigs within the prostate that are often in intimate contact with the walls of ducts and acini.[91] Capsular ganglia are present in 52% of radical prostatectomy specimens, most frequently at the posterolateral aspect of the base. There are no obvious morphologic differences between the capsular and periprostatic ganglia.[92] The posterior capsule has significantly more nerve fibers than the anterior capsule according to S100 protein staining.[91]

Caution is warranted in the interpretation of perineural space invasion as an absolute criterion for the diagnosis of cancer, as rarely this can be seen in benign glands (Fig. 8-16).[23,93]

According to an immunohistochemical survey using S100 protein, innervation of the peripheral zone is significantly greater than in the transition zone, which in turn is significantly more innervated than BPH.[91] The posterior capsule has significantly more nerves than the anterior capsule. The greatest amount of neural tissue is present in the neurovascular bundles and seminal vesicles, with the lowest in the transition zone and BPH. Innervation appears to decrease with age. A recent study of non-nerve-sparing radical prostatectomies revealed that more than 50% of periprostatic nerves are associated with the neurovascular bundles, with up to 25% of nerves situated anterolaterally and laterally; the concentration of nerves was invariably higher at the base than at the apex and mid-prostate.[94]

The blood supply of the prostate is furnished by one of the branches of the internal iliac artery. Veins drain directly into the prostatic plexus, and an extensive arborizing network

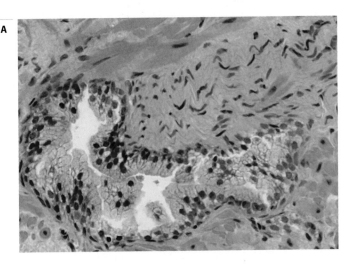
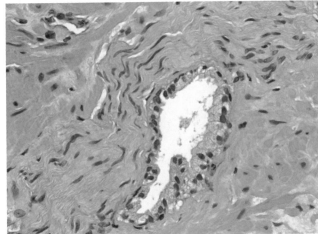

**Fig. 8-16** Perineural abutment by benign glands.

is present in the capsule. The venous drainage empties into the internal iliac vein.

Lymphatics from the prostate drain mainly into the internal iliac lymph nodes, with less drainage into the external iliac and sacral lymph nodes.[2] Antibodies directed against lymphatic vessel endothelial hyaluronan receptor (LYVE-1) revealed that lymphatic density was greater in BPH than carcinoma, whereas microvessel density with anti-CD34 antibodies revealed the opposite.[95]

### Seminal vesicles and ejaculatory ducts

The seminal vesicles arise during the 13th week of development as outpouchings of the lower mesonephric ducts. They are bounded distally by the prostate, anteriorly by the base of the bladder, and posteriorly by Denonvilliers' fascia and the rectum. Their anatomic distribution in this region is variable, and they are occasionally found within the capsule of the prostate gland. The seminal vesicles may be palpable on digital rectal examination and, when intimately associated with the prostate, may be mistaken for prostatic nodularity or induration. Up to 20% of prostate biopsies for nodularity contain fragments of seminal vesicle epithelium, a potential source of diagnostic confusion.[52]

The mucosa displays complex papillary folds and irregular convoluted lumina, and the lining consists of a non-ciliated pseudostratified tall columnar epithelium. The cells are predominantly secretory, with microvesicular lipid droplets and characteristic lipofuscin pigment granules.[96] The pigment is golden-brown and refractile, increasing in amount with age. The muscular wall consists of a thick circumferential coat of smooth muscle and is thought to serve a contractile function. The ducts of the seminal vesicles merge with the vas deferens on each side to form the ejaculatory ducts and then enter the central zone of the prostate and converge prior to termination at the verumontanum and prostatic urethra (Figs 8-17, 8-18).

### Cowper's glands

Cowper's glands are small, paired bulbomembranous urethral glands that may be mistaken for prostatic carcinoma in

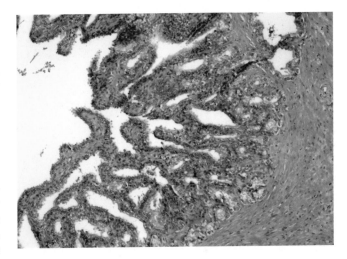

**Fig. 8-17** Ejaculatory duct near origin in the seminal vesicles.

biopsy specimens.[97,98] They are composed of lobules of closely packed uniform acini lined by cytologically benign cells with abundant apical mucinous cytoplasm (Fig. 8-19). Nuclei are small, solitary, punctuate, and basally located, and nucleoli are inconspicuous. Cowper's glands are embedded in smooth muscle, mimicking the infiltrative pattern of prostatic cancer. Misdiagnosis can be avoided if samples display immunoreactivity for mucin and smooth muscle actin and negativity for PSA and prostatic alkaline phosphatase.[99] Carcinoma of Cowper's glands is exceedingly rare, and is characterized by frank anaplasia of tumor cells.

## Immunohistochemistry

The most important immunohistochemical markers in prostate pathology are PSA, PAP, racemase (P504S), high molecular weight keratin 34β-E12, and p63. Androgen receptor immunostaining has not achieved routine clinical utility owing to variable results in many studies. Standardization

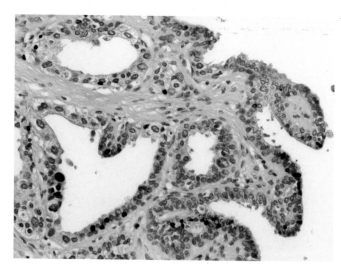

Fig. 8-18 **(A)** Seminal vesicle and **(B)** ejaculatory duct epithelia have similar degrees of severe cytologic atypia, with occasional bizarre giant cells.

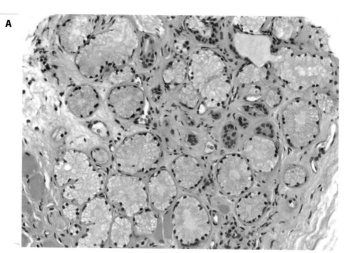
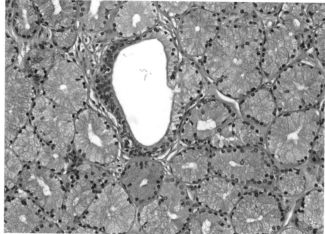

Fig. 8-19 Cowper's gland. **(A)** This lobulated small gland contains multiple small acini with abundant mucinous cytoplasm and small hyperchromatic basal nuclei. **(B)** These acini surround a central duct.

of staining and quantification methods is recommended to avoid technical variation in results reporting.[100]

## Prostate-specific antigen

Immunohistochemical expression of PSA is useful for distinguishing high-grade prostate cancer and urothelial carcinoma, colonic carcinoma, granulomatous prostatitis, and lymphoma.[101–107] PSA also facilitates identifying the site of origin of the tumor in metastatic adenocarcinoma. A list of extraprostatic tissues and tumors that reportedly express PSA immunoreactivity is given in Table 8-2.[108–120]

PSA can be detected in frozen sections, paraffin-embedded sections, cell smears, and in cytologic preparations of normal and neoplastic prostatic epithelium (Fig. 8-20). In the normal and hyperplastic prostate, PSA was uniformly present at the apical portion of the glandular epithelium of secretory cells. The intensity of the staining decreased in poorly differentiated adenocarcinoma.[41,42,107] Staining is invariably heterogeneous. Microwave antigen

Table 8-2 Immunoreactivity of prostate-specific antigen (PSA) in extraprostatic tissues and tumors

| **Extraprostatic tissues** |
| --- |
| Urethra, periurethral glands, male and female |
| Bladder, cystitis cystica and glandularis |
| Urachal remnants |
| Neutrophils |
| Anus, anal glands (male only) |

| **Extraprostatic tumors** |
| --- |
| Mature teratoma |
| Urethra, periurethral gland adenocarcinoma (female) |
| Bladder, villous adenoma and adenocarcinoma |
| Penis, extramammary Paget's disease |
| Salivary gland, pleomorphic adenoma (male only) |
| Salivary gland, carcinoma (male only) |

(Caveat: In many of these tissues and tumors staining may be patchy, weak or equivocal. Many of these reports have not been confirmed or validated. Also, contemporary antibodies to PSA may have different specificity and sensitivity from those used in some of these studies.)

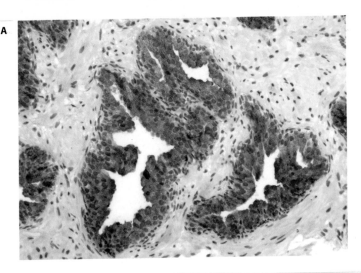

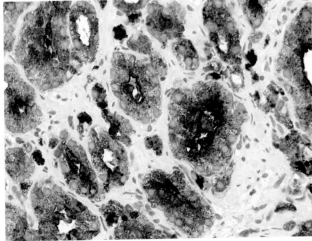

**Fig. 8-20** PSA staining. Normal prostate epithelium labeled with PSA antibody **(A)**. PSA staining in prostate cancer **(B)**.

retrieval is usually not necessary, even in tissues that have been immersed in formalin for years. Formalin fixation is optimal for localization of PSA, and variation in staining intensity is only partially due to fixation and embedding effects.[103] Immunoreactivity is preserved in decalcified specimens, and may be enhanced.

## Prostatic acid phosphatase

When combined with stains for PSA, prostatic acid phosphatase (PAP) is a valuable immunohistochemical marker for identifying prostate cancer.[121,122] In the normal and hyperplastic prostate, PAP was uniformly present at the apical portion of the glandular epithelium of secretory cells. There was more intense and uniform staining of cancer cells and the glandular epithelium of well-differentiated adenocarcinoma, whereas less intense and more variable staining was seen in moderately and poorly differentiated adenocarcinoma. It has been reported that the intensity of PAP immunoreactivity correlated with patient survival, probably owing to greater androgen responsiveness in immunoreactive cancers.[123,124] A list of extraprostatic tissues and tumors that reportedly express PAP immunoreactivity is given in Table 8-3.[107–110,112,115,116,125–130]

Serum PAP is less useful than PSA because of inherent problems in the accuracy of measurement, including the requirement for special handling due to enzyme instability, diurnal fluctuation, variation resulting from prostatic digital examination and biopsy, and cross-reactivity with non-prostatic serum acid phosphatase produced by liver, bone, kidney, and blood cells. At present, serum PAP has little or no clinical utility.

## α-Methylacyl-CoA-racemase/P504S (AMACR, P504S, racemase)

α-Methylacyl-CoA-racemase (racemase) gene product, also referred to as P504S protein, is an enzyme involved in β-oxidation of branched-chain fatty acids. It has recently been identified as a novel tumor marker for several human cancers

**Table 8-3** Immunoreactivity of prostatic acid phosphatase (PAP) in extraprostatic tissues and tumors

**Extraprostatic cells and tissues**
Urethra, periurethral glands, male and female
Bladder, cystitis cystica and glandularis
Pancreas, islet cells
Kidney, renal tubules
Neutrophils
Colon, neuroendocrine cells
Anus, anal glands (male only)
Stomach, parietal cells
Liver, hepatocytes
Breast, ductal epithelial cells

**Extraprostatic tumors**
Bladder, adenocarcinoma
Anus, cloacagenic carcinoma
Rectum carcinoid
Other gastrointestinal carcinoids
Pancreas, islet cell tumor
Mature teratoma
Breast, ductal carcinoma
Salivary gland, pleomorphic adenoma (male only)
Salivary gland, carcinoma (male only)

(Caveat: in many of these tissues and tumors staining may be patchy, weak or equivocal. Many of these reports have not been confirmed or validated. Also, contemporary antibodies to PAP may have different specificity and sensitivity from those used in some of these studies.)

and their precursor lesions, including prostate cancer.[131–136] Initial study showed that racemase was strongly and uniformly positive in 97–100% of prostate cancers. Recent studies suggest that it is positive in 80–100% of small prostate cancers on needle biopsy, and less intense and more heterogeneous in unusual morphologic variants of prostate cancer, including atrophic, foamy gland, and pseudo-hyperplastic cancers (Fig. 8-21) (Table 8-4). We and others found that 91% of irradiated prostate cancers retained racemase immunoreactivity.[137] Androgen deprivation therapy

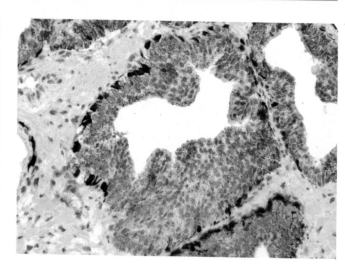

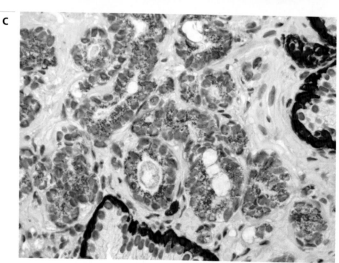

**Fig. 8-21** Racemase/34β-E12/p63 cocktail staining in benign prostatic epithelium **(A)**, high-grade PIN **(B)**, and cancer **(C)**.

**Table 8-4** Immunoreactivity of α-methylacyl-CoA-racemase (AMACR) in the benign and neoplastic prostate

| | Percent immunoreactive cases (range) | Percent immunoreactive acini (range) | Cytoplasmic staining intensity (−, 1+, 2+, 3+) |
|---|---|---|---|
| Benign | 8 (0–10) | 4.6 (0–24.5) | −~1+ |
| Atypical adenomatous hyperplasia | 14 (10–17) | 15.1 (1–50) | −~1+ |
| High-grade PIN | 88 (80–100) | 21.8 (2.7–57.7) | 1+~3+ |
| Cancer | 97 (80–100) | 35.0 (6.2–78.2) | 2+~3+ |

reduces racemase staining in prostate cancer.[43,138] In addition, positive racemase staining is also found in the majority of cases of high-grade prostatic intraepithelial neoplasia, 10–15% of cases of atypical adenomatous hyperplasia, occasional benign glands (Fig. 8-21), and rare seminal vesicle epithelium.[132,133,135,136,139] Nephrogenic metaplasia is an important mimic of malignancy that is strongly positive for racemase; this must be borne in mind in the interpretation of small foci in needle biopsies. Jiang et al.[140] found that the sensitivity and specificity of immunodetection of prostatic adenocarcinoma with racemase were 97% and 92%, respectively; positive and negative predictive values were 95%. The intensity and percentage of racemase immunostaining in prostatic adenocarcinoma was significantly higher than in benign prostatic tissue.

## Keratin 34β-E12 (keratin 903; high molecular weight keratin)

Basal cell-specific anti-keratin 34β-E12 stains virtually all of the normal basal cells of the prostate; there is no staining in the secretory and stromal cells. Basal cell layer disruption is present in 56% of cases of high-grade PIN, more commonly in glands adjacent to invasive carcinoma than in distant glands. The amount of disruption increases with increasing grades of PIN, with loss of more than one-third of the basal cell layer in 52% of foci of high-grade PIN. Early carcinoma occurs at sites of acinar outpouching and basal cell layer disruption.[28] Prostate cancer cells do not react with this antibody, although it may stain other cancers. Basal cell layer disruption also occurs in inflamed acini, atypical adenomatous hyperplasia, and post-atrophic hyperplasia.[14,128,142-152]

Despite the clinical utility of high molecular weight keratin, caution is urged in interpretation because of the need to rely on negative results to separate adenocarcinoma from its mimics. Numerous confounding factors can interfere with staining, including poor tissue preservation and fixation, and lack of enzyme predigestion.[153]

## p63

Recently, p63, a nuclear protein, was shown to be a diagnostically useful basal cell marker. p63 staining was reported to be at least as sensitive and specific for the identification of basal cells in diagnostic prostate specimens as high molecular weight cytokeratin staining (Fig. 8-21).[154] Shah et al.[155] found that p63 was more sensitive than 34β-E12 in staining benign basal cells, particularly in TURP (transurethral resection) specimens, offering a slight advantage over 34β- E12 in diagnostically challenging cases. Zhou et al.[156,157] demonstrated that the basal cell cocktail (34β-E12 and p63) increased the sensitivity of basal cell detection and reduced staining variability. The p63 gene is also expressed in respiratory epithelia, breast and bronchial myoepithelial cells, cytotrophoblast cells of human placenta, in scattered cells of lymph nodes and germinal centers, and in squamous cell carcinoma of the lung.[43,158] Triple staining with racemase, high molecular weight cytokeratin, and p63 is emerging as a standard adjunct for the diagnosis of prostate cancer.[43,152,159-161]

## Combination of racemase, keratin 34β-E12, and p63

Cocktail staining using racemase, high molecular weight cytokeratin, and p63 (basal cell markers) is increasingly being used in the work-up of difficult prostate needle biopsies.[43,151,152,162-166] Negative immunohistochemical staining for basal cells is not diagnostic of carcinoma per se, as occasional benign glands may not show immunoreactivity, so a positive immunohistochemical marker specific for prostate cancer, such as racemase, is of great value in confirming malignancy. Positive racemase staining converts an atypical diagnosis, based on suspicious histology and negative basal cell marker stains, to cancer in approximately 10% of cases thought to be atypical by contributing pathologists, and in approximately 50% of cases thought to be atypical by a specialist in genitourinary pathology. We use the cocktail staining in routine practice, and find it to be very useful for the diagnosis of small prostate cancers (Fig. 8-21). Polyclonal and monoclonal antibodies are available commercially.[167] Optimizing the staining conditions for cocktail antibodies is very important for interpretation.[139,168] Although it has limitations with respect to sensitivity and specificity, racemase has rapidly become a standard adjunctive stain used to reach a definitive diagnosis in prostate biopsies con-

sidered to be atypical but not diagnostic of malignancy on hematoxylin and eosin sections alone.[168-171]

## Prostate-specific membrane antigen

Prostate-specific membrane antigen (PSMA) is a membrane-bound antigen that is highly specific for benign and malignant prostatic epithelium. There is intense cytoplasmic epithelial immunoreactivity for PSMA.[172-175] The number of immunoreactive cells increases from benign epithelium to high-grade PIN and prostatic adenocarcinoma. The most extensive and intense staining for PSMA was observed in high-grade carcinoma, with immunoreactivity in virtually every cell in Gleason primary patterns 4 or 5 (Table 8-5).[176] Extraprostatic expression of PSMA is highly restricted, and non-prostatic cancer is invariably negative for PSMA, including renal cell carcinoma, urothelial carcinoma, and colonic adenocarcinoma. In a cohort of organ-confined margin-negative cancers treated by surgery, PSMA immunoreactivity in cancer cells was not predictive of PSA biochemical failure or recurrence;[177] these findings differ from serum studies, in which elevated concentration of PSMA indicated surgical treatment failure.[178-180] PSMA is clinically useful for diagnostic and therapeutic applications. It is expressed in lymph node[172,181] and bone marrow metastases of prostate cancer (Fig. 8-22), emphasizing its utility in identifying cancers from unknown primary sites. Serum PSMA was of prognostic significance, especially in the presence of metastases, and correlated well with cancer stage in a screened population. Despite its potential utility, PSMA immunohistochemistry is virtually never undertaken in routine practice.

## Human glandular kallikrein 2 (hK2)

The human kallikrein family consists of three members: hK1, hK2, and hK3.[1] The mRNA for hK2 and PSA are located predominantly in prostatic epithelium and are regulated by androgens.[182-185] In addition, hK2 has 78% amino acid homology with PSA and is expressed predominantly in the prostate, suggesting that it may be a clinically useful marker for the diagnosis and monitoring of prostate cancer.[184-187] The intensity and extent of hK2 expression was greater in cancer than in PIN, which in turn was greater than in benign epithelium. Gleason primary grade 4 and 5 cancers showed

**Table 8-5** Comparative immunoreactivity of PSMA and PSA in the benign and neoplastic prostate in 184 radical prostatectomies

| | Percent immunoreactive cells + SD (range) |
|---|---|
| **PSMA** | |
| Benign | 69.5 + 17.3 (20–90) |
| High-grade PIN | 77.9 + 13.7 (30–100) |
| Cancer | 80.2 + 13.7 (30–100) |
| **PSA** | |
| Benign | 81.3 + 11.8 (20–90) |
| High-grade PIN | 64.8 + 17.3 (10–90) |
| Cancer | 74.2 + 16.2 (10–90) |

SD, standard deviation.

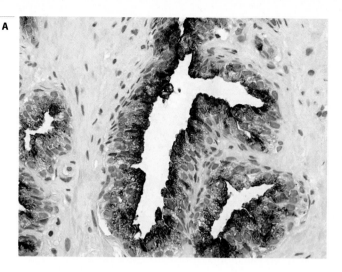

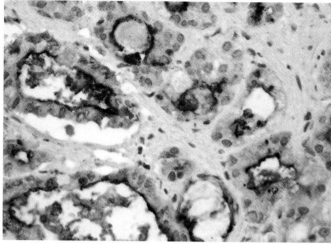

**Fig. 8-22** PSMA Staining. **(A)** Normal prostate epithelium labeled with PSMA antibody. **(B)** PSMA staining in prostate cancer.

hK2 staining in almost every cell, whereas there was greater heterogeneity of staining in lower grades of cancer.[188] In marked contrast to hK2, PSA and PAP immunoreactivity was most intense in benign epithelium and stained to a lesser extent in PIN and carcinoma.[188,189] The number of cells immunoreactive for hK2 and PSA was not predictive of cancer recurrence.[190] Tissue expression of hK2 appears to be regulated independently of PSA and PAP.[191]

## Other markers of basal cells

Numerous immunohistochemical markers have recently been identified in the prostate, and many of these are found preferentially in the basal cell layer of the epithelium (Table 8-6).

Basal cells display immunoreactivity at least focally for keratins 5, 10, 11, 13, 14, 16, and 19; of these, only keratin 19 is also found in secretory cells.[28,143,142,144–146,148,158,192–195] Keratins found exclusively in the secretory cells include 7, 8, and 18. Expression of S100-A6 (calcyclin), a calcium-binding protein, is restricted in the prostate to the basal cells of benign glands, but not in cancer.[196,197]

## Androgen receptors

Androgen receptors are present in both androgen-responsive and -unresponsive cells in prostatic adenocarcinoma. These receptors are widely distributed in the nuclei of the basal cell layer of the normal prostate, hyperplasia,[198] and localized and metastatic prostatic carcinoma.[199,200] The percentage of cancer cells with androgen receptors is not predictive of time to progression after androgen-deprivation therapy;[201,202] however, there is greater heterogeneity of receptor immunoreactivity in adenocarcinoma that responds poorly to therapy.[200,203,204]

Androgen receptor expression in small cell carcinoma appears to predict poor outcome, in contrast to typical adenocarcinoma, which shows no correlation. Androgen receptor gene mutations are present in up to 100% of cases of metastatic hormone-refractory prostate cancer.[205] At present, there is no established role for androgen receptor assays in the diagnosis and treatment of prostate cancer, although this is under active investigation.[206,207]

## Neuroendocrine markers

Neuroendocrine cells are part of the widely dispersed diffuse neuroendocrine regulatory system, also known as endocrine–paracrine cells. Most neuroendocrine cells of the prostate contain serotonin,[208] chromogranin A,[209–211] protein tyrosine phosphatase PTP1B,[212] and other neuroendocrine markers that are not consistently expressed. In humans, there are three patterns of neuroendocrine differentiation in prostatic carcinoma: (1) infrequent small cell neuroendocrine carcinoma (Fig. 8-23); (2) rare carcinoid-like cancer; and (3) conventional prostatic cancer with focal neuroendocrine differentiation. Virtually all prostatic adenocarcinomas contain at least a small number of neuroendocrine cells, but special studies such as histochemistry and immunohistochemistry are usually necessary to identify them.[48,210–221] Neuroendocrine differentiation typically consists of scattered cells that are inapparent by light microscopy but revealed by immunoreactivity for one or more markers. Neuroendocrine cells in prostate cancer are malignant, and lack androgen receptor expression.[210,214,218,219,221–223] According to most reports, neuroendocrine cells have no apparent clinical or prognostic significance in benign epithelium, primary prostatic adenocarcinoma, or lymph node metastases.[44,49,210,211,213,215,219,221,222,224–239] Benign neuroendocrine cells are negative for racemase, whereas malignant cells are positive.[221,240]

## Prostate sampling techniques

### Needle biopsy

The introduction of the automatic spring-driven core biopsy gun in the late 1980s began a new era in the sampling of the prostate for histologic diagnosis (Fig 8-24). The new 18-gauge needle offered important advantages over the older

**Table 8-6** Immunophenotype of prostatic basal cells

| Biomarker | Function | Findings |
|---|---|---|
| PCNA | Cell proliferation marker | Up to 79% of labeled cells are basal cells |
| MIB 1 | Cell proliferation marker | Up to 77% of labeled cells are basal cells |
| Ki-67 | Cell proliferation marker | Up to 81% of labeled cells are basal cells |
| Androgen receptors | Nuclear receptors that are necessary for prostatic epithelial growth | Strong immunoreactivity; also present in cancer cells |
| Prostate-specific antigen | Enzyme that liquefies the seminal coagulum | Present in rare basal cells; mainly in secretory luminal cells |
| Keratin 8.12 | Keratins 13, 16 | Strong immunoreactivity |
| Keratin 4.62 | Keratin 19 | Moderate immunoreactivity |
| Keratin PKK1 | Keratins 7, 8, 17, 18 | Moderate immunoreactivity |
| Keratin 312C8-1 | Keratin 14 | Strong immunoreactivity |
| Keratin 34B-E12 | Keratins 5, 10, 11 | Strong immunoreactivity; most commonly used for diagnostic purposes |
| p63 | A member of the p53 gene family | Strong immunoreactivity; most commonly used for diagnostic purposes |
| S100A6 | Calcium-binding protein | Strong immunoreactivity |
| Epidermal growth factor receptor | Membrane bound 170-kDa glycoprotein that mediates the activity of EGF | Strong immunoreactivity; rare in cancer |
| CuZn-superoxide dismutase | Enzyme that catalyzes superoxide anion radicals | Strong immunoreactivity |
| Type IV collagenase | Enzyme involved in extracellular matrix degradation | Strong immunoreactivity; decreased in cancer |
| Type VII collagen | Part of the hemidesmosomal complex | Strong immunoreactivity; lost in cancer |
| Integrins $\alpha$1, 2, 4, 6, and v; $\beta$1 and 4 | Extracellular matrix adhesion molecules | Strong immunoreactivity; decrease in most with cancer, although $\alpha$6 and $\beta$1 are retained |
| Estrogen receptors | Hormone receptor | Moderate immunoreactivity |
| bcl-2 | Oncoprotein that suppresses apoptosis | Strong immunoreactivity; also found in most cancers |
| c-erbB2 | Oncogene protein in the EGF family | Strong immunoreactivity; also found in most cancers |
| Glutathione *S*-transferase gene (GSTP1) | Enzyme that inactivates electrophilic carcinogens | Strong immunoreactivity; rare in cancer |
| C-CAM | Epithelial cell adhesion molecule | Strong immunoreactivity; absent in cancer |
| TGF-$\beta$ | Growth factor that regulates cell proliferation and differentiation | Strong immunoreactivity; absent in cancer |
| Cathepsin B | Enzyme that degrades basement membranes; may be involved in tumor invasion and metastases | Present in many basal cells, and rarely in luminal secretory cells; also found in cancer cells |
| Progesterone receptors | Hormone receptor | Moderate immunoreactivity |

PCNA, proliferating cell nuclear antigen; TGF, transforming growth factor.

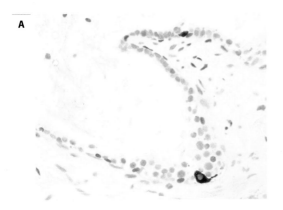

A

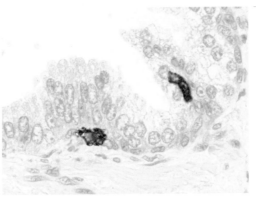

B

**Fig. 8-23** Immunoreactivity of chromogranin A in **(A)** benign prostatic epithelium and **(B)** high-grade PIN.

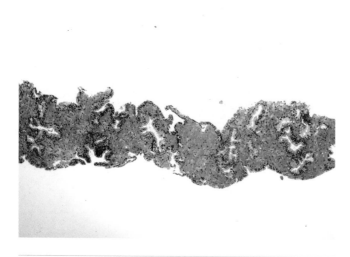

**Fig. 8-24** Prostatic needle biopsy core (18-gauge).

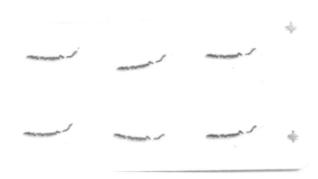

**Fig. 8-25** Six sections of a prostate needle biopsy mounted on one slide.

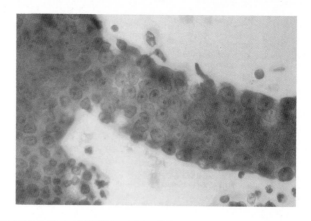

**Fig. 8-26** Adenocarcinoma in fine needle aspiration. Note cohesive cells with prominent nucleolomegaly (Courtesy of Dr John Maksem, Orlando, FL.).

14-gauge needle. The rate of post-biopsy infection declined from 7–39% to 0.81%, and hemorrhage with urinary clot retention fell from 3.2% to less than 1%.[241] The false negative rate declined from 11–25% to 11%, and the quality of the tissue sample improved, usually with little or no compression artifact at the edges of the specimen. The 18-gauge needle also allowed sextant biopsies (six cores, usually including three from each side at the apex, midportion, and base) or more cores, and seminal vesicle biopsies with minimal discomfort.[242,243,244] Saturation biopsy using the 18-gauge core biopsy gun significantly increases the cancer detection rate.[245–248] The main disadvantage of the 18-gauge needle is that it provides less than half as much tissue per core for pathologic examination as the traditional 14-gauge biopsy. A greater number of biopsies in recent years contain less than 10% cancer, owing to the success of early detection efforts in identifying smaller tumors at earlier stages. Frequently, we encounter small suspicious foci in biopsies from asymptomatic young men who have no palpable abnormality and only slight elevation of serum PSA concentration; this issue is discussed in Chapter 9.

Inking the needle biopsy is useful for identifying the tissue cores in paraffin blocks, but this is infrequently performed. There is variation between laboratories in the number of serial sections obtained from prostate tissue blocks for routine examination; we routinely obtain six sections on each slide from three levels (two sections per level)

(Fig. 8-25). We have two slides prepared routinely. Slide 1 is submitted for hematoxylin and eosin staining, and slide 2 is retained for special studies such as immunohistochemistry for keratin 34β-E12/p63/racemase or digital image analysis for DNA ploidy analysis. In our experience, recutting the block for additional levels is useful in about half of cases, with usually no more than four additional slides before the tissue specimen is exhausted.

## Fine needle aspiration

Fine needle aspiration remains popular for cytologic examination of the prostate in parts of Europe and around the world, but in the United States interest in this method has dropped precipitously because of the ease of acquisition and interpretation of the 18-gauge needle core biopsy. Both techniques have similar sensitivity in the diagnosis of prostatic adenocarcinoma, and both are limited by small sample size; they are best considered as complementary techniques.[249–254] Complications of fine needle aspiration occur in less than 2% of patients, and are similar to those with needle core biopsy, including epididymitis, transient hematuria, hemospermia, fever, and sepsis.

Fine needle aspiration produces clusters and small sheets of epithelial cells without stroma (Fig. 8-26).[253] This enrichment for epithelium allows the evaluation of single cells and the architectural relationship between cells. Benign and hyperplastic prostatic epithelium consists of orderly sheets of cells with distinct margins creating a honeycomb-like pattern. Benign nuclei are uniform, with finely granular chromatin and indistinct nucleoli; basal cells are often present at the edge. Prostatic carcinoma is distinguished from benign epithelium by increased cellularity, loss of cell adhesion, variation in nuclear size and shape, and nucleolar enlargement. Fine needle aspiration is not currently used as a screening test for prostate cancer. However, the specimen obtained can be used for other diagnostic and prognostic tests, such as morphometric analysis, DNA ploidy, cytogenetic studies, and molecular diagnostics.[255–257]

## Transurethral resection

The regions of the prostate sampled by transurethral resection and needle biopsy tend to be different.[258–260] Transure-

**Table 8-7** Glandular zones of the prostate: implications for disease

| | Central zone | Transition zone | Peripheral zone |
|---|---|---|---|
| **Tissue Sampling Techniques** | | | |
| Transurethral resection | Poor | Good | Poor |
| Needle biopsy | Variable | Poor | Good |
| **Involvement with Pathological Processes** | | | |
| Atrophy | Infrequent | Variable | Frequent |
| Nodular hyperplasia | Rare | Frequent | Rare |
| Prostatitis | Infrequent | Variable | Frequent |
| Carcinoma (% of prostate cancers) | Infrequent (5) | Frequent (25) | Frequent (70) |

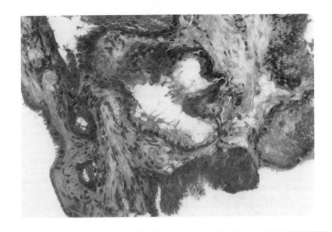

**Fig. 8-27** Artifactual drying of prostatic biopsy with chromatin smearing; this specimen is insufficient for diagnosis.

thral resection specimens usually consist of tissue from the transition zone, urethra, periurethral area, bladder neck, and anterior fibromuscular stroma (Table 8-7). Studies of radical prostatectomies performed after transurethral resection show that the resection does not usually include tissue from the central or peripheral zone, and not all of the transition zone is removed.[261] Most needle biopsy specimens consist only of tissue from the peripheral zone, seldom including the central or transition zones.

Well-differentiated adenocarcinoma found incidentally in transurethral resection chips has usually arisen in the transition zone.[258,259,262] These tumors are frequently small and may be completely resected by transurethral resection. Poorly differentiated adenocarcinoma in transurethral resection chips usually represents part of a larger tumor that has invaded the transition zone from the peripheral zone.[262,263]

The optimal number of chips to submit for histologic evaluation from a transurethral resection specimen remains controversial, with some experts advocating complete submission even with large specimens that would require many cassettes.[264-268] The College of American Pathologists recommends a minimum of six cassettes for the first 30 g of tissue and one cassette for every 10 g thereafter.[269]

## Tissue artifacts

Cautery artifact is frequently extensive in transurethral resection specimens and often limits interpretation, particularly at the edges of the chips. The epithelium usually shows more damage than the stroma, with separation from the basement membrane, cellular disruption, loss of integrity of nuclear membranes, and homogenization of the chromatin, creating featureless dark nuclei. In severely affected chips coagulation necrosis is present, including tissue devitalization with loss of cell membranes and indistinct smeared chromatin.[263,270]

Delayed fixation and air-drying commonly result in separation of the epithelium and the underlying basement membrane, as well as chromatin smearing and smudging (Fig. 8-27) This artifactual change is more prominent in malignant than in benign acini, but both may be affected. Cell clusters floating in empty lumina may be mistaken for microvascular invasion.

Degenerating lymphocytes and stromal myocytes may show vacuolization that mimics signet-ring cell carcinoma.[271] In difficult cases immunohistochemical stains are useful, with immunoreactivity for leukocyte common antigen in lymphocytes and smooth muscle actin in myocytes; both are negative for keratin AE1/AE3, PSA, and PAP.

## Prostatic inflammation

Patchy mild acute and chronic inflammation is present in most adult prostates and is probably a normal finding.[272] When the inflammation is severe, extensive, or clinically apparent, the term 'prostatitis' is warranted.[273] There is a wide spectrum of prostatitides, many of which are rare and poorly understood.[274,275] Stamey[276] considers prostatitis to be a 'wastebasket of clinical ignorance' owing to significant variations in terminology, diagnostic criteria, and treatment.

Inflammation has been implicated in the pathogenesis of BPH. Patients with inflammation have significantly larger prostates, higher serum PSA concentrations, and a greater risk of urinary retention according to the Medical Therapy of Prostate Symptoms study,[277] although this has been refuted.[278] There is elevated expression of proinflammatory cytokines in BPH; IL-6, IL-8 and IL-17 may perpetuate a chronic immune response in BPH and induce fibromuscular growth by an autocrine or paracrine loop or via induction of COX-2 expression. Immune reaction may be activated via Toll-like receptor signaling and mediated by macrophages and T cells. Conversely, anti-inflammatory factors such as macrophage inhibitory cytokine-1 decreased in symptomatic BPH.[277]

## Acute bacterial prostatitis

Patients with acute bacterial prostatitis present with sudden onset of fever, chills, irritative voiding symptoms, and pain in the lower back, rectum, and perineum.[275,279-281] The prostate is swollen, firm, tender, and warm. Microscopically, acute inflammation in the prostate is often intraluminal, with a few scattered neutrophils or aggregates. There are sheets of neutrophils surrounding prostatic glands, often with marked tissue destruction and cellular debris (Fig. 8-28). The stroma is edematous and hemorrhagic, and microabscesses may be present. Diagnosis is based on culture of urine and expressed prostatic secretions; biopsy is contraindicated because of the potential for sepsis. Most cases of acute prostatitis are caused by bacteria responsible for other urinary tract infections, including *Escherichia coli* (80% of infections), other *Enterobacteriaceae, Pseudomonas, Serratia, Klebsiella* (10–15%), and *enterococci* (5–10%). Gonococcal prostatitis due to *Neisseria gonorrhea* was common in the pre-antibiotic era, but is rare today. Most cases of acute prostatitis respond to antibiotics.[275,280,281]

Abscess is a rare complication, usually occurring in immunocompromised patients such as those with AIDS. Transrectal ultrasonography is a valuable method for preoperative diagnosis. Many patients with abscesses are treated by transurethral resection and antibiotics.

## Chronic prostatitis

Chronic bacterial prostatitis is a common cause of relapsing urinary tract infection, and is usually caused by *E. coli*. Clinical diagnosis is difficult, often requiring multiple urine cultures obtained after massage of the prostate.[275,280–282] Treatment is also vexing because of the inability of most intravenous antibiotics to enter the prostate and prostatic fluids when the organ is overrun with a chronic inflammatory infiltrate (Fig. 8-29). Also, prostatic calculi may contain bacteria embedded in the mineral matrix, and this serves as a nidus of recurring infection. The secretory products of the inflamed prostate are alkaline, with low levels of zinc, citric acid, spermine, cholesterol, antibacterial factors, and certain enzymes.

Chronic abacterial prostatitis is more common than bacterial prostatitis, and rarely follows infection elsewhere in the urinary tract. Patients often complain of painful ejaculation. Cultures of urine and expressed prostatic secretions are negative. The etiologic agent is unknown, but *Chlamydia, Ureaplasma,* and *Trichomonas* have been proposed. This form of prostatitis has a prolonged indolent course with relapses and remissions. There appears to be no relationship between chronic prostatitis and the pathogenesis of benign prostatic hyperplasia.[283,284] Microscopically, several patterns of chronic inflammation have been described, including segregated glandular inflammation, periglandular inflammation, diffuse stromal inflammation, intraepithelial lymphocytes, isolated stromal lymphoid nodules, and single scattered lymphocytes (Fig. 8-29).[285]

A recent proposal was made to classify chronic prostatic inflammation according to location, extent, and grade (Table 8-8). If more than one grade of inflammation is present for a given anatomic location, the dominant and most severe grade will be specified, e.g. multifocal mild acinar inflammation, focal mild peri-acinar inflammation, diffuse mild stromal inflammation and focal severe stromal inflammation.[286]

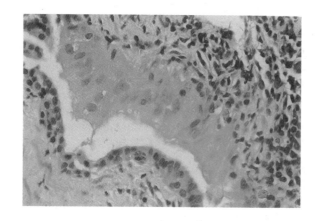

**Fig. 8-29** Inflammatory atypia in the setting of chronic inflammation. Note metaplastic changes adjacent to the inflammation. This was initially misinterpreted as high-grade PIN.

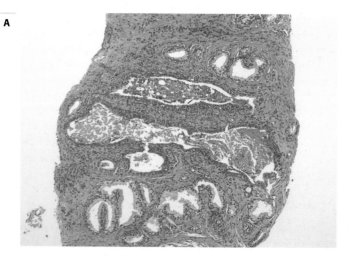

A

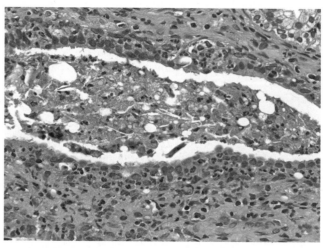

B

**Fig. 8-28** Acute inflammation. **(A)** There is a dense acute and chronic inflammation which obscures the acinar epithelium. **(B)** Constipated acinus with circumferential acute and chronic inflammation.

**Table 8-8** Histologic classification of prostatic inflammation

| Feature | Details |
| --- | --- |
| Anatomic location | Histologic pattern |
| Acini | Inflammation within duct/acinar epithelium and/or lumina |
| Periacinar | Inflammation within stroma, are centered around ducts/acini, and approach ducts/acini within 50 μm |
| Stroma | Inflammation within stroma, but not centered around ducts/acini, and lie ≥50 μm away |
| Extent | Tissue area involved by inflammation |
| Focal | <10% |
| Multifocal | 10–50% |
| Diffuse | >50% |
| Grade | Morphologic description (typical inflammatory cell density, cells/mm²) |
| 1/Mild | Individual inflammatory cells, most of which are separated by distinct intervening spaces (<100) |
| 2/Modearte | Confluent sheets of inflammatory cells with no tissue destruction or lymphoid nodule/follicle formation (100–500) |
| 3/Severe | Confluent sheets of inflammatory cells with tissue destruction or lymphoid nodule/follicle formation (>500) |

**Table 8-9** Classification of granulomatous prostatitis

I Infectious
  **A. Bacterial**
    Tuberculosis
    Brucellosis
    Syphilis
  **B. Fungal**
    Coccidioidomycosis
    Cryptococcosis
    Blastomycosis
    Histoplasmosis
    Paracoccidiodomycosis
  **C. Parasite**
    Schistosomiasis
    Echinococcus
    Enterobius
    Linguatula
  **D. Viral**
    Herpes zoster

II Iatrogenic
  **A. Postsurgical**
  **B. Postradiation**
  **C. BCG-associated**
  **D. Teflon-associated**

III Malakoplakia

IV Systemic granulomatous disease
  **A. Allergic ('eosinophilic')**
  **B. Sarcoidosis**
  **C. Rheumatoid**
  **D. Autoimmune/vascular**
    Wegener's granulomatosis
    Polyarteritis nodosa
    Benign lymphocytic angiitis and granulomatosis (BLAG)
    Churg–Strauss vasculitis

V Idiopathic ('non-specific')

## Granulomatous prostatitis

Granulomatous prostatitis is a group of morphologically distinct forms of chronic prostatitis, the pathogenesis of which often cannot be determined. Causes include infection, tissue disruption following biopsy, BCG therapy, and others listed in Table 8-9.[276-290] The majority of patients have a prior history of urinary tract infection. The prostate is hard, fixed, and nodular, and cancer is usually suspected clinically. Urinalysis often shows pyuria and hematuria. Granulomatous prostatitis is probably caused by blockage of prostatic ducts and stasis of secretions, regardless of its etiology. The epithelium is destroyed, and cellular debris, bacterial toxins, and prostatic secretions, including corpora amylacea, sperm, and semen, escape into the stroma, eliciting an intense localized inflammatory response (Figs 8-29, 8-30, 8-31). This process is similar to intraprostatic sperm granuloma formation. Tissue eosinophilia may be prominent in prostates infested with parasites, systemic allergic or autoimmune disease, iatrogenic post-TURP prostatitis, or non-specific granulomatous prostatitis.

Granulomatous prostatitis accounted for 1.2% of all prostate specimens at the University of Arizona.[291]

## Granulomatous infection

Infectious granulomatous prostatitis is rare, and may be caused by bacteria, fungi, parasites, and viruses. *Mycobacterium tuberculosis* infection of the prostate only occurs after pulmonary infection or miliary dissemination. Small (1–2 mm) caseating granulomas coalesce within the prostatic parenchyma, forming yellow nodules and streaks. Caseation and cavitation can be extensive. Brucellosis may mimic tuberculosis both clinically and pathologically.

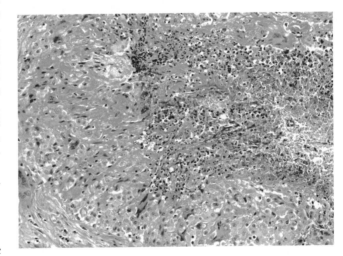

**Fig. 8-30** Necrotizing granulomatous prostatitis. The necrosis is surrounded by histiocytes and reactive stromal cells.

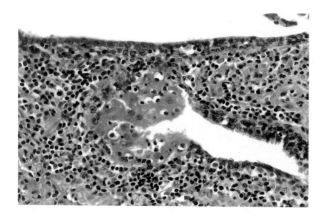

**Fig. 8-31** Granulomatous prostatitis with eosinophilic metaplasia of the epithelium.

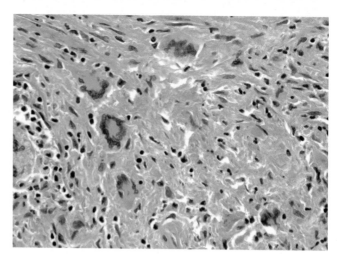

**Fig. 8-32** Granulomatous prostatitis following TURP, characterized by aggregates of multinucleated giant cells.

Predisposing conditions for fungal infection include immunosuppression, prolonged antibiotic use, diabetes mellitus, malignancy, and an indwelling bladder catheter. Mycotic infections of the prostate such as that caused by *Coccidioidomycosis*[291] are rare and invariably follow fungemia. Most of the deep mycoses induce necrotizing and non-necrotizing granulomas and fibrosis; *Candida albicans* is usually only associated with acute inflammation.[291,292]

Granulomas caused by *Schistosoma hematobium* are frequently found in the prostate as well as the bladder and seminal vesicles in endemic areas such as Egypt. The organisms lodge in vesicular and pelvic venous plexuses as the final habitat. The adult female schistosome migrates into the submucosa of the urinary bladder and prostatic stroma, where she lays eggs that induce granuloma formation and fibrosis. Adenocarcinoma[293] and squamous cell carcinoma[294] of the prostate are rarely associated with schistosomiasis.[293]

Herpes zoster infection may be associated with granulomatous prostatitis.

## Postsurgical granulomatous prostatitis

Postsurgical granulomatous prostatitis can be identified years after TURP owing to cauterization and surgical disruption of tissues (Figs 8-32, 8-33).[295,296] The granulomas are characteristically circumscribed and rimmed by palisading histiocytes with central fibrinoid necrosis.[297] A rim of lymphocytes (that mark as T cells) is present outside the palisaded cell layer. Multinucleated giant cells are frequently present. The striking histologic resemblance of postsurgical granulomatous prostatitis to rheumatoid nodules suggests a hypersensitivity reaction or cell-mediated immune response. Tissue eosinophilia is present in many cases. Treatment is unnecessary.

## BCG-induced granulomatous prostatitis

Bacillus Calmette–Guérin (BCG)-induced granulomatous prostatitis occurs in virtually all patients treated with intravesicular BCG immunotherapy for superficial urothelial carcinoma of the bladder.[298] The granulomas are characteristically discrete, with or without necrosis, and often

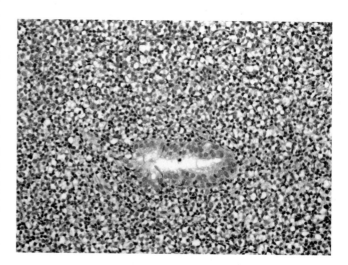

**Fig. 8-33** Non-neoplastic focally dense lymphocytic inflammation surrounding benign acinus. This was an incidental finding in a TURP specimen.

contain numerous acid-fast bacilli. Grossly, the cut surface of the prostate with BCG-induced granulomatous prostatitis shows multiple, firm, white nodules or soft, yellow-gray nodules with granular centers, central caseation, and focal cavitation. Microscopically, the granulomas, particularly the large ones, are typical caseating, tuberculoid type. Smaller granulomas consist predominantly of histiocytes and may lack caseous necrosis and giant cells. No therapy is required.

## Teflon-induced granulomatous prostatitis

Periurethral and submucosal bladder injections of Teflon (polytetrafluoroethylene) have been used in the past for the treatment of urinary incontinence, but this foreign substance may migrate into the prostate and other sites, inducing a florid granulomatous response.[299–302] Teflon in the prostate is basophilic, simulating neoplastic mucin dissecting through the prostatic stroma. Teflon tends to be more basophilic than mucin, and appears filamentous and birefringent. The adjacent prostatic epithelium is rarely intact, and there are scattered or prominent multinucleated cells and other features of granulomatous prostatitis.

## Malakoplakia

Malakoplakia is a granulomatous disease associated with defective intracellular lysosomal digestion of bacteria. It occasionally occurs in the prostate,[274] presenting as a diffuse indurated mass that is clinically suggestive of prostatic carcinoma. *E. coli* is commonly isolated from urine cultures. Microscopically, the prostate is effaced by sheets of macrophages admixed with lymphocytes and plasma cells. Intracellular and extracellular Michaelis–Gutmann bodies are identified, appearing as sharply demarcated spherical structures with concentric 'owl's eyes' measuring 5–10 μm in diameter. The Michaelis–Gutmann bodies represent calcified bacterial debris within phagolysosomes. PAS stain is useful for identifying non-mineralized forms, and von Kossa stain for mineralized forms.

## Allergic (eosinophilic) granulomatous prostatitis

Allergic granulomatous prostatitis is a component of Churg–Strauss syndrome.[303] It should be diagnosed only in a patient with history of asthma or allergy with peripheral eosinophilia and systemic lesions. Histologically, it consists of granulomatous prostatitis with infiltrates of eosinophils, fibrinoid necrosis, and vasculitis.[288,304] Treatment is with steroids.

## Wegener's granulomatosis

Prostatic involvement occurs in up to 7.4% of men with Wegener's granulomatosis, usually causing urinary obstruction, infection, hematuria, and acute retention.[304] The prostate is diffusely enlarged and often indurated. Urinalysis reveals microhematuria, red cell casts, and proteinuria, features indicating renal involvement. The erythrocyte sedimentation rate is frequently elevated. The prostatic urethral mucosa is ragged and friable, and biopsy reveals necrotizing granulomatous inflammation with vasculitis (Fig. 8-34). Stellate and geographic granulomas are present, rimmed by palisading histiocytes and occasional multinucleated giant cells. Vasculitis involves small arteries and veins. Special stains for organisms are negative. Symptomatic prostatic involvement usually responds to chemotherapy,[305,306] similar to pulmonary and renal involvement; TURP may also be helpful.

## Other rare forms of granulomatous prostatitis

Other rare forms of granulomatous prostatitis include sarcoidosis, rheumatoid nodule, polyarteritis nodosa, and silicone-induced prostatitis (Fig. 8-35). Giant cell arteritis also rarely occurs in the prostate, sometimes without systemic involvement.[307]

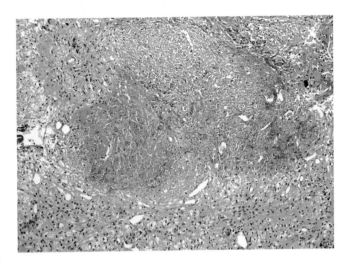

**Fig. 8-34** Wegener's granulomatosis with serpiginous necrosis rimmed by histiocytes mimicking post-TURP granulomatous prostatitis. This middle-aged man was subsequently found to have lung and kidney involvement.

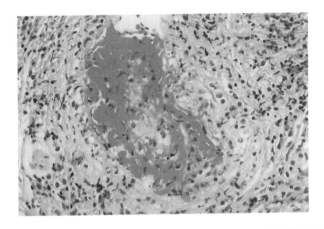

**Fig. 8-35** Churg–Strauss vasculitis with fibrin deposition. This prostate biopsy was the first evidence of systemic vasculitis.

## Idiopathic prostatitis

Idiopathic (non-specific) granulomatous prostatitis ('of unknown cause') comprises the majority of cases of granulomatous prostatitis (69%).[290,308] The granulomas are usually non-caseating and associated with parenchymal loss and marked fibrosis. Classification of eosinophilic and non-eosinophilic types is probably of no clinical value. It is important to recognize the wide variety of inciting agents of granulomatous prostatitis and the histologic clues that allow distinction of these different entities, but most cases elude definitive classification (Fig. 8-36). The spectrum of morphologic abnormalities of idiopathic granulomatous prostatitis includes nodular granulomas centered around ducts and acini, central duct and acinar disruption, mixed granulomatous inflammation, and stromal sclerosis. The cellular infiltrate in granulomatous prostatitis is mixed, with epithelioid histiocytes, lymphocytes, neutrophils, eosinophils, plasma cells, and multinucleated giant cells.

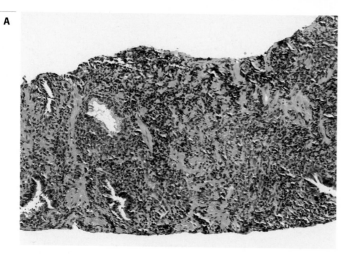

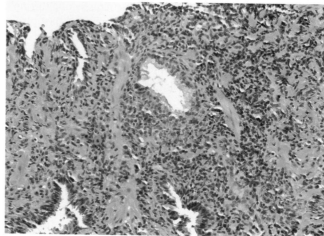

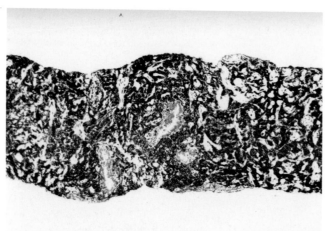

**Fig. 8-36** Idiopathic granulomatous prostatitis misinterpreted as poorly differentiated adenocarcinoma. **(A)** At low magnification there is a dense cellular infiltrate. **(B)** At high magnification there is dense chronic inflammation surrounding benign acini. **(C)** The inflammatory cells are strongly positive for LCA.

Induration may persist on physical examination for years, even when there are no specific clinical symptoms. Up to 10% of patients with idiopathic granulomatous prostatitis do not respond to conservative management, developing severe urethral obstruction that requires TURP. However, transurethral resection is unsuccessful in up to 50% of cases, with some patients requiring multiple procedures.

## Xanthoma and xanthogranulomatous prostatitis

Xanthoma is a rare form of idiopathic granulomatous prostatitis that consists of a localized collection of cholesterol-laden histiocytes; it may also be seen in patients with hyperlipidemia (Fig. 8-37).[309] Xanthoma occurs in older men, and is usually an incidental finding in patients undergoing transurethral resection or needle biopsy, although it may appear as a palpable nodule.[310] Rare cases contain areas of typical granulomatous prostatitis, and in such cases the term xanthogranulomatous prostatitis is appropriate. Distinction from clear cell carcinoma ('hypernephroid' pattern) may be difficult, and immunohistochemical stains for PSA,

PAP and CD68 often assist with this diagnostic concern (Table 8-10).[311]

## AIDS-related prostatitis

Patients infected with human immunodeficiency virus (HIV) are susceptible to opportunistic infections, including prostatitis, due partly to abnormalities of T- and B-lymphocyte function. Infectious prostatitis occurs in 14% of patients with AIDS, and in 3% of those with AIDS-related complex (ARC) or asymptomatic HIV infection. In these patients prostatitis may be due to a variety of pathogens, including *E. coli, Klebsiella, Enterobacter, Serratia, Pseudomonas, Hemophilus parainfluenza, Cryptococcus neoformans, Mycobacterium tuberculosis, Cytomegalovirus, Histoplasma, Candida,* adenovirus,[312] and *Pneumocystis.*[313,314] Microscopically, organisms can be identified in expressed prostatic secretions, prostate needle biopsy, or prostates from postmortem examinations. The prostatic response to infection in patients with AIDS varies from none to necrosis or abscess formation.

Patients with AIDS-related prostatitis may be asymptomatic or present with acute prostatitis, chronic prostatitis, or

A 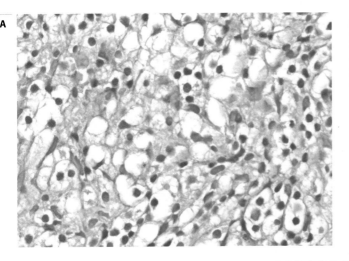 B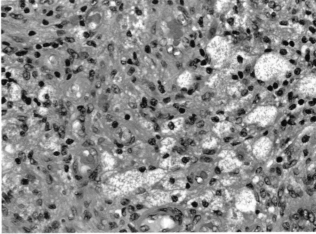

**Fig. 8-37** Xanthoma. **(A)** The needle core contains a collection of cells with clear cytoplasm mimicking signet ring cell carcinoma. **(B)** The foamy histiocytes have small round to oval hyperchromatic nuclei.

**Table 8-10** Clear cell proliferations of the prostate: differential diagnosis

**Benign**
    Atypical adenomatous hyperplasia with clear cell change
    Basal cell hyperplasia with clear cell change
    Cowper's glands
    Mucinous metaplasia
    Paraganglia
    Storage disease
    Stromal nodular hyperplasia with myxoid matrix
    Xanthogranulomatous prostatitis
    Xanthoma

**Malignant**
    Clear cell adenocarcinoma pattern of the prostate
    Transition zone cancer with clear cell pattern
    Cancer with androgen deprivation therapy effect ('nucleolus-poor' clear cell carcinoma)
    Mucinous carcinoma
    Signet ring-cell carcinoma
    Epithelioid leiomyoma and leiomyosarcoma
    Secondary malignancies
        Clear cell carcinoma of the bladder
        Metastatic renal cell carcinoma, clear cell pattern
        Lymphoma with artifactual signet ring-cell like pattern

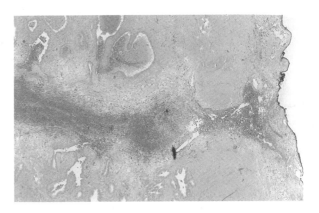

**Fig. 8-38** Line of hemorrhage denotes the needle track beneath the prostatic capsule on the right. This radical prostatectomy was obtained 2 weeks after sextant 18-gauge needle biopsies.

abscess. Relapses are common despite prolonged antibiotic therapy.

# Pathologic changes following needle biopsy

Contemporary transrectal 18-gauge needle biopsy of the prostate induces a predictable inflammatory response along a very narrow track.[241] The biopsy track consists of a partially collapsed cavity, often filled with red blood cells, rimmed by mixed acute and chronic inflammation, including lymphocytes, macrophages, and occasional eosinophils (Fig. 8-38). There is a variable amount of hemosiderin pigment, granulation tissue, and fibrosis, usually limited to the edge of the cavity. Venous thrombosis and foreign body giant cell reaction are seen infrequently. Although tumor cells are frequently enmeshed in fibrous connective tissue, they are not seen within the cavity following 18-gauge needle biopsy.[241] Conversely, tumor is occasionally identified in the track following the wider 14-gauge biopsy, particularly with perineal biopsy.[315-321]

Biopsy tracks in prostatectomies obtained 4–6 weeks after biopsy show fewer red blood cells and less acute inflammation than in those obtained earlier, but no other histologic differences are noted. There is no evidence of florid granulomatous prostatitis or fibrinoid necrosis that is often seen after transurethral resection. Biopsies involving benign prostatic tissue and cancer are histologically similar.

# Non-neoplastic metaplasia

The prostatic epithelium has an interesting but limited repertoire of responses to injury. These include a variety of metaplastic and proliferative lesions that may mimic adenocarcinoma (Table 8-11).

**Table 8-11** Metaplastic changes of the prostate

| Diagnosis | Features |
|---|---|
| Squamous metaplasia | Intraductal aggregates of flattened cells with eosinophilic cytoplasm, usually at edge of infarcts |
| Mucinous metaplasia | Mucin-producing columnar or goblet cells in the prostate epithelium or urothelium |
| Neuroendocrine cells with eosinophilic granules | Isolated cells or small cell clusters with prominent eosinophilic cytoplasmic granules |
| Urothelial metaplasia | Urothelium within ducts and acini of the prostate; difficult to identify because of variable location of the normal urothelial–columnar junction |
| Nephrogenic metaplasia | Inflamed papillary mass of cystic or solid tubules in the urethra; rare |

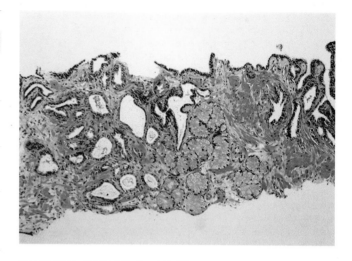

**Fig. 8-40** Mucinous metaplasia.

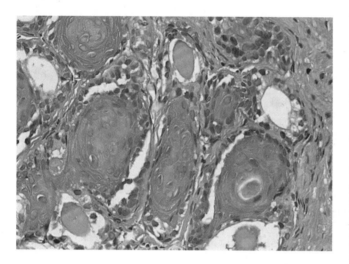

**Fig. 8-39** Squamous metaplasia. This syncytial aggregate of basal cells is whorled, with distinct cell borders. Note oval to elongate nuclei with central linear grooves (right).

## Squamous metaplasia

Squamous metaplasia results from a variety of insults to the prostate, including acute inflammation, infarction, radiation therapy, and androgen deprivation therapy.[294,322–326] The changes may be focal or diffuse, appearing as intraductal syncytial aggregates of flattened cells with abundant eosinophilic cytoplasm, or cohesive aggregates of glycogen-rich clear cells with shrunken hyperchromatic nuclei (Fig. 8-39). Keratinization is unusual except at the edge of infarcts or areas of acute inflammation. Acini may be partially or completely involved by squamous metaplasia. Squamous metaplasia commonly involves the prostatic urethra in patients with an indwelling catheter.

## Mucinous metaplasia

Mucinous metaplasia refers to clusters of tall columnar cells or goblet cells having cytoplasm filled with blue-gray mucin that are infrequently observed in the prostatic acinar epithelium of all ages (Fig. 8-40).[61,327] This finding is invariably microscopic, and can also be seen in the urothelium of large periurethral prostatic ducts, foci of urothelial metaplasia, atrophy, nodular hyperplasia, basal cell hyperplasia, and post-atrophic hyperplasia. The cells contain acid mucin that stains with Mayers' mucicarmine, Alcian blue (pH 2.7), and PAS following diastase predigestion;[328] luminal secretions with similar staining are usually present.

The differential diagnosis of mucinous metaplasia includes Cowper's glands and adenocarcinoma. Unlike Cowper's glands, mucinous metaplasia is usually focal within a small number of acini, lacking complete involvement of a lobular aggregate of acini.[254] The nuclei of the mucinous metaplastic cells are small, dark, and basally situated. There is no immunoreactivity for PSA and PAP. An intact basal cell layer can be confirmed by keratin 34β-E12 and/or p63 stains.

## Neuroendocrine cells with eosinophilic granules (NCEG; Paneth cell-like change)

Neuroendocrine cells with eosinophilic granules (NCEG) are considered a distinct form of neuroendocrine differentiation in the prostatic epithelium and may represent a normal finding rather than metaplasia.[329–344] It is characterized by isolated cells or small groups of cells with prominent eosinophilic cytoplasmic granules, present by routine hematoxylin and eosin-stained sections in 10% of serially sectioned radical prostatectomies. It is usually present focally, but is occasionally prominent and multifocal. NCEG is also present in isolated tumor cells or in continuous groups of cells, sometimes replacing an entire acinus. The distribution of NCEG is always patchy, and they can be found in usual acinar carcinoma as well as cribriform, papillary, and mucinous areas. The nuclei of NCEG are vesicular with prominent nucleoli, similar to other tumor cells. Luminal mucin is more common in cancer with NCEG than in cancer without NCEG. NCEG invariably display intense cytoplasmic immunoreactivity for chromogranin, neuron-specific enolase, and serotonin.[221,240] Many of these cells also express PSA and PAP.[238,239] Lysozyme is negative.

NCEG is not associated with any factors predictive of aggressive behavior of prostate cancer, including tumor stage, serum PSA concentration, and tumor grade, suggesting that this pattern of neuroendocrine differentiation is not indicative of a poor prognosis.[44]

NCEG account for only a small percentage of cells with neuroendocrine differentiation in benign prostatic acini and adenocarcinoma. Most neuroendocrine cells have small granules that are not apparent on H&E-stained sections.

## Urothelial metaplasia

Urothelial metaplasia consists of urothelium within ducts and acini of the prostate beyond the normal transitional–columnar junction, arising apparently as a result of metaplastic change (Fig. 8-41). This junction is variable in location, creating difficulty in distinguishing metaplasia from normal urothelium in fragmented specimens such as transurethral resections and needle biopsies. Consequently, the diagnosis of metaplasia may be overused. Microscopically, usually only a few glands are involved in a single focus, but extensive involvement may also be observed. The glands exhibit proliferation of elongated urothelial cells beneath a bland-appearing luminal secretory cell layer.[333] Urothelial metaplasia is benign and easily distinguished from PIN by its characteristic architectural and cytologic features.

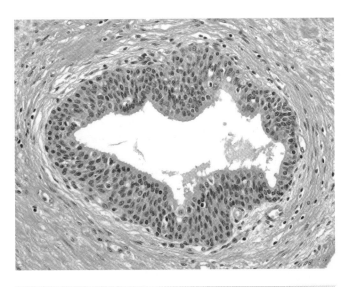

**Fig. 8-41** Urothelial metaplasia. This focus of thickened urothelium was found deep within the prostate in a radical prostatectomy specimen. Note the presence of columnar epithelium indicating the junction with the urothelium.

## Nephrogenic metaplasia (nephrogenic adenoma)

Nephrogenic metaplasia most often occurs in adult patients in the urinary bladder, renal pelvis, ureter, and urethra; prostatic urethral involvement is rare, and extension into the prostatic parenchyma may create diagnostic confusion with adenocarcinoma (Fig. 8-42). It usually follows instrumentation, urethral catheterization, infection, or calculi. Patients present with lower urinary tract symptoms, including hematuria, dysuria, obstruction, and urethral mass.[334–338] Although the term nephrogenic adenoma is commonly used, it is a misnomer; this process is thought to be a reactive and metaplastic response to chronic inflammation or instrumentation and is not neoplastic.

Nephrogenic metaplasia appears as an exophytic papillary mass of cystic and solid tubules protruding from the urethral mucosa. The tubules may extend into the underlying prostate as a proliferation of small round to oval tubules, sometimes filled with colloid-like material. The lining consists of flattened or simple cuboidal cells, often with a distinctive hobnail appearance. Nuclei display finely granular uniform chromatin with inconspicuous nucleoli; occasional prominent nucleoli are observed. There is frequently chronic

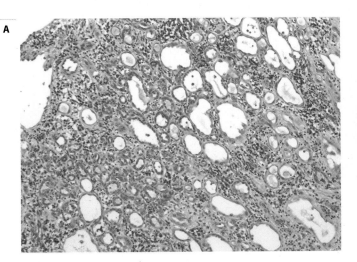
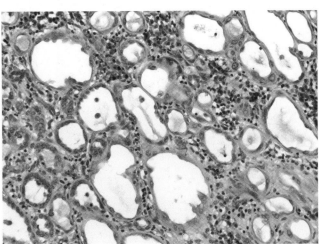

**Fig. 8-42** Nephrogenic metaplasia of the prostatic urethra. **(A)** At low power there is a localized proliferation of irregular tubular structures immediately beneath the urethral epithelium (top right). **(B)** At high magnification the small tubules are lined by flattened or hobnail cells. The stroma is chronically inflamed.

inflammation and edema of the stroma, but no desmoplasia is present.

The tubules contain scant or moderate mucin that is positive with Alcian blue and PAS stains. The basement membrane is accentuated with PAS stain. Epithelial membrane antigen is positive in the tubular epithelial cells, and high molecular weight keratin 34β-E12 and/or p63 stain many of the basal cells. PSA, PAP, and CEA are negative.[20] About 58% of nephrogenic metaplasia cases are strongly positive for racemase (P504) (Fig. 8-42).[337–339] Nephrogenic metaplasia with substantial cytologic atypia (atypical nephrogenic metaplasia) is occasionally encountered and is a benign finding; awareness of the spectrum of cytologic changes within this entity is critical to prevent overdiagnosis of cancer and avoid unnecessary treatment. There is no direct evidence linking atypical nephrogenic metaplasia to cancer.[340]

Some investigators suggested that nephrogenic metaplasia is neither metaplastic nor neoplastic in nature. Nephrogenic metaplasia in renal-transplant recipients is apparently derived from tubular cells of the transplant and is not a metaplastic proliferation of the recipient's bladder urothelium.[338,339,341] Whether this pathogenetic mechanism applies for non-transplant-associated cases awaits further study.

## Hyperplasia and nodular hyperplasia

Enlargement of the prostate, also known as nodular hyperplasia or benign prostatic hyperplasia (BPH), consists of overgrowth of the epithelium and fibromuscular tissue of the transition zone and periurethral area. Symptoms are caused by interference with muscular sphincteric function and by obstruction of urine flow through the prostatic urethra. These symptoms, referred to as lower urinary tract symptoms (LUTS), include urgency, difficulty in starting urination, diminished stream size and force, increased frequency, incomplete bladder emptying, and nocturia.[342–345]

## Usual acinar and stromal hyperplasia

Development of nodular hyperplasia includes three pathologic changes: nodule formation, diffuse enlargement of the transition zone and periurethral tissue, and enlargement of nodules.[150,346] In men under 70 diffuse enlargement predominates; in older men, epithelial proliferation and expansile growth of existing nodules predominates, probably as the result of androgenic and other hormonal stimulation. The proportion of epithelium to stroma increases as symptoms become more severe.[347,348]

Grossly, nodular hyperplasia consists of variably sized nodules that are soft or firm, rubbery, and yellow-gray, and bulge from the cut surface on transection. If there is prominent epithelial hyperplasia in addition to stromal hyperplasia, the abundant luminal spaces create soft and grossly spongy nodules that ooze a pale-white watery fluid. If the nodular hyperplasia is predominantly fibromuscular, there may be diffuse enlargement or numerous trabeculations without prominent nodularity. Degenerative changes include calcification and infarction. Nodular hyperplasia usually involves the transition zone, but occasionally nodules arise from the periurethral tissue at the bladder neck. Protrusion of bladder neck nodules into the bladder lumen is referred to as median lobe hyperplasia (Fig. 8-43).

Microscopically, nodular hyperplasia is composed of varying proportions of epithelium and stroma (fibrous connective tissue and smooth muscle). The most common are

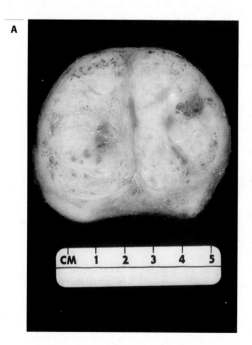

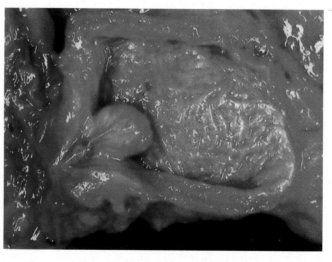

**Fig. 8-43** Nodular hyperplasia, gross appearance. **(A)** Transverse section of the prostate shows massive nodular hyperplasia with small foci of hemorrhagic infarction. A focus of adenocarcinoma forms an ill-defined mass in the peripheral zone at the lower right of the specimen. **(B)** Hyperplasia of the median lobe of the prostate has created an exophytic mass which protrudes into the bladder.

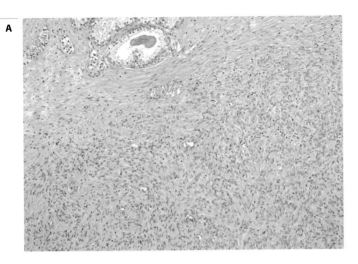

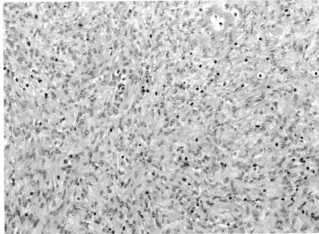

**Fig. 8-44** Pure stromal nodule of nodular hyperplasia. **(A)** This circumscribed nodule is uniform and circumscribed. **(B)** The nodule consists of stromal fibroblasts with scattered lymphocytes.

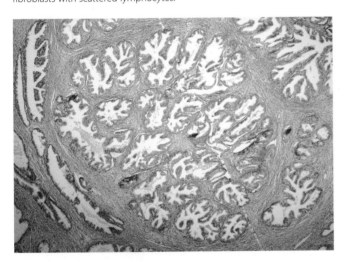

**Fig. 8-45** Mixed epithelial–stromal nodule of nodular hyperplasia. Note the dilated peripheral sinus which forms the boundary of the nodule with the transition zone stroma. This sinus often goes in and out of the plane of section, and may appear incomplete.

adenomyofibromatous nodules that contain all elements (Figs 8-44, 8-45). The total area, luminal area, and epithelial height of the acini are greater in BPH than in benign epithelium, but the number of acini is similar.[29]

The diagnosis of nodular hyperplasia is often used by pathologists in needle biopsy specimens when only normal benign peripheral zone prostatic tissue is present. The transition zone is infrequently sampled by needle biopsies unless the urologist specifically targets this area or there is massive nodular hyperplasia that compresses the peripheral zone. We require the presence of at least part of a nodule for the diagnosis of nodular hyperplasia in needle biopsies. Narrow 18-gauge biopsies virtually never contain the entire nodule unless it is very small and fortuitously sampled. Casual use of the term nodular hyperplasia for benign prostatic tissue may mislead the urologist into believing that a palpable nodule or hypoechoic focus of concern has been sampled and histologically evaluated; it is of clinical value for the

pathologist to correlate the light microscopic findings with the clinical impression.[349] Variants of nodular hyperplasia are compared in Table 8-12.

Vascular insufficiency probably accounts for infarction of hyperplastic nodules, seen in up to 20% of resected cases. The center of the nodule undergoes hemorrhagic necrosis, often with reactive changes in the residual epithelium at the periphery, including squamous metaplasia and urothelial metaplasia.

Nodular hyperplasia is not a precursor of cancer, but there are a number of similarities between the two.[350] Both display a parallel increase in prevalence with patient age according to autopsy studies, although cancer lags by 15–20 years. Both require androgens for growth and development, and both may respond to androgen deprivation treatment. Most cancers arise in patients with concomitant nodular hyperplasia, and cancer is found incidentally in a significant number (10%) of transurethral prostatectomy specimens. Nodular hyperplasia may be related to prostate cancer arising in the transition zone, perhaps in association with certain forms of hyperplasia.[350,351] The pathogenesis of nodular hyperplasia is still poorly understood; it is presumed that there is no single mechanism, but rather a synergistic effect of multiple events in biological communication systems (neural, endocrine, and immune) during aging.[73]

## Atrophy and post-atrophic hyperplasia (postinflammatory hyperplasia; partial atrophy; post-sclerotic hyperplasia)

Atrophy is a common microscopic finding, consisting of small distorted glands with flattened epithelium, hyperchromatic nuclei, and stromal fibrosis.[352-354] It is usually idiopathic, and the prevalence increases with advancing age. At low magnification atrophy may be confused with adenocarcinoma, owing to the prominent acinar architectural distortion and cytoplasmic basophilia. At high magnification, atrophy usually lacks significant nuclear and nucleolar enlargement except in cases of post-atrophic hyperplasia (see below). The nuclear/cytoplasmic ratio is high because of

**Table 8-12** Histopathological variants of nodular hyperplasia

| Variant | Microscopic features | Usual location |
|---|---|---|
| Atypical adenomatous hyperplasia | Localized proliferation of small acini in association with BPH nodule which architecturally mimics adenocarcinoma but lacks cytological features of malignancy | Transition zone |
| Basal cell hyperplasia | Proliferation of basal cells, two or more cells in thickness; may have prominent nucleoli (atypical basal cell hyperplasia) or form a nodule (basal cell adenoma) | Transition zone |
| Cribriform hyperplasia | Acini with distinctive cribriform pattern, often with clear cytoplasm; easily mistaken for proliferative acini of the central zone | Transition zone |
| Hyperplasia of mesonephric remnants | Rare benign lobular proliferation of colloid-like material in the lumina; may mimic nephrogenic metaplasia focally; acini do not apparently express PSA or PAP | All zones (very rare) |
| Postatrophic hyperplasia | Atrophic acini with epithelial proliferative changes; easily mistaken for adenocarcinoma due to architectural distortion | All zones |
| Sclerosing adenosis | Circumscribed proliferation of small acini in a dense spindle cell stroma without significant atypia; usually solitary and microscopic | Transition zone |
| Stromal hyperplasia with atypical giant cells | Stromal nodules in the setting of cellularity and nuclear atypia | Transition zone |
| Verumontanum mucosal gland hyperplasia | Small benign acinar proliferation | Verumontanum |

**Table 8-13** Post-atrophic hyperplasia versus low-grade carcinoma

| | Post-atrophic hyperplasia | Low-grade adenocarcinoma |
|---|---|---|
| Architecture low power | Lobular small acinar proliferation, usually with central large dilated acini or acinus | May be lobular and circumscribed |
| Acinar contours | Irregular, 'atrophic' | May be rounded or smooth |
| Basal cell layer light microscopy | Usually intact; may be inconspicuous | Absent |
| High-molecular-weight keratin (34βE12) immunoreactivity | Intact or fragmented | Absent |
| Stromal changes | Smooth muscle atrophy, often with dense periacinar sclerosis | With or without stromal changes |
| Cytology<br>  Nuclei<br>  Nucleoli | <br>Mild enlargement<br>Usually inconspicuous | <br>Enlarged<br>Usually prominent |
| Cytoplasm | Basophilic | Usually pale due to greater amount of cytoplasm |
| Basophilic mucin | Rare | May be present |
| Crystalloids | Rare | May be present |
| Adjacent acini | Often atrophic | Variable |

scant cytoplasm, and nuclei are dark. The atrophic changes in benign epithelium induced by radiation therapy and androgen deprivation therapy are discussed at the end of this chapter.

Atrophy usually has regenerative features, particularly in the luminal secretory cells, accounting for properties typically associated with high-grade prostatic intraepithelial neoplasia and carcinoma, including immunoreactivity for bcl-2, glutathione S-transferase π (GSTP1),[39] androgen receptors, PSA, PAP, Ki-67,[96] the cyclin-dependent kinase inhibitor p15/CDKN2,[355] COX-2,[39,356] and low NKX3.1 protein,[357] versican,[358] and p27 expression.[359] Racemase immunoreactivity is present in up to 31% of foci of atrophy, and is usually weak or moderate in intensity.[360] However, in isolation this marker is insufficient to reliably distinguish atrophy and the atrophic pattern of adenocarcinoma.[361] Atrophy is enriched with a large number of highly proliferating intermediate cells (phenotypically intermediate between basal cells and secretory cells).[36]

Genetic abnormalities in atrophy included loss of 8p22 in 21% of cases and gain of 8p24 in 19%, slightly higher than benign epithelium (16% and 10%, respectively) and lower than in high-grade PIN (25% and 21%, respectively).[362] These findings were refuted by another report that found no gains or losses of 8p, 8 centromere, or 8q24 (C-myc) in atrophy.[357]

Clusters of atrophic prostatic acini that display proliferative epithelial changes are referred to as post-atrophic hyperplasia[363] (Fig. 8-46).[364,150] PAH is at the extreme end of the morphologic continuum of acinar atrophy that most closely mimics adenocarcinoma (Table 8-13). This continuum varies from mild acinar irregularity with a flattened

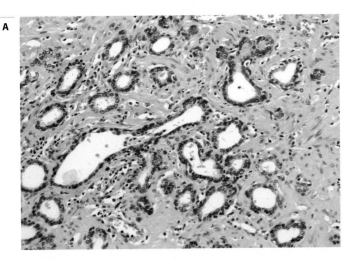

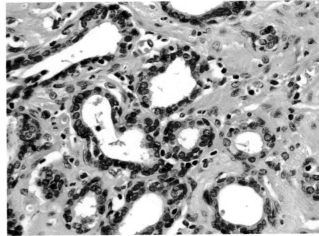

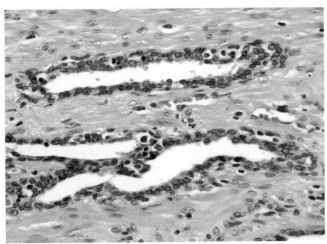

**Fig. 8-46** Post-atrophic hyperplasia. **(A)** The acini are variable in size and shape, set in a fibrous stroma. Part of the epithelium is flattened, indicating atrophy, but other areas show low cuboidal epithelium and luminal secretory blebs. **(B)** The epithelial lining is irregular, with hyperchromatic nuclei. **(C)** These elongate acini have enlarged nuclei with hyperchromasia. Nucleoli are inconspicuous.

layer of attenuated cells containing scant cytoplasm to that of PAH, in which the lining cells are low cuboidal with moderate cytoplasm. There is no sharp division in this continuum between atrophy and PAH, challenging the utility of PAH as a distinct entity. However, the morphologic similarity of PAH and carcinoma creates the potential for misdiagnosis, sometimes resulting in unnecessary prostatectomy.[364,365] To avoid this potentially tragic misinterpretation, the pathologist should have an understanding of this extreme morphologic variant of atrophy. We believe that PAH is a diagnostic category for atrophic acini that most closely mimic adenocarcinoma, recognizing that this is merely a descriptive term.

PAH consists of a microscopic lobular cluster of five to 15 small acini with distorted contours reminiscent of atrophy. One or more larger dilated acini are usually present within these round to oval clusters, and the small acini appear to bud off of the dilated acinus, imparting a lobular appearance to the lesion. The small acini are lined by a layer of cuboidal secretory cells with mildly enlarged nuclei and an increased nuclear/cytoplasmic ratio compared to adjacent benign epithelial cells. The nuclei contain evenly distributed and finely granular chromatin, and nucleoli are usually small, although mildly enlarged basophilic nucleoli are focally present in 39% of cases. The cytoplasm is often basophilic or finely granular to clear, and luminal cytoplasmic apocrine-like blebs are present in 33% of cases. Luminal mucin is occa-

sionally present in PAH. Corpora amylacea are present in 75% of cases of PAH, but crystalloids are rare.

The basal cell layer is usually present in PAH, but is often inconspicuous by routine light microscopy. Basal cell hyperplasia is rarely seen in foci of PAH. Immunohistochemical stains for high molecular weight keratin (antibody 34β-E12) reveal a focally fragmented basal cell layer in some cases. Adjacent prostatic acini always show at least focal atrophy. MIB-1 staining reveals a greater proliferative rate in PAH than in simple atrophy.[366]

Stromal changes are always present in PAH, ranging from smooth muscle atrophy to dense sclerosis with compression of acini. In cases with sclerosis, the acinar lumina are compressed and showed marked distortion. Subtyping of PAH into lobular and post-sclerotic subtypes is useful only to allow recognition of PAH and distinguish it from mimics such as low-grade adenocarcinoma, and we prefer not to subtype PAH. Also, PAH is often associated with patchy chronic inflammation; infrequently, dilated acini contain luminal neutrophils. Elastosis is another distinctive microscopic feature of some cases of PAH.[367]

PAH is distinguished from carcinoma by its characteristic lobular architecture, intact or fragmented basal cell layer, inconspicuous or mildly enlarged nucleoli, and adjacent acinar atrophy with stromal fibrosis or smooth muscle atrophy (Table 8-13). Low-grade adenocarcinoma is the most important differential diagnostic consideration. PAH usually has a lobular pattern on low power, similar to Gleason pattern 2 and 3 adenocarcinoma. However, the lobular pattern in PAH is less distinct in cases with abundant stromal sclerosis, and there may be a pseudoinfiltrative growth pattern with fibrous entrapment of acini. Nucleolar changes are also useful in separating PAH and carcinoma, although some cases of low-grade carcinoma have only scattered large nucleoli or even micronucleoli. Mildly enlarged nucleoli may be present in PAH, but only focally, and the majority of cells have micronucleoli. The separation of PAH from carcinoma is most difficult in needle biopsy specimens in which only a portion of the lesion is sampled, and awareness of this entity assists in this distinction. There may occasionally be genetic changes in chromosome 8 in atrophic epithelium.[368] These changes were present at a similar or higher frequency in high-grade prostatic intraepithelial neoplasia and carcinoma.[96]

Is PAH associated with cancer? Wheeler and colleagues[369] assessed a large series of radical prostatectomy and cystoprostatectomy specimens and found PAH in respectively 32% and 27% of cases. PAH was located in the peripheral zone (91% of cases), transition zone (8%), and central zone (1%), and had no apparent spatial association with cancer. The European Randomized Study of Screening for Prostate Cancer prospectively studied a cohort of 202 random sextant biopsies from men with at least 8 years of follow-up, and found atrophy in 94%; extensive atrophy was observed in 5% of biopsies.[370] Only 4.7% had a subsequent diagnosis of prostate cancer, and the authors concluded that atrophy is a very common lesion in biopsy cores and was not associated with a greater risk of high-grade PIN or cancer.

The term 'partial atrophy' was suggested to describe acini '. . . with relatively scant cytoplasm, yet the glands are not fully atrophic in that they do not appear basophilic at low magnification.'[371] However, we find this description to be inadequate to separate these findings from typical atrophy; also, there is no clinical utility to this designation: it is not used by us or others in routine practice, and was apparently abandoned in most subsequent writings by the originators.[359,366]

The presence of proliferative changes in atrophic acini has spawned the concept of atrophy as a precursor of high-grade PIN and cancer. The term 'proliferative inflammatory atrophy' was proposed,[359] but this is not a clinicopathologic entity and appears to be an inherently redundant term, as all patterns of atrophy have some proliferative/regenerative features according to the original report.[359] Some authors have erroneously equated this concept with PAH.[36] Often there is no inflammation present, despite claims to the contrary in the original description,[359] so the term 'inflammatory atrophy' is actually a misnomer, and we discourage its use. An effort to separate inflammation-associated atrophy and non-inflamed atrophy revealed that both were common findings, with a slightly greater incidence of the former with cancer.[372] Efforts to identify a morphologic continuum between atrophy and high-grade PIN were not convincing despite claims to the contrary,[373] and this concept has been refuted by multiple reports. Billis[352] has proposed ischemia

as a possible causative factor in atrophy, and this is considered a plausible hypothesis.

A recent report classified prostatic atrophy into four bins: simple atrophy, simple atrophy with cyst formation, partial atrophy, and post-atrophic hyperplasia. However, this classification has no clinical significance, is of questionable pathologic utility, and is not used in practice.

Atrophy may also affect prostatic stromal cells, but the heterogeneity of this compartment masks the changes. In the dog model, prostatic myocytes and fibroblasts diminished and underwent serial atrophy and apoptosis after castration; the atrophic cells were filled with intracellular lipofuscin.[374] The expression of myosin declined after castration, coincidentally with the increase in TGF-$\beta$ mRNA and decline in bFGF mRNA.

## Prostatic stromal hyperplasia with atypia (PSHA)

Stromal hyperplasia with atypia consists of stromal nodules in the transition zone with increased cellularity and nuclear atypia (Figs 8-47, 8-48).[375-378] These may appear as solid stromal nodules (often erroneously referred to as atypical leiomyoma) or with atypical cells interspersed with benign glands.

There are two histologic patterns of PSHA.[378] The most common, the infiltrative pattern, consists of one or more ill-defined hyperplastic stromal nodules with variable numbers of atypical bizarre giant cells infiltrating between acini. The stroma is a hypocellular loose myxoid matrix with ectatic hyalinized vessels and mild to moderate chronic inflammation. The less common pattern, the leiomyoma-like pattern, consists of a solid circumscribed expansile stromal nodule with abundant smooth muscle and variable numbers of atypical bizarre giant cells. There are no mitotic figures or necrosis. PSHA has no malignant potential, and the atypical cells are degenerative myofibroblasts. Local recurrence was seen in 25% (7/28) of our cases, with a mean follow-up of 6.3 years (range, 2 months to 16 years), similar to that seen with typical nodular hyperplasia.[378]

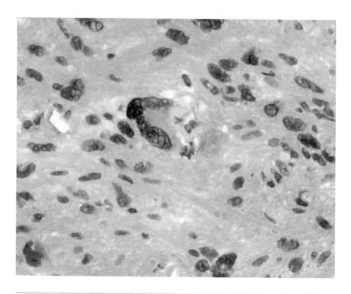

**Fig. 8-47** Prostatic stromal hyperplasia with atypia (PSHA).

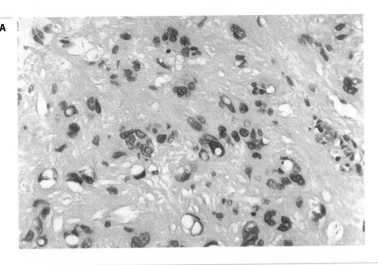
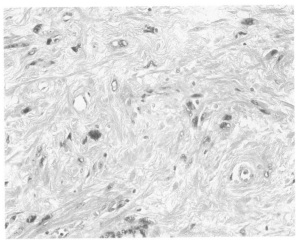

**Fig. 8-48** Prostatic stromal hyperplasia with atypia (PSHA). **(A)** Symplastic changes of many of the myocytes, including nuclear and cytoplasmic vacuolization. **(B)** In another case there is focal crowding of myocytes, with variation in nuclear size. No mitotic figures were observed in either of these cases despite exhaustive sectioning.

**Table 8-14** Basal cell proliferations of the prostate: diagnostic criteria and immunohistochemical profile

|  | Normal basal cell layer | Basal cell hyperplasia (BCH) | Atypical basal cell hyperplasia | Basal cell adenoma | Adenoid cystic basal cell carcinoma |
|---|---|---|---|---|---|
| Architecture | Near–continuous single single cell layer | Small cell nests (solid or cystic), usually in nodular hyperplasia, two cell layer minimum | Same as BCH | Round circumscribed nodule of BCH | Infiltrating 'adenoid cystic' pattern or basaloid pattern; myxoid stroma |
| Cytology | Small elongate cells, ovoid nuclei, scant cytoplasm | Large ovoid nuclei, indistinct nucleoli, scant cytoplasm, may have clear cytoplasm | Same as BCH, but with nucleolomegaly | Same as BCH, may have nucleolomegaly | Basaloid cells with large nuclei |
| Immuonohistochemical findings Basal-cell-specific keratin 34BE12 | + | + | + | + | + (patchy) |
| Prostate specific antigen | − | + (patchy) | + (patchy) | + (focal) | + |
| Prostate acid phosphatase | − | + (patchy) | + (patchy) | + (focal) | + |
| Chromogranin | − | + | + | + | − |
| S100 protein | − | + | + | + | − |
| Neuron-specific enolase | − | + | + | − | − |

+, <5% of cells were positive.

Some authors have suggested the acronym PSPUMP (prostatic stromal proliferation of uncertain malignant potential),[379] later modified to STUMP (stromal tumor of uncertain malignant potential),[380,381] which lumps PSHA (benign entity)[378] with phyllodes tumor[382] and stromal sarcoma (both of the latter entities are malignant). We strongly discourage the use of this terminology, based on differences between these entities according to differences in light microscopic appearances, immunophenotypes, and clinical outcomes.

## Basal cell hyperplasia and basal cell proliferations

There are three patterns of benign basal cell hyperplasia, including typical basal cell hyperplasia, atypical basal cell hyperplasia, and basal cell adenoma (Table 8-14).[383–390] These findings may be particularly challenging in needle biopsies because of limited sampling.[391] Neoplastic basal cell proliferations, referred to as adenoid basal cell tumor, adenoid cystic carcinoma, and basal cell carcinoma, are described in Chapter 9.

## Basal cell hyperplasia

Basal cell hyperplasia (BCH) consists of a proliferation of basal cells two or more cells thick at the periphery of prostatic acini (Fig. 8-49).[383,385,392,393] It sometimes appears as small nests of cells surrounded by compressed stroma, often associated with chronic inflammation. The nests may be solid or cystically dilated, and occasionally are punctuated by irregular round luminal spaces, creating a cribriform pattern.[391] Basal cell hyperplasia frequently involves only part of an acinus, and sometimes protrudes into the lumen, retaining the overlying secretory cell layer; less commonly, there is symmetric duplication of the basal cell layer at the periphery of the acinus. The proliferation may protrude into the acinar lumen, retaining the overlying secretory luminal epithelium. Symmetric circumferential thickening of the basal cell layer is less frequent than eccentric thicken-

ing, and these changes do not result from tangential sectioning.

BCH resembles prostate acini seen in the fetus, accounting for the synonyms 'fetalization' and 'embryonal hyperplasia.' BCH may be composed of basal cell nests with areas of luminal differentiation resembling similar lesions of the salivary gland. This is denoted as the adenoid basal form of BCH. The basal cells in basal cell hyperplasia are enlarged, ovoid or round, and plump (epithelioid), with large pale ovoid nuclei, finely reticular chromatin, and a moderate amount of cytoplasm. Nucleoli are usually inconspicuous (<1 μm in diameter) except in atypical BCH (see below).

Sclerosing basal cell hyperplasia is identical to typical basal cell hyperplasia except for the presence of delicate lace-like fibrosis or dense irregular sclerotic fibrosis and hyperplastic smooth muscle surrounding and distorting hyperplastic basal cell aggregates. It is not associated with carcinoma, but occasionally may be confused with malignancy.

Clear cell change is common in basal cell hyperplasia, often with a cribriform pattern; cribriform pattern without clear cell change is rare. Squamous metaplasia is infrequent, usually associated with infarction. Chronic inflammation is a common association, but is non-specific. Occasional nuclear grooves and nuclear 'bubble' artifact are observed. Focal calcification is evident in some cases, and may be present within the basal cell nests (Table 8-14).

## BCH with florid appearance (florid basal cell hyperplasia)

Florid basal cell hyperplasia consists of compact glandular proliferation with solid nests (Fig. 8-50).[160,394] The cytology in some areas looks disturbing because the basaloid cells have moderately enlarged nuclei, often with prominent nucleoli; a few mitotic figures are present; the intervening stroma is scant and cellular; the lesion is not well circumscribed; and basaloid structures are intermingled with the surrounding glands, giving the impression of 'infiltration' (this is also called diffuse type). The proliferation of basal cells involves more than 100 small crowded acini (per section) forming a nodule.[388]

## Atypical basal cell hyperplasia

Atypical basal cell hyperplasia (ABCH) is identical to basal cell hyperplasia except for the presence of large prominent nucleoli (Fig. 8-51). These are round to oval and lightly eosinophilic, similar to those seen in acinar adenocarcinoma of the prostate (their mean diameter is 1.96 μm). There is chronic inflammation in the majority of cases, suggesting that nucleolomegaly is a reflection of reactive atypia. A morphologic spectrum of nucleolar size is observed in basal cell proliferations, and only those with more than 10% of cells exhibiting prominent nucleoli are considered atypical.[385] This lesion is significant because of the potential for misdiagnosis as adenocarcinoma[333] and high-grade prostatic intraepithelial neoplasia (PIN).

## Basal cell adenoma

Basal cell adenoma is identical to typical BCH, although the proliferating basal cell masses are usually large and circum-

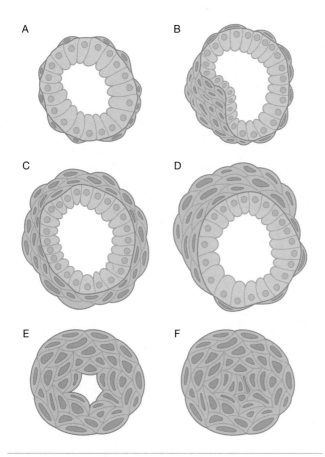

**Fig. 8-49** Schematic illustration of basal cell hyperplasia in the prostate. **(A)** Normal prostatic gland with thin peripheral layer of basal cells and overlying columnar secretory luminal cell layer. **(B)** Focal basal cell proliferation with mild distortion of the glandular luminal contour. **(C)** Symmetric circumferential proliferation of basal cells, at least two cells thick. **(D)** Eccentric focus of atypical basal cell hyperplasia with prominent nucleoli, eccentric pattern. **(E)** Basal cell hyperplasia with loss of secretory cell layer (note retention of glandular lumen). Compare with **(F):** 'solid' pattern of basal cell hyperplasia, with absence of lumen. (Reprinted with permission from Devaraj LT, Bostwick DG. Atypical basal cell hyperplasia of the prostate. Immunophenotypic profile and proposed classification of basal cell proliferations. Am J Surg Pathol 1993; 17: 645–659.)

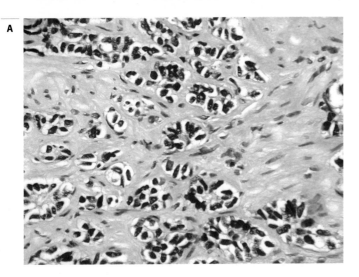

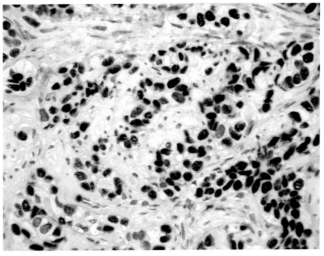

**Fig. 8-50** Florid basal cell hyperplasia. Florid BCH acini mimicking prostate cancer **(A)**. These acini are positive for p63 **(B)**.

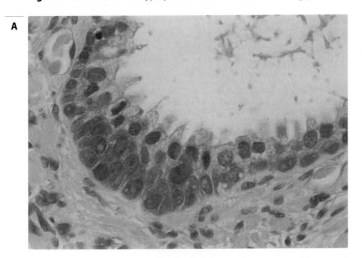

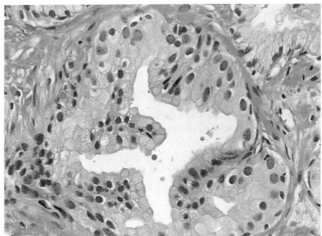

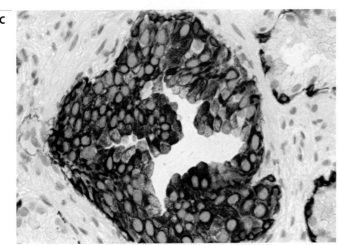

**Fig. 8-51** Atypical basal cell hyperplasia. **(A)** The basal cell nuclei are enlarged and round, with central enlarged nucleoli. Note the secretory cell layer at the surface, consisting of cells with pale finely vacuolated cytoplasm and darkly staining nuclei with irregular nuclear outlines. **(B)** In another case, the basal cell nuclei are slightly enlarged, with punctate dark nucleoli. **(C)** These cells are positive for Keratin 34β-E12.

scribed, with a nodular or adenoma-like pattern. Basal cell adenoma consists of one or more large, round, usually solitary circumscribed nodule of acini with basal cell hyperplasia in the setting of nodular hyperplasia.[395] The nodules contain uniformly spaced aggregates of hyperplastic basal cells that form small solid nests or cystically dilated acini. Condensed stroma is seen at the periphery and often tra-

verses the adenomatous nodules, creating incomplete lobulation in some cases. The stroma is normal or slightly increased in density and may be basophilic without myxoid change adjacent to cell nests.

The basal cells in basal cell adenomas are plump, with large nuclei, scant cytoplasm and inconspicuous nucleoli, although large prominent nucleoli are rarely observed. Many cells are cuboidal or 'epithelioid,' particularly near the center of the cell nests, and some contain clear cytoplasm. Prominent calcific debris is often present within acinar lumina.

Multiple basal cell adenomas are referred to as basal cell adenomatosis. Basal cell adenoma invariably arises in association with nodular hyperplasia and appears to be a variant with no malignant potential. In contrast to basal cell carcinoma, basal cell adenoma is well circumscribed, lacks necrosis, and the stroma between the basal cell nests is similar to that of the surrounding normal prostatic stroma.

## Immunohistochemical findings

Basal cell hyperplasia (typical and atypical forms) displays intense cytoplasmic immunoreactivity in virtually all of the cells with high molecular weight keratin 34β-E12 and p63 (Table 8-14). The combination of 34β-E12 and p63 improves

the sensitivity for basal cell detection over either marker alone (Fig. 8-51).[396] In the majority of cases immunoreactivity for PSA, PAP, chromogranin, S100 protein, α-smooth muscle actin and neuron-specific enolase is present in rare basal cells.

## Differential diagnosis

The differential diagnosis of basal cell proliferation includes a wide variety of benign and malignant lesions (Table 8-15).[397] Atypical adenomatous hyperplasia may be confused with basal cell hyperplasia but does not usually have a prominent basal cell layer and displays a fragmented keratin 34β-E12-immunoreactive basal cell layer.[398] Sclerosing adenosis may be difficult to separate from sclerosing basal cell hyperplasia, and these lesions may coexist; however, sclerosing adenosis has no smooth muscle in the sclerotic stroma and

**Table 8-15** Basal cell hyperplasia (BCH) (ordinary, atypical, and florid): differential diagnoses. Morphological criteria and major immunohistochemical findings

| Differential diagnosis | Architecture | Cytology | Keratin 34β-E12 | p63 | PSA | S100 protein | SMA |
|---|---|---|---|---|---|---|---|
| BCH (typical, florid, and atypical) | Cell nests, two cell layers minimum, solid or cystic | Small to medium sized nuclei, nucleoli may be prominent in some forms | + | + | ± | − to ± | − to ± |
| High grade PIN | Ducts and acini with various architectural patterns, ranging from flat to cribriform | Cells with enlarged nuclei, with a prominent nucleolus, similar to those in adenocarcinoma | ± (basal cells) | ± (basal cells) | + | − | − |
| Adenocarcinoma | Acini of various sizes, either separated or fused, with different architectural patterns, such as flat or monolayered or cribriform | Cells with enlarged nuclei, with prominent nucleoli | − | − | + | − | − |
| Sclerosing adenosis | Acinar structures, predominantly small, lined by bilayered epithelium | Small to medium sized nuclei, inconspicuous nucleoli | + (basal cells) | + (basal cells) | + | + | + |
| Benign seminal vesicle/ejaculatory duct epithelium | Ducts lined by a bilayered epithelium | Prominent nuclear atypia and pleomorphism | + | + | − | − | − |
| Squamous metaplasia | Ducts and acini lined by multilayered epithelium similar to epidermis | Cells with small to medium sized nuclei; inconspicuous nucleoli; keratinization often prominent | + | + | − | − | − |
| Urothelial metaplasia | Ducts and acini lined by multilayered epithelium similar to urothelium | Small to medium sized nuclei, inconspicuous nucleoli; luminal cells larger than those in the intermediate and basal layers | + | + | − to ± (scattered luminal cells) | − | − |

BCH, basal cell hyperplasia; PIN, high-grade prostatic intraepithelial neoplasia; PSA, prostate specific antigen; SMA, α-smooth muscle actin.

displays myoepithelial differentiation (intense cytoplasmic immunoreactivity with keratin 34β-E12, S100 protein, and muscle-specific actin, as well as ultrastructural evidence of cytoplasmic myofilaments).

Seminal vesicle and ejaculatory duct epithelium may also be confused with basal cell hyperplasia and adenoma, particularly in small specimens such as needle biopsies, and rarely in TURP specimens. The proliferation and stratification of lining cells with cytologic atypia may resemble small foci of solid basal cell hyperplasia. Seminal vesicular epithelium is distinguished by the presence of secretory luminal cells, significant cytologic atypia (particularly in the senile seminal vesicle), and distinctive abundant yellow to golden brown lipochrome pigment.

The normal urothelium of the prostatic urethra and periurethral ducts resembles basal cell hyperplasia both histologically and immunohistochemically. Also, transitional metaplasia may occur in the medium-sized and small ducts in the prostate, sometimes in association with inflammation and reactive atypia with mild nucleolomegaly.

Urethral polyp, although uncommon, may be confused with basal cell hyperplasia and adenoma, particularly in small cystoscopic specimens and needle biopsies. Urethral polyp includes proliferative papillary urethritis, ectopic prostatic tissue, nephrogenic metaplasia, and inverted papilloma.

Prostatic intraepithelial neoplasia may be mistaken for atypical basal cell hyperplasia, and is distinguished by the presence of cytologic abnormalities in secretory luminal cells of medium-sized to large acini, intense cytoplasmic PSA, PAP and α-methylacyl-CoA-racemase (P504S) immunoreactivity in the abnormal cells, and an intact or fragmented keratin 34β-E12-immunoreactive basal cell layer.[399] The nuclei of basal cells in BCH tend to be round, and at times, the cells form small, solid basaloid nests. In contrast, the cells in PIN tend to appear pseudo-stratified or stratified and columnar, and do not occlude the acinar lumen.[285,386,399] In

areas of BCH atypical basal cells can be seen underlying the surmounting benign secretory cells. PIN has full-thickness cytological atypia, with the nuclei usually oriented perpendicular to the basement membrane.[285,399]

Well-differentiated adenocarcinoma is distinguished from BCH by the presence of PSA and PAP-immunoreactive luminal secretory cells with nucleolomegaly, frequent luminal crystalloids, and absence of a keratin 34β-E12-immunoreactive basal cell layer. Similar criteria allow separation of the cribriform variant of adenocarcinoma, adenoid basal cell tumor, basal cell hyperplasia with or without clear cell change, and clear cell cribriform hyperplasia.

In contrast to basaloid carcinoma, basal cell adenoma is well circumscribed, lacks necrosis, and the stroma between the basaloid nests is similar to that of the surrounding normal prostatic stroma (see Chapter 9).

## Cribriform hyperplasia

Cribriform hyperplasia, including clear cell cribriform hyperplasia, consists of a nodule of glands arranged in a distinctive cribriform pattern (Fig. 8-52).[400–403] The cells from such glands usually have pale to clear cytoplasm and small uniform nuclei with inconspicuous nucleoli.[401,403] The basal cell layer in cribriform hyperplasia may have enlarged nuclei, and this lesion should be distinguished from high-grade PIN and carcinoma by the lack of prominent nucleoli in acinar cells.

## Atypical adenomatous hyperplasia (AAH; atypical hyperplasia; adenosis)

Atypical adenomatous hyperplasia[317] is a localized proliferation of small acini within the prostate that may be mistaken for carcinoma (Figs 8-53 to 8-58).[23,404,405] It varies in incidence from 20% (transurethral resection specimens) to 24% (autopsy series in 20–40 year-old men)[406] and can be found throughout the prostate but is usually present near the apex

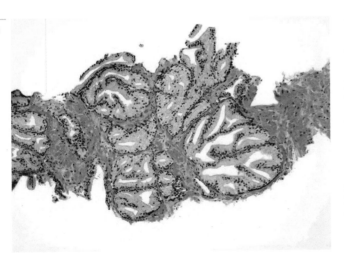 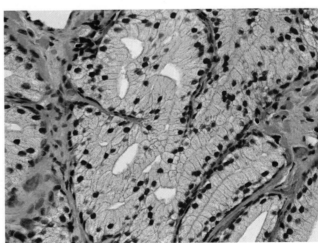

**Fig. 8-52** Clear cell cribriform hyperplasia. **(A)** At low magnification, the fenestrations are irregular in size and shape, and are contained within expanded acini. **(B)** At high magnification epithelial cells contain pale finely vacuolated cytoplasm, uniform nuclei with open chromatin pattern, and small inconspicuous nucleoli.

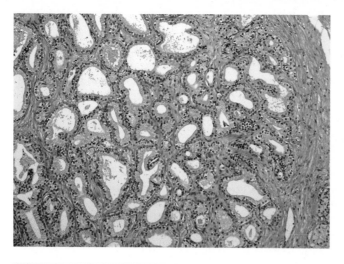

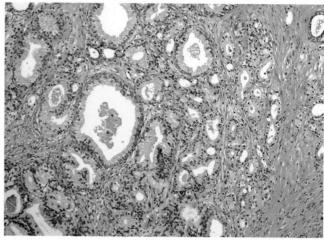

**Fig. 8-53** Atypical adenomatous hyperplasia. The small acinar proliferation shows variation in size, shape, and spacing in a moderately cellular stroma.

**Fig. 8-54** Atypical adenomatous hyperplasia. One edge of this nodule of nodular hyperplasia consists of a proliferation of small pale acini set in a cellular stroma.

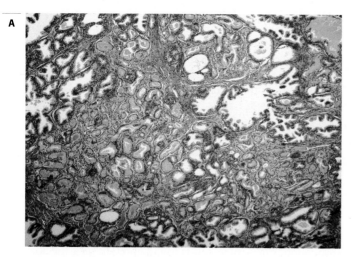

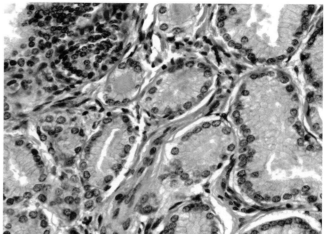

**Fig. 8-55** Atypical adenomatous hyperplasia. **(A)** A group of small acini architecturally mimics well-differentiated adenocarcinoma. **(B)** The acini lack cytologic features of malignancy without significant nuclear or nucleolar enlargement.

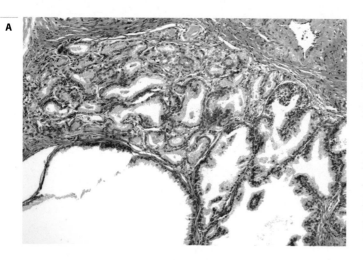

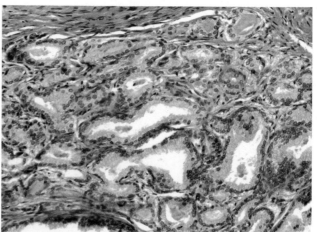

**Fig. 8-56** Atypical adenomatous hyperplasia. **(A)** At the edge of a hyperplastic nodule, there is a minute nest of small acini with pale cytoplasm. **(B)** At high magnification, the small acini contain uniform small nuclei and punctate nucleoli without significant enlargement.

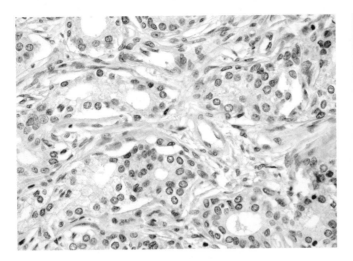

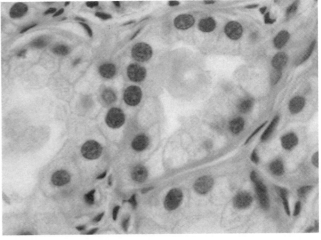

**Fig. 8-57** Atypical adenomatous hyperplasia. The closely packed cluster of acini contains small nuclei and minute punctate nucleoli.

**Fig. 8-59** Atypical adenomatous hyperplasia. Note uniform round nuclei without prominent nucleoli.

A

B

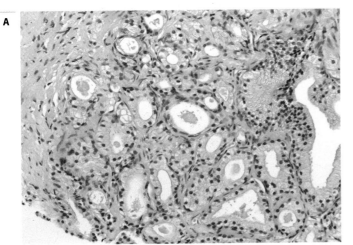

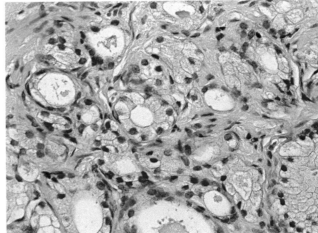

**Fig. 8-58** Atypical adenomatous hyperplasia on needle biopsy. Although very rare on needle biopsy, AAH is occasionally observed, consisting of a small acinar proliferation in intimate association with larger acini of nodular hyperplasia. We require that most or all of the focus be present on the biopsy to diagnose AAH in order to avoid underdiagnosis of adenocarcinoma.

and in the transition zone and periurethral area.[407] The mean size of AAH is 0.03 cm³.

AAH is distinguished from well-differentiated carcinoma by inconspicuous nucleoli, a fragmented basal cell layer, and infrequent crystalloids (Table 8-16). All measures of nucleolar size allow separation of AAH from adenocarcinoma, including mean nucleolar diameter, largest nucleolar diameter, and percentage of nucleoli >1 μm in diameter. There is apparently widespread acceptance of Gleason's criterion of nucleolar diameter >1 μm for separating well-differentiated cancer (Gleason primary grades 1 and 2) from other proliferative lesions such as AAH.[408] Despite the utility of these features, the absolute distinction between AAH and carcinoma is still difficult in some cases. Other morphologic features are not useful in distinguishing AAH from adenocarcinoma, including lesion shape, circumscription, multifocality, mean acinar size, variation in acinar size and shape, chromatin pattern, and the amount and tinctorial quality of

the cytoplasm. Both AAH and cancer contain acidic mucin in the majority of cases.[60,61]

Immunohistochemistry is often useful in the diagnosis of AAH. The basal cell layer is characteristically discontinuous and fragmented in AAH but absent in cancer, a feature that can be demonstrated in routine formalin-fixed sections with basal cell-specific anti-keratin 34β-E12 and or p63 (Figs 8-59, 8-60). AAH is often positive for racemase (P504s), so this marker may not be useful for distinguishing AAH from malignancy.[139,152,168]

Histologic mimics of AAH include nodular hyperplasia without atypia, simple lobular atrophy (Fig. 8-61), post-atrophic hyperplasia, sclerosing atrophy, basal cell hyperplasia, atypical basal cell hyperplasia, and metaplastic changes associated with radiation, infarction, mesonephric remnant hyperplasia, and prostatitis. Many mimics display architectural and cytologic atypia, including nucleolomegaly, and caution is warranted in the interpretation of scant speci-

**Table 8-16** Atypical adenomatous hyperplasia versus well-differentiated adenocarcinoma

| Architectural and associated features | Atypical adenomatous hyperplasia | Carcinoma (Gleason grades 1 and 2) |
|---|---|---|
| Low power | Circumscribed or limited infiltration | Circumscribed or limited infiltration |
| Lesion size | Variable | Variable |
| Gland size | Variable | Less variable |
| Gland shape | Variable | Less variable |
| Crystalloids | Infrequent (16%) | Frequent (75%) |
| Corpora amylacea | Frequent (32%) | Infrequent (13%) |
| Basophilic mucin | Infrequent | Frequent |
| **Nuclear features** | | |
| Nuclear size variation | Less variable | Variable |
| Chromatin | Uniform/granular | Uniform or variable |
| Parachromatin clearing | Infrequent | Frequent |
| Nucleoli | Inconspicuous | Prominent |
| Nucleoli (largest) | 2.5 μ (rare) | 3.0 μm |
| Nucleoli (mean) | <1.0 μm | 1.8 μm |
| Nucleoli >1 μ | 18% | 77% |
| **Basal cell layer** | | |
| Hematoxylin and eosin stain | Inconspicuous | Absent |
| Antikeratin stain (high molecular weight) | Fragmented | Virtually absent |

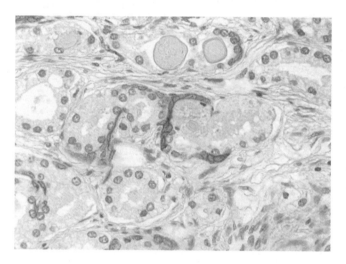
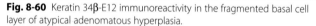

**Fig. 8-60** Keratin 34β-E12 immunoreactivity in the fragmented basal cell layer of atypical adenomatous hyperplasia.

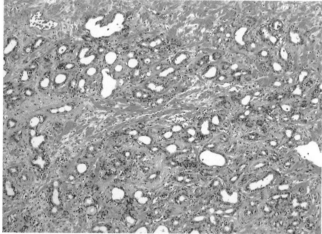

**Fig. 8-61** Simple lobular atrophy mimicking atypical adenomatous hyperplasia.

mens, cauterized or distorted specimens, and specimens submitted with an incomplete patient history. AAH is uncommonly associated with sclerosis, but further study is needed to determine the relationship to sclerosing adenosis. Sclerosing adenosis differs from AAH by displaying myoepithelial features of the basal cells and an exuberant stroma of fibroblasts and loose ground substance. AAH should also be distinguished from lobular atrophy and post-atrophic hyperplasia. Simple atrophy consists of shrunken acini that demonstrate strong basal cell-specific anti-keratin immunoreactivity. Post-atrophic hyperplasia may be difficult to separate from AAH as proliferating luminal cells with small amounts of clear cytoplasm may occur in an atrophic back-

ground. These cells may demonstrate cytologic atypia, sometimes with luminal mucin. Both may have a fragmented basal cell layer.

There are two unanswered clinical questions regarding AAH. First, does Gleason primary grade 1 adenocarcinoma represent overdiagnosed AAH. These lesions are uncommon; most agree that Gleason primary grade 2 adenocarcinoma (infiltrating acini) is malignant, but what is the true biologic potential of the uniform circumscribed proliferation of Gleason primary grade 1 adenocarcinoma? The majority of Gleason pattern 1 cancers are now thought to represent foci of AAH. Second, is AAH a precursor of adenocarcinoma?

AAH may be linked to a subset of prostate cancers that arise in the transition zone, but the evidence is circumstantial: increased incidence in association with carcinoma (15% in 100 prostates without carcinoma at autopsy, and 31% in 100 prostates with cancer at autopsy), topographic relationship with small-acinar carcinoma, age peak incidence that precedes that of carcinoma, increasing silver-staining nucleolar organized region (AgNOR) count, increased nuclear area and diameter, and a proliferative cell index that is similar to that of small-acinar carcinoma but significantly higher than that of normal and hyperplastic prostatic epithelium.[409] Expression of racemase in some cases of AAH has suggested a possible premalignant status to some authors.[139,152,168]

A small but significant number of cases of AAH have genetic instability. A total of 9% of cases of AAH were abnormal using fluorescence in situ hybridization with centromere-specific probes for chromosomes 7, 8,10, 12, and Y.[409,410] Up to 60% of AAH cases had highly variable allelic imbalance at chromosome 8p arm, compared to up to 90% of prostate cancers.[411] Conversely, other studies reported that AAH does not seem to be linked closely to prostate cancer and should not be considered as an obligate premalignant lesion.[412,413]

When AAH is encountered in prostatic specimens we believe that all tissue should be embedded and made available for examination; serial sections of suspicious foci may be useful. Needle biopsies rarely contain AAH, and we require that most or all of the focus be present for diagnosis, recognizing the potential for sampling AAH-like areas in adenocarcinoma. The triple stain (keratin 34β-E12, p63, and racemase) is useful in difficult cases. The identification of AAH should not influence or dictate therapeutic decisions; however, the clinical importance of these lesions is not fully understood, and close surveillance and follow-up may be indicated.

## Sclerosing adenosis

Sclerosing adenosis of the prostate, originally described as adenomatoid or pseudo-adenomatoid tumor, consists of a benign circumscribed proliferation of small acini set in a dense spindle cell stroma.[41,44,154,164,174,184,194] It is an incidental finding in TURP specimens for benign prostatic hyperplasia, present in about 2% of cases; rare cases are associated with elevated serum PSA concentration. Sclerosing adenosis is usually solitary and microscopic, but may be multifocal and extensive.

The acini in sclerosing adenosis are predominantly well formed and small to medium in size but may form minute cellular nests or clusters with abortive lumina (Figs 8-62, 8-63). The cells lining the acini display a moderate amount of clear to eosinophilic cytoplasm, often with distinct cell margins. The basal cell layer may be focally prominent and hyperplastic, particularly in acini thickly rimmed by cellular stroma (Figs 8-62, 8-63). In some areas the acini merge with the exuberant stroma of fibroblasts and loose ground substance. The finding of a cellular stroma with myxoid features may play a role in distinguishing sclerosing adenosis from

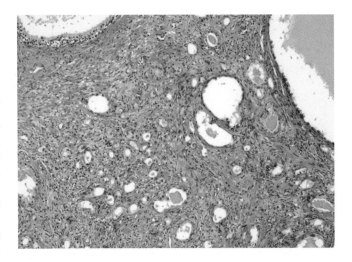

**Fig. 8-62** Sclerosing adenosis with benign acini set in a cellular stroma.

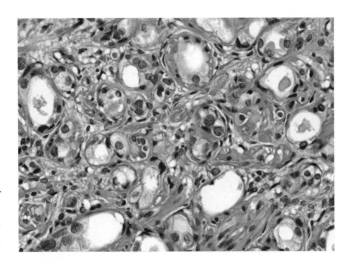

**Fig. 8-63** Sclerosing adenosis. Note prominent periacinar basement membrane thickening.

carcinoma.[421] There is usually no significant cytologic atypia of the epithelial cells or stromal cells, but some cases may show moderate atypia.

The unique immunophenotype of sclerosing adenosis is a valuable diagnostic clue that distinguishes it from adenocarcinoma (Table 8-17). The basal cells show immunoreactivity for S100 protein and muscle-specific actin, unlike normal prostatic epithelium or carcinoma;[146] consequently, sclerosing adenosis is considered a form of metaplasia (Fig. 8-64). In sclerosing adenosis the basal cell layer is intact or fragmented and discontinuous, as demonstrated with immunohistochemical stains for high molecular weight keratin 34β-E12 (Fig. 8-65), compared to the absence of staining in carcinoma. PSA and PAP are present within secretory luminal cells. Ultrastructural studies demonstrate myoepithelial differentiation in sclerosing adenosis, with collections of thin filaments and dense bodies.[420]

Sclerosing adenosis should be distinguished from lobular atrophy and post-atrophic hyperplasia. Both of these lesions

**Table 8-17** Sclerosing adenosis versus adenocarcinoma

| | Sclerosing adenosis | Adenocarcinoma |
|---|---|---|
| Architecture | Lobular small acinar proliferation; may form cell nests or clusters; prominent cellular stroma | May be lobular and circumscribed |
| Acini | Round and smooth; appear to merge with stroma due to pale staining | May be rounded or smooth |
| Basement membrane | Prominent thickening | Inconspicuous |
| Basal cell layer | | |
|   Light microscopy | Usually intact and often hyperplastic | Absent |
|   High-molecular-weight keratin (34BE12) immunoreactivity | Intact or discontinuous | Absent |
| Stromal changes | Prominent cellular stroma without atypia | Without or without stromal sclerosis |
| Cytology | | |
|   Nuclei | Mild enlargement | Enlarged |
|   Nucleoli | Usually inconspicuous | Usually prominent |
| Cytoplasm | Clear or eosinophilic | Usually pale due to greater amount of cytoplasm |
| Immunoreactivity | | |
|   S100 protein | Yes (basal cells) | No |
|   Actin | Yes (basal cells) | No |

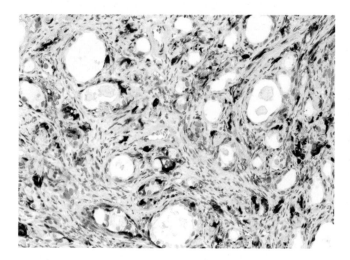

**Fig. 8-64** S100 protein stain in sclerosing adenosis. There is prominent immunoreactivity in most basal cells.

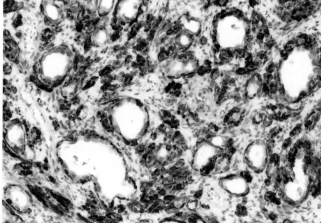

**Fig. 8-65** Keratin 34β-E12 stain in sclerosing adenosis. There is intense cytoplasmic immunoreactivity in most basal cells.

tend to be lobulated. Simple atrophy consists of shrunken acini, whereas post-atrophic hyperplasia contains proliferating luminal cells with small amounts of clear cytoplasm. The cells may demonstrate some degree of cytologic atypia, and luminal mucin may be identified. Other histologic mimics of sclerosing adenosis include sclerosing atrophy, basal cell hyperplasia, atypical basal cell hyperplasia, and metaplastic changes associated with radiation, infarction, and prostatitis.

AAH is occasionally associated with sclerosis but lacks the dense periacinar hyalinized fibrosis sometimes seen in sclerosing adenosis. Immunohistochemical studies reveal a fragmented and discontinuous basal cell layer in AAH, whereas sclerosing adenosis usually retains an intact basal cell layer. The myoepithelial differentiation of sclerosing adenosis is distinctive. Both lesions arise chiefly in the transition zone and are usually incidental findings in TURP specimens with nodular hyperplasia.

Sclerosing adenosis can be distinguished from adenocarcinoma by a distinctive fibroblastic stroma that is rarely seen in carcinoma; benign cytology, with epithelial cells and stromal cells that lack the prominent nucleomegaly and nucleolomegaly usually seen in prostatic carcinoma; hyalinized periacinar stroma occasionally seen in sclerosing adenosis; an intact basal cell layer; a frequent association with nodular hyperplasia; and an immunophenotype of S100 protein and actin immunoreactivity.

## Verumontanum mucosal gland hyperplasia

The epithelial lining of the verumontanum may become abundant and proliferative, rarely causing infertility,[422] but criteria for separating normal and hyperplastic mucosa are not well defined.[423] This is an uncommon form of small acinar hyperplasia that mimics well-differentiated adenocarcinoma (Table 8-18).[423] It is invariably small (<1 mm), often

**Table 8-18** Verumontanum mucosal gland hyperplasia (VMGH) versus adenocarcinoma

| | VMGH | Adenocarcinoma |
|---|---|---|
| Location | Verumontanum | Anywhere in prostate |
| Size | Small (<1 mm) | Any size |
| Architecture | Lobular small acinar proliferations; may be multifocal | May be lobular and circumscribed; usually multifocal |
| Basal cell layer<br>  Light microscopy<br>  High-molecular-weight keratin (34β-E12) immunoreactivity | Usually intact; may be inconspicuous<br>Usually intact | Absent<br>Absent |
| Stromal changes | With or without stromal sclerosis | With or without stromal sclerosis |
| Cytology<br>  Nuclei<br>  Nucleoli | Mild enlargement<br>Usually inconspicuous | Enlarged<br>Usually prominent |
| Cytoplasm | Basophilic or clear on low power | Usually pale due to greater amount of cytoplasm |
| Basophilic mucin | Rare | May be present |
| Crystalloids | Rare | May be present |

**Table 8-19** Mesonephric remnants versus adenocarcinoma

| | Mesonephric remnants | Adenocarcinoma |
|---|---|---|
| Architecture | Lobular small acinar proliferation<br>Two patterns:<br>(1) Small acini with colloid-like material;<br>(2) Small acini with empty lumina or solid nests | May be lobular and circumscribed |
| Acinar contours | May be rounded or smooth; may be atrophic or contain intraluminal micropapillary projections lined by cuboidal cells | May be rounded or smooth |
| Basal cell layer<br>  Light microscopy<br>  High-molecular-weight keratin (34BE12) immunoreactivity | Usually intact; may be inconspicuous<br>Intact | Absent<br>Absent |
| Stromal changes | With or without stromal sclerosis | With or without stromal sclerosis |
| Cytology<br>  Nuclei<br>  Nucleoli | Mild enlargement<br>Usually inconspicuous | Enlarged<br>Usually prominent |
| Cytoplasm | Basophilic or clear on low power | Usually pale due to greater amount of cytoplasm |
| Luminal contents | Often with colloid-like material | May have basophilic mucin |
| Immunoreactivity<br>  PSA<br>  PAP | No<br>No | Yes<br>Yes |

multifocal, and limited anatomically to the verumontanum, utricle, ejaculatory ducts, and adjacent prostatic urethra and ducts. The acini are small and closely packed, with an intact basal cell layer, small uniform nuclei, and inconspicuous nucleoli. The basal cells display immunoreactivity for high molecular weight keratin, and are S100 protein negative. Although verumontanum mucosal gland hyperplasia and atypical adenomatous hyperplasia appear histologically distinct and arise in different areas of the prostate, it appears that each is more likely to be found in prostates if the other is also present in radical prostatectomy specimens.[77] This lesion is rare in needle biopsies, and is almost never sampled in TURP specimens because this procedure spares the verumontanum.[77]

## Hyperplasia of mesonephric remnants

Hyperplasia of mesonephric remnants in the prostate and periprostatic tissues is a rare and benign mimic of adenocarcinoma that is usually identified in TURP specimens (Table 8-19).[19,21,22,424] It shares many features with mesonephric hyperplasia of the female genital tract, including apparent infiltration of the stroma and neural spaces, lobular arrangement of small acini or solid nests lined by a single cell layer, prominent nucleoli, and eosinophilic intratubular material. In one reported case the lobular pattern was lost and the acini were infiltrative.[424]

There are two histopathologic patterns of mesonephric remnant hyperplasia, both with a lobular pattern and cuboidal cell lining. One pattern consists of small acini that contain colloid-like material reminiscent of thyroid follicles (Fig. 8-66). The lining consists of a single layer of cuboidal cells without significant cytologic atypia. The second pattern consists of small acini or solid nests of cells with empty lumina, reminiscent of nephrogenic metaplasia (Fig. 8-66). Acini may be atrophic or exhibit micropapillary projections lined by cuboidal cells. Prominent nucleoli are usually absent but are present in rare cases, compounding the diagnostic confusion.

The diagnosis may be confirmed by cellular immunoreactivity for keratin 34β-E12 (Fig. 8-67) and lack of immunoreactivity for PSA and PAP. One of the original cases was misdiagnosed as adenocarcinoma, resulting in unnecessary prostatectomy. In addition to cancer, mesonephric remnants should be distinguished from other benign small acinar proliferations of the prostate. Differential diagnostic considerations include atypical adenomatous hyperplasia, atrophy,

post-atrophic hyperplasia, basal cell hyperplasia, sclerosing adenosis, verumontanum mucosal gland hyperplasia, and atypical small acinar proliferation suspicious for but not diagnostic of malignancy.

## Benign non-neoplastic conditions

### Amyloidosis

Localized amyloidosis is rarely present in the prostate or urethra[425] but is common in the seminal vesicles (senile seminal vesicle amyloidosis), observed at autopsy in 5–8% of men between 46 and 60 years of age, 13–23% between 61 and 75 years, and 21–34% over 75 years.[426–431] It often extends bilaterally along the ejaculatory ducts, forming linear or massive nodular subepithelial deposits of amorphous eosinophilic fibrillar material (Fig. 8-68). Basement membrane thickening is observed, and deposits may be seen within the vesicular lumina, occasionally causing significant luminal narrowing.

Special stains that confirm the diagnosis of amyloid include Congo red, which appears red by light microscopy with apple-green polarization birefringence; methylene blue,

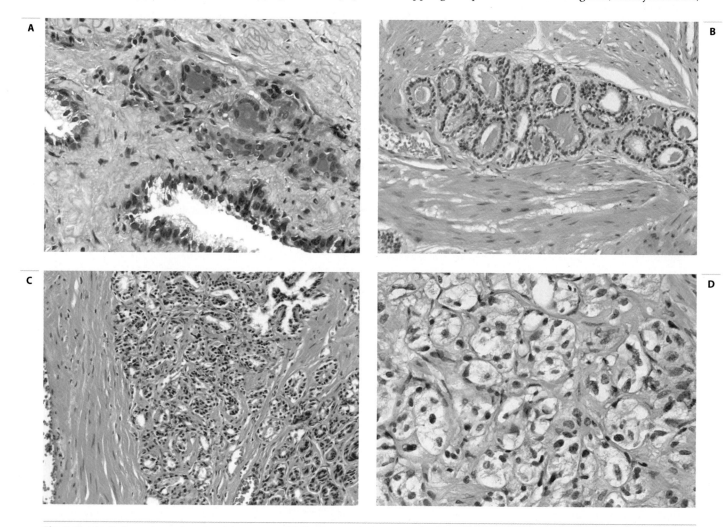

**Fig. 8-66** Histologic spectrum of mesonephric remnants. **(A)** Closely spaced acini arranged in lobules. **(B)** Dilated tubules filled with eosinophilic colloid-like material. **(C)** Infiltrating growth pattern. **(D)** Small closely spaced acini with clear cytoplasm.

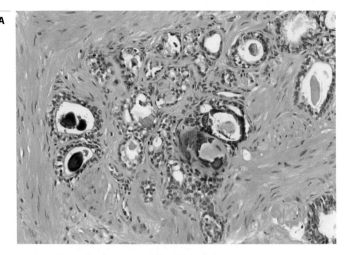

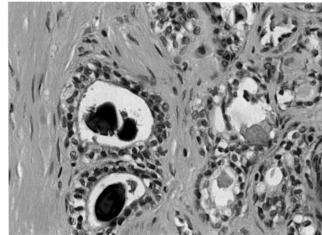

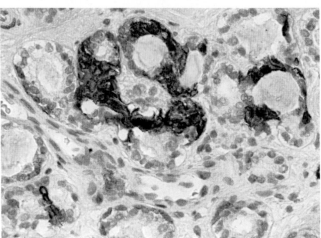

**Fig. 8-67** Mesonephric remnants in transurethral resection. **(A)** Mesonephric remnants consist of a proliferation of closely spaced acini arranged in lobules or infiltrating between muscle bundles without stromal response. Some acini show dilated tubules filled with eosinophilic colloid-like material. **(B)** High-power field shows acini lined by a single layer of small to medium-sized cuboidal cells with scant amounts of eosinophilic or amphophilic cytoplasm. **(C)** Immunohistochemistry reveals strong positive staining for high molecular weight keratin (34β-E12).

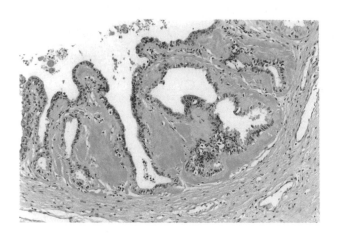

**Fig. 8-68** Amyloidosis of the ejaculatory ducts.

which reveals green polarization birefringence; crystal violet and toluidine blue, which impart a metachromatic appearance to the deposits; and periodic acid–Schiff (PAS) and sulfated Alcian blue stains, which are weakly to moderately positive. The composition of localized seminal vesicle and ejaculatory duct amyloid is histochemically unique (permanganate-sensitive, non-AA, non-B2M, non-prealbumin type), apparently derived from secretory protein of the epithelium; amyloid at other sites is derived from light chains or serum amyloid protein.[432]

## Melanosis

The prostate contains two distinct types of pigment: the common melanin-like lipofuscin-like pigment present in benign prostate epithelium,[433–435] high-grade PIN[54,436] and prostatic adenocarcinoma,[437–439] and melanin, which is rare and found only in prostatic melanocytic lesions such as melanosis, blue nevus and malignant melanoma (see Chapter 9). Melanin-like lipofuscin-like pigment is common in the normal prostate, present in the epithelium in 89% of cases and in the stroma in 78% (Fig. 8-69).[52] It is widely distributed, including the transition zone (67%), central zone (56–100%),[440] peripheral zone (89%), and periurethral glands (56%). This pigment is most commonly seen in the basal portion of the secretory luminal cells but is variable in location and amount. The reported incidence in the normal prostate varies from 4% to 70%.[441,433,434]

Pigment in the prostate has some resemblance to pigment in the seminal vesicular and ejaculatory duct epithelium, particularly when it is present in abundance, and may cause diagnostic confusion in scant specimens such as needle biopsies or TURP specimens, which may contain foci with cytologic atypia.[442] However, the pigment granules tend to be less

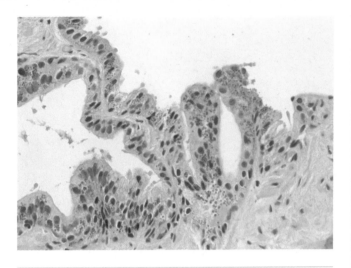

**Fig. 8-69** Prostatic epithelial pigmentation. Note granular pigment within the epithelium, reminiscent of that seen in the seminal vesicles.

**Table 8-20** Histologic features of androgen deprivation therapy in the benign prostate*

| |
| --- |
| Secretory cell layer |
|    Prominent acinar atrophy |
|    Decreased ratio of acini to stroma |
|    Enlargement and clearing of cytoplasm |
|    Prominent clear cell change |
| Basal cell layer |
|    Hyperplasia |
|    Prominent component of benign acini |
|    Squamous metaplasia |
| Stroma |
|    Edema in early stages; fibrosis in late stages |
|    Patchy condensation, resulting in focal hypercellularity |
|    Focal chronic inflammation (lymphohistiocytic) |

*There is variability in these changes, depending on the method of treatment.

coarse and refractile, and have a unique histochemical profile that allows them to be distinguished from seminal vesicular tissue: melanin-like (Fontana–Masson stain-positive and potassium permanganate bleaching-sensitive) and lipofuscin-like (prolonged Ziehl–Neelsen stain-positive and S100-negative); unlike pigment in seminal vesicle epithelium that is not melanin-like (Fontana–Masson stain-negative).

These findings suggest that this pigment is different from typical cutaneous melanin: the lipofuscin-like material ('wear and tear' or 'old age' pigment) is probably an endogenous cellular byproduct of prostate epithelium rather than melanocytic in origin. Its only significance is to be aware of its distribution, as epithelium or stroma with pigment is not necessarily of seminal vesicle origin.

## Endometriosis

Endometriosis is a very rare finding in the prostate, with fewer than a dozen cases reported, invariably following years of estrogen therapy for prostate cancer.[443–445] Patients present with hematuria and obstructive symptoms.

## Treatment-associated changes

Treatment-associated changes in the benign and cancerous prostate create a diagnostic challenge in pathologic interpretation, particularly in needle biopsy specimens. It is critical that the clinician provide the pertinent history of androgen deprivation or radiation therapy to assist the pathologist in rendering the correct diagnosis. This section summarizes therapy-related pathologic findings in the prostate, with emphasis on the recognition of treated adenocarcinoma.

### Androgen deprivation therapy

One of the most popular forms of treatment for prostate cancer – androgen-deprivation therapy – has been in use for more than five decades. Contemporary therapies have varying mechanisms of action, including combined andro-gen blockage (gonadotrophin-releasing hormone – GnRH – agonists (e.g., goserelin and leuprolide) combined with an androgen receptor antagonists (e.g., flutamide, bicalutamide, and nilutamide)), GnRH antagonists (e.g., abarelix), and 5α-reductase inhibitors (e.g., finasteride and dutasteride). These agents are used for preoperative tumor shrinkage, symptomatic relief of metastases, cancer prophylaxis,[446–448] and the treatment of hyperplasia.[449,450]

To achieve total androgen deprivation, therapy should be effective in eliminating both testicular and adrenal hormones. Typical side effects of androgen deprivation therapy include hot flashes, loss of libido, and impotence. There are several methods of achieving androgen deprivation.

The histopathologic effects of most agents are similar (Table 8-20).[451–459] All modes of hormonal treatment alter the benign and cancerous prostatic epithelium, inducing programmed apoptosis characterized by fragmentation of tumor DNA, the appearance of apoptotic bodies, and inhibition of cell growth. The altered epithelium displays involution and acinar atrophy, cytoplasmic clearing, nuclear and nucleolar shrinkage, and chromatin condensation, although changes with 5α-reductase inhibitors appear to be much less pronounced and variable than with other agents (see below).

Following androgen deprivation therapy, benign and hyperplastic prostatic acini are atrophic and collapsed, typically with prominent basal cell hyperplasia and epithelial vacuolization. In some areas the lining epithelium has scant or moderate cytoplasm that is darkly eosinophilic and coarsely granular or clear. The majority of nuclei are small, with condensed chromatin and inconspicuous nucleoli (Fig. 8-70). Luminal secretions are inspissated, resembling corpora amylacea, but usually lack discrete laminations or angulations; multinucleated cells are infrequently present at the periphery. Squamous metaplasia is not significantly increased with contemporary forms of androgen deprivation therapy, but is prominent with estrogen treatment and orchidectomy. Lipofuscin pigment may be observed in scattered benign epithelial and stromal cells, and, rarely, in tumor cells.

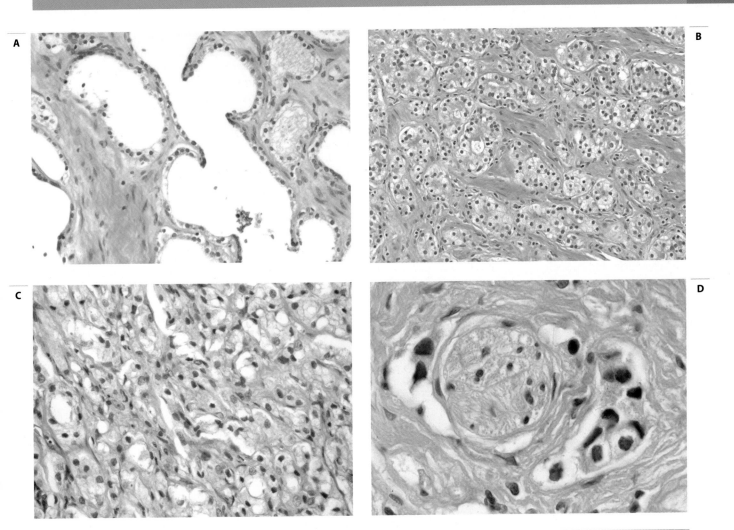

**Fig. 8-70** Androgen deprivation therapy effect. **(A)** Benign prostatic epithelium shows abundant clear cytoplasm, nuclear shrinkage and small dark nuclei. **(B, C)** Androgen derivation therapy in prostatic adenocarcinoma reveals prominent cytoplasmic clearance and small hyperchromatic nuclei. **(D)** Perineural invasion may be mistaken for stromal lymphocytes or myocytes.

## Histopathologic findings after 5α-reductase inhibitors

The primary nuclear androgen responsible for the maintenance of epithelial function and the most potent is dihydrotestosterone.[460,461] By inhibiting DHT synthesis, 5α-reductase inhibitors reduce the androgen drive to hyperplastic and malignant prostate cells while maintaining testosterone levels. Finasteride inhibits only the type 2 isoenzyme of 5α-reductase, thereby partly blocking the conversion of testosterone. Unlike finasteride, dutasteride is a dual inhibitor of both 5α-reductase isoenzymes,[462] resulting in the suppression of serum DHT by more than 90% compared to the 70% seen with finasteride.[460,463] Finasteride is somewhat less effective than other forms of androgen deprivation therapy in altering the histology of the benign and neoplastic prostate (Fig. 8-70), although some changes have been described in all but one report.

Shrinkage of the benign prostate by 5α-reductase inhibitors has been documented in many preclinical[464,465] and clinical[455,466–471] studies (Table 8-21). Similarly, in the benign and hyperplastic prostate, finasteride reduced volume by 20–30%, with an increase in the ratio of stroma to epithelium compared to untreated matched controls.[455,466,468,469] The ducts and acini were variable in size, and some ducts and acini retained a bistratified epithelium (Fig. 8-70); Marks et al.[469] found a 55% decline in epithelial content after 6 months of treatment, and this decline correlated with a reduction in prostate volume. By 24 months the epithelium had involuted further, contracting from 19.2% to 6.4% of mean tissue composition (6.0 mL vs 2.0 mL overall mean epithelial volume; stroma/epithelial ratio from 3.2 to 17.4).[469] In another study, after 24 months of treatment the epithelial involution was similar in different zones of the prostate.[468] The treated secretory cells displayed shrunken nuclei, condensed chromatin, inconspicuous nucleoli and cytoplasmic clearing, and basal cells became prominent. Apoptotic bodies were occasionally present in the epithelial cells and lumina, but there were no mitotic figures. Conversely, one prospective study of needle biopsies from 25 patients treated for up to 4 years and 25 untreated controls found no significant differences in benign epithelium.[472] The cause of these conflicting findings is uncertain, but may be

**Table 8-21** Pathologic changes following finasteride in the benign and hyperplastic human prostate

### Atrophy and involution

Rittmaster RS, et al. J Clin Endocrinol Metab 1996; 81:814

Montironi R, et al. J Urol Pathol 1996; 4:123

Montironi R, et al. J Clin Pathol 1996; 49:324

Civantos F, et al. J Urol Pathol 1997; 6:1

Marks LS, et al. J Urol 1997; 157:2171

Saez C, et al. Prostate 1998; 37:84

Marks LS, et al. Urology 1999; 53:574

Pomante R, et al. Anal Quant Cytol Histol 1999; 21:63

Thomas LN, et al. Prostate 2000; 43:203

### Smaller nuclei and nucleoli

Montironi R, et al. J Urol Pathol 1996; 4:123

Pomante R, et al. Anal Quant Cytol Histol 1999; 21:63

### Increased apoptosis

Montironi R, et al. J Urol Pathol 1994; 2:161

Rittmaster RS, et al. J Clin Endocrinol Metab 1996; 81:814

Glassman DT, et al. Prostate 2001; 46:45

### Decreased microvessel density

Hochberg DA, et al. J Urol 2002; 1731

Pareek G, et al. J Urol 2003; 169:20

### No increase in cell proliferation

Montironi R, et al. J Urol Pathol 1996; 4:123

Glassman DT, et al. Prostate 2001; 46:45

### No effect

Yang XJ et al. Urology 53:696, 1999

attributable to sampling variation with the needle biopsy study approach.

Iczkowski et al.[473] found that the regressive changes in benign epithelium with dutasteride treatment were more marked in the peripheral zone than in other areas of the prostate, and these changes were greater than those observed in cancer. A significant decrease in epithelial height was observed only in benign epithelium, although similar trends were noted in cancer and high-grade PIN. Andriole et al.[474] noted a similar degree of reduction in epithelial cell size in the peripheral and transition zones following dutasteride treatment. The greater sensitivity of the peripheral zone to dutasteride may be attributed to its higher density of androgen receptors compared to the transition zone, as shown by saturation binding assays with a competitive inhibitor.[475–477] Nuclear androgen receptors have been estimated to be present at twice the density[476] and in 71% versus 39% of peripheral versus transition zone specimens studied from 38 prostates.[477]

These results are concordant with other studies of androgen deprivation, emphasizing the limited repertoire of responses to androgen deprivation of the prostate. Finaste-

ride treatment in rats[465,467] and dogs[478] induced prostatic atrophy and involution, similar to humans, although the atrophy was often patchy and incomplete, suggesting differential sensitivity within the gland. Prahalada et al.[465] reported that chronic administration of finasteride resulted in a reduction in the weight of the rat prostate compared to controls, and this finding correlated with a decrease in the total number of epithelial and stromal cells per acinus throughout the treated rat prostate, although they found no qualitative differences in prostatic morphology between the control and finasteride-treated groups.

## Immunohistochemical findings after androgen deprivation therapy

Prostate-specific antigen,[1] prostatic acid phosphatase (PAP), and racemase are retained in benign and neoplastic cells after 3 months of therapy, but decline with longer duration of therapy;[479] keratin 34β-E12 and p63 remain negative, regardless of duration, indicating an absent basal cell layer in carcinoma.[479] No differences were found in the expression of neuroendocrine differentiation markers such as chromogranin, neuron-specific enolase, β-HCG, and serotonin following androgen deprivation therapy.

Proliferating cell nuclear antigen (PCNA) immunoreactivity declines after androgen deprivation therapy, indicating that androgens regulate cyclically expressed proteins involved in cell proliferation.[480–482]

## Radiation therapy

The difficulty of biopsy interpretation after radiation is multifactorial and includes the separation of carcinoma from its many mimics, the identification of small foci of carcinoma, and separation of treatment effects in normal tissue from recurrent or persistent carcinoma. As more patients choose radiotherapy, particularly brachytherapy, and as these patients are observed for longer periods, pathologists bear an increasing burden to discriminate irradiated benign acini from irradiated adenocarcinoma.

The degree of histologic change caused by radiation in benign or hyperplastic acini varies with the dose and duration of irradiation and the interval from the start of therapy (Table 8-22). Changes include acinar atrophy, distortion with loss of cytoplasm, and a reduced ratio of acini to stroma (Fig. 8-71). Nuclear changes include enlargement (86% of cases) and prominent nucleoli (50%).[483] Acinar secretory cells are more sensitive to irradiation necrosis than are basal cells: the basal cell layer is the proliferative compartment in benign acini. Consequently, atypical basal cell hyperplasia, often with an absent secretory cell layer, is seen in 57% of cases,[483] defined as basal cell proliferation with prominent nucleoli in more than 10% of cells. Stroma may be fibrotic, with paucicellular scarring, and vascular changes include intimal thickening and medial fibrosis (Table 8-22). Pathologists must be aware of these changes because they preclude the usual reliance on nuclear and nucleolar size to help identify prostate cancer.

The changes following three-dimensional conformal therapy are similar to those after conventional external beam

**Table 8-22** Histopathologic findings in benign post-irradiation prostate needle biopsies at the time of PSA (biochemical) failure

| Histopathologic findings | % cases |
|---|---|
| Inflammation | 39 |
| Atrophy | 79 |
| Post-atrophic hyperplasia | 18 |
| Acinar distortion | 54 |
| Decreased acinar/stromal ratio | 86 |
| Basal cell hyperplasia | 68 |
| Atypical basal cell hyperplasia | 57 |
| Hyperplastic (proliferative change) | 11 |
| Squamous metaplasia | 0 |
| Eosinophilic metaplasia | 21 |
| Stromal changes | |
|    Stromal fibrosis | 93 |
|    Stromal edema | 21 |
|    Stromal calcification | 21 |
|    Hemosiderin deposition | 0 |
|    Atypical fibroblasts | 25 |
|    Necrosis | 0 |
|    Granulation tissue formation | 0 |
| Myointimal proliferation | 11 |
| Cytologic changes | |
|    Nuclear pyknosis | 75 |
|    Nuclear enlargement | 86 |
|    Prominent nucleoli | 50 |
|    Bizarre nuclei | 54 |
|    Cytoplasmic vacuolization | 29 |
| Intraluminal contents | |
|    Crystalloids | 0 |
|    Mucin | 4 |
|    Eosinophilic granular secretions | 39 |
|    Corpora amylacea | 32 |

therapy.[484] The addition of androgen deprivation therapy has no appreciable histopathologic effect on the radiation-altered prostate.[484]

## Cryoablation therapy (cryosurgery)

Cryosurgical ablation refers to freezing of the prostate. Multiple cryoprobe needles filled with circulating liquid nitrogen transform the prostate into an iceball, resulting in substantial tissue destruction and the death of benign and malignant cells. The flow of liquid nitrogen through the probes is adjusted to create the desired freezing pattern and extent of tissue destruction in the prostate; no liquid nitrogen comes into contact with the tissue.

Following cryosurgery the prostate shows typical features of repair, including marked stromal fibrosis and hyalinization, basal cell hyperplasia with ductal and acinar regeneration, squamous metaplasia, urothelial metaplasia, stromal hemorrhage (Fig. 8-72), and hemosiderin deposition (Fig. 8-72).[485–489] Coagulative necrosis is present between 6 and 30 weeks of therapy (Fig. 8-72), but patchy chronic inflammation is more common after that (Fig. 8-72). Focal granulomatous inflammation is associated with epithelial disruption due to corpora amylacea. Dystrophic calcification is infrequent and usually appears in areas with the greatest reparative response.

In some cases the benign prostate appears unchanged, with no definite evidence of tissue or immune response, indicating lack of inclusion of that area in the ablation killing zone. As the postoperative interval increases, biopsy is more likely to contain unaltered benign prostatic tissue.

## Hyperthermia

All forms of hyperthermia (e.g., high-intensity focused ultrasound (HIFU), microwave thermotherapy, laser therapy, and hot water balloon thermotherapy) result in sharply circumscribed hemorrhagic coagulative necrosis that soon organizes with granulation tissue; the pattern and extent of injury is determined by the method of thermocoagulation employed, the duration of treatment, tissue perfusion factors, and the ratio of epithelium to stroma in the tissue being

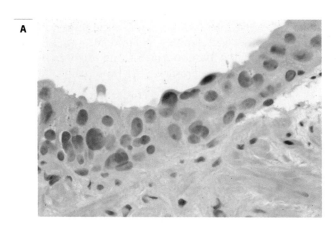

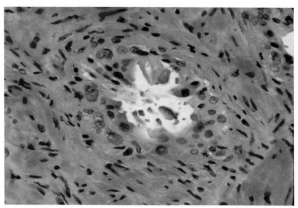

**Fig. 8-71** Radiation changes. **(A)** Prostatic epithelium mimicking high-grade PIN. There are marked nuclear abnormalities, including variation in size and shape and hyperchromasia. **(B)** Prostatic epithelium showing nuclear abnormalities involving the basal cell and secretory cell layers.

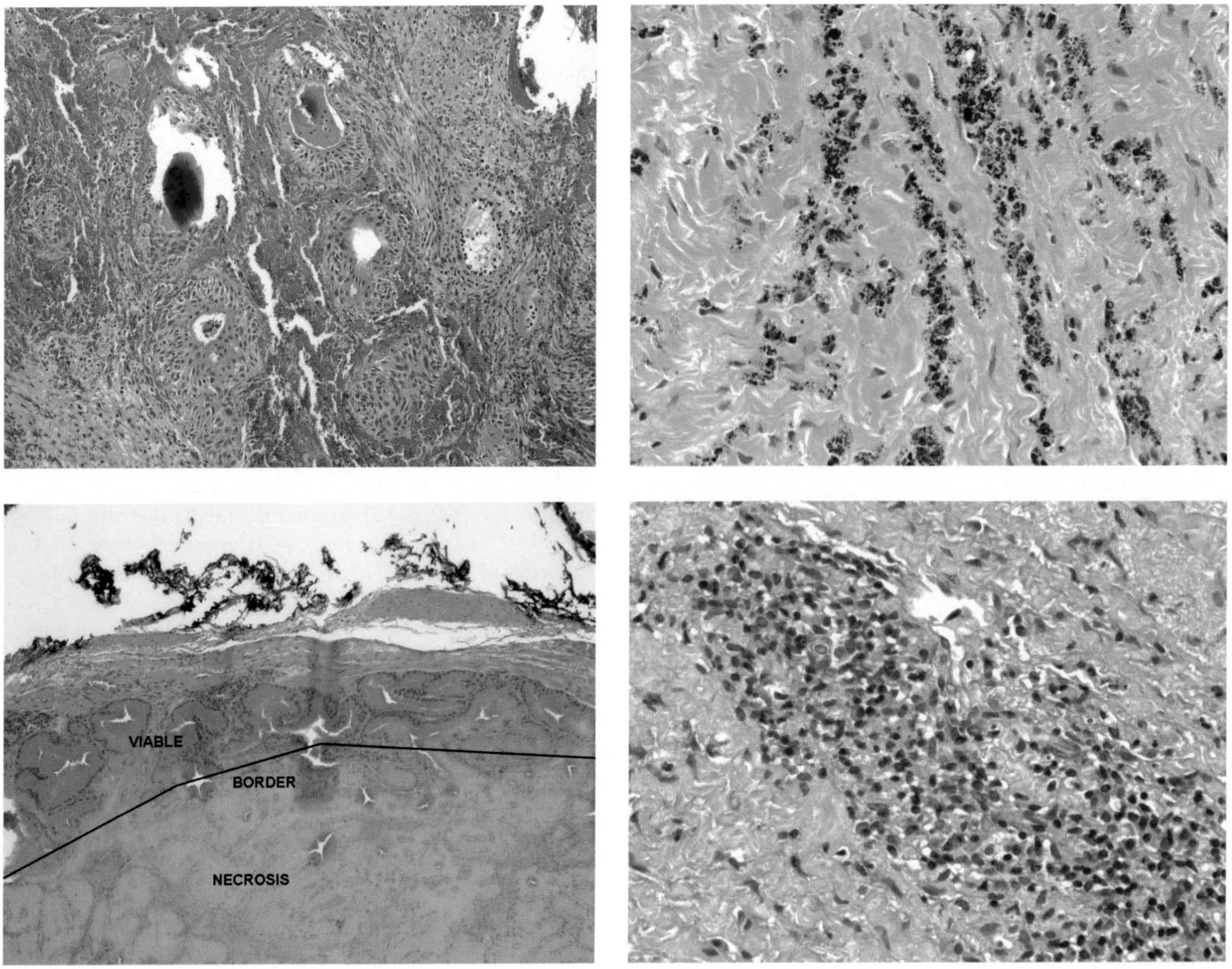

**Fig. 8-72** Cryoablation effects. **(A)** Stromal hemorrhage with residual viable epithelium following prostatic cryoablation (human). **(B)** Hemosiderin deposition (ochre pigment) within the stoma after cryosurgery (human). **(C)** Coagulative necrosis (bottom of image) with devitalization and a thin rim of subcapsular viable tissue (top) following cryosurgery (dog prostate). **(D)** Patchy chronic inflammation within prostatic stroma is a common finding following cryoablation (human).

treated.[490-495] Transurethral methods may be safer and more effective than transrectal methods because they appear to avoid injury to the rectal mucosa. When delivered transurethrally, laser thermocoagulation and microwave hyperthermia do not usually involve the peripheral zone or neighboring structures, presumably because of differences in tissue perfusion.[491,496] Coagulation necrosis is greater in areas of predominantly epithelial nodular hyperplasia rather than predominantly stromal hyperplasia and the dense fibromuscular tissue of the bladder neck. Confluent coagulation necrosis occurs when multiple laser lesions are created in a single transverse plane. Correlation with histopathologic findings showed gadolinium-enhanced MRI to be useful for determining the location, pattern, and extent of necrosis caused within the prostate by minimally invasive techniques.[497]

# REFERENCES

1. Marker P, Donjacour AA, Dahiya R, Cunha GR. Hormonal, cellular, and molecular control of prostatic development. Dev Biol. 2003 253 (2): 165–174.

2. McNeal J. Prostate. In: Sternberg SS, ed. Histology for pathologists, 2nd edn. Philadelphia: Lippincott-Raven, 1997; 997–1097.

3. Shapiro E. Prostatic morphogenesis, stromal–epithelial interactions, zonal anatomy, and quantitative morphometry. In: Fitzpatrick JM, ed. The prostate. New York: Churchill Livingstone, 1989; 8–16.

4. Wong YC, Wang XH, Ling MT. Prostate development and carcinogenesis. Int Rev Cytol 2003; 227: 65–130.

5. Timms BG, Lee CW, Aumuller G, Seitz J. Instructive induction of prostate growth and differentiation by a defined urogenital sinus mesenchyme. Microsc Res Tech 1995; 30: 319–332.

6. Zhuang TN, Ly LP, Cumming RG, Handelsman DJ. Growth and

development during early manhood as determinants of prostate size in later life. J Clin Endocrinol Metab 2005; 90: 6055–6063.

7. Matsuda T, Fujime M, Suda K. Relationship between the prostatic tissue components and natural history of benign prostatic hyperplasia. Anal Quant Cytol Histol 2006; 28: 121–124.

8. Mong A, Bellah R. Imaging the pediatric prostate. Radiol Clin North Am 2006; 44: 749–756, ix.

9. Xing JP, Dang JG, Wu DP, et al. [Papillary cystadenocarcinoma in a Mullerian duct cyst: report of a case with literature review]. Zhonghua Nan Ke Xue 2006; 12: 218–221.

10. Kato H, Hayama M, Furuya S, et al. Anatomical and histological studies of so-called Mullerian duct cyst. Int J Urol 2005; 12: 465–468.

11. Furuya S, Kato H. A clinical entity of cystic dilatation of the utricle associated with hemospermia. J Urol 2005; 174: 1039–1042.

12. Yanai T, Okazaki T, Yamataka A, et al. Cysts of the ejaculatory system: a report of two cases. Pediatr Surg Int 2005; 21: 939–942.

13. Moudouni SM, Tligui M, Doublet JD, et al. Laparoscopic excision of seminal vesicle cyst revealed by obstruction urinary symptoms. Int J Urol 2006; 13: 311–314.

14. Pimpalwar A, Chowdhary S, Huskisson J, Corkery JJ. Cysts of the ejaculatory system – a treatable cause of recurrent epididymo-orchitis in children. Eur J Pediatr Surg 2002; 12: 281–285.

15. Gozen AS, Alagol B. Endoscopic management of seminal-vesical cyst with right renal agenesis causing acute urinary retention: Case report. J Endourol 2006; 20: 919–922.

16. Kosan M, Tul M, Inal G, et al. A large seminal vesicle cyst with contralateral renal agenesis. Int Urol Nephrol 2006; 17: 591–592.

17. Chuang KL, Lai WI, Chiang YJ. Giant seminal vesicle cyst resembling megaureter with hydronephrosis. Arch Androl 2005; 51: 367–369.

18. Mitterberger M, Frausche F, Strasser H, et al. Giant seminal vesicle cyst. Wien Klin Wochenschr 2005; 117: 18.

19. Val-Bernal JF, Gomez-Ortega JM. Hyperplasia of prostatic mesonephric remnants: a potential pitfall in the evaluation of prostate gland biopsy. J Urol 1995; 154: 1138–1139.

20. Malpica A, Ro JY, Troncoso P, et al. Nephrogenic adenoma of the prostatic urethra involving the prostate gland: a clinicopathologic and immunohistochemical study of eight cases. Hum Pathol 1994; 25: 390–395.

21. Andersen CB, Horn T, Rasmussen F, Larsen S. Mesonephric remnants involving renal pelvis and prostatic urethra: a diagnostic problem towards adenocarcinoma. Scand J Urol Nephrol 1994; 157: 119–122.

22. Gikas PW, Del Buono EA, Epstein JI. Florid hyperplasia of mesonephric remnants involving prostate and periprostatic tissue. Possible confusion with adenocarcinoma. Am J Surg Pathol 1993; 17: 454–460.

23. Bostwick DG, Qian J, Schlesinger C. Contemporary pathology of prostate cancer. Urol Clin North Am 2003; 30: 181–207.

24. McNeal JE, Bostwick DG. Anatomy of the prostate: Implications for disease. In: Bostwick DG, ed. Pathology of the prostate. New York: Churchill Livingstone, 1990; 1–14.

25. Shapiro E, Huang H, McFadden DE, et al. The prostatic utricle is not a Mullerian duct remnant: immunohistochemical evidence for a distinct urogenital sinus origin. J Urol 2004; 172: 1753–1756; discussion 1756.

26. Bostwick DG. Normal anatomy and histology. In: Bostwick DG, Dundore P, eds. Biopsy pathology of the prostate. London: Chapman & Hall, 1997: 1–26.

27. Grenier N, Devonec M. [Imaging of normal, hyperplastic and inflammatory prostate gland]. J Radiol 2006; 87: 165–187.

28. Bostwick DG, Brawer MK. Prostatic intra-epithelial neoplasia and early invasion in prostate cancer. Cancer 1987; 59: 788–794.

29. Babinski MA, Chagas MA, Costa WS, Sampaio FJ. Prostatic epithelial and luminal area in the transition zone acini: morphometric analysis in normal and hyperplastic human prostate. BJU Int 2003; 92: 592–596.

30. Zhao H, Ramos CF, Brooks JD, Peehl DM. Distinctive gene expression of prostatic stromal cells cultured from diseased versus normal tissues. J Cell Physiol 2007; 210: 111–121.

31. van der Heul-Nieuwenhuijsen L, Hendriksen PJ, van der Kwast TH, Jenster G. Gene expression profiling of the human prostate zones. BJU Int 2006; 98: 886–897.

32. Shapiro E, Huang H, Masch RJ, et al. Immunolocalization of estrogen receptor alpha and beta in human fetal prostate. J Urol 2005; 174: 2051–2053.

33. Bostwick DG. Progression of prostatic intraepithelial neoplasia to early invasive adenocarcinoma. Eur Urol 1996; 30: 145–152.

34. Bostwick DG, Aquilina JW. Prostatic intraepithelial neoplasia (PIN) and other prostatic lesions as risk factors and surrogate endpoints for cancer chemoprevention trials. J Cell Biochem 1996; 25: 156–164.

35. Bostwick DG, Pacelli A, Lopez-Beltran A. Molecular biology of prostatic intraepithelial neoplasia. Prostate 1996; 29: 117–134.

36. Schalken JA, van Leenders G. Cellular and molecular biology of the prostate: stem cell biology. Urology 2003; 62: 11–20.

37. Signoretti S, Loda M. Defining cell lineages in the prostate epithelium. Cell Cycle 2006; 5: 138–141.

38. Maygarden SJ, Strom S, Ware JL. Localization of epidermal growth factor receptor by immunohistochemical methods in human prostatic carcinoma, prostatic intraepithelial neoplasia, and benign hyperplasia. Arch Pathol Lab Med 1992; 116: 269–273.

39. Karaivanov M, Todorova K, Kuzmanov A, Hayrabedyan S. Quantitative immunohistochemical detection of the molecular expression patterns in proliferative inflammatory atrophy. J Mol Histol 2007; 38: 1–11.

40. Molinie V, Herve JM, Lebret T, et al. [Value of the antibody cocktail anti p63+anti p504s for the diagnosis of prostatic cancer]. Ann Pathol 2004; 24: 6–16.

41. Hameed O, Humphrey PA. Immunohistochemistry in diagnostic surgical pathology of the prostate. Semin Diagn Pathol 2005; 22: 88–104.

42. Hameed O, Sublett J, Humphrey PA. Immunohistochemical stains for p63 and alpha-methylacyl-CoA racemase, versus a cocktail comprising both, in the diagnosis of prostatic carcinoma: a comparison of the immunohistochemical staining of 430 foci in radical prostatectomy and needle biopsy tissues. Am J Surg Pathol 2005; 29: 579–587.

43. Sung MT, Jiang Z, Montironi R, et al. Alpha-methylacyl-CoA racemase (P504S)/34betaE12/p63 triple cocktail stain in prostatic adenocarcinoma after hormonal therapy. Hum Pathol 2007; 38: 332–341.

44. Adlakha H, Bostwick DG. Paneth cell-like change in prostatic adenocarcinoma represents neuroendocrine differentiation: Report of 30 cases. Hum Pathol 1994; 25: 135–139.

45. Yuan TC, Veeramani S, Lin FF, et al. Androgen deprivation induces human prostate epithelial neuroendocrine differentiation of androgen-sensitive LNCaP cells. Endocr Relat Cancer 2006; 13: 151–167.

46. Abrahamsson PA, Wadstrom LB, Alumets J, et al. Peptide-hormone- and serotonin-immunoreactive tumour cells in carcinoma of the prostate. Pathol Res Pract 1987; 182: 298–307.

47. Abrahamsson PA, Alumets J, Wadstrom LB, et al. Peptide hormones, serotonin, and other cell differentiation markers in benign hyperplasia and in carcinoma of the prostate. Prog Clin Biol Res 1987; 243A: 489–502.

48. Bostwick DG, Qian J, Pacelli A, et al. Neuroendocrine expression in node positive prostate cancer: correlation with systemic progression and patient survival. J Urol 2002; 168: 1204–1211.

49. Aprikian AG, Cordon-Cardo C, Fair WR, Reuter VE. Characterization of

neuroendocrine differentiation in human benign prostate and prostatic adenocarcinoma. Cancer 1993; 71: 3952–3965.

50. Di Sant'Agnese PA. Neuroendocrine differentiation in prostatic carcinoma. Recent findings and new concepts. Cancer 1995; 75: 1850–1859.

51. Daneshmand S, Dorff TB, Quek ML, et al. Ethnic differences in neuroendocrine cell expression in normal human prostatic tissue. Urology 2005; 65: 1008–1012.

52. Amin MB, Bostwick DG. Pigment in prostatic epithelium and adenocarcinoma: a potential source of diagnostic confusion with seminal vesicular epithelium. Mod Pathol 1996; 9: 791–795.

53. Farid MK, Gahukamble LD. Melanosis of the prostate in an elderly patient – a case report. Cent Afr J Med 1995; 41: 101–102.

54. Brennick JB, O'Connell JX, Dickersin GR, et al. Lipofuscin pigmentation (so-called 'melanosis') of the prostate. Am J Surg Pathol 1994; 18: 446–454.

55. Cohen RJ, McNeal JE, Redmond SL, et al. Luminal contents of benign and malignant prostatic glands: correspondence to altered secretory mechanisms. Hum Pathol 2000; 31: 94–100.

56. Silva LC, Saldiva PH, Ellinger F, et al. Quantitation of conventional histologic parameters and biologic factors in prostatic needle biopsy are useful to distinguish paramalignant from malignant disease. Pathol Res Pract 2004; 200: 599–608.

57. Christian JD, Lamm TC, Morrow JF, Bostwick DG. Corpora amylacea in adenocarcinoma of the prostate: incidence and histology within needle core biopsies. Mod Pathol 2005; 18: 36–39.

58. Mathur SK, Gupta S, Marwah N, et al. Significance of mucin stain in differentiating benign and malignant lesions of prostate. Indian J Pathol Microbiol 2003; 46: 593–595.

59. Allsbrook WC Jr, Simms WW. Histochemistry of the prostate. Hum Pathol 1992; 23: 297–305.

60. Epstein JI, Fynheer J. Acidic mucin in the prostate: can it differentiate adenosis from adenocarcinoma? Hum Pathol 1992; 23: 1321–1325.

61. Goldstein NS, Qian J, Bostwick DG. Mucin expression in atypical adenomatous hyperplasia of the prostate. Hum Pathol 1995; 26: 887–891.

62. Ro JY, Grignon DJ, Troncoso P, Ayala AG. Mucin in prostatic adenocarcinoma. Semin Diagn Pathol 1988; 5: 273–283.

63. Cozzi PJ, Wang J, Delprado W, et al. MUC1, MUC2, MUC4, MUC5AC and MUC6 expression in the progression of prostate cancer. Clin Exp Metastasis 2005; 22: 565–573.

64. O'Connor JC, Julian J, Lim SD, Carson DD. MUC1 expression in human prostate cancer cell lines and primary tumors. Prostate Cancer Prostatic Dis 2005; 8: 36–44.

65. Xiang ST, Zhou SW, Guan W, et al. [Tumor infiltrating dendritic cells and Mucin1 gene expression in benign prostatic hyperplasia and prostate cancer]. Zhonghua Nan Ke Xue 2003; 9: 497–500.

66. Singh AP, Chauhan SC, Bafna S, et al. Aberrant expression of transmembrane mucins, MUC1 and MUC4, in human prostate carcinomas. Prostate 2006; 66: 421–429.

67. Leroy X, Ballereau C, Villers A, et al. MUC6 is a marker of seminal vesicle-ejaculatory duct epithelium and is useful for the differential diagnosis with prostate adenocarcinoma. Am J Surg Pathol 2003; 27: 519–521.

68. Seaman AR. Cytochemical observations on the corpora amylacea of the human prostate gland. J Urol 1956; 76: 99–106.

69. Magura CE, Spector M. Scanning electron microscopy of human prostatic corpora amylacea and corpora calculi, and prostatic calculi. Scan Electron Microsc 1979; 3: 713–720.

70. Humphrey PA VR. Corpora amylacea in adenocarcinoma of the prostate: prevalence in 100 prostatectomies and clinicopathologic correlations. Surg Pathol 1990; 3: 133–141.

71. Morales E, Polo LA, Pastor LM, et al. Characterization of corpora amylacea glycoconjugates in normal and hyperplastic glands of human prostate. J Mol Histol 2005; 36: 235–242.

72. Shakya G, Malla S, Shakya KN. Salient and co-morbid features in benign prostatic hyperplasia: a histopathological study of the prostate. Kathmandu Univ Med J 2003; 1: 104–109.

73. Untergasser G, Madersbacher S, Berger P. Benign prostatic hyperplasia: age-related tissue-remodeling. Exp Gerontol 2005; 40: 121–128.

74. Fulmer BR, Turner TT. Effect of inflammation on prostatic protein synthesis and luminal secretion in vivo. J Urol 1999; 162: 248–253.

75. Woods JE, Soh S, Wheeler TM. Distribution and significance of microcalcifications in the neoplastic and nonneoplastic prostate. Arch Pathol Lab Med 1998; 122: 152–155.

76. Humphrey P. Prostate gland development and anatomic structure. In: Humphrey P, ed. Prostate pathology. Hong Kong: American Society for Clinical Pathology, 2003; 3–29.

77. Muezzinoglu B, Gurbuz Y. Stromal microcalcification in prostate. Malays J Pathol 2001; 23: 31–33.

78. Kovi J, Rao MS, Heshmat MY, et al. Incidence of prostatic calcification in blacks in Washington, DC, and selected African cities. Correlation of specimen roentgenographs and pathologic findings. Cooperative Prostatic Research Group. Urology 1979; 14: 363–369.

79. Chen X, Zhao J, Salim S, Garcia FU. Intraprostatic spermatozoa: zonal distribution and association with atrophy. Hum Pathol 2006; 37: 345–351.

80. Schowinsky JT, Epstein JI. Distorted rectal tissue on prostate needle biopsy: a mimicker of prostate cancer. Am J Surg Pathol 2006; 30: 866–870.

81. Ayala AG, Ro JY, Babaian R, et al. The prostatic capsule: does it exist? Its importance in the staging and treatment of prostatic carcinoma. Am J Surg Pathol 1989; 13: 21–27.

82. Kiyoshima K, Yokomizo A, Yoshida T, et al. Anatomical features of periprostatic tissue and its surroundings: a histological analysis of 79 radical retropubic prostatectomy specimens. Jpn J Clin Oncol 2004; 34: 463–468.

83. Hong H, Koch MO, Foster RS, et al. Anatomic distribution of periprostatic adipose tissue: a mapping study of 100 radical prostatectomy specimens. Cancer 2003; 97: 1639–1643.

84. Cohen RJ, Stables S. Intraprostatic fat. Hum Pathol 1998; 29: 424–425.

85. Billis A. Intraprostatic fat: does it exist? Hum Pathol 2004; 35: 525.

86. Sung MT, Eble JN, Cheng L. Invasion of fat justifies assignment of stage pT3a in prostatic adenocarcinoma. Pathology 2006; 38: 309–311.

87. Kuo T, Gomez LG. Monstrous epithelial cells in human epididymis and seminal vesicles. A pseudomalignant change. Am J Surg Pathol 1981; 5: 483–490.

88. Madara JL, Haggitt RC, Federman M. Intranuclear inclusions of the human vas deferens. Arch Pathol Lab Med 1978; 102: 648–650.

89. Kovi J, Jackson MA, Akberzie ME. Unusual smooth muscle change in the prostate. Arch Pathol Lab Med 1979; 103: 204–205.

90. Walsh PC, Lepor H, Eggleston JC. Radical prostatectomy with preservation of sexual function: anatomical and pathological considerations. Prostate 1983; 4: 473–485.

91. Powell MS, Li R, Dai H, et al. Neuroanatomy of the normal prostate. Prostate 2005; 65: 52–57.

92. Sakamoto N, Hasegawa Y, Koga H, et al. Presence of ganglia within the prostatic capsule: ganglion involvement in prostatic cancer. Prostate 1999; 40: 167–171.

93. Ali TZ, Epstein JI. Perineural involvement by benign prostatic glands on needle biopsy. Am J Surg Pathol 2005; 29: 1159–1163.

94. Eichelberg C, Erbersdobler A, Michl U, et al. Nerve distribution along the prostatic capsule. Eur Urol 2007; 51: 105–110; discussion 110–101.

95. Trojan L, Michel MS, Rensch F, et al. Lymph and blood vessel architecture in benign and malignant prostatic tissue:

lack of lymphangiogenesis in prostate carcinoma assessed with novel lymphatic marker lymphatic vessel endothelial hyaluronan receptor (LYVE-1). J Urol 2004; 172: 103–107.

96. Shah RB, Lee MW, Giraldo AA, Amin MB. Histologic and histochemical characterization of seminal vesicle intraluminal secretions. Arch Pathol Lab Med 2001; 125: 141–145.

97. Chughtai B, Sawas A, O'Malley RL, et al. A neglected gland: a review of Cowper's gland. Int J Androl 2005; 28: 74–77.

98. Srigley JR. Benign mimickers of prostatic adenocarcinoma. Mod Pathol 2004; 17: 328–348.

99. Saboorian MH, Huffman H, Ashfaq R, et al. Distinguishing Cowper's glands from neoplastic and pseudoneoplastic lesions of prostate: immunohistochemical and ultrastructural studies. Am J Surg Pathol 1997; 21: 1069–1074.

100. Varma M, Berney DM, Jasani B, Rhodes A. Technical variations in prostatic immunohistochemistry: need for standardisation and stringent quality assurance in PSA and PSAP immunostaining. J Clin Pathol 2004; 57: 687–690.

101. Nadji M, Tabei SZ, Castro A, et al. Prostatic-specific antigen: an immunohistologic marker for prostatic neoplasms. Cancer 1981; 48: 1229–1232.

102. Stein BS, Vangore S, Petersen RO, Kendall AR. Immunoperoxidase localization of prostate-specific antigen. Am J Surg Pathol 1982; 6: 553–557.

103. Sinha AA, Hagen KA, Sibley RK, et al. Analysis of fixation effects on immunohistochemical localization of prostatic specific antigen in human prostate. J Urol 1986; 136: 722–727.

104. Keillor JS, Aterman K. The response of poorly differentiated prostatic tumors to staining for prostate specific antigen and prostatic acid phosphatase: a comparative study. J Urol 1987; 137: 894–896.

105. Ordonez NG, Ro JY, Ayala AG. Application of immunocystochemistry in pathology. In: Bostwick DG, ed. Pathology of the prostate. New York: Churchill Livingstone, 1990; 137–160.

106. Brawn PN, Foster DM, Jay DW, et al. Characteristics of prostatic infarcts and their effect on serum prostate-specific antigen and prostatic acid phosphatase. Urology 1994; 44: 71–75.

107. Bostwick DG. Prostate-specific antigen. Current role in diagnostic pathology of prostate cancer. Am J Clin Pathol 1994; 102: S31–37.

108. Tepper SL, Jagirdar J, Heath D, Geller SA. Homology between the female paraurethral (Skene's) glands and the prostate. Immunohistochemical demonstration. Arch Pathol Lab Med 1984; 108: 423–425.

109. Pollen JJ, Dreilinger A. Immunohistochemical identification of prostatic acid phosphatase and prostate specific antigen in female periurethral glands. Urology 1984; 23: 303–304.

110. Nowels K, Kent E, Rinsho K, Oyasu R. Prostate specific antigen and acid phosphatase-reactive cells in cystitis cystica and glandularis. Arch Pathol Lab Med 1988; 112: 734–737.

111. Golz R, Schubert GE. Prostatic specific antigen: immunoreactivity in urachal remnants. J Urol 1989; 141: 1480–1482.

112. Kamoshida S, Tsutsumi Y. Extraprostatic localization of prostatic acid phosphatase and prostate-specific antigen: distribution in cloacogenic glandular epithelium and sex-dependent expression in human anal gland. Hum Pathol 1990; 21: 1108–1111.

113. Spencer JR, Brodin AG, Ignatoff JM. Clear cell adenocarcinoma of the urethra: evidence for origin within paraurethral ducts. J Urol 1990; 143: 122–125.

114. Frazier HA, Humphrey PA, Burchette JL, Paulson DF. Immunoreactive prostatic specific antigen in male periurethral glands. J Urol 1992; 147: 246–248.

115. van Krieken JH. Prostate marker immunoreactivity in salivary gland neoplasms. A rare pitfall in immunohistochemistry. Am J Surg Pathol 1993; 17: 410–414.

116. Cote RJ, Taylor CR. Prostate, bladder, and kidney. In: Taylor CR, Cote RJ, eds. Immunomicroscopy: a diagnostic tool for the surgical pathologist, 2nd edn. Philadelphia: WB Saunders, 1994; 256–276.

117. Elgamal AA, Van de Voorde W, Van Poppel H, et al. Immunohistochemical localization of prostate-specific markers within the accessory male sex glands of Cowper, Littre, and Morgagni. Urology 1994; 44: 84–90.

118. Sleater JP, Ford MJ, Beers BB. Extramammary Paget's disease associated with prostate adenocarcinoma. Hum Pathol 1994; 25: 615–617.

119. Mhawech P, Uchida T, Pelte MF. Immunohistochemical profile of high-grade urothelial bladder carcinoma and prostate adenocarcinoma. Hum Pathol 2002; 33: 1136–1140.

120. Olsson AY, Bjartell A, Lilja H, Lundwall A. Expression of prostate-specific antigen (PSA) and human glandular kallikrein 2 (hK2) in ileum and other extraprostatic tissues. Int J Cancer 2005; 113: 290–297.

121. Lowe FC, Trauzzi SJ. Prostatic acid phosphatase in 1993. Its limited clinical utility. Urol Clin North Am 1993; 20: 589–595.

122. Varma M, Jasani B. Diagnostic utility of immunohistochemistry in morphologically difficult prostate cancer: review of current literature. Histopathology 2005; 47: 1–16.

123. Hammond ME, Sause WT, Martz KL, et al. Correlation of prostate-specific acid phosphatase and prostate-specific antigen immunocytochemistry with survival in prostate carcinoma. Cancer 1989; 63: 461–466.

124. Sakai H, Yogi Y, Minami Y, et al. Prostate specific antigen and prostatic acid phosphatase immunoreactivity as prognostic indicators of advanced prostatic carcinoma. J Urol 1993; 149: 1020–1023.

125. Choe BK, Pontes EJ, Rose NR, Henderson MD. Expression of human prostatic acid phosphatase in a pancreatic islet cell carcinoma. Invest Urol 1978; 15: 312–318.

126. Shaw LM, Yang N, Brooks JJ, et al. Immunochemical evaluation of the organ specificity of prostatic acid phosphatase. Clin Chem 1981; 27: 1505–1512.

127. Epstein JI, Kuhajda FP, Lieberman PH. Prostate-specific acid phosphatase immunoreactivity in adenocarcinomas of the urinary bladder. Hum Pathol 1986; 17: 939–942.

128. Kimura N, Sasano N. Prostate-specific acid phosphatase in carcinoid tumors. Virchows Arch A [Pathol Anat Histopathol] 1986; 410: 247–251.

129. Azumi N, Traweek ST, Battifora H. Prostatic acid phosphatase in carcinoid tumors. Immunohistochemical and immunoblot studies [see comments]. Am J Surg Pathol 1991; 15: 785–790.

130. Bandivdekar AH, Gopalkrishnan K, Garde SV, et al. Antifertility effects in rats actively immunized with 80 kDa human semen glycoprotein. Indian J Exp Biol 1992; 30: 1017–1023.

131. Evans AJ. Alpha-methylacyl CoA racemase (P504S): overview and potential uses in diagnostic pathology as applied to prostate needle biopsies. J Clin Pathol 2003; 56: 892–897.

132. Jiang Z, Woda BA, Rock KL, et al. P504S: a new molecular marker for the detection of prostate carcinoma. Am J Surg Pathol 2001; 25: 1397–1404.

133. Jiang Z, Fanger GR, Woda BA, et al. Expression of alpha-methylacyl-CoA racemase (P504s) in various malignant neoplasms and normal tissues: a study of 761 cases. Hum Pathol 2003; 34: 792–796.

134. Jiang Z, Wu CL, Woda BA, et al. P504S/alpha-methylacyl-CoA racemase: a useful marker for diagnosis of small foci of prostatic carcinoma on needle biopsy. Am J Surg Pathol 2002; 26: 1169–1174.

135. Wu CL, Yang XJ, Tretiakova M, et al. Analysis of alpha-methylacyl-CoA racemase (P504S) expression in high-grade prostatic intraepithelial neoplasia. Hum Pathol 2004; 35: 1008–1013.

136. Magi-Galluzzi C, Luo J, Isaacs WB, et al. Alpha-methylacyl-CoA racemase: a variably sensitive immunohistochemical marker for the diagnosis of small prostate cancer foci on needle biopsy. Am J Surg Pathol 2003; 27: 1128–1133.

137. Yang XJ, Laven B, Tretiakova M, et al. Detection of alpha-methylacyl-

coenzyme A racemase in postradiation prostatic adenocarcinoma. Urology 2003; 62: 282–286.

138. Tang X, Serizawa A, Tokunaga M, et al. Variation of alpha-methylacyl-CoA racemase expression in prostate adenocarcinoma cases receiving hormonal therapy. Hum Pathol 2006; 37: 1186–1192.

139. Yang XJ, Wu CL, Woda BA, et al. Expression of alpha-Methylacyl-CoA racemase (P504S) in atypical adenomatous hyperplasia of the prostate. Am J Surg Pathol 2002; 26: 921–925.

140. Jiang Z, Wu CL, Woda BA, et al. Alpha-methylacyl-CoA racemase: a multi-institutional study of a new prostate cancer marker. Histopathology 2004; 45: 218–225.

141. Brawer MK, Peehl DM, Stamey TA, Bostwick DG. Keratin immunoreactivity in the benign and neoplastic human prostate. Cancer Res 1985; 45: 3663–3667.

142. Nagle RB, Ahmann FR, McDaniel KM, et al. Cytokeratin characterization of human prostatic carcinoma and its derived cell lines. Cancer Res 1987 1; 47: 281–286.

143. Guinan P, Shaw M, Targonski P, et al. Evaluation of cytokeratin markers to differentiate between benign and malignant prostatic tissue. J Surg Oncol 1989; 42: 175–180.

144. Hedrick L, Epstein JI. Use of keratin 903 as an adjunct in the diagnosis of prostate carcinoma. Am J Surg Pathol 1989; 13: 389–396.

145. O'Malley FP, Grignon DJ, Shum DT. Usefulness of immunoperoxidase staining with high-molecular-weight cytokeratin in the differential diagnosis of small-acinar lesions of the prostate gland. Virchows Arch A [Pathol Anat Histopathol] 1990; 417: 191–196.

146. Srigley JR, Dardick I, Hartwick RW, Klotz L. Basal epithelial cells of human prostate gland are not myoepithelial cells. A comparative immunohistochemical and ultrastructural study with the human salivary gland. Am J Pathol 1990; 136: 957–966.

147. Nagle RB, Brawer MK, Kittelson J, Clark V. Phenotypic relationships of prostatic intraepithelial neoplasia to invasive prostatic carcinoma. Am J Pathol 1991; 138: 119–128.

148. Shah IA, Schlageter MO, Stinnett P, Lechago J. Cytokeratin immunohistochemistry as a diagnostic tool for distinguishing malignant from benign epithelial lesions of the prostate. Mod Pathol 1991; 4: 220–224.

149. Okada H, Tsubura A, Okamura A, et al. Keratin profiles in normal/hyperplastic prostates and prostate carcinoma. Virchows Arch A [[Pathol Anat Histopathol]] 1992; 421: 157–161.

150. Cheville JC, Bostwick DG. Postatrophic hyperplasia of the prostate. A histologic mimic of prostatic adenocarcinoma.

Am J Surg Pathol 1995; 19: 1068–1076.

151. Ananthanarayanan V, Deaton RJ, Yang XJ, et al. Alpha-methylacyl-CoA racemase (AMACR) expression in normal prostatic glands and high-grade prostatic intraepithelial neoplasia (HGPIN): association with diagnosis of prostate cancer. Prostate 2005; 63: 341–346.

152. Molinie V, Herve JM, Lugagne PM, et al. Diagnostic utility of a p63/alpha-methyl coenzyme A racemase (p504s) cocktail in ambiguous lesions of the prostate upon needle biopsy. BJU Int 2006; 97: 1109–1115.

153. Martens MB, Keller JH. Routine immunohistochemical staining for high-molecular weight cytokeratin 34-beta and alpha-methylacyl CoA racemase (P504S) in postirradiation prostate biopsies. Mod Pathol 2006; 19: 287–290.

154. Weinstein MH, Signoretti S, Loda M. Diagnostic utility of immunohistochemical staining for p63, a sensitive marker of prostatic basal cells. Mod Pathol 2002; 15: 1302–1308.

155. Shah RB, Zhou M, LeBlanc M, et al. Comparison of the basal cell-specific markers, 34betaE12 and p63, in the diagnosis of prostate cancer. Am J Surg Pathol 2002; 26: 1161–1168.

156. Zhou M, Shah R, Shen R, Rubin MA. Basal cell cocktail (34betaE12+p63) improves the detection of prostate basal cells. Am J Surg Pathol 2003; 27: 365–371.

157. Wu HH, Lapkus O, Corbin M. Comparison of 34betaE12 and P63 in 100 consecutive prostate carcinoma diagnosed by needle biopsies. Appl Immunohistochem Mol Morphol 2004; 12: 285–289.

158. Reis-Filho JS, Simpson PT, Martins A, et al. Distribution of p63, cytokeratins 5/6 and cytokeratin 14 in 51 normal and 400 neoplastic human tissue samples using TARP-4 multi-tumor tissue microarray. Virchows Arch 2003; 443: 122–132.

159. Signoretti S, Waltregny D, Dilks J, et al. p63 is a prostate basal cell marker and is required for prostate development. Am J Pathol 2000; 157: 1769–1775.

160. Yang XJ, McEntee M, Epstein JI. Distinction of basaloid carcinoma of the prostate from benign basal cell lesions by using immunohistochemistry for bcl-2 and Ki-67. Hum Pathol 1998; 29: 1447–1450.

161. Parsons JK, Gage WR, Nelson WG, De Marzo AM. p63 protein expression is rare in prostate adenocarcinoma: implications for cancer diagnosis and carcinogenesis. Urology 2001; 58: 619–624.

162. Zhou M, Aydin H, Kanane H, Epstein JI. How often does alpha-methylacyl-CoA-racemase contribute to resolving an atypical diagnosis on prostate needle biopsy beyond that provided by

basal cell markers? Am J Surg Pathol 2004; 28: 239–243.

163. Iczkowski KA. Current prostate biopsy interpretation: criteria for cancer, atypical small acinar proliferation, high-grade prostatic intraepithelial neoplasia, and use of immunostains. Arch Pathol Lab Med 2006 Jun; 130: 835–843.

164. Nassar A, Amin MB, Sexton DG, Cohen C. Utility of alpha-methylacyl coenzyme A racemase (p504s antibody) as a diagnostic immunohistochemical marker for cancer. Appl Immunohistochem Mol Morphol 2005 Sep; 13: 252–255.

165. Jiang Z, Li C, Fischer A, Dresser K, Woda BA. Using an AMACR (P504S)/34betaE12/p63 cocktail for the detection of small focal prostate carcinoma in needle biopsy specimens. Am J Clin Pathol 2005 Feb; 123: 231–236.

166. Browne TJ, Hirsch MS, Brodsky G, Welch WR, Loda MF, Rubin MA. Prospective evaluation of AMACR (P504S) and basal cell markers in the assessment of routine prostate needle biopsy specimens. Hum Pathol 2004 Dec; 35: 1462–1468.

167. Sanderson SO, Sebo TJ, Murphy LM, Neumann R, Slezak J, Cheville JC. An analysis of the p63/alpha-methylacyl coenzyme A racemase immunohistochemical cocktail stain in prostate needle biopsy specimens and tissue microarrays. Am J Clin Pathol 2004 Feb; 121: 220–225.

168. Kunju LP, Chinnaiyan AM, Shah RB. Comparison of monoclonal antibody (P504S) and polyclonal antibody to alpha methylacyl-CoA racemase (AMACR) in the work-up of prostate cancer. Histopathology 2005 Dec; 47: 587–596.

169. Vanguri VK, Woda BA, Jiang Z. Sensitivity of P504S/alpha-methylacyl-CoA racemase (AMACR) immunohistochemistry for the detection of prostate carcinoma on stored needle biopsies. Appl Immunohistochem Mol Morphol 2006 Sep; 14: 365–368.

170. Tacha DE, Miller RT. Use of p63/P504S monoclonal antibody cocktail in immunohistochemical staining of prostate tissue. Appl Immunohistochem Mol Morphol 2004 Mar; 12: 75–78.

171. Carswell BM, Woda BA, Wang X, Li C, Dresser K, Jiang Z. Detection of prostate cancer by alpha-methylacyl CoA racemase (P504S) in needle biopsy specimens previously reported as negative for malignancy. Histopathology 2006 May; 48: 668–673.

172. Troyer JK, Beckett ML, Wright GL, Jr. Detection and characterization of the prostate-specific membrane antigen (PSMA) in tissue extracts and body fluids. Int J Cancer 1995; 62: 552–558.

173. Zaviacic M, Ruzickova M, Blazekova J, Zaviacic T, Itoh Y, Okutani R, et al.

Immunohistochemical distribution of rabbit polyclonal antiurinary protein 1 antibody in the female (Skene's gland) and male prostate: new marker for neuroendocrine cells? Acta Histochem 1997; 99: 267–275.

174. Lopes AD, Davis WL, Rosenstraus MJ, Uveges AJ, Gilman SC. Immunohistochemical and pharmacokinetic characterization of the site- specific immunoconjugate CYT-356 derived from antiprostate monoclonal antibody 7E11-C5. Cancer Res 1990; 50: 6423–6429.

175. Birtle AJ, Freeman A, Masters JR, Payne HA, Harland SJ. Tumour markers for managing men who present with metastatic prostate cancer and serum prostate-specific antigen levels of <10 ng/mL. BJU international 2005 Aug; 96: 303–307.

176. Marchal C, Redondo M, Padilla M, Caballero J, Rodrigo I, Garcia J, et al. Expression of prostate specific membrane antigen (PSMA) in prostatic adenocarcinoma and prostatic intraepithelial neoplasia. Histol Histopathol 2004 Jul; 19: 715–718.

177. Sweat SD, Pacelli A, Murphy GP, Bostwick DG. Prostate-specific membrane antigen expression is greatest in prostate adenocarcinoma and lymph node metastases. Urology 1998; 52: 637–640.

178. Murphy GP, Elgamal AA, Su SL, Bostwick DG, Holmes EH. Current evaluation of the tissue localization and diagnostic utility of prostate specific membrane antigen. Cancer 1998; 83: 2259–2269.

179. Ross JS, Sheehan CE, Fisher HA, Kaufman RP, Jr., Kaur P, Gray K, et al. Correlation of primary tumor prostate-specific membrane antigen expression with disease recurrence in prostate cancer. Clin Cancer Res 2003 Dec 15; 9: 6357–6362.

180. Schmidt B, Anastasiadis AG, Seifert HH, Franke KH, Oya M, Ackermann R. Detection of circulating prostate cells during radical prostatectomy by standardized PSMA RT-PCR: association with positive lymph nodes and high malignant grade. Anticancer Res 2003 Sep–Oct; 23(5A): 3991–3999.

181. Zaviacic M, Danihel L, Ruzickova M, Blazekova J, Itoh Y, Okutani R, et al. Immunohistochemical localization of human protein 1 in the female prostate (Skene's gland) and the male prostate. Histochem J 1997; 29: 219–227.

182. Partin AW, Catalona WJ, Finlay JA, Darte C, Tindall DJ, Young CY, et al. Use of human glandular kallikrein 2 for the detection of prostate cancer: preliminary analysis. Urology 1999; 54: 839–845.

183. Tremblay RR, Deperthes D, Tetu B, Dube JY. Immunohistochemical study suggesting a complementary role of kallikreins hK2 and hK3 (prostate-specific antigen) in the functional analysis of human prostate tumors. Am J Pathol 1997; 150: 455–459.

184. Darson MF, Pacelli A, Roche P, Rittenhouse HG, Wolfert RL, Young CY, et al. Human glandular kallikrein 2 (hK2) expression in prostatic intraepithelial neoplasia and adenocarcinoma: a novel prostate cancer marker. Urology 1997 Jun; 49: 857–862.

185. Darson MF, Pacelli A, Roche P, Rittenhouse HG, Wolfert RL, Saeid MS, et al. Human glandular kallikrein 2 expression in prostate adenocarcinoma and lymph node metastases. Urology 1999 May; 53: 939–944.

186. Steuber T, Niemela P, Haese A, Pettersson K, Erbersdobler A, Felix Chun KH, et al. Association of free-prostate specific antigen subfractions and human glandular kallikrein 2 with volume of benign and malignant prostatic tissue. Prostate 2004 Sep 17.

187. Obiezu CV, Diamandis EP. Human tissue kallikrein gene family: applications in cancer. Cancer Lett 2005 Jun 16; 224: 1–22.

188. Haese A, Graefen M, Steuber T, Becker C, Noldus J, Erbersdobler A, et al. Total and Gleason grade 4/5 cancer volumes are major contributors of human kallikrein 2, whereas free prostate specific antigen is largely contributed by benign gland volume in serum from patients with prostate cancer or benign prostatic biopsies. J Urol 2003 Dec; 170(6 Pt 1): 2269–2273.

189. Civantos F. Difficulties in interpreting specimens after neoadjuvant hormonal therapy and radiation with illustration of neuroendocrine differentiation. Mol Urol 2000 Fall; 4: 117–121; discussion 123.

190. Vaisanen V, Eriksson S, Ivaska KK, Lilja H, Nurmi M, Pettersson K. Development of sensitive immunoassays for free and total human glandular kallikrein 2. Clin Chem 2004 Sep; 50: 1607–1617.

191. Fuessel S, Sickert D, Meye A, Klenk U, Schmidt U, Schmitz M, et al. Multiple tumor marker analyses (PSA, hK2, PSCA, trp-p8) in primary prostate cancers using quantitative RT-PCR. International Joncology 2003 Jul; 23: 221–228.

192. Kitajima K, Tokes ZA. Immunohistochemical localization of keratin in human prostate. Prostate 1986; 9: 183–190.

193. Purnell DM, Heatfield BM, Anthony RL, Trump BF. Immunohistochemistry of the cytoskeleton of human prostatic epithelium. Evidence for disturbed organization in neoplasia. Am J Pathol 1987; 126: 384–395.

194. Dhom G, Seitz G, Wernert N. Histology and immunohistochemistry studies in prostate cancer. Am J Clin Oncol 1988; 11(Suppl 2): S37–42.

195. Wernert N, Luchtrath H, Seeliger H, Schafer M, Goebbels R, Dhom G. Papillary carcinoma of the prostate, location, morphology, and immunohistochemistry: the histogenesis and entity of so-called endometrioid carcinoma. Prostate 1987; 10: 123–131.

196. Rehman I, Cross SS, Azzouzi AR, Catto JW, Deloulme JC, Larre S, et al. S100A6 (Calcyclin) is a prostate basal cell marker absent in prostate cancer and its precursors. Br J Cancer 2004 Aug 16; 91: 739–744.

197. Abrahams NA, Bostwick DG, Ormsby AH, Qian J, Brainard JA. Distinguishing atrophy and high-grade prostatic intraepithelial neoplasia from prostatic adenocarcinoma with and without previous adjuvant hormone therapy with the aid of cytokeratin 5/6. Am J Clin Pathol 2003 Sep; 120: 368–376.

198. Bonkhoff H, Remberger K. Widespread distribution of nuclear androgen receptors in the basal cell layer of the normal and hyperplastic human prostate. Virchows Arch A [Pathol Anat Histopathol] 1993; 422: 35–38.

199. Ruizeveld de Winter JA, Janssen PJ, Sleddens HM, Verleun-Mooijman MC, Trapman J, Brinkmann AO, et al. Androgen receptor status in localized and locally progressive hormone refractory human prostate cancer. Am J Pathol 1994; 144: 735–746.

200. Sadi MV, Barrack ER. Image analysis of androgen receptor immunostaining in metastatic prostate cancer. Heterogeneity as a predictor of response to hormonal therapy. Cancer 1993 Apr 15; 71: 2574–2580.

201. Sadi MV, Barrack ER. Androgen receptors and growth fraction in metastatic prostate cancer as predictors of time to tumour progression after hormonal therapy. Cancer Surv 1991; 11: 195–215.

202. Sadi MV, Walsh PC, Barrack ER. Immunohistochemical study of androgen receptors in metastatic prostate cancer. Comparison of receptor content and response to hormonal therapy. Cancer 1991; 67: 3057–3064.

203. Schafer W, Funke PJ, Kunde D, Rausch U, Wennemuth G, Stutzer H. Intensity of androgen and epidermal growth factor receptor immunoreactivity in samples of radical prostatectomy as prognostic indicator: correlation with clinical data of long-term observations. J Urol 2006 Aug; 176: 532–537.

204. Inoue T, Segawa T, Shiraishi T, Yoshida T, Toda Y, Yamada T, et al. Androgen receptor, Ki67, and p53 expression in radical prostatectomy specimens predict treatment failure in Japanese population. Urology 2005 Aug; 66: 332–337.

205. Taplin ME, Bubley GJ, Shuster TD, Frantz ME, Spooner AE, Ogata GK, et al. Mutation of the androgen-receptor gene in metastatic androgen-independent prostate cancer. N Engl J Med 1995 May 25; 332: 1393–1398.

206. Strom SS, Gu Y, Zhang H, Troncoso P, Babaian RJ, Pettaway CA, et al. Androgen receptor polymorphisms and

risk of biochemical failure among prostatectomy patients. Prostate 2004 Sep 1; 60: 343–351.

207. Ricciardelli C, Choong CS, Buchanan G, Vivekanandan S, Neufing P, Stahl J, et al. Androgen receptor levels in prostate cancer epithelial and peritumoral stromal cells identify non-organ confined disease. Prostate 2005 Apr 1; 63: 19–28.

208. di Sant'Agnese PA, de Mesy Jensen KL, Churukian CJ, Agarwal MM. Human prostatic endocrine-paracrine (APUD) cells. Distributional analysis with a comparison of serotonin and neuron-specific enolase immunoreactivity and silver stains. Arch Pathol Lab Med 1985; 109: 607–612.

209. McCormick DL, Rao KV. Chemoprevention of hormone-dependent prostate cancer in the Wistar- Unilever rat. Eur Urol1999; 35(5–6): 464–467.

210. Pruneri G, Galli S, Rossi RS, Roncalli M, Coggi G, Ferrari A, et al. Chromogranin A and B and secretogranin II in prostatic adenocarcinomas: neuroendocrine expression in patients untreated and treated with androgen deprivation therapy. Prostate 1998; 34: 113–120.

211. Abrahamsson PA, Falkmer S, Falt K, Grimelius L. The course of neuroendocrine differentiation in prostatic carcinomas. An immunohistochemical study testing chromogranin A as an 'endocrine marker.' Pathol Res Pract 1989; 185: 373–380.

212. Wu C, Zhang L, Bourne PA, Reeder JE, di Sant'Agnese PA, Yao JL, et al. Protein tyrosine phosphatase PTP1B is involved in neuroendocrine differentiation of prostate cancer. Prostate 2006 Aug 1; 66: 1125–1135.

213. Falkmer S, Askensten U, Grimelius L, Abrahamsson PA. Cytochemical markers and DNA content of neuroendocrine cells in carcinoma of the prostate gland during tumour progression. Acta Histochem Suppl 1990; 38: 127–132.

214. Bonkhoff H, Stein U, Remberger K. Endocrine-paracrine cell types in the prostate and prostatic adenocarcinoma are postmitotic cells [see comments]. Hum Pathol 1995; 26: 167–170.

215. McWilliam LJ, Manson C, George NJ. Neuroendocrine differentiation and prognosis in prostatic adenocarcinoma. Br J Urol 1997; 80: 287–290.

216. Umbas R, Isaacs WB, Bringuier PP, Xue Y, Debruyne FM, Schalken JA. Relation between aberrant alpha-catenin expression and loss of E- cadherin function in prostate cancer. Int J Cancer 1997; 74: 374–377.

217. Guy L, Begin LR, Al-Othman K, Chevalier S, Aprikian AG. Neuroendocrine cells of the verumontanum: a comparative immunohistochemical study. Br J Urol 1998; 82: 738–743.

218. Helpap B, Kollermann J. Undifferentiated carcinoma of the prostate with small cell features: immunohistochemical subtyping and reflections on histogenesis. Virchows Arch 1999; 434: 385–391.

219. Helpap B, Kollermann J, Oehler U. Neuroendocrine differentiation in prostatic carcinomas: histogenesis, biology, clinical relevance, and future therapeutic perspectives. Urol Int 1999; 62: 133–138.

220. Bostwick DG, Alexander EE, Singh R, Shan A, Qian J, Santella RM, et al. Antioxidant enzyme expression and reactive oxygen species damage in prostatic intraepithelial neoplasia and cancer. Cancer 2000; 89: 123–134.

221. Huang J, Yao JL, di Sant'Agnese PA, Yang Q, Bourne PA, Na Y. Immunohistochemical characterization of neuroendocrine cells in prostate cancer. Prostate 2006 Sep 15; 66: 1399–1406.

222. Chen X, Okada H, Gotoh A, Arakawa S, Kamidono S. Neuroendocrine cells in the prostatic carcinomas after neoadjuvant hormonal therapy. Kobe J Med Sci 1997; 43: 71–81.

223. Krijnen JL, Janssen PJ, Ruizeveld de Winter JA, van Krimpen H, Schroder FH, van der Kwast TH. Do neuroendocrine cells in human prostate cancer express androgen receptor? Histochemistry 1993; 100: 393–398.

224. Abrahamsson PA, Cockett AT, di Sant'Agnese PA. Prognostic significance of neuroendocrine differentiation in clinically localized prostatic carcinoma. Prostate Suppl 1998; 8: 37–42.

225. Angelsen A, Syversen U, Haugen OA, Stridsberg M, Mjolnerod OK, Waldum HL. Neuroendocrine differentiation in carcinomas of the prostate: do neuroendocrine serum markers reflect immunohistochemical findings? Prostate 1997; 30: 1–6.

226. Angelsen A, Syversen U, Stridsberg M, Haugen OA, Mjolnerod OK, Waldum HL. Use of neuroendocrine serum markers in the follow-up of patients with cancer of the prostate. Prostate 1997; 31: 110–117.

227. Berner A, Waere H, Nesland JM, Paus E, Danielsen HE, Fossa SD. DNA ploidy, serum prostate specific antigen, histological grade and immunohistochemistry as predictive parameters of lymph node metastases in T1-T3/M0 prostatic adenocarcinoma. Br J Urol 1995; 75: 26–32.

228. Bubendorf L, Sauter G, Moch H, Jordan P, Blochlinger A, Gasser TC, et al. Prognostic significance of Bcl-2 in clinically localized prostate cancer. Am J Pathol 1996; 148: 1557–1565.

229. Casella R, Bubendorf L, Sauter G, Moch H, Mihatsch MJ, Gasser TC. Focal neuroendocrine differentiation lacks prognostic significance in prostate core needle biopsies. J Urol 1998; 160: 406–410.

230. Frkovic-Grazio S, Kraljic I, Trnski D, Tarle M. Immunohistochemical staining and serotest markers during development of a sarcomatoid and small cell prostate tumor. Anticancer Res 1994; 14(5B): 2151–2156.

231. Krupski T, Petroni GR, Frierson HF, Jr., Theodorescu JU. Microvessel density, p53, retinoblastoma, and chromogranin A immunohisto-chemistry as predictors of disease-specific survival following radical prostatectomy for carcinoma of the prostate. Urology 2000; 55: 743–749.

232. Aaltomaa S, Lipponen P, Eskelinen M, Ala-Opas M, Kosma VM. Prognostic value and expression of p21(waf1/cip1) protein in prostate cancer. Prostate 1999; 39: 8–15.

233. Mucci NR, Akdas G, Manely S, Rubin MA. Neuroendocrine expression in metastatic prostate cancer: evaluation of high throughput tissue microarrays to detect heterogeneous protein expression. Hum Pathol 2000; 31: 406–414.

234. Noordzij MA, van Weerden WM, de Ridder CM, van der Kwast TH, Schroder FH, van Steenbrugge GJ. Neuroendocrine differentiation in human prostatic tumor models. Am J Pathol 1996; 149: 859–871.

235. Oesterling JE, Hauzeur CG, Farrow GM. Small cell anaplastic carcinoma of the prostate: a clinical, pathological and immunohistological study of 27 patients. J Urol 1992; 147(3 Pt 2): 804–807.

236. Van de Voorde W, Van Poppel H, Haustermans K, Baert L, Lauweryns J. Mucin-secreting adenocarcinoma of the prostate with neuroendocrine differentiation and Paneth-like cells. Am J Surg Pathol 1994; 18: 200–207.

237. Weinstein MH, Partin AW, Veltri RW, Epstein JI. Neuroendocrine differentiation in prostate cancer: enhanced prediction of progression after radical prostatectomy. Hum Pathol 1996; 27: 683–687.

238. Dizeyi N, Bjartell A, Nilsson E, Hansson J, Gadaleanu V, Cross N, et al. Expression of serotonin receptors and role of serotonin in human prostate cancer tissue and cell lines. Prostate 2004 May 15; 59: 328–336.

239. Theodoropoulos VE, Tsigka A, Mihalopoulou A, Tsoukala V, Lazaris AC, Patsouris E, et al. Evaluation of neuroendocrine staining and androgen receptor expression in incidental prostatic adenocarcinoma: prognostic implications. Urology 2005 Oct; 66: 897–902.

240. Evans AJ, Humphrey PA, Belani J, van der Kwast TH, Srigley JR. Large cell neuroendocrine carcinoma of prostate: a clinicopathologic summary of 7 cases of a rare manifestation of advanced prostate cancer. Am J Surg Pathol 2006 Jun; 30: 684–693.

241. Bostwick DG, Vonk, J. Picado, A. Pathologic changes in the prostate

following contemporary 18-gauge needle biopsy: No apparent risk of local cancer seeding. J Urol Pathol 1994; 2: 203–212.

242. Terris MK, McNeal JE, Stamey TA. Detection of clinically significant prostate cancer by transrectal ultrasound-guided systematic biopsies. J Urol 1992 Sep; 148: 829–832.

243. Hammerer P, Huland H, Sparenberg A. Digital rectal examination, imaging, and systematic-sextant biopsy in identifying operable lymph node-negative prostatic carcinoma. Eur Urol1992; 22: 281–287.

244. Stamey TA, Freiha FS, McNeal JE, Redwine EA, Whittemore AS, Schmid HP. Localized prostate cancer. Relationship of tumor volume to clinical significance for treatment of prostate cancer. Cancer 1993 Feb 1; 71(3 Suppl): 933–938.

245. Boccon-Gibod LM, de Longchamps NB, Toublanc M, Boccon-Gibod LA, Ravery V. Prostate saturation biopsy in the reevaluation of microfocal prostate cancer. J Urol 2006 Sep; 176: 961–963; discussion 963–964.

246. Descazeaud A, Rubin M, Chemama S, Larre S, Salomon L, Allory Y, et al. Saturation biopsy protocol enhances prediction of pT3 and surgical margin status on prostatectomy specimen. World J Urol 2006 Dec; 24: 676–680.

247. Walz J, Graefen M, Chun FK, Erbersdobler A, Haese A, Steuber T, et al. High incidence of prostate cancer detected by saturation biopsy after previous negative biopsy series. Eur Urol2006 Sep; 50: 498–505.

248. Chrouser KL, Lieber MM. Extended and saturation needle biopsy for the diagnosis of prostate cancer. Curr Urol Rep 2004 Jun; 5: 226–230.

249. Stilmant MM, Freedlund MC, de las Morenas A, Shepard RL, Oates RD, Siroky MB. Expanded role for fine needle aspiration of the prostate. A study of 335 specimens. Cancer 1989 Feb 1; 63: 583–592.

250. Maksem JA, Galang CF, Johenning PW, Park CH, Tannenbaum M. Aspiration biopsy of the prostate gland: a brief review of collection, fixation, and pattern recognition with special attention to benign and malignant prostatic epithelium. Diagnostic cytopathology 1990; 6: 258–266.

251. Maksem JA. Performance and processing of prostate aspiration biopsies: A strategy to ensure optimum cellularity and fixation. J Urol Pathol 1995; 3: 347–354.

252. Maksem JA, Johenning PW. Is cytology capable of adequately grading prostate carcinoma? Matched series of 50 cases comparing cytologic and histologic pattern diagnoses. Urology 1988 May; 31: 437–444.

253. Maksem J. Fine Needle Aspiration of the prostate. In: Foster C, Bostwick, D. G., ed. Pathology of the Prostate. Philadelphia: WB Saunders 1997.

254. Perez-Guillermo M, Acosta-Ortega J, Garcia-Solano J. Pitfalls and infrequent findings in fine-needle aspiration of the prostate gland. Diagnostic cytopathology 2005 Aug; 33: 126–137.

255. Buhmeida A, Kuopio T, Collan Y. Nuclear size and shape in fine needle aspiration biopsy samples of the prostate. Anal Quant Cytol Histol 2000 Aug; 22: 291–298.

256. Matsuyama H, Pan Y, Oba K, Yoshihiro S, Matsuda K, Hagarth L, et al. The role of chromosome 8p22 deletion for predicting disease progression and pathological staging in prostate cancer. Aktuelle Urol 2003 Jul; 34: 247–249.

257. Buhmeida A, Backman H, Collan Y. DNA cytometry in diagnostic cytology of the prostate gland. Anticancer Res 2002 Jul–Aug; 22: 2397–2402.

258. McNeal JE, Price HM, Redwine EA, Freiha FS, Stamey TA. Stage A versus stage B adenocarcinoma of the prostate: morphological comparison and biological significance. J Urol 1988 Jan; 139: 61–65.

259. McNeal JE, Redwine EA, Freiha FS, Stamey TA. Zonal distribution of prostatic adenocarcinoma. Correlation with histologic pattern and direction of spread. Am J Surg Pathol 1988 Dec; 12: 897–906.

260. Puppo P, Introini C, Calvi P, Naselli A. Role of transurethral resection of the prostate and biopsy of the peripheral zone in the same session after repeated negative biopsies in the diagnosis of prostate cancer. Eur Urol2006 May; 49: 873–878.

261. Radhakrishnan S, Dorkin TJ, Sheikh N, Greene DR. Role of transition zone sampling by TURP in patients with raised PSA and multiple negative transrectal ultrasound-guided prostatic biopsies. Prostate Cancer Prostatic Dis 2004; 7: 338–342.

262. Kitamura H, Masumori N, Tanuma Y, Yanase M, Itoh N, Takahashi A, et al. Does transurethral resection of the prostate facilitate detection of clinically significant prostate cancer that is missed with systematic sextant and transition zone biopsies? Int J Urol 2002 Feb; 9: 95–99.

263. Talic RF, Al Rikabi AC. Transurethral vaporization-resection of the prostate versus standard transurethral prostatectomy: comparative changes in histopathological features of the resected specimens. Eur Urol2000 Mar; 37: 301–305.

264. Rohr LR. Incidental adenocarcinoma in transurethral resections of the prostate. Partial versus complete microscopic examination. Am J Surg Pathol 1987 Jan; 11: 53–58.

265. Murphy WM, Dean PJ, Brasfield JA, Tatum L. Incidental carcinoma of the prostate. How much sampling is adequate? Am J Surg Pathol 1986 Mar; 10: 170–174.

266. Bostwick DG. The pathology of incidental carcinoma. Cancer Surv 1995; 23: 7–18.

267. Eble JN, and Tejada, E. Cost implications of sampling strategies for prostatic transurethral resection specimens: Analysis of 549 cases. Am J Clin Pathol 1986; 85: 382.

268. Vollmer RT. Prostate cancer and chip specimens: complete versus partial sampling. Hum Pathol 1986 Mar; 17: 285–290.

269. Henson DE, Hutter RV, Farrow G. Practice protocol for the examination of specimens removed from patients with carcinoma of the prostate gland. A publication of the cancer committee, college of american pathologists. Task Force on the Examination of Specimens Removed From Patients With Prostate Cancer. Arch Pathol Lab Med 1994 Aug; 118: 779–783.

270. Naspro R, Freschi M, Salonia A, Guazzoni G, Girolamo V, Colombo R, et al. Holmium laser enucleation versus transurethral resection of the prostate. Are histological findings comparable? J Urol 2004 Mar; 171: 1203–1206.

271. Alguacil-Garcia A. Artifactual changes mimicking signet ring cell carcinoma in transurethral prostatectomy specimens. Am J Surg Pathol 1986; 10: 795–800.

272. Blumenfeld W, Tucci S, Narayan P. Incidental lymphocytic prostatitis. Selective involvement with nonmalignant glands. Am J Surg Pathol 1992; 16: 975–981.

273. Lee SW, Cheah PY, Liong ML, Yuen KH, Schaeffer AJ, Propert K, et al. Demographic and clinical characteristics of chronic prostatitis: prospective comparison of the University of Sciences Malaysia Cohort with the United States National Institutes of Health Cohort. J Urol 2007 Jan; 177: 153–157; discussion 158.

274. Lopez-Plaza I Bostwick, DG Prostatitis. In: Bostwick DG, ed. Pathology of the Prostate. New York, NY: Churchill Livingstone 1990.

275. Naide Y, Ishikawa K, Tanaka T, Ando S, Suzuki K, Hoshinaga K. A proposal of subcategorization of bacterial prostatitis: NIH category I and II diseases can be further subcategorized on analysis by therapeutic and immunological procedures. Int J Urol 2006 Jul; 13: 939–946.

276. Stamey TA. Urinary infections in males. In: TA S, ed. Pathogenesis and Treatment of Urinary Tract Infections. Baltimore, MD: Williams & Wilkins 1980: 1.

277. Kramer G, Marberger M. Could inflammation be a key component in the progression of benign prostatic hyperplasia? Curr Opin Urol 2006 Jan; 16: 25–29.

278. Chang SG, Kim CS, Jeon SH, Kim YW, Choi BY. Is chronic inflammatory change in the prostate the major cause of rising serum prostate-specific antigen in patients with clinical suspicion of prostate cancer? Int J Urol 2006 Feb; 13: 122–126.

279. Krieger JN. Prostatitis revisited: new definitions, new approaches. Infect Dis Clin North Am 2003 Jun; 17: 395–409.

280. Weidner W, Naber KG. [Prostatitis syndrome: consensus of the 6th International Consultation in Paris, 2005]. Aktuelle Urol 2006 Jul; 37: 269–271.

281. Hua VN, Williams DH, Schaeffer AJ. Role of bacteria in chronic prostatitis/ chronic pelvic pain syndrome. Curr Urol Rep 2005 Jul; 6: 300–306.

282. Cheah PY, Liong ML, Yuen KH, Teh CL, Khor T, Yang JR, et al. Chronic prostatitis: symptom survey with follow-up clinical evaluation. Urology 2003 Jan; 61: 60–64.

283. Helpap B. Histological and immunohistochemical study of chronic prostatic inflammation with and without benign prostatic hyperplasia. J Urol Pathol 1994; 2: 49–64.

284. Naber KG. Experience with the new guidelines on evaluation of new anti-infective drugs for the treatment of urinary tract infections. Int J Antimicrob Agents 1999 May; 11(3–4): 189–196; discussion 213–186.

285. Montironi R, Vela Navarrete R, Lopez-Beltran A, Mazzucchelli R, Mikuz G, Bono AV. Histopathology reporting of prostate needle biopsies 2005 update. Virchows Arch 2006 Jul; 449: 1–13.

286. Nickel JC, True LD, Krieger JN, Berger RE, Boag AH, Young ID. Consensus development of a histopathological classification system for chronic prostatic inflammation. BJU international 2001 Jun; 87: 797–805.

287. Stillwell TJ, Engen DE, Farrow GM. The clinical spectrum of granulomatous prostatitis: a report of 200 cases. J Urol 1987 Aug; 138: 320–323.

288. Epstein JI, Hutchins GM. Granulomatous prostatitis: distinction among allergic, nonspecific, and post-transurethral resection lesions. Hum Pathol 1984 Sep; 15: 818–825.

289. Crawford BE, Daroca PJ, Davis R. Periprostatic subendothelial intravascular granulomatosis: a mimic of high-grade intravascular prostatic adenocarcinoma. International Jsurgical pathology 2004 Jan; 12: 75–78.

290. Mohan H, Bal A, Punia RP, Bawa AS. Granulomatous prostatitis – an infrequent diagnosis. Int J Urol 2005 May; 12: 474–478.

291. Yurkanin JP, Ahmann F, Dalkin BL. Coccidioidomycosis of the prostate: a determination of incidence, report of 4 cases, and treatment recommendations. J Infect 2006 Jan; 52: e19–25.

292. Sohail MR, Andrews PE, Blair JE. Coccidioidomycosis of the male genital tract. J Urol 2005 Jun; 173: 1978–1982.

293. Ma TK, Srigley JR. Adenocarcinoma of prostate and schistosomiasis: a rare association. Histopathology 1995 Aug; 27: 187–189.

294. Al Adnani MS. Schistosomiasis, metaplasia and squamous cell carcinoma of the prostate: histogenesis of the squamous cancer cells determined by localization of specific markers. Neoplasma 1985; 32: 613–622.

295. Mies C, Balogh K, Stadecker M. Palisading prostate granulomas following surgery. Am J Surg Pathol 1984 Mar; 8: 217–221.

296. Kopolovic J, Rivkind A, Sherman Y. Granulomatous prostatitis with vasculitis. A sequel to transurethral prostatic resection. Arch Pathol Lab Med 1984 Sep; 108: 732–733.

297. Jacob S, Mammen K. Necrotising prostatic granulomas following transurethral resection – a case report. Indian J Pathol Microbiol 2003 Jul; 46: 480–481.

298. Oates RD, Stilmant MM, Freedlund MC, Siroky MB. Granulomatous prostatitis following bacillus Calmette-Guerin immunotherapy of bladder cancer. J Urol 1988 Oct; 140: 751–754.

299. Mahizia AA, Reiman, H. H., Myers, R. P. Migration and granulomatous reaction after periurethral injection of polytef (Teflon). JAMA 1984; 215: 3277–3281.

300. Politano VA. Transurethral polytef injection for post-prostatectomy urinary incontinence. Br J Urol 1992 Jan; 69: 26–28.

301. McKinney CD, Gaffey MJ, Gillenwater JY. Bladder outlet obstruction after multiple periurethral polytetrafluoroethylene injections. J Urol 1995 Jan; 153: 149–151.

302. Orozco RE, and Peters, R. L. Teflon granuloma of the prostate mimicking adenocarcinoma. Report of two cases. J Urol Pathol 1995; 3: 365–368.

303. Kiyokawa H, Koyama M, Kato H. Churg-Strauss syndrome presenting with eosinophilic prostatitis. Int J Urol 2006 Jun; 13: 838–840.

304. Stillwell TJ, DeRemee RA, McDonald TJ, Weiland LH, Engen DE. Prostatic involvement in Wegener's granulomatosis. J Urol 1987 Nov; 138: 1251–1253.

305. Heldmann F, Brandt J, Schoppe H, Braun J. [A 46-year-old-patient with granulomatous prostatitis, arthralgia and haemorrhagic rhinitis]. Dtsch Med Wochenschr 2006 Jan 5; 131(1–2): 22–25.

306. Gaber KA, Ryley NG, Macdermott JP, Goldman JM. Wegener's granulomatosis involving prostate. Urology 2005 Jul; 66: 195.

307. Bretal-Laranga M, Insua-Vilarino S, Blanco-Rodriguez J, Caamano-Freire M, Mera-Varela A, Lamas-Cedron P. Giant cell arteritis limited to the prostate. J Rheumatol 1995 Mar; 22: 566–568.

308. Pavlica P, Barozzi L, Bartolone A, Gaudiano C, Menchi M, Veneziano S. Nonspecific granulomatous prostatitis. Ultraschall Med 2005 Jun; 26: 203–208.

309. Sebo TJ, Bostwick DG, Farrow GM, Eble JN. Prostatic xanthoma: a mimic of prostatic adenocarcinoma. Hum Pathol 1994; 25: 386–389.

310. Rafique M, Yaqoob N. Xanthogranulomatous prostatitis: a mimic of carcinoma of prostate. World J Surg Oncol 2006; 4: 30.

311. Presti B, Weidner N. Granulomatous prostatitis and poorly differentiated prostate carcinoma. Their distinction with the use of immunohistochemical methods. Am J Clin Pathol 1991; 95: 330–334.

312. Dikov D, Chatelet FP, Dimitrakov J. Pathologic features of necrotizing adenoviral prostatitis in an AIDS patient. International Jsurgical pathology 2005 Apr; 13: 227–231.

313. Shah RD, Nardi PM, Han CC. Histoplasma prostatic abscess: rare cause in an immunocompromised patient. AJR Am J Roentgenol 1996 Feb; 166: 471.

314. Mastroianni A, Coronado O, Manfredi R, Chiodo F, Scarani P. Acute cytomegalovirus prostatitis in AIDS. Genitourin Med 1996 Dec; 72: 447–448.

315. Greenstein A, Merimsky E, Baratz M, Braf Z. Late appearance of perineal implantation of prostatic carcinoma after perineal needle biopsy. Urology 1989 Jan; 33: 59–60.

316. Moul JW, Miles BJ, Skoog SJ, McLeod DG. Risk factors for perineal seeding of prostate cancer after needle biopsy. J Urol 1989 Jul; 142: 86–88.

317. Baech J, Gote H, Raahave D. Perineal seeding of prostatic carcinoma after Trucut biopsy. Urol Int 1990; 45: 370–371.

318. Haddad FS. Re: Risk factors for perineal seeding of prostate cancer after needle biopsy. J Urol 1990 Mar; 143: 587–588.

319. Ryan PG, Peeling WB. Perineal prostatic tumour seedling after 'Tru-Cut' needle biopsy: case report and review of the literature. Eur Urol1990; 17: 189–192.

320. Bastacky SS, Walsh PC, Epstein JI. Needle biopsy associated tumor tracking of adenocarcinoma of the prostate. J Urol 1991 May; 145: 1003–1007.

321. Blight EM, Jr. Seeding of prostate adenocarcinoma following transrectal needle biopsy. Urology 1992 Mar; 39: 297–298.

322. Petraki CD, Sfikas CP. Histopathological changes induced by therapies in the benign prostate and prostate adenocarcinoma. Histol Histopathol 2007 Jan; 22: 107–118.

323. Lager DJ, Goeken JA, Kemp JD, Robinson RA. Squamous metaplasia of the prostate. An immunohistochemical study. Am J Clin Pathol 1988; 90: 597–601.

324. Miralles TG, Rodriguez-Perez JA, Alonso de la Campa JM. Squamous metaplasia of the prostate: a potential pitfall in fine needle aspiration cytology. Acta Cytol 1988 Mar-Apr; 32: 272–274.

325. Kastendieck H, Altenahr E. [Morphogenesis and significance of epithelial metaplasia in the human prostate gland. An electron-microscopic study (author's transl)]. Virchows Arch A Pathol Anat Histol 1975; 365: 137–150.

326. Kastendieck H, Altenahr E. [Proceedings: Ultrastructural findings on squamous epithelial metaplasia in the human prostate]. Verh Dtsch Ges Pathol 1974; 58: 572.

327. Grignon DJ, O'Malley FP. Mucinous metaplasia in the prostate gland. Am J Surg Pathol 1993 Mar; 17: 287–290.

328. Gal R, Koren R, Nofech-Mozes S, Mukamel E, His Y, Zajdel L. Evaluation of mucinous metaplasia of the prostate gland by mucin histochemistry. Br J Urol 1996 Jan; 77: 113–117.

329. Haratake J, Horie A, Ito K. Argyrophilic adenocarcinoma of the prostate with Paneth cell-like granules. Acta Pathol Jpn 1987 May; 37: 831–836.

330. Frydman CP, Bleiweiss IJ, Unger PD, Gordon RE, Brazenas NV. Paneth cell-like metaplasia of the prostate gland. Arch Pathol Lab Med 1992 Mar; 116: 274–276.

331. Weaver MG, Abdul-Karim FW, Srigley J, Bostwick DG, Ro JY, Ayala AG. Paneth cell-like change of the prostate gland. A histological, immunohistochemical, and electron microscopic study. Am J Surg Pathol 1992; 16: 62–68.

332. Weaver MG, Abdul-Karim FW, Srigley JR. Paneth cell-like change and small cell carcinoma of the prostate. Two divergent forms of prostatic neuroendocrine differentiation. Am J Surg Pathol 1992; 16: 1013–1016.

333. Luebke AM, Schlomm T, Gunawan B, Bonkhoff H, Fuzesi L, Erbersdobler A. Simultaneous tumour-like, atypical basal cell hyperplasia and acinar adenocarcinoma of the prostate: a comparative morphological and genetic approach. Virchows Arch 2005 Mar; 446: 338–341.

334. Martin SA, Santa Cruz DJ. Adenomatoid metaplasia of prostatic urethra. Am J Clin Pathol 1981 Feb; 75: 185–189.

335. Carcamo Valor PI, San Millan Arruti JP, Cozar Olmo JM, Garcia-Matres MJ, Echevarria C, Martinez-Pineiro L, et al. [Nephrogenic adenoma of the upper and lower urinary tract. Apropos of 22 cases]. Arch Esp Urol 1992 Jun; 45: 423–427.

336. Young RH. Nephrogenic adenomas of the urethra involving the prostate gland: A report of two cases of a lesion that may be confused with prostatic adenocarcinoma. Mod Pathol 1992; 5: 617–620.

337. Gupta A, Wang HL, Policarpio-Nicolas ML, Tretiakova MS, Papavero V, Pins MR, et al. Expression of alpha-methylacyl-coenzyme A racemase in nephrogenic adenoma. Am J Surg Pathol 2004 Sep; 28: 1224–1229.

338. Xiao GQ, Burstein DE, Miller LK, Unger PD. Nephrogenic adenoma: immunohistochemical evaluation for its etiology and differentiation from prostatic adenocarcinoma. Arch Pathol Lab Med 2006 Jun; 130: 805–810.

339. Bonkhoff H. [Differential diagnosis of prostate cancer: impact of pattern analysis and immunohistochemistry]. Pathologe 2005 Nov; 26: 405–421.

340. Cheng L, Cheville JC, Sebo TJ, Eble JN, Bostwick DG. Atypical nephrogenic metaplasia of the urinary tract: a precursor lesion? Cancer 2000 Feb 15; 88: 853–861.

341. Mazal PR, Schaufler R, Altenhuber-Muller R, Haitel A, Watschinger B, Kratzik C, et al. Derivation of nephrogenic adenomas from renal tubular cells in kidney-transplant recipients. N Engl J Med 2002 Aug 29; 347: 653–659.

342. Wasserman NF. Benign prostatic hyperplasia: a review and ultrasound classification. Radiol Clin North Am 2006 Sep; 44: 689–710, viii.

343. Cabelin MA, Te AE, Kaplan SA. Benign prostatic hyperplasia: challenges for the new millennium. Curr Opin Urol 2000 Jul; 10: 301–306.

344. Lowe FC, Batista J, Berges R, Chartier-Kastler E, Conti G, Desgrandchamps F, et al. Risk factors for disease progression in patients with lower urinary tract symptoms/benign prostatic hyperplasia (LUTS/BPH): a systematic analysis of expert opinion. Prostate Cancer Prostatic Dis 2005; 8: 206–209.

345. Chen W, Yang CC, Chen GY, Wu MC, Sheu HM, Tzai TS. Patients with a large prostate show a higher prevalence of androgenetic alopecia. Arch Dermatol Res 2004 Nov; 296: 245–249.

346. McNeal JE. The pathobiology of nodular hyperplasia. In: Bostwick DG, ed. Pathology of the Prostate. new York, NY: Churchill Livingstone 1990: 31–36.

347. Shapiro E, Becich MJ, Hartanto V, Lepor H. The relative proportion of stromal and epithelial hyperplasia is related to the development of symptomatic benign prostate hyperplasia. J Urol 1992 May; 147: 1293–1297.

348. Aoki Y, Arai Y, Maeda H, Okubo K, Shinohara K. Racial differences in cellular composition of benign prostatic hyperplasia. Prostate 2001 Dec 1; 49: 243–250.

349. Bierhoff E, Vogel J, Benz M, Giefer T, Wernert N, Pfeifer U. Stromal nodules in benign prostatic hyperplasia. Eur Urol 1996; 29: 345–354.

350. Bostwick DG, Cooner WH, Denis L, Jones GW, Scardino PT, Murphy GP. The association of benign prostatic hyperplasia and cancer of the prostate. Cancer 1992 Jul 1; 70(1 Suppl): 291–301.

351. Leav I, McNeal JE, Ho SM, Jiang Z. Alpha-methylacyl-CoA racemase (P504S) expression in evolving carcinomas within benign prostatic hyperplasia and in cancers of the transition zone. Hum Pathol 2003 Mar; 34: 228–233.

352. Billis A. Prostatic atrophy: an autopsy study of a histologic mimic of adenocarcinoma. Mod Pathol 1998 Jan; 11: 47–54.

353. Billis A, Magna LA. Inflammatory atrophy of the prostate. Prevalence and significance. Arch Pathol Lab Med 2003; 127: 840–844.

354. Meirelles LR, Billis A, Cotta AC, et al. Prostatic atrophy: evidence for a possible role of local ischemia in its pathogenesis. Int Urol Nephrol 2002; 34: 345–350.

355. Faith D, Han S, Lee DK, et al. p16 Is upregulated in proliferative inflammatory atrophy of the prostate. Prostate 2005; 65: 73–82.

356. Wang W, Bergh A, Damber JE. Chronic inflammation in benign prostate hyperplasia is associated with focal upregulation of cyclooxygenase-2, Bcl-2, and cell proliferation in the glandular epithelium. Prostate 2004; 61: 60–72.

357. Bethel CR, Faith D, Li X, et al. Decreased NKX3.1 protein expression in focal prostatic atrophy, prostatic intraepithelial neoplasia, and adenocarcinoma: association with Gleason score and chromosome 8p deletion. Cancer Res 2006; 66: 10683–10690.

358. Banerjee AG, Liu J, Yuan Y, et al. Expression of biomarkers modulating prostate cancer angiogenesis: differential expression of annexin II in prostate carcinomas from India and USA. Mol Cancer 2003; 2: 34.

359. De Marzo AM, Marchi VL, Epstein JI, Nelson WG. Proliferative inflammatory atrophy of the prostate: implications for prostatic carcinogenesis. Am J Pathol 1999; 155: 1985–1992.

360. Adley BP, Yang XJ. Alpha-methylacyl coenzyme A racemase immunoreactivity in partial atrophy of the prostate. Am J Clin Pathol 2006; 126: 849–855.

361. Farinola MA, Epstein JI. Utility of immunohistochemistry for alpha-methylacyl-CoA racemase in distinguishing atrophic prostate cancer from benign atrophy. Hum Pathol 2004; 35: 1272–1278.

362. Yildiz-Sezer S, Verdorfer I, Schafer G, et al. Assessment of aberrations on chromosome 8 in prostatic atrophy. BJU Int 2006; 98: 184–188.

363. Schambeck CM, Schmeller N, Stieber P, et al. Methodological and clinical comparison of the ACS prostate-specific antigen assay and the Tandem-E prostate-specific antigen assay in prostate cancer. Urology 1995; 46: 195–199.

364. Franks LM. Atrophy and hyperplasia in the prostate proper. J Pathol Bacteriol 1954; 68: 617–621.

365. Amin MB, Tamboli P, Varma M, Srigley JR. Postatrophic hyperplasia of the prostate gland: a detailed analysis of its morphology in needle biopsy

specimens. Am J Surg Pathol 1999; 23: 925–931.

366. Ruska KM, Sauvageot J, Epstein JI. Histology and cellular kinetics of prostatic atrophy. Am J Surg Pathol 1998; 22: 1073–1077.

367. Billis A, Magna LA. Prostate elastosis: a microscopic feature useful for the diagnosis of postatrophic hyperplasia. Arch Pathol Lab Med 2000; 124: 1306–1309.

368. Shah R, Mucci NR, Amin A, et al. Postatrophic hyperplasia of the prostate gland: neoplastic precursor or innocent bystander? Am J Pathol 2001; 158: 1767–1773.

369. Anton RC, Kattan MW, Chakraborty S, Wheeler TM. Postatrophic hyperplasia of the prostate: lack of association with prostate cancer. Am J Surg Pathol 1999; 23: 932–936.

370. Postma R, Schroder FH, van der Kwast TH. Atrophy in prostate needle biopsy cores and its relationship to prostate cancer incidence in screened men. Urology 2005; 65: 745–749.

371. Oppenheimer JR, Wills ML, Epstein JI. Partial atrophy in prostate needle cores: another diagnostic pitfall for the surgical pathologist. Am J Surg Pathol 1998; 22: 440–445.

372. Tomas D, Kruslin B, Rogatsch H, et al. Different types of atrophy in the prostate with and without adenocarcinoma. Eur Urol 2007; 51: 98–103; discussion 103–104.

373. Putzi MJ, De Marzo AM. Morphologic transitions between proliferative inflammatory atrophy and high-grade prostatic intraepithelial neoplasia. Urology 2000; 56: 828–832.

374. Niu Y, Xu Y, Zhang J, et al. Proliferation and differentiation of prostatic stromal cells. BJU Int 2001; 87: 386–393.

375. Leong SS, Vogt PJ, Yu GS. Atypical stromal smooth muscle hyperplasia of prostate. Urology 1988; 31: 163–167.

376. Eble JN, Tejada E. Prostatic stromal hyperplasia with bizarre nuclei. Arch Pathol Lab Med 1991; 115: 87–89.

377. Wang XB, Bostwick DG. Prostatic stromal hyperplasia with atypia. A study of 11 cases. J Urol Pathol 1997; 12: 15–26.

378. Hossain D, Meiers I, Qian J, et al. Prostatic stromal hyperplasia with atypia (PSHA): Follow-up study of 28 cases of a histologic mimic of sarcoma. Arch Pathol Lab Med 2007 (in press).

379. Gaudin PB, Rosai J, Epstein JI. Sarcomas and related proliferative lesions of specialized prostatic stroma: a clinicopathologic study of 22 cases. Am J Surg Pathol 1998; 22: 148–162.

380. Hansel DE, Herawi M, Montgomery E, Epstein JI. Spindle cell lesions of the adult prostate. Mod Pathol 2007; 20: 148–158.

381. Herawi M, Epstein JI. Specialized stromal tumors of the prostate: a clinicopathologic study of 50 cases. Am J Surg Pathol 2006; 30: 694–704.

382. Bostwick DG, Hossain D, Qian J, et al. Phyllodes tumor of the prostate: long-term followup study of 23 cases. J Urol 2004; 172: 894–899.

383. Grignon DJ, Ro JY, Ordonez NG, et al. Basal cell hyperplasia, adenoid basal cell tumor, and adenoid cystic carcinoma of the prostate gland: an immunohistochemical study. Hum Pathol 1988; 19: 1425–1433.

384. Epstein JI, Armas OA. Atypical basal cell hyperplasia of the prostate. Am J Surg Pathol 1992; 16: 1205–1214.

385. Devaraj LT, Bostwick DG. Atypical basal cell hyperplasia of the prostate. Immunophenotypic profile and proposed classification of basal cell proliferations. Am J Surg Pathol 1993; 17: 645–659.

386. Montironi R, Mazzucchelli R, Stramazzotti D, et al. Basal cell hyperplasia and basal cell carcinoma of the prostate: a comprehensive review and discussion of a case with c-erbB-2 expression. J Clin Pathol 2005; 58: 290–296.

387. McKenney JK, Amin MB, Srigley JR, et al. Basal cell proliferations of the prostate other than usual basal cell hyperplasia: a clinicopathologic study of 23 cases, including four carcinomas, with a proposed classification. Am J Surg Pathol 2004; 28: 1289–1298.

388. Yang XJ, Tretiakova MS, Sengupta E, et al. Florid basal cell hyperplasia of the prostate: a histological, ultrastructural, and immunohistochemical analysis. Hum Pathol 2003; 34: 462–470.

389. Thorson P, Swanson PE, Vollmer RT, Humphrey PA. Basal cell hyperplasia in the peripheral zone of the prostate. Mod Pathol 2003; 16: 598–606.

390. Rioux-Leclercq NC, Epstein JI. Unusual morphologic patterns of basal cell hyperplasia of the prostate. Am J Surg Pathol 2002; 26: 237–243.

391. Hosler GA, Epstein JI. Basal cell hyperplasia: an unusual diagnostic dilemma on prostate needle biopsies. Hum Pathol 2005; 36: 480–485.

392. Dermer GB. Basal cell proliferation in benign prostatic hyperplasia. Cancer 1978; 41: 1857–1862.

393. Cleary KR, Choi HY, Ayala AG. Basal cell hyperplasia of the prostate. Am J Clin Pathol 1983; 80: 850–854.

394. van de Voorde W, Baldewijns M, Lauweryns J. Florid basal cell hyperplasia of the prostate. Histopathology 1994; 24: 341–348.

395. Atik E, Unsal I. Basal cell adenoma of prostate. Urol Res 2004; 32: 421–422.

396. Zhou M, Magi-Galluzzi C, Epstein JI. Prostate basal cell lesions can be negative for basal cell keratins: a diagnostic pitfall. Anal Quant Cytol Histol 2006; 28: 125–129.

397. Bostwick DG, Chang L. Overdiagnosis of prostatic adenocarcinoma. Semin Urol Oncol 1999; 17: 199–205.

398. Lopez-Beltran A, Qian J, Montironi R, et al. Atypical adenomatous hyperplasia (adenosis) of the prostate: DNA ploidy analysis and

immunophenotype. Int J Surg Pathol 2005; 13: 167–173.

399. Bostwick DG, Qian J. High-grade prostatic intraepithelial neoplasia. Mod Pathol 2004; 17: 360–379.

400. Mehlhorn J. [Frequency and differential diagnosis of cribriform structures of the prostate]. Zentralbl Pathol 1991; 137: 349–354.

401. Frauenhoffer EE, Ro JY, el-Naggar AK, et al. Clear cell cribriform hyperplasia of the prostate. Immunohistochemical and DNA flow cytometric study. Am J Clin Pathol 1991; 95: 446–453.

402. Cribriform hyperplasia of prostate. Am J Surg Pathol 1987; 11: 488–491.

403. Ayala AG, Srigley JR, Ro JY, et al. Clear cell cribriform hyperplasia of prostate. Report of 10 cases. Am J Surg Pathol 1986; 10: 665–671.

404. Bostwick DG, Algaba F, Amin MB, et al. Consensus statement on terminology: recommendation to use atypical adenomatous hyperplasia in place of adenosis of the prostate. Am J Surg Pathol 1994; 18: 1069–1070.

405. Bostwick DG, Srigley J, Grignon D, et al. Atypical adenomatous hyperplasia of the prostate: morphologic criteria for its distinction from well-differentiated carcinoma [see comments]. Hum Pathol 1993; 24: 819–832.

406. Brawn PN, Speights VO, Contin JU, et al. Atypical hyperplasia in prostates of 20 to 40 year old men. J Clin Pathol 1989; 42: 383–386.

407. Bostwick DG, Qian J. Atypical adenomatous hyperplasia of the prostate. Relationship with carcinoma in 217 whole-mount radical prostatectomies. Am J Surg Pathol 1995; 19: 506–518.

408. Gleason DF. Atypical hyperplasia, benign hyperplasia, and well-differentiated adenocarcinoma of the prostate. Am J Surg Pathol 1985; 9: 53–67.

409. Qian J, Jenkins RB, Bostwick DG. Chromosomal anomalies in atypical adenomatous hyperplasia and carcinoma of the prostate using fluorescence in situ hybridization. Urology 1995; 46: 837–842.

410. Cheng L, Shan A, Cheville JC, et al. Atypical adenomatous hyperplasia of the prostate: a premalignant lesion? Cancer Res 1998; 58: 389–391.

411. Doll JA, Zhu X, Furman J, et al. Genetic analysis of prostatic atypical adenomatous hyperplasia (adenosis). Am J Pathol 1999; 155: 967–971.

412. Bettendorf O, Schmidt H, Eltze E, et al. Cytogenetic changes and loss of heterozygosity in atypical adenomatous hyperplasia, in carcinoma of the prostate and in non-neoplastic prostate tissue using comparative genomic hybridization and multiplex-PCR. Int J Oncol 2005; 26: 267–274.

413. Rekhi B, Jaswal TS, Arora B. Premalignant lesions of prostate and their association with nodular

hyperplasia and carcinoma prostate. Indian J Cancer 2004; 41: 60–65.

414. Chen KT, Schiff JJ. Adenomatoid prostatic tumor. Urology 1983; 21: 88–89.

415. Hulman G. 'Pseudoadenomatoid' tumour of prostate. Histopathology 1989; 14: 317–319.

416. Young RH, Clement PB. Sclerosing adenosis of the prostate. Arch Pathol Lab Med 1987; 111: 363–366.

417. Sakamoto N, Tsuneyoshi M, Enjoji M. Sclerosing adenosis of the prostate. Histopathologic and immunohistochemical analysis. Am J Surg Pathol 1991; 15: 660–667.

418. Jones EC, Clement PB, Young RH. Sclerosing adenosis of the prostate gland. A clinicopathological and immunohistochemical study of 11 cases. Am J Surg Pathol 1991; 15: 1171–1180.

419. Collina G, Botticelli AR, Martinelli AM, et al. Sclerosing adenosis of the prostate. Report of three cases with electronmicroscopy and immunohistochemical study. Histopathology 1992; 20: 505–510.

420. Grignon DJ, Ro JY, Srigley JR, et al. Sclerosing adenosis of the prostate gland. A lesion showing myoepithelial differentiation. Am J Surg Pathol 1992; 16: 383–391.

421. Luque RJ, Lopez-Beltran A, Perez-Seoane C, Suzigan S. Sclerosing adenosis of the prostate. Histologic features in needle biopsy specimens. Arch Pathol Lab Med 2003; 127: e14–16.

422. Perimenis P, Gyftopoulos K, Ravazoula P, et al. Excessive verumontanum hyperplasia causing infertility. Urol Int 2001; 67: 184–185.

423. Gagucas RJ, Brown RW, Wheeler TM. Verumontanum mucosal gland hyperplasia. Am J Surg Pathol 1995; 19: 30–36.

424. Bostwick DG, Qian J, Ma J, Muir TE. Mesonephric remnants of the prostate: incidence and histologic spectrum. Mod Pathol 2003; 16: 630–635.

425. Singh SK, Wadhwa P, Nada R, et al. Localized primary amyloidosis of the prostate, bladder and ureters. Int Urol Nephrol 2005; 37: 495–497.

426. Pitkanen P, Westermark P, Cornwell GG 3rd, Murdoch W. Amyloid of the seminal vesicles. A distinctive and common localized form of senile amyloidosis. Am J Pathol 1983; 110: 64–69.

427. Seidman JD, Shmookler BM, Connolly B, Lack EE. Localized amyloidosis of seminal vesicles: report of three cases in surgically obtained material. Mod Pathol 1989; 2: 671–675.

428. Khan SM, Birch PJ, Bass PS, et al. Localized amyloidosis of the lower genitourinary tract: a clinicopathological and immunohistochemical study of nine cases. Histopathology 1992; 21: 143–147.

429. Coyne JD, Kealy WF. Seminal vesicle amyloidosis: morphological, histochemical and immunohistochemical observations. Histopathology 1993; 22: 173–176.

430. Ramchandani P, Schnall MD, LiVolsi VA, et al. Senile amyloidosis of the seminal vesicles mimicking metastatic spread of prostatic carcinoma on MR images. AJR Am J Roentgenol 1993; 161: 99–100.

431. Lawrentschuk N, Pan D, Stillwell R, Bolton DM. Implications of amyloidosis on prostatic biopsy. Int J Urol 2004; 11: 925–927.

432. Esslimani M, Serre I, Granier M, et al. [Urogenital amyloidosis: clinico-pathological study of 8 cases]. Ann Pathol 1999; 19: 487–491.

433. Guillan RA, Zelman S. The incidence and probable origin of melanin in the prostate. J Urol 1970; 104: 151–153.

434. Seman G, Gallager HS, Johnson DE. Melanin-like pigment in the human prostate. Prostate 1982; 3: 59–72.

435. Muzaffar S, Aijaz F, Pervez S, Hasan SH. Melanosis of the prostate: a rare benign morphological entity. Br J Urol 1995; 76: 265–266.

436. Bostwick DG, Amin MB, Dundore P, et al. Architectural patterns of high-grade prostatic intraepithelial neoplasia. Hum Pathol 1993; 24: 298–310.

437. Ro JY, Grignon DJ, Ayala AG, et al. Blue nevus and melanosis of the prostate. Electron-microscopic and immunohistochemical studies. Am J Clin Pathol 1988; 90: 530–535.

438. Rios CN, Wright JR. Melanosis of the prostate gland: report of a case with neoplastic epithelium involvement. J Urol 1976; 115: 616–617.

439. Aguilar M, Gaffney EF, Finnerty DP. Prostatic melanosis with involvement of benign and malignant epithelium. J Urol 1982; 128: 825–827.

440. Egevad L. Cytology of the central zone of the prostate. Diagn Cytopathol 2003; 28: 239–244.

441. Tannenbaum M. Differential diagnosis in uropathology. III. Melanotic lesions of prostate: blue nevus and prostatic epithelial melanosis. Urology 1974; 4: 617–621.

442. Leung CS, Srigley JR. Distribution of lipochrome pigment in the prostate gland: biological and diagnostic implications. Hum Pathol 1995; 26: 1302–1307.

443. Beckman EN, Pintado SO, Leonard GL, Sternberg WH. Endometriosis of the prostate. Am J Surg Pathol 1985; 9: 374–379.

444. Martin JD Jr, Hauck AE. Endometriosis in the male. Am Surg 1985; 51: 426–430.

445. Schrodt GR, Alcorn MO, Ibanez J. Endometriosis of the male urinary system: a case report. J Urol 1980; 124: 722–723.

446. Thompson CA. Finasteride may prevent prostate cancer. Am J Health Syst Pharm 2003; 60: 1511.

447. Taneja SS, Smith MR, Dalton JT, et al. Toremifene – a promising therapy for the prevention of prostate cancer and complications of androgen deprivation therapy. Expert Opin Invest Drugs 2006; 15: 293–305.

448. Brawley OW. Hormonal prevention of prostate cancer. Urol Oncol 2003; 21: 67–72.

449. Lowe FC, McConnell JD, Hudson PB, et al. Long-term 6-year experience with finasteride in patients with benign prostatic hyperplasia. Urology 2003; 61: 791–796.

450. Vaughan D, Imperato-McGinley J, McConnell J, et al. Long-term (7 to 8-year) experience with finasteride in men with benign prostatic hyperplasia. Urology 2002; 60: 1040–1044.

451. Vailancourt L, Ttu B, Fradet Y, et al. Effect of neoadjuvant endocrine therapy (combined androgen blockade) on normal prostate and prostatic carcinoma. A randomized study. Am J Surg Pathol 1996; 20: 86–93.

452. Civantos F, Marcial MA, Banks ER, et al. Pathology of androgen deprivation therapy in prostate carcinoma. A comparative study of 173 patients. Cancer 1995; 75: 1634–1641.

453. Ellison E, Chuang S-S, Zincke H, et al. Prostate adenocarcinoma after androgen deprivation therapy: A comparative study of morphology, morphometry, immunohistochemistry, and DNA ploidy. Pathol Case Rev 1996; 2: 36–46.

454. Montironi R, Bartels PH, Thompson D, et al. Androgen-deprived prostate adenocarcinoma: evaluation of treatment-related changes versus no distinctive treatment effect with a Bayesian belief network. A methodological approach. Eur Urol 1996; 30: 307–315.

455. Montironi R, Diamanti L, Santinelli A, et al. Effect of total androgen ablation on pathologic stage and resection limit status of prostate cancer. Initial results of the Italian PROSIT study. Pathol Res Pract 1999; 195: 201–208.

456. Murphy WM, Soloway MS, Barrows GH. Pathologic changes associated with androgen deprivation therapy for prostate cancer. Cancer 1991; 68: 821–828.

457. Reuter VE. Pathological changes in benign and malignant prostatic tissue following androgen deprivation therapy. Urology 1997; 49: 16–22.

458. Montironi R, Schulman CC. Pathological changes in prostate lesions after androgen manipulation. J Clin Pathol 1998; 51: 5–12.

459. Grignon DJ BD, Civantos F, Garnick MB, et al. Pathologic handling and reporting of prostate tissue specimens in patients receiving neoadjuvant hormonal therapy: report of the Pathology Committee. Mol Urol 1999; 3: 193–198.

460. Clark RV, Gabriel H, et al. Effective suppression of dihydrotestosterone

(DHT) by GI198745, a novel, dual 5 alpha reductase inhibitor. J Urol 1999; 161: 268; [abstract 1037].

461. Wright AS, Thomas LN, Douglas RC, et al. Relative potency of testosterone and dihydrotestosterone in preventing atrophy and apoptosis in the prostate of the castrated rat. J Clin Invest 1996; 98: 2558–2563.

462. Bramson HN, Hermann D, Batchelor KW, et al. Unique preclinical characteristics of GG745, a potent dual inhibitor of 5AR. J Pharmacol Exp Ther 1997; 282: 1496–1502.

463. McConnell JD, Wilson JD, George FW, et al. Finasteride, an inhibitor of 5 alpha-reductase, suppresses prostatic dihydrotestosterone in men with benign prostatic hyperplasia. J Clin Endocrinol Metab 1992; 74: 505–508.

464. Rittmaster RS, Norman RW, Thomas LN, Rowden G. Evidence for atrophy and apoptosis in the prostates of men given finasteride. J Clin Endocrinol Metab 1996; 81: 814–819.

465. Prahalada S, Rhodes L, Grossman SJ, et al. Morphological and hormonal changes in the ventral and dorsolateral prostatic lobes of rats treated with finasteride, a 5-alpha reductase inhibitor. Prostate 1998; 35: 157–164.

466. Montironi R, Valli M, Fabris G. Treatment of benign prostatic hyperplasia with 5-alpha-reductase inhibitor: morphological changes in patients who fail to respond. J Clin Pathol 1996; 49: 324–328.

467. Rittmaster RS, Manning AP, Wright AS, et al. Evidence for atrophy and apoptosis in the ventral prostate of rats given the 5 alpha-reductase inhibitor finasteride. Endocrinology 1995; 136: 741–748.

468. Marks LS, Partin AW, Dorey FJ, et al. Long-term effects of finasteride on prostate tissue composition. Urology 1999; 53: 574–580.

469. Marks LS, Partin AW, Gormley GJ, \ et al. Prostate tissue composition and response to finasteride in men with symptomatic benign prostatic hyperplasia. J Urol 1997; 157: 2171–2178.

470. Civantos F, Watson RB, Pinto JE, et al. Finasteride effect on benign prostatic hyperplasia and prostate cancer. A comparative clinico-pathologic study of radical prostatectomies. J Urol Pathol 1997; 6: 1–8.

471. Montironi R, Diamanti L. Morphologic changes in benign prostatic hyperplasia following chronic treatment with a 5-a-reductase inhibitor Finasteride. Comparison with combination endocrine therapy. J Urol Pathol 1996; 4: 123–135.

472. Yang XJ LK, Short K, Gottesman J, et al. Does long-term finasteride therapy affect the histologic features of benign prostatic tissue and prostate can cer on needle biopsy? PLESS Study Group. Proscar Long-Term Efficacy and Safety Study. Urology 1999; 53: 696–700.

473. Iczkowski KA, Qiu J, Qian J, et al. The dual 5-alpha-reductase inhibitor dutasteride induces atrophic changes and decreases relative cancer volume in human prostate. Urology 2005; 65: 76–82.

474. Andriole GL, Humphrey P, Ray P, et al. Effect of the dual 5alpha-reductase inhibitor dutasteride on markers of tumor regression in prostate cancer. J Urol 2004; 172: 915–919.

475. Feneley MR, Puddefoot JR, Xia S, et al. Zonal biochemical and morphological characteristics in BPH. Br J Urol 1995; 75: 608–613.

476. Sanchez-Visconti G, Herrero G, Rabadan M, et al. Ageing and prostate: age-related changes in androgen receptors of epithelial cells from benign hypertrophic glands compared with cancer. Mech Ageing Dev 1995; 82: 19–29.

477. Bowman SP BD, Blacklock NJ, Sullivan PJ. Regional variation of cytosol androgen receptors throughout the diseased human prostate gland. Prostate 1986; 8: 167–80.

478. Sirinarumitr K, Sirinarumitr T, Johnston SD, et al. Finasteride-induced prostatic involution by apoptosis in dogs with benign prostatic hypertrophy. Am J Vet Res 2002; 63: 495–498.

479. Patterson RF, Jones EC, Zubovits JT, et al. Immunohistochemical analysis of radical prostatectomy specimens after 8 months of neoadjuvant hormonal therapy. Mol Urol 1999; 3: 277–286.

480. Polito M, Muzzonigro G, Minardi D, Montironi R. Effects of neoadjuvant androgen deprivation therapy on prostatic cancer. Eur Urol 1996; 30: 26–31; discussion 38–29.

481. Minardi D, Galosi AB, Giannulis I, et al. Comparison of proliferating cell nuclear antigen immunostaining in lymph node metastases and primary prostate adenocarcinoma after neoadjuvant androgen deprivation therapy. Scand J Urol Nephrol 2004; 38: 19–25.

482. Moritz R, Srougi M, Ortiz V, et al. [Prostate cancer dedifferentiation following antiandrogen therapy: a morphological finding or an increased tumor aggressiveness?]. Rev Assoc Med Bras 2005; 51: 117–120.

483. Cheng L, Cheville JC, Bostwick DG. Diagnosis of prostate cancer in needle biopsies after radiation therapy. Am J Surg Pathol 1999; 23: 1173–1183.

484. Gaudin PB, Zelefsky MJ, Leibel SA, et al. Histopathologic effects of three-dimensional conformal external beam radiation therapy on benign and malignant prostate tissues. Am J Surg Pathol 1999; 23: 1021–1031.

485. Petersen DS, Milleman LA, Rose EF, et al. Biopsy and clinical course after cryosurgery for prostatic cancer. J Urol 1978; 120: 308–311.

486. Shabaik A, Wilson S, Bidair M, et al. Pathologic changes in prostate biopsies following cryoablation therapy of prostate carcinoma. J Urol Pathol 1995; 3: 183–94.

487. Borkowski P, Robinson MJ, Poppiti RJ Jr, Nash SC. Histologic findings in postcryosurgical prostatic biopsies. Mod Pathol 1996; 9: 807–811.

488. Falconieri G, Lugnani F, Zanconati F, et al. Histopathology of the frozen prostate. The microscopic bases of prostatic carcinoma cryoablation. Pathol Res Pract 1996; 192: 579–587.

489. Shuman BA, Cohen JK, Miller RJ Jr, et al. Histological presence of viable prostatic glands on routine biopsy following cryosurgical ablation of the prostate. J Urol 1997; 157: 552–555.

490. Susani M, Madersbacher S, Kratzik C, et al. Morphology of tissue destruction induced by focused ultrasound. Eur Urol 1993; 23: 34–38.

491. Orihuela E, Motamedi M, Pow-Sang M, et al. Histopathological evaluation of laser thermocoagulation in the human prostate: optimization of laser irradiation for benign prostatic hyperplasia. J Urol 1995; 153: 1531–1536.

492. Corica AG, Qian J, Ma J, et al. Fast liquid ablation system for prostatic hyperplasia: a new minimally invasive thermal treatment. J Urol 2003; 170: 874–878.

493. Seitz C, Djavan B, Marberger M. Morphological and biological predictors for treatment outcome of transurethral microwave thermotherapy. Curr Opin Urol 2002; 12: 25–32.

494. Tucker RD, Platz CE, Huidobro C, Larson T. Interstitial thermal therapy in patients with localized prostate cancer: histologic analysis. Urology 2002; 60: 166–169.

495. Larson BT, Bostwick DG, Corica AG, Larson TR. Histological changes of minimally invasive procedures for the treatment of benign prostatic hyperplasia and prostate cancer: clinical implications. J Urol 2003; 170: 12–19.

496. Bostwick DG, Larson TR. Transurethral microwave thermal therapy: pathologic findings in the canine prostate. Prostate 1995; 26: 116–122.

497. Larson BT, Collins JM, Huidobro C, et al. Gadolinium-enhanced MRI in the evaluation of minimally invasive treatments of the prostate: correlation with histopathologic findings. Urology 2003; 62: 900–904.

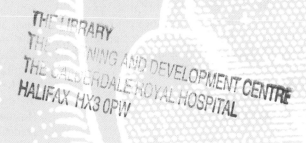

CHAPTER **9**

# Neoplasms of the prostate

David G. Bostwick, Isabelle Meiers

THE LIBRARY
THE LEARNING AND DEVELOPMENT CENTRE
THE CALDERDALE ROYAL HOSPITAL
HALIFAX HX3 0PW

Prostate cancer is the most common cancer of men in the United States and is second only to lung followed by colorectal cancer as a cause of cancer death. In 2008, 28 660 Americans will die of prostate cancer and 186 320 new cases will be diagnosed.[1] The probability of developing clinically detected prostate cancer rose from 1 in 39 in men between 40 and 59 years of age to 1 in 14 for men between 60 and 69 years and 1 in 7 for men 70 and older; for all men, the overall probability was 1 in 6.[1] Despite prevalence at autopsy of up to 80% by age 80 years,[2] the clinical incidence is much lower, indicating that most men die with, rather than of, prostate carcinoma. Little is known about the causes of prostate cancer despite its high incidence and prevalence. This chapter reviews the pathology of adenocarcinoma of the prostate and other prostatic tumors. Issues of grading and staging are addressed, and diagnostic and prognostic markers are discussed.

## Epithelial neoplasms

### Prostatic intraepithelial neoplasia (PIN)

Prostatic intraepithelial neoplasia refers to the preinvasive end of the continuum of cellular proliferations within the lining of prostatic ducts, ductules, and acini. High-grade prostatic intraepithelial neoplasia (PIN) is the earliest accepted stage in carcinogenesis, possessing most of the phenotypic, biochemical, and genetic changes of cancer without invasion into the fibromuscular stroma.[3,4] Recently, the World Health Organization reaffirmed its position that PIN is the only demonstrated preinvasive lesion for prostate cancer.[5] Other potential but unproven candidates for premalignancy in the prostate include atypical adenomatous hyperplasia (Chapter 8), malignancy-associated changes arising in normal-appearing epithelium,[6–8] and atrophy (Chapter 8).

Initial references to the lesion we now know as PIN were apparently made by early authors such as Kastendieck and Helpap,[9] but they did not provide reproducible criteria and distinguish their findings from mimics of PIN. In 1965, McNeal emphasized the possible premalignant nature of

proliferative changes in the prostatic epithelium, but his description included a variety of findings. More than 30 years later, McNeal and Bostwick[10] described, for the first time, reproducible diagnostic criteria for the recognition of what they referred to as 'intraductal dysplasia,' and introduced a three-grade classification system. The following year, Bostwick and Brawer[11] proposed the term prostatic intraepithelial neoplasia – PIN – as a replacement for intraductal dysplasia, and this new term was promulgated in 1989 at a workshop on prostate preneoplastic lesions sponsored by the American Cancer Society and National Cancer Institute,[12] and subsequently endorsed at numerous multiple multidisciplinary and pathology consensus meetings.[5,13–18] Terms such as intraductal dysplasia, severe dysplasia, large acinar atypical hyperplasia, duct–acinar dysplasia, and intraductal carcinoma were discouraged and have ceased to be used in routine practice.[13]

The 1989 conference also recommended compression of the PIN classification into two grades: low-grade (formerly PIN grade 1) or high-grade PIN (formerly PIN grades 2 and 3) (Table 9-1).[12] The clinical significance of high-grade PIN was considered substantial at that time, whereas low-grade PIN was considered largely inconsequential, a belief that was reinforced over subsequent decades and persists today.

Interobserver agreement between pathologists for high-grade PIN is 'good to excellent.'[19–21] However, this is not true for low-grade PIN; also, it has a much lower predictive value for cancer that limits its clinical utility[21–28] (Table 9-2), and most do not routinely report this finding today except in research studies.[18] Thus, most investigators now use the term PIN interchangeably with high-grade PIN. High-grade PIN is considered a standard diagnosis that must be included as part of the reported pathologic evaluation of biopsies, transurethral resections, and radical prostatectomy specimens.[18] Its diagnostic utility when cancer is already present is uncertain, but 69% of urologic pathologists still report PIN in this setting.[21]

### Epidemiology of PIN

The mean reported incidence of isolated high-grade PIN is 9% (range, 4–24%) of prostate biopsies (Tables 9.3, 9.4),

**Table 9-1** Diagnostic criteria for PIN

| | Low-grade PIN (formerly PIN 1) | High-grade PIN (formerly PIN 2 and 3) |
|---|---|---|
| Architecture | Epithelial cells crowding and stratification, with irregular spacing | Similar to low-grade PIN; more crowding and stratification; four patterns: tufting, micropapillary, cribriform, and flat |
| Cytology<br>  Nuclei<br>  Chromatin<br>  Nucleoli | Enlarged, with marked size variation<br>Normal<br>Rarely prominent* | Enlarged; some size and shape variation<br>Increased density and clumping<br>Prominent |
| Basal cell layer | Intact | May show some disruption |
| Basement membrane | Intact | Intact |

*Fewer than 10% of cells have prominent nucleoli.

**Table 9-2** Cancer risk in patients with low- vs high-grade PIN*

| Reference | Low-grade PIN | | High-grade PIN | |
|---|---|---|---|---|
| | No. of men with repeat biopsy or biopsies | Cancer risk (%) | No. of men with repeat biopsy or biopsies | Cancer risk (%) |
| Brawer et al. 1991[22] | 11 | 18 | 8 | 100 |
| Aboseif et al. 1995[23] | 12 | 17 | 24 | 79 |
| Langer et al. 1996[24] | 5 | 40 | 48 | 27 |
| Raviv et al. 1996[25] | 45 | 14 | 48 | 48 |
| Shepherd et al. 1996[26] | 21 | 24 | 45 | 58 |
| Goeman et al. 2003[27] | 43 | 30 | 69 | 27 |
| De Matteis et al. 2005[28] | 50 | 30 | 22 | 45 |
| Range | | 14–40 | | 27–100 |

*Includes only those studies simultaneously reporting low-grade and high-grade PIN.

similar to our personal experience in Virginia in 2007 (data not shown). Given that 1 300 000 prostate biopsies are performed annually, a reasonable estimate is that there are 115 000 new cases annually of high-grade PIN without cancer[29,30] and a prevalence of more than 16 million (Table 9-5).

The incidence of PIN varies according to the population of men under study (Tables 9.3–9.5).[31,32] The lowest likelihood is in men participating in PSA screening and early detection studies, with an incidence ranging from 0.7% to 20%.[31,32]

Men seen by urologists in practice have PIN in 4.4–25% of biopsies. Those undergoing transurethral resection have the highest likelihood of PIN, varying from 2.8% to 33% (Table 9-4).[22,33,34] In such cases all tissue should be examined, but serial sections of suspicious foci are usually not necessary. Unfortunately, needle biopsy specimens fail to show the suspicious focus at deeper levels in about half of cases, often precluding assessment by immunohistochemistry and compounding the diagnostic dilemma.

The prevalence and extent of PIN increase with patient age (Table 9-5).[35] An autopsy study of step-sectioned whole-mount prostates from older men showed that the prevalence of PIN in prostates with cancer increased with age, predating the onset of carcinoma by more than 5 years.[14,36,37] A similar study revealed that PIN is first seen in men in their 20s and 30s (9% and 22% frequency, respectively), and preceded the onset of carcinoma by more than 10 years.[36] Most foci of PIN in young men were low grade, with increasing frequency and volumes of high-grade PIN with advancing age.[38]

Race and geographic location also appear to influence the incidence of PIN after controlling for patient age.[39] For example, African-American men had a greater prevalence of PIN than Caucasians in the 50–60-year age group, the decade that precedes the detection of most prostate cancers.[14,40] African-American men also had the highest incidence of cancer (about 50% more than Caucasians).[2,14,41,42] In contrast, Japanese men living in Osaka, Japan, had a signifi-

cantly lower incidence of PIN than those residing in the United States, and Asians had the lowest clinically detected rate of prostate cancer.[43,44] Interestingly, Japanese men diagnosed with PIN also had an increased likelihood of developing prostate cancer, indicating that PIN is also a precursor of clinical prostate cancer in Asian men.[45] Differences in the frequency of PIN in the 50–60 age group across races essentially mirror the rates of clinical prostate cancer observed in the 60–70-year age group.[43,46]

The likely causal association of PIN with prostatic adenocarcinoma is supported by the observation that the prevalence of both increases with patient age, and that PIN precedes the onset of prostate cancer by less than one decade (Table 9-6).[2,36,46,47] The severity and frequency of PIN in prostates with cancer are greatly increased (73% of 731 specimens) compared to prostates without cancer (32% of 876 specimens).[35,48,49] When high-grade PIN was found on sextant needle biopsy, there was a 50% risk of finding carcinoma on subsequent biopsies within 3 years,[50] although this risk was lower when more than six cores are obtained; this decline in predictive value is expected, given the increased sampling for cancer with a greater number of core biopsies (see below).

### Diagnostic criteria for PIN

There are four main patterns of high-grade PIN: tufting, micropapillary, cribriform, and flat (Figs 9-1-9-3).[51] The tufting pattern is the most common, present in 97% of cases, although most have multiple patterns. There are no known clinically important differences between the architectural patterns, and their recognition appears to be only of diagnostic utility. Sporadic retrospective reports have suggested that the cribriform or micropapillary patterns may indicate a higher risk of coexistent cancer, but this has been repeatedly refuted. Other unusual patterns of PIN include the signet ring-cell pattern, small cell neuroendocrine (oat cell) pattern, mucinous pattern, microvacuolated (foamy gland) pattern, inverted (hobnail) pattern,[52] and PIN with squa-

**Table 9-3** Incidence of isolated high-grade PIN in prostatic needle biopsies

| Reference | Patient population | No. of patients | Incidence of PIN (%) |
|---|---|---|---|
| **Screening Programs** | | | |
| Mettlin et al. 1991[1247] | American Cancer Society National Prostate Cancer Detection Project | 327 | 5.2 |
| Feneley et al. 1997[1248] | Screening population in Gwent, England, 1991–1993 | 212 | 19.8 |
| Hoedemaeker et al. 1999[1249] | PSA screening study in Rotterdam, The Netherlands | 1824 | 0.7 |
| Postma et al. 2004[1250] | Screening population in Rotterdam, The Netherlands (first round) | 4117 | 0.8 |
| Postma et al. 2004[1250] | Screening population in Rotterdam, The Netherlands (second round, performed at a 4-year interval from the first ) | 1840 | 2.5 |
| Picone et al. 2006 | Screening population from Southern Italy | 1008 | 3.0 |
| **Urology Practice** | | | |
| Lee et al. 1989[243] | Consecutive biopsies of hypoechoic lesions at St. Joseph Mercy Hospital | 256 | 11 |
| Bostwick et al. 1995[1251] | Consecutive biopsies at Mayo Clinic | 200 | 16.5 |
| Bostwick et al. 1995[1251] | Consecutive biopsies at Glendale Hospital (CA.) | 200 | 10.5 |
| Langer et al. 1996[24] | Consecutive biopsies at University of Pennsylvania Med. Ctr. | 1275 | 4.4 |
| Wills et al. 1997[302] | Consecutive biopsies at Johns Hopkins Hospital | 439 | 2.7 |
| Feneley et al. 1997[1248] | Consecutive biopsies at University College London Hospitals, 1988–1994 | 1205 | 10.9 |
| Feneley et al. 1997[1248] | Consecutive biopsies of symptomatic men at St. Bartholomew's Hospital, London, 1993–1994 | 118 | 24.6 |
| Skjorten et al. 1997[33] | Consecutive biopsies from 1974–1975 at Ullevaal and Lovisenberg Hospitals, Oslo, Norway | 79 | 7.6 |
| Perachino et al. 1997[32] | Consecutive biopsies | 148 | 14.1 |
| O'Dowd et al. 2000[65] | Consecutive biopsies at UroCor Inc., Oklahoma City, 1994–1998 | 132426 | 3.7 |
| Borboroglu et al. 2001[321] | Consecutive biopsies | 1391 | 5.5 |
| Lefkowitz et al. 2001[1252] | Consecutive biopsies at the Manhattan Veterans Administration Medical Center | 619 | 16.6 |
| San Francisco et al. 2003[1253] | Consecutive biopsies 1996–1997 | 387 | 12.6 |
| Roscigno et al. 2004[56] | Consecutive biopsies at San Raffaele Hospital, Milan, Italy | 2314 | 3.9 |
| Abdel-Khalek et al. 2004[1254] | Consecutive biopsies at Urology and Nephrology Center, Mansoura University, Mansoura, Egypt, 1997–2002 | 3081 | 2.7 |
| Alsikafi et al. 2001[331] | Consecutive biopsies at Section of Urology, University of Chicago, 1998–1999 | 485 | 4.3 |
| Gupta et al. 2004[295] | Consecutive biopsies at St. John Hospital and Medical Center, Detroit, 2001–2002 | 933 | 12.3 |
| Gupta et al. 2004[295] | Consecutive biopsies at St John Hospital and Medical Center, Detroit, 1998–2000 | 515 | 13.5 |
| Kobayashi et al. 2004[300] | Consecutive biopsies at Hamamatsu Rosai Hospital, Hamamatsu, Japan | 104 | 20.2 |
| Naya et al. 2004[301] | Consecutive biopsies at University of Texas MD Anderson Cancer Center, Houston, 1997–2003 | 1086 | 8.7 |
| Moore et al. 2005[322] | Consecutive biopsies at Albany Medical College and Stratton Veterans Administration Medical Center 1998–2003 | 1188 | 2.5 |

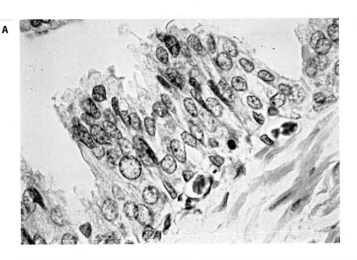
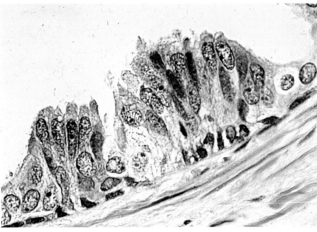

**Fig. 9-1** Prostatic intraepithelial neoplasia. (**A**) Low grade. (**B**) High grade.

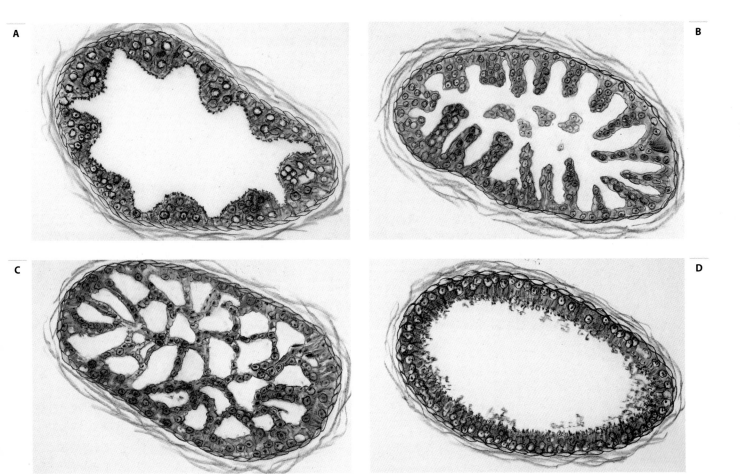

**Fig. 9-2** Architectural patterns of high-grade prostatic, intraepithelial neoplasia. (**A**) Tufting pattern. (**B**) Micropapillary pattern. (**C**) Cribriform pattern. (**D**) Flat pattern. (From Bostwick DG, Amin MB, Dundore P et al. Architectural patterns of high grade prostatic intraepithelial neoplasia, Hum Pathol 1993; 24: 298–310, with permission.)

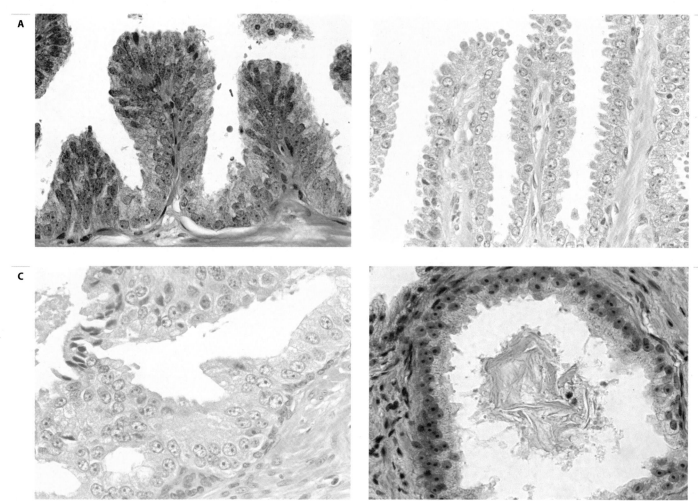

**Fig. 9-3** Architectural patterns of high-grade PIN. Compare with artist's renditions in Figure 9-2. (**A**) Tufting and early micropapillary patterns. (**B**) Micropapillary pattern. (**C**) Cribriform pattern. (**D**) Flat pattern.

**Table 9-4** Incidence of isolated high-grade PIN in transurethral resections

| Reference | Specimen | Patient population | Number of men | Incidence of PIN (%) |
|---|---|---|---|---|
| Gaudin et al. 1997[34] | TURP | Consecutive TURPs without cancer at Johns Hopkins Hospital | 158 | 3.2 |
| Pacelli and Bostwick, 1997[254] | TURP | Consecutive TURPs without cancer at Mayo Clinic | 570 | 2.8 |
| Skjorten et al. 1997[33] | TURP | Consecutive TURPs from 1974–1975 at Ullevaal and Lovisenberg Hospitals, Oslo, Norway | 731 | 33 |

**Table 9-5** Estimated prevalence of high-grade PIN in the United States

| Age | High-grade PIN (%) | US population* (000) | Number of PIN |
|---|---|---|---|
| 40–49 | 15.2 | 20 550 | 3 123 600 |
| 50–59 | 24.0 | 14 187 | 3 404 880 |
| 60–69 | 47.3 | 9 312 | 4 404 576 |
| 70–79 | 58.4 | 6 926 | 4 044 784 |
| 80–89 | 70.0 | 2 664 | 1 864 800 |
| **Total** | | **53 639 000** | **16 842 640** |

**Table 9-6** Evidence for the association of high-grade PIN and prostatic carcinoma

Histology
    Similar architectural and cytologic features

Location
    Both are located chiefly in the peripheral zone and are multicentric
    Close spatial association of PIN and cancer

Correlation with cell proliferation and death (apoptosis)
    Growth fraction of PIN is similar to that of cancer
    Apoptosis-suppressing oncoprotein bcl-2 expression is increased in PIN and cancer

Loss of basal cell layer
    The highest grade of PIN has loss of basal cell layer, similar to cancer

Increased frequency of PIN in the presence of cancer

Increased extent of PIN in the presence of cancer

Increased severity of PIN in the presence of cancer

Immunophenotype
    PIN is more closely related to cancer than benign epithelium
    For some biomarkers there is progressive loss of expression with increasing grades of PIN and cancer, including PSA, neuroendocrine cells, cytoskeletal proteins, and secretory proteins
    For some biomarkers there is progressive increase in expression with increasing grades of PIN and cancer including type IV collagenase, TGF-α, EGF, EGFR, Lewis Y antigen, and c-erB-2 oncogene Morphometry

High-grade PIN and cancer have similar nuclear area, chromatin content and distribution, nuclear perimeter, nuclear diameter, and nuclear roundness
    High-grade PIN and cancer have similar nucleolar number, size, and location
    DNA content
        High-grade PIN and cancer have similar frequency of aneuploidy
    Genetic instability

High-grade PIN and cancer have similar frequency of allelic loss

High-grade PIN and cancer have similar foci of allelic loss
    Microvessel density

Progressive increase in microvessel density from PIN to cancer
    Origin

Cancer found to arise in foci of PIN
    Age

Age incidence peak of PIN precedes cancer
    Predictive value of high-grade PIN

PIN on biopsy has high predictive value for cancer on subsequent biopsy

**Table 9-7** Histologic patterns of high-grade PIN

Usual patterns[51]
    Tufting
    Micropapillary
    Cribriform
    Flat

Signet ring cell

Small cell (neuroendocrine)[53]

Foamy gland (microvacuolated)[1256]

Hobnail (inverted)[52]

Squamous[54]

PIN spreads through prostatic ducts in multiple different patterns, similar to carcinoma. In the first pattern, neoplastic cells replace the normal luminal secretory epithelium, with preservation of the basal cell layer and basement membrane. This pattern often has a cribriform or near-solid appearance. Foci of high-grade PIN are usually indistinguishable from intraductal/intra-acinar spread of carcinoma on routine light microscopy.[59] In the second pattern there is direct invasion through the ductal or acinar wall, with disruption of the basal cell layer. In the third pattern, neoplastic cells invaginate between the basal cell and columnar secretory cell layers ('pagetoid spread'), a very rare finding. The proliferative activity, defined as Ki-67 labeling index, was lower in PIN (mean 6%, range 2–15%) than in ductal adenocarcinoma; the combination of histological features and measurements of cellular proliferation help to distinguish these findings in limited tissue samples.[60,61]

On electron microscopy, high-grade PIN displayed features that were intermediate between those of benign epithelium and adenocarcinoma.[62] These included the presence of cells with a variable number of cytoplasmic secretory vacuoles, luminal apocrine blebs, large nuclei with coarsely clumped chromatin, enlarged nucleoli, prominent apical microvilli, an intact or discontinuous basal cell layer, and intact basement membrane. Occasional acini had luminal cells abutting the basement membrane without interposition of basal cells, and other acini with extremely attenuated basal cell cytoplasmic processes contained sparse bundles of intermediate filaments.

Early stromal invasion, the earliest evidence of carcinoma, occurs at sites of acinar outpouching and basal cell disruption in acini with high-grade PIN (Figs 9-5, 9-6). Such microinvasion is present in about 2% of high-power microscopic fields of PIN, and is seen with equal frequency in all architectural patterns.[39,51]

The mean volume of PIN in prostates with cancer is 1.2–1.32 mL, and increases with increasing pathologic stage, Gleason grade, positive surgical margins, and perineural invasion.[35,63] These findings emphasize the close spatial and biologic relationship of PIN and cancer, and may result from an increase in PIN with increasing cancer volume.

PIN and cancer are usually multicentric.[4,35,51,56] PIN is multicentric in 72% of radical prostatectomies with cancer, including 63% of those involving the non-transition

mous differentiation (Fig. 9-4; Table 9-7).[53,54] The presence of extensive PIN appears to be more predictive of cancer than the more common isolated single acinus with PIN (see below).[55–57] The presence of intraluminal crystalloids in combination with PIN in is a more compelling indication for repeat biopsy than PIN alone.[58]

There is inversion of the normal orientation of epithelial proliferation with PIN. In benign epithelium cell division normally occurs in the basal cell compartment, whereas in PIN the greatest proliferation occurs on the luminal surface, similar to preinvasive lesions in the colon (tubular adenoma) and other sites.

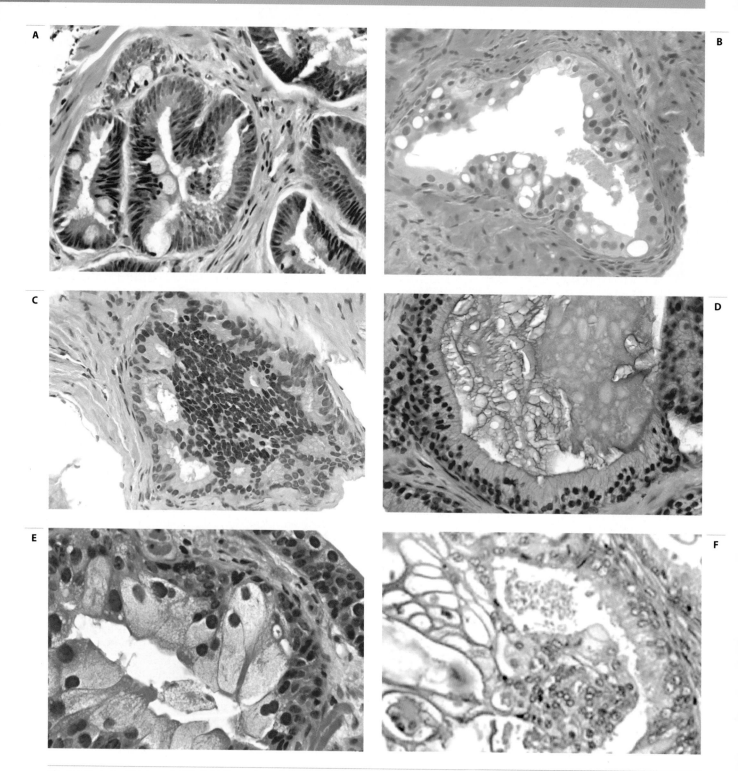

**Fig. 9-4** Variants of high-grade PIN. (**A-B**) Signet ring cell. (**C**) Small cell neuroendocrine. (**D**) Mucinous. (**E**) Foamy gland. (**F**) Squamous.

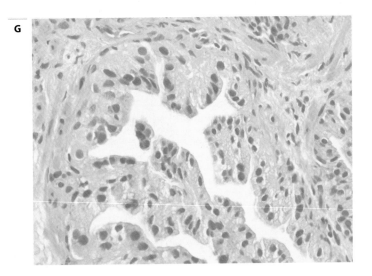

**Fig. 9-4, Cont'd** (**G**) Inverted.

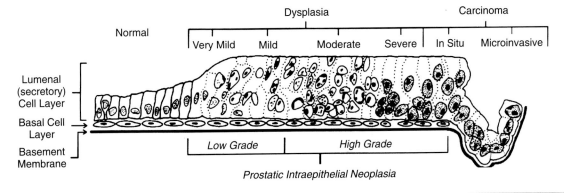

**Fig. 9-5** Morphologic continuum from normal prostatic epithelium through increasing grades of prostatic intraepithelial neoplasia to early invasive carcinoma, according to the disease continuum concept. Low-grade prostatic intraepithelial neoplasia (grade 1) corresponds to very mild to mild dysplasia. High-grade prostatic intraepithelial neoplasia (grades 2 and 3) corresponds to moderate to severe dysplasia and carcinoma in situ. The precursor state ends when malignant cells invade the stroma; this invasion occurs where the basal cell layer is disrupted. Dysplastic changes occur in the superficial (luminal) secretory cell layer, perhaps in response to luminal carcinogens. Disruption of the basal cell layer accompanies the architectural and cytologic features of high-grade PIN, and appears to be a necessary prerequisite for stromal invasion. Basement membrane is retained with high-grade prostatic intraepithelial neoplasia and early invasive carcinoma. (Modified from Bostwick DG, Brawer MK. Prostatic intra-epithelial neoplasia and early invasion in prostate cancer. Cancer 1987; 59: 788–794, with permission.)

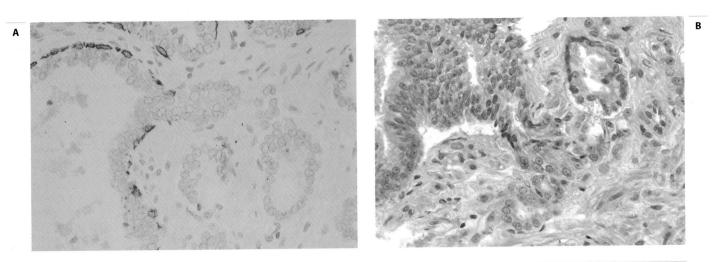

**Fig. 9-6** PIN and microinvasion. (**A**) Basal cell layer disruption in high-grade prostatic intraepithelial neoplasia (left) and absent basal cell layer in cancer (right). The tongue of cells (center) protruding from the large acinar structure with PIN is thought to represent early invasion. (Basal cell-specific anti-keratin 34βE12 imunostain). (**B**) Another case of PIN with invagination suspicious for early invasion.

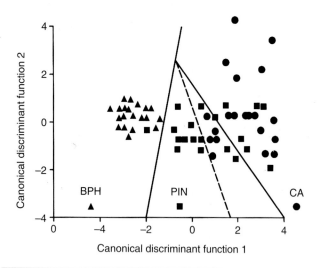

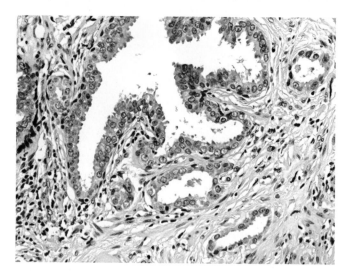

**Fig. 9-7** Scatterplot of the spatial distribution of benign prostatic hyperplasia (BPH), prostatic intraepithelial neoplasia (PIN), and cancer (CA). The cases appear as continuous categories, with overlap mainly between PIN and cancer. The two lines divide the scatterplot into three parts, corresponding to three categories. The part corresponding to PIN is subdivided into two parts (interrupted line), separating low-grade PIN (close to BPH) and high-grade PIN (close to cancer). (Modified from Montironi R, Scarpelli M, Sisti S, et al. Quantitative analysis of prostatic intra-epithelial neoplasia on tissue sections. Anal Quant Cytol Histol 1990; 12: 366–372, with permission.)

**Fig. 9-8** PIN/ASAP. Intermediate-size acini with mild architectural distortion and prominent nuclei and nucleoli in association with high-grade prostatic intraepithelial neoplasia. An unequivocal diagnosis cannot be rendered owing to the small size of this focus. Keratin 34βE12 revealed lack of basal cell staining in the suspicious acini (not shown).

zone and 7% of those involving the transition zone; 2% of cases have concomitant single foci in all zones.[35] The peripheral zone of the prostate, the area in which the majority of cases of prostate cancer occur (70% or more), is also the most common location for PIN.[31,35,36,46,49,51,64,65] Cancer and PIN are frequently multicentric in the peripheral zone, indicating a 'field' effect similar to urothelial carcinoma of the bladder. Central zone cancer is more likely to be associated with PIN in the central zone than the peripheral zone.[66]

High-grade PIN and prostate cancer are morphometrically and phenotypically similar (Fig. 9-7). PIN occurs primarily in the peripheral zone and is seen in areas that are in continuity with prostate cancer.[5,16,35,49,67–70] PIN and prostate cancer are multifocal and heterogeneous.[35,71,72] Increasing rates of aneuploidy and angiogenesis as the grade of PIN progresses are further evidence that high-grade PIN is precancerous.[69,73–75] Prostate cancer and high-grade PIN have similar proliferative and apoptotic indices.[43,73,76–78]

It is often difficult with small foci in needle biopsies to separate cancer from suspicious foci (atypical small acinar proliferation suspicious for but not diagnostic of malignancy – ASAP) when there is coexistent high-grade PIN; the difficulty is based on the inability to separate tangential cutting of the larger pre-existing acini of PIN (that may appear as small separate adjacent acini) from the smaller discrete acini of cancer (Fig. 9-8). In such cases we prefer the term ASAP + PIN (referring to the coexistence of the two lesions in the same high-power microscopic field) to avoid over-diagnosis of tangential cutting of PIN and cancer. PIN usually involves

large or intermediate-sized acini, but occasionally involves smaller ductules and acini.[79]

Recent renewed efforts to introduce the term 'intraductal carcinoma' rely on the abandoned concept that dysplasia (defined here as malignancy arising at that specific site within the epithelium) can be separated reliably from intraductal/intra-acinar spread of cancer (defined here as extension of malignant cells through the pre-existing lumina of the prostate).[80] This concept was rejected by consensus on many occasions owing to lack of reproducible criteria for making the distinction, and the non-committal term intraepithelial neoplasia was internationally adopted and repeatedly reconfirmed as it begs the question of site of origin of the process. Those who persist with the belief that 'intraductal carcinoma' can be diagnosed reproducibly rely on proximity of the epithelial abnormality to invasive cancer, but this criterion is arbitrary and not based on valid objective confirmatory data. Others have defined 'intraductal carcinoma' as malignant epithelial cells filling large acini and prostatic ducts, with preservation of basal cells forming either solid or dense cribriform patterns, or loose cribriform or micropapillary patterns with severe nuclear enlargement (six times normal size) or comedonecrosis.[80] This suggestion remains unvalidated. Most importantly, at present there is no clinical reason to separate dysplasia and intraductal/intra-acinar spread of cancer: even if we could, the clinical response is the same. It is conceivable that future studies may allow diagnostic separation of dysplasia and intraductal/intra-acinar spread of cancer; if so, these steps in the biologic progression of prostate cancer might be shown to have differential predictive values for prostate cancer. Identification of subsets of high-grade PIN that indicate a greater risk of cancer is a clinically important area of investigation, but so far such attempts have not altered clinical practice. The concept of non-invasive ductal carcinoma is discussed below.

Swedish investigators recently stated that PIN should not be diagnosed by fine needle aspiration alone,[81] although this has been refuted.[82]

## Useful immunohistochemical markers for the diagnosis of PIN

Select antibodies such as antikeratin 34βE12 (high molecular weight keratin) and p63 (see below) are used to stain tissue sections for the presence of basal cells,[83,84] recognizing that PIN retains an intact or fragmented basal cell layer whereas cancer does not (Fig. 9-9). In addition, racemase is useful for staining of the dysplastic secretory cells of PIN (see below).

We routinely generate unstained intervening sections of all prostate biopsies for possible future immunohistochemical staining, recognizing that small foci of concern are often lost when the tissue block is recut; one study reported loss of the suspicious focus in 31 of 52 cases.[85]

Monoclonal basal cell-specific antikeratin 34βE12 stains the cytoplasm of most normal basal cells of the prostate, with continuous intact circumferential staining in many instances. There is no staining in secretory and stromal cells.

This marker is the most commonly used immunostain for prostatic basal cells,[86,87] and methods of use with paraffin-embedded sections have been optimized.[88] Keratin 34βE12 is formalin sensitive and requires pretreatment by enzymes or heat if formalin-based fixatives are used. After pepsin predigestion or microwaving, there is progressive loss of immunoreactivity from 1 week or longer of formalin fixation. Heat-induced epitope retrieval with a hot plate yielded consistent results with no decrease in immunoreactivity with as long as 1 month of formalin fixation.[88] The staining intensity was consistently stronger at all periods of formalin fixation when the hot plate method was used, compared to pepsin predigestion or microwaving. Weak immunoreactivity was rarely observed in cancer cells after hot plate treatment, but not with pepsin predigestion or microwave antigen retrieval. Steam EDTA in combination with protease significantly enhanced basal cell immunoreactivity compared with protease treatment alone in benign prostatic epithelium.[89] Non-reactive benign acini were always the most peripheral acini in a lobule, a small cluster of outpouched acini furthest from a large duct, or the terminal end of a large duct.[90] More proximal acini had a discontinuous pattern of immunoreactivity.

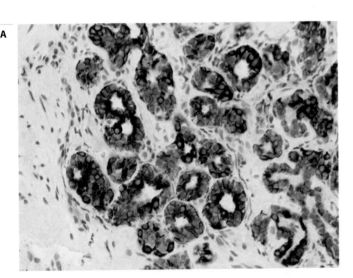

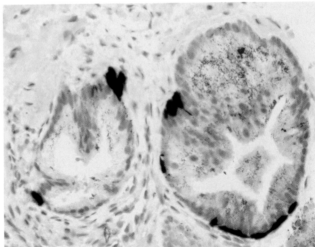

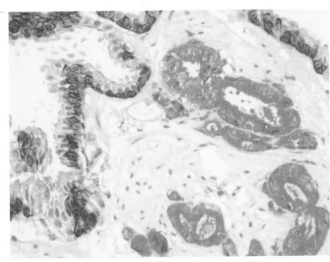

**Fig. 9-9** Immunostain with keratin 34βE12. (**A**) Intact basal cell layer in atrophic acini. (**B**) Basal cell layer is disrupted in high grade PIN; note positive racemase staining (red). (**C**) Absent basal cell layer in cancer; note positive racemase staining (red).

Increasing grades of PIN are associated with progressive disruption of the basal cell layer, according to studies utilizing antikeratin 34βE12. Basal cell layer disruption is present in 56% of cases of high-grade PIN, and is more frequent in acini adjacent to invasive carcinoma than in distant acini. Early invasive carcinoma occurs at sites of glandular outpouching and basal cell discontinuity in association with PIN.[11] The cribriform pattern of PIN may be mistaken for the cribriform pattern of ductal adenocarcinoma, and the use of antikeratin staining is often useful in making this distinction.[91] Cancer cells consistently fail to react with this antibody, although admixed benign acini may be misinterpreted as cancerous staining. Thus, immunohistochemical stains for antikeratin 34βE12 may show the presence or absence of basal cells in a small focus of atypical glands, helping to establish a benign or malignant diagnosis respectively. We believe that this antibody can be employed successfully if one judiciously interprets the results in combination with the light microscopic findings; relying solely on the absence of immunoreactivity (absence of basal cell staining) to render the diagnosis of cancer is without precedent in diagnostic immunohistochemistry and is discouraged.[92] Nonetheless, some studies have noted that the rate of equivocal cases can be reduced considerably,[93] by 68%,[86] or from 5.1% to 1.0%,[94] by addition of this immunohistochemical marker. Evaluation of prostate biopsies following therapy such as radiation may be one of the most useful roles for antikeratin 34βE12 (see below).[95]

In addition to PIN and cancer, basal cell layer disruption or loss also occurs in inflamed acini, atypical adenomatous hyperplasia, and atrophy and post-atrophic hyperplasia, and may be misinterpreted as cancer if one relies exclusively on the immunohistochemical profile of a suspicious focus. Furthermore, basal cells of Cowper's glands may not express keratin 34βE12,[96] although this has been disputed.[97] Rare (0.2%) cases of adenocarcinoma have been reported that focally or weakly express keratin 34βE12, including foci of metastatic high-grade adenocarcinoma.[98]

Basal cell hyperplasia is a histologic mimic of cancer, and use of antikeratin 34βE12 is recommended in any equivocal cases that include this lesion in the differential considerations, as it is invariably positive in that lesion.[99–101]

p63 is a nuclear protein that is at least as sensitive and specific for the identification of basal cells in diagnostic prostate specimens as high molecular weight cytokeratin staining.[83,102–112] Shah et al.[104] found that p63 was more sensitive than keratin 34βE12 in staining benign basal cells, particularly in TURP specimens, offering a slight advantage in diagnostically challenging cases. Zhou et al.[83] demonstrated that a basal cell cocktail (34βE12 and p63) increased the sensitivity of basal cell detection and reduced staining variability, thus rendering basal cell immunostaining more consistent. Triple staining with racemase, high molecular weight cytokeratin, and p63 is emerging as standard for the diagnosis of prostate cancer (Figs 9-10, 9-11).[103,106,109,110,113]

CK5 and CK14 mRNA and protein are expressed in the basal cells of benign acini and PIN, and CK14 mRNA is present in low levels in the luminal cells of the most foci of PIN; thus, if PIN is derived from basal cells, as is currently believed, CK14 translation is depressed and a low level of CK14 mRNA may persist.[114] CK8 mRNA and protein were constitutively expressed in all epithelia of the normal and neoplastic prostate. CK19 mRNA and protein were expressed in both basal and luminal cells of benign acini. CK16 mRNA was expressed in a similar pattern to CK19, but CK16 protein was not detected.[114]

Other markers of basal cells include proliferation markers, differentiation markers, and genetic markers. The preferential localization of many of these markers in basal cells but not in secretory cells suggests that they play a role in growth regulation. p63 is a recently introduced nuclear marker that may be useful for separating PIN and cancer from benign mimics. Basal cells display immunoreactivity at least focally for keratins 5, 10, 11, 13, 14, 16, and 19; of these, only keratin 19 is also found in secretory cells.[115,116] Keratins found exclusively in the secretory cells include 7, 8, and 18.

**A**

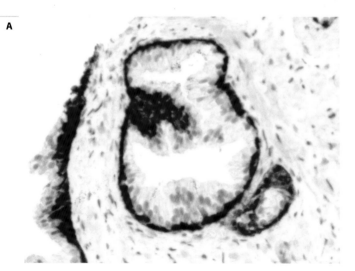

**B**

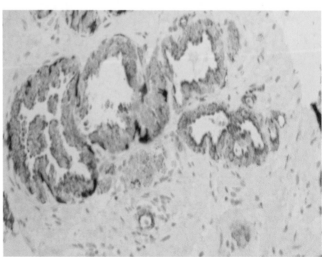

**Fig. 9-10** Triple-antibody cocktail (racemase/keratin 34βE12/p63) staining in (**A**) benign prostatic epithelium, and (**B**) high-grade PIN (left) and cancer (right).

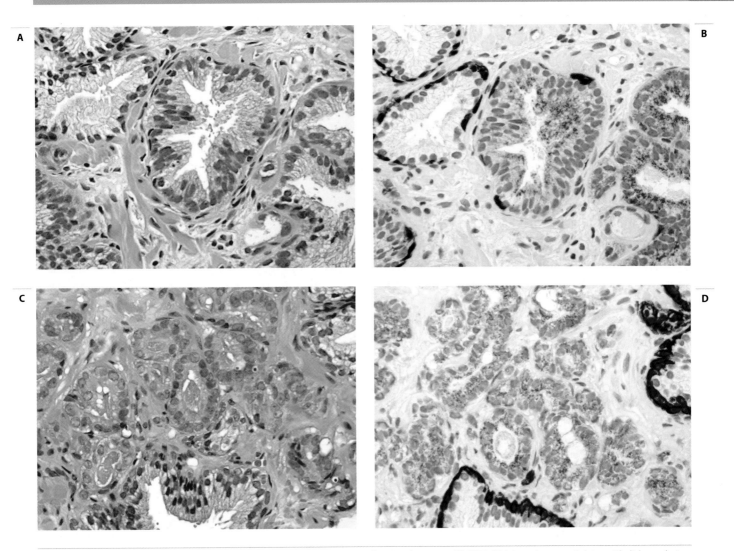

**Fig. 9-11** Comparison of H&E and triple-antibody cocktail (racemase/keratin 34βE12/p63) staining. (**A**) H&E of high-grade prostatic intraepithelial neoplasia (HGPIN) (large central acinus) with adjacent benign acini (left) in a biopsy. Compare with (**B**): immunostain of HGPIN reveals both red cytoplasmic granular staining pattern of racemase and dark brown cytoplasmic (34βE12) and nuclear (p63) staining of basal cells. (**C**) H&E of adenocarcinoma (Gleason 3 + 3 = 6) on biopsy with adjacent benign acini. Compare with (**D**), in which the cancerous glands show epithelial cells with only red cytoplasmic granular staining pattern of racemase, whereas adjacent benign glands show basal cells with only dark brown cytoplasmic (34βE12) and nuclear (p63) staining.

Basal cells usually do not display immunoreactivity for prostate-specific antigen (PSA), prostatic acid phosphatase (PAP), and S100 protein, and only rare single cells stain with chromogranin and neuron-specific enolase. Conversely, the normal secretory luminal cells invariably stain with PSA and PAP. Prostatic basal cells do not usually display myoepithelial differentiation,[117,118] in contrast to basal cells in the breast, salivary glands, pancreas, and other sites.

The molecular marker, racemase (α-methylacyl-CoA racemase, P504S) assists in discriminating between benign and neoplastic acini. This well-characterized enzyme catalyzes the conversion of several (2R)-methyl-branched-chain fatty acyl-CoAs to their (S)-stereoisomers. Analysis of mRNA levels of racemase revealed an average ninefold upregulation of prostate cancer. The gene for α-methylacyl-CoA racemase (AMACR) is greatly overexpressed in prostate cancer cells.[119] Its advantage over antikeratin 34βE12 is its positive granular

cytoplasmic staining in cancer cells, with little or no staining in benign acini. In PIN, monoclonal and polyclonal antibodies to α-methylacyl-CoA racemase (P504S) were positive in 77% and 91%, respectively,[120] consistent with other studies (Fig. 9-11).[119,121–124] As racemase is not specific for prostate cancer and is present in high-grade PIN (>90%), this staining must be interpreted with caution and the diagnosis of PIN or prostate cancer should be rendered only with convincing histologic evidence.[125] Moderate to strong racemase expression in PIN is indicative of an associated adenocarcinoma.[126]

## Chronic inflammation, atrophy, and high-grade PIN

Chronic inflammation has been proposed as a causative mechanism for prostatic carcinogenesis, but the evidence to date is inconclusive or contradictory, probably owing to the ubiquitous presence of inflammation in the prostate (Chapter 8). In a recent study of needle biopsies, chronic inflammation was identified in 7.7% and conferred a protective effect from PIN and cancer even after adjusting for age, digital rectal examination findings, serum PSA, and prostate volume.[127]

## Genetic and molecular changes

High-grade PIN and prostate cancer share similar genetic alterations.[73,128–130] For example, 8p12–21 allelic loss is commonly found in cancer and microdissected PIN.[129] Other genetic changes found in carcinoma that already exist in PIN include loss of heterozygosity (LOH) at 8p22,[131] 12pter-p12, 10q11.2,[14,129] and gain of chromosomes 7, 8[132], 10, and 12[133], and the 8p24[131] and PTEN genes.[134] Loss of heterozygosity frequencies at 13q (one of the most common chromosomal alterations in high-stage cancer) is 0% versus 49% in PIN and clinical prostate cancer, respectively.[135] Alterations in oncogene bcl-2 expression and RER+ phenotype are similar for PIN and prostate cancer.[136,137] Up to 64% of patients with PIN have loss of heterozygosity for the mannose 6-phosphate/insulin-like growth factor 2 receptor (M6P/IGF2R) gene.[138]

PIN is epigenetically similar to carcinoma according to the percentage of methylated alleles for the APC, GSTP1, and RARbeta2 genes.[139] Methylation of the apoptosis-associated ASC promoter region was increased in PIN and cancer.[140] TMPRSS2 exon 1 was fused in-frame with ERG exon 4 in 50% of prostate carcinomas and in 19–21% of cases of PIN, but not in benign prostatic controls, suggesting that the TMPRSS2–ERG fusion molecular rearrangement is an early event that may precede chromosome-level alterations in prostate carcinogenesis.[141,142]

PIN is associated with progressive abnormalities of phenotype and genotype, which are intermediate between normal prostatic epithelium and cancer, indicating impairment of cell differentiation and regulatory control with advancing stages of prostatic carcinogenesis.[143] There is progressive loss of some markers of secretory differentiation, cytoskeletal proteins, and multiple gene products (Table 9-8).[6,115,119,144–163] Other markers show a progressive increase in expression from benign epithelium through PIN to cancer (Table 9-9).[4,6,136,139,145,146,150,153,156,161,162,164–211] A model of prostatic carcinogenesis has been proposed based on the morphologic continuum of PIN and the multistep theory of carcinogenesis.[73,128]

### Microvessel density is increased in PIN

PIN is virtually always accompanied by a proliferation of small capillaries in the stroma, despite separation from the underlying vasculature by a basal cell layer and basement membrane. It is likely that PIN initially co-opts adjacent vessels, similar to other tumors, and that these vessels soon regress, only to be followed by vigorous angiogenesis at the cancer's edge. A critical balance exists between the proangiogenic vascular endothelial growth factor and the angiogenic antagonist angiopoietin-2. Angiogenin is a polypeptide involved in the formation and establishment of new blood

**Table 9-8** Selected markers with progressively reduced expression in PIN and cancer compared to benign epithelium*

| |
|---|
| Activated caspase-3[6] |
| Androgen receptor expression[156] |
| Annexin I[149] |
| Annexin II[119] |
| Blood group antigens |
| CD-10[148] |
| Fibroblast growth factor-2[145] |
| Hepatocyte growth factor activator inhibitor-1[146] |
| Inhibin[147] |
| Insulin-like growth factor-binding protein-3[157,158] |
| Interstitial collagenase (MMP-1)[153] |
| Neuroendocrine cells |
| NKX3.1 homeobox gene-encoded protein[155] |
| Ornithine decarboxylase[154] |
| Prostate-specific antigen |
| Prostatic acid phosphatase |
| p-Cadherin[144] |
| Prostate-specific transglutaminase[163] |
| Telomerase[159] |
| p27KIP1[160,162,195] |
| 5α-reductase type 2[150] |
| 15-lipoxygenase 1[151] and 2[152] |

*The majority of reported results support this conclusion.

vessels necessary for the growth and metastasis of numerous malignant neoplasms, including prostatic cancer. In a recent study, the investigators reported a percentage of cells staining positively for angiogenin in benign prostatic glandular epithelium, high-grade PIN, and prostatic cancer, in 17%, 58%, and 60% of cases, respectively, confirming the potential role that angiogenin plays in neoplastic progression.[212,213]

Microvessel density is higher in high-grade PIN than in adjacent benign prostatic tissue, and the capillaries are shorter, more widely spaced, have more open lumina and curvaceous external contours, and are lined by a greater number of endothelial cells. The degree of microvessel density in PIN is intermediate between benign epithelium and cancer, lending support to the concept of PIN as the precursor of prostate cancer. Microvessel density is significantly higher in cases with PIN associated with prostate cancer than in those with isolated PIN or benign prostatic hyperplasia alone.[196] Inhibition of angiogenesis may be an effective method of chemoprevention for men at high risk, such as those who have high-grade PIN. It should be well tolerated in most adults because under typical conditions angiogenesis is needed only for reproduction and wound healing.[214]

**Table 9-9** Selected markers with progressively increased expression in PIN and cancer compared to benign epithelium*

| | |
|---|---|
| Amphiregulin[1257] | Metallothionien isoform II[194] |
| Aneuploidy[156,165,166] | MIB-1 expression[156,195] |
| Apoptotic bodies[136,168,169,1258] | Microvessel density[196] |
| Aurora-A (Aurora 2 kinase, STK-15), a protein found in centrosomes[170] | Minichromosome maintenance protein-2 (Mcm-2)[6] |
| bcl-2 oncoprotein[172,173,1086] | Mitochondrial protein MAGMAS[197] |
| Cell growth regulatory protein LIM domain only 2 (LMO2)[174] | Mitotic figures[1258] |
| Cell proliferation-associated protein Cdc46[175] | mTOR signaling pathway markers 4E-BP1 and p-4E-BP1[198] |
| Centrosome-associated protein Aurora-A (Aurora 2 kinase, STK-15)[170] | Mutator (RER (+)) phenotype[136] |
| c-erbB-2 (Her-2/neu)[176] and c-erbB-3 oncoproteins[145,177] | Neuropeptide Y (NPY)[192] |
| c-met proto-oncogene | NOS-1 and NOS-2[180] |
| Cyclo-oxygenase-2 (COX-2)[178–180] | Osteopontin[199] |
| Cysteine-rich secretory protein 3 (CRISP-3)[181] | Polo-like kinase-1 (PLK-1)[178] |
| Dentin sialophosphoprotein[182] | Prolactin receptor[200] |
| Ep-Cam transmembrane glycoprotein[183] | Promoter methylation of GSTP1 gene[139] |
| Epidermal growth factor and epidermal growth factor receptor[145] | Prostate-specific membrane antigen[201,202] |
| Estrogen receptor α[184] | Prothymosin-α[203] |
| FAS-related apoptosis signaling pathway markers FADD-FAS associating protein with death Domain, pro-caspase-8, and caspase-8[185] | Rac-specific guanine nucleotide exchange factor Tiam1[204] |
| Gelatinase B (MMP-9), matrilysin-1 (MMP-7) and the membrane-type 1-MMP (MT1-MMP)[153] | RNase III endonuclease Dicer[205] |
| G-protein coupled receptor PSGR2[186] | Serine/threonine kinase Pim-1[206,207] |
| G1 cell cycle arrest regulator p16(INK4a)[187] | Tenascin-C[208] |
| Heat shock protein-90[180,188] | TGF-α |
| Human glandular kallikrein 2 (hK2)[189,190] | Tissue inhibitor of metalloproteinases-4 (TIMP-4)[193] |
| Hypoxia-inducible factor 1α (HIF-1α)[191] | TXA(2) synthase and TXA(2) receptors[179] |
| IL-6 and IL-10[188] | Type IV collagenase |
| Insulin-like growth factor-binding protein IGFBP-rP1 | Vascular endothelial growth factor (VEGF)[191] |
| Ki-67 expression[6] | p21[162] |
| Lewis Y antigen | p53[209,210] |
| Macrophage inhibitory cytokine-1 (MIC-1)[192] | p62 sequestosome 1 (SQSTM1) gene product[211] |
| Matriptase, a type II transmembrane serine protease[146] | 5α-reductase type 1[150] |
| Matrix metalloproteinase-26 (MMP-26)[193] | |

*The majority of reported results support this conclusion.

## Animal models of PIN and prostate cancer

Several different animal models of prostate cancer, including mouse, rat, and dog models, have shown that high-grade PIN is in the direct causal pathway to prostate cancer.[215–217]

The transgenic mouse model of prostate cancer (TRAMP) mimics human prostate cancer.[218,219] In this model, the Pro-basin promoter-SV40 large T antigen (PB-Tag) transgene is expressed specifically in epithelial cells of the murine prostate under the control of the androgen-dependent probasin promoter. As a result, this model has several advantages over others:

- Mice develop progressive forms of prostatic epithelial hyperplasia and high-grade PIN as early as 10 weeks of age, and invasive prostate adenocarcinoma around 18 weeks.[219]

- The pattern of metastatic spread of prostate cancer mimics that of human prostate cancer, common sites of metastases being the lymph nodes, lung, kidney, adrenal gland and bone.

- The development and progression of prostate cancer can be followed within a relatively short period of 10–30 weeks.

- Spontaneous prostate tumors arise with 100% frequency.

- Animals may be screened for the presence of the prostate cancer transgene prior to the onset of clinical prostate cancer.

Another animal model is the transgenic mouse model, which contains a probasin promoter that controls the ECO: R1 gene. This gene product has been implicated in the induction of genomic instability.[220] These animals were followed prospectively from 4 to 24 months of age and showed progressive growth of mild to severe hyperplasia, low-grade PIN, high-grade PIN, and then well-differentiated adenocarcinoma.[220] Transgenic mice that have prostatic overexpression of AR protein develop focal areas of high-grade PIN.[221] Also, when TRAMP mice were treated in a chemopreventive manner with the DNA methyltransferase inhibitor 5-aza-2′-deoxycytidine, none developed prostate cancer at 24 weeks of age compared to 54% of control-treated mice who developed poorly differentiated prostate cancer.[222]

Another transgenic mouse model was recently described in which an oncogenic Neu cDNA (Neu*) driven by the probasin gene promoter was overexpressed in the mouse prostate and caused the development of PIN that progressed to invasive carcinoma.[223]

The mechanism of prostate carcinogenesis may involve estrogenic signaling. Wang et al.[224] treated wildtype mice with testosterone propionate and estradiol for 4 months. These mice developed prostatic hyperplasia, high-grade PIN, and invasive prostate cancer. When a-ERKO mice (mice that have the ERa genetically knocked out) were treated the same way, they developed prostatic hyperplasia but not high-grade PIN or invasive prostate cancer.[224]

The formation of PIN in mutant mice is associated with increased oxidative damage of DNA and progression to adenocarcinoma, as occurred in compound mutant mice lacking Nkx3.1 as well as the Pten tumor suppressor, and was correlated with further deregulation of antioxidants, including superoxide dismutase enzymes, and profound accumulations of oxidative damage to DNA and protein.[225]

Marked increase of luminal epithelial cell proliferation reminiscent of PIN was observed in the Etk transgenic mouse prostate that may be attributed to elevated activity of Akt and signal transducers and activators of transcription 3 (STAT3).[226]

Overexpression of the post-translational modification simulation-specific protease SENP1 in transgenic mice induced PIN at an early age. Interestingly, SENP1 is induced by chronic exposure to androgens, and its effects are associated with upregulation of androgen receptor transcriptional activity.[227]

The dog is the only non-human species in which spontaneous prostate cancer occurs, and, as in humans, the rate of canine prostate cancer increases with age.[228,229] High-grade PIN has been also observed in the prostates of these animals.[229,230] Canine high-grade PIN shows cytological features identical to the human counterpart, including cell crowding, loss of polarity, and nuclear and nucleolar enlargement. Like prostatic adenocarcinoma, PIN also increases with age.[229] High-grade PIN appears to represent an early event in prostate carcinogenesis that occurs with a high frequency in the prostates of pet dogs sharing the same environment as humans. In this model, high-grade PIN was determined to be an intermediate step between benign epithelium and invasive carcinoma. Thus, like the transgenic mouse models, the canine model supports high-grade PIN as part of a continuum in the progression of prostate cancer.

## Animal models of PIN and chemoprevention

In a transgenic mouse model the COX-2 inhibitor celecoxib reduced or eliminated PIN and cancer in a dose-dependent manner.[231]

Sustained delivery of 1,25 D(3) (vitamin D) to Nkx3.1; Pten mutant mice resulted in a significant reduction in the formation of PIN while having no apparent effect on the control mice; this inhibition of PIN was coincident with upregulation of vitamin D receptor expression in the prostatic epithelium of the mutant mice, while having no effect on androgen receptor expression or androgen receptor signaling.[232]

A prospective, placebo-controlled study of TRAMP mice treated with the antiestrogen Toremifene (Acapodene) was performed to pharmacologically antagonize ERa.[233] These Toremifene-treated TRAMP mice had a reduction in high-grade PIN, a significant reduction in cancer incidence, and an increase in survival. Thus, estrogenic signalling through ERa may play a key role in prostatic carcinogenesis; high-grade PIN was observed to be in the direct causal pathway to cancer.

Treatment of male Sprague–Dawley rats with testosterone and N-methyl N-nitroso urea (MNU) induced prostatic carcinogenesis in a multistep process that included hyperplasia and PIN. Additional administration of diallyl disulfide, a major component of garlic (*Allium sativum*) significantly inhibited the formation of PIN.[234]

## Clinical significance of PIN

### PIN does not elevate PSA

Biopsy remains the definitive method for detecting PIN and early invasive cancer. Serum PSA concentration may be elevated in some patients with PIN,[235] but these results have been refuted in most published reports.[236–238] There is a poor correlation of PIN and PSA density according to studies of radical prostatectomy specimens and preoperative serum concentration.[237] Mean PSA increased from 8.4 to 11.6 ng/mL in patients with PIN who developed cancer within 2 years; those with PIN who did not develop cancer during this interval had an increase in PSA from 4.8 to 5.9 ng/mL or a decrease from 5.1 to 4.6 ng/mL. These findings were confirmed in a recent screening study in which the median PSA velocity was significantly greater in men with PIN who were subsequently diagnosed with cancer.[239] A velocity threshold of 0.75 ng/mL/yr predicted which men with high-grade PIN would ultimately be diagnosed with cancer, and velocity was the only significant predictor of subsequent cancer detection on multivariate analysis.[239]

The ratio of free to total PSA is the same for patients with high-grade PIN and cancer, unlike low-grade PIN and hyperplasia.[235,238,240,241] Many patients in these studies were later found to have cancer, so the elevation in serum PSA concentration and its derivatives may have resulted from undetected cancer.

Mean insulin-like growth factor-1 (IGF-1) and IGF-3 concentrations in men with PIN (130.2 and 2394 ng/mL, respectively) were significantly higher than in controls (118.8 and 2276 ng/mL, respectively), but these assays are not routinely available.[242]

### Transrectal ultrasound and magnetic resonance imaging (MRI) cannot detect PIN

On transrectal ultrasound PIN may be hypoechoic, as is carcinoma, although these findings have not been confirmed.[243,244] Most urologists and radiologists do not believe that PIN is detectable by transrectal ultrasound because PIN is a microscopic finding which is below the detection threshold for this form of imaging. Likewise, MRI failed to accurately identify PIN.[245]

### PIN increases the risk of prostate cancer

The clinical importance of recognizing PIN is based on its strong association with prostatic carcinoma. PIN has a high predictive value as a marker for adenocarcinoma, so its identification in biopsy specimens warrants further search for concurrent invasive carcinoma (Table 9-10).[246] If all procedures fail to identify coexistent carcinoma, close surveillance and follow-up are indicated.

The presence of isolated PIN in a set of sextant needle biopsies carries a risk ratio of 14.9 for cancer; this level of risk is considerably lower in men undergoing biopsies with a greater number of cores owing to greater sampling. PIN is a stronger predictor for subsequent cancer than the independent predictors of patient age (>65 years vs = 65 years) and serum PSA concentration (4 ng/mL vs = 4 ng/mL); for these, the respective risk ratios are 3.5 and 3.64.[247]

PIN coexists with cancer in more than 85% of cases, according to studies employing whole-mounted totally embedded prostates. In one report the likelihood of finding cancer increased with the biopsy time interval. The investigators reported a 32% incidence of cancer on repeat biopsy performed within 1 year, compared to a 38% incidence in biopsies obtained after 1 year.[247] Other series have also found a high predictive value of PIN for cancer,[248] although recent reports based on obtaining a greater number of cores shows a lower predictive value (Table 9-10).[24,105,247,249] These data emphasize the strong association between PIN and adenocarcinoma, and indicate that vigorous diagnostic follow-up is needed.

Follow-up biopsy is suggested for patients with PIN within 1 year.[247,250] Some urologists perform 'saturation' biopsies, consisting of more than 16 biopsies in one session, often under brief general anesthesia in the operating theatre, in an effort to definitively exclude cancer. Most authors agree that identification of PIN in the prostate should not influence or

dictate therapeutic decisions.[250] We are aware of 21 radical prostatectomies that were deliberately (three cases) or inadvertently performed (18 cases) in patients whose biopsies contained only high-grade PIN; all but two of the cases contained adenocarcinoma in the surgical specimen (Bostwick, personal communication, 2007).

Several factors account for the decline in the predictive accuracy of high-grade PIN for cancer. The main factor is the use of extended biopsy techniques that result in more thorough prostate sampling and higher cancer detection rates; thus, there is a smaller pool of patients with an isolated diagnosis of PIN.[251] Another factor is the lower detection rate for, and difficulty in the detection of, the remaining small cancers; larger significant tumors may also escape detection. These factors lead to a higher frequency of negative repeat biopsies, and may reflect a new steady state and a new low plateau in the predictive accuracy of this marker. In a recent report, the investigators demonstrated that with six-core biopsies for both the initial and the re-biopsy the risk of cancer was 14.1%, compared to 31.9% in the group that had an initial six-core biopsy and eight cores or more on follow-up. The risk of cancer on biopsy within 1 year following a diagnosis of PIN (13.3%) is relatively low if good sampling (eight or more cores) is performed initially.[252]

High-grade PIN in transurethral resection specimens is also an important predictive factor for prostate cancer.[34,253–255] Among 14 patients with PIN and BPH followed for up to 7 years (mean, 5.9 years), three (21.4%) developed prostatic cancer.[254] Mean serum PSA concentration was higher than in those who did not develop cancer (8.1 vs 4.6 ng/mL, respectively). All subsequent cancers apparently arose in the peripheral zone and were detected by needle biopsy. Thus, all tissue should be submitted by the pathologist for examination when high-grade PIN is found in TURP specimens. The high predictive value of PIN for the development of subsequent cancer warrants reporting the presence of PIN in TURP specimens, according to the Cancer Committee of the College of American Pathologists. Conversely, PIN in the transition and central zones of Norwegian men was not predictive of subsequent cancer development.[253]

The extent of PIN in needle biopsies is another strong predictor of cancer on subsequent biopsy.[55,57,256] The positive predictive value of PIN was 64%, with a sensitivity of 28% and a specificity of 81%. Cancer detection was significantly greater in patients with multifocal high-grade PIN than in those with unifocal PIN (70% vs 10%, respectively).[56,256] When four or more cores contain PIN, the predictive value for cancer on subsequent biopsy was 39%.[257]

Short telomere length in PIN and the surrounding stroma was associated with an increased risk of cancer.[258] Telomere length was also predictive of time from the original biopsy to diagnosis of cancer.[259] Overexpression of p4EBP1 predicted cancer with a sensitivity and specificity of 63% and 100%, respectively.[260]

### Clinical response to high-grade PIN

As PIN progresses, the risk of basal cell layer disruption and stromal invasion increases, similar to carcinoma in situ (CIS)

**Table 9-10** Cancer risk in patients with high-grade PIN according to number of needle biopsy cores obtained

| Reference | No. of cores | No. of subjects with repeat biopsy or biopsies | PIN cases with cancer at follow-up (%) |
|---|---|---|---|
| Davidson et al. 1995[247] | 1–8 | 100 | 35 |
| Raviv et al. 1996[25] | NS | 48 | 48 |
| Langer et al. 1996[24] | F | 53 | 27 |
| Shepherd et al. 1996[26] | 4 | 66 | 47 |
| Kamoi et al. 2000[1259] | Mixed | 45 | 22 |
| O'Dowd et al. 2000[65] | Mixed | 1,306 | 23 |
| Kronz et al. 2001[1260] | NS | 245 | 32 |
| Alsikafi et al. 2001[331] | NS | 21 | 14 |
| Maatman et al. 2001[1261] | 6 | 86 | 16 |
| Borboroglu et al. 2001[321] | 6 | 45 | 44 |
| Lefkowitz et al. 2001[1252d] | 12 | 43 | 2 |
| Roscigno et al. 2004[56] | 10–12 | 47 | 45 |
| San Francisco et al. 2003[1253] | EXT | 47 | 24 |
| Goeman et al. 2003[27] | 6 | 63 | 27 |
| Naya et al. 2004[301] | EXT | 47 | 11 |
| Bishara et al. 2004[1262] | 4–15 | 132 | 29 |
| Rabets et al. 2004[105] | 20 | 38 | 18 |
| Abdel-Khalek et al. 2004[1254] | 11 | 83 | 36 |
| Postma et al. 2004[1250] | 6 | 101 | 13 |
| Moore et al. 2005[322] | EXT | 22 | 5 |
| Schlesinger et al. 2005[316] | 6–18 | 204 | 23 |
| Gokden et al. 2005[1263] | 6 | 190 | 30 |
| El-Fakharany[1264] | 6 or EXT | 585 | 25 |
| Leite et al. 2005[1265] | NS | 142 | 13 |
| Eskicorapci et al. 2006[251] | 6 and 10 | 211 | 57 and 23, respectively |
| Girasole et al. 2006[324] | 2–4 | 358 | 22 |
| Tan et al. 2006[1266] | | 29 | 24 |
| Herawi et al. 2006[252] | 6 | 332 | 21 |
| Herawi et al. 2006[252] | 8–26 | 323 | 13 |
| Rodriguez-Patron Rodriguez et al. 2006[325] | Mixed | 861 | 45 |
| Schoenfield et al. 2007[256] | 24 | 9 | 80 (in those with multifocal PIN) |
| Zhou et al. 2007[249] | 6–9 | 23 | 30 |
| Zhou et al. 2007[249] | >9 | 101 | 34 |

of the urinary bladder. Like PIN, untreated CIS of the urinary bladder may become invasive; however, it is usually treated aggressively.

At present, no routine treatment is available for patients who have high-grade PIN. Prophylactic radical prostatectomy or radiation is not an acceptable treatment for patients who have PIN only.[261] The development and identification of acceptable agents to treat PIN would fill a therapeutic void. As noted above, androgen deprivation therapy and radiation therapy induce acinar atrophy and apoptosis that result in regression of high-grade PIN.[74,261–266]

Chronic therapy, however, would most likely be required to prevent new foci of PIN from invading and becoming clinical prostate cancer. Although more toxicity is likely to be tolerated for the treatment agents targeted to regress or inhibit PIN, compared to treating healthy patients to reduce prostate cancer incidence, androgen deprivation therapy has too many adverse effects in men to be clinically useful. New agents with better safety and lower side-effect profiles are greatly needed, as patients may be taking the agent at least until they attain 70 years of age.[261] Toremifene (Acapodene) is a selective estrogen receptor modulator that eliminates high-grade PIN and reduces the incidence of prostate cancer.

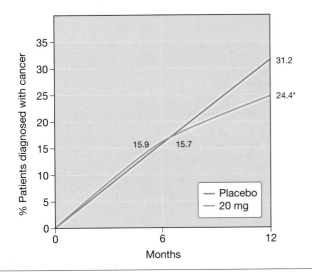

* p = 0.048 versus placebo, Mantel-Cox test stratified for study site

**Fig. 9-12** Toremifene 1-year graph.

After 4 months of toremifene (60 mg/day orally for 4 months), 72% of men treated (vs 17.9% of controls) had no high-grade PIN on subsequent prostate biopsies.[267] In another study the cumulative risk of prostate cancer was reduced in patients taking toremifene 20 mg compared to placebo (24.4% vs 31.2%), with an annualized rate of prevention of 6.8 cancers per 100 men treated (Fig. 9-12).[268] Among patients with no biopsy evidence of cancer at baseline and at 6 months, the 12-month incidence of prostate cancer was reduced by 48.2% with toremifene 20 mg compared to placebo (9.1% vs 17.4%). The 20-mg dose was most effective, but the cumulative and 12-month incidences of prostate cancer were lower with each toremifene dose versus placebo (cumulative risk: 29.2% for 40 mg, 28.1% for 60 mg; 12-month incidence 14.3% for 40 mg, 13.0% for 60 mg).[268]

Green tea catechins (GTCs) also may reduce the incidence of prostate cancer in men with PIN. Catechins are antioxidants in the class of polyphenols called flavonols. After 6 months of green tea catechins (600 mg/day orally), 3.3% of the men with PIN had cancer compared to 30% of those who took placebo.[269]

The potent antioxidant lycopene (4 mg/day)was found in a prospective randomized placebo-controlled 1-year study of 40 men with PIN to significantly reduce the risk of subsequent prostate cancer, with no toxicity and good patient tolerance.[270]

The antioxidants selenium and vitamin E are also under investigation as putative chemopreventive agents in men with PIN.

PIN offers promise as an intermediate endpoint in studies of chemoprevention of prostatic carcinoma. Recognizing the slow growth rate of prostate cancer and the considerable amount of time needed in animal and human studies for adequate follow-up, the non-invasive precursor lesion PIN is a suitable intermediate histologic marker to indicate the subsequent likelihood of cancer.

### PIN does not predict cancer recurrence

PIN was not predictive of PSA (biochemical) failure at 32 months in patients undergoing radical prostatectomy and androgen deprivation therapy.[264]

### Androgen deprivation therapy eliminates PIN

There is a marked decrease in the prevalence and extent of high-grade PIN in cases after androgen deprivation therapy compared to untreated cases.[264,265,271] This decrease is accompanied by epithelial hyperplasia, cytoplasmic clearing, and prominent glandular atrophy, with a decreased ratio of glands to stroma. These findings indicate that the dysplastic prostatic epithelium is hormone dependent. In the normal prostatic epithelium luminal secretory cells are more sensitive to the absence of androgen than are basal cells, and these results indicate that the cells of high-grade PIN share this androgen sensitivity. The loss of some normal, hyperplastic, and dysplastic epithelial cells with androgen deprivation is probably due to acceleration of programmed single cell death. One report suggested that PIN was not substantially decreased after hormonal therapy, but those authors failed to use current criteria for PIN, so the results are not comparable.[272] Further, there is a heterogeneity in the response of PIN to therapy that probably varies further with duration.[273]

Neoadjuvant hormone deprivation using monthly LHRH-agonist leuprolide and anti-androgen flutamide for 3 months resulted in a 50% reduction in high-grade PIN. Longer therapy with 6 months of neoadjuvant androgen deprivation therapy prior to radical prostatectomy in the European Randomized Study of Screening for Prostate Cancer study reduced high-grade PIN even more.[50] Flutamide reduced the prevalence and extent of high-grade PIN and induced epithelial atrophy.[274] There is also evidence that cessation of flutamide therapy resulted in a return of high-grade PIN.[267] Conversely, 60 men with PIN but no evidence of prostate adenocarcinoma were randomized in a double-blind manner to flutamide or placebo and followed with repeat biopsies; at 1 year, 14% of men receiving flutamide and 10% of men receiving placebo had developed prostate adenocarcinoma, indicating no evidence of benefit from 1 year of treatment with flutamide as a chemoprevention agent in men with PIN.[275]

Another anti-androgen, bicalutamide, lowered the mean cancer volume, mean PIN volume, and incidence of PIN after a few months;[276] at radical prostatectomy, Gleason scores were similar to those of the untreated control group.[271] There was no evidence of the emergence of higher-grade cancer after treatment.[271]

The results of 5α-reductase (finasteride) treatment in high-grade PIN are controversial and the cumulative number of cases studied is probably too small to draw firm conclusions.[277] Two reports found no apparent effect on the histologic appearance or extent of high-grade PIN,[278,279] whereas a third study of three cases described atrophy and involution with decreased prevalence.[280]

### Radiation therapy eliminates PIN

The prevalence and extent of PIN are reduced after radiation therapy.[281,282] However, one study paradoxically noted a higher than expected incidence (70%) of PIN after radiation therapy,[283] but the authors failed to employ accepted diagnostic criteria for PIN, so their results are not comparable with others. A report from Memorial Sloan–Kettering Hospital found PIN in 8.8% of biopsies following a course of three-dimensional external beam conformal radiation therapy.[282]

Following radiation therapy, PIN retains the features characteristic of untreated PIN and is readily recognized in tissue specimens. The key pathologic features include nuclear crowding, nuclear overlapping and stratification, nuclear hyperchromasia, and prominent nucleoli. The basal cell layer is present, but often fragmented; racemase shows strong apical to diffuse cytoplasmic staining.[284] The most common patterns of PIN are tufting and micropapillary, similar to those reported in untreated PIN.

The long-term efficacy of radiation treatment may depend on eradication of cancer as well as precancerous lesions that may otherwise lead to the evolution of secondary metachronous invasive cancer. Identification of residual or recurrent cancer portends a worse prognosis. The questions remain whether recurrent cancer after irradiation is due to regrowth of incompletely eradicated tumor or to progression from incompletely eradicated PIN. Further studies of salvage prostatectomy specimens and post-radiation needle biopsies are justified in an attempt to establish the significance of high-grade PIN as a source of long-term treatment failure in these patients. If PIN is associated with treatment failure, adjuvant chemoprevention strategies that ablate this lesion may reduce the risk of late cancer recurrence.

## Differential diagnosis of PIN

The histologic differential diagnosis of PIN includes lobular atrophy, post-atrophic hyperplasia, atypical basal cell hyperplasia, cribriform hyperplasia, and metaplastic changes associated with radiation, infarction, and prostatitis (Tables 9.11, 9.12) (Chapter 8). Many of these display architectural and cytologic atypia, including enlarged nucleoli, and are especially difficult to exclude in small specimens and cauterized or distorted specimens. Cribriform adenocarcinoma, ductal (endometrioid) carcinoma, and urothelial carcinoma involving the prostatic ducts and acini may also be confused with PIN. Biopsies submitted with an incomplete patient history should be interpreted with caution. Proliferative activity, defined as Ki-67 labeling index, was higher in ductal carcinoma than in PIN (33% vs 6%).[60,61] Stratified epithelium in non-cribriform glands of prostate cancer can also resemble high-grade PIN. Recognition of this fact and immunohistochemical evaluation of stratified glands may be indicated to correctly diagnose those glands as prostate cancer.[285]

## Atypical small acinar proliferation (ASAP)

About 4% of contemporary prostate needle biopsies contain collections of small acini that are suspicious for cancer but fall below the diagnostic threshold (Table 9-13).[86,87,286–303] These are reported as atypical small acinar proliferation suspicious for but not diagnostic of malignancy (ASAP) (Figs

**Table 9-11** Prostatic intraepithelial neoplasia: differential diagnosis

Normal anatomic structures and embryonic rests
    Seminal vesicles and ejaculatory ducts
    Cowper's glands
    Paraganglionic tissue
    Mesonephric remnants
    Ectopic prostatic tissue of the urethra

Hyperplasia
    Benign epithelial hyperplasia
    Cribriform hyperplasia

Atypical basal cell hyperplasia

Post-atrophic hyperplasia

Simple lobular atrophy

Sclerosing adenosis

Metaplasia and reactive changes

Urothelial metaplasia

Infarction-induced atypia

Inflammation-induced atypia

Radiation-induced atypia

Nephrogenic adenoma of the prostatic urethra

Carcinoma
    Acinar adenocarcinoma
    Urothelial dysplasia and carcinoma
    Ductal carcinoma

**Table 9-12** Mimics of high-grade PIN (overdiagnosis of PIN) in 60 consecutive cases (From Bostwick DG, Ma J. In press, 2007)

| Mimic of PIN | Number of cases (%) |
|---|---|
| Basal cell hyperplasia | 12 (20) |
| Benign proliferative epithelium (non-central zone) | 10 (17) |
| Low-grade PIN | 10 (17) |
| Reactive changes | 10 (17) |
| Atypical basal cell hyperplasia | 7 (12) |
| Central zone epithelium | 5 (8) |
| Urothelium | 2 (3) |
| Seminal vesicle | 1 (2) |
| Cribriform hyperplasia | 1 (2) |
| Post-atrophic hyperplasia | 1 (2) |
| Atrophy | 1 (2) |

9-13-9-15).[304] Prostate cancer has been identified in subsequent biopsies in the majority of cases of ASAP, indicating that this finding is a significant predictor of cancer (see below). The identification of ASAP warrants repeat biopsy for concurrent or subsequent invasive carcinoma.

The US prevalence of ASAP is estimated to be 2 145 560 men (Table 9-14). It should be noted that ASAP is a diagnostic category but not a true histopathologic entity (most

**Table 9-13** Incidence of ASAP in needle biopsies

| Reference | Patient population | Incidence of ASAP (%) |
|---|---|---|
| Hoedemaeker et al. 1999[289] | Screening population | 2.4 |
| Postma et al. 2004[293] | Screening population | 2.6 |
| Kahane et al. 1995[87] | Urology practice | 0.7 |
| Bostwick et al. 1995[1251,1267] | Urology practice | 1.5 |
| Bostwick et al. 2006[304] | Urology practice | 2.5 |
| Cheville et al. 1997[286] | Urology practice | 4.8 |
| Wills et al. 1997[302] | Urology practice | 4.6 |
| Renshaw et al. 1998[297] | Urology practice | 9.0 |
| Reyes et al. 1998[298] | Urology practice | 23.4 |
| Weinstein et al. 1998[299] | Urology practice | 6.1 |
| Novis et al. 1999[86] | Urology practice | 7.1 |
| O'Dowd et al. 2000[1268] | Urology practice | 2.8 |
| Ouyang et al. 2001[290] | Urology practice | 6.3 |
| Borborgolou et al. 2001[291] | Urology practice | 4.4 |
| Iczkowski et al. 2002[292] | Urology practice | 2.6 |
| Fadare et al. 2004[294] | Urology practice | 1.8 |
| Gupta et al. 2004[295] | Urology practice | 2.8 |
| Naya et al. 2004[301] | Urology practice | 2.9 |
| Kobayshi et al. 2004[300] | Urology practice | 3.8 |
| Brausi et al. 2004[296] | Urology practice | 5.3 |
| Gupta et al. 2004[295] | Urology practice | 6.0 |
| Range | | 2.4–2.6 (Screening) 0.7–23.4 (Urology practice) |

**Table 9-14** Estimated prevalence of ASAP in the United States

| Age | % ASAP* | US population* | Number of ASAP |
|---|---|---|---|
| 40–49 | 4 | 20 550 000 | 822 000 |
| 50–59 | 4 | 14 187 000 | 567 480 |
| 60–69 | 4 | 9 312 000 | 372 480 |
| 70–79 | 4 | 6 926 000 | 177 040 |
| 80–89 | 4 | 2 664 000 | 106 560 |
| **Total** | | **53 639 000** | **2 145 560** |

*The estimated value of 4% is used throughout as the prevalence of ASAP has not been determined as a function of age.

It should be noted that ASAP is not a diagnostic entity but rather a diagnostic category; hence the 'prevalence' shown here represents the theoretical detection level for this histologic finding given current methods of detection if the entire population were to undergo biopsy.

**Table 9-15** Reasons for the diagnosis of ASAP

**Small Size of Focus**

Small number of acini in the focus of concern (invariably fewer than two dozen acini)

Small focus size, average 0.4 mm in diameter

Focus present at core tip or biopsy edge, indicating that the focus is incompletely sampled

Loss of focus of concern in deeper levels

**Conflicting Morphologic Findings**

Distortion of acini raising concern for atrophy

Lack of convincing features of cancer (insufficient nucleomegaly or nucleolomegaly)

Clustered growth pattern mimicking a benign process such as atypical adenomatous hyperplasia

Foamy cytoplasm raising concern for foamy gland carcinoma

**Conflicting Immunohistochemical Findings**

Focally positive high molecular weight cytokeratin

Focally positive p63 staining

Negative racemase immunostaining

**Confounding Findings**

Histologic artifacts such as thick sections or overstained nuclei

Tangential cutting of adjacent high-grade PIN

Architectural or cytologic changes (nucleomegaly and nucleolomegaly) owing to inflammation or other lesions

cases probably represent undersampled adenocarcinoma), so the prevalence data are simply a gauge of the magnitude of the diagnostic problem of ASAP that would be encountered if all men underwent biopsy (biopsy is the only method for detection of ASAP).

## Diagnostic criteria

ASAP represents our inability to render an incontrovertible diagnosis of cancer in a needle biopsy. The focus of concern is invariably no larger than two dozen acini – less than the size of the head of a pin – so the major concern is overdiagnosis of cancer based on insufficient evidence. The diagnostic difficulty with ASAP usually results from one or a combination of the reasons listed in Table 9-15.[305] All of these may hinder a definitive diagnosis of carcinoma, but in such cases the possibility cannot be definitively excluded. The need for this category is based on our 'absolute uncertainty' regarding the diagnosis. That this need exists is manifested by the variety of terms or synonyms currently in use that include the word 'atypical' to describe this diagnosis,

although ASAP is now the term that is most widely used clinically around the world.[306] The diagnosis of ASAP indicates to the clinician that the biopsy in question exhibits histologic features that are neither clearly malignant nor clearly benign, and that follow-up of the patient is warranted.

For pathologists, three questions need to be answered prior to the diagnosis of ASAP or cancer in a small lesion:

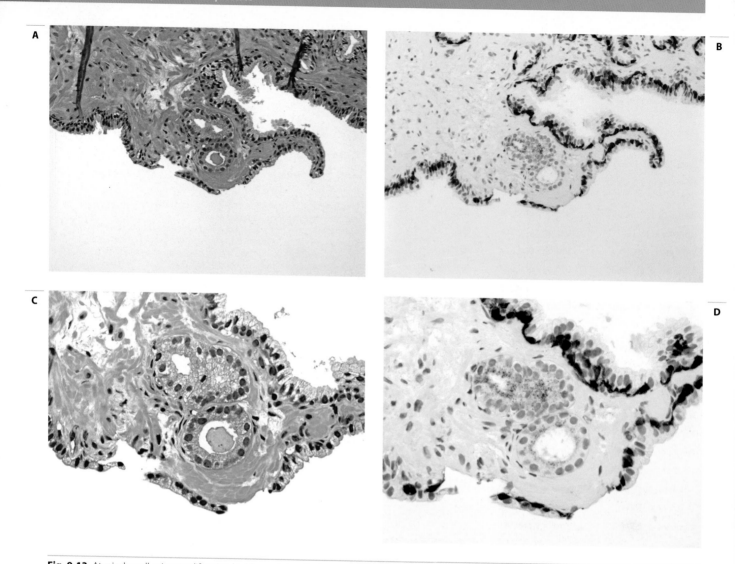

**Fig. 9-13** Atypical small acinar proliferation highly suspicious for but not diagnostic of malignancy (ASAP). This small focus consists of two to three small round to oval acini that stand in contrast to the adjacent benign epithelium; however, there is only slight nucleomegaly and minimal nucleolomegaly. (**A, C**) H&E-stained sections. (**B, D**) Matched triple stains, with strong racemase staining and absence of p63 and keratin 34βE12 immunoreactivity, compounding the suspicion of malignancy. Despite the high level of suspicion, the small size of the focus and the absence of compelling cytologic features warranted diagnosis of ASAP rather than cancer.

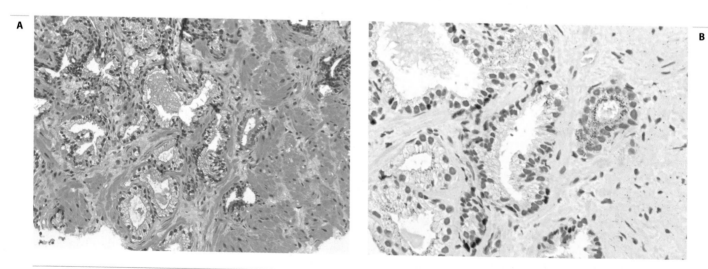

**Fig. 9-14** Atypical small acinar proliferation highly suspicious for but not diagnostic of malignancy (ASAP). (**A**) The proliferation of intermediate-sized acini shows variation in acinar shape and spacing. (**B**) A single acinus displays racemase staining with absence of p63 nuclear immunoreactivity is highly suspicious, but the small size of the focus and the absence of compelling nuclear and nucleolar abnormalities precludes a definite diagnosis of cancer.

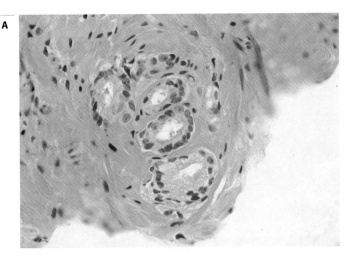

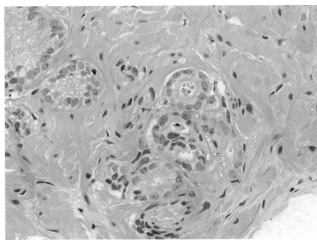

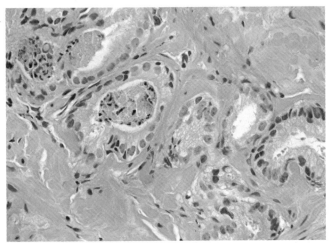

**Fig. 9-15** Atypical small acinar proliferation highly suspicious for but not diagnostic of malignancy (ASAPH). (**A**) The first level through the biopsy reveals a cluster of about half a dozen small to intermediate-sized acini with variation in size and shape and lined by slightly enlarged nuclei with scattered prominent nucleoli. (**B**) The fourth level is similar, with even more prominent nucleoli. (**C**) The seventh tissue slice through the focus of concern reveals luminal necrosis. Despite the high level of suspicion for malignancy, identification of the confounding factor of necrosis (could all of the findings be attributable to inflammation?) small size of the focus, and absence of definitive cytologic features of malignancy, the best diagnosis is ASAPH. Immunostains (not shown) reveal scattered p63 and keratin 34βE12 immunoreactive basal cell nuclei in the focus of concern.

- Would you be absolutely confident of this biopsy diagnosis if it were followed by a negative radical prostatectomy?
- Would another colleague pathologist agree with the diagnosis of cancer?
- Can you confidently support the diagnosis of adenocarcinoma based solely on this biopsy?

If the answer to any of these is 'No,' then we recommend use of the more conservative diagnosis of ASAP. In this setting, we believe that ASAP is a valid diagnostic category as long as it is employed judiciously and that maximum information has been obtained from the available tissue. Other evidence useful in supporting a cancer diagnosis, including patient age, serum PSA concentration, and high molecular weight cytokeratin, p63, and racemase expression, cannot substitute for convincing hematoxylin and eosin-stained microscopic findings. To avoid bias, the above information should be considered only in combination with routine microscopic examination.

The histologic features that most often preclude a definitive diagnosis of malignancy are the small size of the focus (70% of cases), disappearance on step levels (61%), lack of significant cytologic atypia such as nucleolomegaly (55%), and associated inflammation (9%), raising the possibility of one of the many mimics of adenocarcinoma (Fig. 9-16).[287] Other causes include negative high molecular weight cytokeratin or p63 immunostain in the focus, atrophic or inflamed glands lacking a basal cell layer, and the presence of associated PIN.

Immunohistochemical stain for α-methylacyl-coenzyme A-racemase (AMACR, or racemase for short) has greatly facilitated the diagnostic support provided by basal cell specific antikeratin 34βE12 and p63, particularly in equivocal biopsies such as ASAP (Fig. 9-17).[107,108,120,284,307] Performance of these immunostains resolved 76% of atypical small acinar proliferation diagnoses by consensus of three urologic pathologists studied.[308] We routinely use these important techniques in the diagnostic work-up of atypical prostate lesions on needle biopsies, thereby decreasing the incidence of ASAP and reducing the risk of false negatives and the need for additional biopsies, similar to other reports.

Multiple diagnostic criteria differ significantly between ASAP and minimal cancer (Table 9-16).[305,309] First, the mean number of acini and length of the focus of concern in ASAP (11 acini) are about half those for minimal cancer (17 acini). Also, the small size of a focus of concern was the commonest

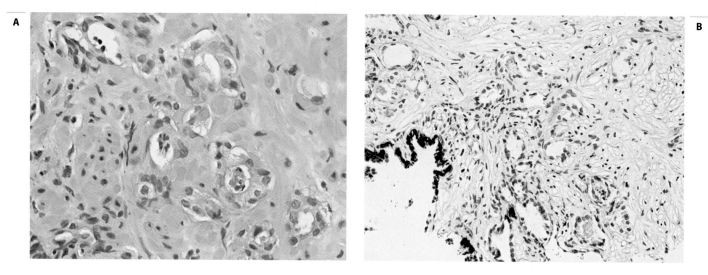

**Fig. 9-16** Atypical small acinar proliferation. (**A**) Luminal neutrophils confound this focus that is highly suspicious for cancer by virtue of the variation in acinar size, shape, and spacing. (**B**) Absence of keratin 34βE12 staining (with internal positive control in adjacent benign epithelium) compounding the suspicion of malignancy.

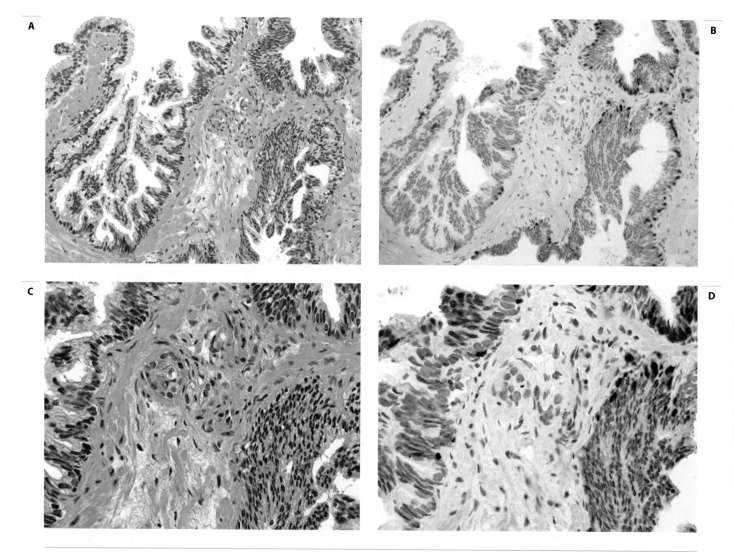

**Fig. 9-17** Atypical small acinar proliferation. (**A, C**) This small focus of two to three acini stands in contrast to the adjacent benign epithelium, but the cytologic features are obscured by the dark staining. (**B, D**) Matched triple stains reveal absence of racemase staining as well as p63 and keratin 34βE12. Absence of racemase staining does little to allay the suspicion for malignancy, but the focus is simply too small and lacks cytologic support for malignancy.

**Table 9-16** Comparative histologic findings in prostate needle biopsies with atypical small acinar proliferation (ASAP) or minimal cancer

| Findings: | ASAP | Minimal cancer |
|---|---|---|
| **Architectural** | | |
| Linear extent (mm), mean ± SD | 0.4 ± 0.3 | 0.8 ± 0.5 |
| Number of acini, mean ± SD | 11 ± 10 | 17 ± 14 |
| Infiltrative growth | 75% | 100% |
| Cytologic | | |
| Nuclear hyperchromasia | 44% | 9% |
| Nuclear enlargement (scale of 0–3), mean ± SD | 1.2 ± 0.8 | 1.8 ± 0.7 |
| Prominent nucleoli in at least 10% of cells | 55% | 100% |
| Mitotic figure(s) | 0% | 10% |
| **Luminal** | | |
| Blue mucin | 6% | 33% |
| Stroma and adjacent acini | | |
| High-grade PIN in same slide | 23% | 57% |
| Moderate–severe atrophy | 59% | 35% |

ASAP, atypical small acinar proliferation, suspicious for malignancy; minimal cancer, adenocarcinoma involving less than 5% of total tissue; PIN, prostatic intraepithelial neoplasia; SD, standard deviation.

source of difficulty in ASAP, accounting for 70% of ASAP diagnoses.[287]

Infiltrative growth is a constant feature of prostate cancer, but also occurred in 68–75% of ASAP cases.[286] All cancers have at least mild nuclear enlargement, but on average the enlargement is moderate, in contrast to mild enlargement in ASAP. When the focus of concern is larger, however, and other architectural and cytologic features are very compelling, one may overlook the lack of prominent nucleoli if they are obscured by nuclear hyperchromasia. This hyperchromasia is more common in ASAP than in minimal cancer, in which the small size of the focus compounds the diagnostic dilemma. Nuclear hyperchromasia is a frequent and confounding staining artifact, and cancer cell nuclei are often more hyperchromatic than those of neighboring benign acini. Reducing the duration of staining with hematoxylin may avoid this problem. The 10% frequency of mitotic figures in cancer stands in contrast to that of benign acini. However, mitotic figures are too rare to be a reliable diagnostic finding in small foci.

Blue-gray luminal mucin is as a significant discriminator between ASAP and minimal cancer (6% vs 33% of cases, respectively). The importance of blue mucin had been recognized previously, with acid mucin occurring in 61% of cancers[310] compared to 42% of ASAP cases.[286] Eosinophilic proteinaceous secretions, although a more common feature of cancer than blue mucin, are non-specific, occurring frequently in ASAP. Eosinophilic secretions were present at least focally in 73% of minimal cancers, compared to 66–74% in cases of ASAP.[286]

Crystalloids[311] are uncommon and non-specific, occurring in 19% of cancers and 16% of cases of ASAP. Prior studies described similar frequencies of 6%,[287] 13%,[312] and 22%[286] of crystalloids in ASAP foci and in 5% of benign biopsy specimens.[313] These data confirm that crystalloids do not pose an increased risk for cancer in subsequent biopsy specimens.[313,314]

Moderate to severe atrophy accompanies more cases of ASAP than cancer. Small foci of post-atrophic hyperplasia (which is invariably associated with typical atrophy and has 'moderately enlarged' nuclei in 39% of cases[286]) and typical atrophy are sometimes interpreted as ASAP.

Obscuring inflammation is responsible for ASAP diagnoses in 30% of cases.[287] However, 20% of minimal cancers have associated acute or chronic inflammation. This is not significantly higher than in ASAP, and indicates that cancer can often be confidently diagnosed despite inflammation.

### Subsets of ASAP

Stratification of ASAP does not increase the predictive accuracy for cancer on repeat biopsy, despite multiple attempts.[315,316] We stratified suspicion in each ASAP case into three levels: ASAPB (atypical small acinar proliferation suspicious for but not diagnostic of malignancy, favor benign); ASAPS (atypical small acinar proliferation suspicious for but not diagnostic of malignancy), and ASAPH (atypical small acinar proliferation highly suspicious for but not diagnostic of malignancy).[316] ASAPB was employed for cases in which we deemed the focus of concern unlikely to be cancer but could not with absolute certainty exclude the possibility. Conversely, ASAPH was employed for cases in which the focus was almost certainly carcinoma, but a confident diagnosis of cancer could not be rendered. ASAPS was employed for cases with intermediate suspicion.

In stratifying ASAP into these levels of suspicion, three criteria emerged as significant. Infiltrative growth was present in just over half of ASAPB cases, but almost all ASAPH cases. ASAPS and ASAPH had a greater degree of nuclear enlargement than in ASAPB, but confounded more frequently by nuclear hyperchromasia. This hyperchromasia, involving over half of cases of ASAPS and ASAPH, often obscured nuclear detail and nucleoli; nevertheless, we noted a non-significant trend toward prominent nucleoli in a higher percentage of the cases as suspicion increased. Two other non-significant trends were noted with increasing suspicion for malignancy: more frequent coexisting high-grade PIN, and less frequent moderate to severe atrophy.

Multiple studies revealed non-significant trends for increasing risk of subsequent cancer with increasing suspicion. Stratification of ASAP also did not predict the normalized percentage of involvement by cancer on positive repeat biopsy.[317] Thus, at present, the level of suspicion should not alter follow-up recommendations.

## ASAP is predictive of cancer on repeat biopsy

Prostate cancer is found in up to 60% of repeat biopsies following the diagnosis of ASAP (Table 9-17).[287,292–294,297,315–326]

ASAP represents undersampled cancer in at least 40% of cases.[292,317,327] Iczkowski et al.[292,317] observed that some men with ASAP in the first set of biopsies and benign findings or high-grade PIN in the second biopsy may still have cancer that was not detected.

False-negative results on repeat sextant biopsy in untreated men with documented adenocarcinoma occurred in 23% of repeat sextant biopsies.[328] These results suggest that the current practice of performing six to 12 biopsies per prostate does not lower the frequency of ASAP. A declining volume of cancer at prostatectomy was noted 5 years ago,[329] and is probably reflective of increased screening and multiple sampling. Thus, as smaller-volume cancers are detected through increased sampling, many will be undersampled and not be resolvable by immunostaining, thereby probably leading to an irreducible rate of ASAP diagnosis.

What prostatic sites should be sampled at repeat biopsy? One study found that sampling only the side or sextant site initially diagnosed as ASAP missed cancer in 39% of patients whose cancer was later detected exclusively at other sites, suggesting that the entire prostate should be rebiopsied.[317]

In a recent provocative report, the investigators recommended immediate radical prostatectomy in patients with a biopsy diagnosis of ASAP. They suggested that the risk of subsequent cancer is 100% in radical prostatectomy specimens.[296] We urge caution in recommending expansion of the indications for prostatectomy to include patients with ASAP.

ASAP is best considered as a diagnostic risk category and not a true entity.

## ASAP in combination with PIN

The combination of high-grade PIN and atypical small acinar proliferation lesions is found in up to 16% of biopsy sets, and has a predictive value for cancer of 33%[316] to 50%.[315] Thus, it is slightly lower or higher than isolated ASAP (37%), but higher than isolated PIN (23%). PIN occurred with ASAP in 17%,[315] 23%,[305] 31%,[286] or 41% of cases with ASAP,[316] but most foci were not adjacent or contiguous.

In a similar investigation, a lesion containing both PIN and ASAP ($n = 51$) was reported to predict cancer in 46% of follow-up biopsies. This lesion was carefully defined, and corresponded to the definition of contiguous PIN/ASAP.[330] Three factors might account for the difference in predictive values (33% vs 46%) seen in our recent report and this study. First, the latter study was restricted to contiguous cases; this type of lesion might have an intrinsically higher predictive value for cancer than in our series, in which the frequency of contiguous lesions was about half. The selection bias present in cases referred for consultation also may have influenced the study results compared with unselected primary cases in another study cohort. Finally, only a modest number of patients were reported in each study, so that the data may have been skewed. In another small study of 12 patients with PIN and adjacent atypical glands (ASAP), 75% had cancer on repeat biopsy.[331] The best available evidence today indicates that the presence of either or both lesions in needle biopsies is still a predictor for concurrent/subsequent cancer compared to patients lacking these lesions.

A novel finding was that high-grade PIN was more than twice as frequent in association with minimal cancer (57%) as ASAP (23%). High-grade PIN accompanied 14%[287] to 31%[286] of ASAP foci, but only 13% of cancers in biopsies.[332] About half of cases of ASAP are probably undersampled cancer, and the smaller mean size of the foci in contemporary specimens reduces the likelihood of sampling accompanying high-grade PIN.

# Adenocarcinoma

Adenocarcinoma accounts for about 95% of prostatic malignancies.

## Epidemiology

Prostate cancer poses a greater risk for American men, especially African-American men, than any other non-skin cancer. This veritable epidemic of prostate cancer has resulted partly from successful efforts at early detection with the use of the serum PSA test, thereby narrowing the still-enormous gap between the clinical incidence (8% lifetime risk) and the autopsy-based prevalence (80% by age 80 years) (Fig. 9-18). Most men die *with* prostate cancer rather than *from* it, yet physicians are unable to accurately stratify patients into those who will have progressive cancer and those who will not. An equally great problem is determining which men are at the greatest risk of developing clinically apparent prostate cancer.

**Table 9-17** Cancer risk in patients with ASAP

| Reference | # Men with repeat biopsy(ies) | Risk of Cancer (%) |
|---|---|---|
| Cheville et al. 1997[318] | 25 | 60 |
| Iczkowski et al. 1997[287] | 33 | 45 |
| Iczkowski et al. 1998[317] | 295 | 42 |
| Renshaw et al. 1998[297] | 59 | 34 |
| Chan et al. 1999[319] | 92 | 49 |
| Park et al. 2001[320] | 45 | 51 |
| Borboroglu et al. 2001[321] | 48 | 48 |
| Iczkowski et al. 2002[292] | 129 | 45 |
| Fadare et al. 2004[294] | 24 | 38 |
| Postma et al. 2004[293] | 96 | 37 |
| Schlesinger et al. 2005[316] | 78 | 37 |
| Scattoni et al. 2005[315] | | 37 |
| Moore et al. 2005[322] | 53 | 36 |
| Leite et al. 2005[323] | 16 | 44 |
| Girasole et al. 2006[324] | 107 | 51 |
| Rodriguez-Patron Rodriguez et al. 2006[325] | | 40 |
| Mancuso et al. 2007[326] | 31 | 55 |
| Range | | 34–60% |

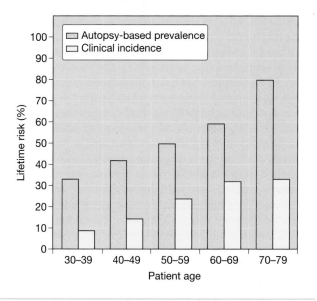

**Fig. 9-18** Autopsy-detected prostate cancer increases with age.

Prostatic adenocarcinoma is rare in patients under 40.[333] Fewer than 50 cases of adenocarcinoma have been reported in each of the following groups: children less than 12 years old, adolescents, and young adults between 20 and 25 years old. In all cases the cancer was poorly differentiated, clinically aggressive, and unresponsive to hormonal therapy and radiation therapy.

Above 40 years of age the incidence rises quickly. Autopsy studies of thoroughly evaluated prostates from men without clinical evidence of cancer have shown a very high level of latent cancer. The incidence of prostatic adenocarcinoma is much higher in men of African ancestry (100 per 100 000) than in men of European ancestry (70.1 per 100 000), and men of African ancestry in the United States have the world's highest mortality rate from prostatic adenocarcinoma.[334] The prevalence of clinically occult cancer is similar in different geographic and ethnic groups despite wide variations in the incidence of clinically apparent adenocarcinoma. The incidence is low in American Indians, Hispanics, and Orientals, but high in American men of African and European ancestry.

Prostate cancer mortality varies considerably from country to country. High rates have been reported in the US, particularly among African-Americans, whereas low rates have been found in China and Japan. There are advantages and disadvantages in using mortality data to examine the underlying risk of prostate cancer. Incidence data are often unavailable, so mortality is a commonly used surrogate. However, mortality is a function of both incidence and survival. International differences in mortality may reflect differences in the underlying risk of developing prostate cancer, but may also reflect differences in survival or ascertainment/reporting (death certificate) bias.

## Latent carcinoma

The age-specific prevalence of latent cancer at autopsy is constant across countries and ethnic groups. Data from the Connecticut (USA) Tumor Registry estimated the age-standardized prevalence rate to be 841.6 per 100 000 in 1994, an increase of 126% over the 1982 rate.[335]

Incidental prostate cancer is less aggressive than clinically apparent prostate cancer according to stage, surgical margin status, and Gleason score. Totally sampled cystoprostatectomy specimens with bladder cancer also contain clinically undetected incidental prostate cancer in about 42% of cases (range, 23–68%).[336]

Cystoprostatectomies with prostate cancer have a lower stage and lower Gleason score than radical prostatectomy cases. Incidental prostate cancer in cystoprostatectomy cases is usually stage pT2a or pT2b (59% and 29%, respectively).[336] Incidental prostate cancer is usually low grade (Gleason score 5 and 6 in 25% and 46% of cases, respectively), much lower than for clinical prostate cancer (5% and 21%, respectively). Only 9% of incidental cancers are Gleason score 8–10. The frequency of positive margins in incidental prostate cancer is lower than in clinical prostate cancer (7% vs 52%).

The relationship between incidental, latent, and clinical prostate cancer may be explained by two hypotheses.[337] One contends that incidental and latent carcinoma are histologically identical to lethal cancer, but are predestined never to acquire biologically aggressive features. The other contends that clinically innocuous cancers are simply the smallest tumors, and cancer acquires the capacity to metastasize as a function of the passage of time, increasing volume, and 'biological tumor progression,' a function of the mutational instability of all cancer, which becomes manifest in proportion to the number of mitotic events. We agree with Selman[338] that the term latent carcinoma is a medical misnomer and should not be used.

## Etiology and pathogenesis

Risk factors can be classified as endogenous or exogenous, although some are not exclusively one or the other (e.g., race, aging, oxidative stress).[334] For the purposes of this chapter, an environmental factor is considered an exogenous factor or exposure. There are numerous endogenous risk factors for prostate cancer, including family history, hormones, race, aging and oxidative stress (Table 9-18).

### Family history

In epidemiologic studies family history is significantly associated with prostate cancer risk, but may be influenced by detection bias. A man's risk is twofold higher if a first-degree relative such as a father or brother has prostatic adenocarcinoma, and five to 11 times higher if two or three first-degree relatives have cancer. The clinical and pathologic features of familial cancer are similar to those of non-familial cancer.

### Hormones

Androgens significantly alter prostate cancer growth rates, and progression from preclinical to clinically significant cancer may result in part from altered androgen metabolism. Elevated concentrations of testosterone and its metabolite dihydrotestosterone, over many decades, may increase risk, but results have been inconsistent.

**Table 9-18** Risk factors for prostate cancer

| |
|---|
| Family history |
| Diet |
| Fat |
| Cadmium |
| Zinc |
| Obesity |
| Alcohol |
| Hormones |
| Smoking |
| Sexual activity |
| Early sexual activity |
| Multiple sexual partners |
| Occupational exposure |
| Agricultural fertilizers and pesticides |
| Rubber |
| Ionizing radiation |
| Venereal diseases |
| Herpes virus type 2 |
| Cytomegalovirus |
| Vasectomy |
| Benign prostatic hyperplasia |
| Prostatic intraepithelial neoplasia |
| Atypical small acinar proliferation |

### Race

Racial differences in prostate cancer risk may reflect three factors: exposure differences, differences in detection, and biological differences. The highest incidence rate in the world is among African-American men, who have a higher risk of prostate cancer than white Americans. However, racial differences may reflect differences in access to care, differences in the decision-making process as to whether to seek medical attention and follow-up, and differences in allelic frequencies of microsatellites at the androgen receptor locus or polymorphic variation.

### Aging and oxidative stress

Prostate cancer may theoretically result from an increase in oxidative stress, but supportive evidence is limited.[334] Clinical studies indicate that intake of antioxidants such as selenium, α-tocopherol (vitamin E), and lycopene (a carotenoid) offers protection against prostate cancer. Our current knowledge of the relationship between aging and pro-oxidation–antioxidation homeostasis of the human prostate remains virtually non-existent.

There are numerous exogenous risk factors for prostate cancer,[334] including diet, endocrine-disrupting chemicals, occupation, and other factors.

*Diet* A wide variety of dietary factors have been implicated in the development of prostate cancer according to descriptive epidemiologic studies of migrants, geographic variations, and temporal studies. Fat consumption, especially of polyunsaturated fats, shows a strong positive correlation with prostate cancer incidence and mortality, perhaps resulting from fat-induced alterations in hormonal profiles, the effect of fat metabolites as protein or DNA-reactive intermediates, or fat-induced elevation of oxidative stress. Retinoids, including vitamin A, help regulate epithelial cell differentiation and proliferation, with a positive association with prostate cancer risk. Vitamin C is a scavenger of reactive oxygen species (ROS) and free radicals, but there is no consistent association of intake and prostate cancer risk. Vitamin D deficiency may be a risk factor for prostate cancer; the hormonal form, 1-25-dihydroxyvitamin D, inhibits invasiveness and has antiproliferative and antidifferentiative effects on prostate cancer. Vitamin E (α-tocopherol) is an antioxidant that inhibits prostate cancer cell growth through apoptosis, and daily intake decreased the risk of prostate cancer by 32% in a large controlled clinical trial from Finland.[339] Zinc concentration is higher in the prostate than any other organ in the body, although it is reduced more than 90% in prostates with cancer; the relationship of dietary zinc and prostate cancer risk is uncertain. Selenium is an essential trace element that inhibits viral and chemical carcinogen-induced tumors in animals; a chemopreventive role for selenium is plausible, but the evidence in humans is limited. Cadmium is a significant environmental contaminant that has been linked to prostatic cancer in some epidemiological studies; interestingly, the carcinogenic potential of cadmium may be modified by zinc. Alcohol intake has no significant association with prostate cancer risk. Consumption of cruciferous vegetables is associated with a reduced risk of many cancers, but there is no evidence of a protective effect for prostate cancer. Lycopene, an abundant constituent of tomato-based products and the most efficient carotenoid antioxidant, has a significant protective effect.

*Endocrine disrupting chemicals (EDC)* An EDC can be defined as a chemical that positively or negatively alters hormone activity and thereby affects reproduction and development. Exposure to EDCs via ingestion of food, water, or air may influence or mediate carcinogenesis. Some men may have chronic exposure over many years to low doses of EDCs that may contribute to prostate cancer. These include certain pesticide residues on foods, and phytoestrogens in soy and other plant products. EDCs may be of particular relevance to individuals with relatively high endogenous estrogen or androgen concentrations (serum or prostate tissue levels), as exposure to EDCs would effectively add or subtract from those concentrations.

*Occupation and other factors* Many industrial and occupational exposures have been studied in relation to prostate cancer risk, but the findings are inconclusive; of the greatest concern is farming, and, to a lesser extent, working in the rubber industry. Numerous other factors have shown inconsistent results, a negative association, or have very limited data on prostate cancer risk, including smoking, energy intake, sexual activity, marital status, vasectomy, social factors (lifestyle, socioeconomic factors, and education), physical activity, and anthropometry.

The mechanism of action that results in prostate cancer is uncertain, but may be classified as genotoxic or non-genotoxic.[334]

*Genotoxic* Genetic mutations may be inherited as a result of familial or racial predilection, or may be induced by a wide variety of agents; it is probable that molecular cloning of activated oncogenes from human prostate cancer and sequencing mutations will provide information on whether specific mutational spectra occur in particular genes. One possible genotoxic trigger could be continuous cell division, driven by hormones such as testosterone, resulting in the accumulation of spontaneous mutations and thereby activating select oncogenes and inactivating tumor suppressor genes. Another possible trigger could be small amounts of dietary carcinogens, such as PhiP in cooked fish and meat, cause mutations in prostate tissue over a lifetime. If this finding is confirmed in humans, it would suggest that lifetime consumption of foods containing PhiP may result in the consumption of a substantial prostate carcinogen. Because PhiP is mutagenic, forms DNA adducts, and is carcinogenic in the rat prostate, this could provide evidence for a genotoxic mechanism of human prostate carcinogenesis. However, there is currently no strong evidence that chemical carcinogens or endocrine disrupting chemicals play a role in the induction or evolution of human prostate cancer.

*Non-genotoxic* One hypothesis proposes that testosterone plays a significant role in the evolution of human prostate cancer by acting as a stimulus for prostate cell growth. It may function as a mitogen or a tumor promoter. Testosterone induces cell division, and, over a lifetime, the large number of cell divisions may result in the accumulation of spontaneous mutations in prostate cells. Testosterone is at least a necessary factor for prostatic carcinogenesis, but may serve as a cofactor rather than the ultimate trigger. Another trigger could be oxidative stress induced by smoldering long-standing chronic inflammation and the unique biochemical milieu of the prostate (e.g., high citrate and zinc levels), ultimately resulting in mitogenesis.

## Prostate cancer and BPH

Prostatic hyperplasia is frequently seen in association with prostatic adenocarcinoma and there are a number of compelling similarities, including increasing incidence and prevalence with age, concordant natural history, and hormonal requirements for growth and development, but no causal relationship has been established or seriously suggested.[334]

### Signs and symptoms

Prostatic adenocarcinoma has no specific presenting symptoms and is usually clinically silent, although it may cause urinary obstructive symptoms mimicking nodular hyperplasia. As a consequence, cancer is occasionally initially manifest in metastatic sites such as cervical lymph nodes and bone. The diagnosis may be made in the following clinical instances:

- If, in routine surveillance for prostatic adenocarcinoma in men over 40 years of age, digital rectal examination shows a nodular or diffusely enlarged prostate (clinical stage T2, T3, or T4); serum PSA level is greater than 2.5 or 4 ng/mL (clinical stage T1c); or transrectal ultrasound and biopsies are positive for malignancy (lesion-directed, random, or systematic sextant needle biopsies).
- Incidental carcinoma in transurethral resection specimens (clinical stage T1a and T1b carcinoma).
- Metastatic adenocarcinoma of unknown primary.
- Carcinoma of the prostate presenting as a rectal mass (prostate carcinoma very rarely produces an eccentric or circumferential rectal and perirectal mass with or without mucosal involvement of the rectum).

## Tissue methods of detection

### Needle core biopsy

The introduction of the fine needle for transrectal biopsy of the prostate in the 1980s, together with the use of serum PSA, revolutionized early detection efforts for prostate cancer. These two advances were mutually beneficial, feeding off each other to effectively replace the large-bore transperineal needles and exclusive reliance on digital rectal examination for cancer detection. The rate of post-biopsy infection with the fine needle declined from 7–39% to 0.81%, and hemorrhage with urinary clot retention fell from 3.2% to less than 1%. The false negative rate declined from 11–25% to 11%, and there was an improvement in the quality of the tissue sample obtained, usually with little or no compression artifact at the lateral edges of the specimens. Also, the 18-gauge needle allows multiple biopsies of the prostate with minimal discomfort, particularly with the use of topical anesthetics such as lidocaine. Today, it is hard to imagine practicing urology and urologic pathology without PSA and multiple biopsies, yet such was not the case less than 20 years ago.

A greater number of prostate biopsies are obtained now and more biopsy cores are submitted than ever before, creating a huge interpretive burden for the pathologist. It is estimated that more than 1 000 000 biopsies are performed annually in the US, with each biopsy consisting on average about 10 cores, creating an estimated 10 million tissue samples for the pathologist to interpret.

This burden is compounded by a number of factors which have increased the difficulty of interpretation. First, many patients now undergo biopsy for elevated serum PSA with no other clinical evidence of cancer, resulting in an enormous number of biopsies that often contain only a small or microscopic suspicious focus. Second, numerous diagnostic pitfalls and mimics of prostate cancer have recently been described or refined, including atypical adenomatous hyperplasia, post-atrophic hyperplasia, and PIN (see above and Chapter 8). The great number of prostate biopsy specimens being generated magnifies the risk of encountering rare or unusual lesions and the potential for misinterpretation of small foci. The concept of atypical small acinar proliferation suspicious for but not diagnostic of malignancy (ASAP) was only introduced a decade ago by Iczkowski and colleagues,[340] accounting for about 2% of biopsy diagnoses. Finally, 10 or more biopsies (five or more from each side) have largely replaced the single bilateral cores of 15 years ago, providing multiple specimens from each patient.

## Detecting cancer: factors that influence diagnostic yield in biopsies

How can we improve the yield of cancer from prostate needle biopsies? Table 9-19 describes the known variables that influence the diagnostic yield of prostate biopsies. Fixed, uncontrolled factors included patient-related factors and prostate-related factors; however, biopsy method-related factors are controllable by the urologist and pathologist to increase the diagnostic yield of cancer, and are thus deserving of additional consideration.

### Number of needle cores obtained

The increase from six to 12 cores improved the detection of prostate cancer by 29%, and all were greater than 0.5 mL in volume.[341,342] Eskicorapci et al.[343,344] noted that 10-, 12-, and 13-core biopsy strategies increased the cancer detection rate by respectively 25.5%, 22%, and 35%. Mathematical models demonstrate that more biopsy cores increase the chance of detecting prostate cancer.[345]

### Method of biopsy

The technical aspects of prostate biopsy are not standardized. The diagnostic yield is improved by ultrasound 'targeted' biopsies, but the magnitude of the increase in accuracy remains controversial. Use of a 29 mm cutting length increased cancer yield 18% above that from a 19 mm cutting length.[346] The combination of six transperineal and six transrectal biopsies resulted in a cancer detection rate of 48.5%,

and this rate increased significantly by respectively 7.2% and 8.5% compared to the transperineal and transrectal groups alone.[347]

### Location of biopsy

Lateral mid-gland and lateral base biopsy cores had the highest cancer detection rates for all prostate volumes, perhaps owing to extensive sampling of the peripheral zone by lateral biopsies. However, mid-gland and base biopsy cores had a relatively low yield, especially in small prostates, owing to sampling of the central zone in these prostates, where the prostate cancer incidence is known to be low.[343] A computer-based model suggests that the cancer detection rate increases 23% with a modified sextant protocol by directing the needles only into the more lateral aspect.[345] Conversely, ultrasound-directed lesion biopsies may be omitted when using 10-core biopsy protocols, as the yield of these biopsies was less than 2%.[343]

### Amount of tissue obtained

The detection rate of cancer in sextant needle biopsies is higher as longer single cores are sampled, particularly at the apex.[348] For example, a 20-mm core from the right apex provides a 0.27 probability of cancer detection versus a probability 0.18 for 10 mm; 0.5% of single-core sextant biopsies were larger than 20 mm. The amount of tissue obtained by biopsy varies widely, and we found an overall tissue sample (likely to be inadequate) of less than 50 mm in up to 4% of biopsies.[348] The dependence of diagnosis on tissue length was strongest at the apex.

### Histotechnologist's skill in processing and cutting prostate biopsies

Prostate biopsies are particularly difficult to embed and cut, owing to their small size and tendency to fragment and curve. Flat embedding of the biopsy cores enhances the amount of tissue that is examined by the pathologist. Laboratories that process prostate biopsies with other tissues of differing densities and consistencies (for example breast biopsies with abundant fatty tissue) usually handle all specimens the same way, optimizing results for some tissues but often resulting in prostate biopsies that are too thick to interpret or are over-stained. Excessively thick tissue specimens are two or three cells thick rather than the optimal one to two cells, thereby precluding adequate assessment of nuclear and cytoplasmic details in foci of concern. Similarly, over-stained sections (the most common problem in our consultation practice) contain obscured nuclear chromatin without recognizable nucleoli. These problems are compounded in biopsies with small foci that are suspicious for malignancy and in younger patients (those in their 40s and 50s) who have abundant proliferative epithelium that may mimic malignancy. The problems noted here apply doubly to the interpretation of high-grade prostatic intraepithelial neoplasia, accounting for both overdiagnosis (the most common mistake in current practice, in our experience) and underdiagnosis. We recommend separate processing of the delicate prostate needle cores to avoid these problems, similar to the recommendations of the European Society of Uropathology.[349]

**Table 9-19** Factors that influence the detection rate of cancer in contemporary prostate needle biopsies

### Uncontrolled Factors

Patient risk factors
    Patient population (e.g., screening population vs urologic practice)
    Patient symptoms
    Serum PSA
    Clinical stage
    Patient age
    Patient race
    Prior biopsy findings (e.g., PIN, ASAP)
        Prostate-related factors
            Prostate volume
            TRUS and other imaging findings

### Controlled Factors

Urologist-controlled factors
    Number of needle cores obtained
    Method of biopsy (e.g., random, ultrasound guided, etc.)
    Location of biopsy (e.g., laterally directed biopsies vs. midline, etc.)
    Amount of tissue obtained (e.g., biopsy 'gun' employed; operator skill)

Pathologist-controlled factors
    Histotechnologist's skill in processing and cutting prostate biopsies
    Number of needle cores embedded per cassette
    Number of tissue cuts obtained per specimen
    Pathologist's skill in prostate biopsy interpretation

### Number of needle cores embedded per cassette

Multiple needle biopsies submitted in one to two containers tend to entangle and fragment and are difficult to embed in a single plane during processing. The resulting loss of tissue surface area makes a definitive diagnosis difficult in many cases, resulting in equivocal pathology reports.[295] If multiple cores are embedded in one cassette, it is necessary to take care that all are separated from each other.

### Number of tissue cuts obtained per specimen

There are variations between laboratories in the number of serial tissue cuts obtained from each needle core for routine examination. To avoid the serious problem of undersampling, we routinely obtain six separate cuts (two adjacent sections from three separate levels) from the paraffin block for hematoxylin and eosin staining; additional intervening sections are placed on another slide and saved for immunohistochemical stains or special studies (Fig. 9-19). We consider the recommendation of the European Randomized Study of Screening for Prostate Cancer to be inadequate (they recommend only two cuts in total)[350], probably missing up to 3% of cancers with such limited sampling.[351] In our experience, recutting the block for additional levels with small suspicious foci is useful in about half of cases, with usually no more than four additional slides before the tissue specimen is exhausted.

Rogatsch et al.[352] compared biopsy cores submitted floating free in formalin with those that were stretched and oriented at biopsy and before formalin fixation, and found that the diagnostic rate of cancer increased from 23.6% to 30.8%.

## Future trends in prostate biopsies

Select future trends in prostate biopsy handling and clinical significance are presented in Table 9-20. More precise localization of prostate cancer by site-specific labeling and three-dimensional mapping of extended saturation biopsies may enable the use of focal therapy such as cryosurgery, a controversial approach that is currently under active investigation.[353–355] Future quality assurance measures in urology and urologic pathology should focus on the quantity and quality of biopsy samples. The ultimate goal of all of our efforts in cancer detection – prediction of outcome for the individual patient – will be augmented by advanced methods of database analysis, such as neural networks.[334,356] Further, a solution is needed for dealing with the definition and treatment of insignificant cancer. Finally, molecular biology will probably revolutionize the field of diagnostic pathology in the next decade.

### Fine needle aspiration

Interest in this method in the United States is minimal because of the ease of acquisition and interpretation of the 18-gauge needle core biopsy. Both techniques have similar sensitivity in the diagnosis of prostatic adenocarcinoma, and both are limited by small sample size; they are best considered as complementary techniques. Complications of fine needle aspiration occur in less than 2% of cases and are similar to those of needle core biopsy, including epididymitis, transient hematuria, hemospermia, fever, and sepsis.

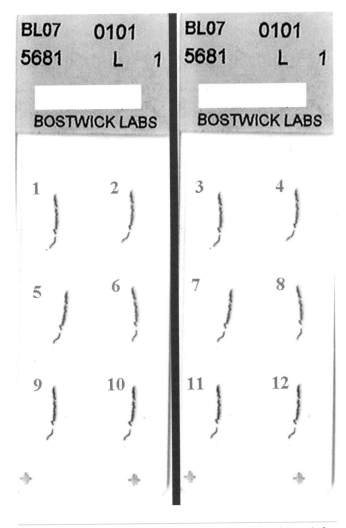

**Fig. 9-19** Bostwick Laboratories' prostate biopsy slide protocol. A total of two slides are obtained, each with six tissue slices. One is stained with H&E and the second is held unstained for subsequent immunostain or – as in this case – a second H&E-stained section. The red numbers indicate the order in which the sections are placed on the slides to ensure optimal comparison of each of the two slides and standardization in every case.

**Table 9-20** Selected future trends in prostate needle biopsy reporting and clinical application

| |
|---|
| Location of prostate cancer |
|    Site-specific labeling |
|    3D mapping |
|    Focal therapy |
| Quality assurance in urology |
|    Quality of biopsies |
|    Number of biopsies |
|    Quality assurance in urologic pathology |
| Personal outcome predictions |
|    Use of neural networks and advanced measures of outcome |
|    Improved understanding of 'clinically insignificant' cancer |
| Molecular diagnostics from needle biopsies |

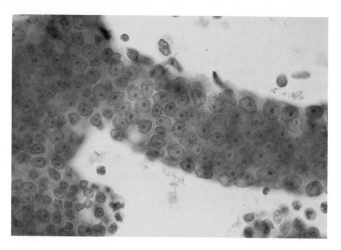

**Fig. 9-20** Moderately differentiated prostatic adenocarcinoma on fine needle aspiration. (Courtesy of Dr John Maksem.)

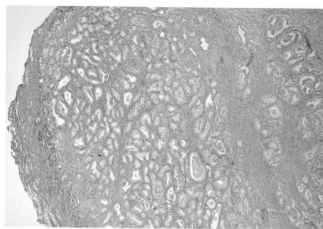

**Fig. 9-21** Gleason grade 1 adenocarcinoma (pseudohyperplastic pattern) in transurethral resection.

Fine needle aspiration produces clusters and small sheets of epithelial cells without stroma.[357] This enrichment for epithelium allows evaluation of single-cell morphology and the relationship between cells. Benign and hyperplastic prostatic epithelium consist of orderly sheets of cells with distinct margins, creating a honeycomb-like pattern. Benign nuclei are uniform with finely granular chromatin and indistinct nucleoli; basal cells are often present at the edge. Prostatic carcinoma is distinguished from benign epithelium by increased cellularity, loss of cell adhesion, variation in nuclear size and shape, and nucleolar enlargement (Fig. 9-20).

### Transurethral resection (TURP)

The regions of the prostate sampled by transurethral resection and needle biopsy tend to be different. Transurethral resection specimens usually consist of tissue from the transition zone, urethra, periurethral area, bladder neck, and anterior fibromuscular stroma. Occasionally, TURP specimens may also contain small portions of seminal vesicle tissue. Studies of radical prostatectomies performed after transurethral resection show that the resection does not usually include tissue from the central or peripheral zones, and not all of the transition zone is removed. Most needle biopsy specimens consist only of tissue from the peripheral zone, and seldom includes the central or transition zones. The role of TURP in dealing with urinary obstructive symptoms has declined in the past decade owing to the introduction of ablative techniques such as the YAG laser, as well as prostate-reducing medications such as 5α-reductase inhibitors (e.g., finasteride, dutasteride).

Well-differentiated adenocarcinoma found incidentally in transurethral resection chips has usually arisen in the transition zone (Fig. 9-21). These tumors are frequently small and may be completely resected transurethrally. Poorly differentiated adenocarcinoma in TURP chips usually represents part of a larger tumor that has invaded the transition zone after arising in the peripheral zone.

The optimal number of chips to submit for histologic evaluation is a minimum of six cassettes for the first 30 g of tissue and one cassette for every 10 g thereafter.[358]

### Prostatic enucleation (suprapubic prostatectomy; adenectomy)

In patients with massive benign hyperplasia, open surgical enucleation may be preferred to transurethral resection. The specimen usually consists exclusively of transition zone tissue and periurethral tissue with grossly visible nodules.

### Radical prostatectomy

There are two main surgical approaches to radical prostatectomy. The first, retropubic prostatectomy, is the most popular approach in the US, allowing staging of lymph node biopsies with frozen section evaluation prior to removal of the prostate. The second approach, perineal prostatectomy, does not allow lymph node biopsy during the same operation because of the anatomic approach employed. Refinements in technique include nerve-sparing prostatectomy, robotic prostatectomy, and laparoscopic prostatectomy.

The completeness of pathologic examination of prostatectomy specimens affects the determination of pathologic stage.[359–369] There was a significant increase in positive surgical margins (12% vs 59%) and pathologic stage with complete sectioning compared to limited sampling (sections of palpable tumor and two random sections of apex and base).[370] Desai and colleagues[371] found that complete sectioning showed higher detection rates of extraprostatic extension (34% vs 55%) and seminal vesicle invasion (8% vs 15%) than with lesser methods of sampling. Complete sectioning also correlated with greater 3-year cancer-free survival in organ-confined and specimen-confined cases. Sehdev and colleagues[362] compared 10 different methods of prostatectomy sampling using complete sectioning as the gold standard, and favored two partial sampling methods that balanced the extra time and expense of additional sections against the risk of missing important predictive information:

- Submit every posterior section plus one mid-anterior section from right and left sides; if either of these anterior sections shows sizeable tumor, all ipsilateral anterior slides are examined. This method detects 98% of tumors with Gleason score ≥7, 100% of positive margins, and 96% of cases with extraprostatic extension (mean 27 slides).

- The above method, but only obtain sections ipsilateral to the previous positive needle biopsy. This method detects 92% of tumors with Gleason score ≥7, 93% of positive margins, and 85% of cases with extraprostatic extension (mean 17 slides).

The presence and extent of extraprostatic extension in clinical stage T2 adenocarcinoma (and hence clinical staging error) is also related to the number of blocks processed. Current guidelines for the evaluation of radical prostatectomy specimens emphasize information that should be included in the pathology report, but leave the decision regarding partial or complete sampling to the pathologist.[334,364,372]

All methods begin with weighing the specimen when fresh and measuring in three dimensions. For ultrasonographic measurements, radiologists often describe the shape of the prostate as a prolate ellipsoid (length × height × width × 0.523), but this is only a rough estimate and shows considerable variability. Separate measurements are made of the attached seminal vesicles.

Subsequent handling can be performed when the specimen is fresh or fixed. The fresh (or fixed) prostate is inked by brief immersion in a small container of India ink, or by painting the surface with different colors of ink to allow unequivocal identification of left and right sides. Subsequently, the wet specimen is briefly immersed in acetone or Bouin's fixative and air dried or blotted dry. Some pathologists use different colors of ink for the anterior and posterior prostate, apex, and base in order to ensure proper orientation.

The apex and base are amputated at a thickness of about 3 mm, and these margins are submitted as 4 mm thick conization slices in the vertical parasagittal plane. Alternatively, some pathologists prefer 1–2 mm thick shave margins. For conization, the apex usually requires quadrant sectioning, and we routinely use abbreviations for the right anterior apex (RAX), left anterior apex (LAX), right posterior apex (RPX), and left posterior apex (LPX). Similarly, the base is

sampled, usually into left and right halves as left bladder base (LBB) and right bladder base (RBB), respectively. The remaining specimen is serially sectioned at 4–5 mm thickness by knife to create transverse sections perpendicular to the long axis of the prostate from its apex to the tip of the seminal vesicles. Partial and complete sampling differ by the amount of prostate tissue submitted after this point.

The Bostwick Laboratories protocols for preparing and reporting radical prostatectomy specimens are shown in Figures 9-22 and 9-23 and Tables 9-21 and 9-22. Complete and careful submission of tissue for histologic evaluation allows the following:

**Table 9-21** Sample surgical pathology report

**Tissue description**
Prostate (5.5 – 3.8 – 3.5 cm) and seminal vesicles (4 – 3.2 – 1 cm) are submitted and weigh 40 and 15 g, respectively. Tumor is identified grossly involving both sides of the prostate extensively, chiefly on the right. Pelvic lymphadenectomy tissue (right, 5.5 – 3 – 1 cm and 3 – 1 – 1 cm; left 4.5 – 2 – 1 cm and 3 – 0.5 – 0.5 cm) submitted separately.

**Diagnosis**
Radical retropubic prostatoseminovesiculectomy–adenocarcinoma (Gleason grade 4 + 3 = 7) Gleason pattern 4 comprises 60% of the cancer. Tertiary pattern 5 comprises 5% of the cancer
Size: about 27.72 mL
Location: bilateral peripheral zone and transition zone
Resection margins: negative
Perineural invasion: extensive
Involvement of capsule: bilateral invasion and extensive multifocal right-sided extraprostatic extension
Premalignant change: patchy high-grade PIN
Pelvic lymph nodes: metastases to 2 of 9 right and 1 of 6 left pelvic lymph nodes
Apex: involvement of the right anterior and posterior and left posterior quadrants without extension to the margin
Bladder base: negative
Seminal vesicles: positive on the right side
Vascular/lymphatic invasion: extensive
Other: nodular hyperplasia focal papillary growth in the peripheral zone cancer
DNA content (flow cytometry): tetraploid (block C8; 60% cancer)
TNN (2002 revision) stage (pathologic): T3bN1Mx ('M' best determined by review of clinical chart)

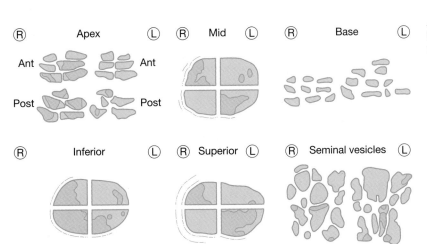

**Fig. 9-22** Partial sampling protocol for preparing and reporting radical prostatectomy specimens.

**Table 9-22** Protocol for processing radical prostatectomies

**Frozen sections of lymph nodes during surgery** This is optional and at the discretion of the treating surgeon. If frozen sections are requested, then all lymph nodes and perinodal adipose tissue is submitted for evaluation. Permanent sections of all frozen tissue should be obtained.

**Radical prostatoseminovesiculectomy** Each prostate is weighed, measured in three dimensions, and inked. Inking is performed by coating with India ink (or another preferred color) and rapid (1–2 s) immersion in acetone to create ink adherence to the tissue.

**Apex and base** Conization or shave margins are acceptable at the discretion of the pathologist; however, each pathologist is encouraged to use only one of these methods for all of their cases. Cancer involving the apex or base is not considered extraprostatic extension even if the margins are positive (exception: when adipose tissue is present and cancer is in contact).

**Conization margins** After fixation, the apex and base are amputated at a thickness of about 4 mm. The apical slice is divided into four quadrants, and each is serially sectioned at 3 mm intervals in the vertical parasagittal plane, similar to a cervical conization specimen, and submitted separately. The section from the bladder base is sectioned in a similar manner, although the amount of tissue was usually less, with divisions as hemispheres rather than quadrants. Cancer touching ink is considered a positive margin. For conization the apex usually requires quadrant sectioning, and we routinely use abbreviations for the right anterior apex (RAX), left anterior apex (LAX), right posterior apex (RPX), and left posterior apex (LPX). Similarly, the base is sampled, usually into left and right halves as left bladder base (LBB) and right bladder base (RBB), respectively. Advantages include greater localization of the cancer and determination of proximity to the margin when the margin is negative.

**Shave margins** A thin translucent shaving of the entire face of the apex and face of the bladder should be taken. Any evidence of cancer in these specimens indicates a positive margin. Advantages include encompassing the entire surface of the apex and base for analysis.

**Seminal vesicles** The seminal vesicles are amputated from the prostate at the junction of the two organs without incising the prostate itself; a slice encompassing each seminal vesicle at this junction should be submitted for routine histologic examination. If cancer is identified in the seminal vesicles or adjacent soft tissues, then the seminal vesicles should be serially sectioned in a manner similar to the prostate and submitted entirely for histologic review.

**Prostate** The prostate is serially sectioned as thinly as possible (about 4–5 mm thick sections) by knife in a coronal plane perpendicular to the long axis of the gland from the apex of the prostate to the site of the amputated seminal vesicles. Orientation and ordering of the slices is maintained throughout to allow spatial reconstruction later of the prostate. The transverse sections are submitted in total for routine processing through neutral buffered formalin (or equivalent alternative fixative) and sectioning as whole mount sections (preferred) or after subdivision into two parts, four parts, or more, depending on the size of each slice. A record should be maintained so that the prostate can be reconstructed at histologic review. Routine sections should be stained with hematoxylin and eosin.

**Protocol for results reporting of radical prostatectomies**

**Volume of prostate** The volume of the prostate is calculated using the formula for a prolate ellipsoid, defined as length × height × width × 0.523 (correction factor for a prolate ellipsoid); no shrinkage correction factor is necessary as these measurements are made in fresh specimens.

**Cancer and ablated tissue volume, location, and extent** On each slide, the exact outlines of carcinoma and ablated tissue are dotted in different-colored inks. The area of extraprostatic extension is measured by an ink line drawn along the prostatic surface, and sites of positive surgical margins are indicated with + sign.

Cancer volume is calculated by the grid method. Briefly, a transparent grid of premeasured squares is placed over the slides, and the number of squares overlying carcinoma is counted; the total number of squares per case is multiplied by the area of each square, and the sum is multiplied by the thickness of each slice of the prostatectomy. Slice thickness is calculated by dividing the fresh tissue measurement of the long axis of the prostate minus 4 mm for conization (accounts for apical section amputation) (2 mm for shave margins) by the total number of slices of the prostate. In order to include the volume of cancer in the apical and basal sections, the number of grids overlying cancer from these sections is multiplied by $0.09 \text{ cm}^2$ and then by 0.5 cm (section thickness). To account for tissue shrinkage due to fixation, final cancer volume is multiplied by 1.25.

The area of extraprostatic extension (EPE) for each case is calculated as the sum of measured line lengths on traced slides multiplied by the section thickness. The volume of tumor in the seminal vesicles is calculated by multiplying the number of grids overlying tumor in the muscular wall of the seminal vesicles by the section thickness. Positive surgical margins are defined as ink touching tumor cells (or foci of ablation); the number of separate foci with positive surgical margins is evaluated. Determinants of pathologic staging include evaluation of seminal vesicle involvement (unilateral or bilateral, as well as volume of tumor), extraprostatic extension (unilateral or bilateral, as well as sites of perforation and area of EPE), and lymph node involvement (unilateral or bilateral, as well as number of nodes involved).

The orientation of the long axis of the tumor is determined, as well as the greatest diameter of the predominant tumor nodule. Tumor location and ablated tissue location is recorded as transition zone and/or non-transition zone, with no attempt to determine precise site of tumor origin due to significant overlap of tumor and multifocality. The number of tumor foci and ablated tissue foci is counted; tumor greater than 2 mm from a tumor nodule is considered a separate focus by convention. Perineural invasion and vascular/lymphatic invasion are considered focal (present in fewer than three separate foci when evaluated by 400–microscopic fields) or extensive (three or more foci involved).

**Cancer grade** The following variables are evaluated: Gleason primary pattern, Gleason secondary pattern, and Gleason score (sum of the primary and secondary patterns). The percentages of Gleason primary pattern 4, primary pattern 5, and the sum of primary patterns 4 and 5 are estimated in 10% increments.

- Unequivocal orientation of specimen and tumor (left, right; transition zone, peripheral zone; anterior, mid, posterior; apex, base, etc.).
- Evaluation of the extent and location of positive surgical margins; assessment and quantification of the extent and location of extraprostatic extension and seminal vesicle invasion.
- Quality control data for the surgeon, particularly with regard to surgical margins in nerve-sparing prostatectomy.
- Postoperative measurement of tumor volume for correlation with imaging studies, as desired.
- Evaluation of tumor grade (percentage of poorly differentiated adenocarcinoma).

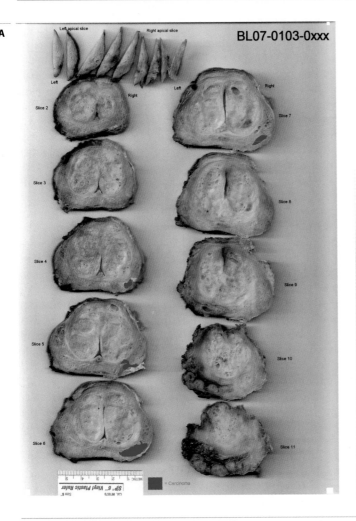
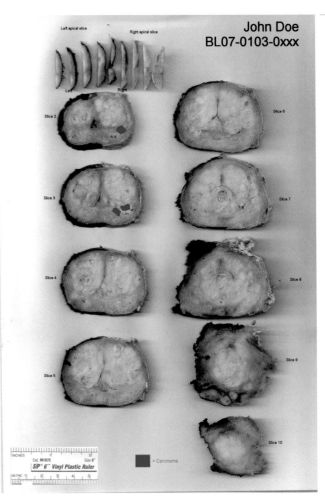

**Fig. 9-23** Sample prostate cancer maps for radical prostatectomy specimens with complete sampling and whole-mount sections. Cancer is marked in red. (**A**) Unilateral, unifocal, organ-confined cancer (pathologic stage T2aN0M0, TNM 2002 classification). (**B**) Unilateral, multifocal (apparently), organ-confined cancer (pathologic stage T2aN0M0).

- Fulfillment of all recommendations by the Cancer Committee of the College of American Pathologists.[367-369]
- Comparison of results with published studies.

Standard protocols are useful because of the frequent multifocality of prostatic adenocarcinoma, the inability to fully identify the location and extent of tumor by examining randomly chosen tissue slices, and the inability to grossly identify positive surgical margins and capsular perforation. Despite our personal preference for complete submission, most pathologists undertake partial submission, and this is practical for most cases, does not require special processing, and provides all necessary clinical information.

### Gross pathology

Gross identification of prostatic adenocarcinoma is often difficult or impossible, and definitive diagnosis requires microscopic examination. In transurethral resection specimens adenocarcinoma is rarely grossly identified unless extensive, owing to the confounding macroscopic features of nodular hyperplasia. In prostatectomies, adenocarcinoma tends to be multifocal, with a predilection for the peripheral zone. Grossly apparent tumor foci are at least 5 mm in greatest dimension and may appear yellow-white with a firm consistency, owing to stromal desmoplasia (Fig. 9-24). Some tumors appear as yellow granular masses, which contrast sharply with the normal spongy prostatic parenchyma. Mucinous (colloid) carcinoma may have a variegated appearance and are often softer than the adjacent prostate. Similar gross findings may be caused by tuberculosis, granulomatous prostatitis, and acute and chronic prostatitis.

### Microscopic pathology

Microscopically, most prostatic adenocarcinomas are composed of small acini arranged in one or more patterns. Diagnosis relies on a combination of architectural and cytologic findings and may be aided by ancillary studies such as immunohistochemistry.

Architectural features are assessed at low- to medium-power magnification, with variations in the size, shape, and

C

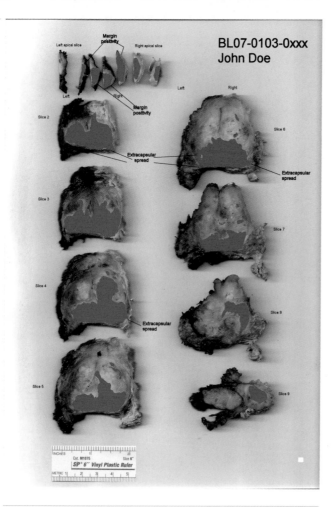

**Fig. 9-23, Cont'd** (**C**) Bilateral, multifocal cancer with multifocal bilateral extraprostatic extension, seminal vesicle invasion, and multiple positive apical surgical margins (pathologic stage T3bN0M0) (Courtesy of Dr Michael Jarmulowicz, Bostwick Laboratories.)

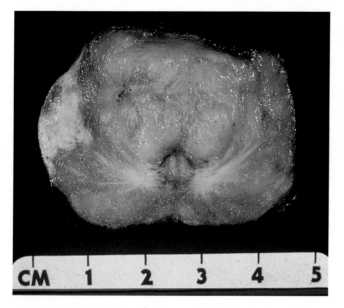

**Fig. 9-24** Gross appearance of prostatic adenocarcinoma. A large, firm, yellow tumor mass is grossly visible on one side, but microscopic foci were present throughout the peripheral zone bilaterally. The yellow color is due to abundant cytoplasmic lipid in tumor cells, which was confirmed histochemically.

spacing of acini (Fig. 9-25). The acini in suspicious foci are usually small or medium sized, with irregular or elongated contours that stand in contrast with the smooth contours of normal prostatic acini. Variable acinar size is of value, particularly when there are small irregular abortive acini with primitive lumina at the periphery. Comparison with adjacent benign prostatic acini is always of value. The arrangement of the acini is diagnostically useful: malignant acini often have an irregular haphazard arrangement, sometimes splitting or distorting muscle fibers in the stroma, with variable spacing between acini. The stroma frequently contains young collagen that appears lightly eosinophilic, and desmoplasia may be prominent, although this is an uncommon and potentially unreliable feature when assessed in isolation. An understanding of the Gleason grading system is valuable in the interpretation of small foci because of its reliance on architectural patterns (see below). Gleason taught that prostate cancer could usually be identified by its pattern at low to intermediate (scanning) magnification, and that high-power magnification (e.g. typical 40× or 60× objectives) were best employed to confirm the diagnosis and avoid misdiagnosis of mimics by the identification of telltale cytologic and luminal features (Bostwick, personal communication).

Cytologic features of adenocarcinoma include nuclear and nucleolar enlargement, and these features are important for the diagnosis of malignancy (Fig. 9-26). Enlarged nuclei are typically present in the majority of adenocarcinoma cells, and enlarged nucleoli are present in many. Every cell has a nucleolus, so one searches for 'prominent' nucleoli, which are at least 1.25–1.50 μm in diameter or larger; of greatest importance is the ratio of nucleolus to nucleus and comparison with adjacent benign acini. The identification of two or more nucleoli is virtually diagnostic of malignancy (or PIN), particularly when the nucleoli are eccentrically located in the nucleus abutting the chromatinic rim. Over-staining of nuclei and other artifacts may obscure the nucleoli, creating diagnostic difficulty.

The basal cell layer is absent in adenocarcinoma, an important feature that may be difficult to evaluate in sections stained with hematoxylin and eosin. Compressed stromal fibroblasts may mimic basal cells but are usually only seen focally at the periphery of acini. An intact basal cell layer is present at the periphery of benign acini, whereas carcinoma entirely lacks a basal cell layer. Sometimes, small foci of adenocarcinoma cluster around larger acini that have intact basal cell layers, compounding the difficulty. In difficult cases it may be useful to employ monoclonal antibodies directed against high molecular weight cytokeratin (e.g., clone 34βE12) and p63 to evaluate the basal cell layer.

## Cancer-associated pathologic findings

### Luminal mucin

Acidic sulfated and non-sulfated mucin is often seen in the acini of adenocarcinoma, appearing in routine sections as amorphous or delicate thread-like basophilic secretions (Fig. 9-27).[373–376] This mucin stains with Alcian blue and is best demonstrated at pH 2.5, whereas normal prostatic epithe-

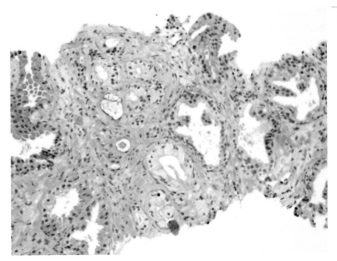

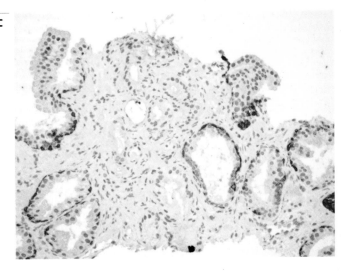

**Fig. 9-25** Minimum criteria for the diagnosis of cancer on needle biopsy. (**A**) Microscopic focus contains acini with variation in size, shape, and spacing. Triple immunostain (not shown) revealed racemase staining as well as absence of p63 and keratin 34βE12 staining. (**B**) Irregular loose cluster of small to intermediate acini, including a few with foamy cytoplasm (bottom) that stands in contrast to the adjacent benign acini. This was diagnosed as 'foamy gland PIN' at another medical center without obtaining immunostains. Compare with **C** (triple immunostain), in which there is absence of racemase staining as well as p63 and keratin 34βE12, with intense immunoreactivity for adjacent benign acini (internal positive control). This immunoprofile effectively excludes PIN from consideration, and, in combination with the architectural abnormalities, is diagnostic of adenocarcinoma (Gleason 3 + 3 = 6) with focal foamy gland pattern.

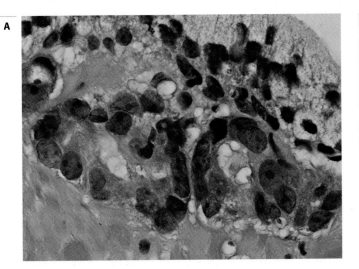

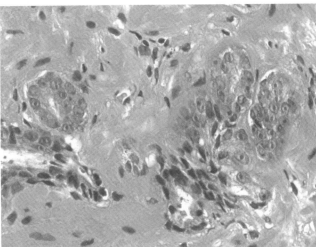

**Fig. 9-26** (**A, B**) Nuclear and nucleolar enlargement in prostate cancer. The focus of adenocarcinoma (left) displays marked nuclear and nucleolar enlargement when compared with adjacent benign epithelium (right).

lium contains periodic acid–Schiff-reactive neutral mucin. Acidic mucin is not specific for carcinoma, and may be found in PIN and rarely in BPH.[377] The predominant acidic mucin is sialomucin, and O-acetylation expression of these mucins is inversely correlated with cancer grade.[378] Expression of episialin, also known as MUC1, may or may not correlate with Gleason grade and microvessel density.[379,380]

### Luminal proteinaceous secretions

Ill-formed secretions are more often found in the lumen of suspicious and cancerous acini than in benign acini, and vary from lightly pink and scant to brightly eosinophilic and extensive (Fig. 9-27).[317] Although a non-specific finding, the abundance of luminal secretions in prostate cancer is often distinctive and should spur the search for other cytologic features of malignancy. Proteinaceous secretions are often found in association with crystalloids and corpora amylacea.

### Crystalloids

Crystalloids are sharp rhomboid or needle-like eosinophilic structures that are often present in the lumen of well- and moderately differentiated carcinoma (Fig. 9-27).[110,311,381,287] They are not specific for carcinoma, and can be found in other conditions such as atypical adenomatous hyperplasia.[382] The presence of crystalloids in metastatic adenocarcinoma of unknown site of origin is strong presumptive evidence of prostatic origin, although it is an uncommon finding.[383,384]

The pathogenesis of crystalloids is uncertain, but they probably result from abnormal protein and mineral metabolism within benign and malignant acini, including loss of acidity.[385] Ultrastructurally, they are composed of electron-dense material that lacks the periodicity of crystals, and X-ray microanalysis reveals abundant sulfur, calcium, and phosphorus, and a small amount of sodium.[311] In many cases seminal vesicles also contain inspissated secretions, including 24% of cases with predominantly crystalloid morphology.[385]

### Collagenous micronodules

Collagenous micronodules are a specific but infrequent and incidental finding in prostatic adenocarcinoma, consisting of microscopic nodular masses of paucicellular eosinophilic

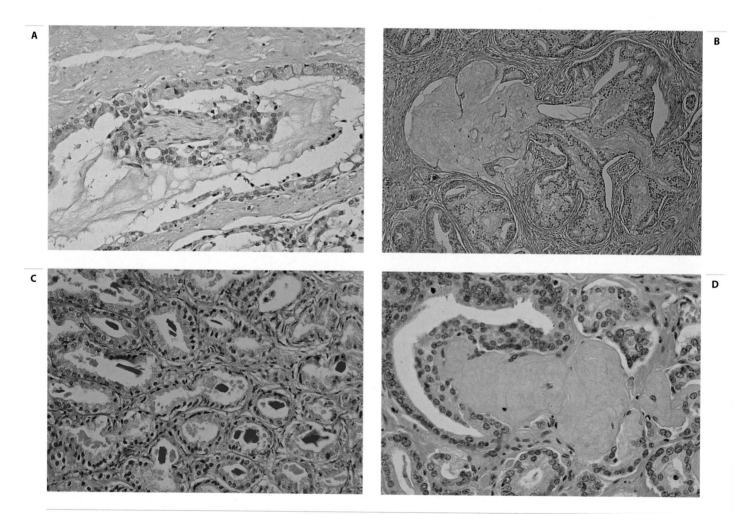

**Fig. 9-27** Ancillary histologic features of prostate cancer. (**A**) Perineural invasion. (**B**) Mucin production. (**C**) Crystalloids. (**D**) Collagenous micronodules.

fibrillar stroma that impinge on acinar lumina (Fig. 9-27).[386] They are usually present in mucin-producing adenocarcinoma, and result from extravasation of acidic mucin into the stroma. Collagenous micronodules are present in 2–13% of cases of adenocarcinoma, and are not observed in benign epithelium, nodular hyperplasia, or PIN.[387] They are an infrequent finding, present in 0.6% of needle biopsies and 12.7% of prostatectomies.[386,387] They are composed predominantly of collagen fragments admixed with basement membrane material.[388]

Ultrastructurally, they consist of fragmented banded collagen fibrils surrounded by the basement membrane material. Collagenous micronodules are formed by subepithelial accumulations of fragmented collagen fibers, possibly related to the digestion by collagenase produced by prostatic adenocarcinoma cells. The term mucinous fibroplasia has been erroneously applied by some to collagenous micronodules, but these micronodules are often not associated with mucin, so this term should be abandoned.

## Perineural invasion

Perineural invasion is the major mechanism of cancer spread outside the prostate, and is present in 17%,[389] 20%,[387] and 38%[390] of biopsies; in some cases it is the only evidence of malignancy (Fig. 9-28). This finding is strong presumptive evidence of cancer, but is not pathognomonic because it occurs rarely with benign acini. Complete circumferential growth, intraneural invasion, and ganglionic invasion are almost always limited to cancer. However, benign acini can rarely mimic cancer with perineural indentation, tracking, wrapping, or even intraneural spread, so caution is warranted in relying on this feature to the exclusion of all others.[391] Perineural invasion usually indicates tumor spread along the path of least resistance, and does not represent lymphatic invasion. Perineural cancer cells acquire a survival and growth advantage using the NFκB survival pathway, and targeting perineural invasion might retard local cancer spread and possibly influence survival.[392] Neural cell adhesion molecular (N-CAM) is upregulated in nerves with perineural invasion.[393]

Routine light microscopy is usually sufficient to identify prostatic nerves.[394] However, in difficult or equivocal cases immunohistochemistry for epithelial membrane antigen (EMA) and S100 protein may be of value in separating perineural invasion from perineural indentation.[395] Normal peripheral nerves are continuously encircled by perineurium which is immunoreactive for EMA. Three patterns of EMA immunoreactivity with perineural invasion were observed in a large series of radical prostatectomies: discontinuity or complete loss of the perineurium (55% of cancers), acini in the perineural space or peripheral nerves (25%) and no changes in the perineurium (20%). In one study, no acini were observed in the perineural space with benign acini.[395]

Half of patients with perineural invasion on biopsy have extraprostatic extension, but perineural invasion has no independent predictive value for stage after consideration of Gleason grade, serum PSA, amount of cancer on biopsy,[390,396,397] or positive surgical margins.[398] Only 24% of experienced

academic urologists use perineural invasion status to guide nerve-sparing surgery.[399]

Perineural invasion was a significant independent adverse predictive factor for patients treated by external beam radiation therapy. However, it was only of value in patients with pretreatment serum PSA < 20 ng/mL, suggesting that the poor prognosis associated with elevated PSA overrides any additional information that perineural invasion may provide.[400,401,402] Perineural invasion was not a significant predictor of biochemical recurrence in patients undergoing brachytherapy for prostate cancer.[389,403] Perineural invasion was predictive of recurrence-free survival after radical prostatectomy in univariate analysis,[404–407] but usually not in multivariate analysis.[408–412] The predictive value of perineural invasion has been recently reviewed.[413]

The diameter of perineural invasion may be an independent predictor of cancer volume[414] and recurrence.[415] It was not predictive of outcome after brachytherapy.[416]

## Vascular and lymphatic invasion

Vascular invasion is present in 38% of radical prostatectomy specimens with cancer, and is commonly associated with extraprostatic extension and lymph node metastases (62% and 67% of cases, respectively; Fig. 9-29).[417] Its presence also correlates with histologic grade[417] and stage.[418] Microvascular invasion appears to be an important predictor of outcome after radical prostatectomy, and carries a fourfold greater risk of tumor progression[419–422] and death.[417,423] However, it may not be an independent predictor of progression when stage and grade are included in the analysis after surgery[417,424] or radiation therapy.[425] Microvascular invasion of the seminal vesicles is also predictive of tumor progression and lymph node metastases.[426]

Lymphovascular invasion is an independent predictor of PSA recurrence and cancer-specific survival after radical prostatectomy.[427–429] Use of antibodies specific for lymphatic endothelial cells (clone D2–40, directed against podoplanin) revealed that intratumoral lymphatic vessel density was significantly lower than that of the peritumoral and normal prostate compartments, and the latter two were not significantly different; peritumoral lymphatic vessel invasion had a better correlation with the presence of lymph node metastases than intratumoral lymphatic vessel invasion.[430] There was no evidence of lymphangiogenesis. The lack of coexpression of podoplanin and VEGF receptor-3 in some lymphatic vessels suggested that there is a heterogeneous population of lymphatic endothelial cells in the prostate.[428]

## Increased microvessel density (angiogenesis)

There is a significant increase in microvessel density in PIN[196] and carcinoma compared to normal prostatic tissue[431–436] or atypical adenomatous hyperplasia (Fig. 9-30).[437] This increase correlates with the expression of angiogenic factors VEGF, bFGF, and the receptors FLK/KDR and Flt-1.[438] Increased microvessel density is probably related to the production of proangiogenic growth factors.[439–441] Transition zone cancer has significantly lower microvessel density than peripheral zone cancer.[442]

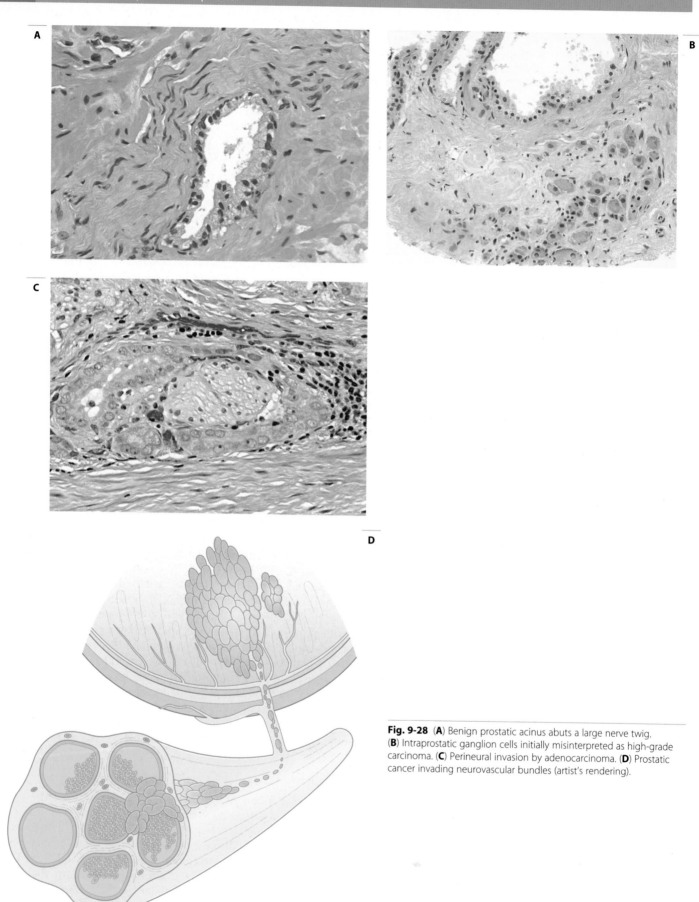

**Fig. 9-28** (**A**) Benign prostatic acinus abuts a large nerve twig. (**B**) Intraprostatic ganglion cells initially misinterpreted as high-grade carcinoma. (**C**) Perineural invasion by adenocarcinoma. (**D**) Prostatic cancer invading neurovascular bundles (artist's rendering).

Mean blood vessel count is higher in tumors with metastases than in those without,[443,444] and most[432–445] but not all[446] studies demonstrate a correlation with pathologic stage. Microvessel density appears to be an independent predictor of cancer progression,[420,421,446–450] but this has been refuted.[417,451] The cumulative data suggest that increased microvessel density contributes to the extraprostatic spread of adenocarcinoma, perhaps by facilitating microvascular invasion, and also promotes the survival of distant metastases because tumor cells can shift angiogenic balance within the distant target. Recent studies found that CD105, Tie-2/Tek and vascular endothelial growth factor receptors were the best markers of neoangiogenesis.[452]

Glomeruloid microvascular proliferation in prostate cancer correlated with microvessel density, aggressive tumor behavior, and reduced survival in multivariate analysis.[453]

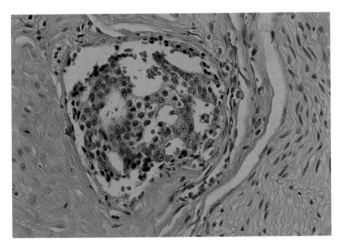

**Fig. 9-29** Microvascular invasion. Note red blood cells at the periphery of the lumen.

## Significant problems in biopsy interpretation and handling

### Atypical small acinar proliferation (ASAP)

In some needle biopsies a proliferation of small acini is found that is highly suggestive of carcinoma but which falls below the diagnostic threshold for adenocarcinoma (Tables 9-21-9-23; see also Chapter 8). This is often caused by the small size of the focus, distorted acini with architectural features of malignancy that lack convincing cytologic features, and acinar atrophy or prominent inflammation in which the adjacent benign acini show distortion and reactive atypia with nuclear and nucleolar enlargement. It may be appropriate to describe such cases as 'small acinar proliferation suspicious for but not diagnostic of malignancy' and to suggest rebiopsy. Such lesions are found in up to 3% of needle biopsy specimens. In view of the serious consequences of the diagnosis of adenocarcinoma, it is prudent to diagnose adenocarcinoma only when one has absolute

**Table 9-23** Differential diagnosis of prostatic adenocarcinoma

| Atrophy |
| --- |
| Postatrophic hyperplasia |
| Basal cell hyperplasia |
| Aypical adenomatous hyperplasia (AAH) |
| Sclerosing adenosis |
| Nephrogenic metaplasia |
| Verumontanum mucosal gland hyperplasia |
| Hyperplasia of mesonephric remnants |
| High-grade PIN |

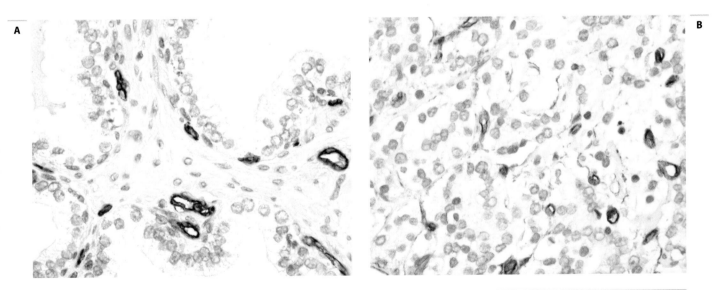

**Fig. 9-30** Microvessel density in benign prostate (**A**) and high-grade adenocarcinoma (**B**). Brown reaction product decorates the delicate vasculature (CD34 immunostain).

confidence in the histologic findings. A wide variety of small acinar proliferations may mimic adenocarcinoma, particularly in small specimens.

## PIN versus large acinar variant of Gleason grade 3 carcinoma

Prostatic intraepithelial neoplasia encompasses the spectrum of dysplastic cytologic abnormalities within preexisting structures in the prostate that are invested with an intact basal cell layer (see above). In contrast, the large acinar variant of Gleason grade 3 carcinoma, including the cribriform variant of ductal carcinoma, does not have a circumferential basal cell layer and is almost always associated with areas of small acinar adenocarcinoma. In equivocal cases diagnosis may be aided by staining with basal cell-specific antibodies to high molecular weight keratin 34βE12.

## Clear cell pattern of carcinoma versus benign acini

Numerous forms of adenocarcinoma contain clear cytoplasm (Fig. 9-31). Adenocarcinoma arising in the transition zone characteristically contains clear cells and is well or moderately differentiated. In contrast, Gleason grades 3 and 4 carcinoma often contain cells with clear cytoplasm, previously referred to as the hypernephroid pattern. In addition, therapy such as androgen deprivation induces abundant clear cell change in benign and carcinomatous acini, and the diagnosis of adenocarcinoma in such cases may be difficult (see discussion later in this chapter). The clear cell pattern of carcinoma may be confused with histiocytes, vacuolated stromal smooth muscle cells, and metaplastic cells.

## 'Vanishing' prostate cancer in radical prostatectomies

Radical prostatectomies have no residual cancer (stage pT0) in up to 0.5% of cases (1 in 200 prostatectomies), and this incidence may be increasing owing to an increase in the number of patients receiving preoperative androgen deprivation therapy (or radiation therapy) that causes an apparent reduction in cancer volume in some cases, and increasing vigilance in screening demonstrates that prostate cancer is now being detected at smaller volumes and lower stages than ever before.[329,454-459] It is highly unlikely that biopsy alone can completely ablate a focus of prostate cancer, although this possibility has been considered.[459] Variance in the handling of radical prostatectomy specimens, including partial submission, may increase the risk of the 'vanishing cancer' phenomenon. When this issue arises, it is recommended that all remaining tissue be submitted for histologic analysis to minimize the concern for incomplete sampling.

Genotypic analysis to verify patient identity in cases of 'vanishing' cancer is becoming increasingly popular and appears prudent to reassure patients.[329,458] The inability to identify residual cancer in radical prostatectomy specimens raises the question of the accuracy of the original diagnosis of cancer. In one report, biopsies were overdiagnosed as cancer in two of four cases with no residual cancer after radical prostatectomy.[329]

In a series of 38 patients with pT0 cancer, we found that none developed clinical evidence of cancer recurrence with a mean follow-up of almost 10 years.[454] Further, those who died of other causes had no evidence of prostate cancer at the time of death. These cumulative data strongly suggest that these patients are cured of cancer and no residual therapy is indicated.

## Grading

Histologic grade is a strong prognostic factor in prostatic adenocarcinoma. Numerous grading systems have been proposed since the pioneering work of Broders more than 80 years ago, and all successfully identify well-differentiated adenocarcinoma, which progresses slowly, and poorly differentiated adenocarcinoma, which progresses rapidly. However, grading systems are less successful in subdividing the majority of moderately differentiated adenocarcinomas which have intermediate clinical and biologic potential. Since 1999, Gleason is the recognized international standard for prostate cancer grading, and in our experience is now employed routinely by most pathologists around the world.[5,372,460]

Problems with grading include inter- and intraobserver variability and imprecise predictive value. In biopsies, these problems are compounded by small sample size, tumor heterogeneity,[461] and undergrading of biopsy samples.[462] Also, significant histologic changes in adenocarcinoma occur as a result of radiation and androgen deprivation therapy. The sections that follow describe the current role of grading in prostatic adenocarcinoma, including possible improvements in grading, correlation of biopsy grade with prostatectomy grade, the influence of treatment on adenocarcinoma grade, and correlation of grade with anatomic and biochemical markers of progression.

### Gleason grading system

The Gleason grading system resulted from the Veterans' Administration Cooperative Urological Research Group study of more than 4000 patients between 1960 and 1975.[463,464] It is based on the degree of architectural differentiation (Table 9-24; Fig. 9-32). Tumor heterogeneity is accounted for by assigning a primary pattern for the dominant grade and a secondary pattern for the non-dominant grade; the histologic score is derived by adding these two patterns together. Early studies described the addition of the clinical stage (1–4 scale) to create the Gleason 'sum,' but this did not achieve widespread use and was abandoned decades ago. Nuclear grade was also originally considered for inclusion by Gleason, but added little or no incremental predictive accuracy for patient outcome beyond the architectural patterns, and was discarded to avoid complexity (Bostwick, personal communication).

The success of the Gleason grading system is due to four factors:

- Histologic patterns are identified by the degree of acinar differentiation without relying on morphogenetic or histogenetic models.
- A simplified and standardized drawing is available.

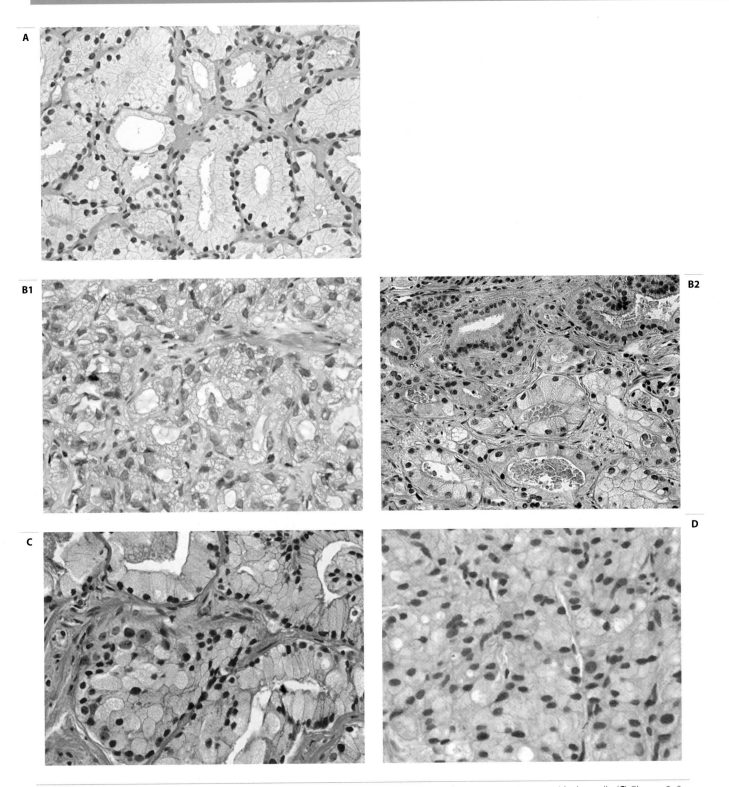

**Fig. 9-31** Clear cell patterns of adenocarcinoma. (**A**) Gleason 2 + 2 = 4 cancer with clear cells. (**B**) Gleason 3 + 3 = 6 cancer with clear cells. (**C**) Gleason 3+3 = 6 with foamy gland pattern. (**D**) 'Hypernephroid' (clear cell) pattern of Gleason 4 + 4 = 8 cancer.

**Table 9-24** Gleason grading system for prostatic adenocarcinoma: histologic patterns

| Pattern | Peripheral borders | Stromal invasion | Appearance of glands | Size of glands | Architecture of glands | Cytoplasm |
|---|---|---|---|---|---|---|
| 1 | Circumscribed pushing, expansible | Minimal | Simple, round, monotonously replicated | Medium, regular | Closely packed rounded masses | Similar to benign epithelium |
| 2 | Less circumscribed; early infiltration | Mild with, definite separation of glands by stroma | Simple, round, some variability in shape | Medium, less regular | Loosely packed rounded masses | Similar to benign epithelium |
| 3A | Infiltration | Marked | Angular, with variation in shape | Medium to large | Variable packed irregular masses | More basophilic than patterns 1 and 2 |
| 3B | Infiltration | Marked | Angular, with variation in shape | Small | Variable packed irregular masses | More basophilic than patterns 1 and 2 |
| 3C | Smooth, rounded | Marked | Papillary and cribriform | Irregular | Round to elongate masses | More basophilic than patterns 1 and 2 |
| 4A | Ragged infiltration | Marked | Microacinar papillary, and cribriform | Irregular | Fused, with chains and cords | Dark |
| 4B | Ragged infiltration | Marked | Microacinar, papillary and cribriform | Irregular | Fused, with chains and cords | Clear (hypernephroid) |
| 5A | Smooth, rounded | Marked | Comedocarcinoma | Irregular | Round to elongate masses | Variable |
| 5B | Ragged infiltration | Marked | Difficulty to identify gland lumina | Irregular | Fused sheets | Variable |

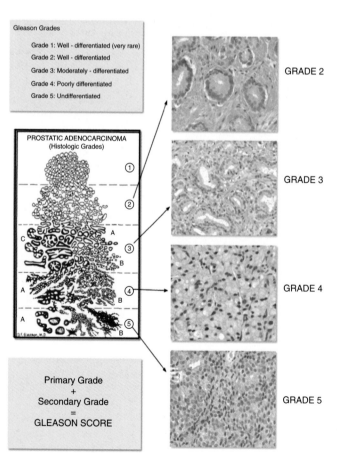

**Gleason Grades**

Grade 1: Well - differentiated (very rare)
Grade 2: Well - differentiated
Grade 3: Moderately - differentiated
Grade 4: Poorly differentiated
Grade 5: Undifferentiated

PROSTATIC ADENOCARCINOMA
(Histologic Grades)

GRADE 2

GRADE 3

GRADE 4

GRADE 5

Primary Grade
+
Secondary Grade
=
GLEASON SCORE

**Fig. 9-32** Gleason grading of prostatic adenocarcinoma.

- The Veterans' Administration study provided abundant prospective information that allowed objective computer-generated development of this self-defining grading system.
- Unlike any other grading system in the body, the Gleason system provided for tumor heterogeneity by identifying primary and secondary patterns.

The Gleason score is a scalar measurement that combines discrete primary and secondary groups into a total of nine discrete groups (scores 2–10). Bibbo et al.[465,466] noted that optimal grading creates a continuum that incorporates the findings of a variety of diagnostic clues, including acinar formation, luminal area, acinar fusion, type of acinar fusion, acinar packing, acinar size, acinar uniformity, thickness of acinar epithelial layer, nuclear size, nuclear variability, nuclear shape, chromatin pattern, and nucleolar size. Using these architectural and nuclear features, Bibbo et al.[466] developed and tested a bayesian belief network for grading prostatic adenocarcinoma and attained agreement with Gleason grading in 241 of 256 microscopic fields.

Common misinterpretations in Gleason grading are presented in Table 9-25.

### Recent trends in grading

Since the introduction of PSA testing, the incidence of low-grade prostate cancer has declined.[467] Interpretive and chronological biases caused expansion of the moderately differentiated category at the expense of well-differentiated cancer and significant deviation in cancer-specific survival curves.[468,469] One report found that Gleason score re-readings

**Table 9-25** Four common misinterpretations in prostate cancer grading

| Misinterpretation | Comment |
|---|---|
| 1. If a biopsied focus of cancer is small, it is Gleason grade 1 or 2, or 'well differentiated' | Unlikely! Most cancers (over 80% in Gleason's original series) are primary grade 3. When the size is too small to call cancer, *suspicious* is the prudent default. Size of the focus of cancer has no bearing on Gleason grade at prostatectomy |
| 2. If a biopsied focus is suspicious for cancer, it is best called Gleason grade 1 or 2, or 'well differentiated' | The prudent diagnosis in the absence of sufficient features for cancer is atypical small acinar proliferation (ASAP). Optimism seems naturally to lead one to consider low Gleason grade; but if there is cancer, it is usually moderately differentiated, since most peripheral zone cancers are moderately differentiated |
| 3. Confusing the large gland variant of Gleason grade 3 cancer with benign acini | Cancer acini occasionally are rounded, and medium to large, like benign acini. Look for microvacuolated cytoplasm, nuclear enlargement, and macronucleoli to diagnose cancer |
| 4. All cribriform acinar formations are Gleason grade 3 | Some cribriform acinar formations are grade 4. These sieve-like spaces lose their round, rigid, punched-out contours, and elongate; the acini collapse into solid areas |

in 2000–2002 were higher than the original readings from 1990–1992 (mean score increased from 5.95 to 6.8).[470] Consequently, the Gleason score-standardized contemporary mortality rate (1.50 deaths per 100 person-years) appeared to be 28% lower than standardized historical rates (2.08 deaths per 100 person-years), even though the overall outcome was unchanged. This decline in the reported incidence of low-grade prostate cancer appeared to be the result of Gleason score reclassification over the past decade, reflecting a statistical artifact known as the Will Rogers phenomenon.[470] Ghani et al.[471] noted that all Gleason 2–4 reports were upgraded to Gleason 5–7 cancer.

## Reproducibility of Gleason grading

Inter- and intraobserver variability has been studied with the Gleason grading system and others. The subjective nature of grading precludes absolute precision, no matter how carefully the system is defined, but significant correlation with virtually every outcome measure attests to the predictive strength and utility of grading in the hands of most investigators.

Intraobserver agreement was exact in up to 78% of cases and +1 score unit in up to 87%.[464,472–478] Melia and eight British uropathology colleagues found a rate of intraobserver

agreement of 77%.[479] Gleason himself noted exact reproducibility of score in 50% of needle biopsies and ± 1 score in 85%.[464]

Interobserver agreement was exact in up to 81% of cases and +1 score unit in up to 86%.[472,473,475,477,478,480–492] Some investigators have expressed concerns with Gleason grading because of the significant incidence of interobserver variability. One study reported a high level of disagreement among three pathologists evaluating 41 cases of well- to moderately differentiated adenocarcinoma.[483] Another report compared the level of interobserver agreement in a consecutive series of 100 prostatic adenocarcinomas and found complete agreement of Gleason score in only 66% of cases.[482] To perform the analysis, the authors compressed the Gleason scores into three grade groups: 2–5, 6–7 and 8–10. Coard and Freeman[493] demonstrated a 60% overall concordance in consensus Gleason scores, which increased to 80% when considered as < 7 versus 7 or more. The greatest discordance seemed to be in distinguishing Gleason score 6 from 7, and was more frequent among biopsy specimens with low cancer volume, particularly among those with less than 30% involvement.

Allsbrook[487] led a group of 10 urologic pathologists who studied 46 needle biopsies and found a κ coefficient ranging from 0.56 to 0.70 (substantial agreement) for Gleason score. The eight 'non-consensus' cases included low-grade cancer, cancer with small cribriform proliferation, and cancer whose histology was on the border between Gleason patterns. When Allsbrook shared the 38 consensus cases with a group of 41 general pathologists, the κ coefficient was 0.44 (moderate agreement), with consistent undergrading of Gleason scores 5–6 (47%), 7 (47%) and, to a lesser extent, 8–10 (25%).[488]

Interobserver reproducibility of percentage grades 4 and 5 was at least as good as that of Gleason score.[494,495] Grading was most difficult when cancer was present in multiple biopsies or contained cribriform or fused patterns.

Reproducibility of the modified Gleason score (primary grade + highest grade) (see below) was as high as that of Gleason score, but there was clustering in odd scores and severe disagreement was more commonly observed than with classic Gleason score.[496] The authors concluded that tertiary Gleason pattern needed to be better defined.

## Concordance of biopsy and prostatectomy grade

There is a significant discordance between biopsy and matched prostatectomy grades. Needle core biopsy underestimates tumor grade in 33–45% of cases and overestimates in 4–32% (Table 9-26).[497–499] Grading errors are common in biopsies with small amounts of tumor and low-grade tumor,[500] probably due to tissue sampling error, tumor heterogeneity, and undergrading of needle biopsies; however, this has been refuted.[498] Men with 'high-risk' cancer (higher PSA concentration or more positive cores) were more likely to have cancer upgraded at prostatectomy, and obtaining more biopsy cores reduced the likelihood of upgrading.[501–505] Biopsy grading error did not correlate with amount of adenocarcinoma on the biopsy[506] or with clinical staging error. In one study the accuracy of biopsy was highest for

**Table 9-26** Concordance of needle biopsy and radical prostatectomy Gleason scores: selected reports

| Authors | No. of patients | Setting | No. pathologists involved in grading | % Exact Gleason correlation | % ± 1 Gleason unit | % > 1 Gleason unit |
|---|---|---|---|---|---|---|
| Bostwick[1269] | 316 | Academic | 1 | 35 | 39 | 26 |
| Spires et al.[1270] | 67 | Academic | Multiple | 58 | 36 | 6 |
| Kojima et al.[1271] | 135 | Academic | 1 | 48 | 43 | 9 |
| Thickman et al.[1272] | 124 | Community | Multiple | 28 | 24 | 38 |
| Cookson et al.[1273] | 226 | Academic | Multiple | 31 | 43 | 26 |
| Steinberg et al.[485] | 499 | Community | Multiple | 34 | 32 | Not available |
| Sved et al.[1274] | 531 with Gleason score 6 | Academic | Multiple | 51 | | |
| Hiseh et al.[1275] | 52 | Community | Multiple | 31 | | |
| King et al.[498] | 371 | Academic | Multiple | 43 | | |
| Tomioka et al.[497] | 223 | Community | Multiple | 37 | 70 | 30 |
| Means | | | | | | |

the primary Gleason pattern, but the secondary pattern on biopsy appeared to be sufficiently accurate in predicting prostatectomy grade to provide useful predictive information, particularly when combined with primary pattern to create the Gleason score (Figs 9-32-9-34).[507] Based on these results, Gleason grading is recommended for all needle biopsies, even those with small amounts of tumor, similar to the original recommendation of Gleason.[462]

Kramer et al.[508] compared the Gleason score in 14-gauge needle biopsies with matched lymph node metastases and found exact correlation in 17 of 42 cases (40%), ±1 in 32 of 42 cases (76%), and ±2 in 40 of 42 cases (95%). The lack of a more anaplastic pattern in the metastatic deposits implied that factors other than loss of differentiation were responsible for the cells' ability to metastasize.

Among patients with Gleason score 8 carcinoma, 45% had a lower Gleason score in the radical prostatectomy specimen and a correspondingly more favorable long-term outcome.[509] Predictors of downgrading were lower clinical stage (T1c) and Gleason score 8 in the biopsy specimen. In another report, clinical stage, serum PSA, and biopsy Gleason score had a predictive accuracy of 0.80 for Gleason sum upgrading between biopsy and prostatectomy.[510,511]

The distribution of cancer grades was not associated with prostate volume.[512] The concordance rate between needle biopsy and radical prostatectomy of the Gleason scores of the greatest tumor percentage in the core, Gleason score of core with maximal tumor length, and the highest Gleason score was 64%, 62%, and 57%, respectively.[513]

Ross and colleagues showed that DNA ploidy analysis of biopsies predicted grade shifting, that it was a more sensitive and specific indicator of final grade at radical prostatectomy than the original needle biopsy grade, and that ploidy status independently predicted postoperative cancer recurrence.[514]

### Proposed modifications to Gleason grading

Numerous modifications have been proposed for Gleason grading to improve its discriminatory capabilities, including the addition of tertiary grading, nuclear grading and mor-

**Table 9-27** Proposed modifications of Gleason grading

| |
|---|
| Grading of tertiary pattern |
| Nuclear grading and morphometric grading |
| Grade compression |
| Amount of high-grade adenocarcinoma (Gleason patterns 4 and 5) |
| Subdivision of Gleason 7 (3 + 4 vs. 4 + 3) |

phometric grading, grade compression, measuring the amount of high-grade adenocarcinoma, and subdividing Gleason score 7 (3 + 4 vs 4 + 3) (Table 9-27).[515,516]

*Tertiary grade* Prostate cancer is heterogeneous for grade. In up to 5% of biopsies three (and very rarely four) separate Gleason grades are encountered. Gleason noted that more than 50% of adenocarcinomas in his series contained two or more patterns.[463,464] Similarly, Aihara et al.[517] found a mean of 2.7 different Gleason grades per case (range, 1–5) in a series of 101 totally embedded prostatectomies, and more than 50% of adenocarcinomas contained at least three different grades. The number of grades increased with greater cancer volume, and the most common finding was high-grade adenocarcinoma within a larger, well- or moderately differentiated adenocarcinoma (53% of cases). Tertiary Gleason pattern 5 was the strongest predictor of an unfavorable outcome in surgically treated patients with Gleason grade 7 carcinoma.[518]

Most urologists want the highest Gleason grade reported by the pathologist, even if this is the tertiary grade (as it almost always is) and accounts for only a small percentage of the cancer volume present in the specimen.[519]

Our group deals with the issue of tertiary grade by providing the classic Gleason score as noted above and simply adding a statement such as: 'In addition, there is a small (5%) component of Gleason grade 5 present.'

The International Society of Urologic Pathology (ISUP) recently proposed modification of the Gleason score to

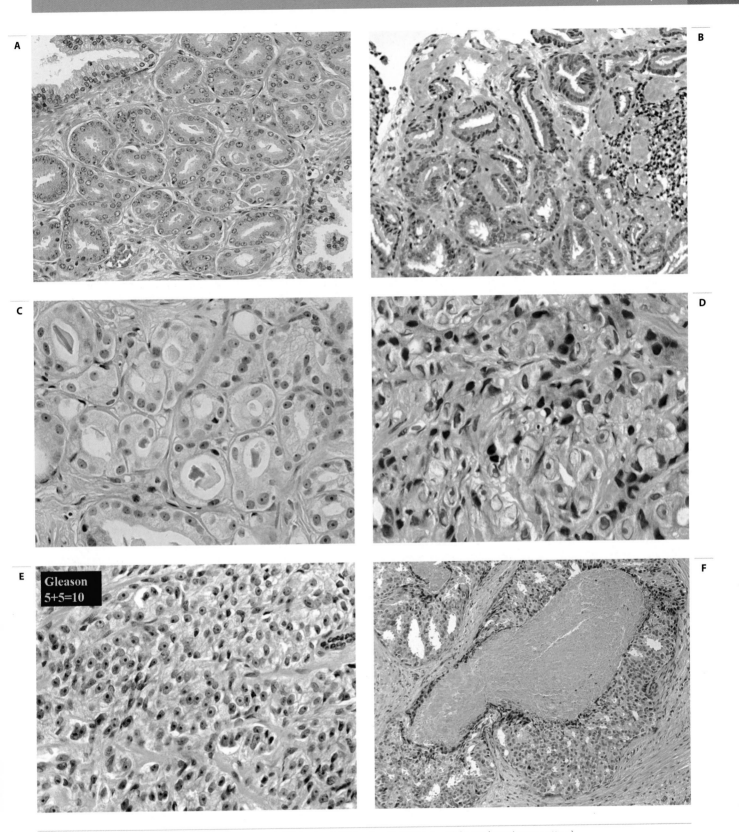

**Fig. 9-33** Gleason grading. (**A**) 2 + 2 = 4. (**B, C**) 3 + 3 = 6. (**D**) 4 + 4 = 8. (**E**) 5 + 5 = 10. (**F**) 5 + 5 = 10 (comedocarcinoma pattern).

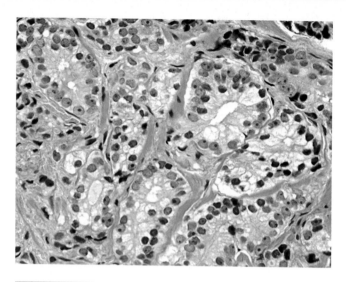

**Fig. 9-34** Gleason pattern 3 adenocarcinoma, large acinar type, consisting of an irregular aggregate of rigid angulated acini with variability of size, shape, and spacing.

include the sum of most common grade and worst grade present to account for cases with three separate Gleason scores.[520] For example, if a radical prostatectomy has 60% Gleason grade 3 cancer, 35% grade 4, and 5% grade 5, the ISUP grade would be 3 (most common) + 5 (worst grade) = score 8; the classic Gleason score would be 3 (most common) + 4 (second most common) = score 7. We believe that this modified system requires the following before acceptance: prospective validation; renaming this new approach (e.g., 'modified Gleason score') to avoid confusion with the classic Gleason scoring system that has remained essentially intact and unaltered for more than 40 years and has been used successfully in more than 3000 published papers; and multidisciplinary discussion and consensus creation.

Patients with a tertiary pattern had a 5-year risk of PSA progression of 37% versus 13% in cases in which no tertiary Gleason pattern was present.[521] There was no prognostic difference between patients with a higher-grade tertiary pattern and those with a lower-grade tertiary pattern. This suggests that tumor multifocality, rather than the presence of a higher-grade tertiary Gleason pattern, has prognostic value.

*Nuclear grading and morphometric grading* Nuclear and nucleolar enlargement are important diagnostic clues for the diagnosis of malignancy. Morphometric methods allow objective evaluation of nuclear size, roundness, shape, chromatin texture, and other features. Numerous investigators have used morphometry to improve the predictive value of Gleason grading, but these methods are not used routinely.[70,460,522–525]

Nuclear roundness has been the subject of considerable interest for more than 20 years, but is not routinely employed.[460,522,523] Mean nuclear roundness accurately predicted prognosis in patients with untreated stage T1b

prostatic adenocarcinoma and other clinical stage adenocarcinomas. However, many of these reports were limited by small sample size (fewer than 30 patients), use of the same patient cohort in multiple publications, failure to describe the morphologic variations and nuclear roundness extremes, and bias in patient selection. Further, significant problems of reproducibility have been encountered, and the results obtained by different digitizing instruments are not comparable. Nuclear roundness identified patients with tumor recurrence following radiation therapy for well-differentiated adenocarcinoma.[526] The good correlation of morphologic nuclear grade in biopsies and prostatectomies is probably due to the large number of cases that fall into the nuclear grade 2 (of 3) category.

Tannenbaum et al.[527,528] compared nucleolar surface area in 40 biopsies and matched prostatectomies with adenocarcinoma, reporting no significant difference in 70% of cases. Nucleolar grading of prostatic adenocarcinoma has also been proposed, but has not been adopted (grade 1: large and prominent nucleoli in virtually every cell; grade 2: intermediate; grade 3: tiny nucleoli that are difficult to find).[529]

*Grade compression* Many authors have simplified the Gleason grading system by compressing (lumping) the scores into groups, usually creating three groups: 2–3–4, 5–6–7, and 8–9–10.[530] Unfortunately, compression diminishes the statistical strength of grading. Further, the choice of grouping is often problematic; the most important 'cut point' is between Gleason scores 6 and 7, owing to the emergence of poorly differentiated adenocarcinoma (pattern 4) in score 7, yet many studies combine these scores. Gleason argued against grade compression, except for studies with a small number of patients in which grouping is unavoidable;[464] in such cases a cut point between scores 6 and 7 is preferred. The probability of lymph node metastases is significantly greater in patients with score 7 adenocarcinoma than in those with score 6.

*Amount of high-grade adenocarcinoma* The volume of high-grade adenocarcinoma appears to be an important prognostic factor: as tumor volume increases, the frequency and volume of high-grade tumor increases. McNeal et al.[531] suggested that the Gleason grade stratifies adenocarcinomas into three subgroups with different levels of aggressiveness. Gleason pattern 1 and 2 adenocarcinomas are almost always small – usually < 1 cm³ – and are indolent, localized, and frequently limited to the transition zone. Grade 3 adenocarcinomas are variable in size and very common. Grade 4 and 5 adenocarcinomas are usually larger and more aggressive than lower-grade tumors, and are likely to extend beyond the prostate or to metastasize. In a study of 209 radical prostatectomies from patients with clinical stage T1 and T2 adenocarcinomas, Gaffney et al.[532] studied the extent of solid undifferentiated carcinoma in 24 cases and found a strong correlation with tumor progression. Bostwick et al.[533] found that Gleason score and the percentage of patterns 4 and 5 adenocarcinoma showed a positive correlation with tumor volume. Vis and colleagues[534] from the European Randomized Study of Screening for Prostate Cancer found that the amount of high-grade cancer (Gleason patterns 4 and 5) was the strongest predictor of biochemical failure after radical prostatectomy, similar to the results of others.[535–537] The cumulative data suggest that the volume of high-grade adenocarcinoma is of prognostic significance,[538] refuting Gleason's contention that prostatic carcinoma behaves according to the average of histologic grades.[464]

*Gleason 7 subdivision (3 + 4 vs. 4 + 3)* Gleason score 7 cancer is common and heterogeneous, and should be considered a specific prognostic category.[539] Most authors claim that it is important to separate predominant pattern 3 from predominant pattern 4. Among patients with Gleason score 7, primary grade 4 indicates a likelihood of higher tumor stage[540] and a higher probability of PSA recurrence after surgery than does primary pattern 3.[518,541,542] However, it does not independently predict a worse outcome after controlling for other known prognostic parameters associated with disease progression,[518,543,544] and appears to be of less value in patients treated by brachytherapy.[545,546] Conversely, Rasiah and colleagues[547] found that patients with primary Gleason grade 4 cancer were more likely to have seminal vesicle involvement and extraprostatic extension and, along with patients with tertiary Gleason grade 5, a significantly shorter time to cancer recurrence.

Of the patients with Gleason pattern 3 + 4 tumors on biopsy, 24% were upgraded to primary pattern 4 or more on final pathologic analysis.[548] Of the patients with Gleason pattern 4 + 3 tumors on biopsy, 47% were downgraded to primary pattern 3 or less on final pathologic analysis.

## Dedifferentiation

Histologic dedifferentiation of prostatic adenocarcinoma has been reported by numerous investigators, but these studies included only cases with more than one resection, probably selecting for adenocarcinomas that are more aggressive and hence more likely to require repeat operation. Brawn[549] reported dedifferentiation in 65% of repeat transurethral resections. Cumming et al.[550] described 74 patients with repeated transurethral resections with a mean interval of 2.4 years: Gleason score remained constant in 12, increased in 49, and decreased in seven, and dedifferentiation occurred in untreated adenocarcinomas and in those subjected to expectant management. Whittemore et al.[551] suggested that dedifferentiation to high-grade adenocarcinoma is unusual in low-grade (Gleason patterns 1–3), small-volume (1 cm³) adenocarcinomas, occurring in only 2.4% of patients in 7 years. Their hypothesis explained the large discrepancy in the incidence of clinical cancer among populations with similar prevalences of occult cancer, and indicates that volume of occult cancer is an important marker of aggressive adenocarcinoma. A recent report followed 67 men with median time to follow-up biopsy of 22 months (range, 7–60), and found that Gleason score was unchanged in 20 patients (30%), upgraded in 19 (28%), and downgraded in 27 (40%); 21 (31%) had no malignancy on follow-up biopsy.[552] They concluded that there was no consistent histologic upgrading on follow-up biopsy at a median of 22 months in untreated,

low to intermediate-grade, clinically localized prostate cancer.[553]

Interestingly, in men over 80 years of age with PSA concentration > 30 ng/mL, at least 97% had cancer and more than 90% had high-grade cancer.[554] Therefore, there may be ascertainment bias if one does not correct for patient age.

Recent epidemiological evidence has revealed that dedifferentiation is a major mechanism of progression in prostate cancer. Tumors may dedifferentiate during the screen-detectable phase; consequently, screening with PSA and early treatment may prevent dedifferentiation.[555]

There was a trend toward histologic dedifferentiation when prostate carcinoma metastasizes to regional lymph nodes.[556] Gleason score in lymph node metastases was higher than in the primary tumor in 45% of cases, lower in 12%, and matched exactly in 43%. The 5-year progression-free survival was significantly lower in patients with histologic dedifferentiation (88% ± 3) and those without dedifferentiation (94% ± 2) (P = 0.04; however, dedifferentiation was not associated with progression when adjusted for lymph node cancer volume).

### Grading after therapy

*Grading after radiation therapy* Grading of specimens after radiation therapy yielded conflicting results, with some observers noting no difference from pre-therapy grade and others finding a substantial increase in grade. Bostwick et al.[557] found no apparent difference in grade before and after external beam therapy in 40 patients. Conversely, Wheeler et al.[558] found an increase in tumor grade following treatment that they attributed to time-dependent tumor progression. Similarly, Siders and Lee[559] evaluated matched tissue specimens from 58 men before therapy and more than 18 months after therapy, and found a significant increase in Gleason score. There was a 24% increase in poorly differentiated adenocarcinoma (scores 8–10) and a shift toward aneuploid DNA content in 31% of pretreatment diploid tumors, indicating increasing histologic and biologic tumor aggressiveness; no outcome data were provided to support this assertion. In grade 4 cancer, radiotherapy may cause the disappearance of glandular lumina, resulting in grade 5 morphology. Despite conflicting results, some investigators recommend grading of specimens after therapy, recognizing that the biologic significance of grade may be different than in untreated cancer. We believe that Gleason grading after radiation therapy is potentially misleading, particularly the risk of overestimation, and we do not report it unless requested to do so and always with the appropriate disclaimer ('Grading of adenocarcinoma after radiation therapy is not validated and may create spurious and misleading higher Gleason grade, so these results may not be predictive of patient outcome and should be interpreted with caution').

Grading systems have been proposed for therapy-induced adenocarcinoma regression, chiefly by German investigators,[560,561] but have not been widely adopted. These systems are considered useful following androgen deprivation therapy and radiation therapy because the histologic changes in cancer cells may be similar. Böcking suggested that reversible cell damage in prostate cancer is characterized by cytoplasmic vacuolization, nuclear shrinkage, and reduction in the number and size of nucleoli, whereas irreversible cell damage is characterized by rupture of the cytoplasm, nuclear pyknosis, and loss of nucleoli.[560]

*Grading after androgen deprivation therapy* Following androgen deprivation therapy (e.g., leuprolide, flutamide) there may be an increase in Gleason grade accompanied by a marked reduction in nuclear and nucleolar size and prominent cytoplasmic clearing.[562] Ellison et al.[563] found a significant increase in Gleason grade, a decrease in nuclear grade, and a decrease in the extent of PIN in a control study of cases treated with androgen deprivation therapy; the 'uncoupling' of the architectural and cytologic pattern was considered vexing owing to identification of small shrunken nuclei within malignant acini. Conversely, there was no significant alteration in Gleason grade following monotherapy with the anti-androgen bicalutamide[271] or the 5α-reductade inhibitors finasteride[277,564,565] and dutasteride.[566]

Despite a potential increase in grade with some agents, adenocarcinoma following androgen deprivation therapy is probably not more clinically aggressive than when untreated; however, no outcome data are available to confirm this assertion. Therefore, we and most investigators conclude that Gleason grading after androgen deprivation therapy is potentially misleading and is not recommended.[562]

## Clinical significance of grading

Grade is one of the strongest predictors of biologic behavior in prostatic adenocarcinoma, including invasiveness and metastatic potential, but is not reliable when used alone to predict pathologic stage or outcome for individual patients. Grade is included among other prognostic factors in therapeutic decision-making, including patient age and health, clinical stage, and serum PSA level. Men with smaller prostates had more high-grade cancer and more advanced disease and were at greater risk of progression after prostatectomy.[567]

## Correlation of grade with recurrence and survival

Virtually every measure of recurrence and survival is strongly correlated with adenocarcinoma grade, including overall survival, tumor-free survival following treatment,[568–573] metastasis-free survival, and cause-specific survival.[574,575] Humphrey et al.[576–578] found that the Gleason score was the strongest predictor of time to recurrence after radical prostatectomy. Biopsy Gleason grade is an integral component of nomograms that predict the 10-year probability of recurrence after radical prostatectomy (in combination with PSA, clinical stage, and number of involved cores).[579]

Schroeder et al.[580] measured the impact on cancer-specific survival of 12 histopathologic characteristics used in grading prostatic adenocarcinoma. In their analysis of 346 patients treated by perineal prostatectomy, they found that four characteristics provided independent predictive value: acinar arrangement (architecture), nuclear size, nuclear shape, and the presence of mitotic figures.

## Correlation of grade and tumor volume

The strong correlation between the Gleason grade and cancer volume has been shown in biopsies,[581] transurethral resections, and radical prostatectomies. McNeal et al.[531] showed that low-grade adenocarcinoma (Gleason patterns 1 and 2) was rarely larger than 1 cm$^3$, whereas high-grade adenocarcinoma (patterns 4 and 5) was almost always larger than 1 cm$^3$. The probability of tumor progression is best indicated by grade and volume; when cancer volume was held constant, grade had residual prognostic value, indicating that it provided additional independent information, although these two prognostic factors are closely linked.

## Correlation of grade and PSA concentration

Adenocarcinoma associated with elevated serum PSA is more likely to be of higher grade, larger volume, and more advanced pathologic stage than adenocarcinoma associated with a normal serum PSA level. Blackwell et al.[582] found a significant positive correlation between serum PSA and primary Gleason grade, the percentage of Gleason patterns 4 and 5, nuclear grade, and DNA content in a large series of totally embedded prostatectomies. Adenocarcinoma with Gleason scores = 7 had a significantly higher median serum PSA and median cancer volume than cancers with lower (<7) Gleason scores. Also, patients with adenocarcinoma consisting of > 30% Gleason patterns 4 and 5 had a significantly higher median serum PSA and cancer volume than those with = 30% Gleason patterns 4 and 5. Further, the median serum PSA level was greater in tumors with Gleason pattern > 3 than in those with Gleason pattern < 3 after controlling for tumor volume in 5 cm$^3$ increments.

Partin et al.[583] found that serum PSA was of limited usefulness for staging localized prostatic adenocarcinoma because of the influence of tumor grade; by controlling for cancer volume but not gland volume (PSA/cancer volume), they found a negative correlation with the Gleason score, suggesting that PSA concentration was determined by multiple confounding factors. However, Blackwell et al.[582] found that combining PSA with gland volume and cancer volume (PSA/cancer density) increased the reliability and predictive value for pathologic stage and tumor grade. Although individual cells in poorly differentiated adenocarcinoma produce less PSA than cells in well- and moderately differentiated adenocarcinoma, they are usually present in such large numbers (greater cancer volume) and replace more of the prostate that serum PSA level is higher.

Serial measurements of PSA suggest that prostatic adenocarcinoma has a constant log-linear growth rate, with mean PSA doubling times of 2.4 years for localized adenocarcinoma and 1.8 years for metastatic adenocarcinoma.[584] Higher Gleason grades are associated with faster doubling times.

## Correlation of grade and pathologic stage

Grade is one of the strongest and most useful predictors of pathologic stage, according to numerous univariate and multivariate studies.[585–587] This predictive ability applies to virtually every measure of pathologic stage, including extraprostatic extension, seminal vesicle invasion, lymph node metastases, and bone metastases. Some investigators claim that a Gleason score of 8 or higher on biopsy is strongly predictive of lymph node metastases and suggest dispensing with staging lymph node dissections in these cases,[588] although this has been refuted.[589] Despite the optimism for grading to predict clinical stage, the predictive value is not high enough to permit its application for individual patients, particularly in those with moderately differentiated adenocarcinoma.

### Correlation of grade and tumor location

Grade may be related to the site of origin of adenocarcinoma within the prostate. Adenocarcinoma arising in the transition zone of the prostate appears to be lower grade and less aggressive clinically than the more common adenocarcinoma arising in the peripheral zone.[442] The majority of transition zone adenocarcinomas arise in foci adjacent to nodular hyperplasia, with one-third actually originating within nodules.[49,366] These adenocarcinomas are better differentiated than those in the peripheral zone, accounting for the majority of Gleason pattern 1 and 2 tumors.

## Variants of prostatic adenocarcinoma and other carcinomas

Variants of adenocarcinoma arising in the prostate raise questions of tumor origin, particularly whether the tumor represents metastasis or contiguous spread from another site. Also, the clinical behavior of morphologic variants may differ from typical adenocarcinoma, carrying a better or a worse prognosis, but data are limited. These tumors are usually associated with typical acinar carcinoma, and rarely occur in pure form. The Gleason grade, pathologic criteria, and clinical significance of variants of prostatic adenocarcinoma and other carcinomas are listed in Table 9-28.

### Adenocarcinoma with endometrioid features (ductal adenocarcinoma)

Ductal carcinoma classically arises as a polypoid, papillary, cribriform, or cystic mass within the prostatic urethra and large periurethral prostatic ducts, and histologically often resembles endometrial adenocarcinoma of the uterus.[59,590–597] Cytologic smears typically showed cells with abundant cytoplasm and oval nuclei arranged in papillary groups or flat and folded sheets, some of which showed peripheral nuclear palisading.[598] In the initial description, Melicow and Pachter[599] suggested that the morphologic appearance and common location of this tumor near the prostatic verumontanum indicated origin from the müllerian (female) remnant of the utriculus masculinus, implying that these tumors are estrogen dependent. The therapeutic importance of estrogen-dependent prostatic carcinoma would be considerable because hormonal (estrogen) therapy would be contraindicated. However, the hypothesis of true uterine ('endometrial') carcinoma arising in the male is now abandoned, and virtually all studies have shown that endometrioid carcinoma is merely a histopathologic variant of prostatic adenocarcinoma; thus, the preferred term is endometrioid carcinoma, or simply ductal carcinoma. The term 'endometrial' should not be used in the prostate.

**Table 9-28** Histologic spectrum of prostatic carcinoma

| |
|---|
| Adenocarcinoma with endometrioid features (Ductal adenocarcinoma) |
|   Non-invasive ductal carcinoma |
|   Papillary (endometrioid) |
|   Cribriform (endometrioid) |
|   Comedocarcinoma |
|   Multicystic |
|   Urothelial-type |
| Mucinous carcinoma |
| Signet ring-cell carcinoma |
| Adenocarcinoma with neuroendocrine differentiation |
| Adenocarcinoma with neuroendocrine differentiation with large eosinophilic granules |
|   Low-grade neuroendocrine carcinoma (Carcinoid) |
|   High-grade neuroendocrine carcinoma (Small cell carcinoma) |
| Sarcomatoid carcinoma (carcinosarcoma) |
| Giant cell carcinoma |
| Adenoid cystic/basal cell carcinoma |
| Lymphoepithelioma-like carcinoma |
| Carcinoma with oncocytic features |
| Comedocarcinoma |
| Cribriform carcinoma |
| Adenocarcinoma with glomeruloid features |
| Adenocarcinoma with atrophic features |
| Adenocarcinoma with microvacuolated cytoplasm (foamy gland carcinoma) |
| Pseudohyperplastic adenocarcinoma |
| Adenosquamous and squamous cell carcinoma |
| Urothelial carcinoma |

Ductal carcinoma accounts for about 0.2–0.8% of cases of prostatic adenocarcinoma.[59] It occurs exclusively in older men, who may have symptoms of hematuria, urinary urgency and frequency, and rarely, acute retention. The clinical symptoms of pure ductal carcinoma and mixed ductal–acinar carcinoma overlap with those of typical acinar carcinoma. In some cases adenocarcinoma is detected by digital rectal examination or PSA elevation in asymptomatic patients, usually in association with peripherally located acinar adenocarcinoma. Cystoscopically, ductal carcinoma may appear as multiple friable polypoid wormlike white masses protruding from ducts at or near the mouth of the prostatic utricle of the verumontanum; more often, however, there are no distinguishing cystoscopic findings. The prostate may be enlarged.

At the time of symptom presentation the majority of patients have tumors confined to the prostate or urethra, with concurrent invasive acinar prostatic adenocarcinoma in at least 77% of cases. Serum concentration of PSA may be normal or elevated at the time of diagnosis.

The tumor is at least focally indistinguishable from uterine carcinoma, consisting of masses of complex papillae or anastomosing glands lined by variably stratified columnar epithelium. The mitotic rate tends to be higher than in typical acinar adenocarcinoma. The histologic spectrum of ductal carcinoma is presented in Table 9-28 (Fig. 9-35). Non-invasive ductal carcinoma is a common finding, but precise histopathologic criteria for separation from high-grade PIN have not yet been defined; nonetheless, all agree that massive expansion of large periurethral prostatic ducts by papillary

and cribriform masses is best diagnosed as non-invasive carcinoma, regardless of the presence or absence of scattered circumferential basal cells (we prefer not to use the term 'intraductal carcinoma' owing to its tainted past and lack of reproducible criteria).[600] The papillary and cribriform patterns of ductal carcinoma coexist in about half of cases, and

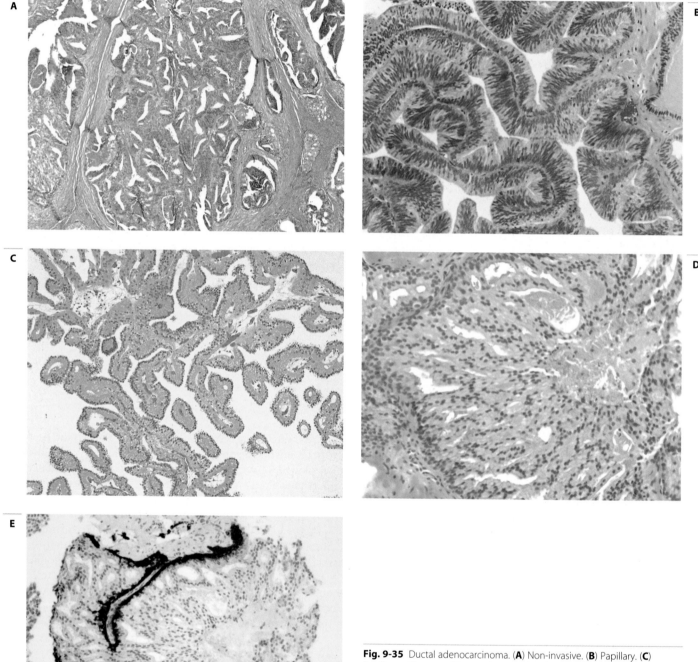

**Fig. 9-35** Ductal adenocarcinoma. (**A**) Non-invasive. (**B**) Papillary. (**C**) Papillary with unusual inverted pattern (nuclei are abluminal rather than typical basal location). (**D**) Cribriform. Compare with **E,** which shows scattered basal cells at the periphery, indicating non-invasive nature of the growth. This papillary proliferation filled the large periurethral prostatic ducts and protruded into the urethra.

both usually display nuclear anaplasia, nucleolomegaly, and frequent mitotic figures, although there is a spectrum of nuclear and nucleolar abnormalities. Comedocarcinoma has the highest level of mitotic activity. Cystic growth is a less common pattern that usually occurs in the peripheral zone,[591,592] often with exophytic papillary and cribriform growth within large accommodating spaces in a manner similar to endometrial tumors expanding within the uterine cavity or ovarian tumors growing within cystic spaces or the peritoneal cavity. The ability to expand potential spaces by adenocarcinoma probably accounts for the distinctive cribriform or papillary growth in large periurethral ducts and the urethra, and thus may merely represent a distinctive growth pattern of acinar adenocarcinoma. Identification of papillary or cribriform growth of cancer in prostate needle biopsies usually represents peripheral zone adenocarcinoma (90% of cases with these patterns) and not periurethral ductal involvement (10%).[59] Consequently, we refer to papillary or cribriform growth of cancer in needle biopsies as the 'ductal subtype' of adenocarcinoma, with a note stating that it is virtually always seen in association with typical acinar adenocarcinoma.

The cribriform pattern of carcinoma is characterized by masses of tumor punctuated by sieve-like spaces. Unlike cribriform PIN, cribriform carcinoma does not have a basal cell layer at the periphery of glands.[80,594,595] McNeal et al. found that up to 70% of cribriform masses were intraductal; however, they described this as cribriform carcinoma and suggested that the cribriform pattern has the same biologic behavior as Gleason pattern 4 cancer. No follow-up information was provided to support their claim, and the number of cases studied (21 cases) was too small to draw conclusions regarding biologic behavior; further, they appear to have mistaken cribriform PIN for carcinoma. Based on the cumulative data, we suggest that the term cribriform carcinoma be used only descriptively, if at all, and should not refer to a specific entity.

Comedocarcinoma is characterized by luminal necrosis within round masses of malignant cells, similar to comedocarcinoma of the breast. This morphologic variant of adenocarcinoma is included in the Gleason grading system as poorly differentiated (grade 5) carcinoma based on the degree of acinar differentiation. Currin et al.[601,602] studied the biologic potential of prostatic comedocarcinoma by flow cytometry and found a high frequency of aneuploidy, suggesting aggressiveness. PAP and PSA were present in the majority of tumor cells.

Comedocarcinoma is invariably found in association with other patterns of adenocarcinoma and does not warrant separation as a clinicopathologic entity.

The least common pattern of ductal carcinoma, urothelial-type adenocarcinoma, is a rare and newly described entity that arises from either the prostatic urethra or proximal ducts, and is most difficult to distinguish histologically from secondary colorectal carcinoma invading the prostate.[603–605] Areas with urothelial-type adenocarcinoma are identified in the intraductal or invasive component of adenocarcinoma. Subtypes include urothelial-like cancer,[593,605,606] mucinous cancer, and intestinal-type mucinous cancer.[607]

The intraductal component usually merges with regions of papillary or cribriform pattern. All prostatic adenocarcinomas having areas with urothelial carcinoma features are high stage, and most have ductal features.

Urothelial-type adenocarcinoma is diffusely positive for cytokeratin 7 and focally positive for keratin 34βE12, thrombomodulin, and cytokeratin 20, consistent with origin from the urothelium of the prostatic urethra or proximal prostatic ducts; interestingly, weak or negative staining for PSA and PAP is also observed. The differential diagnosis includes conventional prostatic adenocarcinoma with mucin production, urothelial carcinoma with glandular differentiation,[608] and secondary adenocarcinoma, usually of colorectal origin. However, mucinous conventional prostatic adenocarcinoma is positive for PSA and PAP, and usually negative for cytokeratin 7, cytokeratin 20, and 34βE12; secondary adenocarcinoma of colonic origin is diffusely cytokeratin 20 positive and either negative or focally positive for cytokeratin 7 and negative for 34βE12.

Ductal carcinoma invariably displays intense cytoplasmic immunoreactivity for PSA and PAP.[596] Nuclear androgen receptor staining is usually strong, whereas estrogen receptor staining is negative. All ductal carcinomas expressed Ki67, whereas expression of Bcl-2 was extensive in well- and moderately differentiated cancer.[609] Focal carcinoembryonic antigen immunoreactivity is observed in a minority of cases. Lee et al.[610] described focal patchy immunoreactivity for estrogen-regulated protein and estrogen receptor-related protein, indicating prostatic origin.

Ultrastructural findings include well-developed acini with distinct basal lamina, luminal microvilli, large nuclei with prominent nucleoli, desmosomes, secretory droplets, lysosomes, and abundant rough endoplasmic reticulum. Two types of tumor cells are distinguished on the basis of cytoplasmic differentiation: light cells are most common, containing secretory droplets, lipid-filled vacuoles, and pinocytotic vesicles; dark cells contain electron-dense cytoplasm with abundant endoplasmic reticulum and free ribosomes. Transitional forms of each of these cell types are present.

Ductal carcinoma must be distinguished from urothelial carcinoma of the prostate, ectopic prostatic tissue, benign polyp, nephrogenic metaplasia, proliferative papillary urethritis, inverted papilloma, and accentuated mucosal folds. There is usually morphologic evidence of glandular differentiation in ductal carcinoma, allowing separation from urothelial carcinoma. In difficult cases or those with small samples, immunohistochemical stains for PSA and PAP are useful (positive in ductal carcinoma and negative in urothelial carcinoma). Benign mimics are distinguished from ductal carcinoma by the absence of nuclear abnormalities.

Subclassification of ductal carcinoma based on location is not performed in routine practice. Primary duct (large duct) and secondary duct prostatic adenocarcinoma are indistinguishable from each other, and most authors consider these a single entity, abandoning this artificial separation. There are no clinical or pathological criteria for the separation of ductal carcinoma into utricular and non-utricular types.

Ductal carcinoma appears to have a less favorable prognosis than typical acinar adenocarcinoma, although conflicting results have been found.[597] Up to 36% of cases have metastases at the time of diagnosis, similar to acinar carcinoma. Bostwick et al.[611] reported 13 patients, seven of whom died of metastases within 6 years of diagnosis. Ro et al.[612] noted that seven of eight patients followed for more than 8 years died of metastases. The 5-year survival rates range from 15% to 43%. The pattern of metastases is identical to that of the typical acinar prostatic adenocarcinoma. Metastases usually reveal a tumor histologically similar to ductal carcinoma, even when coexistent acinar carcinoma is present in the prostate, suggesting that the endometrioid pattern is more aggressive.

Androgen deprivation therapy provides palliative relief in many cases but does not appear to influence survival. In the study by Ro et al.,[612] seven patients responded to orchiectomy or estrogen therapy with marked symptomatic improvement. Radiation therapy has been used to palliate voiding difficulty and hematuria, as well as to control bone pain, and these tumors appear to be sensitive to treatment with radiation. Nonetheless, the prognosis is poor.[594]

### Mucinous (colloid) carcinoma

Fewer than 200 cases of mucinous carcinoma of the prostate have been reported, but the incidence is probably higher.[310,613–617] The signs and symptoms are similar to those of typical acinar carcinoma. There are no apparent differences in patient age, stage at presentation, cancer volume, or serum PSA level. Typical acinar adenocarcinoma may produce mucin following high-dose estrogen therapy.

Focal mucinous differentiation is observed in at least one-third of cases of prostatic carcinoma, but the diagnosis of mucinous carcinoma requires that at least 25% of the tumor consist of pools of extracellular mucin (Fig. 9-36).[614,617,618] Mucinous carcinoma consists of tumor cell nests and clusters floating in mucin, similar to mucinous carcinoma of the breast. In small specimens such as needle biopsies, rare cases consist only of mucin pools without identifiable tumor cells, although serial sectioning usually reveals carcinoma cells on deeper levels. Three patterns of mucinous carcinoma have been described: acinar carcinoma with luminal distension, cribriform carcinoma with luminal distension, and 'colloid carcinoma' with cell nests embedded in mucinous lakes.[614]

Other histologic patterns of adenocarcinoma are typically present in association with mucinous carcinoma, including cribriform and comedocarcinoma patterns. The cells of mucinous carcinoma usually have enlarged nuclei and display the entire spectrum of cytologic abnormalities observed in typical adenocarcinoma. In some cases the nuclei have low-grade cytologic findings, with uniform finely granular chromatin and inconspicuous nucleoli, but their presence within mucin pools is diagnostic of malignancy. Signet ring cells are usually not seen in mucinous carcinoma, although numerous cases have been reported in which such cells were abundant.[619] A unique case of mucinous carcinoma arose in the transition zone in association with large numbers of neuroendocrine cells with large eosinophilic granules. Collagenous micronodules are often an incidental finding in mucin-producing carcinoma that probably result from extracellular acid mucin.[386] The number of collagenous micronodules is correlated with mucin production by the tumor, including luminal mucin and extra-acinar mucin; there is a weak negative correlation of collagenous micronodules with the percentage of tumor composed of signet ring cells.

Prostatic mucin stains with periodic acid–Schiff, Alcian blue, and mucicarmine. Most studies have found neutral mucin in benign acini and acidic mucin in malignant acini, although benign acini rarely produce small quantities of acidic mucin. Based on these findings, some have suggested that acidic mucin is a useful supportive feature in the diag-

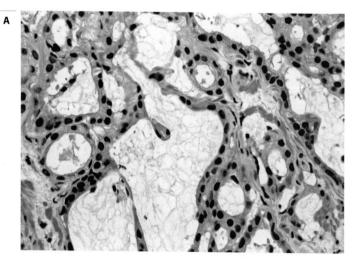
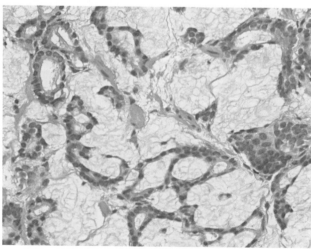

**Fig. 9-36** Mucinous (colloid) carcinoma. (**A, B**) Abundant luminal mucin expands the malignant acinar lumina.

nosis of adenocarcinoma, being present in about 60% of cases.[310,613-615] In adenocarcinoma, sialomucins predominate over sulfomucins. Well- and moderately differentiated non-colloid tumors have non-O-acylated sialomucins. Poorly differentiated tumors contained mono-O-acylated (C9) sialomucins, and colloid-type tumors secreted mono-, di-, and tri-O-acylated sialoglycoproteins. Acidic mucins, mainly sialomucins, constitute the major secretory component in prostatic adenocarcinoma, and Saez and colleagues[378] showed that O-acylation of these sialoglycoproteins correlates inversely with differentiation. Well-differentiated and moderately differentiated tumors are not O-acylated, whereas poorly differentiated cancer characteristically has O-acylated sialomucins in C9. Mucinous adenocarcinoma is the most heavily O-acylated of the variants.[378] Acidic mucin has also been described in atypical adenomatous hyperplasia, mucinous metaplasia, PIN, sclerosing adenosis, and basal cell hyperplasia.

The cells of mucinous carcinoma express PSA and PAP, but usually do not produce CEA unless there is prominent signet ring-cell differentiation.[620] In one case, neuron-specific enolase immunoreactivity was observed, confirming histochemical results with the Grimelius stain.

Ultrastructurally, tumor cells are joined by zonula adherens junctions and set in an amorphous background. Microvilli and cytoplasmic projections are prominent. Nuclei are compressed to one side of the cells, with cytoplasmic organelles and mucinogen granules filling the remainder of the cells.

The pattern of metastases of mucinous carcinoma of the prostate is similar to that of typical prostatic adenocarcinoma. Early reports suggested that these tumors were less aggressive and of lower stage than other forms of prostatic adenocarcinoma, with no tendency for bone metastasis, but recent studies with long-term survival have effectively refuted this claim.[621-623] Patients have been treated with radiation therapy, hormonal therapy, or both. Five of eight patients reported by Ro et al.[614] died from tumor within 7 years, and the remaining three are alive with tumor up to 15 months. Likewise, Saito et al.[624] reported that 50% of patients survived 3 years and 25% survived 5 years. Conversely, a contemporary series of 14 patients revealed survival with a median of 6.4 years, similar to acinar adenocarcinoma.[617]

Mucinous carcinoma of the rectum and urinary bladder may invade the prostate, mimicking mucinous carcinoma of the prostate. Similarly, Cowper's gland carcinoma displays prominent mucinous differentiation. Prostatic ductal adenocarcinoma may also rarely exhibit prominent mucin production,[607] as can urethral adenocarcinoma.[603,604] These distinctions are important because of significant differences in treatment and prognosis.

Pseudomyxoma ovarii-like change is a rare mimic of mucinous carcinoma that consists of extravasated acid mucin, lacks prostatic basal cells, often occurs in intimate association with residual prostatic adenocarcinoma in post-treatment radical prostatectomy specimens, and probably represents tumor regression as a result of tumor cell attrition secondary to androgen ablation.[625] Minute to large pools of extravasated secretions dissect through the prostatic stroma,

with an infiltrative appearance when viewed at low power. Secretions were basophilic in routine sections and contained occasional degenerated cells. Rare pancytokeratin positive cells were seen at the secretion–stroma interface with uniformly negative staining for the high molecular weight keratin 34βE12. The secretions were periodic acid–Schiff positive after diastase digestion and mucicarminophilic and reactive with Alcian blue at a pH of 2.5. There was no correlation between the presence of pseudomyxoma-like change and dose or duration of neoadjuvant therapy, post-prostatectomy clinical follow-up, original or final Gleason score, or pathologic stage.

### Signet ring-cell carcinoma

Signet ring-cell carcinoma of the prostate is rare, with fewer than 200 reported cases.[619,626-634] The characteristic cytoplasmic clearing is rarely mucicarminophilic, in contrast to mucicarmine-positive signet ring-cell carcinoma of the bladder, urachus, stomach, and other sites.

The presenting signs and symptoms of signet ring-cell carcinoma are similar to those of typical acinar adenocarcinoma. Rectal examination of the prostate may reveal stony-hard induration.

The diagnosis of signet ring-cell carcinoma requires that 25% or more of the tumor be composed of signet ring-cells, although some authors require 50% (Fig. 9-37). Tumor cells show distinctive nuclear displacement by clear cytoplasm. Signet ring cells are present in 2.5% of cases of acinar adenocarcinoma, but rarely in sufficient numbers to be considered signet ring-cell carcinoma. Almost all reported cases are associated with other forms of poorly differentiated prostatic adenocarcinoma, including cribriform carcinoma, comedocarcinoma, and solid (Gleason grade 5) carcinoma. Tumor cells infiltrate diffusely through the stroma, invading perineural and vascular spaces and often perforating the prostatic capsule.

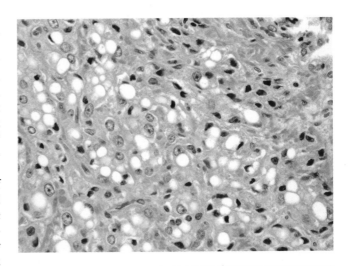

**Fig. 9-37** Signet ring-cell carcinoma with pale blue mucinous luminal secretions.

Histochemical and immunohistochemical stains for mucin, lipid, PSA, PAP, and carcinoembryonic antigen have provided variable results, suggesting variants of signet ring-cell carcinoma (Table 9-29). Giltman[635] reported a case of pure signet ring-cell carcinoma that was periodic acid–Schiff positive and diastase resistant but negative for acid mucin and fat (mucicarmine, Alcian blue, and oil red O). In another case tumor cells were shown to stain with Sudan black, indicating the presence of intracellular lipid. Mucin stains are variably positive. Ro et al.[636] reported eight cases in which the tumor cells did not stain for Alcian blue, mucicarmine, or periodic acid–Schiff with or without diastase. PSA, PAP, and keratin immunoreactivity were observed within signet ring cells and the non-signet ring-cell component, but no carcinoembryonic antigen staining was detected, similar to the findings of Catton et al.[637] Conversely, Remmele et al.[638] reported one case with carcinoembryonic antigen immunoreactivity that was negative for PSA and PAP, and others have reported carcinoembryonic antigen staining with PSA and PAP staining. The signet ring-cell appearance results from different factors in different cases, including cytoplasmic lumina, mucin granules, and fat vacuoles, thus accounting for the contradictory histochemical and immunohistochemical results.

Ultrastructurally, signet ring cells contain cytoplasmic vacuoles and intracytoplasmic lumina, sometimes lined by microvilli and containing no demonstrable mucin or lipid vacuoles. Occasional rod-shaped intraluminal crystalloids are observed in metastatic sites, similar to crystalloids observed in typical acinar adenocarcinoma.

All reported patients have clinical stage T3 or N+ adenocarcinoma. Treatment is variable, including hormonal therapy, radiation therapy, or both. Five of eight patients reported by Ro et al.[636] died between 32 and 60 months after diagnosis, and two were alive with less than 12 months of follow-up. According to Saito and colleagues,[624] patients with primary signet ring-cell carcinoma had a 27.3% 3-year survival rate; none survived 5 years.

Signet ring-cell carcinoma should be distinguished from similar tumors arising in other sites, particularly the gastrointestinal tract and stomach. A prostatic origin should be considered in metastatic signet ring-cell carcinoma of supraclavicular lymph nodes that exhibit negative mucin staining; PSA and PAP immunostaining may be useful. There have been no reported cases of signet ring-cell lymphoma involving the prostate.

Artifactual changes mimicking signet ring-cell carcinoma have been described in transurethral resection specimens, with lymphocytes and vacuolated smooth muscle cells causing diagnostic difficulty.[639,640] In these cases, PSA and PAP staining of the suspicious cells is negative, although leukocyte common antigen immunoreactivity is observed within the inflammatory cells.

### Adenocarcinoma with neuroendocrine differentiation

Neuroendocrine differentiation is present at least focally in virtually all cases of prostatic adenocarcinoma, although the number of cells varies according to the tissue fixative employed, the antibody and the method of staining used,

and the number of tissue sections examined.[641–664] Abrahamsson and colleagues identified neuroendocrine-immunoreactive cells in 92% of prostate cancers fixed in formalin and embedded routinely in paraffin.[659,662,663] Aprikian and associates[665] found neuroendocrine cells in 77% of untreated prostate cancers, 60% of hormone-refractory cancers, and 52% of metastases, with a small number of dispersed positive cells in each of these cases.

Neuroendocrine differentiation typically consists of scattered cells that are inapparent by light microscopy but revealed by immunoreactivity for one or more markers. Chromogranin and serotonin are the best markers of neuroendocrine cells in formalin-fixed sections of the prostate (Fig. 9-38). Neuroendocrine cells in cancer are malignant, and lack androgen receptor expression. Neoplastic neuroendocrine cells devoid of nuclear androgen receptors constitute an androgen-insensitive cell population in prostate cancer. The absence of proliferative and apoptotic activity may endow these tumor cells with relative resistance to cytotoxic drugs and radiation therapy.[666]

About 10% of adenocarcinomas contain unique neuroendocrine cells with distinctive large eosinophilic granules (formerly referred to as adenocarcinoma with Paneth cell-like change; see below).

Neuroendocrine cells have no apparent clinical or prognostic significance in benign epithelium, primary prostate cancer, and lymph node metastases, according to most reports (Table 9-30). Aprikian and colleagues found no correlation of neuroendocrine differentiation with pathologic stage or metastases.[665,667] We found no apparent relationship between the number of immunoreactive neuroendocrine cells in PIN and cancer and a variety of clinical and pathologic factors, including stage.[652] Allen et al.[668] studied 120 patients and found no significant association between neuroendocrine differentiation and patient prognosis. Theodorescu et al.[669] showed that neuroendocrine differentiation predicted patient survival, but this was only true for the analysis with one variable model. Krijnen et al.[670,671] reported that neuroendocrine differentiation was associated with early hormone therapy failure, indicating that these cells are androgen independent. Their findings suggested that the presence of large numbers of neuroendocrine cells in cancer may indicate a poor prognosis, perhaps owing to insensitivity to hormonal growth regulation, but this has been refuted by most studies. We determined the expression of chromogranin A and serotonin in patients with node-positive prostate cancer and found that immunoreactivity was greatest in benign prostatic epithelium, with less expression in primary cancer and lymph node metastases.[652] There was no consistent association between the expression of chromogranin A or serotonin and survival. The cumulative findings reveal no apparent consistent association of neuroendocrine differentiation in typical adenocarcinoma and any clinical outcome variable.[672]

### Adenocarcinoma with neuroendocrine cells with large eosinophilic granules (Paneth cell-like change)

Cells with large eosinophilic granules (Paneth cell-like change) represent an uncommon but distinct form of neu-

**Table 9-29** Signet ring-cell carcinoma of the prostate: laboratory findings

| | Number of cases | Preoperative serum PAP | Preoperative serum PSA | PAS | Lipid stain | Alcian blue | Muci-carmine | PSA | PAP | CEA | Other findings |
|---|---|---|---|---|---|---|---|---|---|---|---|
| Lipid-rich Kums and van Helsdingen, 1985[1276] | 2 | | | – | 1/2 | – | – | – | – | – | |
| Glycogen or mucin-rich Giltman, 1981[635] | 1 | | | 1/1 | 0/1 | 0/1 | 0/1 | – | – | – | |
| Remmele et al. 1988[638] | 1 | | | 1/1 | – | 1/1 | 1/1 | 0/1 | 0/1 | 1/1 | |
| Uchijima et al. 1990[1277] | 1 | | | 0/1 | – | 1/1 | – | 1/1 | – | – | |
| Alline and Cohen, 1992[1278] | 1 | Normal | 5.2 | 0/1 | – | 1/1 | 1/1 | 0/1 | 0/1 | 1/1 | |
| Catton et al. 1992[637] | 1 | 33.6 | – | – | – | 0/1 | 0/1 | 0/1 | 1/1 | 0/1 | |
| Segawa and Kakehi, 1993[1279] | 1 | Normal | <4.0* | 1/1 | – | – | 1/1 | 0/1 | 0/1 | 1/1 | |
| Skodras et al. 1993[1280] | 1 | | | 1/1 | – | 1/1 | 1/1 | 1/1 | 1/1 | 1/1 | |
| Guerin et al. 1993[627] | 5 | 2.4/1.5/21.9 | 4.6* | 5/5 | 0/1 | 5/5 | – | 5/5 | 5/5 | 1/2 | CA19-9 positive |
| Smith et al. 1994[1281] | 1 | 1.7 | | 1/1 | – | – | 1/1 | 1/1 | 1/1 | 1/1 | Diploid primary; aneuploid metastases; |
| Torbenson et al. 1998[631] | 12 | | | 9/10 | – | 6/10 | 5/10 | – | | | |
| Kuroda et al. 1999[630] | 1 | | | 1/1 | – | 1/1 | 1/1 | 1/1 | – | – | |
| Lipid, glycogen, or mucin-Poor Ro et al. 1988[636] | 8 | | | 0/8 | – | 0/8 | 0/8 | 4/4 | 1/1 | | |
| Fujita et al. 2004[1282] | 1 | 9.3 | | 0/1 | – | 0/1 | – | 1/1 | 4/4 | 0/4 | |
| Jiang et al. 2002[1283] | 10 | | | 0/10 | – | 0/10 | 0/10 | 1/1 | 1/1 | 0/1 | |

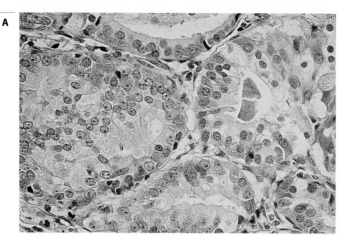 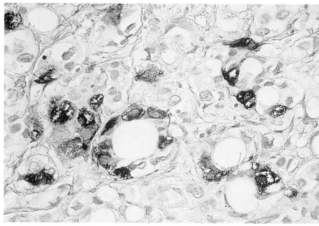

**Fig. 9-38** Prostatic cancer with neuroendocrine differentiation. (**A**) Adenocarcinoma with large eosinophilic granules. (**B**) Another case, with serotonin-immunoreactive cells corresponding to the cells with granules.

roendocrine differentiation in the prostate (Fig. 9-38). This finding is more common than previously believed (10% prevalence), but usually consists of only rare foci of scattered cells and small clusters that may be overlooked.[656,673–680] Although cells with large eosinophilic granules in benign epithelium and adenocarcinoma resemble Paneth cells of the intestine on light microscopy, they are distinguished by the identification of neuroendocrine differentiation and the absence of lysozyme immunoreactivity. They display intense cytoplasmic immunoreactivity for chromogranin, neuron-specific enolase, and serotonin, and are analogous to 'eosinophilic argentaffin cells' of the appendix, uterine cervical glandular mucosa, colonic adenoma, and Sertoli cells of the testis.

A larger number of cells than those with large eosinophilic granules stain with neuroendocrine markers, suggesting that there are neuroendocrine cells with smaller granules that are not apparent on H&E-stained sections.[673,675] Most reports on neuroendocrine differentiation in the benign and malignant prostate have described only scattered cells which are inapparent on routine stain, but which are immunoreactive for neuroendocrine markers.[656,673–679,681] Thus, large eosinophilic granules represent a distinct form of neuroendocrine differentiation.

PSA and PAP immunoreactivity is also observed in cells with large eosinophilic granules, similar to other benign and neoplastic neuroendocrine cells in the prostate.[675] Azumi et al. and others have identified concomitant PSA and neuroendocrine marker immunoreactivity in prostatic carcinoid and other prostatic tumors.[682,683] Abrahamsson et al.[659] showed androgen receptor immunoreactivity in cells with neuroendocrine differentiation. It appears that select cells in the prostate coexpress glandular and neuroendocrine differentiation. This differs from pure neuroendocrine carcinoma of the prostate, in which clonal proliferation and lack of PSA expression is common.

The presence of cells with large eosinophilic granules was not associated with any factors predictive of aggressive

behavior of prostate cancer, including higher tumor stage, serum PSA production, and tumor grade, suggesting that this pattern of neuroendocrine differentiation is not indicative of a poor prognosis.[673,675] We disagree with the suggestion[673] that cancer containing such cells should not be included in the Gleason grading, recognizing that grade is reflective of architectural pattern and cytologic findings. The significance of the cribriform pattern is uncertain. Although the functional role of prostatic cells with neuroendocrine differentiation is unknown, they appear to be important in regulation of growth, differentiation, and secretion.[659,684–686]

### Low-grade neuroendocrine carcinoma (carcinoid)

A spectrum of neuroendocrine differentiation can be seen in prostatic adenocarcinoma, varying from the rare carcinoid-like pattern (low-grade neuroendocrine carcinoma) to the unusual but more common small cell undifferentiated (oat cell) carcinoma (high-grade neuroendocrine carcinoma; see below).[687–694] Carcinoid tumor of the prostate shares similar morphologic and immunophenotypic features with its counterpart in other organs. The differential diagnosis includes metastatic carcinoid tumor from the colon or another site,[695] paraganglioma, and nested variants of urothelial carcinoma. Correlation of the clinical presentation and histopathologic features (including the immunohistochemical profile) ensures accurate diagnosis.

### High-grade neuroendocrine carcinoma (small cell carcinoma)

Most cases of neuroendocrine carcinoma have typical signs and symptoms of prostatic adenocarcinoma, and serum PSA level usually varies according to cancer volume and stage; however, some cases of pure small cell carcinoma may progress without detectable PSA concentration.[696,697] Rare cases are gigantic, enlarging the prostate to more than 500 g.[698] In addition, paraneoplastic syndromes are frequent in patients with small cell carcinoma and carcinoid of the prostate.[699] Cushing's syndrome is most common, invariably in association with adrenocorticotropic hormone immunoreactivity in tumor cells. Other clinical conditions include malignant

**Table 9-30** Predictive value of neuroendocrine differentiation by immunohistochemistry in prostatic adenocarcinoma: collected works

| | No. of patients | Patient population | Tissue studied | NE markers | Cancer cases stained (%) | Quantification of NE staining | Outcome variables | Multivariate analysis | Mean length of follow-up | Comments |
|---|---|---|---|---|---|---|---|---|---|---|
| **Not predictive of outcome** | | | | | | | | | | |
| Aprikian et al. 1993[665] | 78 | 31 primary cancers, 16 metastases, 21 diethylstilbestrol treated cancers, 10 hormone-refractory cancers | Radical prostatectomy and TURP specimens | Chromogranin A, NSE, serotonin, calcitonin, ACTH somatostatin gastrin-releasing peptide, TSH | 77% of primary untreated cancer 56% of metastatic lesions | No positive cells (−), Occasionally identified NE cells (+), numerous cells (++), majority of cells (+++) | Recurrence or metastasis hormone-independent, cancer progression | Yes, factors including cancer grade, stage, progression, hormone-independent | Not given | NE cells were not associated with cancer stage or metastasis |
| Cohen et al. 1994[1284] | 38 | Clinical stage II, III | Retropubic prostatectomy specimens | Chromogranin A, NSE | 29% for Chromogranin A; 24% for NSE | No positive cell identified (−), positive cells identified occasionally (+), 1–3 per acinar structure (++), >3 cells per acinar structure (+++) | PSA failure, recurrence or metastasis in tissue biopsy, positive bone scan or X-ray | Yes, cancer grade, stage, NE staining | 4.2 yrs (range, 4–6 yrs) | Chromogranin A is not useful in predicting cancer progression |
| Bostwick et al. 1994[1285] | 26 | 1 stage pT1b, 10 stage pT2a+b, 13 stage pT2c, 1 stage pT3a, 1 stage T3c cancers, No clinical history of androgen-deprivation therapy or radiation therapy prior to surgery | Whole-mounted, totally-embedded, Radical prostatectomy specimens | Chromogranin A, NSE, serotonin, hCG, calcitonin, ACTH TSH, prolactin, glucagon | 92% | Mean percent of positive high power field (x640) | Cancer grade, stage | Yes, stepwise regression, analysis including cancer grade, stage, volume, microvascular invasion | Not given | NE differentiation was downregulated in prostate cancer. No correlation of NE differentiation with various clinical and pathologic factors |
| Noordzij et al. 1995[1286] | 90 | 22 Stage pT2 cancers, 66 stage pT3 cancers, 2 pT4 cancers, 5 stage pN1 cancers, 2 stage PN2 cancers | Radical prostatectomy specimens | Chromogranin A, Chromogranin B | 78% | No positive cell visible (−), a few positive cells, widely scattered (±), some positive cells, more regularly distributed or small clusters (++), numerous positive cells or large clusters (+++) | Histologically local cancer recurrence or metastasis, cancer-specific death | Yes, Cox's regression model which included cancer grade, stage, | 7.2 yrs (range, 0.1–16.9 yr) | NE differentiation was not associated with Gleason sum, pathology stage or cancer-specific death |

**Table 9-30** Predictive value of neuroendocrine differentiation by immunohistochemistry in prostatic adenocarcinoma: collected works—Cont'd

| | No. of patients | Patient population | Tissue studied | NE markers | Cancer cases stained (%) | Quantification of NE staining | Outcome variables | Multivariate analysis | Mean length of follow-up | Comments |
|---|---|---|---|---|---|---|---|---|---|---|
| Allen et al. 1995[668] | 120 | 17 stage T0, 6 Stage T1, 17 Stage T2, 38 Stage T3, 42 Stage T4 cancers | Needle biopsy, TURP, radical prostatectomy specimens | Chromogranin A, NSE | 31% | Positive (any stained cells), negative (no positive cell) | Systemic progression, cancer-specific survival | Yes, factors included grade, stage, survival | >5 yrs (range, not given) | NE cells was not associated with cancer grade, stage, and patient survival |
| Speights et al. 1997[1287] | 33 | 23 high grade cancers; 10 stage T1a low grade cancers; all diagnosed by TURP; some received androgen deprivation therapy | TURP specimens | Chromogranin A, NSE, Synaptophysin (also included MIB-1) | High grade cancers: 'nearly all'; Low grade: 50% | Counted 1000 cells of benign and cancer per marker | PSA failure (not defined), biopsy-proven recurrence; clinical failure or metastases (imaging)–14 of 23 high grade cancers progressed | Yes; Cox regression models which accounted for variable length of follow-up and Gleason scores | 13.4 months for high-grade cancers (range, 1–42 mo.) | Greater number of NE cells and higher proliferative index (MIB-1 staining) in high stage high grade cancer than low grade cancer |
| McWilliam et al 1997[1288] | 92 | 64 stage T1-2, 9 stage T3, 19 stage M1 | TURP specimens | Chromogranin A, NSE | 52% | Positive (>10% tumor cells), Negative (<10% tumor cells) | Cancer-specific survival (33 cases died from cancer), cancer metastasis (5 cases) | Yes; factors including cancer grade, stage, vascular invasion, bone metastasis | 9 yrs (7–13 yrs) | Positive correlation of NE differentiation with worsening tumor differentiation. No association with cancer stage and cancer-specific survival |
| Pruneri et al. 1998[1289] | 64 | 7 Stage A, 13 stage B, 30 stage C, and 14 stage D. 57 cases underwent preoperative hormonal therapy | Prostatectomy (5 cases), Radical prostatectomy (28 cases), TURP (31 cases) | Chromogranin A, chromogranin B, secretogranin II | 86% | Number of positive cells was counted in at least 50 cancer fields | Overall and disease free survival | Yes; Generalized savage analysis which included grade, stage | 3.6 yrs (range, 1.5–7.3 yrs) | NE differentiation was associated with high Gleason score, but no with stage and patient survival |
| Casella et al. 1998[1290] | 105 | T2 and higher; patients selected 'according to availability of follow-up information'; wide variety of treatments | Needle biopsies | Chromogranin A | 25% (limited biopsy samples) | Subjectively as 'few' or 'numerous' | Cancer-specific survival | 3-group analysis of variance; Gleason score and Ki67 index were predictive, but not NE | Not given | NE differentiation was more frequent and intense in hormone-resistant cancer |

| Study | N | Clinical details | Specimen | Marker | % positive | Staining | Outcome | Multivariate | Follow-up | Conclusion |
|---|---|---|---|---|---|---|---|---|---|---|
| Tan et al. 1999[661] | 41 | Clinical stages: A, 6cases; B, 10 cases; C, 1 case; D, 24 cases | Prostatectomy, TURP specimens | Chromogranin A, NSE | 53.6% | No staining (−), Rare scattered individual positive cells (+), Small clusters of stained cells (++), Large sometimes confluent foci of stained cells (+++) | Systemic progression, cancer-specific survival | Yes, parameters including cancer grade, stage, systemic progression | 5 yrs (range not given) | NE differentiation was not associated with high Gleason score, stage and patient survival |
| Bostwick et al. 2002[652] | 196 | Node-positive prostate cancer treated primarily by radical prostatectomy | Single section of radical prostatectomy or lymph node metastasis | Chromogranin A, serotonin | 98.5% for chromogranin A; 94.9% for serotonin | Subjective in 10% increments; intensity measured independently | Systemic progression, cancer-specific survival, and all-cause survival | Yes, Cox proportional hazards models which included cancer grade, ploidy, volume, progression, survival | 6.8 yrs (range, 0.3–11 yr) | No significant association between the level of chromogranin A with cancer-specific or all-cause survival. Level of serotonin expression was associated with cancer-specific survival, but not for all-cause survival |
| Segawas et al. 2001[657] | 42 | Surgically-treated patients | Diagnostic biopsy specimens | | | | | | | |

**Predictive of Patient Outcome**

| Study | N | Clinical details | Specimen | Marker | % positive | Staining | Outcome | Multivariate | Follow-up | Conclusion |
|---|---|---|---|---|---|---|---|---|---|---|
| Abrahamson et al. 1989[291] | 25 | TURP-detected cancer followed by androgen deprivation therapy (stages A1, A2, B1) | TURP or enucleation prostate specimens | Chromogranin A | 92% | Subjectively as negative (0), isolated single cells (±), rather few scattered cells (+), moderate numbers of cells (++), numerous cells (+++) | Cancer grade in subsequent TURP specimens | No | 5.5 yrs (range, 1–11 yrs) | Most of the 25 tumors underwent marked tumor progression, while the number of NE cells concomitantly increased |
| Cohen et al. 1990, 1992[292,1293] | 90 | TURP or Needle biopsy-detected Stages B (22), C (20), and D (48) | TURP or needle biopsy specimens | Chromogranin A NSE | 52% | Negative (no NE cells present), positive (individual cells or groups of NE cells) | Cancer-specific survival | Yes; grade and NE staining were predictive of tumor progression | >4 yrs (range 4–7 yrs) | NE differentiation was a more important prognostic factor than Gleason score |
| Weinstein et al. 1996[1294] | 104 | Clinically-localized prostate cancer (T1–2) treated by radical prostatectomy | Single section of radical prostatectomy | Chromogranin A | 62% | Maximum number of NE cells at per x100 field | PSA failure | Yes; Cox proportional hazards models which included Gleason grade, NE staining, and tumor progression | 8 yrs (range, 7–10 yrs) | NE differentiation may be a prognostic marker for tumors with intermediate Gleason sum |

**Table 9-30** Predictive value of neuroendocrine differentiation by immunohistochemistry in prostatic adenocarcinoma: collected works—Cont'd

| | No. of patients | Patient population | Tissue studied | NE markers | Cancer cases stained (%) | Quantification of NE staining | Outcome variables | Multivariate analysis | Mean length of follow-up | Comments |
|---|---|---|---|---|---|---|---|---|---|---|
| Krijnen et al. 1997[670] | 72 | TURP-detected cancer followed by androgen deprivation therapy; included 12 stage T1b, 3 stageT2, 36 stage T3, and 21 stage T4 cancers | TURP specimens | Chromogranin A | 55% | Number of positive cells and clusters per 1 mm² tumor area | Progression-free survival | Yes; Cox proportional hazards models, grade and NE staining were predictive | 3 yrs (range, 0.1–7.9 yrs) | Density of NE cells and Gleason score were independent prognostic factors for cancer progression |
| Theodorescu et al. 1997[669] | 71 | T1-2 cancer treated by radical prostatectomy without adjuvant treatment until recurrence | Single section of radical prostatectomy specimen | Chromogranin A (also included cathepsin D) | 24% | Subjectively as negative (0), rare positive cancer cells (1), <1% (2), 1–10% (3), 11–25% (4), 26–50% (5), or >50% (6); number of cells counted not given; for analyses, only 2–6 were considered positive | Cancer-specific survival – 51% of patients has recurrence; 24% died of prostate cancer | Yes; Cox proportional hazards models which included Gleason grade, stage, % cancer in specimen | Median follow-up interval of 10.6 yrs; 53% had more than 10 years of follow-up | Chromogranin A significant in univariate analysis and multivariate analysis with one-variable model, but not two-variable model; Cathepsin D was not predictive of survival in univariate or multivariate analysis |
| Borre et al. 2000[1295] | 221 | Patients treated by watchful waiting | Diagnostic biopsy specimens | VEGF and NE markers | | Semiquantitatively scored as weak, moderate, and strong staining | Cancer-specific survival – 57% died of prostate cancer | Yes; models included VEGF expression and microvessel density | Median follow-up of 15 years | NE differentiation significantly correlated with microvessel density, VEGF expression, and survival |
| Yu et al. 2001[1296] | 30 | Patients treated surgically | Diagnostic biopsy specimens | Chromogranin A, NSE, and serotonin | Chromogranin A (80%), NSE (43%), and serotonin (77%) | Positive and negative | Cancer-specific survival | No | Mean follow-up of 3.7 years | NE differentiation (all three markers) predictive of survival |
| Quek et al. 2006[642] | 140 | Lymph metastatic cancer treated surgically | Prostatectomy and lymph node metastases | Chromogranin A | Primary cancer 61%; lymph node metastases: 12% | Positive and negative | 10-year overall and recurrence-free survival | Yes; models included age | Median follow-up of 10.9 years | NE differentiation in the primary cancer and lymph node metastases correlated with poor overall survival; NE differentiation in the primary cancer correlated with recurrence-free survival |

NE, neuroendocrine; NSE, neuron-specific enolase; TURP, transurethral resection of the prostate; VEGF, vascular endothelial growth factor.

hypercalcemia, the syndrome of inappropriate antidiuretic hormone secretion, and myasthenic (Eaton–Lambert) syndrome.[700]

These tumors are morphologically identical to small cell carcinoma of the lung and other sites (Fig. 9-39). Typical acinar adenocarcinoma is present at least focally in about 25% of cases, and transition patterns may be seen. In cases of adenocarcinoma with a solid Gleason 5 pattern suggestive of neuroendocrine carcinoma, immunohistochemical stains are recommended to confirm differentiation; it should be noted that some cases will be non-reactive. Importantly, the majority of cases of Gleason 5 + 5 = 10 contain at least focal small cell carcinoma.[701]

Immunohistochemically, a wide variety of secretory products may be detected within small cell carcinoma cells, including serotonin, calcitonin, adrenocorticotropic hormone, human chorionic gonadotropin, thyroid-stimulating hormone, bombesin, calcitonin gene-related peptide, atachalcin, and inhibin.[702,703] The same cells may express peptide hormones and PSA and PAP.[700]

Ultrastructurally, small cell carcinoma and carcinoid tumor display features similar to their counterparts in the lung.[644] The characteristic finding is variable numbers of round, regular 100–400 nm diameter membrane-bound neurosecretory granules. Well-defined cytoplasmic processes are usually present, with approximately 8–15 granules per process. The cells are small, with dispersed chromatin and small inconspicuous nucleoli. Acinar formation is lacking in the neuroendocrine component, and no tonofilaments are present.

Large cell neuroendocrine carcinoma is an unusual variant of pure neuroendocrine carcinoma that shares with small cell carcinoma a frequent antecedent history of adenocarcinoma treated with hormone therapy, common coexistence with adenocarcinoma, and rapid metastasis and death.[704] It consists of solid sheets and ribbons of cells with abundant pale to amphophilic cytoplasm, large nuclei with coarse chromatin, prominent nucleoli, brisk mitotic activity, and foci of necrosis. Intense immunoreactivity is seen for CD56, CD57, chromogranin A, synaptophysin, racemase, bcl-2, MIB1, and p53, with focal positive staining for PSA and PAP, and negative androgen receptor staining.[705]

Small cell carcinoma is aggressive and rapidly fatal, and was originally classified by Gleason as a variant of pattern 5 carcinoma. Today, most describe the histogenesis of this cancer without applying a Gleason grade, reserving grading for adenocarcinoma and its variants. Androgen receptor expression in small cell carcinoma was predictive of a poorer outcome (median survival 10 months) than in cases without expression (median survival more than 30 months), regardless of treatment.[706]

Treatment is modeled after those for small cell lung carcinoma; one study found that the addition of doxorubicin to the etoposide/cisplatin regimen improved survival,[707] whereas another found higher toxicity and failure to improve outcome.[708]

Although unusual, metastases to the prostate from other sites may mimic carcinoid and small cell carcinoma of the prostate. High-grade carcinoma from the bladder that invades the prostate may be mistaken for neuroendocrine carcinoma. Other rare tumors, such as peripheral neuroectodermal tumor, desmoplastic small round cell tumor, and malignant lymphoma, may be mistaken for prostatic neuroendocrine carcinoma, particularly in extraprostatic sites.

### Sarcomatoid carcinoma (carcinosarcoma)

Sarcomatoid carcinoma is considered by most to be synonymous with carcinosarcoma.[696,709–714] Authors who separate these tumors define sarcomatoid carcinoma as an epithelial tumor showing spindle cell (mesenchymal) differentiation; carcinosarcoma is defined as adenocarcinoma intimately admixed with identifiable malignant soft tissue elements (Fig. 9-40). Tumors containing areas of bone, cartilage, or striated muscle differentiation are sometimes referred to as

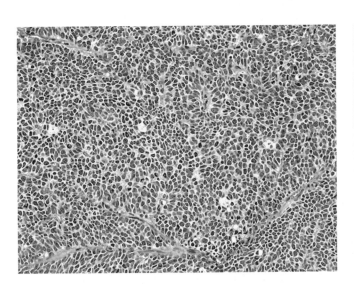

**Fig. 9-39** Small cell undifferentiated (oat cell) carcinoma of the prostate.

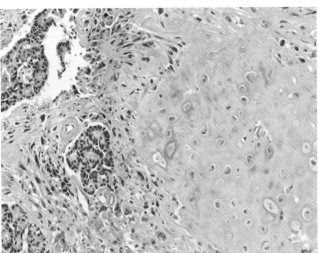

**Fig. 9-40** Sarcomatoid carcinoma (carcinosarcoma) of the prostate, consisting of an intimate admixture of adenocarcinoma and chondroblastic osteosarcoma.

sarcomatoid carcinoma with heterologous elements. Regardless of terminology, these tumors are rare and have a poor prognosis.

Patients tend to be older men who have symptoms of urinary outlet obstruction, similar to typical adenocarcinoma. Serum PSA level may be normal at the time of diagnosis. About half of the patients have a prior history of typical acinar adenocarcinoma treated by radiation therapy or androgen deprivation.[715]

The distinction between sarcomatoid carcinoma and carcinosarcoma is often difficult and of no apparent clinical significance; many authors consider these tumors to be the same entity. In the five cases studied by Shannon and associates, three displayed an intimate mixture of sarcomatoid carcinoma and typical acinar adenocarcinoma, with transition forms.[714] Coexistent adenocarcinoma is almost always high grade (Gleason score 9 or 10). The most common soft tissue elements are osteosarcoma and leiomyosarcoma.[709]

The epithelial component displays cytoplasmic immunoreactivity for keratin, PSA, and PAP, similar to typical prostatic adenocarcinoma. The soft tissue component usually displays immunoreactivity for vimentin, with variable staining for desmin, actin, and S100 protein.

Ultrastructurally, tumor cells within the sarcomatoid areas occasionally display desmosomes and filaments which are apparently cytokeratin. In two cases there was no ultrastructural evidence of epithelial differentiation.[714]

Treatment is variable and has no apparent influence on the poor prognosis. Dundore et al.[709] found a 41% 5-year cancer-specific survival and a 12% 7-year cancer-specific survival in a series of 21 patients from the Mayo Clinic, similar to survival for Gleason score 9 and 10 adenocarcinoma without sarcomatoid features. Of five patients reported by Shannon et al.,[716] three died of tumor within 46 months of diagnosis, one was alive with tumor at 48 months, and one was lost to follow-up after 1 month.[714] Hansel reported that six of seven patients died within 1 year of diagnosis.

Separation of sarcomatoid carcinoma from sarcoma and carcinosarcoma may be difficult and clinically unimportant, although immunohistochemical stains and electron microscopy are helpful. Weak diffuse keratin immunoreactivity has been identified in some cases of leiomyosarcoma, so this finding alone may not be sufficient to determine epithelial differentiation.

### Giant cell carcinoma

Giant cell carcinoma in the prostate is histologically similar to its counterpart in other organs, being composed of pleomorphic giant tumor cells mixed with typical high-grade adenocarcinoma (Fig. 9-41).[717,718] Although exceedingly rare, this variant of prostatic cancer should be considered in the differential diagnosis of metastatic giant cell carcinoma. Patients present with widespread metastases and die soon thereafter; this clinical presentation and aggressive behavior is characteristic of giant cell carcinoma arising in other organs. Giant cell carcinoma is unresponsive to conventional androgen deprivation therapy and is androgen receptor negative by immunohistochemistry. Giant cell carcinoma of the prostate is considered to be Gleason pattern 5.

Controversy exists regarding the histogenesis of giant cell carcinoma. Lopez-Beltran et al.[718] emphasized the importance of radiation therapy and chemotherapy as etiologic factors for spindle cell and giant cell carcinoma in urothelial cancer, and these factors probably apply to this cancer in the prostate.

The most important differential diagnostic considerations of giant cell carcinoma are sarcomatoid carcinoma of the prostate with or without heterologous elements, which occasionally exhibit neoplastic giant cells. By definition, sarcomatoid carcinoma is composed of spindle cells with large, pleomorphic, hyperchromatic nuclei. Other tumors exhibiting giant cells, such as giant cell carcinoma of the bladder, urothelial carcinoma with osteoclast-type giant cells or trophoblastic differentiation should also be considered. Osteoclast-type giant cells have some features of giant cell tumor of bone and are immunoreactive for vimentin and CD68 but not cytokeratin, whereas trophoblastic cells are immunoreactive for β-hCG. Exceptionally, neoplastic giant cells and osteoclast-type cells may be present in the same neoplasm, although this has not been described in the prostate. Immunohistochemical stains for keratin, PSA, and PAP are useful in verifying the epithelial nature of giant cell carcinoma.

### Adenoid cystic/basal cell carcinoma

Grossly, adenoid cystic/basal cell carcinoma is white and fleshy, sometimes with microcysts, unlike acinar carcinoma which is usually yellow. It invariably involved the transition zone with or without peripheral zone involvement.[719,720]

Microscopically, it consists of tumor nests or nodules of various size embedded in a desmoplastic or myxoid stroma (Fig. 9-42). The adenoid pattern is characterized by nests and trabeculae of cells with cribriform growth and microcystic spaces with abundant basement membrane material. The basaloid pattern consists of nests of hematoxyphilic cells with microvacuolated nuclei, scant cytoplasm, and peripheral palisading, virtually identical to basal cell carcinoma of the skin. There is occasional squamous metaplasia with keratinization that may be reminiscent of eccrine spiradenoma, although the latter is lobulated and has never been described in the prostate. Tumor necrosis is uncommon (Table 9-31).

Perineural invasion is often prominent, and rarely intraneural invasion is present. Metastases usually have a predominant adenoid pattern of tumor and are limited to lymph nodes, liver, lung, and bowel (no bone metastases have been reported to date).[719]

Immunohistochemical findings indicate that adenoid cystic/basal cell carcinoma is a biphasic ductal/myoepithelial tumor, similar to its counterpart in the salivary gland.[101,721-725] All cases are at least focally immunoreactive for cytokeratin AE1/3, basal cell cytokeratin 34βE12, and p63 in up to 90% of cells (Table 9-32).[719] Staining with cytokeratin 34βE12 is present in the peripheral but not the luminal cells of the adenoid nests; conversely, staining for

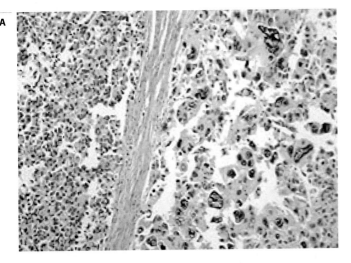

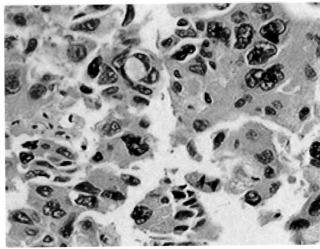

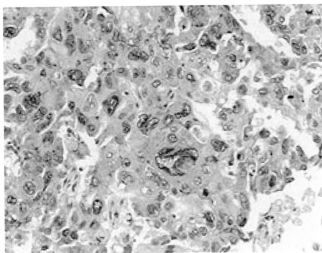

**Fig. 9-41** Giant cell carcinoma. (**A, B**) This unusual cancer is composed of large cells with single or multiple bizarre enlarged hyperchromatic nuclei with adjacent (left) typical high-grade adenocarcinoma. (**C**) PSA immunoreactivity within the majority of cells confirms prostatic origin.

keratin 7 was observed only in luminal cells. No tumors react with keratin 20. Remarkably, cytoplasmic reactivity is noted for S100 protein in a small but significant number of cells (up to 20%) in 63% of cases; α-smooth muscle actin immunoreactivity is present in up to 70% of cells in a minority of cases.[719] There is also strong immunoreactivity in all cases for CD44 and HER-2/neu.[726]

The rarity of immunoreactivity for PSA and PAP (patchy staining limited to luminal cells of adenoid nests with a cribriform pattern) is consistent with the normal preoperative serum PSA usually observed with this variant of adenocarcinoma. No messenger RNA for PSA was detected by in situ hybridization.[723]

Adenoid cystic/basal cell carcinoma has a small but significant potential for late recurrence and metastasis.[719] It often coexists with typical acinar adenocarcinoma, but the absence of transition forms strongly suggests coincidental coexistence or rare collision tumor. Perineural growth is typical, similar to its counterpart in other organs. Prostatic basal cells are not androgen-dependent, unlike typical acinar adenocarcinoma, so adenoic cystic/basal cell carcinoma is considered unresponsive to androgen deprivation therapy.

## Lymphoepithelioma-like carcinoma

Carcinoma accompanied by a dense lymphocytic infiltrate is termed lymphoepithelioma, lymphoepithelioma-like carcinoma, or medullary carcinoma (Fig. 9-43). This histologically distinctive tumor is most common in the head and neck but has rarely arisen in the breast, bladder, and other sites. Rare cases have been reported in the prostate.[712,727] Although prostatic adenocarcinoma may be associated with granulomatous prostatitis or patchy acute and chronic inflammation, it rarely appears as solid islands of epithelial cells punctuating a sheet-like infiltrate of lymphocytes characteristic of lymphoepithelioma-like carcinoma at other sites. The tumor has large areas of typical adenocarcinoma, but the different patterns are not intermingled.

Immunohistochemistry revealed that the lymphocytic infiltrate was composed chiefly of T cells, similar to the lymphocytic response in lymphoepithelioma-like carcinomas at other sites. No atypical lymphocytes were observed, and these were not the features of malignant lymphoma or leukemia involving the prostate. Flow cytometry revealed that the tumor was aneuploid. In situ hybridization was negative for Epstein–Barr virus.

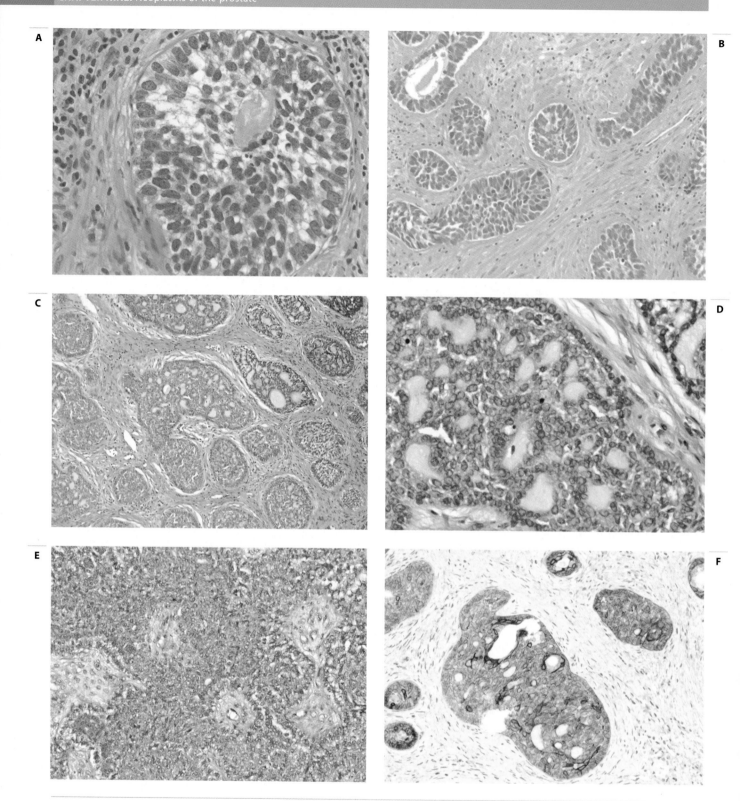

**Fig. 9-42** Adenoid cystic carcinoma of the prostate. (**A, B**) Nests of basaloid cells are punctuated by round punched-out lumina with abundant mucin. (**C, D**) Adenoid cystic pattern. (**E**) Basal cell pattern. (**F**) Strong immunoreactivity fo basal cell-specific keratin 34βE12.

**Table 9-31** Comparative histology of adenoid cystic/basal cell carcinoma with benign basal cell proliferations

|  | Benign basal cell proliferations* | Adenoid cystic/ basal cell carcinoma |
| --- | --- | --- |
| Layers of cells | Multilayered | Multilayered |
| Contour | Rounded, circumscribed nodule | Infiltrative nests or trabeculae |
| Lumen formation | If present, bounded by secretory cells | Present, bounded by basal cells; prominent in adenoid pattern |
| Basement membrane deposits | Absent | Present in lumina |
| Cribriform formations | Absent | Present in adenoid pattern |
| Stroma | Unaltered | Myxoid or desmoplastic |
| Extraprostatic extension | Absent | May be present |
| Perineural invasion | Absent | May be present |
| Macronucleoli | May be present | Present |

*Includes basal cell hyperplasia, atypical basal cell hyperplasia, and basal cell adenoma.

**Table 9-32** Immunohistochemical reactivity of adenoid cystic/basal cell carcinoma

|  | Cases tested | Positive cases | Range of cells positive (%) |
| --- | --- | --- | --- |
| **Prostate Cancer Markers** | | | |
| Cytokeratin 34βE12 | 15 | 15 (100%) | 40–90 |
| p63 | 7 | 6 (86%) | 40–100 |
| P540S/AMACR | 3 | 0 | |
| **Other Markers** | | | |
| CD44 | 10 | 9 (90%) | 100 |
| c-kit | 1 | 1 | 5 |
| Cytokeratin 7 | 12 | 12 (100%)* | 30–90 |
| Cytokeratin 20 | 7 | 0 | |
| Prostate-specific antigen | 10 | 2 (20%)* | <5 |
| Prostatic acid phosphatase | 8 | 1 (14%)* | 1 |
| S100 protein | 8 | 5 (63%) | 2–20 |
| α-Smooth muscle actin | 8 | 2 (25%) | 30–70 |

*In adluminal cells.

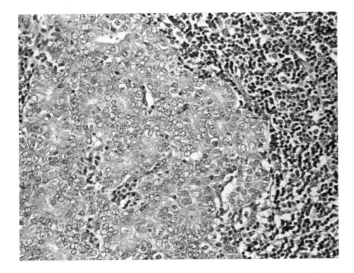

**Fig. 9-43** Lymphoepithelioma-like carcinoma of the prostate.

## Carcinoma with oncocytic features

Rare cases of prostatic adenocarcinoma with diffuse oncocytic change have been reported, characterized by tumor cells with abundant eosinophilic granular cytoplasm reflecting the presence of abundant mitochondria.[728,729] Tumor cells displayed PSA immunoreactivity. The clinical behavior appears to be the same as that of typical acinar adenocarcinoma. Differential diagnosis includes prostatic nodular hyperplasia with oncocytic change (oncocytoma), neuroendocrine carcinoma, and rhabdoid tumor.

### Adenocarcinoma with glomeruloid features

Prostatic cancer with glomeruloid features is characterized by the presence of acinar adenocarcinoma with round to oval epithelial buds (glomerulations) projecting into acinar lumina, architecturally mimicking renal glomeruli (Fig. 9-44).[730] There is an external layer of 'parietal' cells and a conspicuous central tuft of 'visceral' cells. The central tuft sometimes has a cribriform architecture; in other cases a prominent central fibrovascular core is present. Less commonly there is a characteristic concentric infolding of epithelial cells arranged in semicircular rows with delimiting cleft-shaped spaces.

Three percent of needle biopsies and 4.5% of prostatectomies with prostate cancer contain glomeruloid features.[730] A minority of each cancer (up to 20%) consisted of glomeruloid features, and the remaining typical acinar adenocarcinoma was usually Gleason score 6 or 7.[730] The cases were equally divided between the apex and the peripheral zone.

Glomeruloid structures appear to be a specific but uncommon finding in prostate cancer.[21,387,730,731] They are not observed in any benign or hyperplastic processes in radical prostatectomies or needle biopsies. This feature appears to be a useful diagnostic clue for malignancy, and may be valuable in some challenging needle biopsy specimens.

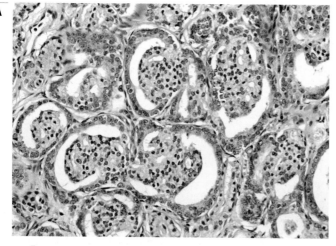

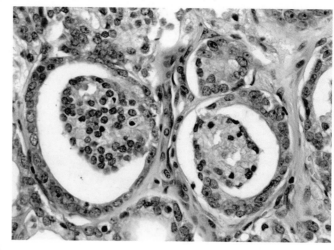

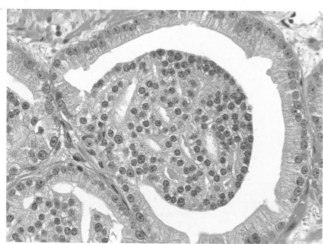

**Fig. 9-44** Adenocarcinoma with glomeruloid features. (**A**) Multiple epithelial buds protrude into acinar spaces, reminiscent of renal glomeruli. (**B**) Each glomerulation shows cribriform growth with a dominant cellular bridge connecting it to the rest of the acinus; in this case, the nuclei in the glomerulation have indistinct nucleoli; compare with **C,** another case in which the nuclei in the glomerulation have prominent nucleoli.

Adenocarcinoma with glomeruloid features may be mistaken for the invasive cribriform pattern of carcinoma. In cribriform carcinoma the cellular bridges around the periphery of the nests are usually relatively evenly spaced and similar in size. In contrast, glomeruloid structures show a distinctive polarity of growth, with a dominant cellular bridge connecting the central cell mass to the periphery. Other cellular bridges may be seen focally, but are thin and few in number. Fibrovascular cores are less common in cribriform carcinoma, and semicircular delimiting concentric cleft-like spaces are lacking. In some cases the glomeruloid and cribriform patterns coexist. It is possible that these two patterns represent a spectrum of differentiation.

Casiraghi and coworkers[732] reported a case of primary Wilms' tumor of the prostate showing glomeruloid structures. This tumor apparently arose from nephrogenic rests in relation to the wolffian duct system, and showed the classic triphasic histological pattern typical of Wilms' tumor. Glomeruloid microvascular proliferations in the prostate are related to increased microvessel density and reduced survival.[453] To our knowledge, no other processes occurring in the prostate possess glomeruloid features.

Adenocarcinoma with glomeruloid features is currently regarded as Gleason grade 3. Further studies are needed to determine the independent prognostic value of the glomeruloid growth pattern and its correlation with Gleason grading.

### Adenocarcinoma with atrophic features

Acinar atrophy and postatrophic hyperplasia in the prostate are commonly confused with adenocarcinoma,[733] and the converse situation also presents a diagnostic dilemma. Cancer acini with round dilated and distorted lumina and flattened lining cells with scant cytoplasm are referred to as 'atrophic' cancer (Fig. 9-45).[390,734] This is an unusual pattern that is easily mistaken for atrophy. All cases had cytologic evidence of malignancy, including nuclear enlargement and prominent nucleoli; these findings could not be attributed to inflammation or treatment effect.[390]

Atrophic features were identified in cancer in 3% of radical prostatectomy specimens and 2% of needle biopsies.[390] The proportion of cancer with atrophic features comprised a mean of 27% of each tumor in the prostatectomy specimens (range 10–60%) and 24% in the needle biopsies (range 10–90%).

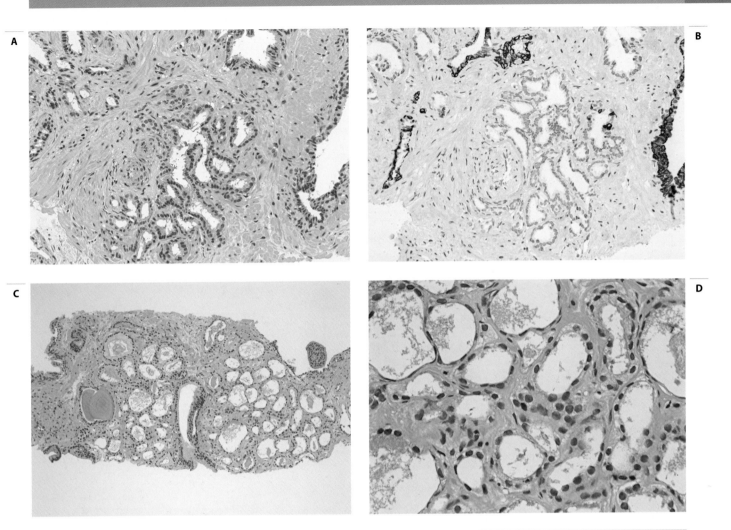

**Fig. 9-45** Atrophic pattern of adenocarcinoma. (**A**) The large irregular acini (center of image) have dilated lumina with modest cytoplasm and hyperchromatic nuclei; at this magnification, it is difficult to distinguish between atrophy and atrophic pattern of cancer. (**B**) The focus of concern lacks basal cells, confirming the suspicion of cancer, with positive internal control indicating benign acini at the periphery (immunohistochemical stain for keratin 34βE12). (**C**) Cancer acini with round dilated and distorted lumina. (**D**) Higher magnification shows acini lined by flattened cells with scant cytoplasm and enlarged nuclei with prominent nucleoli.

Caution is warranted in rendering this difficult diagnosis on needle biopsies with only a small amount of cancer.[390,734] Racemase was expressed in 70% of atrophic prostate cancers compared to weak staining in up to 13% of cases of atrophy; the authors concluded that racemase immunostaining alone was not sufficiently discriminatory by itself, and a panel of immunostains including racemase, keratin 34βE12, and p63 was recommended.[735]

### Adenocarcinoma with microvacuolated cytoplasm (foamy gland carcinoma; xanthomatoid carcinoma)

This adenocarcinoma consists of cells with abundant microvacuoles in the cytoplasm that displace the nuclei basally (Fig. 9-46).[736–741] Patient age is similar to that for typical acinar adenocarcinoma, and preoperative serum PSA level in one study ranged from 2.7 to 37.5 ng/mL (mean, 15.2 ng/mL).[737] Diagnostic difficulty is encountered when this pattern predominates owing to the small size and lack of nuclear hyperchromasia that may be interpreted as benign.[742] Nuclear enlargement and prominent nucleoli were either absent or rare in respectively 61% and 71% of foamy gland carcinomas in a study of needle biopsies.[739]

Foamy gland cancer is negative for mucin and lipid stains, but positive for colloidal iron and Alcian blue stain. About 68% of cases stain with racemase.[736] Ultrastructurally, the foamy cells displayed numerous intracytoplasmic vesicles and numerous polyribosomes.[737]

Patients with foamy gland carcinoma tend to have high-volume bilateral cancer and an aggressive course, although the number of cases with long-term follow-up is very limited.[737,739]

### Pseudohyperplastic adenocarcinoma

At low magnification, this low-grade carcinoma (Gleason primary pattern 2 or 3) may be mistaken for an exuberant hyperplastic nodule.[742–744] It consists of large atypical glands

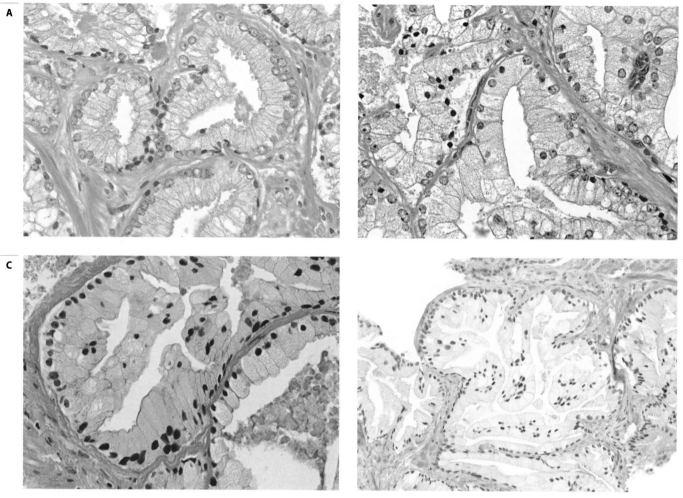

**Fig. 9-46** Foamy gland carcinoma. (**A**) Note pale eosinophilic with finely vacuolated cytoplasm, distinct cell membranes, basal nuclei, and small punctate nucleoli. (**B**) Another case with clear cytoplasm and finely vacuolated cytoplasm. (**C**) A third case with clear finely vacuolated cytoplasm and hyperchromatic nuclei with indistinct nucleoli; compare with **D**, showing absence of immunoreactivity for basal cell-specific keratin 34βE12, immunohistochemical confirmation of the diagnosis of carcinoma.

with branching, papillary infoldings, and corpora amylacea in 20% of cases (Fig. 9-47). The incidence is about 2% in biopsies and 1.3% in transurethral resections.[745] Features most helpful in establishing a malignant diagnosis with this variant are nuclear enlargement (95% of cases), pink amorphous secretions (70%), occasional to frequent nucleoli (45%), and crystalloids (45%),[744] and transition to small acinar pattern of adenocarcinoma.[745] Immunostains for basal cell cytokeratin 34βE12, racemase, and p63 are often required to confirm this lesion as malignant;[285] in our experience the entire focus is negative, in striking contrast to adjacent benign glands. About 77% of cases are positive for racemase.[736] This lesion is histologically distinctive, but it does not warrant separation as a clinicopathologic entity.

### Squamous cell and adenosquamous cell carcinoma

Squamous cell carcinoma is very rare in the prostate, with fewer than 100 published cases.[746–766] Adenosquamous carcinoma refers to the combination of squamous cell carci-

noma and typical acinar carcinoma, and appears to be even more rare than pure squamous cell carcinoma.[766,767]

Presenting signs and symptoms are similar to those of the typical adenocarcinoma, although there is often a history of hormonal or radiation therapy. Patients are more than 50 years of age, with a mean in the seventh decade. PSA and PAP levels are usually normal, even with metastases, and bone metastases are typically osteolytic rather than osteoblastic. Squamous cell carcinoma of the prostate may arise in patients infected with *Schistosoma haematobium*.

Squamous cell carcinoma is histologically similar to its counterpart in other organs, consisting of irregular nests and cords of malignant cells with keratinization and squamous differentiation, rarely with squamous pearls (Fig. 9-48). Keratinizing squamous cell carcinoma usually arises in the periurethral ducts and is very rare; otherwise, the site of origin of squamous cell carcinoma is unknown. Mott[768] required an absence of acinar differentiation for the diagnosis of squamous cell carcinoma, as well as a lack of bladder

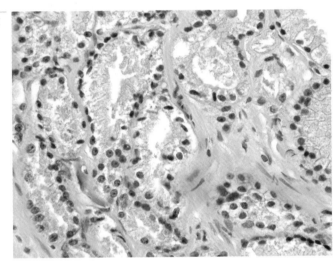

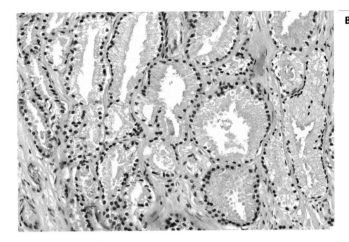

**Fig. 9-47 (A–C)** Pseudohyperplastic carcinoma. Well-differentiated adenocarcinoma (Gleason 1 + 1 = 2) in transurethral resection consists of uniformly spaced acini mimicking hyperplastic epithelium.

involvement; mixed tumors are best classified simply as adenosquamous carcinoma. Mott also required no prior estrogen therapy, but we consider this exclusion unnecessary. Metastases may consist of adenosquamous carcinoma in cases without a squamous component in the primary tumor, perhaps due to sampling error.

Saito et al.[769] identified PAP immunoreactivity in the acinar and squamous components of their case of adenosquamous carcinoma. Conversely, Gattuso et al.[767] found staining only in the acinar component of their case; interestingly, they noted immunoreactivity in the squamous component for high molecular weight keratin AE-3, but not in the acinar component. The adenosquamous carcinoma reported by Devaney et al.[766] showed PSA and PAP immunoreactivity in the acinar component but not in the squamous component; both components were diploid.

The histogenesis of squamous and adenosquamous carcinoma is unknown, but proposed origins include multipotential stem cells, basal cells or reserve cells, columnar secretory cells, prostatic urethral or periurethral urothelial cells, cells of adenocarcinoma, and metaplastic squamous cells. Most contemporary authors believe that the cancer arises from the urothelium of the urethra or large periurethral prostatic ducts.

Squamous cell carcinoma is aggressive, with a mean survival of about 14 months regardless of therapy. These tumors appear to be unresponsive to androgen deprivation therapy.

Squamous cell carcinoma may be confused with squamous metaplasia due to infarction, radiation therapy, and hormonal therapy. Rarely, adenocarcinoma may exhibit benign squamous metaplasia. Squamous cell carcinoma of the bladder may invade the prostate and must be excluded.

## Other epithelial neoplasms

### Urothelial carcinoma

Urothelial carcinoma of the prostate is rarely primary, accounting for less than 4% of tumors originating in the prostate, and usually represents synchronous or metachronous spread from carcinoma in the bladder and urethra (Fig. 9-49).[770–773] It involves the prostate in about 40% of radical cystoprostatectomy specimens for bladder carcinoma. Up to 41% of patients have unsuspected coexistent prostatic adenocarcinoma.[774]

Patients usually have symptoms of hematuria, urinary obstruction, or prostatitis. Serum PSA and PAP levels are not elevated. Clinically, urothelial carcinoma may be mistaken

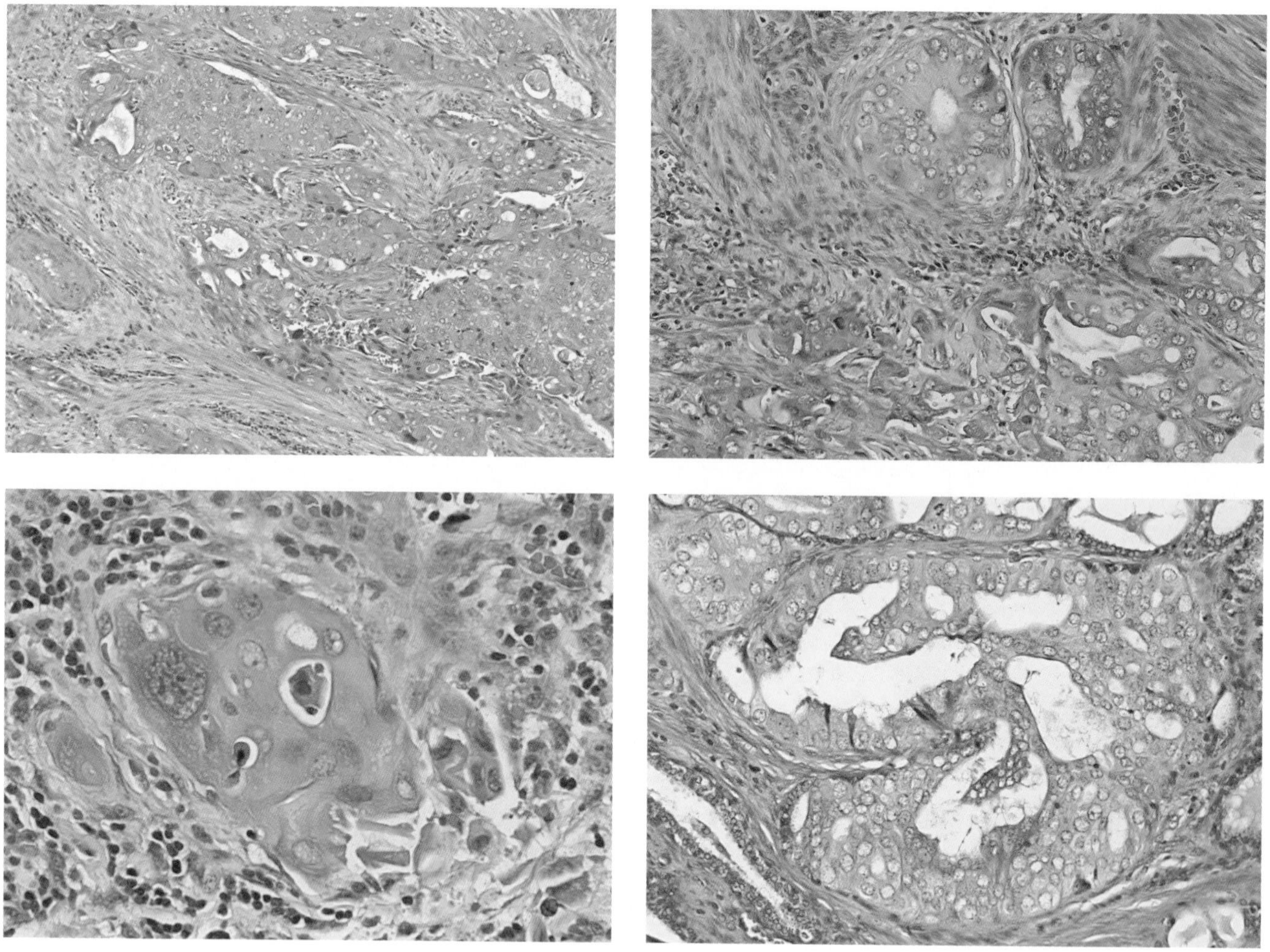

**Fig. 9-48** Adenosquamous cell carcinoma of the prostate. This tumor was identified many years after radiation therapy and androgen deprivation therapy for typical acinar adenocarcinoma. (**A, B**) Mixed glandular and squamous elements. (**C**) High-grade squamous cell carcinoma with keratinization. (**D**) Glandular differentiation.

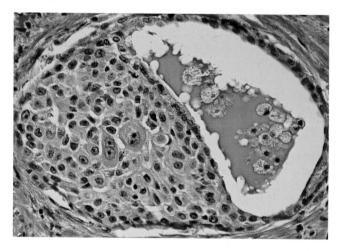

**Fig. 9-49** Urothelial carcinoma showing pagetoid spread through this periurethral prostatic duct.

for prostatitis or nodular hyperplasia. Most clinical findings are due to tumor arising elsewhere in the urothelium.

Urothelial carcinoma involves the periurethral prostatic ducts and acini. A total of 62% of cases diagnosed by needle biopsy consist of urothelial carcinoma in situ of prostatic ducts and acini; 29% consist of both CIS and invasive carcinoma; and 9% have widespread stromal invasion without CIS.[775] Diagnostic criteria are identical to those for urothelial cancer of the bladder; most cancers are moderately or poorly differentiated and usually associated with prominent chronic inflammation. Squamous metaplasia is infrequent.

Sakamoto and colleagues[363] showed that transurethral resection containing prostatic tissue at the 5 and/or 7 o'clock positions of the verumontanum substantially improved the detection of ductal and acinar involvement. Moreover, if superficial glands are involved at these positions, involvement of deeper glands should also be suspected.

Radical cystoprostatectomy is the treatment of choice for invasive urothelial carcinoma of the prostate.[776,777] Bladder cancer extending into the prostate can easily be missed cystoscopically and random biopsies of the prostate are recommended. The 5-year cancer-specific survival rates for the locoregional categories were as follows: CIS of the prostatic urethra and prostatic ducts and acini, 100%; stromal invasion, 45%; extraprostatic extension and seminal vesicle involvement, 0%; and lymph node metastases, 30%.[773]

Distinguishing urothelial carcinoma from adenocarcinoma is clinically important because of the estrogen unresponsiveness of the former; these tumors often coexist coincidentally. On light microscopy adenocarcinoma usually displays some evidence of acinar differentiation, although this may be difficult to identify in high-grade cancers or cases of urothelial carcinoma with pseudoglandular pattern. Immunohistochemical stains for PSA and PAP distinguish these tumors, with immunoreactivity exclusively in adenocarcinoma. Also, keratin 34βE12 is highly specific and sensitive for urothelial carcinoma regardless of grade. Other differential diagnostic considerations include urothelial-type prostatic adenocarcinoma and urothelial differentiation in prostatic carcinosarcoma.[711]

Urothelial carcinoma often arises in patients with previous radiation therapy for prostate cancer, and is usually high grade with a high incidence of sarcomatoid features.[778-780]

## Melanoma

Malignant melanoma of the prostate is histologically identical to its counterpart arising at other sites.[781] A bladder and urethral mucosal origin is much more common.

## Other rare epithelial tumors

A single case of primary Wilms' tumor of the prostate was reported arising in a 32-year-old man with hemospermia and obstructive symptoms.[732] The characteristic triphasic pattern was observed, including blastema, epithelial tubules, and spindled stroma. The patient developed pulmonary metastases 1 year after presentation. Extrarenal Wilms' tumor is thought to arise from embryonic rests of metanephric blastema, explaining the occurrence of this tumor in other urogenital areas, such as the scrotum, spermatic cord, and in an ovotestis. The differential diagnosis includes sarcoma such as rhabdomyosarcoma, sarcomatoid carcinoma, and teratoma.

## Carcinoma metastatic to prostate

Tumors arising in other organs occasionally involve the prostate, usually due to contiguous spread, but metastases are extremely rare, [629,782] with involvement at autopsy in 0.5–2.2% of men dying of malignancies. The most common tumor metastasizing to the prostate is squamous cell carcinoma of the bronchus, which accounts for almost half of all metastases. Malignant melanoma accounts for approximately 27% of prostatic metastases, with an incidence of

prostatic involvement of 1.1% of patients with malignant melanoma at autopsy.[783] An unusual case was reported of tumor-to-tumor metastasis of malignant melanoma to prostatic adenocarcinoma.[783] The remaining 25% of metastases to prostate arise from a variety of sites, including the skin,[784] pancreas, and stomach.

## Treatment changes in prostate cancer

Treatment changes in the cancerous prostate create a diagnostic challenge in pathologic interpretation, particularly in needle biopsy specimens and evaluation of extraprostatic metastases. It is critical that the clinician provide the pertinent history of androgen deprivation or radiation therapy to assist the pathologist in rendering the correct diagnosis.

### Androgen deprivation therapy

One of the most popular forms of treatment for prostate cancer, androgen deprivation therapy, has been in use for more than five decades. Contemporary therapies have varying mechanisms of action, including combined androgen blockage (gonadotropin-releasing hormone (GnRH) agonists (e.g., goserelin and leuprolide) combined with an androgen receptor antagonist such as flutamide, bicalutamide, or nilutamide), GnRH antagonists (e.g., abarelix), and 5α-reductase inhibitors (e.g., finasteride and dutasteride). These agents are used for preoperative tumor shrinkage, symptomatic relief of metastases, cancer prophylaxis,[785,786] and treatment of hyperplasia.[787,788]

To achieve total androgen deprivation, therapy should be effective in eliminating both testicular and adrenal hormones. Typical side effects of androgen deprivation therapy include hot flashes, loss of libido, and impotence.

Pathologic findings after androgen deprivation

The histopathologic effects of most agents are similar (Table 9-33) (Figs 9-50, 9-51).[263,265,278,563,789-793] All modes of hormonal treatment alter the cancerous prostatic epithelium, inducing programmed apoptosis characterized by fragmentation of tumor DNA, the appearance of apoptotic bodies, and inhibition of cell growth. The altered epithelium dis-

**Table 9-33** Androgen deprivation therapy: histologic features in prostatic adenocarcinoma*

| |
|---|
| Loss of glandular architecture |
| Nuclear shrinkage |
| Nuclear hyperchromasia and pyknosis |
| Nucleolar shrinkage |
| Mucinous degeneration |
| Other cytologic changes similar to benign secretory cell layer |

*There is some variability in these changes depending on the treatment method.

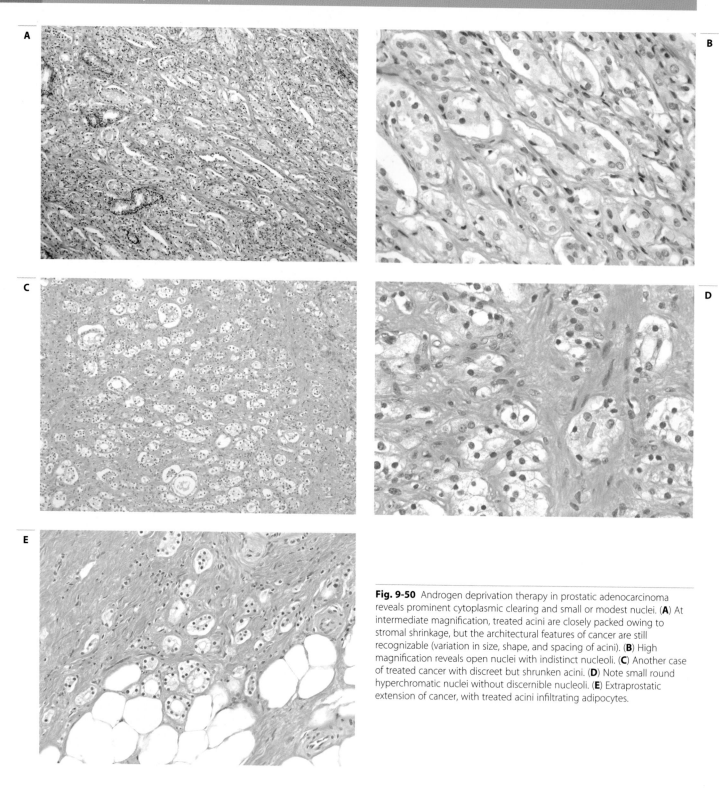

**Fig. 9-50** Androgen deprivation therapy in prostatic adenocarcinoma reveals prominent cytoplasmic clearing and small or modest nuclei. (**A**) At intermediate magnification, treated acini are closely packed owing to stromal shrinkage, but the architectural features of cancer are still recognizable (variation in size, shape, and spacing of acini). (**B**) High magnification reveals open nuclei with indistinct nucleoli. (**C**) Another case of treated cancer with discreet but shrunken acini. (**D**) Note small round hyperchromatic nuclei without discernible nucleoli. (**E**) Extraprostatic extension of cancer, with treated acini infiltrating adipocytes.

plays involution and acinar atrophy, cytoplasmic clearing, nuclear and nucleolar shrinkage, and chromatin condensation, although changes with 5α-reductase inhibitors appear to be much less pronounced and variable than with other agents (see below).

Prostatic adenocarcinoma displays distinctive histologic changes following androgen deprivation therapy. Architec-

turally, the majority of treated cancers have the appearance of Gleason primary grades 4 and 5, with a variety of patterns, including compressed fused glands, sheets of tumor cells, small cell clusters, and single-file ribbons of cells.

Treated tumor cells contain abundant clear vacuolated cytoplasm and central shrunken hyperchromatic nuclei, obscuring the nucleoli and creating a 'nucleolus-poor' appearance in many areas.[794] Anisonucleosis is significantly lower in treated cases than in untreated cases. Longer duration of androgen deprivation further reduces nuclear size. Necrosis and luminal crystalloids are usually absent. The combination of irregular cell clusters and single-file ribbons of tumor cells, cytoplasmic clearing, and shrunken hyperchromatic nuclei is strikingly reminiscent of lobular carcinoma of the breast. This pattern presents similar difficulties in differentiating small tumor foci from treatment-altered benign glands and lymphocytes, particularly in metastatic lymph node deposits. The uncoupling of the architectural and cytologic pattern is vexing owing to the identification of small shrunken nuclei within malignant acini, particularly in lymph nodes submitted for frozen section evaluation.[565] Immunohistochemical studies with basal cell-specific markers and racemase are useful in difficult cases.

Têtu et al.[795] described atypical microacini in treated adenocarcinoma characterized by a single cell layer with large nucleoli, cytoplasmic vacuolation, and a 'hemangiopericytoma-like' arrangement, but this was uncommon.

## Pathologic findings after 5α-reductase inhibitors

The primary nuclear androgen responsible for the maintenance of epithelial function, and the most potent, is dihydrotestosterone (DHT).[796] By inhibiting DHT synthesis, 5α-reductase inhibitors reduce the androgen drive to hyperplastic and malignant prostate cells while maintaining testosterone levels. Finasteride inhibits only the type 2 isoenzyme of 5α-reductase, thereby partially blocking conversion of testosterone. Unlike finasteride, dutasteride is a dual inhibitor of both 5α-reductase isoenzymes,[797] resulting in the suppression of serum DHT by more than 90%, compared to 70% seen with finasteride.[798,799] Finasteride and dutasteride are less effective than other forms of androgen deprivation therapy in altering the histology of the benign and neoplastic prostate (Fig. 9-52), although some changes have been described in all but one report (details below).

Only a few reports have evaluated the histopathology of prostate cancer after 5α-reductase inhibitor treatment.[800–802] Civantos et al.[800] analyzed five radical prostatectomy specimens from patients treated for 3–24 months, and found that the effects of finasteride were more prominent in Gleason primary grades 2 and 3 cancer, making it difficult to recognize at low power and mimicking high Gleason grade cancer. Also, they noted that finasteride did not significantly alter the cribriform pattern of primary grades 3 and 4 cancer, and such foci should also not be overgraded as grades 4 and 5.[800] Conversely, Yang et al.[801] prospectively studied 53 needle biopsy specimens with cancer and found no differences between finasteride-treated and untreated cases for a variety of histopathologic features, including Gleason score, number of cores involved with cancer, extent of cancer in the biopsies, atrophic changes in cancer cells, number of mitotic figures, amount of luminal mucin, and presence of prominent nucleoli. They noted that their results were limited by sampling variation, but cancer was readily identifiable after finasteride treatment.

The Prostate Cancer Prevention trial (PCPT) was the first large-scale study to provide significant evidence for the role of 5α-reductase inhibitors in the chemoprevention of prostate cancer.[803] PCPT demonstrated that treatment with finasteride in a 7-year period was associated with a 24.8% decrease in the prevalence of prostate cancer versus placebo.[804] However, tumors with higher Gleason scores (7–10) were detected significantly more frequently in the treated versus the placebo group (37.0% vs 22.2%),[804] raising concerns that alteration in the androgen milieu by 5α-reductase inhibition may promote the growth of more aggressive tumors. One proven effect of finasteride is shrinkage of the prostate, and it is likely that there is increased detection of cancer (particularly large cancers), probably accounting for the appearance of higher Gleason scores (an example of sampling [detection] bias).[277]

Iczkowski and colleagues[802,805] reported the histopathologic effect in cancer after dutasteride therapy, comparing the pathologic findings in radical prostatectomy specimens from men receiving placebo and those preoperatively treated with a 5–11-week course of the 5α-reductase inhibitor dutasteride.[802] They found that cancer volume was lower in dutasteride-treated men than in the placebo-treated group (15% vs 24%). Also, the percentage of atrophic epithelium was increased and the stroma/gland ratio was doubled. The treatment alteration effect score was doubled and did not correlate with Gleason score changes.[802] These findings indicate that dutasteride probably has a chemopreventive or chemoactive role.

Dutasteride's effect on the development of prostate cancer was studied in 4325 men with benign hyperplasia randomized to 0.5 mg/day dutasteride or placebo.[277] The investigators reported that the incidence of cancer was 51% lower in the dutasteride than in the placebo group (1.2% vs 2.5%) at 27 months.[277] The Reduction by Dutasteride of Prostate Cancer Events (REDUCE) study is a chemoprevention trial designed to determine the effects of 0.5 mg dutasteride daily on the risk of biopsy-detectable prostate cancer. A total of 8000 men were randomized to receive dutasteride or placebo for 4 years.[277] This study should provide definitive data concerning the role of dual 5α-reductase inhibition in chemoprevention, including an understanding of the effects of comprehensive DHT suppression on tumor grade.[277]

## Differential diagnosis

The main differential diagnostic considerations of carcinoma following androgen deprivation therapy are a variety of atrophic and hyperplastic changes in benign glands, including clear cell cribriform hyperplasia, sclerosing adenosis, acinar atrophy, post-atrophic hyperplasia, atypical adenomatous hyperplasia, and atypical basal cell hyperplasia. Significant difficulty may be encountered in separating minute clusters and single-file ribbons of tumor cells after androgen deprivation from lymphocytes, myocytes, and fibroblasts, particularly on a cell-by-cell basis in some foci. Casual low-power scanning of some areas may fail to identify tumor because of the deceptively benign-appearing tinctorial appearance of the cytoplasm and nuclei after therapy. Untreated prostatic adenocarcinoma may have a clear cell pattern, particularly when arising in the transition zone in association with nodular hyperplasia, but it is usually well differentiated (Gleason primary patterns 1 and 2) at that site, exhibits

prominent nucleoli, and is not usually seen with atrophic glands with abundant clear cell change.

### Stage and surgical margins after androgen deprivation therapy

The volume of prostate cancer is reduced by more than 40% after treatment,[265,806] and there is a 20–25% decline in positive margins at radical prostatectomy.[263] Pathologic stage is similar in both untreated and treated prostatic adenocarcinoma, according to retrospective reports of radical prostatectomies, although there is a trend toward lower stage in treated cases.[263,278,807] Occasional cases after therapy display the 'vanishing cancer' phenomenon in which no residual cancer was found in the radical prostatectomy specimen.[455]

### Immunohistochemical findings after androgen deprivation therapy

Expression of PSA, PAP, and racemase is retained in tumor cells after 3 months of therapy, but declines with longer duration of therapy;[808] keratin 34βE12 and p63 remain negative, regardless of duration, indicating an absent basal cell layer[808] (Table 9-34). No differences were found in the expression of neuroendocrine differentiation markers such as chromogranin, neuron-specific enolase, β-hCG, and serotonin following androgen deprivation therapy,[655,809] although some claim a significant increase.[650,810,811] Proliferating cell nuclear antigen (PCNA) immunoreactivity declines after androgen deprivation therapy, indicating that androgens regulate cyclically expressed proteins involved in cell prolif-

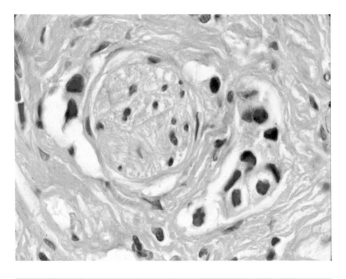

**Fig. 9-51** Perineural invasion by prostatic adenocarcinoma following androgen deprivation therapy.

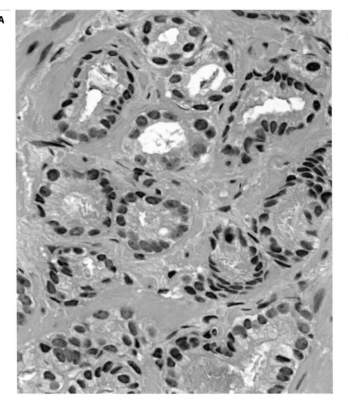

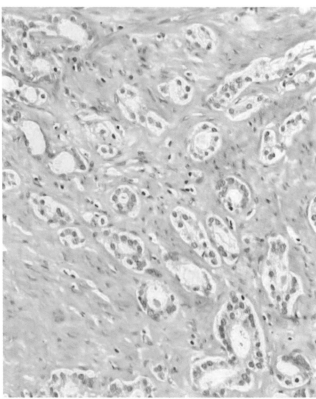

**Fig. 9-52** Dutasteride changes in adenocarcinoma. (**A**) Untreated. (**B**) Three months after treatment.

**Table 9-34** Immunohistochemical changes following androgen deprivation therapy

| Biomarker | Effect of androgen deprivation on cancer* |
|---|---|
| Prostate-specific antigen (PSA) | Unchanged |
| Prostatic acid phosphatase (PAP) | Unchanged |
| Prostate-specific membrane antigen (PSMA) | Unchanged |
| Basal cell-specific keratin 34βE12 | Unchanged |
| Neuroendocrine markers | Unchanged |
| Integrins IL-3, IL-6, M-CSF, TNF-α | Unchanged |
| Estrogen receptors | Increased |
| NM23-H2 | Increased |
| A-80 mucin glycoprotein | Increased |
| Tissue transglutaminase | Increased |
| Oncoprotein bcl-2 | Increased |
| P53 | Increased |
| P21/WAF1/CIP1 | Increased |
| Cytokeratin 5 | Increased |
| TGF-β1 and TGF receptors I and II | Increased |
| Fibroblast growth factor 8 | Increased |
| Insulin-like growth factor-binding protein 2 | Increased** |
| 27-kDa heat shock protein (HSP27) | Increased** |
| Microvessel density | Unchanged or decreased |
| Proliferating cell nuclear antigen (PCNA) | Decreased |
| Ki-67 (MIB-1) | Decreased |
| Integrins Il-1α, Il-1β | Decreased |
| NM23-H1 | Decreased or absent |

*Compared to untreated prostate cancer.
**Studied with cDNA and tissue microarrays.

eration.[812–814] Some investigators reported that after androgen deprivation therapy residual tumoral proliferative activity in lymph nodes, assessed by PCNA staining, was greater than that in primary tumors (4.5% and 1.3%, respectively).[813] This could be attributed to a metastatic phenotype that is less responsive to hormonal therapy than the primary tumor. In another study PCNA was the same for tumors with lower and higher Gleason scores, suggesting that cellular dedifferentiation after neoadjuvant androgen deprivation represents a mere morphologic phenomenon and not a real increase in tumor aggressiveness.[814]

Quantitative comparative genomic hybridization studies of untreated and treated prostate cancer revealed similar level of genetic alterations, suggesting that untreated cancer contains most of the chromosomal changes necessary for recurrence.[815]

The value of immunohistochemistry in predicting outcome after androgen deprivation has not been sufficiently validated to warrant routine clinical use (Table 9-35).

## Radiation therapy

The difficulty of biopsy interpretation after radiation is multifactorial, and includes separation of carcinoma from its many mimics, identification of small foci of carcinoma, and separation of treatment effects in normal tissue from recurrent or persistent carcinoma. As more patients choose radiotherapy, particularly brachytherapy, and as these patients are observed for longer periods, pathologists bear an increasing burden to discriminate irradiated benign acini from irradiated adenocarcinoma.

Most prostate cancers grow slowly and are slow to regress, so histologic changes evolve for about 12 months after the completion of external beam radiation therapy; thus, needle biopsy is of limited value prior to about 12 months owing to ongoing cell death. Slow tumor death is attributed to the fact that radiotherapy causes necrosis only after a prostate cell has gone through cell division. After this period, biopsy is a good method for assessing local tumor control, but complete histologic resolution of cancer may take 2–3 years.[816] Sampling variation is minimized by obtaining multiple specimens.[282,376,558,559,816–818]

Evaluation of local tumor control is assisted by digital rectal examination and transrectal ultrasound. Post-therapy serum PSA correlates with post-therapy biopsy results, including degree of radiation effect.[282,819] Crook et al.[816] diagnosed post-radiotherapy biopsies as indeterminate in 33% of first biopsies (median, 13 months), 24% of second biopsies (28 months), 18% of third biopsies (36 months) and 7% of fourth biopsies (44 months). These figures are higher than the 1.5–9.0%[288,317] of biopsies with atypical indeterminate findings in unselected non-irradiated series, highlighting the increased diagnostic challenge after radiotherapy. The identification of cancer in needle biopsy specimens after radiotherapy has a significant impact on patient management: positive needle biopsies portend a worse prognosis.[282,376,820–823]

The histologic diagnosis of cancer without radiation effect relies on both architectural and cytoplasmic atypia (Figs 9-53, 9-54; Table 9-36). Radiotherapy causes cytologic atypia of benign glands, forcing the pathologist to identify cancer almost totally on architectural findings. Changes vary widely among patients.[282] Radiotherapy causes shrinkage of cancer glands and loss of cytoplasm, although some cases have voluminous foamy cytoplasm. Features most helpful for the diagnosis of cancer after radiotherapy are chiefly architectural: infiltrative growth, perineural invasion, intraluminal crystalloids, blue mucin secretions, the absence of corpora amylacea, and the presence of concomitant high-grade PIN (Fig. 9-54). Paneth cell-like change can be seen in 32% of biopsies.[282] Occasionally cytologic findings such as double nucleoli in a secretory cell may be helpful.

### Differential diagnosis of prostate cancer after radiotherapy

In the authors' experience, following irradiation atypical basal cell hyperplasia most frequently mimics treated cancer. Atypical basal cell hyperplasia is defined as basal cell proliferation with more than 10% of cells exhibiting prominent nucleoli.[101] These cells were present in 57% of cases in the authors' recent study of salvage prostatectomies, and represented a non-specific host response to radiation injury.[824]

**Table 9-35** Prognostic value of immunohistochemical findings in prostate cancer treated by androgen deprivation therapy

| Biomarker | Prognostic value | Reference |
|---|---|---|
| Androgen receptors | Not related to cancer-specific death<br>Predictive of survival in advanced stage<br>Decreased staining is predictive of failure of hormonal therapy | Noordzij et al. 1997[1297]<br>Prins et al. 1998[1298]<br>Shafer et al. 2006[1299]<br>Tilley et al. 1996[1300]<br>Nabi et al. 2004[1301] |
| PSA | Increased expression predicted earlier relapse | Ryan et al. 2006[1302] |
| Neuroendocrine cells | Not predictive of clinical outcome | Pruneri et al. 1998[1289] |
| HER2/neu | Predicts cancer-specific survival<br>Predicts time to biochemical failure<br>Not predictive of cancer-specific survival | Hernes et al. 2004[1303]<br>Osman et al. 2001[1304]<br>Di Lorenzo et al. 2002[1305] |
| Bcl-2 | Not predictive of cancer-specific survival | Noordzij et al. 1997[1297] |
| Ki-67 | Higher values predictive of cancer recurrence | Koivisto et al. 1997[1306] |
| Fibroblast growth factor 8 | Predicts worse survival in patients with androgen independent cancer | Dorkin et al. 1999[1307] |
| Protein kinase C | Predicts decreased survival after relapse | Edwards et al. 2004[1308] |
| BAG-1 | Predicts earlier relapse | Krajewska et al. 2006[1309] |
| p53 immunoreactivity | Predicts androgen receptor gene amplification and cancer progression in patients with androgen independent cancer | Koivisto et al. 1999[1310] |
| P21/WAF1/CIP1 | Predictive of worse clinical outcome | Baretton et al. 1999[1311] |
| Epidermal growth factor receptor | Increased expression predictive of earlier relapse and decreased overall survival | Shafer et al. 2006[1299] |

A

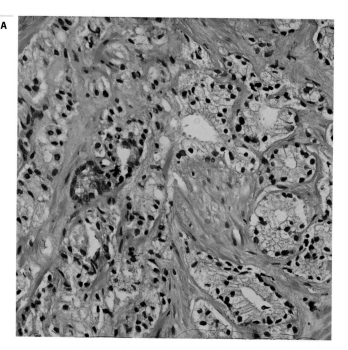

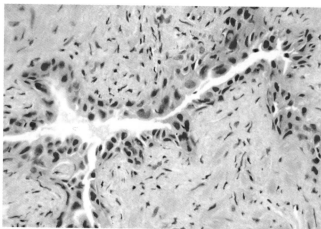

B

**Fig. 9-53** Radiation therapy changes. (**A**) Prostatic adenocarcinoma before (left), and (right) 24 months after external beam radiation therapy. In this case, recurrence is histologically similar to the initial cancer. Compare with **B,** showing acinar atrophy, severe cytologic atypia, and stromal fibrosis without evidence of residual cancer.

Immunohistochemical findings after radiotherapy

PSA, PAP, keratin 34βE12 and racemase expression in the prostatic epithelium are not altered by radiation therapy, and are often of value in separating treated adenocarcinoma and its mimics. Prostate cancer after radiation therapy has increased p53 nuclear accumulation and Ki-67 labeling index associated with a greater risk of distant metastasis and disease-specific survival.[825]

## Cryotherapy

Cryosurgical ablation refers to lethal freezing of the prostate (see Chapter 8). Clinical results with cryoablation for prostate

**Table 9-36** Histopathologic findings in prostatic adenocarcinoma in post-irradiation needle biopsies at the time of PSA (biochemical) failure

| Histopathologic findings | % cases |
|---|---|
| Gleason score | |
| <7 | 17 |
| 7 | 48 |
| >7 | 35 |
| Cancer involvement | |
| ≤10% | 31 |
| 11–40% | 28 |
| 41–80% | 35 |
| 81–100% | 7 |
| No. of cancer foci | |
| 1 | 36 |
| 2–4 | 50 |
| ≥5 | 14 |
| Combined score of radiation effect* | |
| 0–2 (minimal) | 52 |
| 3–4 (moderate) | 38 |
| 5–6 (severe) | 10 |
| Infiltrative growth | 100 |
| Perineural invasion | 31 |
| Atrophic change | 10 |
| Nuclear pykonosis | 72 |
| Nuclear enlargement | 93 |
| Prominent nucleoli | 79 |
| Cytoplasmic vacuolization | |
| <10% | 45 |
| 10–50% | 45 |
| >50% | 10 |
| Inflammation | 0 |
| Stromal desmoplasia | 76 |
| Necrosis | 0 |
| Intraluminal contents | |
| Crystalloids | 3 |
| Mucin | 21 |
| Eosinophilic | 24 |
| Corpora amylacea | 0 |
| Concomitant high-grade PIN† | 7 |

*Radiation effect was quantified using the scoring system described by Crook et al.[816]

†PIN, prostatic intraepithelial neoplasia.

cancer are encouraging, but the method is used only in selected patients.[355,826] Biopsy after cryosurgery may reveal no evidence of recurrent or residual carcinoma in the areas with treatment effect, even in patients with elevated PSA. Some investigators reported residual malignant cells in 7–23% of men, with areas of viable benign glands in 45–70% of patients.[827] Positive biopsy findings were reported in 13% and 18% of patients after cryosurgery with or without androgen deprivation therapy.[353,828] Recently, some authors reported persistence of cancer cells in the 6- and 12- month biopsies in

11% and 5.5% of cases, respectively; all 24-month biopsies were negative,[829] suggesting continued destruction over time, as with radiation therapy. Other authors reported their experience with high-risk patients (defined as either a PSA level > 10 ng/mL, or a Gleason sum score > 8, or both) who were unwilling to undergo radical surgery or radiation therapy. Post-cryosurgical biopsies revealed that 12.5% were positive for cancer.[830] No patient progressed up to the time of last follow-up, and the overall survival rate was 100%.[830] The results for a series of 176 patients who underwent cryosurgery for clinically localized disease were reported by Koppie et al.:[831] 57% of patients had neoadjuvant androgen deprivation. The cancer stage was T1 in 8.7%, T2 in 30%, T3 in 59%, and T4 in 2.3%. The nadir PSA level was undetectable in 49% of patients, 0.1–0.4 in 21%, and > 0.5 ng/mL in 30% after cryosurgery. After 43% of procedures, the serum PSA reached a nadir of < 0.5 ng/mL and did not increase by > 0.2 ng/mL on at least two occasions. However, biopsies were positive after 38% of procedures.[831]

In some cases the cancer appears unchanged, with no change in grade (Fig. 9-55) or no definite evidence of tissue or immune response, indicating lack of inclusion of that area in the ablation killing zone. As the postoperative interval increases, biopsies are more likely to contain unaltered benign prostatic tissue. Bahn et al.[832] demonstrated that outcome was independent of DNA ploidy status. There is no consensus regarding grading after cryoablation therapy, and most pathologists routinely report Gleason grade, including us.

Cryotherapy of the prostate represents a potential treatment for localized recurrent prostate cancer after radiation therapy, and several studies have reported salvage cryotherapy results with biopsy-proven local failure after external beam radiotherapy.[833–838] The most worrisome clinical finding is a positive post-cryotherapy biopsy: the presence of residual or recurrent cancer is considered evidence of inadequate cryotherapy and inadequate radiotherapy. In one study of patients with biopsy-proven local failure after external beam radiotherapy, the combination of neoadjuvant androgen deprivation therapy with salvage cryotherapy resulted in residual cancer, viable benign acini, and viable stroma in 14%, 42%, and 27%, respectively.[834] These biopsy results were obtained with four-core sampling and therefore probably underestimated the true incidence of residual cancer.[834] A cohort of 59 patients who had been previously treated with radiation therapy and had rising PSA underwent salvage cryoablation for localized, histologically proven recurrent cancer.[838] Remarkably, no biopsies (0%) showed evidence of residual or recurrent disease.[838]

No definitive method exists for the assessment of tumor viability after cryoablation. PSA and PAP expression persists in both benign and malignant epithelium, suggesting that tumor cells capable of protein production probably retain the potential for cell division and consequent metastatic spread. Keratin 34βE12, p63, and racemase expression also persists after cryoablation, and is of diagnostic value in separating treated adenocarcinoma and its mimics.

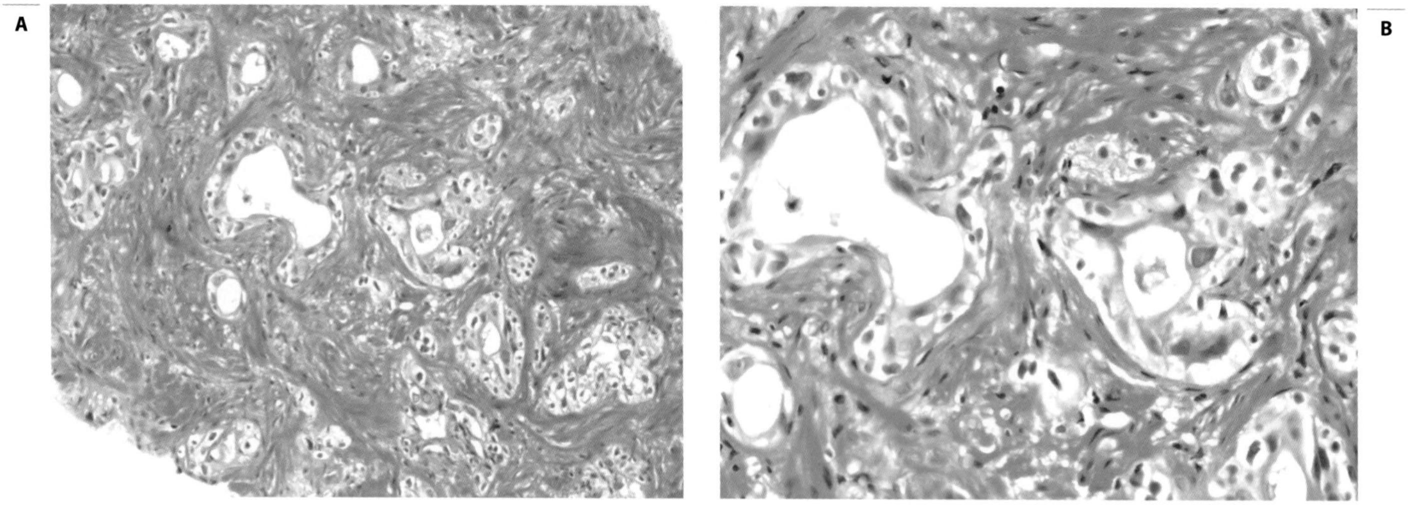

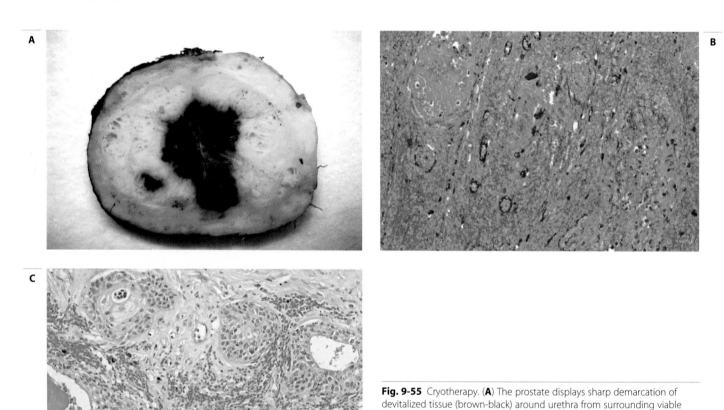

**Fig. 9-54** Radiation therapy changes. (**A, B**) Residual/recurrent prostatic adenocarcinoma 16 months after brachytherapy, with prominent acinar atrophy and cytologic atypia.

**Fig. 9-55** Cryotherapy. (**A**) The prostate displays sharp demarcation of devitalized tissue (brown-black) around urethra from surrounding viable tissue (tan). (**B**) Hemorrhagic necrosis with diffuse devitalized prostatic tissue. (**C**) At the border between treated and untreated tissue there is basal cell hyperplasia with stromal hemorrhage.

There is a strong correlation between magnetic resonance imaging (MRI) with gadolinium defects and the amount of coagulation necrosis caused within the prostate by minimally invasive techniques.[839] However, gadolinium defects were not seen in areas of viable tissue as determined by histopathologic evaluation.[839] However, some investigators reported that the findings of postoperative gadolinium-enhanced MRI were not predictive of 6-month biopsy results or follow-up PSA level.[840]

## Ultrasound hyperthermia, microwave hyperthermia, laser therapy, and hot water balloon therapy

All forms of hyperthermia result in sharply circumscribed hemorrhagic coagulative necrosis that soon organizes with granulation tissue; the pattern and extent of injury are determined by the method of thermocoagulation employed, the duration of treatment, tissue perfusion factors, and the ratio of epithelium to stroma in the tissue being treated.[841,842]

## Predictive factors in prostate cancer

Multifactorial analysis improves prediction of all outcome variables, including pathologic stage, cancer recurrence, and survival.[843] Factors recommended for routine reporting are described in Table 9-37.[372]

### Prostate-specific antigen

Prostate-specific antigen (PSA) is a 34-kDa single-chain glycoprotein of 237 amino acids produced almost exclusively by prostatic epithelial cells. PSA is a serine protease, a member of the kallikrein gene family, and has a high sequence homology with human glandular kallikrein 2. It has chymotrypsin-like, trypsin-like, and esterase-like activity. In the serum, PSA is present mainly as a complex with $\alpha_1$-antichymotrypsin. It is secreted in the seminal plasma and is responsible for gel dissolution in freshly ejaculated semen by proteolysis of the major gel forming proteins semenogelin I and II, and fibronectin. A small amount of PSA in semen is complexed. The free, non-complexed form of PSA constitutes a minor fraction of the serum PSA. Production of PSA appears to be under the control of circulating androgens acting through the androgen receptors. PSA is routinely used for early detection of prostate cancer.

Serum PSA may be elevated by conditions other than cancer, including prostatitis, PIN, acute urinary retention, and renal failure. The value of PSA as a screening tool has been questioned by some investigators because of the overlap of PSA concentration between BPH and prostate cancer.[844-847] PSA is particularly sensitive and accurate in the detection of prostate volume,[848] residual cancer, recurrence, and cancer progression following treatment,[849] irrespective of the treatment modality.[850] PSA accurately predicts cancer status and can detect recurrence several months before detection by any other method.[851]

Multiple derivatives of PSA have been proposed as adjuncts or replacements for total PSA, including free PSA,[852] complex PSA, age-specific reference ranges,[853] PSA density,[854] proPSA,[855] BPSA,[855] and PSA velocity.[239,856] Androgen deprivation therapy predictably reduces serum PSA and hampers its predictive value for cancer.[857]

PSA is a sensitive and specific immunohistochemical marker for tumors of prostatic origin (Fig. 9-56). Staining for PSA is useful in identifying poorly differentiated prostate cancer in close proximity to the bladder and the rectum; it can also verify a prostatic origin of metastatic carcinoma. The intensity of PSA immunoreactivity often varies from field to field within a tumor, and the correlation of staining intensity with tumor differentiation is inconsistent.[285,858,859] PSA expression is generally greater in low-grade than in high-grade tumors, but there is significant heterogeneity from cell to cell. Up to 5% of poorly differentiated cancers are negative for both PSA and PAP.[860,861] The presence of PSA-immunoreactive tumor cells in poorly differentiated carcinoma suggests that these tumors retain subpopulations of cells with properties of normal secretory prostatic epithelial cells. Extraprostatic expression of PSA has been reported in a number of tissues and tumors, including breast tissue,

**Table 9-37** Classification of progostic factors for prostate cancer: recommendations from 1999 Consensus Conferences

**Category 1** Factors that have been proven to be prognostic or predictive based on evidence from multiple published trials, and are recommended for routine reporting.

| 1999 CAP Conference | 1999 WHO Conference |
| --- | --- |
| TNM stage | TNM stage |
| Histologic grade (Gleason) | Histologic grade (Gleason score and WHO nuclear grade) |
| Surgical margin status | Surgical margin status |
| Perioperative PSA | Perioperative PSA |
| | Pathologic effects of treatment |
| | Location of cancer within prostate |

**Category 2** Factors that show promise as predictive factors based upon evidence from multiple published studies but that require further evaluation before recommendation or are recommended despite incomplete data as diagnostic or prognostic markers.

| | |
| --- | --- |
| DNA ploidy | DNA ploidy |
| Histologic type | Histologic type |
| Cancer volume in needle biopsy specimens (recommended) | Cancer volume in needle biopsy specimens (recommended) |
| Cancer volume in radical prostatectomy specimens (recommended) | Cancer volume in radical prostatectomy specimens (recommended) |

**Category 3** Factors that have some scientific evidence to support their adoption as diagnostic or prognostic agents but are not currently recommended; also, factors of uncertain significance.

| 1999 CAP Conference and 1999 WHO Conference |
| --- |
| Prostate-specific membrane antigen |
| Other serum tests (PSM, hK2, IGF, etc.) |
| Perineural invasion |
| Vascular/lymphatic invasion |
| Microvessel density (shows promise, but insufficient data) |
| Stromal factors, including TGF-β, integrins etc. |
| Proliferation markers and apoptosis |
| Nuclear morphometry and karyometric analysis |
| Androgen receptors |
| Neuroendocrine markers |
| Genetic markers (show promise, but insufficient data) |
| All other factors that do not appear in Categories 1 or 2 |

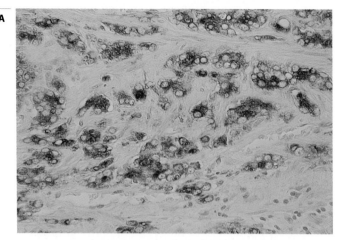

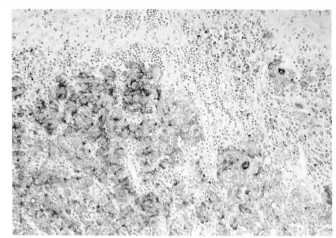

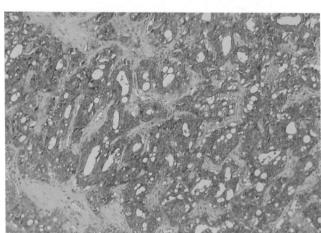

**Fig. 9-56** Prostate-specific antigen immunoreactivity. PSA expression in the cytoplasm of poorly differentiated adenocarcinoma (**A**), metastatic prostatic adenocarcinoma in cervical lymph nodes (**B**), and Skene's gland adenocarcinoma of the female urethra (**C**).

periurethral gland adenocarcinoma in women, rectal carcinoid, and extramammary Paget's disease (Table 9-38).

### Stage

The TNM classification, revised in 2002, is considered the international standard for prostate cancer staging[862] (Fig. 9-57; Table 9-39). The Commission on Cancer of the American College of Surgeons has required it for accreditation since 1995.[863] This staging scheme applies only to adenocarcinoma of the prostate, not to sarcoma and some prostatic carcinoma variants.

Staging of early prostatic adenocarcinoma separates patients into two main groups: those with palpable tumors and those with nonpalpable tumors.[864,865] This reliance on palpability of the tumor as determined by digital rectal examination is unique among organ staging systems and is hampered by the low sensitivity, low specificity, and low positive predictive value of digital rectal examination.

Refinements in staging led to the introduction of a stage of nonpalpable adenocarcinoma detected by elevated serum PSA concentration, referred to as stage T1c; however, this new stage was introduced without supportive clinical evidence, and multiple studies showed that it does not identify a distinct group of patients.[866,867] PSA is responsible for a profound clinical stage migration in newly detected prostate cancer,[868] yet it's measurement is not included in the current staging system.

**Table 9-38** Immunoreactivity of PSA in extraprostatic tissues and tumors

| Extraprostatic tissues |
| --- |
| Urethra, periurethral glands (male and female) |
| Bladder, cystitis cystica and glandularis |
| Urachal remnants |
| Neutrophils |
| Anus, anal glands (male only) |

| Extraprostatic tumors |
| --- |
| Mature teratoma |
| Urethra, periurethral gland adenocarcinoma (female) |
| Bladder, villous adenoma and adenocarcinoma |
| Penis, extramammary Paget's disease |
| Salivary gland, pleomorphic adenoma (male only) |
| Salivary gland, carcinoma (male only) |

The 2002 TNM scheme[862] differs from the 1997 TNM scheme[869] in that it divides T2 disease into T2a, T2b, and T2c subcategories. The 1997 TNM classification had been criticized for compressing the T2 subclassification into T2a and T2b. Evidence shows that, based on the 1992 TNM definitions, T2a and T2b cancers are pathologically and clinically different.[870–872] However, many investigators questioned the existence or utility of the T2b cancer (TNM 2002; unilateral but more than half of one lobe).[873–877] Eichelberger and Cheng[873] recently concluded from a study of prostatectomy

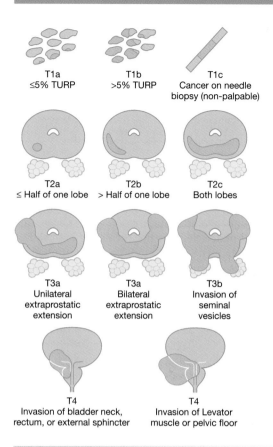

T1a
≤5% TURP

T1b
>5% TURP

T1c
Cancer on needle
biopsy (non-palpable)

T2a
≤ Half of one lobe

T2b
> Half of one lobe

T2c
Both lobes

T3a
Unilateral
extraprostatic
extension

T3a
Bilateral
extraprostatic
extension

T3b
Invasion of
seminal
vesicles

T4
Invasion of bladder neck,
rectum, or external sphincter

T4
Invasion of Levator
muscle or pelvic floor

**Fig. 9-57** Prostate cancer staging using the TNM system, 2002 revision. Black indicates extent of cancer.

**Table 9-39** 2002 TNM staging system

| **Primary Tumor (T)** |
| --- |
| TX: Primary tumor cannot be assessed |
| T0: No evidence of primary tumor |
| T1: Clinically inapparent tumor not palpable nor visible by imaging |
| T1a: Tumor incidental histologic finding in ≤5% of tissue resected |
| T1b: Tumor incidental histologic finding in >5% of tissue resected |
| T1c: Tumor identified by needle biopsy (e.g., because of elevated PSA) |
| T2: Tumor confined within prostate* |
| T2a: Tumor involves 50% of ≤1 lobe or less |
| T2b: Tumor involves >50% of 1 lobe but not both lobes |
| T2c: Tumor involves both lobes |
| T3: Tumor extends through the prostate capsule** |
| T3a: Extracapsular extension (unilateral or bilateral) |
| T3b: Tumor invades seminal vesicle(s) |
| T4: Tumor is fixed or invades adjacent structures other than seminal vesicles: bladder neck, external sphincter, rectum, levator muscles, and/or pelvic wall |
| **Regional Lymph Nodes (N)** |
| NX: Regional lymph nodes were not assessed |
| N0: No regional lymph node metastasis |
| N1: Metastasis in regional lymph node(s) |
| **Distant Metastasis (M)†** |
| MX: Distant metastasis cannot be assessed |
| M0: No distant metastasis |
| M1: Distant metastasis |
| M1a: Nonregional lymph node(s) |
| M1b: Bone(s) |
| M1c: Other site(s) with or without bone disease |

*Tumor that is found in 1 or both lobes by needle biopsy, but is not palpable or reliably visible by imaging, is classified as T1c.
**Invasion into the prostatic apex or into (but not beyond) the prostatic capsule is not classified as T3, but as T2.
†When more than one site of metastasis is present, the most advanced category (pM1c) is used.

specimens that the three-tiered T2 classification system was not necessary, taking into consideration the biology and anatomy of prostate cancer; they preferred the simple unilateral and bilateral classification for stage T2. Chun and colleagues[878] studied more than 1700 patients with stage T2 cancer, and found that all T2 substages were equally predictive of pretreatment PSA, margin status, and Gleason score.

Staging errors vary from 24% to 38%.[879] Reasons for discrepancies included misinterpretation of the digital rectal examination, inappropriate use of TRUS/MRI in staging, stage not assigned at initial diagnosis, misinterpretation of pathology, TNM staging confusion, inappropriate use of biopsy data, disagreement between consultants, and misinterpretation of transurethral resection results. The level of agreement for clinical TNM stage was poor even among experts in the field, according to Campbell and colleagues[880] (T stage, 64%; N stage, 74%; M stage, 77%).

### Pathology of PSA-detected adenocarcinoma (clinical stage T1c)

Prior to the widespread clinical use of PSA, most organ-confined adenocarcinoma was discovered by digital rectal examination[881] or at the time of transurethral resection. Routine use of serum PSA increased the detection rate of prostatic adenocarcinoma and uncovered some cases that would not have been detected by digital rectal examination. There is no pathologic stage equivalent for clinical stage T1c, and such tumors are invariably upstaged at surgery, usually to pathologic stage T2 or T3. Clinical stage T1c, T2a, and T2b adeno-

carcinomas had similar diameters, frequencies of multifocality, tumor grades, DNA content results, pathologic stages, and tumor locations; interestingly, they had different serum PSA values, tumor volumes, positive surgical margins, and prostate gland sizes, with the T1c tumors having higher values for each feature.[882–884] These findings indicate that PSA detects adenocarcinoma that is clinically important, potentially curable, and heterogeneous.[885] Also, PSA-detected tumors that are visible on transurethral ultrasound (TRUS) have similar pathologic features to those that are not visible.[886]

Patients with clinical stage T2 tumor have higher Gleason score and advanced pathological stage than those whose cancer is detected because of high serum PSA concentration (T1c). These results suggest that clinical stage cT1c tumors should be separated from clinical stage T2, but the PSA recurrence rate for both stages is similar, indicating a need for further evaluation and refinement of the current clinical staging system.[883]

### Extraprostatic extension

The term extraprostatic extension (EPE) was accepted at an International Consensus Conference to replace other terms, including capsular invasion, capsular penetration, and capsular perforation.[361] Extension of cancer beyond the edge or capsule of the prostate is diagnostic of EPE. There are three criteria for EPE, depending on the site and composition of the extraprostatic tissue: cancer in adipose tissue; cancer in perineural spaces of the neurovascular bundles; and cancer in anterior muscle (Fig. 9-58). In patients treated by radical prostatectomy for clinically localized cancer, the frequency of EPE (stage pT3 cancer) is 23%,[887] 24%,[820] 41%,[460,888] 43%,[889] 45%,[890] or 52%.[891] There is a strong association of tumor volume with extraprostatic extension and seminal vesicle invasion.[892] An autopsy study showed EPE in 2% of cancers less than 0.46 mL in volume, compared to 52% of larger cancers.[365]

Patients with EPE have a worse prognosis than those with organ-confined cancer.[820,893] Cancer-specific survival 10 years after radical prostatectomy in patients with pT3 cancer was 54%,[894] 62%,[895] 73%,[896] or 80%;[897] at 15 years, survival was 69%.[897] Cancer-specific survival 10 years after definitive radiation therapy in patients with clinical stage T3 was 44%[898] or 59%;[899] at 15 years, survival was 36%,[898] 33%,[900] or 39%.[899]

Many patients with EPE also have positive surgical margins, with a frequency of 41%,[820] 57%,[901] or 81%.[891] The combination of EPE and positive margins predicts a worse prognosis than EPE alone.[902,903] Some investigators reported that a prostate biopsy core with a tumor length of at least 7 mm plus a positive basal biopsy core of any length and tumor grade is predictive of ipsilateral EPE; these criteria might be of value for predicting EPE and selecting patients for nerve-sparing prostatectomy.[904]

Detection of cancer cells within the adipose tissue of needle biopsies is regarded as evidence of EPE despite the very rare presence of intraprostatic fat. Sung et al.[905] reviewed 313 consecutive radical prostatectomy specimens and none of these revealed any adipose tissue components within the most peripheral boundary of normal prostatic acini in the prostate. The authors concluded that the occurrence of fat within the prostate is extremely rare. Accordingly, the finding of carcinoma invading adipose tissue in needle biopsies should continue to be considered as extraprostatic extension and stage pT3a assigned.[905]

### Lymph node metastases

Twenty years ago, the incidence of lymph node metastases in patients with prostate cancer evaluated for surgical treatment was as high as 40%. In the modern era of screening and improved patient selection the incidence is now less than 10%, although most series exclude patients with higher-risk cancer. The risk of lymph node metastases is influenced by cancer stage, PSA concentration, Gleason grade, and the aggressiveness of lymph node dissection.[906,907] Staging pelvic lymph node biopsy is often performed prior to prostatectomy, and urologists may discontinue surgery if metastases are identified. Lymph node dissection is performed by an open or laparoscopic procedure. Radical perineal prostatectomy and lymph node dissection are performed as separate procedures because the surgical approaches are different, whereas radical retropubic prostatectomy and lymphadenectomy are often performed as a single procedure. Results from extended dissection reveal a higher rate of metastases than previously found.[908] Sentinel-guided pelvic lymph node dissection allows detection of even small lymph node metastases.[909,910] The accuracy of sentinel pelvic lymph node dissection is comparable to that of extended pelvic lymph node dissection when the limitations of the method are taken into consideration.[911] A nomogram based on pretreatment PSA, clinical stage, and biopsy Gleason score accurately predicts nodal metastases.[912]

The pathologist should carefully evaluate the fibroadipose tissue obtained by lymphadenectomy, and submit all lymph nodes for pathologic examination. It may not be necessary to submit obvious adipose tissue, although it is our policy

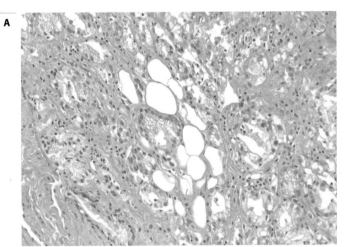
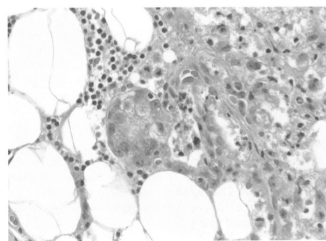

A      B

**Fig. 9-58 (A, B)** Extraprostatic extension with cancer touching adipocytes.

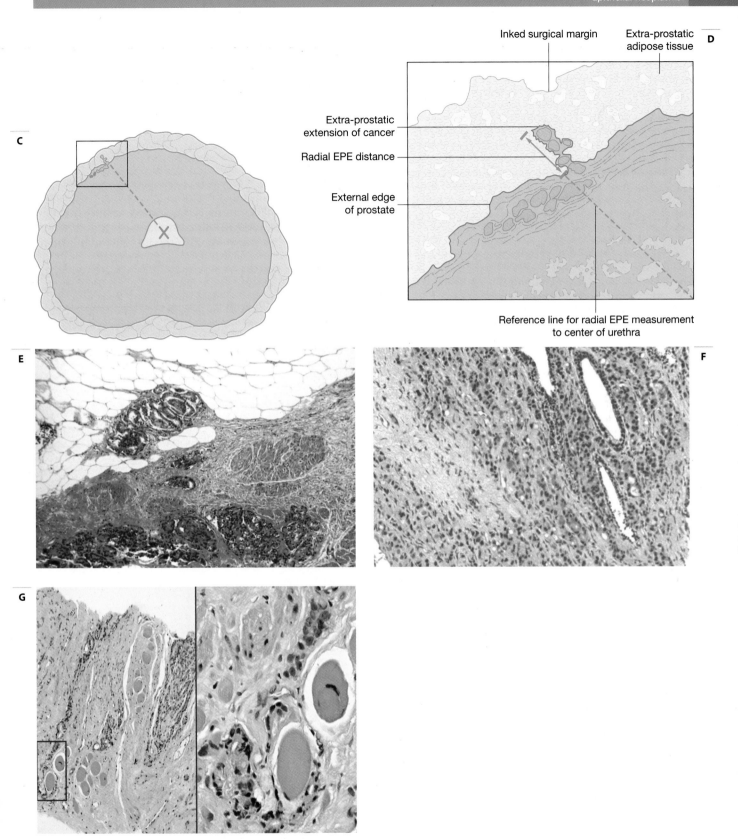

**Fig. 9-58, Cont'd** (**C, D**) Artist's rendering of radial extraprostatic extension. (**E**) Another example of focal extraprostatic extension. (**F**) Seminal vesicle invasion by high-grade adenocarcinoma; note pigmented epithelium. (**G**) Cancer in anterior muscle on needle biopsy (left) with inset (right) is assigned as stage pT3a.

to do so. Sampling error by frozen section accounts for a false negative rate of lymph node metastases of 2–3% in our experience (Bostwick, unpublished observations). The surgical pathology report should include the number and sites of all submitted lymph nodes, as well as sites of involvement and size of cancer foci. Remarkably, a recent report indicated that the development of prostate cancer lymph node metastases is accompanied with smaller lymph node size.[913]

Patients with one or two positive lymph nodes had a clinical recurrence-free survival of respectively 70% and 73% at 10 years, versus 49% in those who had five or more involved lymph nodes.[914] Patients undergoing excision of at least four lymph nodes (node-positive and node-negative patients) or more than 10 nodes (only node-negative patients) had a lower risk of prostate cancer-specific death at 10 years than did those who did not undergo lymphadenectomy.[915] The removal of a greater number of nodes was associated with a greater likelihood of the presence of positive nodes.[915] There was a 3%[916,917] to 13%[918] incidence of occult prostatic carcinoma in pelvic lymph nodes that cannot be detected by routine hematoxylin and eosin staining. The presence of extranodal extension was not associated with unfavorable survival, although nodal cancer volume was predictive of cancer-specific survival.[914] However, in patients treated surgically and with adjuvant androgen deprivation therapy, multivariate analysis identified the presence of micrometastases as an independent factor predicting biochemical recurrence.[919]

Lymph node metastases are heterogeneous and have a close relation to the corresponding primary tumor. Independent predictors of PSA recurrence in lymph node-positive patients include lymphovascular invasion in the lymph nodes and the nuclear grade of the primary tumor.[427,920]

### Distant metastases

The usual sites of metastases are the pelvic lymph nodes, bone (chiefly osteoblastic), and lungs (Fig. 9-59).[921–923] However, many unusual sites of metastases have been described, including kidney, breast, and brain. No important differences are seen in the pattern of metastases at autopsy in Japan and the United States. The number of metastatic sites is similar in those who do and do not receive estrogen therapy, although treated patients were more likely to develop brain metastases. Cluster analysis of metastases revealed a subset of men of African ancestry who developed distant metastases with minimal local spread of cancer.[921]

### Surgical margins

Positive surgical margins are defined as cancer cells that touch the inked surface of the prostate (Fig. 9-60). Surgical margins are not included in pathologic staging.[820] However, many studies have erroneously equated positive margins and extraprostatic extension, particularly in cases in which the surgeon has cut into the prostate and intraprostatic cancer.[361]

The frequency of positive surgical margins has steadily declined in the past decade, probably owing to refinements in surgical technique and earlier detection of cancer at

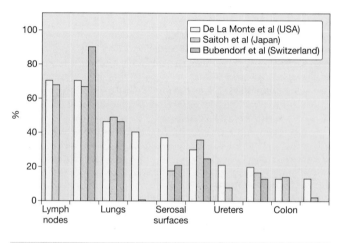

**Fig. 9-59** The 10 most common sites of prostate cancer metastases at autopsy in the United States, Japan, and Switzerland.

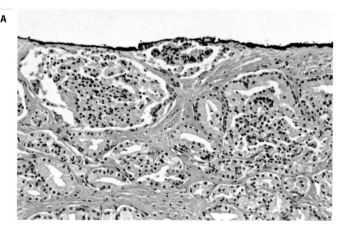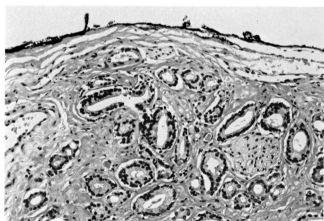

**Fig. 9-60** Surgical margins. (**A**) Positive surgical margin, with cancer touching the inked surface without extraprostatic tissue (surgical incision of the prostate). (**B**) Negative surgical margin. Cancer is close to the surface, but does not make contact. Note perineural invasion on right side.

smaller volumes.[924] Ohori and colleagues[889] found positive surgical margins in 24% of whole-mount radical prostatectomies obtained at their hospital prior to 1987, usually in the posterolateral region near the neurovascular bundles; by modifying surgery to approach the neurovascular bundles laterally and widely dissect the apex of the prostate, they observed a positive surgical margin rate of only 8% within 6 years, despite similar volume grade, and pathologic stage of cancer. Others noted a frequency of positive surgical margins of 8%,[924] 29%,[820] 33%,[925] 46%,[926] and 57%,[927] with no difference in specimens from nerve-sparing and non-nerve-sparing operations.[926,928]

Positive surgical margins are strongly correlated with cancer volume [535,889,892,902,925,929] and number of needle biopsies containing cancer.[930,931] Most positive surgical margins in prostates with cancer smaller than 4 mL are caused by surgical incision.[820,929] Predictors of positive margins include abnormal digital rectal examination, preoperative PSA > 10 ng/mL, biopsy Gleason score > 7, more than one positive biopsy core, and clinical suspicion of extraprostatic extension.[932] Positive margins are located at the apex (48%), rectal and lateral surfaces (24%), bladder neck (16%), and superior pedicles (10%).[925]

Adjuvant radiation therapy in patients with positive surgical margins with or without extraprostatic extension appears to be beneficial.[933,934] Patients had a biochemical failure rate at 5 years of 12%, compared to 41% of patients matched by age, site of positive surgical margins, DNA ploidy status, Gleason score, and PSA who were not given adjuvant radiotherapy.[935]

Surgical margin status was an important predictor of patient outcome after radical prostatectomy;[570,936] it was the only predictor of cancer progression other than Gleason score[866,903] or DNA ploidy[820] in patients without seminal vesicle invasion or lymph node metastases. The actuarial 5- and 10-year biochemical disease-free survival was respectively 71% and 60% for patients with negative and positive surgical margins.[937] The extent of margin positivity correlated with PSA recurrence in univariate analysis, although it had no predictive value independent of Gleason score.[938]

The College of American Pathologists recommends that the presence, extent, and location of each margin reviewed should be specifically reported.[460] However, there is no current agreement or recommendation as to the specific method of quantifying the amount of cancer in these locations.

## Perineural invasion

Perineural invasion is common in adenocarcinoma, present in 11%,[397] 17%,[389] and 38%[939] of biopsies, and may be the only evidence of malignancy in a needle core. Only half of patients with intraprostatic perineural invasion on biopsy have extraprostatic extension. In univariate analysis, perineural invasion was predictive of extraprostatic extension, seminal vesicle invasion, and pathologic stage in patients treated by radical prostatectomy.[939,940] However, in multivariate analysis, perineural invasion had no predictive value after consideration of Gleason grade, serum PSA, and amount of cancer on biopsy.[397,939,941] Perineural invasion was not a

significant predictor of biochemical recurrence in patients undergoing brachytherapy[389] or low-risk patients treated by external beam therapy.[402,942] These findings indicate that there is no value in routinely reporting perineural invasion in biopsy specimens, although this has been refuted.[413] Also, perineural invasion in radical prostatectomy specimens appears to provide no significant prognostic information.[411,412] Immediate treatment rather than watchful waiting may be more appropriate for patients with localized prostatic cancer and perineural invasion.[413]

## Vascular/lymphatic invasion

Microvascular invasion is a strong indicator of malignancy, and its presence correlates with histologic grade, although it is sometimes difficult to distinguish from fixation-associated retraction artifact of acini.[417,418] Microvascular invasion may also be an important predictor of outcome, and carries a fourfold greater risk of tumor progression and death.[417] Immunohistochemical stains directed against endothelial cells such as Factor VIII-related antigen, CD31, CD34, or *Ulex europaeus* may increase the detection rate.[418]

Microvascular invasion is present in 38% of radical prostatectomy specimens, and is commonly associated with extraprostatic extension and lymph node metastases (62% and 67%, of cases, respectively).[417,418] It does not appear to be an independent predictor of progression when stage and grade are included in the multivariate analysis.[417,424] However, Cheng et al.[427] concluded recently on multivariate analysis that lymphovascular invasion is an independent prognosis factor for PSA recurrence and cancer death in patients with prostate cancer, similar to other investigators who showed that the 5-year biochemical-free survival was 87.3% for patients with no lymphovascular invasion and 38.3% with lymphovascular invasion on the radical prostatectomy specimen.[943] By multivariate analysis, lymphovascular invasion and Gleason score were independent predictors of biochemical failure.[943]

## Cancer volume

Biopsy cancer volume depends on multiple factors, including prostate volume, cancer volume, cancer distribution, number of biopsy cores obtained, the cohort of patients being evaluated, and the technical competence of the investigator. The combined results from multiple studies indicate that the biopsy extent of tumor provides some predictive value for extent in radical prostatectomy specimens and should probably be reported, although its predictive value for an individual patient is limited.[866,944–956] Reliance upon this measure alone may often be misleading. There is a fair[949] to good[946] correlation between the amount of cancer reported in biopsies and that subsequently found in radical prostatectomy specimens. This correlation is greatest for large cancers. High cancer burden on needle biopsy is strongly suggestive of large-volume high-stage cancer.[866,944–947]

Unfortunately, low tumor burden on needle biopsy does not necessarily indicate low-volume low-stage cancer. Patients with less than 30% of needle cores replaced by cancer had a mean volume in the radical prostatectomy of 6.1 mL (range, 0.19–16.8 mL), indicating that the amount of tumor on transrectal needle biopsy was not a good predictor of tumor volume.[949] In another report, patients with less than 10% cancer in the biopsy had a 30% risk of positive surgical margins, 27% risk of extraprostatic extension, and 22% risk of PSA biochemical progression; these risks were higher in patients with more than 10% cancer.[955] Patients with less than 3 mm cancer and Gleason score 6 or less on needle biopsy had a 59% risk of cancer volume exceeding 0.5 mL.[945] Those with less than 2 mm of cancer had 26% risk of extraprostatic cancer,[953] and those with less than 3 mm had 52% risk.[952] The CAP recommends that the volume of cancer in needle biopsy should be reported as the percentage of tissue involved by cancer.

Cancer volume should also be recorded in prostatectomy specimens, although there is no accepted universal approach.[358] Methods of cancer volume measurement include computer-assisted morphometric determination,[447,946,957] simple measurement of length × height × section thickness of the cancer (some measure the largest 'index' focus, whereas others report the aggregate volume),[958] greatest cancer dimension,[351,959,960] grid method,[961] and visual estimate of the percentage of cancer.[962–964] Measurements performed on fixed tissue sections may include a formalin shrinkage correction factor which varies from 1.15[965] to 1.5, representing tissue shrinkage of 18–33%; conversely, Schned and colleagues[966] demonstrated that shrinkage correction is unnecessary.

Cancer volume is a critical element in the definition of clinically significant and insignificant prostate cancer.[958,961] Up to 70% of men undergoing radical prostatectomy are found to have multifocal cancer, a finding that is a major theoretical objection to focal ablation (Table 9-40). However, about 80% of incidental tumors are smaller than 0.5 mL, indicating that a significant percentage of multifocal tumors, other than the largest or index cancer identified preoperatively, may not be clinically significant. Until now, however, little attention has been paid to trying to differentiate patients with unifocal and multifocal disease as it had little clinical significance: all treatments are aimed at total gland ablation. Small-volume prostate cancers are often multifocal and bilateral, with a predilection for the peripheral zone. Of these small-volume prostate cases, 16% had Gleason pattern 4 and might therefore be clinically significant.[967] Importantly, Noguchi et al.[538,968] found that secondary cancers in multifocal prostate tumors did not adversely influence prognosis, and they concluded that only the largest (index) cancer was significant.

Cancer volume was usually[535,957,969,970] (but not always[866,971]) predictive of cancer recurrence after radical prostatectomy. In a screening population, median cancer volume in men with biochemical progression after prostatectomy was 2.55 cm$^3$ versus 0.94 cm$^3$ in men who were free of disease 5 years after surgery.[972]

### Location of cancer

The site of origin of cancer appears to be a significant prognostic factor (Table 9-41). Transition zone or anterior cancer tends to be less aggressive than typical peripheral zone acinar adenocarcinoma,[973] although this has been refuted (Fig. 9-61).[974] It is usually lower grade than those in the peripheral zone, accounting for Gleason primary grade 1 and 2 tumors, and has lower rates of extraprostatic extension; conversely, it has a higher positive surgical margins rate.[975] Interestingly, the volume of low-grade transition zone cancer tends to be larger than those arising in the peripheral zone,[975–977] although conflicting findings have been reported.[978] The confinement of transition zone adenocarcinoma to its anatomic site of origin may account in part for the favorable prognosis of clinical stage T1 tumors. Therefore, the prognosis of a patient with prostate cancer is more dependent on the features of cancer in the peripheral zone than in the transition zone.[979] The transition zone boundary probably acts as a relative barrier to tumor extension, as malignant acini appear to frequently fan out along this boundary before invasion into the peripheral and central zones.

Transition zone cancer has a significantly lower rate of positive biopsies in the middle (63% vs 80%) and base (50% vs 80%) of the prostate than peripheral zone cancer.[980] Positive biopsies were exclusively obtained from the apex in

**Table 9-40** Incidence of multifocal prostate cancer in radical prostatectomies

| Publication date | Radical prostatectomy handling | Reference | No. of subjects | Multifocality (%) |
|---|---|---|---|---|
| 1992 | Stanford protocol* | Villers et al.[1312] | 234 | 50 |
| 1994 | Whole-mounted | Miller et al.[1313] | 151 | 56 |
| 1999 | 4-mm specimen sections | Djavan et al.[1314] | 308 | 67 |
| 2003 | Stanford protocol* | Nogushi et al.[968] | 222 | 76 |
| 2003 | Whole-mounted | Song et al.[1315] | 132 | 33 |
| 2004 | Whole-mounted | Ng et al.[412] | 364 | 85 |
| 2004 | Whole-mounted | Eichelberger et al.[873] | 312 | 85 |
| 2004 | 4-mm specimen sections | Horninger et al.[1316] | 80 | 65 |
| 2005 | Whole-mounted | Cheng et al.[1317] | 62 | 69 |
| 2005 | Stanford protocol* | Torlakovic et al.[1318] | 46 | 65 |

*Stanford protocol is using serial transverse sections at 3 mm intervals.[1312,366]

**Table 9-41** Prostatic carcinoma: comparison based on anatomic site of origin*

| | Transition zone cancer | Peripheral zone cancer |
|---|---|---|
| Incidence | | |
| Stage T1a | 75% | – |
| Stage T1b | 79% | – |
| All stage T1 | 78% | – |
| All stages | 24% | 70% |
| Origin | | |
| In or near BPH | Yes | No |
| Near apex | Yes | Yes |
| Detection rate by TURP | 78% | – |
| Pathologic features | | |
| Tumor pattern | Alveolar-medullary | Tubular |
| Tumor grade (primary Gleason grade) | Usually 1 or 2 | Usually 2, 3, or 4 |
| Clear cell pattern | Common | Uncommon |
| Stromal fibrosis | Uncommon | Uncommon |
| Associated putative premalignant changes | AAH or PIN | PIN |
| Aneuploidy[†] | 6% | 31% |
| Clinical behavior | | |
| Extraprostatic extension[†] | 11% | 44% |
| Site of extraprostatic extension | Anterolateral and apical | Lateral |
| Average tumor volume with extraprostatic extension[†] | 4.98 cc | 3.86 mL |
| Risk of seminal vesicle invasion[†] | 0% | 19% |
| Risk of lymph node metastases | Low | High |

[†]Central zone cancer (5–10% of total) excluded.
BPH: benign prostatic hyperplasia; TURP: transurethral resection of the prostate; AAH: atypical adenomatous hyperplasia; PIN: prostatic intraepithelial neoplasia.

20% of transition zone and 5% of peripheral zone cancers. There was exact agreement between Gleason scores of needle biopsies and those of radical prostatectomy specimens in 15% of transition zone and 55% of peripheral zone cancers, respectively.

According to McNeal et al.,[531,981] peripheral zone cancer tended to spread along the prostate capsule and was most extensive transversely. Above 4 mL in volume, bilateral spread, transition zone invasion, and nodularity progressively increased, but dominant growth was toward the base along nerves to the superior pedicle; here extraprostatic extension was most common. Transition zone cancer arose mainly in the anterior-mid transition zone, invading the anterior fibromuscular stroma and, when larger than 4 mL, the anterolateral peripheral zone.

The World Health Organization recommends that prostate biopsy specimens be submitted separately, the anatomic site of each prostate biopsy be labeled, at the discretion of the urologist, and that pathologists report each specimen separately.[372] Thus, the anatomic site, and the amount of high-grade carcinoma within each prostate biopsy should be included in the pathology report and identified in the anatomic area specified by the urologist. The anatomic location of carcinoma in total prostatectomy specimens should also be specified in the pathology report.

### Microvessel density

Microvessel density (MVD) is increased in PIN[196] and cancer compared to benign epithelium,[438,982,983] and its measurement offers promise for predicting pathologic stage and patient outcome in prostate cancer. Most studies found a positive correlation of MVD with Gleason grade[438] and pathologic stage.[431,984,985] MVD in cancer on biopsy showed a positive correlation with matched prostatectomies, and was an independent predictor of extraprostatic extension.[985,986] The bulk of evidence favors the relationship of MVD and cancer stage, although there is variance between methods and patient cohorts.

There is generally good agreement that MVD predicts cancer recurrence.[443,448,987–989] In patients treated by surgery or external beam radiation therapy, MVD[432,443,990] and microvascular invasion[448] predicted biochemical failure.

The 5α-reductase inhibitor finasteride induces prostate apoptosis and reduce tissue vascularity by inhibiting epithelial cell adhesion,[991] and these effects occur within 2 weeks of the onset of therapy.[992]

### DNA ploidy

DNA ploidy analysis of prostate cancer provides important predictive information that supplements histopathologic examination. Patients with diploid tumors have a more favorable outcome than those with aneuploid tumors. Among patients with lymph node metastases treated with radical prostatectomy and androgen deprivation therapy, those with diploid tumors may survive 20 years or more, whereas those with aneuploid tumors die within 5 years.[993] However, the ploidy pattern of prostate cancer is often heterogeneous, creating potential problems with sampling error.[994]

Analysis of multiple biopsies is important for correct preoperative ploidy estimation.[994] A good correlation exists between DNA ploidy and histologic grade,[995] and DNA ploidy adds clinically useful predictive information for some patients.[995–999] The incidence of aneuploidy in high-grade PIN varies from 32% to 68%, and is somewhat lower than carcinoma (55–62%).[1000] There is a high level of concordance of DNA content of PIN and cancer. About 70% of aneuploid cases of PIN are associated with aneuploid carcinoma; conversely, only 29% of cases of aneuploid cancer are associated with aneuploid PIN.[165] DNA ploidy pattern by flow cytometry correlates with cancer grade,[997] volume, and stage.[996,1001] Most low-stage tumors are diploid and high-stage tumors are non-diploid, but numerous exceptions occur.[1002]

The 5-year cancer-specific survival is about 95% for diploid tumors, 70% for tetraploid tumors, and 25% for aneuploid tumors.[1003] Biopsy ploidy status independently

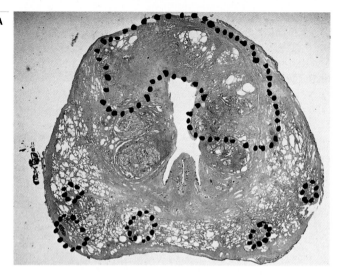
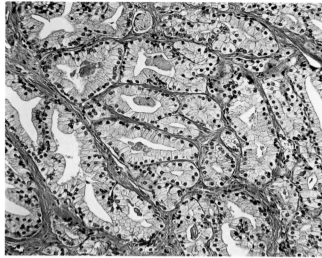

**Fig. 9-61** Transition zone cancer. (**A**) Whole-mount section, showing large transition zone cancer (top) and smaller foci in the peripheral zone (bottom). (**B**) The tumor is well differentiated, with clear cytoplasm and uniform nuclei.

predicted cancer recurrence in patients treated by prostatectomy.[514] Patients with diploid lymph node metastases treated by androgen deprivation therapy alone had longer progression-free and overall survival than those with aneuploid metastases.[1004] Digital image analysis appears to have a high level of concordance (about 85%) with radical prostatectomy specimens evaluated by flow cytometry.[1005] For T1a prostate cancer, DNA ploidy was not predictive of progression or survival, but these patients have a very favorable prognosis.[1006]

### Morphometric markers

Morphometric markers provide useful predictive information in prostate cancer, but are not used routinely and are considered research modalities.[372] Morphometric studies should employ objective, quantitative techniques that are preferably computer assisted. Unfortunately, there are no accepted standards for morphometric analysis, with significant problems of reproducibility, and the results from different digitizing instruments are not comparable.

The most popular morphometric markers are nuclear size,[1007–1009] nuclear shape and roundness,[1008–1010] chromatin texture,[525,1011–1013] size and number of nucleoli,[1014,1015] and number of apoptotic bodies.[262,1008,1014,1016–1025] Volume-weighted mean nuclear volume was independently predictive of cancer-specific survival in combination with Gleason score and clinical stage.[1026] Morphometric alterations demonstrated by quantitative nuclear grade combined with pro-PSA immunohistologic localization independently predicted significant differences between native Japanese and Japanese-American men with prostate cancer,[1027] indicating a basis for biologic and molecular alterations in the benign adjacent and malignant epithelium between these two groups.

### Genetic markers in prostate cancer

Prostate carcinogenesis involves multiple genetic changes, including loss of specific genomic sequences that may be associated with inactivation of tumor suppressor genes and gain of some specific chromosome regions that may be associated with activation of oncogenes. The most common chromosomal aberrations in PIN and carcinoma are TMPRSS2-ETS gene fusions (see below), gain of chromosome 7, (particular 7q31), loss of 8p and gain of 8q, and loss of 10q, 16q and 18q.[75] Fluorescence in situ hybridization[322] studies showed that aneusomy of chromosome 7 is frequent in prostate cancer and associated with higher cancer grade, higher pathologic stage, and early death from prostate cancer.[1028] PCR analysis of microsatellite markers identified frequent imbalance of alleles mapped to 7q31 in prostate cancer.[1029–1031] Allelic imbalance of 7q31 was strongly correlated with cancer aggressiveness, progression, and cancer-specific death.[1032] These findings suggest that genetic alterations of the 7q arm play an important role in the development of prostate cancer.

The chromosome 8p arm is one of the most frequently deleted regions in prostate cancer.[129,135,1033] The rate of 8p22 loss ranged from 29% to 50% in PIN, 32% to 69% in primary cancer, and 65% to 100% in metastatic cancer.[1033] Other frequently deleted 8p regions include 8p21 and 8p12.[129,1033] Emmert-Buck et al.[129] found loss of 8p12-21 in 63% of PIN foci and 91% of cancer foci using microdissected frozen tissue. Bostwick et al.[4] detected loss of 8p21-12 in 37% of PIN foci and 46% of cancer foci. These findings suggest that more than one tumor suppressor gene may be located on 8p, and inactivation of these genes may be important for the initiation of prostate cancer. In addition to loss of the 8p arm, gain of the 8q arm has been reported in prostate cancer.[815,1033–1035] Bova et al.[1036] found gain of 8q in 11% of primary cancers and 40% of lymph-node metastases. Van Den Berg et al.[1037] found amplification of 8q DNA sequences in 75% of cancers metastatic to lymph nodes. Similarly, Visakorpi et al.[1038] found gain of 8q far more frequently in locally recurrent cancer than in primary cancer. Cher et al.[1039] also detected frequent gain of 8q in metastatic and androgen-independent prostate cancers. Four putative target genes for 8q gain have been identified: these are Elongin C at 8q21, as well as EIF3S3, KIAA0196, and RAD21 at 8q23-q24 regions. They seem to be overexpressed and amplified in about 20–30% of the hormone-refractory prostate carcinomas.[1040-1042] Gain of the chromosome 8 centromere or the 8q arm occurs simultaneously with loss of portions of the 8p arm in PIN and carcinoma.[815,1034,1038,1043] One simple genetic mechanism that could explain these observations is the presence of multiple copies of isochromosome 8q in cancer cells. Preliminary simultaneous FISH studies with probes specific for 8p, 8q, and the chromosome 8 centromere support this explanation.

There is also a high frequency of allelic imbalance at 10p and 10q in prostate cancer.[1044,1045] The most commonly deleted region on the 10q arm includes bands 10q23–24, and allelic loss of this region may inactive the MXI-1 gene. Loss of PTEN, a tumor suppressor gene on chromosome 10q23, has been reported in 25–33% of advanced prostate cancers. It has been associated with increased Gleason score and risk of clinical recurrence.[1046]

Chromosome 16 has frequent allelic imbalance in prostate cancer. Allelic imbalance at 16q was present in about 30% of cases of clinically localized prostate cancer,[1047] and there was a high frequency of allelic imbalance at 16q23-q24.[1048] The most commonly deleted region was located at 16q24.1-q24.2, and this deletion was significantly associated with cancer progression.[1048,1049]

The frequency of loss of 18q22.1 varied from 20% to 40%.[1044] Other regions demonstrating frequent allelic imbalance include 3p25–26, 5q12–23, 6q, 13q, 17p31.1, and 21q22.2–22.3.[1049,1050] Loss of 10q, 16q, and 18q has also been reported in PIN.[4,1051]

### TMPRSS2 and ETS-family gene fusions

Recently, gene fusions between the androgen-responsive gene TMPRSS2 and members of the ETS family of DNA-binding transcription factor genes were found in up to 70% of prostate cancers[134,1052-1055] and a lower percentage of cases of high-grade PIN.[141] Recurrent fusions were identified between the 5′ non-coding region of TMPRSS2 and ERG.[1056] These novel gene fusions are the driving mechanism for overexpression of the three members of the ETS transcription factor family, including ERG (21q22.3), ETV1 (7p21.2), and ETV4 (17q21). Considering the high incidence of prostate cancer and the high frequency of this gene fusion, the TMPRSS2-ETS fusion is the most common genetic aberration described to date in human malignancies.

Fusion-positive tumors were associated with higher Gleason grade, higher stage,[1057] and poorer survival than fusion-negative tumors.[1058,1059-1061] Five morphological features were associated with TMPRSS2-ERG fusion prostate cancer: blue-tinged mucin, cribriform growth pattern, macronucleoli, intraductal cancer spread, and signet ring-cell features.[1062] Distinct patterns of hybrid transcripts were found in samples taken from multifocal cancer, suggesting that TMPRSS2-ERG gene fusions are arising independently in different foci.[1063] TMPRSS2: ERG gene fusions were recently detected clinically in the urine of patients with prostate cancer.[1064]

### PCA3

The PCA3 gene, located on chromosome 9q21–22, is greatly overexpressed in more than 90% of prostate cancers, but is not present in the benign prostate.[1065-1068] Moreover, no PCA3 transcripts could be detected in a wide range of human extraprostatic benign and cancerous tissues, indicating that PCA3 is the most specific prostate cancer gene identified to date. The PCA3 mRNA includes a high density of stop codons; thus, it does not have an open reading frame, resulting in a non-coding RNA.

Independent studies showed that this test is a very promising adjunct tool for the early diagnosis of prostate cancer from urine samples.[1065-1068] Radical prostatectomy specimens removed for carcinoma indicate that PCA3 is a significant and independent biomarker of prostate cancer that shows no correlation with cancer volume, location, multifocality, Gleason score, patient age, or pathologic stage.[1069]

### C-myc

Most studies suggest that c-myc plays a role in the regulation of prostate growth and carcinogenesis.[71,1034,1070,1071] C-myc is a well-known oncogene that is activated in many human cancers[1072] and has been shown to be amplified with increasing grade of prostate cancer, particularly in metastases.[1073-1077] C-myc expression correlates with growth of androgen-responsive prostate epithelium.[1078]

### Apoptosis-suppressing oncoprotein bcl-2

bcl-2 is considered to be an apoptosis-suppressor gene. Overexpression of the protein in cancer cells may block or delay the onset of apoptosis, selecting and maintaining long-living cells and arresting cells in the G0 phase of the cell cycle.[1079,1080]

Expression of bcl-2 is usually restricted to the basal cell layer of the normal and hyperplastic prostatic epithelium.[1081,1082] However, bcl-2 is overexpresed in PIN.[6,1081,1083] In cancer, the prevalence and expression pattern of bcl-2 is controversial. Over 70% of prostate carcinomas are bcl-2 negative, 18% have weak expression, and 11% exhibit strong expression.[1084] One study found moderate heterogeneous bcl-2 overexpression in localized cancer[1081] that was inversely correlated with Gleason grade.

Expression of bcl-2 correlated with high stage, high grade,[1070] metastases, and response to therapy.[1085] Androgen deprivation therapy reduced bcl-2 expression in cancer, suggesting that these cells develop resistance to apoptotic signals.[1081,1086,1087] Targeted suppression of bcl-2 anti-apoptotic family members using multitarget inhibition strategies through the effective induction of apoptosis is considered a research modality for the treatment of prostate cancer.[1088]

### p53

Mutant p53 expression is a late event in localized prostate cancer,[1089-1091] usually present in high-grade cancer[1092-1095] and elevated in untreated metastatic cancer,[667,1096,1097] hormone-refractory cancer,[1090,1092,1097] and recurrent cancer.[1096] p53 is an independent predictor of metastatic risk.[1095] Inactivation of p53 (−p53) is associated with progression of prostate cancer and may be a marker of survival in stage T2-3N1-3M0.[1096]

### p21

The WAF1/CIP1 gene encodes a p21 cyclin-dependent kinase inhibitor that plays a role in the regulation of the cell cycle. Upon induction by p53, p21WAF1/CIP1 binds to cyclin-dependent kinase 2, resulting in downregulation of CDK2 activity and G1 growth arrest. Prostatic mutations in the WAF1/CIP1 gene abrogate this apparent tumor suppressor gene activity,[1098] thereby facilitating the escape of G1/S checkpoint control with propagation into S phase and maintenance of malignant potential. There is an increase in WAF1/CIP1 polymorphisms in prostate cancer,[1099] but no correlation exists between WAF1/CIP1 expression and grade, stage, or cancer progression.[1100]

### p27Kip1

The cyclin-dependent kinase inhibitor (p27Kip1) negatively regulates cell proliferation by mediating cell cycle arrest in G1. The decrease in p27Kip1 results from increased proteasome-dependent degradation, which is mediated by its specific ubiquitin ligase subunits S-phase kinase protein 2 and cyclin-dependent kinase subunit 1. Cyclin-dependent kinase subunit 1 is involved in p27Kip1 downregulation and may have an important causative role in the development of aggressive tumor behavior in prostate cancer.[1101] p27Kip1 expression decreases with higher Gleason score and involvement of the seminal vesicles by cancer.[1102] Further, p27Kip1 expression is an independent predictor of treatment failure in node-negative cancer following radical prostatectomy.[1102]

### PSMA

Prostatic membrane antigen (PSMA) is a protein that is expressed in the prostatic epithelium and is a potential marker for studying carcinogenesis and progression of prostate cancer. PSMA overexpression is detected in high-grade PIN and is associated with a higher Gleason score of prostate cancer (Fig. 9-62).[201,1103] In suicide gene therapy, anti-PSMA–liposome complex exerted a significant inhibitory effect on the growth of LNCaP xenograft, in contrast to normal IgG–liposome complex.[1104] A recent study found that PSMA immunoreactivity was predictive of progression after surgery.[1105]

### PCNA

Proliferating cell nuclear antigen[1106] is an auxiliary protein for DNA polymerase which reaches maximal expression during the S phase of the cell cycle.[1107] Hence, PCNA has been widely used as an index of the proliferative activity of cancers. The PCNA labeling index is reported to be lowest in benign normal prostatic epithelium and organ-confined cancer, but to increase progressively from well- to poorly differentiated invasive prostate cancer, although there is wide variance.[1108] The correlation of PCNA index is strong with cancer stage.[1107,1108,1109] Hence, high PCNA labeling indices may indicate progression of prostate cancer,[491,1106,1110] and may be an independent prognostic indicator.[491,1106,1111,1112]

### Androgen receptors

The action of androgens in target cells is mediated by androgen receptors (AR). Mutations of AR are rare in untreated prostate cancer, and are present in up to 25% of cancers from patients treated with anti-androgens.[1113,1114] No amplifications are found in untreated cancer, suggesting that androgen withdrawal selected the gene amplification. The AR gene amplification leads to overexpression of the gene, and almost all hormone-refractory prostate carcinomas express high levels of AR.[1115] It remains unclear what mechanisms exist for AR expression in tumors that do have gene amplification.

A number of molecular events act at the level of the AR and associated co-regulators to influence the natural history of prostate cancer, including deregulated expression, somatic mutation, and post-translational modification.[1116,1117] ERBB[1118] appears to activate AR, especially when androgen levels are low, promoting the survival of prostate cancer

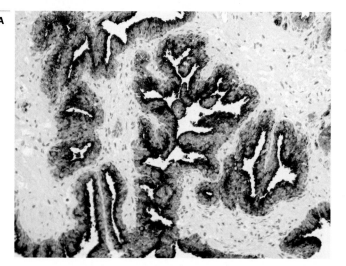
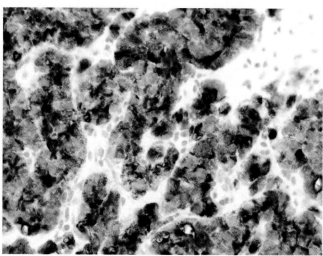

**Fig. 9-62** PSMA immunoreactivity. Intense cytoplasmic and abluminal staining is seen in benign epithelium (**A**) and adenocarcinoma (**B**).

cells. This might be similar to targeting Her-2/neu in hormone-refractory prostate cancer.[1119]

### GSTP1

Glutathione S-transferase class p gene (GSTP1) is the most commonly altered gene in prostate cancer. Silencing of the GSTP1 expression by hypermethylation of the promoter region is present in 90% of prostate cancers and 70% of cases of PIN. Glutathione S-transferases are detoxifying enzymes that catalyze the conjunction of glutathione with harmful electrophilic molecules, either endogenously or exogenously produced, thereby protecting cells from carcinogenic factors.[1120] Detection of hypermethylated GSTP1 may be useful as a diagnostic marker.[1121] High levels of GSTP1 promoter methylation are associated with the transition from PIN to carcinoma.[139]

### Other factors

A wide variety of other predictive factors have been evaluated in prostate cancer, but none are currently recommended for routine use by the College of American Pathologists or the World Health Organization.[369,372,460]

Early prostate cancer antigen EPCA-2 is a novel serum factor with high sensitivity and specificity that differentiates between men with organ-confined and non-organ-confined prostate cancer.[1122]

## Combining multiple predictive factors

The combination of predictive factors provides the greatest accuracy in predicting stage and outcome. The American Joint Committee on Cancer recommends the use of neural network analysis or nomograms to improve survival prediction for prostate cancer.[356]

# Soft tissue neoplasms

Table 9-42 summarizes the current classification of soft tissue tumors of the prostate.

## Benign tumors and tumor-like conditions

Smooth muscle, the dominant tissue in the prostate, accounts for the wide diversity of benign and malignant tumors, most of which have a counterpart in other muscle-rich organs such as the uterus and gastrointestinal system.

**Table 9-42** Soft tissue tumors of the prostate: 2007 new classification

| Benign | Malignant |
|---|---|
| Stromal hyperplasia (stromal subtype of benign nodular hperplasia) | Rhabdomyosarcoma |
| Stromal hyperplasia with atypia | Leiomysarcoma |
| Leiomyoma | Phyllodes tumor |
| Leiomyoma with atypia | Stromal sarcoma |
| Postoperative spindle cell nodule | |
| Inflammatory myofibroblastic tumor | |
| Solitary fibrous tumor | |

Nodular hyperplasia of the prostate (benign prostatic hyperplasia, or BPH) accounts for the majority of tumor-like conditions in the prostate (see Chapter 8). A brief discussion of two variants of hyperplasia – stromal hyperplasia with atypia, and leiomyoma – is presented below owing to the potential for misdiagnosis with malignancy; both are described in greater detail in Chapter 8.

## Stromal hyperplasia (stromal subtype of nodular hyperplasia)

The most common tumor of the prostate, nodular hyperplasia, usually consists of a mixture of epithelial and stromal elements (see Chapter 8). The presence of atypical stromal cells warrants consideration of stromal hyperplasia with atypia (Table 9-43).

In our experience, the stromal subtype of nodular hyperplasia creates the greatest diagnostic difficulty for pathologists in separating it from low-grade leiomyosarcoma, and is the most frequent soft tissue tumor referred for a second opinion. Size alone is usually of great value, as stromal hyperplasia is rarely larger than 1 cm in greatest dimension, whereas leiomyosarcoma is virtually always much larger and is usually high-grade in the prostate.

## Leiomyoma

The distinction between nodular hyperplasia and leiomyoma is often difficult in biopsies or transurethral resection specimens, but this separation appears to have no practical clinical importance. Leiomyoma is defined as a well-circumscribed, encapsulated, solitary smooth muscle nodule greater than 1 cm in diameter (Figs 9-63, 9-64).[1123–1127] It is histologically identical to leiomyoma occurring in the uterus and other sites, and is composed of spindle or epithelioid smooth muscle cells separated by variable amounts of collagen. The tumor cells are often arranged in an orderly pattern of intersecting fascicles. Individual cells have blunt-ended nuclei with evenly distributed nuclear chromatin. Variants of leiomyoma include epithelioid

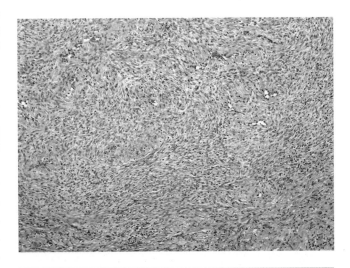

**Fig. 9-63** Stromal nodule. This circumscribed cellular lesion is characterized by vascular and spindle cell proliferation without atypia.

**Table 9-43** Prostatic stromal hyperplasia with atypia (PSHA): differential diagnosis*

| Characteristic features | Stromal hyperplasia with atypia (infiltrative pattern)* | Leiomyoma with atypia (symplastic leiomyoma) | Phyllodes tumor | Leiomyosarcoma |
|---|---|---|---|---|
| Clinical features Mean age (yrs)(range) | 69 (59–80) | 68 (57–80) | 55 (25–86) | 61 (41–78) |
| Presenting symptoms | Urinary obstructive symptoms or incidental finding | Urinary obstructive symptoms or incidental finding | Urinary obstructive symptoms, hematuria, or incidental finding | Urinary obstructive symptoms; perineal pain |
| Cystoscopic/macroscopic | Stromal nodule | Stromal nodule | | Mass measuring 3 to 21 cm in diameter (mean, 9 cm) |
| Serum PSA | Normal range | Normal range | Normal range | Normal range |
| Architecture | Ill-defined hyperplastic stromal nodule with atypical cells diffusely and uniformly infiltrating around typical hyperplasia acini; hypocellular loose myxoid matrix with large ectatic vessels | Solid circumscribed expansile stromal nodule with abundant smooth muscle and atypical stromal cells | Biphasic pattern, including distorted cystically dilated or slit-like epithelial glands, often with leaf-like projections, together with condensed stroma | Large bulky nodular tumor composed of spindle cells |
| Cytology | Bizarre giant stromal cells with vacuolated nuclei and frequent multinucleation; no mitotic figures or necrosis | Bizarre giant stromal cells with vacuolated nuclei and frequent multinucleation; no mitotic figures or necrosis | Benign epithelium; variable number of bizarre stromal cells with vacuolated nuclei and multinucleation; mitotic figures and necrosis indicate higher grade | Spindle or epithelioid tumor cells with variable pleomorphism, mitotic figures, and frequent necrosis |
| Immunohistochemistry | | | | |
| Vimentin | +++ | + | Usually +++ | ++ |
| Desmin | Usually + | +++ | Usually–; rare +++ | Usually –; rare + |
| Actin | + | +++ | + | Usually –; rare + |
| Estrogen receptors | – | – | – | NT |
| *Progesterone | Usually +++ | Usually ++ | Usually –; rare + | NT |
| Receptors | | | | |
| Androgen receptors | +++ | +++ | Usually –; rare ++ | NT |
| Keratin AE1/AE3 | – | – | ++ (epithelium) | Usually – (+ in 27% of cases) |
| Keratin 34βE12 | – | – | ++ (epithelium) | NT |
| PSA | – | – | +++ | – |
| PAP | – | – | +++ | – |
| S100 protein | – | – | – | – |
| Follow-up | Benign; very rare solitary recurrences | Benign; very rare solitary recurrences | Frequent recurrences with late onset of stromal overgrowth | Malignant; mean of 22 months to death (3–72 months) |

*Radiation therapy is also in the differential diagnosis, but can easily be distinguished by clinical history and the diffuse nature of the changes, unlike the focal findings in these neoplasms.

NT, not tested; PAP, prostate acid phosphatase; PSA, prostate-specific antigen.

leiomyoma,[1128] cellular leiomyoma, atypical leiomyoma, and leiomyoblastoma.[1129]

Distinguishing leiomyoma from low-grade leiomyosarcoma is a difficult but uncommon problem in the prostate as most sarcomas are high-grade and easily identified. Infiltrative growth, cellularity, nuclear atypia, tumor necrosis, and increased mitotic activity are the most important distinguishing features, and the diagnosis of sarcoma should be made if at least two or more of these features are present.[1123,1130]

## Pseudosarcomatoid myofibroblastic proliferation (inflammatory myofibroblastic tumor; inflammatory pseudotumor; myofibroblastoma; low-grade inflammatory fibrosarcoma; spindle cell proliferation with no prior operation; pseudosarcoma; nodular fasciitis; pseudosarcomatous fibromyxoid tumor)

This rare benign pathologic entity of unknown etiology (probably reactive) occurs in the bladder, prostate, urethra, and other sites without a history of prior surgery.[1131] Patients

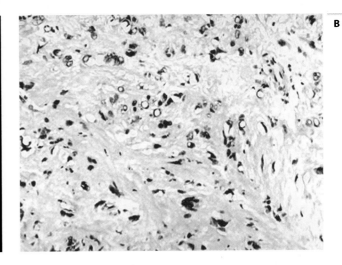

**Fig. 9-64** Leiomyoma. (**A**) Gross of simple prostatectomy with rubbery bulging nodules reminiscent of uterine leiomyoma. (**B**) Stromal hyperplasia with atypical giant cells. Note prominent nuclear vacuolation.

range in age from 16 to 73 years (mean, 41 years), with a slight female predilection in the bladder. Mean tumor size is 3.6 cm, but can measure up to 8 cm in diameter. The stroma is loose, edematous, and myxoid, with abundant small slit-like blood vessels resembling granulation tissue (Figs 9-65, 9-66). Mitotic figures are infrequent, with fewer than 3 per 10 high-power fields; none are atypical. Ulceration and focal necrosis is present in most cases, but is not prominent.

There is intense vimentin immunoreactivity and variable staining for smooth muscle actin, desmin, and keratin; S100 protein and myoglobin are negative. Positivity for anaplastic lymphoma kinase-1 protein (ALK-1) has been reported in some cases of inflammatory myofibroblastic tumor, suggesting a neoplastic rather than a reactive process.[1132–1133] Ultrastructural studies reveal myofibroblastic differentiation, including cytoplasmic microfilaments and dense bodies. Tumors are usually diploid, with a low S-phase fraction.

Recurrences may develop, particularly if incompletely excised, but no reported case in the prostate has metastasized. It should be noted that the clinicopathologic features of lesions associated with (postoperative spindle cell nodule) and without (inflammatory myofibroblastic tumor) instrumentation are similar and inseparable, so many now believe that these are essentially the same entity;[1133,1134] accordingly, Harik et al.[1133] proposed the term pseudosarcomatous myofibroblastic proliferation. Even in the face of atypical histologic features, the prognosis is excellent. Differential diagnostic considerations are identical to those of postoperative spindle cell nodule (Table 9-44).

## Postoperative spindle cell nodule (postoperative inflammatory myofibroblastic tumor)

This rare benign reparative process is considered clinically and histopathologically identical to pseudosarcomatous fibromyxoid tumor except for the antecedent history of surgery or trauma. It occurs 4–12 weeks after surgery, and typically consists of small nodules measuring less than 1 cm

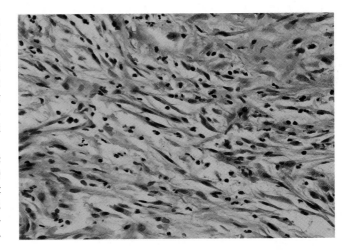

**Fig. 9-65** Pseudosarcomatous fibromyxoid tumor. The loose myxoid stroma contains spindle cells, small, slit-like blood vessels, and inflammatory cells, mainly lymphocytes and plasma cells.

in diameter with spindle cells arranged in fascicles with occasional or numerous mitotic figures (up to 25 per 10 high-power fields).[1135] However, atypical or bizarre mitotic forms have not been reported. The cells have central elongated to ovoid nuclei, small prominent nucleoli, and abundant cytoplasm. There is mild to moderate acute and chronic inflammation. Necrosis may be present, but is usually not a prominent feature.

The cells are strongly positive for vimentin and smooth muscle actin. This immunohistochemical profile cannot differentiate postoperative spindle cell nodule from leiomyoma or low-grade leiomyosarcoma. The key feature in recognizing postoperative spindle cell nodule is the clinical history of surgery or instrumentation in the previous few months. The wide variety of prostatic sarcomas is sufficiently cytologically pleomorphic that differentiation from postoperative spindle cell nodule is usually not a problem. Sarcomatoid

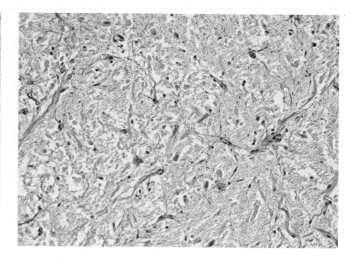

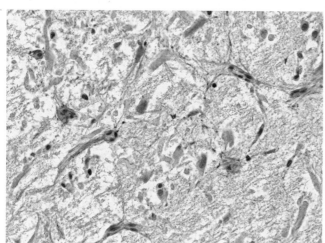

**Fig. 9-66** Pseudosarcomatous fibromyxoid tumor. (**A–C**) This tumor was from a 65-year-old man with a history of prostatitis who underwent transurethral resection of a mass in the prostate protruding into the urethral lumen. The tumor consisted of a loose spindle cell proliferation with abundant granular myxoid background stroma.

carcinoma is also pleomorphic and may display immunoreactivity for cytokeratin and rarely PSA and PAP.[710,714]

### Solitary fibrous tumor

Solitary fibrous tumor is a rare neoplasm that is usually benign but can rarely exhibit malignant behavior. It most commonly arises on serosal surfaces (solitary fibrous mesothelioma) such as the visceral pleura.[1136,1137] Solitary fibrous tumor of the prostate is extremely rare, with fewer than two dozen cases reported to date.[1138,1139]

Solitary fibrous tumor is grossly well circumscribed in the prostate. It is variable in cellularity, consisting of a mixture of haphazard, storiform, or short fascicular patterns of benign-appearing spindle cells with paucicellular dense collagenous bands (Fig. 9-67). A hemangiopericytoma-like growth pattern is typically seen. Positive immunostains for CD34, bcl-2, and CD99 are invaluable in confirming the diagnosis, whereas S100 protein, CD31, and cytokeratin are negative.

### Blue nevus

Blue nevus of the prostate is characterized by the presence of melanin pigment in dendritic bipolar cells in the stroma,[1140–1152] whereas in prostatic melanosis it is chiefly in the epithelium (Fig. 9-68).[1153,1154] Premelanosomes and mela-

nosomes are present ultrastructurally in the cells of prostatic blue nevus, indicating that they are melanocytic. Conversely, only stage IV melanosomes occur in the epithelial cells. S100 protein immunoreactivity was demonstrated in the stromal cells, confirming the ultrastructural findings.[1149]

### Other rare benign soft tissue tumors

A wide variety of other benign tumors that reflect the vast spectrum of mesenchymal tissues may rarely arise in the prostate, including hemangioma,[1155] lymphangioma,[1156] neurofibroma,[1157] neurilemmoma,[1158] chondroma (Fig. 9-69),[1159] gastrointestinal stromal tumor,[1160] hemangiopericytoma,[1161] paraganglioma (pheochromocytoma),[1162] and myxoma.

### Sarcoma

Sarcoma of the prostate accounts for less than 0.1% of prostatic neoplasms. One-third occur in children, and most of these are rhabdomyosarcoma; leiomyosarcoma is most common in adults. Symptoms include prostatism and pelvic pain. Tumors may be 15 cm or more in diameter, and are usually soft with focal necrosis.

In 2004, the World Health Organization held a limited closed meeting that resulted in a new classification of

**Table 9-44** Differential diagnosis of myxoid lesions of the prostate

| | Pseudosarcomatous fibromyxoid tumor | Postoperative spindle cell nodule | Sarcomatoid carcinoma | Myxoid leiomyosarcoma | Myxoid rhabdomyo-sarcoma | Myxoid malignant fibrous histiocytoma |
|---|---|---|---|---|---|---|
| **Light microscopic findings** | | | | | | |
| Cellularity | Variable, often low | Variable, often low | High | Variable | Variable | Variable |
| Growth pattern | Tissue culture-like | Tissue culture-like | Biphasic | Intersecting fasicles | Subepithelial condensation | Storiform |
| Pleomorphism | + | − | +++ | +/− | ++ | +++ |
| Vessels | Slitlike | Unremarkable | Unremarkable | Unremarkable | Unremarkable | Unremarkable |
| Necrosis | +/− | +/− | ++ | ++ | + | ++ |
| Mitotic figures | + | ++ | ++ | + (variable) | ++ | +++ |
| Atypical mitotic figures | + | − | + | + | + | + |
| **IHC findings** | | | | | | |
| Cytokeratin | − (rarely +) | − (rarely +) | + | − (rarely +) | − (rarely +) | − (rarely +) |
| Vimentin | + | + | + | + | + | + |
| Desmin | +/− | +/− | +/− | + | + | − (rarely +) |
| SMA | + | + | +/− | + | − | − |
| S100 | − | − | +/− | − | − | − |
| Myogenin | − | − | − | − | + | − |
| Myoglobin | − | − | − | − | +/− | − |

IHC, immunohistochemical; SMA, smooth muscle actin.

prostatic soft tissue tumors.[1163] Upon publication, the classification was immediately noted to be flawed for including terms such P-STUMP (prostatic stromal tumor of uncertain malignant potential) that erroneously lumped three defined entities together: stromal hyperplasia with atypia, phyllodes tumor, and low-grade stromal sarcoma. Subsequent information has been published regarding these three entities that reaffirmed the clinical necessity to separate them as unique tumors; [1164] we expect P-STUMP to be retired from use in the next WHO consensus meeting.

## Rhabdomyosarcoma

Rhabdomyosarcoma has a peak incidence between birth and 6 years of age, but sporadic cases have been reported in men as old as 80 years. The prostate, bladder, and vagina account for 21% of cases in children, second only to head and neck origin. Serum concentrations of PSA and PAP are normal. Three reported adults had hypercalcemia owing to bone metastases.[1165]

The tumor is usually large and bulky, with a mean diameter up to 9 cm. It often involves the prostate, bladder, and periurethral, perirectal, and perivesicular soft tissues. Urethral involvement may not be apparent cystoscopically. Symptoms include acute or chronic urethral obstruction, bladder displacement, and rectal compression. The prostate may be palpably normal, although large tumors often fill the pelvis and can be palpated suprapubically.

Most are embryonal rhabdomyosarcoma, and the remainder are alveolar, botryoid, and spindle cell subtypes.[1166] Tumor cells are arranged in sheets of immature round to spindle cells set in a myxoid stroma (Figs 9-70, 9-71). Polypoid tumor fragments ('botryoid pattern') may fill the urethral lumen, covered by intact urothelium with condensed underlying tumor cells creating a distinctive cambium layer. Nuclei are usually pleomorphic and darkly staining. Scattered rhabdomyoblasts may be present, with eosinophilic cytoplasmic processes containing cross-striations.

Rhabdomyosarcoma is immunoreactive for markers of muscle differentiation, and myogenin and myo-D1 are the most sensitive and specific.[1167] Tumor cells also display immunoreactivity for myoglobin, desmin, and vimentin, but are negative for PSA and PAP.

Ultrastructural study reveals two cell types, similar to rhabdomyosarcoma at other sites: large oval or elongated tumor cells contain segments of sarcomere with abundant glycogen, and smaller round cells contain abundant cytoplasmic organelles but lack myofibrils. All tumors are aneuploid by flow cytometry.[1168]

Combination chemotherapy, together with surgery and radiotherapy, results in a 3-year survival rate of over 70%,

A

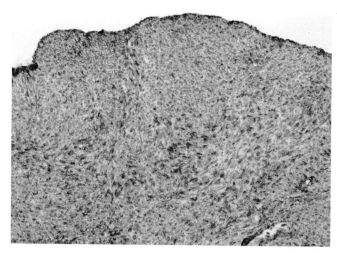

B

C

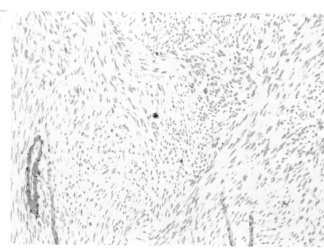

**Fig. 9-67** Solitary fibrous tumor of the prostate. (**A**) The entire biopsy consists of a patternless pattern of bland spindle cells without atypia or mitotic figures. (**B**) Intense cytoplasmic CD34 immunoreactivity is present in every cell. Compare with **C,** showing absence of smooth muscle actin staining (note focal positive blood vessel serving as internal control).

A

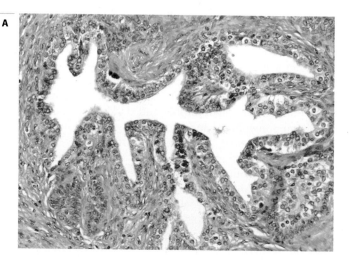

B

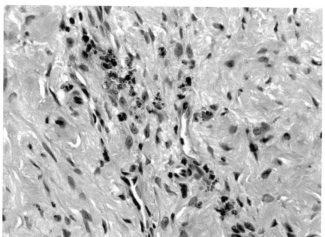

**Fig. 9-68** Prostatic pigment. (**A**) Melanosis, with melanin pigment limited to the benign epithelium. (**B**) Blue nevus, with dusty and granular melanin pigment within myofibroblasts in the stroma.

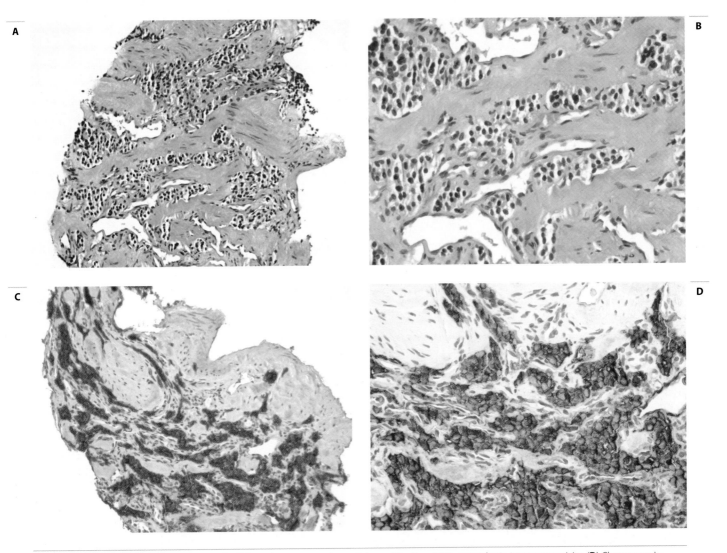

**Fig. 9-69** Paraganglioma on needle biopsy. (**A, B**) Irregular anastomosing cellular proliferation. (**C**) Synaptophysin immunoreactivity. (**D**) Chromogranin immunoreactivity.

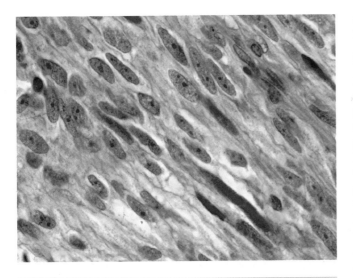

**Fig. 9-70** Rhabdomyosarcoma of the prostate arising in a child.

according to the Intergroup Rhabdomyosarcoma Study.[1169] Long-term survival has been reported.

## Leiomyosarcoma

Leiomyosarcoma is the most common prostatic sarcoma in adults. Patients range in age from 40 to 71 years (mean, 59 years), with sporadic reports in younger patients.[1170] The sarcoma presents as a large bulky mass that replaces the prostate and periprostatic tissues, ranging in size from 3.3 to 21 cm (mean, 9 cm). In our series of 23 cases from the Mayo Clinic, no tumors were grade 1, seven were grade 2, 10 were grade 3, and six were grade 4.[1170] The tumors were histologically similar to leiomyosarcoma at other sites (Fig. 9-72). Prominent sclerotic stroma was noted in two cases. Five tumors had epithelioid features, and one had a focal area reminiscent of neurilemmoma. Necrosis may be extensive. Although the criteria for separating leiomyoma from low-grade leiomyosarcoma have not been precisely defined in the prostate, they are probably similar to those in other organs, including the degree of cellularity, cytologic

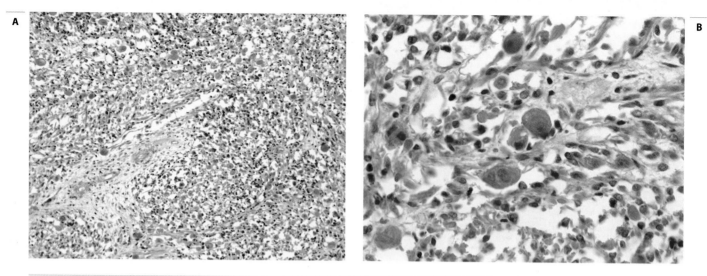

**Fig. 9-71** Rhabdomyosarcoma of the prostate. Rhabdomyoblasts display intensely eosinophilic cytoplasm.

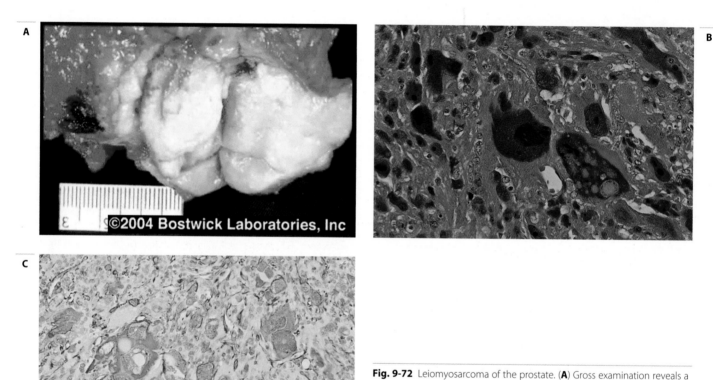

**Fig. 9-72** Leiomyosarcoma of the prostate. (**A**) Gross examination reveals a large fleshy tan mass replacing most of the prostate. (**B**) Bizarre giant cells punctuate this spindle cell proliferation. (**C**) Intense cytoplasmic immunoreactivity for actin in the majority of tumor cells.

anaplasia, number of mitotic figures, amount of necrosis, vascular invasion, and size.

Tumor cells usually display intense cytoplasmic immunoreactivity for smooth muscle-specific actin and vimentin, and weak desmin immunoreactivity. Most are negative for cytokeratin (AE1/AE3) and S100 protein, but exceptions

have been described, particularly in those with epithelioid features in which keratin immunoreactivity may be seen.[1170] Local recurrence and distant metastasis are frequent, and the prognosis is poor. Mean survival after diagnosis was less than 3 years in one series (range, 0.2–6.5 years), and most patients died from sarcoma.[1170]

## Phyllodes tumor (cystic epithelial–stromal tumor; phyllodes type of atypical hyperplasia; cystadenoleiomyofibroma; cystosarcoma phyllodes)

Phyllodes tumor of the prostate is a rare lesion that should be considered a neoplasm rather than atypical hyperplasia owing to frequent early recurrences, infiltrative growth, and its potential for extraprostatic and metastatic spread in some cases.[1164] Dedifferentiation (stromal overgrowth) with multiple recurrences in some cases is further evidence of the potentially aggressive nature of this tumor.[1164] A benign clinical course has been emphasized in early reports, but the cumulative current evidence indicates that a significant number of patients develop local recurrences and metastases.[1164]

Patients with prostatic phyllodes tumor typically present with urinary obstruction, hematuria, and dysuria. There may be severe urinary obstruction, often occurring at a younger age than expected for typical prostatic hyperplasia. Most tumors range in size from 4 to 25 cm. At the time of transurethral resection the urologist may note an unusual spongy or cystic texture of the involved prostate.

The diagnosis of phyllodes tumor is usually made on resected tissue, and it may be overlooked on needle biopsy in which it is difficult to appreciate the pattern of the tumor.

Important diagnostic clues include diffuse infiltration, variably cellular stroma surrounding cysts, and compressed elongated channels that often have a leaf-like configuration (Fig. 9-73). Prostatic phyllodes tumor exhibits a spectrum of histologic features, similar to its counterpart in the breast (Table 9-43).[1164] High-grade prostatic phyllodes tumor has a high stromal–epithelial ratio, prominent stromal cellularity and overgrowth, marked cytologic atypia, and increased mitotic activity. A sarcomatous component may arise within a low-grade tumor over time, invariably after multiple recurrences over many years.[1164] The lining epithelium is benign, but may show various metaplastic and proliferative changes such as basal cell hyperplasia or squamous metaplasia.[1171,1172]

Immunohistochemical studies reveal intense cytoplasmic immunoreactivity in most stromal cells for vimentin and actin, in luminal epithelial cells for PSA, PAP, and keratin AE1/AE3, and in basal epithelial cells for high molecular weight keratin 34βE12; no staining was observed for desmin and S100 protein. Phyllodes tumors of the prostate are clonal, and the epithelial and stromal components have different clonal origins and appear to be true neoplasms.[1173] EGFR and androgen receptor are frequently and strongly expressed in both epithelial and stromal components of prostatic phyllodes tumors.[1174] EGFR gene amplification may account for one of the mechanisms leading to protein

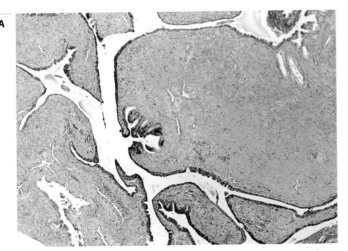

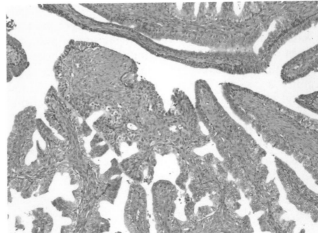

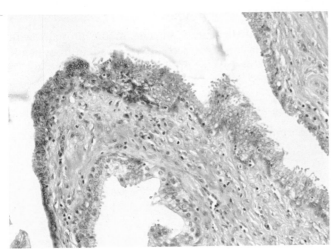

**Fig. 9-73** Phyllodes tumor. (**A, B**) Low-grade prostatic phyllodes tumor with leaf-like intraluminal epithelial-lined stromal projections. (**C**) Low-grade prostatic phyllodes tumor with low cellularity, a low stroma to epithelium ratio, moderate cytologic atypia, and no mitotic figures.

overexpression in some cases. Anti-EGFR and/or anti-andro-gen agents may be potentially useful for management of patients with tumors expressing EGFR and/or androgen receptor.

### Stromal sarcoma

Undifferentiated sarcoma of the prostatic stroma is rare.[1175–1179] Most sarcomas arising in the prostate are classi-fied along the known lines of differentiation for soft tissue sarcomas;[1180] those that do not fit within the known lines of differentiation are simply called stromal sarcoma or sarcoma NOS (not otherwise specified).[1171] Stromal sarcoma may arise in patients of all ages, but is usually seen in adults and the elderly. Prognosis depends on grade and stage, but all are malignant and potentially very aggressive.

Microscopically, stromal sarcoma varies from a diffuse proliferation of round and plump cells (low-grade stromal sarcoma) to spindle cells with a considerable degree of nuclear atypia and hyperchromasia (high-grade stromal sarcoma) (Fig. 9-74). There are invariably more than two mitotic figures per 10 high-power fields, even in needle biop-sies. Areas of necrosis are frequently seen. The cells are arranged in miscellaneous architectural patterns ranging from diffuse sheets to short fascicles that often show a sto-riform pattern.

The neoplastic stromal cells are immunoreactive for vimentin and CD34, but usually negative for smooth muscle actin (SMA), desmin, and S100 protein. Progesterone recep-tors are occasionally positive, whereas estrogen receptors are invariably negative. Some cases showed a similar immuno-histochemical profile: positivity for vimentin and desmin, but negativity for SMA.[1181–1184] In contrast, Yum et al.[1185] reported a case that was positive for vimentin, SMA, and desmin, and classified the tumor as leiomyosarcoma arising in phyllodes tumor.

### Other sarcomas

Other sarcomas reported in the prostate include fibrosar-coma,[1186] osteosarcoma,[1187] malignant fibrous histiocy-toma,[1188] angiosarcoma,[1189] chondrosarcoma,[1190] malignant peripheral nerve sheath tumor,[1191] neurofibrosarcoma, lipo-sarcoma,[1192] and synovial sarcoma.[1193] Regardless of classifi-cation, the prognosis of most adult prostatic sarcomas is poor.

## Other neoplasms and tumor-like proliferations

### Prostatic cysts

Giant multilocular prostatic cystadenoma is a large tumor composed of acini and cysts lined by prostatic-type epithe-lium set in a hypocellular fibrous stroma.[1194–1203] This rare tumor arises in men between ages 28 and 80 years as a large midline prostatic or extraprostatic mass causing urinary obstruction. The epithelial lining displays PSA immuno-reactivity. One case was associated with high-grade PIN.[1204] Surgical excision is usually curative, although the tumor may recur if incompletely excised. The differential diagnosis includes phyllodes tumor, multilocular peritoneal inclusion cyst, multicystic mesothelioma, müllerian duct cyst, seminal vesicle cyst, lymphangioma, and hemangiopericytoma. The light-microscopic appearance of the cyst lining is useful in separating these lesions (Table 9-45).

Other benign unilocular cysts which may be sampled by biopsy include seminal vesicle cyst, ejaculatory duct cyst (Fig. 9-75),[1205–1207] and müllerian duct cyst (Fig. 9-75).[1205,1208] Location is often useful, recognizing that seminal vesicle cyst is typically lateral whereas müllerian duct cyst is midline. Seminal vesicle cysts may contain ectopic prostatic acini[1209] and urothelium.[1210]

Echinococcal cyst is usually associated with prominent inflammation, and organisms are often demonstrable.[1211]

### Ejaculatory duct adenofibroma

A case of benign adenofibroma of the ejaculatory duct was recently reported.[1212] This incidental autopsy finding con-sisted of a small polypoid mass of epithelium and stroma which projected into a cystically dilated duct. Adenomatoid tumor of the ejaculatory duct has also been described.[1213]

### Hematologic malignancies

Hematologic malignancies are rare in the prostate, with primary involvement or secondary spread from systemic lymphoma, leukemia, or myeloma.

**Fig. 9-74** Stromal sarcoma.

**Table 9-45** Prostatic cysts: differential diagnosis

| Type of cyst | Location | Size | Contain sperm |
|---|---|---|---|
| Prostatic cyst | Lateral | Variable | No |
| Seminal vesicle cyst | Lateral | Large | Yes |
| Diverticulum of ejaculatory duct or ampulla | Lateral | Variable | Yes |
| Müllerian duct cyst | Midline | Large | No |

A

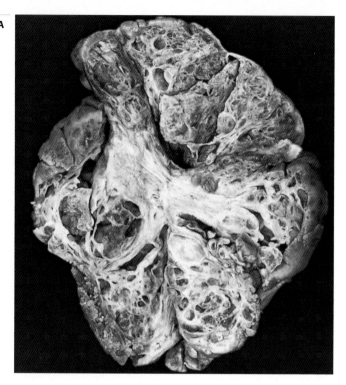

B

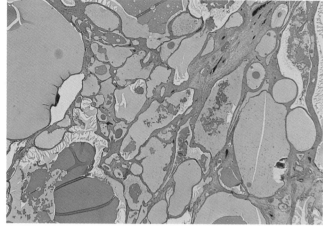

**Fig. 9-75** Cystadenoma of the seminal vesicles. (**A**) Gross. (**B**) Low power. The patient had no recurrence of this 12 cm diameter tumor of the seminal vesicles after 27 years, and died of unrelated causes.

## Leukemia

Chronic lymphocytic leukemia is the most common leukemia involving the prostate, with more than 200 reported cases; many are incidentally discovered during investigation of prostatic enlargement or adenocarcinoma.[681,682,692,1214–1216] The autopsy prevalence of prostatic involvement is about 20% of cases of leukemia. Cachia et al.[1217] followed 46 men with chronic lymphocytic leukemia, and all six who underwent transurethral resection for urinary obstructive symptoms had prostatic involvement. The clinical symptoms and histologic pattern in the prostate are similar to those of malignant lymphoma, and leukemia is distinguished chiefly from lymphoma by the presence of blood involvement. Thalhammer and colleagues[1218] reported an unusual case of late relapse of granulocytic sarcoma (chloroma) detected by urinary obstructive symptoms owing to prostatic enlargement after 9 years of remission; diagnosis was made by transurethral resection. Bladder neck obstruction in patients with leukemia may respond to surgery if chemotherapy is ineffective, although others have successfully used radiation therapy.[1219,1220]

## Malignant lymphoma

Patients with malignant lymphoma involving the prostate are usually older men (mean, 62 years) who have urinary obstructive symptoms, including urinary urgency, urinary frequency, acute urinary retention, urinary tract infections, and hematuria.[1221] Systemic symptoms, including fever, chills, night sweats, and weight loss, are infrequent and are found only in patients with widespread lymphoma. Occasional cases are discovered incidentally at biopsy or radical prostatectomy for

adenocarcinoma.[1214,1216] Grossly, the prostate gland with malignant lymphoma is diffusely enlarged, non-tender, and firm or rubbery. Serum PSA level is usually not elevated.

Primary lymphoma is much less frequent than secondary involvement.[1214,1221,1222] Ewing and others[1223] challenged the existence of primary extranodal lymphoma owing to the paucity of lymphoid tissue in the prostate. However, identification of rudimentary lymphoid nodules in the prostate by Fukase,[1224] the recognition of malignant lymphoma arising in extranodal sites, and histologic documentation of cases with involvement limited to the prostate confirmed the existence of lymphoma apparently arising in the prostate. The prevalence of primary prostatic lymphoma at autopsy is 0.2% of extranodal lymphomas.[1222] Diagnostic criteria that have been proposed for primary lymphoma include symptoms attributable to prostatic enlargement; lymphoma chiefly involving the prostate with or without involvement of adjacent tissues; and lack of liver, spleen, lymph nodes, and peripheral blood involvement within 1 month of diagnosis (sufficient time to allow for typical staging studies).

Microscopically, the lymphomatous infiltrate in the stroma may be diffuse or patchy, with characteristic preservation of prostatic acini (Fig. 9-76); by contrast, granulomatous prostatitis causes acinar destruction.[1221] The infiltrate is usually extensive but may be irregular and patchy, often extending into the extraprostatic soft tissues; involvement of the acinar epithelium is uncommon and rarely includes aggregates in the lumina. The most frequent lymphoma involving the prostate is diffuse non-Hodgkin's lymphoma, including small cleaved-cell, large cell, and mixed-cell types; Hodgkin's disease is very rare, with fewer than five

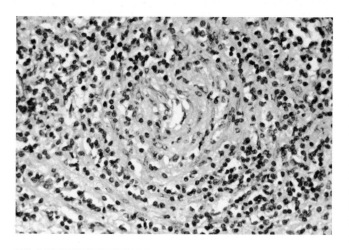

**Fig. 9-76** Malignant lymphoma of the prostate, diffuse small cell type, with prominent angiotropism.

documented cases.[1214,1221] Angiotropic lymphoma has also been described, including one case with spurious immunoreactivity for PAP (PSA was negative) presumably owing to tumor cell absorption from the phosphatase-rich vessel contents.[1225,1226] Mantle zone lymphoma,[1227] Burkitt's lymphoma,[1228] and mucosa-associated lymphoid tissue (MALT) lymphoma[1229,1230] have also been described. Occasional cases of lymphoma have coincidental adenocarcinoma.[1231]

The prognosis of lymphoma involving the prostate is usually poor regardless of patient age, tumor stage, or histologic classification. Lymphoma-specific survival was 64% at 1 year, 33% at 5 years, 33% at 10 years, and 16% at 15 years.[1221] There was no difference in median survival after diagnosis of prostatic involvement between primary and secondary lymphoma (23 months vs 28 months, respectively). Long-term survival is possible with combination chemotherapy, whereas surgery is used chiefly for symptomatic relief of urinary obstruction.

The differential diagnosis of lymphoma includes leukemia, granulomatous prostatitis, chronic prostatitis with follicular hyperplasia, and neuroendocrine carcinoma. A 68-year-old man with prostatic pseudolymphoma was described by Peison et al.[1232] The patient had no prior history of lymphoma and showed symptoms of acute urinary obstruction and a normal blood count. Histologically, there was prominent lymphoid hyperplasia in the transurethral resection specimen without evidence of malignancy. Long-term follow-up was not available. Humphrey and Vollmer[1233] described the first case of extramedullary hematopoiesis of the prostate appearing in a 75-year-old man with a history of myelofibrosis and progressive outlet obstruction. The transurethral resection specimen revealed a diffuse stromal infiltrate of atypical megakaryocytes, immature myeloid elements, and normoblasts; the epithelium was preserved. Chloroacetate esterase staining was useful in confirming the myeloid nature of the infiltrate.

## Multiple myeloma

Multiple myeloma involving the prostate is rare, with fewer than 10 cases reported.[1234] Most are diagnosed at autopsy,

usually after systemic diagnosis. IgD and IgA myelomas have been described and rarely may cause urinary obstructive symptoms. The incidence of prostatic involvement by myeloma is uncertain.

## Germ cell tumors

Rare cases of germ cell tumor apparently arising in the prostate have been reported, invariably with metastases and massive prostatic involvement.[1235-1241] These tumors probably arise from sequestration of germ cells during migration, usually occurring in the midline; this theory also accounts for germ cell tumors in the vagina, mediastinum, liver, retroperitoneum, and liver. Alternatively, some cases probably represent regressed or burned out testicular germ cell tumor with retrovesicular metastasis.

A patient with retroperitoneal seminoma and simultaneous occurrence in the prostate was described by Arai et al.[1242] Michel et al.[1243] reported a 40-year-old with mixed germ cell tumor (embryonal carcinoma and teratoma) who was alive 2 years after treatment. Choriocarcinoma involving the prostate is exceedingly rare.[1244]

The main differential diagnostic considerations include sarcomatoid carcinoma (carcinosarcoma), mucinous carcinoma, typical acinar adenocarcinoma, ductal carcinoma, and metastases from testicular or retroperitoneal primary. The diagnosis of primary germ cell tumor of the prostate should only be considered after all other possibilities are excluded. The usual histologic features of germ cell tumor at other sites are present. For yolk sac tumor, these include Schiller–Duval bodies, hyaline periodic acid–Schiff-positive globules, and elevated serum α-fetoprotein levels; PSA and PAP are normal.

## Rhabdoid tumor

Rhabdoid tumor is a poorly differentiated malignant neoplasm with light-microscopic features of rhabdomyosarcoma that displays epithelial differentiation, including intense cytoplasmic immunoreactivity for keratin proteins and epithelial membrane antigen, rare cell junctions, occasional intracytoplasmic lumina, and distinctive paranuclear aggregates of intermediate filaments. Most cases occur in the kidney, but extrarenal tumors have been identified, including rare cases in the prostate.[1245]

## Other rare tumors and tumor-like conditions

A case of endometriosis of the prostate was documented by Beckman et al.[1246] It arose as a small red-tan raised mass proximal to the internal urethral orifice, which extended into the prostate in a 78-year-old man with a long history of estrogen therapy (chlorotrianisene) for prostatic carcinoma. This case and similar cases reported in the male bladder were invariably associated with hematuria and chlorotrianisene therapy for prostatic adenocarcinoma.

# References

1. Jemal A, Siegel R, Ward E, et al. Cancer statistics, 2008. CA Cancer J Clin 2008; 58: 71–96.

2. Sakr WA, Grignon DJ, Haas GP, et al. Age and racial distribution of prostatic intraepithelial neoplasia. Eur Urol 1996; 30: 138–144.

3. Bostwick DG. Prospective origins of prostate carcinoma. Prostatic intraepithelial neoplasia and atypical adenomatous hyperplasia. Cancer 1996; 78: 330–336.

4. Bostwick DG, Shan A, Qian J, et al. Independent origin of multiple foci of prostatic intraepithelial neoplasia: comparison with matched foci of prostate carcinoma. Cancer 1998; 83: 1995–2002.

5. Bostwick DG, Montironi R, Sesterhenn IA. Diagnosis of prostatic intraepithelial neoplasia: Prostate Working Group/consensus report. Scand J Urol Nephrol 2000; 205: 3–10.

6. Ananthanarayanan V, Deaton RJ, Yang XJ, et al. Alteration of proliferation and apoptotic markers in normal and premalignant tissue associated with prostate cancer. BMC Cancer 2006; 6: 73.

7. Montironi R, Diamanti L, Pomante R, et al. Subtle changes in benign tissue adjacent to prostate neoplasia detected with a Bayesian belief network. J Pathol 1997; 182: 442–449.

8. Montironi R, Mazzucchelli R, Marshall JR, Bartels PH. Prostate cancer prevention: review of target populations, pathological biomarkers, and chemopreventive agents. J Clin Pathol 1999; 52: 793–803.

9. Kastendieck H, Helpap B. Prostatic 'dysplasia/atypical hyperplasia.' Terminology, histopathology, pathobiology, and significance. Urology 1989; 34: 28–42.

10. McNeal JE, Bostwick DG. Intraductal dysplasia: a premalignant lesion of the prostate. Hum Pathol 1986; 17: 64–71.

11. Bostwick DG, Brawer MK. Prostatic intra-epithelial neoplasia and early invasion in prostate cancer. Cancer 1987; 59: 788–794.

12. Drago JR, Mostofi FK, Lee F. Introductory remarks and workshop summary. Urology 1989; 34: 2–3.

13. Montironi R, Bostwick DG, Bonkhoff H, et al. Origins of prostate cancer. Cancer 1996; 78: 362–365.

14. Sakr WA, Grignon DJ, Haas GP, et al. Epidemiology of high grade prostatic intraepithelial neoplasia. Pathol Res Pract 1995; 191: 838–841.

15. Bostwick DG, Grignon DJ, Hammond ME, et al. Prognostic factors in prostate cancer. College of American Pathologists Consensus Statement 1999. Arch Pathol Lab Med 2000; 124: 995–1000.

16. Bostwick DG, Norlen BJ, Denis L. Prostatic intraepithelial neoplasia: the preinvasive stage of prostate cancer. Overview of the prostate committee report. Scand J Urol Nephrol 2000; 205: 1–2.

17. Algaba F, Epstein JI, Aldape HC, et al. Assessment of prostate carcinoma in core needle biopsy – definition of minimal criteria for the diagnosis of cancer in biopsy material. Cancer 1996; 78: 376–381.

18. Egevad L, Allsbrook WC, Epstein JI. Current practice of diagnosis and reporting of prostatic intraepithelial neoplasia and glandular atypia among genitourinary pathologists. Mod Pathol 2006; 19: 180–185.

19. Epstein JI, Grignon DJ, Humphrey PA, et al. Interobserver reproducibility in the diagnosis of prostatic intraepithelial neoplasia. Am J Surg Pathol 1995; 19: 873–886.

20. Allam CK, Bostwick DG, Hayes JA, et al. Interobserver variability in the diagnosis of high-grade prostatic intraepithelial neoplasia and adenocarcinoma. Mod Pathol 1996; 9: 742–751.

21. Egevad L, Allsbrook WC Jr, Epstein JI. Current practice of diagnosis and reporting of prostate cancer on needle biopsy among genitourinary pathologists. Hum Pathol 2006; 37: 292–297.

22. Brawer MK, Bigler SA, Sohlberg OE, et al. Significance of prostatic intraepithelial neoplasia on prostate needle biopsy. Urology 1991; 38: 103–107.

23. Aboseif S, Shinohara K, Weidner N, et al. The significance of prostatic intra-epithelial neoplasia. Br J Urol 1995; 76: 355–359.

24. Langer JE, Rovner ES, Coleman BG, et al. Strategy for repeat biopsy of patients with prostatic intraepithelial neoplasia detected by prostate needle biopsy. J Urol 1996; 155: 228–231.

25. Raviv G, Janssen T, Zlotta AR, et al. Prostatic intraepithelial neoplasia: influence of clinical and pathological data on the detection of prostate cancer. J Urol 1996; 156: 1050–1054; discussion 1054–1055.

26. Shepherd D, Keetch DW, Humphrey PA, et al. Repeat biopsy strategy in men with isolated prostatic intraepithelial neoplasia on prostate needle biopsy. J Urol 1996; 156: 460–462; discussion 462–463.

27. Goeman L, Joniau S, Ponette D, et al. Is low-grade prostatic intraepithelial neoplasia a risk factor for cancer? Prostate Cancer Prostatic Dis 2003; 6: 305–310.

28. De Matteis M, Poggi C, De Martino A, et al. Repeat biopsy in patients with initial diagnosis of PIN. Radiol Med (Torino) 2005; 110: 190–198.

29. Greenlee R, Hill-Harmon M, Murray T, Thun M. Cancer statistics, 2001. CA Cancer J Clin 2001; 51: 15–36.

30. Steiner MS. High grade prostatic intraepithelial neoplasia is a disease. Curr Urol Rep 2001; 2: 195–198.

31. Richie JP, Kavoussi LR, Ho GT, et al. Prostate cancer screening: role of the digital rectal examination and prostate-specific antigen. Ann Surg Oncol 1994; 1: 117–120.

32. Perachino M, di Ciolo L, Barbetti V, et al. Results of rebiopsy for suspected prostate cancer in symptomatic men with elevated PSA levels. Eur Urol 1997; 32: 155–159.

33. Skjorten FJ, Berner A, Harvei S, et al. Prostatic intraepithelial neoplasia in surgical resections: relationship to coexistent adenocarcinoma and atypical adenomatous hyperplasia of the prostate. Cancer 1997; 79: 1172–1179.

34. Gaudin PB, Sesterhenn IA, Wojno KJ, et al. Incidence and clinical significance of high-grade prostatic intraepithelial neoplasia in TURP specimens. Urology 1997; 49: 558–563.

35. Qian J, Wollan P, Bostwick DG. The extent and multicentricity of high-grade prostatic intraepithelial neoplasia in clinically localized prostatic adenocarcinoma. Hum Pathol 1997; 28: 143–148.

36. Sakr WA, Haas GP, Cassin BF, et al. The frequency of carcinoma and intraepithelial neoplasia of the prostate in young male patients. J Urol 1993; 150: 379–385.

37. Soos G, Tsakiris I, Szanto J, et al. The prevalence of prostate carcinoma and its precursor in Hungary: an autopsy study. Eur Urol 2005; 48: 739–744.

38. Stamatiou K, Alevizos A, Agapitos E, Sofras F. Incidence of impalpable carcinoma of the prostate and of non-malignant and precarcinomatous lesions in Greek male population: an autopsy study. Prostate 2006; 66: 1319–1328.

39. Bostwick DG. Prostatic intraepithelial neoplasia. Curr Urol Rep 2000; 1: 65–70.

40. Sakr WA, Grignon DJ, Haas GP. Pathology of premalignant lesions and carcinoma of the prostate in African-American men. Semin Urol Oncol 1998; 16: 214–220.

41. Fowler JE Jr, Bigler SA, Lynch C, et al. Prospective study of correlations between biopsy-detected high grade prostatic intraepithelial neoplasia, serum prostate specific antigen concentration, and race. Cancer 2001; 91: 1291–1296.

42. Angwafo FF 3rd, Zaher A, Befidi-Mengue R, et al. High-grade intra-epithelial neoplasia and prostate cancer in Dibombari, Cameroon.

Prostate Cancer Prostatic Dis 2003; 6: 34–38.

43. Sakr WA. Prostatic intraepithelial neoplasia: A marker for high-risk groups and a potential target for chemoprevention. Eur Urol 1999; 35: 474–478.

44. Watanabe M, Fukutome K, Kato H, et al. Progression-linked overexpression of c-Met in prostatic intraepithelial neoplasia and latent as well as clinical prostate cancers. Cancer Lett 1999; 141: 173–178.

45. Fujita M, Shin M, Yasunaga Y, et al. Incidence of prostatic intra-epithelial neoplasia in Osaka, Japan. Intl J Cancer 1997; 73: 808–811.

46. Sakr WA, Billis A, Ekman P, et al. Epidemiology of high-grade prostatic intraepithelial neoplasia. Scand J Urol Nephrol Suppl 2000: 11–18.

47. Sakr WA, Grignon DJ, Crissman JD, et al. High grade prostatic intraepithelial neoplasia (HGPIN) and prostatic adenocarcinoma between the ages of 20–69: an autopsy study of 249 cases. In Vivo 1994; 8: 439–443.

48. Helpap B, Bonkhoff H, Cockett A, et al. Relationship between atypical adenomatous hyperplasia (AAH), prostatic intraepithelial neoplasia (PIN) and prostatic adenocarcinoma. Pathologica 1997; 89: 288–300.

49. Qian J, Bostwick DG. The extent and zonal location of prostatic intraepithelial neoplasia and atypical adenomatous hyperplasia: relationship with carcinoma in radical prostatectomy specimens. Pathol Res Pract 1995; 191: 860–867.

50. International consultation on prostatic intraepithelial neoplasia pathologic staging of prostatic carcinoma. Rochester M, 3–4 November, 1995. Cancer 1996; 78: 320–381.

51. Bostwick DG, Amin MB, Dundore P, et al. Architectural patterns of high-grade prostatic intraepithelial neoplasia. Hum Pathol 1993; 24: 298–310.

52. Argani P, Epstein JI. Inverted (hobnail) high-grade prostatic intraepithelial neoplasia (PIN): report of 15 cases of a previously undescribed pattern of high-grade PIN. Am J Surg Pathol 2001; 25: 1534–1539.

53. Reyes AO, Swanson PE, Carbone JM, Humphrey PA. Unusual histologic types of high-grade prostatic intraepithelial neoplasia. Am J Surg Pathol 1997; 21: 1215–1222.

54. Melissari M, Lopez Beltran A, Mazzucchelli R, et al. High grade prostatic intraepithelial neoplasia with squamous differentiation. J Clin Pathol 2006; 59: 437–439.

55. Billis A. Widespread high-grade prostatic intraepithelial neoplasia on prostatic needle biopsy: a significant likelihood of subsequently diagnosed adenocarcinoma. Int Braz J Urol 2006; 32: 599–600.

56. Roscigno M, Scattoni V, Freschi M, et al. Monofocal and plurifocal high-grade prostatic intraepithelial neoplasia on extended prostate biopsies: factors predicting cancer detection on extended repeat biopsy. Urology 2004; 63: 1105–1110.

57. Magi-Galluzzi C, Schoenfield L, Reuther AM, et al. Multifocal high-grade prostatic intraepithelial neoplasia on firts-time saturation prostat biopsy is associated with high cancer detection rate on repeat biopsy. Mod Pathol 2007; 20: 162A.

58. Svatek RS, Karam JA, Rogers TE, et al. Intraluminal crystalloids are highly associated with prostatic adenocarcinoma on concurrent biopsy specimens. Prostate Cancer Prostatic Dis 2007; 10: 279–282.

59. Bock BJ, Bostwick DG. Does prostatic ductal adenocarcinoma exist? Am J Surg Pathol 1999; 23: 781–785.

60. Rioux-Leclercq N, Leray E, Patard JJ, et al. The utility of Ki-67 expression in the differential diagnosis of prostatic intraepithelial neoplasia and ductal adenocarcinoma. Hum Pathol 2005; 36: 531–535.

61. Luong A, Chuang ST, Yang XJ. Proliferative activity of prostatic ductal adenocarcinoma. Mod Pathol 2007; 20: 161A.

62. Bostwick DG, Iczkowski KA. Minimal criteria for the diagnosis of prostate cancer on needle biopsy. Ann Diagn Pathol 1997; 1: 104–129.

63. de la Torre M, Haggman M, Brandstedt S, Busch C. Prostatic intraepithelial neoplasia and invasive carcinoma in total prostatectomy specimens: distribution, volumes and DNA ploidy. Br J Urol 1993; 72: 207–213.

64. Sakr WA, Sarkar FH, Sreepathi P, et al. Measurement of cellular proliferation in human prostate by AgNOR, PCNA, and SPF. Prostate 1993; 22: 147–154.

65. O'Dowd G J, Miller MC, Orozco R, Veltri RW. Analysis of repeated biopsy results within 1 year after a noncancer diagnosis. Urology 2000; 55: 553–559.

66. Al-Moghrabi HQ, Belanger EC, Mai KT. Prostatic central zone: High grade prostatic intraepithelial neoplasia and carcinoma. Mod Pathol 2007; 20: 134A.

67. Sakr WA. High-grade prostatic intraepithelial neoplasia: additional links to a potentially more aggressive prostate cancer? J Natl Cancer Inst 1998; 90: 486–487.

68. Montironi R, Scarpelli M, Sisti S, et al. Quantitative analysis of prostatic intraepithelial neoplasia on tissue sections. Anal Quant Cytol Histol 1990; 12: 366–372.

69. Montironi R, Scarpelli M, Sisti S, et al. Morphological and quantitative analyses of intraductal dysplasia of the prostate. Anal Cell Pathol 1990; 2: 277–285.

70. Montironi R, Pomante R, Colanzi P, et al. Diagnostic distance of high grade prostatic intraepithelial neoplasia from normal prostate and adenocarcinoma. J Clin Pathol 1997; 50: 775–782.

71. Qian J, Jenkins RB, Bostwick DG. Detection of chromosomal anomalies and c-myc gene amplification in the cribriform pattern of prostatic intraepithelial neoplasia and carcinoma by fluorescence in situ hybridization. Mod Pathol 1997; 10: 1113–1119.

72. Qian J, Jenkins RB, Bostwick DG. Genetic and chromosomal alterations in prostatic intraepithelial neoplasia and carcinoma detected by fluorescence in situ hybridization. Eur Urol 1999; 35: 479–483.

73. Bostwick DG. Progression of prostatic intraepithelial neoplasia to early invasive adenocarcinoma. Eur Urol 1996; 30: 145–152.

74. Montironi R, Schulman ML. Precursors of prostatic cancer: progression, regression and chemoprevention. Eur Urol 1996; 30: 133–137.

75. Qian J, Jenkins RB, Bostwick DG. Determination of gene and chromosome dosage in prostatic intraepithelial neoplasia and carcinoma. Anal Quant Cytol Histol 1998; 20: 373–380.

76. Sakr WA, Partin AW. Histological markers of risk and the role of high-grade prostatic intraepithelial neoplasia. Urology 2001; 57: 115–120.

77. Qian J, Jenkins RB, Bostwick DG. Potential markers of aggressiveness in prostatic intraepithelial neoplasia detected by fluorescence in situ hybridization. Eur Urol 1996; 30: 177–184.

78. Montironi R, Filho AL, Santinelli A, et al. Nuclear changes in the normal-looking columnar epithelium adjacent to and distant from prostatic intraepithelial neoplasia and prostate cancer. Morphometric analysis in whole-mount sections. Virchows Arch 2000; 437: 625–634.

79. Mai KT, Yazdi HM, Belanger E, et al. High grade prostatic intraepithelial neoplasia involving small ducts and acini. Histopathology 2005; 46: 475–477.

80. Guo ML, Epstein JI. Intraductal carcinoma of the prostate on needle biopsy: Histologic features and clinical significance. Mod Pathol 2006; 19: 1528–1535.

81. Valdman A, Jonmarker S, Ekman P, Egevad L. Cytological features of prostatic intraepithelial neoplasia. Diagn Cytopathol 2006; 34: 317–322.

82. Chen H, Tsuboi N, Nishimura T, et al. Significance of noninvasive diagnosis of prostate cancer with

cytologic examination of prostatic fluid. J Nippon Med Sch 2006; 73: 129–135.

83. Zhou M, Shah R, Shen R, Rubin MA. Basal cell cocktail (34betaE12 + p63) improves the detection of prostate basal cells. Am J Surg Pathol 2003; 27: 365–371.

84. Kruslin B, Tomas D, Cviko A, et al. Periacinar Clefting and p63 Immunostaining in Prostatic Intraepithelial Neoplasia and Prostatic Carcinoma. Pathol Oncol Res 2006; 12: 205–209.

85. Green JS, Knight RJ, Hunter-Campbell P, et al. An investigation into the spatial relationship between prostate intraepithelial neoplasia and cancer. Prostate Cancer Prostatic Dis 2001; 4: 97–100.

86. Novis DA, Zarbo RJ, Valenstein PA. Diagnostic uncertainty expressed in prostate needle biopsies. A College of American Pathologists Q-probes Study of 15,753 prostate needle biopsies in 332 institutions. Arch Pathol Lab Med 1999; 123: 687–692.

87. Kahane H, Sharp JW, Shuman GB, et al. Utilization of high molecular weight cytokeratin on prostate needle biopsies in an independent laboratory. Urology 1995; 45: 981–986.

88. Varma M, Linden MD, Amin MB. Effect of formalin fixation and epitope retrieval techniques on antibody 34betaE12 immunostaining of prostatic tissues. Mod Pathol 1999; 12: 472–478.

89. Iczkowski KA, Cheng L, Crawford BG, Bostwick DG. Steam heat with an EDTA buffer and protease digestion optimizes immunohistochemical expression of basal cell-specific antikeratin 34betaE12 to discriminate cancer in prostatic epithelium. Mod Pathol 1999; 12: 1–4.

90. Goldstein NS, Underhill J, Roszka J, Neill JS. Cytokeratin 34 beta E-12 immunoreactivity in benign prostatic acini. Quantitation, pattern assessment, and electron microscopic study. Am J Clin Pathol 1999; 112: 69–74.

91. Amin MB, Ro JY, Ayala AG. Prostatic intraepithelial neoplasia. Relationship to adenocarcinoma of prostate. Pathol Annu 1994; 29: 1–30.

92. Ramnani DM, bostwick DG. Basal cell-specific anti-keratin antibody 34βE12: optimizing its use in distinguishing benign prostate and cancer. Mod Pathol 1999; 12: 443–444.

93. Shin M, Fujita MQ, Yasunaga Y, et al. Utility of immunohistochemical detection of high molecular weight cytokeratin for differential diagnosis of proliferative conditions of the prostate. Int J Urol 1998; 5: 237–242.

94. Freibauer C. Diagnosis of prostate carcinoma on biopsy specimens improved by basal-cell-specific anti-cytokeratin antibody (34 beta E12).

Wien Klin Wochenschr 1998; 110: 608–611.

95. Brawer MK, Nagle RB, Pitts W, et al. Keratin immunoreactivity as an aid to the diagnosis of persistent adenocarcinoma in irradiated human prostates. Cancer 1989; 63: 454–460.

96. Saboorian MH, Huffman H, Ashfaq R, et al. Distinguishing Cowper's glands from neoplastic and pseudoneoplastic lesions of prostate: immunohistochemical and ultrastructural studies. Am J Surg Pathol 1997; 21: 1069–1074.

97. Cina SJ, Silberman MA, Kahane H, Epstein JI. Diagnosis of Cowper's glands on prostate needle biopsy. Am J Surg Pathol 1997; 21: 550–555.

98. Yang XJ, Lecksell K, Gaudin P, Epstein JI. Rare expression of high-molecular-weight cytokeratin in adenocarcinoma of the prostate gland: a study of 100 cases of metastatic and locally advanced prostate cancer. Am J Surg Pathol 1999; 23: 147–152.

99. Bonkhoff H, Stein U, Remberger K. Multidirectional differentiation in the normal, hyperplastic, and neoplastic human prostate: simultaneous demonstration of cell-specific epithelial markers. Hum Pathol 1994; 25: 42–46.

100. Bonkhoff H, Stein U, Remberger K. The proliferative function of basal cells in the normal and hyperplastic human prostate. Prostate 1994; 24: 114–118.

101. Devaraj LT, Bostwick DG. Atypical basal cell hyperplasia of the prostate. Immunophenotypic profile and proposed classification of basal cell proliferations. Am J Surg Pathol 1993; 17: 645–659.

102. Tacha DE, Miller RT. Use of p63/P504S monoclonal antibody cocktail in immunohistochemical staining of prostate tissue. Appl Immunohistochem Mol Morphol 2004; 12: 75–78.

103. Sung MT, Jiang Z, Montironi R, et al. Alpha-methylacyl-CoA racemase (P504S)/34betaE12/p63 triple cocktail stain in prostatic adenocarcinoma after hormonal therapy. Hum Pathol 2007; 38: 332–341.

104. Shah RB, Kunju LP, Shen R, et al. Usefulness of basal cell cocktail (34betaE12 + p63) in the diagnosis of atypical prostate glandular proliferations. Am J Clin Pathol 2004; 122: 517–523.

105. Rabets JC, Jones JS, Patel A, Zippe CD. Prostate cancer detection with office based saturation biopsy in a repeat biopsy population. J Urol 2004; 172: 94–97.

106. Ng VW, Koh M, Tan SY, Tan PH. Is triple immunostaining with 34betaE12, p63, and racemase in prostate cancer advantageous? A tissue microarray study. Am J Clin Pathol 2007; 127: 248–253.

107. Molinie V, Herve JM, Lugagne PM, et al. Diagnostic utility of a p63/alpha-methyl coenzyme A racemase (p504s) cocktail in ambiguous lesions of the prostate upon needle biopsy. BJU Int 2006; 97: 1109–1115.

108. Molinie V, Fromont G, Sibony M, et al. Diagnostic utility of a p63/alpha-methyl-CoA-racemase (p504s) cocktail in atypical foci in the prostate. Mod Pathol 2004; 17: 1180–1190.

109. Man YG, Zhao C, Chen X. A subset of prostate basal cells lacks the expression of corresponding phenotypic markers. Pathol Res Pract 2006; 202: 651–662.

110. Humphrey PA. Diagnosis of adenocarcinoma in prostate needle biopsy tissue. J Clin Pathol 2007; 60: 35–42.

111. Hameed O, Sublett J, Humphrey PA. Immunohistochemical stains for p63 and alpha-methylacyl-CoA racemase, versus a cocktail comprising both, in the diagnosis of prostatic carcinoma: a comparison of the immunohistochemical staining of 430 foci in radical prostatectomy and needle biopsy tissues. Am J Surg Pathol 2005; 29: 579–587.

112. Davis LD, Zhang W, Merseburger A, et al. p63 expression profile in normal and malignant prostate epithelial cells. Anticancer Res 2002; 22: 3819–3825.

113. Signoretti S, Waltregny D, Dilks J, et al. p63 is a prostate basal cell marker and is required for prostate development. Am J Pathol 2000; 157: 1769–1775.

114. Yang Y, Hao J, Liu X, et al. Differential expression of cytokeratin mRNA and protein in normal prostate, prostatic intraepithelial neoplasia, and invasive carcinoma. Am J Pathol 1997; 150: 693–704.

115. Nagle RB, Brawer MK, Kittelson J, Clark V. Phenotypic relationships of prostatic intraepithelial neoplasia to invasive prostatic carcinoma. Am J Pathol 1991; 138: 119–128.

116. Shah RB, Zhou M, LeBlanc M, et al. Comparison of the basal cell-specific markers, 34betaE12 and p63, in the diagnosis of prostate cancer. Am J Surg Pathol 2002; 26: 1161–1168.

117. Srigley JR, Dardick I, Hartwick RW, Klotz L. Basal epithelial cells of human prostate gland are not myoepithelial cells. A comparative immunohistochemical and ultrastructural study with the human salivary gland. Am J Pathol 1990; 136: 957–966.

118. Howat AJ, Mills PM, Lyons TJ, Stephenson TJ. Absence of S100 protein in prostatic glands. Histopathology 1988; 13: 468–470.

119. Stewart JM, Fleshner N, Cole H, Sweet J. Comparison of annexin II, p63 and AMACR immunoreactivity in prostatic tissue: A tissue microarray

study. J Clin Pathol 2007; 60: 773–780.

120. Kunju LP, Chinnaiyan AM, Shah RB. Comparison of monoclonal antibody (P504S) and polyclonal antibody to alpha methylacyl-CoA racemase (AMACR) in the work-up of prostate cancer. Histopathology 2005; 47: 587–596.

121. Rubin MA, Zhou M, Dhanasekaran SM, et al. Alpha-methylacyl coenzyme A racemase as a tissue biomarker for prostate cancer. JAMA 2002; 287: 1662–1670.

122. Kunju LP, Rubin MA, Chinnaiyan AM, Shah RB. Diagnostic usefulness of monoclonal antibody P504S in the workup of atypical prostatic glandular proliferations. Am J Clin Pathol 2003; 120: 737–745.

123. Murphy AJ, Hughes CA, Lannigan G, et al. Heterogeneous expression of alpha-methylacyl-CoA racemase in prostatic cancer correlates with Gleason score. Histopathology 2007; 50: 243–251.

124. Ananthanarayanan V, Deaton RJ, Yang XJ, et al. Alpha-methylacyl-CoA racemase (AMACR) expression in normal prostatic glands and high-grade prostatic intraepithelial neoplasia (HGPIN): association with diagnosis of prostate cancer. Prostate 2005; 63: 341–346.

125. Gologan A, Bastacky S, McHale T, et al. Age-associated changes in alpha-methyl CoA racemase (AMACR) expression in nonneoplastic prostatic tissues. Am J Surg Pathol 2005; 29: 1435–1441.

126. Helpap B. The significance of the P504S expression pattern of high-grade prostatic intraepithelial neoplasia (HGPIN) with and without adenocarcinoma of the prostate in biopsy and radical prostatectomy specimens. Virchows Arch 2006; 448: 480–484.

127. Karakiewicz PI, Benayoun S, Begin LR, et al. Chronic inflammation is negatively associated with prostate cancer and high-grade prostatic intraepithelial neoplasia on needle biopsy. Int J Clin Pract 2007; 61: 425–430.

128. Bostwick DG, Pacelli A, Lopez-Beltran A. Molecular biology of prostatic intraepithelial neoplasia. Prostate 1996; 29: 117–134.

129. Emmert-Buck MR, Vocke CD, Pozzatti RO, et al. Allelic loss on chromosome 8p12–21 in microdissected prostatic intraepithelial neoplasia. Cancer Res 1995; 55: 2959–2962.

130. Ge K, Minhas F, Duhadaway J, et al. Loss of heterozygosity and tumor suppressor activity of Bin1 in prostate carcinoma. Int J Cancer 2000; 86: 155–161.

131. Yildiz-Sezer S, Verdorfer I, Schafer G, et al. Assessment of aberrations on chromosome 8 in prostatic atrophy. BJU Int 2006; 98: 184–188.

132. Hughes S, Yoshimoto M, Beheshti B, et al. The use of whole genome amplification to study chromosomal changes in prostate cancer: insights into genome-wide signature of preneoplasia associated with cancer progression. BMC Genomics 2006; 7: 65.

133. Qian J, Bostwick DG, Takahashi S, et al. Chromosomal anomalies in prostatic intraepithelial neoplasia and carcinoma detected by fluorescence in situ hybridization. Cancer Res 1995; 55: 5408–5414.

134. Yoshimoto M, Joshua AM, Chilton-Macneill S, et al. Three-color FISH analysis of TMPRSS2/ERG fusions in prostate cancer indicates that genomic microdeletion of chromosome 21 is associated with rearrangement. Neoplasia 2006; 8: 465–469.

135. Lu W TH, Furusato B, Maekawa S, et al. Allelotyping analysis at chromosome arm 8p of high-grade prostatic intraepithelial neoplasia and incidental, latent, and clinical prostate cancers. Genes Chromosomes Cancer 2006; 45: 509–515.

136. Miet SM, Neyra M, Jaques R, et al. RER(+) phenotype in prostate intra-epithelial neoplasia associated with human prostate-carcinoma development. Int J Cancer 1999; 82: 635–639.

137. Baltaci S, Orhan D, Ozer G, et al. Bcl-2 proto-oncogene expression in low- and high-grade prostatic intraepithelial neoplasia. BJU Int 2000; 85: 155–159.

138. Hu CK, McCall S, Madden J, et al. Loss of heterozygosity of M6P/IGF2R gene is an early event in the development of prostate cancer. Prostate Cancer Prostatic Dis 2006; 9: 62–67.

139. Henrique R, Jeronimo C, Teixeira MR, et al. Epigenetic heterogeneity of high-grade prostatic intraepithelial neoplasia: clues for clonal progression in prostate carcinogenesis. Mol Cancer Res 2006; 4: 1–8.

140. Collard RL, Harya NS, Monzon FA, et al. Methylation of the ASC gene promoter is associated with aggressive prostate cancer. Prostate 2006; 66: 687–695.

141. Cerveira N, Ribeiro FR, Peixoto A, et al. TMPRSS2-ERG gene fusion causing ERG overexpression precedes chromosome copy number changes in prostate carcinomas and paired HGPIN lesions. Neoplasia 2006; 8: 826–832.

142. Perez S, Mosquera J-M, Demichelis F, et al. TMPRSS2-ERG fusion prostate cancer: An early molecular event associated with invasion. Mod Pathol 2007; 20: 169A.

143. Nasir A, Copeland J, Gillespie JW, et al. Preneoplastic lesions of the prostate – clinical, pathological and molecular biological aspects. In Vivo 2002; 16: 557–566.

144. Jarrard DF, Paul R, van Bokhoven A, et al. P-cadherin is a basal cell-specific epithelial marker that is not expressed in prostate cancer. Clin Cancer Res 1997; 3: 2121–2128.

145. Harper ME, Glynne-Jones E, Goddard L, et al. Expression of androgen receptor and growth factors in premalignant lesions of the prostate. J Pathol 1998; 186: 169–177.

146. Saleem M, Adhami VM, Zhong W, et al. A novel biomarker for staging human prostate adenocarcinoma: overexpression of matriptase with concomitant loss of its inhibitor, hepatocyte growth factor activator inhibitor-1. Cancer Epidemiol Biomarkers Prev 2006; 15: 217–227.

147. Zhang PJ, Driscoll DL, Lee HK, et al. Decreased immunoexpression of prostate inhibin peptide in prostatic carcinoma: a study with monoclonal antibody. Hum Pathol 1999; 30: 168–172.

148. Bircan S, Kapucuoglu N, Candir O. CD10 expression in prostatic intraepithelial neoplasia and prostatic carcinoma and association with androgen receptor. Mod Pathol 2007; 20: 138A.

149. Patton KT, Chen HM, Joseph L, Yang XJ. Decreased annexin I expression in prostatic adenocarcinoma and in high-grade prostatic intraepithelial neoplasia. Histopathology 2005; 47: 597–601.

150. Thomas LN, Lazier CB, Gupta R, et al. Differential alterations in 5alpha-reductase type 1 and type 2 levels during development and progression of prostate cancer. Prostate 2005; 63: 231–239.

151. Kelavkar UP, Harya NS, Hutzley J, et al. DNA methylation paradigm shift: 15-lipoxygenase-1 upregulation in prostatic intraepithelial neoplasia and prostate cancer by atypical promoter hypermethylation. Prostaglandins Other Lipid Mediat 2007; 82: 185–197.

152. Tang DG, Bhatia B, Tang S, Schneider-Broussard R. 15-lipoxygenase 2 (15-LOX2) is a functional tumor suppressor that regulates human prostate epithelial cell differentiation, senescence, and growth (size). Prostaglandins Other Lipid Mediat 2007; 82: 135–146.

153. Cardillo MR, Di Silverio F, Gentile V. Quantitative immunohistochemical and in situ hybridization analysis of metalloproteinases in prostate cancer. Anticancer Res 2006; 26: 973–982.

154. Young L, Salomon R, Au W, et al. Ornithine decarboxylase (ODC) expression pattern in human prostate tissues and ODC transgenic mice. J Histochem Cytochem 2006; 54: 223–229.

155. Bethel CR, Faith D, Li X, et al. Decreased NKX3.1 protein expression

in focal prostatic atrophy, prostatic intraepithelial neoplasia, and adenocarcinoma: association with Gleason score and chromosome 8p deletion. Cancer Res 2006; 66: 10683–10690.

156. Tsuji M, Kanda K, Murakami Y, et al. Biologic markers in prostatic intraepithelial neoplasia: immunohistochemical and cytogenetic analyses. J Med Invest 1999; 46: 35–41.

157. Liao Y, Abel U, Grobholz R, et al. Up-regulation of insulin-like growth factor axis components in human primary prostate cancer correlates with tumor grade. Hum Pathol 2005; 36: 1186–1196.

158. Hampel OZ, Kattan MW, Yang G, et al. Quantitative immunohistochemical analysis of insulin-like growth factor binding protein-3 in human prostatic adenocarcinoma: a prognostic study. J Urol 1998; 159: 2220–2225.

159. Koeneman KS, Pan CX, Jin JK, et al. Telomerase activity, telomere length, and DNA ploidy in prostatic intraepithelial neoplasia (PIN). J Urol 1998; 160: 1533–1539.

160. Erdamar S, Yang G, Harper JW, et al. Levels of expression of p27KIP1 protein in human prostate and prostate cancer: an immunohistochemical analysis. Mod Pathol 1999; 12: 751–755.

161. Revelos K, Petraki C, Gregorakis A, et al. Immunohistochemical expression of Bcl2 is an independent predictor of time-to-biochemical failure in patients with clinically localized prostate cancer following radical prostatectomy. Anticancer Res 2005; 25: 3123–3133.

162. Doganavsargil B, Simsir A, Boyacioglu H, et al. A comparison of p21 and p27 immunoexpression in benign glands, prostatic intraepithelial neoplasia and prostate adenocarcinoma. BJU Int 2006; 97: 644–648.

163. Dubbink HJ, Hoedemaeker RF, van der Kwast TH, et al. Human prostate-specific transglutaminase: a new prostatic marker with a unique distribution pattern. Lab Invest 1999; 79: 141–150.

164. Bostwick DG, Liu L, Brawer MK, Qian J. High-grade prostatic intraepithelial neoplasia. Rev Urol 2004; 6: 171–179.

165. Baretton GB, Vogt T, Blasenbreu S, Lohrs U. Comparison of DNA ploidy in prostatic intraepithelial neoplasia and invasive carcinoma of the prostate: an image cytometric study. Hum Pathol 1994; 25: 506–513.

166. Zitzelsberger H, Kulka U, Lehmann L, et al. Genetic heterogeneity in a prostatic carcinoma and associated prostatic intraepithelial neoplasia as demonstrated by combined use of laser-microdissection, degenerate oligonucleotide primed PCR and

comparative genomic hybridization. Virchows Arch 1998; 433: 297–304.

167. Montironi R, Bartels PH, Thompson D, et al. Prostatic intraepithelial neoplasia. Quantitation of the basal cell layer with machine vision system. Pathol Res Pract 1995; 191: 917–923.

168. Montironi R, Magi Galluzzi C, Scarpelli M, et al. Occurrence of cell death (apoptosis) in prostatic intra-epithelial neoplasia. Virchows Arch A [Pathol Anat Histopathol] 1993; 423: 351–357.

169. Zeng L, Kyprianou N. Apoptotic regulators in prostatic intraepithelial neoplasia (PIN): value in prostate cancer detection and prevention. Prostate Cancer Prostatic Dis 2005; 8: 7–13.

170. Buschhorn HM, Klein RR, Chambers SM, et al. Aurora-A over-expression in high-grade PIN lesions and prostate cancer. Prostate 2005; 64: 341–346.

171. Colombel M, Dante R, Bouvier R, et al. Differential RNA expression of the pS2 gene in the human benign and malignant prostatic tissue. J Urol 1999; 162: 927–930.

172. Johnson MI, Robinson MC, Marsh C, et al. Expression of Bcl-2, Bax, and p53 in high-grade prostatic intraepithelial neoplasia and localized prostate cancer: relationship with apoptosis and proliferation. Prostate 1998; 37: 223–229.

173. Ramos Soler D, Mayordomo Aranda E, Calatayud Blas A, et al. [Usefulness of bcl-2 expression as a new basal cell marker in prostatic pathology]. Actas Urol Esp 2006; 30: 345–352.

174. Ma S, Guan XY, Beh PS, et al. The significance of LMO2 expression in the progression of prostate cancer. J Pathol 2007; 211: 278–285.

175. Levesque MH, El-Alfy M, Berger L, et al. Evaluation of AIbZIP and Cdc47 as markers for human prostatic diseases. Urology 2007; 69: 196–201.

176. Montironi R, Mazzucchelli R. HER-2 expression and gene amplification in high-grade PIN and prostate cancer. Arch Ital Urol Androl 2006; 78: 135–139.

177. Myers RB, Srivastava S, Oelschlager DK, Grizzle WE. Expression of p160erbB-3 and p185erbB-2 in prostatic intraepithelial neoplasia and prostatic adenocarcinoma. J Natl Cancer Inst 1994; 86: 1140–1145.

178. Denkert C, Thoma A, Niesporek S, et al. Overexpression of cyclooxygenase-2 in human prostate carcinoma and prostatic intraepithelial neoplasia-association with increased expression of polo-like kinase-1. Prostate 2007; 67: 361–369.

179. Dassesse T, de Leval X, de Leval L, et al. Activation of the thromboxane A2 pathway in human prostate cancer correlates with tumor Gleason score and pathologic stage. Eur Urol 2006; 50: 1021–1031; discussion 1031.

180. Khayyata S, Yildirim Kupesiz G, Andea A, et al. Oxidative stress: an

etiologic factor of prostate cancer? A tissue microarray (TMA) and marker study of age, race and neoplastic progression. Mod Pathol 2007; 20: 155A.

181. Bjartell A, Johansson R, Bjork T, et al. Immunohistochemical detection of cysteine-rich secretory protein 3 in tissue and in serum from men with cancer or benign enlargement of the prostate gland. Prostate 2006; 66: 591–603.

182. Chaplet M, Waltregny D, Detry C, et al. Expression of dentin sialophosphoprotein in human prostate cancer and its correlation with tumor aggressiveness. Int J Cancer 2006; 118: 850–856.

183. Poczatek RB, Myers RB, Manne U, et al. Ep-Cam levels in prostatic adenocarcinoma and prostatic intraepithelial neoplasia. J Urol 1999; 162: 1462–1466.

184. Bonkhoff H, Fixemer T, Hunsicker I, Remberger K. Estrogen receptor expression in prostate cancer and premalignant prostatic lesions. Am J Pathol 1999; 155: 641–647.

185. Drewa T, Wolski Z, Skok Z, et al. The FAS-related apoptosis signaling pathway in the prostate intraepithelial neoplasia and cancer lesions. Acta Pol Pharm 2006; 63: 311–315.

186. Weng J, Wang J, Hu X, et al. PSGR2, a novel G-protein coupled receptor, is overexpressed in human prostate cancer. Int J Cancer 2006; 118: 1471–1480.

187. Zhang Z, Rosen DG, Yao JL, et al. Expression of p14ARF, p15INK4b, p16INK4a, and DCR2 increases during prostate cancer progression. Mod Pathol 2006; 19: 1339–1343.

188. Cardillo MR, Ippoliti F. IL-6, IL-10 and HSP-90 expression in tissue microarrays from human prostate cancer assessed by computer-assisted image analysis. Anticancer Res 2006; 26: 3409–3416.

189. Darson MF, Pacelli A, Roche P, et al. Human glandular kallikrein 2 (hK2) expression in prostatic intraepithelial neoplasia and adenocarcinoma: a novel prostate cancer marker. Urology 1997; 49: 857–862.

190. Festuccia C, Angelucci A, Gravina GL, et al. Epithelial and prostatic marker expression in short-term primary cultures of human prostate tissue samples. Int J Oncol 2005; 26: 1353–1362.

191. Wang L, Chen ZJ, Wang QT, et al. [Expression of hypoxia-inducible factor lalpha and vascular endothelial growth factor in prostate cancer and its significance]. Zhonghua Nan Ke Xue 2006; 12: 57–59.

192. Rasiah KK, Kench JG, Gardiner-Garden M, et al. Aberrant neuropeptide Y and macrophage inhibitory cytokine-1 expression are early events in prostate cancer development and are associated with

poor prognosis. Cancer Epidemiol Biomarkers Prev 2006; 15: 711–716.

193. Lee S, Desai KK, Iczkowski KA, et al. Coordinated peak expression of MMP-26 and TIMP-4 in preinvasive human prostate tumor. Cell Res 2006; 16: 750–758.

194. El Sharkawy SL, Abbas NF, Badawi MA, El Shaer MA. Metallothionein isoform II expression in hyperplastic, dysplastic and neoplastic prostatic lesions. J Clin Pathol 2006; 59: 1171–1174.

195. Revelos K, Petraki C, Gregorakis A, et al. p27(kip1) and Ki-67 (MIB1) immunohistochemical expression in radical prostatectomy specimens of patients with clinically localized prostate cancer. In Vivo 2005; 19: 911–920.

196. Sinha AA, Quast BJ, Reddy PK, et al. Microvessel density as a molecular marker for identifying high-grade prostatic intraepithelial neoplasia precursors to prostate cancer. Exp Mol Pathol 2004; 77: 153–159.

197. Li M, Hebert T, Dulou A, et al. Elevated expression of MAGMAS in prostatic neoplasia. Mod Pathol 2007; 20: 159A.

198. Kremer CL, Klein RR, Mendelson J, et al. Expression of mTOR signaling pathway markers in prostate cancer progression. Prostate 2006; 66: 1203–1212.

199. Khodavirdi AC, Song Z, Yang S, et al. Increased expression of osteopontin contributes to the progression of prostate cancer. Cancer Res 2006; 66: 883–888.

200. Leav I, Merk FB, Lee KF, et al. Prolactin receptor expression in the developing human prostate and in hyperplastic, dysplastic, and neoplastic lesions. Am J Pathol 1999; 154: 863–870.

201. Bostwick DG, Pacelli A, Blute M, et al. Prostate specific membrane antigen expression in prostatic intraepithelial neoplasia and adenocarcinoma: a study of 184 cases. Cancer 1998; 82: 2256–2261.

202. Chang SS, Reuter VE, Heston WD, et al. Short term neoadjuvant androgen deprivation therapy does not affect prostate specific membrane antigen expression in prostate tissues. Cancer 2000; 88: 407–415.

203. Suzuki S, Takahashi S, Takahashi S, et al. Expression of prothymosin alpha is correlated with development and progression in human prostate cancers. Prostate 2006; 66: 463–469.

204. Engers R, Mueller M, Walter A, et al. Prognostic relevance of Tiam1 protein expression in prostate carcinomas. Br J Cancer 2006; 95: 1081–1086.

205. Chiosea S, Jelezcova E, Chandran U, et al. Up-regulation of dicer, a component of the MicroRNA machinery, in prostate adenocarcinoma. Am J Pathol 2006; 169: 1812–1820.

206. Cibull TL, Jones TD, Li L, et al. Overexpression of Pim-1 during progression of prostatic adenocarcinoma. J Clin Pathol 2006; 59: 285–288.

207. Valdman A, Fang X, Pang ST, et al. Pim-1 expression in prostatic intraepithelial neoplasia and human prostate cancer. Prostate 2004; 60: 367–371.

208. Xue Y, Smedts F, Latijnhouwers MA, et al. Tenascin-C expression in prostatic intraepithelial neoplasia (PIN): a marker of progression? Anticancer Res 1998; 18: 2679–2684.

209. Yasunaga Y, Shin M, Fujita MQ, et al. Different patterns of p53 mutations in prostatic intraepithelial neoplasia and concurrent carcinoma: analysis of microdissected specimens. Lab Invest 1998; 78: 1275–1279.

210. Haussler O, Epstein JI, Amin MB, et al. Cell proliferation, apoptosis, oncogene, and tumor suppressor gene status in adenosis with comparison to benign prostatic hyperplasia, prostatic intraepithelial neoplasia, and cancer. Hum Pathol 1999; 30: 1077–1086.

211. Kitamura H, Torigoe T, Asanuma H, et al. Cytosolic overexpression of p62 sequestosome 1 in neoplastic prostate tissue. Histopathology 2006; 48: 157–161.

212. Katona TM, Neubauer BL, Iversen PW, et al. Elevated expression of angiogenin in prostate cancer and its precursors. Clin Cancer Res 2005; 11: 8358–8363.

213. Yoshioka Y, Konishi K, Oh RJ, et al. High-dose-rate brachytherapy without external beam irradiation for locally advanced prostate cancer. Radiother Oncol 2006; 80: 62–68.

214. Montironi R, Diamanti L, Thompson D, et al. Analysis of the capillary architecture in the precursors of prostate cancer: recent findings and new concepts. Eur Urol 1996; 30: 191–200.

215. Bostwick DG, Ramnani D, Qian J. Prostatic intraepithelial neoplasia: animal models 2000. Prostate 2000; 43: 286–294.

216. Huang J, Powell WC, Khodavirdi AC, et al. Prostatic intraepithelial neoplasia in mice with conditional disruption of the retinoid X receptor alpha allele in the prostate epithelium. Cancer Res 2002; 62: 4812–4819.

217. Park JH, Walls JE, Galvez JJ, et al. Prostatic intraepithelial neoplasia in genetically engineered mice. Am J Pathol 2002; 161: 727–735.

218. Greenberg NM, DeMayo F, Finegold MJ, et al. Prostate cancer in a transgenic mouse. Proc Natl Acad Sci USA 1995; 92: 3439–3443.

219. Gingrich JR, Barrios RJ, Kattan MW, et al. Androgen-independent prostate cancer progression in the TRAMP model. Cancer Res 1997; 57: 4687–4691.

220. Voelkel-Johnson C, Voeks DJ, Greenberg NM, et al. Genomic instability-based transgenic models of prostate cancer. Carcinogenesis 2000; 21: 1623–1627.

221. Stanbrough M, Leav I, Kwan PW, et al. Prostatic intraepithelial neoplasia in mice expressing an androgen receptor transgene in prostate epithelium. Proc Natl Acad Sci USA 2001; 98: 10823–10828.

222. McCabe NP, Selman SH, Jankun J. Vascular endothelial growth factor production in human prostate cancer cells is stimulated by overexpression of platelet 12-lipoxygenase. Prostate 2006; 66: 779–787.

223. Li Z, Szabolcs M, Terwilliger JD, Efstratiadis A. Prostatic intraepithelial neoplasia and adenocarcinoma in mice expressing a probasin-Neu oncogenic transgene. Carcinogenesis 2006; 27: 1054–1067.

224. Wang Y, Sudilovsky D, Zhang B, et al. A human prostatic epithelial model of hormonal carcinogenesis. Cancer Res 2001; 61: 6064–6072.

225. Ouyang X, DeWeese TL, Nelson WG, Abate-Shen C. Loss-of-function of Nkx3.1 promotes increased oxidative damage in prostate carcinogenesis. Cancer Res 2005; 65: 6773–6779.

226. Dai B, Kim O, Xie Y, et al. Tyrosine kinase Etk/BMX is up-regulated in human prostate cancer and its overexpression induces prostate intraepithelial neoplasia in mouse. Cancer Res 2006; 66: 8058–8064.

227. Cheng J, Bawa T, Lee P, et al. Role of desumoylation in the development of prostate cancer. Neoplasia 2006; 8: 667–676.

228. Aquilina JW, McKinney L, Pacelli A, et al. High grade prostatic intraepithelial neoplasia in military working dogs with and without prostate cancer. Prostate 1998; 36: 189–193.

229. Waters DJ. High-grade prostatic intraepithelial neoplasia in dogs. Eur Urol 1999; 35: 456–458.

230. Waters DJ, Bostwick DG. The canine prostate is a spontaneous model of intraepithelial neoplasia and prostate cancer progression. Anticancer Res 1997; 17: 1467–1470.

231. Narayanan BA, Narayanan NK, Pttman B, Reddy BS. Adenocarcina of the mouse prostate growth inhibition by celecoxib: downregulation of transcription factors involved in COX-2 inhibition. Prostate 2006; 66: 257–265.

232. Banach-Petrosky W, Ouyang X, Gao H, et al. Vitamin D inhibits the formation of prostatic intraepithelial neoplasia in Nkx3.1; Pten mutant mice. Clin Cancer Res 2006; 12: 5895–5901.

233. Steiner MS, Raghow S, Neubauer BL. Selective estrogen receptor modulators for the chemoprevention of prostate cancer. Urology 2001; 57: 68–72.

234. Arunkumar A, Vijayababu MR, Venkataraman P, et al. Chemoprevention of rat prostate carcinogenesis by diallyl disulfide, an organosulfur compound of garlic. Biol Pharm Bull 2006; 29: 375–379.

235. Kilic S, Kukul E, Danisman A, et al. Ratio of free to total prostate-specific antigen in patients with prostatic intraepithelial neoplasia. Eur Urol 1998; 34: 176–180.

236. Ronnett BM, Carmichael MJ, Carter HB, Epstein JI. Does high grade prostatic intraepithelial neoplasia result in elevated serum prostate specific antigen levels? J Urol 1993; 150: 386–389.

237. Alexander EE, Qian J, Wollan PC, et al. Prostatic intraepithelial neoplasia does not appear to raise serum prostate-specific antigen concentration. Urology 1996; 47: 693–698.

238. Xiao LP, Bi XJ, Li YN, et al. [Value of prostate specific antigen in early diagnosis of prostatic cancer]. Nan Fang Yi Ke Da Xue Xue Bao 2007; 27: 107–108, 112.

239. Loeb S, Roehl KA, Yu X, et al. Use of prostate-specific antigen velocity to follow up patients with isolated high-grade prostatic intraepithelial neoplasia on prostate biopsy. Urology 2007; 69: 108–112.

240. Morote J, Raventos CX, Encabo G, et al. Effect of high-grade prostatic intraepithelial neoplasia on total and percent free serum prostatic-specific antigen. Eur Urol 2000; 37: 456–459.

241. Morote J, Encabo G, Lopez M, de Torres IM. Influence of high-grade prostatic intra-epithelial neoplasia on total and percentage free serum prostatic specific antigen. BJU Int 1999; 84: 657–660.

242. Nam RK, Trachtenberg J, Jewett MA, et al. Serum insulin-like growth factor-I levels and prostatic intraepithelial neoplasia: a clue to the relationship between IGF-I physiology and prostate cancer risk. Cancer Epidemiol Biomarkers Prev 2005; 14: 1270–1273.

243. Lee F, Torp-Pedersen ST, Carroll JT, et al. Use of transrectal ultrasound and prostate-specific antigen in diagnosis of prostatic intraepithelial neoplasia. Urology 1989; 34: 4–8.

244. Ozden E, Gogus C, Karamursel T, et al. Transrectal sonographic features of prostatic intraepithelial neoplasia: correlation with pathologic findings. J Clin Ultrasound 2005; 33: 5–9.

245. Hom JJ, Coakley FV, Simko JP, et al. High-grade prostatic intraepithelial neoplasia in patients with prostate cancer: MR and MR spectroscopic imaging features – initial experience. Radiology 2007; 242: 483–489.

246. Sofikerim M, Tatlisen A, Karacagil M. Do all patients with high-grade prostatic intraepithelial neoplasia on initial prostatic biopsy eventually progress to clinical prostate cancer? BJU Int 2006; 97: 869–870.

247. Davidson D, Bostwick DG, Qian J, et al. Prostatic intraepithelial neoplasia is a risk factor for adenocarcinoma: predictive accuracy in needle biopsies. J Urol 1995; 154: 1295–1299.

248. Yanke BV, Salzhauer EW, Colon I. Is race a positive predictor of cancer on repeat prostate biopsy? J Urol 2006; 176: 1114–1117.

249. Zhou M, Klein E, Magi-Galluzzi C. Cancer risk associated with high grade prostatic intraepithelial neoplasia (HGPIN) in a contemporary single-institution cohort. Mod Pathol 2007; 20: 186A.

250. Bostwick DG. Prostatic intraepithelial neoplasia (PIN): current concepts. J Cell Biochem 1992; 16H: 10–19.

251. Eskicorapci SY, Guliyev F, Islamoglu E, et al. The effect of prior biopsy scheme on prostate cancer detection for repeat biopsy population: results of the 14-core prostate biopsy technique. Int Urol Nephrol 2007; 39: 189–195.

252. Herawi M, Kahane H, Cavallo C, Epstein JI. Risk of prostate cancer on first re-biopsy within 1 year following a diagnosis of high grade prostatic intraepithelial neoplasia is related to the number of cores sampled. J Urol 2006; 175: 121–124.

253. Harvei S, Skjorten FJ, Robsahm TE, et al. Is prostatic intraepithelial neoplasia in the transition/central zone a true precursor of cancer? A long-term retrospective study in Norway. Br J Cancer 1998; 78: 46–49.

254. Pacelli A, Bostwick DG. Clinical significance of high-grade prostatic intraepithelial neoplasia in transurethral resection specimens. Urology 1997; 50: 355–359.

255. Meyer F, Tetu B, Bairati I, et al. Prostatic intraepithelial neoplasia in TURP specimens and subsequent prostate cancer. Can J Urol 2006; 13: 3255–3260.

256. Schoenfield L, Jones JS, Zippe CD, et al. The incidence of high-grade prostatic intraepithelial neoplasia and atypical glands suspicious for carcinoma on first-time saturation needle biopsy, and the subsequent risk of cancer. BJU Int 2007; 99: 770–774.

257. Netto GJ, Epstein JI. Widespread high-grade prostatic intraepithelial neoplasia on prostatic needle biopsy: a significant likelihood of subsequently diagnosed adenocarcinoma. Am J Surg Pathol 2006; 30: 1184–1188.

258. Joshua AM, Vukovic B, Braude I, et al. Telomere attrition in isolated high-grade prostatic intraepithelial neoplasia and surrounding stroma is predictive of prostate cancer. Neoplasia 2007; 9: 81–89.

259. Meeker AK. Telomeres and telomerase in prostatic intraepithelial neoplasia and prostate cancer biology. Urol Oncol 2006; 24: 122–130.

260. Iglesius C, de Torres I, Rojo F, et al. Overexpression of p4EBP1 in high grade PIN predicts and associates with prostatic cancer. Mod Pathol 2007; 20: 153A.

261. Abbas F, Hochberg D, Civantos F, Soloway M. Incidental prostatic adenocarcinoma in patients undergoing radical cystoprostatectomy for bladder cancer. Eur Urol 1996; 30: 322–326.

262. Montironi R, Pomante R, Diamanti L, Magi-Galluzzi C. Apoptosis in prostatic adenocarcinoma following complete androgen ablation. Urol Int 1998; 60: 25–29; discussion 30.

263. Montironi R, Schulman ML. Pathological changes in prostate lesions after androgen manipulation. J Clin Pathol 1998; 51: 5–12.

264. Balaji KC, Rabbani F, Tsai H, et al. Effect of neoadjuvant hormonal therapy on prostatic intraepithelial neoplasia and its prognostic significance. J Urol 1999; 162: 753–757.

265. Vailancourt L, Ttu B, Fradet Y, et al. Effect of neoadjuvant endocrine therapy (combined androgen blockade) on normal prostate and prostatic carcinoma. A randomized study. Am J Surg Pathol 1996; 20: 86–93.

266. Montironi R, Magi-Galluzzi C, Muzzonigro G, et al. Effects of combination endocrine treatment on normal prostate, prostatic intraepithelial neoplasia, and prostatic adenocarcinoma. J Clin Pathol 1994; 47: 906–913.

267. Steiner MS, Pound CR. Phase IIA clinical trial to test the efficacy and safety of toremifene in men with high-grade prostatic intraepithelial neoplasia. Clin Prostate Cancer 2003; 2: 24–31.

268. Price D, Stein B, Sieber P, et al. Toremifene for the prevention of prostate cancer in men with high grade prostatic intraepithelial neoplasia: results of a double-blind, placebo controlled, phase IIb clinical trial. J Urol 2006; 176: 965–971.

269. Bettuzzi S, Brausi M, Rizzi F, et al. Chemoprevention of human prostate cancer by oral administration of green tea catechins in volunteers with high-grade prostate intraepithelial neoplasia: a preliminary report from a one-year proof-of-principle study. Cancer Res 2006; 66: 1234–1240.

270. Mohanty NK, Saxena S, Singh UP, et al. Lycopene as a chemopreventive agent in the treatment of high-grade prostate intraepithelial neoplasia. Urol Oncol 2005; 23: 383–385.

271. Scattoni V, Montironi R, Mazzucchelli R, et al. Pathological changes of high-grade prostatic intraepithelial

neoplasia and prostate cancer after monotherapy with bicalutamide 150 mg. BJU Int 2006; 98: 54–58.

272. van der Kwast TH, Labrie F, Tetu B. Persistence of high-grade prostatic intra-epithelial neoplasia under combined androgen blockade therapy. Hum Pathol 1999; 30: 1503–1507.

273. Kang TY, Nichols P, Skinner E, et al. Functional heterogeneity of prostatic intraepithelial neoplasia: the duration of hormonal therapy influences the response. BJU Int 2007; 99: 1024–1027.

274. Alers JC, Krijtenburg PJ, Vissers KJ, et al. Interphase cytogenetics of prostatic adenocarcinoma and precursor lesions: analysis of 25 radical prostatectomies and 17 adjacent prostatic intraepithelial neoplasias. Genes Chromosomes Cancer 1995; 12: 241–250.

275. Alberts SR, Novotny PJ, Sloan JA, et al. Flutamide in men with prostatic intraepithelial neoplasia: a randomized, placebo-controlled chemoprevention trial. Am J Ther 2006; 13: 291–297.

276. Bono AV, Mazzucchelli R, Ferrari I, et al. Bicalutamide 50 mg monotherapy in patients with isolated high-grade PIN. Findings in repeat biopsies at six months. J Clin Pathol 2007; 60: 443–446.

277. Andriole G, Bostwick D, Civantos F, et al. The effects of 5alpha-reductase inhibitors on the natural history, detection and grading of prostate cancer: current state of knowledge. J Urol 2005; 174: 2098–2104.

278. Civantos F, Marcial MA, Banks ER, et al. Pathology of androgen deprivation therapy in prostate carcinoma. A comparative study of 173 patients. Cancer 1995; 75: 1634–1641.

279. Yang XJ, Lecksell K, Short K, et al. Does long-term finasteride therapy affect the histologic features of benign prostatic tissue and prostate cancer on needle biopsy? PLESS Study Group. Proscar Long-Term Efficacy and Safety Study. Urology 1999; 53: 696–700.

280. Montironi R, Pomante R, Diamanti L, et al. Evaluation of prostatic intraepithelial neoplasia after treatment with a 5-alpha-reductase inhibitor (finasteride). A methodologic approach. Anal Quant Cytol Histol 1996; 18: 461–470.

281. Bostwick DG. Prostatic intraepithelial neoplasia is a risk factor for cancer. Semin Urol Oncol 1999; 17: 187–198.

282. Gaudin PB, Zelefsky MJ, Leibel SA, et al. Histopathologic effects of three-dimensional conformal external beam radiation therapy on benign and malignant prostate tissues. Am J Surg Pathol 1999; 23: 1021–1031.

283. Arakawa A, Song S, Scardino PT, Wheeler TM. High grade prostatic intraepithelial neoplasia in prostates removed following irradiation failure in the treatment of prostatic adenocarcinoma. Pathol Res Pract 1995; 191: 868–872.

284. Martens MB, Keller JH. Routine immunohistochemical staining for high-molecular weight cytokeratin 34-beta and alpha-methylacyl CoA racemase (P504S) in postirradiation prostate biopsies. Mod Pathol 2006; 19: 287–290.

285. Hameed O, Humphrey PA. Immunohistochemistry in diagnostic surgical pathology of the prostate. Semin Diagn Pathol 2005; 22: 88–104.

286. Cheville JC, Reznicek MJ, Bostwick DG. The focus of 'atypical glands, suspicious for malignancy' in prostatic needle biopsy specimens: incidence, histologic features, and clinical follow-up of cases diagnosed in a community practice. Am J Clin Pathol 1997; 108: 633–640.

287. Iczkowski KA, MacLennan GT, Bostwick DG. Atypical small acinar proliferation suspicious for malignancy in prostate needle biopsies: clinical significance in 33 cases. Am J Surg Pathol 1997; 21: 1489–1495.

288. Iczkowski KA, Bostwick DG. Prostate biopsy 1999: strategies and significance of pathological findings. Semin Urol Oncol 1999; 17: 177–186.

289. Hoedemaeker RF, Kranse R, Rietbergen JB, et al. Evaluation of prostate needle biopsies in a population-based screening study: the impact of borderline lesions. Cancer 1999; 85: 145–152.

290. Ouyang RC, Kenwright DN, Nacey JN, Delahunt B. The presence of atypical small acinar proliferation in prostate needle biopsy is predictive of carcinoma on subsequent biopsy. BJU Int 2001; 87: 70–74.

291. Borboroglu PG, Comer SW, Riffenburgh RH, Amling CL. Extensive repeat transrectal ultrasound guided prostate biopsy in patients with previous benign sextant biopsies. J Urol 2000; 163: 158–162.

292. Iczkowski KA, Chen HM, Yang XJ, Beach RA. Prostate cancer diagnosed after initial biopsy with atypical small acinar proliferation suspicious for malignancy is similar to cancer found on initial biopsy. Urology 2002; 60: 851–854.

293. Postma R, Roobol M, Schroder FH, van der Kwast TH. Lesions predictive for prostate cancer in a screened population: first and second screening round findings. Prostate 2004; 61: 260–266.

294. Fadare O, Wang S, Mariappan MR. Practice patterns of clinicians following isolated diagnoses of atypical small acinar proliferation on prostate biopsy specimens. Arch Pathol Lab Med 2004; 128: 557–560.

295. Gupta C, Ren JZ, Wojno KJ. Individual submission and embedding of prostate biopsies decreases rates of equivocal pathology reports. Urology 2004; 63: 83–86.

296. Brausi M, Castagnetti G, Dotti A, et al. Immediate radical prostatectomy in patients with atypical small acinar proliferation. Over treatment? J Urol 2004; 172: 906–908; discussion 908–909.

297. Renshaw AA, Santis WF, Richie JP. Clinicopathological characteristics of prostatic adenocarcinoma in men with atypical prostate needle biopsies. J Urol 1998; 159: 2018–2021; discussion 2022.

298. Reyes AO, Humphrey PA. Diagnostic effect of complete histologic sampling of prostate needle biopsy specimens. Am J Clin Pathol 1998; 109: 416–422.

299. Weinstein MH, Greenspan DL, Epstein JI. Diagnoses rendered on prostate needle biopsy in community hospitals. Prostate 1998; 35: 50–55.

300. Kobayashi T, Nishizawa K, Watanabe J, et al. Effects of sextant transrectal prostate biopsy plus additional far lateral cores in improving cancer detection rates in men with large prostate glands. Int J Urol 2004; 11: 392–396.

301. Naya Y, Ayala AG, Tamboli P, Babaian RJ. Can the number of cores with high-grade prostate intraepithelial neoplasia predict cancer in men who undergo repeat biopsy? Urology 2004; 63: 503–508.

302. Wills ML, Hamper UM, Partin AW, Epstein JI. Incidence of high-grade prostatic intraepithelial neoplasia in sextant needle biopsy specimens. Urology 1997; 49: 367–373.

303. Bostwick DG, Montironi R. Prostatic intraepithelial neoplasia and the origins of prostatic carcinoma. Pathol Res Pract 1995; 191: 828–832.

304. Bostwick DG, Meiers I. Atypical small acinar proliferation in the prostate: clinical significance in 2006. Arch Pathol Lab Med 2006; 130: 952–957.

305. Iczkowski KA, Bostwick DG. Criteria for biopsy diagnosis of minimal volume prostatic adenocarcinoma: analytic comparison with nondiagnostic but suspicious atypical small acinar proliferation. Arch Pathol Lab Med 2000; 124: 98–107.

306. Kozuka Y, Imai H, Yamanaka M, et al. [Histopathological features of prostate cancer]. Nippon Rinsho 2005; 63: 231–236.

307. Helpap B. [Small suggestive lesions of the prostate. Histological and immunohistochemical analyses – report of the uropathology consultation service]. Pathologe 2005; 26: 398–404.

308. Iczkowski KA. Current prostate biopsy interpretation: criteria for cancer, atypical small acinar proliferation, high-grade prostatic

intraepithelial neoplasia, and use of immunostains. Arch Pathol Lab Med 2006; 130: 835–843.

309. Cavalcanti Fde B, Alves VA, Pereira J, et al. Proliferative lesions of prostate: a multivariate approach to differential diagnosis. Pathol Oncol Res 2005; 11: 103–107.

310. Ro JY, Grignon DJ, Troncoso P, Ayala AG. Mucin in prostatic adenocarcinoma. Semin Diagn Pathol 1988; 5: 273–283.

311. Del Rosario AD, Bui HX, Abdulla M, Ross JS. Sulfur-rich prostatic intraluminal crystalloids: a surgical pathologic and electron probe X-ray microanalytic study. Hum Pathol 1993; 24: 1159–1167.

312. Bostwick DG, Srigley J, Grignon D, et al. Atypical adenomatous hyperplasia of the prostate: morphologic criteria for its distinction from well-differentiated carcinoma. Hum Pathol 1993; 24: 819–832.

313. Anton RC, Chakraborty S, Wheeler TM. The significance of intraluminal prostatic crystalloids in benign needle biopsies. Am J Surg Pathol 1998; 22: 446–449.

314. Henneberry JM, Kahane H, Humphrey PA, et al. The significance of intraluminal crystalloids in benign prostatic glands on needle biopsy. Am J Surg Pathol 1997; 21: 725–728.

315. Scattoni V, Roscigno M, Freschi M, et al. Atypical small acinar proliferation (ASAP) on extended prostatic biopsies: predictive factors of cancer detection on repeat biopsies. Arch Ital Urol Androl 2005; 77: 31–36.

316. Schlesinger C, Bostwick DG, Iczkowski KA. High-grade prostatic intraepithelial neoplasia and atypical small acinar proliferation: predictive value for cancer in current practice. Am J Surg Pathol 2005; 29: 1201–1207.

317. Iczkowski KA, Bassler TJ, Schwob VS, et al. Diagnosis of 'suspicious for malignancy' in prostate biopsies: predictive value for cancer. Urology 1998; 51: 749–757; discussion 757–758.

318. Cheville JC, Reznicek MJ, Bostwick DG. The focus of 'atypical glands, suspicious for malignancy' in prostatic needle biopsy specimens: incidence, histologic features, and clinical follow-up of cases diagnosed in a community practice. Am J Clin Pathol 1997; 108: 633–640.

319. Chan TY, Epstein JI. Follow-up of atypical prostate needle biopsies suspicious for cancer. Urology 1999; 53: 351–355.

320. Park S, Shinohara K, Grossfeld GD, Carroll PR. Prostate cancer detection in men with prior high grade prostatic intraepithelial neoplasia or atypical prostate biopsy. J Urol 2001; 165: 1409–1414.

321. Borboroglu PG, Sur RL, Roberts JL, Amling CL. Repeat biopsy strategy in patients with atypical small acinar proliferation or high grade prostatic intraepithelial neoplasia on initial prostate needle biopsy. J Urol 2001; 166: 866–870.

322. Moore CK, Karikehalli S, Nazeer T, et al. Prognostic significance of high grade prostatic intraepithelial neoplasia and atypical small acinar proliferation in the contemporary era. J Urol 2005; 173: 70–72.

323. Leite KR, Mitteldorf CA, Camara-Lopes LH. Repeat prostate biopsies following diagnoses of prostate intraepithelial neoplasia and atypical small gland proliferation. Int Braz J Urol 2005; 31: 131–136.

324. Girasole CR, Cookson MS, Putzi MJ, et al. Significance of atypical and suspicious small acinar proliferations, and high grade prostatic intraepithelial neoplasia on prostate biopsy: implications for cancer detection and biopsy strategy. J Urol 2006; 175: 929–933; discussion 933.

325. Rodriguez-Patron Rodriguez R, Mayayo Dehesa T, Burgos Revilla FJ, et al. [Prognostic significance of PIN and atypical small acinar proliferation on transrectal ultrasound-guided prostate biopsy]. Actas Urol Esp 2006; 30: 359–366.

326. Mancuso PA, Chabert C, Chin P, et al. Prostate cancer detection in men with an initial diagnosis of atypical small acinar proliferation. BJU Int 2007; 99: 49–52.

327. Walsh PC. Prostate cancer diagnosed after initial biopsy with atypical small acinar proliferation suspicious for malignancy is similar to cancer found on initial biopsy. J Urol 2003; 170: 316.

328. Rabbani F, Stroumbakis N, Kava BR, et al. Incidence and clinical significance of false-negative sextant prostate biopsies. J Urol 1998; 159: 1247–1250.

329. DiGiuseppe JA, Sauvageot J, Epstein JI. Increasing incidence of minimal residual cancer in radical prostatectomy specimens. Am J Surg Pathol 1997; 21: 174–178.

330. Kronz JD, Shaikh AA, Epstein JI. High-grade prostatic intraepithelial neoplasia with adjacent small atypical glands on prostate biopsy. Hum Pathol 2001; 32: 389–395.

331. Alsikafi NF, Brendler CB, Gerber GS, Yang XJ. High-grade prostatic intraepithelial neoplasia with adjacent atypia is associated with a higher incidence of cancer on subsequent needle biopsy than high-grade prostatic intraepithelial neoplasia alone. Urology 2001; 57: 296–300.

332. Epstein JI. Diagnostic criteria of limited adenocarcinoma of the prostate on needle biopsy. Hum Pathol 1995; 26: 223–229.

333. Shimada H, Misugi K, Sasaki Y, et al. Carcinoma of the prostate in childhood and adolescence: report of a case and review of the literature. Cancer 1980; 46: 2534–2542.

334. Bostwick DG, Burke HB, Djakiew D, et al. Human prostate cancer risk factors. Cancer 2004; 101: 2371–2490.

335. Albertsen PC, Fryback DG, Storer BE, et al. Long-term survival among men with conservatively treated localized prostate cancer. JAMA 1995; 274: 626–631.

336. Montironi R, Mazzucchelli R, Santinelli A, et al. Incidentally detected prostate cancer in cystoprostatectomies: pathological and morphometric comparison with clinically detected cancer in totally embedded specimens. Hum Pathol 2005; 36: 646–654.

337. Bostwick DG, Adolfsson J, Burke HB, et al. Epidemiology and statistical methods in prediction of patient outcome. Scand J Urol Nephrol 2005; 216: 94–110.

338. Selman SH. 'Latent' carcinoma of the prostate: a medical misnomer? Urology 2000; 56: 708–711.

339. Heinonen OP, Albanes D, Virtamo J, et al. Prostate cancer and supplementation with alpha-tocopherol and beta-carotene: incidence and mortality in a controlled trial. J Natl Cancer Inst 1998; 90: 440–446.

340. Iczkowski KA, Bassler TJ, Schwob VS, et al. Diagnosis of 'suspicious for malignancy' in prostate biopsies: predictive value for cancer. Urology 1998; 51: 749–757; discussion 757–78.

341. Brossner C, Bayer G, Madersbacher S, et al. Twelve prostate biopsies detect significant cancer volumes (>0.5 mL). BJU Int 2000; 85: 705–707.

342. Elabbady AA, Khedr MM. Extended 12-core prostate biopsy increases both the detection of prostate cancer and the accuracy of Gleason score. Eur Urol 2006; 49: 49–53.

343. Eskicorapci SY, Guliyev F, Akdogan B, et al. Individualization of the biopsy protocol according to the prostate gland volume for prostate cancer detection. J Urol 2005; 173: 1536–1540.

344. Eskicorapci SY, Tuncay L. Re: Diagnostic value of systematic biopsy methods in the investigation of prostate cancer: a systematic review. Eichler K, Hempel S, Wilby J, et al. J Urol 2006; 175: 1605–1612. J Urol 2006; 176: 2745; author reply 2746.

345. Zeng J, Bauer J, Zhang W, et al. Prostate biopsy protocols: 3D visualization-based evaluation and clinical correlation. Comput Aided Surg 2001; 6: 14–21.

346. Fink KG, Hutarew G, Pytel A, Schmeller NT. Prostate biopsy outcome using 29 mm cutting length. Urol Int 2005; 75: 209–212.

347. Watanabe M, Hayashi T, Tsushima T, et al. Extensive biopsy using a combined transperineal and

transrectal approach to improve prostate cancer detection. Int J Urol 2005; 12: 959–963.

348. Iczkowski KA, Casella G, Seppala RJ, et al. Needle core length in sextant biopsy influences prostate cancer detection rate. Urology 2002; 59: 698–703.

349. Boccon-Gibod L, van der Kwast TH, Montironi R, et al. Handling and pathology reporting of prostate biopsies. Eur Urol 2004; 46: 177–181.

350. van der Kwast TH, Lopes C, Santonja C, et al. Guidelines for processing and reporting of prostatic needle biopsies. J Clin Pathol 2003; 56: 336–340.

351. Renshaw AA. Adequate tissue sampling of prostate core needle biopsies. Am J Clin Pathol 1997; 107: 26–29.

352. Rogatsch H, Moser P, Volgger H, et al. Diagnostic effect of an improved preembedding method of prostate needle biopsy specimens. Hum Pathol 2000; 31: 1102–1107.

353. Bahn DK, Lee F, Badalament R, et al. Targeted cryoablation of the prostate: 7-year outcomes in the primary treatment of prostate cancer. Urology 2002; 60: 3–11.

354. Bahn DK, Silverman P, Lee F Sr, et al. Focal prostate cryoablation: initial results show cancer control and potency preservation. J Endourol 2006; 20: 688–692.

355. Onik G. The male lumpectomy: rationale for a cancer targeted approach for prostate cryoablation. A review. Technol Cancer Res Treat 2004; 3: 365–370.

356. Burke HB, Goodman PH, Rosen DB, et al. Artificial neural networks improve the accuracy of cancer survival prediction. Cancer 1997; 79: 857–862.

357. Maksem JA, Johenning PW. Is cytology capable of adequately grading prostate carcinoma? Matched series of 50 cases comparing cytologic and histologic pattern diagnoses. Urology 1988; 31: 437–444.

358. Henson DE, Hutter RV, Farrow G. Practice protocol for the examination of specimens removed from patients with carcinoma of the prostate gland. A publication of the Cancer Committee, College of American Pathologists. Task Force on the Examination of Specimens Removed From Patients With Prostate Cancer. Arch Pathol Lab Med 1994; 118: 779–783.

359. Cohen MB, Soloway MS, Murphy WM. Sampling of radical prostatectomy specimens. How much is adequate? Am J Clin Pathol 1994; 101: 250–252.

360. Hall GS, Kramer CE, Epstein JI. Evaluation of radical prostatectomy specimens. A comparative analysis of sampling methods. Am J Surg Pathol 1992; 16: 315–324.

361. Sakr WA, Wheeler TM, Blute M, et al. Staging and reporting of prostate cancer – sampling of the radical prostatectomy specimen. Cancer 1996; 78: 366–368.

362. Sehdev AE, Pan ML, Epstein JI. Comparative analysis of sampling methods for grossing radical prostatectomy specimens performed for nonpalpable (stage T1c) prostatic adenocarcinoma. Hum Pathol 2001; 32: 494–499.

363. Sakamoto N, Tsuneyoshi M, Naito S, Kumazawa J. An adequate sampling of the prostate to identify prostatic involvement by urothelial carcinoma in bladder cancer patients. J Urol 1993; 149: 318–321.

364. Epstein JI, Amin M, Boccon-Gibod L, et al. Prognostic factors and reporting of prostate carcinoma in radical prostatectomy and pelvic lymphadenectomy specimens. Scand J Urol Nephrol Suppl 2005: 34–63.

365. McNeal JE, Bostwick DG, Kindrachuk RA, Redwine EA, Freiha FS, Stamey TA. Patterns of progression in prostate cancer. Lancet 1986; 1: 60–3.

366. McNeal JE, Redwine EA, Freiha FS, Stamey TA. Zonal distribution of prostatic adenocarcinoma. Correlation with histologic pattern and direction of spread. Am J Surg Pathol 1988; 12: 897–906.

367. Srigley JR. Key issues in handling and reporting radical prostatectomy specimens. Arch Pathol Lab Med 2006; 130: 303–317.

368. Srigley JR, Amin M, Boccon-Gibod L, et al. Prognostic and predictive factors in prostate cancer: historical perspectives and recent international consensus initiatives. Scand J Urol Nephrol 2005; 216: 8–19.

369. Srigley JR, Amin MB, Epstein JI, et al. Updated protocol for the examination of specimens from patients with carcinomas of the prostate gland. Arch Pathol Lab Med 2006; 130: 936–946.

370. Haggman M, Norberg M, de la Torre M, et al. Characterization of localized prostatic cancer: distribution, grading and pT-staging in radical prostatectomy specimens. Scand J Urol Nephrol 1993; 27: 7–13.

371. Desai A, Wu H, Sun L, et al. Complete embedding and close step-sectioning of radical prostatectomy specimens both increase detection of extra-prostatic extension, and correlate with increased disease-free survival by stage of prostate cancer patients. Prostate Cancer Prostatic Dis 2002; 5: 212–218.

372. Bostwick DG, Foster CS. Predictive factors in prostate cancer: current concepts from the 1999 College of American Pathologists Conference on Solid Tumor Prognostic Factors and the 1999 World Health Organization Second International Consultation on Prostate Cancer. Semin Urol Oncol 1999; 17: 222–272.

373. Silva LC, Saldiva PH, Ellinger F, et al. Quantitation of conventional histologic parameters and biologic factors in prostatic needle biopsy are useful to distinguish paramalignant from malignant disease. Pathol Res Pract 2004; 200: 599–608.

374. Mathur SK, Gupta S, Marwah N, et al. Significance of mucin stain in differentiating benign and malignant lesions of prostate. Indian J Pathol Microbiol 2003; 46: 593–595.

375. Cohen RJ, McNeal JE, Redmond SL, et al. Luminal contents of benign and malignant prostatic glands: correspondence to altered secretory mechanisms. Hum Pathol 2000; 31: 94–100.

376. Cheng L, Cheville JC, Bostwick DG. Diagnosis of prostate cancer in needle biopsies after radiation therapy. Am J Surg Pathol 1999; 23: 1173–1183.

377. Goldstein NS, Qian J, Bostwick DG. Mucin expression in atypical adenomatous hyperplasia of the prostate. Hum Pathol 1995; 26: 887–891.

378. Saez C, Japon MA, Conde AF, et al. Sialomucins are characteristically O-acylated in poorly differentiated and colloid prostatic adenocarcinomas. Mod Pathol 1998; 11: 1193–1197.

379. Papadopoulos I, Sivridis E, Giatromanolaki A, Koukourakis MI. Tumor angiogenesis is associated with MUC1 overexpression and loss of prostate-specific antigen expression in prostate cancer. Clin Cancer Res 2001; 7: 1533–1538.

380. Kirschenbaum A, Itzkowitz SH, Wang JP, et al. MUC1 expression in prostate carcinoma: correlation with grade and stage. Mol Urol 1999; 3: 163–168.

381. Christian JD, Lamm TC, Morrow JF, Bostwick DG. Corpora amylacea in adenocarcinoma of the prostate: incidence and histology within needle core biopsies. Mod Pathol 2005; 18: 36–39.

382. Hosler GA, Epstein JI. Basal cell hyperplasia: an unusual diagnostic dilemma on prostate needle biopsies. Hum Pathol 2005; 36: 480–485.

383. Molberg KH, Mikhail A, Vuitch F. Crystalloids in metastatic prostatic adenocarcinoma. Am J Clin Pathol 1994; 101: 266–268.

384. Tressera F, Barastegui C. Intraluminal crystalloids in metastatic prostatic carcinoma. Am J Clin Pathol 1995; 103: 665.

385. Shah RB, Lee MW, Giraldo AA, Amin MB. Histologic and histochemical characterization of seminal vesicle intraluminal secretions. Arch Pathol Lab Med 2001; 125: 141–145.

386. Bostwick DG, Wollan P, Adlakha K. Collagenous micronodules in prostate cancer. A specific but infrequent diagnostic finding. Arch Pathol Lab Med 1995; 119: 444–447.

387. Varma M, Lee MW, Tamboli P, et al. Morphologic criteria for the diagnosis of prostatic adenocarcinoma in needle biopsy specimens. A study of 250 consecutive cases in a routine surgical pathology practice. Arch Pathol Lab Med 2002; 126: 554–561.

388. Arangelovich V, Tretiakova M, SenGupta E, et al. Pathogenesis and significance of collagenous micronodules of the prostate. Appl Immunohistochem Mol Morphol 2003; 11: 15–19.

389. Weight CJ, Ciezki JP, Reddy CA, et al. Perineural invasion on prostate needle biopsy does not predict biochemical failure following brachytherapy for prostate cancer. Int J Radiat Oncol Biol Phys 2006; 65: 347–350.

390. Egan AJ, Lopez-Beltran A, Bostwick DG. Prostatic adenocarcinoma with atrophic features: malignancy mimicking a benign process. Am J Surg Pathol 1997; 21: 931–935.

391. Ali TZ, Epstein JI. Perineural involvement by benign prostatic glands on needle biopsy. Am J Surg Pathol 2005; 29: 1159–1163.

392. Ayala GE, Dai H, Ittmann M, et al. Growth and survival mechanisms associated with perineural invasion in prostate cancer. Cancer Res 2004; 64: 6082–6090.

393. Li R, Wheeler T, Dai H, Ayala G. Neural cell adhesion molecule is upregulated in nerves with prostate cancer invasion. Hum Pathol 2003; 34: 457–461.

394. Zhou M, Patel A, Rubin MA. Prevalence and location of peripheral nerve found on prostate needle biopsy. Am J Clin Pathol 2001; 115: 39–43.

395. Tsuzuki T, Ujihira N, Ando T. Usefulness of epithelial membrane antigen (EMA) to discriminate between perineural invasion and perineural indentation in prostatic carcinoma. Histopathology 2005; 47: 159–165.

396. Kravchick S, Cytron S, Peled R, et al. Colour Doppler ultrasonography for detecting perineural invasion (PNI) and the value of PNI in predicting final pathological stage: a prospective study of men with clinically localized prostate cancer. BJU Int 2003; 92: 28–31.

397. Bismar TA, Lewis JS Jr, Vollmer RT, Humphrey PA. Multiple measures of carcinoma extent versus perineural invasion in prostate needle biopsy tissue in prediction of pathologic stage in a screening population. Am J Surg Pathol 2003; 27: 432–440.

398. Cannon GM Jr, Pound CR, Landsittel DP, et al. Perineural invasion in prostate cancer biopsies is not associated with higher rates of positive surgical margins. Prostate 2005; 63: 336–340.

399. Rubin MA, Bismar TA, Curtis S, Montie JE. Prostate needle biopsy reporting: how are the surgical members of the Society of Urologic Oncology using pathology reports to guide treatment of prostate cancer patients? Am J Surg Pathol 2004; 28: 946–952.

400. Bonin SR, Hanlon AL, Lee WR, et al. Evidence of increased failure in the treatment of prostate carcinoma patients who have perineural invasion treated with three-dimensional conformal radiation therapy. Cancer 1997; 79: 75–80.

401. Beard C, Schultz D, Loffredo M, et al. Perineural invasion associated with increased cancer-specific mortality after external beam radiation therapy for men with low- and intermediate-risk prostate cancer. Int J Radiat Oncol Biol Phys 2006; 66: 403–407.

402. Wong WW, Schild SE, Vora SA, Halyard MY. Association of percent positive prostate biopsies and perineural invasion with biochemical outcome after external beam radiotherapy for localized prostate cancer. Int J Radiat Oncol Biol Phys 2004; 60: 24–29.

403. Merrick GS, Butler WM, Wallner KE, et al. Prognostic significance of perineural invasion on biochemical progression-free survival after prostate brachytherapy. Urology 2005; 66: 1048–1053.

404. Sebo TJ, Cheville JC, Riehle DL, et al. Perineural invasion and MIB-1 positivity in addition to Gleason score are significant preoperative predictors of progression after radical retropubic prostatectomy for prostate cancer. Am J Surg Pathol 2002; 26: 431–439.

405. Ozcan F. Correlation of perineural invasion on radical prostatectomy specimens with other pathologic prognostic factors and PSA failure. Eur Urol 2001; 40: 308–312.

406. D'Amico AV, Wu Y, Chen MH, et al. Perineural invasion as a predictor of biochemical outcome following radical prostatectomy for select men with clinically localized prostate cancer. J Urol 2001; 165: 126–129.

407. Quinn DI, Henshall SM, Brenner PC, et al. Prognostic significance of preoperative factors in localized prostate carcinoma treated with radical prostatectomy: importance of percentage of biopsies that contain tumor and the presence of biopsy perineural invasion. Cancer 2003; 97: 1884–1893.

408. Nelson CP, Rubin MA, Strawderman M, et al. Preoperative parameters for predicting early prostate cancer recurrence after radical prostatectomy. Urology 2002; 59: 740–745; discussion 745–746.

409. O'Malley KJ, Pound CR, Walsh PC, et al. Influence of biopsy perineural invasion on long-term biochemical disease-free survival after radical prostatectomy. Urology 2002; 59: 85–90.

410. Freedland SJ, Csathy GS, Dorey F, Aronson WJ. Percent prostate needle biopsy tissue with cancer is more predictive of biochemical failure or adverse pathology after radical prostatectomy than prostate specific antigen or Gleason score. J Urol 2002; 167: 516–520.

411. Miyake H, Sakai I, Harada K, et al. Limited value of perineural invasion in radical prostatectomy specimens as a predictor of biochemical recurrence in Japanese men with clinically localized prostate cancer. Hinyokika Kiyo 2005; 51: 241–246.

412. Ng JC, Koch MO, Daggy JK, Cheng L. Perineural invasion in radical prostatectomy specimens: lack of prognostic significance. J Urol 2004; 172: 2249–2251.

413. Harnden P, Shelley MD, Clements H, et al. The prognostic significance of perineural invasion in prostatic cancer biopsies: a systematic review. Cancer 2007; 109: 13–24.

414. Sebo TJ, Cheville JC, Riehle DL, et al. Predicting prostate carcinoma volume and stage at radical prostatectomy by assessing needle biopsy specimens for percent surface area and cores positive for carcinoma, perineural invasion, Gleason score, DNA ploidy and proliferation, and preoperative serum prostate specific antigen: a report of 454 cases. Cancer 2001; 91: 2196–2204.

415. Maru N, Ohori M, Kattan MW, et al. Prognostic significance of the diameter of perineural invasion in radical prostatectomy specimens. Hum Pathol 2001; 32: 828–833.

416. Merrick GS, Butler WM, Galbreath RW, et al. Perineural invasion is not predictive of biochemical outcome following prostate brachytherapy. Cancer J 2002; 8: 79–80.

417. Bahnson RR, Dresner SM, Gooding W, Becich MJ. Incidence and prognostic significance of lymphatic and vascular invasion in radical prostatectomy specimens. Prostate 1989; 15: 149–155.

418. Salomao DR, Graham SD, Bostwick DG. Microvascular invasion in prostate cancer correlates with pathologic stage. Arch Pathol Lab Med 1995; 119: 1050–1054.

419. Babaian RJ, Troncoso P, Bhadkamkar VA, Johnston DA. Analysis of clinicopathologic factors predicting outcome after radical prostatectomy. Cancer 2001; 91: 1414–1422.

420. de la Taille A, Rubin MA, Buttyan R, et al. Is microvascular invasion on radical prostatectomy specimens a useful predictor of PSA recurrence for prostate cancer patients? Eur Urol 2000; 38: 79–84.

421. van den Ouden D, Kranse R, Hop WC, et al. Microvascular invasion in prostate cancer: prognostic significance in patients treated by radical prostatectomy for clinically

localized carcinoma. Urol Int 1998; 60: 17–24.

422. Ito K, Nakashima J, Mukai M, et al. Prognostic implication of microvascular invasion in biochemical failure in patients treated with radical prostatectomy. Urol Int 2003; 70: 297–302.

423. Ferrari MK, McNeal JE, Malhotra SM, Brooks JD. Vascular invasion predicts recurrence after radical prostatectomy: stratification of risk based on pathologic variables. Urology 2004; 64: 749–753.

424. Loeb S, Roehl KA, Yu X, et al. Lymphovascular invasion in radical prostatectomy specimens: prediction of adverse pathologic features and biochemical progression. Urology 2006; 68: 99–103.

425. Brooks JP, Albert PS, O'Connell J, et al. Lymphovascular invasion in prostate cancer: prognostic significance in patients treated with radiotherapy after radical prostatectomy. Cancer 2006; 106: 1521–1526.

426. Graham SD Jr, Napalkov P, Watts L, et al. Microvascular invasion of the seminal vesicles in adenocarcinoma of the prostate. Prostate 1996; 28: 359–363.

427. Cheng L, Jones TD, Lin H, et al. Lymphovascular invasion is an independent prognostic factor in prostatic adenocarcinoma. J Urol 2005; 174: 2181–2185.

428. Zeng Y, Opeskin K, Horvath LG, et al. Lymphatic vessel density and lymph node metastasis in prostate cancer. Prostate 2005; 65: 222–230.

429. Shariat SF, Khoddami SM, Saboorian H, et al. Lymphovascular invasion is a pathological feature of biologically aggressive disease in patients treated with radical prostatectomy. J Urol 2004; 171: 1122–1127.

430. Roma AA, Magi-Galluzzi C, Kral MA, et al. Peritumoral lymphatic invasion is associated with regional lymph node metastases in prostate adenocarcinoma. Mod Pathol 2006; 19: 392–398.

431. Wakui S, Furusato M, Itoh T, et al. Tumour angiogenesis in prostatic carcinoma with and without bone marrow metastasis: a morphometric study. J Pathol 1992; 168: 257–262.

432. Weidner N, Carroll PR, Flax J, et al. Tumor angiogenesis correlates with metastasis in invasive prostate carcinoma. Am J Pathol 1993; 143: 401–409.

433. Brawer MK, Deering RE, Brown M, et al. Predictors of pathologic stage in prostatic carcinoma. The role of neovascularity. Cancer 1994; 73: 678–687.

434. Siegal JA, Yu E, Brawer MK. Topography of neovascularity in human prostate carcinoma. Cancer 1995; 75: 2545–2551.

435. Wilson NM, Masoud AM, Barsoum HB, et al. Correlation of power Doppler with microvessel density in assessing prostate needle biopsy. Clin Radiol 2004; 59: 946–950.

436. Stefanou D, Batistatou A, Kamina S, et al. Expression of vascular endothelial growth factor (VEGF) and association with microvessel density in benign prostatic hyperplasia and prostate cancer. In Vivo 2004; 18: 155–160.

437. Lopez-Beltran A, Qian J, Montironi R, et al. Atypical adenomatous hyperplasia (adenosis) of the prostate: DNA ploidy analysis and immunophenotype. Int J Surg Pathol 2005; 13: 167–173.

438. Pallares J, Rojo F, Iriarte J, et al. Study of microvessel density and the expression of the angiogenic factors VEGF, bFGF and the receptors Flt-1 and FLK-1 in benign, premalignant and malignant prostate tissues. Histol Histopathol 2006; 21: 857–865.

439. Trojan L, Thomas D, Friedrich D, et al. Expression of different vascular endothelial markers in prostate cancer and BPH tissue: an immunohistochemical and clinical evaluation. Anticancer Res 2004; 24: 1651–1656.

440. Trojan L, Thomas D, Knoll T, et al. Expression of pro-angiogenic growth factors VEGF, EGF and bFGF and their topographical relation to neovascularisation in prostate cancer. Urol Res 2004; 32: 97–103.

441. Uehara H. Angiogenesis of prostate cancer and antiangiogenic therapy. J Med Invest 2003; 50: 146–153.

442. Erbersdobler A, Fritz H, Schnoger S, et al. Tumour grade, proliferation, apoptosis, microvessel density, p53, and bcl-2 in prostate cancers: differences between tumours located in the transition zone and in the peripheral zone. Eur Urol 2002; 41: 40–46.

443. Hall MC, Troncoso P, Pollack A, et al. Significance of tumor angiogenesis in clinically localized prostate carcinoma treated with external beam radiotherapy. Urology 1994; 44: 869–875.

444. Vesalainen S, Lipponen P, Talja M, et al. Tumor vascularity and basement membrane structure as prognostic factors in T1–2MO prostatic adenocarcinoma. Anticancer Res 1994; 14: 709–714.

445. Epstein JI, Partin AW, Potter SR, Walsh PC. Adenocarcinoma of the prostate invading the seminal vesicle: prognostic stratification based on pathologic parameters. Urology 2000; 56: 283–288.

446. Silberman MA, Partin AW, Veltri RW, Epstein JI. Tumor angiogenesis correlates with progression after radical prostatectomy but not with pathologic stage in Gleason sum 5 to 7 adenocarcinoma of the prostate. Cancer 1997; 79: 772–779.

447. Stamey TA, McNeal JE, Yemoto CM, et al. Biological determinants of cancer progression in men with prostate cancer. JAMA 1999; 281: 1395–1400.

448. McNeal JE, Yemoto CE. Significance of demonstrable vascular space invasion for the progression of prostatic adenocarcinoma. Am J Surg Pathol 1996; 20: 1351–1360.

449. Mehta R, Kyshtoobayeva A, Kurosaki T, et al. Independent association of angiogenesis index with outcome in prostate cancer. Clin Cancer Res 2001; 7: 81–88.

450. Bono AV, Celato N, Cova V, et al. Microvessel density in prostate carcinoma. Prostate Cancer Prostatic Dis 2002; 5: 123–127.

451. Gravdal K, Halvorsen OJ, Haukaas SA, Akslen LA. Expression of bFGF/FGFR-1 and vascular proliferation related to clinicopathologic features and tumor progress in localized prostate cancer. Virchows Arch 2006; 448: 68–74.

452. Sharma S, Sharma MC, Sarkar C. Morphology of angiogenesis in human cancer: a conceptual overview, histoprognostic perspective and significance of neoangiogenesis. Histopathology 2005; 46: 481–489.

453. Straume O, Chappuis PO, Salvesen HB, et al. Prognostic importance of glomeruloid microvascular proliferation indicates an aggressive angiogenic phenotype in human cancers. Cancer Res 2002; 62: 6808–6811.

454. Bostwick DG, Bostwick KC. 'Vanishing' prostate cancer in radical prostatectomy specimens: incidence and long-term follow-up in 38 cases. BJU Int 2004; 94: 57–58.

455. Goldstein NS, Begin LR, Grody WW, et al. Minimal or no cancer in radical prostatectomy specimens. Report of 13 cases of the 'vanishing cancer phenomenon.' Am J Surg Pathol 1995; 19: 1002–1009.

456. Thwaini A, Anjum F, Kalubac J, et al. 'Vanishing' prostate cancer in radical prostatectomy specimens: incidence and long-term follow-up in 38 cases. BJU Int 2004; 94: 1145–1146.

457. Moskaluk CA. Vanishing prostate cancer syndrome: symptom of a larger clinical issue. Am J Surg Pathol 2005; 29: 561–563.

458. Cao D, Hafez M, Berg K, et al. Little or no residual prostate cancer at radical prostatectomy: vanishing cancer or switched specimen?: a microsatellite analysis of specimen identity. Am J Surg Pathol 2005; 29: 467–473.

459. Kommu S. A model to explain the 'vanishing' prostate – the curative biopsy theory. BJU Int 2004; 94: 939–940.

460. Bostwick DG, Grignon DJ, Hammond ME, et al. Prognostic factors in prostate cancer. College of American Pathologists Consensus Statement 1999. Arch Pathol Lab Med 2000; 124: 995–1000.

461. Arora R, Koch MO, Eble JN, et al. Heterogeneity of Gleason grade in multifocal adenocarcinoma of the prostate. Cancer 2004; 100: 2362–2366.

462. Gleason DF. Undergrading of prostate cancer biopsies: a paradox inherent in all biologic bivariate distributions. Urology 1996; 47: 289–291.

463. Gleason DF. Histologic grade, clinical stage, and patient age in prostate cancer. NCI Monogr 1988: 15–18.

464. Gleason DF. Histologic grading of prostate cancer: a perspective. Hum Pathol 1992; 23: 273–279.

465. Bibbo M, Kim DH, Galera-Davidson H, et al. Architectural, morphometric and photometric features and their relationship to the main subjective diagnostic clues in the grading of prostatic cancer. Anal Quant Cytol Histol 1990; 12: 85–90.

466. Bibbo M, Xiao J, Christen R, et al. Use of computer graphic filters for the nuclear grading of hematoxylin and eosin-stained specimens from prostatic lesions. Anal Quant Cytol Histol 1994; 16: 183–188.

467. Endrizzi J, Optenberg S, Byers R, Thompson IM Jr. Disappearance of well-differentiated carcinoma of the prostate: effect of transurethral resection of the prostate, prostate-specific antigen, and prostate biopsy. Urology 2001; 57: 733–736.

468. Kondylis FI, Moriarty RP, Bostwick D, Schellhammer PF. Prostate cancer grade assignment: the effect of chronological, interpretive and translation bias. J Urol 2003; 170: 1189–1193.

469. Freedland SJ, Presti JC Jr, Amling CL, et al. Time trends in biochemical recurrence after radical prostatectomy: results of the SEARCH database. Urology 2003; 61: 736–741.

470. Albertsen PC, Hanley JA, Barrows GH, et al. Prostate cancer and the Will Rogers phenomenon. J Natl Cancer Inst 2005; 97: 1248–1253.

471. Ghani KR, Grigor K, Tulloch DN, et al. Trends in reporting Gleason score 1991 to 2001: changes in the pathologist's practice. Eur Urol 2005; 47: 196–201.

472. Ozdamar SO, Sarikaya S, Yildiz L, et al. Intraobserver and interobserver reproducibility of WHO and Gleason histologic grading systems in prostatic adenocarcinomas. Int Urol Nephrol 1996; 28: 73–77.

473. Bain GO, Koch M, Hanson J. Feasibility of grading prostatic carcinoma. Arch Pathol Lab Med 1982; 106: 265–267.

474. Babian RJ, Grunow WA. Reliability of Gleason grading system in caomparing prostate biopsies with total prostatectomy specimens. Urology 1985; 25: 564–567.

475. Harada M, Mostofi FK, Corle DK. Preliminary studies of histologic prognosis in cancer of the prostate. Cancer Treat Rep 1977; 61: 223–225.

476. Cintra ML, Billis A. Histologic grading of prostatic adenocarcinoma. Intraobserver reproducibility of the Mostofi, Gleason, and Bocking grading systems. Int Urol Nephrol 1991; 23: 449–454.

477. Svanholm H, Mygind H. Prostatic carcinoma. Reproducibility of histologic grading. Acta Pathol Microbiol Immunol Scand 1985; 93: 67–71.

478. Ten Kate FJN, Gallee MPW, Schmitz PIM. Problems in the grading of prostatic carcinoma: Intraobserver reproducibility of five different grading systems. World J Urol 1986; 4: 147–152.

479. Melia J, Moseley R, Ball RY, et al. A UK-based investigation of inter- and intra-observer reproducibility of Gleason grading of prostatic biopsies. Histopathology 2006; 48: 644–654.

480. Guileyardo JM, Sarma DP, Johnson WD, et al. Incidental prostatic carcinoma: tumor extent versus histologic grade. Urology 1982; 20: 40–42.

481. Humphrey P, Vollmer RT. The ratio of prostate chips with cancer: a new measure of tumor extent and its relationship to grade and prognosis. Hum Pathol 1988; 19: 411–418.

482. de las Morenas A, Siroky MB, Merriam J, Stilmant MM. Prostatic adenocarcinoma: reproducibility and correlation with clinical stages of four grading systems. Hum Pathol 1988; 19: 595–597.

483. di Loreto C, Fitzpatrick B, Underhill S, et al. Correlation between visual clues, objective architectural features, and interobserver agreement in prostate cancer. Am J Clin Pathol 1991; 96: 70–75.

484. McLean M, Srigley J, Banerjee D, et al. Interobserver variation in prostate cancer Gleason scoring: are there implications for the design of clinical trials and treatment strategies? Clin Oncol (Roy Coll Radiol) 1997; 9: 222–225.

485. Steinberg DM, Sauvageot J, Piantadosi S, Epstein JI. Correlation of prostate needle biopsy and radical prostatectomy Gleason grade in academic and community settings. Am J Surg Pathol 1997; 21: 566–576.

486. Kronz JD, Silberman MA, Allsbrook WC Jr, et al. Pathology residents' use of a Web-based tutorial to improve Gleason grading of prostate carcinoma on needle biopsies. Hum Pathol 2000; 31: 1044–1050.

487. Allsbrook WC Jr, Mangold KA, Johnson MH, et al. Interobserver reproducibility of Gleason grading of prostatic carcinoma: urologic pathologists. Hum Pathol 2001; 32: 74–80.

488. Allsbrook WC Jr, Mangold KA, Johnson MH, et al. Interobserver reproducibility of Gleason grading of prostatic carcinoma: general pathologist. Hum Pathol 2001; 32: 81–88.

489. Iczkowski KA, Bostwick DG. The pathologist as optimist: Cancer grade deflation in prostatic needle biopsies. Am J Surg Pathol 1998; 21: 566–576.

490. Egevad L. Reproducibility of Gleason grading of prostate cancer can be improved by the use of reference images. Urology 2001; 57: 291–295.

491. Grignon DJ, Hammond EH. College of American Pathologists Conference XXVI on clinical relevance of prognostic markers in solid tumors. Report of the Prostate Cancer Working Group. Arch Pathol Lab Med 1995; 119: 1122–1126.

492. Lessells AM, Burnett RA, Howatson SR, et al. Observer variability in the histopathological reporting of needle biopsy specimens of the prostate. Hum Pathol 1997; 28: 646–649.

493. Coard KC, Freeman VL. Gleason grading of prostate cancer: level of concordance between pathologists at the University Hospital of the West Indies. Am J Clin Pathol 2004; 122: 373–376.

494. Glaessgen A, Hamberg H, Pihl CG, et al. Interobserver reproducibility of percent Gleason grade 4/5 in prostate biopsies. J Urol 2004; 171: 664–667.

495. Glaessgen A, Hamberg H, Pihl CG, et al. Interobserver reproducibility of percent Gleason grade 4/5 in total prostatectomy specimens. J Urol 2002; 168: 2006–2010.

496. Glaessgen A, Hamberg H, Pihl CG, et al. Interobserver reproducibility of modified Gleason score in radical prostatectomy specimens. Virchows Arch 2004; 445: 17–21.

497. Tomioka S, Nakatsu H, Suzuki N, et al. Comparison of Gleason grade and score between preoperative biopsy and prostatectomy specimens in prostate cancer. Int J Urol 2006; 13: 555–559.

498. King CR, McNeal JE, Gill H, et al. Reliability of small amounts of cancer in prostate biopsies to reveal pathologic grade. Urology 2006; 67: 1229–1234.

499. King CR, Long JP. Prostate biopsy grading errors: a sampling problem? Int J Cancer 2000; 90: 326–330.

500. Tsui KH, Shen BY, Sun GH, et al. Probability based diagnostic biopsy specimens as predictors of tumor grade and stage found. Arch Androl 2004; 50: 333–337.

501. Freedland SJ, Kane CJ, Amling CL, et al. Upgrading and downgrading of prostate needle biopsy specimens: risk factors and clinical implications. Urology 2007; 69: 495–499.

502. Pinthus JH, Witkos M, Fleshner NE, et al. Prostate cancers scored as Gleason 6 on prostate biopsy are frequently Gleason 7 tumors at radical prostatectomy: implication on

outcome. J Urol 2006; 176: 979–984; discussion 984.

503. King CR, McNeal JE, Gill H, Presti JC Jr. Extended prostate biopsy scheme improves reliability of Gleason grading: implications for radiotherapy patients. Int J Radiat Oncol Biol Phys 2004; 59: 386–391.

504. Emiliozzi P, Maymone S, Paterno A, et al. Increased accuracy of biopsy Gleason score obtained by extended needle biopsy. J Urol 2004; 172: 2224–2226.

505. San Francisco IF, DeWolf WC, Rosen S, et al. Extended prostate needle biopsy improves concordance of Gleason grading between prostate needle biopsy and radical prostatectomy. J Urol 2003; 169: 136–140.

506. King CR, Patel DA, Terris MK. Prostate biopsy volume indices do not predict for significant Gleason upgrading. Am J Clin Oncol 2005; 28: 125–129.

507. Poulos CK, Daggy JK, Cheng L. Preoperative prediction of Gleason grade in radical prostatectomy specimens: the influence of different Gleason grades from multiple positive biopsy sites. Mod Pathol 2005; 18: 228–234.

508. Kramer SA, Farnham R, Glenn JF, Paulson DF. Comparative morphology of primary and secondary deposits of prostatic adenocarcinoma. Cancer 1981; 48: 271–273.

509. Donohue JF, Bianco FJ Jr, Kuroiwa K, et al. Poorly differentiated prostate cancer treated with radical prostatectomy: long-term outcome and incidence of pathological downgrading. J Urol 2006; 176: 991–995.

510. Chun FK, Steuber T, Erbersdobler A, et al. Development and internal validation of a nomogram predicting the probability of prostate cancer Gleason sum upgrading between biopsy and radical prostatectomy pathology. Eur Urol 2006; 49: 820–826.

511. Chun FK, Briganti A, Shariat SF, et al. Significant upgrading affects a third of men diagnosed with prostate cancer: predictive nomogram and internal validation. BJU Int 2006; 98: 329–334.

512. Kulkarni GS, Al-Azab R, Lockwood G, et al. Evidence for a biopsy derived grade artifact among larger prostate glands. J Urol 2006; 175: 505–509.

513. Park HK, Choe G, Byun SS, et al. Evaluation of concordance of Gleason score between prostatectomy and biopsies that show more than two different Gleason scores in positive cores. Urology 2006; 67: 110–114.

514. Ross JS, Sheehan CE, Ambros RA, et al. Needle biopsy DNA ploidy status predicts grade shifting in prostate cancer. Am J Surg Pathol 1999; 23: 296–301.

515. Maygarden SJ, Pruthi R. Gleason grading and volume estimation in prostate needle biopsy specimens: evolving issues. Am J Clin Pathol 2005; 123: S58–66.

516. Bonkhoff H. [Gleason grading: diagnostic criteria and clinical implications]. Pathologe 2005; 26: 422–432.

517. Aihara M, Wheeler TM, Ohori M, Scardino PT. Heterogeneity of prostate cancer in radical prostatectomy specimens. Urology 1994; 43: 60–66; discussion 66–67.

518. Hattab EM, Koch MO, Eble JN, et al. Tertiary Gleason pattern 5 is a powerful predictor of biochemical relapse in patients with Gleason score 7 prostatic adenocarcinoma. J Urol 2006; 175: 1695–1699; discussion 1699.

519. Descazeaud A, Rubin MA, Allory Y, et al. What information are urologists extracting from prostate needle biopsy reports and what do they need for clinical management of prostate cancer? Eur Urol 2005; 48: 911–915.

520. Epstein JI, Allsbrook WC Jr, Amin MB, Egevad LL. Update on the Gleason grading system for prostate cancer: results of an international consensus conference of urologic pathologists. Adv Anat Pathol 2006; 13: 57–59.

521. van Oort IM, Schout BM, Kiemeney LA, et al. Does the tertiary Gleason pattern influence the PSA progression-free interval after retropubic radical prostatectomy for organ-confined prostate cancer? Eur Urol 2005; 48: 572–576.

522. Aziz DC, Barathur RB. Quantitation and morphometric analysis of tumors by image analysis. J Cell Biochem 1994; 19: 120–125.

523. Partin AW, Walsh AC, Pitcock RV, et al. A comparison of nuclear morphometry and Gleason grade as a predictor of prognosis in stage A2 prostate cancer: a critical analysis. J Urol 1989; 142: 1254–1258.

524. Montironi R, Scarpelli M, Braccischi A, et al. Quantitative analysis of nucleolar margination in diagnostic cytopathology. Virchows Arch A [Pathol Anat Histopathol] 1991; 419: 505–512.

525. Montironi R, Scarpelli M, Mazzucchelli R, et al. Subvisual changes in chromatin organization state are detected by karyometry in the histologically normal urothelium in patients with synchronous papillary carcinoma. Hum Pathol 2003; 34: 893–901.

526. Hurwitz MD, DeWeese TL, Zinreich ES, et al. Nuclear morphometry predicts disease-free interval for clinically localized adenocarcinoma of the prostate treated with definitive radiation therapy. Int J Cancer 1999; 84: 594–597.

527. Tannenbaum M. Prostate cancer grading: light and electron microscopy. Semin Urol 1983; 1: 186–192.

528. Tannenbaum M, Tannenbaum S, deSanctis PN, Olsson CA. Prognostic significance of nucleolar surface area in prostate cancer. Urology 1982; 19: 546–551.

529. Myers RP, Neves RJ, Farrow GM, Utz DC. Nucleolar grading of prostatic adenocarcinoma: light microscopic correlation with disease progression. Prostate 1982; 3: 423–432.

530. Lilleby W, Torlakovic G, Torlakovic E, et al. Prognostic significance of histologic grading in patients with prostate carcinoma who are assessed by the Gleason and World Health Organization grading systems in needle biopsies obtained prior to radiotherapy. Cancer 2001; 92: 311–319.

531. McNeal JE. Cancer volume and site of origin of adenocarcinoma in the prostate: relationship to local and distant spread. Hum Pathol 1992; 23: 258–266.

532. Gaffney EF, O'Sullivan SN, O'Brien A. A major solid undifferentiated carcinoma pattern correlates with tumour progression in locally advanced prostatic carcinoma. Histopathology 1992; 21: 249–255.

533. Bostwick DG, Graham SD Jr, Napalkov P, et al. Staging of early prostate cancer: a proposed tumor volume-based prognostic index. Urology 1993; 41: 403–411.

534. Vis AN, Roemeling S, Kranse R, et al. Should we replace the Gleason score with the amount of high-grade prostate cancer? Eur Urol 2007; 51: 931–939.

535. Chun FK, Briganti A, Jeldres C, et al. Tumour volume and high grade tumour volume are the best predictors of pathologic stage and biochemical recurrence after radical prostatectomy. Eur J Cancer 2007; 43: 536–543.

536. Cheng L, Koch MO, Juliar BE, et al. The combined percentage of Gleason patterns 4 and 5 is the best predictor of cancer progression after radical prostatectomy. J Clin Oncol 2005; 23: 2911–2917.

537. Egevad L, Granfors T, Karlberg L, et al. Percent Gleason grade 4/5 as prognostic factor in prostate cancer diagnosed at transurethral resection. J Urol 2002; 168: 509–513.

538. Wise AM, Stamey TA, McNeal JE, Clayton JL. Morphologic and clinical significance of multifocal prostate cancers in radical prostatectomy specimens. Urology 2002; 60: 264–269.

539. Tefilli MV, Gheiler EL, Tiguert R, et al. Should Gleason score 7 prostate cancer be considered a unique grade

category? Urology 1999; 53: 372–377.

540. Naya Y, Babaian RJ. The predictors of pelvic lymph node metastasis at radical retropubic prostatectomy. J Urol 2003; 170: 2306–2310.

541. Tiguert R, Ravery V, Grignon DJ, et al. [Main grade of Gleason's 7 score of the surgical sample correlated with biologic progression in patients treated for total prostatectomy]. Prog Urol 2002; 12: 31–36.

542. Sakr WA, Tefilli MV, Grignon DJ, et al. Gleason score 7 prostate cancer: a heterogeneous entity? Correlation with pathologic parameters and disease-free survival. Urology 2000; 56: 730–734.

543. Grober ED, Tsihlias J, Jewett MA, et al. Correlation of the primary Gleason pattern on prostate needle biopsy with clinico-pathological factors in Gleason 7 tumors. Can J Urol 2004; 11: 2157–2162.

544. Herman CM, Kattan MW, Ohori M, et al. Primary Gleason pattern as a predictor of disease progression in Gleason score 7 prostate cancer: a multivariate analysis of 823 men treated with radical prostatectomy. Am J Surg Pathol 2001; 25: 657–660.

545. Merrick GS, Butler WM, Wallner KE, et al. The impact of primary Gleason grade on biochemical outcome following brachytherapy for hormone-naive Gleason score 7 prostate cancer. Cancer J 2005; 11: 234–240.

546. Potters L, Purrazzella R, Brustein S, et al. The prognostic significance of Gleason Grade in patients treated with permanent prostate brachytherapy. Int J Radiat Oncol Biol Phys 2003; 56: 749–754.

547. Rasiah KK, Stricker PD, Haynes AM, et al. Prognostic significance of Gleason pattern in patients with Gleason score 7 prostate carcinoma. Cancer 2003; 98: 2560–2565.

548. Gonzalgo ML, Bastian PJ, Mangold LA, et al. Relationship between primary Gleason pattern on needle biopsy and clinicopathologic outcomes among men with Gleason score 7 adenocarcinoma of the prostate. Urology 2006; 67: 115–119.

549. Brawn PN. The dedifferentiation of prostate carcinoma. Cancer 1983; 52: 246–251.

550. Cumming JA, Ritchie AW, Goodman CM, et al. De-differentiation with time in prostate cancer and the influence of treatment on the course of the disease. Br J Urol 1990; 65: 271–274.

551. Whittemore AS, Keller JB, Betensky R. Low-grade, latent prostate cancer volume: predictor of clinical cancer incidence? J Natl Cancer Inst 1991; 83: 1231–1235.

552. Choo R, Do V, Sugar L, et al. Comparison of histologic grade between initial and follow-up biopsy in untreated, low to intermediate grade, localized prostate cancer. Can J Urol 2004; 11: 2118–2124.

553. Epstein JI, Walsh PC, Carter HB. Dedifferentiation of prostate cancer grade with time in men followed expectantly for stage T1c disease. J Urol 2001; 166: 1688–1691.

554. Bott SR, Foley CL, Bull MD, et al. Are prostatic biopsies necessary in men aged > or = 80 years? BJU Int 2007; 99: 335–338.

555. Draisma G, Postma R, Schroder FH, et al. Gleason score, age and screening: modeling dedifferentiation in prostate cancer. Int J Cancer 2006; 119: 2366–2371.

556. Cheng L, Slezak J, Bergstralh EJ, et al. Dedifferentiation in the metastatic progression of prostate carcinoma. Cancer 1999; 86: 657–663.

557. Bostwick DG, Egbert BM, Fajardo LF. Radiation injury of the normal and neoplastic prostate. Am J Surg Pathol 1982; 6: 541–551.

558. Wheeler JA, Zagars GK, Ayala AG. Dedifferentiation of locally recurrent prostate cancer after radiation therapy. Evidence for tumor progression. Cancer 1993; 71: 3783–3787.

559. Siders DB, Lee F. Histologic changes of irradiated prostatic carcinoma diagnosed by transrectal ultrasound. Hum Pathol 1992; 23: 344–351.

560. Bocking A, Sinagowitz E. Histologic grading of prostatic carcinoma. Pathol Res Pract 1980; 168: 115–125.

561. Helpap B, Bocking A, Dhom G, et al. [Classification, histologic and cytologic grading and regression grading of prostate cancer]. Urologe A 1985; 24: 156–159.

562. Grignon DJ, Bostwick DG, Civantos F, et al. Pathologic handling and reporting of prostate tissue specimens in patients receiving neoadjuvant hormonal therapy: report of the Pathology Committee. Mol Urol 1999; 3: 193–198.

563. Ellison E, Chuang SS, Zincke H, et al. Prostate adenocarcinoma after androgen deprivation therapy: A comparative study of morphology, morphometry, immunohistochemistry, and DNA ploidy. Pathol Case Rev 1996; 2: 36–46.

564. Carver BS, Kattan MW, Scardino PT, Eastham JA. Gleason grade remains an important prognostic predictor in men diagnosed with prostate cancer while on finasteride therapy. BJU Int 2005; 95: 509–512.

565. Bostwick DG, Qian J, Civantos F, et al. Does finasteride alter the pathology of the prostate and cancer grading? Clin Prostate Cancer 2004; 2: 228–235.

566. Gleave M, Qian J, Andreou C, et al. The effects of the dual 5alpha-reductase inhibitor dutasteride on localized prostate cancer – results from a 4-month pre-radical prostatectomy study. Prostate 2006; 66: 1674–1685.

567. Freedland SJ, Isaacs WB, Platz EA, et al. Prostate size and risk of high-grade, advanced prostate cancer and biochemical progression after radical prostatectomy: a search database study. J Clin Oncol 2005; 23: 7546–7554.

568. Chun FK, Graefen M, Zacharias M, et al. Anatomic radical retropubic prostatectomy-long-term recurrence-free survival rates for localized prostate cancer. World J Urol 2006; 24: 273–280.

569. Ward JF, Slezak JM, Blute ML, et al. Radical prostatectomy for clinically advanced (cT3) prostate cancer since the advent of prostate-specific antigen testing: 15-year outcome. BJU Int 2005; 95: 751–756.

570. Stephenson AJ, Scardino PT, Eastham JA, et al. Postoperative nomogram predicting the 10-year probability of prostate cancer recurrence after radical prostatectomy. J Clin Oncol 2005; 23: 7005–7012.

571. Patel DA, Presti JC Jr, McNeal JE, et al. Preoperative PSA velocity is an independent prognostic factor for relapse after radical prostatectomy. J Clin Oncol 2005; 23: 6157–6162.

572. D'Amico AV, Chen MH, Roehl KA, Catalona WJ. Identifying patients at risk for significant versus clinically insignificant postoperative prostate-specific antigen failure. J Clin Oncol 2005; 23: 4975–4979.

573. Johnson CW, Anastasiadis AG, McKiernan JM, et al. Prognostic indicators for long term outcome following radical retropubic prostatectomy for prostate cancer involving the seminal vesicles. Urol Oncol 2004; 22: 107–111.

574. Andren O, Fall K, Franzen L, et al. How well does the Gleason score predict prostate cancer death? A 20-year followup of a population based cohort in Sweden. J Urol 2006; 175: 1337–1340.

575. Albertsen PC, Hanley JA, Fine J 20-year outcomes following conservative management of clinically localized prostate cancer. JAMA 2005; 293: 2095–2101.

576. Humphrey PA. Gleason grading and prognostic factors in carcinoma of the prostate. Mod Pathol 2004; 17: 292–306.

577. Humphrey PA, Frazier HA, Vollmer RT, Paulson DF. Stratification of pathologic features in radical prostatectomy specimens that are predictive of elevated initial postoperative serum prostate-specific antigen levels. Cancer 1993; 71: 1821–1827.

578. Humphrey PA, Walther PJ, Currin SM, Vollmer RT. Histologic grade, DNA ploidy, and intraglandular tumor extent as indicators of tumor progression of clinical stage B prostatic carcinoma. A direct

comparison. Am J Surg Pathol 1991; 15: 1165–1170.

579. Stephenson AJ, Scardino PT, Eastham JA, et al. Preoperative nomogram predicting the 10-year probability of prostate cancer recurrence after radical prostatectomy. J Natl Cancer Inst 2006; 98: 715–717.

580. Schroeder FH, Blom JH, Hop WC, Mostofi FK. Grading of prostatic cancer (I): An analysis of the prognostic significance of single characteristics. Prostate 1985; 6: 81–100.

581. Anast JW, Andriole GL, Bismar TA, et al. Relating biopsy and clinical variables to radical prostatectomy findings: can insignificant and advanced prostate cancer be predicted in a screening population? Urology 2004; 64: 544–550.

582. Blackwell KL, Bostwick DG, Myers RP, et al. Combining prostate specific antigen with cancer and gland volume to predict more reliably pathological stage: the influence of prostate specific antigen cancer density. J Urol 1994; 151: 1565–1570.

583. Partin AW, Carter HB, Chan DW, et al. Prostate specific antigen in the staging of localized prostate cancer: influence of tumor differentiation, tumor volume and benign hyperplasia. J Urol 1990; 143: 747–752.

584. Partin AW, Pearson JD, Landis PK, et al. Evaluation of serum prostate-specific antigen velocity after radical prostatectomy to distinguish local recurrence from distant metastases. Urology 1994; 43: 649–659.

585. Haese A, Vaisanen V, Lilja H, et al. Comparison of predictive accuracy for pathologically organ confined clinical stage T1c prostate cancer using human glandular kallikrein 2 and prostate specific antigen combined with clinical stage and Gleason grade. J Urol 2005; 173: 752–756.

586. Augustin H, Eggert T, Wenske S, et al. Comparison of accuracy between the Partin tables of 1997 and 2001 to predict final pathological stage in clinically localized prostate cancer. J Urol 2004; 171: 177–181.

587. Grossfeld GD, Chang JJ, Broering JM, et al. Under staging and under grading in a contemporary series of patients undergoing radical prostatectomy: results from the Cancer of the Prostate Strategic Urologic Research Endeavor database. J Urol 2001; 165: 851–856.

588. Bluestein DL, Bostwick DG, Bergstralh EJ, Oesterling JE. Eliminating the need for bilateral pelvic lymphadenectomy in select patients with prostate cancer. J Urol 1994; 151: 1315–1320.

589. Sands ME, Zagars GK, Pollack A, von Eschenbach AC. Serum prostate-specific antigen, clinical stage, pathologic grade, and the incidence of nodal metastases in prostate cancer. Urology 1994; 44: 215–220.

590. Yamashita S, Inaba Y, Soma F, Katayama Y. Pure prostatic papillary adenocarcinoma with ductal features. Hinyokika Kiyo 2005; 51: 207–209; discussion 210.

591. Zini L, Villers A, Leroy X, et al. [Cystic prostate cancer: a clinical entity of ductal carcinoma]. Prog Urol 2004; 14: 411–413.

592. Kajiwara M, Mutaguchi K, Usui T. [Ductal carcinoma of the prostate with multilocular cystic formation]. Hinyokika Kiyo 2002; 48: 557–560.

593. Ohyama C, Takyu S, Yoshikawa K, et al. Adenocarcinoma arising from the prostatic duct mimicking transitional cell carcinoma. Int J Urol 2001; 8: 408–411.

594. Brinker DA, Potter SR, Epstein JI. Ductal adenocarcinoma of the prostate diagnosed on needle biopsy: correlation with clinical and radical prostatectomy findings and progression. Am J Surg Pathol 1999; 23: 1471–1479.

595. Rubin MA, de La Taille A, Bagiella E, et al. Cribriform carcinoma of the prostate and cribriform prostatic intraepithelial neoplasia: incidence and clinical implications. Am J Surg Pathol 1998; 22: 840–848.

596. Oxley JD, Abbott CD, Gillatt DA, MacIver AG. Ductal carcinomas of the prostate: a clinicopathological and immunohistochemical study. Br J Urol 1998; 81: 109–115.

597. Millar EK, Sharma NK, Lessells AM. Ductal (endometrioid) adenocarcinoma of the prostate: a clinicopathological study of 16 cases. Histopathology 1996; 29: 11–19.

598. Gong Y, Caraway N, Stewart J, Staerkel G. Metastatic ductal adenocarcinoma of the prostate: cytologic features and clinical findings. Am J Clin Pathol 2006; 126: 302–309.

599. Melicow MM, Pachter MR. Endometrial carcinoma of prostatic utricle (uterus masculinus). Cancer 1967; 20: 1715–1722.

600. Samaratunga H, Singh M. Distribution pattern of basal cells detected by cytokeratin 34 beta E12 in primary prostatic duct adenocarcinoma. Am J Surg Pathol 1997; 21: 435–440.

601. Lile R, Thickman D, Miller GJ, Crawford ED. Prostatic comedocarcinoma: correlation of sonograms with pathologic specimens in three cases. AJR Am J Roentgenol 1990; 155: 303–306.

602. Currin SM, Lee SE, Walther PJ. Flow cytometric analysis of comedocarcinoma of the prostate: an uncommon histopathological variant of prostatic adenocarcinoma. J Urol 1988; 140: 96–100.

603. Curtis MW, Evans AJ, Srigley JR. Mucin-producing urothelial-type adenocarcinoma of prostate: report of two cases of a rare and diagnostically challenging entity. Mod Pathol 2005; 18: 585–590.

604. Ortiz-Rey JA, Dos Santos JE, Rodriguez-Castilla M, et al. Mucinous urothelial-type adenocarcinoma of the prostate. Scand J Urol Nephrol 2004; 38: 256–257.

605. Mai KT, Collins JP, Veinot JP. Prostatic adenocarcinoma with urothelial (transitional cell) carcinoma features. Appl Immunohistochem Mol Morphol 2002; 10: 231–236.

606. Ushida H, Koizumi S, Okada Y. [A prostatic duct carcinoma difficult to distinguish from transitional cell carcinoma: a case report]. Hinyokika Kiyo 2004; 50: 535–538.

607. Sakamoto N, Ohtsubo S, Iguchi A, et al. Intestinal-type mucinous adenocarcinoma arising from the prostatic duct. Int J Urol 2005; 12: 509–512.

608. Huang Q, Chu PG, Lau SK, Weiss LM. Urothelial carcinoma of the urinary bladder with a component of acinar/tubular type differentiation simulating prostatic adenocarcinoma. Hum Pathol 2004; 35: 769–773.

609. Tulunay O, Orhan D, Baltaci S, et al. Prostatic ductal adenocarcinoma showing Bcl-2 expression. Int J Urol 2004; 11: 805–808.

610. Lee SS. Endometrioid adenocarcinoma of the prostate: a clinicopathologic and immunohistochemical study. J Surg Oncol 1994; 55: 235–238.

611. Bostwick DG, Kindrachuk RW, Rouse RV. Prostatic adenocarcinoma with endometrioid features. Clinical, pathologic, and ultrastructural findings. Am J Surg Pathol 1985; 9: 595–609.

612. Ro JY, Ayala AG, Wishnow KI, Ordonez NG. Prostatic duct adenocarcinoma with endometrioid features: immunohistochemical and electron microscopic study. Semin Diagn Pathol 1988; 5: 301–311.

613. Pinder SE, McMahon RF. Mucins in prostatic carcinoma. Histopathology 1990; 16: 43–46.

614. Ro JY, Grignon DJ, Ayala AG, et al. Mucinous adenocarcinoma of the prostate: histochemical and immunohistochemical studies. Hum Pathol 1990; 21: 593–600.

615. McNeal JE, Alroy J, Villers A, et al. Mucinous differentiation in prostatic adenocarcinoma. Hum Pathol 1991; 22: 979–988.

616. Teichman JM, Shabaik A, Demby AM. Mucinous adenocarcinoma of the prostate and hormone sensitivity. J Urol 1994; 151: 701–702.

617. Lane BR, Magi-Galluzzi C, Reuther AM, et al. Mucinous adenocarcinoma of the prostate does not confer poor prognosis. Urology 2006; 68: 825–30.

618. Sousa Escandon A, Arguelles Pintos M, Picallo Sanchez J, et al. [Mucinous carcinoma of the prostate: critical review of Elbadawi's criteria]. Actas Urol Esp 2000; 24: 155–162.

619. Gumus E, Yilmaz B, Miroglu C. Prostate mucinous adenocarcinoma with signet ring cell. Int J Urol 2003; 10: 239–241.

620. Furuta A, Naruoka T, Hasegawa N, et al. [Mucinous adenocarcinoma of the prostate: a case report and review of 32 cases on immunohistochemical study of both PSA and CEA]. Nippon Hinyokika Gakkai Zasshi 2003; 94: 570–573.

621. Rhee AC, Olgac S, Ohori M, Russo P. Mucinous adenocarcinoma of the prostate: a case report of long-term disease-free survival and a review of the literature. Urology 2004; 63: 779–780.

622. Tran KP, Epstein JI. Mucinous adenocarcinoma of urinary bladder type arising from the prostatic urethra. Distinction from mucinous adenocarcinoma of the prostate. Am J Surg Pathol 1996; 20: 1346–1350.

623. Olivas TP, Brady TW. Mucinous adenocarcinoma of the prostate: a report of a case of long-term survival. Urology 1996; 47: 256–258.

624. Saito S, Iwaki H. Mucin-producing carcinoma of the prostate: review of 88 cases. Urology 1999; 54: 141–144.

625. Tran TA, Jennings TA, Ross JS, Nazeer T. Pseudomyxoma ovariilike posttherapeutic alteration in prostatic adenocarcinoma: a distinctive pattern in patients receiving neoadjuvant androgen ablation therapy. Am J Surg Pathol 1998; 22: 347–354.

626. Akagashi K, Tanda H, Kato S, et al. Signet-ring cell carcinoma of the prostate effectively treated with maximal androgen blockade. Int J Urol 2003; 10: 456–458.

627. Guerin D, Hasan N, Keen CE. Signet ring cell differentiation in adenocarcinoma of the prostate: a study of five cases. Histopathology 1993; 22: 367–371.

628. Kendall A, Corbishley CM, Pandha HS. Signet ring cell carcinoma in the prostate. Clin Oncol (Roy Coll Radiol) 2004; 16: 105–107.

629. Lin JT, Yu ML, Lee JH, Wu TT. Secondary signet-ring cell carcinoma of the prostate. J Urol 2002; 168: 1492.

630. Kuroda N, Yamasaki I, Nakayama H, et al. Prostatic signet-ring cell carcinoma: case report and literature review. Pathol Int 1999; 49: 457–461.

631. Torbenson M, Dhir R, Nangia A, et al. Prostatic carcinoma with signet ring cells: a clinicopathologic and immunohistochemical analysis of 12 cases, with review of the literature. Mod Pathol 1998; 11: 552–559.

632. Kanematsu A, Hiura M. Primary signet ring cell adenocarcinoma of the prostate treated by radical prostatectomy after preoperative androgen deprivation. Int J Urol 1997; 4: 522–523.

633. Yoshimura K, Fukui I, Ishikawa Y, et al. Locally confined signet-ring cell carcinoma of the prostate: a case report of a long-term survivor. Int J Urol 1996; 3: 406–407.

634. Leong FJ, Leong AS, Swift J. Signet-ring carcinoma of the prostate. Pathol Res Pract 1996; 192: 1232–1238; discussion 1239–1241.

635. Giltman LI. Signet ring adenocarcinoma of the prostate. J Urol 1981; 126: 134–135.

636. Ro JY, el-Naggar A, Ayala AG, et al. Signet-ring-cell carcinoma of the prostate. Electron-microscopic and immunohistochemical studies of eight cases. Am J Surg Pathol 1988; 12: 453–460.

637. Catton PA, Hartwick RW, Srigley JR. Prostate cancer presenting with malignant ascites: signet-ring cell variant of prostatic adenocarcinoma. Urology 1992; 39: 495–497.

638. Remmele W, Weber A, Harding P. Primary signet-ring cell carcinoma of the prostate. Hum Pathol 1988; 19: 478–480.

639. Schned AR. Artifactual signet ring cells. Am J Surg Pathol 1987; 11: 736–737.

640. Wang HL, Humphrey PA. Exaggerated signet-ring cell change in stromal nodule of prostate: a pseudoneoplastic proliferation. Am J Surg Pathol 2002; 26: 1066–1070.

641. Feria-Bernal G, Garcia-Gonzalez VM, Figueroa-Granados V, et al. [Neuroendocrine differentiation and markers of cell proliferation in a group of patients with prostate adenocarcinoma and normal or high serum prostate-specific antigen levels]. Gac Med Mex 2006; 142: 441–446.

642. Quek ML, Daneshmand S, Rodrigo S, et al. Prognostic significance of neuroendocrine expression in lymph node-positive prostate cancer. Urology 2006; 67: 1247–1252.

643. Slovin SF. Neuroendocrine differentiation in prostate cancer: a sheep in wolf's clothing? Nature Clin Pract Urol 2006; 3: 138–144.

644. Hirano D, Jike T, Okada Y, et al. Immunohistochemical and ultrastructural features of neuroendocrine differentiated carcinomas of the prostate: an immunoelectron microscopic study. Ultrastruct Pathol 2005; 29: 367–375.

645. Theodoropoulos VE, Tsigka A, Mihalopoulou A, et al. Evaluation of neuroendocrine staining and androgen receptor expression in incidental prostatic adenocarcinoma: prognostic implications. Urology 2005; 66: 897–902.

646. Bonkhoff H, Fixemer T. [Neuroendocrine differentiation in prostate cancer: an unrecognized and therapy resistant phenotype]. Pathologe 2005; 26: 453–460.

647. Grobholz R, Griebe M, Sauer CG, et al. Influence of neuroendocrine tumor cells on proliferation in prostatic carcinoma. Hum Pathol 2005; 36: 562–570.

648. Song Y, Wu G, Xin DQ, Na YQ. [The influence of neuroendocrine differentiation on the growth and androgen receptor expression of prostate carcinoma cells]. Zhonghua Wai Ke Za Zhi 2004; 42: 1453–1456.

649. Amorino GP, Parsons SJ. Neuroendocrine cells in prostate cancer. Crit Rev Eukaryot Gene Expr 2004; 14: 287–300.

650. Hirano D, Okada Y, Minei S, et al. Neuroendocrine differentiation in hormone refractory prostate cancer following androgen deprivation therapy. Eur Urol 2004; 45: 586–592; discussion 592.

651. Sciarra A, Mariotti G, Gentile V, et al. Neuroendocrine differentiation in human prostate tissue: is it detectable and treatable? BJU Int 2003; 91: 438–445.

652. Bostwick DG, Qian J, Pacelli A, et al. Neuroendocrine expression in node positive prostate cancer: correlation with systemic progression and patient survival. J Urol 2002; 168: 1204–1211.

653. Fernandes RC, Matsushita MM, Mauad T, Nascimento Saldiva PH. Prostate carcinoma with neuroendocrine differentiation: case report and literature review. Rev Hosp Clin Fac Med Sao Paulo 2001; 56: 153–158.

654. Bollito E, Berruti A, Bellina M, et al. Relationship between neuroendocrine features and prognostic parameters in human prostate adenocarcinoma. Ann Oncol 2001; 12: S159–164.

655. Kollermann J, Helpap B. Neuroendocrine differentiation and short-term neoadjuvant hormonal treatment of prostatic carcinoma with special regard to tumor regression. Eur Urol 2001; 40: 313–317.

656. Islam AM, Kato H, Hayama M, et al. Prostatic adenocarcinoma with marked neuroendocrine differentiation. Int J Urol 2001; 8: 412–415.

657. Segawa N, Mori I, Utsunomiya H, et al. Prognostic significance of neuroendocrine differentiation, proliferation activity and androgen receptor expression in prostate cancer. Pathol Int 2001; 51: 452–459.

658. di Sant' Agnese PA. Divergent neuroendocrine differentiation in prostatic carcinoma. Semin Diagn Pathol 2000; 17: 149–161.

659. Abrahamsson PA. Neuroendocrine cells in tumour growth of the prostate. Endocr Relat Cancer 1999; 6: 503–519.

660. Helpap B, Kollermann J, Oehler U. Neuroendocrine differentiation in

prostatic carcinomas: histogenesis, biology, clinical relevance, and future therapeutical perspectives. Urol Int 1999; 62: 133–138.

661. Tan MO, Karaoglan U, Celik B, et al. Prostate cancer and neuroendocrine differentiation. Int Urol Nephrol 1999; 31: 75–82.

662. Abrahamsson PA. Neuroendocrine differentiation in prostatic carcinoma. Prostate 1999; 39: 135–148.

663. Abrahamsson PA, Cockett AT, di Sant'Agnese PA. Prognostic significance of neuroendocrine differentiation in clinically localized prostatic carcinoma. Prostate 1998; 8: 37–42.

664. Bonkhoff H. Neuroendocrine cells in benign and malignant prostate tissue: morphogenesis, proliferation, and androgen receptor status. Prostate 1998; 8: 18–22.

665. Aprikian AG, Cordon-Cardo C, Fair WR, Reuter VE. Characterization of neuroendocrine differentiation in human benign prostate and prostatic adenocarcinoma. Cancer 1993; 71: 3952–3965.

666. Bonkhoff H. Neuroendocrine differentiation in human prostate cancer. Morphogenesis, proliferation and androgen receptor status. Ann Oncol 2001; 12: S141–144.

667. Aprikian AG, Cordon-Cardo C, Fair WR, et al. Neuroendocrine differentiation in metastatic prostatic adenocarcinoma. J Urol 1994; 151: 914–919.

668. Allen FJ, Van Velden DJ, Heyns CF. Are neuroendocrine cells of practical value as an independent prognostic parameter in prostate cancer? Br J Urol 1995; 75: 751–754.

669. Theodorescu D, Broder SR, Boyd JC, et al Cathepsin D and chromogranin A as predictors of long term disease specific survival after radical prostatectomy for localized carcinoma of the prostate. Cancer 1997; 80: 2109–2119.

670. Krijnen JL, Janssen PJ, Ruizeveld de Winter JA, et al. Do neuroendocrine cells in human prostate cancer express androgen receptor? Histochemistry 1993; 100: 393–398.

671. Krijnen JL, Bogdanowicz JF, Seldenrijk CA, et al. The prognostic value of neuroendocrine differentiation in adenocarcinoma of the prostate in relation to progression of disease after endocrine therapy. J Urol 1997; 158: 171–174.

672. Yamada Y, Nakamura K, Aoki S, et al. Is neuroendocrine cell differentiation detected using chromogranin A from patients with bone metastatic prostate cancer a prognostic factor for outcome? Oncol Rep 2006; 15: 1309–1313.

673. Tamas EF, Epstein JI. Prognostic significance of paneth cell-like neuroendocrine differentiation in adenocarcinoma of the prostate. Am J Surg Pathol 2006; 30: 980–985.

674. Soga N, Suzuki R, Komeda Y. [A case report of prostate cancer with Paneth cell-like change]. Hinyokika Kiyo 1995; 41: 891–894.

675. Adlakha H, Bostwick DG. Paneth cell-like change in prostatic adenocarcinoma represents neuroendocrine differentiation: report of 30 cases. Hum Pathol 1994; 25: 135–139.

676. Weaver MG, Abdul-Karim FW, Srigley J, et al. Paneth cell-like change of the prostate gland. A histological, immunohistochemical, and electron microscopic study. Am J Surg Pathol 1992; 16: 62–68.

677. Weaver MG, Abdul-Karim FW, Srigley JR. Paneth cell-like change of the prostate. Arch Pathol Lab Med 1992; 116: 1101–1102.

678. Frydman CP, Bleiweiss IJ, Unger PD, et al. Paneth cell-like metaplasia of the prostate gland. Arch Pathol Lab Med 1992; 116: 274–276.

679. Haratake J, Horie A, Ito K. Argyrophilic adenocarcinoma of the prostate with Paneth cell-like granules. Acta Pathol Jpn 1987; 37: 831–836.

680. Civantos F. Difficulties in interpreting specimens after neoadjuvant hormonal therapy and radiation with illustration of neuroendocrine differentiation. Mol Urol 2000; 4: 117–121; discussion 123.

681. Weaver MG, Abdul-Karim FW, Srigley JR. Paneth cell-like change and small cell carcinoma of the prostate. Two divergent forms of prostatic neuroendocrine differentiation. Am J Surg Pathol 1992; 16: 1013–1016.

682. Azumi N, Traweek ST, Battifora H. Prostatic acid phosphatase in carcinoid tumors. Immunohistochemical and immunoblot studies. Am J Surg Pathol 1991; 15: 785–790.

683. Azumi N, Shibuya H, Ishikura M. Primary prostatic carcinoid tumor with intracytoplasmic prostatic acid phosphatase and prostate-specific antigen. Am J Surg Pathol 1984; 8: 545–550.

684. Hansson J, Abrahamsson PA. Neuroendocrine differentiation in prostatic carcinoma. Scand J Urol Nephrol 2003: 28–36.

685. Di Sant'Agnese PA, Cockett AT. The prostatic endocrine-paracrine (neuroendocrine) regulatory system and neuroendocrine differentiation in prostatic carcinoma: a review and future directions in basic research. J Urol 1994; 152: 1927–1931.

686. di Sant'Agnese PA. Neuroendocrine differentiation in carcinoma of the prostate. Diagnostic, prognostic, and therapeutic implications. Cancer 1992; 70: 254–268.

687. Murali R, Kneale K, Lalak N, Delprado W. Carcinoid tumors of the urinary tract and prostate. Arch Pathol Lab Med 2006; 130: 1693–1706.

688. Zarkovic A, Masters J, Carpenter L. Primary carcinoid tumour of the prostate. Pathology 2005; 37: 184–186.

689. Lim KH, Huang MJ, Yang S, et al. Primary carcinoid tumor of prostate presenting with bone marrow metastases. Urology 2005; 65: 174.

690. Ghannoum JE, DeLellis RA, Shin SJ. Primary carcinoid tumor of the prostate with concurrent adenocarcinoma: a case report. Int J Surg Pathol 2004; 12: 167–170.

691. Tash JA, Reuter V, Russo P. Metastatic carcinoid tumor of the prostate. J Urol 2002; 167: 2526–2527.

692. di Sant'Agnese PA. Neuroendocrine cells of the prostate and neuroendocrine differentiation in prostatic carcinoma: a review of morphologic aspects. Urology 1998; 51: 121–124.

693. Whelan T, Gatfield CT, Robertson S, et al. Primary carcinoid of the prostate in conjunction with multiple endocrine neoplasia IIb in a child. J Urol 1995; 153: 1080–1082.

694. Reyes A, Moran CA. Low-grade neuroendocrine carcinoma (carcinoid tumor) of the prostate. Arch Pathol Lab Med 2004; 128: e166–168.

695. Parr NJ, Grigor KM, Ritchie AW. Metastatic carcinoid tumour involving the prostate. Br J Urol 1992; 70: 103–104.

696. Leibovici D, Spiess PE, Agarwal PK, et al. Prostate cancer progression in the presence of undetectable or low serum prostate-specific antigen level. Cancer 2007; 109: 198–204.

697. Tanaka M, Suzuki Y, Takaoka K, et al. Progression of prostate cancer to neuroendocrine cell tumor. Int J Urol 2001; 8: 431–436; discussion 437.

698. Yashi M, Suzuki K, Tokue A. [A case of giant small cell carcinoma of the prostate]. Hinyokika kiyo 2001; 47: 55–57.

699. Palmgren JS, Karavadia SS, Wakefield MR. Unusual and underappreciated: small cell carcinoma of the prostate. Semin Oncol 2007; 34: 22–29.

700. Kawai S, Hiroshima K, Tsukamoto Y, et al. Small cell carcinoma of the prostate expressing prostate-specific antigen and showing syndrome of inappropriate secretion of antidiuretic hormone: an autopsy case report. Pathol Int 2003; 53: 892–896.

701. Inman BA, DiMarco DS, Slezak JM, et al. Outcomes of Gleason score 10 prostate carcinoma treated by radical prostatectomy. Urology 2006; 68: 604–608.

702. Helpap B. Morphology and therapeutic strategies for neuroendocrine tumors of the genitourinary tract. Cancer 2002; 95: 1415–1420.

703. Yao JL, Madeb R, Bourne P, et al. Small cell carcinoma of the prostate: an immunohistochemical study. Am J Surg Pathol 2006; 30: 705–712.

704. Evans AJ, Humphrey PA, Belani J, et al. Large cell neuroendocrine carcinoma of prostate: a clinicopathologic summary of 7 cases of a rare manifestation of advanced prostate cancer. Am J Surg Pathol 2006; 30: 684–693.

705. Huang J, Yao JL, di Sant'Agnese PA, et al. Immunohistochemical characterization of neuroendocrine cells in prostate cancer. Prostate 2006; 66: 1399–1406.

706. Ferguson J, Zincke H, Ellison E, et al. Decrease of prostatic intraepithelial neoplasia following androgen deprivation therapy in patients with stage T3 carcinoma treated by radical prostatectomy. Urology 1994; 44: 91–95.

707. Petraki C, Vaslamatzis M, Petraki K, et al. Prostate cancer with small-cell morphology: an immunophenotypic subdivision. Scand J Urol Nephrol 2005; 39: 455–463.

708. Papandreou CN, Daliani DD, Thall PF, et al. Results of a phase II study with doxorubicin, etoposide, and cisplatin in patients with fully characterized small-cell carcinoma of the prostate. J Clin Oncol 2002; 20: 3072–3080.

709. Dundore PA, Cheville JC, Nascimento AG, et al. Carcinosarcoma of the prostate. Report of 21 cases. Cancer 1995; 76: 1035–1042.

710. Ordonez NG, Ayala AG, von Eschenbach AC, et al. Immunoperoxidase localization of prostatic acid phosphatase in prostatic carcinoma with sarcomatoid changes. Urology 1982; 19: 210–214.

711. Rogers CG, Parwani A, Tekes A, et al. Carcinosarcoma of the prostate with urothelial and squamous components. J Urol 2005; 173: 439–440.

712. Randolph TL, Amin MB, Ro JY, Ayala AG. Histologic variants of adenocarcinoma and other carcinomas of prostate: pathologic criteria and clinical significance. Mod Pathol 1997; 10: 612–629.

713. Delahunt B, Eble JN, Nacey JN, Grebe SK. Sarcomatoid carcinoma of the prostate: progression from adenocarcinoma is associated with p53 over-expression. Anticancer Res 1999; 19: 4279–4283.

714. Shannon RL, Ro JY, Grignon DJ, et al. Sarcomatoid carcinoma of the prostate. A clinicopathologic study of 12 patients. Cancer 1992; 69: 2676–2682.

715. Perez N, Castillo M, Santos Y, et al. Carcinosarcoma of the prostate: two cases with distinctive morphologic and immunohistochemical findings. Virchows Arch 2005; 446: 511–516.

716. Hansel DE, Epstein JI. Sarcomatoid carcinoma of the prostate: a study of 42 cases. Am J Surg Pathol 2006; 30: 1316–1321.

717. Parwani AV, Herawi M, Epstein JI. Pleomorphic giant cell adenocarcinoma of the prostate: report of 6 cases. Am J Surg Pathol 2006; 30: 1254–1259.

718. Lopez-Beltran A, Eble JN, Bostwick DG. Pleomorphic giant cell carcinoma of the prostate. Arch Pathol Lab Med 2005; 129: 683–685.

719. Iczkowski KA, Ferguson KL, Grier DD, et al. Adenoid cystic/basal cell carcinoma of the prostate: clinicopathologic findings in 19 cases. Am J Surg Pathol 2003; 27: 1523–1529.

720. Begnami MD, Quezado M, Pinto P, et al. Adenoid cystic/basal cell carcinoma of the prostate: review and update. Arch Pathol Lab Med 2007; 131: 637–640.

721. Tulunay O, Orhan D, Gogus C, et al. Adenoid–basal cell tumor of the prostate gland. A case report: histomorphologic and immunohistochemical features. Int Urol Nephrol 2004; 36: 51–53.

722. Schmid HP, Semjonow A, Eltze E, et al. Late recurrence of adenoid cystic carcinoma of the prostate. Scand J Urol Nephrol 2002; 36: 158–159.

723. Minei S, Hachiya T, Ishida H, Okada K. Adenoid cystic carcinoma of the prostate: a case report with immunohistochemical and in situ hybridization staining for prostate-specific antigen. Int J Urol 2001; 8: S41–44.

724. McKenney JK, Amin MB, Srigley JR, et al. Basal cell proliferations of the prostate other than usual basal cell hyperplasia: a clinicopathologic study of 23 cases, including four carcinomas, with a proposed classification. Am J Surg Pathol 2004; 28: 1289–1298.

725. Grignon DJ, Ro JY, Ordonez NG, et al. Basal cell hyperplasia, adenoid basal cell tumor, and adenoid cystic carcinoma of the prostate gland: an immunohistochemical study. Hum Pathol 1988; 19: 1425–1433.

726. Iczkowski KA, Montironi R. Adenoid cystic/basal cell carcinoma of the prostate strongly expresses HER-2/ neu. J Clin Pathol 2006; 59: 1327–1330.

727. Montironi R, Alexander E, Bostwick DG. Prostate pathology case study seminar. Virchows Arch 1997; 430: 83–94.

728. Pinto JA, Gonzalez JE, Granadillo MA. Primary carcinoma of the prostate with diffuse oncocytic changes. Histopathology 1994; 25: 286–288.

729. Ordonez NG, Ro JY, Ayala AG. Metastatic prostatic carcinoma presenting as an oncocytic tumor. Am J Surg Pathol 1992; 16: 1007–1012.

730. Pacelli A, Lopez-Beltran A, Egan AJ, Bostwick DG. Prostatic adenocarcinoma with glomeruloid features. Hum Pathol 1998; 29: 543–546.

731. Baisden BL, Kahane H, Epstein JI. Perineural invasion, mucinous fibroplasia, and glomerulations: diagnostic features of limited cancer on prostate needle biopsy. Am J Surg Pathol 1999; 23: 918–924.

732. Casiraghi O, Martinez-Madrigal F, Mostofi FK, et al. Primary prostatic Wilms' tumor. Am J Surg Pathol 1991; 15: 885–890.

733. Bostwick DG, Chang L. Overdiagnosis of prostatic adenocarcinoma. Semin Urol Oncol 1999; 17: 199–205.

734. Cina SJ, Epstein JI. Adenocarcinoma of the prostate with atrophic features. Am J Surg Pathol 1997; 21: 289–295.

735. Farinola MA, Epstein JI. Utility of immunohistochemistry for alpha-methylacyl-CoA racemase in distinguishing atrophic prostate cancer from benign atrophy. Hum Pathol 2004; 35: 1272–1278.

736. Zhou M, Jiang Z, Epstein JI. Expression and diagnostic utility of alpha-methylacyl-CoA-racemase (P504S) in foamy gland and pseudohyperplastic prostate cancer. Am J Surg Pathol 2003; 27: 772–778.

737. Tran TT, Sengupta E, Yang XJ. Prostatic foamy gland carcinoma with aggressive behavior: clinicopathologic, immunohistochemical, and ultrastructural analysis. Am J Surg Pathol 2001; 25: 618–623.

738. Schindler S, Usman MI, Yokoo H. Foamy gland carcinoma of the prostate. Am J Surg Pathol 1997; 21: 616–618.

739. Nelson RS, Epstein JI. Prostatic carcinoma with abundant xanthomatous cytoplasm. Foamy gland carcinoma. Am J Surg Pathol 1996; 20: 419–426.

740. Llarena Ibarguren R, Lecumberri Castanos D, Padilla Nieva J, et al. [Foamy carcinoma of the prostate]. Arch Esp Urol 2003; 56: 833–835.

741. Cecchi M, Sepich CA, Bertolini L, et al. [Adenoid cystic carcinoma of the prostate. Clinical case]. Minerva Urol Nefrol 2000; 52: 73–75.

742. Carswell BM, Woda BA, Wang X, et al. Detection of prostate cancer by alpha-methylacyl CoA racemase (P504S) in needle biopsy specimens previously reported as negative for malignancy. Histopathology 2006; 48: 668–673.

743. Humphrey PA, Kaleem Z, Swanson PE, Vollmer RT. Pseudohyperplastic prostatic adenocarcinoma. Am J Surg Pathol 1998; 22: 1239–1246.

744. Levi AW, Epstein JI. Pseudohyperplastic prostatic adenocarcinoma on needle biopsy and simple prostatectomy. Am J Surg Pathol 2000; 24: 1039–1046.

745. Arista-Nasr J, Martinez-Benitez B, Valdes S, et al. Pseudohyperplastic prostatic adenocarcinoma in transurethral resections of the prostate. Pathol Oncol Res 2003; 9: 232–235.

746. Inaba M, Boku H, Tanaka S, Fujito A. [Primary squamous cell carcinoma of the prostate: a case report]. Hinyokika Kiyo 2007; 53: 39–41.

747. Di Pietro C, Celia A, De Stefani S, et al. Squamous cell carcinoma of the prostate. Arch Ital Urol Androl 2006; 78: 75–76.

748. John TT, Bashir J, Burrow CT, Machin DG. Squamous cell carcinoma of the prostate – a case report. Int Urol Nephrol 2005; 37: 311–313.

749. Parwani AV, Kronz JD, Genega EM, et al. Prostate carcinoma with squamous differentiation: an analysis of 33 cases. Am J Surg Pathol 2004; 28: 651–657.

750. Mohan H, Bal A, Punia RP, Bawa AS. Squamous cell carcinoma of the prostate. Int J Urol 2003; 10: 114–116.

751. Mayayo Vicente MS, Fernandez Arjona M, Gascon Veguin JP, et al. [Prostatic epidermoid carcinoma: report of a new case an review of the literature]. Arch Esp Urol 2003; 56: 939–943.

752. Majeed F, Javed TA, Khan AU, Koerber RK. Primary squamous cell carcinoma of the prostate: a novel chemotherapy regimen. J Urol 2002; 168: 640.

753. Herrera Puerto J, Barragan Casas JM, Hoyos Fitto C, et al. [Squamous cell carcinoma of the prostate: a further case]. Actas Urol Esp 2002; 26: 366–368.

754. Puyol Pallas M, Badia F, Gomez Parada J. [Squamous carcinoma of the prostate]. Actas Urol Esp 2001; 25: 71–73.

755. Nabi G, Ansari MS, Singh I, et al. Primary squamous cell carcinoma of the prostate: a rare clinicopathological entity. Report of 2 cases and review of literature. Urol Int 2001; 66: 216–219.

756. Okada E, Kamizaki H. Primary squamous cell carcinoma of the prostate. Int J Urol 2000; 7: 347–350.

757. Rahmanou F, Koo J, Marinbakh AY, et al. Squamous cell carcinoma at the prostatectomy site: squamous differentiation of recurrent prostate carcinoma. Urology 1999; 54: 744.

758. Ulloa SA, Iturregui JR, Amezquita M, Ortiz VN. Squamous cell carcinoma of the prostate: case report and review of literature. Bol Asoc Med P R 1997; 89: 192–194.

759. Uchibayashi T, Hisazumi H, Hasegawa M, et al. Squamous cell carcinoma of the prostate. Scand J Urol Nephrol 1997; 31: 223–224.

760. Okamoto T, Ogiu K, Sato M, et al. [Primary squamous cell carcinoma of the prostate: a case report]. Hinyokika Kiyo 1996; 42: 67–70.

761. Miller VA, Reuter V, Scher HI. Primary squamous cell carcinoma of the prostate after radiation seed implantation for adenocarcinoma. Urology 1995; 46: 111–113.

762. Braslis KG, Davi RC, Nelson E, et al. Squamous cell carcinoma of the prostate: a transformation from adenocarcinoma after the use of a luteinizing hormone-releasing hormone agonist and flutamide. Urology 1995; 45: 329–331.

763. Moskovitz B, Munichor M, Bolkier M, Livne PM. Squamous cell carcinoma of the prostate. Urol Int 1993; 51: 181–183.

764. Little NA, Wiener JS, Walther PJ, et al. Squamous cell carcinoma of the prostate: 2 cases of a rare malignancy and review of the literature. J Urol 1993; 149: 137–139.

765. Kuwahara M, Matsushita K, Yoshinaga H, et al. [Primary squamous cell carcinoma of the prostate: a case report]. Hinyokika Kiyo 1993; 39: 77–80.

766. Devaney DM, Dorman A, Leader M. Adenosquamous carcinoma of the prostate: a case report. Hum Pathol 1991; 22: 1046–1050.

767. Gattuso P, Carson HJ, Candel A, Castelli MJ. Adenosquamous carcinoma of the prostate. Hum Pathol 1995; 26: 123–126.

768. Mott LJ. Squamous cell carcinoma of the prostate: report of 2 cases and review of the literature. J Urol 1979; 121: 833–835.

769. Saito R, Davis BK, Ollapally EP. Adenosquamous carcinoma of the prostate. Hum Pathol 1984; 15: 87–89.

770. Yamauchi H, Tsuka H, Muranaka K. [A case of primary urothelial carcinoma of the prostate]. Hinyokika Kiyo 2006; 52: 959–960.

771. Bassi P, De Lisa A, Usai P, et al. [Transitional cell carcinoma involvement of the prostate]. Ann Urol (Paris) 2005; 39 Suppl 5: S113–119.

772. Nixon RG, Chang SS, Lafleur BJ, et al. Carcinoma in situ and tumor multifocality predict the risk of prostatic urethral involvement at radical cystectomy in men with transitional cell carcinoma of the bladder. J Urol 2002; 167: 502–505.

773. Cheville JC, Dundore PA, Bostwick DG, et al. Transitional cell carcinoma of the prostate: clinicopathologic study of 50 cases. Cancer 1998; 82: 703–707.

774. Revelo MP, Cookson MS, Chang SS, et al. Incidence and location of prostate and urothelial carcinoma in prostates from cystoprostatectomies: implications for possible apical sparing surgery. J Urol 2004; 171: 646–651.

775. Oliai BR, Kahane H, Epstein JI. A clinicopathologic analysis of urothelial carcinomas diagnosed on prostate needle biopsy. Am J Surg Pathol 2001; 25: 794–801.

776. Liedberg F, Chebil G, Mansson W. Urothelial carcinoma in the prostatic urethra and prostate: current

controversies. Expert Rev Anticancer Ther 2007; 7: 383–390.

777. Palou J, Baniel J, Klotz L, et al. Urothelial carcinoma of the prostate. Urology 2007; 69: 50–61.

778. Shah SK, Lui PD, Baldwin DD, Ruckle HC. Urothelial carcinoma after external beam radiation therapy for prostate cancer. J Urol 2006; 175: 2063–2066.

779. Sandhu JS, Vickers AJ, Bochner B, et al. Clinical characteristics of bladder cancer in patients previously treated with radiation for prostate cancer. BJU Int 2006; 98: 59–62.

780. Njinou Ngninkeu B, Lorge F, Moulin P, et al. Transitional cell carcinoma involving the prostate: a clinicopathological retrospective study of 76 cases. J Urol 2003; 169: 149–152.

781. Wong JA, Bell DG. Primary malignant melanoma of the prostate: case report and review of the literature. Can J Urol 2006; 13: 3053–3056.

782. Cobo Dols M, Munoz Gallardo S, Pelaez Angulo J, et al. Secondary signet-ring cell tumour of the prostate derived from a primary gastric malignancy. Clin Transl Oncol 2005; 7: 409–412.

783. Grignon DJ, Ro JY, Ayala AG. Malignant melanoma with metastasis to adenocarcinoma of the prostate. Cancer 1989; 63: 196–198.

784. Mack DP, Moussa M, Cook A, Izawa JI. Metastatic Merkel cell tumor to the prostate and bladder. Urology 2004; 64: 156–158.

785. Jacobsen SJ, Roberts RO. Effects of nonsteroidal anti-inflammatory drugs and finasteride on prostate cancer risk. J Urol 2003; 169: 1798–1799.

786. Brawley OW. Hormonal prevention of prostate cancer. Urol Oncol 2003; 21: 67–72.

787. Lowe FC, McConnell JD, Hudson PB, et al. Long-term 6-year experience with finasteride in patients with benign prostatic hyperplasia. Urology 2003; 61: 791–796.

788. Vaughan D, Imperato-McGinley J, McConnell J, et al. Long-term (7 to 8-year) experience with finasteride in men with benign prostatic hyperplasia. Urology 2002; 60: 1040–1044.

789. Montironi R, Bartels PH, Thompson D, et al. Androgen-deprived prostate adenocarcinoma: evaluation of treatment-related changes versus no distinctive treatment effect with a Bayesian belief network. A methodological approach. Eur Urol 1996; 30: 307–315.

790. Montironi R, Diamanti L, Santinelli A, et al. Effect of total androgen ablation on pathologic stage and resection limit status of prostate cancer. Pathol Res Pract 1999; 195: 201–208.

791. Murphy WM SM, Barrows GH. Pathologic changes associated with androgen deprivation therapy for

prostate cancer. Cancer 1991; 68: 821–828.

792. Reuter VE. Pathological changes in benign and malignant prostatic tissue following androgen deprivation therapy. Urology 1997; 49: 16–22.

793. Grignon DJ, Bostwick DG, Civantos F, et al. Pathologic handling and reporting of prostate tissue specimens in patients receiving neoadjuvant hormonal therapy: report of the Pathology Committee. Mol Urol 1999; 3: 193–198.

794. Ellison E, Chuang SS, Zincke H, et al. Prostate adenocarcinoma after androgen deprivation therapy. A comparative study of morphology, morphometry, immunohistochemistry, and DNA ploidy. Pathol Case Rev 1996; 1: 74–83.

795. Tetu B, Srigley JR, Boivin JC, et al. Effect of combination endocrine therapy (LHRH agonist and flutamide) on normal prostate and prostatic adenocarcinoma. A histopathologic and immunohistochemical study. Am J Surg Pathol 1991; 15: 111–120.

796. Wright AS, Thomas LN, Douglas RC, et al. Relative potency of testosterone and dihydrotestosterone in preventing atrophy and apoptosis in the prostate of the castrated rat. J Clin Invest 1996; 98: 2558–2563.

797. Bramson HN, Hermann D, Batchelor KW, et al. Unique preclinical characteristics of GG745, a potent dual inhibitor of 5AR. J Pharmacol Exp Ther 1997; 282: 1496–1502.

798. Clark RV, Gabriel H, et al. Effective suppression of dihydrotestosterone (DHT) by GI198745, a novel, dual 5 alpha reductase inhibitor. J Urol 1999; 161: 268; abstract 1037.

799. McConnell JD, Wilson JD, George FW, et al. Finasteride, an inhibitor of 5 alpha-reductase, suppresses prostatic dihydrotestosterone in men with benign prostatic hyperplasia. J Clin Endocrinol Metab 1992; 74: 505–508.

800. Civantos F, Watson RB, Pinto JE, et al. Finasteride effect on benign prostatic hyperplasia and prostate cancer. A comparative clinico-pathologic study of radical prostatectomies. J Urol Pathol 1997; 6: 1–8.

801. Yang XJ, Tretiakora MS, Sengupta E, et al. Florid basal cell hyperplasia of the prostate: a histological, ultrastructural, and immunohistochemical analysis. Hum Pathol 2003; 34: 462–470.

802. Iczkowski KA, Qiu J, Qian J, et al. The dual 5-alpha-reductase inhibitor dutasteride induces atrophic changes and decreases relative cancer volume in human prostate. Urology 2005; 65: 76–82.

803. Thompson IM, Coltman CA Jr, Crowley J. Chemoprevention of prostate cancer: the Prostate Cancer Prevention Trial. Prostate 1997; 33: 217–221.

804. Thompson IM, Goodman PJ, Tangen CM, et al. The influence of finasteride on the development of prostate cancer. N Engl J Med 2003; 349: 215–224.

805. Andriole GL, Humphrey P, Ray P, et al. Effect of the dual 5alpha-reductase inhibitor dutasteride on markers of tumor regression in prostate cancer. J Urol 2004; 172: 915–919.

806. Armas OA, Aprikian AG, Melamed J, et al. Clinical and pathobiological effects of neoadjuvant total androgen ablation therapy on clinically localized prostatic adenocarcinoma. Am J Surg Pathol 1994; 18: 979–991.

807. Mazzucchelli R, Montironi R, Prezioso D, et al. Surgical pathology examination of radical prostatectomy specimens. Updated protocol based on the Italian TAP study. Anticancer Res 2001; 21: 3599–3607.

808. Patterson RF GM, Jones EC, et al. Immunohistochemical analysis of radical prostatectomy specimens after 8 months of neoadjuvant hormonal therapy. Mol Urol 1999; 3: 277–286.

809. Shimizu S, Kumagai J, Eishi Y, et al. Frequency and number of neuroendocrine tumor cells in prostate cancer: no difference between radical prostatectomy specimens from patients with and without neoadjuvant hormonal therapy. Prostate 2007; 67: 645–652.

810. Tarle M, Ahel MZ, Kovacic K. Acquired neuroendocrine-positivity during maximal androgen blockade in prostate cancer patients. Anticancer Res 2002; 22: 2525–2529.

811. Ismail AH, Landry F, Aprikian AG, Chevalier S. Androgen ablation promotes neuroendocrine cell differentiation in dog and human prostate. Prostate 2002; 51: 117–125.

812. Polito M, Muzzonigro G, Minardi D, Montironi R. Effects of neoadjuvant androgen deprivation therapy on prostatic cancer. Eur Urol 1996; 30: 26–31.

813. Minardi D, Galosi AB, Giannulis I, et al. Comparison of proliferating cell nuclear antigen immunostaining in lymph node metastases and primary prostate adenocarcinoma after neoadjuvant androgen deprivation therapy. Scand J Urol Nephrol 2004; 38: 19–25.

814. Moritz R, Srougi M, Ortiz V, et al. [Prostate cancer dedifferentiation following antiandrogen therapy: a morphological finding or an increased tumor aggressiveness?]. Rev Assoc Med Bras 2005; 51: 117–120.

815. Cher ML, Bova GS, Moore DH, et al. Genetic alterations in untreated metastases and androgen-independent prostate cancer detected by comparative genomic hybridization and allelotyping. Cancer Res 1996; 56: 3091–3102.

816. Crook JM, Bahadur YA, Robertson SJ, et al. Evaluation of radiation effect, tumor differentiation, and prostate specific antigen staining in sequential prostate biopsies after external beam radiotherapy for patients with prostate carcinoma. Cancer 1997; 79: 81–89.

817. Siders DB LF, Mayman DM. Diagnosis of prostate cancer altered by ionizing radiation with and without neoadjuvant antiandrogen hormonal ablation. In: Foster CS, Bostwick DG, eds. Pathology of the prostate. Philadelphia: WB Saunders, 1998; 315–326.

818. Cheng L, Sebo TJ, Slezak J, et al. Predictors of survival for prostate carcinoma patients treated with salvage radical prostatectomy after radiation therapy. Cancer 1998; 83: 2164–2171.

819. Rossi PJ, Clark PE, Papagikos MA, et al. Percentage of positive biopsies associated with freedom from biochemical recurrence after low-dose-rate prostate brachytherapy alone for clinically localized prostate cancer. Urology 2006; 67: 349–353.

820. Cheng L, Darson MF, Bergstralh EJ, et al. Correlation of margin status and extraprostatic extension with progression of prostate carcinoma. Cancer 1999; 86: 1775–1782.

821. Prendergast NJ, Atkins MR, Schatte EC, et al. p53 immunohistochemical and genetic alterations are associated at high incidence with post-irradiated locally persistent prostate carcinoma. J Urol 1996; 155: 1685–1692.

822. Letran JL, Brawer MK. Management of radiation failure for localized prostate cancer. Prostate Cancer Prostatic Dis 1998; 1: 119–127.

823. Kuban DA, el-Mahdi AM, Schellhammer PF. Prognostic significance of post-irradiation prostate biopsies. Oncology 1993; 7: 29–38; discussion 40, 43–44, 47.

824. Cheng L, Cheville JC, Pisansky TM, et al. Prevalence and distribution of prostatic intraepithelial neoplasia in salvage radical prostatectomy specimens after radiation therapy. Am J Surg Pathol 1999; 23: 803–808.

825. Li R, Heydon K, Hammond ME, et al. Ki-67 staining index predicts distant metastasis and survival in locally advanced prostate cancer treated with radiotherapy: an analysis of patients in radiation therapy oncology group protocol 86–10. Clin Cancer Res 2004; 10: 4118–4124.

826. Merrick GS, Wallner KE, Butler WM. Prostate cryotherapy: more questions than answers. Urology 2005; 66: 9–15.

827. Shinohara K. Prostate cancer: cryotherapy. Urol Clin North Am. 30: 725–736.

828. Long JP, Bahn D, Lee F, et al. Five-year retrospective, multi-institutional pooled analysis of cancer-related outcomes after cryosurgical ablation

of the prostate. Urology 2001; 57: 518–523.

829. Escudero Barrilero A AFF, Rodriguez-Patron Rodriguez R, Garcia Gonzalez R. [Cryotherapy III, bibligraphic review. Our experience (II)] Arch Esp Urol 2005; 58: 1003–1029.

830. Prepelica KL, Okeke Z, Murphy A, Katz AE. Cryosurgical ablation of the prostate: high risk patient outcomes. Cancer 2005; 103: 1625–1630.

831. Koppie TM, Shinohara K, Grossfeld GD, et al. The efficacy of cryosurgical ablation of prostate cancer: the University of California, San Francisco experience. J Urol 1999; 162: 427–432.

832. Bahn DK, Silverman P, Lee F Sr, et al. In treating localized prostate cancer the efficacy of cryoablation is independent of DNA ploidy type. Technol Cancer Res Treat 2004; 3: 253–257.

833. Donnelly BJ, Saliken JC, Ernst DS, et al. Role of transrectal ultrasound guided salvage cryosurgery for recurrent prostate carcinoma after radiotherapy. Prostate Cancer Prostatic Dis 2005; 8: 235–242.

834. Chin JL, Touma N, Pautler SE, et al. Serial histopathology results of salvage cryoablation for prostate cancer after radiation failure. J Urol 2003; 170: 1199–1202.

835. Chin JL, Touma N. Current status of salvage cryoablation for prostate cancer following radiation failure. Technol Cancer Res Treat 2005; 4: 211–216.

836. Touma NJ, Izawa JI, Chin JL. Current status of local salvage therapies following radiation failure for prostate cancer. J Urol 2005; 173: 373–379.

837. Ahmed S, Lindsey B, Davies J. Salvage cryosurgery for locally recurrent prostate cancer following radiotherapy. Prostate Cancer Prostatic Dis 2005; 8: 31–35.

838. Bahn DK, Lee F, Silverman P, et al. Salvage cryosurgery for recurrent prostate cancer after radiation therapy: a seven-year follow-up. Clin Prostate Cancer 2003; 2: 111–114.

839. Larson BT, Collins JM, Huidobro C, et al. Gadolinium-enhanced MRI in the evaluation of minimally invasive treatments of the prostate: correlation with histopathologic findings. Urology 2003; 62: 900–904.

840. Donnelly SE, Donnelly BJ, Saliken JC, et al. Prostate cancer: gadolinium-enhanced MR imaging at 3 weeks compared with needle biopsy at 6 months after cryoablation Radiology 2004; 232: 830–833.

841. Susani M, Madersbacher S, Kratzik C, et al. Morphology of tissue destruction induced by focused ultrasound. Eur Urol 1993; 23 Suppl 1: 34–38.

842. Orihuela E, Motamedi M, Pow-Sang M, et al. Histopathological evaluation of laser thermocoagulation in the

human prostate: optimization of laser irradiation for benign prostatic hyperplasia. J Urol 1995; 153: 1531–1536.

843. Vollmer RT, Keetch DW, Humphrey PA. Predicting the pathology results of radical prostatectomy from preoperative information: a validation study. Cancer 1998; 83: 1567–1580.

844. Porter MP, Stanford JL, Lange PH. The distribution of serum prostate-specific antigen levels among American men: implications for prostate cancer prevalence and screening. Prostate 2006; 66: 1044–1051.

845. Pepe P, Panella P, D'Arrigo L, et al. Should men with serum prostate-specific antigen < or = 4 ng/ml and normal digital rectal examination undergo a prostate biopsy? A literature review. Oncology 2006; 70: 81–89.

846. Thompson IM, Ankerst DP, Chi C, et al. Operating characteristics of prostate-specific antigen in men with an initial PSA level of 3.0 ng/ml or lower. JAMA 2005; 294: 66–70.

847. Hosseini SY, Moharramzadeh M, Ghadian AR, et al. Population-based screening for prostate cancer by measuring total serum prostate-specific antigen in Iran. Int J Urol 2007; 14: 406–411.

848. Bohnen AM, Groeneveld FP, Bosch JL. Serum prostate-specific antigen as a predictor of prostate volume in the community: the krimpen study. Eur Urol 2007; 51: 1645–1653.

849. Lilja H, O'Brien F. Can PSA velocity predict risk of death in men with prostate cancer? Nature Clin Pract Urol 2007; 4: 410–411.

850. Freedland SJ, Mangold LA, Walsh PC, Partin AW. The prostatic specific antigen era is alive and well: prostatic specific antigen and biochemical progression following radical prostatectomy. J Urol 2005; 174: 1276–1281; discussion 1281; author reply 1281.

851. Nam RK, Toi A, Trachtenberg J, et al. Making sense of prostate specific antigen: improving its predictive value in patients undergoing prostate biopsy. J Urol 2006; 175: 489–494.

852. Gregorio EP, Grando JP, Saqueti EE, et al. Comparison between PSA density, free PSA percentage and PSA density in the transition zone in the detection of prostate cancer in patients with serum PSA between 4 and 10 ng/mL. Int Braz J Urol 2007; 33: 151–160.

853. Battikhi MN, Hussein I. Age-specific reference ranges for prostate specific antigen-total and free in patients with prostatitis symptoms and patients at risk. Int Urol Nephrol 2006; 38: 559–564.

854. Ohi M, Ito K, Suzuki K, et al. Diagnostic significance of PSA density adjusted by transition zone volume

in males with PSA levels between 2 and 4 ng/ml. Eur Urol 2004; 45: 92–96; discussion 96–97.

855. Filella X, Alcover J, Molina R, et al. Usefulness of proprostate-specific antigen in the diagnosis of prostate cancer. Anticancer Res 2007; 27: 607–610.

856. Krejcarek SC, Chen MH, Renshaw AA, et al. Prediagnostic prostate-specific antigen velocity and probability of detecting high-grade prostate cancer. Urology 2007; 69: 515–519.

857. Thompson IM, Chi C, Ankerst DP, et al. Effect of finasteride on the sensitivity of PSA for detecting prostate cancer. J Natl Cancer Inst 2006; 98: 1128–1133.

858. Varma M, Jasani B. Diagnostic utility of immunohistochemistry in morphologically difficult prostate cancer: review of current literature. Histopathology 2005; 47: 1–16.

859. Varma M, Berney DM, Jasani B, Rhodes A. Technical variations in prostatic immunohistochemistry: need for standardisation and stringent quality assurance in PSA and PSAP immunostaining. J Clin Pathol 2004; 57: 687–690.

860. Kunju LP, Mehra R, Snyder M, Shah RB. Prostate-specific antigen, high-molecular-weight cytokeratin (clone 34betaE12), and/or p63: an optimal immunohistochemical panel to distinguish poorly differentiated prostate adenocarcinoma from urothelial carcinoma. Am J Clin Pathol 2006; 125: 675–681.

861. Mhawech P, Uchida T, Pelte MF. Immunohistochemical profile of high-grade urothelial bladder carcinoma and prostate adenocarcinoma. Hum Pathol 2002; 33: 1136–1140.

862. Greene FL, Balch PD, Fleming ID, et al. Prostate. In: AJCC Cancer Staging Manual, 6th edn. New York: Springer Verlag, 2002; 309–316.

863. Donaldson ES, Glenn JF. The 1995 staging requirement for approved cancer programs. Urology 1996; 47: 455–456.

864. Bostwick DG, Myers RP, Oesterling JE. Staging of prostate cancer. Semin Surg Oncol 1994; 10: 60–72.

865. Schroder FH HP, Denis L, et al. The TNM classification of prostate carcinoma. Prostate 1992; 4: 129–138.

866. Epstein JI, Walsh PC, Carmichael M, Brendler CB. Pathologic and clinical findings to predict tumor extent of nonpalpable (stage T1c) prostate cancer. JAMA 1994; 271: 368–374.

867. Scaletscky R, Koch MO, Eckstein CW, et al. Tumor volume and stage in carcinoma of the prostate detected by elevations in prostate specific antigen. J Urol 1994; 152: 129–131.

868. Jhaveri FM, Klein EA, Kupelian PA, et al. Declining rates of extracapsular extension after radical prostatectomy:

evidence for continued stage migration. J Clin Oncol 1999; 17: 3167–3172.

869. Fleming ID Cooper IS, Henson DE, et al. Prostate. In: AJCCCancer Staging Manual, 5th edn. Philadelphia: Lippincott-Raven, 1997; 305–315.

870. Han M, Walsh PC, Partin AW, Rodriguez R. Ability of the 1992 and 1997 American Joint Committee on Cancer staging systems for prostate cancer to predict progression-free survival after radical prostatectomy for stage T2 disease. J Urol 2000; 164: 89–92.

871. Iyer RV, Hanlon AL, Pinover WH, Hanks GE. Outcome evaluation of the 1997 American Joint Committee on Cancer staging system for prostate carcinoma treated by radiation therapy. Cancer 1999; 85: 1816–1821.

872. Stamey TA, Sozen TS, Yemoto CM, McNeal JE. Classification of localized untreated prostate cancer based on 791 men treated only with radical prostatectomy: common ground for therapeutic trials and TNM subgroups. J Urol 1998; 159: 2009–2012.

873. Eichelberger LE, Cheng L. Does pT2b prostate carcinoma exist? Critical appraisal of the 2002 TNM classification of prostate carcinoma. Cancer 2004; 100: 2573–2576.

874. Quintal MM, Magna LA, Guimaraes MS, et al. Prostate cancer pathologic stage pT2b (2002 TNM staging system): does it exist? Int Braz J Urol 2006; 32: 43–47.

875. Freedland SJ, Presti JC Jr, Terris MK, et al. Improved clinical staging system combining biopsy laterality and TNM stage for men with T1c and T2 prostate cancer: results from the SEARCH database. J Urol 2003; 169: 2129–2135.

876. Koh H, Maru N, Muramoto M, et al. [The 1992 TNM classification of T2 prostate cancer predicts pathologic stage and prognosis better than the revised 1997 classification]. Nippon Hinyokika Gakkai Zasshi 2002; 93: 595–601.

877. May F, Hartung R, Breul J. The ability of the American Joint Committee on Cancer Staging system to predict progression-free survival after radical prostatectomy. BJU Int 2001; 88: 702–707.

878. Chun FK, Briganti A, Lebeau T, et al. The 2002 AJCC pT2 substages confer no prognostic information on the rate of biochemical recurrence after radical prostatectomy. Eur Urol 2006; 49: 273–278; discussion 278–279.

879. Sexton T, Rodrigues G, Brecevic E, et al. Controversies in prostate cancer staging implementation at a tertiary cancer center. Can J Urol 2006; 13: 3327–3334.

880. Campbell T, Blasko J, Crawford ED, et al. Clinical staging of prostate cancer: reproducibility and clarification of issues. Int J Cancer 2001; 96: 198–209.

881. Allen FJ, de Kock ML, de Klerk DP, Heyns CF. Prostate carcinoma – the value of T stage and grade in predicting metastases and prognosis. A cost-effective approach to clinical staging. S Afr J Surg 1991; 29: 15–18.

882. Oesterling JE, Suman VJ, Zincke H, Bostwick DG. PSA-detected (clinical stage T1c or B0) prostate cancer. Pathologically significant tumors. Urol Clin North Am 1993; 20: 687–693.

883. Armatys SA, Koch MO, Bihrle R, et al. Is it necessary to separate clinical stage T1c from T2 prostate adenocarcinoma? BJU Int 2005; 96: 777–780.

884. Jack GS, Cookson MS, Coffey CS, et al. Pathological parameters of radical prostatectomy for clinical stages T1c versus T2 prostate adenocarcinoma: decreased pathological stage and increased detection of transition zone tumors. J Urol 2002; 168: 519–524.

885. Hung AY, Levy L, Kuban DA. Stage T1c prostate cancer: a heterogeneous category with widely varying prognosis. Cancer J 2002; 8: 440–444.

886. Ferguson JK BD, Suman V, Zincke H, Oesterling JE. Prostate-specific antigen detected prostate cancer: pathological characteristics of ultrasound visible versus ultrasound invisible tumors. Eur Urol 1995; 27: 8–12.

887. Theiss M, Wirth MP, Manseck A, Frohmuller HG. Prognostic significance of capsular invasion and capsular penetration in patients with clinically localized prostate cancer undergoing radical prostatectomy. Prostate 1995; 27: 13–17.

888. Bostwick DG, Qian J, Bergstralh E, et al. Prediction of capsular perforation and seminal vesicle invasion in prostate cancer. J Urol 1996; 155: 1361–1367.

889. Ohori M, Wheeler TM, Kattan MW, et al. Prognostic significance of positive surgical margins in radical prostatectomy specimens. J Urol 1995; 154: 1818–1824.

890. McNeal JE, Bostwick DG. Anatomy of the prostate: Implications for disease. In: Bostwick DG, ed. Pathology of the prostate. New York: Churchill Livingstone, 1990; 1–14.

891. Zietman AL, Edelstein RA, Coen JJ, et al. Radical prostatectomy for adenocarcinoma of the prostate: the influence of preoperative and pathologic findings on biochemical disease-free outcome. Urology 1994; 43: 828–833.

892. Bostwick DG. Significance of tumor volume in prostate cancer. Urol Ann 8: 1–22.

893. Epstein JI, Partin AW, Sauvageot J, Walsh PC. Prediction of progression following radical prostatectomy. A multivariate analysis of 721 men with long-term follow-up. Am J Surg Pathol 1996; 20: 286–292.

894. Schellhammer PF. Radical prostatectomy. Patterns of local failure and survival in 67 patients. Urology 1988; 31: 191–197.

895. Stein A, deKernion JB, Dorey F, Smith RB. Adjuvant radiotherapy in patients post-radical prostatectomy with tumor extending through capsule or positive seminal vesicles. Urology 1992; 39: 59–62.

896. Ward JF, Slezak JM, Blute ML, et al. Radical prostatectomy for clinically advanced (cT3) prostate cancer since the advent of prostate-specific antigen testing: 15-year outcome. BJU Int 2005; 95: 751–756.

897. Lerner SE BM, Zincke H. Primary surgery for clinical stage T3 adenocarcinoma of the prostate. In: Vogelzang NJ, Scardino PT, Shipley WU, Coffey DS, eds. Comprehensive textbook of genitourinary oncology. Baltimore: Williams & Wilkins, 1996; 803–811.

898. Scardino PT. Early detection of prostate cancer. Urol Clin North Am 1989; 16: 635–655.

899. Scardino PT, Frankel JM, Wheeler TM, et al. The prognostic significance of post-irradiation biopsy results in patients with prostatic cancer. J Urol 1986; 135: 510–516.

900. Bagshaw MA, Cox RS, Ray GR. Status of radiation treatment of prostate cancer at Stanford University. NCI Monographs Vol 7. 1988: 47–60.

901. Epstein JI, Carmichael M, Partin AW, Walsh PC. Is tumor volume an independent predictor of progression following radical prostatectomy? A multivariate analysis of 185 clinical stage B adenocarcinomas of the prostate with 5 years of followup. J Urol 1993; 149: 1478–1481.

902. Paulson DF MJ, Walther PJ. Radical prostatectomy for clinical stage T1–2N0M0 prostatic adenocarcinoma: long-term results. J Urol 1990; 144: 1180–1184.

903. Epstein JI, Carmichael M, Walsh PC. Adenocarcinoma of the prostate invading the seminal vesicle: definition and relation of tumor volume, grade and margins of resection to prognosis. J Urol 1993; 149: 1040–1045.

904. Kamat AM JK, Troncoso P, Shen Y, et al. Validation of criteria used to predict extraprostatic cancer extension: a tool for use in selecting patients for nerve sparing radical prostatectomy. J Urol 2005; 174: 1262–1265.

905. Sung MT, Eble JN, Cheng L. Invasion of fat justifies assignment of stage pT3a in prostatic adenocarcinoma. Pathology 2006; 38: 309–311.

906. Swanson GP, Thompson IM, Basler J. Current status of lymph node-positive prostate cancer: Incidence and predictors of outcome. Cancer 2006; 107: 439–450.

907. Kawakami J, Meng MV, Sadetsky N, et al. Changing patterns of pelvic lymphadenectomy for prostate cancer: results from CaPSURE. J Urol 2006; 176: 1382–1386.

908. Malmstrom PU. Lymph node staging in prostatic carcinoma revisited. Acta Oncol 2005; 44: 593–598.

909. Corvin S, Schilling D, Eichhorn K, et al. Laparoscopic sentinel lymph node dissection – a novel technique for the staging of prostate cancer. Eur Urol 2006; 49: 280–285.

910. Takashima H, Egawa M, Imao T, et al. Validity of sentinel lymph node concept for patients with prostate cancer. J Urol 2004; 171: 2268–2271.

911. Hacker A, Jeschke S, Leeb K, et al. Detection of pelvic lymph node metastases in patients with clinically localized prostate cancer: comparison of [18F]fluorocholine positron emission tomography-computerized tomography and laparoscopic radioisotope guided sentinel lymph node dissection. J Urol 2006; 176: 2014–2018; discussion 2018–2019.

912. Briganti A, Chun FK, Salonia A, et al. Validation of a nomogram predicting the probability of lymph node invasion among patients undergoing radical prostatectomy and an extended pelvic lymphadenectomy. Eur Urol 2006; 49: 1019–1026; discussion 1026–1027.

913. Gannon PO, Alam Fahmy M, Begin LR, et al. Presence of prostate cancer metastasis correlates with lower lymph node reactivity. Prostate 2006; 66: 1710–1720.

914. Cheng L, Pisansky TM, Ramnani DM, et al. Extranodal extension in lymph node-positive prostate cancer. Mod Pathol 2000; 13: 113–118.

915. Joslyn SA, Konety BR. Impact of extent of lymphadenectomy on survival after radical prostatectomy for prostate cancer. Urology 2006; 68: 121–125.

916. Moul JW, Lewis DJ, Ross AA, et al. Immunohistologic detection of prostate cancer pelvic lymph node micrometastases: correlation to preoperative serum prostate-specific antigen. Urology 1994; 43: 68–73.

917. Gomella LG, White JL, McCue PA, et al. Screening for occult nodal metastasis in localized carcinoma of the prostate. J Urol 1993; 149: 776–778.

918. Pagliarulo V, Hawes D, Brands FH, et al. Detection of occult lymph node metastases in locally advanced node-negative prostate cancer. J Clin Oncol 2006; 24: 2735–2742.

919. Miyake H, Kurahashi T, Hara I, et al. Significance of micrometastases in pelvic lymph nodes detected by real-time reverse transcriptase polymerase chain reaction in patients with clinically localized prostate cancer undergoing radical prostatectomy after neoadjuvant hormonal therapy. BJU Int 2007; 99: 315–320.

920. Hofer MD, Kuefer R, Huang W, et al. Prognostic factors in lymph node-positive prostate cancer. Urology 2006; 67: 1016–1021.

921. de la Monte SM, Moore GW, Hutchins GM. Metastatic behavior of prostate cancer. Cluster analysis of patterns with respect to estrogen treatment. Cancer 1986; 58: 985–993.

922. Bubendorf L, Schopfer A, Wagner U, et al. Metastatic patterns of prostate cancer: an autopsy study of 1,589 patients. Hum Pathol 2000; 31: 578–583.

923. Saitoh H, Hida M, Shimbo T, et al. Metastatic patterns of prostatic cancer. Correlation between sites and number of organs involved. Cancer 1984; 54: 3078–3084.

924. Touijer K, Kuroiwa K, Vickers A, et al. Impact of a multidisciplinary continuous quality improvement program on the positive surgical margin rate after laparoscopic radical prostatectomy. Eur Urol 2006; 49: 853–858.

925. Stamey TA, Villers AA, McNeal JE, et al. Positive surgical margins at radical prostatectomy: importance of the apical dissection. J Urol 1990; 143: 1166–1172; discussion 1172–1173.

926. Jones EC. Resection margin status in radical retropubic prostatectomy specimens: relationship to type of operation, tumor size, tumor grade and local tumor extension. J Urol 1990; 144: 89–93.

927. Catalona WJ, Dresner SM. Nerve-sparing radical prostatectomy: extraprostatic tumor extension and preservation of erectile function. J Urol 1985; 134: 1149–1151.

928. Ward JF, Zincke H, Bergstralh EJ, et al. The impact of surgical approach (nerve bundle preservation versus wide local excision) on surgical margins and biochemical recurrence following radical prostatectomy. J Urol 2004; 172: 1328–1332.

929. Voges GE, McNeal JE, Redwine EA, et al. Morphologic analysis of surgical margins with positive findings in prostatectomy for adenocarcinoma of the prostate. Cancer 1992; 69: 520–526.

930. Ackerman DA, Barry JM, Wicklund RA, et al. Analysis of risk factors associated with prostate cancer extension to the surgical margin and pelvic node metastasis at radical prostatectomy. J Urol 1993; 150: 1845–1850.

931. Schmid HP, Ravery V, Billebaud T, et al. Early detection of prostate cancer in men with prostatism and intermediate prostate-specific antigen levels. Urology 1996; 47: 699–703.

932. Descazeaud A, Zerbib M, Peyromaure M. [Risk factors for positive surgical margins following radical prostatectomy: review]. Ann Urol (Paris) 2006; 40: 342–348.

933. Macdonald OK, Lee RJ, Snow G, et al. Prostate-specific antigen control with low-dose adjuvant radiotherapy for high-risk prostate cancer. Urology 2007; 69: 295–299.

934. Bolla M, van Poppel H, Collette L, et al. Postoperative radiotherapy after radical prostatectomy: a randomised controlled trial (EORTC trial 22911). Lancet 2005; 366: 572–578.

935. Leibovich BC, Engen DE, Patterson DE, et al. Benefit of adjuvant radiation therapy for localized prostate cancer with a positive surgical margin. J Urol 2000; 163: 1178–1182.

936. Swindle P, Eastham JA, Ohori M, et al. Do margins matter? The prognostic significance of positive surgical margins in radical prostatectomy specimens. J Urol 2005; 174: 903–907.

937. Orvieto MA, Alsikafi NF, Shalhav AL, et al. Impact of surgical margin status on long-term cancer control after radical prostatectomy. BJU Int 2006; 98: 1199–1203.

938. Emerson RE, Koch MO, Jones TD, et al. The influence of extent of surgical margin positivity on prostate specific antigen recurrence. J Clin Pathol 2005; 58: 1028–1032.

939. Egan AJ, Bostwick DG. Prediction of extraprostatic extension of prostate cancer based on needle biopsy findings: perineural invasion lacks significance on multivariate analysis. Am J Surg Pathol 1997; 21: 1496–1500.

940. Hassan MO, Maksem J. The prostatic perineural space and its relation to tumor spread: an ultrastructural study. Am J Surg Pathol 1980; 4: 143–148.

941. Algaba F, Arce Y, Oliver A, et al. Prognostic parameters other than Gleason score for the daily evaluation of prostate cancer in needle biopsy. Eur Urol 2005; 48: 566–571.

942. Beard CJ, Chen MH, Cote K, et al. Perineural invasion is associated with increased relapse after external beam radiotherapy for men with low-risk prostate cancer and may be a marker for occult, high-grade cancer. Int J Radiat Oncol Biol Phys 2004; 58: 19–24.

943. May M, Kaufmann O, Hammermann F, et al. Prognostic impact of lymphovascular invasion in radical prostatectomy specimens. BJU Int 2007; 99: 539–544.

944. Hammerer P, Huland H, Sparanberg S. Digital rectal examination, imaging, and systematic-sextant biopsy in identifying operable lymph node-negative prostatic carcinoma. Eur Urol 1992; 22: 281–287.

945. Terris MK, McNeal JE, Stamey TA. Detection of clinically significant prostate cancer by transrectal ultrasound-guided systematic biopsies. J Urol 1992; 148: 829–832.

946. Stamey TA, Freiha FS, McNeal JE, et al. Localized prostate cancer. Relationship of tumor volume to clinical significance for treatment of prostate cancer. Cancer 1993; 71: 933–938.

947. Haggman M, Nybacka O, Nordin B, Busch C. Standardized in vitro mapping with multiple core biopsies of total prostatectomy specimens: localization and prediction of tumour volume and grade. Br J Urol 1994; 74: 617–625.

948. Irwin MB, Trapasso JG. Identification of insignificant prostate cancers: analysis of preoperative parameters. Urology 1994; 44: 862–867; discussion 867–868.

949. Cupp MR, Bostwick DG, Myers RP, Oesterling JE. The volume of prostate cancer in the biopsy specimen cannot reliably predict the quantity of cancer in the radical prostatectomy specimen on an individual basis. J Urol 1995; 153: 1543–1548.

950. Daneshgari F, Taylor GD, Miller GJ, Crawford ED. Computer simulation of the probability of detecting low volume carcinoma of the prostate with six random systematic core biopsies. Urology 1995; 45: 604–609.

951. Humphrey PA, Baty J, Keetch D. Relationship between serum prostate specific antigen, needle biopsy findings, and histopathologic features of prostatic carcinoma in radical prostatectomy tissues. Cancer 1995; 75: 1842–1849.

952. Weldon VE, Tavel FR, Neuwirth H, Cohen R. Failure of focal prostate cancer on biopsy to predict focal prostate cancer: the importance of prevalence. J Urol 1995; 154: 1074–1077.

953. Bruce RG, Rankin WR, Cibull ML, et al. Single focus of adenocarcinoma in the prostate biopsy specimen is not predictive of the pathologic stage of disease. Urology 1996; 48: 75–79.

954. Goto Y, Ohori M, Arakawa A, et al. Distinguishing clinically important from unimportant prostate cancers before treatment: value of systematic biopsies. J Urol 1996; 156: 1059–1063.

955. Ravery V, Schmid HP, Toublanc M, Boccon-Gibod L. Is the percentage of cancer in biopsy cores predictive of extracapsular disease in T1-T2 prostate carcinoma? Cancer 1996; 78: 1079–1084.

956. Boccon-Gibod LM, Dumonceau O, Toublanc M, et al. Micro-focal prostate cancer: a comparison of biopsy and radical prostatectomy specimen features. Eur Urol 2005; 48: 895–899.

957. Noguchi M, Stamey TA, McNeal JE, Yemoto CE. Assessment of morphometric measurements of prostate carcinoma volume. Cancer 2000; 89: 1056–1064.

958. Babian RJ TP, Steelhammer LC, Lloreta-Trull J, Ramirez EI. Tumor volume and prostate specific antigen: implications for early detection and defining a window of curability. J Urol 1995; 154: 1808–1812.

959. Renshaw AA, Richie JP, Loughlin KR, Jiroutek M, et al. The greatest dimension of prostate carcinoa is a simple inexpensive predictor of prostate specific antigen failure in radical prostatectomy specimens. Cancer 1998; 83: 748–752.

960. Mizuno R, Nakashima J, Mukai M, et al. Maximum tumor diameter is a simple and valuable index associated with the local extent of disease in clinically localized prostate cancer. Int J Urol 2006; 13: 951–955.

961. Dugan JA, Bostwick DG, Myers RP, et al. The definition and preoperative prediction of clinically insignificant prostate cancer. JAMA 1996; 275: 288–294.

962. Humphrey PA VRPcaamoptsirptMPA-.

963. Carvalhal GF HP, Thorson P, Yan et al. Visual estimate of percentage of cancer is an independent predictor. Cancer 2000; 89: 1308–1314.

964. Bettendorf O, Oberpenning F, Kopke T, et al. Implementation of a map in radical prostatectomy specimen allows visual estimation of tumor volume. Eur J Surg Oncol 2007; 33: 352–357.

965. Jonmarker S, Valdman A, Lindberg A, et al. Tissue shrinkage after fixation with formalin injection of prostatectomy specimens. Virchows Arch 2006; 449: 297–301.

966. Schned AR, Wheeler KJ, Hodorowski CA, et al. Tissue-shrinkage correction factor in the calculation of prostate cancer volume. Am J Surg Pathol 1996; 20: 1501–1506.

967. Cheng L JT, Lin H, Eble JN, et al. Lymphovascular invasion is an independent prognostic factor in prostatic adenocarcinoma. J Urol 2005; 174: 2181–2185.

968. Noguchi M, Stamey TA, McNeal JE, Nolley R. Prognostic factors for multifocal prostate cancer in radical prostatectomy specimens: lack of significance of secondary cancers. J Urol 2003; 170: 459–463.

969. Nelson BA, Shappell SB, Chang SS, et al. Tumour volume is an independent predictor of prostate-specific antigen recurrence in patients undergoing radical prostatectomy for clinically localized prostate cancer. BJU Int 2006; 97: 1169–1172.

970. Miyake H, Sakai I, Harada K, et al. Prognostic significance of the tumor volume in radical prostatectomy specimens after neoadjuvant hormonal therapy. Urol Int 2005; 74: 27–31.

971. Wheeler TM, Dillioglugil O, Kattan MW, et al. Clinical and pathological significance of the level and extent of capsular invasion in clinical stage T1–2 prostate cancer. Hum Pathol 1998; 29: 856–862.

972. Berger AP, Deibl M, Strasak A, et al. Relapse after radical prostatectomy correlates with preoperative PSA velocity and tumor volume: results from a screening population. Urology 2006; 68: 1067–1071.

973. Shannon BA, McNeal JE, Cohen RJ. Transition zone carcinoma of the prostate gland: a common indolent tumour type that occasionally manifests aggressive behaviour. Pathology 2003; 35: 467–471.

974. Augustin H, Hammerer PG, Blonski J, et al. Zonal location of prostate cancer: significance for disease-free survival after radical prostatectomy? Urology 2003; 62: 79–85.

975. Koppie TM, Bianco FJ Jr, Kuroiwa K, et al. The clinical features of anterior prostate cancers. BJU Int 2006; 98: 1167–1171.

976. Sakai I, Harada K, Kurahashi T, et al. Analysis of differences in clinicopathological features between prostate cancers located in the transition and peripheral zones. Int J Urol 2006; 13: 368–372.

977. Cheng L, Jones TD, Pan CX, et al. Anatomic distribution and pathologic characterization of small-volume prostate cancer (<0.5 ml) in whole-mount prostatectomy specimens. Mod Pathol 2005; 18: 1022–1026.

978. Chen ME, Johnston DA, Tang K, et al. Detailed mapping of prostate carcinoma foci: biopsy strategy implications. Cancer 2000; 89: 1800–1809.

979. Ohori M, Kattan M, Scardino PT, Wheeler TM. Radical prostatectomy for carcinoma of the prostate. Mod Pathol 2004; 17: 349–359.

980. Augustin H, Erbersdobler A, Graefen M, et al. Differences in biopsy features between prostate cancers located in the transition and peripheral zone. BJU Int 2003; 91: 477–481.

981. McNeal JE, Haillot O. Patterns of spread of adenocarcinoma in the prostate as related to cancer volume. Prostate 2001; 49: 48–57.

982. Fedida S, Fishman D, Suzlovich Z, et al. Impaired access of lymphocytes to neoplastic prostate tissue is associated with neoangiogenesis in the tumour site. Br J Cancer 2007; 96: 980–985.

983. Kaygusuz G, Tulunay O, Baltaci S, Gogus O. Microvessel density and regulators of angiogenesis in malignant and nonmalignant prostate tissue. Int Urol Nephrol 2007; 39: 841–850.

984. Deering RE, Bigler SA, Brown M, Brawer MK. Microvascularity in benign prostatic hyperplasia. Prostate 1995; 26: 111–115.

985. Rogatsch H, Hittmair A, Reissigl A, et al. Microvessel density in core biopsies of prostatic adenocarcinoma: a stage predictor? J Pathol 1997; 182: 205–210.

986. Bostwick DG, Wheeler TM, Blute M, et al. Optimized microvessel density

analysis improves prediction of cancer stage from prostate needle biopsies. Urology 1996; 48: 47–57.

987. Vesalainen SL, Lipponen PK, Talja MT, et al. Proliferating cell nuclear antigen and p53 expression as prognostic factors in T1–2M0 prostatic adenocarcinoma. Int J Cancer 1994; 58: 303–308.

988. Gettman MT, Bergstralh EJ, Blute M, et al. Prediction of patient outcome in pathologic stage T2 adenocarcinoma of the prostate: lack of significance for microvessel density analysis. Urology 1998; 51: 79–85.

989. Mehta R, Kyshtoobayeva A, Kurosaki T, et al. Independent association of angiogenesis index with outcome in prostate cancer. Clin Cancer Res 2001; 7: 81–88.

990. Fregene TA, Khanuja PS, Noto AC, et al. Tumor-associated angiogenesis in prostate cancer. Anticancer Res 1993; 13: 2377–2381.

991. Sutton MT, Yingling M, Vyas A, et al. Finasteride targets prostate vascularity by inducing apoptosis and inhibiting cell adhesion of benign and malignant prostate cells. Prostate 2006; 66: 1194–1202.

992. Donohue JF, Hayne D, Karnik U, et al. Randomized, placebo-controlled trial showing that finasteride reduces prostatic vascularity rapidly within 2 weeks. BJU Int 2005; 96: 1319–1322.

993. Zincke H, Bergstralh EJ, Larson-Keller JJ, et al. Stage D1 prostate cancer treated by radical prostatectomy and adjuvant hormonal treatment. Evidence for favorable survival in patients with DNA diploid tumors. Cancer 1992; 70: 311–323.

994. Haggarth L, Auer G, Busch C, et al. The significance of tumor heterogeneity for prediction of DNA ploidy of prostate cancer. Scand J Urol Nephrol 2005; 39: 387–392.

995. Bantis A, Gonidi M, Athanassiades P, et al. Prognostic value of DNA analysis of prostate adenocarcinoma: correlation to clinicopathologic predictors. J Exp Clin Cancer Res 2005; 24: 273–278.

996. Lorenzato M, Rey D, Durlach A, et al. DNA image cytometry on biopsies can help the detection of localized Gleason 3+3 prostate cancers. J Urol 2004; 172: 1311–1313.

997. Nativ O, Winkler HZ, Raz Y, et al. Stage C prostatic adenocarcinoma: flow cytometric nuclear DNA ploidy analysis. Mayo Clin Proc 1989; 64: 911–919.

998. Konchuba AM, Schellhammer PF, Kolm P, et al. Deoxyribonucleic acid cytometric analysis of prostate core biopsy specimens: relationship to serum prostate specific antigen and prostatic acid phosphatase, clinical stage and histopathology. J Urol 1993; 150: 115–119.

999. Shankey TV, Kallioniemi OP, Koslowski JM, et al. Consensus

1000. Amin MB, Schultz DS, Zarbo RJ, et al. Computerized static DNA ploidy analysis of prostatic intraepithelial neoplasia. Arch Pathol Lab Med 1993; 117: 794–798.

1001. Jones EC, McNeal J, Bruchovsky N, de Jong G. DNA content in prostatic adenocarcinoma. A flow cytometry study of the predictive value of aneuploidy for tumor volume, percentage Gleason grade 4 and 5, and lymph node metastases. Cancer 1990; 66: 752–757.

1002. Tribukait B. DNA flow cytometry in carcinoma of the prostate for diagnosis, prognosis and study of tumor biology. Acta Oncol 1991; 30: 187–192.

1003. Deitch AD, de Vere-White RW. Flow cytometry as a predictive modality in prostate cancer. Hum Pathol 1992; 23: 352–359.

1004. Pollack A, Zagars GK. External beam radiotherapy dose response of prostate cancer. Int J Radiat Oncol Biol Phys 1997; 39: 1011–1018.

1005. Takai K, Goellner JR, Katzmann JA, et al. Static image and flow DNA cytometry of prostatic adenocarcinoma: Studies of needle biopsy and radical prostatectomy specimens. J Urol Pathol 1994; 2: 39–48.

1006. Abaza R DLJ, Laskin WB, Pins MR. Prognostic value of DNA ploidy, bcl-2 and p53 in localized prostate adenocarcinoma incidentally discovered at transurethral prostatectomy. J Urol 2006; 176: 2701–2705.

1007. Lopez-Beltran A, Artacho-Perula E, Luque-Barona RJ, Roldan-Villalobos R. Nuclear volume estimates in prostatic atypical adenomatous hyperplasia. Anal Quant Cytol Histol 2000; 22: 438–444.

1008. Buhmeida A, Kuopio T, Collan Y. Nuclear size and shape in fine needle aspiration biopsy samples of the prostate. Anal Quant Cytol Histol 2000; 22: 291–298.

1009. Choi NG, Sohn JH, Park HW, Jung TY. Apoptosis and nuclear shapes in benign prostate hyperplasia and prostate adenocarcinoma: comparison with and relation to Gleason score. Int J Urol 1999; 6: 13–18.

1010. Mohler JL, Figlesthaler WM, Zhang XZ, et al. Nuclear shape analysis for the assessment of local invasion and metastases in clinically localized prostate carcinoma. Cancer 1994; 74: 2996–3001.

1011. Mohamed MA, Greif PA, Diamond J, et al. Epigenetic events, remodelling enzymes and their relationship to chromatin organization in prostatic intraepithelial neoplasia and prostatic adenocarcinoma. BJU Int 2007; 99: 908–915.

1012. Huisman A, Ploeger LS, Dullens HF, et al. Discrimination between benign and malignant prostate tissue using chromatin texture analysis in 3-D by confocal laser scanning microscopy. Prostate 2007; 67: 248–254.

1013. Weyn B, Jacob W, da Silva VD, et al. Data representation and reduction for chromatin texture in nuclei from premalignant prostatic, esophageal, and colonic lesions. Cytometry 2000; 41: 133–138.

1014. Aydin H, Zhou M, Herawi M, Epstein JI. Number and location of nucleoli and presence of apoptotic bodies in diagnostically challenging cases of prostate adenocarcinoma on needle biopsy. Hum Pathol 2005; 36: 1172–1177.

1015. Bostwick DG. Practical clinical application of predictive factors in prostate cancer. A review with an emphasis on quantitative methods in tissue specimens. Anal Quant Cytol Histol 1998; 20: 323–342.

1016. Fine SW, Epstein JI. Minute foci of Gleason score 8–10 on prostatic needle biopsy: a morphologic analysis. Am J Surg Pathol 2005; 29: 962–968.

1017. Bostwick DG, Aquilina JW. Prostatic intraepithelial neoplasia (PIN) and other prostatic lesions as risk factors and surrogate endpoints for cancer chemoprevention trials. J Cell Biochem Suppl 1996; 25: 156–164.

1018. Aihara M, Truong LD, Dunn JK, et al. Frequency of apoptotic bodies positively correlates with Gleason grade in prostate cancer. Hum Pathol 1994; 25: 797–801.

1019. Wheeler TM, Rogers E, Aihara M, et al. Apoptotic index as a biomarker in prostatic intraepithelial neoplasia (PIN) and prostate cancer. J Cell Biochem 1994; 19: 202–207.

1020. Venkataraman G, Ananthanarayanan V, Paner GP, et al. Morphometric sum optical density as a surrogate marker for ploidy status in prostate cancer: an analysis in 180 biopsies using logistic regression and binary recursive partitioning. Virchows Arch 2006; 449: 302–307.

1021. Martinez-Jabaloyas JM, Ruiz-Cerda JL, Hernandez M, et al. Prognostic value of DNA ploidy and nuclear morphometry in prostate cancer treated with androgen deprivation. Urology 2002; 59: 715–720.

1022. Maffini MV, Ortega HH, Stoker C, et al. Bcl-2 correlates with tumor ploidy and nuclear morphology in early stage prostate carcinoma. A fine needle aspiration biopsy study. Pathol Res Pract 2001; 197: 487–492.

1023. Buhmeida A, Kujari H, Collan Y. Nucleolar morphometry in fine needle aspiration biopsies of the prostate. Anal Quant Cytol Histol 2001; 23: 185–192.

1024. Zhang YH, Kanamaru H, Oyama N, et al. Prognostic value of nuclear morphometry on needle biopsy from patients with prostate cancer: is volume-weighted mean nuclear volume superior to other morphometric parameters? Urology 2000; 55: 377–381.

1025. Veltri RW, O'Dowd GJ, Orozco R, Miller MC. The role of biopsy pathology, quantitative nuclear morphometry, and biomarkers in the preoperative prediction of prostate cancer staging and prognosis. Semin Urol Oncol 1998; 16: 106–117.

1026. Fujikawa K, Sasaki M, Arai Y, et al. Prognostic criteria in patients with prostate cancer: Gleason score versus volume-weighted mean nuclear volume. Clin Cancer Res 1997; 3: 613–618.

1027. Veltri RW, Khan MA, Marlow C, Miller MC, et al. Alterations in nuclear structure and expression of proPSA predict differences between native Japanese and Japanese-American prostate cancer. Urology 2006; 68: 898–904.

1028. Das K Lau W, Sivaswaren C, et al. Chromosomal changes in prostate cancer: a fluorescence in situ hybridization study. Clin Genet 2005; 68: 40–47.

1029. Latil A, Cussenot O, Fournier G, et al. Loss of heterozygosity at 7q31 is a frequent and early event in prostate cancer. Clin Cancer Res 1995; 1: 1385–1389.

1030. Takahashi S, Shan AL, Ritland SR, et al. Frequent loss of heterozygosity at 7q31.1 in primary prostate cancer is associated with tumor aggressiveness and progression. Cancer Res 1995; 55: 4114–4119.

1031. Jenkins RB, Qian J, Lee HK, et al. A molecular cytogenetic analysis of 7q31 in prostate cancer. Cancer Res 1998; 58: 759–766.

1032. Takahashi S, Qian J, Brown JA, et al. Potential markers of prostate cancer aggressiveness detected by fluorescence in situ hybridization in needle biopsies. Cancer Res 1994; 54: 3574–3579.

1033. Macoska JA, Trybus TM, Benson PD, et al. Evidence for three tumor suppressor gene loci on chromosome 8p in human prostate cancer. Cancer Res 1995; 55: 5390–5395.

1034. Jenkins RB, Qian J, Lieber MM, Bostwick DG. Detection of c-myc oncogene amplification and chromosomal anomalies in metastatic prostatic carcinoma by fluorescence in situ hybridization. Cancer Res 1997; 57: 524–531.

1035. MacGrogan D, Levy A, Bostwick D, et al. Loss of chromosome arm 8p loci in prostate cancer: mapping by quantitative allelic imbalance. Genes Chromosomes Cancer 1994; 10: 151–159.

1036. Bova GS, Fox WM, Epstein JI. Methods of radical prostatectomy specimen processing: a novel technique for harvesting fresh prostate cancer tissue and review of processing techniques. Mod Pathol 1993; 6: 201–207.

1037. Van den Berg C, Guan XY, Von Hoff D, et al. DNA sequence amplification in human prostate cancer identified by chromosome microdissection: potential prognostic implications. Clin Cancer Res 1995; 1: 11–18.

1038. Visakorpi T, Kallioniemi AH, Syvanen AC, et al. Genetic changes in primary and recurrent prostate cancer by comparative genomic hybridization. Cancer Res 1995; 55: 342–347.

1039. Cher ML, MacGrogan D, Bookstein R, et al. Comparative genomic hybridization, allelic imbalance, and fluorescence in situ hybridization on chromosome 8 in prostate cancer. Genes Chromosomes Cancer 1994; 11: 153–162.

1040. Nupponen NN, Porkka K, Kakkola L, et al. Amplification and overexpression of p40 subunit of eukaryotic translation initiation factor 3 in breast and prostate cancer. Am J Pathol 1999; 154: 1777–1783.

1041. Porkka K, Saramaki O, Tanner M, Visakorpi T. Amplification and overexpression of Elongin C gene discovered in prostate cancer by cDNA microarrays. Lab Invest 2002; 82: 629–637.

1042. Porkka KP TT, Vessella RL, Visakorpi T. RAD21 and KIAA0196 at 8q24 are amplified and overexpressed in prostate cancer. Genes Chromosomes Cancer 2004; 39: 1–10.

1043. Joos S, Bergerheim US, Pan Y, et al. Mapping of chromosomal gains and losses in prostate cancer by comparative genomic hybridization. Genes Chromosomes Cancer 1995; 14: 267–276.

1044. Gray IC, Phillips SM, Lee SJ, et al. Loss of the chromosomal region 10q23–25 in prostate cancer. Cancer Res 1995; 55: 4800–4803.

1045. Ittman M, Mansukhani A. Expression of fibroblast growth factors (FGFs) and FGF receptors in human prostate. J Urol 1997; 157: 351–356.

1046. Halvorsen OJ HS, Akslen LA. Combined loss of PTEN and p27 expression is associated with tumor cell proliferation by Ki-67 and increased risk of recurrent disease in localized prostate cancer.Clin Cancer Res 2003; 9: 1474–1479.

1047. Carter BS, Epstein JI, Isaacs WB. ras gene mutations in human prostate cancer. Cancer Res 1990; 50: 6830–6832.

1048. Latil A, Cussenot O, Fournier G, et al. Loss of heterozygosity at chromosome 16q in prostate adenocarcinoma: identification of three independent regions. Cancer Res 1997; 57: 1058–1062.

1049. Cunningham JM, Shan A, Wick MJ, et al. Allelic imbalance and microsatellite instability in prostatic adenocarcinoma. Cancer Res 1996; 56: 4475–4482.

1050. Bergheim USR, Kunimi K, Collins VP, Ekman P. Deletion of chromosome 8, 10 and 16 in human prostatic carcinoma. Genes, Chromosomes Cancer 1991; 3: 215–220.

1051. Sakr WA, Macoska JA, Benson P, et al. Allelic loss in locally metastatic, multisampled prostate cancer. Cancer Res 1994; 54: 3273–3277.

1052. Ahlers CM, Figg WD. ETS-TMPRSS2 fusion gene products in prostate cancer. Cancer Biol Ther 2006; 5: 254–255.

1053. Soller MJ, Isaksson M, Elfving P, et al. Confirmation of the high frequency of the TMPRSS2/ERG fusion gene in prostate cancer. Genes Chromosomes Cancer 2006; 45: 717–719.

1054. Tomlins SA, Mehra R, Rhodes DR, et al. TMPRSS2: ETV4 gene fusions define a third molecular subtype of prostate cancer. Cancer Res 2006; 66: 3396–3400.

1055. Rubin MA, Chinnaiyan AM. Bioinformatics approach leads to the discovery of the TMPRSS2: ETS gene fusion in prostate cancer. Lab Invest 2006; 86: 1099–1102.

1056. Winnes M, Lissbrant E, Damber JE, Stenman G. Molecular genetic analyses of the TMPRSS2-ERG and TMPRSS2-ETV1 gene fusions in 50 cases of prostate cancer. Oncol Rep 2007; 17: 1033–1036.

1057. Mehra R, Tomlins SA, Shen R, et al. Comprehensive assessment of TMPRSS2 and ETS family gene aberrations in clinically localized prostate cancer. Mod Pathol 2007; 20: 538–544.

1058. Demichelis F, Fall K, Perner S, et al. TMPRSS2: ERG gene fusion associated with lethal prostate cancer in a watchful waiting cohort. Oncogene 2007; 26: 4596–4599.

1059. Nam RK, Sugar L, Wang Z, et al. Expression of TMPRSS2 ERG gene fusion in prostate cancer cells is an important prognostic factor for cancer progression. Cancer Biol Ther 2007; 6 [e-pub ahead of print].

1060. Wang J, Cai Y, Ren C, Ittmann M. Expression of variant TMPRSS2/ERG fusion messenger RNAs is associated with aggressive prostate cancer. Cancer Res 2006; 66: 8347–8351.

1061. Perner S, Demichelis F, Beroukhim R, et al. TMPRSS2: ERG fusion-associated deletions provide insight into the heterogeneity of prostate cancer. Cancer Res 2006; 66: 8337–8341.

1062. Mosquera JM, Perner S, Demichelis F, et al. Morphological features of TMPRSS2-ERG gene fusion prostate cancer. J Pathol 2007; 212: 91–101.

1063. Clark J, Merson S, Jhavar S, et al. Diversity of TMPRSS2-ERG fusion transcripts in the human prostate. Oncogene 2007; 26: 2667–2673.

1064. Laxman B, Tomlins SA, Mehra R, et al. Noninvasive detection of TMPRSS2: ERG fusion transcripts in the urine of men with prostate cancer. Neoplasia 2006; 8: 885–888.

1065. Marks LS, Fradet Y, Deras IL, et al. PCA3 molecular urine assay for prostate cancer in men undergoing repeat biopsy. Urology 2007; 69: 532–535.

1066. Kirby R. PCA3 improves diagnosis of prostate cancer. Practitioner 2007; 251: 18, 21, 23.

1067. Groskopf J, Aubin SM, Deras IL, et al. APTIMA PCA3 molecular urine test: development of a method to aid in the diagnosis of prostate cancer. Clin Chem 2006; 52: 1089–1095.

1068. Tinzl M, Marberger M, Horvath S, Chypre C. DD3PCA3 RNA analysis in urine – a new perspective for detecting prostate cancer. Eur Urol 2004; 46: 182–186; discussion 188.

1069. Bostwick DG, Gould VE, Qian J, et al. Prostate cancer detected by uPM3: radical prostatectomy findings. Mod Pathol 2006; 19: 630–633.

1070. Iacopino F, Angelucci C, Lama G, et al. Apoptosis-related gene expression in benign prostatic hyperplasia and prostate carcinoma. Anticancer Res 2006; 26: 1849–1854.

1071. Bastacky S, Cieply K, Sherer C, et al. Use of interphase fluorescence in situ hybridization in prostate needle biopsy specimens with isolated high-grade prostatic intraepithelial neoplasia as a predictor of prostate adenocarcinoma on follow-up biopsy. Hum Pathol 2004; 35: 281–289.

1072. Pelengaris S, Khan M, Evan G. c-MYC: more than just a matter of life and death. Nature Rev Cancer 2002; 2: 764–776.

1073. Sato K, Qian J, Slezak JM, et al. Clinical significance of alterations of chromosome 8 in high-grade, advanced, nonmetastatic prostate carcinoma. J Natl Cancer Inst 1999; 91: 1574–1580.

1074. Sato H, Minei S, Hachiya T, et al. Fluorescence in situ hybridization analysis of c-myc amplification in stage TNM prostate cancer in Japanese patients. Int J Urol 2006; 13: 761–766.

1075. Dvorackova J, Uvirova M. A molecularly genetic determination of prognostic factors of the prostate cancer and their relationships to expression of protein p27kip1. Neoplasma 2007; 54: 149–154.

1076. Prowatke I, Devens F, Benner A, et al. Expression analysis of imbalanced genes in prostate carcinoma using tissue microarrays. Br J Cancer 2007; 96: 82–88.

1077. Williams K, Fernandez S, Stien X, et al. Unopposed c-MYC expression in benign prostatic epithelium causes a cancer phenotype. Prostate 2005; 63: 369–384.

1078. Kokontis J, Takakura K, Hay N, Liao S. Increased androgen receptor activity and altered c-myc expression in prostate cancer cells after long-term androgen deprivation. Cancer Res 1994; 54: 1566–1573.

1079. Lebedeva IV, Su ZZ, Sarkar D, et al. Melanoma differentiation-associated gene-7, mda-7/interleukin-24, induces apoptosis in prostate cancer cells by promoting mitochondrial dysfunction and inducing reactive oxygen species. Cancer Res 2003; 63: 8138–8144.

1080. Reed JC. Mechanisms of Bcl-2 family protein function and dysfunction in health and disease. Behring Inst Mitt 1996; 97: 72–100.

1081. Hockenbery DM, Zutter M, Hickey W, et al. BCL2 protein is topographically restricted in tissues characterized by apoptotic cell death. Proc Natl Acad Sci USA 1991; 88: 6961–6965.

1082. Foster CS, Ke Y. Stem cells in prostatic epithelia. Int J Exp Pathol 1997; 78: 311–329.

1083. Tu H, Jacobs SC, Borkowski A, Kyprianou N. Incidence of apoptosis and cell proliferation in prostate cancer: relationship with TGF-beta1 and bcl-2 expression. Int J Cancer 1996; 69: 357–363.

1084. Lipponen P, Vesalainen S. Expression of the apoptosis suppressing protein bcl-2 in prostatic adenocarcinoma is related to tumour malignancy. Prostate 1997; 32: 9–16.

1085. Nagaoka A, Kubota Y, Kurosu S, et al. Absence of Bcl-2 expression favors response to the short-term administration of diethylstilbestrol diphosphate in prostate Cancer. Prostate 2006; 66: 1779–1787.

1086. Colombel M, Symmans F, Gil S, et al. Detection of the apoptosis-suppressing oncoprotein bcl-2 in hormone-refractory human prostate cancers. Am J Pathol 1993; 143: 390–400.

1087. Colecchia M, Frigo B, Del Boca C, et al. Detection of apoptosis by the TUNEL technique in clinically localised prostatic cancer before and after combined endocrine therapy. J Clin Pathol 1997; 50: 384–388.

1088. Yamanaka K, Rocchi P, Miyake H, Fazli L, et al. Induction of apoptosis and enhancement of chemosensitivity in human prostate cancer LNCaP cells using bispecific antisense oligonucleotide targeting Bcl-2 and Bcl-xL genes. BJU Int 2006; 97: 1300–1308.

1089. Ittman M, Wieczorek R, Heller P, et al. Alterations in the p53 and MDC-2 genes are infrequent in clinically localized stage B prostate adenocarcinomas. Am J Pathol 1994; 145: 287–293.

1090. Hall MC, Navone NM, Troncoso P, et al. Frequency and characterization of p53 mutations in clinically localized prostate cancer. Urology 1995; 45: 470–475.

1091. Mottaz AE, Markwalder R, Fey MF, et al. Abnormal p53 expression is rare in clinically localized human prostate cancer: comparison between immunohistochemical and molecular detection of p53 mutations. Prostate 1997; 31: 209–215.

1092. Navone NM, Troncoso P, Pisters LL, et al. p53 protein accumulation and gene mutation in the progression of human prostate carcinoma. J Natl Cancer Inst 1993; 85: 1657–1669.

1093. Kallakury BV, Figge J, Ross JS, et al. Association of p53 immunoreactivity with high Gleason tumor grade in prostate adenocarcinoma. Hum Pathol 1994; 25: 92–97.

1094. Fan K, Dao DD, Schutz M, Fink LM. Loss of heterozygosity and overexpression of p53 gene in human primary prostatic adenocarcinoma. Diagn Mol Pathol 1994; 3: 265–270.

1095. Petrescu A ML, Codreanu O, Niculescu L. Immunohistochemical detection of p53 protein as a prognostic indicator in prostate carcinoma. Rom J Morphol Embryol 2006; 47: 143–146.

1096. Moul JW, Bettencourt MC, Sesterhenn IA, et al. Protein expression of p53, bcl-2, and KI-67 (MIB-1) as prognostic biomarkers in patients with surgically treated, clinically localized prostate cancer. Surgery 1996; 120: 159–166; discussion 166–167.

1097. Heidenberg HB, Sesterhenn IA, Gaddipati JP, et al. Alternation of tumor suppressor gene p53 in a high fraction of hormone refractory prostate cancer. J Urol 1995; 154: 414–421.

1098. Gao X, Chen YQ, Wu N, et al. Somatic mutations of the WAF1/CIP1 gene in primary prostate cancer. Oncogene 1997; 11: 1395–1398.

1099. Facher EA, Becich MJ, Deka A, Law JC. Association between human cancer and two polymorphisms occurring in the p21WAF1/CIP1 cyclin-dependent kinase inhibitor gene. Cancer 1997; 79: 2424–2429.

1100. Byrne RL, Horne CH, Robinson MC, et al. The expression of waf-1, p53 and bcl-2 in prostatic adenocarcinoma. Br J Urol 1997; 79: 190–195.

1101. Shapira M, Ben-Izhak O, Slotky M, et al. Expression of the ubiquitin ligase subunit cyclin kinase subunit 1 and its relationship to S-phase kinase protein 2 and p27Kip1 in prostate cancer. J Urol 2006; 176: 2285–2289.

1102. Tsihlias J, Kapusta LR, DeBoer G, et al. Loss of cyclin-dependent kinase inhibitor p27Kip1 is a novel prognostic factor in localized human prostate adenocarcinoma. Cancer Res 1998; 58: 542–548.

1103. Marchal C, Redondo M, Padilla M, et al. Expression of prostate specific membrane antigen (PSMA) in prostatic adenocarcinoma and prostatic intraepithelial neoplasia. Histol Histopathol 2004; 19: 715–718.

1104. Ikegami S, Yamakami K, Ono T, et al. Targeting gene therapy for prostate cancer cells by liposomes complexed with anti-prostate-specific membrane antigen monoclonal antibody. Hum Gene Ther 2006; 17: 997–1005.

1105. Perner S, Hofer MD, Kim R, et al. Prostate-specific membrane antigen expression as a predictor of prostate cancer progression. Hum Pathol 2007; 38: 696–701.

1106. Taftachi R AA, Ekici S, Ergen A, Ozen H. Proliferating-cell nuclear antigen (PCNA) as an independent prognostic marker in patients after prostatectomy: a comparison of PCNA and Ki-67. BJU Int 2005; 95: 650–654.

1107. Nemoto R, Kawamura H, Miyakawa I, et al. Immunohistochemical detection of proliferating cell nuclear antigen (PCNA)/cyclin in human prostate adenocarcinoma. J Urol 1993; 149: 165–169.

1108. Limas C, Frizelle SP. Proliferative activity in benign and neoplastic prostatic epithelium. J Pathol 1994; 174: 201–208.

1109. Carroll PR, Waldman FM, Rosenau W, et al. Cell proliferation in prostatic adenocarcinoma: in vitro measurement by 5-bromodeoxyuridine incorporation and proliferating cell nuclear antigen expression. J Urol 1993; 149: 403–407.

1110. Idikio HA. Expression of proliferating cell nuclear antigen in node-negative human prostate cancer. Anticancer Res 1996; 16: 2607–2611.

1111. Miyamoto S, Ito K, Kurokawa K, et al. Clinical validity of proliferating cell nuclear antigen as an objective marker for evaluating biologic features in patients with untreated prostate cancer. Int J Urol 2006; 13: 767–772.

1112. Cappello F, Ribbene A, Campanella C, et al. The value of immunohistochemical research on PCNA, p53 and heat shock proteins in prostate cancer management: a review. Eur J Histochem 2006; 50: 25–34.

1113. Taplin ME, Bubley GJ, Shuster TD, et al. Mutation of the androgen-receptor gene in metastatic androgen-independent prostate cancer. N Engl J Med 1995; 332: 1393–1398.

1114. Haapala K, Hyytinen ER, Roiha M, et al. Androgen receptor alterations in prostate cancer relapsed during a combined androgen blockade by orchiectomy and bicalutamide. Lab Invest 2001; 81: 1647–1651.

1115. Linja MJ, Savinainen KJ, Saramaki OR, Tammela TL, et al. Amplification and overexpression of androgen receptor gene in hormone-refractory prostate cancer. Cancer Res 2001; 61: 3550–3555.

1116. Chmelar R, Buchanan G, Need EF, Tilley W, Greenberg NM. Androgen receptor coregulators and their involvement in the development and progression of prostate cancer. Int J Cancer 2007; 120: 719–733.

1117. Burd CJ, Morey LM, Knudsen KE. Androgen receptor corepressors and prostate cancer. Endocr Relat Cancer 2006; 13: 979–994.

1118. Iczkowski KA, McLennan GT, Bostwick DG, et al. Adenoid cystic/basal cell carcinoma of the prostate expresses HER-2/neu. [Abstract]. Mod Pathol 2005; 18: 147A.

1119. Berger R, Lin DI, Nieto M, et al. Androgen-dependent regulation of Her-2/neu in prostate cancer cells. Cancer Res 2006; 66: 5723–5728.

1120. Henrique R, Jeronimo C. Molecular detection of prostate cancer: a role for GSTP1 hypermethylation. Eur Urol 2004; 46: 660–669; discussion 669.

1121. Reibenwein J, Pils D, Horak P, et al. Promoter hypermethylation of GSTP1, AR, and 14–3–3sigma in serum of prostate cancer patients and its clinical relevance. Prostate 2007; 67: 427–432.

1122. Leman ES, Cannon GW, Trock BJ, et al. EPCA-2: a highly specific serum marker for prostate cancer. Urology 2007; 69: 714–720.

1123. Regan JB BM, Wold LE. Giant leiomyoma of the prostate. Arch Pathol Lab Med 1987; 111: 381–382.

1124. Cohen MS, McDonald DF, Smith JH. Solitary leiomyoma of the prostate presenting as an encrusted intravesical mass. J Urol 1978; 120: 641–642.

1125. Yilmaz F, Sahin H, Hakverdi S, et al. Huge leiomyoma of the prostate. Scand J Urol Nephrol 1998; 32: 223–224.

1126. Prabhu GG, Rao MS, Venugopai N. Conservatively managed symptomatic leiomyoma of the prostate. J Indian Med Assoc 1995; 93: 209.

1127. Leonard A, Baert L, Van Praet F, et al. Solitary leiomyoma of the prostate. Br J Urol 1988; 62: 184–185.

1128. Schumacher S, Moll R, Muller SC, et al. Epithelioid leiomyoma of the prostate. Eur Urol 1996; 30: 125–126.

1129. Persaud V, Douglas LL. Bizarre (atypical) leiomyoma of the prostate gland. West Indian Med J 1982; 31: 217–220.

1130. Tetu B SJ, Bostwick DG. Soft tissue tumors. In: Bostwick DG, ed. Pathology of the prostate. New York: Churchill Livingstone, 1990; 117–135.

1131. Ro JY, el-Naggar AK, Amin MB, Ayala AG. Inflammatory pseudotumor of the urinary bladder. Am J Surg Pathol 1993; 17: 1193–1194.

1132. Freeman A, Geddes N, Munson P, et al. Anaplastic lymphoma kinase (ALK 1) staining and molecular analysis in inflammatory myofibroblastic tumours of the bladder: a preliminary clinicopathological study of nine cases and review of the literature. Mod Pathol 2004; 17: 765–771.

1133. Harik LR, Merino C, Coindre JM, et al. Pseudosarcomatous myofibroblastic proliferations of the bladder: a clinicopathologic study of 42 cases. Am J Surg Pathol 2006; 30: 787–794.

1134. Montgomery EA, Shuster DD, Burkart AL, et al. Inflammatory myofibroblastic tumors of the urinary tract: a clinicopathologic study of 46 cases, including a malignant example inflammatory fibrosarcoma and a subset associated with high-grade urothelial carcinoma. Am J Surg Pathol 2006; 30: 1502–1512.

1135. Huang WL, Ro JY, Grignon DJ, et al. Postoperative spindle cell nodule of the prostate and bladder. J Urol 1990; 143: 824–826.

1136. Krishnadas R, Froeschle PO, Berrisford RG. Recurrence and malignant transformation in solitary fibrous tumour of the pleura. Thorac Cardiovasc Surg 2006; 54: 65–67.

1137. Magdeleinat P, Alifano M, Petino A, et al. Solitary fibrous tumors of the pleura: clinical characteristics, surgical treatment and outcome. Eur J Cardiothorac Surg 2002; 21: 1087–1093.

1138. Ishii T, Kuroda K, Nakamura K, Sugiura H. Solitary fibrous tumor of the prostate. Hinyokika Kiyo 2004; 50: 405–407.

1139. Pacios Cantero JC, Alonso Dorrego JM, Cansino Alcaide JR, de la Pena Barthel JJ. [Solitary fibrous tumor of the prostate] Actas Urol Esp 2005; 29: 985–988.

1140. Block NL, Weber D, Schinella R. Blue nevi and other melanotic lesions of the prostate: report of 3 cases and review of the literature. J Urol 1972; 107: 85–87.

1141. Cuervo Pinna C, Godoy Rubio E, Parra Escobar JL, et al. [Prostatic blue nevus. Terminology standardization of prostatic pigmented lesions]. Actas Urol Esp 2001; 25: 245–247.

1142. Jao W, Fretzin DF, Christ ML, Prinz LM. Blue nevus of the prostate gland. Arch Pathol 1971; 91: 187–191.

1143. Kovi J, Jackson AG, Jackson MA. Blue nevus of the prostate: ultrastructural study. Urology 1977; 9: 576–578.

1144. Langley JW, Weitzner S. Blue nevus and melanosis of prostate. J Urol 1974; 112: 359–361.

1145. Martinez Martinez CJ, Garcia Gonzalez R, Castaneda Casanova AL. Blue nevus of the prostate: report of two new cases with immunohistochemical and electron-microscopic studies. Eur Urol 1992; 22: 339–342.

1146. Nigogosyan G, Delapava S, Pickren JW, Woodruff MM. Blue nevus of the prostate gland. Cancer 1963; 16: 1097–1099.

1147. Nogueras Gimeno MA, Sanz Anquela JM, Espuela Orgaz R, et al. [Blue nevus of the prostate]. Actas Urol Esp 1993; 17: 130–131.

1148. Redondo Martinez E, Rey Lopez A, Diaz Cascajo C. [Blue nevus of the prostate. Differential diagnosis of prostatic pigmented lesions]. Arch Esp Urol 1998; 51: 286–289.

1149. Ro JY, Grignon DJ, Ayala AG, et al. Blue nevus and melanosis of the prostate. Electron-microscopic and immunohistochemical studies. Am J Clin Pathol 1988; 90: 530–535.

1150. Scarani P, Lorenzini P. [Blue nevus of the prostate]. Pathologica 1979; 71: 563–568.

1151. Tannenbaum M. Differential diagnosis in uropathology. III. Melanotic lesions of prostate: blue nevus and prostatic epithelial melanosis. Urology 1974; 4: 617–621.

1152. Vesga Molina F, Acha Perez M, Llarena Ibarguren R, Pertusa Pena C. [Intraprostatic blue nevus]. Arch Esp Urol 1995; 48: 985–986.

1153. Farid MK, Gahukamble LD. Melanosis of the prostate in an elderly patient – a case report. Cent Afr J Med 1995; 41: 101–102.

1154. Salinas Sanchez AS, Iniguez de Onzono Martin L, Fernandez Millan I, et al. [Prostatic melanosis]. Arch Esp Urol 1993; 46: 818–820.

1155. Fiorelli RL KH, Klaus RL. Use of polyvinyl alcohol in treatment of bladder and prostatic hemangioma. Urology 1991; 38: 480–482.

1156. Kim SH, Kim YI, Paick JS. Cavernous lymphangioma of prostate: radiological findings. Urol Radiol 1992; 13: 197–199.

1157. Chung AK, Michels V, Poland GA, et al. Neurofibromatosis with involvement of the prostate gland. Urology 1996; 47: 448–451.

1158. Jiang R, Chen JH, Chen M, Li QM. Male genital schwannoma, review of 5 cases. Asian J Androl 2003; 5: 251–254.

1159. Sloan SE, Rapoport JM. Prostatic chondroma. Urology 1985; 25: 319–321.

1160. Herawi M, Montgomery EA, Epstein JI. Gastrointestinal stromal tumors (GISTs) on prostate needle biopsy: A clinicopathologic study of 8 cases. Am J Surg Pathol 2006; 30: 1389–1395.

1161. Reyes JW, Shinozuka H, Garry P, Putong PB. A light and electron microscopic study of a hemangiopericytoma of the prostate with local extension. Cancer 1977; 40: 1122–1126.

1162. Li QK, MacLennan GT. Paraganglioma of the prostate. J Urol 2006; 175: 314.

1163. Eble JN, Santer G, Epstein JI, et al. (eds) Tumours of the urinary system and male genital organs. In: WHO classification of tumours. Lyon, France: IARC Press, 2004; 209–211.

1164. Bostwick DG, Hossain D, Qian J, et al. Phyllodes tumor of the prostate:

long-term followup study of 23 cases. J Urol 2004; 172: 894–899.

1165. Waring PM, Newland RC. Prostatic embryonal rhabdomyosarcoma in adults. A clinicopathologic review. Cancer 1992; 69: 755–762.

1166. Asmar L, Gehan EA, Newton WA, Webber BL, et al. Agreement among and within groups of pathologists in the classification of rhabdomyosarcoma and related childhood sarcomas. Report of an international study of four pathology classifications. Cancer 1994; 74: 2579–2588.

1167. Nigro KG, MacLennan GT. Rhabdomyosarcoma of the bladder and prostate. J Urol 2005; 173: 1365.

1168. Moroz K, Crespo P, de las Morenas A. Fine needle aspiration of prostatic rhabdomyosarcoma. A case report demonstrating the value of DNA ploidy. Acta Cytol 1995; 39: 785–790.

1169. Raney RB Jr, Gehan EA, Hays DM, et al. Primary chemotherapy with or without radiation therapy and/or surgery for children with localized sarcoma of the bladder, prostate, vagina, uterus, and cervix. A comparison of the results in Intergroup Rhabdomyosarcoma Studies I and II. Cancer 1990; 66: 2072–2081.

1170. Cheville JC, Dundore PA, Nascimento AG, et al. Leiomyosarcoma of the prostate. Report of 23 cases. Cancer 1995; 76: 1422–1427.

1171. Gaudin PB, Rosai J, Epstein JI. Sarcomas and related proliferative lesions of specialized prostatic stroma: a clinicopathologic study of 22 cases. Am J Surg Pathol 1998; 22: 148–162.

1172. Sauder KJ, MacLennan GT. Phyllodes tumor of the prostate. J Urol 2005; 174: 2373.

1173. McCarthy RP, Zhang S, Bostwick DG, et al. Molecular genetic evidence for different clonal origins of epithelial and stromal components of phyllodes tumor of the prostate. Am J Pathol 2004; 165: 1395–1400.

1174. Wang X, Jones TD, Zhang S, et al. Amplifications of EGFR gene and protein expression of EGFR, Her-2/neu, c-kit, and androgen receptor in phyllodes tumor of the prostate. Mod Pathol 2007; 20: 175–182.

1175. Rammeh Rommani S, Zermani R, Sfaxi M, et al. [Prostatic stromal sarcoma]. Prog Urol 2006; 16: 381–383.

1176. Probert JL, O'Rourke JS, Farrow R, Cox P. Stromal sarcoma of the prostate. Eur J Surg Oncol 2000; 26: 100–101.

1177. Ma J, Huang S, Zhang C. [Pathological observation of 16 cases with non-epithelial tumor and tumor-like lesions of the prostate]. Zhonghua Bing Li Xue Za Zhi 2001; 30: 264–267.

1178. Herawi M, Epstein JI. Specialized stromal tumors of the prostate: a clinicopathologic study of 50 cases. Am J Surg Pathol 2006; 30: 694–704.

1179. Chang YS, Chuang CK, Ng KF, Liao SK. Prostatic stromal sarcoma in a young adult: a case report. Arch Androl 2005; 51: 419–424.

1180. Russo P, Brady MS, Conlon K, et al. Adult urological sarcoma. J Urol 1992; 147: 1032–1036; discussion 1036–1037.

1181. Young JF JP, Wiley CA. Malignant phyllodes tumor of the prostate. A case report with immunohistochemical and ultrastructural studies. Arch Pathol Lab Med 1992 Mar; 116: 296–299.

1182. Kevwitch MK, Walloch JL, Waters WB, Flanigan RC. Prostatic cystic epithelial–stromal tumors: a report of 2 new cases. J Urol 1993; 149: 860–864.

1183. Yamamoto S, Ito T, Miki M, et al. Malignant phyllodes tumor of the prostate. Int J Urol 2000; 7: 378–381.

1184. Kim HS, Lee JH, Nam JH, et al. Malignant phyllodes tumor of the prostate. Pathol Int 1999; 49: 1105–1108.

1185. Yum M, Miller JC, Agrawal BL. Leiomyosarcoma arising in atypical fibromuscular hyperplasia (phyllodes tumor) of the prostate with distant metastasis. Cancer 1991; 68: 910–915.

1186. Chen HJ, Xu M, Zhang L, et al. [Prostate sarcoma: a report of 14 cases]. Zhonghua Nan Ke Xue 2005; 11: 683–685.

1187. Nishiyama T, Ikarashi T, Terunuma M, Ishizaki S. Osteogenic sarcoma of the prostate. Int J Urol 2001; 8: 199–201.

1188. Shen Z, Wang H, Chen S. [Malignant fibrous histiocytoma of the prostate: one case report]. Zhonghua Nan Ke Xue 2004; 10: 202–204.

1189. Smith DM, Manivel C, Kapps D, Uecker J. Angiosarcoma of the prostate: report of 2 cases and review of the literature. J Urol 1986; 135: 382–384.

1190. Dogra PN, Aron M, Rajeev TP, et al. Primary chondrosarcoma of the prostate. BJU Int 1999; 83: 150–151.

1191. Rames RA, Smith MT. Malignant peripheral nerve sheath tumor of the prostate: a rare manifestion of neurofibromatosis type 1. J Urol 1999; 162: 165–166.

1192. Bostwick DG, Dundore PA. Biopsy pathology of the prostate. London: Chapman & Hall, 1997.

1193. Fritsch M, Epstein JI, Perlman EJ, et al. Molecularly confirmed primary prostatic synovial sarcoma. Hum Pathol 2000; 31: 246–250.

1194. Lim DJ, Hayden RT, Murad T, et al. Multilocular prostatic cystadenoma presenting as a large complex pelvic cystic mass. J Urol 1993; 149: 856–859.

1195. Kobayashi H, Kumagai J, Ono S, et al. [A case of prostatic cystadenoma]. Nippon Hinyokika Gakkai Zasshi 2005; 96: 462–465.

1196. Choi YL, Kang SY, Choi JS, et al. Aberrant hypermethylation of RASSF1A promoter in ovarian borderline tumors and carcinomas. Virchows Arch 2006; 448: 331–336.

1197. Hauck EW, Battmann A, Schmelz HU, et al. Giant multilocular cystadenoma of the prostate: a rare differential diagnosis of benign prostatic hyperplasia. Urol Int 2004; 73: 365–369.

1198. Levy DA, Gogate PA, Hampel N. Giant multilocular prostatic cystadenoma: a rare clinical entity and review of the literature. J Urol 1993; 150: 1920–1922.

1199. Maluf HM, King ME, DeLuca FR, et al. Giant multilocular prostatic cystadenoma: a distinctive lesion of the retroperitoneum in men. A report of two cases. Am J Surg Pathol 1991; 15: 131–135.

1200. Morimoto S, Okuno T, Masuda H, et al. [A case of prostatic cystadenoma]. Hinyokika kiyo 1994; 40: 629–631.

1201. Rusch D, Moinzadeh A, Hamawy K, Larsen C. Giant multilocular cystadenoma of the prostate. AJR Am J Roentgenol 2002; 179: 1477–1479.

1202. Seong BM, Cheon J, Lee JG, et al. A case of multilocular prostatic cystadenoma. J Korean Med Sci 1998; 13: 554–558.

1203. Tuziak T, Spiess PE, Abrahams NA, et al. Multilocular cystadenoma and cystadenocarcinoma of the prostate. Urol Oncol 2007; 25: 19–25.

1204. Allen EA, Brinker DA, Coppola D, et al. Multilocular prostatic cystadenoma with high-grade prostatic intraepithelial neoplasia. Urology 2003; 61: 644.

1205. Furuya S, Kato H. A clinical entity of cystic dilatation of the utricle associated with hemospermia. J Urol 2005; 174: 1039–1042.

1206. Yanai T, Okazaki T, Yamataka A, et al. Cysts of the ejaculatory system: a report of two cases. Pediatr Surg Int 2005; 21: 939–942.

1207. Pryor JP, Hendry WF. Ejaculatory duct obstruction in subfertile males: analysis of 87 patients. Fertil Steril 1991; 56: 725–730.

1208. Hendry WF, Pryor JP. Mullerian duct (prostatic utricle) cyst: diagnosis and treatment in subfertile males. Br J Urol 1992; 69: 79–82.

1209. Yamazaki K, Orikasa H. A seminal vesicle cyst complicated with a tumor like nodular mass of benign proliferating prostatic tissue: a case report with ultrastructural and immunohistochemical studies. J Submicrosc Cytol Pathol 2003; 35: 209–214.

1210. Aslan DL, Pambuccian SE, Gulbahce HE, et al. Prostatic glands and urothelial epithelium in a seminal vesicle cyst: report of a case and review of pathologic features and prostatic ectopy. Arch Pathol Lab Med 2006; 130: 194–197.

1211. Deklotz RJ. Echinococcal cyst involving the prostate and seminal vesicles: a case report. J Urol 1976; 115: 116–117.

1212. Mai KT, Walley VM. Adenofibroma of the ejaculatory duct. J Urol Pathol 1994; 2, 301–305.

1213. Fan K, Johnson DF. Adenomatoid tumor of ejaculatory duct. Urology 1985; 25: 653–654.

1214. Chu PG, Huang Q, Weiss LM. Incidental and concurrent malignant lymphomas discovered at the time of prostatectomy and prostate biopsy: a study of 29 cases. Am J Surg Pathol 2005; 29: 693–699.

1215. Ballario R, Beltrami P, Cavalleri S, et al. An unusual pathological finding of chronic lymphocitic leukemia and adenocarcinoma of the prostate after transurethral resection for complete urinary retention: case report. BMC Cancer 2004; 4: 95.

1216. Weir EG, Epstein JI. Incidental small lymphocytic lymphoma/chronic lymphocytic leukemia in pelvic lymph nodes excised at radical prostatectomy. Arch Pathol Lab Med 2003; 127: 567–572.

1217. Cachia PG, McIntyre MA, Dewar AE, Stockdill G. Prostatic infiltration in chronic lymphatic leukaemia. J Clin Pathol 1987; 40: 342–345.

1218. Thalhammer F, Gisslinger H, Chott A, et al. Granulocytic sarcoma of the prostate as the first manifestation of a late relapse of acute myelogenous leukemia. Ann Hematol 1994; 68: 97–99.

1219. Wazait HD, Al-Buheissi SZ, Dudderidge T, et al. Rare case of primary lymphoma of the prostate: giving the patient the benefit of the doubt. Urol Int 2003; 71: 338–340.

1220. Ghose A, Baxter-Smith DC, Eeles H, et al. Lymphoma of the prostate treated with radiotherapy. Clin Oncol (Roy Coll Radiol) 1995; 7: 134.

1221. Bostwick DG, Iczkowski KA, Amin MB, et al. Malignant lymphoma involving the prostate: report of 62 cases. Cancer 1998; 83: 732–738.

1222. Fell P, O'Connor M, Smith JM. Primary lymphoma of prostate presenting as bladder outflow obstruction. Urology 1987; 29: 555–556.

1223. Ewing J. Neoplastic diseases. Philadelphia: WB Saunders, 1940.

1224. Fukase N. Hyperplasia of the rudimentary lymph nodes of the prostate. Surg Gynecol Obstet 1922; 35: 131–136.

1225. Banerjee SS, Harris M. Angiotropic lymphoma presenting in the prostate. Histopathology 1988; 12: 667–670.

1226. Ben-Ezra J, Sheibani K, Kendrick FE, et al. Angiotropic large cell lymphoma of the prostate gland: an immunohistochemical study. Hum Pathol 1986; 17: 964–967.

1227. Chim CS, Loong F, Yau T, et al. Common malignancies with uncommon sites of presentation: case 2. Mantle-cell lymphoma of the prostate. J Clin Oncol 2003; 21: 4456–4458.

1228. Boe S, Nielsen H, Ryttov N. Burkitt's lymphoma mimicking prostatitis. J Urol 1981; 125: 891–892.

1229. Jhavar S, Agarwal JP, Naresh KN, et al. Primary extranodal mucosa associated lymphoid tissue (MALT) lymphoma of the prostate. Leuk Lymphoma 2001; 41: 445–449.

1230. Tomaru U, Ishikura H, Kon S, et al. Primary lymphoma of the prostate with features of low grade B-cell lymphoma of mucosa associated lymphoid tissue: a rare cause of urinary obstruction. J Urol 1999; 162: 496–497.

1231. Lopez JI, Elorriaga K, Irizar E, Bilbao FJ. Adenocarcinoma and non-Hodgkin's lymphoma involving the prostate. Histopathology 2000; 36: 373–374.

1232. Peison B, Benisch B, Nicora B, Lind E. Acute urinary obstruction secondary to pseudolymphoma of prostate. Urology 1977; 10: 478–479.

1233. Humphrey PA, Vollmer RT. Extramedullary hematopoiesis in the prostate. Am J Surg Pathol 1991; 15: 486–490.

1234. Estrada PC, Scardino PL. Myeloma of the prostate: a case report. J Urol 1971; 106: 586–587.

1235. Farnham SB, Mason SE, Smith JA Jr. Metastatic testicular seminoma to the prostate. Urology 2005; 66: 195.

1236. Han G, Miura K, Takayama T, Tsutsui Y. Primary prostatic endodermal sinus tumor (yolk sac tumor) combined with a small focal seminoma. Am J Surg Pathol 2003; 27: 554–559.

1237. Hayman R, Patel A, Fisher C, Hendry WF. Primary seminoma of the prostate. Br J Urol 1995; 76: 273–274.

1238. Khandekar JD, Holland JM, Rochester D, Christ ML. Extragonadal seminoma involving urinary bladder and arising in the prostate. Cancer 1993; 71: 3972–3974.

1239. Kimura F, Watanabe S, Shimizu S, et al. [Primary seminoma of the prostate and embryonal cell carcinoma of the left testis in one patient: a case report]. Nippon Hinyokika Gakkai Zasshi 1995; 86: 1497–1500.

1240. Motley RC, Utz DC, Farrow GM, Earle JD. Testicular seminoma metastatic to the prostate. J Urol 1986; 135: 801–802.

1241. Plummer ER, Greene DR, Roberts JT. Seminoma metastatic to the prostate resulting in a rectovesical fistula. Clin Oncol (Roy Coll Radiol) 2000; 12: 229–230.

1242. Arai Y, Watanabe J, Kounami T, Tomoyoshi T. Retroperitoneal seminoma with simultaneous occurrence in the prostate. J Urol 1988; 139: 382–383.

1243. Michel F, Gattegno B, Roland J, et al. Primary nonseminomatous germ cell tumor of the prostate. J Urol 1986; 135: 597–599.

1244. Minamino K, Adachi Y, Okamura A, et al. Autopsy case of primary choriocarcinoma of the urinary bladder. Pathol Int 2005; 55: 216–222.

1245. Ekfors TO, Aho HJ, Kekomaki M. Malignant rhabdoid tumor of the prostatic region. Immunohistological and ultrastructural evidence for epithelial origin. Virchows Arch A [Pathol Anat Histopathol] 1985; 406: 381–388.

1246. Beckman EN, Pintado SO, Leonard GL, Sternberg WH. Endometriosis of the prostate. Am J Surg Pathol 1985; 9: 374–379.

1247. Mettlin C, Lee F, Drago J, Murphy GP. The American Cancer Society National Prostate Cancer Detection Project. Findings on the detection of early prostate cancer in 2425 men. Cancer 1991; 67: 2949–2958.

1248. Feneley MR, Busch C. Precursor lesions for prostate cancer. J Roy Soc Med 1997; 90: 533–539.

1249. Hoedemaeker RF, Kranse R, Rietbergen JB, et al. Evaluation of prostate needle biopsies in a population-based screening study: the impact of borderline lesions. Cancer 1999; 85: 145–152.

1250. Postma R, Roobol M, Schroder FH, van der Kwast TH. Lesions predictive for prostate cancer in a screened population: first and second screening round findings. Prostate 2004; 61: 260–266.

1251. Bostwick DG, Qian J, Frankel K. The incidence of high grade prostatic intraepithelial neoplasia in needle biopsies. J Urol 1995; 154: 1791–1794.

1252. Lefkowitz GK, Sidhu GS, Torre P, et al. Is repeat prostate biopsy for high-grade prostatic intraepithelial neoplasia necessary after routine 12-core sampling? Urology 2001; 58: 999–1003.

1253. San Francisco IF, Olumi AF, Kao J, et al. Clinical management of prostatic intraepithelial neoplasia as diagnosed by extended needle biopsies. BJU Int 2003; 91: 350–354.

1254. Abdel-Khalek M, El-Baz M, Ibrahiem el H. Predictors of prostate cancer on extended biopsy in patients with high-grade prostatic intraepithelial neoplasia: a multivariate analysis model. BJU Int 2004; 94: 528–533.

1255. Tunc M, Sanli O, Kandirali E, et al. Should high-grade prostatic intraepithelial neoplasia change our approach to infravesical obstruction? Urol Int 2005; 74: 332–336.

1256. Berman DM, Yang J, Epstein JI. Foamy gland high-grade prostatic intraepithelial neoplasia. Am J Surg Pathol 2000; 24: 140–144.

1257. Bostwick DG, Qian J, Maihle NJ. Amphiregulin expression in prostatic intraepithelial neoplasia and adenocarcinoma: a study of 93 cases. Prostate 2004; 58: 164–168.

1258. Montironi R, Magi-Galluzzi C, Fabris G. Apoptotic bodies in prostatic intraepithelial neoplasia and prostatic adenocarcinoma following total androgen ablation. Pathol Res Pract 1995; 191: 873–880.

1259. Kamoi K, Troncoso P, Babaian RJ. Strategy for repeat biopsy in patients with high grade prostatic intraepithelial neoplasia. J Urol 2000; 163: 819–823.

1260. Kronz JD, Allan CH, Shaikh AA, Epstein JI. Predicting cancer following a diagnosis of high-grade prostatic intraepithelial neoplasia on needle biopsy: data on men with more than one follow-up biopsy. Am J Surg Pathol 2001; 25: 1079–1085.

1261. Maatman TJ, Papp SR, Carothers GG, Shockley KF. The critical role of patient follow-up after receiving a diagnosis of prostatic intraepithelial neoplasia. Prostate Cancer Prostatic Dis 2001; 4: 63–66.

1262. Bishara T, Ramnani DM, Epstein JI. High-grade prostatic intraepithelial neoplasia on needle biopsy: risk of cancer on repeat biopsy related to number of involved cores and morphologic pattern. Am J Surg Pathol 2004; 28: 629–633.

1263. Gokden N, Roehl KA, Catalona WJ, Humphrey PA. High-grade prostatic intraepithelial neoplasia in needle biopsy as risk factor for detection of adenocarcinoma: current level of risk in screening population. Urology 2005; 65: 538–542.

1264. El-Fakharany MM, Wojno KJ. Significance of high-grade prostatic intraepithelial neoplasia in the era of extended prostatic needle biopsies. Mod Pathol 2005; 18: 138A.

1265. Leite KRM MC, Camara-Lopes LH. Prostate biopsies following the diagnosis of PIN and ASAP: numbers and findings in the Brazilian population [Absract]. Mod Pathol 2005; 18: 152A.

1266. Tan PH, Tan HW, Tan Y, et al. Is high-grade prostatic intraepithelial neoplasia on needle biopsy different in an Asian population: a clinicopathologic study performed in Singapore. Urology 2006; 68: 800–803.

1267. Bostwick DG. Clinical utility of prostatic intraepithelial neoplasia. Mayo Clin Proc 1995; 70: 395–396.

1268. O'Dowd G J, Miller MC, Orozco R, Veltri RW. Analysis of repeated biopsy results within 1 year after a noncancer diagnosis. Urology 2000; 55: 553–559.

1269. Bostwick DG. Gleason grading of prostatic needle biopsies. Correlation with grade in 316 matched prostatectomies. Am J Surg Pathol 1994; 18: 796–803.

1270. Spires SE, Cibull ML, Wood DP Jr, et al. Gleason histologic grading in prostatic carcinoma. Correlation of 18-gauge core biopsy with prostatectomy. Arch Pathol Lab Med 1994; 118: 705–708.

1271. Kojima M, Troncoso P, Babaian RJ. Use of prostate-specific antigen and tumor volume in predicting needle biopsy grading error. Urology 1995; 45: 807–812.

1272. Thickman D, Speers WC, Philpott PJ, Shapiro H. Effect of the number of core biopsies of the prostate on predicting Gleason score of prostate cancer. J Urol 1996; 156: 110–113.

1273. Cookson MS, Fleshner NE, Soloway MS, Fair WR. Correlation between Gleason score of needle biopsy and radical prostatectomy specimen: Accuracy and clinical implications. J Urol 1997; 157: 559–562.

1274. Sved PD, Gomez P, Manoharan M, et al. Limitations of biopsy Gleason grade: implications for counseling patients with biopsy Gleason score 6 prostate cancer. J Urol 2004; 172: 98–102.

1275. Hsieh TF, Chang CH, Chen WC, et al. Correlation of Gleason scores between needle-core biopsy and radical prostatectomy specimens in patients with prostate cancer. J Chin Med Assoc 2005; 68: 167–171.

1276. Kums JJ, van Helsdingen PJ. Signet-ring cell carcinoma of the bladder and the prostate. Report of 4 cases. Urol Int 1985; 40: 116–119.

1277. Uchijima Y, Ito H, Takahashi M, Yamashina M. Prostate mucinous adenocarcinoma with signet ring cell. Urology 1990; 36: 267–268.

1278. Alline KM, Cohen MB. Signet-ring cell carcinoma of the prostate. Arch Pathol Lab Med 1992; 116: 99–102.

1279. Segawa T, Kakehi Y. Primary signet ring cell adenocarcinoma of the prostate: a case report and literature review. Hinyokika kiyo 1993; 39: 565–568.

1280. Skodras G, Wang J, Kragel PJ. Primary prostatic signet-ring cell carcinoma. Urology 1993; 42: 338–342.

1281. Smith C, Feddersen RM, Dressler L, et al. Signet ring cell adenocarcinoma of prostate. Urology 1994; 43: 397–400.

1282. Fujita K, Sugao H, Gotoh T, et al. Primary signet ring cell carcinoma of the prostate: report and review of 42 cases. Int J Urol 2004; 11: 178–181.

1283. Jiang Z, Zhang H, Chen J, et al. [Pathologic diagnosis and histogenesis of primary signet ring cell carcinoma of the prostate]. Chin J Pathol 2002; 31: 514–517.

1284. Cohen MK, Arber DA, Coffield KS, et al. Neuroendocrine differentiation in prostatic adenocarcinoma and its relationship to tumor progression. Cancer 1994; 74: 1899–1903.

1285. Bostwick DG, Dousa MK, Crawford BG, Wollan PC. Neuroendocrine differentiation in prostatic intraepithelial neoplasia and adenocarcinoma. Am J Surg Pathol 1994; 18: 1240–1246.

1286. Noordzij MA, van der Kwast TH, van Steenbrugge GJ, et al. The prognostic influence of neuroendocrine cells in prostate cancer: results of a long-term follow-up study with patients treated by radical prostatectomy. Int J Cancer 1995; 62: 252–258.

1287. Speights VO Jr, Cohen MK, Riggs MW, et al. Neuroendocrine stains and proliferative indices of prostatic adenocarcinomas in transurethral resection samples. Br J Urol 1997; 80: 281–286.

1288. McWilliam LJ, Manson C, George NJ. Neuroendocrine differentiation and prognosis in prostatic adenocarcinoma. Br J Urol 1997; 80: 287–290.

1289. Pruneri G, Galli S, Rossi RS, et al. Chromogranin A and B and secretogranin II in prostatic adenocarcinomas: neuroendocrine expression in patients untreated and treated with androgen deprivation therapy. Prostate 1998; 34: 113–120.

1290. Casella R, Bubendorf L, Sauter G, et al. Focal neuroendocrine differentiation lacks prognostic significance in prostate core needle biopsies. J Urol 1998; 160: 406–410.

1291. Abrahamsson PA, Falkmer S, Falt K, Grimelius L. The course of neuroendocrine differentiation in prostatic carcinomas. An immunohistochemical study testing chromogranin A as an 'endocrine marker.' Pathol Res Pract 1989; 185: 373–380.

1292. Cohen RJ, Glezerson G, Haffejee Z. Prostate-specific antigen and prostate-specific acid phosphatase in neuroendocrine cells of prostate cancer. Arch Pathol Lab Med 1992; 116: 65–66.

1293. Cohen RJ, Glezerson G, Haffejee Z, Afrika D. Prostatic carcinoma: histological and immunohistological factors affecting prognosis. Br J Urol 1990; 66: 405–410.

1294. Weinstein MH, Partin AW, Veltri RW, Epstein JI. Neuroendocrine differentiation in prostate cancer: enhanced prediction of progression after radical prostatectomy. Hum Pathol 1996; 27: 683–687.

1295. Borre M, Nerstrom B, Overgaard J. Association between immunohistochemical expression of vascular endothelial growth factor (VEGF), VEGF-expressing neuroendocrine- differentiated tumor cells, and outcome in prostate cancer patients subjected to watchful waiting. Clin Cancer Res 2000; 6: 1882–1890.

1296. Yu DS, Hsieh DS, Chen HI, Chang SY. The expression of neuropeptides in hyperplastic and malignant prostate tissue and its possible clinical implications. J Urol 2001; 166: 871–875.

1297. Noordzij MA, Bogdanowicz JF, van Krimpen C, et al. The prognostic value of pretreatment expression of androgen receptor and bcl-2 in hormonally treated prostate cancer patients. J Urol 1997; 158: 1880–1884; discussion 1884–1885.

1298. Prins GS, Sklarew RJ, Pertschuk LP. Image analysis of androgen receptor immunostaining in prostate cancer accurately predicts response to hormonal therapy. J Urol 1998; 159: 641–649.

1299. Schafer W, Funke PJ, Kunde D, et al. Intensity of androgen and epidermal growth factor receptor immunoreactivity in samples of radical prostatectomy as prognostic indicator: correlation with clinical data of long-term observations. J Urol 2006; 176: 532–537.

1300. Tilley WD, Buchanan G, Hickey TE, Bentel JM. Mutations in the androgen receptor gene are associated with progression of human prostate cancer to androgen independence. Clin Cancer Res 1996; 2: 277–285.

1301. Nabi G, Seth A, Dinda AK, Gupta NP. Computer based receptogram approach: an objective way of assessing immunohistochemistry of androgen receptor staining and its correlation with hormonal response in metastatic carcinoma of prostate. J Clin Pathol 2004; 57: 146–150.

1302. Ryan CJ, Smith A, Lal P, et al. Persistent prostate-specific antigen expression after neoadjuvant androgen depletion: an early predictor of relapse or incomplete androgen suppression. Urology 2006; 68: 834–839.

1303. Hernes E, Fossa SD, Berner A, et al. Expression of the epidermal growth factor receptor family in prostate carcinoma before and during androgen-independence. Br J Cancer 2004; 90: 449–454.

1304. Osman I, Scher HI, Drobnjak M, et al. HER-2/neu (p185neu) protein expression in the natural or treated history of prostate cancer. Clin Cancer Res 2001; 7: 2643–2647.

1305. Di Lorenzo G, Tortora G, D'Armiento FP, et al. Expression of epidermal growth factor receptor correlates with disease relapse and progression to androgen-independence in human prostate cancer. Clin Cancer Res 2002; 8: 3438–3444.

1306. Koivisto P, Kononen J, Palmberg C, et al. Androgen receptor gene amplification: a possible molecular mechanism for androgen deprivation therapy failure in prostate cancer. Cancer Res 1997; 57: 314–319.

1307. Dorkin TJ, Robinson MC, Marsh C, et al. aFGF immunoreactivity in prostate cancer and its co-localization with bFGF and FGF8. J Pathol 1999; 189: 564–569.

1308. Edwards J, Krishna NS, Mukherjee R, Bartlett JM. The role of c-Jun and c-Fos expression in androgen-independent prostate cancer. J Pathol 2004; 204: 153–158.

1309. Krajewska M, Turner BC, Shabaik A, et al. Expression of BAG-1 protein correlates with aggressive behavior of prostate cancers. Prostate 2006; 66: 801–810.

1310. Koivisto PA, Rantala I. Amplification of the androgen receptor gene is associated with P53 mutation in hormone-refractory recurrent prostate cancer. J Pathol 1999; 187: 237–241.

1311. Baretton GB, Klenk U, Diebold J, et al. Proliferation- and apoptosis-associated factors in advanced prostatic carcinomas before and after androgen deprivation therapy: prognostic significance of p21/WAF1/CIP1 expression. Br J Cancer 1999; 80: 546–555.

1312. Villers A, McNeal JE, Freiha FS, Stamey TA. Multiple cancers in the prostate. Morphologic features of clinically recognized versus incidental tumors. Cancer 1992; 70: 2313–2318.

1313. Miller GJ, Cygan JM. Morphology of prostate cancer: the effects of multifocality on histological grade, tumor volume and capsule penetration. J Urol 1994; 152: 1709–1713.

1314. Djavan B, Susani M, Bursa B, et al. Predictability and significance of multifocal prostate cancer in the radical prostatectomy specimen. Tech Urol 1999; 5: 139–142.

1315. Song SY, Kim SR, Ahn G, Choi HY. Pathologic characteristics of prostatic adenocarcinomas: a mapping analysis of Korean patients. Prostate Cancer Prostatic Dis 2003; 6: 143–147.

1316. Horninger W, Berger AP, Rogatsch H, et al. Characteristics of prostate cancers detected at low PSA levels. Prostate 2004; 58: 232–237.

1317. Cheng L, Poulos CK, Pan CX, et al. Preoperative prediction of small volume cancer (less than 0.5 ml) in radical prostatectomy specimens. J Urol 2005; 174: 898–902.

1318. Torlakovic G, Torlakovic E, Skovlund E, et al. Volume-related sequence of tumor distribution pattern in prostate carcinoma: importance of posterior midline crossover in predicting tumor volume, extracapsular extension, and seminal vesicle invasion. Croat Med J 2005; 46: 429–435.

# CHAPTER 10

# Seminal vesicles

David G. Bostwick

The seminal vesicles were described by the Italian anatomist Berengario a Carpi in 1521. These paired androgen-dependent accessory sex glands were first regarded simply as storage sites for semen, but their milky alkaline secretions are now known to constitute the majority of the ejaculate, promoting sperm function and providing a variety of potent antibacterial factors to the male genital tract.[1-3] In the seminal vesicles, infections, cysts, and neoplasms are rare, in sharp contrast to their anatomic neighbor, the prostate.

## Embryology and anatomy

Under the influence of testosterone, the seminal vesicles appear during the 13th week of development as outpouchings of the lower mesonephric ducts. They are bounded by the prostate distally, the base of the bladder anteriorly, and Denonvilliers' fascia and the rectum posteriorly. Their anatomic position in this region is variable, and they are sometimes found within or adherent to the posterior capsule of the prostate gland.[2-4] The seminal vesicles may be palpable on digital rectal examination, and, when adherent to the prostate, may be mistaken for prostatic nodularity or induration. Approximately 5% of prostate biopsies for nodularity contain fragments of seminal vesicle epithelium, a potential source of diagnostic confusion (Fig. 10-1).[5,6] In adults, the seminal vesicles average 6 cm long and 2 cm wide, with a capacity of up to 4.5 mL, although there is wide variation in size, shape, and volume.[4]

The muscular wall of the seminal vesicles consists of a thick circumferential coat of smooth muscle that contracts during ejaculation. Contraction is regulated by excitatory adrenergic and modulatory neuropeptide-Y-encephalin-peptidergic nerve fibers.[4] Tangential cuts through this wall frequently reveal irregular clusters of epithelial tubules that may be mistaken for adenocarcinoma.

The ducts of the seminal vesicles merge with the ampullae of the vasa deferentia on each side to form the ejaculatory ducts, and these structures compose a functional unit that develops slowly until the onset of puberty.[4] These ducts immediately enter the central zone of the prostate and converge as they approach their outlets at either side of the verumontanum in the prostatic sinus of the prostatic urethra. Unlike the seminal vesicles, the ejaculatory ducts lack a thick muscular wall, surrounded by a collagenous stroma. Luminal and wall dimensions are remarkably uniform among adult men, with diameter greater than 2.3 mm the cut point for dilatation.[7]

Histologically, the seminal vesicular mucosa consists of complex papillary folds and irregular convoluted lumina lined by non-ciliated, pseudostratified tall columnar epithelium. The cells are predominantly secretory, containing microvesicular lipid droplets and characteristic lipofuscin pigment granules.[8] The pigment is golden-brown and refractile, increasing in amount with age; similar pigment may be seen in prostatic epithelium, but is usually less conspicuous and abundant.[9] These cells also contain androgen receptors, similar to the prostatic epithelium. Secretory products include glycoproteins, protein kinase inhibitor, protein C inhibitor, fructose, prostaglandins, ascorbic acid, sperm motility factor, transferrin, lactoferrin, lysozyme, and metallothionein. Secretion is regulated by nerves from the pelvic plexus that are cholinergic postganglionic, sympathetic, and possibly parasympathetic.[4,10,11] Up to 85% of the seminal fluid originates in the seminal vesicles, and the volume of semen varies from 2 to 5 mL. It takes 3 days for the epithelium to refill the seminal vesicles after ejaculation.

MUC6 is selectively expressed in benign seminal vesicle epithelium, in contrast to benign prostate and adenocarcinoma.[12]

## Age-associated changes

In the seventh decade of life, the seminal vesicles begin to shrink.[13] The tall columnar cells lining the mucosa in young men are replaced over time by flattened cuboidal cells, comprising only 50% of the epithelium in men in the fifth decade, and 2% in octogenarians. With advancing age, the stroma of the seminal vesicles becomes hyalinized and fibrotic.

The flattening of the epithelium is accompanied by striking nuclear abnormalities, and highly atypical cells are present in about 75% of older men (Fig. 10-2).[14-21] These cells have large irregular hyperchromatic nuclei with coarse chromatin and prominent nucleoli. Multinucleated cells are also present, as well as giant ring-shaped nuclei with large intranuclear cytoplasmic inclusions. Mitotic figures are absent. These nuclear abnormalities, not observed before age 20, are probably degenerative changes reflecting hormonal influences. When encountered in needle biopsies, such 'pseudomalignant' cytologic atypia may lead to a mistaken diagnosis of prostate cancer.[22] Difficulty may also be encountered in cytologic evaluation of fluids obtained by prostatic massage because seminal vesicular cells are frequently shed intact into the lumina. The distinctive lipochrome pigment aids in their recognition.[16-18,20] Cells in prostatic aspirates derived from the seminal vesicles and ejaculatory ducts may

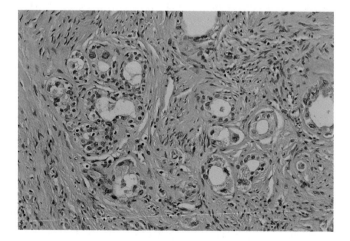

**Fig. 10-1** Tangential needle biopsy through the seminal vesicles which may be mistaken for adenocarcinoma.

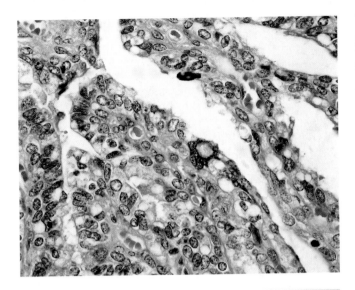

**Fig. 10-2** Seminal vesicle from an 80-year-old man showing distinctive highly atypical epithelial cells.

**Table 10-1** Differential diagnosis of seminal vesicle cyst

| Type of cyst | Location | Size | Contains sperm? |
| --- | --- | --- | --- |
| Seminal vesicle cyst | Lateral | Large | Yes |
| Diverticulum of ejaculatory duct of ampulla | Lateral | Variable | Yes |
| Prostatic cyst | Lateral | Variable | No |
| Müllerian duct cyst | Midline | Large | No |

be cytologically indistinguishable. DNA ploidy analysis reveals aneuploidy in up to 48% of seminal vesicles.[14,23] Consequently, if prostate cancer specimens are contaminated by seminal vesicle tissue, DNA analysis may yield false-positive results. It is uncertain why there is such a low level of aneuploidy in an organ with frequent and substantial cytologic atypia.

Seminal vesicular cells are found as contaminants of cervical smears in 10% of specimens with spermatozoa, and may be diagnostically confusing.[24] These cells contain foamy cytoplasm, scant pigment, vesicular hyperchromatic nuclei, a sieve-like chromatin pattern, and mild anisokaryosis.

## Congenital and acquired malformations

Malformations of the seminal vesicles are frequently associated with abnormal development of other mesonephric derivatives, although isolated hypoplasia, agenesis, and cysts have been reported.[25,26] Unilateral absence of one seminal vesicle may be associated with ipsilateral prostatic central zone agenesis,[27] renal agenesis, or vas deferens anomalies or agenesis.[28] Unilateral agenesis is often associated with reduced semen volume, hypospermia or azoospermia, impaired sperm motility, acidic ejaculate, and absence of fructose and coagulation activity. Up to 37.5% of these men are infertile, implying that the single vas is abnormal. Bilateral dilation or absence of the seminal vesicles is sometimes observed in patients with cystic fibrosis, reportedly caused by an unexplained failure of development.[29] Unilateral duplication of the seminal vesicles is an unusual anomaly. Seminal vesicle surgery is usually undertaken for evaluation of congenital malformations.

Maldevelopment of the ureteric bud results in ureteral ectopy, with the ureters terminating in the seminal vesicles, prostatic urethra, vas deferens, epididymis, or ejaculatory ducts.[30–44] Ureteral ectopy is frequently seen in association with ipsilateral renal dysgenesis or contralateral renal hypertrophy, and the seminal vesicles become enlarged and dilated with accompanying ureterocele.

## Cysts

Seminal vesicle cysts are rare and may be congenital or acquired.[45–48] Symptoms are vague, including perineal pain during ejaculation or defecation, dysuria, urinary retention, and recurrent epididymitis. Congenital cysts are associated with ipsilateral renal agenesis in 80% of cases and commonly with ureteral ectopia or agenesis (Zinner's syndrome), with more than 100 reported cases.[30,47,49–59] These paired anomalies are caused by the close association of the ureteric bud and mesonephric duct during embryogenesis; the ureteric bud is more cephalad, and the elongated ureter may fail to connect with and stimulate the differentiation of the nephrogenic blastema. Other cases of congenital cyst are associated with ipsilateral absence of the testis[34] or hemivertebra.[60] Congenital cysts of the seminal vesicle are usually detected in patients between 18 and 41 years of age, the period of maximal sexual and reproductive activity; most have arisen in white patients.[61] Cyst may be asymptomatic or cause ill-defined lower urinary tract symptoms.[62] Magnetic resonance imaging (MRI) is useful for detecting cyst and associated urogenital tract anomalies.[63]

The cyst is usually unilateral and unilocular, lateral to the midline, up to three times larger than the normal seminal vesicle, and considerably smaller than müllerian duct cyst (Table 10-1), although rarely the cyst is gigantic[64,65] and may cause rectal obstruction.[66] Enlargement is caused by insufficient drainage with accumulation of seminal fluid. The unilocular cyst contains viscous pale white fluid, similar to the usual secretions of the seminal vesicles, and is lined by cuboidal or flattened epithelium with a fibrous wall of variable thickness. Rarely, there may be intracystic papillary adenoma.[67] Massive enlargement has been called hydrocele or hydrops.[68] Bilateral congenital cysts are rare and may be associated with absent vasa deferentia.[69]

Acquired cyst is usually associated with inflammation and obstruction of the ejaculatory ducts and seminal vesicles (Fig. 10-3). This fluctuant cyst may be palpable on digital rectal examination, and often contains red cells, white cells, and spermatozoa. The epithelial lining is inflamed or sloughed, depending on the duration and severity of inflammation. In one case, endoscopic removal of a small calculus lodged at the orifice of the ipsilateral ejaculatory duct caused complete resolution of a 14 cm seminal vesicle cyst, evidence for an obstructive etiology and demonstration of the utility of preoperative imaging techniques to detect stones.[70] One unique case presented as an inguinal hernia, with the cyst extending through the inguinal canal.[71]

Echinococcal (hydatid) cyst can occur in the retrovesicular region, invariably in association with infection in another organ; cyst excision is curative.[72–76] Megavesicles are characterized by marked dilation of the seminal vesicles. The cause of megavesicles is unknown, but this condition is sometimes seen in diabetics.[77] Cystadenoma is a benign neoplasm mimicking acquired cyst (see below).

The differential diagnosis of seminal vesicle cyst includes prostatic cyst,[78] ejaculatory duct diverticulum, and cystic dilation of wolffian and müllerian duct remnants (see Table 10-1).[77,79,80] The cysts may produce hydronephrosis caused by displacement of the lower ureter toward the midline with obstruction. Radiographic evaluation of seminal vesicle cyst includes vasoseminovesiculography, ultrasonography, computed tomography (CT), and MRI.[55,81] Aspiration of congenital or acquired cysts relieves

symptoms, but surgical removal or marsupialization is preferred.

## Ectopic prostatic tissue

Benign ectopic prostatic tissue rarely arises in seminal vesicle tissue and may be mistaken for extraprostatic adenocarcinoma.[82] Ectopia may involve prostatic or urothelial tissue, and most frequently is identified in the wall of a seminal vesicle cyst, sometimes forming a nodular mass.[83,84] The intimate spatial coexistence of endoderm-derived prostatic tissue and mesonephric duct-derived seminal vesicle tissue is rare.[85]

# Non-neoplastic abnormalities

## Amyloidosis

Localized amyloidosis of the seminal vesicles (senile seminal vesicle amyloidosis) is observed at autopsy in 5–8% of men between 46 and 60 years of age, in 13–23% between 61 and 75 years, and in 21–34% of those over 75 years.[86–88] The clinical incidence in men with hemospermia is 33%;[89] at radical prostatectomy the incidence is 1.1%.[90] There may be an association with prior androgen deprivation therapy for prostate cancer,[91] but this has been refuted.[90]

Amyloidosis often extends bilaterally along the ejaculatory ducts, forming linear or massive nodular subepithelial deposits of amorphous eosinophilic fibrillar material (Fig. 10-4). Basement membrane thickening is observed, and deposits may be seen within the vesicular lumina, occasionally causing significant luminal narrowing. Rare cases are associated with calcification or a florid foreign body giant cell reaction.[92] By contrast, systemic amyloidosis infrequently affects the seminal vesicles, involving the vascular walls, smooth muscle, and stroma.[93] Vesicular amyloidosis is usually asymptomatic, but may cause hematospermia, chronic perineal pain, or mimic seminal vesiculitis.[94,95] It is best visualized by MRI, and may mimic tumor invasion from

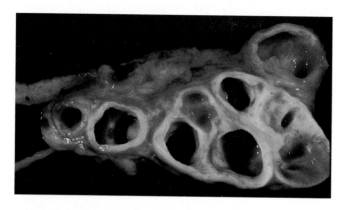

**Fig. 10-3** Incidental acquired cyst of the seminal vesicles found at autopsy in a 70-year-old man.

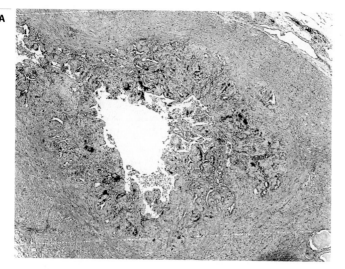

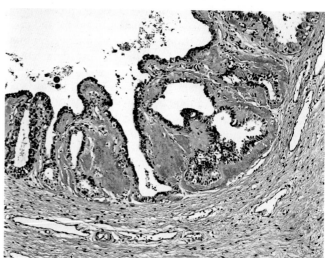

**Fig. 10-4** Amyloidosis of **(A)** seminal vesicles and **(B)** ejaculatory ducts.

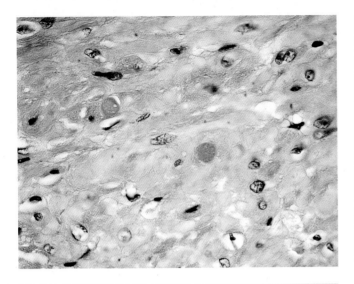

**Fig. 10-5** Stromal hyaline bodies within the muscular wall of the seminal vesicles.

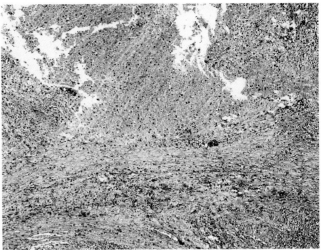

**Fig. 10-6** Patchy acute seminal vesiculitis.

bladder or prostate cancer.[89,96–98] Localized and systemic amyloidosis may coexist.[99]

Special stains that confirm the diagnosis of amyloid include Congo red, which appears red by light microscopy with apple-green polarization birefringence; methylene blue, which reveals green polarization birefringence; crystal violet and toluidine blue, which impart a metachromatic appearance to the deposits; and periodic acid–Schiff (PAS) and Alcian blue stains, which are weakly to moderately positive. The composition of localized seminal vesicle amyloid is histochemically unique (permanganate sensitive, lactoferrin and amyloid P component positive, and non-AA, non-B2M, non-κ or λ, non-prealbumin type[89]), apparently derived from secretory protein of the seminal vesicles; amyloid at other sites is derived from light chains or serum amyloid protein.[88,92,99–101]

## Stromal hyaline bodies

Small (15–20 μm) eosinophilic hyaline bodies are sometimes observed within the muscular wall of the seminal vesicles, vas deferens, and prostate, and are designated stromal hyaline bodies (Fig. 10-5).[19,102,103] These round to oval structures probably result from degeneration of smooth muscle fibers, and transition forms can be seen arising from smooth muscle cells. They stain red with Masson trichrome and pink with PAS, but fail to stain with PTAH, methyl green pyronine, Feulgen, Alcian blue at pH 2.5, or Congo red.

## Fibrosis

Rarely, seminal vesicle fibrosis may be associated with retroperitoneal fibrosis and mediastinal fibrosis.[104]

## Inflammation

Seminal vesiculitis is associated with infection and inflammation of adjacent organs, including the prostate, bladder, ejaculatory ducts, vas deferens, and epididymis.[105] Acute vesiculitis is usually caused by retrograde infection with or without indwelling catheter, ureteral or ejaculatory duct stenosis or anatomic anomaly, calculi, or surgical trauma (Fig. 10-6). Studies in rats have shown that the seminal vesicles are highly resistant to infection unless their secretory capability is reduced, as occurs with androgen deprivation.[106] Antibiotic therapy is usually effective, employing the same agents used for acute prostatitis; biopsies are rarely obtained in such cases and may be contraindicated because of complications of abscess formation and stricture. Protracted acute and chronic seminal vesiculitis results in atrophy and ejaculatory duct stricture. Abscess presents with irritative voiding symptoms, fever, and pain in the scrotum, testis, perineum, or rectum; purulent ejaculation may also occur.[107] Ultrasonography, coaxial CT scans, and MRI are useful in verifying the diagnosis and directing transurethral incision and drainage.[108,109]

Chronic vesiculitis is associated with chronic prostatitis, and both respond poorly to antibiotic therapy. Before the antibiotic era, the most common cause of vesiculitis was tuberculosis, which resulted in perineal fistula, fibrous adhesions, ejaculatory duct stricture, and massive circumferential calcification of the walls of the seminal vesicles at the site of previous necrotizing granulomas. Malakoplakia should be excluded.[110] Seminal vesicle dilation and congestion may occur after prostatectomy, resulting in persistent dysuria.[111]

Schistosomiasis, usually secondary to *Schistosoma haematobium* infection of the bladder, involves the seminal vesicles more commonly than the prostate. Viruses (e.g., cytomegalovirus[112]), fungi, and parasites are rare causes of seminal vesiculitis. Echinococcal cysts of the seminal vesicles and prostate have been reported.[72] Rare cases of localized necrotizing vasculitis have been described.[113]

Surgery for seminal vesiculitis is unnecessary unless complicated by abscess, fistula, or stricture. In the early 1900s, the seminal vesicles were thought to be the cause of inflammatory rheumatoid disease, and perineal seminal vesiculotomy was popular at that time. This was also the treatment of choice for vesicular tuberculosis until the advent of antibiotic therapy.

## Calcification and calculi

Calcification often follows seminal vesiculitis, particularly with tuberculosis. Patients with a history of diabetes mellitus or uremia also develop dystrophic calcification of the seminal vesicles and other mesonephric derivatives. Most foci of calcification are idiopathic and asymptomatic, and imaging studies of the pelvis may detect them incidentally (Fig. 10-7). Calcification may be unilateral or bilateral and usually coexists with calcification of the vas deferens.[114–122] Calcification is present within the muscular wall, often forming concentric rings; the mucosa is rarely involved. Osseous metaplasia is also rarely observed in the wall (see Fig. 10-7).

Calculi are more frequent in the seminal vesicles than in the vas deferens, appearing as variable numbers of brown stones up to 1 cm in diameter (Fig. 10-8). They usually consist of phosphate and carbonate salts. The mechanism of formation is uncertain, but may be due to reflux of urine up the ejaculatory ducts.[123,124] Cutaneous fistula is a rare complication that can be treated by fulguration and lithotripsy.[125]

## Radiation changes

Radiation therapy for prostatic carcinoma causes atrophy and fibrosis of the seminal vesicles and perivesicular fat in

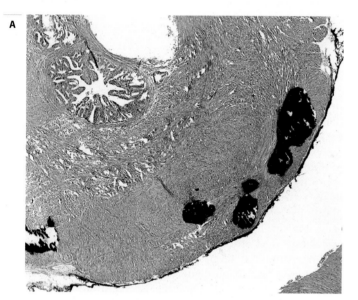
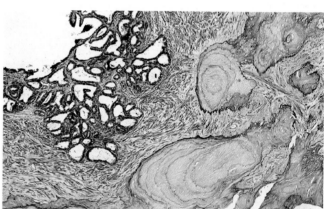

**Fig. 10-7 (A)** Idiopathic mural calcification of the seminal vesicle in a patient undergoing radical prostatoseminovesiculectomy for prostatic adenocarcinoma. **(B)** Osseous metaplasia.

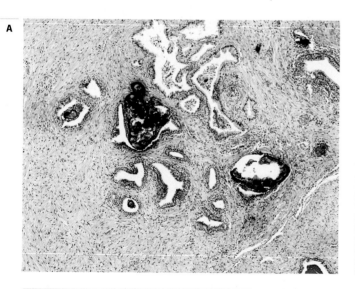
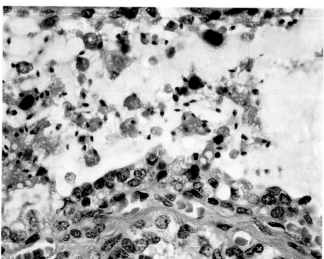

**Fig. 10-8 (A)** Calculi within the seminal vesicular lumen. **(B)** Sperm within the seminal vesicular lumina.

89% of patients.[126] The golden-brown lipochrome pigment characteristic of the seminal vesicle epithelium is retained. MRI shows decreased luminal fluid and stromal fibrosis in about 37% of cases.[127]

# Neoplasms

The seminal vesicles are frequently involved secondarily by tumors originating elsewhere, particularly prostatic carcinoma. However, fewer than 1000 primary neoplasms of the seminal vesicles have been reported. Clinical documentation of many is poor, and the pathologic diagnosis is often questionable.

## Adenocarcinoma

Adenocarcinoma is the most common primary malignancy of the seminal vesicles but is extremely rare, with fewer than 100 acceptable cases reported.[115,128-137] Mean patient age is 62 years (range, 17–90 years), and presenting symptoms include urinary obstruction and hematospermia.[132,133,136] Seminovesiculography and CT are useful in identifying these tumors.

The diagnosis of seminal vesicle adenocarcinoma requires the following: (1) tumor located primarily in the seminal vesicle; (2) no evidence of carcinoma in the prostate, bladder, or colon; (3) architectural features of adenocarcinoma, usually with papillary or sheet-like growth and mucinous differentiation; (4) in situ adenocarcinoma in the adjacent seminal vesicle epithelium; (5) cytoplasmic immunoreactivity for carcinoembryonic antigen (CEA); and (6) absence of staining for prostate-specific antigen (PSA) and prostatic acid phosphatase (PAP).[138] In addition, immunoreactivity for CA-125 may distinguish seminal vesicle adenocarcinoma from a prostatic primary.[139] Some may display weak or focal immunoreactivity for PSA and PAP, so appropriate controls should always be run in parallel.[138] MUC6 is an immunohistochemical marker of seminal vesicle epithelium

(negative in benign prostatic epithelium and adenocarcinoma), but has not been studied in seminal vesicle malignancy.[12] With high-stage poorly differentiated adenocarcinoma, the precise site of origin may be impossible to determine.

Tumor cells may be hobnail, columnar, or polygonal, with clear cytoplasm and rarely lipofuscin. Radical surgery and external beam radiation therapy have been employed in many cases, but the prognosis is poor. Androgen deprivation therapy may also be of value.[140,141]

Two cases of non-invasive well-differentiated adenocarcinoma were reported within seminal vesicle cysts, including one in a 19-year-old with an acquired cyst[132] and another in a 17-year-old with a congenital cyst and ipsilateral renal agenesis.[142] A case of combined seminal vesicle adenocarcinoma, prostatic adenocarcinoma, and carcinosarcoma was reported with autopsy documentation.[143] Primary adenocarcinoma expresses CA-125 immunoreactivity, and serologically fluctuates with growth and recurrence.[144]

Adenocarcinoma of the seminal vesicles and prostate can be induced experimentally in Lobund–Wistar rats using a combination of testosterone propionate and nitrosamine compounds. A recently described system for grading these tumors stratifies them into three groups: in situ, invasive without desmoplasia, and invasive with desmoplasia.[145]

## Metastasis and contiguous spread

Involvement of the seminal vesicles by prostatic adenocarcinoma is common, observed in about 12% of contemporary radical prostatectomy specimens from patients with cancer clinically confined to the prostate (Fig. 10-9). There are three patterns of seminal vesicle invasion: direct spread along the ejaculatory duct complex into the seminal vesicles; prostatic capsular perforation followed by extension into the periprostatic soft tissues and spread into the seminal vesicles; and isolated deposits of cancer in the seminal vesicles (see Chapter 9).[146-149] Endorectal coil MRI is accurate in detecting seminal vesicle invasion according to radical prostatectomy

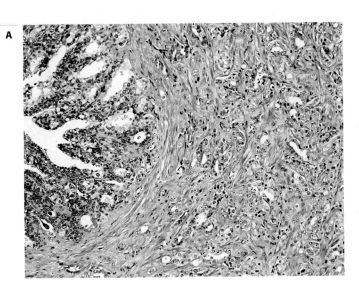
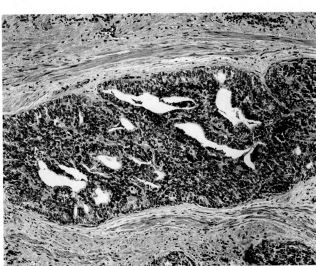

A             B

**Fig. 10-9** Prostatic adenocarcinoma **(A)** invading the seminal vesicles and **(B)** filling the ejaculatory ducts.

correlation studies, with loss of architectural contour as a dominant feature.[150]

Urothelial carcinoma of the bladder may also invade the seminal vesicles by direct extension or mucosal spread,[151] occurring in up to 28% of patients undergoing radical cystectomy.[152] Direct extension is usually observed in cancer of the trigone and inferoposterior wall and indicates pathologic stage T4 cancer. Mucosal involvement by in situ urothelial carcinoma is rare, present in only 1% of cases. It spreads along the mucosa of the prostatic urethra, the prostatic and ejaculatory ducts, and seminal vesicles by intraepithelial replacement and pagetoid spread along the basement membrane.[153] Five-year recurrence-free survival for seminal vesicle involvement was significantly worse than for prostatic involvement (14% vs 68%, respectively).[152]

Rectal adenocarcinoma occasionally invades the seminal vesicles and prostate, and may cause diagnostic difficulty. Metastases to the seminal vesicles and retrovesicular space from other organs are rare, including renal cell carcinoma,[154] seminoma,[155] and malignant thymoma.[156]

## Soft tissue and other tumors

A variety of benign soft tissue tumors have been described in the seminal vesicles, including leiomyoma,[157–160] fibroma, schwannoma,[161,162] paraganglioma[163,164] and solitary fibrous tumor.[165–167] There is a spectrum of mixed epithelial–stromal neoplasms arising in the seminal vesicle, analogous to fibroadenoma and phyllodes tumor in the breast and prostate, and these have been referred to as cystadenoma,[168–173] cystomyoma,[174] low-grade phyllodes tumor,[175] benign mesenchymoma,[176] adenomyosis,[177] and mesonephric hamartoma.[178] Cystadenoma is a rare benign tumor composed of cysts lined by a simple columnar epithelium having chronically inflamed loose fibrous stroma or fibromuscular stroma (Fig. 10-10). The cysts are grossly multiloculated, ranging in size from 5 to 15 cm in diameter. Ultrasound and CT scans reveal a characteristic 'honeycombing' pattern.[179] The patients' average age is 60 years, and most cases are incidental findings at autopsy.[168–171] One case of cystadenoma did not recur in the 25 years after the initial resection (Bostwick, unpublished observation).[171]

Phyllodes tumor consists of a mixture of variably cellular stroma and glandular elements (Fig. 10-11). The density and cytologic features of the stroma determine whether the tumor is a fibroadenoma,[180] low-grade phyllodes tumor, or high-grade phyllodes tumor (cystosarcoma phyllodes).[181] Features considered predictive of malignancy of phyllodes tumor in the breast may apply in the seminal vesicles, including infiltrating margins, stromal atypia, increased numbers of mitotic features, and overgrowth of glands by stroma; however, too few cases have been reported in the seminal vesicles to determine prognosis based on histologic features alone. One case of low-grade phyllodes tumor displayed stromal pleomorphism without mitotic activity; two years after excision the tumor recurred in the pelvis, but did not recur with 18-month follow-up after a second excision.[182] Another report described a benign tumor consisting of glands with epithelium arranged in leaf-like clefts and slits with subepithelial stromal condensation.[171] Fewer than a dozen cases of cystosarcoma phyllodes have been reported,

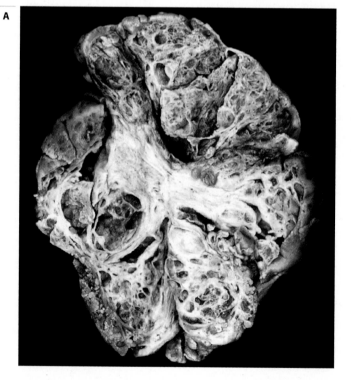

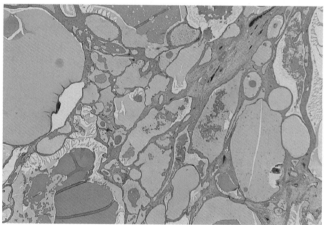

**Fig. 10-10** Cystadenoma of the seminal vesicles. **(A)** Gross. **(B)** Low power.

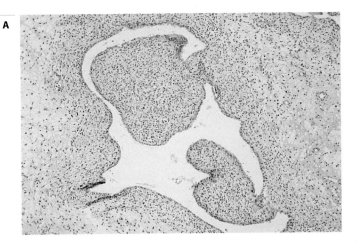
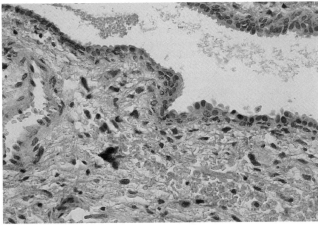

**Fig. 10-11** Cystosarcoma phyllodes of the seminal vesicle. **(A)** At low magnification, there is a proliferation of slit-like epithelial spaces with a cellular stroma. **(B)** At high magnification, the stromal cells display varying degrees of cytologic atypia.

including one that metastasized to the lungs after 5 years despite radical surgery.[175,183,184] This tumor was considered malignant because of its expansive and destructive growth pattern, densely cellular stroma, moderate stromal atypia, focal hemorrhage and necrosis, and numerous mitotic figures. Heterologous differentiation was not apparent histologically or ultrastructurally, although desmin reactivity was observed in 30% of the stromal cells, particularly in the looser myxoid regions, suggesting muscular differentiation.[175] The TRAMP mouse model consistently develops low-grade phyllodes tumor of the seminal vesicles.[185]

Other sarcomas of the seminal vesicle are also rare, including leiomyosarcoma, and usually present with symptoms of pelvic pain, urinary obstruction, rectal obstruction, and symptoms from distant metastases.[186,187] Unlike prostatic sarcoma, seminal vesicle sarcoma rarely presents with hematuria unless the tumor is large and advanced. These tumors grow locally and compress adjacent pelvic organs such as the prostate, bladder, and rectum.[188] Schned et al.[189] reviewed 11 reported cases of primary sarcoma of the seminal vesicle, including leiomyosarcoma, fibrosarcoma, liposarcoma colliding with prostatic carcinoma, 'primary sarcoma,' 'large cell alveolar sarcoma,' 'pleomorphic cell sarcoma,' 'malignant myoblastoma,' leiomyoma of vascular origin with 'some suggestion of malignant potential,' 'round cell sarcoma,' and 'fibrosarcoma with evidence of smooth muscle differentiation by electron microscopy.' Amirkhan et al.[190] reported a high-grade leiomyosarcoma of the right seminal vesicle arising in a 68-year-old man with urinary obstructive symptoms, low back pain, and impending rectal obstruction. The tumor appeared to arise from the muscular wall of the seminal vesicle and displayed immunoreactivity for muscle-specific actin and smooth muscle actin, and focally for keratin AE1/AE3. The patient was well 13 months after radical surgery. Other malignant soft tissue tumors of the seminal vesicle include angiosarcoma,[191,192] fibrosarcoma,[157] and rhabdomyosarcoma.[193,194]

Rare primary germ cell tumors have been reported in the seminal vesicles, presumably caused by midline entrapment of primitive germ cells in the fetus. Primary choriocarcinoma was reported in a 28-year-old, forming a hemorrhagic 12 cm diameter mass; at autopsy, the testes were normal on serial sectioning and no other primary site was found.[195] Primary seminoma was found in a 48-year-old who required cystoprostatectomy; the testes were clinically normal.[196] Primary carcinoid tumor has also been reported in the seminal vesicles.[21] Recurrent adnexal tumor of probable wolffian origin arose in a 20-year-old man.[197]

Primary squamous cell carcinoma was described in a 69-year-old man presenting with a seminal vesicle cyst.[198]

## REFERENCES

1. Aumuller G, Schmitt J, Enderle U, Seitz J. [Immunohistochemical identification of functional relationships in the accessory sex glands]. Anat Anz 1985; 160: 123–131.

2. Clavert A, Cranz C, Bollack C. Functions of the seminal vesicle. Andrologia 1990; 22: 185–192.

3. Ramchandani P, Banner MP, Pollack HM. Imaging of the seminal vesicles. Semin Roentgenol 1993; 28: 83–91.

4. Aumuller G, Riva A. Morphology and functions of the human seminal vesicle. Andrologia 1992; 24: 183–196.

5. Coyne JD, Kealy WF, Annis P. Seminal vesicle epithelium in prostatic needle biopsy specimens. J Clin Pathol 1987; 40: 932.

6. Ibarrola de Andres C, Castellano Megias VM, Perez Barrios A, et al. Seminal vesicle epithelium as a potential pitfall in the cytodiagnosis of presacral masses. A report of two cases. Acta Cytol 2000; 44: 399–402.

7. Nguyen HT, Etzell J, Turek PJ. Normal human ejaculatory duct anatomy: a study of cadaveric and surgical specimens. J Urol 1996; 155: 1639–1642.

8. Shidham VB, Lindholm PF, Kajdacsy-Balla A, et al. Prostate-specific antigen expression and lipochrome pigment granules in the differential diagnosis of prostatic adenocarcinoma versus seminal vesicle-ejaculatory duct epithelium. Arch Pathol Lab Med 1999; 123: 1093–1097.

9. Amin MB, Bostwick DG. Pigment in prostatic epithelium and adenocarcinoma: a potential source of diagnostic confusion with seminal vesicular epithelium. Mod Pathol 1996; 9: 791–795.

10. Lange W, Unger P. Peptidergic innervation with the prostate gland and seminal vesicles. Urol Res 1990; 18: 337–340.

11. Suzuki T, Yamanaka H, Nakajima K. Immunohistochemical study of metallothionein in human seminal vesicles. Tohoku L Exp Med 1992; 167: 127–134.

12. Leroy X, Ballereau C, Villers A, et al. MUC6 is a marker of seminal vesicle-ejaculatory duct epithelium and is useful for the differential diagnosis with prostate adenocarcinoma. Am J Surg Pathol 2003; 27: 519–521.

13. Teraski T, Watanabe H, Kamoi K. Seminal vesicle parameters at 10-year intervals measured by transrectal ultrasonography. J Urol 1993; 150: 914–916.

14. Arber DA, Speights VO. Aneuploidy in benign seminal vesicle epithelium: an example of the paradox of ploidy studies. Mod Pathol 1991; 4: 687–689.

15. Arias-Stella J, Takano-Moron J. Atypical epithelial changes in the seminal vesicle. Arch Pathol 1958; 66: 761–766.

16. Droese M, Voeth C. Cytologic features of seminal vesicle epithelium in aspiration biopsy smears of the prostate. Acta Cytol 1976; 20: 120–125.

17. Droese M, Voeth C, Konetzke C. [The role of cells originating from seminal vesicles in aspiration biopsy smears of the prostate (author's transl)]. Urologe A 1976; 15: 18–20.

18. Koivuniemi A, Tyrkko J. Seminal vesicle epithelium in fine-needle aspiration biopsies of the prostate as a pitfall in the cytologic diagnosis of carcinoma. Acta Cytol 1976; 20: 116–119.

19. Kuo T, Gomez LG. Monstrous epithelial cells in human epididymis and seminal vesicles. A pseudomalignant change. Am J Surg Pathol 1981; 5: 483–490.

20. Mesonero CE, Oertel YC. Cells from ejaculatory ducts and seminal vesicles and diagnostic difficulties in prostatic aspirates. Mod Pathol 1991; 4: 723–726.

21. Soyer P, Rougier P, Gad M, Roche A. Primary carcinoid tumor of the seminal vesicles: CT and MR findings. J Belge Radiol 1991; 74: 117–119.

22. O'Donovan E, Crotty TB, Malone DE, Gibbons D. Seminal vesicle epithelium as a potential pitfall in the cytodiagnosis of presacral masses. Acta Cytol 2001; 45: 893–894.

23. Wojcik EM, Bassler TJ Jr, Orozco R. DNA ploidy in seminal vesicle cells. A potential diagnostic pitfall in urine cytology. Analytical and quantitative cytology and histology. International Academy of Cytology [and] American Society of Cytology. Anal Quant Cytol Histol 1999; 21: 29–34.

24. Meisels A, Ayotte D. Cells from the seminal vesicles: contaminants of the V-C-E smear. Acta Cytol 1976; 20: 211–219.

25. Dominguez C, Boronat F, Cunat E, et al. Agenesis of seminal vesicles in infertile males: ultrasonic diagnosis. Eur Urol 1991; 20: 129–132.

26. Patel B, Gujral S, Jefferson K, et al. Seminal vesicle cysts and associated anomalies. BJU Int 2002; 90: 265–271.

27. Argani P, Walsh PC, Epstein JI. Analysis of the prostatic central zone in patients with unilateral absence of wolffian duct structures: further evidence of the mesodermal origin of the prostatic central zone. J Urol 1998; 160: 2126–2129.

28. Wu HF, Qiao D, Qian LX, et al. Congenital agenesis of seminal vesicle. Asian J Androl 2005; 7: 449–452.

29. Olson JR, Weaver DK. Congenital mesonephric defects in male infants with mucoviscidosis. J Clin Pathol 1969; 22: 725–730.

30. Schnitzer B. Ectopic ureteral opening into seminal vesicle: a report of four cases. J Urol 1965; 93: 576–581.

31. Tokuhara M, Nishio T, Mori Y. [Ectopic ureteral opening into seminal vesicle: Report of a case]. Hinyokika Kiyo 1969; 15: 620–625.

32. Orquiza CS, Bhayani BN, Berry JL, Dahlen CP. Ectopic opening of the ureter into the seminal vesicle: report of case. J Urol 1970; 104: 532–535.

33. Amar E, Trotot P, Baviera E, et al. [Ectopic ureter ending in the seminal vesicle in adults. Apropos of a case and review of the literature]. J Urol Nephrol (Paris) 1979; 85: 113–135.

34. Das S, Amar AD. Ureteral ectopia into cystic seminal vesicle with ipsilateral renal dysgenesis and monorchia. J Urol 1980; 124: 574–575.

35. Williams JL, Sago AL. Ureteral ectopia into seminal vesicle: embryology and clinical presentation. Urology 1983; 22: 594–596.

36. Otani T, Kobayashi M, Kondo A, et al. [Ectopic ureterocele of an adult male]. Hinyokika Kiyo 1984; 30: 1467–1470.

37. Morote Robles J, Palou Redorta J, Conejero Sugranes J, Soler Rosello A. [Ectopic ureter opening into a seminal vesicle]. Actas Urol Esp 1985; 9: 199–200.

38. Pretti G, Minocci D, Monesi G. [Ureteral ectopia in cysts of the seminal vesicle and renal agenesis. Description of a case]. Minerva Urol Nefrol 1988; 40: 171–173.

39. Soler Fernandez JM, Dominguez Bravo C, Herrera Puerto J, et al. [Ectopic ureter in seminal vesicle with cystic dysplasia. A clinical case and review of the literature]. Actas Urol Esp 1990; 14: 447–450.

40. Bittard H, Allouc H, Debiere F, Le Mouel A. [Hydrospermatocyst with ectopic junction of the ureter and ipsilateral renal agenesis. Diagnostic difficulties and contribution of magnetic resonance imaging]. J Urol (Paris) 1995; 101: 97–100.

41. Matsuki M, Matsuo M, Kaji Y, Okada N. Ectopic ureter draining into seminal vesicle cyst: usefulness of MRI. Radiat Med 1998; 16: 309–311.

42. Cabay JE, Lamy S, Dondelinger RF. Ectopic ureter associated with renal dysplasia. JBR-BTR 1999; 82: 228–230.

43. Giglio M, Medica M, Germinale F, Carmignani G. Renal dysplasia associated with ureteral ectopia and ipsilateral seminal vesicle cyst. Int J Urol 2002; 9: 63–66.

44. Radhia S, Samira F, Mounir T, Hamadi S. [Seminal vesicle cyst associated with renal agenesis and ipsilateral ectopic ureter. Report of a case]. Ann Urol (Paris) 2002; 36: 381–383.

45. Heller E, Whitesel JA. Seminal vesicle cysts. J Urol 1963; 90: 305–307.

46. Heetderks DR Jr, Delambre LC. Cyst of the seminal vesicle. J Urol 1965; 93: 725–728.

47. Reddy YN, Winter CC. Cyst of the seminal vesicle: a case report and review of the literature. J Urol 1972; 108: 134–135.

48. Tramoyeres Galvan A, Canovas Ivorra JA, Sanchez Ballester F, et al. [Seminal vesicle cyst. Report of one case and bibliography review]. Arch Esp Urol 2004; 57: 165–168.

49. Beeby DI. Seminal vesicle cyst associated with ipsilateral renal agenesis: case report and review of literature. J Urol 1974; 112: 120–122.

50. Donohue RE, Greenslade NF. Seminal vesicle cyst and ipsilateral renal agenesis. Urology 1973; 2: 66–69.

51. Ejeckam GC, Govatsos S, Lewis AS. Cyst of seminal vesicle associated with ipsilateral renal agenesis. Urology 1984; 24: 372–374.

52. Fuselier HA Jr, Peters DH. Cyst of seminal vesicle with ipsilateral renal agenesis and ectopic ureter: case report. J Urol 1976; 116: 833–835.

53. Juhl M, Larsen KE, Nielsen HV. Bilateral cystic seminal vesicles associated with unilateral renal agenesis. Eur Urol 1983; 9: 319–320.

54. Karamcheti A, Berg G. Seminal vesicle cyst associated with ipsilateral renal agenesis. Urology 1978; 12: 572–574.

55. King BF, Hattery RR, Lieber MM, et al. Seminal vesicle imaging. Radiographics 1989; 9: 653–676.

56. Rappe BJ, Meuleman EJ, Debruyne FM. Seminal vesicle cyst with ipsilateral renal agenesis. Urol Int 1993; 50: 54–56.

57. Zinner A. Ein Fall von Intraavesikaler Samenblasenzyste. Wien Med Wochenschr 1914; 64: 605–607.

58. Verswijvel G, Janssens F, Deroo F, et al. Ureteral ectopy in the seminal vesicle associated with cyst formation and renal dysplasia: contribution of 3D-MRI. JBR-BTR 2004; 87: 175–179.

59. Pascual Samaniego M, Egea Camacho J, Cortinas Gonzalez JR, et al. [Right renal agenesis and ureter ectopic abouchement in cystic dilation of seminal vesicle]. Actas Urol Esp 2004; 28: 688–693.

60. Sheih CP, Li YW, Liao YJ, Hung CS. Bilateral congenital cysts of the seminal vesicle with bilateral duplex kidneys. J Urol 1998; 160: 184–185.

61. Rajfer J, Eggleston JC, Sanders RC, Walsh PC. Fever and prostatic mass in a young man. J Urol 1978; 119: 555–558.

62. Navalon Verdejo P, Pallas Costa Y, Canovas Ivorra JA, et al. [Diagnosis and management of cystic dysplasia of the seminal vesicle]. Actas Urol Esp 2006; 30: 152–158.

63. Chen HW, Huang SC, Li YW, et al. Magnetic resonance imaging of seminal vesicle cyst associated with ipsilateral urinary anomalies. J Formos Med Assoc 2006; 105: 125–131.

64. Mitterberger M, Frausche F, Strasser H, et al. Giant seminal vesicle cyst. Wien Klin Wochenschr 2005; 117: 18.

65. Chuang KL, Lai WI, Chiang YJ. Giant seminal vesicle cyst resembling megaureter with hydronephrosis. Arch Androl 2005; 51: 367–369.

66. Altunrende F, Kim ED, Klein FA, Waters WB. Seminal vesicle cyst presenting as rectal obstruction. Urology 2004; 63: 584–585.

67. Kluckert JT, Zaunbauer W, Diener PA. [Congenial seminal vesicle cyst with an intracystic papillary adenoma associated with ipsilateral renal agenesis]. Radiologe 2002; 42: 837–839.

68. Hart JB. A case of cyst or hydrops of the seminal vesicle. J Urol 1961; 86: 137–141.

69. Ornstein MH, Kershaw DR. Cysts of the seminal vesicle are Mullerian in origin. J Roy Soc Med 1985; 78: 1050–1051.

70. Conn IG, Peeling WB, Clements R. Complete resolution of a large seminal vesicle cyst – evidence for an obstructive aetiology. Br J Urol 1992; 69: 636–639.

71. Inoue K, Higaki Y, Yoshida H. Inguinal hernia of seminal vesicle cyst. Int J Urol 2004; 11: 1039–1040.

72. Deklotz RJ. Echinococcal cyst involving the prostate and seminal vesicles: a case report. J Urol 1976; 115: 116–117.

73. Safioleas M, Stamatakos M, Zervas A, Agapitos E. Hydatid disease of the seminal vesicle: a rare presentation of hydatid cyst. Int Urol Nephrol 2006; 38: 287–289.

74. Papathanasiou A, Voulgaris S, Salpiggidis G, et al. Hydatid cyst of the seminal vesicle. Int J Urol 2006; 13: 308–310.

75. Vasileios R, Athanasios P, Stavros T. Echinococcal cyst of the seminal vesicles: a case-report and literature review. Int Urol Nephrol 2002; 34: 527–530.

76. Emir L, Karabulut A, Balci U, et al. An unusual cause of urinary retention: a primary retrovesical echinococcal cyst. Urology 2000; 56: 856.

77. Pryor JP, Hendry WF. Ejaculatory duct obstruction in subfertile males: analysis of 87 patients. Fertil Steril 1991; 56: 725–730.

78. Furuya S, Kato H. A clinical entity of cystic dilatation of the utricle associated with hemospermia. J Urol 2005; 174: 1039–1042.

79. Hendry WF, Pryor JP. Mullerian duct (prostatic utricle) cyst: diagnosis and treatment in subfertile males. Br J Urol 1992; 69: 79–82.

80. Hendry WF, Rickards D, Pryor JP, Baker LR. Seminal megavesicles with adult polycystic kidney disease. Hum Reprod 1998; 13: 1567–1569.

81. Gevenois PA, Van Sinoy ML, Sintzoff SA Jr, et al. Cysts of the prostate and seminal vesicles: MR imaging findings in 11 cases. AJR Am J Roentgenol 1990; 155: 1021–1024.

82. Salem CE, Gibbs PM, Highshaw RA, et al. Benign ectopic prostatic tissue involving the seminal vesicle in a patient with prostate cancer: recognition and implications for staging. Urology 1996; 48: 490–493.

83. Yamazaki K, Orikasa H. A seminal vesicle cyst complicated with a tumor like nodular mass of benign proliferating prostatic tissue: a case report with ultrastructural and immunohistochemical studies. J Submicrosc Cytol Pathol 2003; 35: 209–214.

84. Fulton RS, Rouse RV, Ranheim EA. Ectopic prostate: case report of a presacral mass presenting with obstructive symptoms. Arch Pathol Lab Med 2001; 125: 286–288.

85. Aslan DL, Pambuccian SE, Gulbahce HE, et al. Prostatic glands and urothelial epithelium in a seminal vesicle cyst: report of a case and review of pathologic features and prostatic ectopy. Arch Pathol Lab Med 2006; 130: 194–197.

86. Bursell S. Beitrag zur Kenntis der Para-amyloidose in urogenitalen System unter besonderer Berucksichtigung der Sog Senilen Amyloidose in den Samem blaschen und ihres Verhaltnisses zum Samenblaschen-pigment. Ups Lakaref Forh 1942; 47: 313–326.

87. Goldman H. Amyloidosis of seminal vesicles and vas deferens. Primary localized cases. Arch Pathol 1963; 75: 94–98.

88. Pitkanen P, Westermark P, Cornwell GG 3rd, Murdoch W. Amyloid of the seminal vesicles. A distinctive and common localized form of senile amyloidosis. Am J Pathol 1983; 110: 64–69.

89. Furuya S, Masumori N, Furuya R, et al. Characterization of localized seminal vesicle amyloidosis causing hemospermia: an analysis using immunohistochemistry and magnetic resonance imaging. J Urol 2005; 173: 1273–1277.

90. Harvey I, Tetu B. [Amyloidosis of the seminal vesicles: a local condition with no systemic impact.]. Ann Pathol 2004; 24: 236–240; quiz 27.

91. Unger PD, Wang Q, Gordon RE, et al. Localized amyloidosis of the seminal vesicle. Possible association with hormonally treated prostatic adenocarcinoma. Arch Pathol Lab Med 1997; 121: 1265–1268.

92. Khan A, Ahmed M, Talati J. Seminal vesicle cystic dilatation masquerading as proctalgia fugax. Br J Urol 1989; 64: 428–429.

93. Suess K, Moch H, Epper R, et al. [Heterogeneity of seminal vesicle amyloid. Immunohistochemical detection of lactoferrin and amyloid of the prealbumin-transthyretin type]. Pathologe 1998; 19: 115–119.

94. Carris CK, McLaughlin AP 3rd, Gittes RF. Amyloidosis of the lower genitourinary tract. J Urol 1976; 115: 423–426.

95. Krane RJ, Klugo RC, Olsson CA. Seminal vesicle amyloidosis. Urology 1973; 2: 70–72.

96. Kaji Y, Sugimura K, Nagaoka S, Ishida T. Amyloid deposition in seminal vesicles mimicking tumor invasion from bladder cancer: MR findings. J Comput Assist Tomogr 1992; 16: 989–991.

97. Ramchandani P, Schnall MD, LiVolsi VA, et al. Senile amyloidosis of the seminal vesicles mimicking metastatic spread of prostatic carcinoma on MR images. AJR Am J Roentgenol 1993; 161: 99–100.

98. Terris MK, Pham TQ, Issa MM, Kabalin JN. Routine transition zone and seminal vesicle biopsies in all patients undergoing transrectal ultrasound guided prostate biopsies are not indicated. J Urol 1997; 157: 204–206.

99. Coyne JD, Kealy WF. Seminal vesicle amyloidosis: morphological, histochemical and immunohistochemical observations. Histopathology 1993; 22: 173–176.

100. Cornwell GG 3rd, Westermark GT, Pitkanen P, Westermark P. Seminal vesicle amyloid: the first example of exocrine cell origin of an amyloid fibril precursor. J Pathol 1992; 167: 297–303.

101. Seidman JD, Shmookler BM, Connolly B, Lack EE. Localized amyloidosis of seminal vesicles: report of three cases in surgically obtained material. Mod Pathol 1989; 2: 671–675.

102. Kovi J, Jackson MA, Akberzie ME. Unusual smooth muscle change in the prostate. Arch Pathol Lab Med 1979; 103: 204–205.

103. Madara JL, Haggitt RC, Federman M. Intranuclear inclusions of the human vas deferens. Arch Pathol Lab Med 1978; 102: 648–650.

104. Taniguchi T, Kobayashi H, Fukui S, et al. A case of multifocal fibrosclerosis involving posterior mediastinal

fibrosis, retroperitoneal fibrosis, and a left seminal vesicle with elevated serum IgG4. Hum Pathol 2006; 37: 1237–1239; author reply 9.

105. Krishnan R, Heal MR. Study of the seminal vesicles in acute epididymitis. Bri J Urol 1991; 67: 632–637.

106. Maglione M, Nardi A, Cranz C, et al. Acute vesiculitis and its prostatic complications caused by E. coli in the rat. Urol Res 1986; 14: 265–266.

107. Monzo JI, Lledo Garcia E, Cabello Benavente R, et al. [Primary seminal vesicle abscess: diagnosis and treatment by transrectal ultrasound]. Actas Urol Esp 2005; 29: 523–525.

108. Chandra I, Doringer E, Sarica K, et al. Bilateral seminal vesicle abscesses. Eur Urol 1991; 20: 164–166.

109. Fox CW Jr, Vaccaro JA, Kiesling VJ Jr, Belville WD. Seminal vesicle abscess: the use of computerized coaxial tomography for diagnosis and therapy. J Urol 1988; 139: 384–385.

110. Sanchez Chapado M, Angulo Cuesta J, Guil Cid M, et al. [Malakoplakia of the prostate and seminal vesicle. Ultrastructural study and review of the literature]. Arch Esp Urol 1995; 48: 775–778.

111. Cytron S, Baniel J, Kessler O, et al. Seminal vesicle congestion as a cause of postprostatectomy dysuria. Eur Urol 1993; 24: 327–331.

112. Kimura M, Maekura S, Satou T, Hashimoto S. [Cytomegaloviral inclusions detected in the seminal vesicle, ductus deferens and lungs in an autopsy case of lung cancer]. Rinsho Byori 1993; 41: 1059–1062.

113. Argani P, Carter HB, Epstein JI. Isolated vasculitis of the seminal vesicle. Urology 1998; 52: 131–133.

114. Bacic J, Kuzmic M. Spermolithiasis. Int Urol Nephrol 1975; 7: 235–239.

115. Camiel MR. Calcification of vas deferens associated with diabetes. J Urol 1961; 86: 634–636.

116. Culver GJ, Tannenhaus J. Calcification of the vas deferens in diabetes. JAMA 1960; 173: 648–651.

117. George S. Calcification of the vas deferens and the seminal vesicles. JAMA 1906; 47: 103–105.

118. Grunebaum M. The calcified vas deferens. Israel J Med Sci 1971; 7: 311–314.

119. Kretschmer HL. Calcification of the seminal vesicles. J Urol 1992; 7: 67–71.

120. Marks JH, Ham DP. Calcification of the vas deferens. Am J Roentgenol 1942; 47: 859–863.

121. Silber SJ, McDonald FD. Calcification of the seminal vesicles and vas deferens in a uremic patient. J Urol 1971; 105: 542–544.

122. Wilson JL, Marks JH. Calcification of the vas deferens; its relation to diabetes mellitus and arteriosclerosis. N Engl J Med 1951; 245: 321–325.

123. Li YK. Diagnosis and management of large seminal vesicle stones. Br J Urol 1991; 68: 322–323.

124. Wilkinson AG. Case report: calculus in the seminal vesicle. Pediatr Radiol 1993; 23: 327.

125. Modi PR. Case report: endoscopic management of seminal vesicle stones with cutaneous fistula. J Endourol 2006; 20: 432–435.

126. Bostwick DG, Egbert BM, Fajardo LF. Radiation injury of the normal and neoplastic prostate. Am J Surg Pathol 1982; 6: 541–551.

127. Chan TW, Kressel HY. Prostate and seminal vesicles after irradiation: MR appearance. J Magn Reson Imaging 1991; 1: 503–511.

128. Vainberg ZS, IuN I. [Carcinoma of the seminal vesicle (a case report).]. Vopr Onkol 1964; 10: 117–119.

129. Smith BA Jr, Webb EA, Price WE. Carcinoma of the seminal vesicle. J Urol 1967; 97: 743–750.

130. Saidinejad H. [Primary seminal vesicle carcinoma]. Zeitschr Urol Nephrol 1970; 63: 697–702.

131. Tanaka T, Takeuchi T, Oguchi K, et al. Primary adenocarcinoma of the seminal vesicle. Hum Pathol 1987; 18: 200–202.

132. Atobe T, Naoe S, Taguchi K, et al. [Primary seminal vesicle carcinoma in a 19-year-old male]. Gan No Rinsho 1984; 30: 205–214.

133. Benson RC Jr, Clark WR, Farrow GM. Carcinoma of the seminal vesicle. J Urol 1984; 132: 483–485.

134. Chinoy RF, Kulkarni JN. Primary papillary adenocarcinoma of the seminal vesicle. Indian J Cancer 1993; 30: 82–84.

135. Dalgaard JB, Giertsen JC. Primary carcinoma of the seminal vesicle; case and survey. Acta Pathol Microbiol Scand 1956; 39: 255–267.

136. Thiel R, Effert P. Primary adenocarcinoma of the seminal vesicles. J Urol 2002; 168: 1891–1896.

137. Oxley JD, Brett MT, Gillatt DA, Burton P. Seminal vesicle carcinoma. Histopathology 1999; 34: 562–563.

138. Varma M, Morgan M, O'Rourke D, Jasani B. Prostate specific antigen (PSA) and prostate specific acid phosphatase (PSAP) immunoreactivity in benign seminal vesicle/ejaculatory duct epithelium: a potential pitfall in the diagnosis of prostate cancer in needle biopsy specimens. Histopathology 2004; 44: 405–406.

139. Ormsby AH, Haskell R, Jones D, Goldblum JR. Primary seminal vesicle carcinoma: an immunohistochemical analysis of four cases. Mod Pathol 2000; 13: 46–51.

140. Gohji K, Kamidono S, Okada S. Primary adenocarcinoma of the seminal vesicle. Br J Urol 1993; 72: 514–515.

141. Williamson RC, Slade N, Feneley RC. Seminal vesicle tumours. J Roy Soc Med 1978; 71: 286–288.

142. Okada Y, Tanaka H, Takeuchi H, Yoshida O. Papillary adenocarcinoma in a seminal vesicle cyst associated with ipsilateral renal agenesis: a case report. J Urol 1992; 148: 1543–1545.

143. Zenklusen HR, Weymuth G, Rist M, Mihatsch MJ. Carcinosarcoma of the prostate in combination with adenocarcinoma of the prostate and adenocarcinoma of the seminal vesicles. A case report with immunocytochemical analysis and review of the literature. Cancer 1990; 66: 998–1001.

144. Ohmori T, Okada K, Tabei R, et al. CA125-producing adenocarcinoma of the seminal vesicle. Pathol Int 1994; 44: 333–337.

145. Slayter MV, Anzano MA, Kadomatsu K, et al. Histogenesis of induced prostate and seminal vesicle carcinoma in Lobund–Wistar rats: a system for histological scoring and grading. Cancer Res 1994; 54: 1440–1445.

146. Epstein JI, Partin AW, Potter SR, Walsh PC. Adenocarcinoma of the prostate invading the seminal vesicle: prognostic stratification based on pathologic parameters. Urology 2000; 56: 283–288.

147. Mukamel E, deKernion JB, Hannah J, et al. The incidence and significance of seminal vesicle invasion in patients with adenocarcinoma of the prostate. Cancer 1987 15; 59: 1535–1538.

148. Ohori M, Scardino PT, Lapin SL, et al. The mechanisms and prognostic significance of seminal vesicle involvement by prostate cancer. Am J Surg Pathol 1993; 17: 1252–1261.

149. Villers AA, McNeal JE, Redwine EA, et al. Pathogenesis and biological significance of seminal vesicle invasion in prostatic adenocarcinoma. J Urol 1990; 143: 1183–1187.

150. Sala E, Akin O, Moskowitz CS, et al. Endorectal MR imaging in the evaluation of seminal vesicle invasion: diagnostic accuracy and multivariate feature analysis. Radiology 2006; 238: 929–937.

151. Ro JY, Ayala AG, el-Naggar A, Wishnow KI. Seminal vesicle involvement by in situ and invasive transitional cell carcinoma of the bladder. Am J Surg Pathol 1987; 11: 951–958.

152. Daneshmand S, Stein JP, Lesser T, et al. Prognosis of seminal vesicle involvement by transitional cell carcinoma of the bladder. J Urol 2004; 172: 81–84.

153. Montie JE, Wojno K, Klein E, et al. Transitional cell carcinoma in situ of the seminal vesicles: 8 cases with discussion of pathogenesis, and clinical and biological implications. J Urol 1997; 158: 1895–1898.

154. Yamamoto S, Mamiya Y, Noda K, et al. [A case of metastasis to the seminal vesicle of renal cell carcinoma]. Nippon Hinyokika Gakkai Zasshi 1998; 89: 563–566.

155. Adachi Y, Rokuiyo M, Kojima H. Nagashima K. Primary seminoma of the seminal vesicle: report of a case. J Urol 1991; 146: 857–859.

156. Tas F, Agan M, Tenekeci N, Topuz E. Retrovesical soft-tissue metastasis of malignant thymoma: case report. Am J Clin Oncol 2003; 26: 366–368.

157. Buck AC, Shaw RE. Primary tumours of the retro-vesical region with special reference to mesenchymal tumours of the seminal vesicles. Br J Urol 1972; 44: 47–50.

158. Gentile AT, Moseley HS, Quinn SF, et al. Leiomyoma of the seminal vesicle. J Urol 1994; 151: 1027–1029.

159. Tambo M, Fujimoto K, Hoshiyama F, et al. [A case of retrovesical leiomyoma]. Hinyokika Kiyo 2004; 50: 497–499.

160. Vigano P, Bonacina P, Strada GR. Leiomyoma of the seminal vesicles. Arch Ital Urol Androl 2003; 75: 230–231.

161. Latchamsetty KC, Elterman L, Coogan CL. Schwannoma of a seminal vesicle. Urology 2002; 60: 515.

162. Iqbal N, Zins J, Klienman GW. Schwannoma of the seminal vesicle. Conn Med 2002; 66: 259–260.

163. Ali-el-Dein B, el-Sobky E, el-Baz M, Shaaban AA. Abdominal and pelvic extra-adrenal paraganglioma: a review of literature and a report on 7 cases. In Vivo 2002; 16: 249–254.

164. Taue R, Takigawa H, Sinotou K, et al. A case of pelvic malignant paraganglioma. Int J Urol 2001; 8: 715–718.

165. Wiessner D, Dittert DD, Manseck A, Wirth MP. Large solitary fibrous tumor of the seminal vesicle. Urology 2003; 62: 941.

166. Westra WH, Grenko RT, Epstein J. Solitary fibrous tumor of the lower urogenital tract: a report of five cases involving the seminal vesicles, urinary bladder, and prostate. Hum Pathol 2000; 31: 63–68.

167. Morin G, Houlgatte A, Camparo P, et al. [Solitary fibrous tumor of the seminal vesicles: apropos of a case]. Prog Urol 1998; 8: 92–94.

168. Damjanov I, Apic R. Cystadenoma of seminal vesicles. J Urol 1974; 111: 808–809.

169. Lundhus E, Bundgaard N, Sorensen FB. Cystadenoma of the seminal vesicle. A case report. Scand J Urol Nephrol 1984; 18: 341–342.

170. Mazzucchelli L, Studer UE, Zimmermann A. Cystadenoma of the seminal vesicle: case report and literature review. J Urol 1992; 147: 1621–1624.

171. Soule EH, Dockerty MB. Cystadenoma of the seminal vesicle, a pathologic curiosity. Report of a case and review of the literature concerning benign tumors of the seminal vesicle. Mayo Clinic Proc 1951; 26: 406–414.

172. Santos LD, Wong CS, Killingsworth M. Cystadenoma of the seminal vesicle: report of a case with ultrastructural findings. Pathology 2001; 33: 399–402.

173. Baschinsky DY, Niemann TH, Maximo CB, Bahnson RR. Seminal vesicle cystadenoma: a case report and literature review. Urology 1998; 51: 840–845.

174. Plaut A. Cystomyoma of the seminal vesicle. Ann Surg 1944; 199: 253–261.

175. Fain JS, Cosnow I, King BF, et al. Cystosarcoma phyllodes of the seminal vesicle. Cancer 1993; 71: 2055–2061.

176. Islam M. Benign mesenchymoma of seminal vesicles. Urology 1979; 13: 203–205.

177. Fujisawa M, Ishigami J, Kamidono S, Yamanaka N. Adenomyosis of the seminal vesicle with hematospermia. Hinyokika Kiyo 1993; 39: 73–76.

178. Kinas H, Kuhn MJ. Mesonephric hamartoma of the seminal vesicle: a rare cause of a retrovesical mass. NY State Med 1987; 87: 48–49.

179. Lagalla R, Zappasodi F, Lo Casto A, Zenico T. Cystadenoma of the seminal vesicle: US and CT findings. Abdom Imag 1993; 18: 298–300.

180. Zanetti GR, Gazzano G, Trinchieri A, et al. A rare case of benign fibroepithelial tumor of the seminal vesicle. Arch Ital Urol Androl 2003; 75: 164–165.

181. Son HJ, Jeong YJ, Kim JH, Chung MJ. Phyllodes tumor of the seminal vesicle: case report and literature review. Pathol Int 2004; 54: 924–929.

182. Mazur MT, Myers JL, Maddox WA. Cystic epithelial–stromal tumor of the seminal vesicle. Am J Surg Pathol 1987; 11: 210–217.

183. Laurila P, Leivo I, Makisalo H, et al. Mullerian adenosarcoma-like tumor of the seminal vesicle. A case report with immunohistochemical and ultrastructural observations. Arch Pathol Lab Med 1992; 116: 1072–1076.

184. Abe H, Nishimura T, Miura T, et al. Cystosarcoma phyllodes of the seminal vesicle. Int J Urol 2002; 9: 599–601.

185. Tani Y, Suttie A, Flake GP, et al. Epithelial–stromal tumor of the seminal vesicles in the transgenic adenocarcinoma mouse prostate model. Vet Pathol 2005; 42: 306–314.

186. Agrawal V, Kumar S, Sharma D, et al. Primary leiomyosarcoma of the seminal vesicle. Int J Urol 2004; 11: 253–255.

187. Muentener M, Hailemariam S, Dubs M, et al. Primary leiomyosarcoma of the seminal vesicle. J Urol 2000; 164: 2027.

188. Tripathi VN, Dick VS. Primary sarcoma of the urogenital system in adults. J Urol 1969; 101: 898–904.

189. Schned AR, Ledbetter JS, Selikowitz SM. Primary leiomyosarcoma of the seminal vesicle. Cancer 1986; 57: 2202–2206.

190. Amirkhan RH, Molberg KH, Wiley EL, et al. Primary leiomyosarcoma of the seminal vesicle. Urology 1994; 44: 132–135.

191. Chiou RK, Limas C, Lange PH. Hemangiosarcoma of the seminal vesicle: case report and literature review. J Urol 1985; 134: 371–373.

192. Lamont JS, Hesketh PJ, de las Morenas A, Babayan RK. Primary angiosarcoma of the seminal vesicle. J Urol 1991; 146: 165–167.

193. Sanghvi DA, Purandare NC, Jambhekar NA, et al. Primary rhabdomyosarcoma of the seminal vesicle. Br J Radiol 2004; 77: 159–160.

194. Berger AP, Bartsch G, Horninger W. Primary rhabdomyosarcoma of the seminal vesicle. J Urol 2002; 168: 643.

195. Fairey AE, Mead GM, Murphy D, Theaker J. Primary seminal vesicle choriocarcinoma. Br J Urol 1993; 71: 756–757.

196. Adachi Y, Rokujyo M, Kojima H, Nagashima K. Primary seminoma of the seminal vesicle: report of a case. J Urol 1991; 146: 857–859.

197. Middleton LP, Merino MJ, Popok SM, et al. Male adnexal tumour of probable Wolffian origin occurring in a seminal vesicle. Histopathology 1998; 33: 269–274.

198. Tabata K, Irie A, Ishii D, et al. Primary squamous cell carcinoma of the seminal vesicle. Urology 2002; 59: 445.

# CHAPTER 11

# Urethra

Victor E. Reuter

THE LIBRARY
THE LEARNING AND DEVELOPMENT CENTRE
THE CALDERDALE ROYAL HOSPITAL
HALIFAX HX3 0PW

# Embryologic development and normal anatomy

The urethra conveys urine from the urinary bladder to the exterior through the external urethral meatus. In males, it also serves as a conduit for semen. The epithelium of the urethra is derived from the urogenital sinus, which is formed when the endodermal cloaca divides into the rectum dorsally and the urogenital sinus ventrally, separated by the urorectal septum.[1] In females, the epithelium of the urethra is derived from endoderm of the urogenital sinus, and the surrounding connective tissue and smooth muscle arise from splanchnic mesenchyme. In males, the epithelium also is derived from the urogenital sinus, except in the fossa navicularis, where it is derived from ectodermal cells migrating from the glans penis. As in females, the connective tissue and smooth muscle surrounding the male urethra is derived from splanchnic mesenchyme.

In men, the urethra is 15–20 cm long and is divided into three anatomic segments (Fig. 11-1). The prostatic urethra is approximately 3–4 cm long and begins at the internal orifice at the bladder neck and extends through the prostate to the prostatic apex.[2] Most prostatic ducts open along the posterior and lateral walls of the prostatic urethra adjacent to the urethral crest, the longitudinal ridge along the dorsal wall of the prostatic urethra. In the central part of the urethral crest is an eminence called the verumontanum or colliculus seminalis. The verumontanum contains a slit-like opening that leads to an epithelial-lined sac called the prostatic utricle, a müllerian vestige. The ejaculatory ducts empty into the urethra on either side of the prostatic utricle. The membranous urethra is the shortest segment, only 1 cm long. It extends from the prostatic apex to the bulb of the penis, traversing the musculature of the urethral sphincter and inferior fascia of the urogenital diaphragm. Cowper's glands, small paired bulbomembranous urethral glands, are located on the left and right sides of the membranous urethra and secrete into it.[2–6] The penile urethra is the longest segment (10–15 cm) and extends from the lower surface of the urogenital diaphragm to the urethral meatus in the glans penis. The orifices of the bulbomembranous urethral glands are located on the lateral surfaces of the proximal (bulbous) portion of the penile urethra. The penile urethra is surrounded by the corpus spongiosum along its length. Scattered mucus-secreting periurethral glands (Littré glands) are present at the periphery of the penile urethra except anteriorly.

The female urethra is approximately 4 cm long (Fig. 11-2). At its periphery are paraurethral glands (Skene's glands), which empty into the urethra through two ducts near the external urethral orifice.

The type of epithelium lining the urethra varies along its length.[2–4] In general, urothelium lines the prostatic urethra; pseudostratified columnar epithelium lines the membranous segment and most of the penile urethra; and non-keratinized stratified squamous epithelium lines the fossa navicularis and external urethral orifice. In females, the proximal one-third of the urethra is lined by urothelium and the distal two-thirds by non-keratinized stratified squamous epithelium. However, it should be remembered that most urethral tissue submitted for surgical pathologic examination is diseased or altered by instrumentation, both of which may cause metaplastic changes.

The lymphatic drainage of the male urethra arises from a rich mucosal network that extends the entire length of the urethra.[5] This network is continuous proximally with that of the prostate and urinary bladder, and distally with that of the penis. The lymphatics of the prostatic and bulbomembranous segments drain to the obturator and medial external iliac lymph nodes, whereas those of the distal penile urethra drain to the superficial inguinal nodes. In females, the proximal urethra drains to the external iliac, hypogastric, and obturator lymph nodes. The distal urethral lymphatics communicate freely with vulvar lymphatics and drain to the superficial inguinal nodes.

# Congenital anomalies

## Urethral valves

Several congenital anomalies may affect the urethra, but are rarely encountered by surgical pathologists. Urethral valves

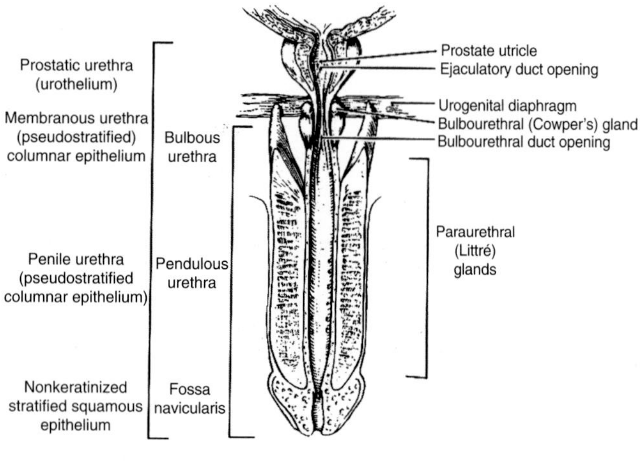

**Fig. 11-1** Anatomy of the male urethra.

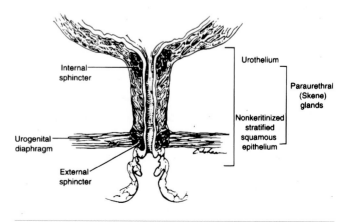

**Fig. 11-2** Anatomy of the female urethra.

are mucosal folds that project into the urethral lumen and may cause obstruction, hematuria, or inflammatory symptoms; although they are usually asymptomatic.[7,8] Urethral valves are usually covered by normal urothelium but may be inflamed. The submucosa may also be inflamed and edematous. The so-called posterior urethral valves, usually seen in adult males, are associated with bladder neck hypertrophy.[7] A recent study reported prenatal diagnosis in monochorionic twins.[9]

## Urethral diverticula

Urethral diverticula are uncommon and often overlooked or misinterpreted. The overwhelming majority occur in women.[10–13] They may be asymptomatic, but can present with irritative symptoms or dribbling, sometimes with localized pain. On physical examination, diverticula present as a paraurethral mass that can sometimes be palpated through the vagina. It is thought that urethral diverticula may be either acquired or congenital, but there are no clear morphologic criteria to make this distinction. The majority of urethral diverticula in adults are acquired as sequelae of infection, trauma, calculus,[14] obstruction, dilation, or inflammation of a paraurethral gland.[12,13,15]

Diverticula are usually lined by urothelium, although this often undergoes squamous or glandular metaplasia. Nephrogenic adenoma may also arise in diverticula.[16] The submucosa is often edematous and inflamed. Most patients with clinically apparent urethral diverticula have a major complication such as infection, stricture,[17] lithiasis with subsequent obstruction, or carcinoma (Fig. 11-3).[12,18] The percentage of urethral diverticula that develop cancer is unclear, with reported incidences ranging from 2% to 15% of symptomatic diverticula.[19,20] Carcinoma that develops in this setting is usually squamous cell carcinoma or adenocarcinoma, but may also be urothelial.[21] Adenocarcinoma may be of the conventional type[22,23] or the clear cell type (see section on clear cell adenocarcinoma later in this chapter).

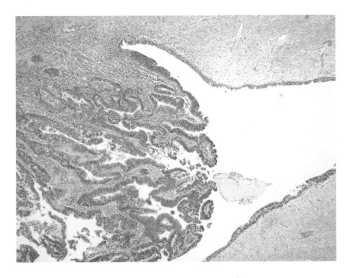

**Fig. 11-3** Adenocarcinoma arising in a urethral diverticulum. Note transition from normal urothelium to adenocarcinoma in situ.

The main differential consideration for diverticulum is urethral cyst.[24,25] An unusual case of endometriosis presented in a woman as a diverticulum.[26]

## Duplication of the urethra

Duplication of the urethra is rare and usually comes to the attention of the surgical pathologist at autopsy.[27–29] The first description of a case of duplication of the urethra is attributed to Aristotle. Duplication may be complete, extending from the bladder to the dorsum of the penis,[28] or partial, extending from the dorsal surface or, less commonly, the ventral surface of the penis and ending blindly. Only 15% of cases of duplicated urethra, whether complete or partial, connect with the functional urethra. Most cases are asymptomatic, but the most common complication is infection. Patients may have urinary obstruction caused by compression of the functional urethra by a mass of desquamated material in the blind accessory urethra. In other cases, patients may complain of incontinence or double urinary stream.

## Congenital urethral polyp

Also known as fibroepithelial polyp, congenital urethral polyp, a rare lesion, occurs almost exclusively in males.[30–38] Patients usually come to clinical attention between the ages of 3 and 9 years, but may rarely present during infancy or adulthood.[7] For this reason, it has been suggested that congenital urethral polyp is secondary to a poorly understood congenital defect in the urethral wall. Congenital urethral polyp usually arises in the prostatic urethra adjacent to the verumontanum (posterior urethral polyp). Signs and symptoms include hematuria, difficulty voiding, urinary retention, and infection. Symptoms are similar to those of other obstructing urethral lesions, including urethral valve, stricture, and lithiasis.

Morphologically, congenital urethral polyp is covered by urothelium that may be inflamed, ulcerated, or exhibit squamous metaplasia. This differs from the more common prostatic urethral polyp occurring in adults that is covered by prostatic epithelium (see section entitled Ectopic prostatic tissue and prostatic urethral polyp, below).

Anterior urethral polyp is extremely rare and arises in the membranous or penile urethra.[36] It produces the same symptoms and has the same morphology as posterior polyp. The subepithelial stroma consists of loose fibrous tissue that may be highly vascular and may contain a few fascicles of smooth muscle. If it has a long stalk, it may 'telescope' into the bladder and produce bladder outlet obstruction.

Polyps in prepubertal girls and women probably arise from prolapsing urothelium that has evolved into a polyp.[39]

## Non-neoplastic diseases

### Urethritis

Urethritis is defined morphologically as an inflammatory response within the urethra. Men are often asymptomatic, and the diagnosis is made by the presence of a urethral discharge and the finding of neutrophils in the urethral smear. Women are often symptomatic; the symptoms are similar to those of cystitis, including dysuria, urinary urgency, and urinary frequency.[40,41] A urethral smear will also aid the diagnosis in women. Urethritis may be caused by sexually transmissible agents such as *Neisseria gonorrhoeae*, *Chlamydia trachomatis*, *Gardnerella vaginalis*, *Ureaplasma urealyticum*, *Mycoplasma hominis*, *Trichomonas vaginalis*, and *Candida* species. In women, urethritis secondary to *Neisseria*, *Trichomonas* or *Candida* rarely occurs without concomitant cervical infection.[41]

Reiter's syndrome is characterized by the triad of urethritis, conjunctivitis, and arthritis.[42] The etiology is uncertain, but it is usually preceded by an enteric or venereal infection. The syndrome occurs predominantly in men between the ages of 18 and 40, but women are occasionally affected. Urethritis is the most common initial symptom. Other urologic manifestations of Reiter's syndrome include prostatitis and hemorrhagic cystitis. In the acute phase the mucosa appears congested and may contain shallow ulcers. Symptoms commonly subside within 2–4 weeks, but recur at irregular intervals in 50–75% of cases. It is important to recognize that not all involved organ systems may be symptomatic at the same time, so this syndrome should always be included in the differential diagnosis of urethritis in young adults.

## Caruncle

Urethral caruncle is a pedunculated or sessile polypoid lesion located in the distal urethra near the meatus in women. Grossly it has a fleshy, pink-red appearance and bleeds readily (Fig. 11-4). Patients may be asymptomatic, although commonly they experience dysuria, urinary frequency, or obstructive symptoms.[43–45] Three histologic subgroups are described: papillomatous, angiomatous, and granulomatous. This separation is based on the most prominent component (surface epithelial, vascular, and inflammatory, respectively); but this distinction has no apparent clinical relevance. The surface epithelium may be transitional or squamous and is invariably inflamed (Fig. 11-5); caruncles covered by metaplastic columnar epithelium have been reported. The epithelium may be hyperplastic and constitute the bulk of the lesion. The underlying stroma is richly vascular and inflamed, occasionally containing glandular elements thought to be derived from Skene's glands.

Rarely, the stroma of urethral caruncle may contain atypical mesenchymal cells, mimicking sarcoma (pseudosarcomatous fibromyxoid lesion) (Fig. 11-6).[46] The mixed inflammatory infiltrate and rich vascularity, combined with the clinical setting, should establish the correct diagnosis. Pseudosarcomatous fibromyxoid lesion may appear spontaneously or follow a pelvic surgical procedure by weeks or months (postoperative spindle cell nodule) and present not only as a polypoid lesion but also as a paraurethral mass.[47] As with other pseudosarcomatous lesions involving the urothelial tract, the atypical spindle cells are reactive myofibroblasts, which may display cytokeratin, actin, and ALK[48] immunoreactivity. Epithelial membrane antigen is invari-

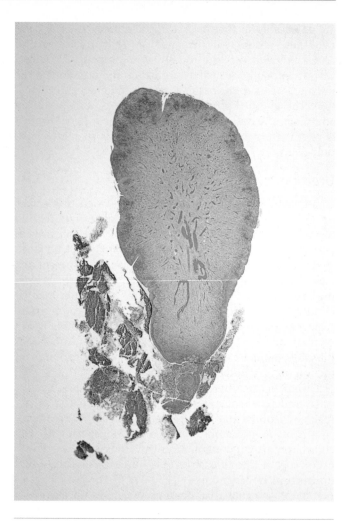

**Fig. 11-4** 'Whole-mount' appearance of caruncle. This reactive erythematous polypoid mass may be confused with a true neoplasm at the time of urethroscopy.

ably negative. Electron microscopy is very helpful in establishing the myofibroblastic component.

## Polypoid urethritis

Polypoid urethritis is the urethral counterpart of polypoid cystitis, although an association with indwelling catheter has not been noted with urethral lesions.[49,50] Polypoid urethritis is a non-neoplastic inflammatory lesion that usually resolves spontaneously after removal of the inflammatory stimulus. It is commonly found in the prostatic urethra near the verumontanum, appearing as single or multiple polypoid or papillary growths. Morphologically, it is characterized by abundant edematous stroma containing distended blood vessels and a chronic inflammatory infiltrate (Fig. 11-7). The overlying urothelium may be ulcerated or exhibit metaplastic and proliferative changes, such as squamous metaplasia, Brunn's nests, or urethritis cystica.[49,50]

Polypoid urethritis does not usually recur after resection unless the cause of the irritation persists. At the time of urethroscopy it may be confused with papillary urothelial

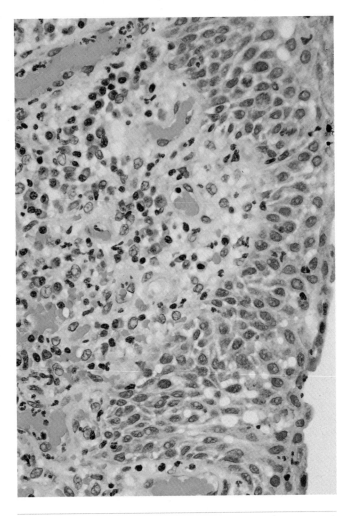

**Fig. 11-5** Caruncle. Inflamed mucosa and lamina propria with extravasated red blood cells and prominent vascularity.

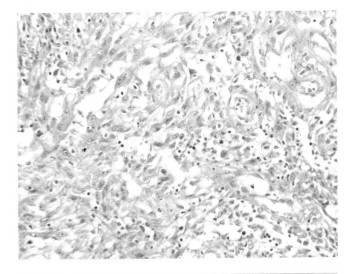

**Fig. 11-6** Pseudosarcomatous fibromyxoid lesion (postoperative spindle cell nodule). The patient developed a hemorrhagic polypoid mass several months after an endoscopic procedure. Note myofibroblasts with epithelioid nuclei and abundant eosinophilic cytoplasm, scattered inflammatory cells, and prominent vascularity.

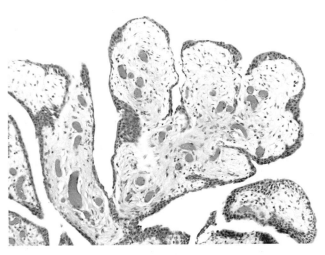

**Fig. 11-7** Polypoid urethritis. This reactive fibroepithelial lesion results from chronic local insult.

tumor, although experienced urologists will recognize it as a benign, reactive, or low-grade lesion and rarely confuse it with high-grade, aggressive neoplasms.

## Nephrogenic adenoma (metaplasia)

Similar to Brunn's nests and urethritis cystica, nephrogenic adenoma is a reactive, proliferative lesion that may occur anywhere along the urothelial tract as a consequence of local irritation.[51-54] It is most common in the urinary bladder, but occasionally arises in the urethra. Nephrogenic adenoma is thought to arise through metaplasia of the urothelium in response to an inflammatory stimulus or local injury, and some researchers prefer the term nephrogenic metaplasia. Often this lesion is an incidental finding at surgery for other reasons. The most common symptom is hematuria. Grossly it appears as flattened, erythematous areas or as discrete papillae. Microscopically, the latter architecture consists of complex papillary structures covered by cuboidal epithelium with basophilic or eosinophilic cytoplasm which may be vacuolated. The nuclei are round to oval, hyperchromatic, centrally located, and may contain small nucleoli. Mitotic figures are uncommon. The same epithelium may form discrete tubules in the underlying stroma. These have distinct lumina that are usually empty but which may contain deeply eosinophilic secretions or pale basophilic material (Fig. 11-8). These tubules are thought to arise through a process of invagination from the surface epithelium, much like Brunn's nests. Each is surrounded by a distinct basement membrane.[51] Infrequently, cuboidal cells are present in the stroma, either singly or in small groups lacking a visible lumen, or they may have a signet ring cell appearance. The luminal secretions may be periodic acid–Schiff positive, diastase resistant, or mucicarminophilic, but intracytoplasmic mucin is less frequent. In a study of 26 cases of nephrogenic adenoma involving the prostatic urethra, Allan et al.[55] found that 77% of cases extended into smooth muscle – not surprising, given the anatomy of this site. The lesion often appears

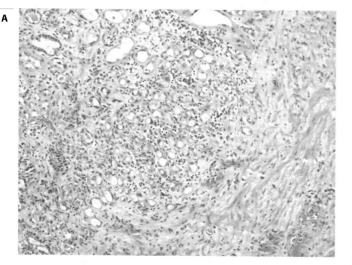

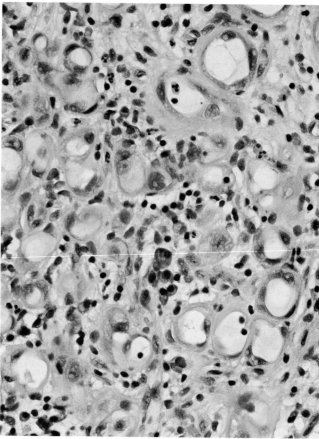

**Fig. 11-8** Nephrogenic 'adenoma.' (**A**) Low-power magnification. (**B**) High-power magnification. Note the small tubules, which may be confused with adenocarcinoma.

infiltrative and may be confused with adenocarcinoma, especially in cases lacking a papillary component and composed primarily of tubules in the stroma. The surrounding stroma may be edematous and inflamed, but there is no desmoplastic reaction to the epithelial cells. Allan et al. reported focal immunoreactivity for PSA and PAP in 36% and 55% of cases, respectively. However, strong cytokeratin 7 positivity, combined with attention to the cytomorphological features, should be sufficient to arrive at the correct diagnosis.[55]

There is no convincing evidence that nephrogenic adenoma is a pre-neoplastic condition, although rare cases coincidentally coexist with or precede the develop-ment of carcinoma.[53] Nevertheless, it is possible that the two have common predisposing conditions and consequently may develop independently. For example, nephrogenic adenoma and adenocarcinoma have been reported in association with urethral diverticulum.[16] Like other proliferative lesions of the urothelium, nephrogenic adenoma may recur after resection if the inflammatory stimulus is not removed.

## Malakoplakia

Malakoplakia is a rare condition that mainly affects the urothelial tract but has also been described in other sites, such as the testes, gastrointestinal tract, and retroperitoneum.[56–58] Although it may occur anywhere along the urothelial mucosa, most cases occur in the urinary bladder and urethral involvement is rare.[59,60] Women are affected more often than men at a ratio of 4:1. Patients usually present with irritative symptoms or urinary obstruction, and endoscopy may reveal an erythematous plaque-like lesion or polypoid or nodular mass that is clinically suggestive of neoplasm. Microscopically, malakoplakia is characterized by a mixed inflammatory infiltrate dominated by histiocytes with abundant granular, eosinophilic cytoplasm (von Hansemann cells). The cytoplasm contains Michaelis–Gutmann bodies, laminated calcospherites that are basophilic and targetoid in appearance, measuring 5–10 μm in diameter. These stain for iron as well as calcium and may occasionally be found within the stroma. The overlying urothelium may be ulcerated, hyperplastic, or metaplastic. In chronic lesions the characteristic infiltrate may be replaced by fibrosis and scar.

The etiology of malakoplakia is unknown, although current knowledge suggests that it is an unusual response to infection, perhaps the result of a disturbed immune response or abnormal macrophage or lysosomal function in the host.[56–58]

## Amyloidosis

The urothelial tract can be involved in cases of systemic amyloidosis but is rarely the primary site of disease.[61-64] In descending order of frequency, amyloid deposits have been described in the urinary bladder, ureter, renal pelvis, and urethra. The usual clinical presentation is hematuria, although dysuria, partial obstruction, or a deviated urinary stream have also been reported. At cystoscopy the lesion may appear anywhere along the urethra as an elevated plaque or mass that is commonly confused with neoplasm. The overlying mucosa may be ulcerated or hyperemic. The amyloid deposits appear as eosinophilic, homogeneous material within the lamina propria, often extending into the underlying muscle and connective tissue. Perivascular amyloid deposits are uncommon in tumoral amyloidosis but common in systemic amyloidosis. Inflammation is usually absent except adjacent to ulcerated mucosa. Special stains, such as Congo red, crystal violet or van Gieson's solution of trinitrophenol and acid fuchsin, are useful in establishing the diagnosis. Localized lesions may be managed by transurethral resection, but cases with diffuse involvement and intractable symptoms may require radical surgery.[65]

## Condyloma acuminatum

Condyloma acuminatum is a common, sexually transmitted infectious squamoproliferative growth caused by human papillomavirus that is not related to squamous papilloma.[66] It usually occurs on the mucocutaneous surfaces of the external genitalia, perineum or anus, but extension into the urethra occurs in up to 20% of cases.[67-70] It is often multifocal or diffuse. Macroscopically, condyloma is smooth, pink-tan, and often papillary. Flat condylomata may be difficult to visualize cystoscopically. Microscopically, it consists of papillary fronds or flat mucosa containing hyperplastic squamous epithelium that may be hyperkeratotic. The squamous epithelial cells typically have clear perinuclear haloes and the nuclei are eccentrically placed, hyperchromatic, pleomorphic (koilocytic atypia) (Fig. 11-9). Many cases can be diagnosed by these morphologic features alone, although in subtle cases the diagnosis can be confirmed by immunohistochemistry, viral culture, in situ hybridization, or polymerase chain reaction.[71-74] The antibodies currently available to identify human papillomavirus are rather insensitive; in situ hybridization and polymerase chain reaction are more sensitive and specific than morphology, even from paraffin-embedded sections.[75] The human papillomavirus serotypes most commonly found in urothelial condylomata are 6, 11, 16, and 18, although high-risk serotypes usually predominate.[70] These often coincide with the type in the patient's sexual partner.[70,73,76]

Condyloma of the urinary tract may cause hematuria and irritative symptoms. Surgical management may include transurethral resection, laser, or cryotherapy, or a more radical procedure, depending on the extent of disease. It is important to remember that condylomata may undergo transformation to verrucous or infiltrating squamous cell carcinoma.[69,72,73]

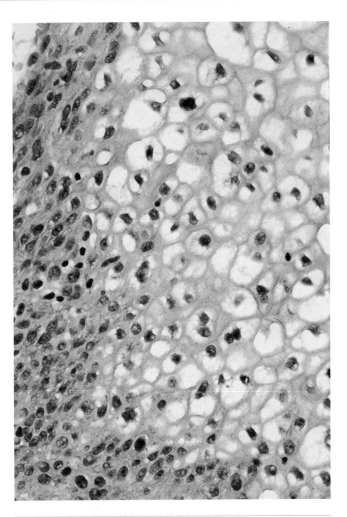

**Fig. 11-9** Condyloma acuminatum. Cells contain vacuolated cytoplasm and irregular nuclei with perinuclear halos.

## Metaplasia of the urothelium

Urothelium frequently undergoes squamous or glandular metaplasia as a response to chronic inflammatory stimuli, such as urinary tract infection, diverticula, calculi, or repeated instrumentation (see Fig. 11-3). This is very common and per se is not pre-neoplastic. Nevertheless, under certain conditions carcinoma may arise in metaplastic epithelium, as in adenocarcinoma or squamous carcinomas arising in diverticula. Glandular metaplasia is more common in the urinary bladder, but may occur along the urethra. The morphology of the metaplastic urothelium is usually tall columnar with goblet cells, strikingly similar to enteric epithelium.

## Ectopic prostatic tissue and prostatic urethral polyp

Prostatic acinar epithelium may line the urothelial tract focally. This is seen mostly in adult men, but occasionally occurs at younger ages.[77-82] This process is most common in the prostatic urethra (prostatic urethral polyp), but has also been described at the bladder neck and in the bulbous and penile urethra.[83-85] This ectopic tissue is usually asymptomatic and discovered at urethroscopy for other causes. Hema-

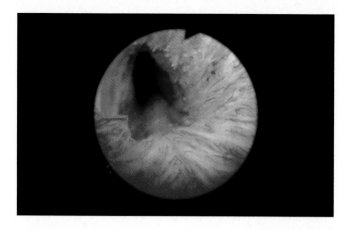

**Fig. 11-10** Prostatic urethral polyp. Endoscopically, the small papillae are clearly identifiable.

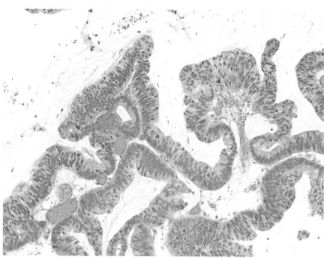

**Fig. 11-12** Urethral implant from urachal adenocarcinoma. After partial cystectomy the patient developed urethral mucosal implants, which were treated by transurethral resection. Given the low-grade appearance of this lesion, it was confused with a prostatic urethral polyp until the pathologist compared it with the original lesion and performed immunohistochemical stains for prostate-specific antigen, which were negative.

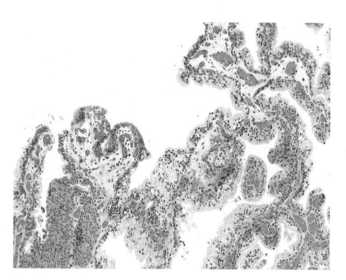

**Fig. 11-11** Prostatic urethral polyp. The urothelium of the prostatic urethra is replaced by papillary fronds lined by benign prostatic acinar cells.

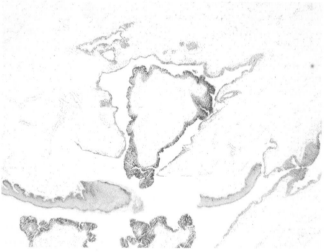

**Fig. 11-13** Benign polyp arising at the fossa navicularis. Immunohistochemical stain for prostate-specific antigen.

turia is the most common symptom. Cystoscopically, the lesions appear as discrete small papillary growths that may be solitary or extensive, producing a velvety coating on the mucosa (Fig. 11-10). The papillary fronds contain a thin fibrovascular core and are covered by prostatic acinar epithelium with abundant clear or faintly eosinophilic apical cytoplasm and small basally located round or oval nuclei without visible nucleoli (Fig. 11-11). Occasionally, foci of residual urothelium are intermingled with the prostatic epithelium. Immunohistochemical stains for prostate-specific antigen are positive.[79,81,83]

The etiology of this phenomenon is controversial. Prostatic urethral polyp probably results from hyperplasia and overgrowth of the overlying urothelium by prostatic acinar epithelium. It is important to examine the underlying prostatic urethral tissue carefully because there may be an associated acinar-type prostatic adenocarcinoma. Also, the cytological features of epithelial cells must be evaluated, as prostatic adenocarcinoma may extend to the mucosal surface

and take on a papillary growth pattern. Rarely, low-grade papillary adenocarcinoma of the bladder or urachus may seed the prostatic urethra, mimicking prostatic urethral polyp (Fig. 11-12). The origin of ectopic prostatic tissue in the penile urethra is less clear and may represent implantation, metaplasia, or an embryologic abnormality (Fig. 11-13). These lesions are benign and, if symptomatic, should be managed conservatively by urethroscopic resection or electrocautery. Urologists commonly see these lesions during endoscopic evaluation for other causes and seldom perform biopsies on them unless they believe they are the source of the patient's symptoms.

# Neoplastic diseases

## Benign neoplasms

### Papilloma

Papilloma, like other papillary urothelial tumors, rarely arises de novo within the urethra. The definition of papilloma has evolved over the years.[86–89] This benign tumor is characterized by discrete exophytic papillary projections with thin fibrovascular cores covered by urothelium indistinguishable from normal urothelium. The urothelial cells maintain their polarity perpendicular to the basement membrane and exhibit abundant eosinophilic cytoplasm, which commonly contains perinuclear vacuoles. Nuclei are elongated or round, depending on the plane of sectioning; they may be slightly enlarged compared to normal urothelium, but show little or no pleomorphism. The chromatin pattern is homogeneous, and nucleoli are absent or small and sparse. Mitotic figures are usually absent, although a few normal mitotic figures may be observed in the basal layer. The thickness of the epithelium (the number of cell layers) is variable owing to the plane of sectioning. Umbrella cells may be prominent and hyperchromatic.[86,87,89]

The main feature of papilloma is its discrete nature and lack of cytologic features of malignancy. Papilloma may rarely recur as carcinoma. Nevertheless, it is incapable of invasion (progression) without showing definitive cytologic and architectural evidence of malignancy. Urothelial papilloma should be managed with transurethral resection alone. Although clinical surveillance is warranted, the optimum interval between visits and the duration of surveillance are not established.

### Inverted papilloma

Inverted papilloma rarely occurs along the urethra, but when it does it shares all the morphologic features of the more common vesicular inverted papilloma.[90,91] Patients usually have hematuria, and on urethroscopy the lesions appear as a polypoid or nodular growth with a smooth, glistening surface. It ranges up to 2.5 cm in diameter[92,93] and is easily confused with carcinoma, even by experienced endoscopists. Microscopically, it is covered by compressed benign invaginated interconnected cords and nests of urothelium that proliferate and expand the lamina propria, giving the lesion its characteristic bulging or polypoid gross appearance.[92] The urothelial cells are cytologically benign but more closely packed than normal because of the endophytic growth pattern. Some cells may be spindle shaped, especially near the center of the cords (Fig. 11-14). Occasionally, the centers of the cords become dilated, forming microcysts lined by flattened or cuboidal cells. Rarely, there is focal squamous metaplasia. The anastomosing cords of urothelium that make up this lesion result from invagination rather than invasion. There is no reactive fibrosis in the surrounding stroma. Mitotic figures are rare and, if present, are normal in the basal layer. Inverted papilloma is well circumscribed.

The etiology of this lesion is controversial. Most investigators conclude that they are neoplasms, but others suggest

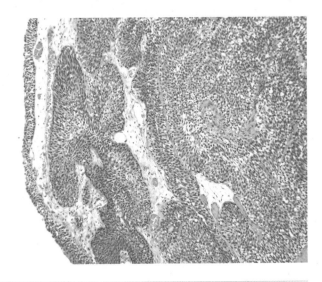

**Fig. 11-14** Inverted papilloma. Anastomosing nests and cords of urothelial cells extend into the periurethral tissue but lack cytologic or architectural evidence of malignancy.

that they are an unusual reactive, proliferative response to inflammation. They are not premalignant, although a few cases have been coincidentally associated with carcinoma.[93] Management of inverted papilloma should be limited to transurethral resection.

## Malignant neoplasms

### Urothelial carcinoma in association with carcinoma of the urinary bladder

Secondary involvement of the urethra by urothelial carcinoma of the bladder is much more common than primary urethral carcinoma. As with vesicular neoplasms, it occurs more often in men. The reported incidence of urethral involvement varies according to the study design and the patient population. For example, an autopsy study by Gowing[94] reported an incidence of 20% in patients who had been treated with cystectomy for bladder cancer. Clinical series have reported the incidence of urethral involvement in patients with bladder cancer to be between 8% and 22%.[95–102] Liedberg and colleagues[103] concluded that the incidence of urothelial carcinoma in the prostatic urethra and prostate is probably underestimated. Recurrent urethral involvement by carcinoma is not an issue in females as total urethrectomy is part of the cystectomy procedure. In males, total urethrectomy is not performed routinely because of the increased morbidity caused by this procedure. It is standard to leave the membranous, bulbous, and penile urethra intact. Recurrence is possible in the immediate postoperative period or as late as 9 years after cystectomy. For this reason, it is important for the clinician to routinely evaluate the urethra by urethroscopy, cytology, flow cytometry, or a combination.[104,105] Most patients with invasive urethral recurrences die within 5 years. Urologists routinely assess the status of the prostatic urethra prior to cystectomy, as most believe that patients with prostatic urethral involvement are not candidates for a 'urethra-sparing' procedure.[101]

**Table 11-1** TNM pathologic staging of primary urethral tumors (male and female)*

| TNM | |
|-----|---|
| pTis | Carcinoma in situ |
| pTa | Non-invasive papillary, polypoid or verrucous carcinoma |
| pT1 | Invasion of submucosa |
| pT2 | Invasion of any of the following structures: corpus spongiosum, prostate, periurethral muscle |
| pT3 | Invasion of any of the following structures: corpus cavernosum, beyond the prostate capsule, anterior vagina, bladder neck |
| pT4 | Invasion into other adjacent organs |

*Pathologic staging refers to the histologic examination and confirmation of extent of disease at the time of attempted total resection. Clinical staging refers to the estimation of the extent of disease by radiographic imaging, cystourethroscopy, palpation, and biopsy or cytology performed prior to definitive extirpative surgery.[108]

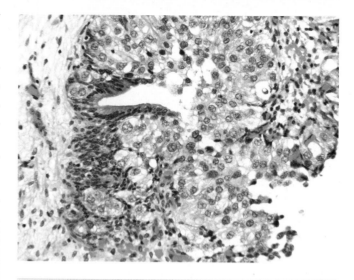

**Fig. 11-15** Urothelial carcinoma of the urinary bladder extending into the urethra. The tumor partially replaces the benign urothelium.

Multifocal papillary carcinoma and multifocal carcinoma in situ in the bladder predispose the patient to urethral involvement or subsequent recurrence. In a study of male patients, DePaepe et al.[106] reported that nine of 20 (45%) cases had involvement of the prostatic duct by urothelial carcinoma at the time of cystoprostatectomy. Carcinoma in situ of the bladder was observed in each of the nine. In a similar study dealing with female patients, four of 22 (18%) had carcinoma in situ in the urethra. These four patients represented 24% of the patients with multifocal carcinoma in situ in the bladder.[107] Interestingly, three of these patients had carcinoma in situ extending into the periurethral glands and 17% of patients with invasive disease in the bladder also had stromal invasion in the urethra. This fact confirms that urethrectomy should be performed along with cystectomy in female patients. Pathologic staging of urothelial carcinoma that involves the prostatic urethra and prostate differs from staging for primary urethral neoplasms (Table 11-1).[108] Microscopically, secondary urethral involvement by urothelial carcinoma may take the form of papillary carcinoma or carcinoma in situ (Fig. 11-15). The tumors may be single or multiple, and may occur at the surgical stump or anywhere along the urethra, including the meatus.[106,107,109]

Papillary urothelial carcinoma is characterized by papillary fronds lined by epithelial cells that show little or no orientation in relation to their basement membrane. The cells are crowded and have variable amounts of eosinophilic cytoplasm with an increased nuclear to cytoplasmic ratio. Nuclei are irregular and contain nucleoli. Mitotic figures may be present, are sometimes atypical, and may be located well above the basal layer. Carcinoma in situ is characterized by flat mucosa containing similarly atypical cells occupying virtually the entire thickness of the mucosa (for a more complete description of papillary and flat urothelial carcinoma please refer to the appropriate section in Chapter 5). Carcinoma in situ may extend into periurethral ducts and glands along the entire length of the urethra as well as into prostatic ducts (Fig. 11-16).[110] It is important for the pathologist to

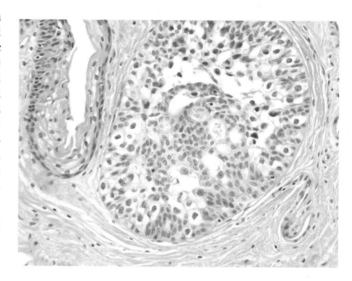

**Fig. 11-16** Urothelial carcinoma extending into periurethral ducts. Duct involvement must be distinguished from stromal invasion.

distinguish between ductal involvement and stromal invasion, as extension into periurethral glands does not affect prognosis, whereas periurethral or prostatic stromal invasion confers a worse prognosis.[95] Although controversial, some investigators advocate transurethral resection with or without instillations with Bacillus Calmette–Guérin as sufficient treatment for patients with intramucosal or periurethral prostatic duct involvement.[111] It is generally agreed that total urethrectomy is the treatment of choice in cases with periurethral involvement.

A subtle but important morphologic pattern of urothelial carcinoma in the urethra is intramucosal pagetoid spread (Fig. 11-17). This pattern occurs most frequently in association with multifocal carcinoma in situ of the bladder and is characterized by individual or small groups of carcinoma cells percolating through an otherwise benign urothe-

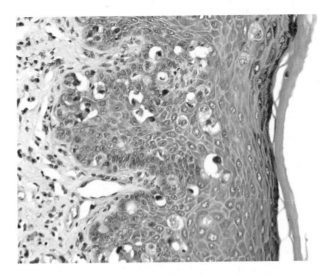

**Fig. 11-17** Pagetoid intramucosal spread of urothelial carcinoma in the membranous urethra. This pattern of spread is most commonly seen in association with multifocal urothelial carcinoma in situ in the urinary bladder.

**Table 11-2** TNM pathologic staging of urothelial carcinoma of the prostate[108]

| | | |
|---|---|---|
| Tis | pu | Carcinoma in situ, involvement of the prostatic urethra |
| Tis | pd | Carcinoma in situ, involvement of the prostatic ducts |
| T1 | | Tumor invades subepithelial connective tissue |
| T2 | | Tumor invades any of the following: prostatic stroma, corpus spongiosum, periurethral muscle |
| T3 | | Tumor invades any of the following: corpus cavernosum, beyond prostatic capsule, bladder neck (extraprostatic extension) |
| T4 | | Tumor invades other adjacent organs (invasion of the bladder |

pu, prostatic urethra; pd, prostatic ducts.

lium.[107,112,113] The carcinoma cells may have minimal or abundant cytoplasm, but have large round or irregular hyperchromatic nuclei with prominent nucleoli that closely resemble the cells of Paget's disease of the breast. The surrounding urothelium often undergoes squamous metaplasia. The tumor cells are unreactive for S100 protein and prostate-specific antigen (PSA). Occasionally, they may be weakly mucicarmine positive. This variant of carcinoma in situ may be seen in the surface urothelium, metaplastic squamous epithelium, or periurethral or prostatic ducts. It is rare in primary urethral carcinoma. For this reason, when this pattern is encountered in a urethral biopsy the differential diagnosis should include urothelial carcinoma arising in the urinary bladder, malignant melanoma, and periurethral or prostatic adenocarcinoma.[114]

### Primary urethral carcinoma

Primary carcinoma of the urethra is rare. The incidence is higher in women than in men[89,99,115,116] and the age distribution is similar to that of other urothelial carcinomas (mean incidence in the seventh decade of life). In general, tumors arising in the proximal (prostatic urethra in males, proximal third in females) have the morphology of typical urothelial cancer, whereas distal carcinomas (membranous, bulbous or penile in men, distal two-thirds in women) are likely to be squamous cell carcinoma. These findings coincide with the epithelial lining in those sites, although it must be remembered that the morphology and anatomic distribution of normal mucosa may be quite variable. This is especially true in patients with irritative symptoms, in whom squamous and glandular metaplasia is quite common. Moreover, it may be morphologically impossible to differentiate moderate to high-grade urothelial carcinoma from non-keratinizing squamous carcinoma. Adenocarcinoma may arise anywhere along the urethra but is most commonly associated with diverticula, prostatic adenocarcinoma, or,

in women, may arise in periurethral glands and extend to the urethral mucosa secondarily. The last is rarely seen in men. Because the incidences of histologic types are different, primary carcinoma in males and females will be discussed separately.

Primary urethral carcinoma is rare in males, a finding emphasized by the paper from Memorial Sloan–Kettering Cancer Center (an institution that treats hundreds of new bladder cancers each year) that reported only 23 urethral tumors in a series spanning 30 years.[98] Two were adenocarcinomas and the rest were either urothelial or squamous cell carcinomas. The symptoms are usually dysuria, hematuria, reduced urinary stream, urinary obstruction, or fistula.[98,99,109] A history of infection, diverticulum, fistula, or stricture is common. Ray et al.[98] found that prognosis correlated with the anatomic location and pathologic stage of the primary, but not with grade or histologic subtype (Tables 11-1, 11-2). Stage for stage, cancer arising in the distal (bulbous and pendulous) urethra had a better prognosis than cancer arising in the membranous or prostatic urethra. In the former group, six of nine patients (67%) survived 5 years, whereas only three of 14 (21%) of the latter survived 5 years. Tumors arising in the distal urethra are commonly diagnosed at an earlier stage. Well-differentiated squamous cell or verrucous carcinoma is common in the distal urethra (Fig. 11-18). Invasion into vascular spaces of the corpus spongiosum (Fig. 11-19) or corpora cavernosa is common, and metastases, if present, involve the inguinal lymph nodes. Wide dissemination at the time of presentation is rare. Partial penectomy and inguinal lymph node dissection is usually the treatment of choice.

Tumors arising in the proximal urethra in males commonly present at a higher stage and can infiltrate into the prostatic stroma or pelvic soft tissues to the point that establishing adequate surgical margins of resection may be difficult (Fig. 11-20).[99] In these tumors, the histologic distinction is difficult to ascertain between high-grade urothelial carcinoma and non-keratinizing squamous cell carcinoma (Fig. 11-21). Metastases may be to inguinal or pelvic lymph nodes, and, if operable, treatment usually requires a cysto-

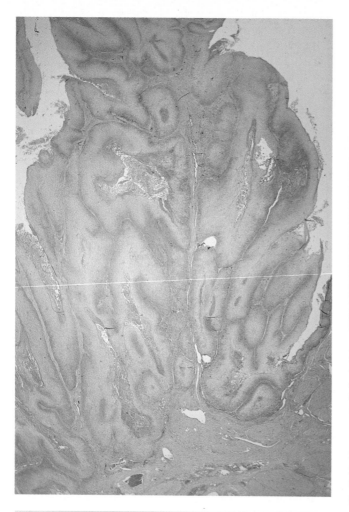

**Fig. 11-18** Verrucous carcinoma. Tall compressed mucosal papillae with a broad infiltrative base. These lesions tend to arise in the distal urethra.

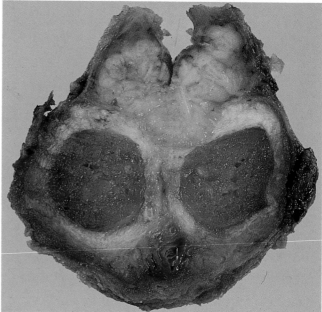

**Fig. 11-19** Squamous carcinoma of the penile urethra. The tumor invades through the corpus spongiosum into the septum but spares the corpora cavernosa (pT2). (From Reuter VE, Melamed M. The lower urinary tract. In: Sternberg S, ed. Diagnostic surgical pathology, 2nd edn. New York: Raven Press, 1994; with permission).

prostatectomy and urethrectomy. If the scrotal skin, soft tissues, or deep pelvic tissues are involved, total emasculation may be required, although heroic surgical procedures rarely ensure long-term survival.

### Urethral carcinoma in women

Primary urethral carcinoma in women is rare, albeit more common than in men.[117-120] The histories and symptoms of these patients are similar to those seen in male patients. In women, urethral carcinoma is frequently initially misdiagnosed as caruncle. For this reason, biopsy should be performed on any presumed caruncle that fails to respond to therapy or is associated with persistent bleeding. Approximately 75% of cases of urethral carcinoma in women are non-keratinizing or keratinizing squamous carcinoma, and the remaining 25–30% are split between urothelial carcinoma and adenocarcinoma. Tumors arising in the distal third of the female urethra are commonly low-grade squamous cell or verrucous carcinoma (Fig. 11-18). If invasive, metastases are usually to inguinal lymph nodes. Treatment usually consists of distal urethrectomy and inguinal lymph node dissection. Cancer arising in the proximal urethra is usually urothelial, and typically metastasizes to pelvic lymph nodes. Treatment includes total urethrectomy as well as inguinal and pelvic lymph node dissection. Wide dissemination at presentation is quite rare, although metastases to regional lymph nodes are common. In two large series approximately 28% of patients who underwent inguinal lymphadenectomy and approximately 50% of those who underwent pelvic lymphadenectomy had metastases.[118,121] Histologic type and grade were not significant predictive factors when corrected for stage.

### Adenocarcinoma

Urethral adenocarcinoma is more common in women than in men.[99,122-127] Stage for stage, it has the same prognosis as squamous cell and urothelial carcinoma of the urethra. Adenocarcinoma may arise from the surface mucosa through metaplasia or from periurethral glands (Figs 11-22, 11-23).[128-132] Those arising from the surface urothelium are usually associated with a chronic inflammatory insult, such as stricture, diverticulum, infection, or fistula (see Fig. 11-3), and present with irritative symptoms, hematuria or urinary obstruction. On urethroscopy, adenocarcinoma appears as papillary or polypoid masses. Microscopically, it is composed of simple or pseudostratified columnar epithelium with apical cytoplasm and basally located hyperchromatic nuclei. Occasionally, the cytoplasm is vacuolated and contains mucin, giving the tumor a colonic appearance. Rarely, urethral adenocarcinoma is frankly mucinous.[133] High-grade lesions exhibit greater pleomorphism and numerous mitotic figures. Glandular metaplasia, urethritis cystica and urethritis glandularis are often present in the adjacent mucosa. This tumor does not react with antibodies

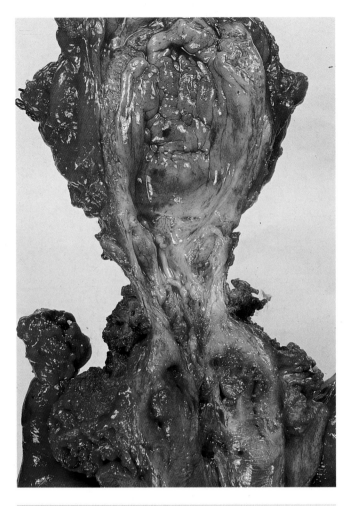

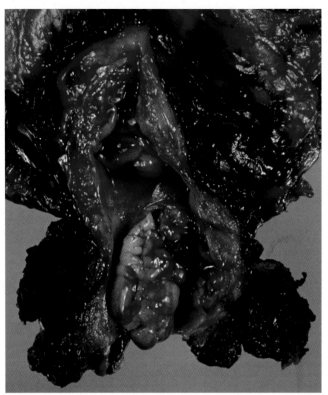

**Fig. 11-22** Adenocarcinoma of the female urethra presenting as an exophytic mass. It is easy to understand how a lesion such as this can lead to dysuria, hematuria and urinary obstruction.

**Fig. 11-20** Squamous cell carcinoma arising in the bulbomembranous urethra. Tumors that arise at this site tend to be at an advanced stage at diagnosis. This lesion infiltrated the cavernous urethra, periurethral, and periprostatic soft tissues, requiring cystoprostaturethrectomy and total emasculation.

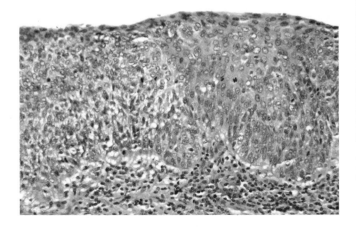

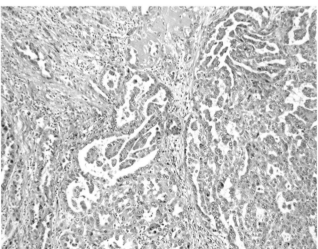

**Fig. 11-23** Adenocarcinoma arising in periurethral (Skene's) glands. The tumor is predominantly papillary and exhibits high nuclear grade.

**Fig. 11-21** Squamous carcinoma in situ of the penile urethra. The full thickness of the mucosa is replaced by neoplastic cells with significant cytologic and architectural disorder.

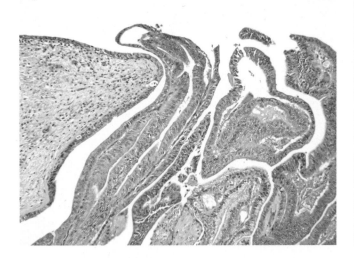

**Fig. 11-24** Prostatic adenocarcinoma, ductal type, extending through periurethral ducts and into the urethra. This phenomenon may be confused with a primary urethral neoplasm.

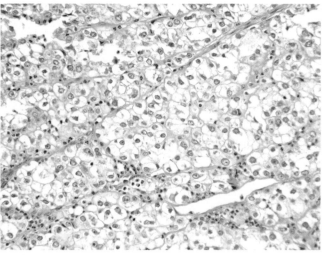

**Fig. 11-25** Clear cell adenocarcinoma. This tumor may arise from the surface mucosa or periurethral glands. Morphologically, it may be difficult to differentiate from clear cell adenocarcinomas arising in the female genital tract or metastatic from the kidney.

to PSA. It must be distinguished from intraurethral papillary prostatic (ductal) adenocarcinoma[134] (Fig. 11-24) which usually arises adjacent to the verumontanum.[79] Papillary prostatic adenocarcinoma tends to have prominent eosinophilic nucleoli and is associated with typical prostatic adenocarcinoma in the underlying periurethral tissue. Extension of other adenocarcinomas into the urethra, such as rectal adenocarcinoma in males or rectal, endometrial, endocervical, vaginal or Bartholin's gland adenocarcinoma in females, must be considered in the differential diagnosis.

### Adenocarcinoma of accessory glands

In males, there are a few reports of adenocarcinoma arising in Cowper's glands and Littré glands.[128–131,135] These diagnoses are very difficult because the tumor has usually destroyed the local anatomic landmarks and extended to or ulcerated the overlying mucosa. Adenocarcinoma arising in Cowper's glands is located in the bulbomembranous region, whereas that arising from Littré's glands tends to originate in the distal portion of the penile urethra but may arise at any point along its length. Both present with hematuria, dysuria, and progressive urinary obstruction. It is common for these patients to be treated for urethritis before the proper diagnosis is established. Microscopically, these neoplasms share features with adenocarcinoma arising from the urethral mucosa. The tumor may have a tubular or micropapillary growth pattern, and tumor cells are either cuboidal or columnar with clear or eosinophilic cytoplasm and large, hyperchromatic nuclei. Intracytoplasmic mucin vacuoles or a frank mucinous component are uncommon. Cytoplasmic clearing, if present, is usually due to glycogen production (see the description on clear cell adenocarcinoma in the following section).

In women, adenocarcinoma arising from periurethral or Skene's glands displays the same symptoms as that in the accessory gland in men (Fig. 11-22).[99,126,132] It may arise at any point in the urethra, but is more common distally. In that location, patients often have a perineal mass that may

be confused with an infected cyst or uterine prolapse. Microscopically, tumors may have a glandular, papillary, or micropapillary architecture, and the tumor cells are either columnar or cuboidal with eosinophilic or clear cytoplasm (Fig. 11-23). Cytoplasmic clearing is usually caused by glycogen deposition or, less frequently, intracytoplasmic mucin. Intraluminal mucin is common. The nuclei are large and hyperchromatic and often exhibit prominent nucleoli. It should be borne in mind that the diagnosis of adenocarcinoma arising in periurethral glands is usually very difficult because of extension or ulceration of the overlying urethral mucosa and obliteration of anatomic landmarks.[99,126] The best indication of periurethral gland origin is partial involvement of recognizable periurethral glands. Even then, this may represent downward extension from the surface. The prognosis in all cases of urethral adenocarcinoma, whether of surface or periurethral gland origin, is determined by pathologic stage at the time of presentation rather than the site of origin.

### Clear cell adenocarcinoma

Clear cell adenocarcinoma is an unusual variant of urethral adenocarcinoma that may arise from the mucosa or from periurethral glands.[126,136–141] It is also called mesonephric adenocarcinoma[138] and glycogen-rich carcinoma.[141] Its morphologic features are identical to those of clear cell adenocarcinoma of the genital tract. Nevertheless, several authors[136,142] have concluded that urethral clear cell adenocarcinoma arises through metaplasia of the surface mucosa or from periurethral glands, rather than from müllerian or mesonephric remnants.

Microscopically, clear cell adenocarcinoma may have tubular, papillary, micropapillary, acinar, or diffuse growth pattern (Fig. 11-25). Commonly, it exhibits a combination of growth patterns. The cells often have abundant clear or eosinophilic cytoplasm that contains glycogen and little or no mucin. Mucicarmine positivity is usually evident only in the luminal secretions. In a few cases, PSA and prostatic acid phosphatase (PAP) immunoreactivity has been demonstrated in clear cell adenocarcinoma in women.[143–146] The nuclei are large, pleomorphic, and hyperchromatic. Luminally located nucleus give the tubules a distinct hobnail appearance. Several cases have presented with paraneoplastic hypercalcemia similar to that seen with other clear cell tumors, such as renal cell carcinoma.[136] Clear cell adenocarcinoma of the urethra is distinguished from gynecologic clear cell carcinoma and metastatic renal cell carcinoma by clinical history and diagnostic workup. Gynecologic clear cell adenocarcinoma tends to occur in younger patients exposed to non-steroidal estrogens before birth. Cantrell et al.[147] reported a case of papillary prostatic adenocarcinoma occupying the prostatic urethra and exhibiting clear cell features. The diffuse pattern may be confused with amelanotic melanoma. Also, clear cell adenocarcinoma must be distinguished from nephrogenic adenoma.[142,148] The latter lacks the nuclear pleomorphism and hyperchromasia and infiltrative and destructive growth pattern seen in adenocarcinoma. Mitotic figures are rare in nephrogenic adenoma but usually are readily apparent in clear cell adenocarcinoma. This distinction may be difficult to establish on small biopsy.

The prognosis of clear cell adenocarcinoma of the urethra is uncertain because of the rarity of this tumor and limited follow-up in reported series. A series from MD Anderson Hospital suggests that these patients may have a somewhat better prognosis than those with other types of adenocarcinoma, although the numbers did not reach statistical significance.[126] In general, prognosis correlates with pathologic stage at presentation. Clinical management has varied, including transurethral resection, radical excision, and radiation therapy or, a combination of these.

## Other histologic types of carcinoma

Other epithelial neoplasms arising within the urethra include adenosquamous carcinoma,[149] adenoid cystic carcinoma,[150] carcinoid,[151] and so-called cloacogenic carcinoma.[152,153] All cases have been single-case reports with limited follow-up. Their morphologic features are similar to their counterparts arising at other sites.

### Malignant melanoma

Although rare, the urethra is the most common site of origin of malignant melanoma in the urinary tract.[154–166] In 1988, Manivel and Fraley[155] reviewed the literature and found only 26 cases. The urethra is more commonly involved by spread from melanoma arising in the glans penis and vulva. Urethral melanoma occurs in both males and females and has been described in black patients.[157,159] The tumor may be associated with melanosis, although precursor lesions are rarely identified. The majority of cases occur in older patients. Begun et al.[154] reported a 13-year-old boy who developed melanoma of the penis.

Patients usually present with hematuria, dysuria, a deviated urinary stream, or urinary obstruction. Melanuria is an uncommon finding. Endoscopic examination reveals a nodular mucosal mass or masses that are usually pigmented and frequently ulcerated. As with other mucosal melanomas the growth pattern is commonly lentiginous, although all other patterns may be represented (Fig. 11-26). Mucosal melanoma is more likely to be amelanotic than cutaneous. Extensive radial growth is common, accounting for the frequency of local recurrence. Metastasis is usually to inguinal and pelvic lymph nodes and common in advanced lesions. Hematogenous spread to liver, lungs and brain is common.

Treatment is surgical and includes urethrectomy or penectomy with regional lymph node dissection. The role of immunotherapy, radiation therapy and chemotherapy remains uncertain.[160,162] Staging for urethral melanoma has not been standardized, as most reports deal with isolated cases. Prognosis depends on the thickness of the lesion, similar to melanoma at other mucosal sites. Pathologists should carefully evaluate the status of the mucosal margin of resection because local recurrence at the surgical bed is common. Skip lesions involving the urinary bladder and

**A**

**B**

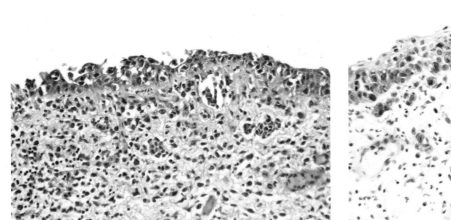
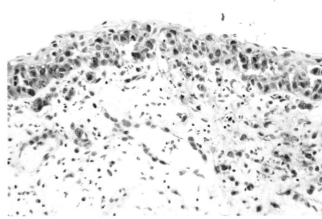

**Fig. 11-26** Urethral malignant melanoma. (**A**) Neoplastic melanocytes occupy the surface mucosa and extend into the submucosa. (**B**) Tumor cells are immunoreactive with S100 protein.

ureter may occur and should be investigated prior to extirpative surgery.

## Soft tissue tumors

Leiomyoma is the most common soft tissue tumor of the urethra, although fewer than 30 cases have been reported.[167-173] Leiomyoma may also involve the paraurethral soft tissue, but the exact site of origin is uncertain. Urethral leiomyoma range in size from 1 to 40 cm and may present as an asymptomatic mass or with dysuria and urinary obstruction.

Other non-epithelial neoplasms are rare in the urethra and periurethral soft tissues. These include hemangioma,[174-177] papillary endothelial hyperplasia,[178] paraganglioma,[179-181] plasmacytoma,[182-184] and neurofibroma.[185] Lymphoma may involve the urethra but is usually a manifestation of systemic disease, with only a few cases asserted to be primary in the urethra.[186,187]

Although sarcoma has been described in the pelvic and paraurethral tissues, it is difficult to establish whether it is truly urethral in origin. Steeper and Rosai[188] described a soft tissue tumor arising in the pelvis and perineal soft tissues of women, termed aggressive angiomyxoma, consisting of vascular fibromyxoid tissue that is locally infiltrative with a tendency to multiple recurrences. These patients present with urinary obstruction or dysuria.

## REFERENCES

1. Moore K. The urinary system. In: Moore K, ed. The developing human, 3rd edn. Philadelphia: WB Saunders, 1982; 267–268.
2. Moore KL. The pelvis and perineum. In: Moore KL, ed. Clinically oriented anatomy, 2nd edn. Baltimore: Williams & Wilkins, 1985; 362–365.
3. Carroll PR, Dixon CM. Surgical anatomy of the male and female urethra. Urol Clin North Am 1992; 19: 339–346.
4. Tanagho E. Anatomy of the lower urinary tract. In: Walsh PCW, Retik AB, Stamey TA, eds. Campbell's urology, 6th edn. Philadelphia: WB Saunders, 1992; 49–54.
5. Herr HW. Surgery of penile and urethral carcinoma. In: Walsh PC W, Retik AB, Stamey TA, eds. Campbell's urology, 6th edn. Philadelphia: WB Saunders, 1992; 3073–3089.
6. Herbut PA. Urological pathology. Philadelphia: Lea & Febiger, 1952.
7. Saraf PG, Valvo JR, Frank IN. Congenital posterior urethral valves in an adult. Urology 1984; 23: 55–57.
8. Williams DI. Discussion on lower urinary obstruction. Arch Dis Child 1962; 37: 132–135.
9. Maruotti GM, Agangi A, Martinelli P, Paladini D. Early prenatal diagnosis of concordant posterior urethral valves in male monochorionic twins. Prenat Diagn 2006; 26: 67–70.
10. Coddington CC, Knab DR. Urethral diverticulum: a review. Obstet Gynecol Surv 1983; 38: 357–364.
11. Newland DE, Patterson JH, Hofsess DW. Urethral diverticulum: a recondite disease. J Urol 1970; 103: 174–175.
12. Davis HJ, Telinde RW. Urethral diverticula: an assay of 121 cases. J Urol 1958; 80: 34–39.
13. Andersen MJ. The incidence of diverticula in the female urethra. J Urol 1967; 98: 96–98.
14. Kaplan M, Atakan IH, Kaya E, et al. Giant prostatic urethral calculus associated with urethrocutaneous fistula. Int J Urol 2006; 13: 643–644.
15. Okeke LI, Aisuodionoe-Shadrach OI, Adekanye AO. Urethral duplication with a perineal opening in a four-year-old boy. J Natl Med Assoc 2006; 98: 284–286.
16. Medeiros LJ, Young RH. Nephrogenic adenoma arising in urethral diverticula. A report of five cases. Arch Pathol Lab Med 1989; 113: 125–128.
17. Fenton AS, Morey AF, Aviles R, Garcia CR. Anterior urethral strictures: etiology and characteristics. Urology 2005; 65: 1055–1058.
18. Bazeed MA, Saad SM, Abou-El-Azm TA. Acquired urethral diverticula in the male. Urol Int 1981; 36: 380–385.
19. Tesluk H. Primary adenocarcinoma of female urethra associated with diverticula. Urology 1981; 17: 197–199.
20. Marshall S, Hirsch K. Carcinoma within urethral diverticula. Urology 1977; 10: 161–163.
21. Srinivas V, Dow D. Transitional cell carcinoma in a urethral diverticulum with a calculus. J Urol 1983; 129: 372–373.
22. Cea PC, Ward JN, Lavengood RW Jr, Gray GF. Mesonephric adenocarcinomas in urethral diverticula. Urology 1977; 10: 58–61.
23. Wheeler JS Jr, Flanigan RC, Hong HY, Walloch JL. Female urethral diverticula with clear cell adenocarcinoma. J Surg Oncol 1992; 49: 66–71.
24. Onaran M, Tan MO, Camtosun A, et al. Parameatal cyst of urethra: a rare congenital anomaly. Int Urol Nephrol 2006; 38: 273–274.
25. Bujons A, Ponce de Leon X, Baez C, et al. [Paraurethral cyst of the Littre's gland: an exceptional case]. Arch Esp Urol 2006; 59: 624–626.
26. Chowdhry AA, Miller FH, Hammer RA. Endometriosis presenting as a urethral diverticulum: a case report. J Reprod Med 2004; 49: 321–323.
27. Gross RE, Moore TC. Duplication of the urethra: report of two cases and summary of the literature. Arch Surg 1950; 60: 749–753.
28. Olsen JG. Complete urethral duplication in a boy. J Urol 1966; 95: 718–720.
29. Ortolano V, Nasrallah PF. Urethral duplication. J Urol 1986; 136: 909–912.
30. Downs RA. Congenital polyps of the prostatic urethra. A review of the literature and report of two cases. Br J Urol 1970; 42: 76–85.
31. Hanani Y, Hertz M, Jonas P. Congenital urethral polyp in children. Urology 1980; 16: 162–164.
32. Youssif M. Posterior urethral polyps in infants and children. Eur Urol 1985; 11: 69–70.
33. Foster RS, Weigel JW, Mantz FA. Anterior urethral polyps. J Urol 1980; 124: 145–146.
34. Bruijnes E, de Wall JG, Scholtmeijer RJ, den Hollander JC. Congenital polyp of the prostatic urethra in childhood. Report of 3 cases and review of literature. Urol Int 1985; 40: 287–291.
35. Murphy DM, Guiney EJ. Polyp of the posterior urethra. Eur Urol 1982; 8: 204–206.
36. Foster RS, Garrett RA. Congenital posterior urethral polyps. J Urol 1986; 136: 670–672.
37. Isaac J, Snow B, Lowichik A. Fibroepithelial polyp of the prostatic urethra in an adolescent. J Pediatr Surg 2006; 41: e29–31.
38. Demircan M, Ceran C, Karaman A, et al. Urethral polyps in children: a review of the literature and report of two cases. Int J Urol 2006; 13: 841–843.
39. Ben-Meir D, Yin M, Chow CW, Hutson JM. Urethral polyps in prepubertal girls. J Urol 2005; 174: 1443–1444.
40. Wallin JE, Thompson SE, Zaidi A, Wong KH. Urethritis in women attending an STD clinic. Br J Vener Dis 1981; 57: 50–54.
41. Swartz SL, Kraus SJ, Herrmann KL, et al. Diagnosis and etiology of nongonococcal urethritis. J Infect Dis 1978; 138: 445–454.
42. Hoffman WW, Cheatum DE. Reiter's disease. Urol Surv 1978; 28: 197–205.

43. Elbadawi A, Malhoski WE, Frank IN. Mucinous urethral caruncle. Urology 1978; 12: 587–590.

44. Jarvi OH, Marin S. Intestinal mucosal heterotopia of an urethral caruncle. Acta Pathol Microbiol Immunol Scand [A] 1982; 90: 213–219.

45. Willett GD, Lack EE. Periurethral colonic-type polyp simulating urethral caruncle. A case report. J Reprod Med 1990; 35: 1017–1018.

46. Young RH, Scully RE. Clear cell adenocarcinoma of the bladder and urethra. A report of three cases and review of the literature. Am J Surg Pathol 1985; 9: 816–826.

47. Proppe KH, Scully RE, Rosai J. Postoperative spindle cell nodules of genitourinary tract resembling sarcomas. A report of eight cases. Am J Surg Pathol 1984; 8: 101–108.

48. Hirsch MS, Dal Cin P, Fletcher CD. ALK expression in pseudosarcomatous myofibroblastic proliferations of the genitourinary tract. Histopathology 2006; 48: 569–578.

49. Walker AN, Mills SE. Papillary and polypoid tumors of the prostatic urethra. In: Damjanov I, Cohen AH, Mills SE, Young RH, eds. Progress in reproductive and urinary tract pathology. New York: Field & Wood, 1989; 113–114.

50. Schinella R, Thurm J, Feiner H. Papillary pseudotumor of the prostatic urethra: proliferative papillary urethritis. J Urol 1974; 111: 38–40.

51. Bhagavan BS, Tiamson EM, Wenk RE, et al. Nephrogenic adenoma of the urinary bladder and urethra. Hum Pathol 1981; 12: 907–916.

52. Odze R, Begin LR. Tubular adenomatous metaplasia (nephrogenic adenoma) of the female urethra. Int J Gynecol Pathol 1989; 8: 374–380.

53. Berger BW, Bhagavan SB, Reiner W, et al. Nephrogenic adenoma: clinical features and therapeutic considerations. J Urol 1981; 126: 824–826.

54. Xiao GQ, Burstein DE, Miller LK, Unger PD. Nephrogenic adenoma: immunohistochemical evaluation for its etiology and differentiation from prostatic adenocarcinoma. Arch Pathol Med 2006; 130: 805–810.

55. Allan CH, Epstein JI. Nephrogenic adenoma of the prostatic urethra: a mimicker of prostate adenocarcinoma. Am J Surg Pathol 2001; 25: 802–808.

56. Lou TY, Teplitz C. Malakoplakia: pathogenesis and ultrastructural morphogenesis. A problem of altered macrophage (phagolysosomal) response. Hum Pathol 1974; 5: 191–207.

57. Damjanov I, Katz SM. Malakoplakia. Pathol Annu 1981; 16: 103–126.

58. Stanton MJ, Maxted W. Malacoplakia: a study of the literature and current concepts of pathogenesis, diagnosis and treatment. J Urol 1981; 125: 139–146.

59. McClure J. A case of urethral malacoplakia associated with vesical disease. J Urol 1979; 122: 705–706.

60. Sharma TC, Kagan HN, Sheils JP. Malacoplakia of the male urethra. J Urol 1981; 125: 885–886.

61. Ordonez NG, Ayala AG, Gresik MV, Bracken RB. Primary localized amyloidosis of male urethra (amyloidoma). Urology 1979; 14: 617–619.

62. Constantian HM, Wyman P. Localized amyloidosis of the urethra: report of a case. J Urol 1980; 124: 728–729.

63. Vasudevan P, Stein AM, Pinn VW, Rao CN. Primary amyloidosis of urethra. Urology 1981; 17: 181–183.

64. Dounis A, Bourounis M, Mitropoulos D. Primary localized amyloidosis of the urethra. Eur Urol 1985; 11: 344–345.

65. Bodner H, Retsky MI, Brown G. Primary amyloidosis of glans penis and urethra: resection and reconstruction. J Urol 1981; 125: 586–588.

66. Cheng L, Leibovich BC, Cheville JC, et al. Squamous papilloma of the urinary tract is unrelated to condyloma acuminata. Cancer 2000; 88: 1679–1686.

67. Debenedictis TJ, Marmar ML, Praiss DE. Intraurethral condylomas acuminata: management and review of the literature. J Urol 1977; 118: 767–769.

68. Murphy WM, Fu YS, Lancaster WD, Jenson AB. Papillomavirus structural antigens in condyloma acuminatum of the male urethra. J Urol 1983; 130: 84–85.

69. Grussendorf-Conen EI, Deutz FJ, de Villiers EM. Detection of human papillomavirus-6 in primary carcinoma of the urethra in men. Cancer 1987; 60: 1832–1835.

70. Aguilar LV, Lazcano-Ponce E, Vaccarella S, et al. Human papillomavirus in men: comparison of different genital sites. Sexually Trans Infect 2006; 82: 31–33.

71. Melchers WJ, Schift R, Stolz E, et al. Human papillomavirus detection in urine samples from male patients by the polymerase chain reaction. J Clin Microbiol 1989; 27: 1711–1714.

72. Del Mistro A, Braunstein JD, Halwer M, Koss LG. Identification of human papillomavirus types in male urethral condylomata acuminata by in situ hybridization. Hum Pathol 1987; 18: 936–940.

73. Wiener JS, Liu ET, Walther PJ. Oncogenic human papillomavirus type 16 is associated with squamous cell cancer of the male urethra. Cancer Res 1992; 52: 5018–5023.

74. Mevorach RA, Cos LR, di Sant'Agnese PA, Stoler M. Human papillomavirus type 6 in grade I transitional cell carcinoma of the urethra. J Urol 1990; 143: 126–128.

75. Nicolau SM, Camargo CG, Stavale JN, et al. Human papillomavirus DNA detection in male sexual partners of women with genital human papillomavirus infection. Urology 2005; 65: 251–255.

76. Giovannelli L, Migliore MC, Capra G, et al. Penile, urethral, and seminal sampling for diagnosis of human papillomavirus infection in men. J Clin Microbiol 2007; 45: 248–251.

77. Remick DG Jr, Kumar NB. Benign polyps with prostatic-type epithelium of the urethra and the urinary bladder. A suggestion of histogenesis based on histologic and immunohistochemical studies. Am J Surg Pathol 1984; 8: 833–839.

78. Craig JR, Hart WR. Benign polyps with prostatic-type epithelium of the urethra. Am J Clin Pathol 1975; 63: 343–347.

79. Walker AN, Mills SE, Fechner RE, Perry JM. 'Endometrial' adenocarcinoma of the prostatic urethra arising in a villous polyp. A light microscopic and immunoperoxidase study. Arch Pathol Lab Med 1982; 106: 624–627.

80. Lubin J, Mark TM, Wirtschafter AR. Papillomas of prostatic urethra with prostatic-type epithelium: report of eight cases. Mt Sinai J Med 1984; 51: 218–221.

81. Satoh S, Ujiie T, Kubo T, et al. Prostatic epithelial polyp of the prostatic urethra. Eur Urol 1989; 16: 92–96.

82. Goldstein AM, Bragin SD, Terry R, Yoell JH. Prostatic urethral polyps in adults: histopathologic variations and clinical manifestations. J Urol 1981; 126: 129–131.

83. Heyderman E, Mandaliya KN, O'Donnell PJ, et al. Ectopic prostatic glands in bulbar urethra. Immunoperoxidase study. Urology 1987; 29: 76–77.

84. Hicks CC, Nicholas EM, Morgan JW. Hematuria from ectopic prostatic tissue in bulbous urethra. Urology 1977; 10: 50–51.

85. Dejter SW Jr, Zuckerman ME, Lynch JH. Benign villous polyp with prostatic type epithelium of the penile urethra. J Urol 1988; 139: 590–591.

86. Reuter VE, Melamed MR. The lower urinary tract. Diagnostic surgical pathology. New York: Raven Press, 1994; 1768–1784.

87. Jordan AM, Weingarten J, Murphy WM. Transitional cell neoplasms of the urinary bladder. Can biologic potential be predicted from histologic grading? Cancer 1987; 60: 2766–2774.

88. Pathology and genetics of tumours of the urinary system and male genital organs. Lyon, France: IARC Press, 2004.

89. Amin MB, Young RH. Primary carcinomas of the urethra. Semin Diagn Pathol 1997; 14: 147–160.

90. Sung MT, Maclennan GT, Lopez-Beltran A, et al. Natural history of urothelial inverted papilloma. Cancer 2006; 107: 2622–2627.

91. Fine SW, Chan TY, Epstein JI. Inverted papillomas of the prostatic urethra. Am J Surg Pathol 2006; 30: 975–979.

92. DeMeester LJ, Farrow GM, Utz DC. Inverted papillomas of the urinary

bladder. Cancer 1975; 36: 505–513.

93. Renfer LG, Kelley J, Belville WD. Inverted papilloma of the urinary tract: histogenesis, recurrence and associated malignancy. J Urol 1988; 140: 832–834.

94. Gowing NF. Urethral carcinoma associated with cancer of the bladder. Br J Urol 1960; 32: 428–439.

95. Schellhammer PF, Whitmore WF Jr. Urethral meatal carcinoma following cystourethrectomy for bladder carcinoma. J Urol 1976; 115: 61–64.

96. Tobisu K, Tanaka Y, Mizutani T, Kakizoe T. Transitional cell carcinoma of the urethra in men following cystectomy for bladder cancer: multivariate analysis for risk factors. J Urol 1991; 146: 1551–1553; discussion 1553–1554.

97. Richie JP, Skinner DG. Carcinoma in situ of the urethra associated with bladder carcinoma: the role of urethrectomy. J Urol 1978; 119: 80–81.

98. Ray B, Canto AR, Whitmore WF Jr. Experience with primary carcinoma of the male urethra. J Urol 1977; 117: 591–594.

99. Schellhammer PF. Urethral carcinoma. Semin Urol 1983; 1: 82–89.

100. Schellhammer PF, Bean MA, Whitmore WF Jr. Prostatic involvement by transitional cell carcinoma: pathogenesis, patterns and prognosis. J Urol 1977; 118: 399–403.

101. Hardeman SW, Soloway MS. Urethral recurrence following radical cystectomy. J Urol 1990; 144: 666–669.

102. Kakizoe T, Tobisu K. Transitional cell carcinoma of the urethra in men and women associated with bladder cancer. Jpn J Clin Oncol 1998; 28: 357–359.

103. Liedberg F, Chebil G, Mansson W. Urothelial carcinoma in the prostatic urethra and prostate: current controversies. Exp Rev Anticancer Ther 2007; 7: 383–390.

104. Wolinska WH, Melamed MR, Schellhammer PF, Whitmore WF Jr. Urethral cytology following cystectomy for bladder carcinoma. Am J Surg Pathol 1977; 1: 225–234.

105. Hermansen DK, Badalament RA, Whitmore WF Jr, et al. Detection of carcinoma in the post-cystectomy urethral remnant by flow cytometric analysis. J Urol 1988; 139: 304–307.

106. De Paepe ME, Andre R, Mahadevia P. Urethral involvement in female patients with bladder cancer. A study of 22 cystectomy specimens. Cancer 1990; 65: 1237–1241.

107. Mahadevia PS, Alexander JE, Rojas-Corona R, Koss LG. Pseudosarcomatous stromal reaction in primary and metastatic urothelial carcinoma. A source of diagnostic difficulty. Am J Surg Pathol 1989; 13: 782–790.

108. Greene F, Page D, Fleming I, et al. AJCC cancer staging manual, 6th edn. New York: Springer Verlag, 2002.

109. Melicow MM, Roberts TW. Pathology and natural history of urethral tumors in males. Review of 142 cases. Urology 1978; 11: 83–89.

110. Velazquez EF, Soskin A, Bock A, et al. Epithelial abnormalities and precancerous lesions of anterior urethra in patients with penile carcinoma: a report of 89 cases. Mod Pathol 2005; 18: 917–923.

111. Orihuela E, Herr HW, Whitmore WF Jr. Conservative treatment of superficial transitional cell carcinoma of prostatic urethra with intravesical BCG. Urology 1989; 34: 231–237.

112. Tomaszewski JE, Korat OC, LiVolsi VA, et al. Paget's disease of the urethral meatus following transitional cell carcinoma of the bladder. J Urol 1986; 135: 368–370.

113. Begin LR, Deschenes J, Mitmaker B. Pagetoid carcinomatous involvement of the penile urethra in association with high-grade transitional cell carcinoma of the urinary bladder. Arch Pathol Lab Med 1991; 115: 632–635.

114. Merino MJ, Livolsi VA, Lytton B. Penile Paget's disease and prostatic carcinoma. J Urol 1978; 120: 121–123.

115. Dalbagni G, Zhang ZF, Lacombe L, Herr HW. Male urethral carcinoma: analysis of treatment outcome. Urology 1999; 53: 1126–1132.

116. Dalbagni G, Zhang ZF, Lacombe L, Herr HW. Female urethral carcinoma: an analysis of treatment outcome and a plea for a standardized management strategy. Br J Urol 1998; 82: 835–841.

117. Grabstald H, Hilaris B, Henschke U, Whitmore WF Jr. Cancer of the female urethra. JAMA 1966; 197: 835–842.

118. Bracken RB, Johnson DE, Miller LS, et al. Primary carcinoma of the female urethra. J Urol 1976; 116: 188–192.

119. Johnson DE, O'Connell JR. Primary carcinoma of female urethra. Urology 1983; 21: 42–45.

120. Roberts TW, Melicow MM. Pathology and natural history of urethral tumors in females: review of 65 cases. Urology 1977; 10: 583–589.

121. Kamat MR, Kulkarni JN, Dhumale RG. Primary carcinoma of female urethra: review of 20 cases. J Surg Oncol 1981; 16: 105–109.

122. Yachia D, Turani H. Colonic-type adenocarcinoma of male urethra. Urology 1991; 37: 568–570.

123. Bostwick DG, Lo R, Stamey TA. Papillary adenocarcinoma of the male urethra. Case report and review of the literature. Cancer 1984; 54: 2556–2563.

124. Loo KT, Chan JK. Colloid adenocarcinoma of the urethra associated with mucosal in situ carcinoma. Arch Pathol Lab Med 1992; 116: 976–977.

125. Lieber MM, Malek RS, Farrow GM, McMurtry J. Villous adenoma of the male urethra. J Urol 1983; 130: 1191–1193.

126. Meis JM, Ayala AG, Johnson DE. Adenocarcinoma of the urethra in women. A clinicopathologic study. Cancer 1987; 60: 1038–1052.

127. Powell I, Cartwright H, Jano F. Villous adenoma and adenocarcinoma of female urethra. Urology 1981; 18: 612–614.

128. Silverman ML, Eyre RC, Zinman LA, Corsson AW. Mixed mucinous and papillary adenocarcinoma involving male urethra, probably originating in periurethral glands. Cancer 1981; 47: 1398–1402.

129. Sacks SA, Waisman J, Apfelbaum HB, et al. Urethral adenocarcinoma (possibly originating in the glands of Littre). J Urol 1975; 113: 50–55.

130. Bourque JL, Charghi A, Gauthier GE, et al. Primary carcinoma of Cowper's gland. J Urol 1970; 103: 758–761.

131. Keen MR, Golden RL, Richardson JF, Melicow MM. Carcinoma of Cowper's gland treated with chemotherapy. J Urol 1970; 104: 854–859.

132. Taylor RN, Lacey CG, Shuman MA. Adenocarcinoma of Skene's duct associated with a systemic coagulopathy. Gynecol Oncol 1985; 22: 250–256.

133. Yvgenia R, Ben Meir D, Sibi J, Koren R. Mucinous adenocarcinoma of posterior urethra. Report of a case. Pathol Res Pract 2005; 201: 137–140.

134. Green JM, Tang WW, Jensen BW, Orihuela E. Isolated recurrence of ductal prostate cancer to anterior urethra. Urology 2006; 68: 428; e413–425.

135. Chughtai B, Sawas A, O'Malley RL, et al. A neglected gland: a review of Cowper's gland. Int J Androl 2005; 28: 74–77.

136. Young RH, Scully RE. Pseudosarcomatous lesions of the urinary bladder, prostate gland, and urethra. A report of three cases and review of the literature. Arch Pathol Lab Med 1987; 111: 354–358.

137. Assimos DG, O'Conor VJ Jr. Clear cell adenocarcinoma of the urethra. J Urol 1984; 131: 540–541.

138. Altwein JE, Schafer R, Hohenfellner R. Mesonephric carcinoma of the female urethra. Eur Urol 1975; 1: 248–250.

139. Rivard DJ, Waisman SS. Primary mesonephric carcinoma of the female urethra. J Urol 1985; 134: 756–757.

140. Tanabe ET, Mazur MT, Schaeffer AJ. Clear cell adenocarcinoma of the female urethra: clinical and ultrastructural study suggesting a unique neoplasm. Cancer 1982; 49: 372–378.

141. Hull MT, Eglen DE, Davis T, et al. Glycogen-rich clear cell carcinoma of the urethra: an ultrastructural study. Ultrastruct Pathol 1987; 11: 421–427.

142. Oliva E, Young RH. Clear cell adenocarcinoma of the urethra: a

clinicopathologic analysis of 19 cases. Mod Pathol 1996; 9: 513–520.

143. Spencer JR, Brodin AG, Ignatoff JM. Clear cell adenocarcinoma of the urethra: evidence for origin within paraurethral ducts. J Urol 1990; 143: 122–125.

144. Svanholm H, Andersen OP, Rohl H. Tumour of female paraurethral duct. Immunohistochemical similarity with prostatic carcinoma. Virchows Arch A [Pathol Anat Histopathol] 1987; 411: 395–398.

145. Ebisuno S, Miyai M, Nagareda T. Clear cell adenocarcinoma of the female urethra showing positive staining with antibodies to prostate-specific antigen and prostatic acid phosphatase. Urology 1995; 45: 682–685.

146. Kawano K, Yano M, Kitahara S, Yasuda K. Clear cell adenocarcinoma of the female urethra showing strong immunostaining for prostate-specific antigen. BJU Int 2001; 87: 412–413.

147. Cantrell BB, Leifer G, DeKlerk DP, Eggleston JC. Papillary adenocarcinoma of the prostatic urethra with clear-cell appearance. Cancer 1981; 48: 2661–2667.

148. Gilcrease MZ, Delgado R, Vuitch F, Albores-Saavedra J. Clear cell adenocarcinoma and nephrogenic adenoma of the urethra and urinary bladder: a histopathologic and immunohistochemical comparison. Hum Pathol 1998; 29: 1451–1456.

149. Saito R. An adenosquamous carcinoma of the male urethra with hypercalcemia. Hum Pathol 1981; 12: 383–385.

150. Aronson P, Ronan SG, Briele HA, et al. Adenoid cystic carcinoma of female periurethral area. Light and electron microscopic study. Urology 1982; 20: 312–315.

151. Sylora HO, Diamond HM, Kaufman M, et al. Primary carcinoid tumor of the urethra. J Urol 1975; 114: 150–153.

152. Diaz-Cano SJ, Rios JJ, Rivera-Hueto F, Galera-Davidson H. Mixed cloacogenic carcinoma of male urethra. Histopathology 1992; 20: 82–84.

153. Lucman L, Vadas G. Transitional cloacogenic carcinoma of the urethra. Cancer 1973; 31: 1508–1510.

154. Begun FP, Grossman HB, Diokno AC, Sogani PC. Malignant melanoma of the penis and male urethra. J Urol 1984; 132: 123–125.

155. Manivel JC, Fraley EE. Malignant melanoma of the penis and male urethra: 4 case reports and literature review. J Urol 1988; 139: 813–816.

156. Weiss J, Elder D, Hamilton R. Melanoma of the male urethra: surgical approach and pathological analysis. J Urol 1982; 128: 382–385.

157. Pow-Sang JM, Klimberg IW, Hackett RL, Wajsman Z. Primary malignant melanoma of the male urethra. J Urol 1988; 139: 1304–1306.

158. Oldbring J, Mikulowski P. Malignant melanoma of the penis and male urethra. Report of nine cases and review of the literature. Cancer 1987; 59: 581–587.

159. Sanders TJ, Venable DD, Sanusi ID. Primary malignant melanoma of the urethra in a black man: a case report. J Urol 1986; 135: 1012–1014.

160. Katz JI, Grabstald H. Primary malignant melanoma of the female urethra. J Urol 1976; 116: 454–457.

161. Yoshida K, Tsuboi N, Akimoto M. Primary malignant melanoma of female urethra: report of a case and review of the literature. Hinyokika Kiyo 1986; 32: 105–111.

162. Nissenkorn I, Servadio C, Avidor I, Marshak G. Malignant melanomas of female urethra. Urology 1987; 29: 562–565.

163. Kim CJ, Pak K, Hamaguchi A, et al. Primary malignant melanoma of the female urethra. Cancer 1993; 71: 448–451.

164. Oliva E, Quinn TR, Amin MB, et al. Primary malignant melanoma of the urethra: a clinicopathologic analysis of 15 cases. Am J Surg Pathol 2000; 24: 785–796.

165. Sanchez-Ortiz R, Huang SF, Tamboli P, et al. Melanoma of the penis, scrotum and male urethra: a 40-year single institution experience. J Urol 2005; 173: 1958–1965.

166. Katz EE, Suzue K, Wille MA, et al. Primary malignant melanoma of the urethra. Urology 2005; 65: 389.

167. Oi RH, Poirier-Brode KY. Leiomyoma of the female urethra. J Reprod Med 1979; 22: 259–260.

168. Mooppan MM, Kim H, Wax SH. Leiomyoma of the female urethra. J Urol 1979; 121: 371–372.

169. Lake MH, Kossow AS, Bokinsky G. Leiomyoma of the bladder and urethra. J Urol 1981; 125: 742–743.

170. Ohtani M, Yanagizawa R, Shoji F, et al. Leiomyoma of the male urethra. Eur Urol 1982; 8: 372–373.

171. Di Cello V, Saltutti C, Mincione GP, et al. Paraurethral leiomyoma in women. Eur Urol 1988; 15: 290–293.

172. Cheng C, Mac-Moune Lai F, Chan PS. Leiomyoma of the female urethra: a

case report and review. J Urol 1992; 148: 1526–1527.

173. Saad AG, Kaouk JH, Kaspar HG, Khauli RB. Leiomyoma of the urethra: report of 3 cases of a rare entity. Int J Surg Pathol 2003; 11: 123–126.

174. Steinhardt G, Perlmutter A. Urethral hemangioma. J Urol 1987; 137: 116–117.

175. Sharma SK, Reddy MJ, Joshi VV, Bapna BC. Capillary haemangioma of male urethra. Br J Urol 1981; 53: 277.

176. Barua R, Munday RN. Intravascular angiomatosis in female urethral mass. Masson intravascular hemangioendothelioma. Urology 1983; 21: 191–193.

177. Tabibian L, Ginsberg DA. Thrombosed urethral hemangioma. J Urol 2003; 170: 1942.

178. Nevin DT, Palazzo J, Petersen R. A urethral mass in a 67-year-old woman. Papillary endothelial hyperplasia (Masson tumor). Arch Pathol Lab Med 2006; 130: 561–562.

179. Badalament RA, Kenworthy P, Pellegrini A, Drago JR. Paraganglioma of urethra. Urology 1991; 38: 76–78.

180. Cholhan HJ, Caglar H, Kremzier JE. Suburethral paraganglioma. Obstet Gynecol 1991; 78: 555–558.

181. Bryant KR, Thompson IM, Ortiz R, Spence CR. Urethral paraganglioma presenting as a urethral polyp. J Urol 1983; 130: 571–572.

182. Witjes JA, De Vries JD, Schaafsma HE, et al. Extramedullary plasmacytoma of the urethra: a case report. J Urol 1991; 145: 826–828.

183. Mark JA, Pais VM, Chong FK. Plasmacytoma of the urethra treated with transurethral resection and radiotherapy. J Urol 1990; 143: 1010–1011.

184. Campbell CM, Smith JA Jr, Middleton RG. Plasmacytoma of the urethra. J Urol 1982; 127: 986.

185. Eidelman A, Reif R. Periurethral myxoid neurofibroma. J Urol 1981; 125: 746–747.

186. Melicow MM, Lattes R, Pierre-Louis C. Lymphoma of the female urethra masquerading as a caruncle. J Urol 1972; 108: 748–749.

187. Touhami H, Brahimi S, Kubisz P, Cronberg S. NonHodgkin's lymphoma of the female urethra. J Urol 1987; 137: 991–992.

188. Steeper TA, Rosai J. Aggressive angiomyxoma of the female pelvis and perineum. Report of nine cases of a distinctive type of gynecologic soft-tissue neoplasm. Am J Surg Pathol 1983; 7: 463–475.

# CHAPTER 12

# Non-neoplastic diseases
of the testis

Manuel Nistal, Ricardo Paniagua

# Embryology and anatomy of the testis

## Embryology

### Development of the testis

*Genetic mechanisms involved in sex determination and testicular differentiation*

Sexual differentiation is the result of complex genetic and endocrine mechanisms that are closely associated with the development of both the genitourinary system and the adrenal glands. Formation of the bipotential gonad and, subsequently, of the ovaries and testes, depends on gene expression in both sex and autosomal chromosomes. Testes secrete steroid and peptidic hormones that are necessary for the development of inner and outer male genitalia. These hormonal actions are mediated by specific receptors that are transcriptional regulators. Alteration of these genetic events leads to sexual dimorphism involving the inner and outer genitalia, and can also hinder the development of other organs.[1]

Chromosomal gender is established at fecundation with formation of an egg with either a 46XY (male) or a 46XX (female) karyotype. Each chromosomal constitution initiates a cascade of genetic events leading to the development of female (ovaries) or male (testes) gonads (gonadal gender). Hormonal secretions from the ovaries or testes are essential for the development of external genitalia (phenotypic gender). The relationship between the individual and the environment determines the social gender.

There are multiple genes involved in the formation of the undifferentiated gonad. The two most important for the proper formation of the bipotential gonad are WT1 (Wilms' tumor gene) and NR5A1 (Fig. 12-1).

WT1 contains 10 exons located on chromosome 11p13, with two alternative splicing loci in introns 5 and 9. Intron 9 splicing can lead to the inclusion or exclusion of three amino acids (KTS: lysine, threonine and serine), giving rise to KTS+ or KTS– isoforms. An adequate KTS+/KTS– balance is crucial for normal expression of the gene. Translation of this gene may generate up to 24 isoforms with several zinc-finger domains. This gene is expressed mainly in the kidneys and gonads, and mediates the transition from stroma to epithelium and morphogenetic differentiation (inhibits those genes that encode proliferative factors and activates those that

enhance epithelial differentiation). WT1 gene anomalies lead to a wide variety of phenotypes; deletions are associated with minimal genitourinary alterations and predisposition to develop Wilms' tumor.[2-4] Missense heterozygous mutations give rise to Denys–Drash syndrome (complete or partial 46XY gonadal dysgenesis, renal disease of early onset with diffuse mesangial sclerosis, and Wilms' tumor (OMIM 19408)).[5] Loss of the KTS+ isoform accounts for Frasier's syndrome (46XY gonadal dysgenesis, renal disease of late onset and absence of Wilms' tumor (OMIM 136680)).[6]

NR5A1 gene product is termed SF-1 (steroidogenic factor 1). The gene has seven exons in chromosome 9q33.3, and is expressed in the urogenital ridge that forms the gonads and adrenal glands. SF-1 promotes the expression of the anti-müllerian hormone (AMH) and joins elements that regulate upstream the AMH gene. SF-1 is first detected in the developing Sertoli cells of sex cords, but later is mainly localized in Leydig cells.[7] A heterozygous deletion causes a female phenotype in patients with 46XY, adrenal failure during the first weeks of extrauterine life, persistence of normal müllerian structures, and gonads consisting of poorly differentiated tubules embedded in abundant connective tissue. These patients do not respond to hCG stimulation.[8] In 46XX patients, ovarian development is not modified by SF-1 mutations, and they present with adrenal failure only.[9]

LIM-1 is another gene involved in the formation of the bipotential gonad and kidneys. It was recently identified in mice that bore homozygous deletions and presented alterations in both organs.[10] FGF-9 (fibroblastic growth factor 9) has also been related to gonadal development.

Both gonosomal and autosomal genes mediate the progression of the bipotential gonad toward testicular differentiation. The signal is triggered by the SRY gene on the distal portion of the short arm of the Y chromosome (sex-determining region of the Y chromosome; Yp11.3), also called TDF (testis determining factor gene).[11] This gene stimulates the differentiation of Sertoli cell precursors and germ cells, is responsible for the production of the anti-müllerian hormone,[12] and regulates other genes of the downstream cascade. These are either activated or inhibited by other genes in such a way that dozens of genes are involved in testicular differentiation.[13]

The SRY gene contains a single exon that encodes a 204 amino acid protein whose central part (79 amino acids) encodes a DNA-binding domain termed HMG (high mobil-

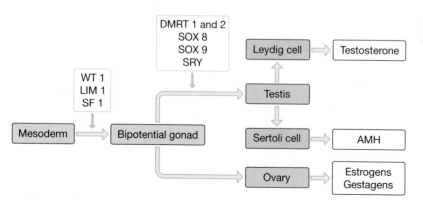

**Fig. 12-1** Genetic mechanisms involved in sex determination and testicular differentiation.

ity group). Immunohistochemical studies have demonstrated expression of the SRY gene in the nuclei of both Sertoli cells and germ cells,[14] suggesting that this gene acts in somatic cells of genital ridge and germ cells. SRY works with the AMH promoter gene and also regulates steroidogenic hormone expression.[15] SRY mutations produce pure gonadal dysgenesis (Swyer's syndrome) or true hermaphroditism; the karyotype of patients with the male phenotype lacking Y chromosome is either 46XX SRY+ (80%) or 46XX SRY– (20%), and all have male external genitalia, testes, azoospermia and no müllerian structures. Some 46XX SRY- patients have SOX-9 duplication.[16]

Following discovery of the SRY gene, the knowledge about genes involved in gonadal formation advanced experimentally with knockout mice and the study of human syndromes. Now, there are numerous reported genes (including SOX-8, SOX-9, DAX-1, LHX-9, LIM-1 and DMRT-1) that encode associated transcription factors.

SOX-8 and SOX-9 (SRYY box 8 and 9 or SRY HMG-BOX gene 9) are related to autosomal genes. SOX-9 is on chromosome 17q24,3q25,1 and is expressed after SRY expression in the same cell type (the pre-Sertoli cell).[17] This gene is also essential for the development of the cartilaginous extracellular matrix. In the mouse gonad, SOX-9 inhibits testicular development or Sertoli cell marker expression, and the gonad acquires an ovarian pattern.[18] SOX-9 haploinsufficiency (loss of a functional allele) causes camptomelic dysplasia (a syndrome characterized by abnormal formation of cartilage) and a 46XY constitution with female phenotype,[17,19] whereas SOX-9 duplication results in 46XX patients with male phenotype.[20]

SOX-8 is other cofactor in AMH regulation and acts by protein–protein interaction with SF-1. Experimental models show that SOX-9 dysfunction results in replacement by SOX-8 expression via a feedback mechanism.[21]

DAX-1 (dosage-sensitive sex-reversal, adrenal hyperplasia, X-linked) gene is involved in the development of testes, ovaries, and adrenal glands. DAX-1, on X chromosome, is expressed during ovarian formation and inhibited by SRY during testicular formation. Duplication of the DAX-1 region in Xp21 results in 46XY gonadal dysgenesis.[22,23] Conversely, DAX-1 mutations decrease gene expression, resulting in absence of adrenal cortex and hypogonadotropic hypogonadism;[10] testicular determination is normal.

Deletions in chromosomes 9p[24] and 10q[25] are associated with the female phenotype in 46XY individuals. Chromosome 9p deletions are also associated with facial malformations, premature closure of the frontal suture, hydronephrosis, and delayed development. Deletions of two genes (DMRT1 and DMRT2) on chromosome 9p24.3 may be found in 46XY females. Terminal deletions in chromosome 10q are associated with genital malformations, multiple phenotypic anomalies, and mental retardation.

## Histological differentiation of genital ridges

In the fourth week of gestation, the urogenital ridges appear as two parallel prominences along the posterior abdominal wall. These give rise to two important pairs of structures: the genital ridges arising from the medial prominences, and the mesonephric ridges from the lateral prominences.

The genital ridges are the first primordium of the gonad and stand out as a pair of prominences about the midline. In 30–32-day embryos, each genital ridge is lateral to the aorta and medial to the mesonephric duct (Fig. 12-2). The celomic epithelium forming the genital ridges grows as cord-like structures to create the primary sex cords. Immediately beneath the celomic epithelium there are several mesonephric ductuli and glomeruli (Fig. 12-3).

The origin of the gonadal blastema results from the junction of two cell types: epithelial cells from the celomic epithelium and mesenchymal cells from the mesonephric region,[26,27] although experimental data are conflicting. One of the earliest effects of SRY expression is induction of mesonephric cell migration toward the genital ridge.[28,29] Histochemical studies revealed that an early event is also disruption of the celomic epithelium basal lamina, permitting the migration of these epithelial cells inside the gonad. If chromosomal constitution is XY, these cells give rise to Sertoli cells.[30] Cells derived from the celomic epithelium are recognized by their pale cytoplasm, large size,

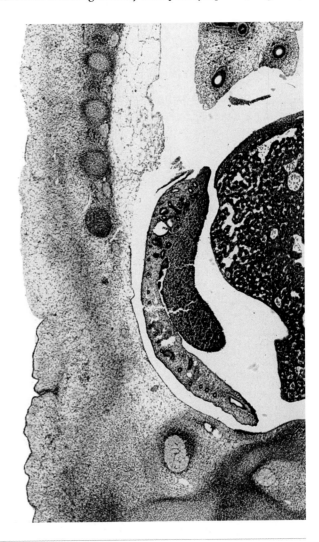

**Fig. 12-2** Longitudinal section of a fetus showing the relationship of the primitive gonad, mesonephros, and metanephros.

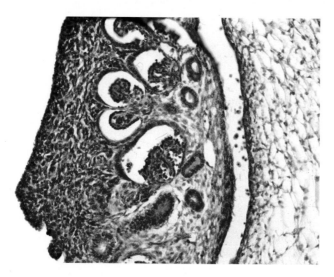

**Fig. 12-3** Longitudinal section of the gonad showing the close relation between the gonadal blastema and mesonephric glomeruli.

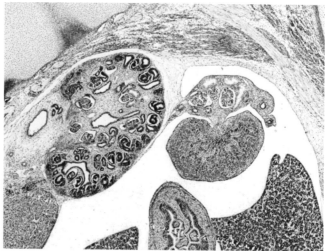

**Fig. 12-4** Transverse section of a fetus showing the relationship between the fetal testis, mesonephros and metanephros.

and ovoid euchromatic nucleus. The cells of mesonephric origin are darker and have a mesenchymal pattern.

Initially, the genital ridges are devoid of germ cells. In the third week, primordial germ cells appear in the extraembryonal mesoderm lining the posterior wall of the yolk sac near the allantoic evagination. They are ovoid, measuring 12–14 µm in diameter, and are easily detected histochemically by a high content of alkaline phosphatase. The nuclei are spherical and possess one or two prominent central nucleoli. The cytoplasm contains mitochondria with tubular cristae, lysosomes, microfilaments, lipid inclusions, numerous ribosomes, and abundant glycogen granules. Attracted by chemotactic factors, the primordial germ cells migrate along the mesenchyma of the mesentery and reach the genital ridge by 32–35 days.

The seminiferous cords arise from the gonadal blastema.[31,32] Many germ cells reach the seminiferous cords, but some degenerate during migration. The seminiferous cords are delimited from the stroma by a basement membrane[33] and lose their connection to the celomic epithelium, which reduces its depth to one or two cell layers only. The intercordal mesenchyma, composed chiefly of cells that migrated from the mesonephric stroma, differentiate later into myoid cells, Leydig cells, fibroblasts, and blood vessels.[34]

Up to the sixth week, the gonads appear similar, although the incipient testes have more numerous blood vessels, more abundant stroma,[35] and a higher total DNA content, suggesting more rapid growth.

Sertoli cells arise from somatic sex cord cells. These cells differentiate at the end of the seventh week from the somatic cells in the cords, develop adherent junctions between them and a basal lamina on the other cord surface, and begin to express AMH.[36]

In the eighth week, Leydig cells differentiate from the intercordal gonadal blastema,[37] and immunohistochemical detection of 3β-HSD is apparently the first step in this process. Leydig cell development peaks during the 18th week, and numbers subsequently decrease progressively.[38]

The rete testis originates from mesonephric remnants of sex cords that are in continuity with the seminiferous cords. The connection between the testis and the mesonephros becomes progressively thinner (Fig. 12-4). The testis has a round transversal section, and remains located between two suspensory ligaments: the cranial and the caudal, the latter of which gives rise to the gubernaculum.

## Development of the urogenital tract

The development of the urogenital tract begins at the stage of the undifferentiated gonad, with the appearance of two different pairs of ducts: the wolffian and the müllerian.

The wolffian ducts are formed in the mesonephros in the third week of gestation, when the cranial region of the segmented intermediate mesoderm gives rise to 10 pairs of tubules (the nephric tubules) that are metamerically arranged. These tubules form the pronephros. On each side of the body, the tubules converge to form a longitudinal duct that opens in the celomic cavity. In the fourth week, the pronephros disappears and is replaced by another tubular system (derived from the intermediate mesoderm, which is not segmented) that forms the mesonephros. The medial ends of the mesonephric tubules do not open to the celomic cavity but are connected to glomeruli at one end and the wolffian duct at the other. At the end of the second month of gestation, the mesonephros is replaced by the metanephros or definitive kidney. However, in the male, the most caudal mesonephric tubules and the wolffian duct persist. The former give rise to the ductuli efferentes, and the latter forms the ductus epididymidis, the ductus deferens, the seminal vesicle, and the ejaculatory duct.

Both müllerian ducts originate from a longitudinal invagination of the celomic epithelium in the anterolateral aspect of the genital ridge. The cranial end of each duct is a funnel that opens in the celomic cavity. Each duct runs parallel and lateral to the respective wolffian duct and, as they pass caudally, the müllerian duct crosses over the wolffian duct and lies medial to it. Finally, the two müllerian ducts fuse into the uterovaginal duct. This elongates caudally up to the posterior aspect of the urogenital sinus, forming the müllerian tubercle. The wolffian ducts terminate at either side of this tubercle.

The remaining structures of the male genital system are derived from the urogenital sinus. Epithelium with endodermal origin forms the prostate, the urethra, and the bulbourethral and periurethral glands. The primitive urogenital sinus derives from the cloaca, a structure that appears at the end of the first month and which consists of a dilation of the terminal portion of the primitive posterior intestine. The cloaca is closed by the cloacal membrane. In the third week, mesenchyma proliferates in the outer aspect of the cloacal membrane to form the cloacal folds and the cloacal eminence. In the sixth week, the cloacal folds enlarge to form the genital (or urethral) tubercle. External to the genital folds, another mesenchymal thickening develops into the genital prominences or genital swellings.

In the fifth week, a septum forms, dividing the cloaca into two compartments. The anterior compartment is the primitive urogenital sinus that is covered by the urogenital membrane. The posterior compartment is the anorectal canal, covered by the anal membrane. The primitive urogenital sinus then divides into two new compartments: superior and inferior. The superior compartment is the vesicourethral canal that later forms the urinary bladder and the urethra. The inferior compartment is the definitive urogenital sinus that will develop later according to the gender.

## Hormonal control

The development of the male genital system is directly influenced by the action of multiple hormones, including anti-müllerian hormone (AMH), dihydrotestosterone (derived from testosterone), and the pituitary hormones follicle-stimulating hormone (FSH) and luteinizing hormone (LH) (Fig. 12-5).

AMH (müllerian inhibitory substance; MIS),[39] secreted by the Sertoli cells, is a glycoprotein polymer consisting of two identical 72 kDa subunits linked by disulfide bonds.[40-42] It belongs to the TGF-β family and is synthesized as a 560 amino-acid precursor protein with proteolytic cleavage at 109 amino acids from the C terminal. Cleavage is necessary to activate the hormone. AMH is encoded by a 2.75 kb gene that comprises five exons and is located on the p13.2 region of chromosome 19.

AMH is secreted by somatic cells only in both sexes: Sertoli cells in males and granulosa cells in females. It is detected by 6–7 weeks of gonadal development (8–9 weeks of gestation), probably as soon as germ cells make contact with pre-Sertoli cells, a week before the müllerian ducts lose their responsiveness.[43,44] AMH is at high concentration in the second trimester, but drops precipitously in the third trimester.[45] Levels rise again during the first year after birth, are detectable during infancy and childhood, and finally drop definitively to undetectable levels at the onset of puberty. The secreted amount of AMH is inversely correlated to the degree of Sertoli cell maturation.

AMH regulation is incompletely understood. Its expression is controlled by steroidogenic factor 1 (SF-1), also called Ad4BP,[46] which is an orphan nuclear receptor that acts as a transcriptional regulator of all steroidogenic genes. AMH regulates SRY expression, which in Sertoli cells is detected

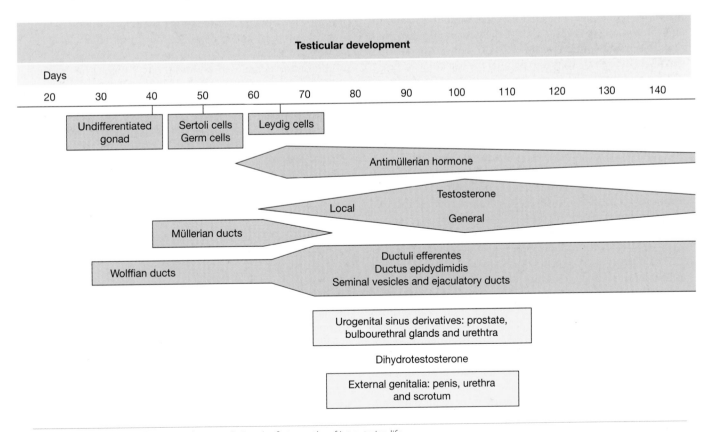

**Fig. 12-5** Development of the genital system during the first months of intrauterine life.

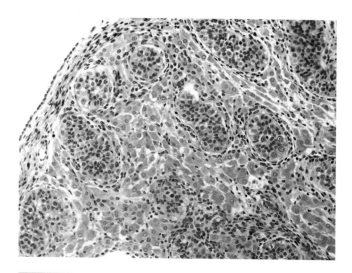

**Fig. 12-6** A 16-week-old fetal testis showing slightly convoluted seminiferous tubules and numerous Leydig cells in the testicular interstitium.

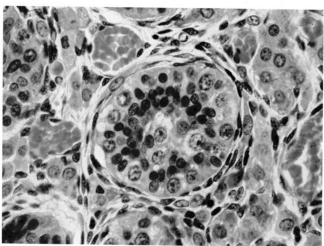

**Fig. 12-7** Testis from a 24-week-old fetus. The seminiferous tubules contain Sertoli cells (small dark nuclei) and gonocytes (spherical cells with larger nuclei and central nucleoli). At this age, the interstitium still contains numerous Leydig cells.

immediately before AMH expression.[47] During puberty, AMH is negatively regulated by androgens.[48]

AMH acts on the testis, genital tract, and extragenital structures. It causes involution of the ipsilateral müllerian duct. Action begins at the caudal testicular pole and progresses rapidly. In adults, remnants of the müllerian ducts include the appendix testis at the cranial end and the prostatic utricle (verumontanum) at the caudal end. AMH also stimulates development of the tunica albuginea, formed by insertion of mesenchyma between the celomic epithelium and primordial sex cords. This mesenchyma is also the origin of collagenized connective tissue, with deposition of collagen fibers in several layers that parallel the testicular surface.[49] AMH also hinders the entry of spermatogonia in meiosis.[50] The best-known function of AMH in the extragonadal system is the maturation of fetal lungs.[51]

Testosterone is synthesized by the Leydig cells. These first appear among the sex cords in the eighth week of gestation, and their number increases to 48 million per pair of testes by the 16th week,[52] occupying about 50% of the testicular volume (Fig. 12-6). The relative number of Leydig cells decreases from the 16th to the 24th week, owing to rapid enlargement of the testis during this period. However, the absolute number of Leydig cells remains constant. From the 24th week to birth, the number of Leydig cells decreases to 18 million per pair of testes. Testosterone synthesis begins after the 56th day of gestation.

Testosterone secretion is regulated by hCG and LH concentrations. hCG peaks between weeks 11 and 17 and drops markedly thereafter; hCG-dependent testosterone is the most important determinant of genital differentiation. Wolffian duct differentiation occurs only as a response to the testosterone secreted by the ipsilateral testis. This secretion stimulates differentiation of the ductus epididymidis, ductus deferens, and seminal vesicle. Anomalies in androgen synthesis lead to incomplete masculinization and cryptorchidism.

Dihydrotestosterone (DHT) derives from testosterone by the action of the enzyme 5α-reductase and is responsible for differentiation of the prostate and the development of the external genitalia, male urethra, penis and scrotum. It induces fusion of the labioscrotal folds in the middle plane to form the scrotum and the middle scrotal raphe. The urethral folds become fused to form the penile urethra. The genital tubercle enlarges to form the glans penis. An ectodermal invagination of the glans tip forms the terminal portion of the urethra. The urogenital sinus gives rise to the urinary bladder, prostatic urethra, and prostate.[53] The initial effects of DHT (labioscrotal fusion) occur on approximately day 70; the urethral groove is closed on about day 74; and the external genitalia are completely developed by week 20.

The actions of these hormones occur at precise moments in development. Failure in the amount or timing of secretion or in the responsiveness of target tissues causes most of the malformations found in intersex conditions.[52]

FSH and LH both play an important role in the last months of gestation. LH appears in the fetal circulation during the 10th week and peaks by the 18th, decreasing progressively and slowly thereafter until birth. LH chiefly regulates androgen production during the second half of fetal life. FSH is an essential mitogen for Sertoli cells that reach the highest mitotic ratio at the end of fetal life (Fig. 12-7).[54,55]

## Testicular descent

Testicular descent is the result of hormonal and mechanical actions that are not fully understood. Three steps are recognized: nephric displacement, transabdominal descent, and inguinal descent. In nephric displacement, the gonad detaches from the metanephros in the seventh week of gestation. Transabdominal descent occurs in the 12th week and consists of the displacement of the testis towards the deep inguinal ring. Inguinal descent occurs between the seventh month and birth.[56] Clinically, the term testicular descent often refers only to this last step, in which the testis passes from the abdominal cavity to the scrotum.

Testicular descent is directed by the gubernaculum testis, a structure that appears in the sixth week as an elongate condensation of mesenchymal cells extending from the genital ridge to the presumptive inguinal region.[57,58] At this level in the abdominal wall, the gubernaculum cells persist as a simple mesenchyma while the remaining abdominal wall cells differentiate into muscle. These mesenchymal cells give rise to the inguinal canal. Thus, the testis lies on a continuous column of mesenchyma limited by the cranial testicular ligament in the upper pole and by the plica gubernaculi that joins the testis to the future scrotal region in the inferior pole. The periphery of this mesenchymal tissue is invaded by the processus vaginalis, which develops from a peritoneal pouch that grows into this mesenchyma. Once the inguinal canal and the plica gubernaculi are formed, development slows. In the seventh month the processus vaginalis undergoes active growth, the cremasteric muscle develops from the mesenchyma outside the processus vaginalis, and the distal end of the gubernaculum enlarges markedly. Gubernacular enlargement occurs from the 16th to the 24th weeks of gestation period and is caused by hyperplasia, hypertrophy, and the absorption of a great volume of water by the glycosaminoglycans of the matrix.[59] The tissue is reminiscent of Wharton's jelly of the umbilical cord. By this time, the testis–epididymis complex is pear-shaped and its largest component is the gubernaculum. The testis and epididymis slide through the inguinal canal behind the gubernaculum. Simultaneously, development of the processus vaginalis is completed and the gubernaculum begins to shorten, the epididymis develops further, and the testicular blood vessels and vas deferens lengthen.[60]

Testicular descent is a complex process integrating several essential factors, including normal function of the hypothalamopituitary–testicular axis, normal development of abdominal musculature, gubernaculum and the processus vaginalis,[61,62] and a testis with normal endocrine function.

The critical role of normal hormonal function is supported by clinical and experimental observations: destruction of the hypophysis in laboratory animals impedes testicular descent; anencephalic fetuses usually have undescended testes; many cryptorchid patients have transitory neonatal hypogonadotropic hypogonadism; and some undescended testes descend after treatment with human chorionic gonadotropin or gonadotropin-releasing hormone. Adequate intra-abdominal pressure is another requisite.[63,64] In the prune-belly syndrome, bilateral cryptorchidism is associated with urologic malformations and absence of the abdominal wall musculature. In a variant of this syndrome, termed pseudo-prune-belly syndrome, there is a positive correlation between the development of the abdominal wall musculature and testicular descent. Development of the processus vaginalis also plays a critical role in testicular descent. This structure grows within the gubernaculum; if it is partially replaced by fibrous tissue, the testis will follow other directions in its descent and end in an ectopic location. If fibrous tissue completely replaces the gubernaculum, the processus vaginalis and cremasteric muscle fail to

develop fully, and descent of the testis is mechanically blocked.[62]

The hormonal requirements for testicular descent are not clear.[65] The most important factor in transabdominal descent is the androgen-independent peptide insulin-like factor 3 (INSF-3), a member of the relaxin–insulin family that is produced by fetal Leydig cells. This peptide stimulates gubernaculum cells to initiate gubernaculum swelling, a necessary step for the initiation of testicular descent.[66] Mutations in INSL-3 gene or its receptors LGRB-8 (leucine-rich repeat-containing G protein-coupled receptor 8) or GREAT (G protein-coupled receptor affecting testicular descent) interfere with transabdominal descent and cause cryptorchidism.[67,68] AMH and androgens are also involved in the gubernaculum swelling reaction; androgens also facilitate regression of the cranial suspensory ligament.

Uncertainty exists regarding the mechanism of inguinoscrotal descent and its hormonal control. Androgens and the genitofemoral nerve are two factors strongly implicated in these processes. The role of androgens on the gubernaculum is very limited, because this structure has neither muscular cells[69] nor androgen receptors at the time of testicular descent. Androgenic effects are explained by the hypothesis of the genitofemoral nerve.[70] Androgens appear to act on the nucleus of the genitofemoral nerve in the spinal cord rather than directly on the gubernacula, producing masculinization of the neurons that form this nucleus[71] (these neurons are much more numerous in males than in females) and secreting great amounts of calcitonin gene-related peptide (CGRP). In rats, CGRP causes rapid rhythmic contractions of the gubernaculum and it has been suggested that the gubernaculum might have embryonic cardiac muscle cells. However, it is also possible that CGRP acts on the cremasteric muscle that develops within the gubernaculum and is innervated by the genitofemoral nerve. This hypothesis is supported by the observation of neurogenic atrophy of this muscle in cryptorchid patients.[72]

Other factors involved in testicular descent are estrogens and epidermal growth factor (EGF). During the first trimester of gestation, mothers of cryptorchid infants have free estradiol serum concentrations that are significantly higher than those of controls.[73] Experimental studies have shown that estradiol diminishes gubernacular swelling and stabilizes müllerian ducts. It has been proposed that estradiol inhibits the cell proliferation that causes gubernaculum swelling.[74,75] EGF may facilitate testicular descent throughout the placental–gonadal axis. Maternal EGF levels increase just before fetal masculinization occurs.[76] The placenta has an elevated concentration of EGF receptors, and placental stimulation by EGF might stimulate hCG production, which may also stimulate fetal Leydig cells to produce androgens; hypothetically, these and/or other factors may determine testicular descent.

After birth, the gubernaculum and processus vaginalis regress. The gubernaculum is replaced by fibrous tissue that forms the scrotal ligament. The cephalic segment of the processus vaginalis atrophies after testicular descent. An exaggerated resorption of the processus vaginalis with pulling up of the testis may induce a testis that had descended normally to ascend, resulting in cryptorchidism.[77]

## Prepubertal testis

From birth to puberty the testis is a dynamic structure, an important consideration in interpreting biopsies from children. All testicular components undergo waves of proliferation and differentiation prior to puberty.[78] Three waves of germ cell proliferation occur: during the neonatal period, infancy, and puberty.[79] The last gives rise to complete spermatogenesis. There also are three waves of Leydig cell proliferation (fetal, neonatal, and pubertal); the last corresponds to the pubertal wave of germ cell proliferation.

### Development of the testis from birth to puberty

#### The testis at birth

The newborn testis has a volume of about 0.57 mL[80] and is covered by a thin tunica albuginea from which the intratesticular septa arise. These divide the testis into lobules containing the seminiferous tubules and testicular interstitium (Fig. 12-8). The seminiferous tubules measure 60–65 μm in diameter, with no apparent lumina, and are filled with Sertoli cells and germ cells. Sertoli cells are the most abundant, with 26–28 cells per tubular cross-section (Fig. 12-9).[81] They form a pseudostratified cellular layer and have elongated to oval nuclei with darker chromatin than that of mature Sertoli cells, as well as one or two small peripheral nucleoli. The cytoplasm contains abundant rough endoplasmic reticulum, several Golgi complexes and numerous vimentin filaments, and expresses inhibin B (Fig. 12-10). No specialized intercellular junctions appear between Sertoli cells, but desmosome-like junctions are present between Sertoli cells and germ cells.[82]

Two types of germ cell are present at birth: gonocytes and spermatogonia. Gonocytes are usually located near the center of the tubules, with voluminous nuclei and large central nucleoli.[82] Gonocyte migration is probably facilitated by cell adhesion molecules such as P cadherin, which is expressed by Sertoli cells of immature testes.[83] Spermatogonia are mainly located on the basal lamina, and possess smaller nuclei and less cytoplasm than gonocytes; the nucleoli are peripheral and very small. At birth, most spermatogonia correspond to the adult type A (see discussion on the adult testis below) (Fig. 12-11).

The testicular interstitium contains fetal Leydig cells that resemble adult Leydig cells but lack Reinke's crystalloids (Fig. 12-12).[84,85] Additionally, mast cells, macrophages, and hematopoietic cell are present.[86]

The first wave of testicular development occurs during the neonatal period and involves germ cells and Leydig cells. These changes are caused by a significant increase in secretion of both FSH and LH during the third postnatal month.[87–89] Testicular weight and volume increase. LH stimulates the Leydig cells to produce testosterone,[90,91] which stimulates the transformation of gonocytes to spermatogonia of the Ad type (Fig. 12-13). Afterwards, some of these

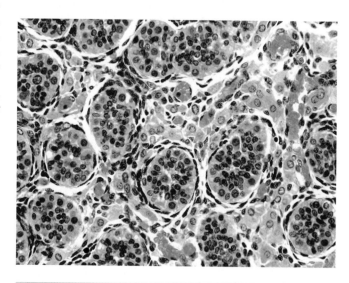

**Fig. 12-9** The seminiferous tubules contain two germ cell types: gonocytes and spermatogonia. The gonocytes have large nuclei with large central nucleoli. The spermatogonia have smaller nuclei and pale cytoplasm. Several Leydig cells are seen in the interstitium.

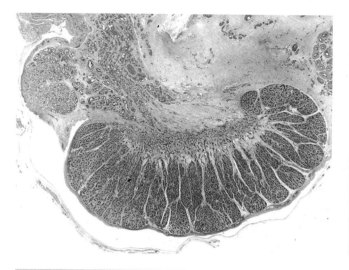

**Fig. 12-8** Longitudinal section of the testis and the epididymis from a newborn. Intratesticular septa split the testis into lobules.

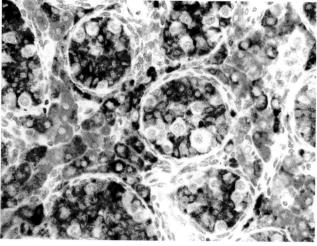

**Fig. 12-10** Newborn testis. Both Sertoli cells and Leydig cells are intensely immunoreactive for inhibin.

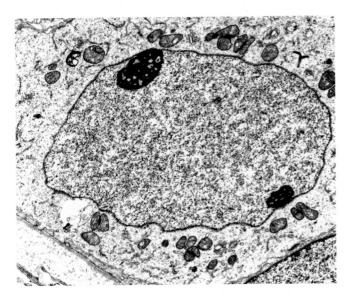

**Fig. 12-11** Spermatogonia show wide cytoplasm and regularly outlined nuclei with eccentric nucleoli. The cytoplasm contains mitochondria joined by electron-dense bars.

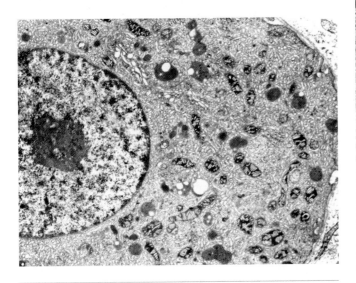

**Fig. 12-12** Leydig cells have eccentric, round nuclei, abundant smooth endoplasmic reticulum and mitochondria, lysosomes, and stacks of rough endoplasmic reticulum cisternae.

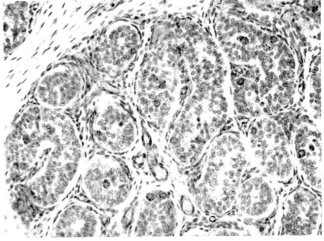

**Fig. 12-13** Testis from a 4-day-old infant. Gonocytes are strongly immunoreactive for c-*kit.*

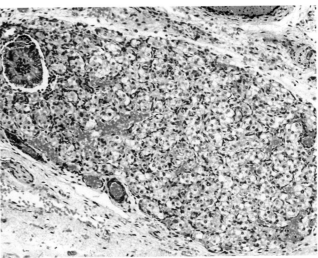

**Fig. 12-14** Newborn epididymis showing a paraganglium around the epididymal duct.

divide to form Ap spermatogonia (see discussion on the adult testis below). Six months after birth, gonocytes are absent, coinciding with the loss of fetal germ cell markers (placental alkaline phosphatase and c-kit).

Paraganglia are often observed in epididymides and spermatic cords from newborns. This is not surprising, as paraganglia are the main source of catecholamine before birth (Fig. 12-14).[92]

### The testis in infancy

From the sixth month to approximately the second half of the third year of life, the testis is in a resting period; this quiescence is broken by the second wave of germ cell proliferation.[93] The number of Ap spermatogonia increases, and B spermatogonia (derived from Ap spermatogonia) appear.

In some normal testes at this age, meiotic primary spermatocytes and round spermatids are observed (Fig. 12-15). This spermatogenic attempt fails and many degenerate germ cells may be present.[94,95] The testis continues to produce AMH (by Sertoli cells)[96] and inhibin B.[97] AMH modulates the number and function of Leydig cells by regulating differentiation of their mesenchymal precursors and the expression of steroidogenic enzymes.[98] Inhibin B plays a role in FSH inactivation during infancy.

The cause of this second wave of germ cell proliferation is unknown; there is no elevation of FSH or LH serum concentrations between 6 months and 10 years of life. After the sixth year, there is a slight increase in adrenal androgens, but testicular testosterone levels increase only after the 10th year.[99,100] By the third year, most Leydig cells have degenerated: from a peak of about 18 million at birth, only 60 000 remain by the age of 6 years. At this age, testosterone levels

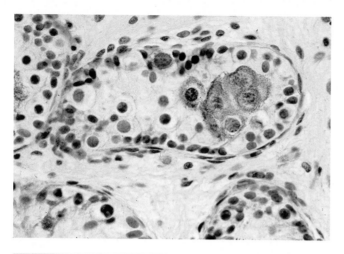

**Fig. 12-15** Testis from a 4-year-old infant. The seminiferous tubules have spermatogonial proliferation and contain a central group of primary spermatocytes.

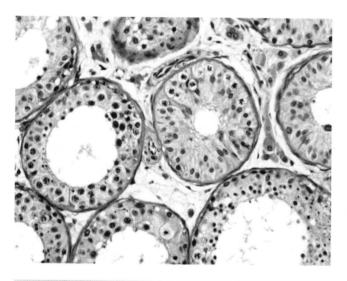

**Fig. 12-16** Testis from an 11-year-old boy. Germ cell development varies from one tubule to another. The number of spermatogonia is lower than that of the adult testes. Residual immature Sertoli cells show elongated nuclei with small nucleoli. Leydig cells are scant.

are similar to those of girls,[99] and most androgens are of adrenal origin.

### The testis in childhood

At about 9 years of age, the third and definitive wave of spermatogenesis begins,[101] coinciding with a significant elevation of LH. This is followed by additional increases in the level of this hormone between 13 and 15 years of age. LH induces fibroblast-like Leydig cell precursors to differentiate into mature Leydig cells.[102] By the end of puberty, the population of Leydig cells per testis has risen to about 786 million.[103] Leydig cells secrete androgens, which, together with the rise in FSH between 11 and 14 years of age, cause Sertoli cell maturation, germ cell development, and the appearance of tubular lumina (Fig. 12-16),[103] increasing the size of the testes between the ages of 11.5 and 12.5 years of life.[104] At 13.5 years, before the testis reaches adult size,

spermatozoa are present, secondary sex characteristics are completely developed, and the epiphyses close.[105]

### Interpretation of testicular biopsy from prepubertal testes

Testicular biopsy in children is useful for diagnosing those with ambiguous genitalia, a history of leukemia or lymphoma whose testes underwent a rapid enlargement, or precocious testicular maturation of unknown cause. In other situations, the value of testicular biopsy is less established. For example, the value of biopsy of cryptorchid testes during orchidopexy is controversial. Evaluation of biopsies of the prepubertal testis should involve the assessment of several features, including tunica albuginea thickness, mean tubular diameter, and the number of germ cells, Sertoli cells, and Leydig cells.

#### Tunica albuginea

The most frequent anomalies of the tunica albuginea include thin, poorly collagenized tunica albuginea with abnormal tubules typical of testicular dysgenesis (see the section on male pseudohermaphrodites with müllerian remnants, below); well-collagenized tunica albuginea containing ectopic seminiferous tubules, a frequent finding in cryptorchidism; and poorly collagenized tunica albuginea containing ovocytes characteristic of true hermaphroditic ovotestes.

#### Mean tubular diameter

The mean tubular diameter is an excellent indicator of the development of the seminiferous epithelium. In the prepubertal testis, tubular diameter depends principally on the Sertoli cells and thus indicates whether they are adequately stimulated by FSH. Tubular diameter varies throughout, being smallest in the end of the third year of life, slowly enlarging up to 9 years of age, and rapidly enlarging thereafter up to 15 years (Fig. 12-17).

The most frequent abnormality in the prepubertal testis is a low mean tubular diameter. This is seen in undescended testes as well as in hypogonadotropic or hypergonadotropic hypogonadism. In the latter, the lesion results from anomalous Sertoli cell responsiveness to FSH.[106]

There are three levels of severity of low tubular diameter: slight tubular hypoplasia (up to 10% reduction in relation to the diameter normal for the age); marked tubular hypoplasia (from 10% to 30% reduction); and severe tubular hypoplasia (more than 30% reduction). Many testicular biopsies show malformed seminiferous tubules that vary from straight or branched tubules up to ring-shaped. These are megatubules formed by either tight spiral or bell-shaped tubules. The presence of these malformations suggests the child will be infertile in adulthood.

Diffuse increase in mean tubular diameter may be unilateral or bilateral. Unilateral increase is found in monorchidism (compensatory testicular hypertrophy) and some testes that are contralateral to cryptorchid testes. Most frequently, diffuse enlargement occurs with benign idiopathic macroorchidism or macroorchidism associated with fragile X chromosome, familial testotoxicosis, hypothyroidism, or different forms of precocious puberty. Focal increases in mean tubular

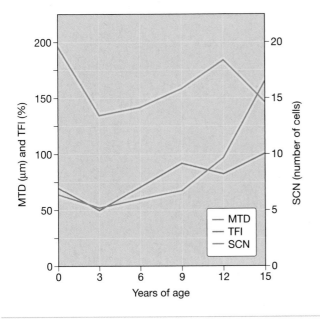

**Fig. 12-17** Changes in mean tubular diameter (MTD), tubular fertility index (TFI), and Sertoli cell number per cross-sectioned tubule (SCN) from birth to puberty.

diameter are usually associated with precocious maturation of the seminiferous epithelium layers, and occur at the periphery of some Sertoli cell and Leydig cell tumors.

### Germ cell number

Germ cells can be counted in two ways: calculation of the number of cells per tubular cross-section, or determination of the tubular fertility index. The former counts the number of germ cells in a light microscopic field and divides this by the number of cross-sectioned tubules in the same field. In the first 6 months of postnatal life the normal testis has two germ cells per cross-sectioned tubule. This number drops to 1.5 at the end of the first year and to 0.5 at the end of the third year. The number of germ cells increases to 1.8 cells at the age of 3–4 years, which coincides with the appearance of spermatocytes in some tubules.

The tubular fertility index reflects the percentage of tubular sections containing germ cells. In newborns, 68% of tubular sections contain at least one germ cell. From birth to 3 years this decreases to 50%, followed by a progressive increase to 100% at puberty.[93] If the numbers of gonocytes and spermatogonia are calculated separately, it is possible to determine when the transformation of gonocytes to spermatogonia occurs. The most accurate measure is calculation of total germ cell numbers per testis. This is more difficult because it requires morphometric assessment of intratubular volume and careful clinical measurement of the three axes of the testis.

Congenital decrease of germ cells occurs in numerous conditions, including trisomies 13, 18, and 21, some forms of primary hypogonadism such as Klinefelter's syndrome, anencephaly, many cryptorchid testes, and in patients with posterior urethral valves and severe obstruction of the urinary ducts.[107] An increased number of germ cells may be seen at the periphery of germ cell tumor, gonadal–stromal tumor,

and paratesticular sarcoma. At the periphery of Leydig cell tumor, seminiferous tubular cellular maturation may be complete.

Three levels of severity of germinal hypoplasia are recognized: slight (tubular fertility index >50), marked (tubular fertility index between 50 and 30), and severe (tubular fertility index <30) (Fig. 12-17). Marked and severe germinal hypoplasia is usually associated with marked or severe tubular hypoplasia, in most cases resulting from tubular dysgenesis. It also is useful to determine whether the seminiferous tubules devoid of germ cells are randomly distributed. If they are grouped, they probably belong to the same lobule or group of lobules that never will develop normally.

Other germ cells observed are multinucleate or hypertrophied spermatogonia and gonocyte-like cells; these latter may require immunohistochemical studies to exclude intratubular germ cell neoplasia.

### Sertoli cell number

The number of Sertoli cells per tubular cross-section varies during childhood as a result of slow proliferation from 4 years to 12 years[108] and the redistribution of Sertoli cells as the seminiferous tubules become longer and broader. The pseudostratified cellular pattern characteristic of Sertoli cells at birth changes slowly to a columnar pattern at puberty (Fig. 12-17). Testicular biopsies may reveal hypoplasia or hyperplasia of Sertoli cells; hyperplasia is usually pronounced and a sign of tubular dysgenesis, often detected during the first year of life or the beginning of puberty.[109] Some biopsies reveal one or several tubular sections containing Sertoli cells with eosinophilic and granular cytoplasm that is positive to CD68 and $\alpha_1$-antitrypsin. These oncocytic changes are the result of lysosomal accumulation.[110]

### Leydig cell number

Calculation of Leydig cell numbers during childhood is difficult because at this age the population is scant.[102] Semi-thin sections or immunohistochemistry to detect testosterone-containing cells may be helpful.[111] Selection of the appropriate denominator to express the Leydig cell population is another problem. The most frequent measures are Leydig cell number per tubular section, per unit area, or total number per testis.[104]

Low numbers of Leydig cell are observed in undescended testes, hypogonadotropic hypogonadism, some variants of male pseudohermaphroditism caused by a defect in the LH receptor, and in anencephalic fetuses. High numbers of Leydig cells occur in congenital Leydig cell hyperplasia,[112] triploid fetuses,[113] variants of precocious puberty, several syndromes such as leprechaunism and Beckwith–Wiederman syndrome, and in most male pseudohermaphroditisms.

### Intertubular connective tissue

An apparent increase in loose connective tissue is found in patients with marked tubular hypoplasia; in addition, disordered thick fusiform cell bundles are seen in patients with androgen insensitivity. Other alterations include the presence of excessively developed lymphatic vessels (lymphangiectasis), focal hematopoiesis, leukemic infiltration, and the presence of cells similar to those of the adrenal cortex (tumors of the adrenogenital syndrome).

## Adult testis

### Anatomy

The adult testis is an egg-shaped organ that hangs in the scrotum from the spermatic cord, the retroepididymal surface, and the scrotal ligament. Mean weight in Caucasian men is 21.6 ± 0.4 g for the right testis and 20 ± 0.4 g for the left. Mean testicular diameter is 4.6 cm (range, 3.6–5.5 cm) for the longest axis and 2.6 cm (range, 2.1–3.2 cm) for the shortest.[114–117] Testicular volume varies from 15 to 25 mL.

### Supporting structures

The tunica albuginea and interlobular septa make up the connective tissue framework of the testis. The tunica albuginea consists of three connective tissue layers and an outer surface covered by mesothelium. From the outer to the inner layers, the amount of collagen fibers decreases while the number of cells increases. The fibers and cells in the two outermost layers form planes parallel to the testicular surface; cell types include fibroblasts, myofibroblasts, and mast cells. Myofibroblasts are more numerous in the posterior portion of the testis. The thickness of the tunica albuginea increases with age from 400–450 μm in young men to more than 900 μm in elderly men.[118] It acts as a semipermeable membrane that produces the fluid of the vaginal cavity. The presence of many contractile cells showing high concentrations of GMP suggests that the tunica albuginea undergoes impulses of contraction and relaxation. These cells might regulate testicular size[119] and favor the transport of spermatozoa into the epididymis.[120]

The innermost layer, the tunica vasculosa, consists of loose connective tissue containing blood and lymphatic vessels. The interlobular septa consist of fibrous connective tissue with blood vessels supplying the testicular parenchyma. The interlobular septa divide the testis into approximately 250 pyramidal lobules with their bases at the tunica albuginea and vertices at the mediastinum testis. Each lobule contains two to four seminiferous tubules and numerous Leydig cells.[121]

### Seminiferous tubules

Adult seminiferous tubules are 180–200 μm in diameter and 30–80 cm long. The total combined length of the seminiferous tubules is about 540 m (range, 299–981 m).[122] They are highly convoluted and tightly packed within the lobules. The seminiferous tubules comprise about 80% of testicular volume. The tubular lining of germ cells and Sertoli cells is surrounded by a lamina propria (tunica propria) (Fig. 12-18).

#### Sertoli cells

Sertoli cells are columnar cells that extend from the basal lamina to the tubular lumen, with 10–12 cells per cross-sectioned tubule. They are easily identified by their nuclear characteristics. The nucleus is located near the basal lamina and has a triangular shape with indented outline, pale chromatin, and a large central nucleolus (Fig. 12-19). Charcot–Böttcher's crystals and lipid droplets often are visible in the cytoplasm.[123–126]

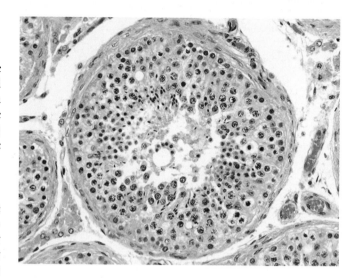

**Fig. 12-18** Seminiferous tubule with complete spermatogenesis.

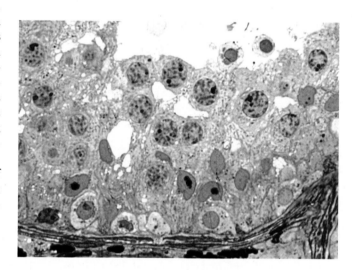

**Fig. 12-19** Germ cell development progresses from the basal lamina towards the lumen of the tubule. Each germ cell type forms a different layer in the seminiferous tubules and may be identified by its nuclei. Spermatogonia are basal cells with pale cytoplasm, round nuclei, and eccentric nucleoli. Above these cells, the Sertoli cell nuclei may be recognized by their large central nucleoli. The inner layers consist of primary spermatocytes showing the chromatin pattern characteristic of meiosis. (Semi-thin section.)

Ultrastructurally, Sertoli cells have characteristic nucleoli, plasma membranes, and cytoplasmic components. The nucleolus has a tripartite structure with a round fibrillar center, a compact granular portion, and a three-dimensional net composed of intermingled fibrillar and granular portions.[127–129] The plasma membrane has two types of intercellular junction which develop at puberty: junctions between adjacent Sertoli cells, and junctions between Sertoli cells and germ cells.[130] The inter-Sertoli cell junctions are tight-junction complexes. The adjacent cytoplasm has numerous actin filaments and parallel-arranged smooth endoplasmic reticula cisternae. In adjacent plasma membranes there are adhesion molecules, including connexin-43. Between the plasma membrane and the adjacent endoplasmic reticulum cisterna there are many molecules, including those required for actin filament anchorage, vinculin, zonula occludens-1, plakoglobin, and radixin. The inter-Sertoli cell junctions are the morphologic basis for the blood–testis barrier and divide the seminiferous epithelium into two compartments: the basal compartment (which contains spermatogonia and newly formed primary spermatocytes) and the adluminal compartment (which contains meiotic primary spermatocytes, secondary spermatocytes and spermatids). These junctions permit each compartment to have its own microenvironment for spermatogenic development.[131–133] The Sertoli cell–germ cell junctions persist from the primary spermatocyte stage through spermatozoon release. These junctions are desmosomes and gap-type junctions. The adhesion among Sertoli cells and germ cells is mediated by N-cadherin. These junctions have also occasionally been observed between spermatogonia.[134]

Sertoli cell cytoplasm contains abundant smooth endoplasmic reticulum, elongated mitochondria, annulate lamellae, lysosomes, residual bodies, glycogen granules, microtubules, vimentin filaments around the nucleus (Fig. 12-20),[135] actin filaments in both inter-Sertoli cell junctions and ectoplasmic specializations that surround germ cells,[136] lipid droplets in amounts that vary with the seminiferous tubular cycle,[137] Charcot–Böttcher crystals (structures several micrometers long, formed of multiple parallel laminae of protein), and scant rough endoplasmic reticulum and ribosomes.[138]

The number of Sertoli cells decreases with age, from about 250 million per testis in young men to 125 million in men over 50 years.[139,140] There is a positive correlation between the number of Sertoli cells and daily sperm production.[141] Sertoli cells are the target of FSH[142,143] and androgen action (Fig. 12-21).[144] In adulthood, they produce testicular fluid through an active transport mechanism, and synthesize multiple products to ensure the nutrition, proliferation and maturation of germ cells, to stimulate other cells such as Leydig cells and peritubular cells,[145] and to contribute to hormonal regulation (inhibin secretion) (Table 12-1). The transport of small molecules (<600–700 Da) such as pyruvate, lactate, and probably choline from the Sertoli cell, to germ cells occurs through gap junctions. Large or small soluble molecules are transported by proteins that are synthesized by the Sertoli cell, and include androgen-binding protein, transferrin, ceruloplas-

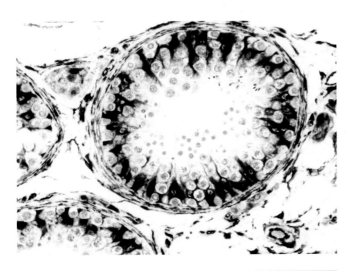

**Fig. 12-20** Cross-section of seminiferous tubule showing Sertoli cells that are intensely immunoreactive for vimentin.

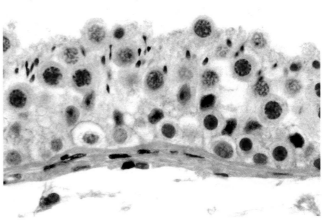

**Fig. 12-21** Sertoli cell nuclei immunostained for androgen receptors.

**Table 12-1** Sertoli cell–Leydig cell regulatory interactions

| Paracrine factor | Origin | Receptor | Action |
|---|---|---|---|
| Androgens | Leydig cell | Sertoli cell | Regulate/maintain function and differentiation |
| Pro-opiomelanocortin peptides | Leydig cell | Sertoli cell | Decrease FSH actions |
| β-endorphin | Leydig cell | Sertoli cell | Decrease steroidogenesis |
| GnRH-like factor | Sertoli cell | Leydig cell | Decrease steroidogenesis |
| Estrogens | Sertoli cell | Leydig cell | Decrease steroidogenesis |
| TGF-α | Sertoli cell | Leydig cell | Decrease steroidogenesis |
| IL-1 | Sertoli cell | Leydig cell | Decrease steroidogenesis |
| IGF-1 | Sertoli cell | Leydig cell | Increase steroidogenesis |

min, sulfated glycoproteins, $\alpha_2$-macroglobulin, and $\gamma$-glutamyl transpeptidase.[146] Activin and inhibin are Sertoli cell-secreted proteins that induce the proliferation and differentiation of germ cells. Whereas activin stimulates FSH production and, subsequently, spermatogonial proliferation, inhibin B inhibits FSH secretion, and is an important marker of spermatogenesis.[147] Other Sertoli cell secretions are interleukins, mainly IL-1,[148] and growth factors such as transforming growth factor-$\beta$ (TGF-$\beta$), insulin growth factors 1 and 2 (IGF-1 and IGF-2), and seminiferous growth factor (SGF) or stem cell factor (SCF). Some of these growth factors, such as TGF-$\alpha$, TGF-$\beta$, and IGF-1, are involved in the regulation of Leydig cell function. Other secreted substances include clusterin, the steroid 3-$\alpha$-4-pregnen-20-one (3HP), and prostaglandin D synthase (Table 12-2).

Sertoli cells are also involved in migration of differentiating germ cells towards the tubular lumen. This movement leads to a continuous remodeling of the plasma membrane and requires synthesis of several proteases, including urokinase, tissue-type plasminogen activator, cyclic protein 2, collagenase IV, other metalloproteins, and several antiproteases, such as cystatin C, tissue inhibitor of metalloproteinase type 2, and $\alpha_2$-macroglobulin.[149] The Sertoli cell also regulates germ cell apoptosis by the production of Fas-ligand, which binds to the Fas-ligand receptor (APO-1, CD95) in germ cell plasma membranes. In addition, Sertoli cells possess receptors for several factors such as the nerve growth factor (NGF) produced by spermatocytes and young spermatids, emphasizing the complexity of the Sertoli cell–germ cell relationship. Sertoli cells also produce some steroid hormones (estradiol and testosterone) and several components of the seminiferous tubule wall, including laminin, type IV collagen, and heparin sulfate-rich proteoglycans.

### Germ cells

The germ cells of the adult testis include spermatogonia, primary and secondary spermatocytes, and spermatids (Fig. 12-18).

*Spermatogonia* There are two types of spermatogonia: A and B. Type A are about 12 μm in diameter, rest on the basal lamina, and are surrounded by the cytoplasm of the adjacent Sertoli cells. The nuclei of type A spermatogonia are spherical, contain several peripheral nucleoli, and have four different patterns: Ad (dark), Ap (pale), Al (long), and Ac (cloudy).[150,151] The cytoplasm of these spermatogonia contains a moderate number of ribosomes, small ovoid mitochondria joined by electron-dense bars, and Lubarsch's crystals. These are several micrometers long and are composed of numerous 8–15 nm parallel filaments intermingled with ribosome-like granules.

Ad spermatogonia are thought to be stem cells in spermatogenesis. Some of them replicate DNA and, during replication, acquire the Al pattern. Afterwards, they divide to make another Ad (maintaining the stem cell reservoir) and an Ap spermatogonium. During replication, Ap spermatogonia become Ac and then divide to form two type B spermatogonia.[152–154]

Type B spermatogonia are the most numerous, and their contact with the basal lamina is less extensive than that of type A. The nuclei usually are more distant from the basal lamina than those of type A spermatogonia and contain one or two large central nucleoli. The cytoplasm contains more ribosomes than type A spermatogonia and intermitochondrial bars are usually not observed. Type B spermatogonia divide to form primary spermatocytes.

*Primary spermatocytes* Interphase primary spermatocytes lose contact with the basal lamina and inhabit cavities formed by the Sertoli cell cytoplasm. Their cytoplasm contains more rough endoplasmic reticulum than that of spermatogonia, and the Golgi complex is more developed.[155] Meiotic primary spermatocytes are readily identified by their chromatin pattern. The leptotene spermatocyte, with filamentous chromatin, leaves the basal compartment, migrates to an intermediate compartment and then to the adluminal compartment. In the zygotene spermatocyte, chromosomes are shorter and pairing of homologous chromosomes begins.

**Table 12-2** Major Sertoli cell secretory products

| Products | Functions and/or characteristics |
| --- | --- |
| **Transport-Binding Proteins** | |
| Androgen-binding protein (ABP) | Androgen transport |
| Transferrin | Iron transport |
| Ceruloplasmin | Copper transport |
| Sulfated glycoprotein-1 | Sphingolipid binding |
| **Regulatory Proteins** | |
| Inhibin | Endocrine-paracrine agent |
| Müllerian duct inhibitory agent | Development |
| Sulfated glycoprotein-2 | Sperm coating-immunosuppressant |
| **Growth Factors** | |
| TGF-$\alpha$ | Growth stimulation |
| TGF-$\beta$ | Growth inhibition |
| IGF-1 | Maintain growth/differentiation |
| IL-1 | Growth regulation |
| **Metabolites** | |
| Lactate-pyruvate | Energy metabolites |
| Estrogens | Steroid hormone–endocrine–paracrine |
| Proteases/inhibitors | |
| Plasminogen activator | Plasminogen activation |
| Cyclic protein-2 | Cathepsin activity |
| $\alpha_2$-Macroglobulin | Protease inhibitor |
| **Extracellular Matrix Components** | |
| Laminin | |
| Collagens I and IV | |
| Proteoglycans | |

TGF, transforming growth factor; IGF-1, insulin-like growth factor; IL-1, interleukin.

Ultrastructural studies show coarse chromatin masses in which synaptonemal complexes and sex pairs may be present. The nucleolus acquires a peculiar appearance, with segregation of the fibrillar and granular portions. Associated with the nucleolus is the round body that contains proteins but no nucleic acids.[128] In the pachytene spermatocyte, homologous chromosomes are completely paired, and on electron microscopy the chromatin masses appear larger and less numerous than in the zygotene spermatocyte. In the diplotene spermatocyte, paired homologous chromosomes begin to separate and remain joined by the points of interchange (chiasmata); neither synaptonemal complexes nor sex pairs are observed. The diakinesis spermatocyte shows maximal chromosome shortening and the chiasmata begin to resolve by displacement towards the chromosomal ends. The nuclear envelope and the nucleolus disintegrate. The spermatocyte completes the other phases of the first meiotic division (metaphase, anaphase and telophase), forming two secondary spermatocytes; the first meiotic division lasts 24 days.[156]

Secondary spermatocytes are haploid cells, smaller than primary spermatocytes, and show coarse chromatin granules and abundant rough endoplasmic reticulum cisternae.[157] These cells rapidly undergo the second meiotic division and within 8 hours give rise to two spermatids. The newly formed spermatids differ from secondary spermatocytes, having smaller nuclei with homogeneously distributed chromatin. *Spermiogenesis* The transformation of spermatids into spermatozoa is called spermiogenesis. During this process pronounced changes occur in the nucleus and cytoplasm.[158] The nucleus becomes progressively darker and elongated.[159] The cytoplasm develops the acrosome and flagellum,[160] the mitochondria cluster around the first portion of the spermatozoon tail, and the remaining cytoplasm is phagocytosed by Sertoli cells.[161,162] By electron microscopy, there are four tran-

sient stages of spermatid development: Golgi, cap, acrosome, and maturation. These correspond to those defined by light microscopy of nuclear morphology: Sa, Sb, $Sb_1$, $Sb_2$, Sc, $Sd_1$ and $Sd_2$.[163,164] These phases may be grouped as early (or round) spermatids that comprise the stages with round nuclei (Sa and Sb), and as late (or elongated) spermatids that comprise the stages with elongated nuclei (Sc and Sd). Mature spermatids ($Sd_2$) are the spermatozoa that are released into the tubular lumen (spermiation). All the germ cells derived from the same stem cell remain interconnected by cytoplasmic bridges that ensure synchronous maturation during the spermatogenic process.[165]

*Cycle of the seminiferous epithelium* At first glance, the arrangement of the germ cells in the seminiferous tubules appears disorderly. However, closer study reveals that these cells are grouped into six successive associations, designated I–VI. In contrast to other mammals, in humans the volume occupied by each association is small, so that several associations may be observed in the same tubular cross-section. Stereological studies have shown that the successive associations are organized helically along the length of the seminiferous tubule.[126,165–167] Each association persists for a specific number of days (I, 4.8 days; II, 3.1 days; III, 1 day; IV, 1.2 days; V, 5 days; and VI, 0.8 days), and each successively transforms into the following one. Finally, at the end of association VI, the cycle is repeated; the spermatogenic process requires 4.6 cycles.[168] Because each cycle lasts 15.9 days, the transformation of spermatogonium into spermatozoon takes 74 days (Fig. 12-22).

The succession of different associations probably depends on cyclic Sertoli cell activity. Cyclic changes in the mitochondria, rough endoplasmic reticulum, Golgi complex, lysosomes, and lipid droplets have been reported.[169–171] This cyclic activity is probably regulated by germ cell signals.[172] The yield of human spermatogenesis is lower than that of

**Fig. 12-22** The six different germ cell associations of the seminiferous tubules and the sequence of spermatogenesis. Completion of spermatogenesis requires more than four cycles and lasts for approximately 74 days. Each association is indicated by Roman numerals with its corresponding duration. Ad: dark type of A spermatogonia; Ap: pale type of a spermatogonia; B: B spermatogonia; I: interphase primary spermatocyte; L: leptotene primary spermatocyte; Z: zygotene primary spermatocyte; P: pachytene primary spermatocyte; II: secondary spermatocyte (only in stage VI). $S_a$, $S_{b1}$, $S_{b2}$, $S_c$, $S_{d1}$, and $S_{d2}$ represent the progressive stages of spermatid differentiation into spermatozoa.

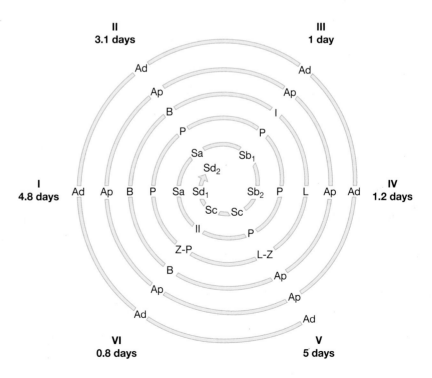

**Table 12-3** Major peritubular cell secretory products

| Products | Functions |
|---|---|
| P-mod-S | Paracrine regulatory agent |
| Plasminogen activator inhibitor | Inhibition of plasminogen activator activity |
| Fibronectin | Extracellular matrix component |
| Collagen I | Extracellular matrix component |
| Proteoglycans | Extracellular matrix component |
| TGF-α | Growth stimulation/EGF-like |
| TGF-β | Growth inhibition |
| IGF-1 | Maintenance growth/differentiation |

TGF, transforming growth factor; IGF-1, insulin-like growth factor.

most mammalian species, including primates, with maximal cell degeneration occurring at the end of meiosis.[173]

### Tunica propria

The seminiferous tubule is surrounded by a 6 μm thick lamina propria (tunica propria) consisting of a basement membrane, myofibroblasts, fibroblasts, collagen and elastic fibers, and extracellular matrix.[174,175]

The basement membrane measures 100–200 nm in thickness, and displays three layers: lamina lucida (beneath the Sertoli cells), lamina densa (basal lamina), and lamina reticularis (a discontinuous layer containing fibers). The basal lamina contains laminin, type IV collagen, entactin (nidogen), and heparan sulfate.[176] External to the basal lamina there are five to seven layers of flattened, elongated peritubular cells that have important secretory functions (Table 12-3).[177] The cells forming the three to five innermost layers are myofibroblasts containing numerous actin, myosin, and desmin filaments. These cells play an important role in the rhythmic tubular contractions that propel spermatozoa toward the rete testis.[178,179] The two outermost cell layers consist of fibroblasts without desmin filaments, and with less actin and myosin than the myofibroblasts.

Collagen fibers are present among the peritubular cells and are abundant between the basal lamina and the peritubular cells. Elastic fibers are located mainly at the periphery of peritubular cells. Because elastic fibers appear at puberty, their absence in adults is a sign of tubular immaturity or dysgenesis.[180] The extracellular matrix contains proteoglycans and fibronectin. In addition, the tubular wall contains capillaries and Leydig cells. These are very similar to the interstitial Leydig cells and are named peritubular Leydig cells.

The most important functions of myofibroblasts are contraction of seminiferous tubules and control of Sertoli cells.[181] Myofibroblasts have α and β adrenergic and muscarinic receptors.[182] Contractility depends on several factors produced in the testis (endothelin-1, vasopressin, oxytocin, and TGF-β) and prostaglandins. Relaxation can be facilitated by the NO/cGMP system because myofibroblasts are also able to synthesize nitric oxide. Sertoli cell control by myofibroblasts is facilitated by the production of P-Mod-S, which

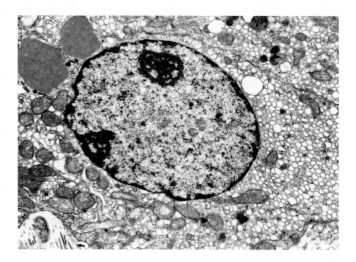

**Fig. 12-23** Leydig cells with round nuclei, abundant smooth endoplasmic reticulum, and Reinke's crystalloids.

activates aromatase activity, inhibin production, and the secretion of androgen-binding protein and transferrin.

### Testicular interstitium

The interstitium between the seminiferous tubules contain Leydig cells, macrophages, neuron-like cells, mast cells, blood vessels, lymphatic vessels, and nerves, accounting for 12–20% of testicular volume.[183]

### Connective tissue cells

The most numerous connective tissue cells are fibroblasts and myofibroblasts. The former are also known as interstitial dendritic cells or CD34-positive stromal cells. They display a network around the seminiferous tubules and Leydig cells, and also form the outermost layers of the tubular wall.[184] This distribution begins in fetal life. Some of these cells are in contact with typical macrophages, so it has been suggested that they might be involved in immune surveillance. Myofibroblasts, in addition to their presence in the inner layer of the tubular wall, are numerous in the tunica albuginea.

### Leydig cells

Leydig cells are distributed single or in clusters, and form about 3.8% of testicular volume. Most are in the testicular interstitium, although they may also be found in the tubular tunica propria, mediastinum testis, tunica albuginea, epididymis, and spermatic cord. Extratesticular Leydig cells are usually seen within or near nerve trunks.[185–187]

Leydig cells have spherical eccentric nuclei with one or two eccentric nucleoli and prominent nuclear lamina. The cytoplasm is abundant, eosinophilic, and contains lipid droplets and lipofuscin granules (residual bodies) (Fig. 12-23). Reinke's crystalloids are found only in the Leydig cells of adults and, although it was believed that these crystals were present exclusively in humans, they have also been observed in the wild bush rat. Reinke's crystalloids are up to 20 μm long and 2–3 μm wide, consisting of a complicated meshwork of 5 nm filaments with a trigonal lattice arrangement. Depending on the plane of section, three basic aspects of this lattice can be discerned. Frequently, the crystalloids display pale lines, con-

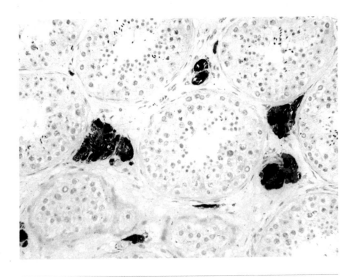

**Fig. 12-24** Leydig cells form small intertubular clusters that are immunostained for calretinin.

**Table 12-4** Major Leydig cell secretory products

| Products | Functions and/or characteristics |
| --- | --- |
| Androgens | Steroid hormone/endocrine–paracrine agent |
| Pro-opiomelanocortin peptides | Opiates/pro-opiomelanocortin regulatory agents |
| Inhibin | Endocrine–paracrine regulatory agent |
| IGF-1 | Maintenance growth/differentiation |

IGF-1, insulin-like growth factor.

sidered to be potential planes of cleavage. The filaments are grouped into 19 nm-wide hexagons visible on cross-section. In some areas there are aggregates of electron-dense, rod-shaped structures. Some Leydig cells contain other types of paracrystalline inclusion, the most common of which consists of multiple parallel-folded laminae.[188]

Leydig cells contain abundant well-developed smooth endoplasmic reticulum, pleomorphic mitochondria with tubular cristae, lysosomes, and peroxisomes. Leydig cells react with antibodies to S100 protein and neuron-specific enolase.[189]

Leydig cells immunoreact to LH receptors, 3-β-hydroxy-steroid dehydrogenase (3-β-HSD), relaxin-like factor,[190] inhibin, and ghrelin.[191] Relaxin-like factor, also known as insulin-like factor 3 (INSF-3), is a peptide that is involved in testicular descent and can be found in serum. Its concentration is a maker of the Leydig cell functional status. As occurs with testosterone, INSF-3 production is associated with that of LH.[192] Leydig cells immunoreact with calretinin, a 29 kDa calcium-binding protein that has a buffering effect to avoid abnormal increases in intracellular calcium.[193] Calretinin is a more sensitive marker than inhibin, albeit less specific (Fig. 12-24).[194] Leydig cells also contain VEGF and its two receptors (Flt-1 and KDR), and endothelin and its two receptors (α and β). VEGF and endothelin are involved in paracrine and autocrine control of Leydig cells. Leydig cells near seminiferous tubules show immunoreactivity for glial fibrillar acid protein (GFAP)[195] (Fig. 12-24). The demonstration of several substances that are characteristic of nerve cells, such as substance P, neurofilament triplet proteins (NF-L, NF-M and NF-H), and the ultrastructural observation of microtubules, intermediate filaments, and clear and dense core vesicles, qualifies Leydig cells for inclusion within the family of the diffuse endocrine system or paraneurons.[196,197]

Leydig cells of the adult testis originate from fibroblastic precursor cells at puberty under LH stimulation.[198] Experimental studies in rats have shown that adult Leydig cells differentiate from peritubular cells (myofibroblasts and blood capillary pericytes). Precursor Leydig cells are reminiscent of neural stem cells because they express nestin and eventually acquire properties of neurons and glial cells.[199]

The human testis contains about 200 million Leydig cells. This number decreases with age: the testes of 60-year-old men contain about half as many as those of 20-year-old men.[202–203] Mitotic figures are seen occasionally in normal Leydig cells.[204]

Leydig cells are the target cell of LH, in response to which they produce testosterone and other androgens necessary for the maintenance of spermatogenesis and many structures of the male genital tract, as well as other tissues such as bone, muscle, and skin.[205–208] Testosterone acts on the Sertoli cells, either directly[209] or via the P-mod-S factor secreted by the myofibroblasts in the tunica propria.[210–212] Leydig cells also secrete numerous non-steroidal factors, including oxytocin, which acts on myofibroblasts and stimulates seminiferous tubule contraction; β endorphin, which inhibits Sertoli cell proliferation and function; EGF, which regulates spermatogenesis; and other factors with less known actions, such as angiotensin, pro-opiomelanocortin, and α-melanotropic stimulating hormone (Table 12-4). Together with Sertoli cells, peritubular cells, and endothelial cells, Leydig cells produce nitric oxide, which has a relaxing effect on smooth muscle.[213]

Leydig cells are associated with cholinergic and adrenergic nerve fibers.[186] Varicosities containing synaptic vesicles in the proximity of Leydig cells and nerve endings in direct contact with Leydig cells have been reported, although the functional significance of this innervation is unknown.[214,215]

### Macrophages, neuron-like cells, and mast cells

Macrophages are a normal component of the testis[216–218] and can be classified into two groups: resident and activated. Resident macrophages are an essential cell type of the testicular interstitium (about 25% of interstitial cells in mouse testis).[219] In young adult men, there is one macrophage per 10–15 Leydig cells, and this number increases with age. Macrophages are closely related to Leydig cells and play a role in proliferation and differentiation of Leydig cell fibroblastic precursors.[220] Interaction between macrophages and Leydig cells is an example of paracrine function. In the rat, testicular macrophages produce 25-hydroxycholesterol (25-HC) and express 25-hydroxylase, which transforms cholesterol into 25-HC.[221,222]

Activated macrophages produce interleukins 1 and 6 (IL-1 and IL-6), tumor necrotizing factor-α (TNF-α), and transforming growth factor-α (TGF-α).

Immunohistochemical techniques have demonstrated neuron-like cells in the testicular interstitium.[223] These cells are an important source of intratesticular cate-cholamines, which appear to be increased in some disorders such as the Sertoli cell-only syndrome, and hypospermatogenesis.

Mast cells are a normal component of the testicular interstitium, where they are often found near blood vessels. Their number increases in several diseases.[224]

### Blood and lymphatic vessels

The testis is supplied by the testicular artery, which arises from the abdominal aorta. In the spermatic cord, the testicular artery gives rise to two or three branches that obliquely penetrate the tunica albuginea testis and to multiple branches that run along the intralobular septa of the testis.[225] These centripetal arteries lead to the mediastinum testis. Along their course, the centripetal arteries give off branches that abruptly reverse direction; these are called centrifugal arteries. At puberty, both the centripetal and the centrifugal arteries develop a pronounced spiral architecture.[226,227] The centrifugal arteries develop additional branches in the testicular interstitium, giving rise to arterioles and capillaries that form intertubular plexuses, some of which are apposed to the tunica propria.[228,229] Capillaries are of the continuous type, except for the seminiferous tubule capillaries, which are partially fenestrated,[230] and their endothelial cells are similar to those of brain capillaries, with scant pinocytosis, intercellular junctions of the fascia adherens type, and low permeability. The mediastinum testis is poorly vascularized.

The inner two-thirds of the testicular parenchyma is drained by veins that follow the interlobular septa to the mediastinum testis (centripetal veins). The outer third is drained by veins that lead to the tunica albuginea (centrifugal veins). Both centripetal and centrifugal veins join to form the pampiniform plexus, which drains the testis via the spermatic cord.

Lymphatic vessels are poorly developed in the testis and limited to the tunica vasculosa and interlobular septa,[231] where they accompany arterioles and venules. Prelymphatic vessels have been reported in the interstitium and probably drain interstitial fluid into the true interlobular lymphatic vessels.

### Nerves

Efferent innervation of the testis is mainly supplied by neurons of the pelvic ganglia, where contralateral and bilateral neural connections occur. Postganglionic nerve fibers enter the testis via the pelvic nerves, extend throughout the tunica vasculosa, and follow the interlobular septa to reach the interstitium. These nerve fibers end in the wall of arterioles, the wall of seminiferous tubules, and the Leydig cells.[232] Adrenergic nerve fibers innervate the tunica albuginea and the blood vessels of the tunica vasculosa.[233] Peptidergic nerve endings are uncommon. Afferent nerve endings form corpuscles similar to those of Meissner and Pacini in the tunica albuginea.

## Rete testis

The rete testis is a network of channels and cavities that connects the seminiferous tubules with the ductuli efferentes. Differences in the configuration and size of channels and cavities distinguish three portions of the rete testis: septal (intralobular), composed of the tubuli recti; mediastinal, composed of a network of interconnected channels; and extratesticular, composed of dilated cavities (up to 3 mm in diameter) termed the bullae retis.

The tubuli recti are short tubules (0.5–1 mm long) that connect the seminiferous tubules to the mediastinal rete, although some seminiferous tubules may connect directly to the mediastinal rete, principally those in the central region of the testis. The tubuli recti are lined by cuboidal epithelium. There are approximately 1500 tubuli recti (or their analogous seminiferous tubule segments). The tubuli recti in the cranial, central, and anterior testis are perpendicular to the mediastinal rete testis channel into which they drain, and those in the caudal testicular region are parallel to their respective channels. The transitional segments between the seminiferous tubules and the tubuli recti are formed by modified Sertoli cells.[234]

The epithelium of the mediastinal rete testis consists of flattened cells interspersed with small areas of columnar cells. Both cell types have single centrally located cilia and numerous microvilli on their free surfaces, and contain keratin and vimentin filaments.[235] There are interdigitations between adjacent cells. The epithelium rests on a basal lamina, surrounded by a layer of myofibroblasts and a more peripheral layer of fibroblasts and collagen and elastic fibers.

The rete channels and cavities are traversed by the chordae rete, columns from 15 μm to 100 μm long and from 5 μm to 40 μm wide, arranged obliquely to the long axis of the cavity. The chordae consist of fibrous connective tissue with fibroblasts and are covered by flattened epithelium; the widest contain capillaries. The rete testis probably has the following functions: damping differences in pressure between the seminiferous tubules and ductuli efferentes; reabsorption of protein and potassium from tubular fluid; and, occasionally, phagocytosis of spermatozoa.

# Congenital anomalies of the testis

## Alterations in number, size and location

### Anorchidism

#### Types

Anorchidism refers to the absence of one (monorchidism) or both testes (testicular regression syndrome). Monorchidism is estimated to occur in about 4.5% of cryptorchid testes,[236] 40% of the testes that are impalpable in physical examination,[237] or 1 in 5000 males. Bilateral anorchidism occurs in approximately 1 in 20 000 males.[238]

*Monorchidism* The hormonal pattern in prepubertal patients with monorchidism does not differ from that of normal children, whereas children lacking both testes have elevated levels of gonadotropins and fail to respond to stimulation

**Table 12-5** Testicular regression syndromes

|  | Embryonal period | | Fetal period | | |
|---|---|---|---|---|---|
|  | Early | Late | Early | Middle | Late |
| Müllerian structures | Vestigial | Differentiated | Differentiated/vestigial | Vestigial | Vestigial |
| Wolffian structures | Vestigial | Vestigial | Vestigial/differentiated | Differentiated | Differentiated |
| External genitalia | Female | Female | Ambiguous | Ambiguous–male | Male |

with hCG.[238–240] Although the hCG stimulation test is often positive in children with bilateral cryptorchidism, it is negative in some children with bilateral intra-abdominal cryptorchidism and this further complicates the differential diagnosis between anorchidism and cryptorchidism.[241]

For unknown reasons, the left testis is more frequently absent (68.7%) than the right. In such cases the contralateral scrotal testis undergoes compensatory hypertrophy and its volume increases to more than 2 mL.[242] Compensatory hypertrophy has also been reported in association with abdominal cryptorchid testis.[243]

The absence of testicular parenchyma should be confirmed before diagnosing monorchidism. At exploration, the finding of a vas deferens ending near or in a hypoplastic epididymis is not sufficient for the diagnosis of monorchidism. The only acceptable finding is blind-ending spermatic vessels. If inguinoscrotal exploration fails to identify these vessels, intra-abdominal exploration is required to insure against an undescended testis and avoid the development of a testicular tumor.[224] All remnants found at exploration should be removed.[245]

*Testicular regression syndrome* Testicular regression syndrome refers to a variety of conditions, including agonadism, anorchidism, testicular agenesis, rudimentary testes, hypoplastic testes, and embryonal testicular dysgenesis.[246] Each of these syndromes shares a complete absence or involution of both testes[247] but differ in the time of testicular disappearance during development. The most frequently observed are Swyer's syndrome (see discussion on gonadal dysgenesis below), true agonadism, rudimentary testes, bilateral anorchidism, vanishing testes syndrome, and Leydig cell-only syndrome (Table 12-5).

*True agonadism (46XY gonadal agenesis syndrome)* Patients with true agonadism have ambiguous external genitalia, fusion of the labia, and a short vagina, reflecting very early testicular regression (between the eighth and 12th weeks of embryonal development). The internal genitalia consist of a uterus and two uterine tubes, although both müllerian and wolffian derivatives may be absent. No gonads (not even in an ectopic location) are found. Patients are phenotypically girls, and the male gender may be discovered only at the time of referral for other symptoms.[248] Both sporadic and familial cases with associated extragenital anomalies have been reported. In some cases the cause is a heterozygous mutation of WT1.[249] In most familial cases inheritance is either recessive autonomic or X-linked, and the cause seems to be either unknown anomalies in the WT1 gene or known anomalies in other genes involved in development.[250] A SRY molecular defect has never been observed.[251] Agonadism may be associ-

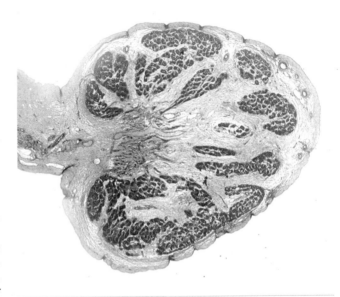

**Fig. 12-25** Cross-sectioned rudimentary testis from a 2-year-old infant. Testicular lobules are separated by wide septa and contain scant seminiferous tubules.

ated with several syndromes, including those of PAGOD (hypoplasia of lungs and pulmonary artery, agonadism, omphalocele/diaphragmatic defect, dextrocardia),[252] Kennerknecht,[253] Seckel,[254] and CHARGE.[255]

*Rudimentary testes syndrome* Patients with rudimentary testes have a normal male phenotype. Müllerian remnants are absent and wolffian derivatives usually are found. The testes are cryptorchid and very small, less than 0.5 cm long. Seminiferous tubules are few (Fig. 12-25). The testicular regression occurs between the 14th and 20th weeks of gestation. This syndrome has been reported in several members of the same family,[256] suggesting genetic transmission, but this is not a constant feature.[257,258]

*Congenital bilateral anorchidism* Congenital bilateral anorchidism occurs in 1 in 20 000 newborns. The patients have male external genitalia, but the internal genitalia consist only of normal wolffian derivatives without müllerian derivatives, suggesting that the testes were present and functionally active up to approximately the 20th week of gestation. Patients have male external genitalia with hypoplasia of both the scrotum and penis. The karyotype is the normal male. The disorder may be associated with other malformations, such as anal atresia, rectourethral and rectovaginal fistula, and urinary exstrophy. Patients diagnosed at adulthood have male phenotype, androgen insufficiency symptoms, and elevated levels of both FSH and LH.[259,260]

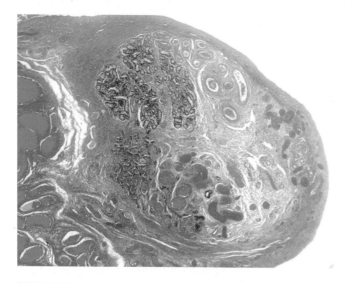

**Fig. 12-26** Vanishing testis, consisting of a small group of seminiferous tubules, the rete testis, and numerous blood vessels.

Familial incidence in some cases suggests SRY gene mutation, but this has not been confirmed.[261,262]

*Vanishing testes syndrome* This term refers to the disappearance of one or both testes between the last months of intrauterine life and the beginning of puberty.[263–265] As testicular regression occurs after the seventh month, exploration finds the vas deferens in the inguinal canal or high in the scrotum; it may be accompanied by the epididymis and, less frequently, by testicular remnants consisting of small groups of seminiferous tubules (Fig. 12-26). Patients lacking both testes develop hypergonadotropic hypogonadism after puberty, with gynecomastia, infantile phallus, hypoplastic scrotum, and impalpable prostate. The condition is usually secondary to a perinatal scrotal torsion,[266] although rarely there is a genetic cause.[267,268]

*Leydig cell-only syndrome* Patients with Leydig cell-only syndrome have agonadism without eunuchoidism and a normal male phenotype, although meticulous surgical exploration fails to find testicular remnants. Study of serial sections from the spermatic cord reveals clusters of Leydig cells.[269] Detection of testosterone in spermatic vein blood indicates that these ectopic Leydig cells are functionally active and synthesize testosterone in amounts sufficient to induce a rudimentary male phenotype but insufficient to support the complete development of secondary sex characteristics.

### Macroscopic and microscopic findings

The morphology of spermatic cord remnants is similar in monorchidism and testicular regression syndrome occurring after the 20th week of gestation.[270–272] Grossly, a small, firm mass is found at the end of the cord (Fig. 12-27). Histologic examination reveals vas deferens, epididymis, or small groups of seminiferous tubules in 69–83% of cases.[273] Vas deferens is the most constant finding (79%), followed by epididymis (36%) and seminiferous tubules (5–13%). The spermatic vessels are abnormally small in 83% of cases.[245,274] Areas of dystrophic calcification, hemosiderin deposition, and giant cell reaction may be found within the mass in place of the testis. Other findings include arterial and venous

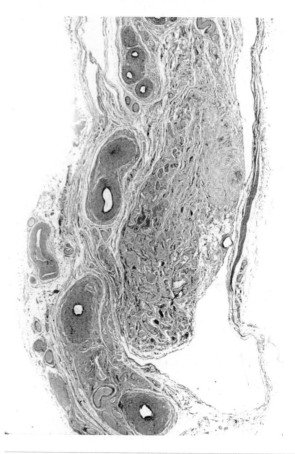

**Fig. 12-27** Spermatic cord in anorchidism. Fibrous connective tissue with dystrophic calcification surrounds the distal end of the vas deferens and replaces the testis.

vessels (88%), fat (44%), and nerves that may resemble traumatic neuroma (56%).

The minimal requirement to diagnose vanishing testis is to find either a vascularized fibrous nodule with calcification or hemosiderin, or a fibrous nodule with cord elements.[275] It has been proposed that removal of the testicular nubbin in this syndrome may not be required because the percentage of seminiferous tubules is very low and the presence of germ cells low, and thus the probability of a tumor is minimal.[276,277] The general recommendation is scrotal exploration as a first step, reserving laparoscopy for cases in which either the atrophic remnant cannot be identified during scrotal exploration or has a patent vaginal process.[266]

### Etiology

The histologic findings suggest that most cases of unilateral and bilateral anorchidism are produced during the fetal period after the testis has inhibited the müllerian ducts and induced differentiation of wolffian duct derivatives. Two hypotheses account for the disappearance of the testes: primary anomaly of the gonad; and atrophy secondary to a vascular lesion such as thrombosis or intrauterine torsion. The presence of macrophages with hemosiderin and dystrophic calcification supports the latter. Absence of one testis may be associated with malformations of the urogenital system, such as absence of the kidney, cystic seminal vesicles, and ipsilateral renal dysgenesis.[278,279]

## Micro-orchidism

This clinical term refers to diverse conditions (Klinefelter's syndrome, hypogonadotropic hypogonadism, rudimentary testes syndrome, bilateral cryptorchidism, etc.) that share small testicular size.[280,281]

A peculiar case is presented by some patients with Kenny–Caffey syndrome: short stature, cortical thickening and medullary stenosis of long bones, delayed closure of anterior fontanelles, hypoparathyroidism, and several ocular alterations. FSH serum levels are elevated, but only in some cases, whereas LH and testosterone are normal. Adult testes are small, with seminiferous tubules showing complete but diminished spermatogenesis. Leydig are hyperplastic. Unlike patients with the rudimentary testes syndrome, micro-orchidism patients have a normal-sized penis and no epididymal or prostatic atrophy.[282]

## Polyorchidism

Polyorchidism is a rare condition, with approximately 100 reported cases.[283,284] It was first described in a postmortem study in 1880,[285] and the first case treated surgically and confirmed histologically was reported in 1895.[286] Although three testes are the most common,[287] four testes have been reported in six patients,[288–292] and five in one case but without histologic confirmation.[293] Age of diagnosis varies from newborn to 74 years, with a mean of 17 years. Testicular duplication is usually an incidental finding during surgery for inguinal hernia, cryptorchidism, or testicular torsion, but has also been detected in patients with infertility or unexplained fertility after bilateral vasectomy.[294] The extra testis is often intrascrotal (75%) and less frequently inguinal (20%), abdominal,[295] or retroperitoneal (5%).[296,297] Duplication is three times more frequent on the left than on the right.[298] High-resolution ultrasound is the appropriate diagnostic technique.[284,299] Testicular maldescent (40%), inguinal hernia (30%), hydrocele, varicocele, and contralateral cryptorchidism are the most frequently associated anomalies.[300–302] Testicular torsion (13%)[303] and testicular cancer (5.4%) are occasional complications. Although the extra testis may be histologically normal,[304–306] usually it is not,[300,307] and displays lesions such as Sertoli cell-only tubules, hypospermatogenesis, or maturation arrest. The lack of spermatogenesis has been attributed to the anomalous location of the testis and the absence of communication between the testis and excretory ducts.[308]

The embryologic origin of polyorchidism remains uncertain, and the following have been proposed to account for the variety of findings in different cases (Fig. 12-28):

- Longitudinal division of all the structures of the genital ridge and mesonephric ducts. Each of the two testes resulting from the duplication has an excretory duct and develops active spermatogenesis.[286,294,309–311]
- Longitudinal division of the genital ridge. Of the two resulting testes, the medial loses its connection with the mesonephric ducts and undergoes atrophy.
- High transverse division of the genital ridge. The two resulting portions are in continuity with the mesonephric ducts that give rise to the ductuli

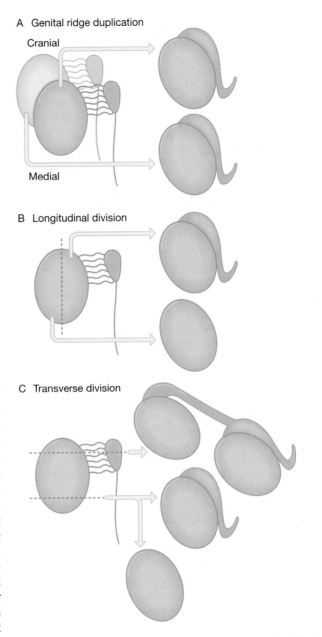

**Fig. 12-28** Possible mechanisms of polyorchidism. **(A)** Genital ridge duplication gives rise to two testes with their respective epididymides. **(B)** Longitudinal division of the genital ridge. The testis derived from the medial region has no epididymis. **(C)** Transverse division of the genital ridge. The resulting testes either share a single epididymis or one testis is devoid of epididymis.

efferentes. Each testis has its own ductus epididymidis or shares a common one, but there is a single vas deferens for both.[302,312]

- Low transverse division of the genital ridge. The more caudal testis has no excretory ducts.[302]

The clinical differential diagnosis of polyorchidism includes most of pathologic conditions that enlarge the scrotum and spermatic cords: spermatocele, hydrocele, cysts and tumors of the spermatic cord, crossed testicular ectopia, adrenal cortical ectopia, and splenogonadal fusion. Orchidectomy used to be the treatment of choice for all atrophic and non-scrotal testes. Today, most surgeons undertake fixation of the testis to the scrotal pouch and the re-creation of a 'simple testis' if it is permitted by the anatomical condition and malignancy has been precluded. This treatment may allow spermatogenesis as well as additional psychologic and cosmetic benefits.[313] Intrascrotal rhabdomyosarcoma, testicular teratoma, and seminoma have been reported in patients with polyorchidism.[314,315]

## Testicular hypertrophy (macroorchidism)

Macro-orchidism may be uni- or bilateral and be associated with chromosomal anomalies or endocrine alterations. An increase in the testicular parenchyma occurs in several conditions,[316] including congenital Leydig cell hyperplasia, compensatory hypertrophy, benign idiopathic macroorchidism, bilateral megalotestes with low gonadotropins, fragile X chromosome, and the testicular hypertrophy observed in juvenile hypothyroidism.

### Congenital Leydig cell hyperplasia

Congenital Leydig cell hyperplasia is uncommon and may be diffuse or nodular. The diagnosis of diffuse Leydig cell hyperplasia requires quantification of Leydig cells by morphometry, using normal newborn testes as controls (Fig. 12-29). Nodular Leydig cell hyperplasia is characterized by the presence of non-encapsulated Leydig cell nodules in the mediastinum testis, adjacent testicular parenchyma and connective tissue among the ductuli efferentes (Fig. 12-30).

The differential diagnosis of nodular Leydig cell hyperplasia includes intratesticular adrenal rests and bilateral Leydig cell tumor. Except for patients with adrenogenital syndrome, intratesticular adrenal rests are rare. These rests are encapsulated, with the exception of the adrenogenital tumors, and consist of radially arranged cells with vesicular nuclei and small nucleoli displacing the rete testis or seminiferous tubules. Leydig cell tumors may be bilateral, poorly circumscribed, and surrounded by testicular parenchyma, features making it difficult to distinguish from Leydig cell hyper-

plasia. However, Leydig cell tumors are rarely congenital, whereas those occurring at infancy often induce precocious maturation of the adjacent seminiferous tubules and early macrogenitosomia.

Leydig cell hyperplasia is caused by large quantities of hCG entering the fetal circulation. Diabetic mothers, particularly those with hypertension, may develop hyperplacentosis; the resulting edema in the placental villi alters the vascular permeability and allows the passage of hCG to the fetus. Congenital Leydig cell hyperplasia decreases rapidly during the first months of postnatal life, after maternal human chorionic gonadotropin is gone. Combined diffuse and nodular Leydig cell hyperplasia occurs in several malformative syndromes, such as Beckwith–Wiederman, leprechaunism, triploid fetuses, fetuses with Rh isoimmunization,[317] and in several complications of pregnancy.

### Compensatory hypertrophy of the testis

Compensatory hypertrophy has been observed in monorchidism,[318] cryptorchidism[319] (Fig. 12-31), varicocele,[320] and after testicular injury. Hypertrophy persists and may increase during childhood and puberty, but ceases thereafter; the hypertrophied testis then becomes normal or remains slightly enlarged.[321,322] The degree of hypertrophy is determined by three factors: the volume of the remaining testicular parenchyma, the age at which the injury occurred, and the functional ability of the descended testis.[323] Compensatory hypertrophy results from an alteration in the hypophyseal hormonal feedback mechanism, followed by an increase in secretion of FSH, evidence that the contralateral testis is normal. In monorchidism, the testis is initially normal.[237] When a 50% reduction of testicular mass occurs (probably before birth), the endocrine feedback changes and the resulting secretion of FSH (before or immediately after birth) causes accelerated growth of the contralateral testis. In cryptorchidism, the reduction in testicular mass is less severe than in monorchidism, and the scrotal testis may also be abnormal, inducing a lesser compensatory hypertrophy. Compen-

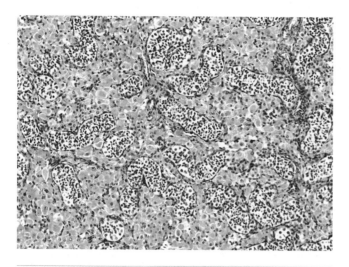

**Fig. 12-29** Congenital Leydig cell hyperplasia. Multiple nodules of Leydig cells are present in the mediastinum testis as well as deep in the parenchyma.

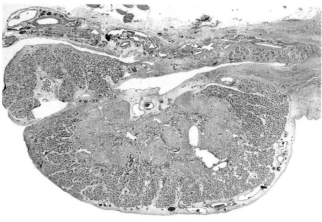

**Fig. 12-30** Congenital Leydig cell hyperplasia. Fetal Leydig cells form large clusters surrounding groups of seminiferous tubules.

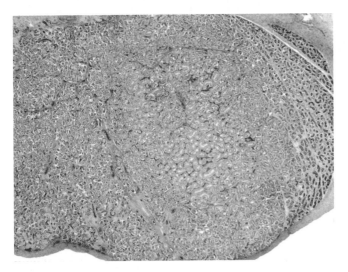

**Fig. 12-31** Contralateral scrotal testis from a cryptorchid patient showing a group of large seminiferous tubules that stands out from the surrounding small tubules.

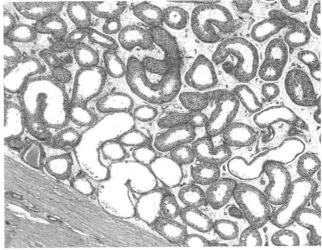

**Fig. 12-32** Martin–Bell syndrome (fragile X chromosome). The seminiferous tubules show variable degrees of dilatation and marked hypospermatogenesis.

satory hypertrophy develops between birth and 3 years of age, and the testis may reach a volume twice normal when the other testis is absent.[243]

### Idiopathic benign macroorchidism

Some prepubertal and pubertal patients have pronounced unilateral[324] or bilateral[325-327] testicular hypertrophy in the absence of other pathologic findings. This probably results from hormonal receptivity in the testicular parenchyma. Morphometric studies have shown that the testicular enlargement is chiefly due to an increase in the length of the seminiferous tubules, although increases in tubular diameter and Sertoli cell numbers have also been observed. Elevated FSH serum levels, reported in some cases, or hyperactive FSH receptors might be the cause of the excessive Sertoli cell proliferation and the lengthening and thickening of seminiferous tubules.[328-330] In addition, Leydig cell hyperplasia and deficient spermatogenesis are frequent findings in adult life. As the development of the two testes may be asynchronous during puberty, some unilateral macroorchidisms may represent cases in which these differences are unusually exaggerated.

### Bilateral megalotestes with low gonadotropins

About 2% of adults with fertility problems have enlarged testes, with volumes over 25 mL, and low levels of FSH, LH, testosterone, prolactin, and estradiol.[331] Despite the important hormonal changes, sperm concentrations and total numbers of spermatozoa are higher than normal. Low FSH levels may be attributable to increased inhibin secretion because the number of Sertoli cells is elevated in these testes, but no explanation for the reduction in the other hormone levels has been found.

### Fragile X chromosome; Martin–Bell syndrome

Fragile X chromosome is the best-known form of inherited mental retardation, with an incidence of 1 in 1500 males and 1 in 2500 females.[332] In addition to facial dysmorphia (large ears, prognathism, high forehead, and arched palate), macroorchidism (Martin–Bell syndrome) is often an associated finding.[333-337] The impaired gene (FMR1 gene) is mapped to Xq27,3 which is genetically fragile. The gene alteration is due to a lengthening of a trinucleotide CGG repeat that results in FMR1 gene silencing. If the CGG sequence is repeated fewer than 200 times, the disorder is considered a premutation and males show no symptoms; if the number of repetitions exceeds 200, mutation is complete and all show the disorder.[338-340] In men with this syndrome, the average testicular volume is more than 70 mL (four times greater than normal). The penis also is larger than normal, and both anomalies are apparent in infancy. The scrotum is also enlarged and prematurely pigmented. This precocious genital development is difficult to explain because the hypothalamopituitary axis is normal, but it may be caused by increased sensitivity to stimulation by FSH.[341]

Testicular biopsies from adults may be normal or show interstitial edema and hypospermatogenesis (Fig. 12-32). Usually, there is normal testicular parenchyma with focal reduced spermatogenesis and Sertoli cell hyperplasia (Fig. 12-33) or tubules containing only immature Sertoli cells. Morphometry indicates that testicular enlargement is chiefly the result of lengthening of seminiferous tubules.[328] The low number of spermatids is attributed to atrophy caused by compression of the seminiferous epithelium by marked increase in intratubular fluid.[342] Meiotic anomalies have been excluded.[343] The fragile X syndrome is second in frequency only to Down's syndrome as a cause of mental retardation.[344-346] However, this chromosomal anomaly is not always associated with mental retardation or macroorchidism, and there are men with fragile X syndrome who are otherwise normal.[347]

The terms 'fragile X-negative Martin–Bell syndrome' or 'mental retardation–macro-orchidism' refer to X-linked (MRMO) or XLMR+MO patients who have the Martin–Bell syndrome phenotype but do not present the fragile X site. The gene responsible for this disorder is mapped to Xq12-q21.[348]

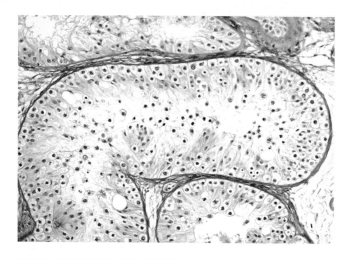

**Fig. 12-33** Martin–Bell syndrome (fragile X chromosome). The seminiferous tubules show marked hypospermatogenesis. Several groups of dysgenetic Sertoli cells are seen near the lumen.

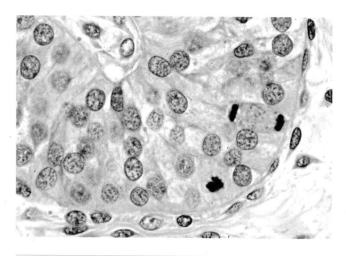

**Fig. 12-34** Macroorchidism in a 3-year-old infant with hypothyroidism. The Sertoli cells have spherical nuclei which contain small heterochromatin granules. Two mitotic figures are seen. The testicular interstitium has no Leydig cells.

## Other testicular hypertrophies

Testicular hypertrophy appears associated with FSH-secreting pituitary adenoma,[349] hyperprolactinemia, hypoprolactinemia, and hypothyroidism.[350,351] The most frequent association of testicular hypertrophy is with hypothyroidism. Children with hypothyroidism often show testicular enlargement without virilization.[350] About 80% have macroorchidism,[352] most have elevated FSH levels, and half have increased LH levels.[353,354] Testosterone levels are normal during infancy. The response of FSH and LH to GnRH is altered and no pulsatile LH release occurs (Fig. 12-34).[355]

Testicular biopsies before puberty show an accelerated development of the testis with pubertal maturation of seminiferous tubules but not Leydig cells. Testicular biopsies in untreated adults show tubular and interstitial hyalinization with few Leydig cells.[356,357] Testicular size in this type of macroorchidism diminishes as soon as the substitutive therapy

starts.[353,358,359] The etiopathogenesis has been explained by three hypotheses: an increase in gonadotropin secretion caused by TRH stimulation of gonadotropic cells;[360,361] a direct TSH effect on the testis due to the structural similarity between TSH receptors and FSH receptors present in the testis;[362] and a lack of steroid hormones that are required for testicular maturation (in their absence, Sertoli cell proliferation is excessive, giving rise to testicular enlargement).[363–366]

### Precocious puberty

Precocious puberty is defined by onset of secondary sex characteristics at a chronologic age that is below the mean middle age for the population. For practical purposes, this is considered to be before 8 years of age in girls and 9 years in boys. The incidence is estimated at between 1 in 5000 and 1 in 10 000, with a female:male ratio higher than 20:1. In boys, the first symptom is rapid testicular enlargement followed by growth of pubic and axillary hair, enlargement of the penis, and acceleration of skeletal growth.[367]

According to hypothalamopituitary–gonadal axis function, precocious puberty can be classified into three groups: central or gonadotropin-dependent, which results from the activation of this axis; peripheral or gonadotropin-independent, mediated by sex steroid hormones secreted by the testis or adrenal glands; and a mixed group that first appears as peripheral precocious puberty and thereafter, because of the secondary response of the hypothalamus, becomes gonadotropin dependent.

Other possible causes of precocious puberty are hypoprolactinemia, pituitary tumor, and alteration of testicular steroid metabolism.

***Central precocious puberty (CPP)*** Central precocious puberty, also known as true precocious puberty, is isosexual. It is the most common form of precocious puberty in girls and accounts for more than 50% of cases in boys. The age of presentation is between 4 and 10 years.[368] The cause is only known in 60% of cases; most are related to lesions in the central nervous system, whereas the others are usually idiopathic.

Lesions in the central nervous system that causes CPP share alterations of specific areas, including the posterior hypothalamus (eminencia media and tuber cinereum), mammillary bodies, the bottom of the third ventricle, or the pineal gland.[369,370] The most frequent causes are:

- Tumor of the hypothalamus (astrocytoma, ganglioneuroma, ganglioglioma, craniopharyngioma, cyst of the third ventricle, and suprasellar cyst of the arachnoid space),[371–373] hamartoma (gangliocytoma) of the tuber cinereum and mammillary body, tumor of the pineal gland (teratoma and pinealoma), tumor of the optic nerve (glioma), and cerebral and cerebellar astrocytoma.
- Cerebral trauma (including postpartum and accidental trauma) that stimulates the extrahypothalamic areas responsible for hypothalamic activation.[374–376]
- Infections such as meningitis, encephalitis, toxoplasmosis, and syphilis.
- Cerebral malformations, including hydrocephaly, microcephaly, and craniosynostosis.[377]

- Hereditary diseases as neurofibromatosis and tuberous sclerosis. Children with type I neurofibromatosis often have also optic pathway tumors.
- Cerebral irradiation, as occurs in hypothalamopituitary selective irradiation,[378] prophylactic irradiation in children with acute lymphoblastic leukemia,[379] and irradiation of cerebral tumor that is far from the hypothalamopituitary region.

The diagnosis of central precocious puberty is easy if the hormonal findings show elevated gonadotropin levels (both basal values and in response to GnRH), associated with high testosterone levels and an increase in either LH/FSH ratio or in LH and FSH values after stimulation with GnRH agonists. However, in some cases it is necessary to measure nocturnal LH secretion to find secretion pulses before a dynamic test can reveal the pubertal pattern.

Knowledge of the etiology in males has improved with the use of CT and MRI.[380,381] One of the most important contributions of these techniques is the finding of a high number of hamartomas in children with precocious puberty.[382-384] These lesions, also known as gangliocytomas, consist of abnormally located neurons and glial cells. Lesions are usually multiple, small, and located on the hypothalamus between the anterior part of the mammillary body and the posterior part of the tuber cinereum. These neurons contain LHRH-positive neurosecretory granules, suggesting that this hormone can be released into the blood draining the hypophyseal portal system and reach the gonadotropic cells.[385]

Precocious puberty owing to cerebral tumors usually occurs with advanced stage of the tumor, preceded by cerebral symptoms such as hydrocephaly, papillary edema, or psychic alterations. The same occurs when precocious puberty results from cerebral inflammation or cerebral malformation.

Although pineal gland tumor is rare in children, 30% produce precocious puberty, principally in boys. This tumor is usually a teratoma or non-parenchymatous tumor that destroys the pineal gland, hindering its antigonadotropic action and initiating puberty.[386] In contrast, pinealocyte-derived tumor secretes great amounts of melatonin that delay the onset of puberty.

*Peripheral precocious puberty (PPP)* Peripheral precocious puberty is also known as precocious pseudopuberty. It may be caused by a primary testicular disorder, a lesion in other endocrine glands, or hormonal treatment. Primary testicular disorders causing precocious pseudopuberty include familial testotoxicosis, functioning testicular tumor, excessive aromatase activity, or Leydig cell hyperplasia with focal spermatogenesis. The principal secondary anomalies include adrenal cortical anomaly (congenital adrenal hyperplasia, virilizing tumor of the adrenal, and Nelson's syndrome), and lesion secondary to hCG-secreting tumor (hepatoblastoma accounts for half of precocious pseudopuberty cases, and testicular germ cell tumor and the tumors of the retroperitoneum, mediastinum, and pineal gland are responsible for the other half of cases).[387]

*Familial testotoxicosis: gonadotropin-independent precocious puberty (GIPP) or familial male-limited precocious puberty*

*(FMPP)* Familial testotoxicosis is a form of male sexual precocity characterized by early differentiation of Leydig cells and the initiation of spermatogenesis in the absence of stimulation by pituitary gonadotropin. This is a primary testicular abnormality with autosomal dominant inheritance.[388,389] Ultrastructural studies confirm an adult Leydig cell pattern and complete spermatogenesis, although many spermatids are abnormal.[390] The cause of familial testotoxicosis is a constitutive activating mutation of the LH receptor gene.[391] This gene comprises 11 exons and has been mapped to 2p21. Hormonal measurements show elevated serum levels of testosterone, and low levels of dihydroepiandrosterone sulfate, androstenedione, 17-hydroxyprogesterone, gonadotropin-releasing hormone (GRH), and LH, as well as absence of a pulsatile pattern. In addition, serum levels of inhibin B appear elevated before the normal age of onset of puberty.[392] In some patients, a mutation in LH receptor induces Leydig cell adenoma.[393]

*Precocious puberty secondary to functioning testicular tumor* A syndrome of precocious puberty can be the result of different tumors, including Leydig cell tumor, sex cord tumor, adrenal cortex virilizing carcinoma, and extratesticular hCG-secreting germ cell tumor.

Leydig cell tumor may cause precocious puberty. The testis is enlarged owing to tumor growth and maturation of the seminiferous tubules adjacent to the tumor; such maturation results from androgen secretion by tumor cells (Fig. 12-35). In most cases, the contralateral testis is not enlarged.[394,395]

Sex cord tumor with annular tubules and large cell calcifying Sertoli cell tumor may give rise to precocious pseudopuberty that is isosexual (development of musculature and axillary and pubic hair) and heterosexual (gynecomastia). This precocious testicular maturation and the development of the tumor itself cause testicular enlargement. It has been suggested that tumor cells stimulate Leydig cells to produce androgens that are aromatized to estrogens by the tumor cells themselves, thus accounting for the clinical

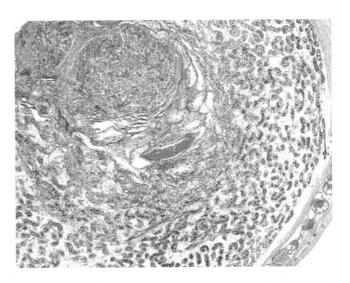

**Fig. 12-35** Precocious maturation of seminiferous tubules, which surround a virilizing Leydig cell tumor.

symptoms. These tumors are frequently observed in Peutz–Jeghers syndrome[396,397] and Carney's complex.[398]

Most infants with adrenal cortex virilizing tumors have small testes, but some cases of testicular hypertrophy have also been observed.[399] Testicular development in these cases is attributed to adrenal androgenic action on seminiferous tubules.[400] In untreated (or maltreated) congenital adrenal hyperplasia, both testes can be enlarged because they contain growing masses of adrenal cortex-like cells.[401] A similar condition is observed in Nelson's syndrome.

Testicular enlargement is modest in paraneoplastic precocious pseudopuberty secondary to hepatoblastoma[402] or extratesticular hCG-secreting germ cell tumor, although nodular or diffuse precocious maturation has been occasionally reported.[403]

*Precocious pseudopuberty secondary to excessive aromatase activity* Biosynthesis of C18 estrogens from C19 androgens occurs by three consecutive oxidative reactions that are catalyzed by an enzymatic complex known as estrogen synthetase or aromatase.[404] This complex has two components: P450 arom (a product from the CYP19 gene located on 15p21.1),[405] which joins C19 substrate and catalyzes the insertion of oxygen in C19 to form C18 estrogens; and NADPH-cytochrome P450 reductase, a ubiquitous flavoprotein that conveys reducing equivalents to any form of cytochrome P450 it meets.

Aromatase is in the endoplasmic reticulum of estrogen-synthesizing cells and expressed in placenta, ovarian granulosa, Sertoli cells, Leydig cells, adipose tissue, and several central nervous system regions, including the hypothalamus, amygdala, and hippocampus. Excessive aromatase causes excessive conversion of androgens to estrogen,[406] and is a heterogeneous genetic disorder with an autosomal dominant inheritance. The disorder leads to heterosexual precocious pseudopuberty with gynecomastia in males, and to isosexual precocity and macromastia in females. Ultimately, patient stature is short because of the potent ability of androgens to accelerate epiphyseal closure. Most males are fertile and have normal libido.[407] Generally, the inhibitory estrogenic effect on testicular function is less than that observed with estrogen-producing tumors or in patients treated with exogen estrogens.

Excessive aromatase caused by P450 mutation induces alterations in both males and females. In females lacking estrogens owing to desmolase deficiency, excessive aromatase leads to pseudohermaphroditism and progressive virilization at puberty; conversely, pubertal development is normal in males. In children, FSH and LH levels and gonadotropin response to GnRH are normal, suggesting that the role of estrogens in pituitary regulation is weak during infancy.[408] In both genders, epiphyseal closure is delayed and a eunuchoid habitus results. Adult males have small testes, severe oligozoospermia, and complete asthenozoospermia; FSH and LH levels are high, testosterone levels are normal, and serum estrogen levels are very low.

All patients with excessive aromatase have short stature, with continuing linear growth into adulthood, unfused epiphyses, osteoporosis, bilateral genu valgum, and eunuchoid proportions. The testes show macroorchidism with normal testicular consistency in some cases,[409] and are small with severe oligozoospermia and 100% immotile spermatozoa in other cases.[410]

A syndrome similar to that of excessive aromatase production is found in patients with estrogen resistance caused by disruptive mutations of the ER gene. These patients show macroorchidism, elevated testosterone levels, and increased levels of FSH, LH, estradiol, and estrona.[411]

*Precocious pseudopuberty secondary to Leydig cell hyperplasia with focal spermatogenesis* This entity can present with clinical symptoms similar to those of a functioning Leydig cell tumor; this is a precocious pseudopuberty with ipsilateral testicular enlargement.[412] The testes contains hypertrophic Leydig cell nests in association with normal spermatogenesis. No tumoral mass is seen. Leydig cells do not contain Reinke's crystalloids and do not compress the seminiferous tubules. There is a clear delimitation between tubules with spermatogenesis and infantile immature tubules. The differential diagnosis between this entity and Leydig cell tumor with precocious pseudopuberty is based on the histological pattern. Open excisional testicular biopsy is recommended; if there is Leydig cell tumor, or the diagnosis by frozen section is not conclusive, removal is advisable.[413] There are no data to suggest that this hyperplasia might develop into Leydig cell tumor.

*Mixed precocious puberty* The best known form is the McCune–Albright syndrome (MAS), characterized by the association of 'coffee and milk' pigmentary lesions in the skin, bone lesions (polyostotic fibrous dysplasia), enlarged testes, prepubertal size of the penis, and absence of pubic and axillary hair. Although testicular enlargement is usually bilateral, unilateral macroorchidism may be the first symptom.[414] An interesting finding is that the onset of testicular maturation is induced by the testis itself, which produces steroid secretion due to autonomous hyperfunction of Sertoli cells without evidence of Leydig cell involvement.[415] This secretion causes early maturation of the hypothalamo-pituitary–testicular axis and, subsequently, true precocious puberty.[416] Serum levels of testosterone are low, but those of inhibin B and AMH are abnormally increased. This syndrome is caused by mutations that activate the GNAS-1 gene, which encodes the α subunit of the trimeric G-protein. Because mutations are lethal in the uterus, those subjects producing AMH bear a mosaicism chromosomal constitution for this deficiency.

## Testicular ectopia and testicular fusion

### Testicular ectopia

A testis is ectopic when it is in a location outside the normal path of descent. Unlike cryptorchid testes, ectopic testes are nearly normal in size and are accompanied by a spermatic cord that is normal or even longer than normal, and by a normal scrotum.[417]

Testicular ectopia is classified according to location;[418–422] in decreasing order of frequency, the major types are:

- *Interstitial or inguinal superficial ectopia.* This is the most frequent form and may be confused with inguinal cryptorchidism. After passing through the outer genital opening, the testis ascends to the anterosuperior iliac spine and remains on the aponeurosis of the major oblique muscle. These testes often are more nearly normal histologically than are cryptorchid testes.

- *Femoral or crural ectopia.* After passing through the inguinal canal, the testis lodges in the high crural cone in Scarpa's triangle.
- *Perineal.* The testis is located between the raphe and the genitocrural fold.
- *Transverse or crossed ectopia.* Both testes descend through the same inguinal canal and lodge in the same scrotal pouch. Each possesses its own vascular supply, epididymis, and vas deferens. In addition, there is ipsilateral hernia.[423–430] Between 20% and 40% of patients with this ectopia have persistent müllerian duct syndrome[431–432] and show a high incidence of testicular germ cell tumor.[433]
- *Pubopenile ectopia.* The ectopic testis is on the back of the penis near the symphysis pubis.[434]
- *Pelvic ectopia.* The testis is in the pelvis, usually in the depth of Douglas' cul-de-sac.
- Other unusual testicular ectopias include *retroumbilical, craniolateral to the inner inguinal opening* between the outer and inner oblique muscles, and *subumbilical.*[435] Rarely, the testis and its spermatic cord may protrude through a defect in the scrotal skin, a condition called *testicular exstrophy.*[436]

The term *testicular dislocation* refers to testes that secondarily disappear from the scrotum and lodge around the superficial inguinal ring, within the inguinal ring, or inside the abdominal cavity as a result of testicular trauma. The formation of canalicular and intra-abdominal dislocation requires the presence of previous inguinal hernia.[437]

### Testicular fusion

Testicular fusion is a rare anomaly characterized by fusion of the testes to form a single structure, usually in the midline. Each has its own epididymis and vas deferens. This anomaly is often associated with other malformations, such as fusion of the adrenal glands or horseshoe kidney.

## Hamartomatous testicular lesions

### Cystic dysplasia

Cystic dysplasia of the testis is a congenital lesion characterized by cystic transformation of an excessively developed rete testis that may extend to the tunica albuginea of the opposite pole.[438] To date, fewer than 40 cases have been reported.[439,440] The seminiferous tubules may be dilated and atrophic; this is more evident after puberty. Ultrasound images are characteristic.[441,442] Cysts arise in the septal and mediastinal rete testis (Fig. 12-36); they are interconnected and contain acellular, eosinophilic, periodic acid–Schiff-positive material. They are lined by cuboidal cells that resemble those of the normal rete testis.[443–445] The connective tissue between the cysts is scant and histologically similar to the interstitial connective tissue. There may be small groups of cysts limited to the region of the mediastinum testis, or cysts extending throughout the entire testis. In extensive

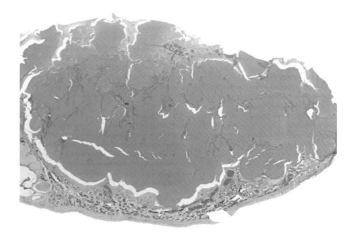

**Fig. 12-36** Cystic dysplasia of the testis. There is cystic transformation of the rete testis and adjacent seminiferous tubules.

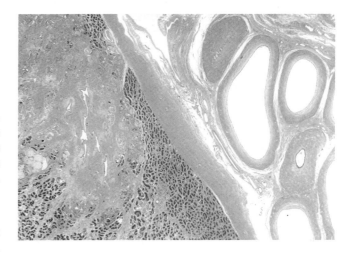

**Fig. 12-37** Marked luminal dilation of the ductus epididymidis in an infant with cystic dysplasia of the rete testis.

cases, residual seminiferous tubules occupy only a small crescent beneath the tunica albuginea and the testis is grossly spongy. Cystic dysplasia occurs in normally descended and cryptorchid testes in children and adults, and may affect one or both testes.[446] In adults, the residual parenchyma often shows complete tubular sclerosis or hypospermatogenesis with intratubular accumulation of spermatozoa and Leydig cell pseudohyperplasia.

In most cases the epididymis is altered.[447] The head of the epididymis is small and contains few ductuli efferentes with irregular, usually dilated lumina. The ductus epididymidis is dilated, has an atrophic epithelium, and thick connective tissue replaces the muscular layer (Fig. 12-37).

Testicular cystic dysplasia is frequently associated with severe anomalies of the urinary system. Renal agenesis,[446–449] renal dysplasia,[446] hydroureter, and urethral stenosis[450] have been reported ipsilateral to cystic dysplasia. The clinical differential diagnosis should consider all cystic testicular lesions impairing prepubertal testes, including epidermoid cyst,

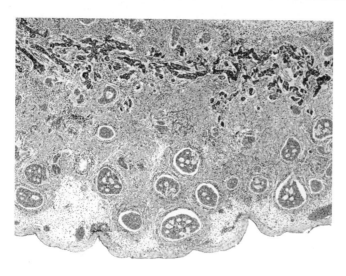

**Fig. 12-38** Gonadoblastoid testicular dysplasia. Several nodules are present at the periphery of the testicular parenchyma.

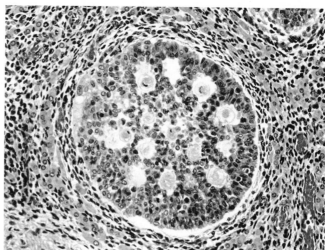

**Fig. 12-39** Gonadoblastoid testicular dysplasia. A nodule contains numerous Sertoli-like cells, Call–Exner bodies, and isolated germ cells. The nodule is surrounded by two cell layers: fusiform cells (inner layer) and Leydig cells (outer layer).

cystic teratoma, juvenile granulosa cell tumor, testicular lymphangiectasis, and simple cyst of the testis.[451] The presence of ipsilateral renal anomalies during ultrasound exploration provides an important diagnostic clue.[452] Previously, orchidectomy was the treatment of choice, but testis-sparing surgery[453] is now recommended.[454,455]

The etiology and pathogenesis of cystic dysplasia are uncertain. Given that the rete testis is a mesonephric derivative and most of the associated renal malformations are apparently caused by failure in the induction of renal blastema by the mesonephros, cystic dysplasia is considered to be the result of an abnormal mesonephros.

During childhood, the normal rete testis has no lumina, and these form during puberty. The adult rete testis is a conduit for the passage of tubular fluid and spermatozoa and also actively reabsorbs part of this fluid while adding ions, proteins and steroids to it. Malfunction of the rete testis cells may cause the formation of excessive fluid of abnormal composition, resulting in a condition morphologically similar to cystic dysplasia of the rete testis induced in fowl by sodium intoxication or the administration of the salt-retaining hormone deoxycorticosterone acetate.

### Gonadoblastoid testicular dysplasia

Gonadoblastoid testicular dysplasia refers to an abnormally differentiated testicular parenchyma beneath the tunica albuginea.[456] The anomaly consists of large tubular or nodular structures within a dense stroma, reminiscent of ovarian stroma (Fig. 12-38). Each structure is composed of three cell types: cells with vesicular nuclei and vacuolated cytoplasm; cells with hyperchromatic nuclei; and germ cell-like cells. The former two types are arranged at the periphery, forming a pseudostratified epithelium. The third type resembles fetal spermatogonia and are fewer in number. These structures contain eosinophilic, periodic acid–Schiff-positive material, similar to Call–Exner bodies (Fig. 12-39). There may be continuity between these structures and normal seminiferous tubules. The differential diagnosis includes conditions showing anomalous seminiferous tubules at the gonadal periphery, including testicular dysgenesis and gonadoblastoma. Testicular dysgenesis also presents tubular or cord-like structures, but these are differentiated (some form true seminiferous tubules) and may also be present within a poorly collagenized tunica albuginea; patients with testicular dysgenesis are male pseudohermaphrodites with müllerian remnants. Gonadoblastoma usually appears in a streak gonad or dysgenetic gonad and contains granulosa–Sertoli cells and germ cells that are similar to those of dysgerminoma or seminoma; these cells are absent in gonadoblastoid testicular dysplasia. Several cases with this disorder have been reported in patients with Walker–Warburg syndrome.[457,458]

### Sertoli cell nodule (hypoplastic zones or dysgenetic tubules)

This disorder refers to the presence, in an adult testis, of one or several foci of infantile (immature) seminiferous tubules. Each group of tubules appears well delimited but unencapsulated. Nodule size varies from microscopic to 5 mm. On section, each nodule is distinguished by its whitish color. Sertoli cell nodule is found in most adult cryptorchid testes, regardless of when the testes descended. It is also present in 22% of normal scrotal testes in some series,[459] and is an occasional finding in males with idiopathic infertility.

The seminiferous tubules have a prepubertal diameter and may be anastomotic. The epithelium is columnar or pseudostratified, devoid of lumina, and usually consists only of Sertoli cells (Fig. 12-40). The cells have elongated hyperchromatic nuclei with one or several peripherally placed small nucleoli.[459] The interstitium varies from scant to well collagenized. Leydig cells are usually absent in these areas and, if present, their numbers are low. Study of serial sections reveals continuity between some of these tubules and normal tubules. Sertoli cell nodule changes with advancing age. The Sertoli cells produce large amounts of basal lamina

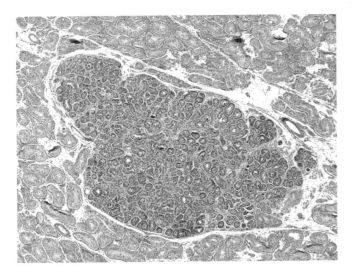

**Fig. 12-40** Sertoli cell nodule. This adult cryptorchid testis contains compact groups of small seminiferous tubules with pseudostratified cell layers without lumina.

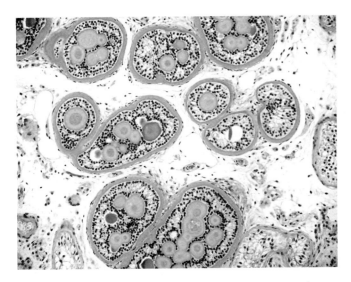

**Fig. 12-41** Sertoli cell nodule. Sertoli cell-produced material, similar to the basal lamina material, forms fingerlike protrusions inside the hypoplastic tubules. The Sertoli cells are arranged in a ring around this material.

that protrudes inside the hypoplastic tubules. In transverse and oblique sections, these protrusions might be misinterpreted as intratubular accumulations of basal lamina material (Fig. 12-41). This material can undergo calcification to form microliths. Immunohistochemical study reveals two basic components of the basal lamina (collagen IV and laminin), confirming its extracellular origin; the protrusions consist mainly of laminin, whereas collagen IV delimits the outer profile of the seminiferous tubules. So, while the amount of collagen IV is uniform around the tubules, the depth of laminin varies within the same tubule.

Tubular hypoplasia is assumed to be a primary testicular lesion, and refers to the presence of seminiferous tubules that are unable to undergo pubertal development despite the same hormonal stimuli of adjacent normal tubules. This dysgenesis includes immature Sertoli cell pattern, low inhibin secretion, absence of androgen receptors,[460] and lack of maturation of peritubular myoid cells that fail to synthesize elastic fibers. The presence of hypoplastic zones in a testicular biopsy is an adverse prognostic sign for fertility.

The differential diagnosis includes tubular hamartoma in androgen insensitivity syndrome, sex cord tumor with annular tubules, and mixed atrophy of the testis. Tubular hamartoma in androgen insensitivity syndrome is multiple, similar to the hypoplastic zones of tubular hypoplasia; however, the Sertoli-like cells of hamartoma have spherical nuclei (rather of elongated nuclei), form a cuboidal epithelium, and contain numerous Leydig cells among the tubules (see Androgen insensitivity syndrome, below). Sex cord tumor with annular tubules may present with multiple foci of intratubular neoplasia, similar in distribution to that of hypoplastic zones; however, sex cord tumor appears in undescended testes, and in patients with Peutz–Jeghers syndrome, and consists of cuboidal or spherical cells that express cytokeratins that are not expressed in hypoplastic tubules.

It is possible that hypoplastic tubules contain some germ cells that may be spermatogonia or gonocytes. There are scant spermatogonia that fail to display signs of maturation or proliferation. Also, some of the tubules contain intratubular undifferentiated germ cell neoplasia that usually also appears in the adjacent, non-hypoplastic seminiferous tubules. The histologic picture is similar to that of gonadoblastoma, but such a tumor can be easily excluded because it arises in malformed gonads (gonadal dysgenesis and testicular dysgenesis) characteristic of intersex stages, unlike patients with tubular hypoplasia.

## Congenital testicular lymphangiectasis

Congenital testicular lymphangiectasis is characterized by abnormal and excessive development of lymphatic vessels in the tunica albuginea, mediastinum testis, interlobular septa, and testicular interstitium.[461–463] Ultrastructurally these dilated vessels are similar to normal lymphatic capillaries, although some are markedly dilated and the testicular interstitium is slightly edematous (Fig. 12-42). Testicular lymphangiectasis occurs in both cryptorchid and scrotal testes; in one of the latter cases, the patient had Noonan's syndrome. The disease does not seem to affect the seminiferous tubules, and low numbers of spermatogonia and reduced tubular diameters are observed only in cryptorchid testes. The epididymis and spermatic cord are not affected, and congenital testicular lymphangiectasis is not associated with pulmonary, intestinal, or systemic lymphangiectasis. During fetal life, lymphatic vessels are visible only immediately beneath the tunica albuginea and in the interlobular septa.[464] During childhood, the number and size of the septal lymphatic vessels decreases;[465] by adulthood they are inconspicuous.[466] In lymphangiectasis, the septal lymphatic vessels are large and often massively dilated. Testicular lymphangiectasis occurs only in the childhood testis, suggesting that these dilated vessels undergo involution at puberty or that pubertal development of the seminiferous tubules masks the lymphangiectasis. One exceptional case of epididymal lymphangiectasis, with dilated epididymal blood vessels,

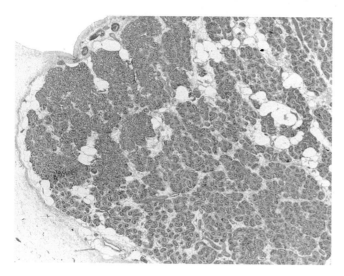

**Fig. 12-42** Congenital testicular lymphangiectasis. Ectatic lymphatic vessels are seen in the tunica vasculosa and interlobular septa, as well as among the seminiferous tubules, causing compression.

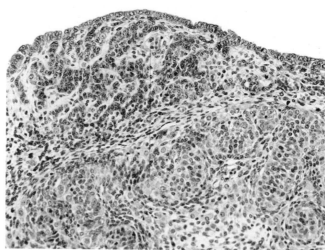

**Fig. 12-44** Persistent testicular blastema in a newborn. The blastema forms anastomosic cord-like formations which connect to the superficial cells. Several gonocytes are observed at the periphery of the blastema.

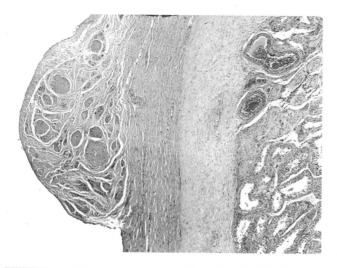

**Fig. 12-43** Smooth muscle hamartoma within enlarged tunica albuginea.

was reported in a 59-year-old man.[467] The vessels distort the architecture of the ductuli efferentes, which in turn become irregularly dilated by mechanical compression.

### Other hamartomatous testicular lesions

Other hamartomas of the testis include hamartoma of the rete testis and smooth muscle hamartoma. Hamartoma of the rete testis is a disordered proliferation of tubular structures in a loose connective tissue.[468] Cystic transformation of the rete testis associated with proliferation of smooth muscle cells and abundant myxoid stroma was reported in a 26-year-old man.[469]

Smooth muscle hamartoma is located in the inferior testicular pole, the cauda of the epididymis, and the proximal segment of the vas deferens (Fig. 12-43),[470] and is similar to that reported in the digestive and respiratory tracts.[471,472] Smooth muscle hyperplasia also occurs in the androgen insensitivity syndrome, forming nodules up to 1 cm in diameter. The muscular proliferation is located in the lower testicular pole, and involves the tunica albuginea and adjacent soft tissues.

## Testicular ectopia

### Gonadal blastema ectopia

This infrequent finding has been observed in newborns and consists of gonadal blastema in otherwise normal testes. The blastema is located in the vicinity of the upper testicular pole, near the implantation of the caput of the epididymis, displays a crescent shape, and extends throughout the depth of the tunica albuginea and the adjacent testicular parenchyma.

The blastema consists of epithelial cords of cells or solid masses in continuity with the mesothelium (Fig. 12-44). These cells are intermingled with others that are larger, with pale cytoplasm, vesicular nuclei, and prominent nucleoli. The blastematous epithelial cells display immunoreactivity for vimentin, laminin, type IV collagen, and cytokeratin; the expression of the latter in the most superficial cells is similar to that of mesothelial cells and decreases in intensity in the deeper cells. This suggests that these may be pre-Sertoli cells. The cord-like structures are delimited by laminin and type IV collagen. The second larger cell type is immunoreactive for placenta-like alkaline phosphatase (PLAP) on the surface, suggesting that it is related to the gonocyte. Leydig cells have not been observed among the cords of gonadal blastema.

The differential diagnosis of gonadal blastema ectopia is with ovotestes. The small size of the gonocytes distinguishes them from ovocytes, which are several times larger. In addition, no intersex condition is observed.

### Seminiferous tubule ectopia

The presence of seminiferous tubules within the tunica albuginea is rare and usually an incidental histologic finding.[473] Ectopic tubules are present in approximately 0.8% of pediatric autopsies and 0.3% of adult autopsies. The lower inci-

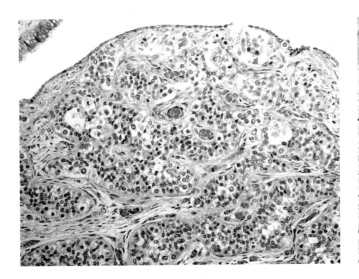

**Fig. 12-45** Testis from 2-month-old infant showing ectopic seminiferous tubules within the tunica albuginea in the upper testicular pole.

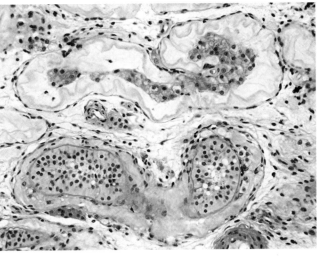

**Fig. 12-46** Ectopic Leydig cells inside a hyalinized seminiferous tubule. This picture contrasts with that of dysgenetic Sertoli-cell-only tubule, which shows a patent basal membrane located between the dysgenetic Sertoli cells and the tubular wall.

dence in adults may be explained by proportionally less sampling. The lesion ranges from microscopic size to a few millimeters in diameter, and may be visible as minute bulges in which multiple small vesicles protrude through a thin tunica albuginea.[474] Histologically there are groups of seminiferous tubules in the tunica albuginea, sometimes accompanied by Leydig cells. In children, the ectopic tubules appear normal (Fig. 12-45), whereas in adults they are usually slightly dilated, although some may be hyalinized. Serial sections reveal continuity with the intraparenchymatous seminiferous tubules.

Ectopia of the seminiferous tubule is probably congenital, although it has been found in elderly men.[475] It does not appear to be the result of trauma. The malformation probably arises in the sixth week of gestation, when the primordial sex cords have formed and are branching toward the gonadal surface, and the developing testes is covered by only one to three layers of celomic epithelium. Later, the tunica albuginea forms around the sex cords and under the celomic epithelium. Failure of insertion of the tunica albuginea between the sex cords and celomic epithelium may entrap seminiferous tubules.

Ectopia differs from testicular dysgenesis, a distinctive form of male pseudohermaphroditism with müllerian remnants. Numerous features, characteristic of ectopic seminiferous tubules, distinguish it from other conditions, including normal thickness and collagenization of the tunica albuginea, absence of interstitial tissue resembling ovarian stroma (characteristic of testicular dysgenesis), and clear delimitation of the tunica albuginea and testicular parenchyma (see discussion on male pseudohermaphroditism with müllerian remnants, below).

In a unique case, there were multiple clusters of seminiferous tubules in the wall of a hernia sac that accompanied an undescended testis removed from an adult man. The ectopic tubules were not surrounded by tunica albuginea and were similar to those in cryptorchid testicular parenchyma with only dysgenetic Sertoli cells.

### Leydig cell ectopia

Leydig cells occur normally in the testicular interstitium (interstitial Leydig cells) and in the wall of the seminiferous tubules (peritubular Leydig cells). However, clusters of Leydig cells are often observed in other locations in the testis, or in the epididymis or spermatic cord.[476]

Ectopic Leydig cells may be found in the interlobular septa,[477-479] rete testis, tunica albuginea,[480-482] or within hyalinized seminiferous tubules.[478,483-485] Intratubular Leydig cells are found only in tubules with advanced atrophy and marked thickening of the tunica propria, including the tubules in adult cryptorchid testes, those of men with Klinefelter's syndrome, and in some other primary hypogonadisms (Fig. 12-46). Immunohistochemical studies suggest that the endocrine function of these Leydig cells is low.[486] Several theories have been offered to account for these ectopic cells, including in situ differentiation, migration from the testicular interstitium, and trapping of peritubular Leydig cells in the tunica propria during its thickening.[487] Leydig cells are commonly found in the epididymis[487] and spermatic cord;[488,489] 26 of 64 autopsies had such foci.[490] Extratesticular Leydig cells usually form small groups within or adjacent to nerves (Fig. 12-47).[477,490]

The occurrence of ectopic Leydig cells in the albuginea, epididymis, or spermatic cord may account for the rare cases of Leydig cell tumor in these paratesticular structures. Ectopic Leydig cells should not be misinterpreted as tumor cells (infiltration or metastasis) when malignancy of a testicular Leydig cell tumor is suspected.

### Other ectopias

Other rare forms of ectopia are found within and outside the testis. Intratesticular ectopia includes adrenal cortical ectopia, osseous and adipose tissue heterotopia, and ectopia of the ductus epididymidis. Extratesticular ectopia includes splenic ectopia (splenogonadal fusion), hepatic ectopia (hepatotes-

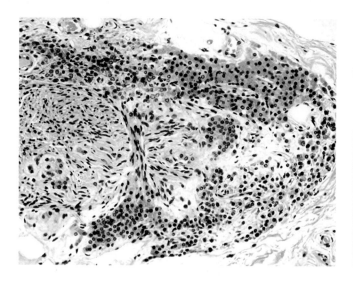

**Fig. 12-47** Ectopic Leydig cells around and inside a spermatic cord nerve.

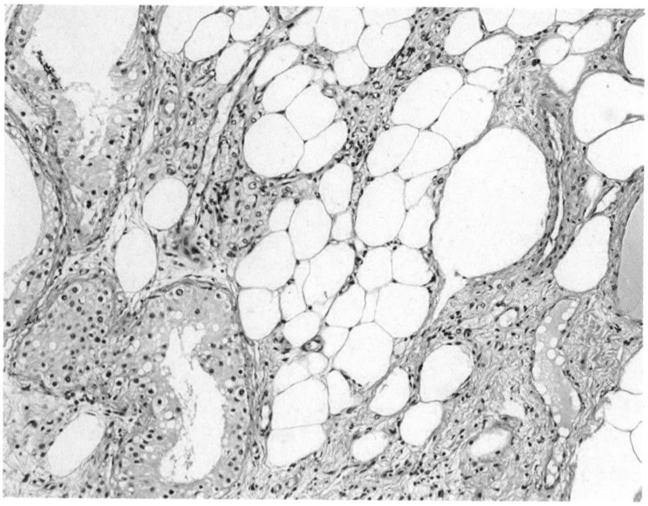

**Fig. 12-48** Adult cryptorchid testis showing metaplastic fat cells between the seminiferous tubules and the rete testis.

ticular fusion), and renal blastema ectopia (see discussion in Chapter 12).

Adrenal cortical ectopia may be important in two conditions that develop tumoral masses: adrenogenital syndrome and Nelson's syndrome. Tumors in adrenogenital syndrome appear in 8.2% of patients with congenital adrenal hyperplasia, appearing as bilateral testicular masses of synchronous growth. These tumors consist of well delimited but non-encapsulated yellow nodules, several centimeters long, composed of large microvacuolated cells. The cause seems to be prolonged stimulation by elevated ACTH secretion. The differential diagnosis includes Leydig cell tumor. The diagnosis of tumors in adrenogenital syndrome is supported by a family or personal history of salt-lost syndrome or hypertension, demonstration of 11 β-hydroxysteroids (a specific marker for adrenal cortex) in spermatic vein blood, or a rapid positive response of tumor to corticoid treatment. Nelson's syndrome occurs in patients who, after adrenalectomy for treatment of Cushing's syndrome, develop an ACTH-secreting pituitary adenoma. These patients may develop testicular tumor growth similar to that in adrenogenital syndrome. Most Nelson's syndrome tumors do not respond to dexametasone treatment.

Cartilaginous heterotopia may be found in the caput of the epididymis and has been attributed to metaplasia of metanephric rests. Osseous heterotopia (testicular osteoma) is a metaplasia occurring in areas of the testicular parenchyma with fibrosis or ischemia.[491] Adipose metaplasia is frequent in undescended testis, elderly men, and those with Cowden's syndrome (Fig. 12-48).[492] Groups of tubular formations that resembles the epididymis have been reported inside the testicular parenchyma in testes with marked tubular atrophy, and probably represent a rare form of metaplasia.[493]

## Undescended testes

Testicular descent is not always complete at birth, and about 3.2% of full-term newborns have incompletely descended testes. Most of these descend within 3 months, and only 0.8% of infants have incompletely descended testes 12 months after birth. Spontaneous testicular descent is exceptional after the first year. In recent decades, a significant increase in the incidence of cryptorchidism has been detected.[494]

Only 5% of patients with impalpable testes are actually devoid of testes. Other causes include true cryptorchidism, testicular ectopia, and retractile testes. True cryptorchidism includes abdominal, inguinal, and high scrotal testes that cannot be moved to the scrotum. Ectopic testes are those located out of the normal path of testicular descent; the most frequent site is the superficial inguinal pouch. Other rare locations of ectopia include the abdominal wall, the upper thigh, the perineum, and the base of the penis. Retractile testes may be moved to the scrotum at exploration and account for about one third of undescended testes.

### True cryptorchidism

Patients with true cryptorchidism account for about 25% of cases of empty scrotum. These testes most frequently are found in the inguinal canal or upper scrotum; arrest within the abdomen is less frequent. Cryptorchidism is slightly more frequent on the right than the left, and in approximately 18% of cases is bilateral. There is a family history of cryptorchidism in 14% of cases.[495] The cryptorchid testis is usually smaller than the contralateral one, and this difference is often discernible at 6 months of age.[496] One-third of cryptorchid testes are soft.

#### Etiology

Several conditions are predictive of high risk of cryptorchidism, including increased maternal age, maternal obesity, pregnancy toxemia, bleeding during late pregnancy, and smoking, tallness, subfertility antecedents, cesarean birth, low birthweight, preterm newborn, twin birth, hypospadias[497] and other congenital malformations, and children born from September to November, and in May and

June.[498,499] Of these associations, low birth weight seems to be the most important.[500]

There are two types of cryptorchidism: congenital and acquired.

## Congenital cryptorchidism

This cryptorchidism is caused by anomalies in anatomic development or hormonal mechanisms involved in testicular descent (described above). Impalpable undescended testes are infrequent because the transabdominal phase follows the simple mechanism of relative movement of the testis, whereas displacement of the ovary is more complex.[501] Conversely, palpable undescended testes are more frequent because the second phase of testicular descent is more complex. Unilateral cryptorchidism may be caused by androgen failure, which leads to either an ipsilateral lesion in the development of genitofemoral nerve neurons or a defect in CGRP release that hinders normal migration of the gubernaculum.

## Acquired cryptorchidism

A normally descended testis may become cryptorchid and locate even in the abdominal cavity. Two categories of acquired undescended testis have been described.

The *postoperative trapped testis*[502] is a normally descended testis that leaves the scrotal pouch after surgery owing to an inguinal hernia or hydrocele.[503–505] This iatrogenic cryptorchidism occurs in 1.2% of children after herniotomy. Adherence of the testis or the cremasteric muscle to the surgical incision causes testicular ascent when the incision heals and undergoes retraction.

*Spontaneous ascent* from unknown causes. Various mechanisms have been proposed, including inability of the spermatic blood vessels to grow adequately,[506] anomalous insertion of the gubernaculum,[507] failure in reabsorption of the vaginal process[508,509] and failure in postnatal elongation of the spermatic cord.[510,511] The spermatic cord measures 4–5 cm at birth and reaches 8–10 cm at 10 years of age. This growth does not occur if the peritoneal–vaginal duct has become a fibrous remnant. The cause might be a defect in postnatal CGRP release by the genitofemoral nerve.[501,512,513]

## Pathogenesis

The most frequent findings in congenital and acquired cryptorchidism at infancy are decreased germ cell numbers and diminished tubular diameter.[514,515] There are multiple causes of testicular maldescent, including anatomical anomalies of the gubernaculum testis, hormonal dysfunction (hypogonadotropic hypogonadism), mechanical impairment (insufficient intra-abdominal pressure, short spermatic cord, underdeveloped processus vaginalis), dysgenetic (primary anomaly of the testis), and heredity.

Most cryptorchidism appears to be caused by either a deficit of fetal androgens or an excess of maternal estrogens. Androgen insufficiency seems to be slight and transient because anomalies other than hypoplasia of the epididymis are not seen. Elevated maternal estrogens level could cause diminution of FSH secretion by the fetal pituitary, inducing low müllerian-inhibiting hormone production that would hinder testicular descent.[516]

Three mechanisms seem to be involved in the process:

- *Primary testicular anomaly.* Cryptorchid testes may bear an anomalous germ cell population, as suggested many years ago.[517] More than 40% of cryptorchid patients have a marked decrease in the tubular fertility index,[518] even with nearly normal numbers of spermatogonia; these cells also have abnormal DNA content.[519]

- *Lesions secondary to transient perinatal hypogonadotropic hypogonadism.* Cryptorchid patients do not have gonadotropin elevation, which normally occurs between 60 and 90 days after birth, and this deficiency of LH could cause Leydig cell involution. The subsequent androgen deficiency could account for failure of gonocytes to differentiate into spermatogonia.[520–522]

- *Injury caused by increased temperature.* This was suggested in the past on the basis of experimental studies in laboratory animals. In follow-up biopsies from testes that were descended surgically or with hormonal treatment, the sole parameter that improved during childhood was tubular diameter. Because this depends on Sertoli cells, it may be that temperature is more important for Sertoli cells than for spermatogonia.[518]

In the normal testis there is transient formation of spermatocytes at 4–5 years of age. This meiotic attempt is probably an androgenic event that does not occur in cryptorchid testes and agrees with the characteristic low numbers of spermatogonia in the prepubertal age.[523]

### Histology of cryptorchid testes

**Prepubertal testes** Undescended testes are usually smaller than the contralateral ones. This difference is already significant at 6 months of age.[524,525] Although there have been a number of biopsy studies in the first years of life, there is no agreement about the severity of damage or the time of its onset.[523,526,527] Based on the tubular fertility index (TFI) and mean tubular diameter (MTD), most testicular biopsies from cryptorchid testes of children can be classified into one of three groups:

- *Type I (testes with slight alterations).* The tubular fertility index is higher than 50, and the mean tubular diameter is normal or slightly (<10%) decreased. Approximately 31% of cryptorchid testes are in this group (Fig. 12-49).

- *Type II (testes with marked germinal hypoplasia).* Tubular fertility index is between 30 and 50, and mean tubular diameter is 10–30% lower than normal. The spermatogonia are distributed irregularly and most are in tubular sections that are grouped in the same testicular lobule. These testes comprise approximately 29% of cryptorchid testes (Fig. 12-50).[528]

- *Type III (testes with severe germinal hypoplasia).* Tubular fertility index is less than 30, and mean tubular diameter less than 30% of normal. Many of the spermatogonia are giant with dark nuclei (Fig. 12-51). These testes often contain ring-shaped tubules,

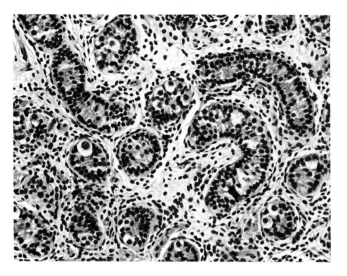

**Fig. 12-49** Cryptorchidism. Seminiferous tubules with type I lesions show slightly decreased diameters and a normal tubular fertility index.

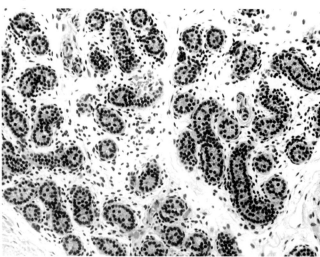

**Fig. 12-51** Cryptorchidism. Seminiferous tubules with type III lesions show severe reduction in both tubular diameter and tubular fertility index.

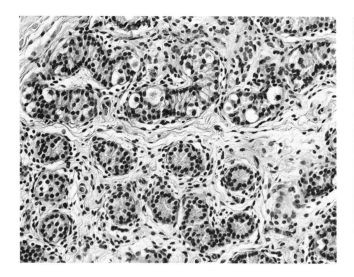

**Fig. 12-50** Cryptorchidism. Seminiferous tubules with type II lesions show markedly decreased diameters and an irregular distribution of germ cells.

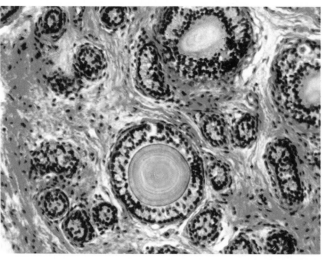

**Fig. 12-52** Microlithiasis in an infant cryptorchid testis. The seminiferous tubules show type III lesions and contain numerous microliths.

megatubules (with or without eosinophilic bodies or microliths) (Fig. 12-52), and focal granular changes in the Sertoli cells (Fig. 12-53). The testicular interstitium is wide and edematous. These comprise about 40% of cryptorchid testes.

About 8% of tests with type I lesions show many multinucleated spermatogonia (with three or more nuclei) (Fig. 12-54).[529] The seminiferous tubules of testes with types II or III lesions have a thickened lamina propria during childhood and, at puberty, Sertoli cell hyperplasia.[526] Patients with bilateral cryptorchidism have a higher incidence of type II and III lesions than those with unilateral cryptorchidism.

Type I lesions are comparable to those seen in experimental cryptorchidism; normal testes in which lesions were induced by increased temperature.[527] Testes with type II or III lesions bear variable degrees of dysgenesis that, in addition to germ cells, involve Sertoli cells, peritubular myofibroblasts, and Leydig cells. The dysgenesis of these other cell types is evident only after puberty. In about 25% of cases the contralateral scrotal testis also has histologic lesions of variable severity. This finding supports the hypothesis of a bilateral defect in many cases of unilateral cryptorchidism. Microdeletions in the long arm of the Y chromosome are present in 27% of patients with corrected unilateral cryptorchidism who present with azoospermia or severe oligospermia.[530] These findings are similar to those observed in patients with azoospermia or severe idiopathic oligospermia. Unilateral cryptorchidism with a normal contralateral testis could be due to an end-organ failure.[531] In cryptorchidism secondary to spontaneous ascent, lesions are similar to

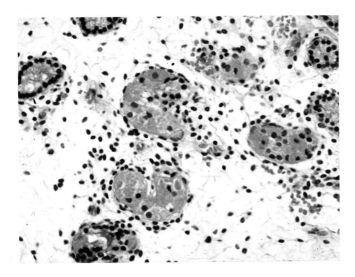

**Fig. 12-53** Cryptorchidism. Type III lesions, in which the interstitium is expanded by edema. The cytoplasm of the Sertoli cells contains numerous eosinophilic granules of variable size.

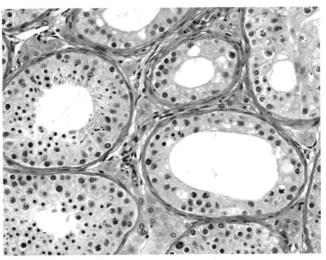

**Fig. 12-55** Adult ex-cryptorchid testis which was surgically descended at the age of 2 years. Tubular sections show a pattern varying from spermatogonial maturation arrest to complete, although decreased, spermatogenesis.

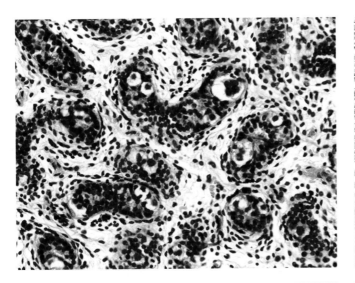

**Fig. 12-54** Prepubertal cryptorchid testis. The seminiferous tubules have Sertoli cells with elongated nuclei, pseudostratified growth pattern, and isolated spermatogonia, some of which are multinucleate or contain hypertrophic nuclei.

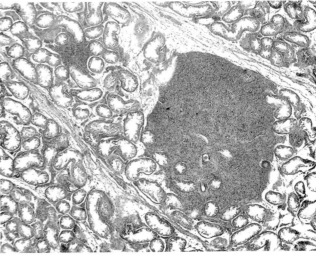

**Fig. 12-56** Nodular Leydig cell hyperplasia in an adult ex-cryptorchid testis.

those of congenital cryptorchidism, whereas in cryptorchidism secondary to herniotomy, germ cell depletion is slight[532] and becomes important only after 5 years of age.[533]

*Adult testes* Most pubertal and adult cryptorchid testes have anomalies in all testicular structures. The seminiferous tubules have decreased diameters and deficient spermatogenesis. In decreasing order of frequency, the most common germ cell lesions are tubules with Sertoli cell and spermatogonia-only pattern; tubules with Sertoli cells (dysgenetic) only; tubular hyalinization; and mixed atrophy. The lamina propria has scant elastic fibers and increased collagen fibers.[534] Sertoli cells are present in increased numbers and do not mature normally except in tubules with germ cells (Fig. 12-55).[528,535] Often, groups of tubules containing only

Sertoli cells with a prepubertal pattern (very small diameter and total absence of maturation) are present and are considered hypoplastic, dysgenetic, or hamartomatous. Areas of apparent Leydig cell hyperplasia are frequent, and many of these cells contain vacuolated lipid-laden cytoplasm (Fig. 12-56).

The rete testis is hypoplastic in most cases and is lined by columnar epithelium with rare areas of flattened cells. Cystic dilation is common, and adenomatous hyperplasia has been found in some cases. Near the rete testis, the testicular parenchyma frequently contains metaplastic fat. In some cryptorchid testes, several tubular segments are destroyed by inflammation that probably has an autoimmune cause (focal orchitis).[536] Epididymal tubules are poorly developed and peritubular tissue is immature.

Blood flow is associated with testicular histology. For example, testicular volume, histologic pattern, and testicular artery resistive index are lower in undescended testes than in controls, and testicular artery resistive index is inversely proportional to testicular histology score in undescended testes.[537] There is also an apparent correlation between testicular size, spermiogram, and hormone levels. Assuming that a significant reduction in testicular size (>12 mL) is only observed in 9.3% of cases, and that serum levels of FSH, LH, and testosterone are normal, an inverse correlation is seen between FSH and testicular volume, sperm concentration, sperm motility, and normally shaped sperm. In addition, there is a direct relation between testicular volume and sperm concentration, sperm motility, and normally shaped sperm. These findings indicate the cause of tubular impairment in young men operated on in childhood for cryptorchidism.[538]

### Obstructed testes

Obstructed testes are located in the superficial inguinal pouch (Denis–Browne pouch) and are considered ectopic by some authors and cryptorchid by others.[539,540] Histologic studies reveal that most obstructed testes bear the same lesions as true cryptorchid testes. Type I lesions are observed in half, type II in more than one-third, and the remainder show type III lesions. The higher proportion of type I lesions suggests a better prognosis than in true cryptorchid testes.

### Retractile testes

Some authors assume that retractile testes are normal and exclude them from studies of cryptorchidism.[541,542] However, these testes may present important lesions and many consider them to be a form of cryptorchidism.[543–545] Retractile testes may not always be movable to the lower scrotum (70–75 mm from the pubic tubercle) and in 50% of cases are smaller than scrotal testes. Approximately 50% of retractile testes remain high after age 6 years, when cremasteric activity declines.[546] Retractile testes have a 32% risk of becoming ascending or acquired undescended testes. The risk is higher in boys younger than 7 years, or when the spermatic cord is tight or inelastic.[547] During childhood, tubular diameter and tubular fertility index decrease.[544] Adults with retractile testes that descended spontaneously but late may be fertile[548] or infertile.[549] Usually there is germ cell atrophy that varies in severity from lobule to lobule.[544] Regular examination of retractile testes is advisable during childhood and, if complete testicular descent does not occur, orchidopexy is indicated.

### Congenital anomalies associated with undescended testes

Most cryptorchid patients have a patent processus vaginalis, and 65–75% have a hernia sac, although most hernias are not clinically visible. Urologic anomalies are present in 10.5% of patients, the most frequent being hypospadias, complete duplication of the urinary tract, non-obstructive ureteral dilatation, kidney malrotation, and posterior urethral valves. Cryptorchidism is more frequent in patients with microcephaly, myelomeningocele, bifid spine, omphalocele, gastroschisis, micropenis, and imperforate anus.

Cryptorchidism may appear isolated or associated with congenital anomalies, endocrine dysfunction, chromosomal disorders, or intersex conditions. Thus, cryptorchidism is found in the Kallmann, Prader–Willi, Klinefelter, Noonan, Smith–Lemli–Opitz, Aarskog–Scott, Rubinstein–Taybi, prune belly, and caudal regression syndromes, anomalies of the androgen receptor, absence of anti-müllerian hormone, CHARGE association, and trisomies 13, 18, and 21.

Sperm excretory duct anomalies occur in 9–36% of cryptorchid patients,[550,551] and are classified into three types:[552]

- *Ductal fusion anomalies* (25% of cases). These consist of anomalous fusion of the caput of the epididymis to the testis or segmental atresia of the epididymis and vas deferens. This is chiefly associated with intra-abdominal or high scrotal cryptorchid testes.
- *Ductal suspension anomalies* (59% of cases). The caput of the epididymis is attached to the testis, whereas the corpus and the cauda of the epididymis are separated from the testis by a mesentery. A variant consists of an excessively long cauda of the epididymis that descends along the inguinal duct to the scrotum.
- Anomalies associated with absent or vanishing testes (16% of cases).

Cryptorchidism is part of the testicular dysgenesis syndrome. This consists of abnormal testicular development that predisposes to cryptorchidism, hypospadias, spermatogenetic alterations, and testicular cancer. The association of these disorders with cryptorchidism has been corroborated by numerous clinical, epidemiological and genetic studies. The least severe form of this syndrome is a defect in spermatogenesis; the most severe is testicular cancer. A constellation of histologic lesions is common in the testes of men with testicular dysgenesis; these lesions include Sertoli cell-only pattern, mixed atrophy, hypoplastic tubules (Sertoli cell nodules), microlithiasis, malformed tubules, granular changes in Sertoli cells, nodular Leydig cell hyperplasia, and intratubular germ cell neoplasia. It is assumed that there is a prenatal development of the lesions as a result of several genetic, environmental, or endocrine disruptor factors that would interfere with the estrogen/androgen ratio.[553–556]

### Complications of cryptorchidism

The main complications of cryptorchidism are testicular cancer, infertility, testicular torsion, and psychological problems.

#### Testicular cancer

Approximately 0.8% of 1-year-old males have cryptorchidism, and about 10% of testicular cancer patients had cryptorchidism. The risk of testicular cancer in cryptorchid males is four to 10 times higher than that of the general population. Testes with elevated number of multinucleated spermatogonia seem to have a higher risk of cancer and adulthood.[557] About 5% of biopsies in children contain cells similar to those seen in undifferentiated intratubular germ cell neoplasia, and these cells may evolve toward germ cell tumor (Fig. 12-57).[558] The most frequent tumor in undescended testes is seminoma.[559,560] Regardless of timing, orchidopexy does not

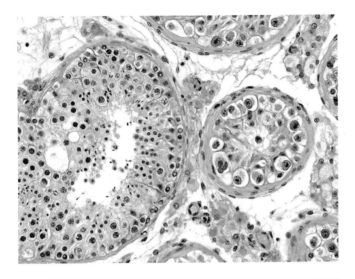

**Fig. 12-57** Adult ex-cryptorchid testis which was surgically descended at infancy. The patient was infertile. The smallest seminiferous tubule shows intratubular germ cell neoplasia, undifferentiated type. The relative tumor cell homogeneity contrasts with the variety in shape and size of the cells in the adjacent seminiferous tubule.

reduce the risk of cancer, although it facilitates early detection as the intrascrotal testis is palpable. One in five testicular tumors arises in properly descended testes contralateral to cryptorchid testes, suggesting that there is a primary bilateral testicular anomaly in cryptorchidism. Intra-abdominal testes also have a higher incidence of tumors.[560]

### Infertility

Infertility is the most frequent problem caused by cryptorchidism. In a series of patients with infertility, nearly 9% had cryptorchidism.[561] Infertility is influenced by several factors, including bilaterality, number of germ cells, location and size of the testis, and age at time of orchidopexy. The most important risk factors are bilaterality and germ cell number. Only 16%[562] to 25%[563] of men with bilateral cryptorchidism have normal sperm counts (20 million/mL or more). The highest sperm counts occur with testes in the superficial inguinal pouch. Patients with bilaterally impalpable testes are usually azoospermic.[563] Fertility rates in unilateral cryptorchidism vary from 25% to 81%.[564]

The number of germ cells per cross-sectioned tubule is the most important prognostic factor. Patients with no increase in inhibin B during the postoperative period usually have a low number of spermatogonia per cross-sectioned tubule and a low tubular fertility index. In unilateral cryptorchidism, fertility depends on the number of spermatogonia in the contralateral testis. However, if the number of germ cells per cross-sectioned tubule in the cryptorchid testis is lower than 1% of normal, the risk of infertility is 33%. In bilateral cryptorchidism the risk of infertility rises from 75% to 100% when one or both testes have less than 1% of germ cells per cross-sectioned tubule. Neither the preoperative location of the testis in patients with unilateral cryptorchidism nor the small size of the testis at the time of orchidopexy is relevant for fertility.[565-567] An important fertility factor is the permeability of sperm excretory ducts. The age at orchidopexy may also influence fertility, although this has not been proven. In patients over 4 years of age orchidopexy does not enhance fertility.[568,569]

### Benefit of testicular biopsy in patients with cryptorchidism

Testicular biopsies of infantile testes at orchidopexy are useful for determining baseline germ cell status and whether surgery should be completed with hormonal treatment.[570] However, even if biopsy supplies important data, it is not considered a routine procedure.

Even in the best cases when the number of spermatogonia is nearly normal, spermatogenesis may never occur owing to deficient spermatogonium development during childhood, failure of spermatogenesis at puberty, and, if complete spermatogenesis occurs, this might be associated with obstruction of sperm excretory ducts.

In childhood, the chance of a biopsy finding an occult cancer or precancer is low because intratubular germ cell neoplasia is not diffusely distributed throughout the testis. Testicular biopsy is recommended in patients with intra-abdominal testes, abnormal external genitalia, or abnormal karyotype.[571] The situation is different in adults because intratubular germ cell neoplasia is present in 2–3% of cases and is diffuse.[572,573] When intratubular germ cell neoplasia is detected in a child, further examination of the testis and rebiopsy after puberty are recommended.[574] In adults, if intratubular germ cell neoplasia is unilateral orchidectomy should be performed, but if it is bilateral, radiation may be used to eradicate the neoplasia while maintaining Leydig cell function.[575]

### Testicular microlithiasis

Testicular microlithiasis (TM) is characterized by the presence of numerous calcifications diffusely distributed throughout the testicular parenchyma. The number and size of the calcifications often is great enough to be detected radiographically or by ultrasound.[576] Isolated microliths have been reported in undescended testes, prepubertal Klinefelter's syndrome, male pseudohermaphroditism, and otherwise normal children and patients studied for other diseases.[577] In adults, microliths are frequently observed in cryptorchid and ex-cryptorchid testes,[578] seminiferous tubules located at the periphery of germ cell tumor,[579] infertile patients,[580-582] and in some patients complaining of orchialgia[583,584] or testicular asymmetry.[585]

Testicular microlithiasis occurs in 0.3% of cryptorchid testes and is slightly more common in prepubertal than adult testes. In adults, it usually is diagnosed when men seek help for infertility, pain, or testicular asymmetry.[581] Microlithiasis has been observed in 1.4–2% of testicular echographies of different disorders.[586,587] In infertile patients the incidence is slightly higher. Microlithiasis is present in 35% of testis having a malignant tumor.[588]

Ultrasound studies reveal two types of microlithiasis: classic TM, in which the number of microliths is five or more; and limited TM, when there are fewer than five microliths (Fig. 12-58). The incidences of TM in these studies are lower than 1% in infants, 5.6% in the general population aged between 18 and 35 years (bilateral in 66% of patients

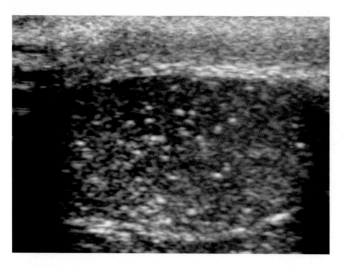

**Fig. 12-58** Testicular microlithiasis showing the characteristic 'snowstorm' pattern.

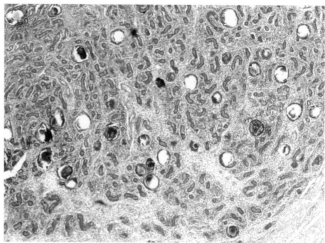

**Fig. 12-59** Testicular microlithiasis. Infantile cryptorchid testis with type III lesions and numerous microliths within the seminiferous tubules.

showing microliths,[589] 0.68–4.1% in patients with other disorders,[586,587,590–592] from 4.6%[593] to 20%[594] in subfertile patients, 9.52% in ex-cryptorchid testes,[595] and more than 30% in adult testes with germ cell tumors).[588,596–599] Several cases of testicular microlithiasis have also been observed in infant testes with germ cell tumor or gonadal stroma tumor.[600,601] The incidence is higher in whites than in blacks.

Pain is the most common clinical symptom in patients without a palpable testicular mass, and has been attributed to dilation of seminiferous tubules secondary to obstruction by microliths.

Microliths are made by hydroxyapatite, according to X-ray diffraction studies[602] and Raman spectroscopy.[603] In the pre-pubertal testis, microliths are surrounded by a double layer of Sertoli cells and measure up to 300 μm in diameter. When they are very large, the seminiferous epithelium may be destroyed and the microlith is surrounded by peritubular cells (Fig. 12-59). Testes with microliths have subnormal mean tubular diameters and tubular fertility index.[604] In adult testes with microliths there is incomplete spermatogenesis. Some seminiferous tubules with microliths are cystically dilated (Fig. 12-60). Microliths arise as extratubular eosinophilic bodies that mineralize and pass into the tubular lumina.[605] Microlithiasis may be a disorder of the tunica propria. Also, testicular microlithiasis is occasionally associated with pulmonary microlithiasis and with calcifications in the parasympathetic nervous system.[606,607]

The association of microlithiasis and testicular cancer is controversial.[608,609] Although the development of testicular cancer has been observed in several patients whose testicular microlithiasis had been previously diagnosed by ultrasound studies,[610–614] it is also thought that patients with testicular microlithiasis not associated with other disorder do not require any follow-up.[615] When microlithiasis is associated with infertility the incidence of cancer varies according to the unilaterality or bilaterality of microlithiasis:[594] subfertile patients with unilateral microlithiasis show no intratubular germ cell neoplasia, whereas this is present in 20% of those

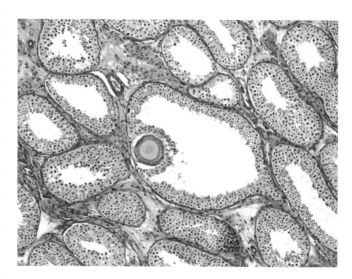

**Fig. 12-60** Testicular microlithiasis. Seminiferous tubules with dilated lumina in a patient biopsied for infertility. The central tubule contains a microlith which developed in the tubular wall and protrudes into the lumen.

with bilateral microlithiasis. The risk of malignancy is higher in classic than in limited TM.[616] The nexus between microlithiasis and cancer does not seem to be the predisposition of one disorder towards the other but rather the predisposition of both to develop in abnormal testes. This may also explain the association between microlithiasis and infertility.

Yearly ultrasound examination, perhaps with testicular biopsy, is recommended in those with testicular microlithiasis associated with cryptorchidism, infertility, atrophic testes, or contralateral testis bearing germ cell tumor.[617]

Microlithiasis also occurs in the rete testis or sperm excretory ducts. Epididymal rupture and extravasation of microliths into the interductal tissue may cause a histiocytic reaction resembling malakoplakia (Fig. 12-61). The disorder is asymptomatic and not associated with testicular cancer.[618]

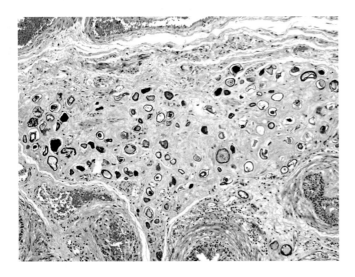

**Fig. 12-61** Epididymal microlithiasis. Numerous microliths displaying a psammoma body-like appearance are set in hyalinized stroma.

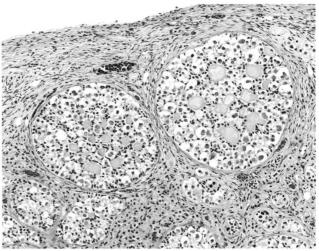

**Fig. 12-63** Frasier's syndrome in a 16-year-old patient. The two streak gonads contain gonadoblastoma.

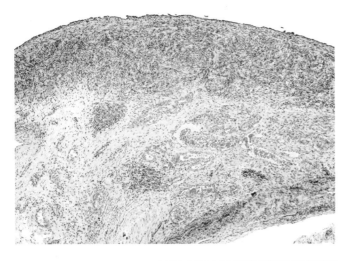

**Fig. 12-62** Gonadal dysgenesis. The elongate formation consists of an outer cellular part devoid of ovarian follicles and a central part with numerous blood vessels.

## Gonadal dysgenesis

Gonadal dysgenesis refers to disorders characterized by amenorrhea and streak gonads in phenotypically female patients. In adults, streak gonads are elongated masses of fibrous tissue resembling ovarian stroma (Fig. 12-62). They may contain hilar cells and rete or epithelial cords with variable degrees of maturation, and may result from failure in gonad formation, failure of gonadal differentiation to ovary, or failure of gonadal differentiation to testis. Some streak gonads contain a few ovocytes or primordial follicles, but all germ cells disappear at puberty. Patients with streak gonads have a hypoplastic uterus and fallopian tubes. Four types of gonadal dysgenesis have been described: 46XY pure, 46XX pure, 45X0, and mixed.

## 46XY Gonadal dysgenesis

46XY gonadal dysgenesis (Swyer's syndrome) is characterized by female phenotype, absence of Turnerian stigmata, and female external genitalia, sometimes with fused labia majora, a hypertrophic clitoris, and hypospadias. The breasts develop at puberty. Sexual infantilism persists in adulthood, and eunuchoidism and amenorrhea appear. These patients have elevated serum gonadotropin levels and low serum estradiol.

There are two types of gonadal dysgenesis: complete and incomplete. Patients with the complete type have female external genitalia and classic streak gonads, although cases with ovarian tissue have been reported. The cause is unknown in about 80% of cases,[619] and is due to alterations in the SRY gene in the remainder (a mutation in 10–15% of cases, and a SRY deletion as a result of an aberrant X/Y interchange in 10–15%).[620] The consequence of failure is very early gonadal alteration (sixth to eighth week of gestation). With the subsequent absence of müllerian inhibiting factor, testosterone, and dihydrotestosterone, a female phenotype develops.

Patients with incomplete 46XY gonadal dysgenesis have ambiguous external genitalia and variable degree of development of the müllerian and wolffian structures. Although they have streak gonads, testicular development is usually observed. This gonadal dysgenesis does not seem to be caused by SRY alterations.[621] These findings suggest that in the first type ovarian differentiation was canceled, and that in the second type testicular differentiation failed. The first is similar to the gonad of 45X0 Turner's syndrome, whereas the second resembles the gonad of mixed gonadal dysgenesis.[622] The clitoromegaly may be caused by androgens secreted by hyperplastic Leydig cells in the streak gonad.

Some patients with 46XY gonadal dysgenesis present with extragonadal anomalies and multiple syndromes, including camptomelic dysplasia and renal disorder,[623] myotonic dystrophy and terminal renal disease,[624] progressive renal insufficiency and gonadoblastoma (Frasier's syndrome) (Figs 12-63 and 12-64),[625-629] mental retardation with[630] or

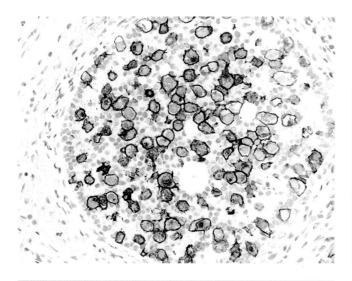

**Fig. 12-64** Frasier's syndrome. The cell surface and Golgi zone of the atypical gonadoblastoma germ cells are immunoreactive for *c-kit*.

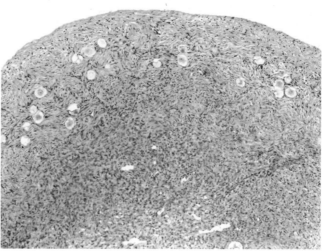

**Fig. 12-65** 46XX gonadal dysgenesis. The streak gonads contain isolated ovocytes.

without[631] facial anomalies or short stature,[632] renal insufficiency and Wilms' tumor (Denys–Drash syndrome), the combination of cleft palate, micrognathia, kyphosis, scoliosis, and clubfoot (Gardner–Silengo–Wachtel syndrome or genitopalatocardiac syndrome),[633] pterygium multiple syndrome,[634] Graves' disease,[635,636] and congenital universalis alopecia, microcephaly, cutis marmorata, and short stature.[637,638]

Most cases are sporadic,[639] although the syndrome has been reported in several members of the same family,[640–643] and several forms of inheritance (X-linked, autosomal recessive, and male-limited autosomal dominant) have been proposed.[644] In addition to infertility, patients with 46XY gonadal dysgenesis have a high risk of germ cell tumor. This risk is about 5% in the first decade of life, and 25–30% overall,[645–648] and, thus, prophylactic gonadectomy is recommended.

## 46XX Gonadal dysgenesis

Patients with 46XX gonadal dysgenesis have normal stature, female phenotype, well-developed external genitalia, and hypoplastic ovaries rather than streak gonads (Fig. 12-65). The anomaly is usually detected when patients present with primary amenorrhea or infertility. This syndrome is sporadic and familial, and it may be linked to recessive autosomal inheritance.[649,650] Patients have no predisposition to gonadal neoplasia. Associated somatic anomalies such as neurosensory hearing loss (Perrault's syndrome) are rare.

Some familial cases have shown a balanced translocation of the X chromosome (from the long arm to the short arm)[651,652] or between chromosomes 1 and 11.[653] Because the development of ovarian follicles requires FSH, mutations have been sought in the FSHR gene. Mutations have been detected in familial cases and also in unrelated patients,[654,655] whereas other patients have shown no mutations in this gene.[656] The incidence of tumors in these patients is very low, and the most common is dysgerminoma.[657–659]

## 45X0 Gonadal dysgenesis

This is one of the most common chromosomal anomalies (from 1/2500 to 1/5000 in female newborns),[660] although 99% of zygotes with this karyotype are aborted in the first stages of embryonal development.[661]

Patients with 45XO gonadal dysgenesis have characteristic stigmata of Turner's syndrome, including short stature, pterygium coli, lymphedema, and cardiac malformations. The external genitalia are female and infantile; the gonads are typical streak gonads. Today, Turner's syndrome is defined by the combination of physical features and the complete or partial absence of one of both X chromosomes, frequently associated with mosaicism. Turnerian stigmata may be classified into four groups:[662] skeletal anomalies such as cubitus valgus, shortening of the fourth metacarpal and Madelund's deformity characteristic of Leri–Weill dyschondrosteosis; soft tissue anomalies such as webbed neck, low posterior hair line, and puffy hands and feet; visceral anomalies such as aortic coarctation, horseshoe kidney, polycystic kidney, urethral stenosis and vesicourethral reflux; and miscellaneous anomalies such as nevus pigmentosus.[663]

During embryonic life, these gonads show normal germ cell numbers up to the third month, when germ cell proliferation ceases.[665,666] Ovogenesis stops in meiosis I, usually before the pachytene stage. The cause seems to be generalized meiotic pairing errors with the start of an apoptotic mechanism to avoid the formation of abnormal gametes.[667] Massive apoptosis of ovocytes occurs between the 15th and the 20th weeks.[668] Surviving germ cells disappear throughout fetal life, and their numbers at birth are usually low (Fig. 12-66).[669]

Patients with mosaicism have fewer anomalies than pure 45X0 individuals; 12% have menstruation (compared to 3% of pure 45X0 patients), and 18% have breast development (compared to 5% of pure 45X0 patients). In 10–20% of

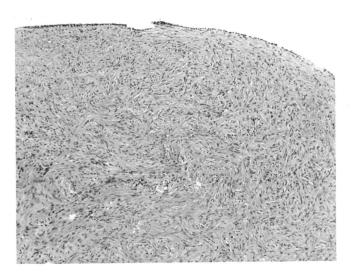

**Fig. 12-66** Gonadal dysgenesis. Streak fibroblastic stroma resembling ovarian cortex.

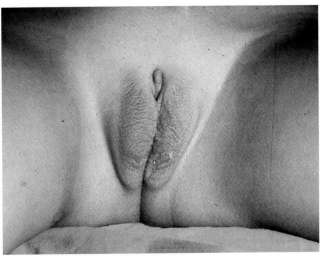

**Fig. 12-67** True hermaphrodite showing external genitalia which display transverse folds and a slightly hypertrophic clitoris.

45X0 patients the SRY gene is demonstrable by in-situ hybridization. It has been proposed that patients with SRY expression should undergo gonadectomy, because this gene is also a marker of gonadoblastoma.[670] These patients may develop gonadoblastoma, dysgerminoma, and mixed germ cell tumor.[670,671]

### Mixed gonadal dysgenesis

Mixed gonadal dysgenesis is characterized by the presence of a streak gonad and a contralateral testis (often cryptorchid) or streak testis (see discussion on male pseudohermaphroditism with müllerian remnants, below).

### True hermaphroditism

True hermaphroditism is a disorder of gonadal differentiation characterized by the presence in the same individual of both testicular and ovarian tissue. This condition is rare and usually difficult to diagnose, so only 25% of male hermaphrodites are diagnosed before age 20.[672] Failure to recognize this disorder may lead to surgical intervention for hernia repair or orchidopexy. Most hermaphrodites raised as males display symptoms for the first time at puberty because of breast development[673] (95% of hermaphrodites have some degree of gynecomastia), periodic hematuria[674] (if they have a uterus ending in the urinary tract), or cryptorchidism.[675] Hermaphrodites raised as females initially present with irregular menstruation or clitoromegaly. True hermaphroditism should be suspected in all children with ambiguous sex characteristics (Fig. 12-67). The gonads of these patients are ovotestes, ovaries, or testes, with all possible combinations.[676] True hermaphroditism can be (1) unilateral, if there are both testicular and ovarian tissues (forming one ovotestes or two separated gonads) on one side, and a testis or an ovary in the other side; if there is no gonadal tissue in this latter side, unilateral hermaphroditism is incomplete; (2) bilateral, if testicular and ovarian tissues are present on both sides of the body; and (3) alternate, if there is a testis on one side, and an ovary on the other side.

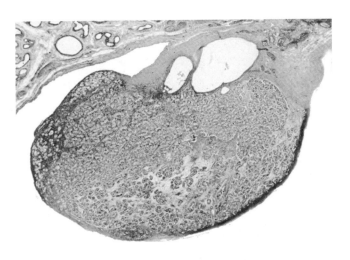

**Fig. 12-68** True hermaphroditism. The ovotestis contains ovarian follicles arranged in a crescent. There is cystic transformation of the rete testis. The epididymis is hypoplastic.

Ovotestis is the most frequent gonadal type in true hermaphroditism. It is more frequent on the right side and is located in the abdomen (50% of cases), labioscrotal folds, inguinal canal, or the external inguinal ring. The ovotestis has a bilobated or ovoid shape (Fig. 12-68). In the bilobated ovotestis the testis and ovary are connected by a pedicle, whereas in the ovoid ovotestis the ovarian tissue forms a crescent capping the testicular parenchyma. The proportion of ovary to testis varies widely (Fig. 12-69). At adulthood, the ovarian follicles mature and corpora lutea or corpora albicantia may be seen. The seminiferous tubules rarely develop complete spermatogenesis. The interstitium usually contains Leydig cells. Ovotestis is associated with a fallopian tube in 65% of cases, and with a vas deferens in the remainder. If the patient has ovotestis/ovary, a completely developed uterus is present. If the patient has bilateral ovotestis (13%), uterine agenesis is frequent (Fig. 12-70).[677]

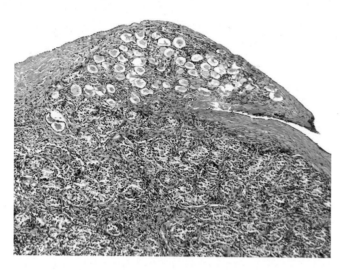

**Fig. 12-69** True hermaphroditism. Ovotestis from a 2-year-old. The ovarian and testicular tissues are sharply demarcated.

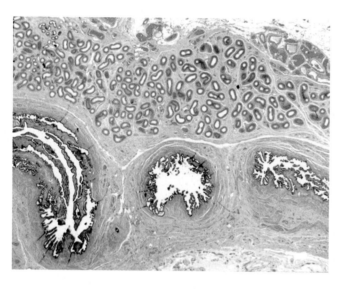

**Fig. 12-70** True hermaphroditism. Epididymis and fallopian tube in an adult hermaphrodite raised as a female.

The testis of hermaphrodites is most often on the right side (60%) and is located anywhere from the abdomen to the scrotum. These testes have low tubular fertility indices during childhood. After puberty, the seminiferous tubules remain small, often containing only dysgenetic Sertoli cells, similar to the tubules of cryptorchid testes. Incomplete spermatogenesis has been reported, but complete spermatogenesis is exceptional. The ovary of hermaphrodites is most frequently on the left side (63%) and usually is hypoplastic with few primordial follicles. However, in occasional patients the ovary is histologically and functionally normal.

The most frequent karyotype is 46XX (60%), followed by several mosaicisms (33%) which, in decreasing order of frequency, are 46XX/46XY, 46XY/47XXY, 45X0/46XY, 46XX/47XXY. The 46XY karyotype is the least common (7%). There is variation in the incidence of some karyotypes

around the world. Mosaicism is found in 40.5% of European cases, but in only 21% of North America cases. Conversely, most African true hermaphrodites (97%) have 46XX karyotype. The karyotype 46XY is rare and its frequency is similar in Europe, Asia, and North America.[678,679] Most cases are sporadic, and families with several affected members also have 46XX males. This finding suggests that both genetic anomalies are alternative forms of a single genetic defect.[680] The following mechanisms[681,682] have been proposed to explain the occurrence of testicular parenchyma: true hermaphroditism 46XX, a hidden mosaicism with a cell line having a Y chromosome; transfer from a Y chromosome fragment (including SRY gene) to the X chromosome; autosomal mutation of variable penetrance; and X-linked mutation coupled with rare X inactivation or X mutation that permits testicular differentiation in the absence of SRY. Some 46XX hermaphrodites with SRY-negative leukocytes are positive for this gene in DNA from the testicular parenchyma in the ovotestis.[683] Over 22 pregnancies in true hermaphrodites have been reported,[684] in contrast to the exceptional cases of paternity. Ovules may arise from the ovotestes or the ovary.

Management of true hermaphroditism depends on the patient's age at the time of diagnosis, the nature and location of the gonads, and the developmental stage of the external genitalia. Although bilateral castration may be justified in order to avoid the risk of neoplasia, gonadal preservation may be desirable until adulthood. In this case, if the patient is raised as a girl, puberty will occur spontaneously and there is a small chance of fertility.[685] However, the high risk of malignancy (estimated at 4.6%) should be taken into account. The most frequent tumors are gonadoblastoma, dysgerminoma, and yolk sac tumor.[676] The risk of cancer may be reduced if some precautions are taken, including removal of the testis if it has not descended and surveillance of the residual gonad with periodic ultrasound studies, especially in cases of chromosomal mosaicisms.

## Male pseudohermaphroditism

Normal male development requires adequate differentiation of the testes in the fetal period, synthesis and secretion of testicular hormones, and proper response of target organs to these hormones. Anti-müllerian hormone produced by Sertoli cells inhibits the development of müllerian derivatives that would otherwise form the uterus and fallopian tubes. Testosterone produced by Leydig cells stimulates differentiation of the wolffian ducts into male genital ducts. The conversion of testosterone into dihydrotestosterone by the enzyme 5α-reductase ensures the development of male external genitalia. Alterations in these processes may cause male pseudohermaphroditism.

### Impaired Leydig cell activity

#### Androgen synthesis deficiencies

These autosomal recessive syndromes are characterized by an error in testosterone synthesis that results in incomplete or absent virilization. Cholesterol is the source for the synthesis of androgens, estrogens, and other steroid hormones through multiple steps. First, the steroidogenic acute regulatory protein (StAR) generates cholesterol into mitochondria; StAR gene mutations cause congenital lipoid adrenal hyperplasia. Second, within mitochondria, the cholesterol side-chain cleavage enzyme P450scc transforms cholesterol into pregnenolone; a disorder in this enzyme is rare because it is highly lethal in embryonic life. Third, pregnenolone undergoes 17α-hydroxylation by microsomal P450c17; deficiency in 17α-hydroxylase causes female sexual infantilism and hypertension. Fourth, 17-OH-pregnenolone is converted into DHEA by 17,20-lyase activity of P450c17. The ratio of 17,20-lyase to 17α-hydroxylase activity of P450c17 determines the ratio of C21 to C19 steroids produced. The ratio is regulated by at least three factors, including the electron-donating protein P450 oxidoreductase (POR), cytochrome b5, and serine phosphorylation of P450c17. Mutations in POR are present in the Antley–Bixler skeletal dysplasia syndrome as well as a variant of polycystic ovarian syndrome. Figure 12-71 shows the enzymes involved in the abovementioned steps. The enzyme 3β-hydroxysteroid dehydrogenase transforms DHEA to androstenedione, and the enzymatic complex called aromatase transforms androstenedione into estrone and testosterone into estradiol.

In some patients cholesterol synthesis is also impaired, and congenital adrenal hyperplasia is superimposed on androgen deficiency. Deficient testosterone synthesis may result from abnormalities in the enzymes involved in pregnenolone formation (congenital lipoid adrenal hyperplasia), including 3β hydroxysteroid dehydrogenase, 17α-hydroxylase, 17,20-desmolase, and 17β-hydroxysteroid dehydrogenase (Fig. 12-71).

*Congenital lipoid adrenal hyperplasia* Congenital lipoid adrenal hyperplasia is the most severe form of congenital adrenal hyperplasia.[686] The disorder is characterized by a deficit in steroid hormone synthesis in the adrenal cortex and gonads, producing a female phenotype with severe salt-loss syndrome. Conversion of cholesterol to pregnenolone requires the enzymes 20α-hydroxylase, 20,22-desmolase, and 22α-hydroxylase. Failure of any of these leads to deficits in cortisol, aldosterone, and testosterone.[687]

The enzymatic defect is usually is caused by a deficit in the steroidogenic acute regulatory (StAR) protein; in other cases, the deficit is in P450ssc. The mitochondrial protein StAR promotes cholesterol transfer from the outer to inner mitochondrial membrane, where cholesterol serves as a substrate for P450scc and initiates steroidogenesis. More than 35 different mutations in the StAR gene have been identified.[690] As a result, cholesterol is not converted to pregnenolone, which is required for the synthesis of mineralocorticoids, glucocorticoids, and sex hormones.

The disorder is rare in most countries, but is common in Japan, Korea, and the Arabian countries.[691,692] Patients usually present with salt-losing crisis in the first 2 months of life.[693,694] In most cases, males have female or ambiguous external genitalia and a blind-sac vagina, hypoplastic wolffian derivatives, absence of müllerian structures, and cryptorchidism.[695] The adrenals usually appear enlarged and contain lipid accumulations,[696,697] but these diminish with age and the adrenals shrink.

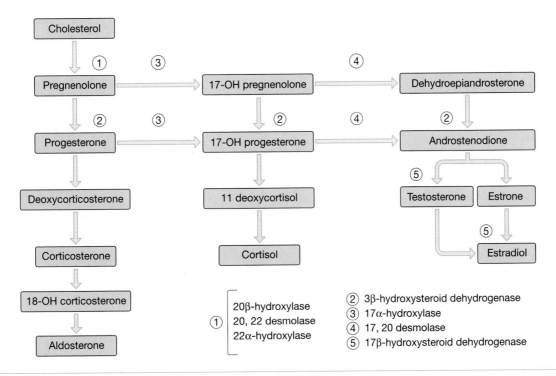

**Fig. 12-71** Enzymatic defects in impaired testosterone biosynthesis.

In the testes, lipid accumulations may be present or absent in Leydig cells[686,696,698–702] or Sertoli cells.[703] An 8-year-old child had partially hyalinized seminiferous tubules with Sertoli cell-only pattern.[704] The testes of pubertal patients are usually normal for age.[701,702] Intratubular germ cell neoplasia has been reported in one case.[705]

Most patients die from adrenal insufficiency. Survivors have female phenotype[704] and require the administration of glucocorticoids, mineralocorticoids, and gonadal steroids.[703]

*3β-Hydroxysteroid dehydrogenase deficiency* Patients with this defect have two main problems: salt-loss syndrome produced by reduced aldosterone secretion, and incomplete virilization.[706] At puberty, virilization increases and gynecomastia develops.[707,708]

The enzyme 3BHSD catalyzes the conversion of 5-3β-hydroxysteroids such as pregnenolone, 17-hydroxypregnenolone, and dehydroepiandrosterone into respectively 4-3β-ketosteroid, progesterone, 17-hydroxyprogesterone, and androstenedione.[709] There are two 3BHSD genes located on the p11-p13 region of chromosome 1. The type I gene is expressed in the placenta, kidney, and skin, whereas the type II gene 3BHSD is expressed only in the gonads and adrenal glands. Complete absence of the 3BHSD gene is lethal; therefore, most reported cases have only partial 3BHSD deficits.[710–712] It is assumed that these deficits account for 10% of cases of congenital adrenal hyperplasia.

The classic form of salt-losing 3BHSD deficit is diagnosed in the first months of life because of insufficient aldosterone synthesis and subsequent loss of salt. The other 3BHSD deficit, without salt loss, is due to mutations in the type II 3BHSD gene[708] and its diagnosis may be delayed until puberty.

Severe forms of 3BHSD deficiency are associated with deficits in aldosterone, cortisol, and estradiol. Symptoms may vary widely, as enzymatic activity in the adrenal gland is not the same as in the testis. Most patients show salt loss and adrenal crisis; they have incomplete masculinization and may develop spontaneous puberty and gynecomastia.[706,707,713] Patients with mild forms have normal genitalia and normal mineralocorticoid levels. Some patients have only hypospadias[714] or micropenis.[715] The testes are smaller and softer than normal.

*17α-Hydroxylase deficiency* The cause of deficits in the enzymes 17α-hydroxylase and 17,20-lyase are mutations of the CYP17 gene that encodes cytochrome P450c17.[716] The CYP17 gene is located on chromosome 10q24-q25,[717] and 50 different mutations have been described.[718] P450c17 catalyzes the 17α-hydroxylation of pregnenolone to 17OH-pregnenolone and of progesterone to 17α-OH-progesterone. This enzyme also catalyzes 17,20-lyase activity, transforming 17OH-pregnenolone to DHEA. The classic form of 17α-hydroxylase deficit is caused by severe deficiencies in CYP17; less severe defects give rise to the isolated 17,20-lyase deficit. 17α-Hydroxylase deficit impairs the synthesis of both cortisol and testosterone.[719] Low cortisol levels stimulate ACTH secretion, causing hypersecretion of aldosterone precursors and the development of hypokalemic hypertension and male pseudohermaphroditism in males.[720] Patients

usually have hypospadias and develop gynecomastia at puberty.[721]

*17,20-Desmolase deficiency* The enzyme 17,20-desmolase cleaves the side chain of 17-hydroxypregnenolone and 17-hydroxyprogesterone to form dehydroepiandrosterone and androstenedione, respectively. Varying degrees of 17,20-desmolase deficiency are seen, resulting in varied development of external genitalia, ranging from female phenotype to virilization with microphallus, bifid scrotum, and perineal hypospadias. In childhood, the testes contain reduced numbers of spermatogonia (Figs 12-72, 12-73).[722,723] The cause may be mutations in one of the genetic loci encoding P450c17, flavoprotein OR or b5.[724]

*17β-Hydroxysteroid dehydrogenase deficiency* This enzyme transforms androstenedione into testosterone and also converts estrone into estradiol. The enzymatic defects are sex-linked. Most patients have female phenotype at birth and

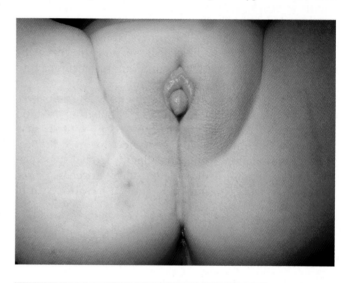

**Fig. 12-72** Male pseudohermaphrodite with androgen synthesis deficiency. The external genitalia are ambiguous.

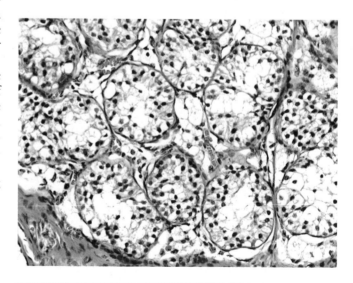

**Fig. 12-73** Intense Leydig cell vacuolation in an infant with androgen synthesis deficiency.

are raised as girls, but at puberty undergo virilization.[725] One or both testes may be cryptorchid or are located in the labia majora. Normal spermatogenesis has never been observed. The most common testicular patterns are hypoplasia or absence of germ cells and Leydig cell hyperplasia.[726] The germ cell injury was initially attributed to cryptorchidism, but it is now thought to be a primary testicular lesion because even very young patients lack germ cells.[727] This deficit is due to mutations in the HSD17B3 gene located on 9q22.[728,729]

### Leydig cell hypoplasia

This variant of male pseudohermaphroditism is defined by insufficient testosterone secretion[422] and the following characteristics: predominance of female external genitalia; absence of male secondary sex characteristics at puberty; absence of uterus and fallopian tubes and the presence of epididymis and vas deferens; 46XY karyotype; lack of response to human chorionic gonadotropin stimulation; absence of an enzymatic defect in testosterone synthesis; and small undescended testes that are gray and mucous on section.[730–733] Age at diagnosis varies from 4 months to 35 years. The syndrome is sporadic and familial.[734,735]

The best-known cause of Leydig cell hypoplasia is inactivating mutation of the LH receptor in these cells.[736–738] During fetal life, there is an inadequate response to placental hCG initially and to pituitary LH subsequently. Phenotypes vary widely according to the presence of complete or partial loss of receptor function. These changes range from male pseudohermaphroditism with female external genitalia (type I of Leydig cell hypoplasia) to male phenotype with micropenis, hypospadias, pubertal delay, and primary hypogonadism (type II of Leydig cell hypoplasia).

In type I hypoplasia, the testes contain small seminiferous tubules with Sertoli cells, spermatogonia, and thickened basement membranes. Leydig cells are rare or absent, in contrast to Leydig cell hyperplasia seen in other types of male pseudohermaphroditism, such as those arising from defects in androgen synthesis or androgen action on peripheral tissues.[739,740] Leydig cell hypoplasia accounts for low serum testosterone levels, lack of virilization, and lack of spermatogenesis. The absence of müllerian derivatives suggests a normal function of Sertoli cells, which synthesize müllerian inhibiting factor. In type II hypoplasia, adult testes show maturation arrest of spermatogonia and a few incompletely differentiated Leydig cells.[741,742]

## Impaired androgen metabolism in peripheral tissues

### Androgen insensitivity syndromes

Resistance to androgen stimulation is the cause of several syndromes with phenotypes varying from complete testicular feminization[743] to normal male.[744,745] These syndromes are caused by partial or complete lack of response of the target organs to androgens[746] due to the absence, diminution, or impairment of androgen receptors or postreceptor anomaly.[740] The gene for the androgen receptor is located on the X chromosome (Xq11-q12), and X-linked transmission occurs in two-thirds of cases. The karyotype is usually 46XY, but 47XXY and several mosaicisms have been observed.[747]

These syndromes affect 1:20 000–1:40 000 newborns. The diverse phenotypes associated with androgen insensitivity may be classified as: complete androgen insensitivity syndrome (CAIS) or testicular feminization syndrome; partial androgen insensitivity syndrome (PAIS) or partial testicular feminization syndrome, which includes the syndromes of Lubs, Gilbert–Dreyfus, Reifenstein, and Rossewater; and mild androgen insensitivity syndrome (MAIS), infertile men with light androgen insensitivity, and Kennedy's disease.

***Complete androgen insensitivity syndrome (complete testicular feminization syndrome)*** This form of male pseudohermaphroditism is characterized by female phenotype with testes. Complete testicular feminization syndrome is rarely diagnosed during childhood except in patients who present with hernia, inguinal tumor, or with a family history of pseudohermaphroditism. Primary amenorrhea is the principal presentation in adults.

The testes may be in the abdomen, inguinal canal, or labia majora, and during the first year of life may be normal histologically except for reduced tubular diameter and low tubular fertility index. After the first year, decreased germ cell numbers become evident and the few remaining spermatogonia are concentrated in clusters of seminiferous tubules. The testicular interstitium contains numerous spindle cells arranged in bundles, and during the first year of life has Leydig cells with abundant eosinophilic or vacuolated cytoplasm. At puberty, patients have female external genitalia, a short blind-ended vagina, feminine breast development; and scarce pubic and axillary hair. Serum testosterone is at the normal male level and LH is markedly increased.

In adults, the testes vary in size from small to large, are tan-brown, and contain small seminiferous tubules without lumina which usually contain only Sertoli cells.[748,749] In one-third of patients both Sertoli cells and spermatogonia are present.[750] Ultrastructurally, Sertoli cells lack Charcot–Böttcher crystals and annulated lamellae; inter-Sertoli cell specialized junctions are not well developed, and in cryofracture studies the arrangement of membrane particles has an immature pattern.[751] Leydig cells are abundant, but few contain Reinke's crystalloids. Often, there are areas resembling ovarian stroma in the testicular interstitium.

In about two-thirds of cases the testes contain grossly visible white nodules that stand out from the surrounding testicular parenchyma (Figs 12-74, 21-75). Histologically, the nodules consist of clusters of small seminiferous tubules with immature Sertoli cells, hyalinized lamina propria, numerous Leydig cells, and an absence of elastic fibers (Fig. 12-76). These have been referred to as Sertoli–Leydig cell hamartoma. About 25% of testes have Sertoli cell adenoma, sometimes very large, consisting of tubules resembling infantile testis but lacking in germ cells and peritubular myofibroblasts. No Leydig cells are present between the tubules (Figs 12-77, 12-78).[752] Other benign tumors include Sertoli cell tumor (large cell calcifying Sertoli cell tumor and sex cord tumor with annular tubules), Leydig cell tumor, leiomyoma, and fibroma.[746]

Approximately 60% of cases have small cystic structures closely apposed to the testes, and about 80% of patients have thick bundles of smooth muscle fibers resembling myo-

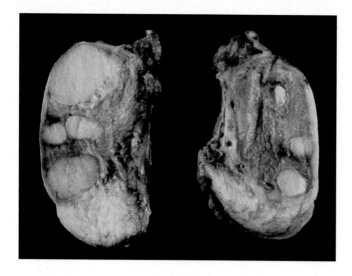

**Fig. 12-74** Testicular feminization syndrome. Both testes are enlarged and contain several gray-white nodules.

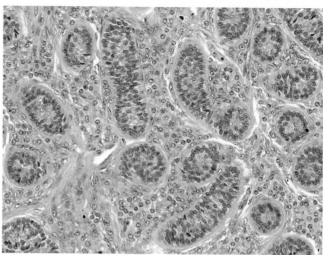

**Fig. 12-76** Testicular feminization syndrome. Small seminiferous tubules with immature Sertoli cells surrounded by thick basement membranes and numerous Leydig cells.

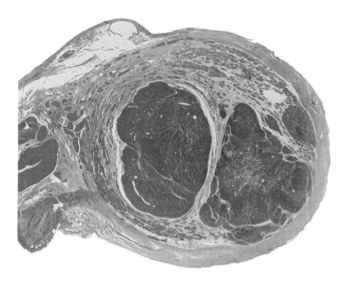

**Fig. 12-75** Testicular feminization syndrome. Cross-sectioned testis with multiple well-demarcated nodules.

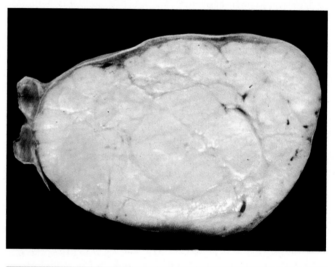

**Fig. 12-77** Large Sertoli cell adenoma in an abdominal testis from a 65-year-old patient with testicular feminization syndrome.

metrium near the testis. True myometrium has been demonstrated in only one case. Hypoplastic fallopian tubes are present in about one-third of cases. In about 70% of patients the epididymis and vas deferens are rudimentary; the only explanation for this is residual activity of the mutated androgen receptor.[753] Approximately 10% of testes from patients with testicular feminization syndrome develop cancer. The frequency increases with age, but tumors rarely appear before puberty. These tumors include intratubular germ cell neoplasia (Fig. 12-79),[749] several types of germ cell tumor,[750,754] and sex cord tumor.[441] Thus, the gonads should be removed immediately after puberty.[755]

***Partial androgen insensitivity syndrome (partial testicular feminization syndrome)*** The phenotype of patients with partial testicular feminization varies from normal female to normal male. The disorder includes four classic syndromes:

Lubs' syndrome,[756] characterized by partial fusion of labioscrotal folds, a definitive introitus, clitoromegaly, pubic and axillary hair, and poor breast development;[757] Gilbert–Dreyfus syndrome, characterized by progressively greater male phenotypic features that include small phallus, hypospadias, incomplete development of wolffian derivatives, and gynecomastia;[758] Reifenstein's syndrome, characterized by hypospadias, weak or absent virilization, testicular atrophy, gynecomastia, azoospermia, and infertility;[759] and Rosewater–Gwinup–Hamwi syndrome, characterized by infertile men whose only abnormal feature is gynecomastia.[760]

***Mild androgen insensitivity syndrome*** Spermatogenesis requires high levels of intratesticular testosterone. A minor form of androgen insensitivity may be observed in some patients with male phenotype who present with infertility.[761]

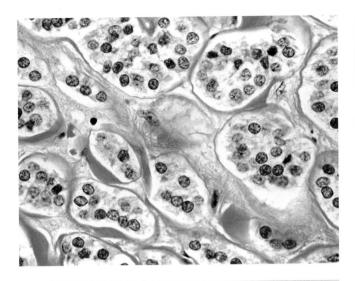

**Fig. 12-78** Sertoli cell adenoma showing tubular clusters with a hyalinized wall in a stroma devoid of Leydig cells.

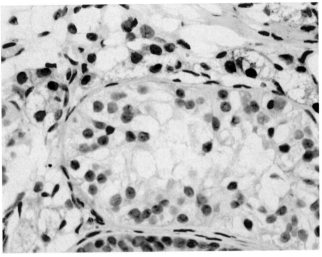

**Fig. 12-80** Testis from an infant with 5α-reductase deficiency showing hyperplastic Leydig cells that have marked cytoplasmic vacuolation and surround a seminiferous tubule lacking germ cells. (Immunostain for calretinin.)

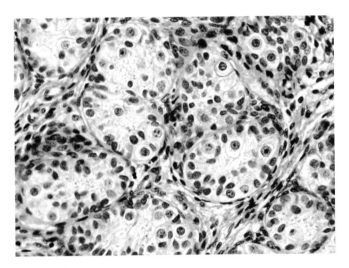

**Fig. 12-79** Intratubular germ cell neoplasia, undifferentiated type, in a phenotypically female patient with inguinal testes. The tumor cells stand out by virtue of their large size, pale cytoplasm, and prominent nucleoli.

The frequency of androgen resistance among azoospermic and oligozoospermic men is estimated at about 19%[762] or lower.[763,764] Some patients have lost exon 4[765] or mutated exons 6[764] or 7.[766]

**Kennedy's disease** Kennedy's disease (spinal and bulbar muscular atrophy, SBMA) is an X-linked recessive disorder of the adult male[767,768] characterized by loss of motor neurons in the spinal cord and brain stem and associated with less important loss of sensory neurons and atrophy caused by skeletal muscle denervation.[767,769] Disease onset around 20 years of age includes muscular weakness, cramps, and fasciculations.[770] In most cases the male reproductive system is impaired.[770-772] The testes may be normal in the initial stages of the disease, and many patients are fertile; however, with progression, there is onset of secondary testicular atrophy and gynecomastia. Testosterone levels are decreased in some cases.

The disease results from mutations in the first exon of the androgen receptor (AR) gene.[773] The SMBA gene, located on Xq11-12, has expansion of a repetitive CAG sequence in exon A. The number of CAG repeats is 21 (range, 17–26) in control men and more than 40 in men with Kennedy's disease.[768,774-777]

### 5α-Reductase deficiency

This disorder is a variant of male pseudohermaphroditism caused by a lack of the enzyme 5α-reductase with failure of conversion of testosterone to dihydrotestosterone.[778] In patients with the 46XY karyotype there are two isoenzymes: isoenzyme 1 is encoded by the gene SRD5A, located on 5p15, and isoenzyme 2 is encoded by the gene SRD5A2 on 2p23. Most reported cases result from defects in SRD5A2.[779] Many mutations in different exons have been reported.[780-784]

During childhood, patients have a clitoriform penis, bifid scrotum, urogenital sinus, and testes in the inguinal canal or labioscrotal folds (Fig. 12-80). Müllerian derivatives are absent. At puberty they acquire the male phenotype, with development of the penis and scrotum. Adults have erections, ejaculations, and normal libido, scant body hair and a thin beard, a very small prostate, and lack of temporal hairline recession (male pattern baldness). Serum levels of FSH, LH, and testosterone are increased, but dihydrotestosterone is decreased.[785,786]

The disorder is autosomal recessive and has been observed in many consanguineous families from the Dominican Republic.[787]

### Defective regression of müllerian ducts

This group of male pseudohermaphrodites is characterized by the presence of müllerian derivatives and unilateral or bilateral testicular dysgenesis. These two features depend on anti-müllerian hormone gene mutations and end-organ insensitivity.[788-791]

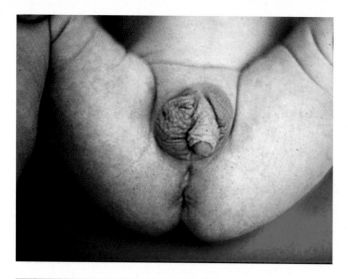

**Fig. 12-81** Mixed gonadal dysgenesis in a 3-year-old infant with ambiguous external genitalia, hypoplastic uterus, testicular dysgenesis on the right side, and streak gonad on the left side.

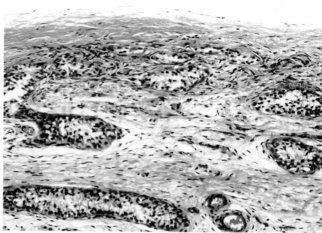

**Fig. 12-82** Testicular dysgenesis. Several irregularly shaped seminiferous tubules are observed within a thin, poorly collagenized tunica albuginea.

In normal development, anti-müllerian hormone is responsible for inhibition of the ipsilateral müllerian ducts and collagenization of the tunica albuginea. Patients with deficient secretion of this hormone may also have androgen deficiency. Three variants of defective müllerian duct regression have been reported: mixed gonadal dysgenesis, dysgenetic male pseudohermaphroditism, and persistent müllerian duct syndrome.

### Mixed gonadal dysgenesis

Mixed gonadal dysgenesis (asymmetric gonadal differentiation) is characterized by the presence of a testis on one side of the body and a streak gonad on the other.[792] If the gonads are intra-abdominal, the labioscrotal folds may appear as either normal labia or empty scrotal sacs (Fig. 12-81). In the former, the syndrome cannot be recognized in the newborn unless a peniform clitoris is present. If the gonad is descended, it is usually a testis. Müllerian derivatives such as fallopian tubes are usually associated with streak gonad (95% of cases), but may also be associated with testicular tissue (74%). Ipsilateral to the testis there is one epididymis and one vas deferens. On the contralateral side, no gonad or a streak gonad and a fallopian tube are present. A hypoplastic uterus and a poorly developed vagina are frequent findings.

This syndrome accounts for about 15% of intersex conditions. Some patients are raised as males, although their external genitalia are usually ambiguous as a result of fetal virilization. The penis is clitoriform, and the urethra opens in the perineum. Most have cryptorchid testes and are raised as girls, becoming virilized at puberty. Infertility is a common symptom.[793] The etiology is heterogeneous:[794] one-third of patients have turnerian features, in accordance with the presence of the 45X0/46XY karyotype in more than 50% of patients. Other observed karyotypes are 46XY and 45X0/47XYY. Approximately 81% of patients have one Y chromosome. Mutation in the SRY gene has not been found.[795]

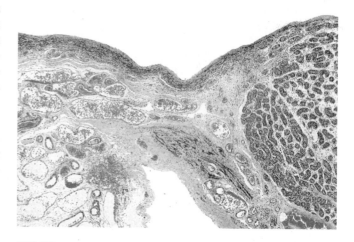

**Fig. 12-83** Streak testis consisting of a streak gonad connected to a testis which shows the characteristic lesions of testicular dysgenesis.

The testes can show two different patterns: testicular dysgenesis and streak testis. *Testicular dysgenesis* is characterized by a tunica albuginea that varies in width and is reminiscent of ovarian stroma by the storiform distribution of cells and fibers; there are also malformed seminiferous tubules (Fig. 12-82) that are small, usually lack lumina, and contain only immature Sertoli cells. In adults, spermatogenesis has been observed occasionally. The testicular interstitium contains increased numbers of Leydig cells.

*Streak testes* are complex gonads in which testicular dysgenesis is associated with a fibrous streak. Most of the gonad consists of a testis showing the characteristic lesions of testicular dysgenesis. In a pole of the gonad, or in continuity with it, there is a fibrous streak whose structure may correspond to any of the varieties mentioned above (Fig. 12-83). This peculiar gonad can also be observed in some dysgenetic male pseudohermaphrodites as well as in the persistent mül-

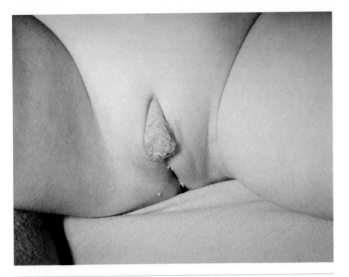

**Fig. 12-84** Male pseudohermaphrodite with bilateral testicular dysgenesis.

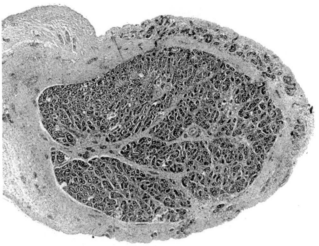

**Fig. 12-85** Testicular dysgenesis. The gonad has a central portion showing a testicular pattern and a peripheral band consisting of poorly collagenized connective tissue that contains seminiferous tubules that reach the gonadal surface.

lerian duct syndrome. In these cases, the streak contains no ovocytes. Light microscopy indicates a wide spectrum of testicular lesions, ranging from those of patients with 46XY pure gonadal dysgenesis to true hermaphroditism. Differentiation of the ovocyte-containing streak testis and ovotestis remains controversial.[796,797]

The testes in mixed gonadal dysgenesis are incapable of müllerian duct inhibition and allow complete differentiation of wolffian derivatives, virilization of external genitalia, and, in most cases, testicular descent. The risk of germ cell neoplasia reaches 50% in the third decade of life, usually beginning with gonadoblastoma. The testes should be removed after puberty.

### Dysgenetic male pseudohermaphroditism

Dysgenetic male pseudohermaphroditism is a disorder of sexual differentiation characterized by bilateral dysgenetic testes or streak testis, persistent müllerian structures, and cryptorchidism. This syndrome is considered a variant of mixed gonadal dysgenesis (Fig. 12-84).[791,798] The karyotype may be 46XY or 45X0/46XY, and turnerian stigmata may be present. The uterus and fallopian tubes are present and both are usually hypoplastic (Fig. 12-85).[799] The testes show lesions characteristic of testicular dysgenesis, with few germ cells during childhood (Fig. 12-85).[799] In adults, spermatogenesis is poorly developed and the testicular interstitium shows Leydig cell hyperplasia. About 25% of patients develop gonadoblastoma.[800]

### Persistent müllerian duct syndrome

Persistent müllerian duct syndrome has many names, including male with uterus, tubular hermaphroditism, persistent oviduct syndrome, and hernia uteri inguinalis.[801] It is a rare form of pseudohermaphroditism, with müllerian derivatives in an otherwise phenotypically normal male, and is the most characteristic form of isolated anti-müllerian hormone deficiency.

The molecular basis of this syndrome is heterogeneous. Three hypotheses have been proposed, including a defect in anti-müllerian hormone synthesis, caused by mutation in the anti-müllerian hormone gene (45% of cases); resistance

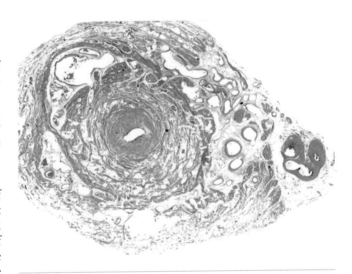

**Fig. 12-86** Persistent müllerian duct syndrome. Cross sectioned hypoplastic uterus. In its tunica adventitia and parallel to it, a folded ductus deferens is seen.

of target organs to this hormone, caused by mutation in the receptor II for this hormone (39% of cases); and failure in the action of this hormone immediately before the eighth week of gestation (16% of cases).[802]

Although the external genitalia are male, one (35% of cases) or both testes (75% of cases) are cryptorchid. The syndrome usually also includes inguinal hernia contralateral to the undescended testis, with a uterus and fallopian tubes within the hernia sac (Figs 12-86, 12-87).[803] Several cases with transverse testicular ectopia and persistent müllerian duct structures have been reported.[804,805] Patients usually have inguinal hernia, but others have cryptorchidism, infertility,[806] and testicular tumor.[807]

In childhood, the testes have a low tubular fertility index and decreased tubular diameter. In adults, the tunica albu-

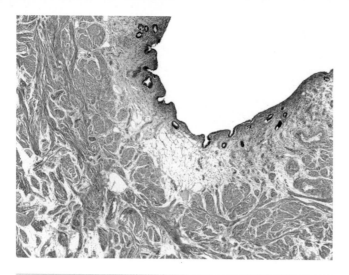

**Fig. 12-87** Persistent müllerian duct syndrome. Uterus with atrophic endometrium and hypoplastic myometrium within a hernia sac.

ginea is variably thickened, contains connective tissue resembling ovarian stroma, and may contain tubular structures – alterations typical of testicular dysgenesis. The seminiferous tubules are usually atrophic and hyalinized. Tubules with reduced spermatogenesis or patterns suggesting mixed atrophy (seminiferous tubules with spermatogenesis intermingled with Sertoli cell-only tubules) have also been reported. The Leydig cells appear hyperplastic. Azoospermia or oligozoospermia are common, and paternity is exceptional.[808]

The syndrome is sporadic or familial, with autosomal recessive or X-linked inheritance.[809,810] These patients have a higher risk of testicular tumor than that attributed to cryptorchidism,[811] and all types of germ cell tumor have been observed.[812,813]

## Other forms of male pseudohermaphroditism

Of the dysmorphic syndromes associated with incomplete virilization of external genitalia, the best-known are those of RSH, Denys–Drash, WAGR, Opiz, camptomelic dysplasia, ATR-X, Gardner–Silengo–Wachtel, Meckel, branchioskeletal–genital, Down's, and other trisomies.

RSH (Smith–Lemli–Opitz) syndrome is a malformative recessive autosomal syndrome caused by mutations in the gene encoding for 7-dehydrocholesterol reductase (DHCR7), responsible for the synthesis of cholesterol from its immediate precursor 7-dehydrocholesterol.[814–816] The disorder is common in Europe and rare in other countries.[817]

The most severe form is lethal before birth. Fetuses show postaxial oligodactyly (instead of polydactyly) and sometimes severe hydrops.[818] Non-lethal forms are characterized after birth by severe growth failure; a semi-obtunded state; absence of psychomotor development; microcephaly; congenital cataracts; peculiar facies; broad anteriorly rugose alveolar ridges with cleft palate, edema of the nape of the neck, and unilobulate lungs; male pseudohermaphroditism or female external genitalia in 46,XY patients; postaxial polydactyly of the hands and feet; congenital heart defects; and

renal anomalies.[819] Hepatic and renal insufficiencies are frequent.[820]

The less severe forms in the male have genital anomalies (70%) varying from normal genitalia to severe hypospadias with or without cryptorchidism, and numerous small anomalies whose collection characterizes the syndrome. Most patients also show mental retardation and severe behavioral problems.[821]

The DHCR7 gene maps to chromosome 11q12-13. Its product is a microsomal, membrane-bound protein. Many different missense, nonsense, and splice-site mutations as well as duplications and deletions have been reported.[822–827] Prenatal diagnosis is possible by relating ultrasound and cytogenetic studies and carrying out a biochemical analysis in the second trimester in those pregnant women who have low levels or no conjugated estriol.[828]

In Denys–Drash syndrome, male pseudohermaphroditism is associated with nephroblastoma and renal insufficiency.[829] The pseudohermaphroditism is usually either mixed gonadal dysgenesis, dysgenetic male pseudohermaphroditism, 46XY pure gonadal dysgenesis, or true hermaphroditism.[830] The most common nephropathy is diffuse mesangial sclerosis.[831] Most patients have mutations in the WT-1 gene,[832] which is expressed in the genital ridge in the sixth week of gestation and gives rise to either streak gonads or testicular dysgenesis, but, if a delay in testicular determination occurs, normal testes are formed.[833]

The term WAGR syndrome refers to Wilms' tumor, aniridia, genital anomalies, and mental retardation. Prevalence is estimated at between 0.75% and 2% of Wilms' tumor patients. The syndrome is related to the syndrome of Denys–Drash and that of Frasier (a variety of 46,XY gonadal dysgenesis).[834,835] All have in common mutations in the WT-1 gene located on chromosome 11 (11p13).

WT-1 product is a transcription factor expressed in different tissues that participates in embryogenesis and cell differentiation. Mutations lead to the production of an anomalous protein that causes alterations in renal function, gonadal anomalies, and the loss of tumor suppressor function. Six variants of alleles have been described: isolated Wilms' tumor, mesothelioma, isolated diffuse mesangial sclerosis, Denis–Drash syndrome, Frasier syndrome, and WAGR syndrome. Frasier syndrome is caused by mutations in the donor zone of the intron 9 link, with the subsequent loss of the +KTS isoform (the patient has an imbalance in KTS isoforms), whereas large deletions or loss of genetic material that comprises the WT-1 gene and other contiguous genes (PAX6 or AN) lead to the WAGR syndrome.[836,837]

Patients with Opitz's syndrome are mainly boys with hypertelorism and, in the severe forms, unilateral or bilateral lip cleft, laryngeal cleft, severe dysphagia with more or less life-threatening aspiration, hypospadias and, occasionally, imperforate anus. The most important internal anomalies are those in the tracheobronchial tree, cardiovascular system (defects in cardiac septation), and gallbladder, with a subjacent defect of the developing embryonal ventral midline. The syndrome is genetically heterogeneous and consists of two entities that were described as different in the past: ADOS, or autosomal dominant Opitz syndrome or G syndrome[838] with a mutated gene that maps to 22q11.2; and XLOS, or X-linked Opitz syndrome or BBB syndrome[839] with a mutated gene that maps to Xp22.3.[840,841]

Camptomelic dysplasia is an autosomal dominant syndrome with multiple osseous malformations. Patients have 46XY karyotype and external genitalia that are ambiguous or female. Gonadal histology varies from testes to dysgenetic ovaries with primary follicles. The cause is a haploinsufficiency of SOX9, located on 17q.[842] The incidence of gonadoblastoma is low.

ATR-X syndrome is characterized by mild α-thalassemia, mental retardation, facial dysmorphism, and hypospadias.[843,844] The disorder is X-linked, and is caused by mutation in the ART-X gene (synonymous XNP, HX2).[845]

# Infertility

## Testicular biopsy

Testicular biopsy to diagnose infertility began in the 1940s,[846,847] and most of the diagnostic terms used today were created then.[848] These terms are usually descriptive and, except for a few (normal testes, Sertoli cell-only tubules, tubular hyalinization, for example), do not specify the degree of tubular abnormality that is evaluated by each pathologist subjectively. The terms maturation arrest and hypospermatogenesis have been applied to biopsies in more than 50% of cases of infertility,[849–851] but the criteria for these vary widely among pathologists.

Two forms of maturation arrest have been described: spermatogenic arrest, and spermatocytic arrest, or its equivalent, meiotic arrest. True spermatogenic arrest is rare because germ cell maturation usually does not arrest at the level of a defined germ cell type.[852] To avoid confusion the term irregular hypospermatogenesis has been proposed[853] for testicular biopsies with decreased numbers of germ cells, subclassified as slight, moderate, or severe. However, this diagnosis is of little help to clinicians. The reported frequency of spermatocytic (meiotic) arrest in infertile men varies from 12%[854] to 32.1%[855] and is present in one or both testes of about 18% of oligozoospermic or azoospermic patients.[856] If observed in only one testis, the contralateral testis may show histologic changes ranging from normal spermatogenesis to hyalinized tubules.

Disorganization of the seminiferous tubular cell layers is another frequent diagnosis in testicular biopsies,[848,857,858] but this term is rejected by many pathologists. Actual disorganization of the seminiferous tubular cells is unlikely and has not been demonstrated in ultrastructural studies. In most cases, the apparent disorganization is an artifact induced by handling or fixation.[859,860]

The term tubular blockage was introduced by Meinhard and co-workers[858] for testes with at least 50% of seminiferous tubules devoid of a central lumen and showing spatial disorganization of germ cells. This morphology was found in 28% of testicular biopsies from infertile men, mainly those with obstructive azoospermia.[861] Although this appearance can result from improper fixation,[862] the accumulation of Sertoli cells and immature germ cells in the centers of tubules suggests a specific lesion, a variant of germ cell sloughing.

Diagnostic confusion decreased the interest and trust of urologists and andrologists in the study of testicular biopsies. Subsequent studies attempted to correlate semen spermatozoa concentration with testicular size and biochemical findings such as serum levels of FSH, and testicular biopsies were undertaken in only a limited number of oligozoospermic and azoospermic patients.[859,862,863] However, these studies were also discouraging because FSH was found to correlate poorly with numbers of spermatozoa in the semen but better with numbers of spermatogonia in the seminiferous tubules,[864] and normal numbers of spermatozoa can be produced by relatively small testes whereas some large testes have no spermatogenesis. In recent years, serum levels of inhibin B have been shown to have a positive correlation with spermatozoon numbers and serum FSH level.[865,866]

The development of morphometry caused a resurgence of interest in biopsies. Many semiquantitative[853,867–869] and quantitative[870–875] studies were carried out. The greatest achievements of these studies were enhancement of the reproducibility of results and better evaluation of the reversibility of lesions. Morphometry emerged as the best method to objectively evaluate the seminiferous tubular cells.[876] The scoring method of Johnsen,[868] estimation of the germ cell/Sertoli cell ratio for each germ cell type,[871] and calculation of germ cell number per unit length of seminiferous tubules[870] are reliable and useful.

Several methods are available to evaluate the Leydig cell population, including the mean number of cells per seminiferous tubule and per cell cluster; the mean number of Leydig cell clusters per seminiferous tubule; the ratio of Leydig cell area to seminiferous tubule area;[877] and the ratio of Leydig cells to Sertoli cells.[878] These methods have shown that the appearance of Leydig cell hyperplasia described in many conditions is false, and that true Leydig cell hyperplasia is extremely rare.

Optimal interpretation of testicular biopsies depends on the surgical technique by which the tissue sample is taken, the care and delicacy with which the specimen is manipulated, and proper fixation and processing of the tissue. The size of the biopsy should not be greater than a grain of rice: that is, no diameter should be greater than 3 mm. This amounts to about 0.12% of testicular volume (normal volume is approximately 20 mL). The biopsy should be bilateral because in more than 28% of patients the findings differ between the testes. At the time of biopsy, the testicular axes should be measured as the basis of quantitative studies. The tissue should be taken opposite to the rete testis through a 4–5 mm incision in the tunica albuginea. This parenchyma herniates through the incision and can be carefully snipped off. If only light microscopy is to be performed, the specimen should be fixed in Bouin's fluid for 24 hours. If electron microscopy is indicated, a small biopsy fragment should be fixed in glutaraldehyde–osmium tetroxide or a similar fixative. To perform meiotic studies, testicular biopsy should be processed by air-drying or surface-spreading methods. The examination of testicular biopsies includes qualitative and quantitative evaluation of the testis and correlation between the biopsy and spermiogram.

## Qualitative and quantitative evaluation of testicular biopsy

Light microscopy immediately reveals whether the lesion is focal or diffuse. If focal, the percentage of tubules showing each lesion (Sertoli cell-only, hyalinization, tubular hypoplasia, etc.) should be calculated. It is useful to evaluate elastic fibers with a special stain because this highlights groups of small tubules that may be missed with hematoxylin and eosin. A minimum of 30 cross-sectioned tubules should be studied (this is usually possible when five or six histological sections are available). The diameter of each tubule should be measured, and the number of spermatogonia, primary spermatocytes, young spermatids (also called round spermatids or $S_a + S_b$ spermatids), mature spermatids (also called elongated or $S_c + S_d$ spermatids), Sertoli cells, and, in some cases, peritubular cells counted. The presence of tubular diverticula,[879,880] the maturation of Sertoli cells, and morphologic anomalies in germ cells should also be noted. Evaluation of the testicular interstitium should include the number of Leydig cells per tubule (or number of Leydig cell clusters per tubule), the presence of angiectasis (phlebectasis), and the occurrence of peritubular or perivascular inflammation. Normal values are tabulated in Table 12-6. For a clear and rapid understanding of the results, data can be presented using cartesian axes (see Figs 12-96 and 12-103).

## Common lesions

The most frequently observed lesions are Sertoli cell-only tubules, tubular hyalinization, alterations in spermatogenesis in either the adluminal or the basal compartments of seminiferous tubules, and mixed tubular atrophy.

## Sertoli cell-only syndrome

Sertoli cell-only syndrome includes all azoospermias in which the seminiferous epithelium consists only of Sertoli cells. To better understand this syndrome, it is necessary to consider the morphological and functional changes induced in the Sertoli cell by hypophyseal gonadotropin secretion during puberty. During childhood, Sertoli cells are pseudostratified and their nuclei are dark, small, and round or elongated, with regular outlines and one or two small peripherally placed nucleoli. The cytoplasm lacks specialized organelles.[881] Adult Sertoli cells have characteristically pale, triangular nuclei with irregular, indented outlines. The nucleoli are large and have tripartite structures. The cytoplasm contains abundant smooth endoplasmic reticulum and specialized structures, including annulate lamellae, Charcot–Böttcher crystals, and specialized junctional complexes with other Sertoli cells. The pubertal increase in length and width of the seminiferous tubules replaces the infantile pseudostratified pattern with a simple columnar distribution.

Five variants of the Sertoli cell-only syndrome are identified by Sertoli cell morphology, the degree of development of the seminiferous tubules, and the presence or absence of interstitial lesions.[882] These variants are designated by the appearance of the predominant Sertoli cell population: immature Sertoli cells, dysgenetic Sertoli cells, adult Sertoli cells, involuting Sertoli cells, and dedifferentiated Sertoli cells (Fig. 12-88). Each type is associated with other tubular and interstitial alterations (Table 12-7).

The most frequent types of Sertoli cell-only syndrome in infertility patients are dysgenetic Sertoli cells, adult Sertoli cells, and involuting Sertoli cells. The clinical manifestations are similar, including normal external genitalia, well-developed secondary male characteristics, azoospermia, elevated serum FSH level, normal or elevated serum LH level, and normal or slightly low testosterone. These clinical and

**Table 12-6** Testicular parameters in normal adult testes (means ± SD)

| Values per cross-sectioned tubule | Means ± SD |
|---|---|
| **Seminiferous Tubules** | |
| Mean tubular diameter (μm) | 193 ± 8 |
| Number of spermatogonia | 21 ± 4 |
| Number of primary spermatocytes | 31 ± 6 |
| Number of young ($S_a + S_b$) spermatids | 37 ± 7 |
| Number of mature ($S_c + S_d$) spermatids | 25 ± 4 |
| Number of Sertoli cells | 10.4 ± 2 |
| Number of Sertoli cell vacuoles | 0.8 ± 0.3 |
| Lamina propria thickness (μm) | 5.3 ± 1 |
| Number of peritubular cells | 21 ± 4 |
| **Testicular Interstitium** | |
| Number of Leydig cell clusters per tubule | 1.2 ± 0.3 |
| Number of Leydig cells per tubule | 5 ± 0.2 |

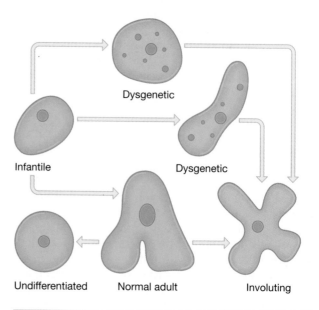

**Fig. 12-88** Sertoli cell types.

**Table 12-7** Variants of Sertoli cell-only syndrome

| Testis pattern | Variants of the Sertoli cell-only syndrome | | | | |
|---|---|---|---|---|---|
| | Immature Sertoli cells | Dysgenetic Sertoli cells | Adult Sertoli cells | Involuting Sertoli cells | Dedifferentiated Sertoli cells |
| Tubular diameter | Very decreased | Decreased | Decreased | Decreased | Decreased |
| Tubular lumen | Small or absent | Small or absent | Normal | Normal | Normal |
| Lamina propria thickness | Thin | Enlarged | Normal or enlarged | Normal or enlarged | Enlarged |
| Elastic fibers in lamina propria | Absent | Decreased | Normal | Normal | Normal |
| Sertoli cells | | | | | |
| Number | Very increased | Increased | Normal or increase | Normal or increased | Increased |
| Distribution | Pseudostratified | Pseudostratified | Columnar | Columnar | Columnar or pseudostratified |
| Nuclear shape | Ovoid | Round or ovoid | Triangular | Lobated | Round |
| Nuclear outline | Regular | Regular | Few indented | Very indented | Regular |
| Chromatin | Dark | Pale with granules | Pale | Pale | Pale |
| Nucleolus | Small, peripheral | Developed, central | Developed, central | Developed, central | Small, central or peripheral |
| Vacuoles | Absent | Present | Present | Abundant | Abundant |
| Lipids | Absent | Absent | Decreased | Abundant | Abundant |
| Vimentin filaments | Basal | Basal | Basal and perinuclear | Basal and perinuclear | Basal |
| Antimüllerian hormone | Present | Present | Absent | Absent | Absent |
| Interstitium | Scanty | Increased | Normal | Normal/fibrosis | Fibrosis |
| Leydig cells | Absent | Pleomorphic, vacuolated, increased or decreased | Normal | Decreased, many lipofuscin granules | Decreased, many lipofuscin granules |
| Clinical symptoms | Hypogonadotropic hypogonadism | Infertility | Infertility, orchitis | Infertility, hypergonadotropic hypogonadism, chemo- or radiotherapy | Treatment with estrogens, antiandrogens or cisplatinum, chronic hepatopathy |

histologic features were long thought to constitute a single syndrome, Del Castillo's syndrome, but recent ultrastructural, histochemical, immunohistochemical, and cytogenetic studies have shown that this results from a variety of syndromes that may have primary or secondary causes (Table 12-7).[883–887]

Some patients with the adult or dysgenetic Sertoli cell-only syndrome variants have a few spermatozoa in their spermiograms. This discrepancy between oligozoospermia and the biopsy histology is caused by the presence of some seminiferous tubules with complete spermatogenesis elsewhere in the testicular parenchyma.

*Sertoli cell-only syndrome with immature Sertoli cells* Sertoli cells in adult testes with this variant of Sertoli cell-only syndrome have an immature prepubertal appearance with pseudostratification. The number of cells per cross-sectioned tubule is greater than normal. Other tubular and interstitial features suggest immaturity, including small tubular diame-

ters (<80 µm), tubules lacking central lumina, thin lamina propria lacking elastic fibers, and interstitium lacking mature Leydig cells.[888–890]

This syndrome is caused by a deficiency of both FSH and LH which begins in childhood and is responsible for the lack of maturation of the Sertoli cells, tubular walls, and interstitium. Subsequently, there is no renewal or differentiation of germ cells, and these eventually disappear. When these patients are treated with hormones, the biopsy may show some degree of spermatogenesis or thickening and hyalinization of the tubular basement membrane.

*Sertoli cell-only syndrome with dysgenetic Sertoli cells* Dysgenetic Sertoli cells begin pubertal differentiation but variably deviate from normal maturation, so that the morphology of dysgenetic Sertoli cells differs among tubules and even among Sertoli cells within the same tubule. Nuclei usually have both mature features (pale chromatin and a centrally located, tripartite nucleolus) and features of immaturity

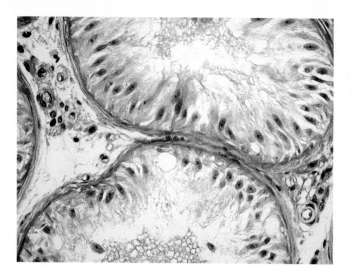

**Fig. 12-89** Sertoli cell-only syndrome with dysgenetic Sertoli cells. Seminiferous tubules show slightly thickened tunica propria. The Sertoli cells are increased in number and have elongated nuclei and abundant apical cytoplasm.

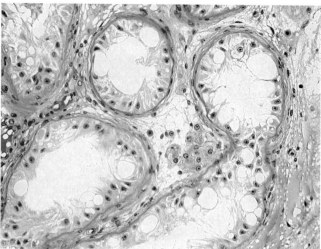

**Fig. 12-90** Sertoli cell-only syndrome with mature Sertoli cells. The seminiferous tubules are lined by normal adult Sertoli cells, many with cytoplasmic vacuoles.

(ovoid or round shape; regular outline; and small, dense chromatin granules) (Fig. 12-89).[891] In addition to vimentin, Sertoli cells immunoexpress anti-müllerian hormone (AMH)[892] and cytokeratin 18.[893] Immunoreaction to these two substances is assumed to be a sign of immaturity, as under normal conditions it is not detected after puberty. Other signs of immaturity are poor development of the hematotesticular barrier[894] and the absence of tubular lumina.

Tubular lumina are very small or absent in most dysgenetic Sertoli cell-containing tubules, because the ability to produce testicular fluid is greatly reduced. Sertoli cell numbers per cross-sectioned tubule are very high, and mean tubular diameter is lower than 120 μm. The tubular walls have few elastic fibers,[534] and most tubules show a variable degree of tunica propria hyalinization.

Completely hyalinized tubules are frequent. The testicular interstitium contains a variable number of Leydig cells (normal, decreased, or apparently increased), many of which are pleomorphic with abundant paracrystalline inclusions.[895,896]

Most patients have normal or slightly subnormal testosterone level and elevated levels of FSH and LH. This syndrome can be observed in men with cryptorchid testes, at the periphery of germ cell tumors, in men with idiopathic infertility,[897] and in men with Y chromosome anomalies.[898]

*Sertoli cell-only syndrome with mature Sertoli cells* In this variant, most Sertoli cells appear mature but are present in increased numbers (14 ± 0.8 per cross-sectioned tubule). The seminiferous tubules have small diameters, but are still larger than in the two variants described above, and central lumina are visible. The cytoplasm contains abundant vacuoles that communicate with the tubular lumina (Fig. 12-90). The lateral cell surfaces have many unfolding and extensive specialized junctions with other Sertoli cells (from the basement membrane to the apical cytoplasmic portion). Lipid

droplets, usually derived from phagocytosis of spermatid tubulobulbar complexes and dead germ cells, are scant.[884] Vimentin filaments are abundant in the basal and perinuclear cytoplasm.[899] The lamina propria is normal or slightly thickened. Leydig cells are normal.

Serum testosterone level is normal or nearly normal, and FSH and LH levels are elevated.[900–902] This syndrome is probably caused by failure of migration of primordial germ cells from the primitive yolk sac to the gonadal ridge.[903] This failure may be due to a deletion in the AZFa region in Yq11[904] or a mutation in the genes that encodes c-KIT or its ligand (stem cell factor), responsible for migration, proliferation, and survival of germ cells.

*Sertoli cell-only syndrome with involuting Sertoli cells* Testes with this variant of Sertoli cell-only syndrome have numerous changes. Sertoli cell nuclei may have lobulated shapes with irregular outlines, coarse chromatin granules, and inconspicuous nucleoli. Seminiferous tubules have central lumina, decreased diameters, and variable thickening of the basement membrane (Fig. 12-91). Elastic fibers are present in normal or diminished amounts. Leydig cells are variably involuted.

This syndrome may be a primary disorder or secondary to irradiation or cytotoxic therapy, such as cancer chemotherapy or treatment for nephrotic syndrome.[905] It is not usually possible to determine the etiology from the biopsy findings alone. Changes in the tubular walls are more pronounced in patients with a history of cyclophosphamide treatment, combination chemotherapy, or radiotherapy. The testicular interstitium may be fibrotic in patients treated with *cis*-platinum or cyclophosphamide.[906] Some syndromes with involuting Sertoli cells, mainly those associated with decreased number of elastic fibers, probably express a primary testicular anomaly with involuting and dysgenetic Sertoli cells within the same tubule.

*Sertoli cell-only syndrome with dedifferentiated Sertoli cells* The presence of immature-appearing Sertoli cells in

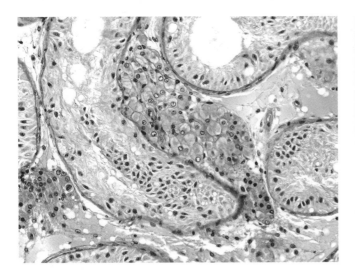

**Fig. 12-91** Sertoli cell-only syndrome with involuting Sertoli cells. The Sertoli cell nuclei are hyperchromatic and have irregular outlines.

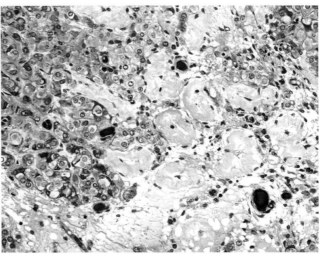

**Fig. 12-92** Dysgenetic hyalinization. Fully hyalinized seminiferous tubules and a few peritubular cells among Leydig cell clusters.

otherwise mature tubules is the most striking feature of this variant of Sertoli cell-only syndrome. Sertoli cells appear abnormally numerous due to shortening of the tubule, and nuclei are either round or elongated. Round nuclei have single, small, central or peripheral nucleoli, whereas elongated nuclei have dense clumped chromatin and small peripheral nucleoli.

The tubular wall is thickened and contains elastic fibers, increased amounts of collagen fibers, and elevated numbers of peritubular cells as a result of tubular shortening. Mean tubular diameter is markedly decreased to less than 90 μm. The testicular interstitium contains few Leydig cells, and these appear dedifferentiated or contain an increased amount of lipofuscin.

This variant has been observed in surgical specimens from patients receiving androgen deprivation therapy for prostatic cancer, estrogen treatment for transsexuality, and cancer chemotherapy with *cis*-platinum. There is a correlation between the degree of Sertoli cell dedifferentiation and the dose and timing of treatment with estrogens or anti-androgens. Brief treatment induces germ cell loss and inconspicuous Sertoli cell changes; long-term treatment causes pronounced Sertoli cell changes, including initial nuclear rounding followed by nuclear elongation and the development of dark chromatin masses.[907] Eventually, the nuclei come to resemble those of infantile Sertoli cells, including pseudostratification. At the same time, the tubules become hyalinized and peritubular cells increase whereas Leydig cells disappear.[908,909]

Estrogens act on the pituitary by inhibiting LH secretion, and on Leydig cells.[910] The action of gonadotropin-releasing hormone agonist analogs is only on the pituitary, whereas *cis*-platinum acts only on the testis.

### Tubular hyalinization

A few azoospermic patients have diffuse hyalinization of seminiferous tubules. The incidence of this lesion is difficult to estimate, as these patients usually are not biopsied because their testes are small. Hyalinization of seminiferous tubules is the endpoint of tubular atrophy and includes the absence of both germ cells and Sertoli cells with alterations in the lamina propria and Leydig cells. Etiology can be determined from several histologic features and clinical data, including:

- *General histologic appearance*: extent and topography of the hyalinized tubules and presence of isolated tubules containing germ cells or Sertoli cells only (dysgenetic, adult, involuting, or dedifferentiated).
- *Appearance of atrophic tubules, all showing the same pattern or variable degrees of atrophy*: tubular diameter; trophism of peritubular cells; presence of elastic fibers; degree of collagenization of the lamina propria, and the presence of cell remnants or unusual cells in the tubules.
- *Appearance of the interstitium*: number and morphology of Leydig cells; vascular lesions; and lymphoid infiltrate.
- *Chronology of testicular shrinkage*.

The most common causes of tubular hyalinization include dysgenetic hyalinization, hormonal deficit, ischemia, obstruction, inflammation, and physical or chemical agents. The differential diagnosis is given in Table 12-8.

*Dysgenetic hyalinization* Dysgenetic hyalinization is a diffuse lesion in which most tubules are uniformly hyalinized (Fig. 12-92). Tubules lack seminiferous tubular cells and have a reduced number of peritubular cells. The few preserved tubules usually contain only Sertoli cells, although rarely a few with spermatogenesis are present. Dysgenetic hyalinization is seen in Klinefelter's syndrome, testes that remain cryptorchid through puberty, and some hypergonadotropic hypogonadisms associated with myopathy. Focal lesions are seen in mixed atrophy of the testis.

Tubular hyalinization is pronounced in Klinefelter's syndrome, and from infancy the seminiferous tubules are small, containing reduced numbers of Sertoli cells and few or no spermatogonia. At puberty, the dysgenetic Sertoli cells fail to

**Table 12-8** Differential diagnosis of tubular hyalinization

| | Dysgenetic | Hormonal deficit | Ischemia | Excretory duct obstruction | Postinflammatory hyalinization | Physical or chemical agents |
|---|---|---|---|---|---|---|
| Hyalinized tubule size | Minimum | Minimum | Minimum | Very decreased | Minimum | Very decreased |
| Tubular lumen | Absent | Absent | Absent | Present | Absent | Absent |
| Peritubular cells | Decreased | Decreased | Decreased | Increased | Decreased or increased | Decreased |
| Elastic fibers | Decreased | Normal | Normal | Normal | Normal | Normal |
| Leydig cells | Increased or decreased, pleomorphic | Absent | Absent | Normal | Pseudo-hyperplasia | Decreased |
| FSH | Increased | Decreased | Increased | Increased | Increased | Increased |
| LH | Increased | Decreased | Increased | Increased | Increased | Increased |
| Testosterone | Normal or decreased | Decreased | Normal or decreased | Normal | Normal | Normal or decreased |

mature and soon disappear. The tubules collapse, giving the appearance of phantom tubules.[911] Peritubular cells fail to differentiate and their number is low.[912] They form a discontinuous ring around the hyalinized tubules and are incapable of synthesizing elastic fibers and other components of the lamina propria. Dysgenesis also involves the interstitium: Leydig cells exhibit a characteristic adenomatous pattern, although their total number is decreased. The morphology of the Leydig cell is not uniform, and there are shrunken, normal, and large forms. Most contain reduced amounts of lipofuscin granules and lipid droplets. Reinke's crystalloids are uncommon, and paracrystalline inclusions are abundant.[896] In spite of the hyperplastic adenomatous appearance of the Leydig cells, testosterone secretion is markedly decreased, and the resulting hypogonadism is the most important clinical feature of Klinefelter's syndrome.

Tubular hyalinization in the cryptorchid testis is also dysgenetic. However, in contrast to the atrophic collapse seen in Klinefelter's syndrome, cross-sections of the hyalinized tubules in cryptorchidism are targetoid. This results from the arrangement of the peritubular cells into two layers, suggesting an atrophic process that has evolved over a longer period than in Klinefelter's syndrome, or a lower degree of dysgenesis.[913] Elastic fibers are diminished.[534] In the interstitium Leydig cells appear hyperplastic, forming large aggregates, although their absolute numbers are decreased. Leydig cell pleomorphism is less intense than in Klinefelter's syndrome. Many Leydig cells have abundant vacuolated cytoplasm. Whereas tubular hyalinization in Klinefelter's syndrome is secondary to the effect of pubertal gonadotropin secretion on dysgenetic tubules, tubular hyalinization in cryptorchidism probably results from the effect of increased temperature on the dysgenetic tubules. However, other mechanisms are also involved in cryptorchid tubular hyalinization, including obstruction of sperm excretory ducts (anomalies in these ducts are frequent in cryptorchidism) and ischemia (principally in testes that could only be incompletely descended by surgery).

*Hyalinization caused by hormonal deficit* Hormonal deficit causes diffuse tubular hyalinization, although the tubules may be recognized for a time as cellular cords surrounded by hyaline material. Sertoli cell, a few spermatogonia, and rare primary spermatocytes may be identified in these cords. When hyalinization is complete, only the elastic fibers in the lamina propria indicate the structure of the previously normal adult testis. Peritubular myofibroblasts decrease in number and form a ring at the periphery of the lamina propria. Leydig cells disappear as hyalinization progresses, and the few that remain have pyknotic nuclei and shrunken cytoplasm with abundant lipofuscin granules.

This process manifests clinically as postpubertal hypogonadotropic hypogonadism and is usually caused by a lesion in or near the pituitary, such as pituitary adenoma, craniopharyngioma, and trauma to the cranial base or sella turcica (see discussion on hypogonadotropic hypogonadism in this chapter).

*Ischemic hyalinization* Ischemic atrophy is usually caused by torsion of the spermatic cord, vascular injury during inguinal surgery,[914] polyarteritis nodosa, and severe arteriosclerosis.[915] Except for cases caused by torsion of the cord, these patients usually are not referred to infertility clinics.

Torsion of the spermatic cord often is not listed as a cause in large series of infertile patients. However, follow-up of men with torsion reveals marked alteration in their spermiograms. Several hypotheses have been offered to explain the low number of sperm produced by the contralateral normal testis; the most promising include response to the release of antigens by the ischemic testis, and primary lesions of the contralateral testis[916] (see discussion on testicular torsion in this chapter).

Testicular anoxia caused by torsion rapidly produces severe lesions that are irreversible without adequate treatment. Eight hours after torsion, there is intense hemorrhagic infarction of the seminiferous tubular cells. Chronic anoxia leads to tubular hyalinization and loss of Leydig cells (Fig. 12-93).

Testicular atrophy secondary to inguinal hernia surgery occurs in 0.03–0.5% of patents in the first repair, and in 0.8–5% in surgery for recurrent hernia. Atrophy is most fre-

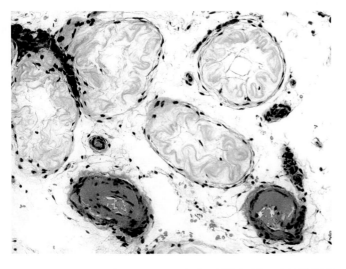

**Fig. 12-93** Ischemic tubular hyalinization. Fully hyalinized seminiferous tubules are surrounded by peritubular cells. The testicular interstitium lacks Leydig cells and shows arteriolar hyalinization.

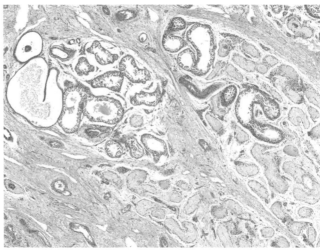

**Fig. 12-94** Post-obstructive hyalinization. Seminiferous tubules with marked ectasis with hyalinized tubules. Leydig cell clusters are seen among the hyalinized tubules.

quent in cases that require extensive dissection of the spermatic cord.

***Postobstructive hyalinization*** Obstruction of sperm excretory ducts may cause atrophy of seminiferous tubules. In order to produce tubular hyalinization, the obstruction must be close to the testis because the ductuli efferentes in the caput epididymis absorb about 90% of tubular fluid and protect the testis from excessive intratubular pressure. Obstructive tubular hyalinization is usually focal and secondary to varicocele and other disorders involving dilation of the channels of the rete testis. These may be congenital, as in epididymis–testis dissociation, or acquired, as in rete testis dilation secondary to epididymal atrophy caused by arteritis, arteriosclerosis, or androgen insufficiency. Obstructive tubular hyalinization also occurs in the seminiferous tubules at the periphery of the testis in patients who have had orchitis.[917]

Obstructive hyalinization has a mosaic distribution: lobules of completely hyalinized tubules are intermingled with lobules of normal tubules (Fig. 12-94). The diameter of the hyalinized tubules is not as small as in other causes of hyalinization, and the tubules occasionally contain Sertoli cells. In the centers of many of the tubules there is a small lumen or vacuole, the latter in the cytoplasm of a residual Sertoli cell.[918] The lamina propria is thick and contains hypertrophic peritubular cells and abundant extracellular material. Finally, the peritubular cells dedifferentiate and only fibroblasts remain.[919] The interstitium contains a normal number of Leydig cells forming small clusters, some of which are among hyalinized tubules. This is not seen in other patterns such as ischemic hyalinization. In addition, dilated veins with eccentrically hyalinized walls can be seen in testes associated with varicocele. This lobular pattern of tubular atrophy causes a peculiar ultrasound image which has been described as a striated pattern.[920,921]

***Postinflammatory hyalinization*** Many infections of the testis cause irreversible lesions in the seminiferous tubules. In bacterial infection the epididymis is usually involved, resulting

in obstructive azoospermia. In viral infection the testis is often affected, even without symptoms. Two types of viral orchitis often cause infertility, including mumps orchitis and Coxsackie B orchitis.

Tubular atrophy caused by viral infection has a mosaic topography in which hyalinized and normal tubules are intermingled. In fully hyalinized tubules, the only recognizable cells are peritubular cells that form an incomplete, peripheral ring around the hyalinized material. The presence of elastic fibers in these tubules distinguishes this from dysgenetic hyalinization. Leydig cells form clusters of variable size, but their total number is normal. In bacterial infection the pattern of tubular hyalinization is variable.

Tubular atrophy of unknown etiology may be caused by an autoimmune response. This appears to occur in hypogonadism associated with disorders in other endocrine glands, such as Addison's disease associated with gonadal insufficiency; adrenal–thyroid–gonadal insufficiency; and the association of diabetes, hypogonadism, adrenal insufficiency, and hypothyroidism. The testicular lesions are morphologically similar to those seen in the seminiferous tubules at the periphery of germ cell tumor and in testes with burn-out germinal cancer. In the initial stages of hyalinization associated with germ cell neoplasm, the tubules are small, contain intratubular germ cell neoplasia and dedifferentiating Sertoli cells, and the lamina propria is infiltrated by macrophages, lymphocytes, and plasma cells. In the final stages, the intratubular cells have degenerated, the inflammation has disappeared, and the seminiferous tubules are replaced by areas of hypocellular or acellular fibrosis (Fig. 12-95). It should be noted that autoimmune hyalinization is not the most common type of hyalinization associated with testicular tumors: the obstructive, ischemic, and dysgenetic variants are more common.

***Hyalinization caused by physical or chemical agents*** Radiation and a wide variety of chemicals cause tubular hyalinization. Lengthy cancer chemotherapy combined with

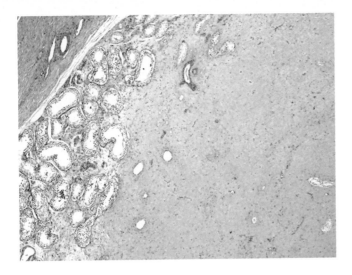

**Fig. 12-95** Post-inflammatory hyalinization. Most of the testis consists of cicatricial tissue with no recognizable seminiferous tubules.

radiotherapy invariably causes hyalinization. Children's testes are more sensitive to radiation than those of adults. Radiation for testicular leukemia frequently causes tubular hyalinization. In addition, radiation induces dense interstitial fibrosis and loss of peritubular cells, obscuring the borders between the interstitium and the tubules. This makes the tubules hard to see in hematoxylin–eosin-stained sections. Leydig cells are atrophic and decreased in number. Ischemia secondary to radiation-induced vascular injury also contributes to hyalinization.

In tubular hyalinization associated with cancer chemotherapy, in addition to the direct toxicity of drugs on seminiferous tubular cells (see discussion on Sertoli cell-only syndrome with involuting Sertoli cells in this chapter), nutritional deficiencies cause hypogonadotropic hypogonadism.[922,923]

### Diffuse lesions in spermatogenesis

Histophysiological studies have distinguished two compartments in the seminiferous tubules: basal and adluminal. The blood–testis barrier separates these, and each contains different cell types with diverse hormonal and nutritional requirements. On this basis, lesions may be classified as involving only the adluminal compartment or both the basal and the adluminal compartments. The following discussion of spermatogenic lesions uses this new concept of tubular pathophysiology, conserving as much as possible of the classic terminology.

***Lesions in the adluminal compartment of seminiferous tubules*** This category includes all infertile testes with normal numbers of spermatogonia per cross-sectioned tubule, normal or decreased numbers of spermatocytes and young spermatids, and variable numbers of adult spermatids. A descriptive term for this disorder is immature germ cell sloughing.

A few immature germ cells are normally found in the lumina of the seminiferous tubules,[923] a finding that correlates with their presence in the ejaculates of fertile men.[924]

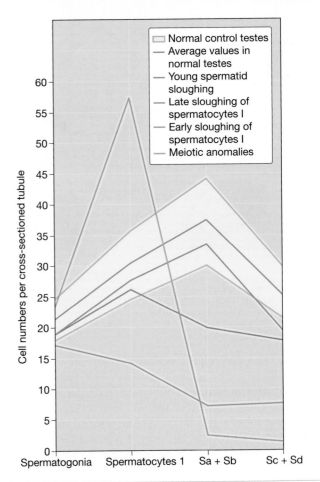

**Fig. 12-96** Germ cell number per cross-sectioned tubule in patients with lesions in the adluminal compartment of the seminiferous tubules.

When these cells make up more than 4% of the cells in the ejaculate, it is abnormal and the result of premature sloughing of spermatids and, in some cases, of spermatocytes.[925,926] Some authors have attempted to establish a correlation between the number of sloughed immature germ cells and the severity of lesions of the seminiferous tubules using light[927] and electron[928] microscopy.

Lesions in the adluminal compartment are classified according to the most abundant type of germ cell whose maturation is arrested and which then sloughs: young spermatids, late primary spermatocytes, or early primary spermatocytes (Fig. 12-96).

***Young spermatid sloughing*** Young spermatid sloughing is present when the ratio of elongated ($S_c + S_d$) spermatids to round ($S_a + S_b$) spermatids is lower than normal. The implication of this pattern is that many round spermatids are incapable of further differentiation and are sloughed (Fig. 12-97).

***Late primary spermatocyte sloughing*** In this condition, spermatogenesis develops normally up to the level of interphase primary spermatocytes, and these are present in normal numbers. Afterwards, these spermatocytes degenerate without achieving meiosis and slough into the tubular lumen. All types of spermatid are greatly reduced in number.

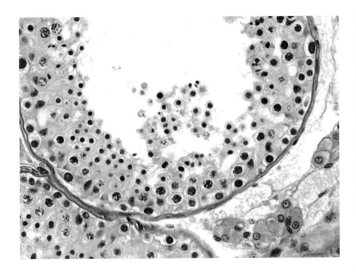

**Fig. 12-97** Seminiferous tubule with dilated lumen and moderate young spermatid sloughing.

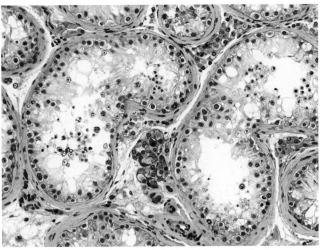

**Fig. 12-99** Seminiferous tubule with dilated lumen, apical vacuolation of Sertoli cells, normal number of spermatogonia, and decreased number of other germ cell types.

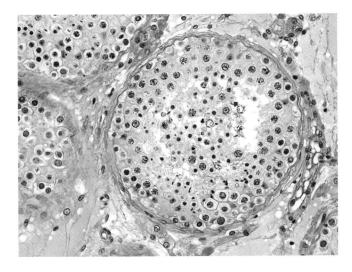

**Fig. 12-98** Seminiferous tubule with sloughing of both primary spermatocytes and young spermatids.

When biopsies of these testes are not properly fixed, the seminiferous tubules may have a target-like appearance, with numerous cells in the lumen. This appearance sometimes has been referred to as tubular blockage. Another descriptive term, spermatogenic arrest, also has been applied to this morphology. The latter term is inadequate in most cases, because some spermatids are present, and the number of primary spermatocytes is usually not increased as would occur if the transformation of spermatocyte into spermatid were blocked (Fig. 12-98). Late spermatocyte sloughing is a more accurate term for this condition and is preferred. Primary spermatocyte sloughing occurs at the pachytene or diplotene stage of meiosis.

*Early primary spermatocyte sloughing* This lesion is characterized by the presence of a normal number of spermatogonia and decreased numbers of primary spermatocytes (Fig. 12-99). The seminiferous tubules may contain a few spermatids.

The term early primary spermatocyte sloughing does not necessarily imply an early meiotic lesion, which is quite rare.[856,926] Rather, it refers to the sloughing of newly formed spermatocytes. The Sertoli cells may show vacuolation of the apical cytoplasm as an expression of germ cell loss. This lesion is more severe than that in testes with late primary spermatocyte sloughing, and is considered to result from failure of the Sertoli cells to maintain the adluminal compartment.

*Etiology* The mechanisms causing adluminal compartment lesions can be classified into obstructive and non-obstructive. Obstruction is present in more than 70% of cases, and is characterized by variability of involvement among lobules and the presence of at least two of the following abnormalities: enlargement of tubular diameter and a lumen with remarkable differences among lobules; Sertoli cells with adherens germ cells protruding into the lumen, giving an indented outline; intense apical vacuolation of Sertoli cell cytoplasm; accumulation of spermatozoa in the lumen of some tubules; or number of spermatids $S_c + S_d$ is higher that that of $S_a + S_b$ (see Testicular lesions resulting from obstruction of sperm excretory ducts).[929]

The three levels of severity of adluminal compartment lesions emphasized by the terms young spermatid sloughing, later primary spermatocytes sloughing, and early primary spermatocyte sloughing, depend on the degree (total or partial) of obstruction and the level of sperm excretory duct obstruction: as the obstruction gets nearer to the testis, the greater the severity. Obstruction may be extratesticular (epididymis, vas deferens, and ejaculatory ducts) or intratesticular (rete testis or any level of the seminiferous tubule length). The most frequent causes of extratesticular excretory duct obstruction are vasectomy, inflammation (epididymitis, prostatitis), mucoviscidosis (congenital bilateral absence of vas deferens), and testis–epididymis dissociation.

*Rete testis obstruction.* Varicocele is the most frequent cause of obstruction of the rete testis. More than 50% of testes with

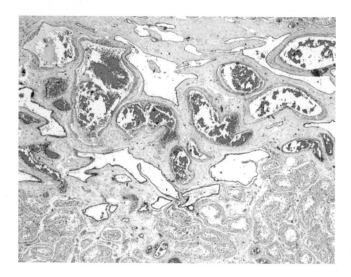

**Fig. 12-100** Mediastinum testis from a young man with varicocele. Marked venous dilation (intratesticular varicocele) disrupts and compresses the rete testis cavities, causing partial obstruction of the tubuli recti.

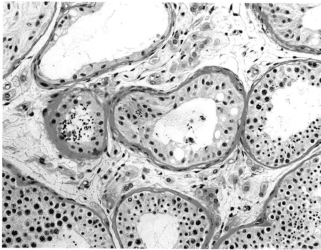

**Fig. 12-101** Segmentary dysgenesis of seminiferous tubules. The two central tubules, which only display dysgenetic Sertoli cells, contain numerous spermatozoa from adjacent seminiferous tubules with normal spermatogenesis.

varicocele have a mosaic pattern of tubular lesions, together with marked dilation and eccentric mural fibrosis of intratesticular veins. In normal testes, the walls of veins are extremely thin and the lumina nearly collapsed. Varicocele patients also often have spermatozoa with characteristically elongated heads with thin bases.[930] Initially, abnormalities are confined to the testis ipsilateral to the varicocele, but eventually both testes are affected, although abnormalities are more severe in the ipsilateral testis. Elevated pressure in the pampiniform plexus is transmitted to the veins within the testes, principally to the centripetal veins that cross the testicular mediastinum and drain most of the testicular parenchyma (Fig. 12-100).[931] The dilated centripetal veins compress the intratesticular sperm excretory ducts, explaining the mosaic distribution of the tubular lesions.[932]

*Seminiferous tubule obstruction.* Obstruction at the level of the seminiferous tubules can be dysgenetic or post-orchitic. A dysgenetic cause may be suspected in specimens with a mosaic distribution of lesions and seminiferous tubules with small diameters, thickened lamina propria, and an unusual seminiferous tubular cell layer consisting of cuboidal Sertoli cells and spermatozoa that clog the lumina (Fig. 12-101). The diagnosis is confirmed if study of serial sections demonstrates continuity between these tubules and those with conserved spermatogenesis. The structure of seminiferous tubules has been observed with scanning microscopy at such points of continuity.[858,933] Tubular stenosis appears to be due to a primary anomaly of Sertoli cells and peritubular cells.

Post-orchitic obstruction should be suspected in cases of tubular atrophy with a mosaic pattern without dysgenetic tubules or varicocele. Some patients have a history of orchitis associated with parotiditis;[934] in others the only findings are oligozoospermia and small testes. Testicular biopsy, sampling only the testicular periphery, reveals only the consequences of obstruction, lesions similar to those observed with varicocele. However, some postinflammatory changes

should also be present, including hyalinized tubules, dilated tubules lined by cuboidal Sertoli cells, or complete spermatogenesis. Occasionally, there is modest perivascular or peritubular inflammation and angiectasis.[935,936]

About 30% of testes with lesions in the adluminal compartment have no obstruction, and most have primary anomalies of germ cells. This claim is supported by the following: pronounced decrease of germ cell type when the preceding type is greatly increased in number; normal correlation between the number of mature spermatids in biopsy and number of spermatozoa in the spermiogram; and the presence of numerous malformed germ cells in the adluminal compartment.

Decrease in the number of a germ cell type may be so important that spermatogenesis is arrested, with subsequent azoospermia. In some cases, maturation arrest is only partial and results in severe oligozoospermia. This maturation arrest is observed mainly in primary spermatocytes and young spermatids.

Primary spermatocyte sloughing may also be owing to meiotic anomalies (Fig. 12-102). The observation of increased numbers of spermatocytes arrested in preleptotene–leptotene[926] or, more frequently, pachytene[856] suggests the diagnosis. The lesion is always bilateral. Spermatocytes arrested in pachytene are usually increased in size and later degenerate. In addition, some spermatids have large, diploid, spherical, hyperchromatic nuclei. The anomaly does not always affect all spermatocytes, and then a higher number of spermatids are produced.[856]

Young spermatid sloughing not associated with obstruction may be due to either meiotic anomalies or defective spermiogenesis. The former gives rises to the appearance of many multinucleate, polyploid, hyperchromatic young spermatids. In the second cause, young spermatids are incapable of transforming into mature spermatids, and only round spermatids appear in the ejaculate.

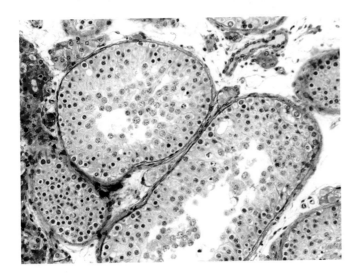

**Fig. 12-102** Meiotic abnormalities. The seminiferous tubules contain normal number of spermatogonia and disproportionately high number of primary spermatocytes which do not complete meiosis. No spermatids are seen.

***Lesions in basal and adluminal compartments of seminiferous tubules*** Lesions in the basal and adluminal compartments of seminiferous tubules are the most frequent histological findings in testicular biopsies from infertile men. These testes may be classified into two major subgroups: hypospermatogenesis and spermatogonial maturation arrest (Fig. 12-103).

*Hypospermatogenesis: Types and etiology* Hypospermatogenesis is defined as a reduced number of spermatogonia and primary spermatocytes, with primary spermatocytes outnumbering the spermatogonia. Most seminiferous tubules contain few spermatids. About 8% of patients with hypospermatogenesis have focal tubular hyalinization.[937] Two variants of hypospermatogenesis have been quantitatively distinguished: pure hypospermatogenesis, and hypospermatogenesis associated with sloughing of primary spermatocytes.

*Pure hypospermatogenesis* is defined as a proportionate decrease in the number of all types of germ cell. The number of spermatogonia per cross-sectioned tubule is less than 17 and usually more than 10. The number of primary spermatocytes is equal to or higher than that of spermatogonia. The number of round spermatids is higher than that of primary spermatocytes, and the number of elongated spermatids is similar to that of spermatogonia (Fig. 12-104).

*Hypospermatogenesis associated with primary spermatocyte sloughing* is characterized by two features: low numbers of spermatogonia and primary spermatocytes (with spermatocytes more numerous than spermatogonia), and degeneration and sloughing of many primary spermatocytes. The remaining spermatocytes give rise to the few spermatids observed in the tubules (Fig. 12-105).

*Etiology of hypospermatogenesis.* Hypospermatogenesis may result from hormonal dysfunction, congenital germ cell deficiency, Sertoli cell dysfunction, Leydig cell dysfunction,

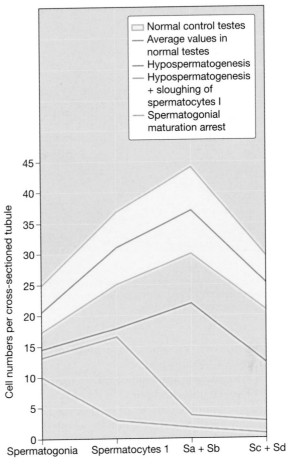

**Fig. 12-103** Germ cell number per cross-sectioned tubule in patients with lesions in the basal and adluminal compartments of the seminiferous tubules.

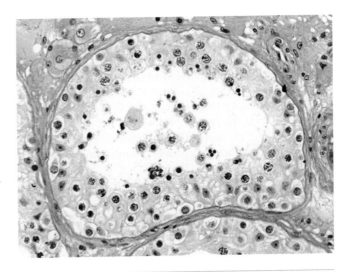

**Fig. 12-104** Pure hypospermatogenesis in a patient with severe oligozoospermia. The seminiferous tubule shows slight ectasis and a proportionate decrease of all germ cell types.

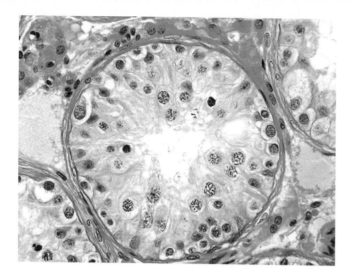

**Fig. 12-105** Hypospermatogenesis associated with primary spermatocyte sloughing in an azoospermic patient. Spermatogonia and primary spermatocytes are the sole germ cell types.

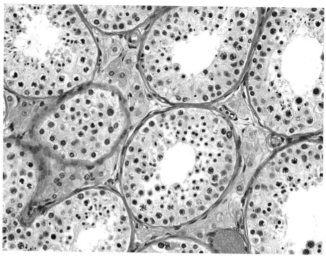

**Fig. 12-106** Hypospermatogenesis due to androgen receptor defect. The seminiferous tubules show hypospermatogenesis associated with diffuse Leydig cell hyperplasia.

androgen insensitivity, exposure to chemical or physical agents, and vascular malfunction.

*Hormonal dysregulation.* Although complete spermatogenesis may be observed in men with low levels of FSH and LH, the production of a normal number of spermatozoa requires normal gonadotropin levels. Hypospermatogenesis has been reported in patients with abnormal pulsatile secretion of FSH and LH,[938] low gonadotropin secretion,[939] biologically inactive gonadotropins, mutation in the gonadotropin β subunit,[940] inactivating mutation of FSH receptor gene,[941] hyperprolactinemia, and adrenal and thyroid dysfunction (see discussion on hypogonadisms secondary to endocrine gland dysfunction in this chapter).

*Congenital germ cell deficiency.* Biopsy of cryptorchid patients after orchidopexy reveals that spermatogonia proliferation is decreased and germ cell development is insufficient in adulthood even if the number of spermatogonia was normal in infancy. Is it likely that this poorly understood primary anomaly of germ cells is present in some cases of hypospermatogenesis.

*Sertoli cell dysfunction.* For many years, primary germ cell deficiency was considered the most common cause of hypospermatogenesis; today, it is known that Sertoli cell failure is the cause of many cases of germ cell deficiency. This conclusion is based on several findings. Sertoli cells in many infertile patients are markedly abnormal, with an increase in the number of glycogen granules[942] and acid phosphatase activity;[884] a decrease in the number of lipid droplets; and alterations in the cytoskeleton,[943] the nucleus,[944] and cytoplasmic organelles.[945] In some cases Sertoli cells have abnormal maturation, with elongated nuclei containing coarse clumped chromatin instead of triangular-shaped nuclei with pale chromatin. Anomalies in Sertoli cell FSH receptors may be present in idiopathic oligozoospermia associated with elevated levels of FSH.[946] Serum inhibin B concentration may be used as a marker to estimate Sertoli cell function.[947]

*Leydig cell dysfunction.* Testosterone synthesis by Leydig cells is necessary for normal spermatogenesis,[948] and abnormal Leydig cell function is a frequent finding in idiopathic oligozoospermia.[949-951] Leydig cell dysfunction should be suspected when the cells appear diffusely hyperplastic. Patients have elevated serum LH level with depletion of rapid-release testosterone, revealing a lack of early response of Leydig cells to gonadotropin-releasing hormone stimulation. The ratio of testosterone to LH in the plasma indicates the degree of Leydig cell dysfunction. Decreased ratio with normal testosterone level suggests compensated dysfunction. Patients with a ratio of less than 1:5 and normal other parameters may have complete spermatogenesis.[951]

*Androgen insensitivity.* Some patients with severe oligozoospermia or azoospermia have a defect in androgen receptor responsiveness, similar to that in Reifenstein's syndrome.[952-954] The abnormality may arise from a genetic defect in the eight exons that code for this receptor, mapped to Xq11-12,[955] or from post-translational errors.[956,957] This defect is also referred to as infertile male syndrome and mild androgen insensitivity, and the patients have male phenotype with somatic features of slight androgen deficit.[958] Histologically, the testis is similar to that observed with Leydig cell dysfunction or mixed atrophy, although the mechanism causing the Leydig cell hyperplasia is quite different (Fig. 12-106). Peripheral resistance to testosterone action alters regulation of the hypothalamohypophyseal–testicular axis, and LH and testosterone levels are elevated. Androgen insensitivity causes between 10%[959] and 40%[960] of all cases of severe oligozoospermia or azoospermia. In such cases spermatogenesis improves with the administration of tamoxifen citrate,[960] clomiphene citrate, or androgen therapy.[961,962] Calculation of the index of androgen insensitivity can be helpful: plasma LH (mIU/mL) × plasma testosterone levels (ng/mL). In patients with androgen insensitivity, the index is higher than 200 (normal is about 102).

*Physical and chemical agents.* The number of chemicals implicated in infertility increases daily. A detailed history is invaluable in evaluating these patients. The same is true of physical agents such as prolonged exposure to heat, ionizing radiation, or microwave radiation.[963]

*Etiology of hypospermatogenesis associated with primary spermatocyte sloughing.* Most testes with primary spermatocyte sloughing have varicocele, and this is commonly associated with infertility.[964–967] Varicocele is found in 15% of the general population, and is present in 30–40% of infertile men. The mechanism by which varicocele affects fertility is unknown. Clinical varicocele may occur without a testicular lesion (or only phlebectasis), and subclinical varicocele may be associated with severe spermatogenic lesions. Increased testicular temperature[968,969] and compression of intratesticular sperm excretory ducts by dilated veins[932] are the most plausible mechanisms. In other cases, primary spermatocyte sloughing results from anomalies of primary spermatocytes and spermatids, suggesting a meiotic anomaly. Finally, in some patients the cause may be the presence of involuting Sertoli cells.

*Spermatogonial maturation arrest* Spermatogonial maturation arrest is a disorder defined by the presence of fewer than 17 spermatogonia per cross-sectioned tubule and even fewer primary spermatocytes. Spermatids are usually absent. There have been attempts to correlate the etiology of spermatogonial maturation arrest with the Sertoli cell type present.[970] Immature Sertoli cells are characteristic of hypogonadotropic hypogonadism and some syndromes with androgen insensitivity (Fig. 12-107). Mature Sertoli cells, if their presence is unilateral, are observed in varicocele, epididymitis, and ipsilateral testicular traumatism, but if they appear in both testes the etiology is unknown. Involuting Sertoli cells are usually present bilaterally; some cases are idiopathic, whereas others are associated with a history of alcoholism or chemotherapy. Dedifferentiated Sertoli cells

are found in spermatogonial maturation arrest caused by gonadotropin inhibition in treatment with estrogen, -releasing hormone agonist, or anti-androgen.[971]

### Focal lesions in spermatogenesis (mixed atrophy)

Mixed atrophy is a descriptive term for the coexistence, in the same testis, of tubules containing only Sertoli cells and tubules with complete or incomplete spermatogenesis.[972] This disorder includes patchy failure of spermatogenesis and partial del Castillo's syndrome.

The extent of Sertoli cell-only tubules varies widely. Tubules with spermatogenesis may be normal or partially atrophic. Tubular hyalinization is occasionally seen (Fig. 12-108). Mixed atrophy is more common than suggested by the literature, and many cases are included under other diagnoses, such as 'hypospermatogenesis with a severe germ cell depletion in such a way that some Sertoli cell-only tubules are seen,'[859] and 'Sertoli cell-only syndromes with focal spermatogenesis.'[973]

Serial sections from testes with mixed atrophy reveal that the two different types of tubule are grouped according to their histologic pattern, suggesting that the distribution is by testicular lobules. In cases of mixed atrophy, the percentage of tubules with spermatogenesis, the degree of spermatogenic development in the tubules, and the type of Sertoli cell present should be reported. Correlation of the first two with the spermiogram gives an indication of prognosis, and the Sertoli cell types identifies the nature (primary or secondary) of the lesion.[974]

Mixed atrophy (probably primary) is observed in idiopathic infertility, cryptorchidism (even if orchidopexy was done at infancy, in both the cryptorchid and the contralateral descended testis), retractile testes, macroorchidism, intravaginal torsion of the spermatic cord (in both twisted and contralateral testis), and chromosomal anomalies such as Down's syndrome, 47/XYY karyotype, 46/XX karyotype,

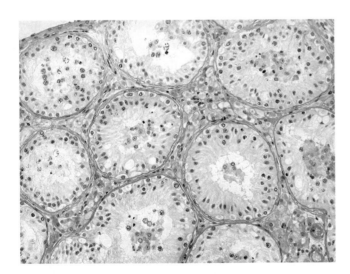

**Fig. 12-107** Spermatogonial maturation arrest. The seminiferous tubules have increased numbers of Sertoli cells and nearly normal number of spermatogonia, while the remaining germ cell types are scant. The testicular interstitium shows diffuse Leydig cell hyperplasia.

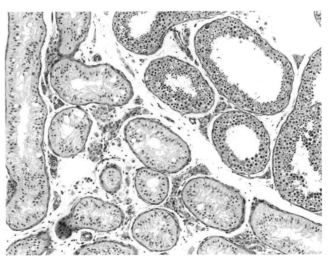

**Fig. 12-108** Mixed atrophy. Seminiferous tubules with slight ectasis and complete spermatogenesis adjacent to Sertoli-cell-only pattern. The tubular lesions probably belong to different lobules.

giant Y chromosome, Klinefelter's syndrome with chromosomal mosaicism, partial androgen insensitivity, and some male pseudohermaphrodites. Secondary mixed atrophy may be seen in patients undergoing chemotherapy, corticoid therapy,[975] or in those with a history of viral orchitis.

## Germ cell anomalies in infertile patients

In addition to anomalies in the seminiferous tubules, examination of the biopsy should include a description of the morphology of the germ cells.

### Giant spermatogonia

Giant spermatogonia are a normal component of the seminiferous epithelium. These cells may be altered spermatogonia in the S or G$_2$ phases of the cell cycle. They rest on the basal lamina and have pale cytoplasm and an ovoid nucleus measuring at least 13 μm in diameter. The frequency of these cells in normal and infertile men is about 0.65 cells per 50 cross-sectioned tubules, although their number is usually higher in mixed atrophy. These cells should not be mistaken for intratubular germ cell neoplasia; they are also present in normal numbers in tubules at the periphery of germ cell tumor (Fig. 12-109).[976]

### Multinucleate spermatogonia

Multinucleate spermatogonia are a common finding in cryptorchid testes that were surgically corrected, infertile patients, and old men. Nuclei of both Ad and Ap spermatogonial types may be seen within the same cell.

### Dislocated spermatogonia

Normally, spermatogonia are present only in the transition zone between the seminiferous tubule basal layer and the tubuli recti. Dislocated spermatogonia have been found throughout the testis in old age,[977] in infertile patients with a variety of lesions, after long-term estrogen therapy,[978] and in seminiferous tubules with intratubular germ cell neoplasia.[979]

### Megalospermatocytes

Megalospermatocytes are large primary spermatocytes arrested in the leptotene stage (Fig. 12-110)[980] that exhibit asynapsis of chromosomes.[981] Joined by cytoplasmic bridges, they form small groups. These cells may be clones of synchronously degenerating spermatocytes.[982] They are frequently found in elderly men and are a non-specific finding in infertile patients.

### Multinucleated spermatids

The presence of spermatids with multiple nuclei (from 2 to 86) is frequent is old age.[983] Similar cells with fewer nuclei have also been reported in infertility due to cryptorchidism,[984] hyperprolactinemia, and idiopathic infertility (Fig. 12-111).

### Malformed spermatids

There are at least four teratozoospermic syndromes that may be easily identified by testicular biopsy, although in most

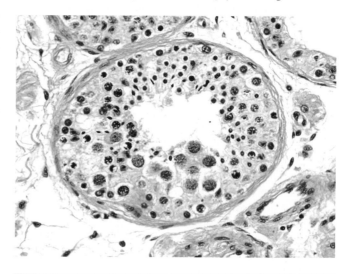

**Fig. 12-110** Megalospermatocytes. The seminiferous tubule contains a group of very large primary spermatocytes displaying fine chromatin and eosinophilic cytoplasm.

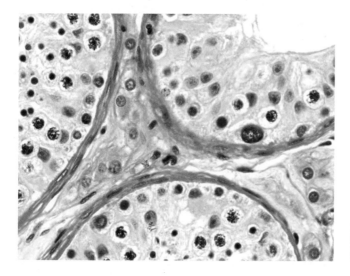

**Fig. 12-109** Hypertrophic spermatogonia in a seminiferous tubule showing marked decrease in the number of spermatogenetic cells.

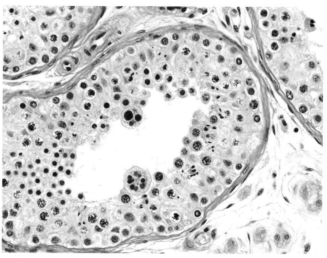

**Fig. 12-111** Multinucleation of both spermatids and spermatocytes.

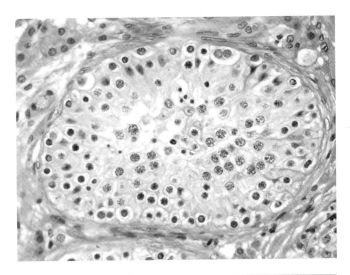

**Fig. 12-112** Testicular biopsy showing spermatids with small spherical nuclei, a finding characteristic of round spermatozoa lacking acrosomes. The remaining germ cells are morphologically normal.

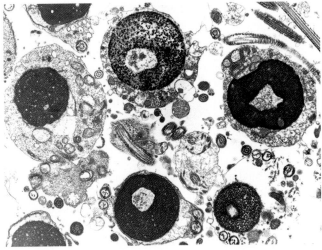

**Fig. 12-114** Microcephalic spermatozoa with a spherical nucleus lacking an acrosome and poorly condensed chromatin. Ultrastructural anomalies are observed.

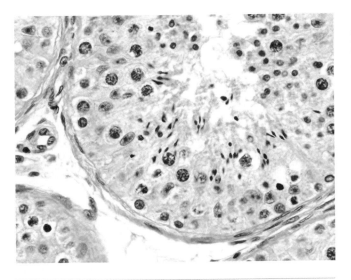

**Fig. 12-113** Elongated spermatids showing bell-clapper nuclei in a patient with varicocele.

the diagnosis previously relied on morphologic study of the spermiogram: (1) round-headed spermatids (characteristic of spermatozoa lacking acrosomes) (Fig. 12-112), (2) $S_c + S_d$ spermatids with a very elongated head (characteristic of varicocele) (Fig. 12-113), (3) macrocephalic $S_c + S_d$ spermatids whose DNA content suggests an anomaly in the first meiotic division, and (4) $S_c + S_d$ spermatids with voluminous eosinophilic cytoplasmic droplets (syndrome of spermatozoa with short thick flagella[985] or fibrous sheath dysplasia).

In some patients, $S_a + S_b$ spermatids rest in these initial phases of spermiogenesis and eventually become sloughed in the tubular lumina.[986] In other testes there are macrocephalic $S_c$ and $S_d$ spermatids with anomalous DNA content, suggesting an anomaly in the first meiotic division.

### Morphologically abnormal spermatozoa

Ultrastructural study of spermatozoa is sometimes necessary to determine the cause of male infertility. A number of mor-
phologically abnormal spermatozoa are present in all semen samples, including those from fertile men, but abnormal spermatozoa are very numerous in infertile patients. Ultrastructural study is advised in all cases of asthenozoospermia, in teratozoospermia when the number of spermatozoa showing the same morphological anomaly is high, and in cases with apparently normal spermatozoa that fail to fertilize in vitro.[987] The classification of ultrastructural anomalies in spermatozoa is based on light microscopy findings[988] of lesions in the head and tail.

*Anomalies of the spermatozoal head* These are defined by changes in the shape of the head, and usually involve both the nucleus and the acrosome. Some anomalies, such as pear-shaped, candle-shaped, or egg-shaped heads,[989,990] are regarded as minor variants of normal. More significant abnormalities are the elongated, microcephalic, macrocephalic, and crater-defect forms.

The most frequent abnormal head shape is elongated with a narrow base (tapered head spermatozoa). This anomaly is frequently associated with varicocele.[991]

Microcephalic spermatozoa have spherical (globozoospermia) or irregularly shaped heads. The former have spherical nuclei with poorly condensed chromatin and lack acrosomes, postacrosomal sheaths, and a nuclear ring (Fig. 12-114). Most cases are sporadic, but this lesion was also reported in two pairs of infertile brothers.[992,993] Microcephalic spermatozoa with irregularly shaped heads have small and irregularly shaped acrosomes that usually are not in contact with the nucleus. This anomaly may be congenital, as in Aarskog–Scott syndrome,[994] or secondary to heat exposure or hashish smoking. In both types of microcephaly loss of connection between the acrosomal vesicle and the spermatozoal head is attributed to a deficiency in basic proteins of the sperm perinuclear theca that promotes nuclear envelope organization and adhesion of the acrosomal vesicle.[995] Acrosin is reduced or absent in spermatozoa lacking acrosomes and those with small acrosomes.[996] Motility may be normal. The occurrence of aneuploidy[997] and disomy of sex chromosomes[998,999] in some cases should be evaluated before performing intracytoplasmic sperm injection (ICSI).

The cause of round-headed spermatozoa might be the lack of Golgi-associated protein known in male mice as Golgi-associated PDZ- and coiled-coil motif-containing protein (GOPC). This protein is principally localized in the *trans*-Golgi region in round spermatids, and its loss produces globozoospermia. The primary defect consists of an inability of acrosomal vesicles to fuse to each other to create the acrosome.[1000]

Macrocephalic spermatozoa (macronuclear spermatozoa) have enlarged, irregularly shaped heads and deficient chromatin condensation. There are two types (multiple tails[1001,1002] and aflagellate), both of which have abnormal DNA content (many are tetraploid), suggesting a meiotic anomaly.[1003,1004]

Irregularly shaped spermatozoa are characterized by irregularity in the shape of the nucleus or acrosome.[1005] In the crater defect syndrome, there is invagination of the nuclear envelope in which the acrosome penetrates. The tail is morphologically normal, and motility is only slightly reduced. In spermatozoa with spoon-shaped nuclei, the defect is probably genetic. Other anomalies include double-headed spermatozoa with two nuclei sharing a single acrosome.[1006]

***Anomalies in the spermatozoal tail*** Spermatozoal tail anomalies are classified as generalized anomalies of the tail or anomalies in defined tail components, such as the connecting piece, the axoneme, or the periaxonemal structure.[1007]

*Generalized anomalies in the tail Cytoplasmic remnants.* The presence of cytoplasmic droplets is normal during spermiogenesis. An elevated number of spermatozoa with cytoplasmic droplets in semen is associated with premature sloughing of spermatozoa, as occurs in varicocele, and should not be misinterpreted as spermatozoa with excess residual cytoplasm.[1008] These spermatozoa are very often abnormal and the residual cytoplasm may be located around the intermediate piece or surrounding the head. These spermatozoa also have other flagellar anomalies.

*Bent tail.* A bend in the tail may occur at the level of the connecting piece or the intermediate piece. In bends of the connecting piece, the tail is laterally implanted and forms an angle with a nucleus that displays a thin base. Bends of the intermediate piece are associated with cytoplasmic droplets, malposition of mitochondria, and loss of the parallel arrangement of the dense outer fibers.

*Coiled tail.* Spermatozoa with a coiled tail are a frequent finding in centrifuged semen, but they may also be a true abnormality. These spermatozoa have a perinuclear cytoplasmic remnant containing a flagellum that is coiled around the nucleus and along the middle or principal pieces (Fig. 12-115). This is frequently associated with abnormalities of the periaxonemal structures.

*Tail stump (short-tail spermatozoa).* The presence of many spermatozoa with short, thick tails in semen represents a well-defined teratozoospermic syndrome.[1009] Ultrastructural examination reveals hypertrophy and hyperplasia of the fibrous sheath,[1010] hence this syndrome has also been termed 'fibrous sheath dysplasia.'[1011] Additional axonemal malformations, including absence of the central pair of microtu-

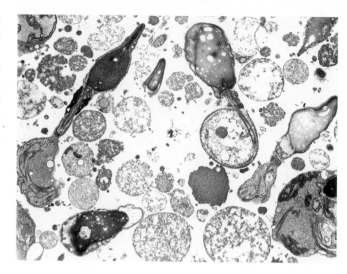

**Fig. 12-115** Spermatozoa with coiled tails. The anomaly occurs in the principal pieces. The intermediate pieces show variable lengths, absence of parallelism in the outer dense fibers, and large cytoplasmic droplets. This teratozoospermia was found in two infertile brothers.

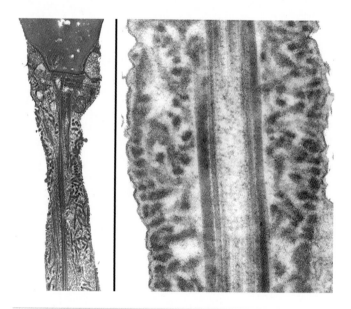

**Fig. 12-116** Tail-stump spermatozoal malformation. Longitudinal section of two spermatozoa showing a marked thickening of the principal piece with both hypertrophy and hyperplasia of the fibrous sheath. One of them also shows a very short intermediate piece.

bules (Fig. 12-116)[1012] and, less frequently, lack of dynein arms, are observed in 50% of cases. About 24% of patients have respiratory disease, such as rhinosinusitis, bronchitis, and bronchiectasis from an early age. Similar findings have been reported in the cilia of the upper respiratory tract, and thus a relationship between fibrous sheath dysplasia and immotile cilia syndrome has been assumed. Clinical presentation may be sporadic or familial. The cause of fibrous sheath dysplasia and the subsequent lack of motility in these spermatozoa is probably related to the occurrence of deletions in Akap3 and Akap4 genes, as well as the absence of Akp4 protein in the fibrous sheath.[1013]

*Multiple tails.* The presence of more than two tails is associated with macrocephalic spermatozoa.[1014]

*Sperm tail agenesis.* Teratozoospermia with 100% sperm tail agenesis has been reported in patients with a high degree of consanguinity. These spermatozoa also have defects in chromatin condensation and residual cytoplasmic droplets.[1015]

*Anomalies of the connecting piece* Anomalies of the connecting piece are classified as acephalic spermatozoa, deficient organization of the connecting piece, and separation between the head and the tail.

Acephalic spermatozoa are known as 'pin-headed,' although they lack a true head; the small cephalic knob-like thickening is actually a cytoplasmic droplet with a variable degree of mitochondrial organization giving rise to a variable degree of motility.[1016] This anomaly is due to an early failure in spermiogenesis. It may be familial in some cases.[1017,1018] Spermatozoa with deficient organization of the connecting piece have narrowing at this level, with loss of alignment of the head and flagellum axes. Spermatozoa with a separated head and flagellum, known as decapitated and decaudated spermatozoa, are also the result of an anomaly in spermiogenesis, but the separation between heads and tails can occur during spermiation or at any level of the sperm excretory ducts.[1019,1020]

*Anomalies in axoneme* Abnormalities of the axoneme are classified as numerical anomalies, microtubular ectopia, and immotile cilia syndrome.

The most common numerical anomalies are the absence of one or both microtubules of the central pair and complete lack of the axoneme. Spermatozoa lacking the central microtubule pair also lack the central sheath and are immotile, although they are normal by light microscopy. Familial cases have been reported.[1021] This anomaly may be associated with ciliary dyskinesia.[1022]

Immotile cilia syndrome (primary ciliary dyskinesia)[1023] refers to patients having low mucociliary clearance associated with otitis, sinusitis, bronchitis, bronchiectasis, and immotile spermatozoa. Most patients have the same defect in the axoneme and cilia of the respiratory mucosa. The frequency of this syndrome is estimated at between 1 in 20 000 and 1 in 60 000 men. Clinical symptoms consist of reduced clearance of ciliary mucus in the airway, with onset at infancy. In order to prevent the later development of bronchiectasis, ultrastructural study of the respiratory mucosa is advisable if other disorders have been excluded, including cystic fibrosis, allergy and other immune disorders, $\alpha_1$-antitrypsin deficiency, and cardiovascular and metabolic diseases.[1024] The most frequent anomalies of this syndrome are the absence of microtubule doublets and peripheral junctions, the central microtubule pair, the outer dynein arms, the central junctions, the two dynein arms, and the inner dynein arm plus the peripheral junctions (Fig. 12-117). Spermatozoa lacking the two dynein arms or the peripheral junctions are immotile. Reduced motility is seen in spermatozoa with only one dynein arm. Kartagener's syndrome is a variant of the immotile cilia syndrome characterized by the classic triad of situs inversus, bronchiectasis, and chronic sinusitis. The syndrome has autosomal recessive

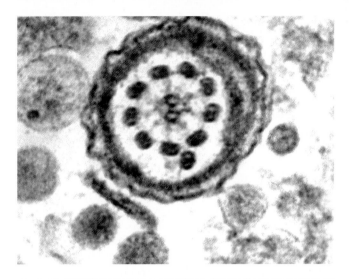

**Fig. 12-117** Cross-section of the intermediate piece from a spermatozoon lacking dynein arms and showing a supernumerary microtubule doublet.

inheritance[1025] and is found in 20–25% of patients with situs inversus.[1026]

*Anomalies in periaxonemal structures* Periaxonemal abnormalities include mitochondrial sheath defects,[1027] malposition of the annulus, alteration in number, shape, or length of the outer dense fibers, and absence, thickening, or disruption of the fibrous sheath.[1011,1028]

Many cases of asthenozoospermia, present in 30% of infertile men, may be attributable to deficient mitochondrial function, possibly caused by mutations in their DNA.[1029] Abnormalities of the dense fibers are associated with deficient motility. Abnormalities of the fibrous sheath include, in addition to the abovementioned dysplasia of the fibrous sheath, absence of the fibrous sheath, and redundant fibrous sheath material associated with a deficit or lack of mitochondria.[1030] The three defects are probably inherited.

## Presence of intratubular germ cell neoplasia

The incidence of intratubular germ cell neoplasia (IGCN) in infertile patient is 0.4% in England,[1031] 0.7% in Spain,[1932] 0.73% in Germany,[1033] and 1.1% in Denmark.[1034] A higher risk occurs in patients with severe oligozoospermia (fewer than 10 million spermatozoa per milliliter), azoospermia associated with unilaterally or bilaterally diminished testicular volume,[1035] a history of testicular maldescent,[1036,1037] or unilateral testicular cancer.[1038]

The cells of IGCN are located in seminiferous tubules with decreased tubular diameter and lacking spermatogenesis. These cells are large and have pale cytoplasm and large and irregularly outlined nuclei, with one or several prominent nucleoli. They stain intensely with periodic acid–Schiff and express placenta-like alkaline phosphatase, *c-kit*, and the cell adhesion molecule CD44.[1039]

## Anomalies in Leydig cells

A reduction in the number or absence of Leydig cells is infrequent in infertility, and only occurs in hypogonadotropic hypogonadism secondary to LH deficit and in patients with biologically inactive LH. Leydig cell hyperplasia is very common,[1040] and has been observed in Klinefelter's syndrome, cryptorchidism, male pseudohermaphroditism, minor androgen insensitivity, infertility secondary to Leydig cell dysfunction, varicocele, after treatment with 5α-reductase inhibitors or non-steroidal anti-androgens, and in some elderly men. Such hyperplasia may give rise to hypoechoic or hyperechoic images that may be misdiagnosed as tumor.[1041]

## Mast cells

There is a close relationship between testicular dysfunction and elevated mast cell numbers in the testis. An increase in interstitial and peritubular mast cells occasionally occurs in infertile patients.[1042,1043] This increase is higher than that observed in inflammatory or neoplastic process.[1044] Daily administration of ketotifen, an antihistamine-like drug with a mast cell-stabilizing effect, significantly improves the spermiogram parameters in some patients.[1045]

## Correlation between testicular biopsy and spermiogram

For effective therapy, it is important to know whether or not the azoospermia or oligozoospermia is the result of obstruction.[863,1046]

### Obstructive azoospermia and oligozoospermia

Azoospermia caused by obstruction is usually easily diagnosed, but this determination is more difficult with oligozoospermia. Obstruction of the ductal system should be suspected when there are more than 20 mature spermatids ($S_c + S_d$) per cross-sectioned tubule and fewer than 10 million spermatozoa in the spermiogram (Fig. 12-118).[1047,1048] Obstructive azoospermia is implicated in 7.4–14.3% of cases of male infertility.

*Classification of obstructive azoospermia by location* Obstruction is classified as proximal, distal, and mixed, according to the distance from the testis to the point of obstruction in the ductal system.

*Proximal obstruction* Obstruction is considered proximal when the lesion lies between the seminiferous tubules and the distal end of the ampulla of the vas deferens. Epididymal obstruction, principally of the caput-corpus transition zone, accounts for 66% of cases. Rarely, there is a defective connection between the rete testis and epididymal ductuli efferentes. Because the seminal vesicles are normal, men with proximal obstruction have a normal volume of semen (the testicular contribution to semen is about 5% of the total volume). When obstruction is in the cauda of the epididymis, epididymal markers, including carnitine, glycerophosphorylcholine and α-glycosidase are low.[1049] The nearer the obstruction is to the caput of the epididymis, the higher the level of these markers.

*Distal obstruction* Distal obstruction is located between the ampulla of the vas deferens and the junction of the ejaculatory ducts and urethra. These patients present with sacral, perineal, or scrotal pain on ejaculation. Rectal examination often reveals enlarged seminal vesicles. The volume of semen is low and consists of watery fluid that fails to

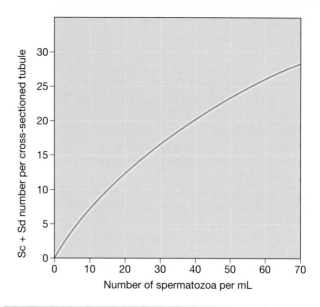

**Fig. 12-118** Power curve showing the correlation between the number of spermatozoa in the spermiogram and the number of mature spermatids (Sc + Sd) per cross-sectioned tubule. If the number of mature spermatids is correlated to that of spermatozoa in spermiogram, the oligozoospermia is of the pure secretory type. If the number of mature spermatids is higher than that of spermatozoa in spermiogram, the disorder is either an obstructive azoospermia with 'normal' testicular biopsy or a mixed obstructive secretory oligozoospermia.

coagulate. Seminal vesicle secretions are lacking. The concentration of prostatic secretions, such as acid phosphatase and citric acid, is increased owing to the lack of semen dilution. Vasography may help in diagnosis, as higher segments fail to fill.[1050] Transrectal ultrasonography is the most accurate imaging modality for the diagnosis of ejaculatory duct obstruction. Needle aspiration of seminal vesicle fluid may show spermatozoa that have entered the seminal vesicles by reflux.

*Mixed obstruction* Mixed obstruction refers to lack of patency of the vas deferens or the epididymis and alterations in the ejaculatory ducts or seminal vesicles (low ejaculate volume, and absence of fructose). The most frequent cause is mucoviscidosis. One-third of patients with congenital bilateral absence of the vas deferens have agenesis or hypoplasia of the seminal vesicles. The cause of epididymal obstruction in patients with anomalies of the prostate–vesiculo–deferential junctions is difficult to determine.

*Etiology of obstructive azoospermia* Obstructive azoospermia may be caused by congenital or acquired lesions.

*Congenital azoospermia* The most frequent anomalies associated with congenital azoospermia are testis–epididymis dissociation, epididymal malformation in cryptorchidism, bilateral absence of the vas deferens, congenital unilateral absence of the vas deferens associated with pathology of the contralateral testis or its sperm excretory ducts, seminal vesicle agenesis, and ejaculatory duct obstruction (Table 12-9).

*Agenesis of all mesonephric duct derivatives.* Agenesis of all mesonephric duct derivatives is a rare disorder that gives rise to varied anatomical anomalies, depending on the stage of

**Table 12-9** Congenital anomalies of the male mesonephric ducts

I. Agenesis of all mesonephric duct derivatives

II. Epididymis
   Agenesis of the epididymis
   Testis–epididymis dissociation
   Failure in the connection between ductuli efferentes and ductus epididymidis
   Cysts of the epididymis
   Anomalies in epididymal configuration
      Elongated epididymis
      Angulated epididymis
      Free epididymis

III. Vas deferens
   Agenesis of the vas deferens
   Persistent mesonephric duct

IV. Seminal vesicle
   Agenesis of the seminal vesicle
   Cysts of the seminal vesicle
   Opening of the ureter into the seminal vesicle

V. Ejaculatory duct
   Agenesis of the ejaculatory duct

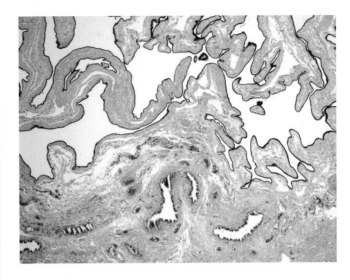

**Fig. 12-119** Infertile patient with bilateral epididymal cysts. The cystic wall appears collapsed and folded on the epididymis.

embryonic development at which the mesonephric duct derivatives disappear. If failure occurs before the fourth week the ipsilateral kidney and ureter are absent, although the testis may be present, or there may be other renal anomalies. If failure occurs in the fourth week, and the ureteral bud is already formed, the ureter and kidney may develop normally. If failure occurs between the fourth and the 13th weeks, there is a variable constellation of anomalies that most frequently include normal development of the testis and globus major and hypoplasia of the other excretory duct segments, or agenesis of an excretory duct segment (epididymis, vas deferens, or seminal vesicle).

*Epididymal anomalies.* The most frequent epididymal anomalies are absence of the epididymis, testis–epididymis dissociation, defective connection of the vas deferens and epididymis, epididymal cyst, and anatomical abnormalities of the epididymis.

Complete absence of the epididymis is frequent in monorchidism and anorchidism. The epididymis is replaced by a small mass of cellular connective tissue with abundant blood vessels at the blind end of the vas deferens.

Partial absence of the epididymis is more frequent than complete absence. Absence of the corpus of the epididymis gives rise to a characteristic malformation called bilobated epididymis. This varies from simple strangulation to complete separation of the caput and cauda. These anomalies are often associated with absence of the vas deferens.

Testis–epididymis dissociation is found in 1% of cases of obstructive azoospermia and is usually associated with cryptorchidism.

Defects in connection between the ductuli efferentes and the ductus epididymidis are rarely complete. In the incomplete form, some of the five to 30 ductuli efferentes in the epididymis are short and end blindly.

Epididymal cysts usually arise from blind-ended ductuli efferentes and contain spermatozoa. These spermatoceles

retain their epithelial lining, although it becomes atrophic (Fig. 12-119). Spermatozoa may be obtained from these cysts. Some epididymal cysts arise from embryonic remnants, do not contain spermatozoa, and are lined by columnar or pseudostratified epithelium. Wolffian cyst, unlike müllerian cyst, is immunoreactive in the apical border of epithelial cells with CD10.[1051] Cyst lined by clear cells with or without papillae raises concern for von Hippel–Lindau disease.[1052] Large epididymal cyst requires removal and must be excised with great care to avoid damaging the ductuli efferentes and resulting in obstruction. Epididymal cyst is present in about 5% of males, and the incidence is high (21%) in those exposed to diethylstilbestrol during gestation. The incidence of epididymal cyst in those with hepatorenal polycystosis is similar to that in the general population.[1053]

Anomalies in epididymal configuration, altering its shape and location, are frequent in men with cryptorchidism and uncommon with descended testes. The most common malformations are elongated epididymis, angulated epididymis, and free epididymis. Elongated epididymis is found in approximately 68% of undescended testes. The length of the epididymis may be several times that of the testis, and, in abdominal or inguinal cryptorchidism, the epididymis extends several centimeters below the testis. Angulated epididymis is characterized by a long epididymis that has a sharp bend in the corpus with or without stenosis. With free epididymis, all or part of the epididymis is unattached to the testis. The most common variant is epididymis with free cauda.

*Vas deferens anomalies.* The most frequent anomalies are of the vas deferens are congenital absence, segmental aplasia, ectopia, duplication, diverticula, and crossed dystopia.[1054]

Congenital absence is defined as unilateral or bilateral absence of either the whole vas deferens or only a segment. Obviously, azoospermia occurs with bilateral absence. The frequency of this malformation varies among populations. At autopsy, the prevalence is 0.5%, but the clinical incidence is 1–1.3% in infertile men[1055] and 10–25% in patients with obstructive azoospermia. Unilateral complete absence is three times more frequent than bilateral absence, and absence of only a segment is even more frequent. The affected segment may be absent or reduced to a fibrous cord. Absence of the vas deferens may be associated with other malformations of the sperm excretory ducts or urinary system. The most frequent malformations of the excretory ducts are absence of the ejaculatory ducts (33% of cases) and, less frequently, absence of the seminal vesicles. About 71% of patients with bilateral absence of the vas deferens have partial aplasia of the epididymis. The most frequent malformations of the urinary system are absence of the ipsilateral kidney and other renal anomalies. Complete or partial absence of the vas deferens occurs frequently in patients with cystic fibrosis.

Persistent mesonephric duct consists of the ureter joined to the vas deferens, forming a single duct that opens in an ectopic orifice between the trigone and the verumontanum. This malformation may be associated with cystic transformation or absence of the seminal vesicle. The kidney may be normal or dysplastic.

*Anomalies of seminal vesicle and ejaculatory duct.* The most frequent anomalies are agenesis of the seminal vesicles or ejaculatory ducts, cyst of the seminal vesicle, and ectopic opening of the ureter into the seminal vesicle. The last is the most common and often is associated with ipsilateral renal dysplasia.

*Acquired azoospermia* Inflammation and trauma are the main causes of acquired azoospermia. Epididymitis is a frequent cause; *Chlamydia trachomatis*[1056,1057] and *Escherichia coli* are the most common infectious causes in developed countries.[1958] Infections with *Neisseria gonorrheae* and mycobacteria are also implicated, and non-specific epididymitis is important.[1059] Apart from elective vasectomy, the most frequent traumatic causes of azoospermia are surgical accidents during herniorrhaphy in chidren,[1060] orchidopexy, varicocelectomy, hydrocelectomy, deferentography,[1061] and removal of epididymal cyst. Obstructive azoospermia may also result from blockage of the ejaculatory ducts following transurethral resection, or as a result of chronic urethral catheterization.

***Testicular and epididymal lesions resulting from obstruction of sperm excretory ducts*** Lesions of the testis and epididymis may result from obstructed sperm excretory ducts, depending on the location, origin (congenital or acquired), and duration of the obstruction.

*Location of obstruction* Obstruction at the level of the ampulla of the vas deferens, seminal vesicles, or ejaculatory ducts does not usually cause significant lesions in the testis or epididymis. More proximal obstruction at the level of the vas deferens, epididymis, or testis–epididymis junction usually causes severe lesions in both the sperm excretory ducts and the testicular parenchyma. Obstruction of the vas deferens causes increased pressure within the ductus epididymis. As a result, epididymal lumina dilate, the epithelium atrophies, and fluid containing few spermatozoa and some spermiophages accumulates in the lumen (Fig. 12-120). The most dilated epididymal segment is the caput. The

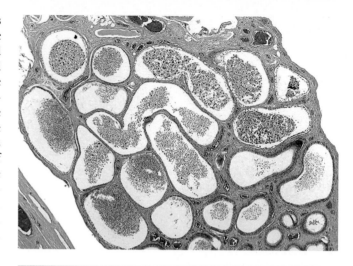

**Fig. 12-120** Obstructive azoospermia in a patient with history of epididymitis. The caput epididymidis shows marked dilation of the ductuli efferentes with numerous spermatozoa.

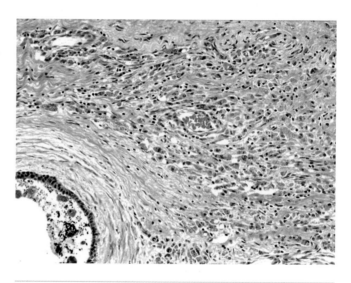

**Fig. 12-121** Ceroid granuloma in a patient with history of sperm excretory duct obstruction.

ductuli efferentes often become cystically dilated and filled with spermatozoa and macrophages. From reabsorption and lysosomal degradation of this protein-rich fluid, the epithelium accumulates lipofuscin granules or aquires apical eosinophilic granules (Paneth cell-like change).[1062] Rupture of the vas deferens gives rise to microgranulomas and ceroid granuloma (Fig. 12-121). Macrophages and lymphocytes are often present in the intertubular connective tissue.[1063]

The most frequent testicular lesions in proximal obstruction involve the adluminal compartment, and are the result of the negative effect of hydrostatic pressure on the seminiferous tubular cell layers and, in particular, on the Sertoli cell (Figs 12-122–12-124).

*Etiology of obstruction* Obstruction secondary to congenital absence of the vas deferens usually causes little testicular injury, mainly dilation of the seminiferous tubules and an increase in the number of mature ($S_c + S_d$) spermatids.[1064]

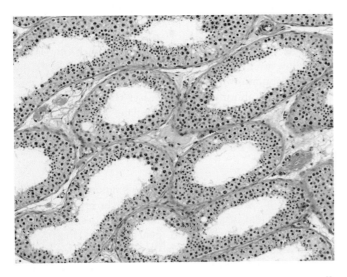

**Fig. 12-122** Seminiferous tubules with marked luminal dilation, moderate decrease in cellularity, and occasional vacuolation of Sertoli cell cytoplasm.

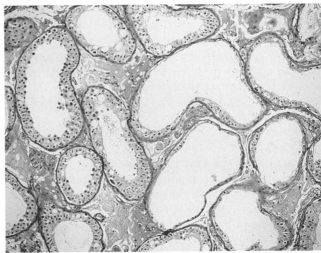

**Fig. 12-124** Seminiferous tubules with marked ectasis and atrophy of the seminiferous epithelium in a patient with epididymal obstruction.

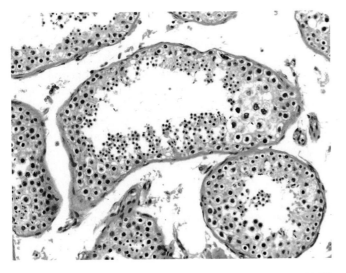

**Fig. 12-123** Seminiferous tubules with slight luminal dilation. The seminiferous tubular cell layers have a 'toothed' pattern. Degenerating megalospermatocytes can be seen in the seminiferous epithelium.

Lesions resulting from vasectomy are more important. Increased intraluminal pressure in the epididymis[1065] may give rise to pain (late post-vasectomy syndrome).[1066] Testicular lesions depend on the surgical technique used: they are slight if the proximal end of the vas deferens is not ligated or sperm granuloma forms at the site of vasectomy. The spermatogenic rhythm in the testis is slower than before vasectomy, and lesions characteristic of testicular obstruction develop, including thickening of the lamina propria and fibrosis of the interstitium.[1067,1068] In testicular obstruction secondary to herniorrhaphy in infancy, testicular lesions are mild. Testicular lesions may be important if the epididymis is damaged by hydrocelectomy, and consist mainly of primary spermatocyte sloughing. In addition to these lesions, hyalinized tubules may be observed when obstruction is caused by inflammation.

*Duration of obstruction* In acquired obstruction the testicular lesions worsen with time. Obstruction in the caput of the epididymis leads to disappearance of all germ cells in the adluminal compartment of seminiferous tubules. The tubules become dilated and Sertoli cells appear vacuolated. Testicular alterations after vasectomy may not be related to the duration of the obstruction but rather to the initial injury, and may disappear with time as the intraluminal pressure decreases.[1069] However, if a significant amount of time has elapsed after vasectomy, the possibility of attaining a normal spermiogram with vasovasostomy is very low. Vasal patency is restored in most cases of reanastomosis, but paternity rates are markedly lower (25–51%)[1069] than normal (85%).[1070]

Functional azoospermia and oligozoospermia

Some azoospermic patients have testicular biopsy with minimal histologic abnormality or minor tubular dilation without detectable excretory duct obstruction. These findings are characteristic of two main conditions: Young's syndrome, and alterations in spermatozoal transport.

*Young's syndrome* Young's syndrome is defined by the following constellation of findings: azoospermia, sinusitis, bronchitis or bronchiectasis, and normal spermatozoal flagella.[1071] The incidence is probably higher than that recorded in the literature, and Young's syndrome should be suspected in all patients with obstructive azoospermia without a history of epididymitis or scrotal trauma. These patients have a lesion at the junction of the caput and corpus of the epididymis that gives the epididymis a characteristic gross appearance. The caput of the epididymis is distended, the ductuli efferentes contain yellowish fluid and numerous spermatozoa, and the remaining epididymal segments are normal. The ductus epididymidis is blocked by thick fluid.[1072] Young's syndrome should be distinguished from other causes of infertility also associated with chronic sinusitis and pulmonary infections, including ciliary dyskinesia and cystic fibrosis. Ciliary dyskinesia consists of morphological, biochemical, and functional alterations in cilia and flagella, and includes several diseases such as the immotile cilia syndrome, Kartagener's syndrome, and miscellaneous syndromes characterized by imperfectly defined abnormalities of cilia and flagella.[1073] In Young's syndrome, sinusitis and pulmonary infections develop in childhood and stabilize or improve in adolescence; in other conditions, the pulmonary damage increases with age and the cilia and flagella are ultrastructurally abnormal.[1074]

*Alterations in spermatozoon transport* Normally, spermatozoa detach from the Sertoli cells and are transported through the intratesticular and extratesticular excretory ducts, where they are stored, mainly in the cauda of the epididymis, and finally released from the corpus by ejaculation or eliminated by phagocytosis. Only about 50% of spermatozoa are ejaculated. Whereas the release of spermatozoa from the corpus is intermittent, their transport through the sperm excretory ducts is continuous. Transport is accomplished by the myofibroblasts in the wall of the seminiferous tubules and ductuli efferentes and the smooth muscle cells in the wall of the ductus epididymidis and vas deferens. These cells cause peristaltic contraction, propelling spermatozoa along the length of the epididymis in a mean of 12 days (range, 1–21 days). The walls of the seminiferous tubules and extratesticular excretory ducts are under hormonal and neural control. The myofibroblasts in the seminiferous tubules have oxytocinic, $\alpha_1$-$\beta$-adrenergic, and muscarinic receptors. Unmyelinated nerve fibers penetrate the tubular lamina propria, pass among the myofibroblasts, and end near the Sertoli cells.[1075] Along their length these nerve fibers have varicosities containing sympathetic vesicles.

The ductus epididymis is innervated by sympathetic adrenergic nerve fibers that end among the smooth muscle cells. Several hormones, including oxytocin, endothelin-1, vasopressin, and prostaglandins, act on the musculature of the ductus epididymis. The peristaltic contractions begin in the caput and propagate toward the cauda. The frequency and amplitude of contractions vary from region to region, being higher in frequency near the caput and of maximal amplitude in the initial portion of the cauda. The progressive increase in amplitude parallels the progressive increase in thickness of the muscular wall and the requirement for greater force to propel the fluid as it becomes progressively more viscous with a higher concentration of spermatozoa. The distal portion of the cauda is unusually at rest because it is the main reservoir of spermatozoa between ejaculations. Several times daily, vigorous contractions of the distal cauda impel the spermatozoa from the cauda toward the vas deferens.[1076]

Several drugs that favor contraction of the muscular wall ($\alpha_1$ blocking and $F_{2\alpha}$ prostaglandins) have been successfully used in the treatment of alterations in the spermatozoon transport.[1077]

## Infertility and chromosomal anomalies

Knowledge of the incidence of chromosomal abnormalities in male infertility has progressed in parallel with advances in technology: karyotypic studies in peripheral blood, meiotic and chromosomal studies of testicular biopsies, analysis of chromosomes in spermatozoa, and analysis of DNA in blood and spermatozoa for the detection of chromosome Y deletions.[1078] The incidence of chromosomal anomalies in infertile men is 2.2–6.6%, whereas in the general population it is lower than 0.5%. The frequency of chromosomal abnormalities increases with the decrease in number of spermatozoa in the ejaculate.[1079]

### Abnormalities of sex chromosomes

#### Klinefelter's syndrome

*Genetic and clinical aspects* Klinefelter's syndrome is characterized by an abnormal number of X chromosomes and primary gonadal insufficiency. The original description was of a man with eunuchoidism, gynecomastia, small testes, mental retardation, and elevated level of serum gonadotropins.[1080] The frequency of this syndrome varies according to the population studied: 1 in 1000 to 1 in 1400 surviving newborns; 1 in 100 patients in mental institution; 3.4 in 100 infertile men; and 11% of patients who are azoospermic.[1081]

In 80% of cases, the karyotype is 47XXY. The remaining 20% have chromosomal mosaicism with at least two X chromosomes. The most common are XY/XXY, XY/XXXY, XX/XXY, XXY/XX/XY, XY/XO/XXY, XX/XXY/XXXY, and XXXY/XXXXY. The 47XXY lesion is due to non-disjunction in sex chromosome migration during the first or second meiotic division of the spermatocyte or ovule, or during the first meiotic division of the zygote.[1082] Study of the Xg antigen in blood revealed that the extra X chromosome is from the mother in 73% of cases. Advanced maternal age increases the incidence of children with the 47XXY karyotype.

In 47XXY patients, the most common clinical findings are:[1083]

- Eunuchoid phenotype with increased stature.
  The increased height is due to a disproportionate lengthening of the lower extremities. The ratio of span to height is less than 1.
- Incomplete virilization. This is variable and ranges from normal development to absence of secondary sex characteristics.
- Gynecomastia, usually bilateral, present in 50% of patients.
- Mental retardation.

Other commonly associated conditions include chronic bronchitis; varicose veins; cervical rib; kyphosis; scoliosis or pectus excavatum; and a high incidence of hypothalamic, hypophyseal, thyroid, and pancreatic dysfunction.[1084]

The external genitalia usually are normally developed. The testes are usually less than 2.5 cm long, although in some cases of chromosomal mosaicism they are of normal size.[1085] The incidence of cryptorchidism is low in 47XXY patients but increased in mosaicism.[1086]

Supernumerary X-chromosome material is associated with a reduction of gray matter in the left temporal lobe, a finding correlated with verbal and language deficits.[1087]

Histologically, the testes show the classic picture of tubular dysgenesis with small hyalinized seminiferous tubules

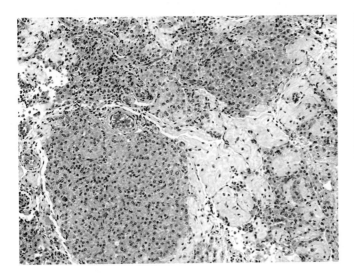

**Fig. 12-125** Klinefelter's syndrome. Leydig cell nodules mingle with hyalinized tubules.

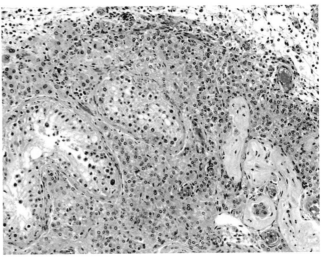

**Fig. 12-127** Klinefelter's syndrome mosaicism showing focal spermatogenesis in two seminiferous tubules located within a Leydig cell nodule.

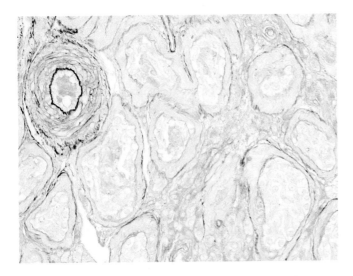

**Fig. 12-126** Klinefelter's syndrome. Most seminiferous tubules, even those with Sertoli cell only, have scant elastic fibers that can be demonstrated with orcein stain. The intense staining observed in the inner elastic lamina of arterioles provides a positive control.

lacking elastic fibers and pseudoadenomatous clustering of Leydig cells (Figs 12-125, 12-126).[1080] Most biopsies show some tubules with a few Sertoli cells.[1088] These cells may be dysgenetic (pseudostratified distribution of nuclei that are dark and elongate and contain small peripherally placed nucleoli in tubules without apparent lumina). Sex chromatin may only be observed in dysgenetic Sertoli cells.[1089] This suggests that either there is testicular mosaicism of the X chromosome, or that both X chromosomes are heterochromatinized. In mosaicism, Sertoli cell-only tubules may be more numerous than hyalinized ones.

The reduced testicular volume gives an appearance of Leydig cell hyperplasia,[1090] although quantitative studies have shown that the total number of Leydig cells is lower than normal.[1091] Many of the Leydig cells are pleomorphic

and some are multivacuolated. Immature fibroblast-like Leydig cells may be present. The abnormally differentiated Leydig cells have nuclei with coarse masses of dense chromatin, deep unfolding of the nuclear envelope, multiple paracrystalline inclusions instead of Reinke's crystalloids, multilayered concentric cisternae of smooth endoplasmic reticulum, large masses of microfilaments, and scant lipid droplets.[1092] Sex chromatin is apparent in 40–70% of Leydig cells. Leydig cell function is insufficient and androgen levels are less than 50% of normal. Basal FSH and LH are markedly increased.[1084,1093,1094] In a few patients the testicular damage is less severe, with some tubules showing spermatogenesis and less prominence of Leydig cells.[1095] Exceptionally, complete spermatogenesis and even paternity have been reported.[1096]

The XY/XXY karyotype is the most frequent variant of Klinefelter's syndrome with chromosomal mosaicism. In this condition, the clinical abnormalities may be attenuated. Gynecomastia is present in 33% of cases, compared to a frequency of 55% in men with the 47XXY karyotype. Azoospermia is found in 50% of cases (93% in XXY men). The testes are larger and spermatogenesis is more developed in men with XXY (Fig. 12-127). Patients with the 47XXY karyotype who have spermatozoa in seminiferous tubules are bearers of 46XY spermatogonia and also of 47XXY spermatogonia, whereas those who have no spermatozoa have 47XXY spermatogonia only; these 47XXY spermatogonia may include some spermatozoa with 23X or 23Y chromosomal complement, elevated numbers of both 24XY and 24XX spermatozoa, and also a high frequency of spermatozoa with 21 disomy; this could be an important risk for gonosomy[1097] and also for trisomy 21.[1098] Genetic counseling is advisable in patients seeking intracytoplasmic sperm injection therapy. Genetic diagnosis before implantation of the zygote or prenatal diagnosis have been recommended, except for parents who assume the risk of gonosomy.

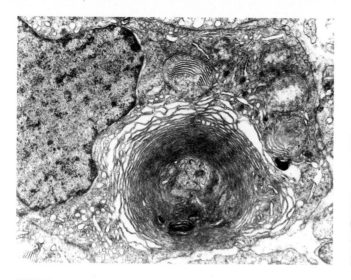

**Fig. 12-128** 48XXYY Klinefelter's syndrome showing a Leydig cell that contains giant mitochondria and a wheel of smooth endoplasmic reticulum.

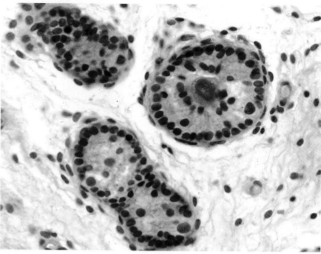

**Fig. 12-129** Klinefelter's syndrome at infancy. Seminiferous tubules showing decreased diameters, isolated germ cells, and a ring-shaped tubule that contains a microlith.

The incidence of the 48XXYY karyotype is estimated to be 0.04 per 1000 live births.[1099-1102] This karyotype may be associated with aggressive character, antisocial behavior, more severe mental retardation, and a higher frequency of congenital malformations than the 47XXY karyotype. Men with the 48XXYY karyotype also have characteristic dermatoglyphics with an increase in arches, a decrease in total finger ridge count, and ulnar triradiuses associated with changes in the hypothenar region.[1103] Concentric lamellae of smooth endoplasmic reticulum in Leydig cells are a characteristic finding (Fig. 12-128).[1104] Men with the 48XXXY or 49XXXYY karyotype often have skeletal malformations, principally radioulnar synostosis, and cryptorchidism.[1105] In addition to the characteristic symptoms of 47XXY Klinefelter's syndrome,[1106] men with the 49XXXXY karyotype have other abnormalities, including severe mental retardation, hypoplasia of external genitalia, cardiac malformations, radioulnar synostosis, microcephaly, and a high arched palate.[1107]

*Association of Klinefelter's syndrome with malignancy* Patients with Klinefelter's syndrome have a higher incidence of malignancy than the general population. The association was first discovered with breast carcinoma,[1108] which had an incidence 20 times greater than in the general male population,[1109] and is related to hormonal stimulation.[1110] Although testicular germ cell tumor is rare in these patients,[1111] extragonadal germ cell tumor is 30–40 times more frequent than in the general population. Most occur in the mediastinum (about 71%) and are less frequent in the pineal gland, central nervous system, and retroperitoneum. The most frequent types are teratoma and choriocarcinoma; embryonal carcinoma and seminoma are rare.[1112-1114] The extragonadal origin of germ cell tumors has been attributed to abnormal germ cell migration from the yolk sac. The high incidence has been attributed to elevated hormone levels and chromosomal anomaly.[1115] In a patient with the XY/XXY chromosomal mosaic and bronchogenic carcinoma, cultured XXY fibroblasts transformed three times more frequently when exposed to SV40 virus than did fibroblasts from normal men.[1116]

Other tumors reported in patients with Klinefelter's syndrome (lymphoma, leukemia, bronchogenic carcinoma, urothelial carcinoma of the bladder, adrenal carcinoma, prostatic adenocarcinoma, testicular Leydig cell tumor, and epidermoid cyst) do not appear to have a higher incidence than in the general population.[1117-1120]

*Occurrence of Klinefelter's syndrome in childhood* Early identification of this syndrome is possible with systematic cytogenetic study of newborns with positive sex chromatin or mental retardation.[1121] Several clinical symptoms suggest Klinefelter's syndrome. Initial symptoms include decreased muscle tone, delayed speech, and poor language skills with an increased incidence of reading difficulties and dyslexia.[1122] Later, there may be recognition of mental retardation,[1123] psychiatric problems, excessive stature for age, disproportionately long legs, micropenis, and small testes.[1124-1127] Androgen deficiency is an early finding.[1128] Testicular biopsy reveals scant or absent germ cells. Quantitative studies indicate that the number of germ cells in 47XXY fetuses is significantly lower than in normal 46XY fetuses. The seminiferous tubules have reduced diameter, particularly those devoid of germ cells. The number of Sertoli cells per cross-sectioned tubule is reduced. Megatubules, ring-shaped tubules, and intratubular eosinophilic bodies are common (Fig. 12-129). In some cases of Klinefelter's syndrome associated with Down's syndrome, tubular hyalinization is observed in childhood.[1129] The interstitium is wide and contains few Leydig cell precursors. If one testis is undescended, its histology does not differ from that of the contralateral testis. The testicular pattern remains constant through childhood.[1130] At puberty, before maturation of the tunica propria occurs, the seminiferous tubules rapidly hyalinize and Leydig cell precursors differentiate into Leydig cells.[1131]

*Association of Klinefelter's syndrome with precocious puberty* Although precocious puberty is not a characteristic finding in Klinefelter's syndrome, karyotyping in older boys with mental retardation, gynecomastia, small testes, and precocious puberty is advisable. In most cases, the cause of precocious puberty is a hCG-secreting germ cell tumor in the mediastinum.[1132] Infrequently, precocious puberty is idiopathic, and only in isolated cases is there a hamartoma in the third ventricle.[1133]

*Association of Klinefelter's syndrome with hypogonadotropic hypogonadism* Klinefelter's syndrome is often associated with pituitary disorders such as panhypopituitarism[1134] or incomplete hypopituitarism.[1135] Deficits in FSH,[1136] LH,[1137] or both[1138,1139] have been reported. The cause of this association is unknown, and diverse etiologies such as trauma, immunologic disorders, and genetic deficiencies have been postulated. Alternatively, it may be due to exhaustion of pituitary gonadotropin-secreting cells after years of gonadotropin-releasing hormone stimulation.[1135]

In patients deficient in both gonadotropins, testicular biopsy shows diffuse tubular hyalinization and a marked reduction in or absence of Leydig cells. The histological picture is similar to that of hypogonadotropic hypogonadism occurring after puberty, except for the presence of isolated tubules containing only dysgenetic Sertoli cells and absence of elastic fibers in the hyalinized tubular wall (Fig. 12-130).[1139] Biopsy of patients with a deficit only in FSH is similar to that of the dysgenetic Sertoli cell variant of the Sertoli cell-only syndrome, although some hyalinized tubules are present. The testicular biopsy of patients deficient only in LH resembles that of men with classic 47XXY Klinefelter's syndrome.

*46XX males* The 46XX karyotype may be present in three phenotypes: male phenotype, including normal external genitalia; male pseudohermaphrodites, with a variable degree of ambiguity in external genitalia, ranging from hypospadias to micropenis; and true male hermaphrodites.

*46XX males with male phenotype and normal external genitalia* Men with the 46XX karyotype having male phenotype and normal external genitalia have clinical features similar to those of Klinefelter's syndrome, including small testes, small or normal penis, azoospermia, gynecomastia, and minimal development of secondary sex characteristics. However, these men have harmonious body proportions, normal or slightly low stature, and normal intelligence.[1140] The incidence of 46XX males varies from 1:10 000 to 1:25 000 live births, accounting for about 0.2% of infertile men.[1141,1142] Males with 46XX karyotype have hypergonadotropic hypogonadism with elevated serum levels of FSH and, to a lesser degree, elevated LH, with normal or slightly decreased testosterone. Familial cases have been reported.[1143]

During childhood, biopsy of 46XX males reveals decreased numbers of germ cells.[1144,1145] Biopsies from adults show one of three patterns: histology similar to that of 47XXY men, including diffuse tubular hyalinization with prominent Leydig cells;[1146] Sertoli cell-only tubules;[1147,1148] and both patterns intermingled with less prominent Leydig cells. The last is the most frequent (Fig. 12-131). Ultrastructural studies reveal an increase in intermediate filaments, absence of annulate lamellae in Sertoli cells,[1149] absence of Reinke's crystalloids, and abundance of intracytoplasmic and intranuclear paracrystalline inclusions in Leydig cells.[1147]

*46XX males with ambiguous external genitalia* Some patients with the 46XX karyotype have ambiguous external genitalia or hypospadias and are assumed to have a variation of male pseudohermaphroditism.[1150] These males, together with true hermaphrodites, may be found in the same family, suggesting that both disorders are different manifestations of the same genetic defect.

*Etiology of 46XX males* The origin of 46XX males may be difficult to determine. However, as testicular differentiation requires genes located on the Y chromosome, 46XX males have been classified by cytogenetics as those having the SRY gene, those lacking the SRY gene, and XX/XY mosaicism. Males with the SRY gene comprise 80% of 46XX males.[1151] It is likely that this occurs when the genetic material from

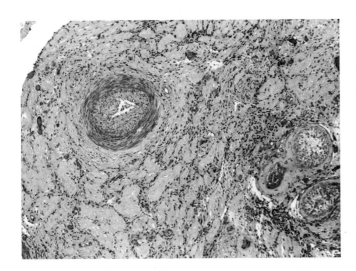

**Fig. 12-130** Klinefelter's syndrome with hypogonadotropic hypogonadism showing diffuse tubular hyalinization associated with absence of Leydig cells. Only tubules with dysgenetic Sertoli cells are present.

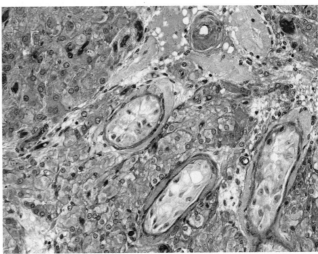

**Fig. 12-131** Testis from a 46XX male showing Sertoli-cell-only tubules together with hyalinized tubules, and nodular and diffuse Leydig cell hyperplasia.

the short arm of the Y chromosome is translocated to the X chromosome.[1152] During paternal meiosis, the homolog pseudoautosomal regions of chromosomes X and Y interchange the terminal portions of their short arms, giving rise to an X chromosome with the SRY gene but lacking the azoospermia factor.[1153–1158] Alternatively, the SRY region may be inserted in an autosome.[1159] Most 46XX patients who are SRY positive have a normal male phenotype. About 10% of 46XX males are SRY negative and most have ambiguous genitalia. Some patients have a normal male phenotype[1161] and only infertility.[1162] Although SRY is assumed to be the most important regulator factor of testicular determination, these patients may have mutation of one of the downstream non-Y testis-determining genes.[1163–1166] About 10% of 46XX males have XX/XY mosaicism or other karyotype with the chromosomal complement Y. In these cases, detection of the specific DNA sequences of Y chromosome may be difficult because this chromosome may be only in some tissues and in a small number of cells.[1160]

*47XYY syndrome* The 47XYY syndrome was first described in 1961 in the father of a girl with Down's syndrome.[1167] The only clinical findings were excessive height and pustular acne. Study of other cases suggests that these men are predisposed to a psychopathic personality and antisocial behavior, although most have a normal personality and are socially adapted. The incidence of 47XYY patients is estimated to be 0.01% of the general population, 0.7–0.9% of men in prison, and 1.8% of sexual homicide criminals.[1168] The extra Y chromosome originates from non-disjunction during the paternal second meiotic division.

In the past decade, many cases have been diagnosed prenatally. From birth, the patients have weight, stature and cephalic circumference above mean values and a higher risk for delayed language and/or motor development. About 50% of children have psychological and psychiatric problems such as autism; although their intelligence is normal, many patients are referred to special education programs.[1169] As adults, they have normal external genitalia and secondary sex characteristics. Fertility is reduced,[1170] although many have been fathers. Usually, testicular biopsy reveals mixed atrophy characterized by tubules with spermatogenesis associated with Sertoli cell-only tubules (Fig. 12-132).[1171,1172] Those tubules with spermatogenesis may show normal spermatogenesis or have lesions in the adluminal or basal compartments. In these tubules, many XXY spermatocytes degenerate during meiosis. About 64 % of pachytene cells have three sex chromosomes.[1173] The number of normal spermatozoa in the ejaculate is low. There is a high incidence of both YY and XY spermatozoa and disomy 18.

The variability in germ cell development is apparently due to elimination of germ cells that could not pair their sex chromosomes during the first or second meiotic divisions[1174] or, later, during the round spermatid stage.[1175] Spermatocytes that succeed in forming trivalent chromosomes are initially viable.[1176] The ultimate trivalent chromosome segregation yields aneuploid and euploid cells in equal numbers. Sertoli cell-only tubules are attributed to either spermatogonial damage by substances released from degenerated spermatocytes[1177] or absence of testicular colonization

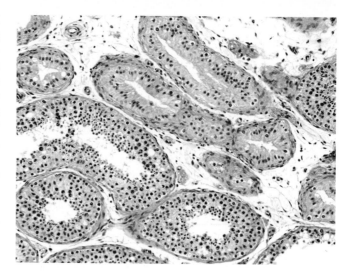

**Fig. 12-132** 47/XYY syndrome. The testis show tubules with complete spermatogenesis, Sertoli-cell-only tubules, and tubules with spermatogonial maturation arrest.

by primordial germ cells. These men have normal serum levels of testosterone and LH. The latter may be slightly increased in 47XYY men with severe spermatogenic alterations.[1178]

47XYY men with mosaicism (47XYY/46XY) have a higher risk of fathering children with hyperdiploid chromosomal constitution, and spermatozoa should be studied genetically to evaluate the risk of intracytoplasmic sperm injection.[1179]

Men with three and four Y chromosomes have been reported. Men with the 48XYYY karyotype are tall and have normal male phenotype, slight mental retardation, azoospermia and, during childhood, frequent infections of the upper respiratory tract.[1180] Testicular biopsy shows Sertoli cell-only tubules, severe hyalinization of tubular basement membrane, and diffuse Leydig cell hyperplasia. The chromosomal complement of parents can be normal.[1181] Men with 49XYYYY also have no significant phenotypic abnormalities (except for cases of chromosomal mosaicism). Slight mental retardation, infertility, and antisocial behavior are the most significant clinical findings.[1182] Rarely patients have facial dysmorphism and various skeletal abnormalities.[1183]

Structural anomalies of the Y chromosome

The Y chromosome is essential for gender determination and spermatogenesis, and abnormalities often lead to infertility. The relationship between Y chromosome abnormalities and infertility is best understood in azoospermic men with alterations in Yq11, the distal region of the euchromatic part of the long Y arm, the location of a male fertility gene complex called azoospermia factor. Infertility may result from deletion of any of four subregions in which the azoospermia factor has been divided (AZFa, AZFb, AZFc and AZFd).[1184,1185] The best-known Y chromosome genes involved in spermatogenesis are RBM. DAZ, DFFRY, CDY, SMCY, and ZFY. Six different partial deletions of this region have been found in azoospermic patients (Table 12-10). Other genes related to spermatogenesis are BPY2, PRY, TTY1, TTY2, and VCY.[1186]

**Table 12-10** Pathologic findings in infertile men with Y chromosome anomalies in the $Y_Q11$ region

| Karyotype | External genitalia | Testicular lesions | Associated anomalies |
|---|---|---|---|
| $46XY_q$ | Small testes | Tubular hyalinization, Sertoli cell-only, spermatogenetic maturation arrest | Low stature, mental retardation, gynecomastia |
| $46XY_{nf}$ / 45X0 | Small and soft testes, small penis, ambiguous genitalia, cryptorchidism, hypospadias | Tubular hyalinization, Sertoli cell-only, Leydig cell hyperplasia, decreased spermatid number | Low stature, gynecomastia |
| $46Xr(Y)$ / 45X0 | Small testes, cryptorchidism, hypospadias | Sertoli cell-only, spermatogenetic arrest in premeiotic spermatocytes | Low stature |
| $46Xt(Y_p11,Y_q11)$ / 45X0 | Small and soft testes, hypospadias | Spermatogenetic arrest in premeiotic spermatocytes, decreased spermatid number | Low stature |
| $46Yt(X_p22,Y_q11)$ | Small testes, small penis | Spermatogenetic arrest in premeiotic spermatocytes | Mental retardation, digital anomalies, facial dysmorphism |
| $46XY_qt(Y_q11\text{-}qter,A)$ | Normal or small testes | Spermatogenetic arrest in premeiotic spermatocytes | |
| $46Xt(Y_q11\text{-}pter,A)$ | Normal or hypoplastic testes, cryptorchidism, hypospadias | Sertoli cell-only, immature seminiferous tubules | |

*Monocentric deleted Yq chromosome* Partial deletion of the distal portion of the Yq11 euchromatic region is associated with azoospermia owing to loss of the azoospermia factor. These men have normal external genitalia except for small testes,[1187] normal testosterone and LH serum levels, and increased FSH serum level. The most frequent histological finding is Sertoli cell-only pattern, although many other patterns have been reported.[1188] The number of Leydig cells is normal or increased. These findings suggest that the azoospermia factor is required for early spermatogenesis.[1189] If the breakpoint of Yq11 is proximal to the centromere, patients are short because the gene that controls stature is close to that for the azoospermia factor.[1190]

*Dicentric Yq isochromosomes* Sterility is frequent in men with dicentric Yq isochromosomes.[1191] This anomaly is usually associated with a 45X cell line. The proportion of this line varies between patients and between cell types (fibroblasts or lymphocytes). When the point of breakage and fusion of the two Y chromosomes is in the distal region Yq11, and the second centromere is inactivated, the Y isochromosome is normal in size but does not stain with quinacrine, and thus is called non-fluorescent Y chromosome (Ynf). As the breakpoint is in the Yq11 region, the azoospermia factor function is altered. Development of external genitalia varies from ambiguous to normal, and is probably related to the extent of XO present.[1192] Testicular biopsies are similar to those of men with monocentric deleted Yq chromosomes (Fig. 12-133).[1193,1194]

*Ring Y chromosome* Men with ring Y chromosomes have normal male phenotype, azoospermia, and, in some cases, short stature. Most have mosaic karyotype with a 45X line. In some cases, testicular biopsy resembles that of men with monocentric deleted Yq chromosome, but in others there is premeiotic arrest of spermatocyte maturation.[1195] This is attributed to difficulty in pairing the X and Y chromosomes during meiosis. Many patients have deletion of some AZF regions.[1196,1197]

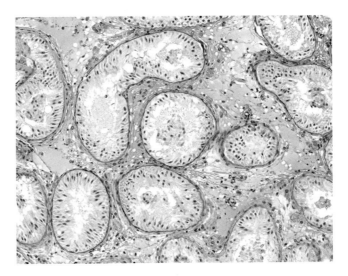

**Fig. 12-133** Testis from a male with dicentric Yq isochromosome showing seminiferous tubules with Sertoli cell-only pattern and slight Leydig cell hyperplasia.

*Y/Y translocation chromosome* Patients with this anomaly have small soft testes and primary spermatocyte maturation arrest owing to defective pairing of the X and Y chromosomes. The karyotype may be mosaic with a 45X line.[1198]

*Translocation of Y chromosome to X chromosome* Most frequently this translocation is cytogenetically undetectable, and patients present with infertility and are found to have 46XX karyotype.[1199] The phenotype is similar to that of men with Klinefelter's syndrome except for shorter stature, absence of mental retardation, and smaller teeth. Testicular biopsy shows Sertoli cell-only pattern. Men with cytogenetically detectable translocations have short stature, small testes, tubular hyalinization, and prominent clustered Leydig cells similar to Klinefelter's syndrome.

*Autosomal translocation of Y chromosome* Translocation of the distal heterochromatic portion of the Y chromosome to the short arm of an acrocentric chromosome occurs occasionally. The most frequent are translocations to chromosomes 5, 18, 13, 15, and 22. The fertility of these men depends on the point of breakage.[1200,1201] If this occurs in the Yq12 heterochromatic region, the patient has a male phenotype and is fertile. If the point of breakage is in the Yq11 region, the patient is infertile and has small testes. Seminiferous tubules may show only Sertoli cells, spermatogenetic arrest in early stages of meiosis, or an infantile pattern.[1202,1203]

*Interstitial microdeletion in Yq11* Yq11 microdeletion is the most frequent congenital cause of infertility. The frequency of Y chromosome microdeletion in infertile patients varies widely (1–35%).[1204] In azoospermic men, the frequency is between 18%[1205] and 37%.[1206] In oligozoospermic males the incidence drops. Most microdeletions are in the AZFc subregion.[1207,1208] Testicular biopsy shows only Sertoli cells, maturation arrest, or mixed atrophy. There is no correlation between site of AZF subregion alteration and histological pattern.[1209] There is no exact correlation between genotype and phenotype,[1209] but most microdeletions in AZFa are associated with azoospermia, most microdeletions in AZFb are associated with maturation arrest, and most microdeletions of AZFc are associated with spermatid maturation arrest or mixed testicular atrophy. Partial deletion of AZFc has a mild effect on fertility.[1210]

### Structural anomalies of the X chromosome

External genitalia in 46XY patients with duplication of distal Xp vary from male, ambiguous, to female, and gonadal dysgenesis is frequent. If the patient has male genitalia, these are usually hypoplastic with hypogonadotropic hypogonadism and, frequently, multiple congenital anomalies and mental retardation.[1211]

Males with translocation of the X chromosome to an autosome may have disturbed spermatogenesis with subfertility or infertility.[1212,1213] 47XXX males show mental retardation, gynecomastia, normal stature, hypoplastic scrotum, a well-configured but small penis, small testes, and poorly developed pubic hair. Serum testosterone levels are very low. Seminiferous tubules appear severely hyalinized. 47XXX males result from an abnormal X–Y interchange during paternal meiosis and X–X non-disjunction during maternal meiosis.[1214]

### Anomalies in autosomes

There have been many reports on the relationship between autosomal anomalies and infertility, although the causes are not fully understood because the same anomaly is associated with infertility in some patients but not in others.

### Chromosomal translocations and inversions

Robertsonian translocations are found in 0.7% of infertile men (8.5% higher than in the normal population) and are more frequent in oligozoospermic than in azoospermic men. The most frequent translocations are 13;14 and 14;21.

The incidence of reciprocal translocations in infertile patients is 0.5% (0.1% in the general population) and increases to 0.8% in patients with azoospermia or severe oligozoospermia.[1215] The most frequent in infertile men are 11;22 and 17;21.

Paracentric and pericentric inversions (except for the pericentric inversion of the heterochromatic region in chromosome 9) are eight times greater in infertile patients (0.16%) than in the general population. The highest risk for infertility occurs in the pericentric inversion of chromosome 1.[1216,1217]

The most common testicular lesions in men with autosomal anomalies are spermatogonial maturation arrest, primary spermatocyte sloughing sometimes associated with hypospermatogenesis, and Sertoli cell-only pattern.[1218]

### Down's syndrome

The only autosomal anomaly with prolonged survival is Down's syndrome. In addition to trisomy of chromosome 21 and the characteristic appearance, patients with Down's syndrome usually have cryptorchidism, small testes, hypoplasia of the penis and scrotum, and hypospadias.[1219] Adults have oligozoospermia or azoospermia secondary to primary testicular deficiency. Levels of FSH and LH are elevated, but testosterone is normal or slightly diminished.[1220] Isolated cases of paternity have been reported.[1221,1222]

In utero, there is marked delay in germ cell development.[1223] Histologic studies of prepubertal testes at autopsy reveal decreased tubular diameter and tubular fertility index. Eosinophilic bodies or microliths may be present in some tubules (Fig. 12-134). Adult testes have deficient spermatogenesis and mixed atrophy, with some tubules showing complete spermatogenesis and others containing Sertoli cell-only pattern.[1224]

## Other syndromes associated with hypergonadotropic hypogonadism

Hypergonadotropic hypogonadism is found in several myopathies (myotonic dystrophy and progressive muscular

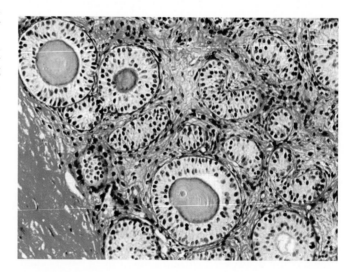

**Fig. 12-134** Prepubertal testis in Down's syndrome. There are megatubules, ring-shaped tubules, and small tubules. Germ cell number is very low in all these tubules. Eosinophilic bodies or microliths are present in some tubules.

dystrophy) and dermopathies (Bloom's, Rothmund–Thomson, Werner's, Cockayne's, and Tay's syndromes), with testicular histology that resembles that of Klinefelter's syndrome. Hypogonadism is also observed in Noonan's syndrome, cerebellar ataxia (with milder testicular lesions), and a miscellaneous group of syndromes with variable histological findings.[1225]

*Myotonic dystrophy* accounts for approximately 30% of men with muscular disorders, and about 80% have testicular atrophy. The estimated incidence is 1 in 8000 live births. The abnormality involves the distal muscles of the extremities. In addition, patients may have premature baldness, posterior subcapsular cataracts, cardiac conduction defects, impotence, gynecomastia (rarely), and dementia (at later stages). Myotonic dystrophy is an autosomal dominant inherited disease with variable penetrance. Two loci are associated with the disease phenotype: DM1 in 19q13.3, and DM2 in chromosome 3. Mutation in DM1 results in a serine/threonine protein kinase deficiency that causes expansion of a CTG repeat (from 50 to several hundred repeats) located on the 3'-untranslated region of the dystrophy myotonic-protein kinase gene. The number of repeats is positively correlated to severity of the disease and negatively correlated to age of clinical onset.[1226–1228] DM2 is caused by a mutation in 3q21.3 of the ZNF9 gene and accounts for CCTG-repeat expansion (from 75 to 11 000 repeats) in intron 1 of this gene. The common clinical symptoms are due to gain of function of RNA mechanism in CUG and CCUG repeats altering cellular function, including alternative splicing of various genes.[1229] The severity of the disease increases in the successive generations.[1230] The number of CTG repeats is not associated with male subfertility.[1231]

Hypogonadism is hypergonadotropic in most cases and is not related to the number of CTG repeats.[1232] Testicular lesions probably begin late because 65% of patients are fathers. Testicular biopsy shows different degrees of severity, ranging from nearly normal to fully hyalinized seminiferous tubules, with the number of Leydig cells varying from increased to decreased. In some patients the hypogonadism is hypogonadotropic, and the testes show an infantile pattern. Infertility may be the first symptom of myotonic dystrophy.[1233]

*Progressive muscular dystrophy* is a multisystemic X-linked disease. It is usually associated with gonadal atrophy caused by a defective locus in chromosome 19. Patients rarely live more than 20 years. The incidence is approximately 1 in 4000 live births. In both Duchenne and Becker forms the cause is a defect in the dystrophin gene.[1234,1235]

*Bloom's, Rothmund–Thomson, and Werner's syndromes* are caused by a homozygous defect in human RECEQ helicases in chromosome 15. Of the five members of this gene family (RECQ1, BLM, WRN, RECQ4, and RECQ5), three produce autosomal recessive inherited diseases. Mutations of BLM have been identified in patients with Bloom's syndrome, WRN has been shown to be mutated in Werner's syndrome, and mutations of RecQ4 have been associated with Rothmund–Thomson syndrome.[1236,1237] Despite the close genetic origin of the three syndromes, symptoms are very different. *Bloom's syndrome* is characterized by short stature, narrow face with prominent nose, facial 'patchy' skin color changes that become more marked with sunlight exposure, and increased susceptibility to respiratory diseases, cancer and leukemia. Severe oligozoospermia and azoospermia are common. Leydig cell function is conserved.[1238] *Rothmund–Thomson syndrome* presents with poikiloderma, juvenile cataracts, sparse hair, short stature, skeletal defects, dystrophic teeth and nails, and hypogonadism. These patients are predisposed to cancer and osteogenic sarcoma.[1239] *Werner's syndrome (progeria)* is characterized by short stature, prematurely graying hair, baldness, cataracts, atrophy and calcification of muscle and fat, wrinkling of the skin, keratosis, osteoporosis, telangiectasis, atheroma, diabetes mellitus, gynecomastia, and hypergonadotropic hypogonadism. The lifespan of fibroblasts and other cells is shortened in this syndrome. The mutation is in the RECQ3 helicase gene.

*Cockayne's syndrome* is a rare autosomal recessive neurodegenerative disorder. Signs and symptoms include infantile failure to thrive, short stature, poorly developed trunk, premature aging, neurological alterations, retinitis pigmentosa, optic atrophy, cataract, deafness, microcephaly, micrognathia, photosensitivity, delayed eruption of primary teeth, congenital absence of some permanent teeth, partial macrodontia, atrophy of the alveolar process and caries, limited articular movements in elbows, knees, and fingers,[1240] abnormally small eccrine glands,[1241] and hypergonadotropic hypogonadism. It may be caused by two gene mutations: CNK1 (ERCC8) and ERCC6, located respectively on chromosomes 5 and 10, and causing two variations of Cockayne's syndrome, including CS-A, secondary to a ERCC8 mutation, and CS-B with ERCC6 mutation. CS-B patients have hypersensitivity to ultraviolet light secondary to a DNA repair defect.[1242]

*Tay's syndrome* (trichothiodystrophy) has two presentations: IBSD (ichthyosis, brittle hair, impaired intelligence, short stature) and IBISD (photosensitivity, ichthyosis, brittle hair, impaired intelligence, short stature). In both forms, patients have decreased fertility. One case of hypergonadotropic hypogonadism has been reported.[1243]

*Noonan's syndrome* is characterized by multiple malformations reminiscent of Turner's syndrome, including short statute, pterygium coli, and cubitus valgus, although there is normal male karyotype. The disease has an incidence of 1 in 1000 to 1 in 2500 live births and autosomal dominant inheritance, with sporadic occurrence in about 50% of cases. A locus for dominant forms has been mapped to 12q24.1.[1244] Mutation in PTPN11 (protein–tyrosine phosphatase, nonreceptor-type 11) accounts for half of cases, although similar germline mutations also cause Leopard's syndrome and certain pediatric hematopoietic malignancies.[1245] Cryptorchidism is present in about 70% of cases and is usually bilateral. During childhood, testicular biopsy shows a low tubular fertility index. Puberty is often delayed, and, at adulthood, hypogonadotropic or hypergonadotropic hypogonadism occurs. Ultrastructural studies reveal morphologic anomalies in germ cells.[1246] Although spermatogenesis is generally impaired, some patients have been fertile (Fig. 12-135).

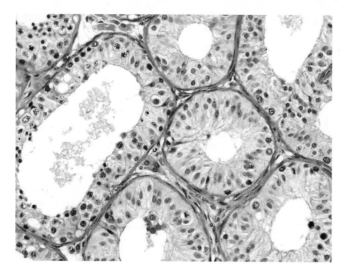

**Fig. 12-135** Testis from a 15-year-old boy with Noonan's syndrome. Most seminiferous tubules are small and contain Sertoli cells and isolated spermatogonia. The most dilated tubules have complete although quantitatively decreased spermatogenesis.

*Cerebellar atrophy* may be associated with hypogonadism. Patients are infertile and have moderate ataxia without endocrine disorder. Infertility is due to morphological abnormalities of spermatozoa caused by decreased expression of MAP2 (the most important microtubule-associated protein), and a defect in erythroid ankyrin.[1247,1248]

Many other syndromes also present with primary hypogonadism. The best known are Alström's, Weinstein's, Borjenson-Forssman-Lehmann, Marinesco-Sjögren, Richards-Rundle, Robinow's, and Silver-Russell syndromes.

## Secondary idiopathic hypogonadism

Hypogonadotropic hypogonadism or hypogonadism of hypothalamo–hypophyseal origin is classified according to whether the hypothalamo–hypophyseal failure occurs before or after puberty. Eunuchoidism, present only in the former group, is the basis of the distinction. The most frequent types of hypogonadism caused by hypothalamo–hypophyseal failure are those caused by a deficit of gonadotropin-releasing hormone, bioinactive FSH and LH, deficit in growth hormone, those associated with Prader–Willi syndrome, and Laurence–Moon–Rozabal–Bardet–Biedl syndrome.

### GnRH deficit

The onset and maintenance of the hypothalamo–hypophyseal–gonadal axis is due to pulsatile gonadotropin-releasing hormone (GnRH) secretion by neurons of the nucleus arcuatus hypothalamus, with release into the pituitary portal system and subsequent stimulation of gonadotropin-releasing hormone receptors on the surface of gonadotropin-secreting cells. The GnRH gene is located on 4q13.[1249]

Patients with GnRH deficit have partial or complete absence of GnRH-induced pulsatile LH secretion, and normalization of pituitary and gonadal secretions after exogenous GnRH administration. Imaging studies of the hypothalamo–hypophyseal region are normal. Clinical

symptoms vary with age at presentation (congenital or acquired) and severity (complete or partial deficit). Clinical presentations include delayed puberty, idiopathic hypogonadotropic hypogonadism (isolated gonadotropin deficit), Kallmann's syndrome, isolated FSH deficit, and isolated LH deficit (fertile eunuch syndrome).

### Constitutional delayed puberty

Constitutional delayed puberty is assumed to be a minor form of GnRH deficit,[1250] and is characterized by delayed sexual maturation in otherwise healthy males. Patients are short and usually have a family history of delayed puberty. Puberty usually begins at 13–14 years of age and progresses over 2 years. If a 14-year-old boy has not begun pubertal changes (testicular enlargement, growth in height, and development of secondary sex characteristics), delayed puberty should be suspected.[1251] Simple pubertal delay that is overcome naturally in a short time without treatment must be distinguished from hypogonadotropic hypogonadism. The latter should be suspected when any of the following symptoms are present in the patient or his family: a midline defect, anosmia, or pubic hair without testicular development. Hormone assays may also assist in diagnosis. If a patient between 16 and 18 years old has prepubertal gonadotropin levels, he probably has hypogonadotropic hypogonadism.

### Isolated gonadotropin deficit

A variant of hypogonadotropic hypogonadism, isolated gonadotropin deficit is characterized by defects in the synthesis or release of FSH and LH; other hypophyseal functions are normal. Patients have eunuchoid phenotype, with small testes and penis, scanty body hair and beard, a high-pitched voice, and poorly developed muscles. Presentation may be sporadic, autosomal dominant, autosomal recessive, or X-linked. The cause might be a mutation in the GnRH receptor gene.[1252] Patients have very low levels of FSH, LH, testosterone, and estrogen. Clomiphene citrate treatment fails to stimulate hormonal secretion.[1253] Pulsatile administration of GnRH is useful to promote both androgen production and spermatogenesis. The LH–Leydig cell–testosterone axis is normal in most cases, but normalization of the FSH–Sertoli cell–inhibin axis is not achieved in all cases. Basal inhibin levels higher than 60 pg/mL and absence of cryptorchidism are favorable predictor factors for the acquisition of normal testicular size and acceptable spermatogenesis.[1254]

Testicular biopsy reveals an immature pattern. The seminiferous tubules have neither lumina nor elastic fibers (Fig. 12-136). Sertoli cells are immature, and no differentiated Leydig cells are seen. Spermatogonia are rare. In some patients the pattern is similar to that of Sertoli cell-only testes with immature Sertoli cells.[1255]

### Hypogonadism associated with anosmia

Hypogonadism associated with anosmia is also known as Maestre de San Juan,[1256] Kallman,[1257] or De Morsier[1258] syndromes. The two most important features are hypogonadotropic hypogonadism and anosmia. Members of affected families may have both features or only one. Associated

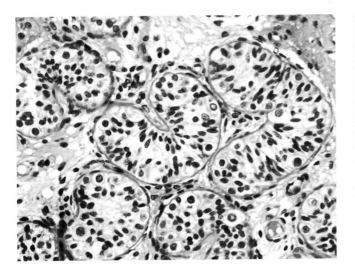

**Fig. 12-136** Isolated gonadotropin deficit. The seminiferous tubules have prepubertal diameter, pseudostratified distribution of the Sertoli cells, and several spermatogonia per tubular section.

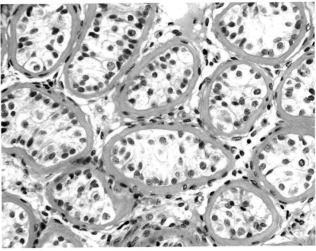

**Fig. 12-137** Hypogonadism associated with anosmia in a previously treated patient. The testis shows marked hyalinization of the tubular wall. Some spermatogonia can be observed among the Sertoli cells. The testicular interstitium lacks Leydig cells.

abnormalities include olfactory bulb agenesis, cryptorchidism, mental retardation, color blindness, facial asymmetry, nerve deafness, epilepsy, shortening of the fourth metacarpal, tarsal navicular fibrous dysplasia, familial cerebellar ataxia, diabetes mellitus, hyperlipidemia, gynecomastia, cleft lip, maxillary or palate, unilateral renal aplasia, and cardiovascular abnormalities. The syndrome may be X-linked or autosomal. The gene for the X-linked form is mapped to Xp22.3 and may have different mutations (termed Kal-X, KALIG-1, and ADMLX), complete deletion, and point mutations. This gene encodes the protein anosmin-1, which is similar to other nerve cell adhesion molecules and is involved in axonal growth and development. KAL protein, secreted by mitral cells, permits the passage of olfactory neurons into the olfactory bulbs and is lacking in Kallmann's syndrome. This failure also inhibits migration of neuroblasts from the olfactory epithelium to the hypothalamus to form GnRH-secreting neurons.[1259] The autosomal dominant presentation (occurring in 10% of cases) is due to loss of function of fibroblastic growth factor receptor 1 (FGFR1).[1260] Interaction between KAL1 and FGFR1 is required for neuronal migration.[1261]

Patients are classified into two groups according to the partial or complete absence of GnRH. Partial absence of GnRH is diagnosed by the presence of spontaneous pulses of LH, FSH, and testosterone during a 24-hour period. Complete absence is diagnosed by the absence of spontaneous pulses of LH, FSH, and testosterone during a 24-hour period. These patients show an increase in FSH only after GnRH administration.[1262] Testes are histologically infantile; the tubules have a small diameter, lack lumina, and contain immature Sertoli cells and isolated spermatogonia.[1263] The interstitium is wide and consists of acellular connective tissue with no recognizable Leydig cell precursors (Fig. 12-137).[1264]

Autopsy studies in patients with anosmia and hypogonadism reveal agenesis of the olfactory bulbs that may be partial or complete and unilateral or bilateral, together with an apparently normal hypophysis and normal or hypoplastic hypothalamus. This syndrome is the least severe form of holoprosencephaly–hypopituitarism complex, a spectrum of developmental anomalies associated with impaired midline cleavage of the embryonic forebrain, aplasia of the olfactory bulbs and tracts, and midline dysplasia of the face. Testicular seminoma has been reported in a patient with anosmia with hypogonadotropic hypogonadism.[1265]

## Isolated FSH deficiency

This rare syndrome is characterized by azoospermia or oligozoospermia in normally virilized patients with normal sexual potency. Serum levels of LH and testosterone are normal, but FSH levels are very low or undetectable. The clomiphene stimulation test gives variable results. The GnRH test induces a normal response only of LH. Mutations in the FSH-β gene are exceptional.[1266,1267]

Testicular biopsy shows maturation arrest at the spermatocyte level, hypospermatogenesis, or partial Sertoli cell-only pattern.[1268] Gonadotropin treatment increases spermatozoal numbers in most cases, and fertility may be induced.

## Isolated LH deficiency

Isolated LH deficiency, also known as Pasqualini's or fertile eunuch syndrome,[1269,1270] is characterized by hypogonadism secondary to LH deficit with preservation of spermatogenesis. Patients have eunuchoid habitus, small testes, decreased libido, female distribution of pubic hair, and a high-pitched voice. Other frequent findings include gynecomastia, anosmia, ocular lesions, and pituitary tumor.[1271] FSH level is normal, but LH and testosterone levels are very low. Mutations in the LH-β subunit gene[1272] and the GnRH receptor have been reported.[1273]

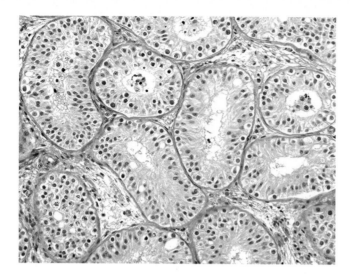

**Fig. 12-138** Isolated deficiency of luteinizing hormone. Most seminiferous tubules have a central lumen, numerous spermatogonia, and increased number of Sertoli cells. Spermatocytes and spermatids are observed only in isolated tubules. The testicular interstitium lacks Leydig cells.

The clomiphene test is usually negative, and GnRH stimulation increases LH and, to a lesser degree, FSH. Testicular biopsy shows seminiferous tubules with normal or slightly decreased diameters and complete spermatogenesis; however, the number of all germ cell types is below normal. Leydig cells are rare or absent (Fig. 12-138). Maintenance of spermatogenesis in the absence of Leydig cells and serum testosterone can only be explained by assuming the occurrence of testosterone secretion sufficient for spermatogenesis but not to be detectable in the blood.

## Bioinactive FSH and LH

In addition to adequate hypothalamic function, spermatogenesis requires that FSH and LH are biologically active. LH is a heterodimer, composed of two subunits: α (common to FSH and LH) and β (specific for LH). The genes for the β subunit are on 19q13.32. If both alleles are mutated for this subunit, the LH produced in biologically inactive although it may be detectable in standard hormone assay. Homozygous patients have elevated serum level of LH and low testosterone levels, lack of puberty, and infantile testes. Heterozygous patients are only infertile.[1274] Patients with mutation in the β subunit of the FSH gene are oligozoospermic or azoospermic.[1275]

## Mutations in gonadotropin receptor genes

Activating and inactivating mutations of gonadotropin receptor genes have been reported. Activating mutation of the LH/human chorionic gonadotropin receptor gene causes familial precocious puberty (see discussion on familial testotoxicosis, below). Inactivating mutation of this gene causes male pseudohermaphroditism (see discussion on Leydig cell hypoplasia in this chapter).

Inactivating mutation of the FSH receptor gene produces only mild spermatogenetic lesions, emphasizing the relative value assumed for FSH in spermatogenesis. Activating muta-

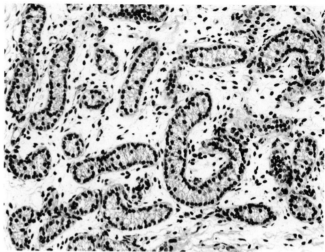

**Fig. 12-139** Testis from a 7-year-old child with Prader–Willi syndrome. The seminiferous tubules have a reduced diameter and lack germ cells.

tion of this gene gives rise to spermatogenesis even in the absence of pituitary function.

## Growth hormone deficit

Patients with isolated growth hormone deficit and those with resistance to growth hormone action may have delayed puberty and hypogonadotropic hypogonadism.[1276] Some patients with spermatogenetic maturation arrest or idiopathic oligozoospermia have a relative deficit of growth hormone. This hormone probably acts on the testis by stimulating local secretion of insulin-like growth factor-1, which cooperates with testosterone.

## Prader–Willi syndrome

Prader–Willi syndrome is characterized by hypogonadism, obesity, muscular hypotonia, mental and physical retardation, and acromicria.[1277] Other frequent findings include strabismus and non-insulin-dependent diabetes mellitus. The incidence is estimated at between 1 in 12 000 and 1 in 15 000 newborns in 25 000 live births, and is higher in males. Patients have low serum levels of LH, testosterone, estradiol, and inhibin B, and high levels of FSH. These hormonal findings suggest the occurrence of a mixed form of central (low LH) and peripheral (low inhibin B and high FSH) hypogonadism.[1278]

The penis and testes are hypoplastic, and cryptorchidism is present in about 70% of cases (bilateral in 45% of cases) (Fig. 12-139).[1279] During infancy and childhood, the testes have reduced tubular diameters; adults have an infantile pattern.[1280] This syndrome is caused by an anomaly of chromosome 15, usually in the 15p11-12 band. Other chromosomal anomalies include Robertsonian translocations, reciprocal translocations, small supernumerary metacentric chromosomes, and partial deletion of the long arm of chromosome 15.

## Bardet–Biedl syndrome

This syndrome is a pleiotropic disorder characterized by obesity, infantilism, short stature, diabetes insipidus, mental retardation, retinitis pigmentosa, polydactyly, and syndactyly. It is more frequent in males than in females. Men with this syndrome are infertile, and about 74% show hypogonadism. The testes are prepubertal, the scrotum is hypoplastic or bifid, and the penis is small. Cryptorchidism is found in 42% of males, and is bilateral in 28%. At least 11 genes responsible for this syndrome have been cloned, and it is probable that additional genes are involved. The function of the products of these gene is to mediate and regulate microtubule-based transport processes.[1281,1282]

## Hypogonadotropic hypogonadism associated with dermatologic diseases

Several dermatopathies are associated with hypogonadotropic hypogonadism, including ichthyosis and Johnson's neuroectodermic syndrome. Most cases of ichthyosis associated with hypogonadism are X-linked. About 15% of these patients have cryptorchidism, small testes, micropenis, and high risk of testicular cancer. The cause is a defective microsomal enzyme, steroid sulfatase, causing the accumulation of cholesterol sulfate that hinders sloughing of the cornified layer of the epidermis. The gene responsible for this enzyme is mapped to Xp22,3. Some of these patients also have anosmia or hyposmia owing to involvement of the neighboring genes, causing a contiguous gene defect.[1283]

Johnson–McMillin neuroectodermic syndrome is a rare autosomal dominant disorder characterized by alopecia, hypogonadotropic hypogonadism, anosmia or hyposmia, deafness, prominent ears, microtia and/or atresia of the external auditory meatus, and a pronounced tendency to dental caries.[1284]

## Hypogonadotropic hypogonadism associated with ataxia

Hypogonadism associated with ataxia is rare. Most patients are the offspring of a consanguineous marriage. Inheritance is autosomal recessive. The most frequent syndromes are Louis–Bar's syndrome (ataxia–telangiectasia) and Friedreich's ataxia.

*Ataxia–telangiectasia* is the most common inherited ataxia and is characterized by cerebellar ataxia that starts in infancy and develops progressively; mucocutaneous telangiectasis; anomalies of the immune system that cause pulmonary infection; hypersensitivity to ionizing radiation owing to impairment of DNA repair; and a high risk of lymphoid neoplasia. The gene responsible is on 11q22-q23.1.[1285] This ataxia results from inactivation of the A-T mutated (ATM) kinase, a critical protein kinase that regulates the response to DNA double-strand breaks by selective phosphorylation of a variety of substrates.[1286]

*Friedreich's ataxia* is a neurodegenerative disorder characterized by degeneration of dorsal root ganglia and spinocerebellar tracts. Hypertrophic myocardiopathy is also observed in many of these patients. The incidence is estimated at 1 in 40 000 children. It is caused by defects in the gene encoding frataxin, a protein required for vesicular traffic in cell and synaptic transmission.[1287] About 95% of patients are homozygous for an unstable trinucleoid (GAA) expansion in intron 18 of STM7 on 9q13. The normal gene has up to 35 or 40 triplet repeats, whereas patients with this ataxia carry 70 to more than 1000 GAA triplets.[1288] The normal gene has seven to 22 GAA repeats, whereas the mutated gene has over 120 repeats. The extent of the expanded allele is directly proportional to the severity of disease, early onset of disease, and development of cardiac abnormalities.

Other ataxias associated with hypogonadism are Kearns–Sayre, Boucher–Neuhauser, and Gordon–Holmes syndromes.

## Other forms of hypogonadotropic hypogonadism

Hypogonadotropic hypogonadism may also be present in Carpenter's, Biemond's, Fraser's, and Moebius' syndromes, and in patients with mental retardation.

## Hypogonadism secondary to endocrine gland dysfunction and other disorders

Maintenance of spermatogenesis requires the harmonious cooperation of several endocrine glands and proper functioning of other tissues. Symptomatic endocrinopathy is present in only 1.7% of infertile men, but over 9% of infertile patients have abnormalities in their endocrine studies.[1289] Hypogonadism may be present in disorders involving the hypothalamus–hypophysis, thyroid, adrenals, pancreas, liver, kidney, and gastrointestinal tract, and may be associated with AIDS, chronic anemia, obesity, lysosomal and peroxisomal diseases, and neoplasia. Hypogonadotropic hypogonadism can also be found in some (usually women) who perform rigorous sports (long-distance runners, swimmers, dancers, and rhythmic gymnasts).[1290]

### Hypothalamus–hypophysis

#### Hypopituitarism

Hypogonadism may result from destruction of the hypothalamus or hypophysis by primary or secondary hypothalamic tumor; granulomatous disease (Fig. 12-140); fracture

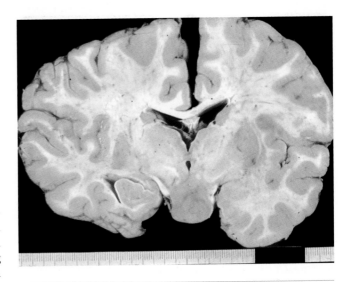

**Fig. 12-140** Frontal section from an 18-year-old patient showing destruction of the hypothalamus caused by Langerhans' cell granulomatosis.

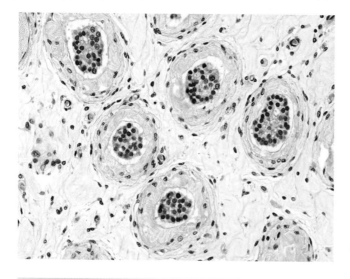

**Fig. 12-141** Tubular hyalinization caused by hormonal deprivation and decreased Leydig cell number in a 28-year-old patient who underwent surgery owing to pituitary adenoma. The seminiferous tubules contain dedifferentiated Sertoli cells and isolated spermatogonia.

of the cranial base; radiotherapy for malignancy of the nasopharynx, central nervous system, or the eye orbit; pituitary adenoma and cyst; aneurysm of the inner carotid artery; and chronic and nutritional disease. Many of these processes cause panhypopituitarism with varied symptoms.[1291]

Clinical manifestations of hypogonadism in patients with pituitary lesions vary according to time of onset (childhood, or after puberty). In prepubertal hypopituitarism the testes retain an infantile appearance into adulthood, and there is rarely proliferation of spermatogonia and the development of primary spermatocytes. Biopsy shows variable hyalinization of tubules. In postpubertal hypopituitarism the appearance ranges from complete spermatogenesis to tubular hyalinization (Fig. 12-141). The presence of elastic fibers in tubular walls indicates that pubertal maturation occurred before the development of hypopituitarism. Leydig cells have pyknotic nuclei and retracted cytoplasm with abundant lipofuscin. In some patients, recovery of spermatogenesis occurs after administration of human chorionic gonadotropin.[1292]

There are cases in which pituitary adenoma secretes both FSH and LH, inducing testosterone hypersecretion and an elevated sperm count.[1293] FSH-secreting pituitary adenoma associated with large testes and increased serum inhibin concentration has been reported.[1294]

### Hyperprolactinemia

Prolactin inhibits GnRH secretion and hence FSH and LH secretion. In addition, prolactin has a direct inhibitory effect on androgens in target tissues. In men, hyperprolactinemia causes impairment of spermatogenesis, impotence, loss of libido, and depressed serum testosterone.[1295] Some patients seek treatment because of oligozoospermia and infertility. Hyperprolactinemia is also associated with dysfunction of prolactin receptors.[1296] Spermiograms usually show oligozoospermia and an elevated level of fructose,[1287] although

not all males with hyperprolactinemia have subnormal testicular function.[1298]

Testicular biopsy reveals variable testicular atrophy. The most frequent lesion is in the tubular adluminal compartment, with degenerative changes in the apical cytoplasm of Sertoli cells, sloughing of young spermatids,[1297] and increased lipid droplets in Leydig cells.[1299] In boys, two different conditions associated with abnormal prolactin secretion have been reported: hyperprolactinemia, testicular enlargement, and primary hypothyroidism; and prolactin deficiency, obesity, and enlarged testes.

### Thyroid gland

Infertility caused by thyroid gland malfunction is rare but reversible. It accounts for about 0.5% of male infertility Testicular function is impaired more by hypo- than by hyperthyroidism. Patients with hyperthyroidism may have gynecomastia, impotence, and infertility. Levels of FSH and LH serum are normal or increased, with elevated sex hormone-binding globulin, increased testosterone concentration, reduced non-sex hormone-binding globulin-bound testosterone, and little or no change in free testosterone.[1300,1301] In Graves' disease there is a pronounced inhibition of gonadal steroidogenesis.[1302] In patients with hyperthyroidism, spermatozoa may be normal or reduced in number, and in both cases progressive motility is low.

Prepubertal hypothyroidism may impair testicular function by causing precocious or delayed puberty. In delayed puberty, hypothyroidism leads to hypogonadotropic hypogonadism, with testes showing incomplete maturation arrest and, in severe myxedematous hypothyroidism, hydrocele.[1303] In experimental hypothyroidism, testicular enlargement is frequently associated with increased spermatid production.[1304] Primary hypothyroidism in adults causes hypergonadotropic, hypogonadotropic, or normogonadotropic hypogonadism,[1305] but testicular function is rarely impaired and patients are usually infertile.[1306] The cause of testicular damage is decreased gonadotropins or hyperprolactinemia.[1307] Children with hypothyroidism usually have precocious pseudopuberty.[1308]

### Adrenals

About 11% of infertile patients reportedly have subclinical adrenal dysfunction, but the true incidence is probably lower. Adrenal disorders most frequently associated with infertility are adrenal hypoplasia, adrenal hyperplasia, and adrenal carcinoma.

### Congenital adrenal hypoplasia

Congenital adrenal hypoplasia with hypogonadotropic hypogonadism is an X-linked recessive disorder that gives rise to adrenal insufficiency in the first months of life. In later presentations, patients have cryptorchidism and delayed puberty.[1309] The responsible gene, DAX1 on Xp21, is expressed in the adrenals, testes, pituitary, and hypothalamus. The resulting hypogonadism may be either pure or mixed (hypophyseal and testicular). In the last case, hypogonadism is partial.[1310] Testicular biopsy from one adult with adrenal hypoplasia showed an apparent primary lesion,

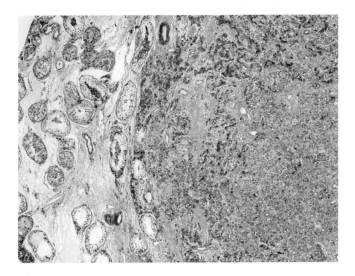

**Fig. 12-142** Intratesticular adrenal choristoma near the rete testis from a newborn. The seminiferous tubules are rejected by the mass. The adrenal cortex cells show bizarre nuclei and eosinophilic cytoplasm.

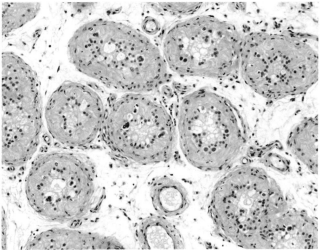

**Fig. 12-143** Hypogonadism caused by estrogen therapy for prostate cancer. The seminiferous tubules contain isolated spermatogonia and dedifferentiated Sertoli cells with spherical nuclei, small nucleoli, and pseudostratified infantile distribution. The interstitium contains scattered Leydig cells.

including tubules with dysgenetic Sertoli cells and others with spermatogonial maturation arrest in associated with hypertrophy and hyperplasia of Leydig cells.[1311]

### Congenital adrenal hyperplasia

Infertility is frequent in patients with minor forms of congenital adrenal hyperplasia. Those with deficiency of 21-hydroxylase[1312] or 11β-hydroxylase usually have complete spermatogenesis but with reduced numbers of all germ cells. The characteristic histologic finding is decreased numbers of Leydig cells.[1313–1316] In untreated patients, the testes become enlarged by 'tumors' of the adrenogenital syndrome that consist of cells similar to adrenal cortical cells (Fig. 12-142).[1316–1319]

### Adrenal cortical carcinoma

Adrenal carcinoma is often associated with excessive secretion of several hormones, causing hyperaldosteronism, Cushing's syndrome, virilization, or feminization. Virilizing tumors in infancy have their own characteristics, which differ from those of the same adult tumors as the infantile form may be associated with other disorders, such as hemihypertrophy and Beckwith–Wiederman syndrome, may be included in the spectrum of 'families with cancer predisposition' (mutations in p53 gene), and produce precocious pseudopuberty syndrome. In adults, adrenal carcinoma may cause marked spermatogenic depletion owing to the conversion of large amounts of dehydroepiandrosterone produced by the tumor into estrogen. Feminizing tumor in infancy causes gynecomastia and pubic hair development.[1320] Feminizing tumor presents more striking clinical characteristics, including progressive loss of secondary sex characteristics and feminization due to elevated estrogen. Testicular atrophy results from the inhibitory effect of estrogen on pituitary gonadotropins. Similar symptoms may be observed in patients with prostatic carcinoma treated with estrogens (Fig. 12-143) and in other conditions with excessive estrogen production, such as Sertoli cell or Leydig cell tumor.

### Cushing's syndrome

Patients with Cushing's syndrome or diseases that require long-term corticoid therapy, such as ulcerous colitis, rheumatoid arthritis, or asthma, have reversible reduction of fertility. The explanation for this is that most testicular receptors for corticoids are in Leydig cells, and thus glucocorticoids are powerful inhibitors of testosterone synthesis.

## Pancreas

### Diabetes mellitus

Alterations in the carbohydrate, lipid and protein metabolism characteristic of diabetes mellitus involve the genital system, although most diabetic patients are fertile. Gonadal impairment depends on the type of diabetes and the time of disease onset (infancy and childhood, puberty, or adulthood).[1321,1322] Testicular lesions in newborns with diabetic mothers are discussed in the section on congenital anomalies of the testis.[317]

Puberty may be delayed in diabetic patients, although the cause is unknown. Other gonadal alterations appear at puberty, and diabetic men who have not been adequately treated may be infertile and have sexual dysfunction. Serum levels of FSH, LH, and testosterone are decreased.[1323] Spermiograms reveal low numbers and poor motility of spermatozoa.[1324] Prolactin levels are increased and testosterone levels low or near normal.

The seminiferous tubules have reduced diameters, thickening of the lamina propria, and alterations in the adluminal compartment. These consist of degenerative changes in the Sertoli cell apical cytoplasm and sloughing of immature germ cells. The major lesion is in the interstitial connective tissue and Leydig cells. Small interstitial blood vessels show diabetic microangiopathy characterized by enlargement and duplication of the basal lamina, pericyte degeneration, and endothelial cell alterations. The number of fibroblasts

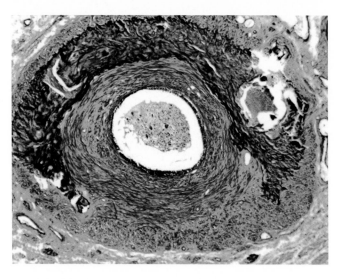

**Fig. 12-144** Diabetic patient with dystrophic calcification in the ductus deferens muscular wall.

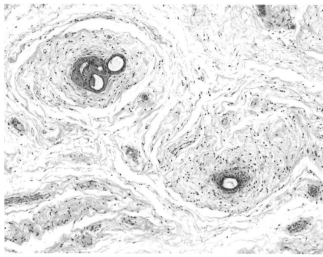

**Fig. 12-145** Epididymis in cystic fibrosis. Sections of the ductus epididymidis show decreased lumen diameter with surrounding concentric rings of loose connective tissue.

and the amount of collagen and ground substance in the interstitial connective tissue are increased.[1325] Leydig cells are decreased in number and show increased amounts of lipid droplets and lysosomes, accounting for the reduced function of these cells.

The tubular lesions are attributed to low serum testosterone, probably owing to deficient Leydig cell stimulation by insulin (or a decrease in insulin-dependent FSH) and abnormal carbohydrate metabolism of Sertoli cells. Sexual dysfunction is present in more than half of patients and consists of impotence, decreased libido, disorders of intercourse, and retrograde ejaculation. The causes of impotence are multiple, including microangiopathy and macroangiopathy, hormonal deficiencies, psychological factors, and autonomic neuropathy affecting the parasympathetic system. Neuropathy is probably chiefly responsible for erectile failure in diabetic men.[1326] Alterations in sperm excretory ducts may be associated with diabetes. The most frequent are enlarged seminal vesicles and calcification of both seminal vesicles and vasa deferentia. Calcifications are found in the muscular layers and display a concentric arrangement (Fig. 12-144).[1327]

### Mucoviscidosis

Although cystic fibrosis (mucoviscidosis) was recognized as a disease prior to 1940, its effects on the male genital system were not recognized until the 1970s. This may be explained by improvements in medical care during childhood, allowing the survival of many patients to adulthood, and the recognition of cystic fibrosis in patients who had been diagnosed with chronic bronchitis and hepatic or digestive dysfunction. In the US, cystic fibrosis is the most lethal congenital disease, with a prevalence of 1 in 2500 children, and a carrier status of 1 in 25 white men.[1328] Lesions in sperm excretory ducts involve (in decreasing order of frequency) the vas deferens (congenital bilateral absence, unilateral absence), ejaculatory ducts (bilateral obstruction), epididymis (diffuse or segmental hypoplasia), and seminal vesicles (incomplete development). Thus, it appears that most patients with cystic fibrosis have infertility due to obstruction.[1329,1330]

Histologic studies in children, even at an early age, reveal that the vas deferens and ductus epididymis are absent or reduced to small ductuli with reduced or absent lumina and thin, poorly muscular walls (Fig. 12-145). The testes are normal during childhood, but show hypospermatogenesis and spermatid malformations by adulthood. The spermiogram is characteristic of obstructive azoospermia, with acid pH, decreased semen volume and fructose concentration, and increased citric acid and acid phosphatase.[1331]

The disease is a genetic disorder with autosomal recessive inheritance. The impaired gene (cystic fibrosis gene) is on chromosome 7 (7q31),[1332] and encodes a protein termed cystic fibrosis transmembrane regulator (CFTR). Alterations in this protein cause cystic fibrosis. Although more than 800 mutations of this gene have been identified,[1333] the most frequent mutation in Caucasians is D-F508, responsible for 70% of cases. Congenital bilateral obstructive azoospermia secondary to bilateral absence of the vas deferens, even in the absence of other symptoms, is often a *forme fruste* of cystic fibrosis.[1334] Before initiating treatment for infertility, the possibility that the patient is a carrier of the cystic fibrosis gene should be evaluated.[1335]

Malformation of the genital system plays the most important role in infertility in cystic fibrosis.[1336] The lesions begin in the 10th week of gestation, when the wolffian duct forms the sperm excretory ducts.[1337] Variable penetrance of the cystic fibrosis gene accounts for the diversity of malformations affecting different regions of the male genital system.

### Liver

The liver has a primary role in metabolism, detoxification, and excretion of sex steroid hormones. Chronic hepatic failure damages the hypothalamo–hypophyseal–testicular axis, and subsequently all related endocrine glands. Hypogonadism is frequent in the final stages of severe chronic liver diseases, including alcoholism, non-alcoholic liver disease, and hemochromatosis.

### Hypogonadism, liver disease, and excessive alcohol consumption

The association of testicular atrophy with gynecomastia and hepatic cirrhosis is well known and is referred to as Silvestrini–Corda syndrome.[1338,1339]

Alcohol has a direct toxic effect on Leydig cells. Acute alcoholic intoxication suppresses serum testosterone in voluntary non-alcoholic men and laboratory animals. Chronic alcohol ingestion, even in the absence of cirrhosis, causes hypogonadism, with symptoms of Leydig cell failure, including testicular atrophy, infertility, decreased libido, impotence, and reduced size of the prostate and seminal vesicles.[1340] Chronic alcoholic patients with cirrhosis also have symptoms of hyperestrogenism, including gynecomastia, female escutcheon, and female fat distribution pattern.

Most chronic alcoholic men, with or without cirrhosis, have significant testicular lesions. The seminiferous tubules have reduced diameters, thickened lamina propria, and decreased or absent germ cells. Leydig cells are reduced in number and contain abundant lipofuscin granules (Fig. 12-146). The epididymis becomes atrophic, mainly in the ductuli efferentes, owing to androgen deprivation. The epithelium of the rete testis becomes cuboidal or columnar due to estrogens. The spermiogram correlates with the variability of histologic findings, usually showing a marked reduction in the number and motility of spermatozoa and an increase in the percentage of morphologically abnormal spermatozoa.[1341,1342] About 20% of patients initially have an increase in serum testosterone; with advanced disease, testosterone level decreases. The initial increase is due to an elevation in sex hormone-binding globulin concentration and reduced testosterone metabolism by the liver.[1343] Serum estrogen level also increases owing to increased conversion of testosterone into estrogen in peripheral adipose and muscular tissue.[1344]

### Non-alcoholic hepatic disease and infertility

Non-alcoholic liver disease impairs gonadal function according to the severity of the disease.[1345] Patients have decreased levels of total and biologically active free testosterone. Hormonal alterations are not as severe as in alcoholic patients, emphasizing the direct action of alcohol on Leydig cells. In $\alpha_1$-antitrypsin deficiency testicular function and fertility are conserved; only in advanced stages of the disease do minor biochemical alterations occur.[1346] In Alagille's syndrome (intrahepatic biliary duct hypoplasia), hypogonadism is associated with cholestasis, frequent vertebral, cardiac, and facial malformations, and mental retardation. Hypogonadism is manifest by small testes, delayed puberty, and, in adults, lack of germ cell development.

### Hemochromatosis and infertility

Hereditary hemochromatosis is the most frequent genetic disease in the northern hemisphere and results from excessive iron absorption and accumulation in multiple tissue and organs, leading to cirrhosis, diabetes, hypogonadism, and arthralgia. Four types of hereditary hemochromatosis have been reported.[1347] Type 1, the most frequent, is caused by mutation in the HFE gene (C282Y), leading to increased intestinal absorption of iron, supersaturation of iron deposits, and damage in multiples organs. The type I hereditary hemochromatosis gene (HFE) is located on the short arm of chromosome 6,[1348,1349] is present in 85–100% of hemochromatosis patients with northern European ancestry, and its protein product is mainly expressed in the epithelium of Lieberkühn crypts. This protein interacts with the transferrin receptor, reducing its affinity for iron-bound transferrin; therefore, HFE becomes a negative regulator of transferrin-bound iron uptake. Type 2 gene is a juvenile form that expresses before the age of 30 years in both sexes, and is associated with severe cardiomyopathy and hypogonadism.[1350] The type 2 hemochromatosis locus is on chromosome 1q21, but this gene has not yet been isolated.[1351,1352] Type 3 is on chromosome 7q22, impairs the transferrin 2 receptor, and its consequences are similar to those of type 1 receptor defect. Type 4 is autosomal dominant, on 2q32, and affects the basolateral iron carrier ferroportin 1, resulting in iron deposition in macrophages. Types 1, 2, and 3 have recessive autosomal inheritance and show a similar distribution pattern of iron deposits. In these three types, alteration of gonadal function has also been reported.

Iron homeostasis depends on many genes that act in a coordinated manner, and their exact function is not well known. It is assumed that normal individuals absorb 1–2 mg/day of iron, whereas homozygous patients with hereditary hemochromatosis absorb up to 3–4 mg/day. Once iron deposits become saturated (cells of liver, pancreas, hypophysis, heart, adrenals, and gastric mucosa), the toxic effects of iron cause dysfunction of the liver (cirrhosis and cancer in 5–10% of patients), the pancreas (diabetes in 80% of patients), the heart (myocardiopathy), musculoskeletal system (arthritis), and hypophysis (hypogonadism) (Fig. 12-147).

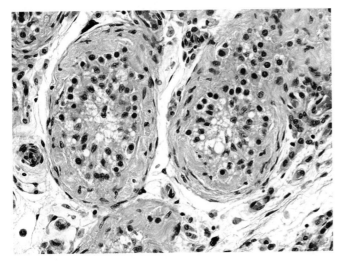

**Fig. 12-146** Testis from a patient with alcoholic cirrhosis. The seminiferous tubules show decreased diameter, thickening of the tubular wall, and spermatogonia, isolated spermatocytes, and Sertoli cells exhibiting intense vacuolation of the adluminal compartment. The testicular interstitium shows marked Leydig cell atrophy and numerous macrophages.

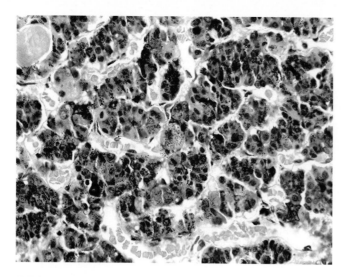

**Fig. 12-147** Perl stains decorates the voluminous iron deposits in cells of the anterior pituitary in a patient with hemochromatosis.

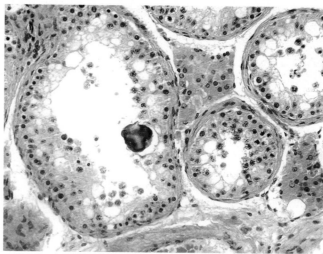

**Fig. 12-148** Testis from a patient with chronic renal insufficiency. The seminiferous tubules show premature sloughing of primary spermatocytes. An intraepithelial microlith is present.

Hypogonadism may be the first sign of disease when it starts in adult life.[1353] With age, hypogonadism becomes hypogonadotropic, with low serum levels of testosterone, LH, and FSH in more than 40% of patients,[1354] except if early treatment is initiated.[1355] The most frequent findings are testicular atrophy with diminished tubular diameter, tubular wall thickening, a progressive decrease in spermatogenesis, and increased lipofuscin granules in Leydig cells. The cause of these testicular disorders might be preferential deposition of iron in gonadotropic cells.[1356] Iron deposits are not observed in the testis. Hypogonadism decreases after aggressive therapy.[1357]

### Kidney

#### Polycystic renal disease

Polycystic renal disease in adults is a dominant autosomal disorder that appears with 1 in 1000 frequency in the general population. Patients with this disease comprise 10% of end-stage renal failure cases.[1358] Infertility is common, even before the beginning of renal insufficiency. Oligoteratozoospermia and necrospermia are frequent findings.[1359,1360] Serum levels of FSH, LH, prolactin, testosterone, and estradiol remain normal for a long time before the onset of renal insufficiency. The causes of spermiogram alterations have been related to partial obstruction of ejaculatory ducts (based on finding cystic dilations in seminal vesicles in 60% of patients) or seminal vesicle cyst.[1361] The incidence of these two disorders in patients with polycystic renal disease is very high compared to andrological patients without this disease (5.2%).[1362]

#### Chronic renal insufficiency

Chronic renal insufficiency is associated with disturbed endocrine function in the pituitary, thyroid, parathyroids, and testes. The associated sexual dysfunction consists of erectile impotence, diminution of libido and semen volume, oligozoospermia or azoospermia, and infertility. In children, skeletal development and puberty are delayed.[1363]

Hormonal studies reveal elevated levels of FSH, LH, and prolactin, but testosterone levels are low.[1364] Testicular biopsy shows seminiferous tubules with reduced diameters and reduced or absent germ cells (Fig. 12-148).[1365,1366] The interstitium contains a normal number of Leydig cells and increased numbers of macrophages. Additionally, patients with chronic renal insufficiency due to glomerulonephritis have thickening of the tubular lamina propria and decreased number of Leydig cells. Patients with end-stage renal disease who undergo dialysis show calcifications in several organs and tissues, including the male genital system (epididymidis, tunica albuginea, and cavernous tissue) in 87% of cases, and, in isolated cases, calcification of the testicular parenchyma and microlithiasis.[1367] Elevated serum levels of phosphorus, increased calcium–phosphorus product, severe hyperparathyroidism secondary to other disorders, older age, and prolonged time on dialysis contribute to this disorder. Uremic calcification is a cell-mediated process in which elevated levels of TGF, vitamin K-dependent proteins such as osteocalcin and atherocalcin, and defects in calcium-regulatory proteins such as fetuin are implicated.[1368] When these patients are dialyzed, accumulations of urate and oxalate crystals are deposited in the rete testes and ductuli efferentes. These crystals are deposited beneath the epithelium and often sloughed into the lumen. Reactive changes in the rete testis, including cystic transformation, are frequent (see Disorders of the rete testis).[1369]

The cause of gonadal dysfunction is unclear and probably involves several factors, including impaired testicular steroidogenesis,[1370] reduced clearance of pituitary hormones,[1371] and secretory defects of the pituitary and hypothalamus.[1372] Dialysis does not improve testicular function. The response to renal transplantation is not immediate and is related to the glomerular filtration rate. Patients with rates lower than 50 mL/min develop atrophy of the seminiferous tubular cells.[1370]

## Chronic inflammatory bowel disease

Hypogonadism is a frequent finding in men with celiac disease, and results in clinical symptoms in 5–10% of untreated patients. Celiac disease causes infertility in some cases. Spermiograms show reduced motility and numerous morphologic anomalies in spermatozoa. Hormonal studies show elevated serum FSH levels in more than 25% of men with celiac disease. LH also is increased in more than 50% of these men. The response of FSH and LH to GnRH stimulation is excessive. The cause of this pituitary derangement is unknown. Sperm anomalies are not always corrected by a gluten-free diet. Studies in patients with ulcerative colitis and regional enteritis reveal a low sperm count, impaired motility, and ultrastructural alterations, including nuclear pleomorphism and chromatin malcondensation and decondensation. Zinc deficit may be responsible for these alterations in Crohn's disease.[1373] The alterations apparently are related to the extent of the intestinal lesions and the severity of symptoms.[1374] Patients with ulcerative colitis treated with salazopyrine,[1375] mesalazine[1376] or fasalazine[1377] present with significant impairment of spermatogenesis and subfertility. Spermiogram parameters improve when treatment ceases.

## Acquired immunodeficiency syndrome (AIDS)

More than 17% of HIV-infected men have hypogonadism,[1378] which can be observed even in those whose viral replication is under control and show normal numbers of CD4 lymphocytes. Patients frequently develop 'early andropause,' marked by dysregulation of the hypothalamopituitary–testicular axis.[1379]

Hypogonadism is more frequent in HIV-infected men with wasting syndrome, and therefore these patients should undergo screening for hypogonadism and, if necessary, physiologic androgen replacement therapy.[1380–1383]

The incidence of hypogonadism in males with AIDS is estimated to be 50%.[1384,1385] According to autopsy studies this increases to 100% in the 3–24 months prior to death.[1386] Histological studies reveal that 28% have complete but quantitatively abnormal spermatogenesis, and the remainder have spermatocytic arrest or Sertoli cell-only pattern.

## Chronic anemia

Patients with chronic anemia requiring multiple transfusions develop iron deposits in the pituitary and polyglandular insufficiency, with atrophy of the thyroid, adrenals, and testes (Fig. 12-149). The most frequent conditions are β-thalassemia and sickle cell anemia (see Fig. 12-119).

β-*Thalassemia* is an autosomal dominant disease with three types: thalassemia trait (heterozygous β-thalassemia), intermediate thalassemia, and major β-thalassemia. The cause is mutation in the β-globin gene resulting in ineffective erythropoiesis, hemolysis, and anemia. Nearly 20% of patients with major thalassemia have delayed puberty,[1387–1389] and 69% have hypogonadotropic hypogonadism.[1390] Gonadal dysfunction persists in most patients after healing of the thalassemia.[1391]

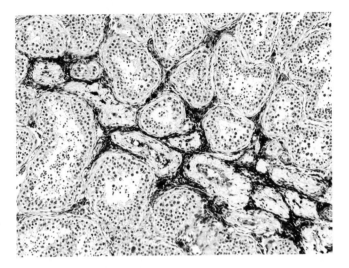

**Fig. 12-149** Major thalassemia in a patient who underwent multiple blood transfusions. The testicular interstitium and atrophic tubules show Perl's stain-positive iron deposits.

*Sickle cell anemia* is an autosomal recessive disorder with a constellation of findings resulting from abnormal synthesis of hemoglobin, with over 90% of hemoglobin being type A. Most patients have hypogonadotropic hypogonadism.[1392]

## Obesity

The majority of people in developed countries are currently overweight, and the incidence of obesity seems to be increasing. Infertility is frequently associated with obesity. Very obese males have increased levels of serum estradiol and decreased levels of free testosterone and inhibin B.[1393] Testosterone reduction is not followed by a compensatory increase in gonadotropins, resulting in hypogonadotropic hypogonadism.[1394,1395] Testicular abnormalities begin with the adluminal compartment and later involve the basal compartment; also, there are Leydig cell atrophy, cuboidal metaplasia of the rete testis, and epididymal atrophy.

## Autoimmune polyglandular syndrome

There are three types of autoimmune polyglandular insufficiency syndrome. Type I is defined by the presence of at least two of three characteristic features: Addison's disease, hypoparathyroidism, and chronic mucocutaneous candidiasis. The AIRE gene (autoimmune regulator), responsible for type I disease, is on 21q22.3,[1396,1397] and the disorder is recessive autosomal. Hypergonadotropic hypogonadism is frequent.[1398] Patients with type I syndrome have antibodies against many autoantigens, intracellular enzymes including the P450 side-chain cleavage enzyme, 17α-hydroxylase[1399,1400] and 21-hydroxylase, glutamic acid decarboxylase 65, aromatic L-amino acid decarboxylase, tyrosine phosphatase-like protein IA-2, tryptophan hydroxylase (TPH), tyrosine hydroxylase, and cytochrome P450 1A2.[1401]

Type II autoimmune polyglandular syndrome is characterized by the presence of diabetes mellitus, hyperthyroid-

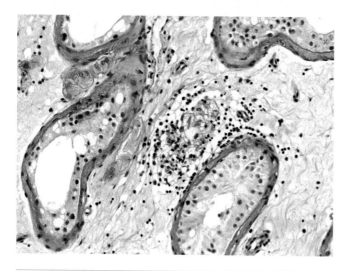

**Fig. 12-150** Testis from a man with autoimmune polyglandular syndrome showing selective lymphoid infiltrates in a Leydig cell cluster. Reinke's crystalloid can be recognized. The seminiferous tubules contain Sertoli cells and isolated spermatogonia.

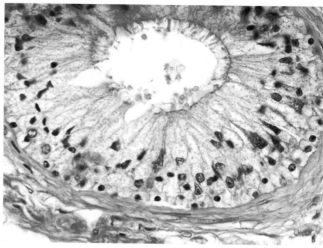

**Fig. 12-151** Fabry's disease. Both basal and principal cells of the epididymis show pale and vacuolated cytoplasms, due to lipid deposits.

ism, Hashimoto's thyroiditis, Addison's disease, vitiligo, alopecia, pernicious anemia, and hypogonadism (listed in decreasing order of frequency). Type III syndrome includes thyroiditis, diabetes mellitus, pernicious anemia, and vitiligo or alopecia. About 14% of patients have hypogonadism owing to autoimmune destruction of the testis or pituitary gonadotropin-secreting cells (Fig. 12-150).[1402,1403]

### Lysosomal and peroxisomal diseases

There are at least four diseases caused by metabolic deposits in lysosomes or peroxisomes associated with testicular alterations, including Fabry's disease, adrenal leukodystrophy, Wolman's disease, and cystinosis.

#### Fabry's disease

Fabry's disease is an X-linked metabolic disorder characterized by intralysosomal deposits of globotriaosylceramide (Gb3) owing to α-galactosidase deficiency. Clinical symptoms begin with painful neuropathy and progressive renal, cardiovascular, and cerebrovascular dysfunction. All endocrine glands may accumulate Gb3 as a result of well-developed vasculature and low rate of cell proliferation.[1404] Testes and sperm excretory ducts are always damaged. Some alterations, including those of endothelial cells, smooth muscle cells, and fibroblasts, are non-specific; others, such as those of myofibroblasts, Leydig cells, and epididymal epithelium, are specific (Figs 12-151, 12-152). Spermatogenesis is deficient.[1405] Enzyme replacement therapy with recombinant human α-galactosidase eliminates existing glycosphingolipid deposits and blocks new ones, and is thus recommended for implementation as soon as possible after diagnosis.[1406–1408]

#### Adrenoleukodystrophy (adrenal testicular myeloneuropathy)

This disorder is caused by mutation in the adrenoleukodystrophy gene on Xq28.[1409] Mutation at this site produces three peroxisomal diseases: adrenoleukodystrophy, adrenomyeloneuropathy, and Addison's disease.

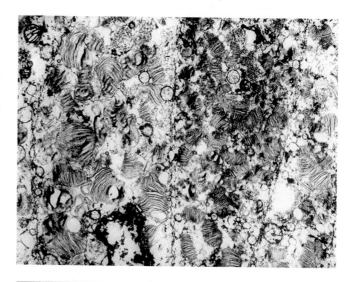

**Fig. 12-152** Fabry's disease. The deposits observed in the ductus epididymidis epithelium consist of multiple, parallelly arranged laminae.

Adrenoleukodystrophy is characterized by progressive demyelinization of the central nervous system, usually in children and young adults, often with adrenal insufficiency and testicular failure. Peroxisomal β-oxidation is deficient and, as a result, very long-chain fatty acids accumulate inside peroxisomes in many tissues, causing the signs and symptoms of the disease.[1410,1411]

Adrenomyeloneuropathy begins at a later age (about 30 years) with progressive paraparesis, peripheral neuropathy, and adrenal cortical failure. Males usually have gonadal dysfunction with oligozoospermia or azoospermia and hypergonadotropic hypogonadism.[1412] Testicular atrophy develops slowly, the seminiferous epithelium disappear, and Leydig cells contain characteristic cytoplasmic lamellar inclusions, with similar inclusions in adrenal cortical cells and cerebral cells.[1413]

### Wolman's disease

Wolman's disease is a rare inherited lysosomal disease characterized by a deficit in acid lipase/cholesteryl ester hydrolase. The genetic mutation has been mapped to 10q23.2-q23.3.[1414] Complete enzymatic deficiency (Wolman's disease) causes death in infancy as a result of the accumulation of cholesterol esters and triglycerides in numerous organs such as the liver, adrenal cortex, and intestines.[1415] Partial deficiency is known as cholesteryl ester storage disease, and the testis accumulates triglycerides and cholesterol in Leydig cells and, to a lesser degree, in interstitial macrophages. Delayed disruption of spermatogenesis by this storage disease probably accounts for the frequent lack of fertility problems in men with this disease.[1416] Early treatment of children with Wolman's disease by transplantation of umbilical cord blood-derived stem cells may successfully restore acid lipase level in some.[1417]

### Cystinosis

Cystinosis is an autosomal recessive metabolopathy characterized by alterations in cystine transport from the lysosomes to the cytosol that results in intralysosomal accumulation of cystine. There are several genes responsible, all on chromosome 17p13. Cystine storage occurs in all body tissues. Deposits in the renal parenchyma cause the main complication of cystinosis, namely renal insufficiency (nephropathic cystinosis). Patients also develop hypergonadotropic hypogonadism. Testicular involvement may be massive, with interstitial macrophages filled with cystine crystals that are visible by polarized light.[1418]

### Niemann–Pick disease

Niemann-Pick disease consists of a heterogeneous group of inherited recessive autosomal diseases characterized by deposition of lipids in macrophages and other tissues. There are four reported types (A, B, C, D). The most common, type A, results from excessive storage of sphingomyelin owing to a mutation in the acid sphingomyelin gene that encodes a lysosomal hydrolase, located on 11p15.1-4 region.[1419]

Interstitial macrophages in the testes have wide eosinophilic, granular cytoplasm. Ultrastructural studies reveal a large number of lysosomes filled with laminate bodies.

## Infertility secondary to physical and chemical agents

Physical and chemical agents may impair testicular function by direct action on the pituitary, the testis, or the sperm excretory ducts. In the pituitary, damage to gonadotropic cells may be caused by estrogen. In the testes, gonadotoxic agents may selectively impair a select cell type, but later, global dysfunction occurs. For example, there is direct toxicity to Sertoli cells by phthalates used as plasticizers, nitroaromatic compounds intermediate in the production of dyes and explosives, and γ-diketones used as solvents. Direct toxicity on spermatogenesis is seen wtih ionizing radiation. Many drugs that impair epididymal fluid or spermatozoon transport damage sperm excretory ducts, with subsequent loss of fertility.[1420]

## Occupational exposure

The relationship between infertility or subfertility and certain professions or exposures to environmental agents is well known.[1421] Adverse effects of the following agents on spermatogenesis has been demonstrated: organic solvents such as chlorinated solvents, aromatic solvents and varnishes, degreasers, thinners, and adhesives; this is also the case with carbon disulfide exposure; pesticides such as DDT, linuron, and polychlorinated biphenyls;[1422] heavy metals such as lead, cadmium, mercury, and copper; industrial wastes such as dioxins and ethylene dibromide; phthalates and polyvinyl chloride; oral contraceptives; exposure to radiation or high temperature; and recreational drugs and doping. There is also a long list of potentially harmful agents that disrupt testicular function.[1423]

### Carbon disulfide

Carbon disulfide is used as a solvent in the production of rayon. Continuous exposure is toxic to the nervous system, and causes a decrease in spermatogenesis and libido and an increase in FSH and LH serum levels.[1424,1425]

### Dibromochloropropane

Dibromochloropropane is used as a soil fumigant to control nematodes. Lengthy exposure causes oligozoospermia, azoospermia, increased FSH and LH levels, and Y-chromosome non-dysjunction.[1426]

### Lead

Of the two natural forms of lead, organic and inorganic, the inorganic form is more dangerous. Exposure to inorganic lead by workers in smelting, battery, and stained-glass plants causes direct spermatogenic damage.[1427] Patients have asthenospermia, teratozoospermia, and oligozoospermia.[1428,1429]

### Oral contraceptive manufacture

Workers in pharmaceutical plants using synthetic estrogens and progestins develop hyperestrogenism with gynecomastia, decreased libido, and impotence.[1430]

Neonatal exposure of males to diethylstilbestrol may induce cryptorchidism, testicular hypoplasia, epididymal cyst, and severe anomalies in semen production.[1431]

### Endocrine-disrupting compounds

There is increasing evidence to suggest that estrogen-like effects are produced by a variety of naturally occurring estrogens (so-called phytoestrogens) and numerous synthetic compounds such as phthalates,[1432] pesticides,[1433] and polychlorinated biphenyls.[1434] The principal methods of contact with potential endocrine-disrupting compounds is dietary ingestion of milk, fish, meat, fruits and vegetables, or environmental exposure.[1435] The increasing incidence of cryptorchidism, hypospadias, testicular cancer, and poor semen quality may be related to the negative influence of environmental factors on the testis during fetal life. The term 'testicular dysgenesis syndrome' has been proposed to designate this constellation of putative syndromes.[1436]

Estrogen exposure in utero may disrupt development of the testes and the entire male reproductive tract. Estrogen may hinder FSH secretion by the fetal pituitary, and also interfere with subsequent Sertoli cell proliferation, and

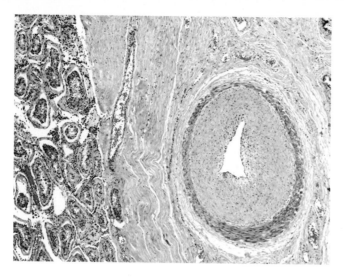

**Fig. 12-153** Testis from a 40-year-old patient who consumed cocaine from the age of 16 years. In the tunica albuginea, a branch of the testicular artery shows intense fibrosis in the tunica intima. The seminiferous tubules have marked germ cell atrophy.

hence the secretion of AMH required for the regression of müllerian ducts. Persistence of müllerian derivatives is associated with lack of testicular descent. Changes in AMH secretion may also account for altered germ cell proliferation during fetal life. Exposure to high concentrations of estrogen might compromise testosterone production as well as masculinization of external genitalia (hypospadias) and inguinal descent of the testis (cryptorchidism). Abnormal development of Sertoli cells and low germ cell numbers could cause diminished spermatozoon production and infertility.[1437]

### Recreational drugs and doping

Marijuana decreases sperm density and motility and increases the number of morphologically abnormal spermatozoa.[1438] Cocaine induces apoptosis in the rat testis (Fig. 12-153).[1439] About 20% of injection drug users have low serum testosterone levels. Consumption of more than 80 g alcohol per day adversely affects spermatogenesis in two-thirds of patients.[1440] Women smoking more than 20 cigarettes per day have fertility problems, neonatal and perinatal mortality, miscarriage, and congenital malformations.[1441] Abuse of anabolic steroids by athletes causes hypogonadotropic hypogonadism and transient azoospermia.[1442]

### Radiation

Ionizing radiation causes alterations in spermatogenesis and hormonal regulation of the testes. Some patients recover fertility a few years after exposure.[1443] The effects of non-ionizing radiation are less severe; however, reduced libido and reduced numbers of spermatozoa have been reported in men exposed to microwaves.[1444]

### Heat

Normal intratesticular temperature is 31–33°C, about 4–6°C lower than core body temperature. Conditions causing higher testicular temperature, such as varicocele and cryptorchidism, also cause testicular damage, with decreased numbers of spermatozoa and an elevated percentage of sper-

matozoa with abnormal forms and low motility.[1445,1446] Primary spermatocytes at the end of the pachytene stage are most sensitive to heat. The mechanism by which heat produces testicular lesions is unknown; hyperthermia affects the activity of enzymes such as ornithine decarboxylase[1447] and carnitine acetyl transferase,[1448] both necessary for metabolism and proliferation of the seminiferous tubular cells.[1449] The synthesis of DNA and RNA by germ cells also depends on temperature. DNA synthesis by spermatogonia and preleptotene primary spermatocytes is higher at 31°C than at 37°C. RNA and protein synthesis are normal at temperatures between 28°C and 37°C, but decrease markedly at 40°C.[1450]

## Testicular trauma

Testicular trauma is especially frequent among athletes. Trauma results in a wide variety of lesions, including contusion with or without hematocele, rupture, dislocation, and eventually spermatogenetic alteration that may lead to infertility. Dislocation involves the displacement of one or both testes to a non-scrotal location[1451,1452] such as the inguinal canal, abdominal cavity, acetabular area, or distant locations such as the perineum, subcutaneous tissues, or superficial to the outer oblique fascia.[1453,1454] Spermatogenetic recovery by orchidopexy has been successfully performed up to 13 years after bilateral traumatic dislocation.[1455]

## Cancer therapy

Sexual dysfunction is found in 25–50% of patients who are treated for cancer.[1456] Testicular cancer, Hodgkin's disease, and leukemia are the most frequent malignancies during the reproductive years. Therefore, preservation of fertility requires careful selection of less gonadotoxic therapeutic regimens; if paternity is planned, cryopreservation of semen before treatment may be considered. The most destructive treatments for gonadal function are radiation therapy and alkylating agents.[1457]

### Radiation therapy

The testicular parenchyma is one of the most radiosensitive tissues of the body, and the germ cells are the most radiosensitive cells of the testis. Experimental irradiation of volunteers with a single dose revealed that late spermatogonia (Ap and B) are more radiosensitive than early (Ad) spermatogonia. Ap and B spermatogonia may be destroyed with doses as low as 0.3 Gy (1 Gy = 100 rad), whereas Ad spermatogonia tolerate doses higher than 4 Gy. Type A spermatogonia, spermatids, and spermatozoa are respectively 100, 200, and 10 000 times less radiosensitive than B spermatogonia. Doses higher than 6 Gy produce a Sertoli cell-only pattern. Leydig cells tolerate up to 8 Gy and Sertoli cells up to 60 Gy, although Sertoli cells show ultrastructural alterations and increased phagocytosis of germ cell remnants after low doses of radiation.

Even with optimal protection, the contralateral testis absorbs from 0.2 to 1.4 Gy in adjuvant therapy for rectal cancer[1458] or when the opposite testis is irradiated,[1459] a dose sufficient to cause temporary azoospermia. Likewise, irradiation of iliac or inguinal lymph nodes for Hodgkin's disease

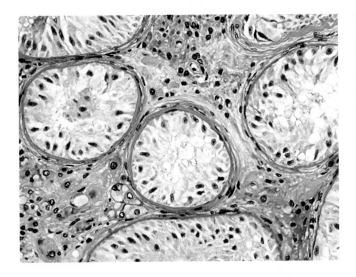

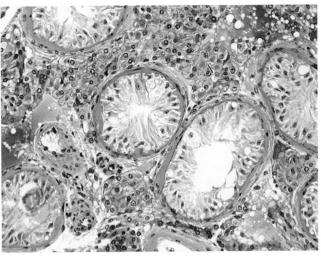

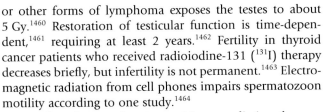

**Fig. 12-154** Testis from a 26-year-old patient who, at the age of 9 years, underwent surgery followed by radiotherapy for paratesticular rhabdomyosarcoma. The testicular biopsy shows post-irradiation lesions, including germ cell aplasia and peritubular and interstitial fibrosis.

**Fig. 12-155** Testis from a patient with Hodgkin's disease after chemotherapy. The seminiferous tubules are small and contain only vacuolated Sertoli cells. The testicular interstitium has pseudohyperplasia of Leydig cells.

or other forms of lymphoma exposes the testes to about 5 Gy.[1460] Restoration of testicular function is time-dependent,[1461] requiring at least 2 years.[1462] Fertility in thyroid cancer patients who received radioiodine-131 ($^{131}$I) therapy decreases briefly, but infertility is not permanent.[1463] Electromagnetic radiation from cell phones impairs spermatozoon motility according to one study.[1464]

Prepubertal testes also are sensitive to radiation therapy. Patients treated for Wilms' tumor may have delayed puberty and, at adulthood, oligoospermia or azoospermia with elevated levels of FSH; this finding suggests that Leydig cells are also damaged. A special case is that of children with acute lymphoblastic leukemia involving the testis. Radiotherapy with doses of 20–25 Gy, either alone or with chemotherapy, causes irreversible damage to the seminiferous tubules and Leydig cells. These patients develop azoospermia and hypogonadotropic hypogonadism with low serum testosterone (Fig. 12-154).

### Chemotherapy

Widespread use of cytotoxic chemotherapy has created a number of adverse side effects, including gonadotoxicity. Combination chemotherapy makes it difficult to ascertain which specific agent is responsible for azoospermia and Leydig cell dysfunction. Comparative studies of chemotherapy for acute lymphoblastic leukemia,[1465] extragonadal solid tumors,[1466] Hodgkin's disease,[1467] Ewing's sarcoma, and other soft tissue sarcomas[1468] in children and pubertal boys have shown that alkylating agents cause the most severe testicular damage. Alkylating agents destroy the seminiferous tubular cells and induce tubular atrophy, shrinking the testis and increasing FSH serum concentration.[1469] These agents also impair Leydig cell function, causing low testosterone, normal or elevated serum levels of LH, and an exaggerated response of LH to GnRH administration.[1470] Testicular damage may be increased by combination with other agents (Fig. 12-155).

Cyclophosphamide appears to be responsible for the greatest number of permanent or temporary cases of azoospermia after chemotherapy. This agent acts directly on the spermatogenic stem cells,[1468] and recovery depends on the number of surviving cells. In children, cyclophosphamide reduces seminiferous tubule diameter and germ cell numbers; in the residual spermatogonia nuclei are enlarged. Puberty may progress, even during treatment, and the adult testis may show a Sertoli cell-only pattern.[1465] In adults, cyclophosphamide treatment may cause irreversible testicular damage. Administered alone, a dose of 20 000 mg/m$^2$ produces permanent azoospermia in 50% of men. If cyclophosphamide is administered with doxorubicin, vincristine, dacarbazine, or dactinomycin (drugs that alone do not cause azoospermia), doses of 7500 mg/m$^2$ cause azoospermia in 50% of patients. Fludarabine, used for the treatment of chronic lymphocytic leukemia, produces testicular damage with diminution of ejaculate volume, oligozoospermia, increase in serum levels of FSH and LH, and decreased testosterone level. DNA in spermatozoa is markedly abnormal, an effect that persists for several months.[1471]

Procarbazine, used to treat Hodgkin's disease, causes permanent azoospermia in 30% of patients, even when not combined with alkylating agents.[1472] Patients treated with a combination of cyclophosphamide and procarbazine in the COPP protocol (cyclophosphamide, vincristine, procarbazine, and prednisone) do not recover spermatogenesis even if the cyclophosphamide dose does not exceed 4800 mg/m$^2$.

Chemotherapy without both alkylating agents and procarbazine, such as the ABVD (dexorubicin, bleomycin, vinblastine and dacarbazine) or VBM (vinblastine, bleomycin and methotrexate) regimens, produces reversible azoospermia in 36% of patients. The alternating use of MOPP (mechlorethamine, vincristine, procarbazine and prednisone) and

ABVD treatments causes testicular dysfunction in 87% of patients, but spermatogenesis recovers in 40%.[1473]

Patients with germ cell cancer who received chemotherapy with BEP regimens (cisplatinum, etoposide, and bleomycin) become azoospermic 7–8 weeks after starting treatment. When the total doses reaches 600 mg/m[2], infertility is irreversible; at lower dosages, fertility might be recovered over a period of about 2 (50% of patients) to 5 (80%) years,[1474] although a high percentage of spermatozoa with DNA abnormalities persists.[1475]

An important consideration in patients with testicular cancer or Hodgkin's disease is the existence of testicular dysfunction before treatment. In some series[1476] dysfunction is present at diagnosis in more than 50% of patients; its cause is unknown. Proposed mechanisms include primary germ cell deficiency, release of toxic substances by tumor cells, and alteration in the hypothalamo–hypophyseal–testicular axis.

### Surgery

Sexual function is often lost in patients who undergo bilateral retroperitoneal lymph node dissection for non-seminomatous testicular cancer. Up to 90% lose antegrade ejaculation, although libido, erection, and orgasm are normal. Loss of antegrade ejaculation results from the removal of or injury to sympathetic ganglia and the hypogastric nervous plexus during surgery. Unilateral surgery, especially if the left side is not operated on, reduces this complication.[1477,1478] Hypospermatogenesis sometimes occurs after surgery for rectal cancer, perhaps due to vascular compromise.

## Infertility in patients with spinal cord injury

Spinal cord injury is a frequent finding, with more than 10 000 cases annually in the US, mostly in young adults.[1479] Fertility is impaired in 90% of males with spinal cord injury. The major sexual dysfunctions in these patients are the lack of erection and ejaculation and poor semen quality.[1480–1485] Failure of ejaculation occurs in 95% of patients. Semen may be obtained by means of vibratory stimulation of the penis or electroejaculation in more than 90%, but its quality is low, with increased numbers of dead spermatozoa, markedly low motility, and reduced fertilization rate.[1486–1488] Possible explanations include genitourinary tract infection, endocrine anomaly, and impaired spermatogenesis. Recurrent infection occurs in 60–70% of patients. Compared to controls, a significant increase in the numbers of neutrophils and macrophages occurs, with a marked increase in the production of reactive oxygen species.[1489,1490] This finding and the presence of elevated cytokine levels[1491] are assumed to be involved in pathogenesis. Endocrine anomalies are transient, and hormonal levels return to normal after a few months. More than 50% of patients have abnormalities of the adluminal compartment of the seminiferous tubules, with variable degrees of immature germ cell sloughing;[1482] in 50% of patients the number of mature spermatids per cross-sectioned tubule is less than 10 (normal >21).

Possible etiologies include an increase in testicular temperature due to vascular dilation, or an alteration in scrotal thermoregulation secondary to impaired sympathetic innervation from prolonged wheelchair restraint; alteration in sperm transport secondary to nerve injury, resulting in sperm stagnation in seminal vesicles, a hostile environment that normally is devoid of spermatozoa;[1493] and abnormal composition of seminal fluid, causing deterioration of spermatozoa that in the epididymis and ductus deferens had good motility.[1494]

More than 25% of patients with spinal cord injury have brown-tinged semen in some ejaculations.[1495] Although the cause is unknown, it might be related to seminal vesicle dysfunction.

When spermatozoa cannot be obtained by electroejaculation or vibratory stimulation, vasal aspiration or testicular biopsy are recommended. Most patients have at least a few mature spermatids in some seminiferous tubules; therefore, testicular sperm extraction followed by intracytoplasmic sperm injection is a reasonable consideration in azoospermic patients.[1492]

# Inflammation and infection

Infectious agents may reach the testis and epididymis through blood vessels, lymphatics, sperm excretory ducts, or directly from a superficial wound. Infection transmitted through the blood mainly affects the testis and causes orchitis, whereas infection ascending through the sperm excretory ducts usually causes epididymitis. Acute inflammation is accompanied by enlargement of the testis or epididymis. The tunica albuginea is covered by a fibrinous exudate, and the testicular parenchyma is yellow or brown. Bacterial infection may cause abscess. In some cases the infection begins to heal, with the deposition of granulation tissue and fibrosis; in others, the infection may persist as an active process for a long time, resulting in chronic orchidoepididymitis.

## Orchitis

### Viral orchitis

The most frequent causes of viral orchidoepididymitis are mumps virus and Coxsackie B virus. Other viral infections that occasionally cause acute orchitis include influenza, infectious mononucleosis, echovirus, lymphocytic choriomeningitis, adenovirus, coronavirus, bat salivary gland virus, smallpox, varicella, vaccinia, rubella, dengue, and phlebotomous fever. Subclinical orchitis probably occurs during other viral infections (Fig. 12-156).

Before vaccination was commonly used, mumps orchidoepididymitis complicated 14–35% of adult mumps cases and was bilateral in 20–25% of cases. Nevertheless, mini-epidemics still occasionally occur.[1496,1497] As expected, the incidence remains high in countries where vaccination is not obligatory.[1498] In about 85% of cases of mumps orchitis the epididymis is also involved, but epididymal involvement alone is rare.[1499] Clinical symptoms of orchitis usually appear 4–6 days after symptoms of parotiditis, but orchitis may also appear without parotid involvement.[1500] Testicular involvement is multifocal, and consists of acute inflammation of

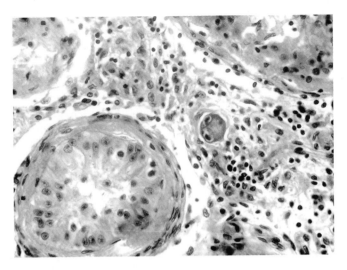

**Fig. 12-156** Orchitis caused by cytomegalovirus in a patient with HIV. The inflammatory infiltrate of the testicular interstitium has two characteristic intranuclear inclusions.

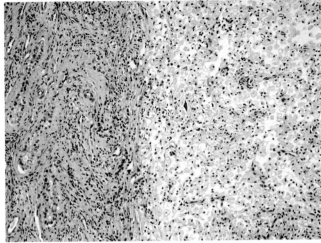

**Fig. 12-157** Xanthogranulomatous orchitis showing a dense infiltrate of macrophages with vacuolated cytoplasm surrounded by atrophic seminiferous tubules.

the interstitium and seminiferous tubules. The tubular lining is destroyed, and eventually only hyalinized tubules and clusters of Leydig cells remain.[1501] With time, the testes shrink and become soft. If the infection is bilateral the patient is usually infertile, with severe oligozoospermia or azoospermia, although biopsy may reveal the presence of mature spermatids in some tubules, allowing sperm extraction for paternity.[1502] If only one testis was affected, the sperm concentration may be normal or slightly decreased and fertility is maintained. Occasionally the testicular damage is so severe that testicular endocrine function is impaired, causing hypergonadotropic hypogonadism, with low testosterone levels and regression of secondary sex characteristics. Mumps orchidoepididymitis is infrequent in childhood.

## Bacterial orchitis

Most bacterial orchitis is associated with bacterial epididymitis. Orchitis secondary to suppurative epididymitis caused by *Escherichia coli* is most common.[1503] On light microscopy, the tubules are effaced by intense acute inflammation. Chronic orchitis with microabscesses is caused by *E. coli*, streptococci, staphylococci, pneumococci, *Salmonella enteritidis*,[1504] and *Actinomyces israeli*.[1505,1506] In some cases of chronic bacterial orchitis, the testis contains an inflammatory infiltrate consisting of numerous histiocytes with foamy cytoplasm (xanthogranulomatous orchitis) (Fig. 12-157),[1507] similar to that of idiopathic granulomatous orchitis but lacking intratubular giant cells. Rarely, as in Whipple's disease, large numbers of bacilli are present in histiocytes in the interstitium, vascular walls, and seminiferous tubules.

The most frequent complications of pyogenic bacterial orchidoepididymitis are scrotal pyocele and chronic draining scrotal sinus. Small fragments of testicular parenchyma may be eliminated through the scrotal skin, known clinically as fungus testis. Another complication is testicular infarct, resulting from compression or thrombosis of the veins of the spermatic cord, in the scrotal neck, or the superficial inguinal ring.

## Granulomatous orchidoepididymitis

Most cases of chronic orchidoepididymitis are associated with granulomas in the testis. Specific causes may require special stains, cultures, or serologic tests, and include tuberculosis, syphilis, leprosy, brucellosis, mycoses, and parasitic diseases. In sarcoidosis and idiopathic granulomatous orchitis, the agent is unknown.

### Tuberculosis

The incidence of tuberculous orchidoepididymitis declined after the development of effective antibiotics, but it has recently undergone a resurgence among people who have emigrated from countries with a high incidence of the disease and the increasing population of immunologically compromised patients.

Most cases of tuberculous orchidoepididymitis are associated with involvement elsewhere in the genitourinary system.[1508] Tuberculous epididymitis is usually the result of ascent from tuberculous prostatitis, which in turn is often secondary to renal or pulmonary tuberculosis. The pattern of spread is different in children: more than half have advanced pulmonary tuberculosis, and the testis is infected through the blood.[1509] More than 50% of patients with renal tuberculosis develop tuberculous epididymitis, and orchitis occurs in approximately 3% of patients with genital tuberculosis, usually secondary to epididymal tuberculosis. It has been suggested that some cases of tuberculous orchidoepididymitis are sexually transmitted.[1510] Tuberculous orchidoepididymitis occurs mainly in adults: 72% of patients are older than 35 years, and 18% are over 65 years. The signs and symptoms may be mild, consisting only of testicular enlargement and scrotal pain. In such cases, fever is infrequent and constitutional symptoms may be absent.[1511]

Histologically, there are typical caseating and non-caseating granulomas that destroy the seminiferous tubules

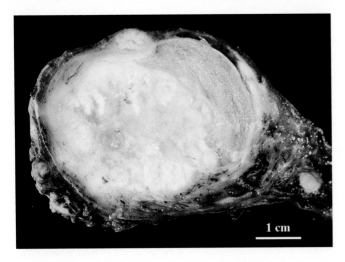

**Fig. 12-158** Tuberculous orchitis in a 38-year-old patient with a white-gray nodule which has a pseudotumoral pattern and caused testicular enlargement.

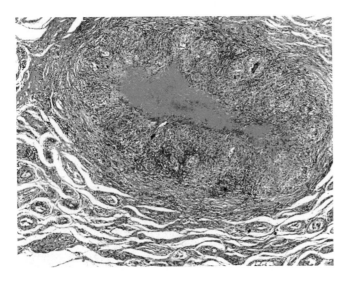

**Fig. 12-159** Tuberculous orchitis showing central necrosis surrounded by numerous granulomas, some of which contain giant cells in their centers.

and interstitium (Figs 12-158, 12-159). In immunosuppressed patients, the granulomas consist of epithelioid histiocytes and a few lymphocytes with rare giant cells. Acid-fast bacilli tend to be more numerous in immunosuppressed patients. Similar lesions may be observed in orchidoepididymitis caused by bacillus Calmette–Guérin, which is usually used for intravesical instillation in patients with vesicular urothelial carcinoma.[1512]

### Syphilis

Syphilitic orchitis may be congenital or acquired. In congenital orchitis, both testes are enlarged at birth. The histological findings are similar to those of the interstitial orchitis of acquired syphilis. If diagnosis is delayed until puberty, the testis often shows retraction and fibrosis. In adults, acquired orchitis is a complication of the tertiary stage of syphilis and

has two characteristic histologic patterns: interstitial inflammation and gumma.

Early in the disease, patients with interstitial orchitis have painless enlargement. Grossly, the parenchyma is gray with translucent areas. Histologically, plasma cells are abundant. The inflammation begins in the mediastinum testis and testicular septa, later extending through the parenchyma as the seminiferous tubules lose their cellular lining and undergo sclerosis. Initially, the arteries show an obliterans type of endarteritis. Small gummas may be observed. Eventually, the inflammation subsides and is replaced by fibrosis. The epididymis is usually not affected.

Gummatous orchitis is characterized by the presence of one or several well-delineated grossly gray-yellow zones of necrosis.[1513] Histologically, ghostly silhouettes of seminiferous tubules are visible within the gumma, surrounded by inflammation consisting of lymphocytes, plasma cells, and scattered giant cells. In most cases spirochetes may be demonstrated histochemically with Warthin–Starry silver stain, but the most specific diagnostic technique is genetic testing.

### Leprosy

The testis may be infected in patients with lepromatous or borderline leprosy. Frequent involvement of the testis in lepromatous leprosy results from the low intrascrotal temperature that promotes growth of the bacilli. Orchitis is usually bilateral, although the degree of involvement may differ between the testes. Occasionally, testicular involvement may be the sole indication of the infection, and the diagnosis may be made by testicular biopsy.[1514]

The histologic findings in the testis vary with the duration of the infection. Initially, there is perivascular lymphocytic inflammation and interstitial macrophages that contain numerous acid-fast bacilli. Later, the seminiferous tubules undergo atrophy, the Leydig cells cluster, and blood vessels show endarteritis obliterans. Finally, the testis is replaced by fibrous tissue with a few lymphocytes and macrophages containing acid-fast bacilli. Most patients with lepromatous leprosy are infertile, even if the orchitis was clinically mild.[1515,1516]

### Brucellosis

Brucellosis is common in some parts of the world, including the Middle East.[1517,1518] Orchitis occurs in some patients and may be the first sign of disease. Brucellosis should be suspected when testicular enlargement occurs in patients with undulating fever, malaise, sweats, weight loss, and headache.[1519] Occasionally this may mimic testicular tumor. Histologically, there is a dense lymphohistiocytic inflammation with occasional non-caseating granulomas in the interstitium. The seminiferous tubules are infiltrated by inflammatory cells and undergo atrophy. Diagnosis is made by clinical and laboratory findings, including blood culture, the Bengal rose test, and high brucella agglutination titers,[1520,1521] or by real-time polymerase chain reaction assay of urine.[1522]

### Sarcoidosis

Sarcoidosis is a systemic granulomatous disease of unknown etiology that preferentially affects young black adults. The genitourinary tract is involved in only 0.5% of clinical cases and 5% of autopsy cases. Fewer than 30 cases of primary epididymal involvement have been reported, and about 12 of these also involved the testis.[1523,1524] Isolated testicular involvement is exceptional.[1523,1525,1526] Testicular sarcoidosis is usually unilateral and nodular.[947] It is often asymptomatic and found at autopsy.[1527] The testis contains non-caseating granulomas similar to sarcoid granulomas at other locations. Before diagnosing testicular sarcoidosis, other granulomatous lesions should be excluded, including tuberculosis, sperm granuloma, granulomatous orchitis, and seminoma. Seminoma often has an intense sarcoid-like reaction, and examination of multiple histologic sections may be necessary to find diagnostic foci of seminoma. An association of mediastinal sarcoidosis and testicular cancer has been reported.[1528] Genital involvement of sarcoidosis may be the cause of intermittent azoospermia that benefits from corticoid therapy.[1529]

## Malakoplakia

Malakoplakia is a chronic inflammatory disease that was initially described in the bladder[1530] and subsequently in many other organs. The testes (alone or together with the epididymis) are involved in 12% of cases involving the urogenital system.[1531,1532] Grossly, the testes are enlarged and have a brown-yellow parenchymous discoloration,[1533] often with abscesses. Malakoplakia causes tubular destruction that is associated with a dense infiltrate of macrophages with granular eosinophilic cytoplasm that often contains Michaelis–Gutmann bodies (Fig. 12-160).[1534,1535]

The differential diagnosis includes idiopathic granulomatous orchitis and Leydig cell tumor. Inflammation in idiopathic granulomatous orchitis includes intratubular multinucleate giant cells; in malakoplakia it is difficult to identify the tubular outlines, and giant cells are usually absent. Leydig cell tumor is not usually associated with

inflammation, but may contain mononucleated or binucleated cells with abundant eosinophilic cytoplasm. Reinke's crystalloids are identified in up to 40% of cases of Leydig cell tumor but absent in malakoplakia, and Michaelis–Gutmann bodies are absent.

## Orchidoepididymitis caused by fungi and parasites

Fungal orchitis is rare; most cases are associated with blastomycosis, coccidiomycosis, histoplasmosis, and cryptococcocis.[1536] The genital tract may be involved in widespread blastomycosis. In decreasing order, the organs most frequently affected are the prostate, epididymis, testis, and seminal vesicles. Grossly, there often are small abscesses that may have caseous centers. Fungi measuring 8–15 µm in diameter with double refringent contours are present in the giant cells in granulomas and stain positively with periodic acid–Schiff and methenamine silver stains.

Coccidioidomycosis is endemic in California, the southwestern United States, and Mexico, and may present as epididymal disease after remission of systemic symptoms.[1537] The granulomas are similar to those of tuberculosis and contain 30–60 µm sporangia with endospores that stain with periodic acid–Schiff. Dissemination of histoplasmosis and cryptococcosis frequently occurs after steroid therapy and may give rise to granulomatous orchitis with extensive necrosis.[1538] Histoplasma capsulatum measures 1–5 µm in diameter and may be demonstrated with silver stain. Cryptococcus is identified by its thick wall that stains with mucicarmine.

Most parasites that reach the genital tract, such as Phyllaria and Schistosoma, are in the spermatic cord, and testicular lesions are secondary to vascular injury.[1539] Testicular infection has also been reported in patients with visceral leishmaniasis, congenital and acquired toxoplasmosis (Fig. 12-161),[1540] Echinococcus infection,[1541] and orchitis due to Trichomonas vaginalis.

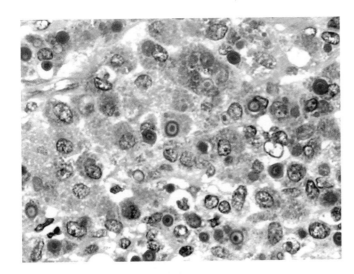

**Fig. 12-160** Malakoplakia of the testis showing macrophages with granular and eosinophilic cytoplasm that contains several Michaelis–Gutmann bodies.

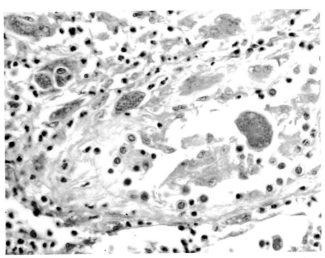

**Fig. 12-161** Orchitis caused by toxoplasmosis. The giant cells in the testicular interstitium and those in the seminiferous tubules or walls contain numerous organisms.

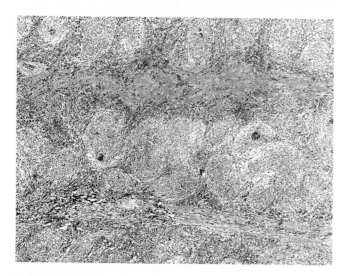

**Fig. 12-162** Idiopathic granulomatous orchitis showing seminiferous tubules with peritubular fibrosis. Numerous lymphocytes and macrophages are present in the interstitium and within seminiferous tubules. Multinucleated giant cells are present in some tubules.

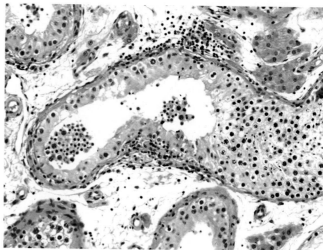

**Fig. 12-163** Focal orchitis showing infiltrates of lymphoid cells and macrophages within a seminiferous tubule. There is persistence of Sertoli cells and isolated spermatogonia.

## Idiopathic granulomatous orchitis

Idiopathic granulomatous orchitis is a chronic inflammatory condition of older adults (mean, 59.2 years). The most prominent clinical symptom is testicular enlargement, suggesting malignancy.[1542] Most patients have a history of scrotal trauma, 66% have symptoms of urinary tract infection with negative cultures, and 40% have sperm granuloma in the epididymis. An autoimmune etiology has been suggested.

The testis is enlarged, with a nodular cut surface and areas of necrosis or infarction. There are two histologic forms, according to whether the lesion is predominantly in the tubules (tubular orchitis) or the interstitium (interstitial orchitis). In tubular orchitis, germ cells degenerate and the Sertoli cells have vacuolated cytoplasm and vesicular nuclei. Plasma cells and lymphocytes infiltrate the walls of the seminiferous tubules, forming concentric rings. Multinucleated giant cells are present in the tubular lumina and sometimes in the interstitium (Fig. 12-162). Vascular thrombosis and arteritis are common. In interstitial orchitis, the inflammation is predominantly interstitial. Ultimately, tubular atrophy and interstitial fibrosis prevail in both forms, which may arise from different immune mechanisms.[1543] Tubular orchitis histologically resembles experimental orchitis caused by injection of serum from animals with orchitis, whereas interstitial orchitis resembles orchitis produced by the transfer of cells from immunized animals.

The differential diagnosis of idiopathic granulomatous orchitis is infectious orchitis caused by bacteria, spirochetes, fungi, or parasites. A useful clue in the tubular form is the presence of giant cells within seminiferous tubules.

## Focal orchitis

The occurrence of focal lymphoid cell infiltrates in the testicular interstitium is common in infertile patients,[1544,1545] patients who have undergone surgery for bilateral inguinal hernia,[1546] vasectomized patients who developed post-infection obstruction,[1547] after testicular piercing,[1548] and cryptorchidism.[1549] Inflammatory infiltrates usually involve the seminiferous tubules, and this suggests the disorder is due to an immunologic response (Fig. 12-163).

## Testicular pseudolymphoma

Pseudolymphoma is a benign reactive process with a lymphoid cell proliferation so intense that it may be mistaken for lymphoma. Testicular pseudolymphoma consists of inflammatory infiltrates with numerous lymphocytes and plasma cells that partially or totally destroy testicular parenchyma.[1550,1551]

The differential diagnosis includes lymphoma, various forms of orchitis, and seminoma. The diagnosis of lymphoma may be excluded by the lack of atypia and polyclonal nature of the inflammation. Syphilitic orchitis also contains a plasma cell-rich inflammatory infiltrate, but pseudolymphoma does not have other characteristic features of syphilitic orchitis, such as endarteritis obliterans; spirochetes cannot be demonstrated by special stains. The lack of granulomas or significant numbers of macrophages, together with the negative results of specific histochemical stains, also helps to exclude idiopathic granulomatous orchitis, tuberculosis, leprosy, sarcoidosis, and fungal infection. Finally, although the presence of a prominent inflammatory infiltrate and, in many cases, numerous lymphoid follicles, may suggest the diagnosis of seminoma, the presence of seminoma cells should be easily demonstrated with Best's carmine stain, periodic acid–Schiff, or placenta-like alkaline phosphatase. The term plasma cell granuloma[1152] refers to a reactive process characterized by the presence of polyclonal adult plasma cells that are absent in testicular plasmacytoma.[1553]

## Histiocytosis with testicular involvement

Sinus histiocytosis with massive lymphadenopathy (Rosai–Dorfman disease) is a benign proliferation of macrophages that uniquely contain numerous lymphocytes in their cytoplasm. The disease was reported in a kidney and testis of a patient in remission from malignant lymphoma in association with monoclonal IgA gammopathy,[1554] and in a second patient with diabetes mellitus who had been previously treated for pulmonary tuberculosis.[1555]

Increased numbers of interstitial macrophages may also be observed in more than two-thirds of autopsies from adult patients, but the cause is unknown. One condition associated with this disorder is treatment with hydroxyethylstarch plasma expander. In this lesion, the interstitial macrophages stand out by virtue of their large size and multivacuolated cytoplasm, suggesting thesaurosis. There is no evidence of mucin glycoproteins, proteoglycans, starch, lipids, glycogen, or foreign body material. Most patients have no clinical symptoms other than pruritus and persistent erythrema.[1556]

## Other testicular and epididymal lesions

### Epididymitis nodosa

Epididymitis nodosa is a proliferation of small irregular ducts whose epithelium lacks the characteristic features of the epididymal epithelium. The disorder is associated with inflammation and fibrosis, similar to vasitis nodosa.[1557]

### Epididymitis induced by amiodarone

In several tissues, including the testis, amiodarone is concentrated up to 300 times its plasma level,[1558] causing testicular atrophy and increased serum levels of FSH and LH in some patients.[1559] The incidence of epididymitis during amiodarone therapy varies from 3% to 11%,[1560,1561] and more than 35 cases (in several cases involvement was bilateral) have been reported, although there are probably many others.[1562,1563] The disorder may occur at any age.[1564] When amiodarone dosage is reduced to 300 mg/day the epididymitis heals within a few weeks.[1565] Autopsy studies show focal areas of fibrosis and lymphoid cell infiltrates not related to infection. Recognition is important to avoid unnecessary antibiotics or aggressive surgery.

### Ischemic granulomatous epididymitis

This term describes a lesion located in the epididymal head characterized by non-infectious necrosis with polypoid masses of inflamed granulation tissue in peripheral ductal structures. Granulomas containing multinucleated giant cells present within efferent ductuli or form sperm microgranulomas with ductal neoformation similar to that of epididymitis nodosa. The cause is unknown, but may result from ischemia.[1566]

### Calculus (stone in the testis)

The terms 'testicular calculus' and 'stone in the testis' have been used to describe a lesion characterized by the presence of nodular testicular calcification that is not related to ischemia, orchitis, vasculitis, hematoma, or tumor.[1567,1568]

## Polyarteritis nodosa

The testicular arteries may be affected by systemic disorders such as Schönlein–Henoch purpura,[1569] Wegener's disease,[1570,1571] Kogan's disease,[1572] Behçet's disease,[1573] relapsing polychondritis, rheumatoid arthritis, and dermatomyositis, but the most frequent involvement is with polyarteritis nodosa.[1574] Approximately 80% of patients with polyarteritis nodosa have testicular or epididymal involvement,[1575] but only 2–18% are diagnosed during life. Rarely, testicular or epididymal polyarteritis nodosa is the first manifestation of the disease. In these cases the symptoms may suggest orchitis, epididymitis, testicular torsion, or tumor.[1576-1578]

The testis usually shows arterial lesions in different stages of evolution, including fibrinoid necrosis, inflammatory reaction, thrombosis, or aneurysm. The parenchyma initially has zones of infarction (Fig. 12-164). Histologic and immunohistochemical findings similar to those of polyarteritis nodosa may occasionally be observed in the testis or the epididymis without lesions elsewhere; this condition is referred to as isolated arteritis of the testis and epididymis,[1579] and differs from classic polyarteritis by a lack of vascular thrombosis, aneurysm, or infarct. The etiology of isolated arteritis is unknown, but the prognosis is excellent.[1580] The histologic findings of necrotizing arteritis in the testis or epididymis should be followed by clinical, hematologic, and biochemical studies to exclude systemic arteritis.[1581,1582]

## Testicular infarct

Torsion of the spermatic cord is the most frequent cause of testicular infarct, followed by trauma, incarcerated inguinal hernia, epididymitis, and vasculitis.

### Spermatic cord torsion

Spermatic cord torsion is a surgical emergency. If repair is delayed more than 8 hours, testicular viability is usually compromised. This disorder may appear at any age, but the

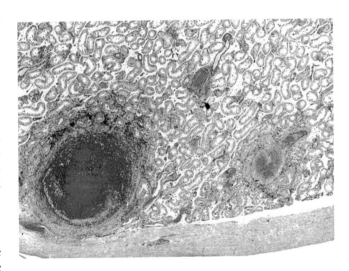

**Fig. 12-164** Polyarteritis nodosa involving several intraparenchymal arteries.

peaks of maximal incidence are the perinatal period and puberty.[1583]

Factors that predispose to testicular torsion are anatomical anomalies in testicular suspension and abnormal position of the testis. Many men with testicular torsion have an abnormally high reflection of the tunica vaginalis, giving rise to the deformity known as 'bell-clapper.' Other anomalies include elongated mesorchium, separation between the epididymis and testis, and absent or very elongated gubernaculum. The frequency of testicular torsion is higher in cryptorchid and retractile testes than in normal testes.

There are two classic anatomic forms of testicular torsion: high (supravaginal or extravaginal) and low (intravaginal). Each appears at a different age. Extravaginal torsion typically occurs in infancy and childhood, whereas intravaginal torsion is more frequent at puberty and adulthood.

Neonatal torsion is bilateral in 12–21% of cases.[1584] Most torsion observed on the first of life is intrauterine.[1585] Pubertal and adult torsion causes testicular pain that may radiate to the abdomen or other sites. About 36% of patients have a previous history of pain or swelling in one or both testes. The differential diagnosis includes all causes of acute scrotum.[1586,1587]

Torsion causes hemorrhagic infarction of the testis (Fig. 12-165). In old neonatal torsion, the histological findings are so advanced that only collagenized tissue containing calcium and hemosiderin deposits is seen. In adults, three degrees of histological lesion may be distinguished.[1588] Degree I (26.5% of adult twisted testes) is characterized by edema, vascular congestion, and focal hemorrhage. Seminiferous tubules are dilated, with sloughed immature germ cells, apical vacuolation of Sertoli cells, and dilated lymphatic vessels.[1589] Degree II (26.5% of testes) has pronounced interstitial hemorrhage and sloughing of all germ cell types in the seminiferous tubules. The lesion is more severe in the center of the testis, and thus biopsy might provide erroneous information (Fig. 12-166). Degree III lesions (45% of testes) are characterized by necrosis of the seminiferous tubular cell layers. There is often a correlation between the time interval of torsion and the degree of the histologic lesion.[1590] Degree I appears in torsion of less than 4 hours' duration, degree II in torsion of between 4 and 8 hours, and degree III in torsion of more than 12 hours. Nevertheless, there are some exceptions that could probably be related, among other factors, to the number of twists in the torsed spermatic cord (degrees of testicular rotation). The testicular salvage rate, defined as testicular growth and development that reflects the age of the patient and the contralateral testis, is around 50% in all cases of testicular torsion.[1591] Testes that do not bleed into the albugineal incision within 10 minutes are assumed to be non-viable and should be removed.[1592]

Little attention has been paid to intermittent testicular torsion. Early orchiopexy may save these testes, but after surgery, the testis becomes small and excessively mobile, and most have the bell-clapper deformity.[1593] Seminiferous tubules are devoid of germ cells and have hyalinized walls.

Some adults with untreated testicular torsion develop lipomembranous fat necrosis of the spermatic cord.[1594] Patients seek help for pain in the high scrotum. At this level, there is a small nodule that corresponds to remnants of the twisted testis. The epididymis and proximal spermatic cord characteristically contain fat necrosis (Fig. 12-167).

Adults with prior spermatic cord torsion often consult for infertility. The mechanism causing spermiogram alteration is controversial, and three hypotheses have been proposed:

- *Autoimmune process.* It has been suggested that the ischemic injury breaks the blood–testis barrier, and antigens released from the necrotic germ cells activate

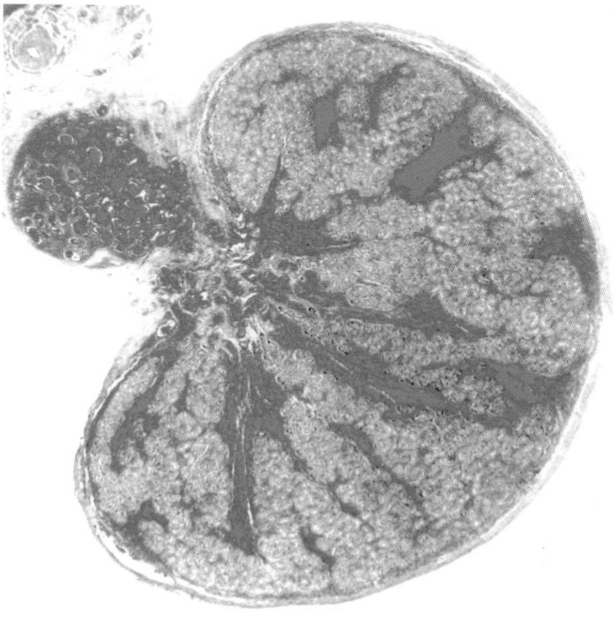

**Fig. 12-165** Hemorrhagic infarct in a newborn testis. The hemorrhagic areas are near the rete testis and follow the course of the centripetal veins.

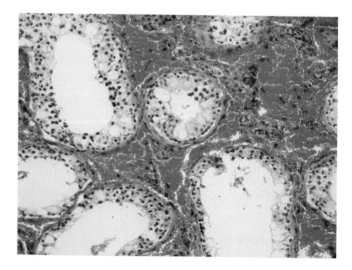

**Fig. 12-166** Hemorrhagic infarct grade II in a 13-year-old boy. There is interstitial hemorrhage, focal sloughing of the seminiferous tubular cells, and intense Sertoli cell vacuolation.

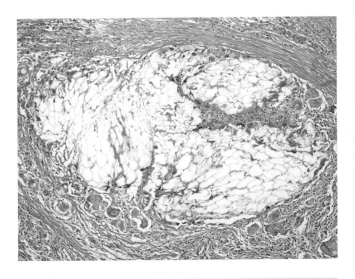

**Fig. 12-167** Lipomembranous fat necrosis in a 14-year-old boy who presented with a history of several weeks of intense scrotal pain. Giant cell granulomatous reaction around the membranes had developed.

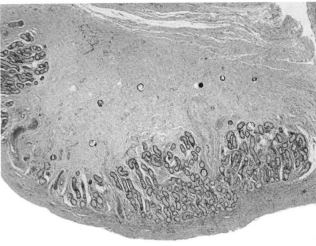

**Fig. 12-168** Longitudinally sectioned testis from a 4-year-old infant who had previously undergone orchidopexy. The testis shows marked fibrosis and numerous calcifications except for the periphery of the testicular parenchyma.

macrophages and lymphocytes in the interstitium, stimulating the formation of antibodies against these antigens. These antibodies that enter in the blood circulation may presumably damage the contralateral testis.[1595]

- *Alterations in microcirculation.* After testicular torsion, blood flow decreases in the contralateral testis, causing an increase in the characteristic products of hypoxia, such as lactic acid and hypoxanthine.[1596] Intense apoptosis involving mainly spermatocytes I and II has been observed.[1597] Long-term effects are yet unknown.

- *Primary testicular lesions.* Many twisted testes have lesions that cannot be formed in a few hours, such as hypoplastic tubules, microlithiasis, and focal spermatogenesis. In addition, more than half of biopsies of the contralateral testis show marked spermatogenetic lesions.[1598] These findings suggest that torsion occurs in testes with congenital lesions.

### Other causes of testicular infarct

Trauma[1599] and lesions of the vessels of the spermatic cord may also cause testicular infarct. Ischemic atrophy is a risk of inguinal surgery, including herniorrhaphy, varicocelectomy, hydrocelectomy, and descent of cryptorchid testis (Fig. 12-168). The incidence of atrophy after inguinal herniorrhaphy varies from 0.06% in primary herniorrhaphy[1600] to 7.9% after surgery for recurrent herna,[1601] depending on the difficulty and extent of the hernia. Atrophy occurs in some cases of thrombosis of the vena cava or spermatic artery.[1602] Focal infarction of the testis is associated with polycythemia, sickle cell disease, trauma,[1603,1604] and laparoscopic inguinal hernia repair.

Focal infarction may also be spontaneous. Clinical symptoms of testicular infarct mimic testicular tumor. Color Doppler ultrasound reveals the diagnosis in most cases.[1605]

## Other testicular diseases

### Cystic malformation

Cystic malformation of the tunica albuginea and testicular parenchyma was first described in the 19th century,[1606] and was long considered rare and mainly present in the tunica albuginea.[1607,1608] With the systematic use of ultrasonography, the incidence of cysts has been found to be much higher:[1609] non-neoplastic cysts are found in 2.1%[1610] to 9.8%[1611] of testes.[1612,1613]

Cyst of the tunica albuginea is usually an incidental finding in patients in the fifth or sixth decade of life. It is located in the anterolateral aspect of the testis and may be unilocular or multilocular,[1614] ranging from 2 to 4 mm and containing clear fluid without spermatozoa. The cyst may be embedded within the connective tissue of the tunica albuginea, protrude from the inner surface of the tunica albuginea into the testicular parenchyma, or protrude from the outer surface forming a blue lump in the tunica albuginea. The epithelium lining the cyst may be simple columnar or stratified cuboidal, and is supported by a thin layer of collagenized connective tissue. The columnar epithelium usually includes some ciliated cells,[1615] and the cuboidal epithelium is composed of two layers of non-ciliated cells (Fig. 12-169).

Cyst of the rete testis is identified by a distinctive epithelial lining of areas of flattened cells intermingled with areas of tall columnar cells. Spermatozoa are frequently found within the cyst,[1616] and hence the cyst is also called intratesticular spermatocele.[1617] It may be associated with cystic transformation of the rete testis and multiple epididymal cysts. Rete testis cyst is not always attached to the rete and may be found at a distance.

Simple cyst of the testis constitutes the remaining intraparenchymal cyst. It is usually lined by cuboidal epithelium and contains no spermatozoa.[1618,1619] Simple cyst ranges

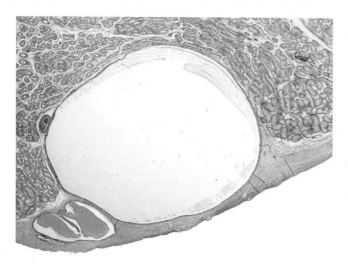

**Fig. 12-169** Multilocular cyst in the tunica albuginea. The largest cavity protrudes into the testicular parenchyma.

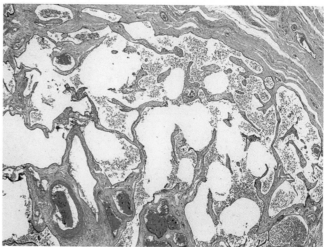

**Fig. 12-170** Cystic transformation of the rete testis secondary to a lesion in the caput epididymidis in a patient with chronic epididymitis.

from 2 nm to 18 mm in diameter.[1620,1621] The disorders occurs at any age, from 5 months to 80 years, with a bimodal distribution with peaks at 8 month and 60 years.[1622] It may occur bilaterally,[1623] and may present as two cysts in the same testis.[1624]

Origin of the three types of testicular cyst is uncertain. Previously, traumatic[1625] and inflammatory[1626] origins were attributed to tunica albuginea cyst, but most now believe that they are derived from embryonal remnants of the mesonephric ducts[1615,1627] or mesothelial cells embedded in the tunica albuginea during embryogenesis.[1614,1628,1629] Simple cyst of the testis may also have a mesothelial origin, but it is possible that some arise from ectopic rete testis epithelium. These cysts are unrelated to epidermoid cyst, differing in the ultrasonographic[1630,1631] and histologic features (see discussion on cystic dysplasia and testicular tumors in the section on hamartomatous testicular lesions). Ultrasound studies indicate that testicular cyst has little potential for growth.[1630,1632] Currently, excision is recommended only in children when the cyst may impair testicular development.[1633]

## Disorders of the rete testis

### Dysgenesis

Dysgenesis of the rete testis is characterized by inadequate maturation and persistence of infantile or pubertal characteristics in adults.[1634] This disorder is frequent in undescended adult testes. The lesion involves the rete testis segments referred to as septal, mediastinal, and extratesticular. There is poor development of the cavities and their epithelial lining, which becomes cuboidal or columnar instead of flattened with areas of columnar cells. The lumina of the rete testis cavities may be completely absent (simple hypoplasia) or, conversely, undergo microcystic dilation (cystic hypoplasia). In a few cases, the rete testis develops papillary, cribriform, or tubular formations (adenomatous hyperplasia).

## Metaplasia

The epithelium of the rete testis is usually flattened, with scattered areas of columnar cells. In estrogen-treated patients, those with chronic hepatic insufficiency, functioning tumor that secretes estrogens or human chorionic gonadotropin, and other disorders that are described as hyperplasia of the rete testis it may undergo diffuse transformation into tall columnar epithelium. Except for the latter group, metaplasia of the rete testis seems to be an estrogen-dependent process, and estrogen receptors are present in the rete testis epithelium.[1635]

## Cystic ectasia of the rete testis (acquired cystic transformation)

Acquired cystic transformation of the rete testis is common, and its incidence increases with age and associated disorders.[1636] Ultrasound[1637,1638] and magnetic resonance[1639] studies reveal characteristic images that may suggest malignancy. The lesion has three forms: simple, associated with epithelial metaplasia, and with crystalline deposits.

Simple cystic transformation consists of dilated cavities with normal epithelium. It results from obstruction of the epididymis or the initial portion of the vas deferens due to ischemia (aging men); compression by epididymal and spermatic cord tumor, or by congestive veins in varicocele; inflammation in patients with previous epididymitis; malformation (testis–epididymis dissociation, malformed epididymis and absence of the vas deferens);[1640] or iatrogenic causes (surgery for epididymoectomy or removal of epididymal cyst) (Fig. 12-170).[1641]

Cystic transformation with epithelial metaplasia is a frequent finding at autopsy.[1369] Its development is probably due to the concurrence of sperm excretory duct obstruction and conditions involved in increased serum estrogen levels, such as chronic liver insufficiency. Another possible cause is inflammation involving the rete testis.

Cystic transformation with crystalline deposits has also been called cystic transformation of the rete testis secondary

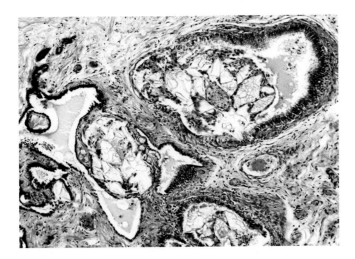

**Fig. 12-171** Changes in the rete testis associated with dialysis. Dilation of the rete testis and initial portion of the ductuli efferentes can be observed. Crystalline structures, mainly rhomboidal in shape, accumulate inside and outside the tubules.

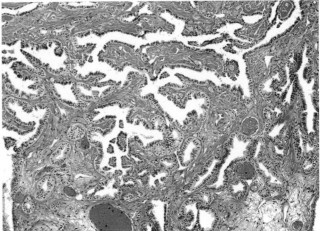

**Fig. 12-173** Adenomatous hyperplasia of the rete testis. The epithelium is columnar and supported by a well-collagenized stroma.

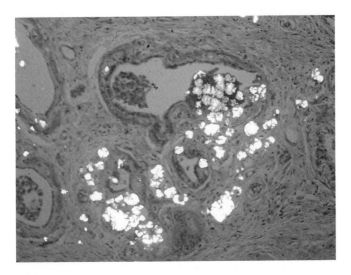

**Fig. 12-172** Renal dialysis-associated cystic transformation of the rete testis with oxalate crystals demonstrated by polarized light.

to renal insufficiency.[1642] It is a bilateral lesion of adult testes characterized by the concurrence of three findings: cystic transformation of the rete testis, cuboidal or columnar metaplasia of its epithelium, and the presence of urate and oxalate crystalline deposits that may be recognized by polarized light. The lesion is pathognomonic of dialyzed patients with chronic renal insufficiency. Crystalline deposits are initially formed beneath the epithelia of the rete testis and ductuli efferentes; later they protrude into the lumina, where they are finally released. Inflammation is absent or slight, although a few giant cells and small fibrotic areas are often seen (Figs 12-171, 12-172).

## Adenomatous hyperplasia

This lesion is characterized by diffuse or nodular proliferation of tubular or papillary structures that are derived from the rete testis[1643] and are observed in cryptorchid or normally descended testes. Cases have been reported in newborns, children, and adults.[1644]

Adenomatous hyperplasia in newborn and infantile testes consists of enlargement of the mediastinum testis by cord-like or tubular structures derived from the rete testis. The lesion may extend up to one-third of testicular volume. Despite excessive development of the rete testis, the normal connections with seminiferous tubules and efferent ductuli remain. Presentation may be unilateral or bilateral. Unilateral presentation is associated with cryptorchidism or vanishing testis. Bilateral cases may also present with bilateral renal dysplasia. Efferent ductuli may show luminal dilation and irregular outlines. The etiopathogenesis might be similar to that of cystic dysplasia of the testis.[1644]

Adenomatous hyperplasia in adults is usually an incidental finding at autopsy,[1645] in cryptorchid testes,[1646] or in testes with germ cell tumor. The rete testis epithelium forms non-encapsulated nodular outgrowths or a diffuse pattern. Nodule size may be large enough to suggest tumor. The epithelium consists of cuboidal cells with ovoid nuclei, deep nuclear folds, and peripheral nucleoli. Atypias and mitotic figures are lacking (Fig. 12-173). The ultrastructure and immunophenotype of the epithelium are similar to those of the normal rete testis. Spermatozoa may be seen inside the cavities in some cases, suggesting that such a proliferation is connected with the seminiferous tubules. Most of the testes show a certain degree of seminiferous tubular atrophy.

In incidental autopsy cases the etiology is unknown, although it may be related to hormonal or chemical agent effects.[1647-1649] In cryptorchid testes and with many testicular tumors, the most probable cause is a primary anomaly that is part of the testicular dysgenesis syndrome.[1650]

Adenomatous hyperplasia should be distinguished from three entities: rete testis pseudohyperplasia, which appears in atrophic testes; primary rete testis tumor; and metastasis of adenocarcinoma. In pseudohyperplasia, lesions are focal, microscopic, and usually located in the septal rete, although the mediastinal rete shows few or no alterations. Benign rete testis tumor such as adenoma (solid and papillary variants)

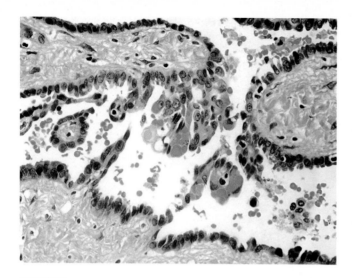

**Fig. 12-174** Rete testis hyperplasia with hyaline globules. The globule-containing cells protrude into the lumina of the rete testis channels.

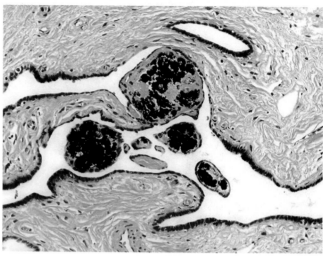

**Fig. 12-175** Nodular proliferation of calcifying connective tissue in the rete testis with large calcium deposits.

and cystoadenoma are isolated and focal,[1651] whereas rete testis hyperplasia is diffuse. Adenocarcinoma of the rete testis is a tumor that displays numerous mitotic figures and infiltrates adjacent structures.[1652] Metastasis of prostatic adenocarcinoma may be excluded because these metastases alter the rete testis architecture and are immunoreactive for prostatic acid phosphatase and PSA.

### Hyperplasia with hyaline globule formation

This reactive lesion is characterized by the presence of intracytoplasmic accumulation of hyaline eosinophilic globules in the epithelial cells of the rete testis. The epithelium may be hyperplastic, but does not contain mitotic figures or nuclear atypia. The globules are up to 15 µm in diameter (Fig. 12-174). This lesion is associated with tumor and inflammatory processes occurring near the mediastinum testis, and can be observed in association with 75% of mixed testicular germ cell tumors, 47% of seminomas, and 20% of non-germ cell testicular tumors, such as epididymal tumor that infiltrates the testis (adenomatoid tumor).[1653] Yolk sac tumor infiltrating the rete testis may closely resemble this type of rete testis hyperplasia. Positive immunoreactions for α-fetoprotein and placenta-like alkaline phosphatase, as

well as nuclear atypia, are helpful to distinguish germ cell neoplasia from this rete testis hyperplasia.[1654]

### Intracavitary polypoid nodular proliferation

This lesion, described as nodular proliferation of calcifying connective tissue in the rete testis, is characterized by the presence of multiple nodules that originate from the rete testis lining and subjacent connective tissue, protruding into the channels of the rete testis. These consist of cellular connective tissue covered by several layers of a fibrin-like material, which in turn is covered by rete testis epithelium. The nodules may be totally or partially calcified (Fig. 12-175).[1655] The lesion is an incidental finding at autopsy in patients with impaired peripheral perfusion.

Selective location of the lesion in the walls of the cavities and chordae rete testis is probably related to poor vascularization of these structures. The etiopathogenetic mechanism may be anoxia, necrosis, fibrin deposition, proliferation of connective tissue, or dystrophic calcification. The intracavitary growth of the lesion might be due to the lower intracavitary pressure and also to the stiff structure of the mediastinum testis.

## REFERENCES

1. Hiort O, Holterhus PM. The molecular basis of male sexual differentiation. Eur J Endocrinol 2000; 142: 101–110.
2. Gessler M, Poustka A, Cavenee W, et al. Homozygous deletions in Wilms' tumours of a zinc-finger gene identified by chromosome jumping. Nature 1990; 343: 774–778.
3. Call, KM, Glaser T, Ito CY, et al. Isolation and characterization of a zinc finger polypeptide gene at the human chromosome 11 Wilms' tumor locus. Cell 1990; 60: 509–520.
4. Kreidberg JA, Sariola H, Loring JM, et al. WT-1 is required for early kidney development. Cell 1993; 74: 679–691.
5. Pelletier J, Bruening W, Kashtan CE, et al. Germline mutations in the Wilms' tumor suppressor gene are associated with abnormal urogenital development in Denys–Drash syndrome. Cell 1991; 67: 437–447.
6. Barbaux S, Niaudet P, Gubler MC, et al. Donor splice-site mutations in WT1 are responsible for Frasier syndrome. Nature Genet 1997; 17: 467–470.
7. Hanley NA, Ball SG, Clement-Jones M, et al. Expression of steroidogenic factor 1 and Wilms' tumour 1 during early human gonadal development and sex determination. Mech Dev 1999; 87: 175–180.
8. Achermann JC, Ito M, Hindmarsh PC, et al. A mutation in the gene encoding steroidogenic factor-1 causes XY sex reversal and adrenal failure in humans. Nature Genet 1999; 22: 125–126.

9. Biason-Lauber A, Schoenle EJ. Apparently normal ovarian differentiation in a prepubertal girl with transcriptionally inactive steroidogenic factor 1 (NR5A1/SF-1) and adrenal cortical insufficiency. Am J Hum Genet 2000; 67: 1563–1568.

10. Lim HN, Hawkins JR. Genetic control of gonadal differentiation, Baillière's Clin Endocrinol Metab 1998; 12: 1–16.

11. Bishop CE, Guellaen G, Gelowerth D, et al. Single-copy DNA sequences specific for the human Y chromosome. Nature 1984; 309: 253–255.

12. McElreavey K, Fellous M. Sex determination and the Y chromosome, Am J Med Genet 1999; 89: 176–185.

13. Blyth B, Duckett JW. Gonadal differentiation: a review of the physiological process and influencing factors based on recent experimental evidence. J Urol 1991; 145: 689–694.

14. Salas-Cortes L, Jaubert F, Barbaux S, et al. The human SRY protein is present in fetal and adult Sertoli cells and germ cells. Int J Dev Biol 1999; 43: 135–140.

15. Haqq CM, King CY, Ukiyama E, et al. Molecular basis of mammalian sexual determination: activation of Müllerian inhibiting substance gene expression by SRY. Science 1999; 266: 1494–1500.

16. Huang B, Wang S, Ning Y, et al. Autosomal XX sex reversal caused by duplication of SOX-9. Am J Med Genet 1999; 87: 349–353.

17. Foster JW, Dominguez-Steglich MA, Guioli S, et al. Campomelic dysplasia and autosomal sex reversal caused by mutations in an SRY-related gene. Nature 1994; 372: 525–530.

18. Chaboissier MC, Kobayashi A, Vidal VI, et al. Functional analysis of Sox8 and Sox9 during sex determination in the mouse. Development 2004; 131: 1891–1901.

19. Wagner T, Wirth J, Meyer J, et al. Autosomal sex reversal and campomelic dysplasia are caused by mutations in and around the SRY-related gene SOX9. Cell 1994; 79: 1111–1120.

20. Zhou R, Liu L, Guo Y, et al. Similar gene structure of two Sox9a genes and their expression patterns during gonadal differentiation in a teleost fish, rice field eel (*Monopterus albus*). Mol Reprod Dev 2003; 66: 211–217.

21. Koopman P. Sex determination: a tale of two Sox genes. Trends Genet 2005; 21: 367–370.

22. Wolf U. The molecular genetics of human sex determination. J Mol Med 1995; 73: 325–331.

23. Baumstark A, Barbi G, Djalali M, et al. X-p duplications with and without sex reversal. Hum Genet 1996; 97: 79–86.

24. Bennett CP, Docherty Z, Robb SA, et al. Deletion 9p and sex reversal. J Med Genet 1993; 30: 518–520.

25. Wilkie AOM, Campbell FM, Daubeney P. Complete and partial XY sex reversal associated with terminal deletion of 10q: report of 2 cases and literature review. Am J Med Genet 1993; 46: 597–600.

26. Merchant-Larios H, Moreno-Mendoza N, Buehr M. The role of the mesonephros in cell differentiation and morphogenesis of the mouse fetal testis. Int J Dev Biol 1993; 37: 407–415.

27. Moreno-Mendoza N, Herrera-Muñoz J, Merchant-Larios H. Limb bud mesenchyme permits seminiferous cord formation in the mouse fetal testis but subsequent testosterone output is markedly affected by the sex of the donor stromal tissue. Dev Biol 1995; 169: 51–56.

28. Tilmann C, Capel B. Mesonephric cell migration induces testis cord formation and Sertoli cell differentiation in the mammalian gonad. Development 1999; 126: 2883–2890.

29. Capel B, Albrecht K, Washburn LL, et al. Migration of mesonephric cells into the mammalian gonad depends on Sry. Mech Dev 1999; 84: 127–131.

30. Karl J, Capel B. Sertoli cells of the mouse testis originate from the coelomic epithelium. Dev Biol 1998; 203: 323–333.

31. Magre S, Jost A. Sertoli cells and testicular differentiation in the rat fetus. J Electron Microsc Tech 1991; 19: 172–188.

32. Wartenberg H, Kinsky I, Viebahn C, Schmolke C. Fine structural characteristics of testicular cord formation in the developing rabbit gonad. J Electron Microsc Tech 1991; 19: 133–157.

33. Satoh M. Histogenesis and organogenesis of the gonad in human embryos. J Anat 1991; 177: 85–107.

34. Merchant-Larios H, Moreno-Mendoza N. Mesonephric stromal cells differentiate into Leydig cells in the mouse fetal testis. Exp Cell Res 1998; 244: 230–238.

35. Merchant-Larios H, Taketo T. Testicular differentiation in mammals under normal and experimental conditions. J Electron Microsc Tech 1991; 19: 158–171.

36. Takedo T. Production of müllerian-inhibiting substance (MIS) and sulfated glycoprtein-2 (SGP-2) associated with testicular differentiation in the XX mouse gonadal graft. In: Robaire B, ed. The male germ cell. Ann NY Acad Sci 1991; 637: 74–89.

37. Byskov AG. Differentiation of the mammalian embryonic gonad. Physiol Rev 1986; 66: 71–117.

38. Haider SG, Laue D, Schwochau G, Hilscher B. Morphological studies on the origin of adult-type Leydig cells in rat testis. Ital J Anat Embryol 1995; 100: 535–541.

39. Lee MM, Donahoe PK. Müllerian inhibiting substance: a gonadal hormone with multiple functions. Endocrinol Rev 1993; 14: 152–164.

40. Picard JY, Josso N. Purification of testicular anti-müllerian hormone allowing direct visualization of the pure glycoprotein and determination of yield and purification factor. Mol Cell Endocrinol 1984; 34: 23–29.

41. Josso N, Picard JY. Anti-müllerian hormone. Physiol Rev 1986; 66: 1038–1090.

42. Behringer RR, Finegold MJ, Cate RL. Müllerian-inhibiting substance function during mammalian sexual development. Cell 1994; 79: 415–425.

43. Tran D, Muesy-Dessole N, Josso N. Anti-müllerian hormone is a functional marker of foetal Sertoli cells. Nature 1977; 269: 411–412.

44. Josso N, Cate RL, Picard JY, et al. Anti-Müllerian hormone, the Jost factor. Recent Prog Hormone Res 1993; 48: 1–59.

45. Schwindt B, Doyle LW, Hutson JM. Serum levels of müllerian inhibiting substance in preterm and term male neonates. J Urol 1997; 158: 610–612.

46. Shen WH, Moore CC, Ikeda Y, et al. Nuclear receptor steroidogenic factor 1 regulates the müllerian inhibiting substance gene: a link to the sex determination cascade. Cell 1994; 77: 651–661.

47. Barbara PS, Moniot B, Poulat F, et al. Steroidogenic factor-1 regulates transcription of the human anti-müllerian hormone receptor. J Biol Chem 1998; 273: 29654–29660.

48. Rey R, Josso N. Regulation of testicular anti-Müllerian hormone secretion. Eur J Endocrinol 1996; 135: 144–152.

49. Jirasek JE. Development of the genital system and male pseudohermaphroditism. Baltimore: Johns Hopkins, 1971.

50. Musnsterberg A, Lovell-Badge R. Expression of the mouse anti-müllerian hormone gene suggests a role in both male and female sexual differentiation. Development 1991; 113: 613–624.

51. Catlin EA, Powell SM, Manganaro TF, et al. Sex-specific fetal lung development and Müllerian inhibiting substance. Am Rev Respir Dis 1990; 141: 466–470.

52. Cunha GR, Alarid ET, Turner T, et al. Normal and abnormal development of the male urogenital tract. Role of androgens, mesenchymal–epithelial interactions, and growth factors. J Androl 1992; 13: 465–475.

53. Larsen WJ. Human embryology. London: Churchill Livingstone, 1993; 247.

54. Orth JM. The role of follicle-stimulating hormone in controlling Sertoli cell proliferation in testes of fetal rats. Endocrinology 1984; 115: 1248–1255.

55. Eskola V, Nikula H, Huhtaniemi I. Age-retated variation of follicle-stimulating hormone stimulated cAMP production, protein kinase C activity and their interactions on the rat testis. Mol Cell Endocrinol 1993; 93: 143–148.

56. Wensing CJ. The embryology of testicular descent. Hormone Res 1988; 30: 144–152.

57. Heyns CF, De Klerk DP. The gubernaculum during testicular descent in the pig fetus. J Urol 1985; 133: 694–699.

58. Heyns CF. The gubernaculum during testicular descent in the human fetus. J Anat 1987; 153: 93–112.

59. Heyns CF, Human HJ, De Klerk DP. Hyperplasia and hypertrophy of the gubernaculum during testicular descent in the fetus. J Urol 1986; 135: 1043–1047.

60. Frey HL, Rajfer J. Incidence of cryptorchidism. Urol Clin North Am 1982; 9: 327–329.

61. Baumans V, Dijkstra G, Wensing CJ. The role of a non-androgenic testicular factor in the process of testicular descent in the dog. Int J Androl 1983; 6: 541–552.

62. Backhouse KM. Mechanism of testicular descent. Karger Prog Reprod Biol Med 1984; 10: 16–23.

63. Backhouse KM. The gubernaculum testis Hunteri, testicular descent and maldescent. Ann Roy Coll Surg Engl 1964; 35: 227–233.

64. Frey HL, Rajfer J. Role of the gubernaculum and intraabdominal pressure in the process of testicular descent. J Urol 1984; 131: 574–579.

65. Hutson JM, Hasthorpe S. Testicular descent and cryptorchidism: the state of the art in 2004. J Pediatr Surg 2005; 40: 297–302.

66. Baker LA, Nef S, Nguyen MT, et al. The insulin-3 Gene: Lack of a genetic basis for human cryptorchidism. J Urol 2002; 167: 2534–2537.

67. Tomiyama H, Hutson JM, Truong A, Agoulnik AI. Transabdominal testicular descent is disrupted in mice with deletion of insulinlike factor 3 receptor. J Pediatr Surg 2003; 38: 1793–1798.

68. Foresta C, Bettella A, Vinanzi C, et al. A novel circulating hormone of testis origin in humans. J Clin Endocrinol Metab 2004; 89: 5952–5958.

69. Yamanaka J, Metcalf SA, Hutson JM, Mendelsohn FA. Testicular descent II. Ontogeny and response to denervation of calcitonin gene-related peptide receptors in neonatal rat gubernaculum. Endocrinology 1993; 132: 280–284.

70. Hutson JM, Beasley SW. The mechanism of testicular descent. Aust Paediatr J 1987; 23: 215–216.

71. Goh DW, Middlesworth W, Farmer PJ, Hutson JM. Prenatal androgen blockade with flutamide inhibits masculinization of the genitofemoral nerve and testicular descent. J Pediatr Surg 1994; 29: 836–838.

72. Tanyel FC, Erdem S, Büyükpamukcu N, Tan E. Cremaster muscles obtained from boys with an undescended testis show significant neurological changes. BJU Int 2000; 85: 116–119.

73. Bernstein L, Pike MC, Depue RH, et al. Maternal hormone levels in early gestation of cryptorchid males: a case-control study. Br J Cancer 1988; 58: 379–381.

74. Spencer JR. The endocrinology of testicular descent. AUA Update Series Lesson 1994; 12: 94–99.

75. Staub C, Rauch M, Ferriere F, et al. Expression of estrogen receptor ESR1 and its 46-kDa variant in the gubernaculum testis. Biol Reprod 2005; 73: 703–707.

76. Cain MP, Kramer SA, Tindall DJ, Husmann DA. Expression of androgen receptor protein within the lumbar spinal cord during ontologic development and following antiandrogen induced cryptorchidism. J Urol 1994; 152: 766–769.

77. Belman AB. Acquired undescended (ascended) testis: Effects of human chorionic gonadotropin. J Urol 1988; 140: 1189–1190.

78. Vilar O. Histology of the human testis from neonatal period to adolescence. Adv Exp Med Biol 1970; 10: 95–111.

79. Müller J, Skakkebaek NE. Fluctuations in the number of germ cells during late foetal and early postnatal periods in boys. Acta Endocrinol 1984; 105: 271–274.

80. Müller J, Skakkebaek NE. Quantification of germ cells and seminiferous tubules by stereological examination of testicles of 50 boys who suffered from sudden death. Int J Androl 1983; 6: 143–156.

81. Cortes D, Müller J, Skakkebaek NE. Proliferation of Sertoli cells during development of the human testis assessed by stereological methods. Int J Androl 1987; 10: 589–596.

82. Nistal M, Abaurrea MA, Paniagua R. Morphological and histometric study of human Sertoli cells from birth to the onset of puberty. J Anat 1982; 134: 351–363.

83. Lin LH, DePhilip RM. Dfferential expression of placental (P)-cadherin in Sertoli cells and peritubular myoid cells during postnatal development of the mouse testis. Anat Rec 1996; 244: 155–164.

84. Prince FP. Ultrastructural evidence of mature Leydig cells and Leydig cell regression in the neonatal human testis. Anat Rec 1990; 228: 405–417.

85. Hadziselimovic F. Ultrastructure of normal and cryptorchid testis development. Adv Anat Embryol Cell Biol 1977; 53: 47–50.

86. Nistal M, Santamaría L, Paniagua R. Mast cells in the human testis and epididymis from birth to adulthood. Acta Anat 1984; 139: 535–552.

87. Faiman C, Reyes FI, Winter JSD. Serum gonadotropin patterns during the perinatal period in man and in the chimpanzee. INSERM 1974; 32: 281–298.

88. Forest mg, Sizonenko PC, Cathiard AM, et al. Hypophyso-gonadal function in humans during the first year of life. 1. Evidence for testicular activity in early infancy. J Clin Invest 1974; 53: 819–824.

89. Bidlingmaier F, Dörr HG, Eisenmenger W, et al. Testosterone and androstenedione concentrations in human testis and epididymis during the first two years of live. J Clin Endocrinol Metab 1983; 57: 311–315.

90. Pelliniemi LK, Kuopio T, Fröjdman K. The cell biology and function of the fetal Leydig cell. In: Payne A., Hardy M, Russel L, eds. The Leydig cell. Vienna, FL: Cache River Press, 1996; 141–174.

91. Codesal J, Regadera J, Nistal M, et al. Involution of human fetal Leydig cells. An immunohistochemical, ultrastructural and quantitative study. J Anat 1990; 172: 103–114.

92. Nistal M. Paraganglios del epidídimo humano. An Anat 1977; 1: 307–316.

93. Müller J, Skakkebaek NE. Quantification of germ cells and seminiferous tubules by stereological examination of testicles from 50 boys who suffered from sudden death. Int J Androl 1983; 6: 143–156.

94. Paniagua R, Nistal M. Morphological and histometric study of human spermatogonia from birth to the onset of puberty. J Anat 1984; 139: 535–552.

95. Codesal J, Santamaría L, Paniagua R, et al. Proliferative activity of human spermatogonia from fetal period to senility measured by cytophotometric DNA quantification. Arch Androl 1989; 22: 209–215.

96. Rey R. Assessment of seminiferous tubule function (anti-müllerian hormone). Baillière's Best Pract Res Clin Endocrinol Metab 2000; 14: 399–408.

97. Andersson AM, Toppari J, Haavisto AM, et al. Longitudinal reproductive hormone profiles in infants: Peak of inhibin B levels in infant boys exceeds levels in adult men. J Clin Endocrinol Metab 1998; 83: 675–681.

98. Racine C, Rey R, Forest MG, et al. Receptors for anti-Müllerian hormone on Leydig cell are responsible for its effects on steroidogenesis and cell differentiation. Proc Natl Acad Sci USA 1998; 95: 594–599.

99. Frasier SD, Horton R. Androgens in the peripheral plasma of prepubertal

children and adults. Steroids 1966; 8: 777–784.

100. Forti G, Santoro S, Andrea-Grisolia G, et al. Spermatic and peripheral plasma concentration of testosterone and androstenedione in prepubertal boys. J Clin Endocrinol Metab 1981; 53: 883–886.

101. Lee VMK, Burger HG. Pituitary testicular axis during puberal development. In: De Kretser DM, Burger HG, Hudson B, eds, The pituitary and testis: Clinical and experimental studies. Heidelberg: Springer Verlag, 1983; 44–70.

102. Mancini RE, Vilar O, Lavieri JC, et al. Development of Leydig cells in the normal human testis. A cytological, cytochemical and quantitative study. Am J Anat 1963; 112: 203–214.

103. Nistal M, Paniagua R, Regadera J, et al. A quantitative morphology study of human Leydig cells from birth to adulthood. Cell Tissue Res 1986; 246: 229–236.

104. Zachmann M, Kind HP, Häfliger H, et al. Testicular volume during adolescence. Cross-sectional and longitudinal studies. Helv Paediatr Acta 1974; 29: 61–72.

105. Daniel WA, Feinstein RA, Howard-Peebles P, et al. Testicular volumes of adolescent. J Pediatr 1982; 101: 1010–1012.

106. Hansen P, With TH. Clinical measurement of the testes in boys and men. Acta Med Scand 1952; 226: 457–465.

107. Orvis BR, Bottle SK, Kogan BA. Testicular histology in fetuses with the prune belly syndrome and posterior urethral valves. J Urol 1988; 139: 335–337.

108. Cortes D, Müller J, Skakkebaek NE. Proliferation of Sertoli cells during development of the human testis assessed by stereological methods. Int J Androl 1987; 10: 589–596.

109. Nistal M, Paniagua R, Abaurrea MA, et al. Hyperplasia and the immature appearance of Sertoli cells in primary testicular disorders. Hum Pathol 1982; 13: 3–12.

110. Nistal M, Garcia-Rodeja E, Paniagua R. Granular transformation of Sertoli cells in testicular disorders. Hum Pathol 1991; 22: 131–137.

111. Nistal M, Paniagua R, Regadera J, et al. A quantitative morphological study of human Leydig cells from birth to adulthood. Cell Tissue Res 1986; 246: 229–236.

112. Nistal M, González-Peramato P, Paniagua R. Congenital Leydig cell hyperplasia. Histopathology 1988; 12: 307–317.

113. Doshi N, Surti UI, Szulman AE. Morphologic anomalies in triploid liveborn fetuses. Hum Pathol 1983; 14: 716–723.

114. Behre HM, Nashan D, Nieschlag E. Objective measurement of testicular volume by ultrasonography: evaluation of the technique and

comparison with orchidometer estimates. J Androl 1989; 12: 395–403.

115. Diamond JM. Ethnic differences. Variation in human testis size. Nature 1986; 320: 488–489.

116. Handelsman DJ, Stara S. Testicular size: The effects of ageing, malnutrition, and illness. J Androl 1985; 6: 144–151.

117. Prader A. Testicular size: assesment and clinical importance. Triangle 1966; 7: 240–243.

118. Sosnik H. Studies of the participation of the tunica albuginea and rete testis (TA and RT) in the quantitative structure of human testis. Gegenbaurs Morphol Jahrb 1985; 131: 347–356.

119. Leeson CR, Forman DE. Postnatal development and differentiation of contractile cells within the rabbit testis. J Anat 1981; 132: 491–511.

120. Middendorff R, Muller D, Mewe M, et al. The tunica albuginea of the human testis is characterized by complex contraction and relaxation activities regulated by cyclic GMP. J Clin Endocrinol Metab 2002; 87: 3486–3499.

121. Trainer TD. Histology of the normal testis. Am J Surg Pathol 1987; 11: 107–171.

122. Lennox B, Ahmad RN, Mack WS. A method for determining the relative total lenght of the tubules in the testis. J Pathol 1970; 102: 229–238.

123. Fawcett DW, Burgos MH. The fine structure of Sertoli cells in the human testis. Anat Res 1956; 124: 401–402.

124. Nagano T. Some observations on the fine structure of the Sertoli cell in the human testis. Zeitschr Zellforsch 1966; 73: 89–106.

125. Schulze C. On the morphology of the human Sertoli cell. Cell Tissue Res 1974; 153: 339–355.

126. Schulze W, Rehder V. Organization and morphogenesis of the human seminiferous epithelium. Cell Tissue Res 1984; 237: 395–407.

127. Fawcett DW. The mammalian spermatozoon. Dev Biol 1975; 44: 394–436.

128. Paniagua R, Nistal M, Amat P, et al. Ultrastructural observations on nucleoli and related structures during human spermatogenesis. Anat Embryol 1986; 174: 301–306.

129. Bustos-Obregón E, Esponda P. Ultrastructure of the nucleus of human Sertoli cells in normal and pathological testes. Cell Tissue Res 1974; 152: 467–475.

130. Sáez JM, Avallet O, Lejeune H, et al. Cell–cell communication in the testis. Hormone Res 1991; 36: 104–115.

131. Dym M. The fine structure of the monkey (Macaca) Sertoli cell and its role in maintaining the blood–testis barrier. Anat Rec 1973; 175: 639–656.

132. Fawcett DW, Leak LV, Heidger PM. Electron microscopic observations on

the structural components of the blood testis barrier. J Reprod Fertil 1979; 22: 105–122.

133. Russell LD, Peterson RN. Sertoli cell junctions: morphological and functional correlates. Int Rev Cytol 1985; 94: 177–211.

134. Russell LD: Morphological and functional evidence for Sertoli-germ cell relationship. In: Russell LD, Griswold MD, eds. The Sertoli cell. Clearwater, FL: Cache River Press, 1993; 365–390.

135. Ritzen EM, Hansson V, French FS. The Sertoli cell. In: Burger H, De Kretser DM, eds. The testis. New York: Raven Press, 1981; 171–194.

136. Pfeiffer DC, Vogl AW. Evidence that vinculin is codistributed with actin bundles in ectoplasmic ('junctional') specializations of mammalian Sertoli cells. Anat Rec 1991; 231: 89–100.

137. Paniagua R, Rodríguez MC, Nistal M, et al. Changes in the lipid inclusion/ Sertoli cell cytoplasm area ratio during the cycle of the human seminiferous epithelium. J Reprod Fertil 1987; 80: 335–341.

138. Bawa SR. Fine structure of the Sertoli cell of the human testis. J Ultrastruct Res 1963; 9: 459–474.

139. Paniagua R, Martín A, Nistal A, et al. Testicular involution in elderly men: comparison of histologic quantitative studies with hormone patterns. Fertil Steril 1987; 47: 671–679.

140. Schulze W, Schulze C. Multinucleate Sertoli cells in aged human testes. Cell Tissue Res 1981; 217: 259–266.

141. Johnson L, Petty CS, Neaves WB. Influence of age on sperm production and testicular weights in men. J Reprod Fertil 1984; 70: 211–218.

142. Bockers TM, Nieschlag E, Kreutz MR, et al. Localization of follicle-stimulating hormone (FSH) immunoreactivity and hormone receptor mRNA in testicular tissue of infertile men, Cell Tissue Res 1994; 278: 595–600.

143. Simoni M, Weinbauer GF, Gromoll J, et al. Role of FSH in male gonadal function, Ann Endocrinol 1999; 60: 102–106.

144. Suarez-Quian CA, Martinez-García F, Nistal M, et al. Androgen receptor distribution in adult human testis. J Clin Endocrinol Metab 1999; 84: 350–358.

145. Lejeune H, Skalli M, Chatelain PG, et al. The paracrine role of Sertoli cells on Leydig cell function. Cell Biol Toxicol 1992; 8: 73–83.

146. Petrie RG, Morales CR. Receptor-mediated endocytosis of testicular transferrin by germinal cells of the rat testis. Cell Tissue Res 1992; 267: 45–55.

147. Anderson RA, Sharpe RM. Regulation of inhibin production in the human male and its clinical applications. Int J Androl 2000; 23: 136–144.

148. Khan SA, Schmidt K, Hallin P, et al. Human testis cytosol an ovarian

follicular fluid contain high amounts of interleukin-1-like factor(s). Mol Cell Endocrinol 1988; 58: 221–230.

149. Parvinen M, Vihko KK, Toppari J. Cell interactions during the seminiferous epithelial cycle. Int Rev Cytol 1986; 104: 115–151.

150. Paniagua R, Nistal M, Amat P, et al. Quantitative differences between variants of A spermatogonia in man. J Reprod Fertil 1986; 77: 669–673.

151. Rowley MJ, Berlin JD, Heller CG. The ultrastructure of the four types of human spermatogonia. Zeitschr Zellforsch 1971; 112: 139–157.

152. Nistal M, Codesal J, Paniagua R, et al. Decrease in the number of Ap and Ad spermatogonia and the Ap/Ad ratio with advancing age. J Androl 1987; 8: 64–68.

153. Paniagua R, Codesal J, Nistal M, et al. Quantification of cell types throughout the cycle of the human seminiferous epithelium and their DNA content. Anat Embryol 1987; 176: 225–230.

154. Schulze W. Normal and abnormal spermatogonia in the human testis. Fortschr Androl 1981; 7: 33–45.

155. Nistal M, Paniagua R, Esponda E. Development of the endoplasmic reticulum during human spermatogenesis. Acta Anat 1980; 108: 238–249.

156. Heller CG, Clermont Y. Kinetics of the germinal epithelium in man. Recent Prog Hormone Res 1964; 20: 545–571.

157. Holstein AF, Roosen-Runge EC. Atlas of human spermatogenesis. Berlin: Grosse-Verlag, 1981.

158. De Kretser DM. Ultrastructural features of human spermiogenesis. Zeitschr Zellforsch 1969; 98: 477–505.

159. Fawcett DW, Anderson WA, Phillips DM. Morphogenetic factors influencing the shape of the sperm head. Dev Biol 1971; 26: 220–251.

160. Fawcett DW, Phillips DM. The fine structure and development of the neck region of the mammalian spermatozoon. Anat Rec 1969; 165: 153–184.

161. Bruecker H, Shafe E, Holstein AF. Morphogenesis and fate of the residual body in human spermiogenesis. Cell Tissue Res 1985; 240: 303–309.

162. Chemes M. The phagocytic function of Sertoli cells. A morphological, biochemical, and endocrinological study of lysosomes and acid phosphatase localization in the rat testis. Endocrinology 1986; 119: 1673–1686.

163. Clermont Y. Renewal of spermatogonia in man. Am J Anat 1966; 118: 509–524.

164. Holstein AF. Ultrastructural observations on the differentiation of spermatids in man. Andrologia 1976; 8: 157–165.

165. Dym M, Fawcet DW. Further observations on the numbers of spermatogonia, spermatocytes and spermatids connected by intercellular bridges in the mammalian testis. Biol Reprod 1971; 4: 195–215.

166. Schulze W. Evidence of a wave of spermatogenesis in the human testis. Andrologia 1982; 14: 200–207.

167. Schulze W, Reimer M, Rehder V, et al. Computeraided three-dimensional reconstructions of the arrangement of primary spermatocytes in human seminiferous tubules. Cell Tissue Res 1986; 244: 1–8.

168. Clermont Y. The cycle of the seminiferous epithelium in man. Am J Anat 1963; 2: 35–51.

169. Ueno H, Mori H. Morphometrical analysis of Sertoli cell ultrastructure during the seminiferous epithelial cycle in rats. Biol Reprod 1990; 43: 769–776.

170. Grandjean V, Sage J, Ranc F, et al. Stage-specific signals in germ line differentiation control of Sertoli cell phagocytic activity by spermatogenic cells. Dev Biol 1997; 184: 165–174.

171. Paniagua R, Rodriguez MC, Nistal, M, et al. Changes in the lipid inclusions/Sertoli cell cytoplasm area ratio during the cycle of the Sertoli cell of the human seminiferous epithelium. J Reprod Fertil 1987; 80: 335–341.

172. Griswold MD. Interaction between germ cells and Sertoli cells in the testis. Biol Reprod 1995; 52: 211–216.

173. Bartke A. Apoptosis of male germ cells, a generalized or a cell type-specific phenomenon? Endocrinology 1995; 136: 3–4.

174. Bustos-Obregón E. Ultrastructure and function of the lamina propia of mammalian seminiferous tubules. Andrologia 1976; 8: 179–185.

175. De Kretser DM, Kerr JB, Paulsen CA. The peritubular tissue in the normal and pathological human testis: an ultrastructural study. Biol Reprod 1975; 12: 317–324.

176. Dym M. Basement membrane regulation of Sertoli cells. Endocrinol Rev 1994, 15: 102–115.

177. Christl HW. The lamina propia of vertebrate seminiferous tubules: A comparative light and electron microscopic investigation. Andrologia 1990; 22: 85–94.

178. Ross MH, Long IR. Contractile cells in human seminiferous tubules. Science 1986; 153: 1271–1273.

179. Virtanen I, Kallojoki M, Narvanen O. Peritubular myoid cells of human and rat testis are smooth muscle cells that contain desmin-type intermediate filaments. Anat Rec 1986; 215: 10–20.

180. De Menczes AP. Elastic tissue in the limiting membrane of the human seminiferous tubules. Am J Anat 1977; 150: 349–374.

181. Gabbiani G. The biology of myofibroblasts. Kidney Int 1992; 41: 530–532.

182. Miyake K, Yamamoto M, Narita H, et al. Evidence for contractility of the human seminiferous tubule confirmed by its response to noradrenaline and acetylcholine. Fertil Steril 1986; 46: 734–737.

183. Johnson L, Petty CS, Neaves WB. Age-related variations in seminiferous tubules in men. A stereologic evaluation. J Androl 1986; 7: 316–322.

184. Kuroda N, Nakayama H, Miyazaki E, et al. Distribution and role of CD34-positive stromal cells and myofibroblasts in human normal testicular stroma. Histol Histopathol 2004; 19: 743–751.

185. Nelson AA. Giant interstitial cells and extraparenchimal interstitial cells of the human testis. Am J Pathol 1938; 14: 831–841.

186. Okkels M, Sand K. Morphological relationship between testicular nerves and Leydig cells in man. J Endocrinol 1940; 2: 38–49.

187. Schulze C. Sertoli cells and Leydig cells in man. Adv Anat Embryol Cell Biol 1984; 88: 1–104.

188. Paniagua R, Amat P, Nistal M, et al. Ultrastructure of Leydig cells in human ageins testes. J Anat 1986; 146: 173–183.

189. Schulze W, Davidoff MS, Ivell R, et al. Neuron-specific enolase-like inmunoreactivity in human Leydig cells. Andrologia 1991; 23: 279–283.

190. Ivell R, Balvers M, Domagalski R, et al. Relaxin-like factor: a highly specific and constitutive new marker for Leydig cells in the human testis. Mol Hum Reprod 1997; 3: 459–466.

191. Barreiro ML, Tena-Sempere M. Ghrelin and reproduction: a novel signal linking energy status and fertility. Mol Cell Endocrinol 2004; 226: 1–9.

192. Foresta C, Bettella A, Vinanzi C, et al. A novel circulating hormone of testis origin in humans. J Clin Endocrinol Metab 2004; 89: 5952–5958.

193. Strauss KI, Isaacs KR, Ha QN, Jacobowitz DM. Calretinin is expressed in the Leydig cells of rat testis. Biochim Biophys Acta 1994; 1219: 435–440.

194. Movahedi-Lankarani S, Kurman RJ. Calretinin, a more sensitive but less specific marker than α-inhibin for ovarian sex cord-stromal neoplasms: an immunohistochemical study of 215 cases. Am J Surg Pathol 2002; 26: 1477–1483.

195. Holash JA, Harik SI, Perry G, Stewart PA. Barrier properties of testis microvessels. Proc Natl Acad Sci USA 1993; 90: 11069–11073.

196. Davidoff MS, Schulze W, Middendorff R, et al. The Leydig cell of the human testis – a new member of the diffuse neuroendocrine system. Cell Tissue Res 1993; 271: 429–439.

197. Davidoff MS, Middendorff R, Pusch W, et al. Sertoli and Leydig cells of the human testis express neurofilament triplet proteins. Histochem Cell Biol 1999; 111: 173–187.

198. Chemes H, Cigorraga S, Bergada C, et al. Isolation of human Leydig cell mesenchymal precursors from patients with the androgen insensitivity syndrome: testosterone production and response to human chorionic gonadotropin stimulation in culture. Biol Reprod 1992; 46: 793–801.

199. Davidoff MS, Middendorff R, Enikolopov G, et al. Progenitor cells of the testosterone-producing Leydig cells revealed. Cell Biol 2004; 167: 935–944.

200. Kaler LW, Neaves WB. Attrition of the human Leydig cell population with advancing age. Anat Rec 1978; 192: 513–518.

201. Kothari LK, Gupta AS. Effect of ageing on the volume, structure and total Leydig cell content of human testis. Int J Fertil 1974; 19: 140–146.

202. Mori H, Hiromoto N, Nakahara M, et al. Stereological analysis of Leydig cell ultrastructure in aged humans. J Clin Endocrinol Metab 1982; 55: 634–641.

203. Nistal M, Santamaría L, Paniagua R, et al. Multinucleate Leydig cells in normal human testes. Andrologia 1986; 18: 268–272.

204. Amat P, Paniagua R, Nistal M, et al. Mitosis in adult human Leydig cells. Cell Tissue Res 1986; 243: 219–221.

205. Neaves WB, Johnson L, Porter JC, et al. Leydig cell numbers, daily sperm production and serum gonadotropin levels in ageing men. J Clin Endocrinol Metab 1984; 55: 756–763.

206. Neaves WB, Johnson L, Petty CS. Age-related change in numbers of other interstitial cells in testes of adult men: evidence bearing on the fate of Leydig cells lost with increasing age. Biol Reprod 1985; 33: 259–269.

207. Sharpe RM, Maddocks S, Millar M, et al. Testosterone and spermatogenesis. Identification of stage-specific, androgen-regulated proteins secreted by adult rat seminiferous tubules. J Androl 1992; 13: 172–184.

208. Parvinen M. Regulation of the semininiferous epithelium. Endocrinol Rev 1982; 3: 404–417.

209. Paniagua R, Rodríguez MC, Nistal M, et al. Changes in surface area and number of Leydig cells in relation to the 6 stages of the cycle of the human seminiferous epithelium. Anat Embryol 1988; 178: 423–427.

210. Anthony CT, Rosselli M, Skinner MK. Actions of the testicular paracrine factor (P-Mod-S) on Sertoli cell transferrin secretion throgout pubertal development. Endocrinology 1991; 129: 353–360.

211. Norton JN, Skinner MK. Regulation of Sertoli cell function and differentiation through the actions of a testicular paracrine factor P-Mod-S. Endocrinology 1989; 124: 2711–2719.

212. Skinner MK. Cell–cell interactions in the testis. Endocrinol Rev 1991; 12: 45–77.

213. Middendorff R, Müller D, Wichers S, et al. Evidence for production and functional activity of nitric oxide in seminiferous tubules and blood vessels of the human testis, J Clin Endocrinol Metab 1997; 82: 4154–4161.

214. Prince FP. Ultrastructural evidence of indirect and direct autonomic innervation of human Leydig cells. Comparison of neonatal, childhood and pubertal ages. Cell Tissue Res 1992; 269: 383–390.

215. Nistal M, Paniagua R. Leydig cell differentiation induced by stimulation with HCG and HMG in two patients affected with hypogonadotropic hypogonadism. Andrologia 1979; 11: 211–222.

216. Miller SC, Bowman BM, Rowland HG. Structure, cytochemistry, endocytic activity, and immunoglobulin (Fc) receptors of rat testicular interstitial-tissue macrophages. Am J Anat 1983; 168: 1–13.

217. Hutson JC. Changes in the concentration and size of testicular macrophages during development. Biol Reprod 1990; 43: 885–890.

218. Hutson JC. Testicular macrophages. Int Rev Cytol 1994; 149: 99–143.

219. Jonsson CK, Setchell BP, Martinelle N, et al. Endotoxin-induced interleukin 1 expression in testicular macrophages is accompanied by downregulation of the constitutive expression in Sertoli cells. Cytokine 2001; 14: 283–288.

220. Gaytan F, Romero JL, Morales C, et al. Response of testicular macrophages to EDS-induced Leydig cell death. Andrologia 1995; 27: 259–65.

221. Afane M, Dubost J-J, Sauvezie B, et al. Modulation of Leydig cell testosterone production by secretory products of macrophages. Andrologia 1998; 30: 71–78.

222. Lukyanenko Y, Chen JJ, Hutson JC. Testosterone regulates 25-hydroxycholesterol production in testicular macrophages. Biol Reprod 2002; 67: 1435–1438.

223. Mayerhofer A, Frungieri MB, Fritz S, et al. Evidence for catecholaminergic, neuron-like cells in the adult human testis: changes associated with testicular pathologies. J Androl 1999; 20: 341–347.

224. Maseki Y, Mikaye K, Mitsuya H, et al. Mastocytosis occurring in testes from patients with idiopathic male infertility. Fertil Steril 1981; 36: 814–817.

225. Jarow JP, Ogle A, Kaspar J, Hopkins M. Testicular artery ramification within the inguinal canal. J Urol 1992; 147: 1290–1292.

226. Kormano M, Suoranta H. Microvascular organization of the adult human testes. Anat Rec 1971; 170: 31–40.

227. Suoranta M. Changes in the small blood vessels of the adult human testis in relation to age and to some pathological conditions. Virchows Arch A [Pathol Anat] 1971; 352: 165–181.

228. Takayama H, Tomoyoshi T. Microvascular architecture of rat and human testes. Invest Urol 1981; 18: 341–344.

229. Suzuki F, Nagano T. Microvasculature of the human testis and excurrent duct system. Resin-casting and scanning electron-microscopic studies. Cell Tissue Res 1986; 243: 79–89.

230. Ergun S, Davidoff M, Holstein AF. Capillaries in the lamina propria of human seminiferous tubules are partly fenestrated. Cell Tissue Res 1996; 286: 93–102.

231. Holstein AF, Orlandini GE, Moller R. Distribution and fine structure of the lymphatic system in the human testis. Cell Tissue Res 1979; 200: 15–27.

232. Nistal M, Paniagua R, Abaurrea MA. Varicose axons bearing 'synaptic' vesicles on the basal lamina of the human seminiferous tubules. Cell Tissue Res 1982; 226: 75–82.

233. Santamaría L, Reoyo A, Regadera J, et al. Histochemistry and ultrastructure of nerve fibres and contractile cells in the tunica albuginea of the rat testis. Acta Anat 1990; 139: 126–133.

234. Jonte G, Holstein AF. On the morphology of the transitional zones from the rete testis into the ductuli efferentes and from the ductuli efferentes into the ductus epididymidis investigations on the human testis and epididymis. Andrologia 1978; 19: 398–412.

235. Dinges HP, Zatloukal K, Schmid C, et al. Co-expression of cytokeratin and vimentin filaments in rete testis and epididymis. An inmunohistochemical study. Virchows Archiv A [Pathol Anat] 1991; 418: 119–127.

236. Kogan SJ. Cryptorchidism. In: Kelalis PP, King LR, Belman AB, eds. Clinical pediatric urology, 2nd edn. Vol 2. Philadelphia: WB Saunders, 1985; 864.

237. Oesch I, Ransley PG. Unilaterally impalpable testis. Eur Urol 1987; 13: 324–325.

238. Levitt SB, Kogan SJ, Schnider KM, et al. Endocrine tests in phenotypic children with bilateral impalpable testes can reliably predict 'congenital' anorchism. Urology 1978; 11: 11–17.

239. Aynsley-Green A, Zachmann M, Illig R, Prader A. Congenital bilateral anorchia in childhood: a clinical

endocrine and therapeutic evaluation of twenty-one cases. Clin Endocrinol 1976; 5: 381–391.

240. Rivarola MA, Bergada C, Cullen M. HCG estimulation test in prepubertal boys with cryptorchidism, in bilateral anorchia and in male pseudohermaphroditism. J Clin Endocrinol Metab 1970; 31: 526–530.

241. Jarow JP, Berkovitz GD, Migeon CJ, et al. Elevation of serum gonadotropins establishes the diagnosis of anorchism in prepubertal boys with bilateral cryptorchidism. J Urol 1986; 136: 277–279.

242. Koff SA. Does compensatory testicular enlargement predict monorchism? J Urol 1991; 146: 632–633.

243. Huff DS, Snyder HM, Hadziselimovic F, et al. An absent testis is associated with contralateral testicular hypertrophy. J Urol 1992; 148: 627–628.

244. Brothers LR, Weber CH, Ball TP. Anorchismus versus cryptorchidism; the importance of a diligent search for intra-abdominal testes. J Urol 1971; 119: 207–209.

245. Plotzker ED, Rushton HG, Belman AB, et al. Laparoscopy for nonpalpable testes in childhood: Is inguinal exploration also necessary when the vas and vessels exit the inguinal ring? J Urol 1992; 148: 635–638.

246. Edman CD, Winter AJ, Porter JC, et al. Embryonic testicular regression: a clinical spectrum of XY agonadal individuals. Obstet Gynecol 1977; 2: 208–217.

247. Coulam CB. Testicular regression syndrome. Obstet Gynecol 1979; 53: 44–49.

248. Maciel-Guerra AT, Farah SB, Garmes HM, et al. True agonadism: report of a case analyzed with Y-specific DNA probes. Am J Med Genet 1991; 41: 444–445.

249. Devriendt K, Deloof E, Moerman P, et al. Diaphragmatic hernia in Denys–Drash syndrome. Am J Med Genet 1995; 57: 97–101.

250. Manouvrier-Hanu S, Besson R, Cousin L, et al. Sex reversal and diaphragmatic hernia in phenotypically female sibs with normal XY chromosomes. J Med Genet 2000; 37: 315–318.

251. Zenteno JC, Jimenez AL, Canto P, et al. Clinical expression and SRY gene analysis in XY subjets lacking gonadal tissue. Am J Med Genet 2001; 99: 244–247.

252. Macayran JF, Doroshow RW, Phillips J, et al. PAGOD syndrome: eighth case and comparison to animal models of congenital vitamin A deficiency. Am J Med Genet 2002; 108: 229–234.

253. Kennerknecht l, Sorgo W, Oberhoffer R, et al. Familial occurrence of agonadism and multiple internal malformations in phenotypically normal girls with 46,XY and 46,XX karyotypes, respectively: a new autosomal recessive syndrome. Am J Med Genet 1993; 47: 1166–1170.

254. Silengo M, Del Monaco A, Linari A, Lala R. Low birth-weight, microcephalic malformation syndrome in a 46,XX girl and her 46,XY sister with agonadism: third report of the Kennerknecht syndrome or autosomal recessive Seckel-like syndrome with previously undescribed genital anomalies. Am J Med Genet 2001; 101: 275–278.

255. Kushnick T, Wiley JE, Palmer SM. Agonadism in a 46,XY patient with CHARGE association. Am J Med Genet 1992; 42: 96–99.

256. Najjar SS, Takla RJ, Nassar VH. The syndrome of rudimentary testes: occurrence in live siblings. J Pediatr 1974; 84: 119–122.

257. Glass AR. Identical twins discordant for the 'rudimentary testes' syndrome. J Urol 1982; 127: 140–141.

258. Acquafredda A, Vassal J, Job JC. Rudimentary testes syndrome revisited. Paediatrics 1987; 2: 209–214.

259. Tzvetkov D, Tzvetkova P, Kanchev L. Congenital anorchism: diagnostic and therapeutic aspects. Arch Androl 1994; 32: 243–249.

260. De Rosa M, Lupoli G, Mennitti M, et al. Congenital bilateral anorchia: clinical, hormonal and imaging study in 12 cases. Andrologia 1996; 28: 281–285.

261. Lobaccaro JM, Medlej R, Berta P, et al. PCR analysis and sequencing of the SRY sex determining gene in four patients with bilateral congenital anorchia. Clin Endocrinol 1993; 38: 197–201.

262. Parigi GB, Bardoni B, Avoltini V, et al. Is bilateral congenital anorchia genetically determined? Eur J Pediatr Surg 1999; 9: 312–315.

263. Tosi SE, Morin LS. The vanishing testis syndrome. Indications for conservative therapy. J Urol 1976; 115: 758.

264. Sparnon A, Guiney EJ, Puri P. The vanishing testis. Pediatr Surg Int 1986; 1: 227–228.

265. Abeyaratne MR, Aherne WA, Scott JES. The vanishing testis. Lancet 1969; 2: 822–824.

266. Belman AB, Rushton HG. Is the vanished testis always a scrotal event? BJU Int 2001; 87: 480–483.

267. Simpson JL, Horwith M, Morrillo-Cucci G. Bilateral anorchia: discordance in monozygotic twins. Birth Defects 1971; 7: 196–200.

268. Vinci G, Anjot MN, Trivin C, et al. An analysis of the genetic factors involved in testicular descent in a cohort of 14 male patients with anorchia. J Clin Endocrinol Metab 2004; 89: 6282–6285.

269. Amelar RD. Anorchism without eunuchoidismn. J Urol 1956; 76: 174.

270. Honoré M Unilateral anorchism. Report of 11 cases with discussion of etiology and pathogenesis. Urology 1978; 11: 251–254.

271. Nistal M, Paniagua R, Regadera J, et al. Hyperplasia of spermatic cord nerves: a sign of testicular absence. Urology 1987; 29: 411–415.

272. Salle B, Hedinger C, Nicole R. Significance of testicular biopsies in cryptorchidism in children. Acta Endocrinol 1968; 58: 67–76.

273. Kogan SJ, Gill B, Bennett B, et al. Human monorchism: A clinicopathological study of unilateral absent testes in 65 boys. J Urol 1986; 135: 758–761.

274. Smith NM, Byard RW, Bourne AJ. Testicular regression syndrome a pathological study of 77 cases. Histopathology 1991; 19: 269–272.

275. Spires SE, Woolums CS, Pulito AR, Spires SM. Testicular regression syndrome: a clinical and pathologic study of 11 cases. Arch Pathol Lab Med 2000; 124: 694–698.

276. Grady RW, Mitchell ME, Carr MC. Laparoscopic and histologic evaluation of the inguinal vanishing testis. Urology 1998; 52: 866–869.

277. Cendron M, Schned AR, Ellsworth PL. Histological evaluation of the testicular nubbin in the vanishing testis syndrome. J Urol 1998; 160: 1161–1163.

278. Das S, Amar AD. Ureteral ectopia into cystic seminal vesicle with ipsilateral renal dysgenesis and monorchia. J Urol 1980; 124: 574–575.

279. Matsuoka LY, Wortsman J, McConnachie P. Renal and testicular agenesis in a patient with Darier's disease. Am J Med 1985; 78: 873–877.

280. Konig MP. Findings: small testicles. Schweiz Med Wschr 1987; 117: 731–735.

281. Margery J, Le Berre JP, Bredin C, et al. Klinefelter's syndrome diagnosed three years after surgery for mediastinal teratoma Presse Med 2005; 34: 1078–1079.

282. Hoffman WH, Kovacs K, Li S, et al. Kenny–Caffey syndrome and microorchidism. Am J Med Genet 1998; 80: 107–111.

283. Thum G. Polyorchidism: case report and review of literature. J Urol 1991; 145: 370–372.

284. Oner AY, Sahin C, Pocan S, Kizilkaya E. Polyorchidism: sonographic and magnetic resonance image findings. Acta Radiol 2005; 46: 769–771.

285. Ahlfeld F. Die Missbildungen des Menschen. Leipzig: Grunow, 1880; 126–127.

286. Lane WA. A case of supernumerary testis. Trans Clin Soc Lond 1895; 28: 59–60.

287. Khetan N, Torkington J, Jamison MH. Polyorchidism presenting as retractile testes. BJU Int 1999; 83: 524.

288. Baker LL, Hajek PC, Burkhard TK, et al. Polyorchidism: evaluation by MR. AJR Am J Roentgenol 1987; 148: 305–307.

289. Singh A, Sobti MK. Polyorchidism. Br J Urol 1988; 61: 458–459.

290. Snow BW, Tarry WF, Duckett JW. Polyorchidism: An unusual case. J Urol 1985; 133: 483–484.

291. Spranger R, Gunst M, Kühn M. Polyorchidism: a strange anomaly with unsuspected properties. J Urol 2002; 168: 198.

292. Deveci S, Aygun C, Agildere AM, Ozkardes H. Bilateral double by testis: evaluation magnetic resonance imaging. Int J Urol 2004; 11: 813–815.

293. Day GH. One man with five testes: report of case. JAMA 1918; 71: 2055–2057.

294. Hakami M, Mosavy SH. Triorchidism with normal spermatogenesis: an unusual cause for failure of vasectomy. Br J Surg 1975; 62: 633.

295. Yeniyol CO, Nergiz N, Tuna A. Abdominal polyorchidism: a case report and review of the literature. Int Urol Nephrol 2004; 36: 407–408.

296. Giyanani VL, McCarthy J, Venable DD, et al. Ultrasound of polyorchidism: Case report and literature review. J Urol 1987; 138: 863–864.

297. Hancock RA, Hodgins TE. Polyorchidism. Urology 1984; 24: 303–307.

298. Abbasoglu L, Salman FT, Gun F, Asicioglu C. Polyorchidism presenting with undescended testis. Eur J Pediatr Surg 2004; 14: 355–357.

299. Chung T-J, Yao W-J. Sonographic features of polyorchidism. J Clin Ultrasound 2002; 30: 106–108.

300. Pelander WM, Luna G, Lilly JR. Polyorchidism: Case report and literature review. J Urol 1978; 119: 705–706.

301. Gandia VM, Arrizabalaga M, Leiva O, et al. Polyorchidism discovered as testicular torsion associated with undescended atrophic contralateral testis. A surgical solution. J Urol 137: 1987; 743–744.

302. Verdú TF, Pérez-Bustamante I, Jiménez CM. Poliorquia. Revisión y aportación de un nuevo caso. Actas Urol Esp 1986; 10: 277–278.

303. Feldman S, Drach GW. Polyorchidism discovered as testicular torsion. J Urol 1983; 130: 976–977.

304. Khan C. Polyorchidism with normal spermatogenesis. Br J Urol 1988; 61: 100–103.

305. Smart RH. Polyorchidism with normal spermatogenesis. J Urol 1972; 107: 278.

306. Nocks BN. Polyorchidism with normal spermatogenesis and equal sized testes. A theory of embryonal development. J Urol 1978; 120: 638–640.

307. Garat JM, Marina S, Sole-Balcells F, et al. Polyorchidie. J d'Urol 1981; 87: 175–176.

308. Mallafre JM, Janeiro MR, Corominas S, et al. Testiculo supernumerario. Comunicación de un caso y revisión de la literatura. Arch Esp Urol 1989; 42: 166–168.

309. Al-Hibbal Z, Izzidien AY. Polyorchidism: case report and review of the literature. J Pediatr Surg 1984; 19: 212–214.

310. Darrow RP, Humes JJ. Polyorchidism: a case report. J Urol 1954; 72: 53–54.

311. Thiessen NW. Polyorchidism: report of a case. J Urol 1943; 49: 710–711.

312. Nistal M, Paniagua R, Martín-Lopez R. Polyorchidism in a newborn: case report and review of the literature. Pediatr Pathol 1990; 10: 601–607.

213. Holland AJ. Polyorchidism: A case report and review of the literature. J Pediatr Surg 2005; 40: 1219.

314. Grechi G, Zampi GC, Selli C, et al. Polyorchidism and seminoma in a child. J Urol 1980; 123: 291–292.

315. Scott KW. A case of polyorchidism with testicular teratoma. J Urol 1980; 124: 930–932.

316. Takihara H, Consentino MJ, Sakatoku J, et al. Significance of testicular size measurement in andrology. II Correlation of testicular size with testicular function. J Urol 1987; 137: 416–418.

317. Nistal M, González-Peramato P, Paniagua R. Congenital Leydig cell hyperplasia. Histopathology 1988; 12: 307–317.

318. Huff DS, Wu HY, Snyder H, et al. Evidence in favor of the mechanical (intrauterine torsion) theory over the endocrinopathy (cryptorchidism) theory in the pathogenesis of testicular agenesis. J Urol 1991; 146: 630–631.

319. Laron Z, Zilka E. Compensatory hypertrophy of testicle in unilateral cnyptorchidism. J Clin Endocrinol Metab 1969; 29: 1409–1413.

320. Ku JH, Son H, Kwak C, et al. Impact of varicocele on testicular volume in young men: significance of compensatory hypertrophy of contralateral testis. J Urol 2002; 168: 1541–1544.

321. Laron Z, Dickerman Z, Prager-Lewin R, et al. Plasma LH and FSH response to LRH in boys with compensatory testicular hypertrophy. J Clin Endocrinol Metab 1975; 40: 977–981.

322. Laron Z, Dickerman Z, Ritterman I, et al. Followup of boys with unilateral compensatory testicular hypertrophy. Fertil Steril 1980; 33: 297–300.

323. Zachman M, Prader A, Kind HP, et al. Testicular volume during adolescence. Helv Paediatr Acta 1974; 29: 61–72.

324. Lee PA, Marshall FF, Greco JM, et al. Unilateral testicular hypertrophy: An apparently benign occurrence without cryptorchidism. J Urol 1982; 127: 329–331.

325. Nisula BC, Loriaux DL, Sherins RJ, et al. Benign bilateral testicular enlargement. J Clin Endocrinol Metab 1974; 38: 440–445.

326. Breen DH, Braunstein GD, Neufeld N, et al. Benign macroorchidism in a pubescent boy. J Urol 1981; 125: 589–591.

327. Truwit CHL, Jackson M, Thompson IM. Idiopathic macroorchidism. J Clin Ultrasound 1989; 17: 200–205.

328. Nistal M, Martínez-García F, Regadera J, et al. Macro-orchidism: light and electron microscopic study of four cases. Hum Pathol 1992; 23: 1011–1018.

329. Somuncu S, Cakmak M, Caglayan F, et al. Idiopathic benign bilateral testicular enlargement in a pubertal boy: a case report and review of literature. J Pediatr Surg 2005; 40: 23–25.

330. Alvarez-Acevedo Garcia M, Molina Rodriguez MA, Gonzalez Casado I, et al. Macroorchidism: a case report. An Pediatr 2006; 64: 89–92.

331. Meschede D, Behre HM, Nieschlag E. Endocrine and spermatological characteristics of 135 patients with bilateral megalotestis. Andrologia 1995; 27: 207–212.

332. Van Esch H. The Fragile X premutation: new insights and clinical consequences. Eur J Med Genet 2006; 49: 1–8.

333. Lubs HA. A marker X chromosome. A J Hum Genet 1969; 21: 231–234.

334. Martin JP, Bell J. A pedigree of mental defect showing sex-linkage. J Neurol Psychiatr 1943; 6: 154–157.

335. Turner G, Eastman C, Casey J, et al. X-linked mental retardation associated with macroorchidism. J Med Genet 1975; 12: 367–371.

336. Cantú JM, Scaglia HE, González-Didi M, et al. Inherited congenital normofunctional testicular hyperplasia and mental deficiency. A corroborative study. Hum Genet 1975; 12: 367–371.

337. Ruvalcaba RHA, Myhre SA, Roosen-Runge EC, et al. X-linked mental deficiency megalotestes syndrome. JAMA 1977; 238: 1646–1650.

338. Sutherland GR, Ashforth PLC. X-linked mental retardation with macroorchidism and the fragile site at Xq 27 or 28. Hum Genet 1979; 48: 117–120.

339. Howard-Peebles PN, Stoddard GR. Familial-X-linked mental retardation with a marker X chromosome and its relationship to macroorchidism. Clin Genet 1980; 17: 125–128.

340. Hecht JT, Moore CM, Scott CI. A recognizable syndrome of sex-linked mental retardation, large testes and

marker X chromosome. South Med J 1981; 74: 1493–1495.

341. Berkowitz GD, Wilson DP, Carpenter NJ, et al. Gonadal function in men with the Martin–Bell (fragile X) syndrome. Am J Med Genet 1986; 23: 227–239.

342. Johannisson R, Rehder H, Wendt V, et al. Spermatogenesis in two patients with the fragile X syndrome. I. Histology: light and electron microscopy. Hum Genet 1987; 76: 141–147.

343. Johannisson R, Froster-Iskenius U, Saadallah N, et al. Spermatogenesis in two patients with the fragile X syndrome. Hum Genet 1988; 79: 231–234.

344. Gerald PS. X-linked mental retardation and an X-chromosome marker. N Engl J Med 1980; 303: 696–697.

345. Webb TP, Bundey SE, Thake AI, et al. Population incidence and segregation ratios in Martin–Bell syndrome. Am J Hum Genet 1986; 23: 573–580.

346. Vuelckel MA, Philip N, Piquet C, et al. Study of a family with a fragile site of the X chromosome at Xq 27–28 without mental retardation. Hum Genet 1989; 81: 353–357.

347. Rudelli RD, Jenkins EC, Wisniewscki K, et al. Testicular size in fetal fragile X syndrome. Lancet 1983; 1: 1221–1222.

348. Johnson JP, Nelson R, Schwartz CE. A family with mental retardation, variable macrocephaly and macro-orchidism, and linkage to Xq12-q21. J Med Genet 1998; 35: 1026–1030.

349. Heseltine D, White MC, Kendall-Taylor P, et al. Testicular enlargement and elevated serum inhibin concentrations occur in patients with pituitary macroadenomas secreting follicle stimulating hormone. Clin Endocrinol 1989; 31: 411–423.

350. Laron Z, Karp M, Dolberg L. Juvenile hypothyroidism with testicular enlargement. Acta Paediatr Scand 1970; 59: 317–322.

351. Cordero GL, Gracia R, Nistal M, et al. Hipotiroidismo y maduración testicular precoz. Rev Clin Esp 1973; 128: 83–88.

352. Hannini EA, Ulisse S, D'Armiento M. Thyroid hormone and male gonadal function. Endocrinol Rev 1995; 16: 443–459.

353. Barnes ND, Hayles AB, Ryan RJ. Sexual maturation in juvenile hypothyroidism. Mayo Clin Proc 1973; 48: 849–856.

354. Castro-Magana M, Angulo M, Canas A, et al. Hypothalamic–pituitary gonadal axis in boys with primary hypothyroidism and macroorchidism. J Pediatr 1988; 112: 397–402.

355. Maran RR. Thyroid hormones: their role in testicular steroidogenesis. Arch Androl 2003; 49: 375–388.

356. De La Balze F, Arrillaga F, Mancini RE, et al. Male hypogonadism in hypothyroidism: A study of six cases. J Clin Endocrinol Metab 1962; 22: 212–222.

357. Hoffman WH, Kovacs KT, Gala RR, et al. Macroorchidism and testicular fibrosis associated with autoimmune thyroiditis. J Endocrinol Invest 1991; 14: 609–616.

358. Franks RC, Stempfel RS. Juvenile hypothyroidism and precocious testicular maturation. J Clin Endocrinol Metab 1963; 23: 805–810.

359. Hopwood NJ, Lockhart LH, Bryan GT. Acquired hypothyroidism with muscular hypertrophy and precocious testicular enlargement. J Pediatr 1974; 85: 233–236.

360. Wierman ME, Bruder JM, Kepa JK. Regulation of gonadotropin-releasing hormone (GnRH) gene expression in hypothalamic neuronal cells. Cell Mol Neurobiol 1995; 15: 79–88.

361. Bruder JM, Samuels MH, Bremner WJ, et al. Hypothyroidism-induced macroorchidism: Use of a gonadotropin-hormone agonist to understand its mechanism and augment adult stature. J Clin Endocrinol 1995; Metab 80: 11–16.

362. Anasti JN, Flack MR, Froehlich J, et al. A potential novel mechanism for precocious puberty in juvenile hypothyroidism. J Clin Endocrinol Metab 1995; 80: 276–279.

363. Van Haaster LH, De Jong FH, Docter R, De Rooij DG. High neonatal triiodothyronine levels reduce the period of Sertoli cell proliferation and accelerate tubular lumen formation in the rat testis, and increase serum inhibin levels. Endocrinology 1993; 133: 755–760.

364. Simorangkir DR, De Kretser DM, Wreford NG. Increased numbers of Sertoli and germ cells in adult rat testes induced by synergistic action of transient neonatal hypothyroidism and neonatal hemicastration. J Reprod Fertil 1995; 104: 207–213.

365. Palmero S, Prati M, Bolla F, Fugassa E. Tri-iodothyronine directly affects rat Sertoli cell proliferation and differentiation. J Endocrinol 1995; 145: 355–362.

366. De Franca LR, Hess RA, Cooke PS, Russell LD. Neonatal hypothyroidism causes delayed Sertoli cell maturation in rats treated with propylthiouracil: evidence that the Sertoli cell controls testis growth. Anat Rec 1995; 242: 57–69.

367. Lee PA. Central precocious puberty. An overview of diagnosis, treatment, and outcome. Endocrinol Metab Clin North Am 1999; 28: 901–918.

368. Colaco P. Precocious puberty. Indian J Pediatr 1997; 64: 165–175.

369. Cloutier MD, Hayles AB. Precocious puberty. Adv Pediatr 1970; 17: 125–138.

370. Bierich JR. Sexual precocity. Clin Endocrinol Metab 1975; 4: 107–142.

371. Brauner R, Pierre-Kahn A, Nemedy-Sandor E, et al. Precocious puberty caused by a suprasellar arachnoid cyst. Analysis of 6 cases. Arch Fr Pediatr 1987; 44: 489–493.

372. Mohn A, Schoof E, Fahlbusch R, et al. The endocrine spectrum of arachnoid cysts in childhood. Pediatr Neurosurg 1999; 31: 316–321.

373. Adan L, Bussieres L, Dinand V, et al. Growth, puberty and hypothalamic–pituitary function in children with suprasellar arachnoid cyst. Eur J Pediatr 2000; 159: 348–355.

374. Bovier-Lapierre M, Sempe M, David M. Aspects étiologiques cliniques et biologiques des pubertés précoces d'origine centrale. Pediatrie 1972; 27: 587–609.

375. Shaul PW, Towbin RB, Chernausek SD. Precocious puberty following severe head trauma. Am J Dis Child 1985; 139: 467–469.

376. Sockalosky JJ, Kriel RL, Krach LE, Sheehan M. Precocious puberty after traumatic brain injury. J Pediatr 110: 373–377, 1987.

377. Morello A, Porcaro S, Lima J, Impallaria P. Endocrine disorder as the only sign of chronic 'non-hypertensive' hydrocephalus. J Neurosurg Sci 2002; 46: 81–84.

378. Brauner R, Czernichow P, Rappaport R. Precocious puberty after hypothalamic and pituitary irradiation in young children. N Engl J Med 1984; 311: 920.

379. Leiper AD, Stanhope R, Kitching P, Chessells JM. Precocious and premature puberty associated with treatment of acute lymphoblastic leukaemia. Arch Dis Child 1987; 62: 1107–1112.

380. Cacciari E, Zucchini S, Carla G, et al. Endocrine function and morphological findings in patients with disorders of the hypothalamo-pituitary area: a study with magnetic resonance. Arch Dis Child 1990; 65: 1191–1202.

381. Fahmy JL, Kaminsky CK, Kaufman F, et al. The radiological approach to precocious puberty. Br J Radiol 2000; 73: 560–567.

382. Shah P, Patkar D, Patankar T, et al. MR imaging features in hypothalamic hamartoma: a report of three cases and review of literature. J Postgrad Med 1999; 45: 84–86.

383. Feuillan PP, Jones JV, Barnes KM, et al. Boys with precocious puberty due to hypothalamic hamartoma: reproductive axis after discontinuation of gonadotropin-releasing hormone analog therapy. J Clin Endocrinol Metab 2000; 85: 4036–4038.

384. De Sanctis V, Corrias A, Rizzo V, et al. Etiology of central precocious puberty in males: the results of the Italian Study Group for Physiopathology of Puberty. J Pediatr Endocrinol Metab 2000; 13: 687–693.

385. Judge DM, Kulin HE, Page R, et al. Hypothalamic hamartoma: a source

of luteinizing-hormone-releasing factor in precocious puberty. N Engl J Med 1977; 296: 7–10.

386. Tandon N, Chopra R, Ghoshal S, et al. Mixed germ cell tumour of the pineal region: a case report. Neurol India 1999; 47: 321–323.

387. Nogueira K, Liberman B, Pimentel-Filho FR, et al. hCG-secreting pineal teratoma causing precocious puberty: report of two patients and review of the literature. J Pediatr Endocrinol Metab 2002; 15: 1195–1201.

388. Wierman ME, Beardsworth DE, Mansfield MJ. Puberty without gonadotropins: A unique mechanism of sexual development. N Engl J Med 1985; 312: 65–72.

389. Rosenthal SM, Grumbach MM, Kaplan SL. Gonadotropin-independent familial sexual precocity with premature Leydig and germinal cell maturation (familial testotoxicosis): Effects of a patent luteinizing hormone-releasing factor agonist and metroxyprogesterone acetate therapy in four cases. J Clin Endocrinol Metab 1983; 57: 571–579.

390. Gondos B, Egli CA, Rosenthal SM, Grumbach MM. Testicular changes in gonadotropin-independent familial male sexual precocity. Familial testotoxicosis. Arch Pathol Lab Med 1985; 109: 990–995.

391. Latronico AC, Shinozaki H, Guerra G Jr, et al. Gonadotropin-independent precocious puberty due to luteinizing hormone receptor mutations in Brazillian boys: A novel constitutively activating mutation in the first transmembrane helix. J Clin Endocrinol Metab 2000; 85: 4799–4805.

392. Soriano-Guillen L, Mitchell V, Carel JC, et al. Activating mutations in the LH receptor gene: a human model of non FSH-dependent inhibin production and germ cell maturation. J Clin Endocrinol Metab 2006; 91: 3041–3047.

393. Canto P, Soderlund D, Ramon G, et al. Mutational analysis of the luteinizing hormone receptor gene in two individuals with Leydig cell tumors. Am J Med Genet 2002; 108: 148–152.

394. Gracia R, Nistal M, Gallego ME, et al. Tumor de células de Leydig con pseudopubertad precoz. An Esp Pediatr 1980; 13: 593–598.

395. Polepalle SK, Shabaik A, Alagiri M. Leydig cell tumor in a child with spermatocyte maturation and no pseudoprecocious puberty. Urology 2003; 62: 55 1–55, vii.

396. Coen P, Kulin H, Ballantine T, et al. An aromatase-producing sex-cord tumor resulting in prepubertal gynecomastia. N Engl J Med 1991; 324: 317–322.

397. Ros P, Nistal M, Alonso M, et al. Sertoli cell tumour in a boy with Peutz–Jeghers syndrome. Histopathology 1999; 34: 84–86.

398. Carney JA. Carney complex: the complex of myxomas, spotty pigmentation, endocrine overactivity, and schwannomas. Semin Dermatol 1995; 14: 90–98.

399. Bonfig W, Bittmann I, Bechtold S, et al. Virilising adrenal cortical tumours in children. Eur J Pediatr 2003; 162: 623–628.

400. Drago JR, Olstein JS, Tesluk H, et al. Virilizing adrenal cortical carcinoma with hypertrophy of spermatic tubules in childhood. Urology 1979; 14: 70–75.

401. Cunnanh D, Perry L, Dacie JA, et al. Bilateral testicular tumours in congenital adrenal hyperplasia: A continuing diagnostic and therapeutic dilemma. Clin Endocrinol 1989; 30: 141–147.

402. Heimann A, White PF, Riely CA, et al. Hepatoblastoma presenting as isosexual precocity. The clinical importance of histologic and serologic parameters. J Clin Gastroenterol 1987; 9: 105–110.

403. Cohgen AR, Wilson JA, Sadeghi-Nejad A. Gonadotropin-secreting pineal teratoma causing precocious puberty. Neurosurgery 1991; 28: 597–602.

404. Nebert DW, Nelson DR, Adesnik M, et al. The P450 gene superfamily: updated listing of all genes and recommended nomenclature for the chromosomal loci. DNA 1989; 8: 1–13.

405. Chen SA, Besman MJ, Sparkes RS, et al. Human aromatase: cDNA cloning, Southern blot analysis, and assignment of the gene to chromosome 15. DNA 1988; 7: 27–38.

406. Martin RM, Lin CJ, Nishi MY, et al. Familial hyperestrogenism in both sexes: clinical, hormonal, and molecular studies of two siblings. J Clin Endocrinol Metab 2003; 88: 3027–3034.

407. Stratakis CA, Vottero A, Brodie A, et al. The aromatase excess syndrome is associated with feminization of both sexes and autosomal dominant transmission of aberrant P450 aromatase gene transcription. J Clin Endocrinol Metab 1998; 83: 1348–1357.

408. Deladoëy J, Flück C, Bex M, et al. Aromatase deficiency caused by a novel P450arom gene mutation: impact of absent estrogen production on serum gonadotropin concentration in a boy. J Clin Endocrinol Metab 1999; 84: 4050–4054.

409. Morishima A, Grumbach MM, Simpson ER, et al. Aromatase deficiency in male and female siblings caused by a novel mutation and the physiological role of estrogens, J Clin Endocrinol Metab 1995; 80: 3689–3698.

410. Carani C, Qin K, Simoni M, et al. Effect of testosterone and estradiol in a man with aromatase deficiency. N Engl J Med 1997; 337: 91–95.

411. Grumbach MM, Auchus RJ. Estrogen: consequences and implications of human mutations in synthesis and action. J Clin Endocrinol Metab 1999; 84: 4677–4694.

412. Wilson BE, Netzloff ML. Primary testicular abnormalities causing precocious puberty Leydig cell tumor, Leydig cell hyperplasia, and adrenal rest tumor. Ann Clin Lab Sci 1983; 13: 315–320.

413. Leung AC, Kogan SJ. Focal lobular spermatogenesis and pubertal acceleration associated with ipsilateral Leydig cell hyperplasia. Urology 2000; 56: 508–509.

414. Arrigo T, Pirazzoli P, De Sanctis L, et al. McCune–Albright syndrome in a boy may present with a monolateral macroorchidism as an early and isolated clinical manifestation. Hormone Res 2006; 65: 114–119.

415. Coutant R, Lumbroso S, Rey R, et al. Macroorchidism due to autonomous hyperfunction of Sertoli cells and G(s)alpha gene mutation: an unusual expression of McCune–Albright syndrome in a prepubertal boy. J Clin Endocrinol Metab 2001; 86: 1778–1781.

416. Giovannelli G, Bernasconi S, Banchini G. McCune–Albright syndrome in a male child: A clinical and endocrinologic enigma. J Pediatr 1978; 92: 220–226.

417. Campbel MF. Anomalies of the testicle. In: Campbell MF, Harrisson JH, eds. Urology, 3rd edn. Philadelphia: WB Saunders, 1970; 1632.

418. Dieckmann KP, Düe W, Fiedler U. Perineale Hodenektopie. Urologe (A) 1988; 27: 358–362.

419. Murphy DM, Butler MR. Preperitoneal ectopic testis: a case report. J Pediatr Surg 1985; 20: 93–94.

420. Paramo PG, Nacarino L, Polo G. Ectopia epidídimo-perineal. Arch Esp Urol 1971; 24: 61–63.

421. Tramoyeres A, Esteve J, Fernández A, et al. Testículo ectópico perineal. Arch Esp Urol 1980; 33: 157.

422. Wattenberg CA, Rape MG, Beare JB. Perineal testicle. J Urol 1949; 62: 858–861.

423. Oludiran OO, Sakpa CL. Crossed ectopic testis: a case report and review of the literature. Pediatr Surg Int 2005; 21: 672–673.

424. Doraiswamy NV. Crossed ectopic testis. Case report and review. Zeitschr Kinder Chir 1983; 38: 264–268.

425. Fujita J. Transverse testicular ectopia. Urology 16: 400–402, 1980.

426. Miura T, Takahashi G. Crossed ectopic testis with common vas deferens. J Urol 1985; 134: 1206–1208.

427. Gornall PG, Pender DJ. Crossed testicular ectopia detected by laparoscopy. Br J Urol 1987; 59: 283.

428. Peters JH, Sing S. Transverse testicular ectopia: a case report. Del Med 1987; J 59: 333–335.

429. Beasley SW, Auldist AW. Crossed testicular ectopia in association with double incomplete testicular descent. Aust NZ J Surg 1985; 55: 301–303.

430. Dogruyol H, Özcan M, Balkan E. Two rare genital abnormalities: Crossed testicular and scroto-testicular ectopia. Br J Urol 1992; 70: 201–203.

431. Tiryaki T, Hucumenoglu S, Atayurt H. Transverse testicular ectopia associated with persistent Müllerian duct syndrome. A case report. Urol Int 2005; 74: 190–192.

432. Josso N, Picard JY, Imbeaud S, et al. The persistent müllerian duct syndrome: a rare cause of cryptorchidism. Eur J Pediatr 1993; 152: S76-S78.

433. Manassero F, Cuttano MG, Morelli G, et al. Mixed germ cell tumor after bilateral orchidopexy in persistent Müllerian duct syndrome with transverse testicular ectopia. Urol Int 2004; 73: 81–83.

434. Middleton GW, Beamon CR, Guillenwater JY. Two rare cases of ectopic testes. J Urol 1976; 115: 445–446.

435. Gaur DD, Purohit KC, Joshi AS, et al. Subumbilical ectopic testis, BJU Int 1999; 84: 887.

436. Heyns CF. Exstrophy of the testis. J Urol 1990; 144: 724–725.

437. O'Donnell C, Kumar U, Kiely EA. Testicular dislocation after scrotal trauma, Br J Urol 1998; 82: 768.

438. Leissring JC, Oppenheimer ROF. Cystic dysplasia of the testis: a unique anomaly studied by microdissection. J Urol 1973; 110: 362–363.

439. Kajo K, Matoska J, Javorka K, et al. Cystic dysplasia of the rete testis. Case report. APMIS 2005; 113: 720–723.

440. Nanni L, Buonuomo V, Gessi M, et al. Cystic dysplasia of the rete testis associated to cryptorchidism: a case report. Arch Ital Urol Androl 2005; 77: 199–201.

441. Cho CS, Kosek J. Cystic dysplasia of the testis: sonographic and pathologic findings. Radiology 1985; 156: 777–778.

442. Garrett JE, Cartwright PC, Snow BW, et al. Cystic testicular lesions in the pediatric population. J Urol 2000; 163: 928–936.

443. Roosen-Runge EC, Holstein AF. The human rete testis. Cell Tissue Res 1978; 189: 409–433.

444. Bustos-Obregón E, Holstein AF. The rete testis in man: Ultrastructural aspects. Cell Tissue Res 1976; 175: 1–15.

445. Dym M. The mammalian rete testis. A morphological examination. Anat Rec 1976; 186: 493–524.

446. Nistal M, Regadera J, Paniagua R. Cystic displasia of the testis: light and electron microscopic study of three cases. Arch Pathol Lab Med 1984; 108: 579–583.

447. Robson WL, Thomason MA, Minette LJ. Cystic dysplasia of the testis associated with multicystic dysplasia of the kidney. Urology 1998; 51: 477–479.

448. Fischer JE, Jewett TC, Nelson ST, et al. Ectasia of the rete testis with ipsilateral renal agenesis. J Urol 1982; 128: 1040–1043.

449. Glantz I, Hansen K, Caldamone A, et al. Cystic dysplasia of the testis. Hum Pathol 1993; 24: 1141–1145.

450. Tesluk H, Blankenberg TA. Cystic dysplasia of testis. Urology 1987; 29: 47–49.

451. Garrett JE, Cartwright PC, Snow BW, Coffin CM. Cystic testicular lesions in the pediatric population. J Urol 2000; 163: 928–936.

452. Bonnet JP, Aigrain Y, Ferkadji L. Cystic dysplasia of the testis with ipsilateral renal agenesis. A case report and review of the literature. Eur J Pediatr Surg 1997; 7: 57–59.

453. Noh PH, Cooper CS, Snyder HM III. Conservative managemet of cystic dysplasia of the testis. J Urol 1999; 162: 2145.

454. Toffolutti T, Gamba PG, Cecchetto G, et al. Testicular cystic dysplasia: evaluation of 3 new cases treated without surgery. J Urol 1999; 162: 2146–2148.

455. Cimador M, Rosone G, Castagnetti M, et al. Cystic dysplasia of rete testis associated with ipsilateral renal agenesis. Case report. Minerva Pediatr 2003; 55: 175–179.

456. Spear GS, Martin CG. Fetal gonadoblastoid testicular dysplasia. Hum Pathol 1986; 17: 531–533.

457. Hung NA, Silver MM, Chitayat D, et al. Gonadoblastoid testicular dysplasia in Walker–Warburg syndrome. Pediatr Dev Pathol 1998;1: 393–404.

458. Nistal M, Rodriguez JI, García-Fernandez E, et al. Fetal gonadoblastoid testicular dysplasia: a focal failure of testicular development. Pediatr Dev Pathol 2007 (in press).

459. Hedinger CE, Huber R, Weber E. Frequency of so-called hypoplastic or dysgenetic zones in scrotal and otherwise normal testes. Virchows Arch [Pathol Anat Physiol Klin Med] 1967; 342: 165–168.

460. Regadera J, Martínez-García F, González-Peramato P, et al. Androgen receptor expression in Sertoli cells as a function of seminiferous tubule maturation in the human cryptorchid testis. J Clin Endocrinol Metab 2001; 86: 413–421.

461. Nistal M, Paniagua R. Congenital testicular lymphangiectasis. Virchows Arch A [Pathol Anat Histol] 1977; 377: 79–84.

462. Nistal M, Paniagua R, Bravo MP. Congenital testicular lymphangiectasis in Noonan's syndrome. J Urol 1984; 131: 759–761.

463. Nistal M, Garcia-Rojo M, Paniagua R. Congenital testicular lymphangiectasis in children with otherwise normal testes. Histopathology 1990; 17: 335–338.

464. Ostroverkhova V G. Macro-microscopischeskoe is sledavanie vnutriorgannoi limfaticheskoi sistemy muzhskoi polovoi zhelezy [Macro/microscopic study of intraorgan lymphatic system of male gonad in man]. Arch Anat Gist Embriol 1960; 39: 59–65.

465. Holstein AF, Orlandini GE, Moller R. Distribution and fine structure of the lymphatic system in the human testis. Cell Tissue Res 1979; 200: 15–27.

466. Fawcett DW, Heidger PM, Leak LV. Lymph vascular system of the interstitial tissue of the testis as revealed by electron microscopy. J Reprod Fertil 1969; 19: 109–119.

467. Kaido M, Iwai S, Ide Y, et al. Epididymal lymphangiectasis. J Urol 1993; 150: 1251–1252.

468. Srigley JR, Hartwick RWJ. Tumors and cysts of the paratesticular region. Pathol Annu 1990; 25: 51–108.

469. Fridman E, Skarda J, Ofek-Moravsky E, Cordoba M. Complex multilocular cystic lesion of rete testis, accompanied by smooth muscle hyperplasia, mimicking intratesticular Leydig cell neoplasm. Virchows Arch 2005; 447: 768–771.

470. Barton JH, Davis CJ Jr, Sesterhenn IA, et al. Smooth muscle hyperplasia of the testicular adnexa clinically mimicking neoplasia. Clinicopathologic study of sixteen cases. Am J Surg Pathol 1999; 23: 903–909.

471. Tanaka N, Seya T, Onda M, et al. Myoepithelial hamartoma of the small bowel: report of a case. Surg Today 1996; 26: 1010–1013.

472. Benisch BM, Wood WG, Kroeger GB, et al. Focal muscular hyperplasia of the trachea. Arch Otolaryngol 1974; 99: 226–227.

473. Nistal M, Paniagua R, León L, et al. Ectopic seminiferous tubules in the tunica albuginea of normal and dysgenetic testes. Appl Pathol 1985; 3: 123–128.

474. Schmidt SS, Minckler TM. Pseudocysts of the tunica albuginea: Benign invasion by testicular tubules. J Urol 1987; 138: 151.

475. Nistal M, Paniagua R. Development of the testis from birth to puberty. In: Nistal M, Paniagua R, eds. Testicular and epididymal pathology. New York: Thieme-Stratton, 1984; 14–25.

476. Regadera J, Cobo O, Martínez-García C, et al. Testosterone immunoexpression in human Leydig cells of the tunica albugiena testis and spermatic cord. A quantitative study in normal fetuses, young adults, elderly men and patients with cryptorchidism. Andrologia 1993; 25: 115–122.

477. Nelson AA. Giant interstitial cells and extraparenchymal interstitial cells of the human testis. Am J Pathol 1938; 14: 831–841.

478. Halley JBW. The infiltrative activity of Leydig cells. J Pathol Bacteriol 1961; 81: 347–353.

479. Halley JBW. Relation of Leydig cells in the human testicle to the tubules and testicular function. Nature 1960; 185: 865–866.

480. McDonald JH, Calams JA. A histological study of extraparenchymal Leydig-like cells. J Urol 1958; 79: 850–858.

481. Berbingler H. Über die Zwischenzellen des Hodens. Verh D Path Ges 1921; 18: 186–197.

482. Brack E. Zur pathologischen Anatomie der Leydig Zelle. Virchows Arch [Pathol Anat Physiol] 1923; 240: 127–143.

483. Schulze C, Holstein AF. Leydig cells within the lamina propria of seminiferous tubules in four patients with azoospermia. Andrologia 1978; 10: 444–452.

484. Mori H, Shiraishi T, Matsumoto K. Ectopic Leydig cells in seminiferous tubules of an infertile human male with a chromosomal aberration. Andrologia 1978; 10: 434–443.

485. Mori H, Tamai M, Fushimi H, et al. Leydig cells within the spermatogenic seminiferous tubules. Hum Pathol 1987; 18: 1227–1231.

486. Regadera J, Codesal J, Paniagua R, et al. Immunohistochemical and quantitative study of interstitial and intratubular Leydig cells in normal men, cryptorchidism, and Klinefelter's syndrome. J Pathol 1991; 164: 299–306.

487. Priesel A. Über das Verhalten von Hoden und Nebenhoden bei angeborenem Fehlen des Ductus deferens, zugleich zur Frage des Vorkommens von Zwischenzellen in menschliche Nebenhoden. Virchows Arch [Pathol Anat Physiol] 1924; 249: 246–304.

488. Berger L. Sur l'existence de glands sympathicotropes dans l'ovaire et le testicule humains; leur rapport avec la glande interstitielle du testicule. Compt Rend Acad Sci Paris 1922; 175: 907–909.

489. Peters KH. Zur Ultrastruktur der Leydigzellen im Funiculus spermaticus des Menschen. Verh Anat Ges 1977; 71: 555–559.

490. Nistal M, Paniagua R. Histogenesis of human extraparenchymal Leydig cells. Acta Anat 1979; 105: 188–197.

491. Lespi PJ, Gregorini SD, De Lasa AT, D'Orazio O. Osteoma testicular. Presentación de un caso y revisión de la literatura. Patologia 1999; 37: 289–290.

492. Woodhouse JB, Delahunt B, English SF, et al. Testicular lipomatosis in Cowden's syndrome. Mod Pathol 2005; 18: 1151–1156.

493. Nistal M, Garcia-Cabezas MA, Castello MC, et al. Age-related epididymis-like intratesticular structures: benign lesions of Wolffian origin that can be misdiagnosed as testicular tumors. J Androl 2006; 27: 79–85.

494. Storgaard L, Bonde JP, Olsen J. Male reproductive disorders in humans and prenatal indicators of estrogen exposure. A review of published epidemiological studies. Reprod Toxicol 2006; 21: 4–15.

495. Suetomi T, Kawai K, Sekido N, et al. Testicular cancers occurring in brothers with cryptorchism. Int J Urol 2002; 9: 67–70.

496. Cendron M, Huff DS, Keating MA, et al. Anatomical, morphological and volumetric analysis: a review of 759 cases of testicular maldescent. J Urol 1993; 149: 570–573.

497. Akre O, Lipworth L, Cnattingius S, et al. Risk factor patterns for cryptorchidism and hypospadias. Epidemiology 1999; 10: 364–369.

498. Hjertkvist M, Dauber JE, Berhg A. Cryptorchidism: a registry based study in Sweden on some factors of some possible etiological importance. J Epidemiol Commun Health 1989; 43: 324–329.

499. Berkowitz GS, Lapinski RH, Godbold JH, et al. Maternal and neonatal risk factors for cryptorchidism. Epidemiology 1995; 6: 127–131.

500. Weidner IS, Moller H, Jensen TK, Skakkebaek NE. Risk factors for cryptorchidism and hypospadias. J Urol 1999; 161: 1606–1609.

501. Hutson JM, Hasthorpe S. Abnormalities of testicular descent. Cell Tissue Res 2005; 322: 155–158.

502. Eardley KC, Saw KC, Whitaker RH. Surgical outcome of orchidopexy II. Trapped and ascending testes. Br J Urol 1994; 73: 204–206.

503. Kaplan GW. Iatrogenic cryptorchidism resulting from hernia repair. Surg Gynecol Obstet 1976; 142: 671–672.

504. Surana R, Puri P. Iatrogenic ascent of the testis: an under-recognized complication of inguinal hernia operation in children. Br J Urol 1994; 73: 580–581.

505. Colodny AH. Iatrogenic ascent of the testis: an underrecognized complication of inguinal hernia operation in children. Br J Urol 1994; 74: 531–532.

506. Docimo SG. Testicular descent and ascent in the first year of life. Urology 1996; 48: 458–460.

507. Rabinowitz R, Hulbert WC Jr. Late presentation of cryptorchidism: The etiology of testicular re-ascent. J Urol 1997; 157: 1892–1894.

508. Atwell JD. Ascent of the testis: fact or fiction. Br J Urol 1985; 57: 474–477.

509. Clarnette TD, Rowe D, Hasthorpe S, Hutson JM. Incomplete disappearance of the processus vaginalis as a cause of ascending testis. J Urol 1997; 157: 1889–1891.

510. Myers NA, Officer CB. Undescended testis: congenital or acquired? Aust Paediatr J 1975; 11: 76–80.

511. Gracia J, Navarro E, Guirado F, et al. Spontaneous ascent of the testis. Br J Urol 1997; 79: 113–115.

512. Schiffer KA, Kogan SJ, Reda EF, et al. Acquired undescended testis. Am J Dis Child 1987; 141: 106–107.

513. Shono T, Zakaria O, Imajima T, et al. Does proximal genitofemoral nerve division induce testicular maldescent or ascent in the rat? BJU Int 1999; 83: 323–326.

514. Konstantinos S, Alevizos A, Anargiros M, et al. Association between testicular microlithiasis, testicular cancer, cryptorchidism and history of ascending testis. Int Braz J Urol 2006; 32: 434–438.

515. Rusnack SL, Wu H-Y, Huff DS, et al. The ascending testis and the testis undescended since birth share the same histopathology. J Urol 2002; 168: 2590–2591.

516. Hadziselimovic F, Geneto R, Emmons LR. Elevated placental estradiol: a possible etiological factor of human cryptorchidism. J Urol 2000; 164: 1694–1695.

517. Farrington GH. Histologic observations in cryptorchidism: the congenital germinal-cell deficiency of the undescended testis. J Pediatr Surg 1969; 4: 606–613.

518. Nistal M, Paniagua R, Díez-Pardo JA. Histologic classification of undescended testes. Hum Pathol 1980; 11: 666–673.

519. Codesal J, Paniagua R, Queizán A, et al. Cytophotometric DNA quantification in human spermatogonia of cryptorchid testes. J Urol 1993; 149: 382–385.

520. Huff DS, Hadziselimovic F, Snyder HMC, et al. Early postnatal testicular maldevelopment in cryptorchidism. J Urol 1991; 146: 624–626.

521. Christiansen P, Müller J, Buhl S, et al. Hormonal treatment of cryptorchidism – hCG or GnRH – a multicentre study. Acta Paediatr 1992; 81: 605–608.

522. Bica DTG, Hadsizelimovic F. Busereline treatment of cryptorchidism: a randomized, double-blind, placebo-controlled study. J Urol 1992; 148: 617–621.

523. Huff DS, Fenig DM, Canning DA, et al. Abnormal germ cell development in cryptorchidism. Hormone Res 2001; 55: 11–17.

524. Cendron M, Huff DS, Keating MA, et al. Anatomical, morphological and volumetric analysis: A review of 759 cases of testicular maldescent. J Urol 1993; 149: 570–573.

525. Nagar H, Haddad R. Impact of early orchidopexy on testicular growth. Br J Urol 1997; 80: 334–335.

526. Kogan S, Tennenbaum S, Gill B, et al. Efficacy of orchiopexy by patient age 1 year for cryptorchidism. J Urol 1990; 144: 508–509.

527. Thorup J, Cortes D, Nielsen H. Clinical and histopathologic evaluation of operated maldescended testes after luteinizing hormone-releasing hormone treatment. Pediatr Surg Int 1993; 8: 419–422.

528. Nistal M, Paniagua R, Riestra ML, et al. Bilateral prepubertad testicular biopsias predict significance of cryptorchisism-associated mixed testicular atrophy, and allow assessment of fertility. Am J Surg Pathol 2007 (in press).

529. Cortes D, Thorup J, Visfeldt J. Multinucleated spermatogonia in cryptorchid boys: a possible association with an increased risk of testicular malignancy. APMIS 2003; 111: 25–30.

530. Foresta C, Moro E, Garolla A, et al. Y chromosome microdeletions in cryptorchidism and idiopathic infertility. J Clin Endocrinol Metab 1999; 84: 3660–3665.

531. Hadziselimovic F, Snyder HM, Huff DS. An unusual subset of cryptorchidism: possible end organ failure. J Urol 1999; 162: 983–985.

532. Mayr J, Rune GM, Holas A, et al. Ascent of the testis in children. Eur J Pediatr 1995; 154: 893–895.

533. Imthurn T, Hadziselimovic F, Herzog B. Impaired germ cells in secondary cryptorchid testis after herniotomy. J Urol 1995; 153: 780–781.

534. Gotoh M, Miyake K, Mitsuya H. Elastic fibers in tunica propria of undescended and contralateral scrotal testes from cryptorchid patients. Urology 1987; 30: 359–363.

535. Nistal M, Paniagua R, Abaurrea MA, Santamaria L. Hyperplasia and the immature appearance of Sertoli cells in primary testicular disorders. Hum Pathol 1982; 13: 3–12.

536. Nistal M, Riestra ML, Paniagua R. Focal orchitis in undescended testes: discussion of pathogenetic mechanisms of tubular atrophy. Arch Pathol Lab Med 2002; 126: 64–69.

537. Atilla MK, Sargin H, Yilmaz Y, et al. Undescended testes in adults: clinical significance of resistive index values of the testicular artery measured by Doppler ultrasound as a predictor of testicular histology. J Urol 1997; 158: 841–843.

538. Vinardi S, Magro P, Manenti M, et al. Testicular function in men treated in childhood for undescended testes. J Pediatr Surg 2001; 36: 385–388.

539. Nistal M, Paniagua R, Queizán A. Histologic lesions in undescended ectopic obstructed testes. Fertil Steril 1985; 43: 455–462.

540. Herzog B, Steigert M, Hadziselimovic F. Is a testis located at the superficial inguinal pouch (Denis Browne pouch) comparable to a true cryptorchid testis? J Urol 1992; 148: 622–623.

541. Huff DS, Hadziselimovic F, Snyder HM III, et al. Histologic maldevelopment of unilaterally cryptorchid testes and their descended partners. Eur J Pediatr 1993; 152: S10–14.

542. Cendron M, Huff DS, Keating MA, et al. Anatomical, morphological and volumetric analysis: a review of 759 cases of testicular maldescent. J Urol 1993; 149: 570–573.

543. Alexandre C. Les testicules oscillants. forme degradée de cryptorchidie? JGynecol Obstet Biol Reprod (Paris) 1977; 6: 71–74.

544. Nistal M, Paniagua R. Infertility in adult males with retractile testes. Fertil Steril 1984; 41: 395–403.

545. Ito H, Katauni Z, Kuwamura K, et al. Changes in the volume and histology of retractile testes in prepubertal boys. Int J Androl 1986; 9: 161–169.

546. Wyllie GW. The retractile testis. Med J Aust 1984; 140: 403–405.

547. Agarwal PK, Diaz M, Elder JS. Retractile testis – is it really a normal variant? J Urol 2006; 175: 1496–1499.

548. Puri P, Nixon HH. Bilateral retractile testes – subsequent effects on fertility. J Pediatr Surg 1967; 12: 563–566.

549. Caroppo E, Niederberger C, Elhanbly S, et al. Effect of cryptorchidism and retractile testes on male factor infertility: a multicenter, retrospective, chart review. Fertil Steril 2005; 83: 1581–1584.

550. Elder JS. Epididymal anomalies associated with hydrocele/hernia and cryptorchidism: implications regarding testicular descent. J Urol 1992; 148: 624–626.

551. Scorer CG, Farrington GH. Congenital deformities of the testis and epididymis, p 136. New York: Appleton-Century-Crofts, 1971.

552. Mollaeian M, Nehrabi V, Elahi V. Significance of epididymal and ductal anomalies associated with undescended testis. Urology 1994; 43: 857–860.

553. Ferlin A, Bogatcheva NV, Gianesello L, et al. Insulin-like factor 3 gene mutations in testicular dysgenesis syndrome: clinical and functional characterization. Mol Hum Reprod 2006; 12: 401–406.

554. Bay K, Asklund C, Skakkebaek NE, Andersson AM. Testicular dysgenesis syndrome: possible role of endocrine disrupters. Best Pract Res Clin Endocrinol Metab 2006; 20: 77–90.

555. Giwercman A, Rylander L, Hagmar L, Giwercman YL. Ethnic differences in occurrence of TDS – genetics and/or environment? Int J Androl 2006; 29: 291–297.

556. Nistal M, Regadera J, Winitzky P, et al. Granular changes in Sertoli cells in children and pubertal patients. Fertil Steril 2005; 83: 1489–99.

557. Cortes D, Visfeldt J, Thorup JM. Erythropoietin may reduce the risk of germ cell loss in boys with cryptorchidism. Hormone Res 2001; 55: 41–45.

558. Engeler DS, Hösli PO, John H, et al. Early orchiopexy: prepubertal intratubular germ cell neoplasia and fertility outcome. Urology 2000; 56: 144–148.

559. Abrat RP, Reddi VB, Sarembock LA. Testicular cancer and cryptorchidism. Br J Urol 1992; 70: 656–659.

560. Giwercman A, Müller J, Skakkebaek NE. Cryptorchidism and testicular neoplasia. Hormone Res 1988; 30: 157–163.

561. Larizza C, Antiba A, Palazzi J, et al. Testicular maldescent and infertility. Andrologia 1990; 22: 285–288.

562. Cortes D, Thorup J. Histology of testicular biopsies taken at operation for bilateral maldescended testis in relation to fertility in adulthood. Brit J Urol 68: 285–291, 1991.

563. Puri P, O'Donnell B. Semen analysis in patients operated on for impalpable testes. Br J Urol 1990; 66: 646–647.

564. Kogan SJ. Fertility in cryptorchidism: an overview in 1987. Eur J Pediatr 1987; 146: S21.

565. Lee PA, Coughlin MT, Bellinger MF. Paternity and hormone levels after unilateral cryptorchidism: association with pretreatment testicular location. J Urol 2000; 164: 1697–1701.

566. Lee PA, Coughlin MT, Bellinger MF. No relationship of testicular size at orchiopexy with fertility in men who previously had unilateral cryptorchidism. J Urol 2001; 166: 236–239.

567. Wilkerson ML, Bartone FF, Fox L, Hadziselimovic F. Fertility potential: a comparison of intra-abdominal and intracanalicular testes by age groups in children. Hormone Res 2001; 55: 18–20.

568. Okuyama A, Nonomure N, Nakamura M, et al. Surgical mangement of undescended testis: retrospective study of potential fertility in 274 cases. J Urol 1989; 142: 749–751.

569. Cendron M, Keating MA, Huff DS, et al. Cryptorchidism, orchiopexy and infertility: a critical long-term retrospective analysis. J Urol 1989; 142: 559–562.

570. Hadziselimovic F, Zivkovic D, Bica DT, Emmons LR. The importance of mini-puberty for fertility in cryptorchidism. J Urol 2005; 174: 1536–1539.

571. Cortes D, Thorup JM, Visfeldt J. Cryptorchidism: aspects of fertility

and neoplasms. A study including data of 1,335 consecutive boys who underwent testicular biopsy simultaneously with surgery for cryptorchidism. Hormone Res 2001; 55: 21–27.

572. Pedersen KV, Boisen P, Zetterlund CG. Experience of screening for carcinoma-in-situ of the testis among young men with surgically corrected maldescended testes. Int J Androl 1987; 10: 181–185.

573. Berthelsen JG, Sakakkebaek NE. Distribution of carcinoma-in-situ in testes from infertile men. Int J Androl 1981; 4: 172–184.

574. Giwercman A, Clausen OPF, Skakkebaek NE. Carcinoma-in-situ of the testis: aneuploid cells in semen. Br Med J 1988; 296: 1762–1764.

575. Giwercman A, Müller J, Skakkebaek NE. Cryptorchidism and testicular neoplasia. Hormone Res 1988; 30: 157–163.

576. Smith SW, Brammer HM, Henry M, et al. Testicular microlithiasis: sonographic features with pathologic correlation. AJR Am J Roentgenol1991; 157: 1003–1004.

577. Kwan DJ, Kirsch AJ, Chang DT, et al. Testicular microlithiasis in a child with torsion of the appendix testis. J Urol 1995; 153: 183–184.

578. Mullins TL, Sant GR, Ucci AA Jr, Doherthy JF. Testicular microlithiasis occurring in a postorchidopexy testis. Urology 1986; 27: 144–146.

579. Ikinger U, Wuster K, Terwey B, Mohring K.: Microcalcifications in testicular malignancy: diagnostic tool in occult tumor? Urology 1982; 19: 525–528.

580. Schantz A, Milsten R. Testicular microlithiasis with sterility. Fertil Steril 1976; 27: 801–805.

581. Sasagawa I, Nakada T, Kazama T, et al. Testicular microlithiasis in male infertility. Urol Int 1988; 43: 368–369.

582. Gonzalez Sanchez FJ, Encinas Gaspar MB, Napal Lecumberri S. Microlitiasis testicular asociada a infertilidad. Arch Esp Urol 1997; 50: 71–74.

583. Duchek M, Bergh A, Oberg L. Painful testicular lithiasis. Scand J Urol Nephrol 1991; 138: 231–233.

584. Jara Rascon J, Escribano Patino G, Herranz Amo F, et al. Testicular microlithiasis: diagnosis associated with orchialgia. Arch Esp Urol 1998; 51: 82–85.

585. Moran JM, Moreno F, Climent V, Nistal M. Idiopathic testicular microlithiasis. Ultrastructural study. Br J Urol 1993; 72: 252–253.

586. Skyrme RJ, Fenn NJ, Jones AR, et al. Testicular microlithiasis in a UK population: its incidence, associations and follow-up. BJU Int 2000; 86: 482–485.

587. Ganem JP, Workman KR, Shaban SF. Testicular microlithiasis is associated with testicular pathology. Urology 1999; 53: 209–213.

588. Berger A, Brabrand K. Testicular microlithiasis – a possibly premalignant condition. Report of five cases and a review of the literature. Acta Radiol 1998; 39: 583–586.

589. Peterson AC, Bauman JM, Light DE, et al. The prevalence of testicular microlithiasis in an asymptomatic population of men 18 to 35 years old. J Urol 2001; 166: 2061–2064.

590. Cast JE, Nelson WM, Early AS, et al. Testicular microlithiasis: prevalence and tumor risk in a population referred for scrotal sonography. Am J Roentgenol 2000; 175: 1703–1706.

591. Miller FN, Rosairo S, Clarke JL, et al. Testicular calcification and microlithiasis: association with primary intra-testicular malignancy in 3,477 patients. Eur Radiol 2007; 17: 363–369.

592. Derogee M, Bevers RF, Prins HJ, et al. Testicular microlithiasis, a premalignant condition: prevalence, histopathologic findings, and relation to testicular tumor. Urology 2001; 57: 1133–1137.

593. Mazzilli F, Delfino M, Imbrogno N, et al. Seminal profile of subjects with testicular microlithiasis and testicular calcifications. Fertil Steril 2005; 84: 243–245.

594. De Gouveia Brazao CA, Pierik FH, Oosterhuis JW, et al. Bilateral testicular microlithiasis predicts the presence of the precursor of testicular germ cell tumors in subfertile men. J Urol 2004; 171: 158–160.

595. Nicolas F, Dubois R, Laboure S, et al. Testicular nicrolithiasis and cryptorchidism: ultrasound analysis after orchidopexy. Prog Urol 2001; 11: 357–361.

596. Miller RL, Wissman R, White S, Ragosin R. Testicular microlithiasis. a benign condition with a malignant association. J Clin Ultrasound 1996; 24: 197–202.

597. Rashid HH, Cos LR, Weinberg E, et al. Testicular microlithiasis: a review and its association with testicular cancer. Urol Oncol 2004; 22: 285–289.

598. Arrigo T, Messina MF, Valenzise M, et al. Testicular microlithiasis heralding mixed germ cell tumor of the testis in a boy. J Endocrinol Invest 2006; 29: 82–85.

599. Zastrow S, Hakenberg OW, Wirth MP. Significance of testicular microlithiasis. Urol Int 2005; 75: 3–7.

600. Drut R. Yolk sac tumor and testicular microlithiasis. Pediatr Pathol Mol Med 2003; 22: 343–347.

601. Leenen AS, Riebel TW. Testicular microlithiasis in children: sonographic features and clinical implications. Pediatr Radiol 2002; 32: 575–579.

602. Smith GD, Steele l, Barnes RB, Levine LA. Identification of seminiferous tubule aberrations and a low

incidence of testicular microliths associated with the development of azoospermia. Fertil Steril 1999; 72: 467–471.

603. De Jong BW, De Gouveia Brazao CA, Stoop H, et al. Raman spectroscopic analysis identifies testicular microlithiasis as intratubular hydroxyapatite. J Urol 2004; 171: 92–96.

604. Priebe CJ, Garret R. Testicular calcification in a 4-year-old boy. Pediatrics 1970; 46: 785–789.

605. Nistal M, Martinez-Garcia C, Paniagua R. The origin of testicular microliths. Int J Androl 1995; 18: 221–229.

606. Nistal M, Paniagua R, Díez-Pardo JA. Testicular microlithiasis in 2 children with bilateral cryptorchidism. J Urol 1979; 121: 535–537.

607. Coetzee T. Pulmonary alveolar microlithiasis with involvement of the sympathetic nervous system and gonads. Thorax 1970; 25: 637–642.

608. Wegner HE, Hubotter A, Andresen R, Miller K. Testicular microlithiasis and concomitant testicular intraepithelial neoplasia. Int Urol Nephrol 1998; 30: 313–315.

609. Holm M, Hoei-Hansen CE, Rajpert-De Meyts E, Skakkebaek NE. Increased risk of carcinoma in situ in patients with testicular germ cell cancer with ultrasonic microlithiasis in the contralateral testicle. J Urol 2003; 170: 1163–1167.

610. Winter TC III, Zunkel DE, Mack LA. Testicular carcinoma in a patient with previously demostrated testicular microlithiasis. J Urol 1996; 155: 648.

611. Frush DP, Kliewer MA, Madden JF. Testicular microlithiasis and subsequent development of metastatic germ cell tumor. Am J Roentgenol 1996; 167: 889–890.

612. Gooding GAW. Detection of testicular microlithiasis by sonography. Am J Roentgenol 1997; 168: 281–282.

613. Golash A, Parker J, Ennis O, et al. The interval of development of testicular carcinoma in a patient with previously demonstrated testicular microlithiasis. J Urol 2000; 163: 239.

614. Hoei-Hansen CE, Sommer P, Meyts ER, et al. A rare diagnosis: testicular dysgenesis with carcinoma in situ detected in a patient with ultrasonic microlithiasis. Asian J Androl 2005; 7: 445–447.

615. Ravichandran S, Smith R, Cornford PA, Fordham MV. Surveillance of testicular microlithiasis? Results of an UK based national questionnaire survey. BMC Urol 2006; 6: 8.

616. Bennett HF, Middleton WD, Bullock AD, Teefey SA. Testicular microlithiasis: US follow-up. Radiology 2001; 218: 359–363.

617. Parra BL, Venable DD, Gonzalez E, et al. Testicular microlithiasis as a predictor of intratubular germ cell

neoplasia. Urology 1996; 48: 797–799.

618. Nistal M, García-Cabezas MA, Regadera J, Castillo MC. Microlithiasis of the epididymis and the rete testis. Am J Surg Pathol 2004; 28: 514–522.

619. Scherer G, Held M, ErdeL M, et al. Three novel SRY mutations in XY gonadal dysgenesis and the enigma of XY dysgenesis cases without SRY mutations. Cytogenetic Cell Genet 1998; 80: 188–192.

620. Bilbao JR, Loridan L, Castaño J. A novel postzygotic nonsense mutation in SRY in familial XY gonadal dysgenesis. Hum Genet 1996; 97: 537–539.

621. Tagliarini EB, Assumpcao JG, Scolfaro MR, et al. Mutations in SRY and WT1 genes required for gonadal development are not responsible for XY partial gonadal dysgenesis. Braz J Med Res 2005; 38: 17–25.

622. Vilain E, Jaubert F, Fellous M, et al. Pathology of 46,XY pure gonadal dysgenesis: absence of testis differentiation associated with mutations in the testis-determining factor. Differentiation 1993; 52: 151–159.

623. Simpson JL, Blagowidow N, Martin AO. XY gonadal dysgenesis: Genetic heterogeneity based upon clinical observations, H-Y antigen status and segregations analysis. Hum Genet 1981; 58: 91–97.

624. Simpson JL, Chaganti RSK, Mouradian J, German J. Chronic renal disease, myotonic dystrophy, and gonadoblastoma in XY gonadal dysgenesis. J Med Genet 1982; 19: 73–76.

625. Harkins PG, Haning RV Jr, Shapiro SS. Renal failure with XY gonadal dysgenesis: Report of the second case. Obstet Gynecol 1980; 56: 751–752.

626. Haning RV, Chesney RW, Moorthy AV, Gilbert EF. A syndrome of chronic renal failure and XY gonadal dysgenesis in young phenotypic females without genital ambiguity. Am J Kidney Dis 1985; 6: 40–48.

627. Machin GA. Atypical presentation of Denys–Drash syndrome in a female with a novel WT1 gene mutation. Birth Defects 1996; 30: 269–286.

628. Perez de Nanclares G, Castaño L, Bilbao JR, et al. Molecular analysis of Frasier syndrome: mutation in the WT1 gene in a girl with gonadal dysgenesis and nephronophthisis. J Pediatr Endocrinol Metab 2002; 15: 1047–1050.

629. Zugor V, Zenker M, Schrott KM, Schott GE. Frasier syndrome: a rare syndrome with WT1 gene mutation in pediatric urology. Aktuelle Urol 2006; 37: 64–66.

630. Hoffman RP, Steele MW, Lee PA, et al. 46,XY siblings with inadequate virilization and CNS deficiency. Hormone Res 1988; 29: 207–210.

631. Schipper JA, Delemarre-vd Waal HA, Hansen M, Sprangers MAJ. Testicular dysgenesis and mental retardation in two incompletely masculinized XY-siblings. Acta Paediatr Scand 1991; 80: 125–128.

632. Tsutsumi O, Iida T, Nakahori Y, Taketani Y. Analysis of the testis-determining gene SRY in patients with XY gonadal dysgenesis. Hormone Res 46 1996; 46 (Suppl 1): 6–10.

633. Greenberg F, Gresik MV, Carpenter RJ, et al. The Gardner–Silengo–Wachtel or genitor–palato–cardiac syndrome: Male pseudohermaphroditism with micrognathia, cleft palate, and conotruncal cardiac defects. Am J Med Genet 1987; 26: 59–64.

634. Angle B, Hersh JH, Yen F, Verdi GD. XY gonadal dysgenesis associated with a multiple pterygium syndrome phenotype. Am J Med Genet 1997; 68: 7–11.

635. Kawamura M, Owada M, Kimura Y, et al. 46,XY pure gonadal dysgenesis: a case with Graves' disease. Intern Med 2001; 40: 740–743.

636. Tanwani LK, Chudgar D, Murphree SS, et al. A case of gonadal dysgenesis, breast development, Graves' disease, and low bone mass. Endocrinol Pract 2003; 9: 220–224.

637. El-Shanti H, Ahmad M, Ajlouni K. Alopecia universalis congenita, XY gonadal dysgenesis and laryngomalacia: a novel malformation syndrome. Eur J Pediatr 2003; 162: 36–40.

638. Teebi AS, Dupuis L, Wherrett D, et al. Alopecia congenita universalis, microcephaly, cutis marmorata, short stature and XY gonadal dysgenesis: variable expression of El-Shanti syndrome. Eur J Pediatr 2004; 163: 170–172.

639. Neri G, Opitz J. Syndromal (and nonsyndromal) forms of male pseudohermaphroditism. Am J Med Genet 1999; 89: 201–209.

640. Kempe A, Engels H, Schubert R, et al. Familial ovarian dysgerminomas (Swyer syndrome) in females associated with 46 XY-karyotype. Gynecol Endocrinol 2002; 6: 107–111.

641. Brosnan PG, Lewandowski RC, Toguri AG, et al. A new familial syndrome of 46 XY gonadal dysgenesis with anomalies of ectodermal and mesodermal structural. J Pediatr 1980; 97: 586–590.

642. Sternberg WH, Barclay DL, Klopfer HW. Familial XY gonadal dysgenesis. N Engl J Med 1968; 278: 695–700.

643. Chemke J, Carmichael R, Stewart JM, et al. Familial XY gonadal dysgenesis. J Med Genet 1970; 7: 105–111.

644. Simpson JL, Blagowidow N, Martin AO. XY gonadal dysgenesis: Genetic heterogeneity based upon clinical observations, H-Y antigen status and

segregations analysis. Hum Genet 1981; 58: 91–97.

645. Mann JR, Corkery JJ, Fisher HJW, et al. The X linked recessive form of XY gonadal dysgenesis with high incidende of gonadal cell tumors: Clinical and genetic studies. J Med Genet 1983; 20: 264–270.

646. Simpson JL, Photopulos G. The relationship of neoplasia to disorders of abnormal sexual diferentiation. Birth Defects 1976; 12: 15–50.

647. Le Caignec C, Baron S, McElreavey K, et al. 46,XY gonadal dysgenesis: evidence for autosomal dominant transmission in a large kindred. Am J Med Genet 2003; 116A: 37–43.

648. Hoepffner W, Horn LC, Simon E, et al. Gonadoblastomas in 5 patients with 46XY gonadal dysgenesis. Exp Clin Endocrinol Diabetes 2005; 113: 231–235.

649. Portuondo JA, Neyro JL, Benito JA, et al. Familial 46,XX gonadal dysgenesis. Int J Fertil 1987; 32: 56–58.

650. Marrakchi A, Belhaj L, Boussouf H, et al. Pure gonadal dysgenesis XX and XY: observations in fifteen patients. Ann Endocrinol (Paris) 2005; 66: 553–556.

651. Carpenter NJ, Say B, Browning D. Gonadal dysgenesis in a patient with an X; 3 translocation: case report and review. J Med Genet 1980; 17: 216–221.

652. Grass FS, Schwartz RP, Deal JO, Parke JC Jr. Gonadal dysgenesis, intra-X chromosomal insertion, and possible position effect in an otherwise normal female. Clin Genet 1981; 20: 28–35.

653. Tullu MS, Arora P, Parmar RC, et al. Ovarian dysgenesis with balanced autosomal translocation. J Postgrad Med 2001; 47: 113–115.

654. Doherty E, Pakarinen P, Tiitinen A, et al. A novel mutation in the FSH receptor inhibiting signal transduction and causing primary ovarian failure. J Clin Endocrinol Metab 2002; 87: 1151–1155.

655. Allen LA, Achermann JC, Pakarinen P, et al. A novel loss of function mutation in exon 10 of the FSH receptor gene causing hypergonadotropic hypogonadism: clinical and molecular characteristics. Hum Reprod 2003; 18: 251–256.

656. De la Chesnaye E, Canto P, Ulloa-Aguirre A, Mendez JP. No evidence of mutations in the follicle-stimulating hormone receptor gene in Mexican women with 46,XX pure gonadal dysgenesis. Am J Med Genet 2001; 98: 125–128.

657. Letterie GS, Page DC. Dysgerminoma and gonadal dysgenesis in a 46,XX female with no evidence of Y chromosomal DNA. Gynecol Oncol 1995; 57: 423–425.

658. Norimura Y, Nishiyama H, Yanagida K, Sato A. Dysgerminoma with syncytiotrophoblastic giant cells

arising from 46,XX pure gonadal dysgenesis. Obstet Gynecol 1998; 92: 654–656.

659. Namavar-Jahromi B, Mohit M, Kumar PV. Familial dysgerminoma associated with 46, XX pure gonadal dysgenesis. Saudi Med J 2005; 26: 872–874.

660. Gravholt CH, Juul S, Naeraa R, Hansen J. Prenatal and postnatal prevalence of Turner's syndrome: a registry study. Br Med J 1996; 312: 16–21.

661. Hook EB, Warburton D. The distribution of chromosomal genotypes associated with Turner's syndrome: livebirth prevalence and evidence for dismissed fetal mortality and severity in genotypes associated with structural X abnormalities or mosaicism. Hum Genet 1983; 64: 24–27.

662. Lippe BM. Primary ovarian failure. In: Kaplan SA, ed. Clinical pediatric endocrinology. Philadelphia: WB Saunders, 1990; 325–366.

663. Ogata T, Matsuo N. Turner syndrome and female sex chromosome aberrations: deduction of the principal factors involved in the development of clinical features. Hum Genet 1995; 95: 607–629.

664. Ranke MB, Saenger P. Turner's syndrome. Lancet 2001; 358: 309–314.

665. Singh RP, Carr DH. The anatomy and histology of XO human embryos and fetuses. Anat Rec 1966; 155: 369–383.

666. Jirasek J. Principles of reproductive embryology. In: Simpson, JL, ed. Disorders of sexual differentiation. New York: Academic Press, 1976; 51–111.

667. Edelmann W, Cohen PE, Kneitz B, et al. Mammalian MutS homologue 5 is required for chromosome pairing in meiosis. Nature Genet 1999; 21: 123–127.

668. Modi DN, Sane S, Bhartiya D. Accelerated germ cell apoptosis in sex chromosome aneuploid fetal human gonads. Mol Hum Reprod 2003; 9: 219–225.

669. Ohno S. Sex chromosomes and sex-linked genes. Berlin: Springer-Verlag, 1967.

670. Tanaka Y, Sasaki Y, Tachibana K, et al. Gonadal mixed germ cell tumor combined with a large hemangiomatous lesion in a patient with Turner's syndrome and 45,X/46,X, + mar karyotype. Arch Pathol Lab Med 1994; 118: 1135–1138.

671. Brant WO, Rajimwale A, Lovell MA, et al. Gonadoblastoma and Turner syndrome. J Urol 2006; 175: 1858–60.

672. Aaronson IA. True hermaphoditism. A review of 41 cases with observations on testicular histology and function. Br J Urol 1985; 57: 775–779.

673. Ouhilal S, Turco J, Nangia A, et al. True hermaphroditism presenting as bilateral gynecomastia in an adolescent phenotypic male. Fertil Steril 2005; 83: 1041.

674. Osorio Acosta VA, Alonso Dominguez FJ. True hermaphroditism. Arch Esp Urol 2004; 57: 856–860.

675. Morel Y, Rey R, Teinturier C, et al. Aetiological diagnosis of male sex ambiguity: a collaborative study. Eur J Pediatr 2002; 161: 49–59.

676. Nichter LS. Seminoma in a 46 XX true hermaphrodite with positive H-Y antigen. A case report. Cancer 1984; 53: 1181–1184.

677. Van Niekert WA, Retief AE. The gonads of human true hermaphrodites. Hum Genet 1981; 58: 117–122.

678. Van Niekert WA. True hermaphroditism. Clinical morphological and cytogenetic aspects. New York: Harper & Row, 1974.

679. Krob G, Braun A, Kuhnle U. True hermaphroditism: geographical distribution, clinical findings, chromosomes and gonadal histology. Eur J Pediatr 1994; 153: 2–10.

680. Yordam N, Alikasifoglu N, Caglar M, et al. True hermaprhoditism: clinical features, genetic variants and gonadal histology. J Pediatr Endocrinol Metab 2001; 14: 421–427.

681. Toublanc JE, Boucekkine C, Abbas N, et al. Hormonal and molecular genetic fundings in 46, XX subjects with sexual ambiguity and testicular differentiation. Eur J Pediatr 1993; 152: S70–S75.

682. Greenfield SP. Familial 46XX males coexisting with familial 46,XX true hermaphrodites in same pedigree. J Pediatr 1987; 110: 244–248.

683. Jimenez AL, Kofman-Alfaro S, Berumen J, et al. Partially deleted SRY gene confined to testicular tissue in a 46,XX true hermaphrodite without SRY in leukocytic DNA. Am J Med Genet 2000; 93: 417–420.

684. Tanaka Y, Fujiwara K, Yamauchi H, et al. Pregnancy in a woman with a Y chromosome after removal of an ovarian dysgerminoma. Gynecol Oncol 2000; 79: 519–521.

685. Nihoul-Fekete C, Lortat-Jacob S, Cachin O, et al. Preservation of gonadal function in true hermaphroditism. J Pediatr Surg 1984; 19: 50–55.

686. Prader A, Gurtner HP. Das syndrom des Pseudohermaphroditismus masculinus bei kongenitaler Nebennierensiden-Hyperplasie ohne Androgenüberproduktion. Helvet Pediatr Acta 1955; 10: 397–412.

687. Kirkland RT, Kirkland JL, Johnson CM, et al. Congenital lipoid adrenal hyperplasia in an eight-year-old phenotype female. J Clin Endocrinol 1973; 36: 488–496.

688. Katsumata N, Kawada Y, Yamamoto Y, et al. A novel compound heterozygous mutation in the steroidogenic acute regulatory protein gene in a patient with congenital lipoid adrenal hyperplasia. J Clin Endocrinol Metab 1999; 84: 3983–3987.

689. Achermann JC, Meeks JJ, Heffs B, et al. Molecular and structural analysis of two novel StAR mutation in patients with lipoid congenital adrenal hyperplasia. Mol Genet Metab 2001; 73: 354–357.

690. Fluck CE, Maret A, Mallet D, et al. A novel mutation L260P of the steroidogenic acute regulatory protein gene in three unrelated patients of Swiss ancestry with congenital lipoid adrenal hyperplasia. J Clin Endocrinol Metab 2005; 90: 5304–5308.

691. Bose HS, Sato S, Aisenberg J, et al. Mutations in the steroidogenic acute regulatory protein (StAR) in six patients with congenital lipoid adrenal hyperplasia. J Clin Endocrinol Metab 2000; 85: 3636–3639.

692. Miller WL. Disorders of androgen synthesis – from cholesterol to dehydroepiandrosterone. Med Princ Pract 2005; 14: 58–68.

693. Chen X, Baker BY, Abduljabbar MA, Miller WL. A genetic isolate of congenital lipoid adrenal hyperplasia with atypical clinical findings. J Clin Endocrinol Metab 2005; 90: 835–840.

694. Bhangoo A, Anhalt H, Ten S, King SR. Phenotypic variations in lipoid congenital adrenal hyperplasia. Pediatr Endocrinol Rev 2006; 3: 258–271.

695. Saenger P. Abnormal sex differentiation. J Pediatr 104: 1–17, 1984.

696. Saenger P, Klonari Z, Black SM, et al. Prenatal diagnosis of congenital lipoid adrenal hyperplasia. J Clin Endocrinol Metab 1995; 80: 200–205.

697. Caron KM, Soo SC, Wetsel WC, et al. Targeted disruption of the mouse gene encoding steroidogenic acute regulatory protein provides insights into congenital lipoid adrenal hyperplasia. Proc Natl Acad Sci USA 1997; 94: 11540–11545.

698. Tsutsui Y, Hirabayashi N, Ito G. An autopsy case of congenital lipoid hyperplasia of the adrenal cortex. Acta Pathol Jpn 20: 227–237,1970.

699. Müller J, Torsson A, Damkjaer Nielsen M, et al. Gonadal development and grown in 46,XX and 46,XY individuals with P450scc deficiency (congenital lipoid adrenal hyperplasia). Hormone Res 1991; 36: 203–208.

700. Saenger P. New developments in congenital lipoid adrenal hyperplasia and steroidogenic acute regulatory

protein. Pediatr Clin North Am 1997; 44: 397–421.

701. Dhom G. Zur Morphologie und Genese der kongenitalen Nebennierenhyperplasie beim männlichen scheinzwitter. Zeitschr Allg Pathol Anat 1958; 97: 346–357.

702. Ogata T, Matsuo N, Saito M, Prader A. The testicular lesion and sexual differentiation in congenital lipoid adrenal hyperplasia. Helv Paediatr Acta 1989; 43: 531–538.

703. Hauffa BP, Miller WL, Grumbach MM, et al. Congenital adrenal lipoid hyperplasia due to deficient cholesterol side-chain cleavage activity (20,22-desmolase) in a patient treated for 18 years. Clin Endocrinol 1985; 23: 481–493.

704. Kirkland RT, Kirkland JL, Johnson CM, et al. Congenital lipoid adrenal hyperplasia in a eight-year-old phenotype female. J Clin Endocrinol 1973; 36: 488–496.

705. Korsch E, Peter M, Hiort O, et al. Gonadal histology with testicular carcinoma in situ in a 15-year old 46,XY female patient with a premature termination in the steroidogenic acute regulatory protein causing congenital lipoid adrenal hyperplasia. J Clin Endocrinol Metab 1999; 84: 1628–1632.

706. Bongiovanni AM. Unusual steroid pattern in congenital adrenal hyperplasia: deficiency of 3β-hydroxydehydrogenase. J Clin Endocrinol 1961; 21: 860–862.

707. Parks GA, Bermudez JA, Anast CS, et al. Pubertal boy with the 3β-hydroxysteroid dehydrogenase defect. J Clin Endocrinol 1971; 33: 269–278.

708. Zhang L, Mason JI, Naiki Y, et al. Characterization of two novel homozygous missense mutations involving codon 6 and 259 of type II 3β-hydroxysteroid dehydrogenase (3βHSD) gene causing, respectively, nonsalt-wasting and salt-wasting 3βHSD deficiency disorder. J Clin Endocrinol Metab 2000; 85: 1678–1685.

709. Griffin JE, Wilson JD. Disorders of sexual differentiation. In: Walsh PC, Retik AB, Stamey TA, et al., eds. Campbell's urology. Vol. 2. Philadelphia: WB Saunders, 1992;1496–1542.

710. Rheaume E, Simard J, Morel Y, et al. Congenital adrenal hyperplasia due to point mutations in the type II 3β-hydroxysteroid dehydrogenase gene. Nature Genet 1992; 1: 239–45.

711. Simard J, Rheaume E, Sanchez R, et al. Molecular basis of congenital adrenal hyperplasia due to 3β-hydroxysteroid dehydrogenase deficiency. Mol Endocrinol 1993; 7: 716–28.

712. Sanchez R, Rheaume E, Laflamme N, et al. Detection and functional characterization of the novel missense mutation Y254D in type II 3β-hydroxysteroid dehydrogenase

(3βHSD) gene of a female patient with nonsalt-losing 3βHSD deficiency. J Clin Endocrinol Metab 1994; 78: 561–567.

713. Pang S, Levine LS, Stoner E, et al. Nonsalt-losing congenital adrenal hyperplasia due to 3β-hydroxysteroid dehydrogenase deficiency with normal glomerulosa function. J Clin Endocrinol Metab 1983; 56: 808–818.

714. Aaronson IA, Carkmak MA, Key LL. Defects of the testosterone biosynthetic pathway in boys with hypospadias. J Urol 1997; 157: 1884–1888.

715. Sapunar J, Vidal T, Bauer K. Abnormalities of adrenal steroidogenesis in Chilean boys with micropenis. Rev Med Chile 2003; 131: 46–54.

716. Lam CW, Arlt W, Chan CK, et al. Mutation of proline 409 to arginine in the meander region of cytochrome p450c17 causes severe 17 alpha-hydroxylase deficiency. Mol Genet Metab 2001; 72: 254–259.

717. Fan YS, Sasi R, Lee C, et al. Localization of the human CYP17 gene (cytochrome P450 (17 alpha)) to 10q24.3 by fluorescence 'in situ' hybridization and simultaneous chromosome banding. Genomics 1992; 14: 1110–1111.

718. Brooke AM, Taylor NF, Shepherd JH, et al. A novel point mutation in P450c17 (CYP17) causing combined 17alpha-hydroxylase/17,20-lyase deficiency. J Clin Endocrinol Metab 2006; 91: 2428–2431.

719. Auchus RJ, Gupta MK. Towards a unifying mechanism for CYP17 mutations that cause isolated 17,20-lyase deficiency. Endocrinol Res 2002; 28: 443–447.

720. Biglieri EG, Herron MA, Brust N. 17 alpha-hydroxylation deficiency in man. J Clin Invest 1966; 45: 1946–1954.

721. Sabage MO, Chausain JL, Evain D, et al. Endocrine studies in male pseudohermaphroditism in childhood and adolescence. Clin Endocrinol 1978; 8: 219–231.

722. Zachmann M, Vollman JA, Hamilton W, et al. Steroid 17,20 desmolase deficiency. Clin Endocrinol 1972; 1: 369–385.

723. Goebelsmann U, Davajan V, Isreal R, et al. Male pseudohermaphroditism consistent with 17–20 desmolase deficiency. Gynecol Invest 1974; 5: 60–64.

724. Gupta MK, Geller DH, Auchus RJ. Pitfalls in characterizing P450c17 mutations associated with isolated 17,20-lyase deficiency. J Clin Endocrinol Metab 2001; 86: 4416–4423.

725. Twesten W, Johannisson R, Holterhus PM, Hiort O. Severe 46,XY virilization deficit due to 17β-hydroxysteroid dehydrogenase

deficiency. Klin Paediatr 2002; 214: 314–315.

726. Millan M, Audi L, Martinez-Mora J, et al. 17 ketosteroid reductase deficiency in an adult patient without gynecomastia but with female psychosexual orientation. Acta Endocrinol 1983; 102: 633–640.

727. Dumic M, Plavsic V, Fattorini I, et al. Absent spermatogenesis despite early bilateral orchidopexy in 17-ketoreductase deficiency. Hormone Res 1985; 22: 100–106.

728. Lindqvist A, Hughes IA, Andersson S. Substitution mutation C268Y causes 17β-hydroxysteroid dehydrogenase 3 deficiency. J Clin Endocrinol Metab 2001; 86: 921–923.

729. Richter-Unruh A, Korsch E, Hiort O, et al. Novel insertion frameshift mutation of the LH receptor gene: problematic clinical distinction of Leydig cell hypoplasia from enzyme defects primarily affecting testosterone biosynthesis. Eur J Endocrinol 2005; 152: 255–259.

730. Brown DM, Markland C, Dehner LP. Leydig cell hypoplasia: A cause of male pseudohermaphroditism. J Clin Endocrinol Metab 1978; 46: 1–7.

731. Eil C, Austin RM, Sesterhenn I, Dunn JF, et al. Leydig cell hypoplasia causing male pseudohermaphroditism: diagnosis 13 year after prepubertal castration. J Clin Endocrinol Metab 1984; 58: 441–448.

732. Lee PA, Rock JA, Brown TR, et al. Leydig cell hypofunction resulting in male pseudohermaphroditism. Fertil Steril 1982; 37: 675–679.

733. Park IJ, Burnett LS, Jones HW, et al. A case of male pseudohemaphroditism associated with elevated LH, normal FSH and low testosterone possibly due to the secretion of an abnormal LH molecule. Acta Endocrinol 1976; 83: 173–181.

734. Pérez-Palacios G, Scaglia HE, Kofman-Alpharo S, et al. Inherited male pseudohermaphroditism due to gonadotropin irresponsiveness. Acta Endocrinol 1981; 98: 148–155.

735. Saldanha PH, Arnhold IJP, Mendonça BB, et al. A clinico-genetic investigation of Leydig cell hypoplasia. Am J Med Genet 1987; 26: 337–344.

736. Latronico AC. Naturally occurring mutations of the luteinizing hormone receptor gene affecting reproduction. Semin Reprod Med 2000; 18: 17–20.

737. Salameh W, Choucair M, Guo TB, et al. Leydig cell hypoplasia due to inactivation of luteinizing hormone receptor by a novel homozygous nonsense truncation mutation in the seventh transmembrane domain. Mol Cell Endocrinol 2005; 229: 57–64.

738. Leung MY, Steinbach PJ, Bear D, et al. Biological effect of a novel mutation in the third leucine-rich repeat of human luteinizing hormone

receptor. Mol Endocrinol 2006; 20: 2493–2503.

739. Wilson JD, Harrod MJ, Goldstein JL, et al. Familial incomplete male pseudohermaphroditism, type I. Evidence for androgen resistance and variable clinical manifestations in a family with the Reifenstein syndrome. N Engl J Med 1974; 290: 1097–1103.

740. Griffin JE, Durrant JL. Quantitative receptor defects in families with androgen resistance; failure of stabilization of the fibroblast cytosol androgen receptor. J Clin Endocrinol Metab 1982; 55: 465–474.

741. Toledo SPA, Arnhold IJP, Luthold W, et al. Leydig cell hypoplasia determining familial hypergonadotropic hypogonadism. Prog Clin Biol Res 1985; 200: 311–314.

742. Arnhold IJP, Mendonça BB, Bloise W, et al. Male pseudohermaphroditism resulting from Leydig cell hypoplasia. J Pediatr 1985; 106: 1057–1060.

743. Morris JM. The syndrome of testicular feminization in male pseudohermaphrodites. Am J Obstet Gynecol 1953; 65: 1192–1211.

744. Nitsche EM, Hiort O. The molecular bases of androgen insensitivity. Hormone Res 2000; 54: 327–333.

745. Brinkmann AO. Molecular basis of androgen insensitivity, Mol Cell Endocrinol 2001; 179: 105–109.

746. Rutgers JL, Scully RE. The androgen insensitivity syndrome (testicular feminization). A clnicopathologic study of 43 cases. Int J Gynecol Pathol 1991; 10: 126–145.

747. Gerli M, Migliorini G, Bocchini V, et al. A case of complete testicular feminization and 47 XXY karyotype. J Med Genet 1979; 16: 480–483.

748. Müller J. Morphometry and histology of gonads from twelve children and adolescents with the androgen insensitivity (testicular feminization) syndrome. J Clin Endocrinol Metab 1984; 59: 485–789.

749. Müller J, Skakkebaek NE. Testicular carcinoma in situ in children with the androgen insensitivity (testicular feminization) syndrome. Br Med J 1984; 288: 1419–1420.

750. Nistal M, De la Roza C, Cano J. Síndrome de feminización testicular completa. Patología 1979; 12: 119–125.

751. Aumuller G, Peter ST. Inmunohistochemical and ultrastructural study of Sertoli cells in androgen insensitivity. Int J Androl 1986; 9: 99–108.

752. Ko HM, Chung JH, Jung IS, et al. Androgen receptor gene mutation associated with complete androgen insensitivity syndrome and Sertoli cell adenoma. Int J Gynecol Pathol 2001; 20: 196–199.

753. Hannema SE, Scott IS, Hodapp J, et al. Residual activity of mutant androgen receptors explains wolffian duct development in the complete androgen insensitivity syndrome. J Clin Endocrinol Metab 2004; 89: 5815–5822.

754. Sakai N, Yamada T, Asao T, et al. Bilateral testicular tumors in androgen insensitivity syndrome. Int J Urol 2000; 7: 390–392.

755. Papadimitriou DT, Linglart A, Morel Y, Chaussain JL. Puberty in subjects with complete androgen insensitivity syndrome. Hormone Res 2006; 65: 126–131.

756. Lubs HA Jr, Vilar O, Bergenstal DM. Familial male pseudohermaphroditism with labial testes and partial feminization: endocrine studies and genetic aspects. J Clin Endocrinol Metab 1959; 19: 1110–1120.

757. Gunasegaram R, Loganath A, Peh KL, et al. Altered hypothalamic–pituitary-testicular function in incomplete testicular feminization syndrome. Aust NZ J Obstet Gynecol 1984; 24: 288–292.

758. Gilbert-Dreyfus S, Sebaoum CIA, Belaisch J. Etude d'un cas familial d'androgynoïdisme avec hypospadias grave, gynécomastie et hyperoestrogénie. Ann Endocrinol 1957; 18: 93–101.

759. Reifenstein EC Jr. Hereditary familial hypogonadism. Clin Res 1947; 3: 86–89.

760. Rosewater S, Gwinup G, Hamwi GJ. Familial gynecomastia. Ann Intern Med 1965; 63: 377–385.

761. Lombardo F, Sgro P, Salacone P, et al. Androgens and fertility. J Endocrinol Invest 2005; 28: 51–55.

762. Morrow AG, Gyorki S, Warne GL, et al. Variable androgen receptor levels in infertile men. J Clin Endocrinol Metab 1987; 64: 1115–1121.

763. Schulster A, Ross L, Scommegna A. Frecuency of androgen insensitivity in infertile phenotypically normal men. J Urol 1983; 130: 699–701.

764. Wang Q, Ghadessy FJ, Yong EL. Analysis of the transactivation domain of the androgen receptor in patients with male infertility. Clin Genet 1998; 54: 185–192.

765. Akin JW, Behzadian A, Tho SPT, McDonough PG. Evidence for partial deletion in the androgen receptor gene in a phenotypic male with azoospermia. Am J Obstet Gynecol 1991; 165: 1891–1894.

766. Giwercman A, Kledal T, Schwartz M, et al. Preserved male fertility despite decreased androgen sensitivity caused by a mutation in the ligand-binding domain of the androgen receptor gene. J Clin Endocrinol Metab 2000; 85: 2253–2259.

767. Kennedy WR, Alter M, Sung JH. Progressive proximal spinal and bulbar muscular atrophy of late onset. A sex-linked recessive trait. Neurology 1968; 18: 671–680.

768. Tanaka F, Doyu M, Ito Y, et al. Founder effect in spinal and bulbar muscular atrophy (SBMA). Hum Mol Genet 1996; 5: 1253–1257.

769. Sobue G, Hashizume Y, Mukai E, et al. X-linked recessive bulbospinal neuronopathy: a clinicopathological study. Brain 1989; 112: 209–232.

770. Harding AE, Thomas PK, Baraitser M, et al. X-linked recessive bulbospinal neuronopathy: a report of ten cases. J Neurol Neurosurg Psychiatry 1982; 45: 1012–1019.

771. Stefanis C, Papapetropoulos T, Scarpalezos S, et al. X-Linked spinal and bulbar muscular atrophy of late onset. A separate type of motor neuron disease? J Neurol Sci 1975; 24: 493–503.

772. Arbizu T, Santamaria J, Gomez JM, et al. A family with adult spinal and bulbar muscular atrophy, X-linked inheritance and associated testicular failure. J Neurol Sci 1983; 59: 371–382.

773. La Spada AR, Wilson EM, Lubahn DB, et al. Androgen receptor gene mutations in X-linked spinal and bulbar muscular atrophy. Nature 1991; 352: 77–79.

774. La Spada AR, Roling DB, Harding AE, et al. Meiotic stability and genotype-phenotype correlation of the tricucleotide repeat in X-linked spinal and bulbar muscular atrophy. Nature Genet 1992; 2: 301–304.

775. Chamberlain NL, Driver ED, Miesfeld RL. The length and location of CAG trinucleotide repeats in the androgen receptor N-terminal domain affect transactivation function. Nucleic Acids Res 1994; 22: 3181–3186.

776. MacLean HE, Choi WT, Rekaris G, et al. Abnormal androgen receptor binding affinity in subjects with Kennedy's disease (spinal and bulbar muscular atrophy). J Clin Endocrinol Metab 1995; 80: 508: 516.

777. Gottlieb B, Lombroso R, Beitel LK, Trifiro MA. Molecular pathology of the androgen receptor in male (in)fertility. Reprod Biomed Online 2005; 10: 42–48.

778. Imperato-McGinley J, Guerrero J, Gautier T, Peterson RE. Steroid 5 alpha-reductase deficiency in man. An inherited form of male pseudohermaphroditism. Science 1974; 186: 1213–1215.

779. Vilchis F, Mendez JP, Canto P, et al. Identification of missense mutations in the SRD5A2 gene from patients with steroid 5alpha-reductase 2 deficiency. Clin Endocrinol 2000; 52: 383–387.

780. Andersson S, Berman DM, Jenkins EP, Russell DW. Deletion of steroid 5 alpha reductase 2 gene in male pseudohermaphroditism. Nature 1991; 354: 159–161.

781. Wilson JD, Griffin JE, Russell DW. Steroid 5 alpha-reductase 2 deficiency. Endocrinol Rev 1993; 14: 577–593.

782. Boudon C, Lumbroso S, Lobaccaro JM, et al. Molecular study of the 5

alpha-reductase type 2 gene in three european families with 5 alpha-reductase deficiency. J Clin Endocrinol Metab 1995; 80: 2149–2153.

783. Skordis N, Patsalis PC, Bacopoulou I, et al. 5alpha-reductase 2 gene mutations in three unrelated patients of Greek Cypriot origin: identification of an ancestral founder effect. J Pediatr Endocrinol Metab 2005; 18: 241–246.

784. Kim SH, Kim KS, Kim GH, et al. A novel frameshift mutation in the 5alpha-reductase type 2 gene in Korean sisters with male pseudohermaphroditism. Fertil Steril 2006; 85: 750; e9–750.e12.

785. Schmidt JA, Schweikert, HU. Testosterone and epitestosterone metabolism of single hairs in 5 patients with 5 alpha-reductase-deficiency. Acta Endocrinol 1986; 113: 588–592.

786. Okon E, Livni N, Rösler A, et al. Male pseudohermaphroditism due to 5 alpha-reductase deficiency. Arch Pathol Lab Med 1980; 104: 363–367.

787. Peterson RE, Imperato-Mcginley J, Gautier T, et al. Male pseudohermaphroditism due to steroid 5 alpha-reductase deficiency. Am J Med 1977; 62: 170–191.

788. Josso N, Fekete C, Cachin O, et al. Persistence of müllerian ducts in male pseudohermaphroditism, and its relationship to cryptorchidism. Clin Endocrinol 1983; 19: 247–258.

789. Josso N, Boussin L, Knebelmann B, et al. Anti-Müllerian hormone and intersex states. Trends Endocrinol Metab 1991; 2: 227–233.

790. Josso N, Cate RL, Picard JY, et al. Anti-Müllerian hormone, the Jost factor. Rec Progr Hormone Res 1993; 48: 1–59.

791. Josso N, Picard JY, Imbeaud S, et al. The persistent müllerian duct syndrome: a rare cause of cryptorchidism. Eur J Pediatr 1993; 152: S76–S78.

792. Sohval AR. Hermaphroditism with atypical or 'mixed' gonadal dysgenesis. Relationship to gonadal neoplasm. Am J Med 1964; 36: 281–292.

793. Zäh W, Kalderon AE, Tucci JR. Mixed gonadal dysgenesis. Acta Endocrinol 1975; 197: 3–39.

794. Konrad D, Sossay R, Winklehner HL, et al. Penoscrotal hypospadias and coarctation of the aorta with mixed gonadal dysgenesis. Pediatr Surg Int 2000; 16: 226–228.

795. Alvarez-Nava F, Soto M, Borjas L, et al. Molecular analysis of SRY gene in patients with mixed gonadal dysgenesis. Ann Genet 2001; 44: 155–159.

796. Robboy SJ, Miller T, Donahoe PK, et al. Dysgenesis of testicular and streak gonads in the syndrome of mixed gonadal dysgenesis. Perspective derived from a clinicopathologic analysis of twenty-one cases. Hum Pathol 1982; 13: 700–716.

797. Berkovitz GD, Fechner PY, Zacur HW, et al. Clinical and pathologic spectrum of 46,XY gonadal dysgenesis: its relevance to the understanding of sex differentiation. Medicine (Baltimore) 1991; 70: 375–383.

798. Rajfer J, Mendelsohn G, Arnheim J, et al. Dysgenetic male pseudohermaphroditism. J Urol 1978; 119: 525–527.

799. Ribeiro-Scolfaro M, Aparecida-Cardinalli l, Gabas-Stuchi-Perez E, et al. Morphometry and histology of gonads from 13 children with dysgenetic male pseudohermaphroditism. Arch Pathol Lab Med 2001; 125: 652–656.

800. Slowikoska-Hilcer J, Szarras-Czapnik M, et al. Testicular pathology in 46,XY dysgenetic male pseudohermaphroditism: an approach to pathogenesis of testis cancer. J Androl 2001; 22: 781–792.

801. Nilson O. Hernia uteri inguinalis beim Manne. Acta Chirurg Scand 1939; 83: 231–240.

802. Belville C, Josso N, Picard JY. Persistence of müllerian derivatives in males. Am J Med Genet 1999; 89: 218–223.

803. Sheehan SJ, Tobbia IN, Ismail MA, et al. Persistent müllerian duct syndrome. Review and report of 3 cases. Br J Urol 1985; 57: 548–551.

804. Beheshti M, Churchill BM, Hardy BE, et al. Familial persistent müllerian duct syndrome. J Urol 1984; 131: 968–969.

805. Mouli K, McCarthy P, Ray P, et al. Persistent müllerian duct syndrome in a man with transverse testicular ectopia. J Urol 1988; 139: 373–375.

806. Hershlag A, Spitz IM, Hochner-Celnikier D, et al. Persistent müllerian structures in infertile male. Urology 1986; 28: 138–141.

807. Malayaman D, Armiger G, D'Arcangues C, et al. Male pseudohermaphroditism with persistent müllerian and wolffian structures complicated by intra-abdominal seminoma. Urology 1984; 24: 67–69.

808. Belville C, Josso N, Picard J-Y. Persistence of müllerian derivatives in males. Am J Med Genet 1999; 89: 218–223.

809. Sloan WR, Walsh PC. Familial persistent müllerian duct syndrome. J Urol 1976; 115: 459–461.

810. Carré-Eusèbe D, Imbeaud S, Harbison M, et al. Variants of the anti-müllerian hormone gene in a compound heterozygote with the persistent müllerian duct syndrome and his family. Hum Genet 1992; 90: 389–394.

811. Nistal M, Paniagua R, Isorna S, et al. Diffuse intratubular undifferentiated germ cell tumor in both testes of a male subject with a uterus and ipsilateral testicular dysgenesis. J Urol 1980; 124: 286–289.

812. Snow BW, Rowland RG, Seal GM, et al. Testicular tumor in patient with persistent müllerian duct syndrome. Urology 1985; 26: 495–497.

813. Dueñas A, Saldivar C, Castillero C, et al. A case of bilateral seminoma in the setting of persistent müllerian duct syndrome. Rev Invest Clin 2001; 53: 193–196.

814. Kelley RI. RSH/Smith–Lemli–Opitz syndrome: mutations and metabolic morphogenesis. Am J Med Genet 1998; 63: 322–326.

815. Angle B, Tint GS, Yacoub OA, Clark AL. Atypical case of Smith–Lemli–Opitz syndrome: implications for diagnosis. Am J Med Genet 1998; 80: 322–326.

816. Nwokoro NA, Wassif CA, Porter FD. Genetic disorders of cholesterol biosynthesis in mice and humans. Mol Genet Metab 2001; 74: 105–119.

817. Witsch-Baumgartner M, Ciara E, Loffer J, et al. Frequency gradients of DHCR7 mutations in patients with Smith–Lemli–Opitz syndrome in Europe: evidence for different origins of common mutations. Eur J Hum Genet 2001; 9: 45–50.

818. Putnam AR, Szakacs JG, Opitz JM, Byrne JL. Prenatal death in Smith–Lemli–Opitz/RSH syndrome. Am J Med Genet A 2005; 138: 61–65.

819. Goldenberg A, Wolf C, Chevy F, et al. Antenatal manifestations of Smith–Lemli–Opitz (RSH) syndrome: a retrospective survey of 30 cases. Am J Med Genet A 2004; 124: 423–426.

820. Bradley LA, Palomaki GE Knight GJ, et al. Levels of unconjugated estriol and other maternal serum markers in pregnancies with Smith–Lemli–Opitz (RSH) syndrome fetuses. Am J Med Genet 1999; 82: 355–358.

821. Neri G, Opitz J. Syndromal (and nonsyndromal) forms of male pseudohermaphroditism. Am J Med Genet 1999; 89: 201–209.

822. Fitzky BU, Witsch-Baumgartner M, Erdel M, et al. Mutations in the delta7-steroid reductase gene in patients with the Smith–Lemli–Opitz syndrome. Proc Natl Acad Sci USA 1998; 95: 8181–8186.

823. Moebius FF, Fitzky BU, Lee JN, et al. Molecular cloning and expression of the human delta7-sterol reductase. Proc Natl Acad Sci USA 1998; 95: 1899–1902.

824. Wassif CA, Maslen C, Kachilele-Linjewile S, et al. Mutations in the human sterol delta7 reductase gene at 11q12-13 cause Smith–Lemli–Opitz syndrome. Am J Hum Genet 1998; 63: 55–62.

825. Waterham HR, Wijburg FA, Hennekam RC, et al. Smith–Lemli–Opitz syndrome is caused by mutations in the 7-dehydrocholesterol reductase gene. Am J Hum Genet 1998; 63: 329–338.

826. Porter FD. RSH/Smith–Lemli–Opitz syndrome: a multiple congenital anomaly/mental retardation syndrome due to an inborn error of cholesterol biosynthesis. Mol Genet Metab 2000; 71: 163–174.

827. Krakowiak PA, Nwokoro NA, Wassif CA, et al. Mutation analysis and description of sixteen RSH/Smith–Lemli–Opitz syndrome patients: polymerase chain reaction-based assays to simplify genotyping. Am J Med Genet 2000; 94: 214–227.

828. Shinawi M, Szabo S, Popek E, et al. Recognition of Smith–Lemli–Opitz syndrome (RSH) in the fetus: utility of ultrasonography and biochemical analysis in pregnancies with low maternal serum estriol. Am J Med Genet A 2005; 138: 56–60.

829. Drash A, Sherman F, Hartmann WH, et al. A syndrome of pseudohermaphroditism, Wilms' tumor, hypertension and degenerative renal disease. J Pediatr 1970; 76: 585–593.

830. Rajfer J. Association between Wilms' tumor and gonadal dysgenesis. J Urol 1981; 125: 388–390.

831. McCoy FE, Franklin WA, Aronson AJ, et al. Glomerulonephritis associated with male pseudohermaphroditism and nephroblastoma. Am J Surg Pathol 1983; 7: 387–395.

832. Royer-Pokora B, Beier M, Henzler M, et al. Twenty-four new cases of WT1 germline mutations and review of the literature: genotype/phenotype correlations for Wilms' tumor development. Am J Med Genet 2004; A 27: 249–257.

833. Heppe RK, Koyle MA, Beckwith JB. Nephrogenic rests in Wilms' tumor patients with the Drash syndrome. J Urol 1991; 145: 1225–1228.

834. Koziell A, Charmandari E, Hindmarsh PC, et al. Frasier syndrome, part of the Denys Drash continuum or simply a WT1 gene associated disorder of intersex and nephropathy? Clin Endocrinol 2000; 52: 519–524.

835. Zugor V, Zenker M, Schrott KM, Schott GE. Frasier syndrome: a rare syndrome with WT1 gene mutation in pediatric urology. Aktuelle Urol 2006; 37: 64–66.

836. Chao LY, Huff V, Strong LC, Saunders GF. Mutation in the PAX6 gene in twenty patients with aniridia. Hum Mutat 15: 332–339, 2000.

837. Fischbach BV, Trout KL, Lewis J, et al. WAGR syndrome: a clinical review of 54 cases. Pediatrics 2005; 116: 984–988.

838. Opitz JM, Frías JL, Gutenberger JE, Pellett JR. The G syndrome of multiple congenital anomalies. Birth Defects 1969; 5: 95–101.

839. Opitz JM, Summitt RL, Smith DW. The BBB syndrome: familial telecanthus with associated congenital anomalies. Birth Defects 1969; 5: 95–101.

840. Berti C, Fontanella B, Ferrentino R, Meroni G. Mig12, a novel Opitz syndrome gene product partner, is expressed in the embryonic ventral midline and co-operates with Mid1 to bundle and stabilize microtubules. BMC Cell Biol 2004; 5: 9.

841. Cho HJ, Shin MY, Ahn KM, et al. X-linked Opitz G/BBB syndrome: identification of a novel mutation and prenatal diagnosis in a Korean family. J Korean Med Sci 2006; 21: 790–793.

842. Giordano J, Prior HM, Bamforth JS, et al. Genetic study of SOX9 in a case of campomelic dysplasia Am J Med Genet 2001; 98: 176–181.

843. Gibbons RJ, Higgs DR. Molecular-clinical spectrum of the ATR-X syndrome. Am J Med Genet 2000; 97: 204–212.

844. Wada T, Fukushima Y, Saitoh S. A new detection method for ATRX gene mutations using a mismatch-specific endonuclease. Am J Med Genet A 2006; 140: 1519–1523.

845. Fichera M, Silengo M, Spalletta A, et al. Prenatal diagnosis of ATR-X syndrome in a fetus with a new G>T splicing mutation in the XNP/ATR-X gene. Prenat Diagn 2001; 21: 747–751.

846. Charny CW. Testicular biopsy, its value in male sterility. JAMA 1940; 115: 1429–1432.

847. Charny CW, Meranze DR. Testicular biopsy. Further studies in male infertility. Surg Gynecol Obstet 1942; 74: 836–842.

848. Nelson WO. Interpretation of testicular biopsy. JAMA 1953; 151: 449–452.

849. Pesce C. Testicular biopsy in the evolution of male infertility. Semin Diagn Pathol 1987; 4: 264–274.

850. Wong TW, Straus FH II, Warner NE. Testicular causes of infertility. Arch Pathol 1973; 95: 151–159.

851. Wong TW, Straus FH II, Warner NE. Pretesticular causes of infertility. Arch Pathol 1974; 98: 1–8.

852. Guarch R, Pesce C, Puras A, et al. A quantitative approach to the classification of hypospermatogenesis in testicular biopsies for infertility. Hum Pathol 1992; 23: 1032–1037.

853. Honoré LJ. Testicular biopsy for infertility: a review of sixty-eight cases with a simplified histologic classification of lesions. Int J Fertil 1979; 24: 49–52.

854. Girgis SM, Etriby A, Ibrahim AA, et al. Testicular biopsy in azoospermia: a review of the last ten years. Experience of over 800 cases. Fertil Steril 1969; 20: 467–477.

855. Wong TW, Straus FH II, Warner NE. Posttesticular causes of infertility. Arch Pathol 1973; 95: 160–164.

856. Söderstrom KO, Suominen J. Histopathology and ultrastructure of meiotic arrest in human spermatogenesis. Arch Pathol Lab Med 1980; 198: 476–482.

857. Charny CW. Reflections on testicular biopsy. Fertil Steril 1963; 14: 610–616.

858. Meinhard E, McRae CU, Chisholm GD. Testicular biopsy in evaluation of male infertility. Br Med J 1973; 3: 577–581.

859. Levin HS. Testicular biopsy in the study of male infertility. Its current usefulness, histologic techniques, and prospects for the future. Hum Pathol 1979; 10: 569–584.

860. Bairati A, Della Morte E, Giarola A, et al. Testicular biopsy of azoospermic men with vas deferens malformation using two different techniques. Arch Androl 1986; 17: 67–78.

861. Narbaitz R, Tolnai G, Jolly E, et al. Ultrastructural studies on testicular biopsies from eighteen cases of hypospermatogenesis. Fertil Steril 1978; 30: 679–686.

862. Fossati P, Asfour M, Blacker C, et al. Serum and seminal gonadotropins in normal and infertile men: correlations with sperm count, prolactinemia, and seminal prolactin. Arch Androl 1979; 2: 247–252.

863. Johnson L, Petty CS, Neaves WB. The relationship of biopsy evaluations and testicular measurements to overall daily sperm production in human testes. Fertil Steril 1980; 34: 36–40.

864. De Kretser DM, Burger HG, Hudson B. The relationship between germinal cells and serum FSH levels in males with infertility. J Clin Endocrinol Metab 1974; 38: 787–793.

865. Jensen TK, Andersson AM, Hjollund NH, et al. Inhibin B as a serum marker of spermatogenesis: correlation to differences in sperm concentration and follicle-stimulating hormone levels. A study of 349 Danish men. J Clin Endocrinol Metab 1997; 82: 4059–4063.

866. Kumanov P, Nandipati K, Tomova A, Agarwal A. Inhibin B is a better marker of spermatogenesis than other hormones in the evaluation of male factor infertility. Fertil Steril 2006; 86: 332–338.

867. Makler A, Abramovici H. The correlation between sperm count and testicular biopsy using a new scoring system. Int J Fertil 1978; 23: 300–304.

868. Johnsen SG. Testicular biopsy score count – a method for registration of spermatogenesis in human testes: Normal values and results in 335 hypogonadal males. Hormones 1970; 1: 2–25.

869. Meyer JM, Roos M, Rumpler Y. Statistical study of a semiquantitative evaluation of testicular biopsies. Arch Androl 1988; 20: 71–71.

870. Steinberger E, Tjioe DY. A method for quantitative analysis of human seminiferous epithelium. Fertil Steril 1968; 19: 960–970.

871. Rowley MJ, Heller CG. Quantitation of the cells of the seminiferous

epithelium of human testis employing Sertoli cells as a constant. Zeitschr Zellforsch 1971; 115: 461–472.

872. Skakkebaek NE, Hammen R, Philip J, et al. Quantification of human seminiferous epithelium. III Histological studies in 44 infertile men with normal chromosome complements. Acta Pathol Microbiol Scand (A) 1973; 81: 97–111.

873. Skakkebaek NE, Hulten M, Philip J. Quantification of human seminiferous epithelium. 4. Histological studies in 17 men with numerical and structural autosomal aberrations. Acta Pathol Microbiol Scand (A) 1973; 81: 112–124.

874. Skakkebaek NE, Heller CG. Quantification of human seminiferous epithelium. I Histological studies in twenty-one fertile men with normal chromosome complements. J Reprod Fertil 1983; 32: 179–189.

875. Zuckerman Z, Rodriguez-Rigau LJ, Weiss DB, et al. Quantitative analysis of the seminiferous epithelium in human testicular biopsies, and the relation of spermatogenesis to sperm density. Fertil Steril 1978; 30: 448.455.

876. Johnson L, Zane RS, Petty CS, et al. Quantification of the human Sertoli cell population: its distribution, relation to germ cell numbers, and age related decline. Biol Reprod 1984; 31: 785–795.

877. Weiss DB, Rodriguez-Rigau L, Smith KD, et al. Quantitation of Leydig cells in testicular biopsies of oligospermic men with varicocele. Fertil Steril 1978; 30: 305–312.

878. Heller CG, Lalli MF, Pearson JE, et al. A method for the quantification of Leydig cells in man. J Reprod Fertil 1971; 25: 177–184.

879. Averback P, Wight DGD. Seminiferous tubule hypercurvature: a newly recognized common syndrome of human male infertility. Lancet 1979; 1: 181–183.

880. Averback P. Branching of seminiferous tubules associated with hypofertility and chronic respiratory infection. Arch Pathol Lab Med 1980; 104: 361–362.

881. Nistal M, Abaurrea MA, Paniagua R. Morphological and histometric study on the human Sertoli cells from birth to the onset of puberty. J Anat 1982; 134: 351–363.

882. Nistal M, Jiménez F, Paniagua R. Sertoli cell types in Sertoli-cell-only syndrome: relationships between Sertoli cell morphology and aetiology. Histopathology 1990; 16: 173–180.

883. Schulze C, Holstein AF, Schirden C, et al. On the morphology of the human Sertoli cells under normal conditions and in patients with impaired fertility. Andrologia 1976; 8: 167–178.

884. Chemes HE, Dym, M, Fawcet DW, et al. Pathophysiological observations of Sertoli cells in patients with germinal aplasia or severe germ cell depletion. Ultrastructural findings and hormone levels. Biol Reprod 1977; 17: 108–128.

885. Terada T, Hatakeyama S. Morphological evidence for two types of idiopathic 'Sertoli-cell-only' syndrome. Int J Androl 1991; 14: 117–126.

886. Goslar HG, Hilscher B, Haider SG, et al. Enzyme histochemical studies on the pathological changes in human Sertoli cells. J Histochem Cytochem 1982; 30: 1268–1274.

887. Fabbrini A, Re M, Spera G. Behaviour of glycogen and related enzymes in the Sertoli cell syndrome. Experientia 1969; 25: 647–651.

888. Nistal M. Testículo humano. Hipoplasia túbulo intersticial difusa (hipogonadismo hipogonadotrópico). Arch Esp Urol 1973; 3: 252–280.

889. Nistal M, Paniagua R. Leydig cell differentiation induced by stimulation with HCG and HMG in two patients affected with hypogonadotropic hypogonadism. Andrologia 1979; 11: 211–222.

890. De Kretser DM. The fine structure of the immature human testis in hypogonadotrophic hypogonadism. Virchows Arch [Cell Pathol] 1968; 1: 283–296.

891. Nistal M, Paniagua R, Abaurrea MA, et al. Hyperplasia and the immature appearance of Sertoli cells in primary testicular disorders. Hum Pathol 1982; 13: 3–12.

892. Steger K, Rey R, Kliesch S, et al. Immunohistochemical detection of immature Sertoli cell markers in testicular tissue of infertile adult men: a preliminary study. Int J Androl 1996; 19: 122–128.

893. Bar-Shira Maymon B, Paz G, Elliott DJ, et al. Maturation phenotype of Sertoli cells in testicular biopsies of azoospermic men. Hum Reprod 2000; 15: 1537–1542.

894. Cavicchia JC, Sacerdote FL, Ortiz L. The human blood–testis barrier in impaired spermatogenesis. Ultrastruct Pathol 1996; 20: 211–218.

895. Steger K, Rey R, Louis F, et al. Reversion of the differentiated phenotype and maturation block in Sertoli cells in pathological human testis.Hum Reprod 1999; 14: 136–143.

896. Paniagua R, Nistal M, Bravo MP. Leydig cell types in primary testicular disorders. Hum Pathol 1984; 15: 181–190.

897. Mack WS, Scott LS, Ferguson-Smith MA, et al. Ectopic testis and the undescended testis: a histological comparison. J Pathol Bacteriol 1961; 82: 439–443.

898. Taniuchi I, Mizutani S, Namiki M, et al. Short arm dicentric Y chromosome in a sterile man: a case report. J Urol 1991; 146: 415–416.

899. Aumuller G, Schulze C, Viebahn C. Intermediate filaments in Sertoli cells. Microsc Res Tech 1992; 20: 50–72.

900. Christiansen P. Urinary gonadotropins in the Sertoli-cell-only syndrome. Acta Endocrinol 1975; 78: 180–191.

901. Hammar M, Berg AA. Impaired Leydig cell function in vitro in testicular tissue from human males with 'Sertoli cell only' syndrome. Andrologia 1985; 17: 37–41.

902. Okuyama A, Nonomura N, Koh E, et al. Testicular FSH and HCG receptors in Sertoli-cell-only syndrome. Arch Androl 1989; 23: 119–124.

903. Del Castillo EB, Trabucco A, De la Balze FA. Syndrome produced by absence of the germinal epithelium without impairment of the Sertoli or Leydig cells. J Clin Endocrinol Metab 1947; 7: 493–497.

904. Blagosklonova O, Fellmann F, Clavequin MC, et al. AZFa deletions in Sertoli cell-only syndrome: a retrospective study. Mol Hum Reprod 2000; 6: 795–799.

905. Rothman MC, Sims SA, Stotts CI. Sertoli cell only syndrome in 1982. Fertil Steril 1982; 38: 388–390.

906. Buchanan JD, Fairley KF, Barrie JU. Return of spermatogenesis after stopping cyclophosphamide therapy. Lancet 1975; 2: 156–157.

907. Decensi AU, Guarneri D, Marroni P, et al. Evidence for testicular impairment after long-term treatment with a luteinizing hormone-releasing hormone agonist in elderly men. J Urol 1989; 142: 1235–1238.

908. Sapino A, Pagani A, Godano A, et al. Effects of estrogens on the testis of transsexuals: a pathological and immunocytochemical study. Virchows Arch A 1987; 411: 409–414.

909. Schulze C. Response of the human testis to long-term estrogen treatment: Morphology of Sertoli cells, Leydig cells and spermatogonial stem cells. Cell Tissue Res 1988; 251: 31–43.

910. Daehlin L, Tomic R, Damber JE. Depressed testosterone release from testicular tissue in vitro after withdrawal of oestrogen treatment in patients with prostatic carcinoma. Scand J Urol Nephrol 1988; 22: 11–13.

911. Söderstrom KD. Tubular hyalinization in human testes. Andrologia 1986; 18: 97–103.

912. Martín R, Santamaría L, Nistal M, et al. The peritubular myofibroblasts in the testes from normal men and men with Klinefelter's syndrome. A quantitative, ultrastructural, and immunohistochemical study. J Pathol 1992; 168: 59–66.

913. Santamaría L, Martínez-Onsurbe P, Paniagua R, et al. Laminin, type IV collagen, and fibronectin in normal

and cryptorchid human testes. An immunohistochemical study. Int J Androl 1990; 13: 470–487.

914. Wantz GI. Testicular atrophy as a sequela of inguinal herniorrhaphy. Int Surg 1986; 71: 159–163.

915. Regadera J, Nistal M, Paniagua R. Testis epididymis, and spermatic cord in elderly men. Correlation of angiographic and histologic studies with systemic arteriosclerosis. Arch Pathol Lab Med 1985; 109: 663–667.

916. Nistal M, Martínez C, Paniagua R. Primary testicular lesions in the twisted testis. Fertil Steril 1992; 57: 381–386.

917. Morgan AD. Inflammation and infestation of the testis and paratesticular structures. In: Puch RCB ed. Pathology of the testis. Oxford: Blackwell, 1976; 79–138.

918. Mirsch IH, Choi H. Quantitative testicular biopsy in congenital and acquired genital obstruction. J Urol 1990; 143: 311–312.

919. Santamaría L, Martín R, Nistal M, et al. The peritubular myoid cells in the testes from men with varicocele. An ultrastructural, immunohistochemical and quantitative study. Histopathology 1992; 21: 423–433.

920. Cohn EL, Watson L, Older R, Moran R. Striated pattern of the testicle on ultrasound: an appearance of testicular fibrosis. J Urol 1996; 156: 180–181.

921. Casalino DD, Kim R. Clinical importance of a unilateral striated pattern seen on sonography of the testicle. AJR Am J Roentgenol 2002; 178: 927–930.

922. Potashnic G, Ben-Aderet N, Israeli R, et al. Suppressive effects of 1,2-dibromo-3-3-chloropropane on human spermatogenesis. Fertil Steril 1978; 30: 444–447.

923. Barton M, Wiesner BP. Significance of testicular exfoliation in male infecundity. Br Med J 1952; 1: 958–962.

924. Belsey MAR, Eliasson AJ, Gallegos KS, et al. Laboratory manual for the examination of human semen and semen–cervical mucus interaction. In: Paulsen CA, Prasac MNR, eds. VHO special program in human reproduction. Singapore: Press Concern, 1980; 74–94.

925. Sigg C, Hornstein OP. Zytologische Klassifikation in reifer Keimzellen im Luftgetrockneten Ejakulatanstrich beim spermatologische Syndrom der vermehrten Desquamation von Zellen der Spermatogenese (VDZS). Andrologia 1987; 19: 378–391.

926. Breucker H, Hofmann N, Holstein AF. Transformed spermatocytes constituting the ejaculate of an infertile man. Andrologia 1988; 20: 526–535.

927. Riedel HH, Schirren C. Studies on the differentiation of round cells in the human ejaculate. Zeitschr Hautkr 1978; 53: 255–267.

928. Holstein C. Morphologie freier unreifer Keimzellen im menschlichen Hoden, Nebenhoden und Ejaculat. Andrologia 1983; 15: 7–25.

929. Nistal M, Gonzalez-Peramato P, Paniagua R. Diagnostic value of differential quantification of spermatids in obstructive azoospermia. J Androl 2003; 24: 721–726.

930. MacLeod J. Seminal cytology in the presence of varicocele. Fertil Steril 1965; 16: 735–757.

931. Takihara M, Sakatoku J, Cockett ATK. The pathophysiology of varicocele in male infertility. Fertil Steril 1991; 55: 861–868.

932. Nistal M, Paniagua R, Regadera J, et al. Obstruction of the tubuli recti and ductuli efferentes by dilated veins in the testes of men with varicocele and its possible role in causing atrophy of the seminiferous tubules. Int J Androl 1984; 7: 309–323.

933. Yamamoto M, Hashimoto J, Takaba H, et al. Scanning electron microscopic study on the shape of infertile seminiferous tubules: A hypothesis of pathogenesis of idiopathic male infertility. Int J Fertil 1988; 33: 265–272.

934. Gall EA. The histopathology of acute mumps orchitis. Am J Pathol 1947; 23: 637–651.

935. Sciurano RB, Rahn MI, Pigozzi MI, et al. An azoospermic man with a double-strand DNA break-processing deficiency in the spermatocyte nuclei: case report. Hum Reprod 2006; 21: 1194–1203.

936. Kostova E, Yeung CH, Luetjens cm, et al. Association of three isoforms of the meiotic BOULE gene with spermatogenic failure in infertile men. Mol Hum Reprod 2007; 13: 85–93.

937. Gulizia S, Vicari E, Aleffi A, et al. Abnormal germ cell exfoliation in semen of hypogonadotrophic patients during a hCG treatment. Andrologia 1981; 13: 74–77.

938. Scaglia HE, Timossi cm, Carrere CA, et al. Altered luteinizing hormone pulsatility in infertile patients with idiopathic oligoasthenozoospermia. Hum Reprod 1998; 13: 2782–2786.

939. Dony JM, Smals AG, Rolland R, et al. Differential effect of luteinizing hormone-releasing hormone infusion on testicular steroids in normal men and patients with idiopathic oligospermia. Fertil Steril 1984; 42: 274–280.

940. Harsch IA, Simoni M, Nieschlag E. Molecular heterogeneity of serum follicle-stimulating hormone in hypogonadal patients before and during androgen replacement therapy and in normal men. Clin Endocrinol 1993; 39: 173–180.

941. Tapanainen JS, Aittomaki K, Min J, et al. Men homozygous for an inactivating mutation of the follicle-stimulating-hormone (FSH) receptor gene present variable suppression of spermatogenesis and fertility. Nature Genet 1997; 15: 205–206.

942. Sigg S. Klassifizierung tubulärer Hodenatrophien bei Sterilitätabklärungen. Schweiz Med Wschr 1979; 35: 1284–1293.

943. Martinova Y, Kantcheva L, Tzvetkov D. Testicular ultrastructure in infertile men. Arch Androl 1989; 22: 103–122.

944. Bustos-Obregón E, Esponda P. Ultrastructure of the nucleus of human Sertoli cells in normal and pathological testes. Cell Tissue Res 1974; 152: 467–475.

945. De Kretser DM, Kerr JB, Paulsen CA. Evaluation of the ultrastructural changes in the human Sertoli cell in testicular disorders and the relationship of the changes to the levels of serum FSH. Int J Androl 1981; 4: 129–144.

946. Namiki M, Koide T, Okuyama A, et al. Abnormality of testicular FSH receptors in infertile men. Acta Endocrinol 1984; 106: 548–555.

947. Kumanov P, Nandipati KC, Tomova A, et al. Significance of inhibin in reproductive pathophysiology and current clinical applications. Reprod Biomed Online 2005; 10: 786–812.

948. Gerris J, Comhaire F, Hellemans P. Placebo-controlled trial of high-dose mesterolone treatment of idiopathic male infertility. Fertil Steril 1991; 55: 603–607.

949. Andersson AM, Jorgensen N, Frydelund-Larsen L, et al. Impaired Leydig cell function in infertile men: a study of 357 idiopathic infertile men and 318 proven fertile controls. J Clin Endocrinol Metab 2004; 89: 3161–3167.

950. Stecker JF, Lloyd JW. Leydig and Sertoli cell function in normal and oligospermic males: a preliminary report. Fertil Steril 1978; 29: 204–208.

951. Giagulli VA, Vermeulen A. Leydig cell function in infertile men with idiopathic oligospermic infertility. J Clin Endocrinol Metab 1988; 66: 62–67.

952. Aiman J, Griffin JE, Gazak JM, et al. Androgen insensitivity as a cause of infertility in otherwise normal men. N Engl J Med 1979; 300: 223–227.

953. Aiman J, Griffin JE. The frequency of androgen receptor deficiency in infertile men. J Clin Endocrinol Metab 1982; 54: 725–732.

954. O'Dowd J, Gaffney EF, Young RH. Malignant sex cord stromal tumor in a patient with the androgen insensitivity syndrome. Histopathology 1990; 16: 279–282.

955. Knoke Y, Jakubiczka S, Lehnert H, et al. A new point mutation of the androgen receptor gene in a patient with partial androgen resistance and severe oligozoospermia. Andrologia 1999; 31: 199–201.

956. Akin JW. The use of clomiphene citrate in the treatment of azoospermia secondary to incomplete androgen resistance. Fertil Steril 1993; 59: 223–224.

957. Akin JW, Behzadian A, Tho, SPT, et al. Evidence for a partial deletion in the androgen receptor gene in a phenotypic male with azoospermia. Am J Obstet Gynecol 1991; 165: 1891–1894.

958. Hiort O, Holterhus PM. Androgen insensitivity and male infertility. Int J Androl 2003; 26: 16–20.

959. Schulster A, Ross L, Scommegna A. Frequency of androgen insensitivity infertile phenotypically normal men. J Urol 1983; 130: 699–701.

960. Gooren L. Improvement of spermatogenesis after treatment with the antiestrogen tamoxifen in a man with the incomplete androgen insensitivity syndrome. J Clin Endocrinol Metab 1989; 68: 1207–1210.

961. Sokol RZ, Steiner BS, Bustillo M, et al. A controlled comparison of the efficacy of clomiphene citrate in male infertility. Fertil Steril 1988; 49: 865–870.

962. Yong EL, Ng SC, Roy AC, et al. Pregnancy after hormonal correction of severe spermatogenic defect due to a mutation in androgen receptor gene. Lancet 1994; 344: 826–827.

963. Schrag SD, Dixon RL. Occupational exposures associated with male reproductive dysfunction. Ann Rev Pharmacol Toxicol 1985; 25: 567–592.

964. Cameron DT, Snydle FE. Ultrastructural surface characteristics of seminiferous tubules from men with varicocele. Andrologia 1982; 14: 425–433.

965. Takihara H, Cosentino MJ, Sakaratoku J, et al. Significance of testicular size measurement in andrology. II. Correlation of testicular size with testicular function. J Urol 1987; 137: 416–419.

966. Chehval MJ, Purcell MH. Deterioration of semen parameters over time in men with untreated varicocele: evidence of progressive testicular damage. Fertil Steril 1992; 57: 174–177.

967. Agger P, Johnsen S. Quantitative evaluation of testicular biopsies in varicocele. Fertil Steril 1978; 29: 52–57.

968. Dubin L, Hotchkiss RS. Testis biopsy in subfertile men with varicocele. Fertil Steril 1969; 20: 50–57.

969. Etriby A, Girgis SM, Hefnawy H, et al. Testicular changes in subfertile males with varicocele. Fertil Steril 1967; 18: 666–671.

970. Nistal M, De Mora JC, Paniagua R. Classification of several types of maturational arrest of spermatogonia according to Sertoli cell morphology: an approach to aetiology. Int J Androl 1998; 21: 317–326.

971. Denis L. Prostate cancer. Primary hormonal treatment. Cancer 1993; 71: 1050–1058.

972. Hatakeyama S, Takizawa T, Kawara Y. Focal atrophy of the seminiferous tubule in the human testis. Acta Pathol Jpn 1979; 29: 901–905.

973. Sigg C, Hedinger C. Quantitative and ultrastructural study on germinal epithelium in testicular biopsies with 'mixed atrophy.' Andrologia 1981; 13: 412–424.

974. Sharpe RM, McKinnell C, Kivlin C, Fisher JS. Proliferation and functional maturation of Sertoli cells, and their relevance to disorders of testis function in adulthood. Reproduction 2003; 125: 769–784.

975. Buchanan JD, Fairley KF, Barrie JU. Return of spermatogenesis after stopping cyclophosphamide therapy. Lancet 1975; 2: 156–157.

976. Sigg C, Hedinger C. The frequency and morphology of 'giant spermatogonia' in the human testis. Virchows Arch B [Cell Pathol] 1983; 44: 115–134.

977. Paniagua R, Nistal M, Amat P, et al. Seminiferous tubule involution in elderly men. Biol Reprod 1987; 36: 939–947.

978. Bergmann M, Nashan D, Nieschlag E. Pattern of compartmentation in human seminiferous tubules showing dislocation of spermatogonia. Cell Tissue Res 1989; 256: 183–190.

979. Holstein AF, Bustos-Obregon E, Hartmann M. Dislocated type-A spermatogonia in human seminiferous tubules. Cell Tissue Res 1984; 236: 35–40.

980. Miething A. Intercellular bridges between megalospermatocytes in the human testis. Andrologia 1991; 23: 91–97.

981. Johannisson R, Schulze W, Holstein AF. Megalospermatocytes in the human testis exhibit asynapsis of chromosomes. Andrologia 2003; 35: 146–151.

982. Holstein AF, Eckmann C. Megalospermatocytes: indicators of disturbed meiosis in man. Andrologia 1986; 18: 601–609.

983. Nistal M. Codesal J, Paniagua R. Multinucleate spermatids in aging human testes. Arch Androl 1986; 16: 125–129.

984. Vegni-Talluri M, Bigliardi E, Soldani P. Unusual incidence of binucleate spermatids in human cryptorchidism. J Submicrosc Cytol 1978; 10: 357–361.

985. Nistal M, Paniagua R. Testicular and epididymal pathology. New York: Thieme-Stratton, 1984; 227–240.

986. Aumüller G, Fuhrmann W, Krause W. Spermatogenetic arrest with inhibition of acrosome and sperm tail development. Andrologia 1987; 19: 9–17.

987. Baccetti B, Capitani S, Collodel G, et al. Recent advances in human sperm pathology. Contraception 2002; 65: 283–287.

988. David G, Bisson JP, Czyglik F, et al. Anomalies morphologiques du spermatozoide humain. Propositions pour un système de classification. J Gynecol Obstetr Biol Reprod 1975; 4: 17–36.

989. Holstein AF. Morphologische Studien an abnormen Spermatiden und Spermatozoen des Menschen. Virchows Arch [Pathol Anat Histol] 1975; 367: 92–112.

990. Holstein AF, Schirren C. Classification of abnormalities in human spermatids based on recent advances in ultrastructural research on spermatid differentiation. In: Fawcett DW, Bedford JM, eds. The spermatozoon. Maturation, mobility, surface properties and comparative aspects. Baltimore: Urban and Schwarzenberg, 1979; 341–353.

991. Portuondo JA, Calabozo M, Echanojauregui AD. Morphology of spermatozoa in fertile man with and without varicocele. J Androl 1983; 4: 312–315.

992. Kullander S, Rausing A. On round headed human spermatozoa. Int J Fertil 1975; 2: 33–40.

993. Nistal M, Paniagua R. Morphogenesis of round headed human spermatozoa lacking acrosomes in a case of severe teratozoospermia. Andrologia 1978; 10: 49–51.

994. Meschede D, Rolf C, Neugebauer D-C, et al. Sperm acrosome defects in a patient with Aarskog–Scott syndrome, Am J Med Genet 1996; 66: 340–342.

995. Escalier D. Failure of differentiation of the nuclear-perinuclear skeletal complex in the round-headed human spermatozoa. Int J Dev Biol 1990; 34: 287–297.

996. Reichart M, Lederman H, Har-Even D, et al. Human sperm acrosin activity with relation to semen parameters and acrosomal ultrastructure. Andrologia 1993; 25: 59–66.

997. Morel F, Douet-Guilbert N, Moerman A, et al. Chromosome aneuploidy in the spermatozoa of two men with globozoospermia. Mol Hum Reprod 2004; 10: 835–838.

998. Martin RH, Greene C, Rademaker AW. Sperm chromosome aneuploidy analysis in a man with globozoospermia. Fertil Steril 2003; 79: 1662–1664.

999. Moretti E, Collodel G, Scapigliati G, et al. 'Round head' sperm defect. Ultrastructural and meiotic segregation study. J Submicrosc Cytol Pathol 2005; 37: 297–303.

1000. Yao R, Ito C, Natsume Y, et al. Lack of acrosome formation in mice lacking a Golgi protein, GOPC. Proc Natl Acad Sci USA 2002; 99: 11211–11216.

1001. German J, Rasch EM, Huang CY, et al. Human infertility due to production of multiple-tailed spermatozoa with excessive amounts of DNA. Am J Hum Genet 1981; 33: 64–74.

1002. Nistal M, Paniagua R, Herruzo A. Multi-tailed spermatozoa in a case with asthenospermia and teratospermia.Virchows Arch B [Cell Pathol] 1977; 26: 111–118.

1003. Escalier D. Human spermatozoa with large heads and multiple flagella: a quantitative ultrastructural study of 6 cases. Biol Cell 1983; 48: 65–74.

1004. Guthauser B, Vialard F, Dakouane M, et al. Chromosomal analysis of spermatozoa with normal-sized heads in two infertile patients with macrocephalic sperm head syndrome. Fertil Steril 2006; 85: 750. e5.

1005. Baccetti B, Burrini AG, Collodel G, et al. Crater defect in human spermatozoa. Gamete Res 1989; 22: 249–255.

1006. Matano Y. Ultrastructural study of human binucleate spermatids. J Ultrastruct Res 1971; 34: 123–134.

1007. Dadoune JP. Ultrastructural abnormalities of human spermatozoa. Hum Reprod 1988; 3: 311–318.

1008. Cooper TG. Cytoplasmic droplets: the good, the bad or just confusing? Hum Reprod 2005; 20: 9–11.

1009. Nistal M, Paniagua R, Herruzo A. Absence de la paire centrale du complexe axonemique dans une tératospermie avec flagelles courts et épais. J Gynecol Obstet Biol Reprod 1979; 8: 47–50.

1010. Alexandre C, Bisson JP, David G. Asthenozoospermie totale avec anomalie ultrastructurale du flagelle dans deux frères stériles. J Gynecol Obstet Biol Reprod 1978; 7: 31–38.

1011. Chemes HE, Brugo Olmedo S, et al. Dysplasia of the fibrous sheath. An ultrastructural defect of human spermatozoa associated with sperm immotility and primary sterility. Fertil Steril 1987; 48: 664–669.

1012. Barthelemy C, Tharanne MJ, Lebos C, et al. Tail stump spermatozoa: morphogenesis of the defect. An ultrastructural study of sperm and testicular biopsy. Andrologia 1990; 22: 417–425.

1013. Baccetti B, Collodel G, Estenoz M, et al. Gene deletions in an infertile man with sperm fibrous sheath dysplasia. Hum Reprod 2005; 20: 2790–2794.

1014. Nistal M, Paniagua R, Herruzo A. Multi-tailed spermatozoa in a case with asthenospermia and teratospermia.Virchows Arch B [Cell Pathol] 1977; 26: 111–118.

1015. Latini M, Gandini L, Lenzi A, Romanelli F. Sperm tail agenesis in a case of consanguinity. Fertil Steril 2004; 81: 1688–1691.

1016. Perotti ME, Giarola A, Gioria M. Ultrastructural study of the decapitates sperm defect in a infertile man. J Reprod Fertil 1981; 63: 543–549.

1017. Baccetti B, Burrini AG, Collodel G, et al. Morphogenesis of the decapitated and decaudated sperm defect in two brothers. Gamete Res 1989; 23: 181–188.

1018. Chemes HE, Puigdomenech ET, Carizza C, et al. Acephalic spermatozoa and abnormal development of the head–neck attachment: a human syndrome of genetic origin. Hum Reprod 1999; 14: 1811–1818.

1019. Zamboni L. Sperm structure and its relevance to infertility. Arch Pathol Lab Med 1992; 116: 325–344.

1020. Toyama Y, Iwamoto T, Yajima M, et al. Decapitated and decaudated spermatozoa in man, and pathogenesis based on the ultrastructure. Int J Androl 2000; 23: 109–115.

1021. Okada H, Fujioka H, Tatsumi N, et al. Assisted reproduction for infertile patients with 9 + 0 immotile spermatozoa associated with autosomal dominant polycystic kidney disease. Hum Reprod 1999; 14: 110–113.

1022. Baccetti B, Burrini AG, Pallini V. Spermatozoa and cilia lacking axoneme in an infertile man. Andrologia 1980; 12: 525–532.

1023. Afzelius BA, Eliasson R, Hoh O, Lindholmer C. Lack of dynein arms in immotile human spermatozoa. J Cell Biol 1975; 66: 225–232.

1024. Holzmann D, Ott PM, Felix H. Diagnostic approach to primary ciliary dyskinesia: a review. Eur J Pediatr 2000; 159: 95–98.

1025. Carlen B, Stenram U. Primary ciliary dyskinesia: a review. Ultrastruct Pathol 2005; 29: 217–220.

1026. Douard R, Feldman A, Bargy F, et al. Anomalies of lateralization in man: a case of total situs inversus. Surg Radiol Anat 2000; 22: 293–297.

1027. Schieferstein G, Wolburg H, Adam W. Stiff-tail-oder Mittelstück-Syndrom. Andrologia 1987; 1: 5–8.

1028. Haidl G, Becker A, Henkel R. Pour development of outer dense fibres as a mayor cause of tail abnormalities in the spermatozoa of asthenoteratozoospermic men. Hum Reprod 1991; 6: 1431–1438.

1029. Ruiz-Pesini E, Lapeña A-C, Díez-Sanchez C, et al. Human mtDNA haplogroups associated with high or reduced spermatozoa motility. Am J Hum Genet 2000; 67: 682–696.

1030. Carra E, Sangiorgi D, Gattuccio F, Rinaldi AM. Male infertility and mitochondrial DNA. Biochem Biophys Res Commun 2004; 322: 333–339.

1031. Pryor JP, Cameron KM, Chilton CP, et al. Carcinoma in situ in testicular biopsies from men presenting with infertility. Br J Urol 1983; 55: 780–784.

1032. Nistal M, Codesal J, Paniagua R. Carcinoma in situ of the testis in infertile men. A histological,

immunocytochemical and cytophotometric study of DNA content. J Pathol 1989; 159: 205–210.

1033. Schütte B. Early testicular cancer in severe oligozoospermia. In: Holstein AF, Leindenberger F, Hölzer KH, Bettendorf G, eds. Carl Schirren Symposium. Advances in andrology. Berlin: Diesbach Verlag, 1988; 188–190.

1034. Skakkebaek NE, Berthelsen JG, Giwercman A, et al. Carcinoma-in-situ of the testis: possible origin from gonocytes and precursor of all types of germ cell tumours except spermatocytoma. Int J Androl 1987; 10: 19–28.

1035. Schutte B. Male subfertility. Continuing diagnostic and therapeutic measures. Ther Umsch 1980; 37: 487–493.

1036. Giwercman A, Grindsted J, Hansen B, et al. Testicular cancer risk in boys with maldescended testis: A cohort study. J Urol 1987; 138: 1214–1216.

1037. Novero V Jr, Goossens A, Tournaye H, et al. Seminoma discovered in two males undergoing successful testicular sperm extraction for intracytoplasmic sperm injection. Fertil Steril 1996; 65: 1051–1054.

1038. Berthelsen JC, Skakkebaek NE, Von Der Maase H, et al. Screening for carcinoma in situ of the contralateral testis in patients with germinal testicular cancer. Br Med J 1982; 285: 1683–1686.

1039. Hadziselimovic F, Herzog B, Emmons LR. The incidence of seminoma and expression of cell adhesion CD44 in cryptorchid boys and infertile men. J Urol 1997; 157: 1895–1897.

1040. Singh R, Shastry PK, Rasalkar AA, et al. A novel androgen receptor mutation resulting in complete androgen insensitivity syndrome and bilateral Leydig cell hyperplasia. J Androl 2006; 27: 510–516.

1041. Olumi AF, Garnick MB, Renshaw AA, et al. Leydig cell hyperplasia mimicking testicular neoplasm. Urology 1996; 48: 647–649.

1042. Hashimoto J, Nagay T, Takaba H, et al. Increased mast cells in the limiting membrane of seminiferous tubules in the testes of patients with idiopathic infertility. Urol Int 1988; 43: 129–132.

1043. Nagai T, Takaba H, Miyake K, et al. Testicular mast cell heterogeneity in idiopathic male infertility. Fertil Steril 1992; 57: 1331–1336.

1044. Kollur SM, Pattankar VL, El Hag IA. Mast cells in testicular lesions. Ups J Med Sci 2004; 109: 239–245.

1045. Oliva A, Multigner L. Ketotifen improves sperm motility and sperm morphology in male patients with leukocytospermia and unexplained infertility. Fertil Steril 2006; 85: 240–243.

1046. Makler A, Geresh I. An attempt to explain occurrence of patent reproductive tract in azoospermic males with tubular spermatogenesis. Int J Fertil 1979; 24: 246–250.

1047. Silber SJ, Rodriguez-Rigau LJ. Quantitative analysis of testicular biopsy: determination of partial obstruction and prediction of sperm count after surgery for obstruction. Fertil Steril 1981; 36: 480–485.

1048. Nistal M, Codesal J, Santamaría L, Paniagua R. Correlation between spermatozoon numbers in spermiogram and seminiferous epithelium histology in testicular biopsies from subfertile men. Fertil Steril 1987; 48: 507–509.

1049. Sandoval L, Diaz M, Rivas F. Alpha-1,4-glucosidase activity and the presence of germinal epithelium cells in the semen for differential diagnosis of obstructive and nonobstructive azoospermia. Arch Androl 1995; 35: 155–158.

1050. Pryor JP, Hendry WF. Ejaculatory duct obstruction in subfertile males: analysis of 87 patients. Fertil Steril 1991; 56: 725–730.

1051. Nistal M, Gonzalez-Peramato P, Serrano A, et al. Paratesticular cysts with benign epithelial proliferations of wolffian origin. Am J Clin Pathol 2005; 124: 245–251.

1052. Sano T, Horiguchi H. Von Hippel–Lindau disease. Microsc Res Tech 2003; 60: 159–164.

1053. Belet U, Danaci M, Sarikaya S, et al. Prevalence of epididymal, seminal vesicle, prostate, and testicular cysts in autosomal dominant polycystic kidney disease. Urology 2002; 60: 138–141.

1054. Vohra S, Morgentaler A. Congenital anomalies of the vas deferens, epididymis, and seminal vesicles. Urology 1997; 49: 313–321.

1055. Dubin L, Amelar RD. Etiologic factors in 1294 consecutive cases of male infertility. Fertil Steril 1971; 22: 469–474.

1056. Auroux M, De Mouy DM, Acar JF. Male fertility and positive chlamydial serology. A study of 61 fertile and 82 subfertile men. J Androl 1987; 8: 197–200.

1057. Hillier SL, Rabe LK, Muller CH, et al. Relationship of bacteriologic characteristics to semen indices in men attending an infertility clinic. Obstet Gynecol 1990; 75: 800–804.

1058. Wagenlehner FM, Naber KG. Treatment of bacterial urinary tract infections: presence and future. Eur Urol 2006; 49: 235–244.

1059. Delavierre D. Orchi-epididymitis: Ann Urol 2003; 37: 322–338.

1060. Sandhu DPS, Osborn DE, Munson KW. Relationship of azoospermia to inguinal surgery. Int J Androl 1992; 15: 504–506.

1061. Ross LS, Flom LS. Azoospermia. A complication of hydrocele repair in a fertile population. J Urol 1991; 146: 852–853.

1062. Schned AR, Memoll VA. Coarse granular cytoplasmic change of the epididymis. An immunohistochemical and ultrastructural study. J Urol Pathol 1994; 2: 213–222.

1063. Rajalakshmi M, Kumar BV, Ramakrishnan PR, Kapur MM. Histology of the epididymis in men with obstructive infertility. Andrologia 1990; 22: 319–326.

1064. Hirsch IH, McCue P, Allen J, et al. Quantitative testicular biopsy in spinal cord injured men: comparison to fertile controls. J Urol 1991; 146: 337–341.

1065. Pardanini DS, Patil NG, Pawar HN. Some gross observations of the epididymides following vasectomy: a clinical study. Fertil Steril 1976; 27: 267–270.

1066. McMahon AJ, Buckley J, Taylor A, et al. Chronic testicular pain following vasectomy. Br J Urol 1992; 69: 188–191.

1067. Jarow JP, Budin RE, Dym M, et al. Quantitative pathologic changes in the human testis after vasectomy. A controlled study. N Engl J Med 1985; 313: 1252–1256.

1068. Jenkins IL, Muir VY, Blacklock NJ, et al. Consequences of vasectomy: an immunological and histological study related to subsequent fertility. Br J Urol 1979; 51: 406–410.

1069. Marmar JL. The status of vasectomy reversals. Int J Fertil 1991; 36: 352–357.

1070. Urry RL, Heaton JB, Moore M, et al. A fifteen-year study of alterations in semen quality occurring after vasectomy reversal. Fertil Steril 1990; 53: 341–345.

1071. Young D. Surgical treatment of male infertility. J Reprod Fertil 1970; 23: 541–542.

1072. Handelsman DJ, Conway AJ, Boylan LM, Turtle JR. Young's syndrome: obstructive azoospermia and chronic sinopulmonary infections. N Engl J Med 1984; 310: 3–4.

1073. Neville E, Brewis RAL, Yeates WK, et al. Respiratory tract disease and obstructive azoospermia. Thorax 1983; 38: 929–930.

1074. Hendry WF, Knight RK, Whitfield HN. Obstructive azoospermia: respiratory function tests, electron microscopy and the results of surgery. Br J Urol 1978; 50: 598–604.

1075. Nistal M, Paniagua R, Abaurrea MA. Varicose axon bearing 'synaptic' vesicles on the basal lamina of the human seminiferous tubules. Cell Tissue Res 1982; 226: 75–82.

1076. Filippi S, Morelli A, Vignozzi L, et al. Oxytocin mediates the estrogen-dependent contractile activity of endothelin-1 in human and rabbit epididymis. Endocrinology 2005; 146: 3506–3517.

1077. Yamamoto M, Hibi H, Miyake, K. Comparison of the effectiveness of placebo and alpha-blocker therapy

for the treatment of idiopathic oligozoospermia. Fertil Steril 1995; 63: 396–400.

1078. Aran B, Blanco J, Vidal F, et al. Screening for abnormalities of chromosomes X, Y, and 18 and for diploidy in spermatozoa from infertile men participating in an vitro fertilization-intracytoplasmic sperm injection program. Fertil Steril 1999; 72: 696–701.

1079. Bertini V, Simi P, Valetto A. Cytogenetic study of 435 subfertile men: incidence and clinical features. J Reprod Med 2006; 51: 15–20.

1080. Klinefelter HF, Reifenstein EC, Albright F. Syndrome characterized by gynecomastia, aspermatogenesis without aleydigism and increased excretion of follicle-stimulating hormone. J Clin Endocrinol 1942; 2: 615–627.

1081. Glander HJ. Infertility in the Klinefelter syndrome. MMW Fortschr Med 2005; 147: 39–41.

1082. Ohno S. Control of meiotic process. In: Troen P, Nankin HR, eds. The testis in normal and infertile men. New York: Raven Press, 1977; 1–8.

1083. Smyth CM, Bremner WJ. Klinefelter syndrome. Arch Intern Med 1998; 158: 1309–1314.

1084. Hsueh WA, Hsu TH, Federman DD. Endocrine features of Klinefelter's syndrome. Medicine 1978; 57: 447–461.

1085. Kamischke A, Baumgardt A, Horst J, Nieschlag E. Clinical and diagnostic features of patients with suspected Klinefelter syndrome. J Androl 2003; 24: 41–48.

1086. Becker KL. Clinical and therapeutic experiences with Klinefelter's syndrome. Fertil Steril 1972; 23: 568–578.

1087. Patwardhan AJ, Eliez S, Bender B, et al. Brain morphology in Klinefelter syndrome: extra X chromosome and testosterone supplementation. Neurology 2000; 54: 2218–2223.

1088. Mor C, Ben-Bassat M, Leiba S. Leydig and Sertoli cells. Their fine structure in three cases of Klinefelter's syndrome. Arch Pathol Lab Med 1982; 106: 228–230.

1089. Frohland A, Skakkebaek NE. Dimorphism in sex chromatin pattern of Sertoli cells in adults with Klinefelter's syndrome: correlation with two types of 'Sertoli-cell-only' tubes. J Clin Endocrinol Metab 1971; 33: 683–687.

1090. Ahmad KW, Dykes JRW, Ferguson-Smith MA, et al. Leydig cell counts in chromatin-positive Klinefelter's syndrome. J Clin Endocrinol Metab 1971; 33: 517–520.

1091. Nistal M, Santamaría L, Paniagua R. Quantitative and ultrastructural study of Leydig cells in Klinefelter's syndrome. J Pathol 1985; 146: 323–331.

1092. Rubin P, Mattei A, Cesarini JP, et al. Etude en microscopie électronique de la cellule de Leydig dans la maladie de Klinefelter en périodes pre, per et postpubertaires. Ann Endocrinol 1971; 32: 671–681.

1093. Gabrilove JC, Freiberg EK, Nicolis GC. Testicular function in Klinefelter's syndrome. J Urol 1980; 124: 825–828.

1094. Wellen JJ, Smals AGH, Rijken JCW, et al. Testosterone and δ4 androstenedione in the saliva of patients with Klinefelter's syndrome. Clin Endocrinol 1983; 18: 51–59.

1095. Gómez-Acebo J, Parrilla R, Abrisqueta JA, et al. Fine structure of spermatogenesis in Klinefelter's syndrome. J Clin Endocrinol Metab 1968; 28: 1287–1292.

1096. Steinberger E, Smith KD, Perloff WH. Spermatogenesis in Klinefelter's syndrome. J Clin Endocrinol Metab 1965; 25: 1325–1330.

1097. Staessen C, Tournaye H, Van Assche E, et al. PDG in 47,XXY Klinefelter's syndrome patients. Hum Reprod Update 2003; 9: 319–330.

1098. Hennebicq S, Pelletier R, Bergues U, Rousseaux S. Risk of trisomy 21 in offspring of patients with Klinefelter's syndrome. Lancet 2001; 357: 2104–2105.

1099. Mudal S, Ockey CH. The 'double male.' A new chromosome constitution in Klinefelter's syndrome. Lancet 1960; 2: 492–493.

1100. Ellis JR, Miller OJ, Penrose LS, et al. A male with XXYY chromosomes. Ann Hum Genet 1961; 25: 145–152.

1101. Borgaonkar DS, Muler E, Char F. Do the 48 XXYY males have a characteristic phenotype? Clin Genet 1970; 1: 272–277.

1102. Bloomgarden ZT, Delozier CD, Cohen MP, et al. Genetics and endocrine findings in a 48 XXYY male. J Clin Endocrinol Metab 1980; 50: 740–743.

1103. Uchida IA, Miller JR, Soltan HC. Dermatoglyphics associated with the XXYY chromosome complement. Ann J Hum Genet 1964; 16: 284–289.

1104. Nistal M, Paniagua R, López-Pajares I. Ultrastructure of Leydig cells in Klinefelter's syndrome with 48 XXYY karyotype. Virchows Arch B [Cell Pathol] 1978; 28: 39–46.

1105. Ferguson-Smith MA, Johnston AW, Handmaker S. Primary amentia and microorchidism associated with an XXXY sex-chromosome constitution. Lancet 1960; 2: 184–187.

1106. Kim HJ, Kim D, Shin JM, et al. 49,XXXXY syndrome with diabetes mellitus. Hormone Res 2006; 65: 14–17.

1107. Fraccaro M, Kaijser K, Lindsten J. A child with 49 chromosomes. Lancet 1960; 2: 899–902.

1108. Jackson AW, Mudal S, Ockey CH, et al. Carcinoma of the male breast in association with Klinefelter's syndrome. Br Med J 1965; 1: 223–225.

1109. Scheike O. Male breast cancer. Acta Pathol Microbiol Scand 1975; 251: 13–35.

1110. Mies R, Fischer H, Pfeiff B, et al. Klinefelter's syndrome and breast cancer. Andrologia 1982; 14: 317–321.

1111. Isurugi K, Imao S, Hirose K, et al. Seminoma in Klinefelter's syndrome with 47 XXY, 15s+ karyotype. Cancer 1977; 39: 2041–2047.

1112. Vanfleteren E, Steeno O. Klinefelter's syndrome and mediastinal teratoma. Andrologia 1981; 13: 573–577.

1113. Gohji K, Goto A, Takenaka A, et al. Extragonadal germ cell tumor in the retrovesical region associated with Klinefelter's syndrome: A case report and review of literature. J Urol 1989; 141: 133–136.

1114. McNeil MM, Leong A, Sage RE. Primary mediastinal embryonal carcinoma in association with Klinefelter's syndrome. Cancer 1981; 47: 343–345.

1115. Sogge MR, McDonald SDM, Cofold PB. The malignant potential of the dysgenetic germ cell in Klinefelter's syndrome. Am J Med 1979; 66: 515–518.

1116. Mukerjee D, Bowen J, Anderson DE. Simian papovavirus 40 transformation of cells from cancer patient with XY/XXY mosaic Klinefelter's syndrome. Cancer Res 1970; 30: 1769–1772.

1117. Pascual J, Liaño F, García-Villanueva A, et al. Isolated primary aldosteronism in a patient with adrenal carcinoma and XY/XXY Klinefelter's syndrome. J Urol 1990; 144: 1454–1456.

1118. Penchansky L, Krause JR. Acute leukemia following a malignant teratoma in a child with Klinefelter's syndrome. Cancer 1982; 50: 684–689.

1119. Keung YK, Buss D, Chauvenet A, Pettenati M. Hematologic malignancies and Klinefelter syndrome. A chance association? Cancer Genet Cytogenet 2002; 139: 9–13.

1120. Hwang JJ, Dharmawardana PG, Uchio EM, et al. Prostate cancer in Klinefelter syndrome during hormonal replacement therapy. Urology 2003; 62: 941.

1121. Ferguson-Smith MA. The prepubertal testicular lesion in chromatin-positive Klinefelter's syndrome (primary micro-orchidism). As seen in mentally handicapped children. Lancet 1959; 1: 219–222.

1122. Samango-Sprouse C. Mental development in polysomy X Klinefelter syndrome (47,XXY; 48,XXXY): effects of incomplete X inactivation. Semin Reprod Med 2001; 19: 193–202.

1123. Khalifa M, Struthers J. Klinefelter syndrome is a common cause for mental retardation of unknown etiology among prepubertal males. Clin Genet 2002; 61: 49–53.

1124. Schibler D, Brook CG, Kind HP, et al. Growth and body proportions in 54 boys and men with Klinefelter's syndrome. Helv Paediatr Acta 1974; 29: 325–333.

1125. Grumbach MM, Conte FA. Disorders of sex differentiation. In: Wilson JD, Foster DW, eds. Williams' textbook of endocrinology, 8th edn. Philadelphia: WB Saunders, 1992;.853–951.

1126. Smyth CM, Bremner WJ. Klinefelter syndrome. Arch Intern Med 1998; 158: 1309–1314.

1127. Visootsak J, Aylstock M, Graham JM Jr. Klinefelter syndrome and its variants: an update and review for the primary pediatrician. Clin Pediatr 2001; 40: 639–651.

1128. Ross JL, Samango-Sprouse C, Lahlou N, et al. Early androgen deficiency in infants and young boys with 47,XXY Klinefelter syndrome. Hormone Res 2005; 64: 39–45.

1129. Lanman JT, Skalarin BS, Cooper HL, et al. Klinefelter's syndrome in a ten month old mongolian idiot. N Engl J Med 1960; 263: 887–888.

1130. Gracia R, Martín-Álvarez L, Figols J, et al. Síndrome de Klinefelter's XXY en el periodo prepuberal. Estudio de ocho observaciones. An Esp Pediatr 1974; 7: 510–523.

1131. Aksglaede L, Wikstrom AM, Rajpert-De Meyts E, et al. Natural history of seminiferous tubule degeneration in Klinefelter syndrome. Hum Reprod Update 2006; 12: 39–48.

1132. Volkl TM, Langer T, Aigner T, et al. Klinefelter syndrome and mediastinal germ cell tumors. Am J Med Genet A 2006; 140: 471–481.

1133. Bertelloni S, Battini R, Baroncelli GL, et al. Central precocious puberty in 48,XXYY Klinefelter syndrome variant. J Pediatr Endocrinol Metab 1999; 12: 459–465.

1134. Maisey DN, Mills IH, Middleton H, et al. A case of Klinefelter's syndrome with acquired hypopituitarism. Acta Endocrinol 1984; 105: 126–129.

1135. Smals AGH, Kloppenborg PWC. Klinefelter's syndrome with hypogonadotropic hypogonadism. Br Med J 1977; 1: 839–839.

1136. Rabinowitz D, Cohen MM, Rosenmann E, et al. Chromatin-positive Klinefelter's syndrome with undetectable peripheral FSH levels. Am J Med 1975; 59: 584–590.

1137. Shirai M, Matsuda S, Mitsukawa S. A case of hypogonadotrophic hypogonadism with an XY/XXY chromosome mosaicism. Tohoku J Exp Med 1974; 114: 131–139.

1138. Carter JN, Wisseman DGH, Lee HB. Klinefelter's syndrome with hypogonadotrophic hypogonadism. Br Med J 1977; 1: 212–212.

1139. Nistal M, Paniagua R, Abaurrea MA, et al. 47,XXY Klinefelter's syndrome with low FSH and LH levels and absence of Leydig cells. Andrologia 1980; 12: 426–433.

1140. Fuse H, Ito H, Minagawa H, et al. A case of XX-male syndrome. Jpn J Fertil Steril 1982; 27: 77–82.

1141. Maeda O, Nakamura M, Namiki M, et al. 45X/46XX boy with hypospadias: case report. J Urol 1986; 135: 1249–1251.

1142. De la Chapelle A, Hortling H, Niemi M, et al. XX sex chromosomes in a human male. First case. Acta Med Scand 1964; 175: 25–38.

1143. Radi O, Parma P, Imbeaud S, et al. XX sex reversal, palmoplantar keratoderma, and predisposition to squamous cell carcinoma: genetic analysis in one family. Am J Med Genet A 2005; 138: 241–246.

1144. De la Chapelle A. Analytic review: Nature and origin of males with XX sex chromosomes. Am J Hum Genet 1972; 24: 71–105.

1145. Kovacs K, Singer W, Casal G. Leydig cell ultrastructure in an XX male. J Urol 1974; 112: 651–654.

1146. Nistal M, Barreiro E, Herruzo A, et al. Varón con cariotipo 46 XX. Arch Esp Urol 1975; 28: 263–272.

1147. Nistal M, Paniagua R. Ultrastructure of testicular biopsy from an XX male. Virchows Arch B [Cell Pathol] 1979; 31: 45–55.

1148. Romani F, Terquem A, Dadoune JP. Le testicule chez l'homme 46, XX: A propos d'une observation ultrastructural. J Gynecol Obstet Biol Rep 1977; 6: 1049–1059.

1149. Sasagawa I, Terada T, Katayama T, et al. Ultrastructure of the testis in an XX male with normal plasma testosterone. Andrologia 1986; 18: 361–367.

1150. Mittwoch U. Sex determination and sex reversal: genotype, phenotype, dogma and semantics. Hum Genet 1992; 89: 467–479.

1151. Marquet F, Verloes A, Beckers A. Clinical case of the month. A male with 46,XX karyotype. Rev Méd Liège 1998; 53: 515–517.

1152. Ferguson-Smith MA. X-Y chromosomal interchange in the etiology of true hermaphroditism and of XX Klinefelter's syndrome. Lancet 1966; 27: 475–476.

1153. Butler MG, Walzak MP, Sanger WG, et al. A possible etiology of the infertile 46 XX male subject. J Urol 1983; 130: 154–156.

1154. Muller U, Donlon T, Schmid M, et al. Deletion mapping of the testis determining locus with DNA probes in 46 XX males and 46 XY and 46 X dic (Y) females. Nucleic Acids Res 1986; 14: 6489–6505.

1155. Fuse H, Satomi S, Kazama T, et al. DNA hybridization study using Y-specific probes in an XX-male. Andrologia 1991; 23: 237–239.

1156. Suzuki Y, Sasagawa I, Yazawa H, et al. Localization of the sex-determining region-Y gene in XX males. Arch Androl 2000; 44: 133–136.

1157. Castineyra G, Copelli S, Levalle O. 46,XX male: clinical, hormonal/genetic findings. Arch Androl 2002; 48: 251–257.

1158. Rigola MA, Carrera S, Ribas I, et al. A comparative genomic hybridization study in a 46,XX male. Fertil Steril 2002; 78: 186–188.

1159. Dauwerse JG, Hansson KB, Brouwers AA, et al. An XX male with the sex-determining region Y gene inserted in the long arm of chromosome 16. Fertil Steril 2006; 86: 463; e1–5.

1160. Yoshida M, Kakizawa Y, Moriyama N, et al. Deoxyribonucleic acid and cytological detection of Y-containing cells in a XX hypospadic boy with polyorchidism. J Urol 1991; 146: 1356–1358.

1161. Abusheikha N, Lass A, Brinsden P. XX males without SRY gene and with infertility. Hum Reprod 2001; 16: 717–718.

1162. Rajender S, Rajani V, Gupta NJ, et al. SRY-negative 46,XX male with normal genitals, complete masculinization and infertility. Mol Hum Reprod 2006; 12: 341–346.

1163. Ferguson-Smith MA, Cooke A, Affara NA, et al. Genotype-phenotype correlations in XX males and their bearing on current theories of sex determination. Hum Genet 1990; 84: 198–202.

1164. McElreavey K, Vilain E, Abbas N, et al. A regulatory cascade hypothesis for mammalian sex determination: SRY represses a negative regulator of male development. Proc Natl Acad Sci USA 1993; 90: 3368–3372.

1165. Seeherunvong T, Perera EM, Bao Y, et al. 46,XX sex reversal with partial duplication of chromosome arm 22q. Am J Med Genet A 2004; 127: 149–151.

1166. Ergun-Longmire B, Vinci G, Alonso L, et al. Clinical, hormonal and cytogenetic evaluation of 46,XX males and review of the literature. J Pediatr Endocrinol Metab 2005; 18: 739–748.

1167. Sanberg AA, Koepf GF, Ishihara T, et al. XYY human male. Lancet 1961; 2: 888.

1168. Briken P, Habermann N, Berner W, Hill A. XYY chromosome abnormality in sexual homicide perpetrators. Am J Med Genet B Neuropsychiatr Genet 2006; 141: 198–200.

1169. Geerts M, Steyaert J, Fryns JP. The XYY syndrome: a follow-up study on 38 boys. Genet Couns 2003; 14: 267–279.

1170. Baghdassarian A, Bayard F, Borgaonkar DS, et al. Testicular function in XYY men. Johns Hopkins Med J 1975; 136: 15–24.

1171. Skakkebaek NE, Hulten M, Jacobsen P, et al. Quantification of human seminiferous epithelium. II. Histological studies in eight 47, XYY men. J Reprod Fertil 1973; 32: 391–401.

1172. Speed RM, Faed MJ, Batstone PJ, et al. Persistence of two Y chromosomes through meiotic prophase and metaphase I in an XYY man. Hum Genet 1991; 87: 416–420.

1173. Rives N, Milazzo JP, Miraux L, et al. From spermatocytes to spermatozoa in an infertile XYY male. Int J Androl 2005; 28: 304–310.

1174. Miklos GL. Sex chromosome pairing and male fertility. Cytogenet Cell Genet 1974; 13: 558–577.

1175. Burgoyne PS, Sutcliffe MJ, Mahadevaiah SK. The role of unpaired sex chromosomes in spermatogenetic failure. Andrologia 1992; 24: 17–20.

1176. Burgoyne PS. Evidence for an association between univalent Y chromosomes and spermatocyte loss in XYY mice and men. Cytogenet Cell Genet 1979; 23: 84–89.

1177. Hulten M. Meiosis in XYY men. Lancet 1970; 1: 717–718.

1178. Nielsen J, Johnsen SG. Pituitary gonadotrophins and 17-ketosteroids in patients with the XYY syndrome. Acta Endocrinol 1973; 72: 191–196.

1179. Lim AST, Fong Y, Yu SL. Analysis of the sex chromosome constitution of sperm in men with a 47,XYY mosaic karyotype by fluorescence in situ hybridization. Fertil Steril 1999; 72: 121–123.

1180. Hori N, Kato T, Sugimura Y, et al. A male subject with 3 Y chromosomes (48,XYYY): A case report. J Urol 1988; 139: 1059–1061.

1181. Venkataraman G, Craft I. Triple-Y syndrome following ICSI treatment in a couple with normal chromosomes: case report. Hum Reprod 2002; 17: 2560–2563.

1182. Sirota L, Zlotogora Y, Shabtai F, et al. 49 XYYYY. A case report. Clin Genet 1981; 19: 87–93.

1183. DesGroseilliers M, Lemyre E, Dallaire L, Lemieux N. Tetrasomy Y by structural rearrangement: clinical report. Am Med Genet 2002; 111: 401–404.

1184. Vogt PH. Human Y chromosome function in male germ cell development (review). Adv Dev Biol 1996; 4: 191–257.

1185. Kent-First M, Muallem A, Shultz J, et al. Defining regions of the Y-chromosome reponsible for male infertility and identification of a fourth AZF region (AZFd) by Y-chromosome microdeletion. Mol Reprod Dev 1999; 53: 27–41.

1186. Stuppia L, Gatta V, Fogh l, et al. Characterization of novel genes in AZF regions. J Endocrinol Invest 2000; 23: 659–663.

1187. Tiepolo L, Zuffardi O. Localization of factors controlling spermatogenesis in the nonfluorescent portion of the human Y chromosome long arm. Hum Genet 1976; 34: 119–124.

1188. Reijo R, Alagappan RK, Patrizio P, et al. Severe oligozoospermia resulting from deletions of azoospermia factor gene on Y chromosome. Lancet 1996; 347: 1290–1293.

1189. Hartung M, Devictor M, Codaccioni JL, et al. Yq deletion and failure of spermatogenesis. Ann Genet 1988; 31: 21–26.

1190. Kosztolanyi G, Trixler M. Yq deletion with short stature, abnormal male development, and schizoid character disorder. J Med Genet 1983; 20: 393–394.

1191. Codina-Pascual M, Oliver-Bonet M, Navarro J, et al. FISH characterization of a dicentric Yq (p11.32) isochromosome in an azoospermic male. Am J Med Genet A 2004; 127: 302–306.

1192. Daniel A. Y isochromosomes and rings. In: Sandber AA, ed. The Y chromosome, Part B. Clinical aspects of Y chromosome abnormalities. New York: Alan R Liss, 1985; 105–135.

1193. Chandley AC, Ambros P, McBeach S, et al. Short arm dicentric Y chromosome with associated statural defect in a sterile man. Hum Genet 1986; 73: 350–353.

1194. Giraud F, Mattei JF, Lucas C, et al. Four new cases of dicentric Y chromosomes. Hum Genet 1977; 36: 249–260.

1195. Chandley AC, Edmond P. Meiotic studies on a subfertile patient with a ring Y chromosome. Cytogenetics 1971; 10: 295–304.

1196. Bertini V, Canale D, Bicocchi MP, et al. Mosaic ring Y chromosome in two normal healthy men with azoospermia. Fertil Steril 2005; 84: 1744.

1197. Lin YH, Lin YM, Lin YH, et al. Ring (Y) in two azoospermic men. Am J Med Genet A 2004; 128: 209–213.

1198. Wahlström J. Y/Y translocations and their cytologic and clinical manifestation. In: Sandberg AA, ed. The Y chromosome Part B: Clinical aspects of Y chromosome abnormalities. New York: Alan R Liss, 1985; 207–212.

1199. Petit C, De la Chapelle A, Levilliers J, et al. An abnormal terminal X-Y interchange accounts for most but not all cases of human XX maleness. Cell 1987; 49: 595–602.

1200. Brisset S, Izard V, Misrahi M, et al. Cytogenetic, molecular and testicular tissue studies in an infertile 45,X male carrying an unbalanced (Y; 22) translocation: case report. Hum Reprod 2005; 20: 2168–2172.

1201. Pinho MJ, Neves R, Costa P, et al. Unique t(Y; 1)(q12; q12) reciprocal translocation with loss of the heterochromatic region of chromosome 1 in a male with azoospermia due to meiotic arrest: a case report. Hum Reprod 2005; 20: 689–696.

1202. Andersson M, Page DC, Pettay D, et al. Y; autosome translocations and mosaicism in the aetiology of 45,X

maleness: assignment of fertility factor to distal Yq ll. Hum Genet 1988; 79: 2–7.

1203. Andersson M, Page DC, Brown LG, et al. Characterization of a (Y; 4) translocation by DNA hybridization. Hum Genet 1988; 78: 377–381.

1204. Vogt P, Keil R, Kohler M, et al. Genome analysis: From sequence to function. Adv Mol Genet 1991; 4: 277–280.

1205. Girardi SK, Mielnik A, Schlegel PN. Submicroscopic deletions in the Y chromosome of infertile men. Hum Reprod 1997; 12: 1635–1641.

1206. Foresta C, Ferlin A, Garolla A, et al. Y-chromosome deletions in idiopathic severe testiculopathies. J Clin Endocrinol Metab 1997; 82: 1075–1080.

1207. Oliva R, Margarit E, Ballesta JL, et al. Prevalence of Y chromosome microdeletions in oligospermic and azoospermic candidates for intracytoplasmic sperm injection. Fertil Steril 1998; 70: 506–510.

1208. Dewan S, Puscheck EE, Coulam CB, et al. Y-chromosome microdeletions and recurrent pregnancy loss. Fertil Steril 2006; 85: 441–445.

1209. Johnson MD, Tho SPT, Behzadian A, et al. Molecular scanning of Yq 11 (interval 6) in men with Sertoli-cell-only syndrome. Am J Obstet Gynecol 1989; 161: 1732–1737.

1210. McElreavey K, Ravel C, Chantot-Bastaraud S, Siffroi JP. Y chromosome variants and male reproductive function. Int J Androl 2006; 29: 298–303.

1211. Telvi LT, Ion A, Carel J-C, et al. A duplication of distal Xp associated with hypogonadotrophic hypogonadism, hypoplastic external genitalia, mental retardation, and multiple congenital abnormalities. Med Genet 1996; 33: 767–771.

1212. Solari AJ, Rahn IM, Ferreyra ME, Carballo MA. The behavior of sex chromosomes in two human X-autosome translocations: failure of extensive -inactivation spreading. Biocell 2001; 25: 155–166.

1213. Ma S, Yuen BH, Penaherrera M, et al. ICSI and the transmission of X-autosomal translocation: a three-generation evaluation of X; 20 translocation: case report. Hum Reprod 2003; 18: 1377–1382.

1214. Ogata T, Matsuo M, Muroya K, et al. 47,XXX male: a clinical and molecular study. Am J Med Genet 2001; 98: 353–356.

1215. Martin RH, Hulten M. Chromosome complements in 695 sperm from three men heterozygous for reciprocal translocations and a review of the literature. Hereditas 1993; 118: 165–175.

1216. Martin RH, Chernos JE, Lowry RB, et al. Analysis of sperm chromosome complements from a man heterozygous for a pericentric

inversion of chromosome 1. Hum Genet 1994; 93: 135–138.

1217. Bache I, Assche EV, Cingoz S, et al. An excess of chromosome 1 breakpoints in male infertility. Eur J Hum Genet 2004; 12: 993–1000.

1218. Shapiro CE. Unbalanced chromosomal translocation associated with Sertoli-cell-only histology. J Urol 1991; 145: 563–564.

1219. Mercer ES, Broecker B, Smith EA, et al. Urological manifestations of Down syndrome. J Urol 2004; 171: 1250–1253.

1220. Sasagawa I, Nakada T, Hasihimoto T, et al. Hormone profiles and contralateral testicular histology in Down's syndrome with unilateral testicular tumor. Arch Androl 1993; 30: 93–98.

1221. Zuhlke C, Thies U, Braulke l, et al. Down syndrome and male fertility: PCR-derived fingerprinting, serological and andrological investigations. Clin Genet 1994; 46: 324–326.

1222. Kim ST, Cha YB, Park JM, Gye MC. Successful pregnancy and delivery from frozen-thawed embryos after intracytoplasmic sperm injection using round-headed spermatozoa and assisted oocyte activation in a globozoospermic patient with mosaic Down syndrome. Fertil Steril 2001; 75: 445–447.

1223. Cools M, Honecker F, Stoop H, et al. Maturation delay of germ cells in fetuses with trisomy 21 results in increased risk for the development of testicular germ cell tumors. Hum Pathol 2006; 37: 101–111.

1224. Johannisson R, Gropp A, Winking H, et al. Down syndrome in the male. Reproductive pathology and meiotic studies. Hum Genet 1983; 63: 132–138.

1225. Nistal M, Paniagua R. Hypogonadism due to primary testicular failure. In: Nistal M, Paniagua R, eds. Testicular and epididymal pathology. New York: Thieme-Stratton, 1984; 145–167.

1226. Tsilfidis C, MacKenzie AE, Mettler G, et al. Correlation between CTG trinucleotide repeat length and frequency of severe congenital myotonic dystrophy. Nature Genet 1992; 1: 192–195.

1227. Harley HG, Rundle SA, MacMillan JC, et al. Size of the unstable CTG repeat sequence in relation to phenotype and prenatal transmission in myotonic dystrophy. Am J Hum Genet 1993; 52: 1164–1174.

1228. Redman JB, Fenwick RG Jr, Fu YH, et al. Relationship between parenteral trinucleotide CTG repeat length and severity of myotonic dystrophy in offspring. JAMA 1993; 269: 1960–1965.

1229. Ranum LP, Day JW. Myotonic dystrophy: clinical and molecular parallels between myotonic dystrophy type 1 and type 2. Curr Neurol Neurosci Rep 2002; 2: 465–470.

1230. Brunner HG, Brüggenwirth HT, Nillesen W, et al. Influence of sex of the transmitting parent as well as of parental allele size on the CTG expansion in myotonic dystrophy (DM). Am J Hum Genet 1993; 53: 1016–1023.

1231. Kunej T, Teran N, Zorn B, Peterlin B. CTG amplification in the DM1PK gene is not associated with idiopathic male subfertility. Hum Reprod 2004; 19: 2084–2087.

1232. Marchini C, Lonigro R, Verriello L, et al. Correlations between individual clinical manifestations and CTG repeat amplification in myotonic dystrophy. Clin Genet 2000; 57: 74–82.

1233. Hauser W, Aulitzky W, Baltaci S, Frick J. Increasing infertility in myotonia dystrophica Curschmann–Steinert. A case report. Eur Urol 1991; 20: 341–342.

1234. Hoffman EP, Fischbeck KH, Brown RH, et al. Dystrophin characterization in muscle biopsies from Duchenne and Becker muscular dystrophy patients. N Engl J Med 1988; 318: 1363–1368.

1235. Ervasti JM. Dystrophin, its interactions with other proteins, and implications for muscular dystrophy. Biochim Biophys Acta 2007; 1772: 108–117.

1236. Kitao S, Ohsugi l, Ichikawa K, et al. Cloning of two new human helicase genes of the RECQ family: biological significance of multiple species in higher eukaryotes. Genomics 1998; 54: 443–452.

1237. Yu CE, Oshima J, Fu YM, et al. Positional cloning of the Werner's syndrome gene. Science 1996; 272: 258–262.

1238. Martin RH, Rademaker A, German J. Chromosomal breakage in human spermatozoa, a heterozygous effect of the Bloom syndrome mutation. Am J Hum Genet 1994; 55: 1242–1246.

1239. Werner SR, Prahalad AK, Yang J, Hock JM. RECQL4-deficient cells are hypersensitive to oxidative stress/damage: Insights for osteosarcoma prevalence and heterogeneity in Rothmund–Thomson syndrome. Biochem Biophys Res Commun 2006; 345: 403–409.

1240. Hamdani M, El Kettani A, Rais L, et al. Cockayne's syndrome with unusual retinal involvement (report of one family). J Fr Ophtalmol 2000; 23: 52–56.

1241. Landing BH, Sugarman G, Dixon LG. Eccrine sweat gland anatomy in cockayne syndrome: a possible diagnostic aid. Pediatr Pathol 1983; 1: 349–353.

1242. Arenas-Sordo M de L, Hernandez-Zamora E, Montoya-Perez LA, Aldape-Barrios BC. Cockayne's syndrome: a case report. Literature review. Med Oral Patol Oral Cir Bucal 2006; 11: e236–238.

1243. McCuaig C, Marcoux D, Rasmussen JE, et al. Trichothiodystrophy associated with photosensitivity, gonadal failure, and striking osteosclerosis. J Am Acad Dermatol 1993; 28: 820–826.

1244. Jamieson CR, Van der Burgt I, Brady AF, et al. Mapping a gene for Noonan syndrome to the long arm of chromosome 12. Nature Genet 1994; 8: 357–360.

1245. Tartaglia M, Gelb BD. Noonan syndrome and related disorders: genetics and pathogenesis. Annu Rev Genomics Hum Genet 2005; 6: 45–68.

1246. Nistal M, Paniagua R, Pallardo LF. Testicular biopsy and hormonal study in a male with Noonan's Syndrome. Andrologia 1983; 15: 415–425.

1247. Peters LL, Birkenmeier CS, Bronson RT, et al. Purkinje cell degeneration associated with erythroid ankyrin deficiency in nb/nb mice. J Cell Biol 1991; 114: 1233–1241.

1248. Harada T, Pineda LL, Nakano A, et al. Ataxia and male sterility (AMS) mouse. A new genetic variant exhibiting degeneration and loss of cerebellar Purkinje cells and spermatic cells. Pathol Int 2003; 53: 382–389.

1249. Kakar SS. Molecular structure of the human gonadotropin-releasing hormone receptor gene. Eur J Endocrinol 1997; 137: 183–192.

1250. Seminara SB, Hayes FJ, Crowley WF Jr. Gonadotropin-Releasing hormone deficiency in the human (idiopathic hypogonadotropic hypogonadism and Kallmann's syndrome): pathophysiological and genetic considerations. Endocrinol Rev 1998; 19: 521–539.

1251. Pallardo LF, Santiago M, Cerdán A, et al. Algunos aspectos del eunucoidismo hipogonadotrópico. Med Clin 1972; 59: 390–396.

1252. Pralong FP, Gomez F, Castillo E, et al. Complete hypogonadotropic hypogonadism associated with a novel inactivating mutation of the gonadotropin-releasing hormone receptor. J Clin Endocrinol Metab 1999; 84: 3811–3816.

1253. Boyar R, Finkelstein J, Roffwang H, et al. Synchronization of augmented luteinizing hormone secretion with sleep during puberty. N Engl J Med 1972; 287: 582–586.

1254. Pitteloud N, Hayes FD, Dwyer A, et al. Predictors of outcome of long-term GnRH therapy in men with idiopathic hypogonadotropic hypogonadism. J Clin Endocrinol Metab 2002; 87: 4128–4136.

1255. Nistal M, Paniagua R. Hypogonadism due to secondary testicular failure. In: Nistal M, Paniagua R, eds. Testicular and epididymal pathology. New York: Thieme-Stratton, 1984; 169–177.

1256. Maestre de San Juan A. Falta total de nervios olfatorios con anosmia en un individuo en quien existía una atrofia congénita de los testículos y miembro viril. Siglo Médico 1856; 131: 211–214.

1257. Kallmann FJ, Shoenfeld WA, Barrera SE. The genetic aspects of primary eunuchoidism. Am J Ment Defic 1944; 48: 203–236.

1258. De Morsier G, Gauthier G. La dysplasie olfacto-génitale. Pathol Biol 1963; 11: 1267–1271.

1259. Yoshida K, Rutishauser U, Crandall JE, et al. Polysialic acid facilitates migration of luteinizing hormone-releasing hormone neurons on vomeronasal axons. J Neurosci 1999; 19: 794–801.

1260. Tsai PS, Gill JC. Mechanisms of disease: Insights into X-linked and autosomal-dominant Kallmann syndrome. Nature Clin Pract Endocrinol Metab 2006; 2: 160–171.

1261. Pitteloud N, Meysing A, Quinton R, et al. Mutations in fibroblast growth factor receptor 1 cause Kallmann syndrome with a wide spectrum of reproductive phenotypes. Mol Cell Endocrinol 2006; 254–255: 60–69.

1262. Happ J, Ditscheid W, Krause U. Pulsatile gonadotropin-releasing therapy in male patients with Kallmann's syndrome or constitutional delay of puberty. Fertil Steril 1985; 43: 599–608.

1263. Enríquez L, Díaz-Rubio M, Zamarrón A, et al. Hipogonadismo hipogonadotrópico con anosmia. Rev Clin Esp 1973; 131: 383–392.

1264. Pervaiz N, Hagedoorn J, Mininberg DT. Electron microscopic studies of testes in Kallmann syndrome. Urology 1979; 14: 267–269.

1265. Albers DD, Males JL. Seminoma in hypogonadotropic hypogonadism associated with anosmia (Kallmann's syndrome). J Urol 1981; 126: 57–58.

1266. Berger K, Souza H, Brito VN, et al. Clinical and hormonal features of selective follicle-stimulating hormone (FSH) deficiency due to FSH β-subunit gene mutations in both sexes. Fertil Steril 2005; 83: 466–470.

1267. Lamminen T, Jokinen P, Jiang M, et al. Human FSH β subunit gene is highly conserved. Mol Hum Reprod 2005; 11: 601–605.

1268. Al-Ansari AAK, Khalil TH, Kelani Y, Mortimer CH. Isolated follicle-stimulating hormone deficiency in men: successful long-term gonadotropin therapy. Fertil Steril 1984; 42: 618–626.

1269. Pasqualini RQ, Bur GE. Síndrome hipoandrogénico con gametogénesis conservada: clasificación de la insuficiencia testicular. Rev Asoc Med Argent 1950; 64: 6–10.

1270. Pasqualini RQ, Bur GE. Hypoandrogenic syndrome with spermatogenesis. Fertil Steril 1955; 6: 144–157.

1271. McCullagh EP, Beck JC, Schaffenburg CA. A syndrome of eunuchoidism with spermatogenesis, normal urinary FSH, and low-normal ICSH ('fertile eunuchs'). J Clin Endocrinol Metab 1953; 13: 489–509.

1272. Shiraishi K, Naito K. Fertile eunuch syndrome with the mutations (Trp8Arg and Ile15Thr) in the β subunit of luteinizing hormone. Endocrinol J 2003; 50: 733–737.

1273. Pitteloud N, Boepple PA, DeCruz S, et al. The fertile eunuch variant of idiopathic hypogonadotropic hypogonadism: spontaneous reversal associated with a homozygous mutation in the gonadotropin-releasing hormone receptor. J Clin Endocrinol Metab 2001; 86: 2470–2475.

1274. Weiss J, Axelrod L, Whitcomb RW, et al. Hypogonadism caused by a single amino acid substitution in the β subunit of luteinzing hormone. N Engl J Med 1992; 326: 179–183.

1275. Layman LC, Porto AL, Xie J, et al. FSH β gene mutations in a female with partial breast development and a male sibling with normal puberty and azoospermia. J Clin Endocrinol Metab 2002; 87: 3702–3707.

1276. Tato L, Zamboni G, Antoniazzi F, et al. Gonadal function and response to growth hormone (GH) in boys with isolated GH deficiency and to GH and gonadotropins in boys with multiple pituitary hormone deficiencies. Fertil Steril 1996; 65: 830–834.

1277. Prader A, Labhart A, Willi H. Ein syndrom von Adipositas, Kleinwuchs, Kryptorchismus, und Oligophrenie nach myotonieartigen Zustand in Neugeborenenalter. Schweiz Med Wschr 1956; 86: 1260–1261.

1278. Eiholzer U, l'Allemand D, Rousson V, et al. Hypothalamic and gonadal components of hypogonadism in boys with Prader–Labhart–Willi syndrome. J Clin Endocrinol Metab 2006; 91: 892–898.

1279. Uehling D. Cryptorchidism in the Prader–Willi syndrome. J Urol 1980; 124: 103–104.

1280. Martín-Zurro A, Sánchez-Franco F, Cerdán-Vallejo A, et al. Síndrome de Prader–Willi. Rev Clin Esp 1972; 125: 5–15.

1281. Young TL, Penney L, Woods MO, et al. A fifth locus for Bardet–Biedl syndrome maps to chromosome 2q31. Am J Hum Genet 1999; 64: 900–904.

1282. Blacque OE, Leroux MR. Bardet–Biedl syndrome: an emerging pathomechanism of intracellular transport. Cell Mol Life Sci 2006; 63: 2145–2161.

1283. Maya-Nuñez G, Torres L, Ulloa-Aguirre A, et al. An atypical contiguous gene syndrome: molecular studies in a family with X-linked Kallmann's syndrome and X-linked ichthyosis. Clin Endocrinol 1999; 50: 157–162.

1284. Cushman LJ, Torres-Martinez W, Weaver DD. Johnson–McMillin syndrome: report of a new case with novel features. Birth Defects Res A Clin Mol Teratol 2005; 73: 638–641.

1285. Savitsky K, Bar-Shira A, Gilad S, et al. A single ataxia telangiectasia gene with a product similar to PI-3 kinase. Science 1995; 268: 1749–1753.

1286. Frappart PO, McKinnon PJ. Ataxia-telangiectasia and related diseases. Neuromol Med 2006; 8: 495–512.

1287. Carvajal JJ, Pook MA, Dos Santos M, et al. The Friedreich's ataxia gene encodes a novel phosphatidylinositol-4-phosphatase 5-kinase. Nature Genet 1996; 14: 157–162.

1288. Pandolfo M. Friedreich ataxia: Detection of GAA repeat expansions and frataxin point mutations. Meth Mol Med 2006; 126: 197–216.

1289. Sigman M, Jarow JP. Endocrine evaluation of infertile men. Urology 1997; 50: 659–664.

1290. Burge MR, Lanzi RA, Skarda ST, et al. Idiopathic hypogonadotropic hypogonadism in a male runner is reversed by clomiphene citrate. Fertil Steril 1997; 67: 783–785.

1291. Veldjuis JB, Hammond JM. Endocrine function after spontaneous infarction of the human pituitary. Report, review and reappraisal. Endocrinol Rev 1980; 1: 100–107.

1292. Tash J, McGovern JH, Schlegel PN. Acquired hypogonadotropic hypogonadism presenting as decreased seminal volume. Urology 2000; 56: 669.

1293. Zárate A, Fonseca ME, Mason M, et al. Gonadotropin-secreting pituitary adenoma with concomitant hypersecretion of testosterone and elevated sperm count. Treatment with LRH agonists. Acta Endocrinol 1986; 113: 29–34.

1294. Heseltine D, White MC, Kendall-Taylor P, et al. Testicular enlargement and elevated serum inhibin concentrations occur in patients with pituitary macroadenomas secreting follicle stimulating hormone. Clin Endocrinol 1989; 31: 411–423.

1295. Corona G, Petrone L, Mannucci E, et al. The impotent couple: low desire. Int J Androl 2005; 28: 46–52.

1296. Bouhdiba M, Leroy-Martin B, Peyrat JP, et al. Immunohistochemical detection of prolactin and its receptors in human testis. Andrologia 1989; 21: 223–228.

1297. Cameron DF, Murray FT, Drylie D. Ultrastructural lesions in testes from hyperprolactinemic men. J Androl 1984; 5: 285–293.

1298. Eggert-Kruse W, Schwalbach B, Gerhard I, et al. Influence of serum prolactin on semen characteristics and sperm function. Int J Fertil 1991; 36: 243–251.

1299. Murray FT, Cameron DF, Ketchum C. Return of gonadal function in men with prolactin-secreting tumors. J Clin Endocrinol Metab 1984; 59: 79–85.

1300. Ford HC, Cooke RR, Keightley EA, et al. Serum levels of free and bound testosterone in hyperthyroidism. Clin Endocrinol 1992; 36: 187–192.

1301. Hudson RW, Edwards AL. Testicular function in hyperthyroidism. J Androl 1992; 13: 117–124.

1302. Willey KP, Hunt N, Castel MA, et al. Graves'autoimmune serum inhibits gonadal steroidogenesis. Development of a Leydig cell bioassay to identify broad spectrum anti-endocrine autoantibodies. J Reprod Immunol 1993; 24: 45–63.

1303. De La Balze F, Arillaga F, Mancini RE, et al. Male hypogonodism in hypothyroidism: A study of six cases. J Clin Endocrinol Metab 1962; 22: 212–222.

1304. Krassas GE, Pontikides N. Male reproductive function in relation with thyroid alterations. Best Pract Res Clin Endocrinol Metab 2004; 18: 183–95.

1305. Donnelly P, White C. Testicular dysfunction in men with primary hypothyroidism; reversal of hypogonadotropic hypogonadism with replacement thyroxine. Clin Endocrinol 2000; 52: 197–201.

1306. Corrales-Hernández JJ, Miralles García JM, García-Díez LC. Primary hypothyroidism and human spermatogenesis. Arch Androl 1990; 25: 21–27.

1307. Buitrago JM, Garía-Díez LC. Serum hormones and seminal parameters in males with thyroid disturbance. Andrologia 1987; 19: 37–41.

1308. Weber G, Vigone MC, Stroppa L, et al. Thyroid function and puberty. J Pediatr Endocrinol Metab 2003; 16: 253–257.

1309. Loke KY, Larry KS, Lee YS, et al. Prepubertal diagnosis of X-linked congenital adrenal hypoplasia presenting after infancy. Eur J Pediatr 2000; 159: 671–675.

1310. Calvari V, Alpigiani mg, Poggi E, et al. X-linked adrenal hypoplasia congenita and hypogonadotropic hypogonadism: report on new mutation of the DAX-1 gene in two siblings. J Endocrinol Invest 2006; 29: 41–47.

1311. Seminara SB, Achermann JC, Gene LM, et al. X-linked adrenal hypoplasia congenita: a mutation in DAX1 expands the phenotypic spectrum in males and females. J Clin Endocrinol Metab 1999; 84: 4501–4509.

1312. Sugino Y, Usui T, Okubo K, et al. Genotyping of congenital adrenal hyperplasia due to 21-hydroxylase deficiency presenting as male infertility: Case report and literature review. J Assist Reprod Genet 2006; 23: 377–380.

1313. Bonaccorsi AC, Adler I, Figueiredo JG. Male infertility due to congenital adrenal hyperplasia: testicular biopsy findings, hormonal evaluation, and therapeutic results in three patients. Fertil Steril 1987; 47: 664–670.

1314. Burke EF, Gilbert E, Uehling DT. Adrenal rest tumors of the testes. J Urol 1973; 109: 649–652.

1315. Oberman AS, Flatau E, Luboshitzki R. Bilateral testicular adrenal rests in a patient with 11-hydroxylase deficient congenital adrenal hyperplasia. J Urol 1993; 149: 350–352.

1316. Cutfield RG, Bateman JM, Odell WD. Infertility caused by bilateral testicular masses secondary to congenital adrenal hyperplasia (21-hydroxylase deficiency). Fertil Steril 1983; 40: 809–814.

1317. Cara JF, Moshang T Jr, Bongiovanni AM, et al. Elevated 17-hydroxyprogesterone and testosterone in a newborn with 3β-hydroxysteroid dehydrogenase deficiency. N Eng l J Med 1985; 313: 618–621.

1318. Sasano H, Masuda T, Ojima M, et al. Congenital 17 alfa-hydroxylase deficiency: A clinico-pathologic study. Hum Pathol 1987; 18: 1002–1007.

1319. Battaglia M, Ditonno P, Palazzo S, et al. Bilateral tumors of the testis in 21-alpha hydroxylase deficiency without adrenal hyperplasia. Urol Oncol 2005; 23: 178–180.

1320. Watanabe T, Yasuda T, Noda H, et al. Estrogen secreting adrenal adenocarcinoma in an 18-month-old boy: aromatase activity, protein expression, mRNA and utilization of gonadal type promoter. Endocrinol J 2000; 47: 723–730.

1321. Dinulovic D, Radonjic G. Diabetes mellitus/male infertility. Arch Androl 1990; 25: 277–293.

1322. Elamin A, Hussein O, Tuvemo T. Growth, puberty, and final height in children with type 1 diabetes. J Diabetes Complications 2006; 20: 252–256.

1323. Ballester J, Munoz MC, Dominguez J, et al. Insulin-dependent diabetes affects testicular function by FSH- and LH-linked mechanisms. J Androl 2004; 25: 706–719.

1324. García-Díez LC, Corrales-Hernández J, Hernández-Díaz J, et al. Semen characteristics and diabetes mellitus: significance of insulin in male infertility. Arch Androl 1991; 26: 219–227.

1325. Cameron DF, Murray FT, Drylie DD. Interstitial compartment pathology and spermatogenic disruption in testes from impotent diabetic men. Anat Rec 1985; 213: 53–62.

1326. Quadri R, Veglio M, Flecchia D, et al. Autonomic neuropathy and sexual impotence in diabetic patients: Analisis of cardiovascular reflexes. Andrologia 1989; 21: 346–352.

1327. Regadera J, Nistal M, Paniagua R. Idiopathic vas deferens calcification. Morfol Normal Patol B 1983; 8: 219–223.

1328. Lemna WK, Feldman GL, Kerem B, et al. Mutation analysis for heterozygote detection and the prenatal diagnosis of cystic fibrosis. N Engl J Med 1990; 322: 291–296.

1329. Stuhrmann M, Dork T. CFTR gene mutations and male infertility. Andrologia 2000; 32: 71–83.

1330. Denning CR, Sommers SC, Herbert J, et al. Infertility in male patients with cystic fibrosis. Pediatrics 1968; 41: 7–17.

1331. Feigelson J, Pecau Y. Anomalies du sperme, des defferents et de l'epididyme dans la mucoviscidose. Presse Med 1986; 15: 523–525.

1332. Osborne L, Knight RA, Santis G, et al. A mutation in the second nucleotide binding fold of the cystic fibrosis gene. Am J Hum Genet 1991; 48: 608–612.

1333. Lewis-Jones Dl, Gazvani MR, Mountford R. Cystic fibrosis in infertility: screening before assisted reproduction: opinion. Hum Reprod 2000; 15: 2415–2417.

1334. Schellen TM, Van Straatten A. Autosomal recessive hereditary congenital aplasia of the vasa deferentia in four siblings. Fertil Steril 1980; 34: 401–404.

1335. Anguiano A, Oates RD, Amos JA, et al. Congenital bilateral absence of the vas deferens. A primary genital form of cystic fibrosis. JAMA 1992; 267: 1794–1797.

1336. Olson JR, Weaver DK. Congenital mesonephric defects in male infants with mucoviscidosis. J Clin Pathol 1969; 22: 725–730.

1337. Holsclaw DS, Perlmutter AD, Jockin H, et al. Genital abnormalities in male patients with cystic fibrosis. J Urol 1971; 106: 568–574.

1338. Silvestrini R. La revivisicenza mammaria nell'uomo affecto da cirrosi del Laennec. Riforma Med 1926; 42: 701–704.

1339. Corda L. Sulla c.d. revivisicenza della mammella maschile nella cirrosi epatica (nota preventiva). Minerva Medica 5: 1064–1067, 1925.

1340. Van Thiel DH, Lester R, Sherins RJ. Hypogonadism in alcoholic liver direase: evidence for a double defect. Gastroenterology 1974; 67: 1188–1199.

1341. Comathi C, Balasubramanian K, Vijayabhanu N, et al. Effect of chronic alcoholism on semen – studies on lipid profiles. Int J Androl 1993; 16: 175–181.

1342. Galvao-Teles A, Goncalves L, Carvalho H, Monteiro E. Alterations of testicular morphology in alcoholic disease. Alcohol Clin Exp Res 1983; 7: 144–149.

1343. Terasaki T, Nowlin DM, Pardridge WM. Differential binding of testosterone and oestradiol to isoforms of sex hormone binding glolulim: selective alteration of estradiol binding in cirrhosis. J Clin

Endocrinol Metab 1988; 67: 639–643.

1344. Gluud, C and the Copenhagen Study Group for Liver Diseases. Serum testosterone concentration in men with alcoholic cirrhosis: background for variation. Metabolism 1987; 36: 373–378.

1345. Zifroni A, Schiavi RC, Schaffner F. Sexual function and testosterone levels in men with nonalcoholic liver disease. Hepatology 1991; 14: 479–482.

1346. Handelsman DJ, Conway AJ, Boylan LM, et al. Testicular function and fertility in men with homozygous alpha-1 antitrypsin deficiency. Andrologia 1986; 18: 406–412.

1347. Niederau C. Hereditary hemochromatosis. Internist 2003; 44: 191–205.

1348. Jazwinska EC, Cullen LM, Busfield F, et al. Haemochromatosis and HLA-H. Nature Genet 1996; 14: 249–251.

1349. Feder JN, Gnirke A, Thomas W, et al. A novel MHC class 1-like gene is mutated in patients with hereditary haemochromatosis. Nature Genet 1996; 13: 399–408.

1350. Rivard SR, Mura C, Simard H, et al. Clinical and molecular aspects of juvenile hemochromatosis in Saguenay-Lac-Saint-Jean (Quebec, Canada). Blood Cells Mol Dis 2000; 26: 10–14.

1351. Roetto A, Totaro A, Cazzola M, et al. Juvenile hemochromatosis locus maps to chromosome 1q. Am J Hum Genet 1999; 64: 1388–1393.

1352. Camaschella C, Roetto A, De Gobbi M. Juvenile hemochromatosis. Semin Hematol 2002; 39: 242–248.

1353. Berent R, Allinger S, Hobling W, et al. A 24-year-old patient with decreased libido and erectile dysfunction as initial manifestations of hemochromatosis. Dtsch Med Wochenschr 2000; 125: 1466–1468.

1354. Paris l, Hermans M, Buysschaert M. Endocrine complications of genetic hemochromatosis. Acta Clin Belg 54: 334–345, 1999.

1355. McDermott JH, Walsh CH. Hypogonadism in hereditary hemochromatosis. J Clin Endocrinol Metab 2005; 90: 2451–2455.

1356. Kontogeorgos G, Handy S, Kovacs K, et al. The anterior pituitary in hemochromatosis. Endocrinol Pathol 1996; 7: 159–164.

1357. Angelopoulos NG, Goula A, Dimitriou E, et al. Reversibility of hypogonadotropic hypogonadism in a patient with the juvenile form of hemochromatosis. Fertil Steril 2005; 84: 1744.

1358. Manno M, Marchesan E, Tomei F, et al. Polycystic kidney disease and infertility: case report and literature review. Arch Ital Urol Androl 2005; 77: 25–28.

1359. Li Vecchi M, Cianfrone P, Damiano R, et al. Infertility in adults with polycystic kidney disease. Nephrol Dial Transplant 2003; 18: 190–191.

1360. Fang S, Baker HW. Male infertility and adult polycystic kidney disease are associated with necrospermia. Fertil Steril 2003; 79: 643–644.

1361. Peces R, Venegas JL. Seminal vesicle cysts and infertility in autosomal dominant polycystic kidney disease. Nefrologia 2005; 25: 78–80.

1362. Behre HM, Kliesch S, Schadel F, et al. Clinical relevance of scrotal and transrectal ultrasonography in andrological patients. Int J Androl 1995; 2: 27–31.

1363. Van Steenbergen MW, Wit JM, Donckerwolcke RA. Testosterone esters advance skeletal maturation more than growth in short boys with chronic renal failure and delayed puberty. Eur J Pediatr 1991; 150: 676–680.

1364. Blackman MR, Weintraub BD, Kourides IA, et al. Discordant elevation of the common alpha subunit of the glycoprotein hormones compared to β subunits in serum of uremic patients. J Clin Endocinol Metab 1981; 53: 39–48.

1365. Holsdsworth S, Atkins RC, De Kretser DM. The pituitary testicular axis in men with chronic renal failure. N Engl J Med 1977; 296: 1245–1249.

1366. Elias AN, Vaziri ND, Farooqui S, et al. Pathology of endocrine organs in chronic renal failure. An autopsy analysis of 66 patients. Int J Artif Organs 1984; 7: 251–256.

1367. Guvel S, Pourbagher MA, Torun D, et al. Calcification of the epididymis and the tunica albuginea of the corpora cavernosa in patients on maintenance hemodialysis. J Androl 2004; 25: 752–756.

1368. Ketteler M, Vermeer C, Wanner C, et al. Novel insights into uremic vascular calcification: role of matrix Gla protein and alpha-2-heremans Schmid glycoprotein/fetuin Blood Purif 2002; 20: 473–476.

1369. Nistal M, Jimenez-Hefferman JA, Garcia-Viera M, et al. Cystic transformation and calcium oxalate deposits in rete testis and efferent ducts in dialysis patients. Hum Pathol 1996; 27: 336–341.

1370. Lim VS, Fang VS. Gonadal dysfunction in uremic men. A study of the hypothalamo-pituitary–testicular axis before and after renal transplantation. Am J Med 1975; 58: 655–662.

1371. Enmanouel DS, Lindheimer MD, Katz AI. Pathogenesis of endocrine abnormalities in uremia. Endocrinol Rev 1980; 1: 28–44.

1372. Cowden EA, Ratcliffe WA, Ratcliffe JG, et al. Hypothalamic–pituitary function in uremia. Acta Endocrinol 1981; 98: 488–495.

1373. El-Tawil AM. Zinc deficiency in men with Crohn's disease may contribute to poor sperm function and male infertility. Andrologia 2003; 35: 337–341.

1374. Hrudka F, Singh A. Sperm nucleomalacia in men with inflamatory bowel disease. Arch Androl 1984; 13: 37–57.

1375. Cosentino MJ, Chey WY, Takihara H, et al. The effects of sulphasalazine on human male fertility potencial and seminal prostaglandins. J Urol 1984; 132: 682–686.

1376. Chermesh I, Eliakim R. Mesalazine-induced reversible infertility in a young male. Dig Liver Dis 2004; 36: 551–552.

1377. Di Paolo MC, Paoluzi OA, Pica R, et al. Sulphasalazine and 5-aminosalicylic acid in long-term treatment of ulcerative colitis: report on tolerance and side-effects. Dig Liver Dis 2001; 33: 563–569.

1378. Hengge UR. Testosterone replacement for hypogonadism: clinical findings and best practices. AIDS Read 2003; 13: S15–21.

1379. Cohan GR. HIV-associated hypogonadism. AIDS Read 2006; 16: 341–345.

1380. Berger D, Muurahainen N, Wittert H, et al. Hypogonadism and wasting in the era of HAART in HIV-infected patients. Twelfth World AIDS Conference, Geneva, Switzerland, 1998 [Abstract 32174].

1381. Rietschel P, Corcoran C, Stanley T, et al. Prevalence of hypogonadism among men with weight loss related to human immunodeficiency virus infection who were receiving highly active antiretroviral therapy. Clin Infect Dis 2000; 31: 1240–1244.

1382. Grinspoon S, Corcoran C, Lee K, et al. Loss of lean body mass and muscle mass correlates with androgen levels in hypogonadal men with acquired immunodeficiency syndrome and wasting. J Clin Endocrinol Metab 1996; 81: 4051–4058.

1383. Grinspoon S, Corcoran C, Stanley T, et al. Effects of hypogonadism and testosterone administration on depression indices in HIV-infected men. J Clin Endocrinol Metab 2000; 85: 60–65.

1384. Wahlstrom JT, Tang A, Cofrancesco J, et al. Gonadal hormone levels in injection drug users. Drug Alcohol Depend 2000; 60: 311–313.

1385. Dobs S, Dempsey MA, Ladenson PW, et al. Endocrine disorders in men infected with human immunodeficiency virus. Am J Med 1988; 84: 611–616.

1386. Salehian B, Jacobson D, Swerdloff RS, et al. Testicular pathologic changes and the pituitary-testicular axis during human immunodeficiency virus infection. Endocrinol Pract 1999; 5: 1–9.

1387. Pintor C, Loche S, Puggioni R, et al. Adrenal and testicular function in boys affected by thalassemia. J Endocrinol Invest 1984; 7: 147–149.

1388. De Sanctis V, Roos M, Gasser T, et al. Italian Working Group on Endocrine Complications in Non-Endocrine Diseases. Impact of long-term iron chelation therapy on growth and endocrine functions in thalassaemia. J Pediatr Endocrinol Metab 2006; 19: 471–480.

1389. Al-Rimawi HS, Jallad MF, Amarin ZO, et al. Pubertal evaluation of adolescent boys with β-thalassemia major and delayed puberty. Fertil Steril 2006; 86: 886–890.

1390. Moayeri H, Oloomi Z. Prevalence of growth and puberty failure with respect to growth hormone and gonadotropins secretion in β-thalassemia major. Arch Iran Med 2006; 9: 329–334.

1391. De Sanctis V. Growth and puberty and its management in thalassaemia. Hormone Res 2002; 58: 72–79.

1392. Soliman AT, El-Zalabany MM, Ragab M, et al. Spontaneous and GnRH-provoked gonadotropin secretion and testosterone response to human chorionic gonadotropin in adolescent boys with thalassaemia major and delayed puberty. J Trop Pediatr 2000; 46: 79–85.

1393. Globerman H, Shen-Orr Z, Karnieli E, et al. Inhibin B in men with severe obesity and after weight reduction following gastroplasty. Endocrinol Res 2005; 31: 17–26.

1394. Norman RJ, Clark AM. Obesity and reproductive disorders: a review. Reprod Fertil Dev 1998; 10: 55–63.

1395. Pasquali R. Obesity, fat distribution and infertility. Maturitas 2006; 20: 363–371.

1396. Boe AS, Knappskog PM, Myhre AG, et al. Mutational analysis of the autoimmune regulator (AIRE) gene in sporadic autoimmune Addison's disease can reveal patients with unidentified autoimmune polyendocrine syndrome type l. Eur J Endocrinol 2002; 146: 519–522.

1397. Meyer G, Badenhoop K. Autoimmune regulator (AIRE) gene on chromosome 21: implications for autoimmune polyendocrinopathy-candidiasis-ectodermal dystrophy (APECED) any more common manifestations of endocrine autoimmunity. J Endocrinol Invest 2002; 25: 804–811.

1398. Smith BR, Furmaniak J. Adrenal and gonadal autoimmune diseases. J Clin Endocrinol Metab 1995; 80: 1502–1505.

1399. Krohn K, Uibo R, Aavik E, et al. Identification by molecular cloning of an autoantigen associated with Addison's disease as steroid 17 alpha-hydroxylase. Lancet 1992; 339: 770–773.

1400. Winqvist O, Gustafsson J, Rorsman F, et al. Two different cytochrome p450 enzymes are the adrenal antigens in autoimmune polyendocrine syndrome type I and Addison's disease. J Clin Invest 1993; 92: 2377–2385.

1401. Soderbergh A, Myhre AG, Ekwall O, et al. Prevalence and clinical associations of 10 defined autoantibodies in autoimmune polyendocrine syndrome type I. Clin Endocrinol Metab 2004; 89: 557–562.

1402. Trence DL, Morley JE, Handwerger BS. Polyglandular autoimmune syndromes. Am J Med 1984; 77: 107–116.

1403. Barkan AL, Kelch RP, Marshall JC. Isolated gonadotrope failure in the polyglandular autoimmune syndrome. N Engl J Med 1985; 312: 1535–1540.

1404. Faggiano A, Pisani A, Milone F, et al. Endocrine dysfunction in patients with Fabry disease. J Clin Endocrinol Metab 2006; 91: 4319–4325.

1405. Nistal M, Paniagua R, Picazo ML. Testicular and epididymal involvement in Fabry's disease. J Pathol 141: 113–124, 1983.

1406. Eng C, Guffon N, Wilcox WR, et al. Safety and efficacy of recombinant human alpha-galactosidase A replacement therapy in Fabry's disease. N Engl J Med 2001; 345: 9–16.

1407. Desnick RJ, Brady R, Barranger J, et al. Fabry disease, an under-recognized multisystemic disorder: expert recommendations for diagnosis, management, and enzyme replacement therapy. Ann Intern Med 2003; 138: 338–346.

1408. Schwarting A, Dehout F, Feriozzi S, et al. Enzyme replacement therapy and renal function in 201 patients with Fabry disease. Clin Nephrol 2006; 66: 77–84.

1409. Mosser J, Douar AM, Sarde CO, et al. Putative X-linked adrenoleukodystrophy gene shares unexpected homology with ABC transporters. Nature 1993; 361: 726–730.

1410. Graham GE, MacLeod PM, Lillicrap DP, et al. Gonadal mosaicism in a family with adreno-leukodystrophy. Molecular diagnosis of carrier status among daughters of a gonadal mosaic when direct detection of the mutation is not possible. J Inherit Metab Dis 1992; 15: 68–74.

1411. Jia Z, Pei Z, Li Y, et al. X-linked adrenoleukodystrophy: role of very long-chain acyl-CoA synthetases. Mol Genet Metab 2004; 83: 117–127.

1412. Libber SM, Migeon CJ, Brown FR, et al. Adrenal and testicular function in 14 patients with adrenoleukodystrophy or adrenomyeloneuropathy. Hormone Res 1986; 24: 1–8.

1413. Powers JM, Schaumburg HH. The testis in adreno-leukodystrophy. Am J Pathol 1981; 102: 90–98.

1414. Anderson RA, Rao N, Byrum RS, et al. In situ localization of the genetic locus encoding the lysosomal acid lipase/cholesteryl esterase (LIPA) deficient in Wolman disease to chromosome 10q23.2-q23.3. Genomics 1993; 15: 245–247.

1415. Contreras F, Alvarez l, Nistal M, et al. Enfermedad de Wolman. Estudio anatomopatológico de dos observaciones. Patología 1974; 7: 189–200.

1416. Elleder M, Chlumská A, Ledvinová J, et al. Testis – a novel storage site in human cholesteryl ester storage disease. Autopsy report of an adult case with a long-standing subclinical course complicated by accelerated atherosclerosis and liver carcinoma. Virchows Arch 2000; 436: 82–87.

1417. Stein J, Garty BZ, Dror Y, et al. Successful treatment of Wolman disease by unrelated umbilical cord blood transplantation. Eur J Pediatr 2007; 166: 663–555.

1418. Chik CL, Friedman A, Merriam GR, et al. Pituitary–testicular function in nephropathic cystinosis. Ann Intern Med 1993; 119: 568–575.

1419. Suzuki K, Suzuki K. Lysosomal diseases. In: Grahan DI, Lantos PL, eds. Greenfield's neuropathology, 7th edn. Oxford: Arnold, 2002; 673–712.

1420. Brinkworth MH, Handelsman DJ. Environmental influences on male reproductive health. In: Nieschlag S, Behre HM, eds. Andrology. Male reproductive health and dysfunction, 2nd edn. Berlin: Springer Verlag, 2000; 253–270.

1421. Schrag SD, Dixon RL. Occupational exposures associated with male reproductive dysfunction. Annu Rev Pharmacol Toxicol 1985; 25: 567–592.

1422. Swan SH. Semen quality in fertile US men in relation to geographical area and pesticide exposure. Int J Androl 2006; 29: 62–68.

1423. De Celis R, Feria-Velasco A, González-Unzaga M, et al. Semen quality of workers occupationally exposed to hydrocarbons. Fertil Steril 2000; 73: 221–228.

1424. Meyer CR. Semen quality in workers exposed to carbon disulfide compared to a control group from the same plant. J Occup Med 1981; 23: 435–439.

1425. Wagar G, Tolonen M, Stenman UH, Helpio E. Endocrinologic studies in men exposed occupationally to carbon disulfide. J Toxicol Environ Health 1981; 7: 363–371.

1426. Kapp RW Jr, Picciano DJ, Jacobson CB. Y-chromosomal nondysjunction in dibromochloropropane exposed workmen. Mutat Res 1979; 64: 47–51.

1427. Naha N, Chowdhury AR. Inorganic lead exposure in battery and paint factory: effect on human sperm structure and functional activity. J UOEH 2006; 28: 157–171.

1428. Lancranjan I, Popescu HI, Gavanescu O, et al. Reproductive ability of workmen occupationally exposed to lead. Arch Environ Health 1975; 30: 396–401.

1429. Cullen MR, Kayne RD, Robins JM. Endocrine and reproductive dysfunction in men associated with occupational inorganic lead intoxication. Arch Environ Health 1984; 39: 431–440.

1430. Harrington JM. Occupational exposure to synthetic estrogens: some methodological problems. Scand J Work Environ Health 1992; 8: 167–171.

1431. Gill WB, Schumacher GFB, Bibbo M, et al. Association of diethylstilbestrol exposure in utero with cryptorchidism, testicular hypoplasia and semen abnormalities. J Urol 1979; 122: 36–39.

1432. Hauser R, Meeker JD, Duty S, et al. Altered semen quality in relation to urinary concentrations of phthalate monoester and oxidative metabolites. Epidemiology 2006; 17: 682–691.

1433. Jurewicz J, Hanke W, Sobala W, et al. Current use of pesticides in Poland and the risk of reproductive disorders. Med Pr 2004; 55: 275–281.

1434. Hauser R. The environment and male fertility: recent research on emerging chemicals and semen quality. Semin Reprod Med 2006; 24: 156–167.

1435. Andersson A-M, Skakkebaek NE. Exposure to exogenous estrogens in food: possible impact on human development and health. Eur J Endocrinol 1999; 140: 477–485.

1436. Skakkebaek NS, Rajpert-De Meyts E, Main KM. Testicular dysgenesis syndrome; an increasingly common developmental disorder with environmental aspects. Hum Reprod 2001; 16: 972–978.

1437. Weber RF, Pierik FH, Dohle GR, Burdorf A. Environmental influences on male reproduction. BJU Int 2002; 89: 143–148.

1438. Whan LB, West MC, McClure N, Lewis SE. Effects of delta-9-tetrahydrocannabinol, the primary psychoactive cannabinoid in marijuana, on human sperm function in vitro. Fertil Steril 2006; 85: 653–660.

1439. Yang GS, Wang W, Wang YM, et al. Effect of cocaine on germ cell apoptosis in rats at different ages. Asian J Androl 2006; 8: 569–575.

1440. Muthusami KR, Chinnaswamy P. Effect of chronic alcoholism on male fertility hormones and semen quality. Fertil Steril 2005; 84: 919–924.

1441. Hassa H, Yildirim A, Can C, et al. Effect of smoking on semen parameters of men attending an infertility clinic. Clin Exp Obstet Gynecol 2006; 33: 19–22.

1442. Karila T, Hovatta O, Seppala T. Concomitant abuse of anabolic androgenic steroids and human chorionic gonadotrophin impairs spermatogenesis in power athletes. Int J Sports Med 2004; 25: 257–263.

1443. Ash P. The influence of radiation on fertility in man. Br J Radiol 1980; 53: 271–278.

1444. Lancrajan I, Maicanescu M, Rafaila E, et al. Gonadal function in workmen with long term exposure to microwaves. Health Phys 1975; 29: 381–383.

1445. Mieusset R, Bujan L, Mansat A, et al. Effects of artificial cryptorchidism on sperm morphology. Fertil Steril 1987; 47: 150–155.

1446. Dada R, Gupta NP, Kucheria K. Spermatogenic arrest in men with testicular hyperthermia. Teratog Carcinog Mutagen 2003; Suppl 1: 235–243.

1447. Peñafiel R, Solano F, Gramdes A. The effect of hyperthermia on ornithine decarboxylase activity in different rat tissue. Biochem Pharmacol 1988; 37: 497–502.

1448. Amendola R, Cordelli E, 'Mauro F, et al. Effects of L-acetylcarnitine (LAC) on the post-injury recovery of mouse spermatogenesis monitored by flow cytometry. Recovery after hyperthermic treatment. Andrologia 1991; 23: 135–140.

1449. Casillas ER, Erickson BJ. The role of carnitine in spermatozoa metabolism. Substrate induced elevations in the acetylation state of carnitine and coenzyme A in bovine and monkey spermatozoa. Biol Reprod 1975; 12: 275–283.

1450. Okuyama A, Koh E, Kondoh N, et al. In vitro temperature sensitivity of DNA, RNA, and protein synthesis throughout puberty in human testis. Arch Androl 1991; 26: 7–13.

1451. Lee JY, Cass AS, Streitz JM. Traumatic dislocation of testes and bladder rupture. Urology 1992; 40: 506–508.

1452. Lopez Alcina E, Martin JC, Fuster A, et al. Testicular dislocation. Report of 2 new cases and review of the literature. Actas Urol Esp 2001; 25: 299–302.

1453. Nagarajan VP, Pranikoff K, Imahori SC, et al. Traumatic dislocation of testis. Urology 1983; 22: 521–524.

1454. Kochakarn W, Choonhaklai V, Hotrapawanond P, et al. Traumatic testicular dislocation a review of 36 cases. J Med Assoc Thai 2000; 83: 208–212.

1455. Yoshimura K, Okubo K, Ichioka K, et al. Restoration of spermatogenesis by orchiopexy 13 years after bilateral traumatic testicular dislocation. J Urol 2002; 167: 649–650.

1456. Arai Y, Kawakita M, Okada Y, et al. Sexuality and fertility in long-term survivors of testicular cancer. J Clin Oncol 1997; 15: 1444–1448.

1457. Nicholson HS, Beyrne J. Fertility and pregnancy after treatment for cancer during childhood or adolescence. Cancer 1993; 71: 3392–3399.

1458. Piroth MD, Hensley F, Wannenmacher M, et al. Male gonadal dose in adjuvant 3-d-pelvic irradiation after anterior resection of rectal cancer. Influence to fertility. Strahlenther Onkol 2003; 179: 754–759.

1459. Hahn EW, Feingold SM, Simpson L, et al. Recovery from aspermia induced by low-dose radiation in seminoma patients. Cancer 1982; 50: 337–340.

1460. Speiser B, Rubin P, Casarett G. Aspermia following lower truncal irradiation in Hodgkin's disease. Cancer 1973; 32: 692–698.

1461. Freund I, Zenzes MA, Muller RP, et al. Testicular function in eight patients with seminoma after unilateral orchidectomy and radiotherapy. Int J Androl 1987; 10: 447–455.

1462. Fossa SD, Almaas B, Jetne V, et al. Paternity after irradiation for testicular cancer. Acta Radiol Oncol 1986; 25: 33–36.

1463. Esfahani AF, Eftekhari M, Zenooz N, Saghari M. Gonadal function in patients with differentiated thyroid cancer treated with (131)I. Hell J Nucl Med 2004; 7: 52–55.

1464. Erogul O, Oztas E, Yildirim I, et al. Effects of electromagnetic radiation from a cellular phone on human sperm motility: an in vitro study. Arch Med Res 2006; 37: 840–843.

1465. Müller J, Hertz H, Skakkebaek NE. Development of the seminiferous epithelium during and after treatment for acute lymphoblastic leukemia in childhood. Hormone Res 1988; 30: 115–120.

1466. Matus-Ridley M, Nicosia SV, Meadows AT. Gonadal effects of cancer therapy in boys. Cancer 1985; 55: 2353–2363.

1467. Brämswig JH, Heimes U, Heiermann E, et al. The effects of different cumulative doses of chemotherapy on testicular function. Cancer 1990; 65: 1298–1302.

1468. Meistrich ML, Wilson G, Brown BW, et al. Impact of cyclophosphamide on long-term reduction in sperm count in men treated with combination chemotherapy for Ewing and soft tissue sarcomas. Cancer 1992; 70: 2703–2712.

1469. Bar-Shira Maymon B, Yogev L, Marks A, et al. Sertoli cell inactivation by cytotoxic damage to the human testis after cancer chemotherapy. Fertil Steril 2004; 81: 1391–1394.

1470. Friedman NM, Plymate SR. Leydig cell dysfunction and gynaecomastia in adult males treated with alkylating agents. Clin Endocrinol 1980; 12: 553–556.

1471. Chatterjee R, Haines GA, Perera DM, et al. Testicular and sperm DNA damage after treatment with fludarabine for chronic lymphocytic leukaemia. Hum Reprod 2000; 15: 762–766.

1472. Howell SJ, Shalet SM. Spermatogenesis after cancer treatment: damage and recovery. J Natl Cancer Inst Monogr 2005; 34: 12–17.

1473. van den Berg H, Furstner F, van den Bos C, Behrendt H. Decreasing the number of MOPP courses reduces gonadal damage in survivors of childhood Hodgkin disease. Pediatr Blood Cancer 2004; 42: 210–215.

1474. Delbes G, Hales BF, Robaire B. Effects of the chemotherapy cocktail used to treat testicular cancer on sperm chromatin integrity. J Androl 2007; 28: 241–249.

1475. Spermon JR, Ramos L, Wetzels AM, et al. Sperm integrity pre- and post-chemotherapy in men with testicular germ cell cancer. Hum Reprod 2006; 21: 1781–1786.

1476. Viviani S, Ragni G, Santoro A, et al. Testicular dysfunction in Hodgkin's disease before and after treatment. Eur J Cancer 1991; 27: 1389–1392.

1477. Fossa SD, Ous S, Byholm T, et al. Posttreatment fertility in patients with testicular cancer. Part 1. Br J Urol 1985; 57: 204–209.

1478. Nijman JM, Schraffordt Koops H, et al. Sexual function after bilateral retroperitoneal lymph node dissection for nonseminomatous testicular cancer. Arch Androl 1987; 18: 255–267.

1479. Bennett CJ, Seager SW, Vasher EA, et al. Sexual dysfunction and electroejaculation in men with spinal cord injury: review. J Urol 1988; 139: 453–457.

1480. Murphy JB, Lipschultz LI, Vervoort SM. Infertilty in the spinal cord injuried male. World J Urol 1986; 4: 83–87.

1481. Perkash I, Martin DE, Warner H, et al. Reproductive biology of paraplegics: Results of semen collection, testicular biopsy and serum hormone evaluation. J Urol 1985; 134: 284–288.

1482. Siösteen A, Steen Y, Forssman L, et al. Auto-immunity to spermatozoa and quality of semen in men with spinal cord injury. Int J Fertil 1993; 38: 117–122.

1483. Leriche A, Berard E, Vauzelle JL, et al. Histological and hormonal testicular changes in spinal cord patients. Paraplegia 1977–1978; 15: 274–279.

1484. Brown DJ, Hill ST, Baker HW. Male fertility and sexual function after spinal cord injury. Prog Brain Res 2006; 152: 427–439.

1485. Kafetsoulis A, Brackett NL, Ibrahim E, et al. Current trends in the treatment of infertility in men with spinal cord injury. Fertil Steril 2006; 86: 781–789.

1486. Holstein AF, Sauerwein D, Schirren U. Spermatogenese bei Patienten mit traumatischer Querschnittähmung. Urologe A 1985; 24: 208–215.

1487. Brindley GS. Deep scrotal temperature and the effect on it of clothing, air, temperature, activity, posture and paraplegia. Br J Urol 1982; 54: 49–55.

1488. Chapelle PA, Roby-Brami A, Yakovleff A, et al. Neurological correlations of ejaculation and testicular size in men with a complete spinal cord section. J Neurol Neurosurg Psychiatry 1988; 51: 197–202.

1489. Aird IA, Vince GS, Bates MD, et al. Leukocytes in semen from men with spinal cord injuries. Fertil Steril 1999; 72: 97–103.

1490. Trabulsi EJ, Shupp-Byrne D, Sedor J, Hirsch IH. Leukocyte subtypes in electroejaculates of spinal cord injured men. Arch Phys Med Rehab 2002; 83: 31–34.

1491. Basu S, Aballa TC, Ferrel SM, et al. Inflammatory cytokine concentrations are elevated in seminal plasma of men with spinal cord injuries. J Androl 2004; 25: 250–254.

1492. Elliott SP, Orejuela F, Hirsch IH, et al. Testis biopsy findings in the spinal cord injured patient. J Urol 2000; 163: 792–795.

1493. Ohl DA, Menge AC, Jarow JP. Seminal vesicle aspiration in spinal cord injured men: insight into poor sperm quality. J Urol 1999; 162: 2048–2051.

1494. Brackett NL, Lynne CM, Aballa TC, et al. Sperm motility from the vas deferens of spinal cord injured men is higher than from the ejaculate. J Urol 2000; 164: 712–715.

1495. Wieder JA, Lynne cm, Ferrell SM, et al. Brown-colored semen in men with spinal cord injury. J Androl 1999; 20: 594–600.

1496. Casella R, Leibundgut B, Lehmann K, et al. Mumps orchitis: report of a mini-epidemic. J Urol 1997; 158: 2158–2161.

1497. Masarani M, Wazait H, Dinneen M. Mumps orchitis. J Roy Soc Med 2006; 99: 573–575.

1498. Duszczyk E, Krynicka-Czech B, Talarek E, Popielska J. Mumps – an underestimated disease. Przegl Epidemiol 2006; 60: 99–104.

1499. Shulman A, Shohat B, Gillis D, et al. Mumps orchitis among soldiers: frequency, effect on sperm quality, and sperm antibodies. Fertil Steril 1992; 57: 1344–1346.

1500. Diehl K, Hondl H. Mumps orchitis: symptoms and treatment possibilities. Zeitschr Urol Nephrol 1990; 83: 243–247.

1501. Charny CW, Meranze DR. Pathology of mumps orchitis. J Urol 1948; 60: 140–146.

1502. Lin YM, Hsu CC, Lin JS. Successful testicular sperm extraction and fertilization in an azoospermic man with postpubertal mumps orchitis. BJU Int 1999; 83: 526–527.

1503. Mikuz G, Damjanov I. Inflammation of the testis, epididymis, peritesticular membranes and scrotum. Pathol Annu 1982; 1: 101–128.

1504. Ejlertsen T, Jensen HK. Orchitis and testicular abscess formation caused by non-typhoid salmonellosis. APMIS 1990; 98: 294–298.

1505. Jani AN, Casibang V, Mufarrij W. Disseminated actinomycosis presenting as a testicular mass. A case report. J Urol 1990; 143: 1012–1014.

1506. Lin CY, Jwo SC, Lin CC. Primary testicular actinomycosis mimicking metastatic tumor. Int J Urol 2005; 12: 519–521.

1507. Nistal M, Gonzalez-Peramato P, Serrano A, Regadera J. Xanthogranulomatous funiculitis and orchiepididymitis: report of 2 cases with immunohistochemical study and literature review. Arch Pathol Lab Med 2004; 128: 911–914.

1508. Almagro UA, Tresp M, Sheth NK. Tuberculous epididymitis occurring 35 years after renal tuberculosis. J Urol 1989; 141: 1204–1205.

1509. Cabral DA, Johnson HW, Coleman GU, et al. Tuberculous epididymitis as a cause of testicular pseudomalignancy in two young children. Pediatr Infect Dis 1985; 4: 59–62.

1510. Wolf JS Jr, McAninch JW. Tuberculous epididymo-orchitis. Diagnosis by fine needle aspiration. J Urol 1991; 145: 836–838.

1511. Stein AL, Miller DB. Tuberculous epididymo-orchitis. A case report. J Urol 1983; 129: 613.

1512. Harada H, Seki M, Shinojima H, et al. Epididymo-orchitis caused by intravesically instilled bacillus Calmette–Guérin: genetically proven using a multiplex polymerase chain reaction method. Int J Urol 2006; 13: 183–185.

1513. Persaud V, Rao A. Gumma of testis. Br J Urol 1977; 49: 142–143.

1514. Akhtar M, Alli MA, Mackey DM. Lepromatous leprosy presenting as orchitis. Am J Clin Pathol 1980; 73: 712–715.

1515. Kumar B, Raina A, Kraur S, et al. Clinicopathological study of testicular involvement in leprosy. Indian J Lepr 1982; 54: 48–55.

1516. Richens J. Genital manifestations of tropical diseases. Sex Transm Infect 2004; 80: 12–17.

1517. Fallatah SM, Oduloju AJ, Al-Dusari SN, Fakunle YM. Human brucellosis in Northern Saudi Arabia. Saudi Med J 2005; 26: 1562–1566.

1518. Yetkin MA, Erdinc FS, Bulut C, Tulek N. Epididymoorchitis due to brucellosis in central Anatolia, Turkey. Urol Int 2005; 75: 235–238.

1519. Romero-Perez P, Navarro-Ibañez V, Amat-Cecilia M, et al. Brucellar orchiepididymitis in acute brucellosis. Actas Urol Esp 1995; 19: 330–332.

1520. Reisman EM, Colquitt LA, Childers J, et al. Brucella orchitis: a rare cause of testicular enlargement. J Urol 1990; 143: 821–822.

1521. Perez Fentes D, Blanco Parra M, Alende Sixto M, et al. Orquioepididimitis brucelosa: A propósito de un caso. Arch Esp Urol 2005; 58: 674–677.

1522. Queipo-Ortuno MI, Colmenero JD, Munoz N, et al. Rapid diagnosis of Brucella epididymo-orchitis by real-time polymerase chain reaction assay in urine samples. J Urol 2006; 176: 2290–2293.

1523. Ryan DM, Lesser BA, Crumley LA, et al. Epididymal sarcoidosis. J Urol 1993; 149: 134–136.

1524. Handa T, Nagai S, Hamada K, et al. Sarcoidosis with bilateral epididymal and testicular lesions. Intern Med 2003; 42: 92–97.

1525. Metcalfe MS, Rees Y, Morgan P, et al. Sarcoidosis presenting as a testicular mass. Br J Urol 1998; 82: 769–770.

1526. Wong JA, Grantmyre J. Sarcoid of the testis. Can J Urol 2006; 13: 3201–3203.

1527. Singer AJ, Gavrell GJ, Leidich RB, et al. Genitourinary involvement of systemic sarcoidosis confined to testicle. Urology 1990; 35: 422–444.

1528. Blacher EJ, Maynard JF. Seminoma and sarcoidosis: an unusual association. Urology 1985; 26: 288–289.

1529. Svetec DA, Waguespack RL, Sabanegh ES Jr. Intermittent azoospermia associated with epididymal sarcoidosis. Fertil Steril 1998; 70: 777–779.

1530. Michaelis L, Gutmann C. Ueber Einschlüsse in Blastumoren. Ztschr Klin Med 1902; 47: 208–215.

1531. McClure J. A case of malacoplakia of the epididymis associated with trauma. J Urol 1980; 124: 934–935.

1532. Kusuma V, Niveditha SR, Krishnamurthy, Ramdev K. Epididymo-testicular malacoplakia – a case report. Indian J Pathol Microbiol 2006; 49: 413–415.

1533. Saraf P, Disant'Agnese P, Valvo J, et al. An unusual case of malakoplakia involving the testis and prostate. J Urol 1983; 129: 149–151.

1534. Díaz-González R, Leiva D, Navas-Palacios JJ, et al. Testicular malacoplakia. J Urol 1982; 127: 325–328.

1535. Nistal M, Rodríguez Echandía EL, Paniagua R. Septate junctions between digestive vacuoles in human malakoplakia. Tissue Cell 1978; 10: 137–142.

1536. Orr WA, Mulholland SG, Walzak Jr MP. Genitourinary tract involvement with systemic mycosis. J Urol 1972; 107: 1047–1150.

1537. Dykes TM, Stone AB, Canby-Hagino ED. Coccidioidomycosis of the epididymis and testis. AJR Am J Roentgenol 2005; 84: 552–553.

1538. James CL, Lomax-Smith JD. Cryptococcal epididymoorchitis complicating steroid therapy for releasing polychondritis. Pathology 1991; 23: 256–258.

1539. Alves LS, Assis BP, Rezende MM. Schistosomal epididymitis. Int Braz J Urol 2004; 30: 413–415.

1540. Nistal M, Santana A, Paniagua R, et al. Testicular toxoplasmosis in two men with the acquired immunodeficiency syndrome (AIDS). Arch Pathol Lab Med 1986; 110: 744–746.

1541. Strohmaier WL, Bichler KH, Wilbert DM, et al. Alveolar echinococcosis with involvement of the ureter and testes. J Urol 1990; 144: 733–734.

1542. Martinez-Rodriguez M, Navarro Fos S, Soriano Sarrio P, et al. Idiopathic granulomatous orchitis: pathologic study of one case. Arch Esp Urol 2006; 59: 725–727.

1543. Sato K, Hirokawa K, Hatakeyana S. Experimental allergic orchitis in mice. Histopathological and immunological studies. Virchows Arch [Pathol Anat] 1981; 392: 147–158.

1544. Lehmann D, Emmons LR. Immunological phenomena observed in the testis and their possible role in infertility. Am J Reprod Immunol 1989; 19: 43–52.

1545. El-Demiry MI, Hargreave TB, Bussuttil A. Immunocompetent cells in human testis in health and disease. Fertil Steril 1987; 48: 470–479.

1546. Suominen JJ. Sympathetic auto-immune orchitis. Andrologia 1995; 27: 213–216.

1547. Hendry WF, Levison DA, Parkinson MC, et al. Testicular obstruction: clinicopathological studies. Ann Roy Coll Surg Engl 1990; 72: 396–407.

1548. Lehmann J, Jancke C, Retz M, et al. Hypoechoic Lesion found on testicular ultrasound after testicular piercing. J Urol 2000; 164: 1651.

1549. Nistal M, Riestra ML, Paniagua R. Focal orchitis in undescended testes: discussion of pathogenetic mechanisms of tubular atrophy. Arch Pathol Lab Med 2002; 126: 64–69.

1550. Jass JR, Farrell MA, Ellis H. Pseudolymphoma of the testis. Br J Urol 1984; 56: 102–103.

1551. Algaba F, Santaularia JM, Garat JM, Cubells J. Testicular pseudolymphoma. Eur Urol 1986; 12: 362–363.

1552. Aksoy PK, Ozdemir BH, Aygun C, Agildere M. Plasma cell granuloma of the testis: unusual localization. J Urol 2001; 166: 1000.

1553. Anghel G, Petti N, Remotti D, et al. Testicular plasmacytoma: report of a case and review of the literature. Am J Hematol 2002; 71: 98–104.

1554. Lossos IS, Okon E, Bogomolski-Yahalom V, et al. Sinus histiocytosis with massive lymphadenopathy (Rosai–Dorfman disease): report of a patient with isolated renotesticular involvement after cure of non-Hodgkin's lymphoma. Ann Hematol 1997; 74: 41–44.

1555. Fernandopulle SM, Hwang JS, Kuick CH, et al. Rosai–Dorfman disease of the testis: an unusual entity that mimics testicular malignancy. J Clin Pathol 2006; 59: 325–327.

1556. Cox NH, Popple AW. Persistent erythema and pruritus, with a confluent histiocytic skin infiltrate, following the use of a hydroxyethylstarch plasma expander. Br J Dermatol 1996; 134: 353–357.

1557. Schned AR, Selikowitz SM. Epididymitis nodosa. An epididymal lesion analogous to vasitis nodosa. Arch Pathol Lab Med 1986; 110: 61–64.

1558. Adams PC, Holt P, Holt DW. Amiodarone in testis and semen. Lancet 1985; 1: 341.

1559. Dobs AS, Sarma PS, Guarnieri T, Griffith L. Testicular dysfunction with amiodarone use. J Am Coll Cardiol 1991; 18: 1328–1332.

1560. Gasparich JP, Mason JT, Green HL, et al. Non-infectious epididymitis associated with amiodarone therapy. Lancet 2: 1211–1212, 1984.

1561. Sadek l, Biron P, Kus T. Amiodarone-induced epididymitis: report of a new case and literature review of 12 cases. Can J Cardiol 1993; 9: 833–836.

1562. Kirkali Z. Amiodarone-induced sterile epididymitis. Urol Int 43: 372–373, 1988.

1563. Gabal-Shehab LL, Monga M. Recurrent bilateral amiodarone induced epididymitis. J Urol 1999; 161: 921.

1564. Hutcheson J, Peters CA, Diamond DA. Amiodarone induced epididymitis in children. J Urol 1998; 160: 515–517.

1565. Hamoud Kaneti J, Smailowitz Z, Lissmer L. Amiodarone-induced epididymitis. Report of 2 cases. Eur Urol 1996; 29: 497–498.

1566. Nistal M, Mate A, Paniagua R. Granulomatous epididymal lesion of possible ischemic origin. Am J Surg Pathol 1997; 21: 951–956.

1567. Ellis H, Hutton PA. A stone in the testicle. Br J Urol 1983; 55: 449.

1568. Dayanc M, Kilciler M, Kibar Y, et al. Testicular calculus. J Urol 2000; 163: 1253–1254.

1569. O'Regan S, Robitaille P. Orchitis mimicking testicular torsion in Henoch–Schönlein's purpura. J Urol 1981; 126: 834–835.

1570. Davenport A, Downey SE, Goel S, et al. Wegener's granulomatosis involving the urogenital tract. Br J Urol 1996; 78: 354–357.

1571. Barber TD, Al-Omar O, Poulik J, McLorie GA. Testicular infarction in a 12-year-old boy with Wegener's granulomatosis. Urology 2006; 67: 846.e9–10.

1572. Vollerten RS, McDonald TJ, Younge BR, et al. Cogan's syndrome: 18 cases and a review of the literature. Mayo Clin Proc 1986; 61: 344–361.

1573. Karlamani VG, Vaiopoulos G, Markomichelakis N, et al. Recurrent epididymo-orchitis in patients with Behçet's disease. J Urol 2000; 163: 487–489.

1574. Nigro KG, Abdul-Karim FW, Maclennan GT. Testicular vasculitis. J Urol 2006; 176: 2682.

1575. Persellin ST, Menke DM. Isolated polyarteritis nodosa of the male reproductive system. J Rheumatol 1992; 19: 985–988.

1576. Mukamel E, AbarbaneL J, Savion M, et al. Testicular mass as presenting symptom of isolated polyarteritis nodosa. Am J Clin Pathol 1995; 103: 215–217.

1577. Dahl EV, Baggenstoss AH, DeWeerd JH. Testicular lesions of periarteritis nodosa, with special reference to diagnosis. Am J Med 1960; 28: 222–226.

1778. Teichman JM, Mattrey RF, Demby AM, Schmidt JD. Polyarteritis nodosa presenting as acute orchitis: A case report and review of the literature. J Urol 1993; 149: 1139–1140.

1579. Kessel A, Toubi E, Golan, TD, et al. Isolated epididymal vasculitis. Isr Med Assoc J 2001; 3: 65–66.

1580. Fraenkel-Rubin M, Ergas D, Sthoeger ZM. Limited polyarteritis nodosa of the male and female reproductive systems: diagnostic and therapeutic approach. Ann Rheum Dis 2002; 61: 362–364.

1581. Huisman TK, Collins WT, Voulgarakis GR. Polyarteritis nodosa masquerading as a primary testicular neoplasm. A case report and review of the literature. J Urol 1990; 114: 1236–1238.

1582. Shurbaji MS, Epstein JI. Testicular vasculitis: Implication for systemic disease. Hum Pathol 1988; 19: 186–189.

1583. Nistal M, Alcoba M, Contreras F. Torsión del cordón espermático. A propósito de 87 nuevos casos. Revisión de la literatura. Arch Esp Urol 1971; 24: 385–398.

1584. Das S, Singer D. Controversies of perinatal torsion of the spermatic cord: a review, survey and recommendations. J Urol 1990; 143: 231–233.

1585. Arena F, Nicotina PA, Romeo C, et al. Prenatal testicular torsion: ultrasonographic features, management and histopathological findings. Int J Urol 2006; 13: 135–141.

1586. Cuckow PM, Frank JD. Torsion of the testis. BJU Int 2000; 86: 349–353.

1587. Davol P, Simmons J. Testicular torsion in a 68-year-old man. Urology 2005; 66: 195.

1588. Mikuz G. Testicular torsion: simple grading for histological evaluation of tissues damage. Appl Pathol 1985; 3: 134–139.

1589. Nistal M, Martinez C, Paniagua R. Primary testicular lesions in the twisted testis. Fertil Steril 1992; 57: 381–386.

1590. Granados EA, Caicedo P, Garat JM. Torsión testicular antes de 6 horas.I. Arch Esp Urol 1998; 51: 971–974.

1591. Tryfonas G, Violaki A, Tsikopoulos G, et al. Late postoperative results in males treated for testicular torsion during childhood. J Pediatr Surg 1994; 29: 553–556.

1592. Arda IS, Ozyaylali L. Testicular tissue bleeding as an indicator of gonadal salvageability in testicular torsion surgery. BJU Int 2001; 87: 89–92.

1593. Johnston BI, Wiener JS. Intermittent testicular torsion. BJU Int 2005; 95: 933–934.

1594. Nistal M, Gonzalez-Peramato P, Paniagua R. Lipomembranous fat necrosis in three cases of testicular torsion. Histopathology 2001; 38: 443–447.

1595. Kosar A, Küpeli B, Alcigir G, et al. Immunologic aspects of testicular torsion: detection of antisperm antibodies in contralateral testicle. Eur Urol 1999; 36: 640–644.

1596. Akgür FM, Kilinç K, Tanyel FC, et al. Ipsilateral and contralateral testicular biochemical acute changes after unilateral testicular torsion and detorsion. Urology 1994; 44: 413–418.

1597. Hadziselimovic F, Geneto R, Emmons LR. Increased apoptosis in the contralateral testes of patients with testicular torsion as a factor for infertility. J Urol 1998; 160: 1158–1160.

1598. Laor E, Fisch S, Tennenbaum S, et al. Unilateral testicular torsion: abnormal histological findings in the contralateral testis. Cause or effect? Br J Urol 1990; 65: 520–523.

1599. Tomomasa H, Oshio S, Ameniya H, et al. Testicular injury. Late results of semen analyses after orchiectomy. Arch Androl 1992; 29: 59–63.

1600. Wantz GE. Testicular atrophy as a sequela of inguinal hernioplasty. Int Surg 1986; 71: 159–163.

1601. Rutledge RH. Cooper's ligament repair for adult growing hernias. Surgery 1980; 87: 601–610.

1602. Roach R, Messing E, Starling J. Spontaneous thrombosis of left spermatic vein: Report of 2 cases. J Urol 1985; 134: 369–373.

1603. Nistal M, Palacios J, Regadera J, et al. Postsurgical focal testicular infarct. Urol Int 1986; 41: 149–151.

1604. Nawrocki JD, Cook AJ. Localised infarction of the testis. Br J Urol 1992; 69: 541.

1605. Sriprasad S, Kooiman GG, Muir GH, Sidhu PS. Acute segmental testicular infarction: differentiation from tumour using high frequency colour Doppler ultrasound. Br J Radiol 2001; 74: 965–967.

1606. Cooper AP. Observations on the structure and diseases of the testis. London: S McDowall, 1930; 79.

1607. Jenkins RH, Deming CL. Cysts of the testicle. N Engl J Med 1935; 213: 57–59.

1608. Sethney HT, Albers DD. Tunica albuginea cyst: rare testicular mass. Urology 1980; 15: 285–286.

1609. Leung ML, Gooding GAW, Williams RD. High-resolution sonography of scrotal contents in asymptomatic subjects. AJR Am J Roentgenol 1984; 143: 161–164.

1610. Haas GP, Shumaker BP, Cerny JC. The high incidence of benign testicular tumors. J Urol 1987; 138: 1219–1220.

1611. Gooding GAW, Leonhardt W, Stein R. Testicular cysts. US findings. Radiology 1987; 163: 537–538.

1612. Rubenstein RA, Dogra VS, Seftel AD, Resnick MI. Benign intrascrotal lesions. J Urol 2004; 71: 1765–1772.

1613. Bhatt S, Rubens DJ, Dogra VS. Sonography of benign intrascrotal lesions. Ultrasound Q 2006; 22: 121–136.

1614. Nistal M, Íñiguez L, Paniagua R. Cysts of the testicular parenchyma and tunica albuginea. Arch Pathol Lab Med 1989; 113: 902–906.

1615. Bryant J. Efferent ductule cyst of tunica albuginea. Urology 1986; 27: 172–173.

1616. Tejada E, Eble JN. Simple cyst of the rete testis. J Urol 1988; 139: 376–377.

1617. Davis RS. Intratesticular spermatocele. Urology 1998; 51: 67–169.

1618. Tosi SE, Richardson J. Simple cyst of the testis: case report and review of literature. J Urol 1975; 114: 473–475.

1619. Schmidt SS. Congenital simple cysts of the testis: a hitherto undescribed lesion. J Urol 1966; 96: 236–238.

1620. Takihara H, Valvo JR, Tokuhara M, et al. Intratesticular cysts. Urology 1982; 20: 80–82.

1621. Hamm B, Fobbe F, Loy V. Testicular cysts: Differentiation with US and clinical findings. Radiology 1988; 168: 19–23.

1622. Ceylan H, Karaca I, Sari I, et al. Simple testicular cyst: A rare cause of scrotal swelling in infancy. Int J Urol 2004; 11: 352–354.

1623. Lam KY. Bilateral intratesticular cysts. A specific entity. Scand J Urol Nephrol 1996; 30: 329–331.

1624. Sahin A, Ozen H, Gedikoglu G, et al. Two simple cysts of the same testis. Br J Urol 1994; 73: 107–108.

1625. Frater K. Cysts of the tunica albuginea (cysts of the testis). J Urol 1929; 21: 135–136.

1626. Arcadi JA. Cysts of the tunica albuginea testis. J Urol 1952; 68: 631–632.

1627. Mennemeyer RP, Mason JT. Non-neoplastic cystic lesions of the tunica albuginea: an electron microscopic and clinical study of 2 cases. J Urol 1979; 121: 373–375.

1628. Mancilla-Jiménez R, Matsuda GT. Cysts of the tunica albuginea: report of 4 cases and review of the literature. J Urol 1975; 114: 730–733.

1629. Warner KE, Noyes DT, Ross JS. Cysts of the tunica albuginea: a report of 3 cases with a review of the literature. J Urol 1984; 132: 131–132.

1630. Köbarth K, Kratzik CH. High resolution ultrasonography in the diagnosis of simple intratesticular cysts. J Urol 1992; 70: 546–549.

1631. Rifkin MD, Jacobs JA. Simple testicular cyst diagnosed preoperatively by ultrasound. J Urol 1983; 129: 982–983.

1632. Kratzik C, Hainz A, Kuber W, et al. Surveillance strategy for intratesticular cysts: preliminary report. J Urol 1990; 143: 313–315.

1633. Altadonna V, Snyder HM, Rosenberg HK, et al. Simple cysts of the testis in children: Preoperative diagnosis by ultrasound and excision with testicular preservation. J Urol 1988; 140: 1505–1507.

1634. Nistal M, Jimenez-Hefferman JA. Rete testis dysgenesis. A characteristic lesion of undescended testes. Arch Pathol Lab Med 1997; 121: 1259–1264.

1635. Lee KH, Hess RA, Bahr JM, et al. Estrogen receptor alpha has a functional role in the mouse rete testis and efferent ductules. Biol Reprod 2000; 63: 1873–1880.

1636. Nistal M, Mate A, Paniagua R. Cystic transformation of the rete testis. Am J Surg Pathol 1996; 20: 1231–1239.

1637. Colangelo SM, Fried K, Hyacinthe LM, et al. Tubular ectasia of the rete testis: an ultrasound diagnosis. Urology 1995; 45: 532–534.

1638. Pascual Mateo C, Fernandez Gonzalez I, Lujan Galan M, et al. Cystic ectasia of the rete testis. Arch Esp Urol 2006; 59: 55–58.

1639. Meyer DR, Huppe T, Lock U, et al. Pronounced cystic transformation of the rete testis. MRI appearance. Invest Radiol 1999; 34: 600–603.

1640. Wilschanski M, Corey M, Durie P, et al. The diversity of reproductive tract abnormalities in males with cystic fibrosis. JAMA 1996; 276: 607–608.

1641. Tchetgen MB, Wolf JS Jr. Postsurgical changes in the testis: a diagnostic dilemma. Urology 1998; 51: 333–334.

1642. Nistal M, Santamaría L, Paniagua R. Acquired cystic transformation of the rete testis secondary to renal failure. Hum Pathol 1989; 20: 1065–1070.

1643. Nistal M, Paniagua R. Adenomatous hyperplasia of the rete testis. J Pathol 1988; 154: 343–346.

1644. Nistal M, Castillo MC, Regadera J, Garcia-Cabezas MA. Adenomatous hyperplasia of the rete testis. A review and report of new cases. Histol Histopathol 2003; 18: 741–752.

1645. Nistal M, García-Villanueva M, Sánchez J. Displasia quística del testículo: anomalia en la diferenciación del parénquima testicular por probable fallo en la conexión entre los conductos de origen mesonéfrico y los cordones testiculares. Arch Esp Urol 1976; 29: 431–444.

1646. Uguz A, Gonlusen G, Ergin M, Tunali N. Adenomatous hyperplasia of the rete testis: report of two cases. Int Urol Nephrol 2002; 34: 87–89.

1647. Channer JL, MacIver AG. Glandular changes in the rete testis: metastatic tumour or adenomatous hyperplasia? [Letter] J Pathol 1989; 157: 81–83.

1648. Srigley JR, Hartwick RW. Tumors and cysts of the paratesticular region. Pathol Annu 1990; 25: 51–108.

1649. Hartwick RW, Ro JY, Srigley JR, et al. Adenomatous hyperplasia of the rete testis. A clinicopathologic study of nine cases. Am J Surg Pathol 1991; 15: 350–357.

1650. Nistal M, Gonzalez-Peramato P, Regadera J, et al. Primary testicular lesions are associated with testicular germ cell tumors of adult men. Am J Surg Pathol 2006; 30: 1260–1268.

1651. Badoual C, Cohen C, Michenet P, et al. Adénome du rete testis. Ann Pathol 1999; 19: 80–81.

1652. Nochomovitz LE, Orenstein JM. Adenocarcinoma of the rete testis: case report, ultrastructural observations, and clinicopathologic correlates. Am J Surg Pathol 1984; 8: 625–634.

1653. Skinnider BF, Young RH. Infarcted adenomatoid tumor: a report of five cases of a facet of a benign neoplasm that may cause diagnostic difficulty. Am J Surg Pathol 2004; 28: 77–83.

1654. Ulbright TM, Gersell DJ. Rete testis hyperplasia with hyaline globule formation. A lesion simulating yolk sac tumor. Am J Surg Pathol 1991; 15: 66–74.

1655. Nistal M, Paniagua R. Nodular proliferation of calcifying connective tissue in the rete testis: A study of three cases. Hum Pathol 1989; 20: 58–61.

THE LIBRARY
THE ... ING AND DEVELOPMENT CENTRE
THE ... HOSPITAL
HALIFAX HX3 0PW

# CHAPTER 13

# Neoplasms of the testis

Thomas M. Ulbright, Robert E. Emerson

Although it weighs only about 19 g,[1] the testis is responsible for a complex array of neoplasms. The rapidly proliferating spermatogenic cells give rise to the majority of testicular tumors, 95% of which are of germ cell derivation. Most are malignant and usually occur in young men, but they can be cured by current therapies; accurate diagnosis is therefore essential. The supporting cells and interstitial cells of the testis may give rise to the uncommon sex-cord stromal tumors that are responsible for a disproportionate number of diagnostic problems. Some of these are associated with clinical syndromes that may be detected from the testicular pathology.[2-7] A number of tumors of soft tissue origin may be identified in the paratestis, and secondary tumors are relatively frequent in both the testis and the paratestis. The spectrum of lesions and the capacity of many tumors to mimic others make testicular neoplasia a continuing challenge to surgical pathologists.

## Staging

The currently recommended staging system for testicular cancer is that of the American Joint Committee on Cancer (AJCC), published in 2002.[8] Its subdivisions are shown in Table 13-1. Serum marker studies play a key role in the evaluation of patients with testicular germ cell tumors, so the values of serum α-fetoprotein (AFP), human chorionic gonadotropin (hCG) and lactate dehydrogenase (LDH) were incorporated into the determination of the stage groupings.

## Patterns of metastasis

Testicular neoplasms usually first metastasize to retroperitoneal lymph nodes. There tends to be selective lymph node involvement with early-stage tumors, which depends on whether the right or left testis is involved. For right-sided tumors the interaortocaval nodes at about the level of the second lumbar vertebra are usually first involved, although right paracaval and precaval involvement may also occur.[9,10] In early-stage involvement from right-sided tumors there is an absence of both suprahilar nodal involvement and involvement of the left para-aortic nodes below the inferior mesenteric artery (Fig. 13-1).[10] For left-sided tumors the left para-aortic nodes, in an area bounded by the left ureter, left renal vein, aorta, and origin of the inferior mesenteric artery, are first involved.[9] Suprahilar nodal metastases may be seen

**Table 13-1** AJCC staging system for testicular cancer

| Stage TNM system | | | | Grouping |
|---|---|---|---|---|
| TX Unknown status of testis | | | | Stage 0 – Tis, N0, M0, S0 |
| T0 No apparent primary (includes scars) | | | | Stage IA – T1, N0, M0, S0 |
| Tis Intratubular tumor, no invasion | | | | Stage IB – T2-T4, N0, M0, S0 |
| T1 Testis and epididymis only; no vascular invasion or penetration of tunica albuginea | | | | Stage IS – any T, N0, M0, S1-S3 |
| T2 Testis and epididymis with vascular invasion or through tunica albuginea to involve tunica vaginalis | | | | Stage IIA – any T, N1, M0, S0-S1 |
| T3 Spermatic cord | | | | Stage IIB – any T, N2, M0, S0-S1 |
| T4 Scrotum | | | | Stage IIC – any T, N3, M0, S0-S1 |
| NX Unknown nodal status | | | | Stage IIIA – any T, any N, M1a, S0-S1 |
| N0 No regional node involvement | | | | Stage IIIB – any T, any N, M0-M1a, S2 |
| N1 Node mass or single nodes ≤2 cm; ≤5 nodes involved; no node >2 cm | | | | Stage IIIC – any T, any N, M0-M1a, S3 |
| N2 Node mass >2 but ≤5 cm; or >5 nodes involved, none >5 cm; or extranodal tumor | | | | any T, any N, M1b, any S |
| N3 Node mass > 5 cm | | | | |
| MX Unknown status of distant metastases | | | | |
| M0 No distant metastases | | | | |
| M1a Non-regional nodal or lung metastases | | | | |
| M1b Distant metastasis other than non-regional nodal or lung | | | | |
| SX No marker studies available | | | | |
| S0 All marker studies normal | | | | |
| | LDH* | hCG (mIU/mL) | AFP(ng/mL) | |
| S1 | <1.5 × N & | <5000 & | <1000 | |
| S2 | 1.5–10 × N or | 5000–50 000 or | 1000–10 000 | |
| S3 | >10 × N or | >50 000 or | >10 000 | |

*LDH levels expressed as elevations above upper limit of normal (N).

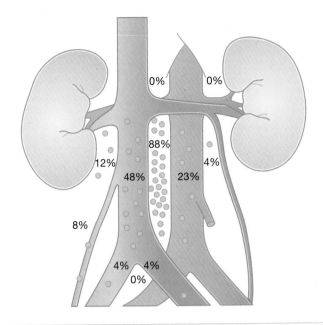

**Fig. 13-1** Pattern of early retroperitoneal lymph node involvement from right-sided testicular tumors. (From Donohue JP. Metastatic pathways of nonseminomatous germ cell tumors. Semin Urol 1984; 2: 217–2290, with permission.)

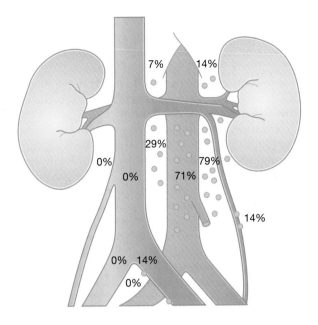

**Fig. 13-2** Pattern of early retroperitoneal lymph node involvement from left-sided testicular tumors. (From Donohue JP. Metastatic pathways of nonseminomatous germ cell tumors. Semin Urol 1984; 2: 217–229, with permission.)

in early-stage disease from left-sided testicular tumors, in contrast to right-sided lesions (Fig. 13-2).[10] As metastases become more widespread, right-sided lesions develop suprahilar and contralateral spread and left-sided tumors develop interaortocaval and precaval involvement, as well as a greater frequency of suprahilar involvement. As the volume of retroperitoneal disease increases, retrograde involvement of iliac and inguinal nodes may be seen.[10] Inguinal nodal involvement may also be seen when the primary tumor has extended to the scrotal skin or a trans-scrotal approach was used for the primary resection. The extension of the primary tumor to the epididymis also correlates with the development of external iliac nodal spread. Eventually, supradiaphragmatic spread occurs to the mediastinum and supraclavicular and cervical lymph nodes, tending to involve the left supraclavicular nodes much more commonly than the right.[11]

Seminoma tends to metastasize in an orderly pattern through lymphatics, whereas choriocarcinoma more frequently spreads by hematogenous routes. The other germ cell tumors, such as embryonal carcinoma, tend to have a lymphatic pattern of spread, although hematogenous spread can also be seen. Hematogenous spread is most commonly reflected by lung, liver, central nervous system, and bone involvement;[12] brain involvement is most common with choriocarcinoma and, perhaps unexpectedly, bone involvement with seminoma.[12]

## Gross examination

Gross examination and proper handling of the orchiectomy specimen are often neglected, and many diagnostic problems at the microscope can be traced to suboptimal processing of the gross specimen. Under the best circumstances,

the testis and accompanying tunics and spermatic cord should be received fresh, dissected, and allowed to fix thoroughly before tissue blocks are submitted. What often happens, however, is that the urologist places the radical orchiectomy specimen intact into fixative, and only hours later is the specimen dissected. The testicular tunics do not permit ready penetration of fixative, so this approach results in autolytic changes. It would be preferable for the urologist to make a single, virtually through-and-through incision in the specimen before placing it into fixative if it is not feasible to send it to the laboratory immediately in the fresh state.

A radical orchiectomy specimen consists of the testis, tunica vaginalis, and a portion of spermatic cord. The specimen should be weighed, measured in three dimensions, and the length of the cord noted. We recommend examination of the spermatic cord next, prior to incision of the testis, to avoid the common contamination by 'buttered' tumor of the cord,[13] with submission of the cord resection margin and a cross-section adjacent to the testis. The tunica vaginalis should then be incised, any abnormalities described, the quantity and nature of any intratunical fluid recorded, and the tunica albuginea carefully inspected and palpated for penetration by neoplasm. The testis should then be bisected in the plane of its long axis, through the testicular hilum, using a long, sharp knife. Fresh tissues may then be harvested for special studies such as cytogenetics, flow cytometry, electron microscopy, and molecular studies, although these are not routinely needed for diagnosis. Photographs may be obtained, and then multiple, serial, parallel cuts at 3 mm intervals should be made, leaving the tunica albuginea intact posteriorly to keep the specimen together. The specimen should then be placed in a generous volume of the pathologist's preferred fixative (10% neutral buffered formalin is quite suitable) and allowed to fix thoroughly prior to further processing. After fixation, the neoplasm should be described and measured, with particular attention paid to the relationships to the tunica albuginea and the testicular hilum. Most examples of extratesticular spread occur by extension through the hilum.[14] Multiple blocks of neoplasm should be submitted, as many tumors are quite heterogeneous. Blocks of all of the different-appearing areas should be made, including hemorrhagic and necrotic areas. A minimum of one block of neoplasm for every centimeter of maximum tumor dimension is a general rule of thumb. However, it is prudent to submit blocks quite generously if the gross appearance suggests seminoma, as the discovery of non-seminomatous elements usually changes therapy. Hence, small seminomas should be submitted totally, and at least 10 blocks of larger tumors, (or one block for every centimeter of maximum tumor dimension, whichever is the larger number) submitted. The non-neoplastic testis should also be sampled, as well as a block to include the testicular hilum. The epididymis should be incised by multiple, parallel cuts perpendicular to its long axis, any abnormalities noted, and the appropriate blocks submitted.

# Germ cell tumors

## Classification

About 95% of testicular neoplasms are of germ cell origin. The classification of testicular germ cell tumors presented in Table 13-2 is a modification of that of the World Health Organization (WHO)[15] and is the recommended one, although a second classification that was developed by the British Testicular Tumour Panel (BTTP)[16] is sometimes used in Europe.

## Histogenesis

The histogenesis of testicular germ cell tumors has been clarified over the past three decades by a number of observations. Perhaps foremost in importance is the recognition that all of the adult germ cell tumors, with the exceptions of spermatocytic seminoma and epidermoid and dermoid cyst, are derived from a common precursor which Skakkebaek originally recognized and described as 'carcinoma in situ' of the testis.[17,18] The preferred term for this lesion, given the non-epithelial nature of the constituent cells, is 'intratubular germ cell neoplasia of the unclassified type' (IGCNU).[19,20] It consists of an initially basilar proliferation of seminoma-like cells with clear cytoplasm and enlarged, hyperchromatic nuclei having one or two prominent nucleoli (Fig. 13-3). In addition it has many features, apart from its light microscopic appearance, that it shares with seminoma, including ultrastructure,[21,22] immunohistochemical reactions with various antibodies ($M_2A$,[23] TRA-1-60,[24] placenta-like alkaline phosphatase (PLAP),[25–27] glutathione-S-transferase (isoenzyme $\pi$),[28] OCT3/4,[29,30] NANOG[31]), DNA content,[32] the number of nucleolar organizer regions,[33] and the lectin-binding patterns.[34]

The strong similarities between IGCNU and seminoma imply that seminoma is also a precursor for other germ cell tumors. This interpretation is supported by a number

**Table 13-2** Classification of testicular tumors

**Germ cell tumors**

Precursor lesion
  Intratubular germ cell neoplasia
    Unclassified type ('carcinoma-in-situ')
    Specific types

Tumors of one histologic type
  Seminoma
  Variant: Seminoma with syncytiotrophoblast cells
  Spermatocytic seminoma
  Variant: Spermatocytic seminoma with a sarcomatous component
  Embryonal carcinoma
  Yolk sac tumor (endodermal sinus tumor)
    Teratoma
    Teratoma with a secondary malignant component
    Monodermal variants
      Carcinoid (pure and with teratomatous elements)
      Primitive neuroectodermal tumor
    Dermoid cyst
    Epidermoid cyst
  Choriocarcinoma and other trophoblastic tumors

Tumors of more than one histologic type
  Mixed germ cell tumors (specify individual components and estimate their amount as a percentage)
    Polyembryoma
    Diffuse embryoma

Regressed ('burnt-out') germ cell tumor

**Sex Cord-Stromal Tumors**

Leydig cell tumor
Sertoli cell tumor
  Not otherwise specified
  Sclerosing
  Large cell calcifying
  Intratubular large cell hyalinizing
Granulosa cell tumor
  Adult
  Juvenile

Tumors in the fibroma–thecoma group

Mixed sex cord-stromal tumors

Unclassified sex cord–stromal tumors

**Mixed Germ Cell/Sex Cord-stromal Tumors**

Gonadoblastoma
Others

**Ovarian-type Tumors**

**Tumors of the Rete Testis**

Adenocarcinoma
Adenoma
Adenomatous hyperplasia

**Tumors of Hematopoietic Origin**

Lymphoma
Plasmacytoma
Leukemia

**Miscellaneous**

Mesenchymal tumors
Metastatic tumors

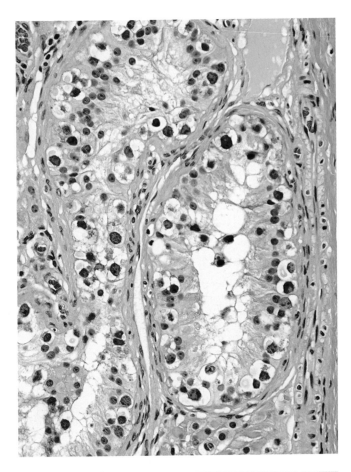

**Fig. 13-3** IGCNU in seminiferous tubules. There are cells with clear cytoplasm and enlarged, hyperchromatic nuclei along the basilar aspect of tubules lacking spermatogenesis. Sertoli cells are displaced luminally.

of observations. First, pure testicular seminoma may subsequently develop non-seminomatous elements, as evidenced by histologic examination or elevation of serum α-fetoprotein (AFP). Autopsy studies of patients who died of metastatic germ cell neoplasm following orchiectomy showing pure testicular seminoma have demonstrated non-seminomatous elements in 30–40% of cases.[12,35] On light microscopy seminoma may appear to transform either to embryonal carcinoma or to yolk sac tumor.[36,37] Also, 10–20% of seminomas contain syncytiotrophoblast cells, and some trophoblastic hormone-containing cells in seminoma are not easily distinguished histologically from the surrounding seminoma cells.[38–40] Ultrastructural studies of seminoma have demonstrated evidence of epithelial differentiation ('seminoma with early carcinomatous features') in some light microscopically typical cases.[41] Furthermore, the DNA content of seminoma is consistently higher than that of non-seminomatous germ cell tumors,[32,42,43] suggesting that non-seminomatous tumors evolve from seminoma as a consequence of gene loss, perhaps due to loss of cancer suppressor genes. Karyotypic analyses have shown a striking tendency for certain chromosomes to be in parallel excess or deficiency in seminoma and the non-seminomatous germ cell tumors,[42] and loss of heterozygosity studies also show similar patterns of allelic imbalance

between coexisting seminoma and non-seminoma in the testis.[44] These data indicate that seminoma may transform to non-seminomatous tumors.

Genetic changes precede the development of an invasive germ cell tumor from IGCNU.[45] Although over-representation of gene sequences from the short arm of chromosome 12, mostly in the form of an isochromosome [i(12p)], is consistent in invasive germ cell tumors of adult patients, such over-representation is not found in the associated IGCNU.[46–48] It is believed that additional 12p sequences are essential for invasive growth by inhibiting apoptosis and thereby permitting survival of invasive tumor cells outside the microenvironment of the seminiferous tubules.[47] On the other hand, there are marked similarities between many of the genetic changes in IGCNU and the associated invasive tumor,[44,45] in support of the precursor role of the former.

Immunohistochemical study has shown that loss of the cell cycle-dependent kinase inhibitors p18 and p21 accompanies invasive growth,[49,50] as does gain of the ubiquitin ligase double minute-2 (mdm-2)[49] and increased production of cyclin E.[50]

Transformation of IGCNU to non-seminomatous tumor may apparently occur at the time of invasion, as pure embryonal carcinoma, yolk sac tumor or choriocarcinoma are associated with IGCNU. The common occurrence of seminoma with non-seminomatous elements also supports transformation from invasive seminoma. IGCNU adjacent to seminoma or non-seminomatous tumors shares certain chromosomal abnormalities with the invasive tumor, and these abnormalities differ depending on whether the adjacent tumor is seminomatous or non-seminomatous,[51] an observation that supports the occurrence of genetic transformation within the tubules before morphological change. Additionally, intratubular malignant germ cells that are not morphologically recognizable as embryonal carcinoma cells may show CD30 reactivity, suggesting early-phase differentiation of IGCNU cells to embryonal carcinoma cells within the tubules, followed by rapid extratubular invasion.[52] These observations lead to a revised model of testicular germ cell tumor histogenesis, based on the tetrahedron model proposed by Srigley and co-workers (Fig. 13-4).[41]

The histogenesis of testicular germ cell tumors in children is different from that of postpubertal patients. Unlike the postpubertal tumors, the examples in children (virtually confined to two types of neoplasm, yolk sac tumor and teratoma[53]) lack any consistent association with IGCNU.[54–57] Furthermore, the teratomas have a diploid DNA content and a normal karyotype, unlike those of postpubertal patients, and the yolk sac tumors lack consistent 12p abnormalities.[58–60] The pediatric germ cell tumors therefore have a fundamentally different pathogenesis. These observations and others have led one group to propose that there are five fundamentally different forms of germ cell tumor:[61] type I represented by the pediatric types; type II consisting of the usual postpubertal germ cell tumors; type III consisting only of spermatocytic seminoma; type IV represented by ovarian dermoid cyst; and type V consisting of gestational choriocarcinoma. Each has its own unique pattern of gene activation and genomic imprinting.

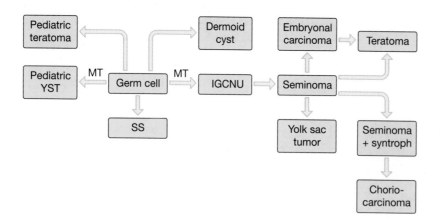

**Fig. 13-4** New model of germ cell tumor histogenesis, based on the tetrahedron model of Srigley et al.[41] In this model, seminoma plays a pivotal role as a precursor for many other forms of germ cell tumor. Note the absence of IGCNU for pediatric teratoma, pediatric yolk sac tumor, dermoid cyst and spermatocytic seminoma. IGCNU, intratubular germ cell neoplasia, unclassified; MT, malignant transformation; SS, spermatocytic seminoma; syntroph, syncytiotrophoblast cells.

## Epidemiology

Germ cell tumors of the testis (with the notable exception of spermatocytic seminoma) occur mostly in young males, with the incidence accelerating rapidly following puberty and peaking close to 30 years of age (Fig. 13-5). There is a small peak in early childhood, but many of the cases of 'testicular cancer' in elderly men correspond to lymphomatous involvement or secondary tumors rather than to germ cell tumors (Fig. 13-5). Whites have a much higher frequency of testicular germ cell tumors than do non-whites, with the exception of the Maori of New Zealand, who have an incidence comparable to that of white populations.[62,63] Native Hawaiians, Native Alaskans, and Native Americans are also at higher risk than other 'non-whites.'[64] Denmark and Switzerland have the highest rates of testicular cancer: about nine cases per 100 000 males per year, compared with the rate in the United States white population of about six per 100 000 males. The rates in Africans and Asians are generally about one per 100 000 males.[65] The incidence of testicular germ cell tumors increased steadily in the United States during the 20th century,[66,67] and a similar trend was noted in several other countries,[68] including Denmark,[69–71] Norway,[72] England,[3–75] Germany,[70] Scotland,[76] New Zealand,[63] Australia,[77] Canada,[78] Iceland,[79] and Japan.[74] Numerous studies have demonstrated a higher frequency of testicular germ cell tumors in professional workers or those of higher socioeconomic class than in laborers or those of lower socioeconomic status;[63,64,80–86] in those with occupational exposure to fertilizers, phenols, heat, smoke, or fumes;[87] in farm workers,[81,88] draftsmen,[81] and those in food manufacture and preparation;[81] in leather workers;[89,90] in pesticide applicators;[91] in those exposed to insect repellants;[88] in metal workers;[92] in policemen exposed to handheld radar;[93] in aircraft repairmen;[94,95] in motor vehicle mechanics;[63] in electrical workers, fishermen, paper and printing workers, and foresters;[80] in men of tall stature;[96] and in physicians.[63] Other studies have suggested other possible etiologies, including in-utero exposure to high estrogen levels,[97–100] dietary iron,[101] testicular trauma,[102] various HLA haplotypes,[103–110] a family history of breast cancer,[111] early puberty,[111,112] early birth order,[97] dizygotic twinship,[113,114] ichthyosis,[115] Marfan's syndrome,[116] the Li–Fraumeni syndrome,[117] and the dysplastic nevus syndrome.[118] One study has shown a correlation between testicular cancer and a variant allele of the glutathione-S-transferase π gene.[119] Another demonstrated increased

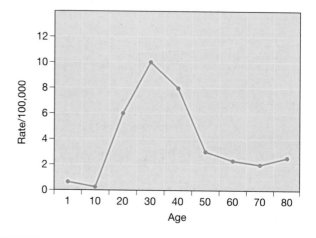

**Fig. 13-5** Incidence of testicular tumors according to patient age. Note a small peak in infancy, nadir at age 10 years, and rapid rise after puberty. The peak incidence occurs at 25–30 years. The cases in older patients correspond to non-germinal tumors, mainly lymphoma. (Data from the Surveillance, Epidemiology and End Results [SEER] Program.)

risk in the sons of fathers who were wood processors, metal workers, or employed in the food product industry.[120] Most of these associations, however, are weak and fail to account for the general increase in testicular germ cell tumors. It is hypothesized that important causative factors in testicular cancer occur in the antenatal period, with a protective effect in European countries for men born during the World War II era.[68,121,122] This protective effect leads to the hypothesis that testicular cancer is causally related to prosperity, probably secondary to its in-utero effects. The use of alcohol and tobacco, prior vasectomy, and radiation exposure have not been associated with testicular germ cell tumors.[62,123–126]

Despite the weak correlation of most etiologic factors with testicular germ cell tumors,[62,127] four contributing factors are proven: cryptorchidism, prior testicular germ cell tumor, family history of testicular germ cell tumors, and certain somatosexual ambiguity syndromes. An estimate of the increased risks associated with these disorders is provided in Table 13-3.

## Cryptorchidism

An increased frequency of cryptorchidism, varying from 6.5% to 14.5%, has been found in patients with testicular germ cell

**Table 13-3** Estimated increased risks of testicular germ cell tumors associated with certain conditions

| Condition | Estimated increased risk | References |
|---|---|---|
| Cryptorchidism | 3.5–5× | 132,134 |
| Prior testicular germ cell tumor | 5–10× | 1,135–138 |
| Family history (first-degree male relative) | 3–10× | 139–142 |
| Gonadal dysgenesis with a Y chromosome | 50×* | 1,143,144 |
| Androgen insensitivity syndrome | 15× | 1,145–148 |

*Includes cases of gonadoblastoma.

tumors,[66,98,128–133] which has led to calculations of 2.5–35 times increased risk among cryptorchid patients.[129–132,134,149–155] Such risk does not manifest prior to 20 years of age[134] and is probably most accurately assessed as 3.5–5.0 times higher over a control population.[132,134] If cryptorchidism is unilateral, the non-cryptorchid testis is also at increased risk for a testicular germ cell tumor, although at a lower rate than the cryptorchid testis.[64,149,151,156–158] Ectopia alone cannot explain the association of cryptorchidism and testicular germ cell tumor, a fact reinforced by the failure of orchidopexy to reduce the risk[133,149,159,160] (although there is probably insufficient experience with orchidopexy in the very young to rule out an ameliorating effect).[64] It is possible that cryptorchidism is a marker of patients with a general defect in genitourinary embryogenesis and that cryptorchid testes are dysgenetic,[161] as supported by abnormalities of the external genitalia or sex chromosomes in some cryptorchid patients with germ cell tumors.[158,162,163] Cryptorchidism may predispose disproportionately to seminoma rather than non-seminomatous tumors.[128,153,164,165] About 2–4% of patients with cryptorchidism have IGCNU,[138,166,167] and at least 50% of such patients develop germ cell tumor within 5 years.[168] Giwercman and co-workers[169] cite a 2.8% frequency of IGCNU in the cryptorchid population, a fourfold increase over the general population of young men. Thus, bilateral testicular biopsy at 18–20 years of age has been recommended for cryptorchid patients.[170] A negative result is good evidence of no increased risk,[166] although there are occasional false negative results.[171,172] A positive biopsy should prompt orchiectomy of the affected testis. In testes with extreme atrophy, the biopsy should be directed to sample the region near the rete testis.[173] Apart from germ cell tumors cryptorchid testes have an increased frequency of nodules composed of small tubules lined by Sertoli cells, often with central deposits of basement membrane (see page 824 Figs 13-131, 13-132). These Sertoli cell nodules have been termed 'Pick's adenoma,' which is something of a misnomer as they are not true neoplasms.[174,175]

## Prior testicular germ cell tumor

A second germ cell tumor occurs in the remaining testis of 1–5% of patients with a previous germ cell tumor.[136,176–186]

The risk of a second tumor is higher in patients with seminoma, especially in men 30 years old or younger.[186] Similarly, there is a 4.5–6.6% frequency of IGCNU in the opposite testis of patients with a germ cell tumor.[135–137,181,187] There is a low risk in the absence of IGCNU on biopsy because of occasional false negative results.[187] In one study, five of 1859 patients (0.3%) who had negative testicular biopsies opposite a germ cell tumor developed a second tumor on follow-up.[172] Sensitivity is improved if three biopsies of the contralateral testis are performed.[188] If the residual testis is either atrophic[187,189] or cryptorchid the risk is even greater,[137] with a 23% frequency of IGCNU.[135] Unfortunately, almost 50% of cases of contralateral IGCNU would be missed if contralateral biopsies were restricted to patients with atrophy or cryptorchidism.[137] One study suggested that atrophy rather than maldescent is the important predictor of contralateral IGCNU.[190] Young age at onset of the first tumor[190] and bilateral cryptorchidism also appear to be associated with an increased risk of bilateral occurrence.[136] It is estimated that biopsy of an atrophic testis opposite a germ cell tumor in a patient younger than 31 years of age will detect IGCNU in one-third of cases.[190] About 50% of second primary tumors of the testis occur 3–5 years after the diagnosis of the initial germ cell tumor,[178,191] with a mean of 5.6–6.5 years,[185,192] but intervals of more than a decade can occur.[186,193] Concordant or discordant neoplastic types may occur, with some tendency for concordance of pure seminoma.[178] The risk of bilateral tumors in patients with a germ cell tumor is increased about fourfold with a positive family history.[194,195] Chemotherapy administered for the treatment of the first tumor reduces the risk of a contralateral tumor,[180,182] but contralateral tumors may occur even in the absence of IGCNU in biopsies of the opposite testis performed at the time of the first germ cell tumor diagnosis.[196] An increased frequency of rare alleles of the Ha-ras1 oncogene is seen in patients with testicular germ cell tumors, and such rare alleles are associated with bilaterality and early age of onset.[197]

Some testicular lesions other than IGCNU have been noted in the testis adjacent to germ cell tumors, including Leydig cell hyperplasia, microlithiasis, angiopathy, Sertoli cell nodules, tubular atrophy, and multinucleated spermatogonia.[198]

## Family history

First-degree male relatives of patients with germ cell tumor of the testis have a 3–10 times greater risk of a testicular germ cell tumor than the general population.[139–142] The risk is highest for brothers (10 times), intermediate for sons (six times) and lowest for fathers (four times).[199] Also, a family history of testicular germ cell tumor is associated with an 8–14% frequency of bilaterality,[139,194,199] compared to the 1–5% frequency in the general population of patients with testicular germ cell tumors.[176–179,186] The occurrence of an unexpected number of testicular germ cell tumors in the relatives of children with soft tissue sarcomas has raised the question of whether testicular germ cell tumors may represent part of the spectrum of the Li–Fraumeni cancer syndrome.[200,201] It appears, however, that neither germline nor somatic p53 mutations occur in these cases.[202,203] Immunohistochemical demonstration of p53 protein[204,205] therefore indicates overexpression of non-mutated protein. Segregation analysis of data regarding familial cases has suggested the presence of a major gene that conveys risk in a recessive model.[206] In one study[207] genetic linkage analysis implicated a susceptibility gene localized to Xq27, but this was not confirmed in a second study.[208]

## Intersex syndromes

Patients with some intersex syndromes are at increased risk for germ cell tumors. Patients with gonadal dysgenesis in the presence of a Y chromosome, including patients with pure 46,XY gonadal dysgenesis (Swyer's syndrome), mixed gonadal dysgenesis, and dysgenetic male pseudohermaphroditism, commonly develop gonadal germ cell tumors.[143,144,209,210] About 25–30% of such patients develop gonadoblastoma,[143,144,210] and this may serve as the precursor lesion for the development of an invasive germ cell tumor (see page 829). IGCNU is also present in about 8% of children and adolescents with gonadal dysgenesis.[211] Because an invasive tumor may develop in childhood, gonadectomy is indicated as soon as the diagnosis is established. Male pseudohermaphrodites with the androgen insensitivity syndrome develop a malignant germ cell tumor in 5–10% of cases overall.[145–148,212] Such patients have been shown to have various mutations in the androgen receptor gene.[213] The tumor usually develops after puberty, and this may permit gonadectomy to be delayed until full feminization has occurred, although this remains controversial because of an occasional case of invasive germ cell tumor developing at an early age. Delay of prophylactic gonadectomy beyond the early postpubescent period in patients with the androgen insensitivity syndrome is risky,[145] with a 22% frequency of malignant germ cell tumor in such patients beyond 30 years of age.[214] Not all testicular masses in patients with the androgen insensitivity syndrome are germ cell tumors; these patients commonly develop hamartomatous nodules composed of Sertoli cell-lined tubules with intervening clusters of Leydig cells in the interstitium, as well as pure Sertoli cell adenomas[143,147,148] (see page 824) and occasional juvenile granulosa cell tumors.[209] Additionally, there is a single report of IGCNU in a male pseudohermaphrodite with a nonsense mutation in the gene for steroidogenic acute regulatory protein.[215]

## Infertility

Patients with infertility have under a 1% frequency of testicular germ cell tumor.[21,135,138,216] It is not clear, however, whether infertility is a risk factor for germ cell tumor that is independent of cryptorchidism or gonadal dysgenesis.[217]

## Intratubular germ cell neoplasia[18]

Grossly, the testis with IGCNU may be unremarkable or appear atrophic and fibrotic. Microscopically, intratubular germ cell neoplasia consists of a proliferation of malignant germ cells, which may be a specific neoplastic type, such as

intratubular embryonal carcinoma or intratubular spermatocytic seminoma, or may consist of undifferentiated germ cells resembling primitive gonocytes. The primitive gonocyte-like form of intratubular germ cell neoplasia is typically confined to the basilar aspect of the seminiferous tubules and is associated with all types of germ cell tumor, except for spermatocytic seminoma and dermoid/epidermoid cyst. It is designated 'intratubular germ cell neoplasia of the unclassified type' (IGCNU). The cells of IGCNU have enlarged, hyperchromatic nuclei, often with one or two prominent nucleoli, thickened nuclear membranes, and clear cytoplasm (Fig. 13-3). The median nuclear diameter of the cells of IGCNU is 9.7 μm, compared to a median nuclear diameter in spermatogonia of 6.5 μm.[218] Spermatogenesis in the affected tubules is usually decreased or absent, and the tubules may have a thickened peritubular basement membrane. Sertoli cells are often displaced luminally (Fig. 13-3). The distribution of IGCNU is characteristically patchy, and adjacent profiles of seminiferous tubules may appear unremarkable, with intact spermatogenesis (Fig. 13-6). Leydig cell hyperplasia may occur in the interstitium. IGCNU often spreads into the rete testis in a pagetoid fashion, intermixing with non-neoplastic epithelium (Fig. 13-7).[219] The strong similarity between the cells of seminoma and those of IGCNU suggests that IGCNU could be termed intratubular

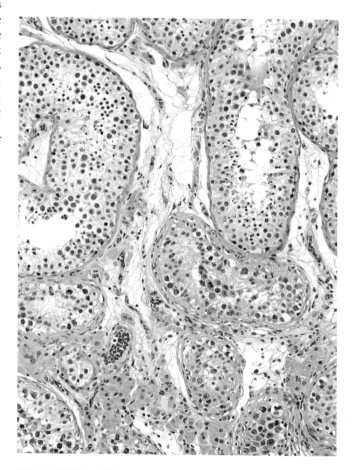

**Fig. 13-6** Patchy distribution of IGCNU. Tubules without IGCNU have spermatogenesis, whereas adjacent tubules with IGCNU lack spermatogenesis.

A

B

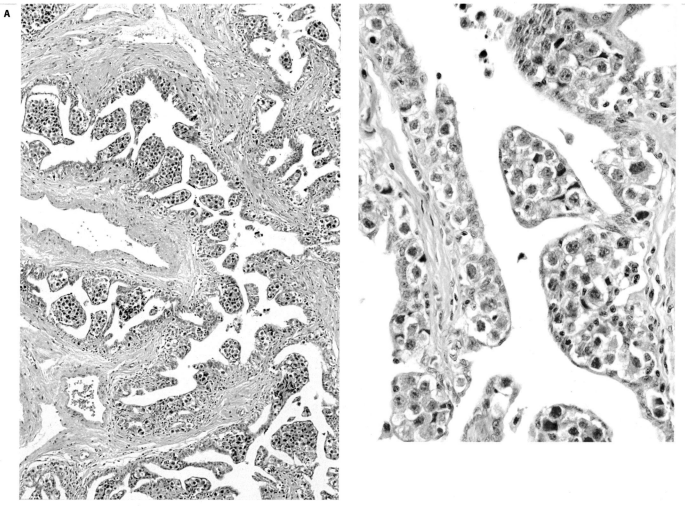

**Fig. 13-7** IGCNU cells have extended in a pagetoid fashion into the rete testis, with a layer of rete epithelium stretched over them.

seminoma; however, this term may falsely connote that IGCNU is the precursor lesion only for seminoma, rather than for virtually all postpubertal germ cell tumors. By convention, the term intratubular seminoma is reserved for those proliferations of IGCNU-like cells that fill and distend seminiferous tubules (Fig. 13-8), although fundamentally such lesions may simply be a more advanced stage of IGCNU.[220]

## Special studies of IGCNU

Glycogen is present in the cytoplasm of 98% of cases of IGCNU[221] (Fig. 13-9), and its demonstration is diagnostically helpful but non-specific because non-neoplastic spermatogonia and Sertoli cells may also contain glycogen.[222] Equally sensitive but more specific for IGCNU are immunostains directed against placental alkaline phosphatase, which highlight a placenta-like alkaline phosphatase (PLAP) with a predominantly cytoplasmic membrane pattern of distribution in virtually every case (Fig. 13-10A).[26,222–224] Only rarely (<1%) are isolated non-neoplastic spermatocytes (which are unlikely to be confused with IGCNU) PLAP positive, with

spermatogonia being PLAP negative.[225] Immunohistochemical staining for OCT3/4, a stem cell factor receptor, is also useful to identify early forms of intratubular germ cell neoplasia, characteristically showing strong nuclear reactivity (Fig. 13-10B).[29,30,226] Immunohistochemical staining for NANOG, a regulatory factor upstream of OCT3/4, similarly marks IGCNU.[31] IGCNU has also been found to react with monoclonal antibodies M₂A (D2-40/gp36/podoplanin),[23,224,227,228] 43-9F,[224,229] TRA-1-60,[24] HB5, HF2, HE11,[230] and with antibodies directed against glutathione-S-transferase, isoenzyme π,[28] the c-kit protein (Fig. 13-10C),[231] angiotensin-converting enzyme,[232] and p53.[233] In contrast to non-neoplastic germ cells it is negative for the RNA-binding motif protein.[234] The positive reactions for PLAP and TRA-1-60 support that IGCNU resembles fetal gonocytes.[24,26,235] By electron microscopy, IGCNU has evenly dispersed chromatin, intricate nucleoli, and sparse cytoplasmic organelles with prominent glycogen deposits. Occasional rudimentary intercellular junctions may be identified.[21,236–239] These features are essentially the same as those of seminoma.[240] The DNA content of IGCNU is similar to that of seminoma – usually in the triploid and hypotetraploid range.[32,241] Some

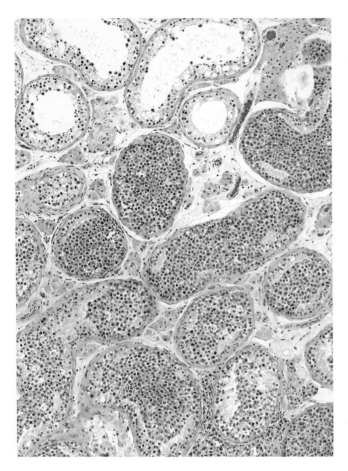

**Fig. 13-8** Distension of seminiferous tubules by seminoma-like cells is referred to as 'intratubular seminoma.'

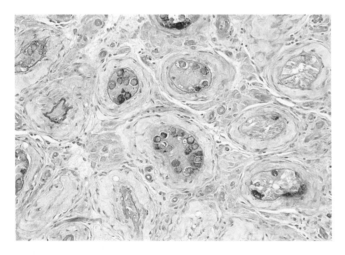

**Fig. 13-9** Cytoplasmic glycogen in IGCNU. (Periodic acid–Schiff stain.)

of the genetic features of IGCNU have already been mentioned (see page 761).

## Differential diagnosis of IGCNU

IGCNU should be distinguished from specific forms of intratubular germ cell neoplasia. Intratubular seminoma fills and distends the tubules, whereas IGCNU is restricted to the basilar area, although the cells are histologically identical. Atypical germ cells that do not resemble IGCNU cells may also occur in seminiferous tubules. These cells may have large nuclei or be multinucleated. They lack the cytoplasmic clarity and nucleolar prominence of IGCNU cells and do not stain for the usual IGCNU markers. Although they may indicate a perturbation in testicular development, as evidence by increased frequency in cryptorchid boys[242] and adjacent to testicular germ cell tumors,[198] their significance is really not clear, unlike IGCNU.

## Prognosis of IGCNU

The practical importance of IGCNU is its progression to an invasive germ cell tumor (either seminomatous or non-seminomatous) in about 50% of cases within 5 years after identification.[243] Also, only a small fraction of patients remain free of an invasive tumor by 7 or 8 years of follow-up (Fig. 13-11),[244] although some may not develop a tumor for more than 15 years.[169] Furthermore, there is no documented case of spontaneous regression of typical IGCNU.[169] IGCNU is identified with increased frequency in patients with cryptorchidism,[21,166,167,170,245] a previous history of a testicular germ cell tumor,[181,187,190,246–248] gonadal dysgenesis,[249,250] androgen insensitivity syndrome[251,252] and infertility.[248,253,254] IGCNU is also identified in the residual seminiferous tubules of virtually every postpubertal patient with an invasive testicular germ cell tumor, with the exceptions of spermatocytic seminoma and dermoid and epidermoid cysts.[168,221,255–257] The pediatric germ cell tumors, as mentioned previously (see page 761), lack a consistent association with IGCNU, although there are a few reports describing the occasional pediatric case.[241,258–260] It is possible that some of these cases of 'IGCNU' represent the reactive enlargement of non-neoplastic germ cells induced by a mass lesion (Fig. 13-12), as described by Hawkins and Hicks,[261] rather than a neoplastic process.

## Biopsy diagnosis of IGCNU

Testicular biopsies are a sensitive method for detecting IGCNU. Fixatives such as Bouin's, B-5, and Stieve's enhance cytological detail and may permit easier detection of IGCNU than with formalin fixation. Formalin, Bouin's and Stieve's fixatives permit immunohistochemical detection of placental alkaline phosphatase, whereas Cleland's fluid yields inconsistent results.[224] Berthelsen and Skakkebaek[262] concluded that one or two 3 mm biopsies of a testis harboring IGCNU will detect virtually every case, although rare false negative results do occur (0.3% in one study of 1859 biopsies that were initially interpreted as negative[172]). Another study supported three biopsies, each 5 mm long, as optimal.[188] In cases of severe atrophy where many tubules are obliterated it may be necessary to sample the region near the hilum, where IGCNU is more frequently preserved within the epithelium of the rete testis.[173] Potential populations for screening biopsies include patients with cryptorchidism (2–4% positivity for IGCNU), a prior testicular germ cell tumor (5% positivity), somatosexual ambiguity (25% positivity), and, less strongly, oligospermic infertility (0–1%

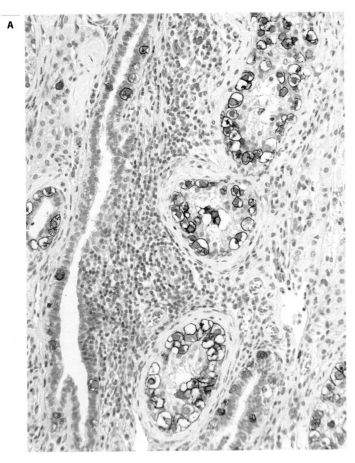

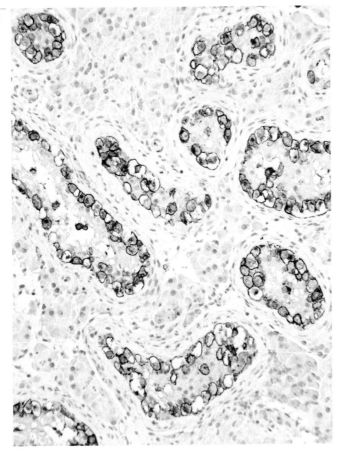

**Fig. 13-10** (**A**) Cytoplasmic membrane positivity for placental alkaline phosphatase in IGCNU cells in seminiferous tubules and rete testis. (**B**) Strong nuclear reactivity for OCT3/4 in IGCNU. (**C**) An identical pattern of positivity for c-kit in IGCNU cells as seen for placental alkaline phosphatase.

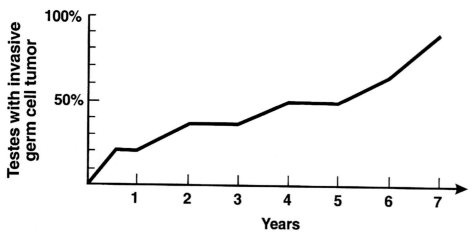

**Fig. 13-11** Follow-up of patients with IGCNU on biopsy. About 90% have invasive tumor after 7 years. (Data from Skakkebaek NE, Berthelsen JG, Visfeldt J. Clinical aspects of testicular carcinoma-in-situ. Int J Androl 1981; 4: 153–162.)

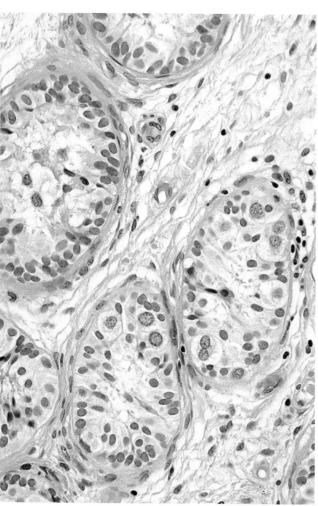

**Fig. 13-12** Atypical germ cells, some binucleated, adjacent to teratoma in a pediatric patient. These cells lack the features of IGCNU.

positivity).[138,169,218] IGCNU in a biopsy from a patient with retroperitoneal germ cell tumor probably indicates the regression of a previous invasive tumor that had metastasized to the retroperitoneum.[263,264] Therefore, a patient with presumed primary germ cell tumor of the retroperitoneum may benefit from testicular biopsy.[169]

### Treatment of IGCNU

Because of the high rate of progression of IGCNU to invasive testicular germ cell tumor, these patients should receive appropriate ablative treatment. Unilateral IGCNU is usually managed by orchiectomy, and bilateral IGCNU may be treated by bilateral orchiectomy or radiation. Chemotherapy, often given to patients with metastatic disease from a contralateral testicular tumor, may ablate IGCNU in the residual testis but is not a consistently effective means of therapy.[218,265–268]

## Seminoma

### Clinical features

Seminoma is the most common form of testicular germ cell tumor, and pure seminoma accounts for about 50% of all cases of testicular germ cell tumor.[269–271] It occurs in patients with an average age of 40 years,[269] which is about 10 years older than those patients with non-seminomatous germ cell tumor;[36,269] African-Americans may have an earlier age of onset.[272] Seminoma is extremely rare before puberty.[273,274] Most patients with seminoma present with a painless testicular mass, but there may be a dull, aching sensation. Up to 11% of seminoma patients have normal-sized or atrophic testes.[275] Occasional patients (2–3%) with seminoma present with symptoms of metastases, usually back pain due to retroperitoneal involvement, but gastrointestinal bleeding, bone pain, central nervous system dysfunction, dyspnea and cough, and other symptoms may rarely be presenting complaints.[9] Gynecomastia may occur as a result of elevation of serum human chorionic gonadotropin (hCG) due to intermingled syncytiotrophoblast elements in seminoma, and is rarely a presenting feature;[276] also, very rarely, a paraendocrine form of exophthalmos can be a presenting complaint,[277,278] as can paraneoplastic hypercalcemia,[279] hemolytic anemia,[280] and limbic encephalopathy.[281] Although symptoms of metastases are unusual presenting complaints in patients with seminoma, about 30% have metastases at the time of diagnosis.[269]

Patients with seminoma usually lack serum AFP and hCG elevations, which occur commonly in patients with non-seminomatous germ cell tumors. AFP levels should be normal, although concomitant liver disease (including seminomatous metastases to the liver) may cause modest AFP elevation,[282] and 'borderline' elevated AFP levels have been seen in some cases without evidence of non-seminomatous elements.[283] Most oncologists regard significant AFP elevation in a patient with apparently pure testicular seminoma as evidence of non-seminomatous elements and treat accordingly. About 10–20% of patients with clinical stage I 'pure' testicular seminoma have elevated serum hCG, and 25% or more with advanced seminoma have hCG elevations.[284] At initial diagnosis, 7–25% of patients with seminoma have elevated hCG.[285–291] If blood is sampled from the testicular vein, 80–85% of patients have elevated hCG.[292,293] Such elevation reflects the presence of intermingled syncytiotrophoblast elements in these tumors, and the elevations are generally modest. Elevations of serum hCG exceeding 40 IU/L have been correlated with a worse prognosis,[294] although this is controversial.[285,295] Peripheral venous elevations of hCG have been correlated with larger tumors,[293] perhaps explaining the relationship of elevated hCG with adverse prognostic features. Elevation of serum levels of lactate dehydrogenase, PLAP, and neuron-specific enolase may also occur in patients with seminoma. Such elevations, however, are neither specific nor especially sensitive,[284,294,296–299] which limits their clinical utility.

## Pathologic findings

Grossly, seminoma is usually cream to tan and often multinodular (Fig. 13-13), with occasional yellow foci of necrosis. Infrequently, necrosis is extensive. In some cases the tumor is diffuse, fleshy, and encephaloid, similar to testicular lymphoma (Fig. 13-14). In contrast to lymphoma, however, only about 10% of seminomas extend into paratesticular structures.[300] Intraparenchymal hemorrhage may cause red discoloration.[20] The cut surface of seminoma usually bulges from the surrounding parenchyma (Fig. 13-13). Punctate

foci of hemorrhage often correspond to intermingled foci of syncytiotrophoblast elements.[301] A fibrous consistency is uncommon but results when prominent fibrous septa develop in the tumor.

Microscopically, seminoma is usually arranged in a diffuse, sheet-like pattern interrupted by branching, fibrous septa containing an inflammatory infiltrate (Fig. 13-15) consisting chiefly of lymphocytes but often containing plasma cells and sometimes eosinophils. Distinct nodules of seminoma may be apparent, sometimes with confluent growth imparting a lobulated pattern. In some cases a prominent cord-like arrangement of cells is present (Fig. 13-16), often at the periphery of nodules showing a sheet-like pattern. Foci of intertubular growth may be seen, with preservation of seminiferous tubules; this pattern is usually most apparent at the periphery of neoplastic nodules and may be associated with rete testis invasion and aggressive behavior.[302] In rare seminomas an intertubular growth pattern may predomi-

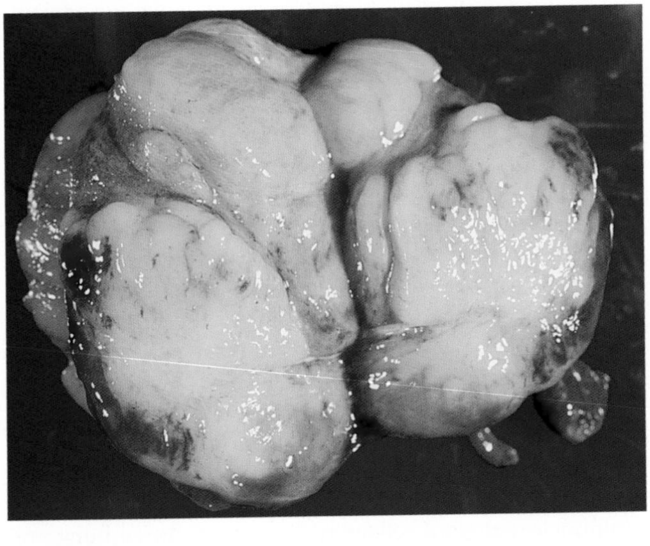

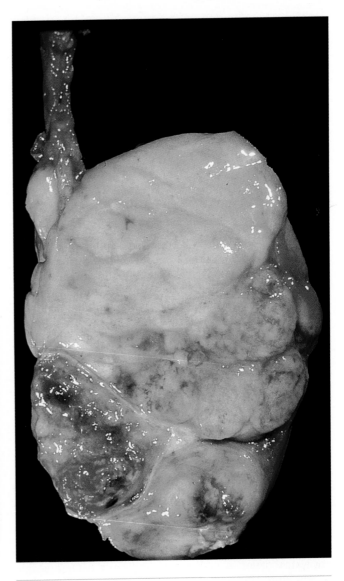

**Fig. 13-13** Cut surface of a seminoma demonstrating a cream-colored, multinodular neoplasm bulging from the surrounding testicular parenchyma.

**Fig. 13-14** Seminoma with a diffusely fleshy, encephaloid appearance and foci of hemorrhage. (Courtesy of Dr RH Young, Harvard Medical School, Boston, MA.)

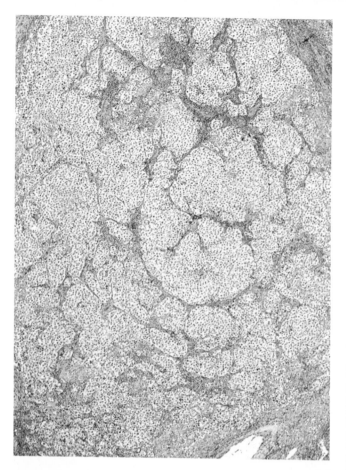

**Fig. 13-15** The sheet-like pattern of seminoma is interrupted by branching, fibrous septa containing lymphocytes.

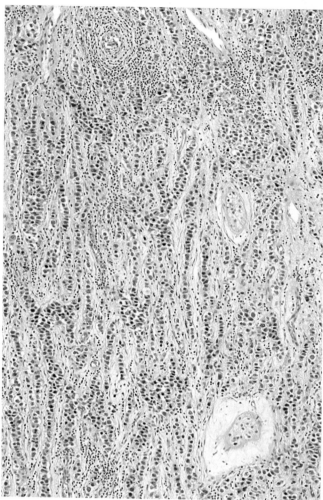

**Fig. 13-16** Prominent cord-like pattern in seminoma.

nate (Fig. 13-17), with well-preserved seminiferous tubules even in the central portions of the neoplasm. Such cases are prone to being overlooked as they do not destroy the seminiferous tubules, and they often do not form a discrete mass.[303] The presence of a lymphocytic infiltrate may be a clue to intertubular seminoma (Fig. 13-17) This growth pattern is much more common, however, in testicular lymphoma (see page 834). With time, many seminomas develop foci of scarring. Hyalinized deposits of collagen may separate the neoplastic cells into small nests resembling solid pseudotubules (Fig. 13-18). Extensive collagen deposits may result in broad scars with only a few scattered neoplastic cells. Calcification and even ossification may rarely occur in hyalinized fibrous trabeculae of seminoma.[304] Rarely, seminoma may show a distinctly tubular pattern in which a palisade-like arrangement of neoplastic cells occurs at the periphery of tubule-like structures which may contain loosely cohesive neoplastic cells in their 'lumina' (Fig. 13-19).[305–308] Seminoma may also develop intercellular edema with separation of neoplastic cells and the formation of microcystic spaces (Fig. 13-20). These spaces are generally (but not always) irregular in outline and frequently contain visible edema fluid and intracystic exfoliated neoplastic cells[309] which contrast with the 'cleaner,' rounder and more regular microcystic spaces commonly identified in yolk sac tumor

(see page 788). Foci of coagulative necrosis are present in about half of seminomas and in a minority of cases may be extensive.[275]

A lymphoid infiltrate is a virtually constant feature of seminoma and is usually most evident in perivascular areas and around fibrous trabeculae, which also contain many capillaries (Fig. 13-21). Lymphocytes are also frequently intermingled with the seminoma cells elsewhere. A florid lymphoid reaction, with formation of germinal centers, occurs in a minority of cases, but most of the lymphocytes in seminomas are T cells.[310–316] Ultrastructural studies have demonstrated a cytolytic effect of the lymphocytes on the seminoma cells,[315] correlating with the observation of some investigators of a better prognosis in cases associated with a prominent lymphocytic reaction.[317]

A variable granulomatous reaction occurs in up to 50% of seminomas. In most cases this reaction consists of small clusters of epithelioid histiocytes scattered among neoplastic cells (Fig. 13-21); Langhans'-type giant cells and other multinucleated giant cells may be present. Intratubular collections of epithelioid histiocytes may also be seen. Rarely, the granulomatous reaction can be extensive and virtually efface the neoplasm (Fig. 13-22); in such cases it may

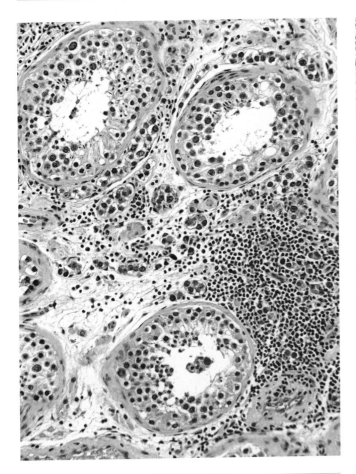

**Fig. 13-17** Intertubular growth of seminoma. There are small nests of seminoma cells between tubules. The lymphocytes are a helpful clue.

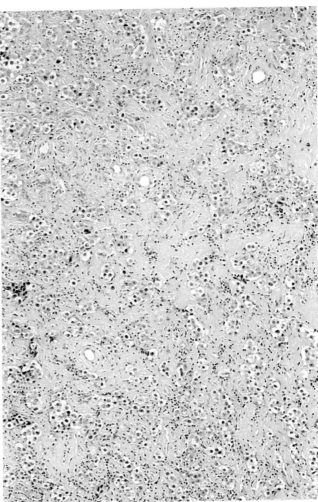

**Fig. 13-18** Scarring in seminoma creates a pattern of small nests and solid pseudotubules separated by hyalinized stroma.

be difficult to distinguish a florid granulomatous reaction in a seminoma from granulomatous orchitis, and careful search for residual seminoma and IGCNU is indicated.

The cells of seminoma are generally clear to lightly eosinophilic, measuring 15–25 μm in diameter. The nuclei are uniform, round to oval, usually central or slightly eccentric, with finely granular chromatin and one or two prominent nucleoli (Fig. 13-23). Often some nuclei have a relatively flat edge that has been described as 'squared-off,' lending them a 'boxy' appearance. The nuclear membranes are irregularly thickened. The cell borders are well defined in adequately fixed specimens (Fig. 13-24). Abundant cytoplasm separates the nuclei so that overlapping nuclei are not seen. Occasionally, seminoma displays foci of increased cellular atypia with less well-defined cytoplasmic boundaries, darker cytoplasm, and enlarged, crowded nuclei (Fig. 13-24). These changes may impart a plasmacytoid appearance to the tumor cells (Fig. 13-25). Such changes may be seen in association with early necrosis and contain pyknotic nuclear fragments. In the absence of distinct epithelial differentiation such isolated foci should not militate against a diagnosis of seminoma.

Mitotic figures in seminoma are prominent, and, in the past, when present in sufficient numbers, were considered as evidence of 'anaplastic seminoma.'[150] Now it is clear that

the practice of using an average of three mitoses per high-power field identified far too many seminomas as 'anaplastic,'[318] and, more importantly, there is evidence that 'high mitotic rate' seminoma behaves no differently from seminoma with a lower mitotic rate.[319,320] Furthermore, there is no immunohistochemical difference between typical and 'anaplastic' seminomas.[320] Use of the term 'anaplastic seminoma' is therefore discouraged. Although some seminomas behave more aggressively than most, it remains unclear whether such cases can be identified prospectively. Tickoo and associates[321] described cases of 'seminoma with atypia' based on nuclear pleomorphism and crowding, paucity of lymphocytes, and darker-staining cytoplasm (Figs 13-24, 13-25). In their experience such tumors were more likely to present at an advanced clinical stage and to focally express CD30 and lose c-kit expression. It remains unclear, however, whether such cases should receive a different therapy.

## Seminoma with syncytiotrophoblast cells

Syncytiotrophoblast cells are present in 10–20% of seminomas.[39] The morphology of these cells is variable, ranging

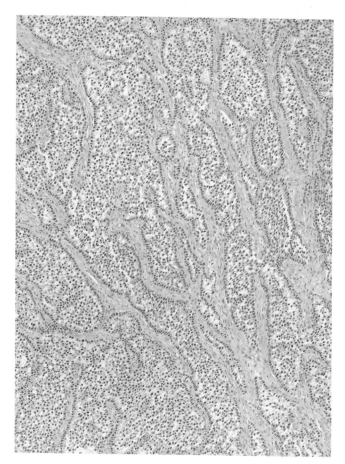

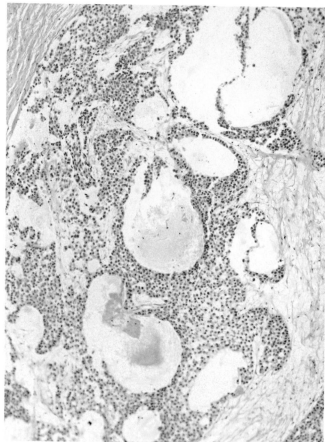

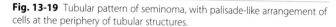

**Fig. 13-19** Tubular pattern of seminoma, with palisade-like arrangement of cells at the periphery of tubular structures.

**Fig. 13-20** Edema in seminoma creating an irregular, microcystic pattern.

from typical syncytiotrophoblast cells having cytoplasmic lacunae and multinucleation (Fig. 13-26) to large mononucleated or binucleated cells which may not be easily distinguished from the background of seminoma cells but which are highlighted by immunostains directed against hCG.[322] Intermediate between these extremes are cells containing multiple nuclei in a 'mulberry' pattern. Syncytiotrophoblast cells are often located close to capillaries, and microhemorrhages may be seen in these foci. Unlike choriocarcinoma, the syncytiotrophoblast cells are not intermingled with a mononucleated trophoblast cell component nor do they form a nodular aggregate of variably differentiated trophoblastic cells. Instead, they are randomly scattered as single cells or very small groups. With hCG immunohistochemistry intratubular trophoblast can be detected in a substantial fraction of seminoma cases, indicating that differentiation toward trophoblastic elements may occur prior to invasion.[323]

### Special studies

Glycogen is usually prominent in seminoma (Fig. 13-27), and most cases show immunoreactivity for PLAP, generally in a peripheral, 'membranous' staining pattern (Fig. 13-28A); cytoplasmic staining may also be identified.[27,222,324,325] In one study[232] angiotensin-converting enzyme was demonstrated in 100% of 91 seminomas. Reactivity for the c-kit protein

occurs in most seminomas, again with a cytoplasmic membrane pattern similar to that of PLAP (Fig. 13-28B).[326,327] Seminomas are also uniformly reactive for OCT3/4 (Fig. 13-28C), a nuclear transcription factor identified in non-neoplastic stem cells and embryonic cells that plays an important role in the maintenance of a pluripotential capacity.[328,329] OCT3/4 staining is also seen in embryonal carcinoma but not in other testicular tumors.[226,328,329] The NANOG protein, a product of a gene located at 12p13, a region frequently amplified in testicular germ cell tumors, is similarly detectable by immunohistochemistry in IGCNU, seminoma, and embryonal carcinoma but not in teratoma or yolk sac tumor.[31,330] Many seminomas also express cytokeratin immunoreactivity, although such staining may only be demonstrable using frozen sections.[331] The most common cytokeratins in seminoma are cytokeratins 7, 8 and 18, although others, including cytokeratins 4, 17, and 19, can occasionally be identified.[331,332] Cytokeratin 20 is negative.[332] Epithelial membrane antigen (EMA) is only rarely expressed in seminoma,[27,300,332] and the combination of positivity for PLAP and negativity for EMA and cytokeratin (AE1/AE3) in formalin-fixed, paraffin-embedded tissue appears to be a relatively specific pattern for seminoma.[333] Vimentin, LDH, and NSE may be present in seminoma[27,331,334] but are not specific findings. A minority of seminomas may stain for Leu-7, $\alpha_1$-antitrypsin, desmin, and neurofilament protein.[27,331] Desmo-

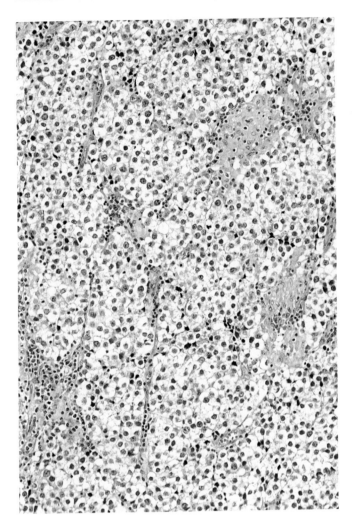

Fig. 13-21 Lymphocytes and epithelioid granulomas in seminoma.

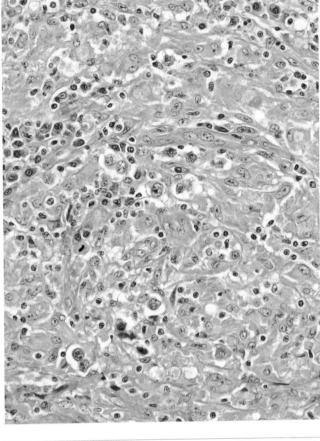

Fig. 13-22 An extensive granulomatous reaction in seminoma, leaving only rare tumor cells.

plakins and desmoglein are usually present in seminoma.[331,335] The syncytiotrophoblast cells that occur in some seminomas contain hCG,[27,38-40,336] and some cells containing hCG may not have an overtly 'syncytiotrophoblastic' appearance in routine sections.[38,39] CD30 is usually negative in seminoma, which contrasts with its virtually uniform presence in embryonal carcinoma,[332] except after chemotherapy, in which case loss of CD30 expression is frequently seen.[337]

Ultrastructurally, seminoma has closely apposed cytoplasmic membranes that usually show only sparse, primitive, intercellular junctions. The cellular organelles consist of scattered mitochondria, occasional cisternae of smooth and rough endoplasmic reticulum, ribosomes and polyribosomes, occasional membrane-bound lysosome-like structures, and occasional Golgi bodies; glycogen may be present in large quantities, but may also be sparse. It is common for the cytoplasmic organelles to be polarized eccentrically in the cytoplasm. The nuclei are round and have evenly dispersed chromatin and intricate, large nucleoli.[41,338,339] Occasional seminomas that are typical-appearing at the light microscopic level may show evidence of epithelial differentiation, with small, extracellular lumina, microvilli, and well-defined junctional complexes.[41] Despite 'transitional'

morphology at the ultrastructural level, such cases appear to behave as typical seminoma.[41]

The DNA content of seminoma is generally in the triploid to hypotetraploid range and is greater than that of non-seminomatous tumors.[32,43,340] The DNA content of seminomas with syncytiotrophoblast cells does not differ from that of seminomas lacking them, supporting their classification as seminoma.[341] Evolution of seminoma to other types of germ cell tumor may occur as a result of gene loss.[32,43,340,342] As in many testicular germ cell tumors, seminoma frequently contains an isochromosome derived from the short arms of chromosome 12-i(12p).[343,344] Numerous other cytogenetic abnormalities have also been described;[343] certain chromosomes are commonly overrepresented (1q, 7, 8, 12, 14q, 15q, 17, 21q, 22q, and X) and others underrepresented (3, 4, 5, 10, 11, 12q, 13q, 16, 18q, and Y).[343,345-347] A number of molecular observations are reported in seminoma, including absence of Fas,[348] loss of p18$^{INK4C}$ and upregulation of cyclin E,[50] cyclin D2 expression,[349] and inactivation of p16$^{INK4}$ by hypermethylation.[350] Activating exon 17 mutations of the c-kit gene are seen in 12–13% of cases[351,352] and about 20% have c-kit gene amplification.[352] Seminomas are reported to have loss of Notch 1, Jagged 2 and Fhit expression,[353,354] show SMAD4 and ras mutations,[355,356] and express DAZL1 protein,[357] hst-1,[358,359] N-myc,[360-362] and MAGE genes.[363]

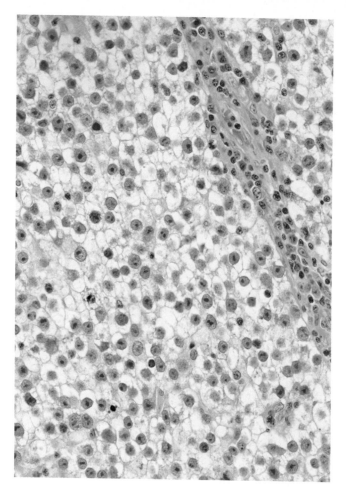

**Fig. 13-23** Seminoma cells with clear cytoplasm, well-defined cell borders, and nuclei with one or two prominent nucleoli. Lymphocytes and plasma cells are admixed, and some tumor nuclei have 'squared-off' edges.

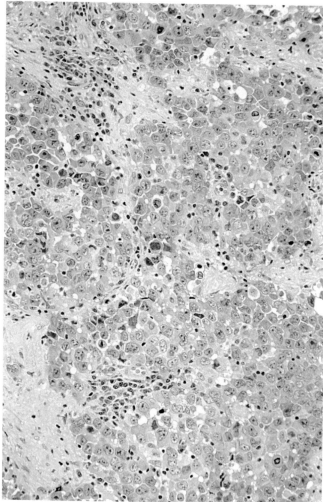

**Fig. 13-24** Seminoma with increased nuclear pleomorphism and crowding and denser cytoplasm than usual.

## Differential diagnosis

Seminoma can be misinterpreted as the solid pattern of embryonal carcinoma, especially in poorly fixed preparations. The formation of glands, true tubules, or papillae argues against the diagnosis of seminoma; the nuclei of seminoma are more uniform, less crowded, and more evenly spaced than those of embryonal carcinoma, which are pleomorphic, irregularly shaped, crowded, and appear to abut or even overlap. The cytoplasmic borders of seminoma are well defined, and those of embryonal carcinoma poorly defined. Embryonal carcinoma lacks the regular fibrous septa of many seminomas. Cytokeratin reactivity is usually weaker and PLAP reactivity stronger in seminoma than in embryonal carcinoma. CD30 reactivity is rare in seminoma and positive in embryonal carcinoma,[332] and CD30 immunohistochemistry may be especially useful in combination with CD117 (c-kit) to distinguish seminoma (CD30–/CD117+) from embryonal carcinoma (CD30+/CD117–).[364] AFP is occasionally positive in embryonal carcinoma and is negative in seminoma. Monoclonal antibody 43-9F is reported to be strongly reactive in embryonal carcinoma and negative or only weakly positive in seminoma,[365] but additional experience is necessary to confirm this finding. Podo-

planin (M2A, D2-40) is typically diffusely positive in seminoma and usually negative or focally reactive in embryonal carcinoma.[227,366]

The distinction of seminoma from spermatocytic seminoma is discussed on page 780.

Yolk sac tumor with a solid pattern may mimic seminoma. Such cases are usually distinguished from seminoma by the presence of typical patterns of yolk sac tumor and the tendency for microcyst formation in the solid areas. Edematous seminoma, however, may also produce a microcystic pattern, but the cystic spaces are usually more irregular and contain edema fluid and exfoliated neoplastic cells, in contrast to those of yolk sac tumor, although there are exceptional seminomas with regular and uniform microcysts.[309] The typical polygonal cells of seminoma in microcystic areas, however, contrast with the flattened cellular profiles and more variable nuclear appearance of yolk sac tumor cells lining microcystic spaces. Hyaline globules and intercellular basement membrane are frequent in yolk sac tumor but are rare in seminoma.[367] Fibrous septa and a lymphoid infiltrate are not usual features of yolk sac tumor. AFP is negative in

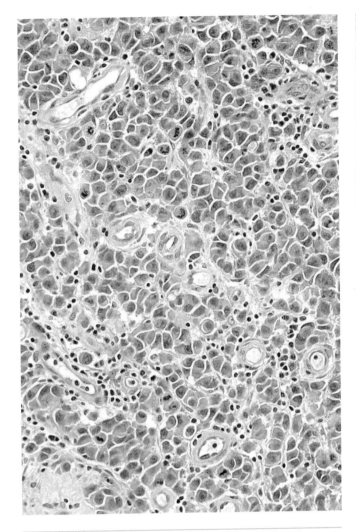

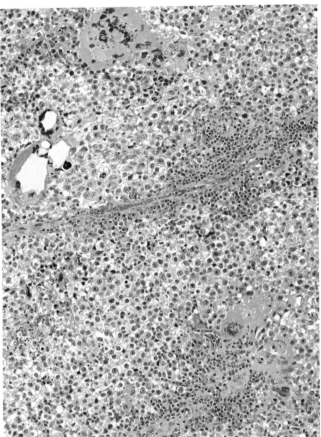

**Fig. 13-26** Seminoma with syncytiotrophoblast cells. Intracytoplasmic lacunae are present in some of the syncytiotrophoblast cells.

**Fig. 13-25** Plasmacytoid seminoma. Many cells have dense cytoplasm and eccentric nuclei.

seminoma and usually positive in yolk sac tumor; cytokeratin is often negative or weak in seminoma (in routinely processed tissues) whereas it is almost always strongly positive in yolk sac tumor. OCT3/4 and CD117 are strongly positive in seminoma but negative in yolk sac tumor.

Lymphoma must be distinguished from seminoma; most patients with testicular lymphoma are over 50 years of age, whereas those with seminoma are usually younger.[368-374] Bilateral involvement is more likely in lymphoma than in seminoma.[369,371-373,375] Lymphoma usually infiltrates the interstitium, preserving the seminiferous tubules,[371,372,376] whereas most seminomas do not show as prominent a degree of intertubular growth, although there are exceptions.[303] IGCNU is seen in seminoma but not lymphoma. Lymphoma often is more pleomorphic than seminoma, and may be composed of cells with cleaved and irregularly shaped nuclei that stand in contrast to the polygonal and relatively uniform nuclei of seminoma. The cytoplasm of lymphoma is usually amphophilic and less distinct than that of seminoma. Immunostains directed against PLAP and OCT3/4 are positive in seminoma and negative in lymphoma, whereas leukocyte common antigen (LCA) shows opposite results.[27,333]

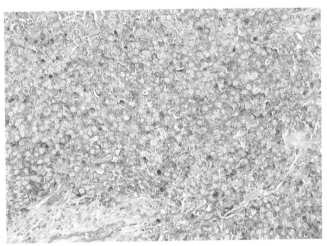

**Fig. 13-27** Periodic acid–Schiff positivity in a seminoma, indicating abundant glycogen.

Rarely, seminoma with a tubular pattern[305,306,308] may be confused with Sertoli cell tumor, a neoplasm that frequently has a tubular architecture.[377] The cytoplasmic clarity in seminoma is due to glycogen, whereas in Sertoli cell tumor lipid is mainly responsible for this appearance. Most Sertoli cell

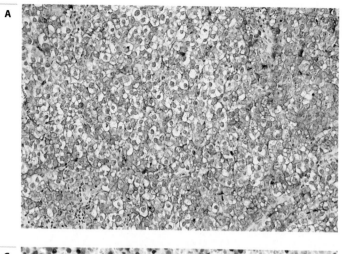

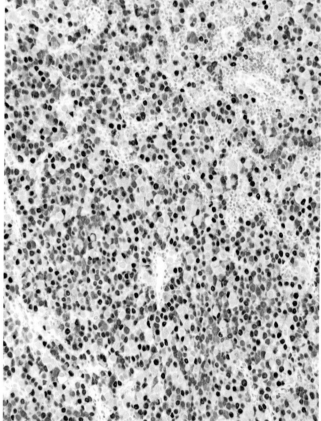

**Fig. 13-28** Seminoma showing a membranous pattern of positivity for (**A**) placental alkaline phosphatase and (**B**) c-kit (CD117). (**C**) Strong nuclear reactivity for OCT3/4 in seminoma.

tumors have low-grade cytological atypia that contrasts with the high-grade atypia of seminoma. IGCNU is present in almost all seminomas but is not associated with Sertoli cell tumor. Tubular patterns in seminoma are usually focal but may be widespread in Sertoli cell tumor.[306] Immunostains for PLAP and OCT3/4 are positive in seminoma but negative in Sertoli cell tumor, whereas inhibin is positive in a substantial proportion (but not all) of Sertoli cell tumors but negative in seminomas. This differential diagnosis may be further complicated by those Sertoli cell tumors that show a mostly diffuse growth pattern, frequently associated with a lymphocytic infiltrate.[378]

## Treatment and prognosis

Patients with early seminoma (clinical stage I or non-bulky stage II) are often treated with orchiectomy and radiation to the para-aortic and paracaval nodes, frequently with ipsilateral pelvic nodal radiation (so-called 'dog-leg' field),[379–381] although the pelvic field component may not be necessary for clinical stage I patients.[382,383] Prophylactic mediastinal radiation is not recommended. More than 95% of patients in clinical stages I and II are cured.[379–381,384,385] Most recurrences arise outside the radiated field, in the mediastinum, cervical lymph nodes, or lungs.[381,386] Surveillance remains a possible option for clinical stage I patients, 20% of whom will undergo relapse.[387] Chemotherapy is currently recommended for patients with bulky retroperitoneal involvement or in more advanced stages. ('Bulky' is defined variously in different studies as metastases greater than 5 cm, 6 cm, or 10 cm in diameter.) There is an 87% progression-free survival for advanced-stage seminoma patients who are initially treated with chemotherapy, whereas such patients who are initially irradiated and then treated with chemotherapy for persistent disease have a 3-year progression-free survival of 69%.[388]

A prominent lymphocytic reaction has been associated with an improved prognosis.[389,390] Elevation of serum hCG levels may indicate a worse prognosis,[288,293,294,391] although there are contradictory results in the literature.[285,291,295,392] It would be useful to identify a subset of seminoma with a poor prognosis at an early stage, as initial treatment with chemotherapy would probably improve the outcome in such a group. It is likely that the poor prognosis relates to the tendency of such cases to transform to non-seminomatous tumors, given the high frequency of non-seminomatous tumors at autopsy in patients who died following resection of pure testicular seminoma.[12,35]

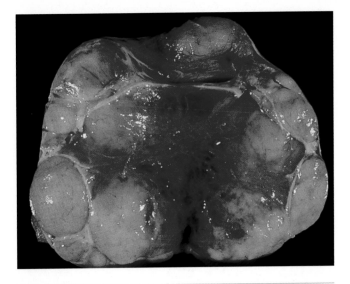

**Fig. 13-29** Cut surface of spermatocytic seminoma showing a multinodular, myxoid tumor. (Courtesy of Dr RH Young, Harvard Medical School, Boston, MA.)

## Spermatocytic seminoma

### Clinical features

Historically, spermatocytic seminoma was considered a variant of seminoma. Today it is recognized as a unique clinicopathologic entity with morphology and clinical features distinct from those of seminoma and other germ cell tumors.[393] Originally described by Masson in 1946,[394] spermatocytic seminoma is an unusual neoplasm that represents only 1–2% of testicular germ cell tumors[269] and occurs 20 times less frequently than seminoma.[395] Unlike other germ cell tumors it occurs only in the testis, more frequently on the right side.[396–398] Also unlike other testicular germ cell tumors, spermatocytic seminoma is not associated with cryptorchidism,[395] IGCNU,[257] or other types of germ cell tumor. It occurs as a pure lesion, except in rare cases in which it is associated with a sarcoma.[397,399–401] Spermatocytic seminoma is bilateral in about 9% of cases,[395] about four times as frequently as seminoma.

Most patients with spermatocytic seminoma are older than those with other types of testicular germ cell tumor. In three series, the average age varied from 52 to 59 years,[269,397,402,403] compared to an average of 40 years for patients with seminoma.[269] Most patients are white, but occurrence in African-Americans and Asians has been reported.[397] Most patients present with painless, often long-standing, testicular enlargement.[395,397] Serum marker studies (AFP, hCG, LDH) are negative.

### Pathologic features

Grossly, spermatocytic seminoma usually ranges from 3 to 15 cm in diameter[395] and has a variable appearance, with zones of fleshy, white tissue, mucoid change, friability, hemorrhage, and cystic change (Fig. 13-29). A multinodular appearance is frequent, and paratesticular extension may uncommonly occur.[397,404] Several patterns may be identified,

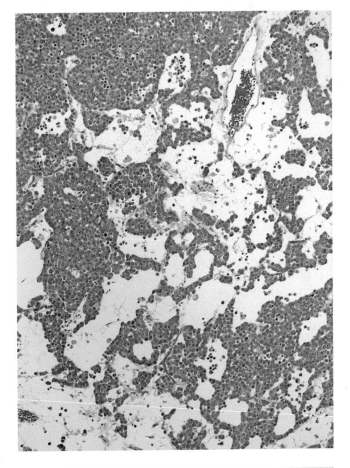

**Fig. 13-30** Sheets of tumor cells are interrupted by edema, creating irregular spaces and cords in a spermatocytic seminoma.

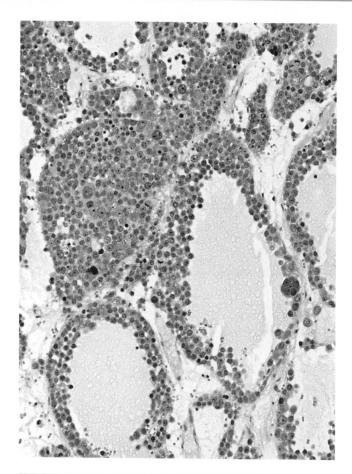

**Fig. 13-31** A pseudoglandular pattern in an edematous spermatocytic seminoma. Note multinucleated tumor giant cell.

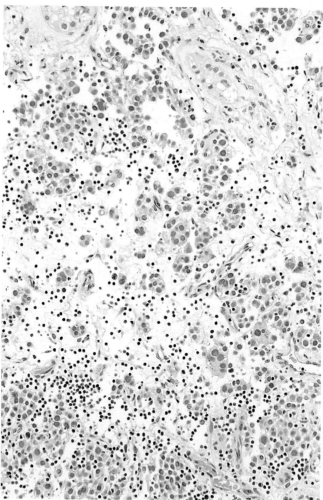

**Fig. 13-32** Small clusters of spermatocytic seminoma cells are separated by edematous stroma. Note admixed lymphocytes, an unusual feature.

frequently including a diffuse, sheet-like pattern that may be interrupted by pseudoglandular or microcystic areas caused by edema (Figs 13-30, 13-31). A well-defined cord-like (Fig. 13-30) or small nested pattern (Fig. 13-32) is most commonly seen in association with edematous areas. A lymphoid infiltrate is rarely seen (Fig. 13-32), and granulomatous reactions are virtually never encountered, unlike with seminoma. The microscopic hallmark of spermatocytic seminoma is a polymorphous population of cells (Fig. 13-33) that consists of three major types: a small, lymphocyte-like cell 6–8 µm in diameter; an intermediate-sized cell averaging 15–20 µm in diameter; and giant cells, some of which may be multinucleated (Fig. 13-31), averaging 50–100 µm in diameter. The smallest cell has smudged, degenerate-appearing chromatin and scant eosinophilic to basophilic cytoplasm. The intermediate-sized cell has a round nucleus, usually with granular chromatin and scant cytoplasm. In some intermediate-sized and giant cells the chromatin has a distinctive filamentous appearance similar to the chromatin of meiotic-phase, non-neoplastic spermatocytes ('spireme' chromatin) (Fig. 13-33). In contrast to seminoma, the borders between the cells are generally indistinct. Intratubular growth is common, and probably gives rise to separate invasive foci that cause the common multinodular or lobulated pattern of the tumor.

An 'anaplastic' variant of spermatocytic seminoma has been described.[405] These tumors have conventional areas but also large areas with a uniform population of cells having vesicular nuclei and prominent nucleoli (Fig. 13-34) that resemble either usual seminoma or embryonal carcinoma. Nonetheless, the immunohistochemical features are those of spermatocytic seminoma (see below), including negativity for PLAP, OCT3/4 and cytokeratins. The available follow-up has been benign.[405] Because the term 'anaplasia' often connotes a tumor with a poor prognosis, and this does not appear to be true for this variant, we prefer to recognize such cases as part of the spectrum of spermatocytic seminoma without designating them separately.

### Special studies

In contrast to seminoma, spermatocytic seminoma lacks glycogen. Most immunohistochemical markers are negative, including OCT3/4, vimentin, actin, desmin, AFP, hCG, NSE, carcinoembryonic antigen, and leukocyte common antigen.[327–329,396,397,405,406] Stains for placental alkaline phosphatase are also generally negative, although focal positivity for PLAP may occur in isolated clusters of cells.[397,406] Cyto-

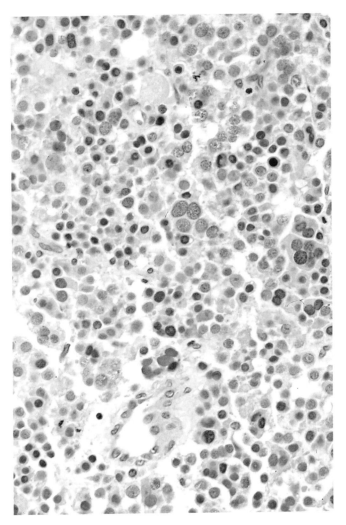

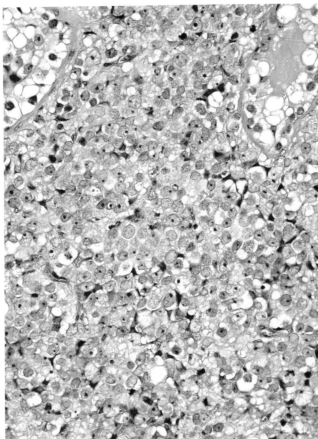

**Fig. 13-34** 'Anaplastic' spermatocytic seminoma. There is a predominance of intermediate-sized cells with prominent nucleoli.

**Fig. 13-33** The characteristic polymorphous cell population of spermatocytic seminoma. Several cells have filamentous chromatin.

keratin stains are also usually negative, although perinuclear dot-like positivity for cytokeratin 18 can be seen infrequently.[331,396] Spermatocytic seminoma expresses proteins (synaptonemal complex protein 1, synovial sarcoma on X chromosome and xeroderma pigmentosa type A) that are characteristic of spermatogonia and spermatocytes,[407] indicating a more 'mature' form of tumor differentiation than classic seminoma.

Ultrastructurally, spermatocytic seminoma may show intercellular bridges similar to those described in spermatocytes, as well as leptotene stage-type chromosomes – i.e., filamentous chromosomes with lateral fibrils.[408,409] These features suggest meiotic-phase differentiation, but their presence and specificity are disputed.[410] Adjacent cells occasionally show macula adherens-type junctions, and a Golgi body is a variably prominent feature. Other features include scattered mitochondria, occasional profiles of rough endoplasmic reticulum, nuclei with prominent nucleoli, and a thin basement membrane surrounding nests of tumor cells.[408,410]

Flow cytometric studies have demonstrated variable DNA content, including hyperdiploidy, peritriploidy, diploidy,

peridiploidy, tetraploidy, and aneuploidy.[257,327,406,410] No haploid population has ever been found, arguing against the concept that spermatocytic seminoma is postmeiotic. These variable results probably reflect the heterogeneous population of these neoplasms, as static cytophotometry of spermatocytic seminoma has demonstrated a diploid or near-diploid DNA content in the small cell component, and a DNA content ranging up to 42C in the giant cell population, with intermediate values in the intermediate-sized cells.[411] One study suggested that the cells of spermatocytic seminoma arise following cycles of polyploidization, refuting the notion of a meiotic-phase tumor.[412] A recent karyotypic and differential gene profiling study (versus usual seminoma) found that spermatocytic seminoma showed consistent gain in chromosome 9, failed to express the stem cell associated genes typical of usual seminoma, and expressed genes associated with prophase of meiosis I.[413] These data support the derivation of spermatocytic seminoma from the primary spermatocyte.

### Treatment and prognosis

There are only two credible cases of metastasizing spermatocytic seminoma,[414,415] and earlier reports of metastases reflect misdiagnoses of testicular lymphoma.[398] As several hundred cases of spermatocytic seminoma have been

**Table 13-4** Comparison of the clinical and pathologic features of spermatocytic seminoma and typical seminoma (Adapted from Scully RE. Spermatocytic seminoma of the testis: a report of 3 cases and review of the literature. Cancer 1961; 14: 788–794; and Damjanov I. Tumors of the testis and epididymis. In: Murphy WM, ed. Urological pathology. Philadelphia: WB Saunders, 1989; 314–379)

| | Spermatocytic seminoma | Typical seminoma |
|---|---|---|
| Mean age | 55 years | 40 years |
| Proportion of germ cell tumors | 2% | 40–50% |
| Sites | Testis only | Testis, ovary (dysgerminoma), mediastinum, pineal, RP |
| Associated with cryptorchidism | No | Yes |
| Bilaterality | 9% | 2% |
| Association with other forms of germ cell tumor | No | Yes |
| Association with IGCNU | No | Yes |
| Association with sarcoma | Rare | No |
| Composition | 3 cell types, with denser cytoplasm, round nuclei | 1 cell type, often clear cytoplasm, 'boxy' nuclei |
| Intercellular edema | Common | Less common |
| Stroma | Scanty | Prominent |
| Lymphoid reaction | Rare to absent | Prominent |
| Granulomas | Virtually never | Often prominent |
| Glycogen | Absent to scant | Abundant |
| PLAP staining | Absent to scant | Prominent |
| OCT3/4 staining | Absent | Prominent |
| hCG staining | Absent | Present in 10% |
| Metastases | Virtually never | Common |

hCG, human chorionic gonadotropin; IGCNU, intratubular germ cell neoplasia, unclassified; PLAP, placental-like alkaline phosphatase; RP, retroperitoneum.

reported in the literature, the frequency of malignant behavior is well under 1%. Therefore, orchiectomy alone is adequate treatment;[395,403] adjuvant therapy is not indicated and may be harmful.

### Differential diagnosis

The major differential diagnosis of spermatocytic seminoma is seminoma. A summary of features helpful in this distinction is listed in Table 13-4. For the 'anaplastic' variant, embryonal carcinoma is a consideration. The presence of the usual triphasic appearance of spermatocytic seminoma, at least in foci, is quite helpful in such cases, as is the round nuclear contour that contrasts with the much more irregularly shaped nuclei of embryonal carcinoma. Strong cytokeratin, OCT3/4, and CD30 reactivity is expected for embryonal carcinoma but is absent in spermatocytic seminoma.[416]

### Spermatocytic seminoma with sarcoma

Several cases of spermatocytic seminoma associated with sarcoma have been reported.[397,399-401] Some of the patients gave a history of a stable testicular mass that underwent rapid enlargement or became painful.[399,400] Some patients had symptoms secondary to metastases.[399] Grossly, many of the tumors were hemorrhagic, necrotic, and had a whorled appearance on the cut surface.[399,400] Microscopically, the sarcoma was often admixed with the spermatocytic

seminoma and usually described as an undifferentiated spindle cell sarcoma or embryonal rhabdomyosarcoma (Fig. 13-35).[397,399-401] In contrast to pure spermatocytic seminoma, over half of the reported cases of spermatocytic seminoma with sarcoma metastasized, frequently with a fatal outcome.[399-401] The metastases were in a hematogenous distribution, with the lung being the most common metastatic site, and consisted solely of sarcoma.

### Embryonal carcinoma

Although very common in mixed germ cell tumors (occurring in 87% of non-seminomatous germ cell tumors[269]), embryonal carcinoma is less frequent as a pure testicular germ cell tumor, comprising only 2.3% of cases in a referral practice[418] and about 10% of testicular tumors in two general series.[269,270] A decline in the reported proportion of pure embryonal carcinoma among testicular germ cell tumors is largely attributable to the recognition of foci of yolk sac tumor in such cases, leading to their categorization as mixed germ cell tumors. This finding reflects the capacity of embryonal carcinoma to differentiate into other forms of testicular neoplasia, as verified by experimental observations, including tissue culture.[419-423] Embryonal carcinoma expresses the stage-specific embryonic antigen (SSEA) indicative of a primitive, undifferentiated stage of development, SSEA-3, but not SSEA-1, which indicates a more mature phenotype.[424]

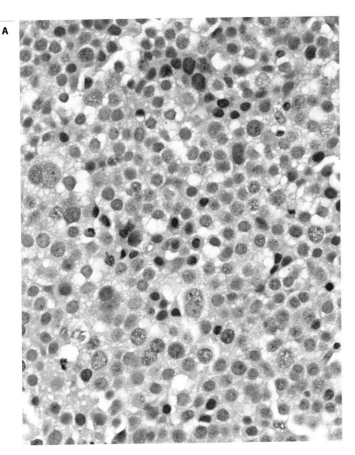
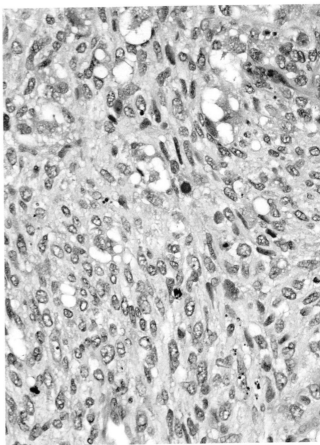

**Fig. 13-35** (**A**) A spermatocytic seminoma with a spindle cell sarcoma component (**B**).

## Clinical features

The peak incidence of embryonal carcinoma occurs at about 30 years of age;[269] it is distinctly rare in prepubertal children.[274,425–427] It usually presents as a testicular mass, with gynecomastia or symptoms of metastases occurring in about 10% of cases each.[428] Rare cases may present with sudden death due to massive tumor thromboemboli to the lungs.[429,430] However, metastases are clinically or radiographically evident in about 40% of patients at presentation, and two-thirds of patients who are pathologically staged have metastases.[428] As in seminoma, limbic encephalopathy may be a rare form of presentation.[281]

Serum AFP elevation in embryonal carcinoma[286] is usually the result of misclassification of mixed germ cell tumor (embryonal carcinoma and yolk sac tumor), and it is uncommon for morphologically pure embryonal carcinoma to be associated with serum AFP elevation.[418] Many embryonal carcinomas are associated with syncytiotrophoblast cells, accounting for serum hCG elevation in 60% of cases.[286] PLAP, LDH and CA19-9 levels may also be elevated.[431,432]

## Pathologic features

Grossly, embryonal carcinoma is usually poorly circumscribed and gray-white, with prominent areas of hemorrhage and necrosis (Fig. 13-36). Microscopically there are three major patterns, all of which are composed of cohesive groups of primitive, anaplastic epithelial cells. In the solid pattern, the cells are arranged in diffuse sheets (Fig. 13-37). In the tubular or glandular pattern, well-defined, gland-like or tubule-like structures are formed by epithelium varying from cuboidal to columnar (Fig. 13-38). The luminal spaces are cleft-like or round. In the papillary pattern, the papillae may or may not have stromal cores (Fig. 13-39). Prominent foci of eosinophilic, coagulative necrosis are common in all forms of embryonal carcinoma. Cells with smudged, hyperchromatic nuclei are distinctive but non-specific (Fig. 13-40). Such cells are considered to be degenerate, but they may be misinterpreted as syncytiotrophoblasts, thereby leading to a misdiagnosis of choriocarcinoma. Unlike syncytiotrophoblast cells, however, these degenerate embryonal carcinoma cells lack hCG and are not usually associated with hemorrhage.

Rarely, embryonal carcinoma has a blastocyst-like pattern with central vesicle-like spaces.[301] A 'double-layered' pattern of embryonal carcinoma has also been described in which a papillary arrangement of embryonal carcinoma is accompanied by a parallel layer of flattened neoplastic epithelium (Fig. 13-41).[433] This pattern, however, is more accurately classified as embryonal carcinoma with yolk sac tumor

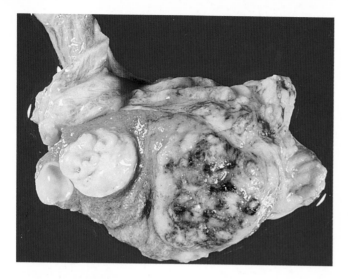

**Fig. 13-36** The large nodule is embryonal carcinoma, showing areas of hemorrhage and necrosis.

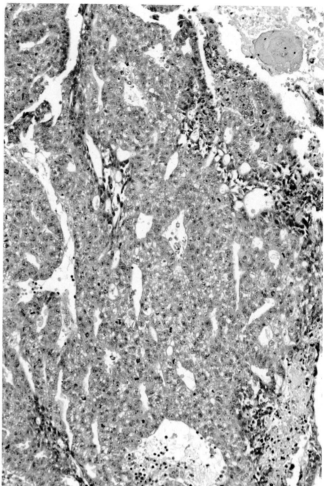

**Fig. 13-38** Embryonal carcinoma, glandular pattern.

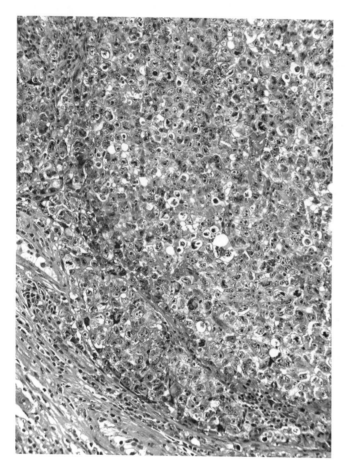

**Fig. 13-37** Solid pattern of embryonal carcinoma.

and should therefore be regarded as a mixed germ cell tumor.

At high magnification the cells have variable staining, abundant cytoplasm and large, vesicular, irregular nuclei with prominent macronucleoli (Fig. 13-42). The cell borders

are ill defined, unlike those of seminoma, and the nuclei are often crowded, appearing to abut or overlap. Karyorrhectic fragments are frequent in the background, and the mitotic rate is high.

The capacity of embryonal carcinoma to form a minor amount of undifferentiated neoplastic stroma (Fig. 13-43) is widely recognized.[15,300] The rationale for this is that embryonal carcinoma is a primitive neoplasm recapitulating an early phase of embryonic development, and the formation of such stroma is consistent with this concept. Nonetheless, there are inconsistencies with respect to diagnosing such cases as embryonal carcinoma or embryonal carcinoma and teratoma.[270] Based on the experience of the BTTP, no significant prognostic difference was noted in embryonal carcinoma with or without a stromal component, but those data were obtained in an era before effective chemotherapy.[16] Because teratoma components in the testis are associated with an increased risk for persistent tumor in metastatic sites following chemotherapy, we believe that a stromal component should be regarded as teratoma rather than 'lumped' under the diagnosis of embryonal carcinoma.

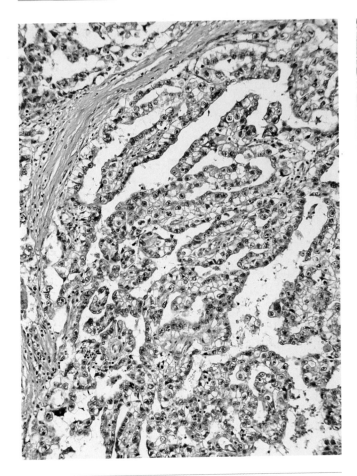

**Fig. 13-39** Embryonal carcinoma, papillary pattern.

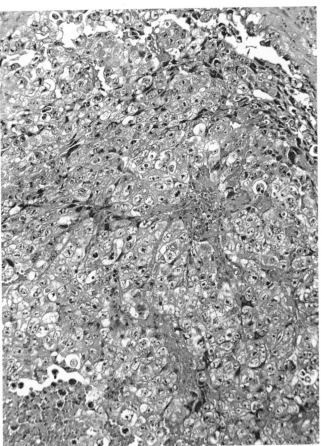

**Fig. 13-40** Solid pattern of embryonal carcinoma with degenerate, smudged cells and focal necrosis.

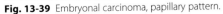

Embryonal carcinoma is often associated with intratubular embryonal carcinoma, which is typically extensively necrotic, having a comedocarcinoma-like appearance (Fig. 13-44). Such necrotic foci may undergo dystrophic calcification, leading to the formation of so-called 'hematoxylin-staining bodies.'[434] Such coarse intratubular calcifications in scarred areas are excellent evidence of a regressed germ cell tumor.[434,435]

The identification of vascular invasion in non-seminomatous germ cell tumors (including embryonal carcinoma) is important in deciding whether patients with clinical stage I tumors are appropriate candidates for 'surveillance only' management (see page 786). In the majority of cases when such invasion is present, embryonal carcinoma is the angio-invasive element. There are some pitfalls in deciding whether vascular invasion is present. First, intratubular neoplasm may closely resemble intravascular neoplasm. The presence of residual Sertoli cells in a possible 'vessel' is good evidence that it is a tubule (Fig. 13-45). Additionally, intratubular tumor is often extensively necrotic, and the tubules are non-branching and relatively similar in caliber, whereas intravascular tumor does not typically show necrosis and may occur in branched vessels of different sizes. Second, stringent criteria must be applied such that invaded tissue spaces are clearly lined by endothelial cells before they are regarded as vessels. Third, germ cell tumors, and especially embryonal

carcinoma, are quite cellular and friable, leading to artifactual, knife-implantation of tumor cells into vascular spaces. Such implants, however, are loosely cohesive and unassociated with vascular thrombosis, whereas legitimate vascular invasion is characterized by neoplasm conforming to the shape of the vessel, which may also show evidence of thrombosis. Commonly, artifactual vascular implants are also associated with implants on the surfaces of tissues. It is usually easiest to appreciate vascular invasion a short distance away from the periphery of the neoplasm (Fig. 13-46).

### Special studies

Only a small percentage of cases of pure embryonal carcinoma demonstrate AFP immunoreactivity, but such positivity is more common in the embryonal carcinoma component of mixed germ cell tumor,[436,437] a fact that probably represents early biochemical transformation to a yolk sac tumor component in cases of mixed germ cell tumor before morphological differentiation. PLAP positivity occurs in 86–97% of cases of embryonal carcinoma[27,225,438] but is usually patchy and weaker than in seminoma. Several different cytokeratin classes are present in embryonal carcinoma, most prominently cytokeratins 8 and 18, but also 19, and occasionally 4 and 17.[439] Most authors therefore report strong and diffuse

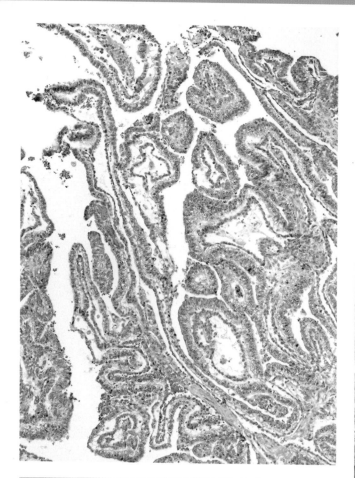

**Fig. 13-41** The 'double-layered' pattern of embryonal carcinoma, consisting of ribbons of embryonal carcinoma with a parallel layer of flattened cells. This is classified as mixed germ cell tumor, sometimes termed 'diffuse embryoma,' and consists of embryonal carcinoma and yolk sac tumor (the flattened layer).

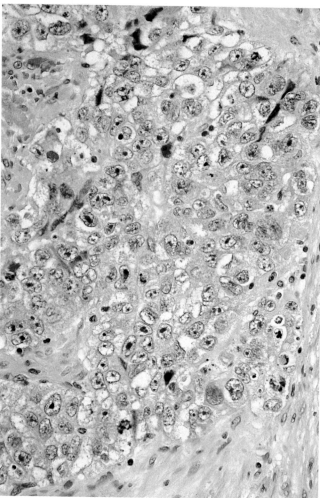

**Fig. 13-42** Embryonal carcinoma. Note the ill-defined cell borders and large, crowded, vesicular nuclei with large nucleoli.

positivity for cytokeratins in the majority of embryonal carcinomas, including routinely processed cases.[27,440] Immunostains for CD30 (Ber-H2, Ki-1) are positive in 84% of cases (Fig. 13-47),[441,442] whereas EMA is negative in almost all embryonal carcinomas.[27] In contrast to seminoma, CD117 is negative or only focally positive in embryonal carcinoma. OCT3/4, a nuclear transcription factor, is highly sensitive and specific for embryonal carcinoma, seminoma, and IGCNU, with no staining observed in other germ cell tumor types or other forms of testicular tumor, and only very rare positivity seen in lung and renal cell carcinomas.[29,329] There is therefore a characteristic immunohistochemical profile: cytokeratin-positive, PLAP-positive, OCT3/4-positive, CD30-positive with EMA-negative and c-kit-negative. This profile can be of great value in distinguishing embryonal carcinoma in an extragonadal site (either a metastasis or an extratesticular primary) from a poorly differentiated carcinoma of non-germinal origin (typically, cytokeratin-positive, PLAP-variable – but most commonly negative – CD30-negative, OCT3/4-negative and EMA-positive).[333] The presence of CD30 in embryonal carcinoma indicates the necessity for caution and additional supportive evidence before accepting a CD30-positive, poorly differen-

tiated malignant neoplasm as an anaplastic large cell lymphoma. Reactivity with monoclonal antibody 43-9F has been reported as positive in embryonal carcinoma, but weak or absent in seminoma, choriocarcinoma, and most cases of yolk sac tumor.[365] Occasionally, embryonal carcinoma will also stain for $\alpha_1$-antitrypsin, Leu-7, vimentin, LDH, human placental lactogen (HPL), and ferritin.[27,334,436,443] The product of the p53 tumor suppressor gene is often identifiable in embryonal carcinoma,[204,205] although the absence of mutations with molecular biologic techniques support that this is the result of non-mutated overexpression.[202,203]

Ultrastructurally, embryonal carcinoma usually resembles a poorly differentiated, primitive adenocarcinoma with ill-defined lumina in solid areas and well-defined, large lumina in glandular areas.[41] The lumina are bordered by cells having well-defined junctional complexes with characteristically long tight junctions.[444] Short microvilli project into the luminal spaces, and the cytoplasm contains ribosomes, a prominent Golgi body, rough endoplasmic reticulum, teleolysosomes, mitochondria, glycogen, and occasional lipid droplets. The nuclei are large, deeply indented, often contain

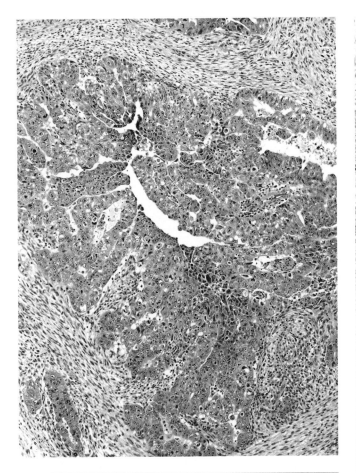

**Fig. 13-43** Neoplastic stroma in an embryonal carcinoma. Classification as embryonal carcinoma and teratoma is recommended, although some regard the neoplastic stroma as being within the spectrum of embryonal carcinoma.

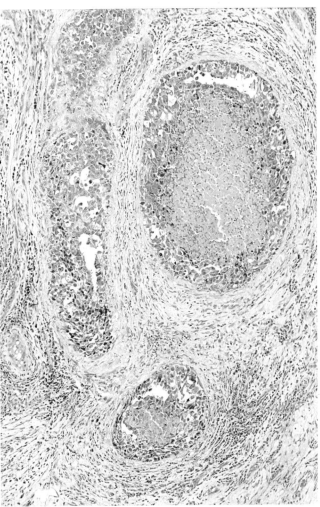

**Fig. 13-44** Intratubular embryonal carcinoma with characteristic abundant necrosis.

cytoplasmic inclusions, and have large nucleoli with complex nucleolonema.[41]

Embryonal carcinoma has a DNA index ranging from 1.4 to 1.6 times normal, which is significantly less than that of seminoma.[32,43] Embryonal carcinoma often contains isochromosome (12p), and increased copy numbers of i(12p) have correlated with a more aggressive clinical course.[344] The presence of i(12p) or other 12p amplifications[445] in a poorly differentiated carcinoma, either metastatic or a primary neoplasm of an extragonadal site, may be a useful means of separating embryonal carcinoma from other poorly differentiated neoplasms.[446] The detection of 12p abnormalities can be accomplished in interphase cells obtained from fresh biopsy samples or in paraffin-embedded tumor by the fluorescence in situ hybridization technique.[447,448]

### Differential diagnosis

The distinction of embryonal carcinoma from seminoma was discussed on page 774. The distinction of embryonal carcinoma from yolk sac tumor depends on the presence, in yolk sac tumor, of one of several distinctive patterns (see page 788), and the larger and more pleomorphic nature of the neoplastic cells in embryonal carcinoma. Yolk sac tumor often contains hyaline globules and intercellular basement membrane, which are almost always lacking in embryonal carcinoma,[367] and AFP is much more likely to be present in yolk sac tumor than in embryonal carcinoma. CD30 positivity is characteristic of embryonal carcinoma and is not usually present in yolk sac tumor.[441] OCT3/4 is positive in embryonal carcinoma and negative in yolk sac tumor.[30,328] Recently, glypican-3 has been identified as an immunohistochemical marker for yolk sac tumor: it is negative in seminoma and positive in only 0–8% of embryonal carcinomas.[449,450] Because embryonal carcinoma may transform into yolk sac tumor, there are foci where the distinction is arbitrary. However, such cases invariably show areas of both neoplastic types. The smudged, degenerate cells common in embryonal carcinoma may be misinterpreted as syncytiotrophoblast cells, causing a misdiagnosis of choriocarcinoma. These cells lack hCG, however, and the background is usually not hemorrhagic, unlike true choriocarcinoma. Large cell lymphoma usually occurs in older patients, lacks the epithelial patterns usually identified in embryonal carcinoma, has an interstitial growth pattern, is not associated with IGCNU, and is PLAP, OCT3/4 and cytokeratin negative and LCA positive, features which contrast with those of embryonal carci-

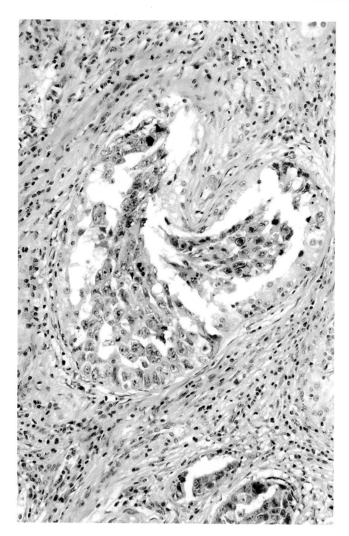

**Fig. 13-45** Intratubular embryonal carcinoma can be reliably distinguished from vascular invasion if there are residual Sertoli cells.

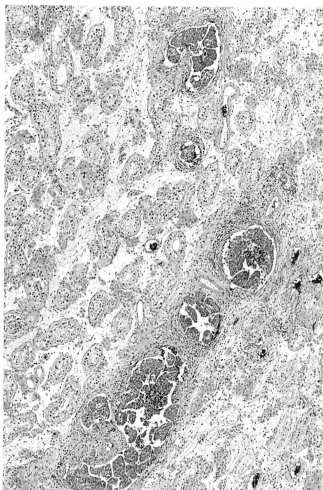

**Fig. 13-46** Vascular invasion that was peripheral to embryonal carcinoma.

noma.[333] The differential with 'anaplastic' spermatocytic seminoma is discussed on page 780.

### Treatment and prognosis

The treatment of non-seminomatous germ cell tumors, including embryonal carcinoma, depends on the clinical stage of the patient; there is a lack of consensus about the best approach in some cases. For patients with clinical stage I tumor, the lack of consensus is most apparent. Orchiectomy is required in all instances for therapy and diagnosis. However, one school of thought advocates nerve-sparing retroperitoneal lymph node dissection (RPLND),[451] tailored to excise the commonly involved nodal groups ipsilateral to the affected testis, in order to verify the absence of retroperitoneal metastases (pathologic stage I).[452] If nodal involvement is not identified by RPLND, no additional treatment is required. Overall, about 10% of such patients relapse, but almost all are salvaged by combination chemotherapy.[452,453] The relapse rate is higher (21%) for those patients who had a predominance of embryonal carcinoma in the orchiec-

tomy specimen.[454] If there are nodal metastases, such patients may either be followed (with the thought that RPLND was both diagnostic and therapeutic) or receive adjuvant chemotherapy, depending on such factors as the extent of nodal involvement and the reliability of the patient. In one series of clinical stage I patients, retroperitoneal lymph node dissection confirmed pathologic stage II disease in 28% of patients.[455] For the pathologic stage II patients who receive no adjuvant chemotherapy, the overall relapse rate is 23%; for those who receive adjuvant chemotherapy it is 0%.[453]

Another school of thought advocates simple follow-up of patients with clinical stage I non-seminomatous germ cell tumor (the 'surveillance only' approach), as only about 30% ultimately relapse (most of whom would have had clinically occult metastases identified on RPLND). Relapse can be detected early by serum marker elevation, and almost all relapsing patients can be salvaged by standard chemotherapy. This approach avoids unnecessary RPLND in the 70–72% of patients who are cured by orchiectomy alone.[455,456] A review of 560 clinical stage I patients managed by surveillance only found that 97% were tumor free and that 72% required no therapy after orchiectomy.[457] However, there may be certain patients with clinical stage I tumors in whom

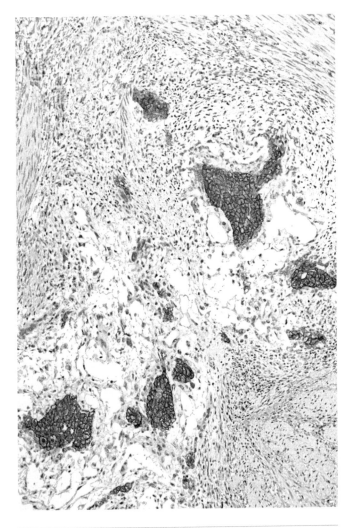

**Fig. 13-47** Immunostaining for CD30 selectively highlights the embryonal carcinoma component in a mixed germ cell tumor also having foci of yolk sac tumor.

expected.[452] For patients with bulky clinical stage II or more advanced tumor, treatment is combination chemotherapy followed by surgical resection of residual masses if the serum markers have normalized. A survival rate of 70–80% is expected.[9,477] Specimens resected after chemotherapy must be carefully evaluated pathologically to determine the need for additional chemotherapy (see page 812).[478]

A number of different studies have been conducted in order to identify prognostic factors in patients with non-seminomatous testicular germ cell tumors. The most important are tumor stage, the extent of serum marker elevation, the age of the patient (older being worse), the presence of choriocarcinoma, and the proliferative fraction by flow cytometry.[477,479–482]

## Yolk sac tumor

Yolk sac tumor is the most recently recognized testicular germ cell tumor. For years, ovarian yolk sac tumor was misclassified, along with ovarian clear cell carcinoma, as 'mesonephroma.' Teilum[483] recognized the similarity between testicular and ovarian yolk sac tumor and the frequent admixture of the testicular lesion with other forms of germ cell tumor. This observation permitted the classification of yolk sac tumor as a form of germ cell neoplasm and the removal of the ovarian lesion from the 'mesonephroma' category. Subsequently, Teilum recognized the resemblance of the mesenchyme of yolk sac tumor to the extraembryonic mesenchyme of development and the glomeruloid structures to the endodermal sinuses of the rat placenta.[484,485]

### Clinical features

In registry series of prepubertal testicular tumors, yolk sac tumor is the most common neoplasm, accounting for 82% of testicular germ cell tumors and the majority of all testicular neoplasms.[274] This dominance, however, is questioned as secondary to reporting bias, as yolk sac tumors represented only 15% of the cases in the combined experience at four centers with testicular tumors in patients less than 12 years of age.[486] It occurs in children from birth to 9 years of age, with a median age of about 18 months.[487,488] Unlike yolk sac tumors in adults, those in children are almost always pure, without other germ cell tumor components. Postpubertal patients with yolk sac tumor fall within the usual spectrum of age for non-seminomatous testicular germ cell tumor, ranging from 15 to 45 years and averaging 25–30 years; rare cases have been reported in elderly patients.[489] Prospective studies of non-seminomatous germ cell tumors have shown that yolk sac tumor elements are present in 44% of cases.[490]

The usual epidemiological associations of testicular germ cell tumor do not apply to childhood yolk sac tumor. There is no association with cryptorchidism, and the predilection for whites over other races is lacking.[491]

Children with yolk sac tumor almost always present with a painless testicular mass; clinical evidence of metastasis is rare at presentation, occurring in only 6% of cases.[487,492] Adults with yolk sac tumor in a mixed germ cell tumor are more likely to have lower-stage disease than those without

the risk of relapse is excessive, making them inappropriate candidates for surveillance only. These patients may be identified by a careful, multifactorial analysis of the orchiectomy specimen. Factors that correlate with relapse or occult retroperitoneal metastases include lymphovascular invasion,[428,455,457–469] a large proportion or volume of embryonal carcinoma,[462,468–471] pure embryonal carcinoma,[461] absence of a yolk sac tumor component,[472] embryonal carcinoma in the absence of teratoma,[457] less than 50% teratoma,[459,462] the presence of choriocarcinoma,[464] high S or $G_2M+S$ phase values as determined by flow cytometry,[471] a high proportion of proliferating tumor cells,[473] and highly aneuploid tumor stemlines.[474,475] Embryonal carcinomas with a high Ki-67 labeling index, low apoptosis, and low p53 expression have a better overall survival.[476] A pre-orchiectomy AFP value exceeding 80 ng/mL[462] and an abnormally slow decline in AFP values following orchiectomy[465] have also correlated with relapse. Patients having clinically apparent, non-bulky retroperitoneal involvement (clinical stage II) are usually managed by RPLND with either close follow-up or a limited course of adjuvant therapy. Survival in excess of 95% is

a yolk sac tumor component, and the absence of a yolk sac tumor component in a mixed germ cell tumor may be a positive predictor of occult metastases with clinical stage I tumors.[466] Almost all patients with yolk sac tumor have significant elevation of serum AFP, typically ranging from hundreds to thousands of nanograms per milliliter.[493,494] Embryonal carcinoma or enteric elements of teratoma may cause minor elevations of serum AFP, but this is unusual.[418,493]

## Pathologic features

Grossly, yolk sac tumor in children appears as solid, gray-white to tan, relatively homogeneous nodules with myxoid or gelatinous cut surfaces (Fig. 13-48); cystic change may be present. In adults the appearance is usually heterogeneous, with frequent areas of hemorrhage, necrosis, and cystic change (Fig. 13-49). Numerous microscopic patterns are seen in yolk sac tumor and commonly include hybrid, incomplete, and transitional forms. The patterns, modified from the enumeration of Talerman,[495] include microcystic (honeycomb, reticular, vacuolated); endodermal sinus (perivascular); papillary; solid; glandular/alveolar; myxomatous; sarcomatoid; macrocystic; polyvesicular vitelline; hepatoid; and parietal.

The microcystic pattern is the most common and is characterized by intracellular vacuoles creating attenuated lengths of cytoplasm connected in a spider-web-like array (Fig. 13-50). The cells often resemble lipoblasts, with compressed nuclei secondary to the vacuoles, although the vacuoles do not contain lipid. In some cases the cells are arranged in cords and surround extracellular spaces, creating a reticular arrangement (Fig. 13-51). The microcystic pattern is often seen with a myxoid stroma and blends with the myxomatous pattern (Fig. 13-52). The solid pattern is also commonly intermingled with the microcystic (Fig. 13-53).

The endodermal sinus pattern consists of a central vessel rimmed by fibrous tissue which in turn is surrounded by malignant epithelium. This structure is contained within a cystic space that is often lined by flattened tumor cells

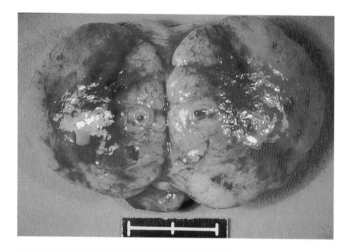

**Fig. 13-48** Infantile yolk sac tumor consists of a myxoid, tan nodule with focal hemorrhage.

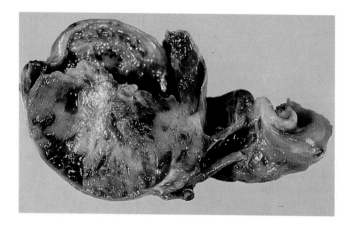

**Fig. 13-49** Adult yolk sac tumor showing hemorrhage, cystic degeneration, and myxoid change. (From Ulbright TM, Roth LM. Testicular and paratesticular neoplasms. In: Sternberg SS, ed. Diagnostic surgical pathology. New York: Raven Press, 1994; 1885–1947, with permission.)

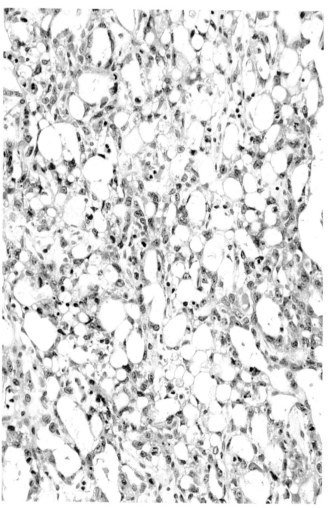

**Fig. 13-50** Microcystic pattern of yolk sac tumor resulting from intracellular vacuoles.

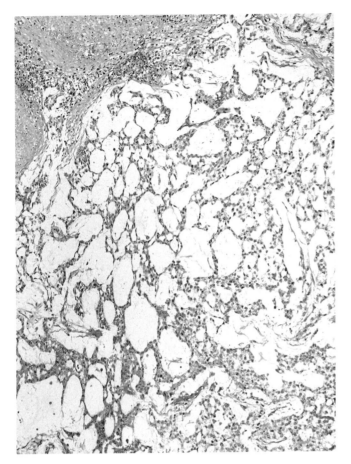

**Fig. 13-51** Microcystic pattern of yolk sac tumor created by cords of cells surrounding extracellular space (also referred to as reticular pattern).

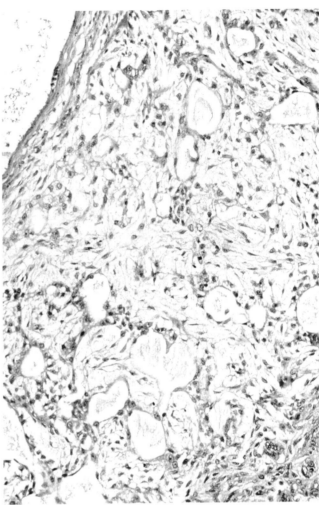

**Fig. 13-52** Blending of microcystic and myxoid patterns of yolk sac tumor. Neoplastic cells appear to 'bud' from microcystic structures and blend into a myxoid stroma.

(Fig. 13-54). Oblique cuts of these structures result in fibrovascular cores of tissue that are 'draped' or 'festooned' by malignant cells with an accompanying complex ('labyrinthine') arrangement of anastomosing extracellular spaces (Fig. 13-55). Some authors designate this a 'perivascular' or a 'festoon' pattern. The endodermal sinus-like structure is sometimes termed a 'glomeruloid' or 'Schiller–Duval' body.[485]

The papillary pattern has papillae, with or without fibrovascular cores, which project into cystic spaces (Fig. 13-56). The cells are often cuboidal to low columnar, with a 'hobnail' configuration due to the nucleus producing an apical cytoplasmic 'bulge.' Exfoliated clusters of neoplastic cells may be present in the cystic spaces. The papillary pattern may blend with the endodermal sinus pattern.

The solid pattern is quite common and may resemble seminoma, consisting of sheets of tumor cells with lightly staining to clear cytoplasm and well-defined borders (Fig. 13-57). However, the lymphoid component and fibrous septa of seminoma are usually absent, and the cells are less uniform than those of seminoma. Some solid patterns have prominent thin-walled blood vessels, and focal microcysts may also be seen in an otherwise solid pattern (Figs 13-53, 13-57). In some cases the solid pattern has small cells with scant cytoplasm resembling blastema (Fig. 13-58); such foci are intimately intermingled with classic patterns of yolk sac tumor.

Well-defined glands, often with enteric features, are common in yolk sac tumor (Fig. 13-59), present in 34% of cases in one series.[367] The glands may be contiguous with vesicles typical of the polyvesicular vitelline pattern, or may appear in a background of myxomatous, microcystic, or solid patterns. Usually the glands are simple, round, and tubular, but may show an elaborate branching pattern or become quite intricate and complex (Fig. 13-60). Unlike the glands of teratoma, the glands of yolk sac tumor are not associated with other teratomatous components and lack the smooth muscle component that is common but not invariable in teratoma.[496] In many cases the nuclei of the glands are more bland than those of the surrounding yolk sac tumor. The glands may show subnuclear vacuolation, reminiscent of the early secretory pattern of the endometrium; and predominantly glandular yolk sac tumor in the ovary has been termed 'endometrioid-like' to emphasize its resemblance to endometrioid carcinoma.[497] Purely or predomi-

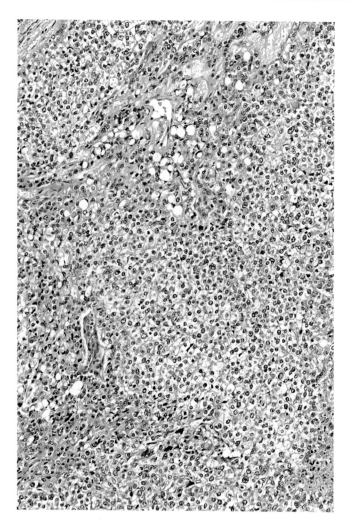

**Fig. 13-53** Mixture of solid and microcystic patterns in yolk sac tumor.

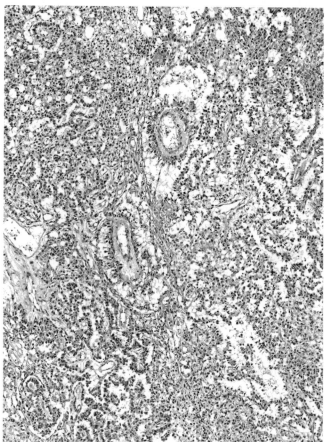

**Fig. 13-54** Endodermal sinus pattern of yolk sac tumor. Several endodermal sinus-like structures are present in this field.

nantly glandular testicular yolk sac tumor is more rare than in the ovary, but may be associated with a high serum AFP.[216] Purely glandular yolk sac tumor is more common following chemotherapy and is therefore usually found in metastases; it is particularly more frequent in late recurrences of yolk sac tumor.[498]

The myxomatous pattern is common, consisting of neoplastic epithelioid to spindle cells dispersed in a stroma that is rich in mucopolysaccharide, staining only lightly with hematoxylin and eosin (Fig. 13-61). A prominent vascular network is common, and Teilum[499] described this pattern as 'angioblastic mesenchyme,' which he felt was homologous with the extraembryonic mesenchyme (the 'magma reticulare') of development. Myxomatous foci commonly merge with other patterns, and hybrids of microcystic and myxomatous patterns are more the rule than the exception. On light microscopy the spindle cells appear to arise from solid or microcystic foci by budding from them and blending into the surrounding myxoid stroma (Fig. 13-52). Intense cytokeratin immunoreactivity within these cells supports derivation from the epithelial component of yolk sac tumor.[500] These cells are, in fact, pluripotential cells with the capacity

to form differentiated mesenchymal tissue such as skeletal muscle, cartilage, and bone,[500] thereby blurring the distinction between yolk sac tumor and teratoma (Fig. 13-62). Classification of such elements as yolk sac tumor is justified by the recognition that the surrounding tissues are typical yolk sac tumor.

The sarcomatoid pattern is uncommon, consisting of a cellular proliferation of spindle cells in continuity with other yolk sac tumor patterns, most commonly the microcystic pattern (Fig. 13-63). The sarcomatoid pattern is distinguished from the solid pattern by the spindle cell nature of the component cells. Despite the sarcomatoid appearance, the spindle cells usually express cytokeratin. It is likely that some embryonal rhabdomyosarcomas arising in testicular germ cell tumors derive from differentiation of sarcomatoid spindle cells to rhabdomyoblastic cells.[501] The occasional intimate admixture of embryonal rhabdomyosarcoma with yolk sac tumor supports this hypothesis. Spindle cell patterns in yolk sac tumor have also been reported in primary mediastinal examples.[502]

The macrocystic pattern appears to arise from coalescence of microcystic spaces to form large, round to irregular cysts (Fig. 13-64), and the surrounding pattern is often microcystic.

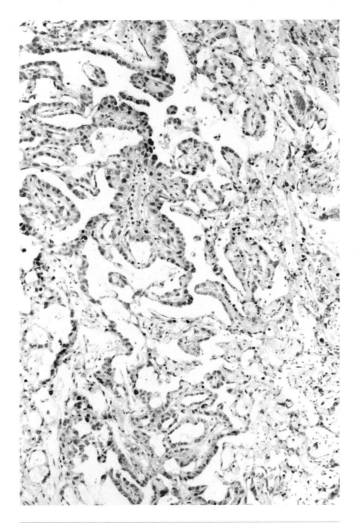

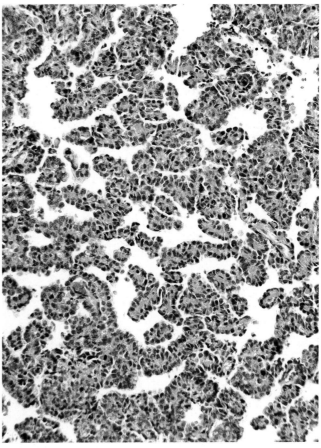

**Fig. 13-56** Papillary yolk sac tumor having a single layer of hobnail-type cells on fibrovascular cores.

**Fig. 13-55** Oblique sections of endodermal sinus-like structures result in ellipsoid configurations with festoons of malignant epithelium at the periphery and a complex, labyrinthine pattern of interconnecting extracellular spaces.

In the polyvesicular vitelline pattern, vesicle-like structures are lined by flattened, innocuous-appearing epithelium, with a myxoid to fibrous stroma (Fig. 13-65). Sometimes the vesicles have a central constriction, resembling a dumbbell or figure-of eight. Teilum[503] compared these vesicles to the embryonic subdivision of the primary yolk sac into the secondary yolk sac. At the point of constriction, the epithelium may change from flattened to cuboidal or columnar; the latter often has enteric features, including an apical brush border. AFP is often present in the lining epithelium of the vesicles, and hyaline globules are occasionally seen within the epithelial cells. In some cases a transition from microcystic pattern to polyvesicular vitelline pattern can be identified. The bland cytological appearance of the polyvesicular vitelline pattern may falsely suggest a benign neoplasm, but the presence of other patterns should prevent this pitfall. The polyvesicular pattern is less common in testicular yolk sac tumor than in its ovarian counterpart.

A hepatoid pattern also occurs in about 20% of yolk sac tumors and consists of small clusters of polygonal, eosino-philic cells arranged in sheets, nests or trabeculae (Fig. 13-66).[367,504] The cells have round, vesicular nuclei with prominent nucleoli and contain abundant AFP; hyaline globules are common in hepatoid foci, as are bile canaliculi, although bile is not present.[301,505] Hepatoid foci are scattered randomly in yolk sac tumor and are usually a minor component; rarely, a more diffuse hepatoid pattern may be seen,[506] although a prominent hepatoid pattern is more common in ovarian tumors[507] and in late recurrences of testicular examples.[498]

The parietal pattern has extensive deposits of extracellular basement membrane, with only scattered neoplastic cells in an abundant, eosinophilic matrix (Fig. 13-67). It is considered the extreme end of parietal differentiation (see below) in which basement membrane is deposited in the extracellular space in a variety of yolk sac tumor patterns. In a true parietal pattern yolk sac tumor the basement membrane deposits efface the underlying yolk sac tumor pattern. This is a very rare pattern, most often seen following chemotherapy,[508] particularly in late recurrences.[498]

The frequency of the different patterns of yolk sac tumor is difficult to determine because of lack of uniformity in classification. The microcystic, solid, and myxomatous patterns are most common, with glandular, macrocystic, endo-

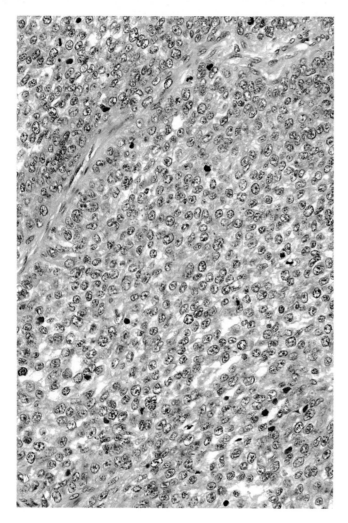

**Fig. 13-57** Solid pattern of yolk sac tumor.

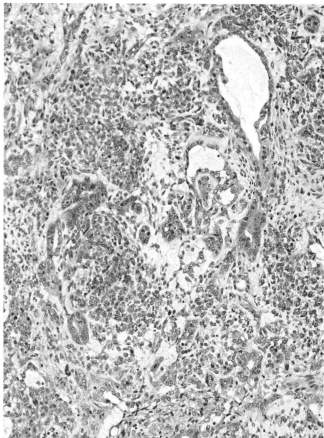

**Fig. 13-58** Solid areas in yolk sac tumor, composed of small, blastematous cells, mixed with microcystic and glandular patterns.

dermal sinus, hepatoid, and papillary patterns also occurring frequently. The polyvesicular vitelline pattern is less common, and sarcomatoid and parietal patterns are unusual. If only four patterns are employed for classification, the frequency of the patterns diminishes from reticular to solid to endodermal sinus to polyvesicular vitelline. Jacobsen noted a 'vacuolated network' in 91% of yolk sac tumors, a microcystic pattern in 67%, myxomatous pattern in 51%, macrocystic pattern in 44%, solid pattern in 27%, hepatoid areas in 23%, labyrinthine formations in 17%, and endodermal sinus-like structures in 9%.[433]

A common feature of yolk sac tumor is the deposition of extracellular basement membrane, identified in 92% of cases.[367] These deposits generally are irregularly shaped, eosinophilic bands between the neoplastic cells (Fig. 13-68) and have been referred to as parietal differentiation because of the synthesis of a thick basement membrane (known as Reichert's membrane) by the parietal layer of the embryonic yolk sac of the rodent.[367,503] Such intercellular basement membrane, although not specific for yolk sac tumor, is characteristic and can be helpful in diagnosis, particularly in small biopsy samples taken from extratesticular tumors.

Another characteristic but non-specific feature in most yolk sac tumors is the presence of intracellular, round, hyaline globules of variable size (from 1 to more than 50 µm in diameter) (Fig. 13-69). These globules are PAS positive and diastase resistant and may be present in the extracellular space following cell necrosis. Occasionally these globules may stain positively for AFP, but most do not. The hyaline globules and basement membrane deposits of yolk sac tumor are separate and distinct findings, although they have sometimes been confused in the literature.

Hematopoietic elements, usually erythroblasts, are present in a minority of testicular yolk sac tumors, usually in vascular spaces or stromal tissues.

### Special studies

Most yolk sac tumors show cytoplasmic AFP positivity on immunostaining; the frequency varies from 50% to 100%, depending on the technique employed and the number of blocks examined.[27,40,436,509] Positivity is characteristically patchy (Fig. 13-70); intense staining is usually present in hepatoid foci. Adult yolk sac tumor stains more frequently for AFP than do childhood cases.[436] Positivity for α$_1$-antitrypsin (AAT) occurs in about 50% of cases,[27,40] and the enteric glands of yolk sac tumor may stain for carcinoembryonic antigen.[27,367,443] Glypican-3, a proteoglycan that

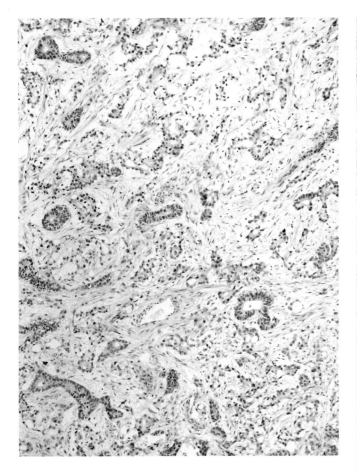

**Fig. 13-59** Glandular structures in a microcystic (reticular) pattern of yolk sac tumor.

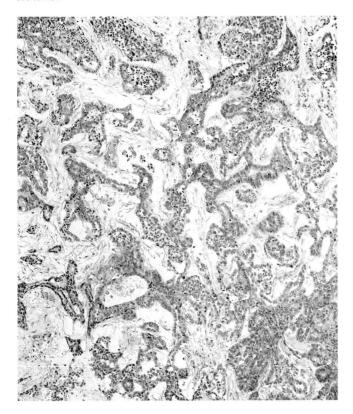

**Fig. 13-60** Complex glands in yolk sac tumor.

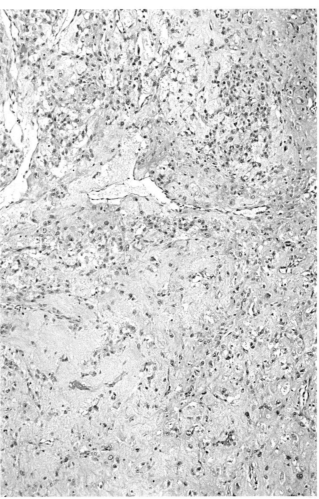

**Fig. 13-61** Stellate and spindle cells are dispersed in a myxoid stroma in the myxomatous pattern of yolk sac tumor.

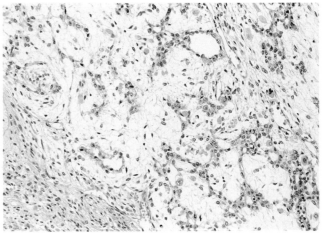

**Fig. 13-62** Rhabdomyoblastic cells intermingle with spindle cells in the myxomatous portion of this yolk sac tumor.

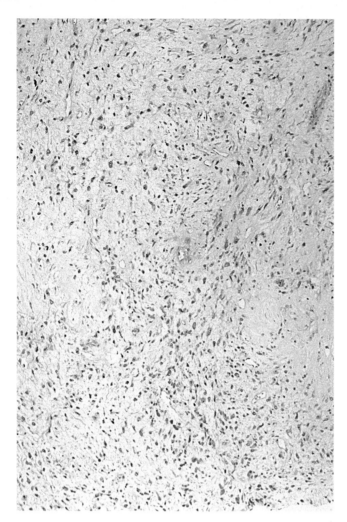

**Fig. 13-63** Sarcomatoid yolk sac tumor with a myxoid background.

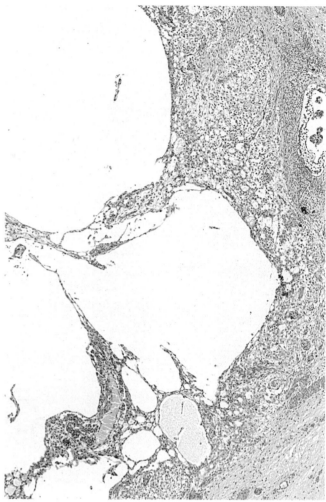

**Fig. 13-64** Macrocystic pattern of yolk sac tumor. Note adjacent microcystic pattern.

plays a role in embryonic growth, is positive in yolk sac tumor and is much less commonly expressed in most other forms of testicular germ cell tumor.[449,450] Cytokeratin is present in virtually all cases,[27,510] and vimentin is present in the spindle cells of myxomatous and sarcomatoid patterns.[510] Positivity with HEA 125, an epithelial marker, occurs in most cases.[511] Albumin, ferritin, neuron-specific enolase, and Leu-7 are present in a variable number of cases.[27,443] Chromogranin reactivity is unusual.[511] From 39% to 85% of yolk sac tumors are reported as positive for PLAP,[27,222,225] and EMA is usually negative,[27] as is CD99.[511] p53 may be identified in yolk sac tumor,[204] and laminin is present in areas of parietal differentiation.[367] We have noted reactivity of hepatoid foci for hepatocyte-specific antigen (HEPPAR1) (clone OCH1E5) (unpublished observations, 2001) and others have reported HEPPAR1 positivity in occasional yolk sac tumors in the absence of light-microscopically evident hepatoid features.[512] Experimental antibodies directed against cell surface antigens of a yolk sac tumor cell line have marked yolk sac tumors.[513]

Ultrastructurally, yolk sac tumor shows clusters of epithelial cells joined by junctional complexes. Glands have microvilli with glycocalyceal bodies and long anchoring rootlets.[367]

Basement membrane material can be identified in the extracellular space, and flocculent material is present within dilated cisternae of endoplasmic reticulum, often with a central lucent zone.[41,367,514,515] Cytoplasmic glycogen may be conspicuous.[514,516] The nuclei are usually irregular, with complex nucleolonema. Densely osmiophilic, cytoplasmic, non-membrane-bound round bodies correspond to the hyaline globules observed at the light-microscopic level.

Unlike adult cases, childhood yolk sac tumor lacks i(12p) on karyotypic analysis.[58,60,517] About 30% of childhood yolk sac tumors are diploid, with peritetraploid values in the remainder,[42] whereas adult tumors are almost invariably non-diploid.[42]

### Differential diagnosis

In the differential diagnosis of yolk sac tumor the solid pattern must be distinguished from seminoma, an issue that has been addressed on page 774. The distinction of yolk sac tumor from embryonal carcinoma has less clinical significance but is based on the distinctive patterns of yolk sac tumor and the less pleomorphic, less atypical nature of the neoplastic cells. CD30, OCT3/4, AFP, and glypican-3 stains

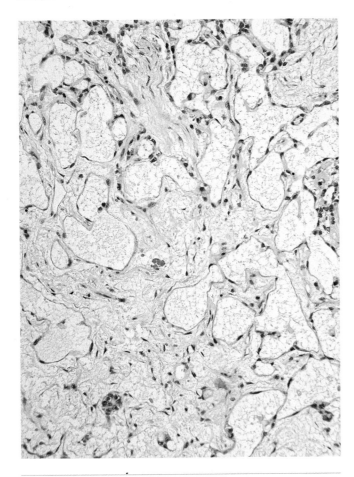

**Fig. 13-65** Polyvesicular vitelline pattern of yolk sac tumor is composed of irregular, often constricted, vesicle-like structures lined by flattened epithelium in a myxoid stroma.

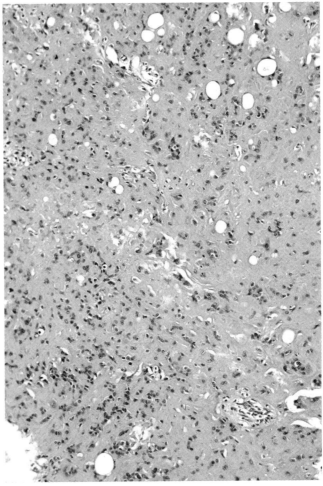

**Fig. 13-67** Diffuse basement membrane deposits characterize the parietal pattern of yolk sac tumor.

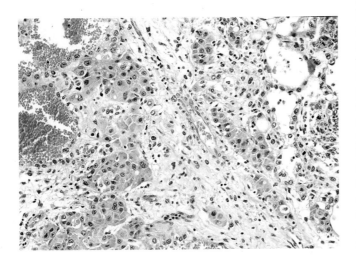

**Fig. 13-66** Hepatoid pattern of yolk sac tumor. Note islands of eosinophilic cells with round nuclei and prominent nucleoli adjacent to microcystic (reticular) pattern.

are helpful; the first two are positive in embryonal carcinoma but not yolk sac tumor, and the latter two are positive in many yolk sac tumors and usually negative in embryonal carcinomas. Embryonal carcinoma probably transforms to yolk sac tumor,[518] so there are transitional forms that are difficult to categorize. Juvenile granulosa cell tumor (see page 827) may mimic yolk sac tumor; both may be seen in very young children, but juvenile granulosa cell tumor usually is seen in children under 5 months of age,[519] whereas yolk sac tumor tends to occur in older children, the peak being at 17–18 months of age.[487,488] Histologically, both tumors may show microcystic, macrocystic, and solid patterns, as well as high mitotic rates and cellular atypia. Follicles lined by multiple layers of tumor cells and a lobular arrangement are key to the recognition of juvenile granulosa cell tumor. The presence of other characteristic patterns is important to recognizing yolk sac tumor; intracellular AFP and PLAP do not occur in juvenile granulosa cell tumor but may be seen in pediatric yolk sac tumor.[20,511] Positivity for inhibin-α and CD99 occurs in juvenile granulosa cell tumor but is not seen in yolk sac tumor.[511] Serum AFP levels may be physiologically 'elevated' in infants under 6 months of age,[520] and should not be overinterpreted to support the

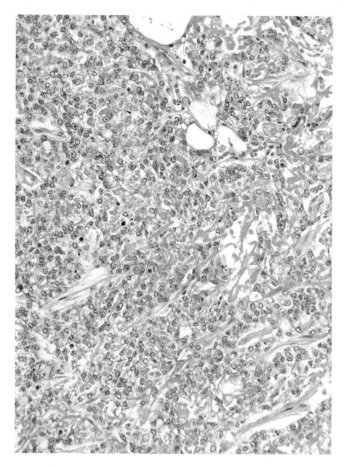

**Fig. 13-68** Bands and irregularly shaped deposits of basement membrane constitute parietal differentiation in this yolk sac tumor.

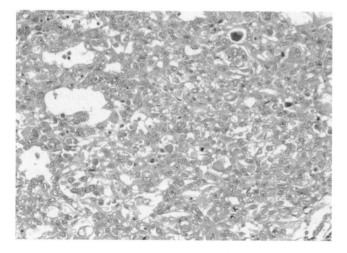

**Fig. 13-69** Solid and microcystic patterns of yolk sac tumor with eosinophilic, hyaline globules.

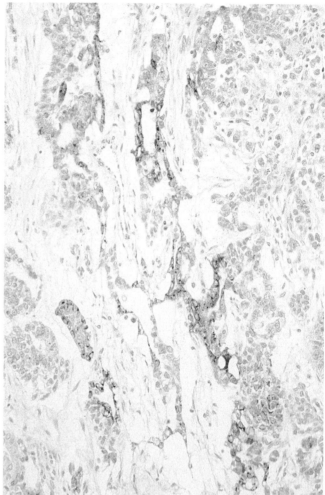

**Fig. 13-70** Patchy immunoreactivity for α-fetoprotein in a yolk sac tumor.

bland nature of the hyperplastic cells should prevent this misinterpretation, although immunostains may also be of value.[521]

### Treatment and prognosis

Adults with yolk sac tumor are treated in a fashion similar to that outlined on pages 786–787, although the presence of a yolk sac tumor component in a patient with clinical stage I tumor has been associated with a reduced likelihood of occult metastases.[466,522] Patients with metastatic yolk sac tumor do not respond as well to chemotherapy as patients with other forms of metastatic non-teratomatous testicular germ cell tumor, and therefore seem to have a worse prognosis.[523] Eighty to 90% of children with testicular yolk sac tumor have pathologic stage I tumor,[487,524] and most patients with clinical stage I tumors (including post-orchiectomy AFP levels) receive surveillance management rather than RPLND.[492,525] RPLND may not be the optimal therapy in children, given an increased frequency of hematogenous metastases to the lung, and the occurrence of retroperitoneal involvement in only 4–14% of cases.[524,526] These data indicate that childhood yolk sac tumor behaves in a more indo-

diagnosis of yolk sac tumor rather than juvenile granulosa cell tumor. A hyperplastic reaction of the rete testis with hyaline globules may be induced by invasion of the rete testis by a neoplasm, thereby simulating yolk sac tumor (Fig. 13-71).[521] The arborizing pattern of the rete testis and the

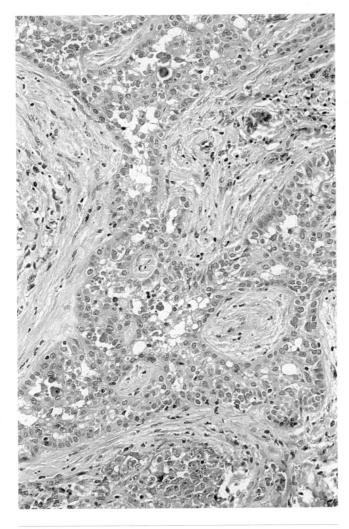

**Fig. 13-71** Rete testis hyperplasia with hyaline globules. Confusion with yolk sac tumor is possible.

lent fashion than non-seminomatous germ cell tumors in adults,[527] although some investigators believe that retroperitoneal involvement is more common than is usually stated in childhood yolk sac tumor, and that dissemination in the absence of AFP elevation may occur more commonly in childhood cases, thereby making early relapse difficult to detect.[528]

The prognosis of childhood yolk sac tumor is good, with a 5-year survival of more than 90%.[426,529] Differences in prognosis with respect to age in children[488] are no longer identified,[426,487] perhaps as a result of contemporary therapies. The greater chemoresistance of yolk sac tumor in adults compared to other forms of germ cell tumor is reflected in a higher frequency of yolk sac tumor metastases at autopsy in the chemotherapeutic era compared to the pre-chemotherapeutic era.[530]

## Teratoma

### Clinical features

Teratoma is the second most common form of testicular germ cell tumor in children (yolk sac tumor is the most common), accounting for 14–18% of cases in registry series[274,488] but a higher proportion (48%) in the combined experience of four pediatric centers.[486] In children, testicular teratoma occurs as a pure neoplasm at a median age of 13 months,[488] and is most commonly found during routine physical examination or by a parent. Testicular teratoma in children older than 4 years is unusual.[488] In contrast, teratoma usually occurs in adults as a component of a mixed germ cell tumor, and is present in more than half of all mixed germ cell tumors and in approximately 25% of all non-seminomatous germ cell tumors.[270,531]

The metastatic potential of pure testicular teratoma has been a source of confusion. Children with pure teratoma are not reported to have metastases,[532–534] with one possible exception.[535] Conversely, postpubertal patients have a definite risk of metastases, even with pure mature teratoma. Hence, there are reports of pure mature teratoma metastasizing as pure mature teratoma[536–539] and, interestingly, pure mature teratoma associated with metastases of non-teratomatous type, such as embryonal carcinoma.[532,540,541] The explanation for these observations is that postpubertal patients with pure, mature teratoma develop their neoplasm by evolution from IGCNU, through an intermediary of invasive, non-teratomatous malignant germ cell tumor.[542] This is supported by the frequent identification of IGCNU in seminiferous tubules adjacent to pure teratoma of the testis in postpubertal patients,[57] and the uncommon occurrence of postpubertal teratoma in isolation. Therefore, non-teratomatous malignant elements are initially a component of postpubertal teratoma, but transformation of such elements to teratoma (or their regression) occurs prior to orchiectomy. Metastasis of non-teratomatous elements with subsequent transformation at the metastatic site to teratomatous elements explains the phenomenon of mature teratoma metastasizing as mature teratoma; failure to transform at the site of metastasis explains mature teratoma of the testis associated with metastases of non-teratomatous type. It is of paramount importance to recognize that a postpubertal patient with a pure, mature testicular teratoma is at risk for metastasis, and the term 'pure, mature teratoma' *cannot* be equated with a benign neoplasm.

The pathogenesis of prepubertal teratomas, on the other hand, appears to be fundamentally different, a supposition supported by the absence (or paucity) of IGCNU.[55,57] These tumors do not develop from an invasive malignant germ cell but probably derive from a benign germ cell in a process more akin to that seen in the usual ovarian teratoma. This pathogenesis is supported by the normal karyotype of prepubertal testicular teratoma[58,59] and its benign outcome.[534] One group has proposed a model where the pediatric teratomas are distinct from the postpubertal germ cell tumors, based partly on differences in their patterns of genomic imprinting.[61]

Most patients with testicular teratoma present with a testicular mass, although postpubertal patients may have symptoms secondary to metastases. Serum marker elevation may occur in postpubertal patients because of admixed yolk sac tumor or syncytiotrophoblast cells; in addition, mild AFP elevation may occur in patients with pure teratoma secondary to synthesis of AFP by endodermal glandular structures of teratomatous type.[38,40,443]

## Pathologic features

Grossly, teratoma has a variable appearance. Mature teratoma often contains multiple cysts, generally less than 1 cm in diameter, which contain watery to mucoid fluid (Fig. 13-72). Semi-translucent nodules of gray-white cartilage may be present, and a fibromuscular stroma may be seen among the cartilaginous and cystic structures. In other areas the tumor may be solid (Fig. 13-73). Fleshy, encephaloid, and hemorrhagic areas usually correspond to foci of immaturity, which, if extensive, may justify a diagnosis of teratoma with a secondary malignant component. Such foci in postpubertal patients may also represent intermixed non-teratomatous elements.

Microscopically, mature teratoma consists of a variety of somatic-type tissues (Fig. 13-74), commonly including cartilage, smooth and skeletal muscle, neuroglia, enteric-type glands (Fig. 13-75), squamous epithelial islands and cysts, respiratory epithelium, and urothelial islands. Less commonly, bone and pigmented choroidal epithelium, and

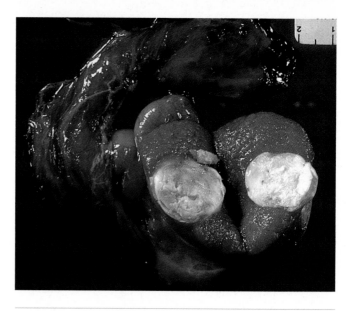

**Fig. 13-73** Teratoma with solid appearance.

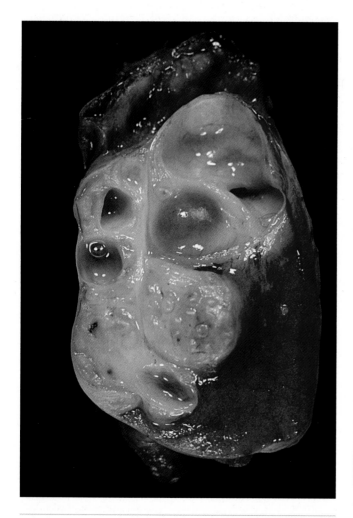

**Fig. 13-72** Teratoma with several cysts and cartilage.

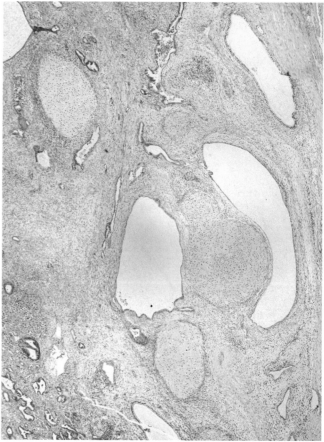

**Fig. 13-74** Teratoma with islands of hyaline cartilage, glandular structures lined by enteric-type epithelium, and fibromuscular stroma.

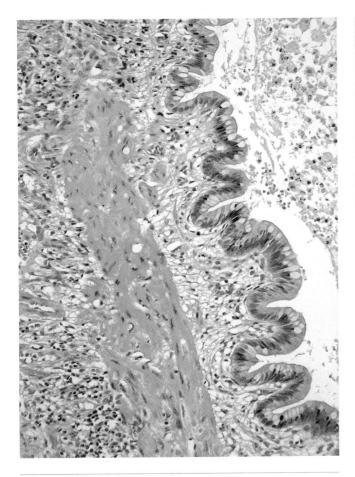

**Fig. 13-75** Mature enteric-type epithelium in teratoma.

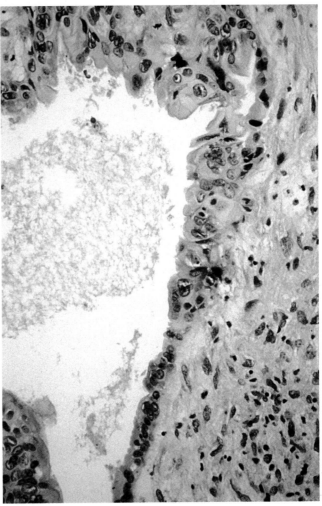

**Fig. 13-76** Cytological atypia of glandular epithelium in teratoma.

rarely kidney, liver, pancreas, thyroid, meninges, choroid plexus or prostatic tissues are present. These tissues are considered mature, but it is quite common to find significant cytological atypia, especially in postpubertal patients (Figs 13-76, 13-77). This atypia correlates with the presence of aneuploidy in mature testicular teratoma.[543] There is no evidence that the grading of the degree of atypia, based on qualitative assessment of nuclear enlargement, hyperchromasia, and mitotic rate, has any prognostic significance.

Immature elements are common but are not known to have any prognostic significance. In fact, the latest edition of the WHO monograph dealing with testicular neoplasms no longer draws a distinction between mature and immature testicular teratomas.[544] Such elements are easily recognized when they consist of highly immature tissues such as neuroepithelium, blastema, or embryonic tubules. Neuroepithelium consists of small, hyperchromatic cells arranged in tubules and rosettes (Fig. 13-78). Blastema consists of nodular collections of oval cells with scant cytoplasm and hyperchromatic nuclei (Fig. 13-79); such blastematous elements may be mixed with embryonic tubules lined by cuboidal cells with scant, inconspicuous cytoplasm. When intermixed, these two components resemble a primitive blastomatous neoplasm such as nephroblastoma or pulmonary blastoma (Fig. 13-79). Lower-grade immature elements may

consist of a hypercellular or a myxomatous, hypocellular mesenchyme (Fig. 13-80). This low-grade immature stroma often is arranged concentrically around islands of epithelium, resembling developing smooth muscle in the embryonic gastrointestinal or respiratory system (Fig. 13-80).

## Special studies

Immunohistochemical staining of teratomatous elements yields results expected for the nature of the particular tissue.[510,511,545] AFP may be present within glands of enteric or respiratory type,[40,443] as well as within liver-like tissue;[38] therefore, pure teratoma may be associated with modestly elevated serum AFP. $\alpha_1$-Antitrypsin, CEA, and ferritin may also be produced by teratomatous epithelium,[443] and PLAP positivity may be expressed in glands of a minority of teratomas.[222,225,324]

Mature postpubertal teratoma often has aneuploid DNA content, frequently in the hypotriploid range.[546–548] The i(12p) marker chromosome is also found in postpubertal cases.[344,548] These data support the derivation of postpubertal teratoma from IGCNU. As mentioned previously, the karyotype of the prepubertal tumors is normal.

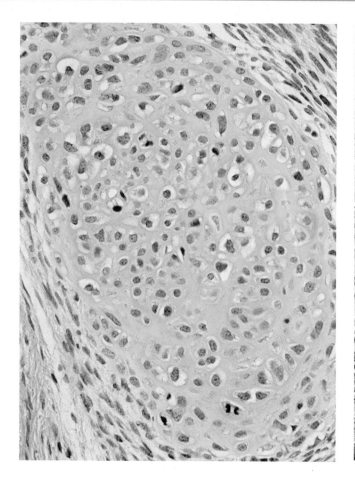

**Fig. 13-77** Cytological atypia of hyaline cartilage in teratoma.

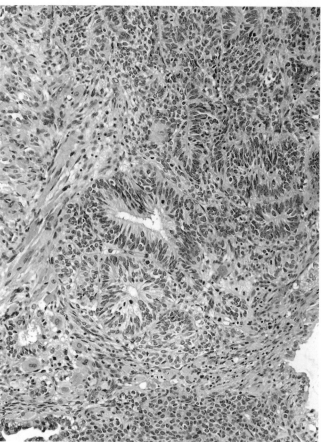

**Fig. 13-78** Neuroepithelium in teratoma.

## Differential diagnosis

It is important to distinguish dermoid and epidermoid cysts from mature teratoma because they are benign.[300,549–553] Dermoid cyst[553] (see page 803) often has grossly evident hair within a largely cystic lesion, unlike typical teratoma. On microscopic examination it has an organotypical arrangement of hair and adnexal structures to an epidermal surface, a feature rarely encountered in mature teratoma. Although it shares with teratoma the presence of diverse tissue types, including intestinal mucosa, cartilage, bone and others, these lack the cytological atypia that may be seen in mature teratoma. Most importantly, dermoid cyst is not associated with IGCNU.[553] Epidermoid cyst (see page 804) is lined by keratinizing squamous epithelium but lacks associated adnexal structures. Unlike mature teratoma in postpubertal patients, epidermoid cysts does not display cytological atypia and there is an absence of IGCNU.[57,554] No immature elements are present in dermoid or epidermoid cyst.

## Treatment and prognosis

The prognosis of patients with pure testicular teratoma is variable. Prepubertal patients are almost invariably cured by orchiectomy, with only a single report of a metastasis in a 6-month-old infant who had an 11 cm teratoma in an intra-abdominal testis resected 3 months previously.[555] Recently, testis-sparing surgery has been advocated for prepubertal boys with pure teratoma.[556] Postpubertal patients with pure mature teratoma have a guarded prognosis. In two referral series of adult patients with pure, mature teratoma, the frequency of metastases was over 40%,[540,541] to some extent reflecting a referral bias. Johnson and co-workers[557] performed orchiectomy and RPLND in 18 patients with mature teratoma, some of whom also had a seminomatous component, and reported 100% 5-year survival. Conversely, two of 12 adult patients with pure teratoma reported by the British Testicular Tumour Panel died of non-teratomatous metastases.[532] Dixon and Moore[558] reported 70% 5-year survival for patients with teratoma, with or without seminoma.

## Teratoma with a secondary malignant component

Teratoma with a secondary malignant component has also been classified as teratoma with malignant transformation. The latter term, however, connotes an unacceptable notion that teratoma in the absence of such transformation is not malignant. A secondary malignant component in a teratoma may have either a mature or an immature appearance. Carcinoma of somatic type, representing the destructive growth of epithelium with a mature phenotype, is recognized by its

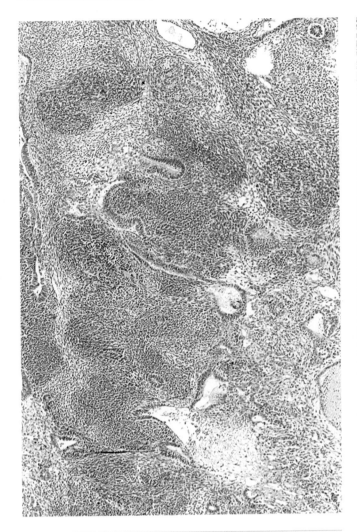

**Fig. 13-79** Cellular nodules of blastema with glands in a teratoma.

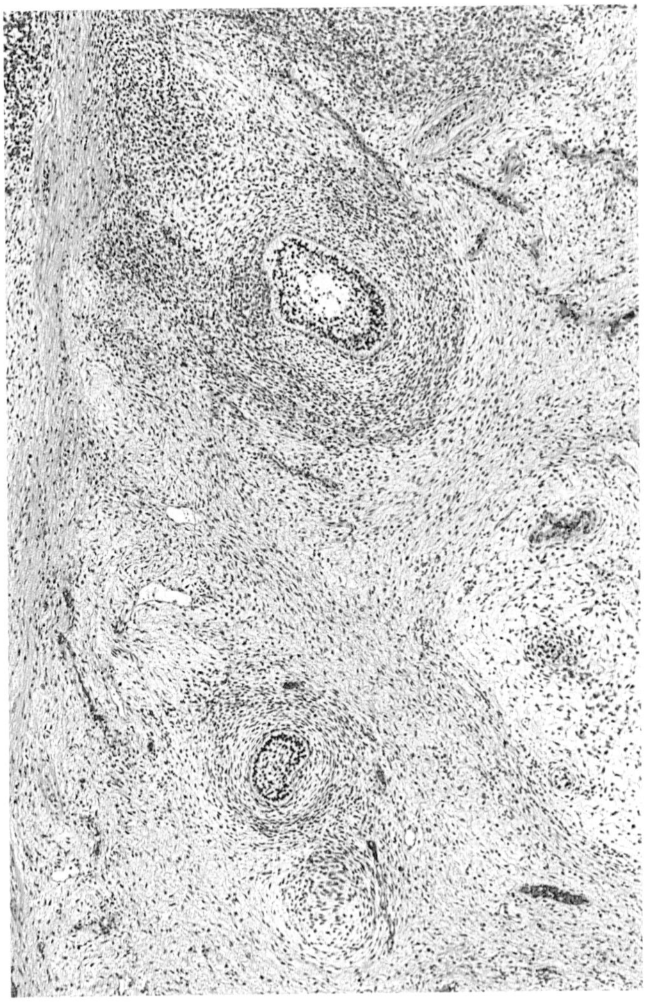

**Fig. 13-80** A lower degree of immaturity in this teratoma compared to that in Figure 13-79, with modestly cellular stroma around islands of epithelium.

invasive features. It forms masses of cytologically malignant epithelium or irregularly configured, infiltrating cords or nests associated with a desmoplastic reaction. Adenocarcinoma, squamous cell carcinoma, and undifferentiated carcinoma may occur. Sarcoma may also occur but, because invasion of mesenchymal elements is not as easily appreciated as with epithelium and may be confused with atypical teratomatous mesenchyme, it seems reasonable that growth beyond a certain size connotes an independently evolving neoplasm, but a threshold has not been established. Our guideline is to diagnose a sarcoma when the majority of a 4X field is occupied by a pure proliferation of a single type of highly atypical mesenchyme, but this is arbitrary. Similarly, 'teratoma with malignant transformation' can be recognized in immature teratoma by the pure overgrowth of immature elements, using the guidelines described above. Thus, it is justifiable to diagnose primitive neuroectodermal tumor with a pure overgrowth of neuroepithelium;[559,560] a blastomatous, Wilms' tumor-like neoplasm with overgrowth of blastema and primitive tubules;[561,562] and embryonal rhabdomyosarcoma with a pure overgrowth of primitive

rhabdomyoblastic cells (Fig. 13-81). Similar primitive elements may be admixed with other teratomatous components, a finding within the spectrum of teratoma; hence the emphasis on a 'pure' proliferation of such elements in this type of overgrowth.

The clinical significance of teratoma with a secondary malignant component in the absence of known metastatic disease is not clear. Patients with such tumors probably more commonly develop chemoresistant 'non-germ cell' neoplasms following chemotherapy.[563,564] Disseminated secondary teratomatous malignancies do not respond to the usually effective treatments for metastatic germ cell tumors;[565] the prognosis is therefore worse for these patients,[563,566,567] especially those whose tumors represent primitive neuroectodermal tumor[559,566] and rhabdomyosarcoma.[563,566] Ahmed and co-workers,[567] however, were unable to document a poor prognosis in five patients with germ cell tumors having 'malignant transformation of teratomatous elements' that were clinically confined to the testis. The secondary malignancies in such cases have been shown to have the abnormalities of chromosome 12p.[565]

**A**
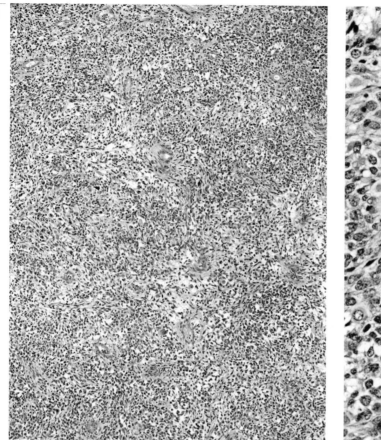

**B**
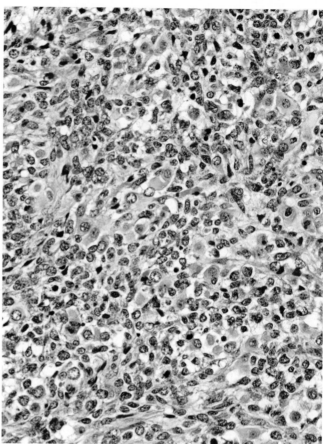

**Fig. 13-81** Embryonal rhabdomyosarcoma in teratoma. (**A**) Low magnification shows tumor overgrowth. (**B**) High magnification shows primitive cells with differentiated rhabdomyoblasts.

## Monodermal teratoma

### Carcinoid tumor

Carcinoid tumor of the testis is considered a monodermal form of teratoma; in support of this concept, about 15–25% of testicular carcinoid tumors are associated with other teratomatous elements.[568–570] These rare tumors constitute 0.17% of testicular tumors in the files at the Armed Forces Institute of Pathology.[569] They occur in older patients than those with other germ cell tumors, with a median age of 45–50 years,[569,570] with some cases reported in elderly men,[568,571] although some occur in the typical age range of most germ cell tumors.[572] Most patients present with a testicular mass; carcinoid syndrome is uncommon (occurring in about 12% of cases) but correlates with increased metastatic potential.[570] It is more common to identify serotonin in tissue or serum, or its metabolites in urine, than for clinical carcinoid syndrome to occur.[570] AFP and hCG levels are normal.

Grossly, testicular carcinoids are solid, yellow to tan, and well circumscribed, varying from 0.8 to 8 cm in diameter (Fig. 13-82).[568,570] Associated cystic spaces may represent a teratomatous component; calcification occurs in about 10% of cases.[570] Microscopically, a pattern of midgut carcinoid tumor is the usual finding, with solid nests and acini of cells in a fibrous to hyalinized stroma (Fig. 13-83). The cells have

eosinophilic, granular cytoplasm and round nuclei with a punctate or 'salt and pepper' chromatin pattern. Vascular invasion or extratesticular extension occur in about 20% of testicular carcinoids, but do not correlate with clinical malignancy in most instances.[570,572] Argyrophil and argentaffin stains are typically positive, and luminal mucin can be identified in some cases. Rarely a trabecular carcinoid pattern may occur.[571] Serotonin, substance P, chromogranin, synaptophysin, neuron-specific enolase, gastrin, vasoactive intestinal polypeptide, neurofilament protein, and cytokeratin have been identified in testicular carcinoid,[570,573–575] and one would expect to find positivity for other substances typical of midgut-type carcinoid tumors[576] in many cases. Ultrastructurally, the tumor cells contain pleomorphic neurosecretory granules typical of midgut carcinoid tumor.[568,570,573] Flow cytometry has demonstrated aneuploid or tetraploid DNA values and variable S-phase fractions.[570,572] Despite the relationship of carcinoid to teratoma, almost all cases lack IGCNU,[575,577,578] with one possible exception,[579] so they have a different pathogenesis from most postpubertal germ cell tumors.

It is prognostically important to differentiate primary carcinoid tumor from metastasis to the testis. The occurrence of other teratomatous elements in some testicular carcinoid tumors is an indication of their primary nature. The occur-

tumor elements as having areas of primitive neuroectodermal tumor with other germ cell tumor components. The distinction of such cases from immature teratoma depends on the overgrowth of a primitive neural component, as previously described (see page 801).

Clinically, these cases occur in the typical age range for germ cell tumors. Gray-white, partially necrotic tumors are identified. Microscopically, the tumors contain small, hyperchromatic, poorly differentiated neural-type cells arranged in rosettes, tubules, or diffusely.[580,582] The tumors typically resemble neuroblastoma and/or medulloepithelioma of the central nervous system.[559] Neurosecretory granules may be identified ultrastructurally.[582] Immunohistochemical studies utilizing neural markers, including chromogranin, synaptophysin and CD99,[559] may be useful. The differential diagnosis includes other small cell tumors, including immature teratoma, metastatic small cell carcinoma, malignant lymphoma, and overgrowth of a blastematous component of immature teratoma. As discussed above, the distinction from immature teratoma is based on the amount of primitive neural tissue. Small cell carcinoma does not form the well-defined tubules and rosettes that occur in most primitive neuroectodermal tumors and usually shows more intense and widespread cytokeratin reactivity that contrasts with the focal, weak or absent reactivity in primitive neuroectodermal tumor. The absence of IGCNU in metastatic small cell carcinoma contrasts with its usual presence in testicular primitive neuroectodermal tumor. Additionally, small cell carcinoma tends to occur in older patients, who often have a history of lung cancer[582] or cancer at another appropriate primary site. The absence of IGCNU, tubules, and rosettes and the tendency for interstitial growth help in the differential from lymphoma, although immunohistochemistry offers a powerful method for distinction. Overgrowth of blastema and epithelium in a teratoma can produce a tumor resembling a nephroblastoma[562] that can easily be confused with a primitive neuroectodermal tumor. Distinction may require immunohistochemistry for neural markers, which are negative in nephroblastoma-like tumors. Ultrastructural or immunohistochemical studies permit separation of the other alternative diagnoses.

Testicular germ cell tumors with primitive neuroectodermal tumor behave more aggressively than germ cell tumors lacking it as a component. Seven of 15 clinical stage I patients with a component of testicular primitive neuroectodermal tumor either had metastases or relapsed on surveillance management.[560] Of the 23 patients who presented with metastatic primitive neuroectodermal tumor who received chemotherapy, only three had a complete response.[560] The mainstay of treatment is therefore complete surgical excision of metastatic lesions.[565]

### Dermoid cyst

Dermoid cyst is very rare and represents a form of teratoma that should be separated from 'mature teratoma' because of its different pathogenesis and benign behavior.[553] Grossly it forms a unicystic mass filled with friable, keratinous debris and may contain hair. There may be some solid foci at the periphery. Analogous to its ovarian counterpart, it may have

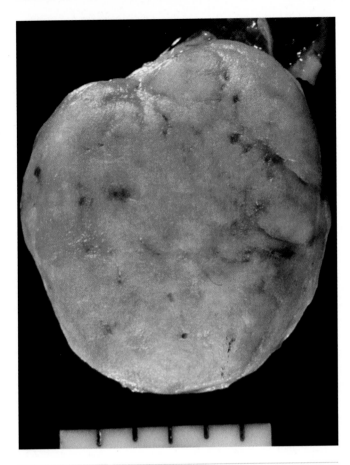

**Fig. 13-82** Testicular carcinoid tumor with a solid, tan appearance. (Courtesy of Dr RH Young, Massachusetts General Hospital, Boston, MA.)

rence of bilateral involvement, multifocal tumor, vascular invasion, or extratesticular spread favor carcinoid tumor metastatic to the testis rather than primary testicular carcinoid. Primary carcinoid has a good prognosis; Berdjis and Mostofi[569] reported metastases in two of 12 patients; Reyes et al.[575] reported malignant behavior in one of five patients with follow-up, and Zavala-Pompa and co-workers[570] reported metastases in 11.6% of patients. Large size (average diameter of metastasizing tumors = 7.3 cm vs average diameter of non-metastasizing tumors = 2.9 cm) and the carcinoid syndrome were the strongest predictors of metastasis,[570] whereas mitotic activity, vascular invasion, and tumor necrosis had no predictive value.[570] Most cases are cured by orchiectomy. The course of patients with metastatic testicular carcinoid tumor is often indolent, and the utility of retroperitoneal lymph node dissection is unknown.

### Primitive neuroectodermal tumor

Primitive neuroectodermal tumor of the testis, like carcinoid tumor, is considered a monodermal form of testicular teratoma. This neoplasm results from overgrowth of neuroepithelial elements that are a common component of immature testicular teratoma. It is best to reserve the term 'primitive neuroectodermal tumor' of the testis for those rare cases that are a pure proliferation of such elements,[20,580–582] and to diagnose cases with residual teratomatous or other germ cell

A

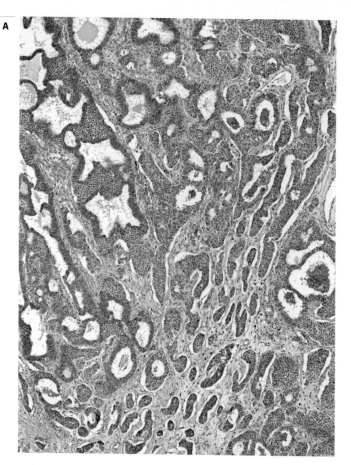

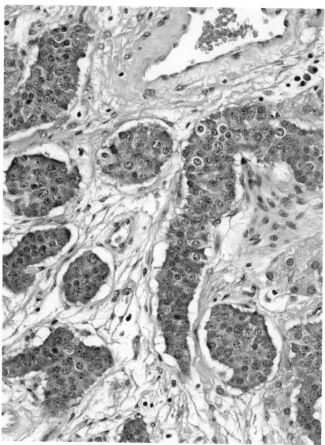

B

**Fig. 13-83** (**A**) Insular, glandular and trabecular patterns in testicular carcinoid tumor. (**B**) Note punctate chromatin and acidophilic granules.

a mural protuberance.[552,583] Microscopically, a cyst, filled with keratin and lined by epidermis and dermis containing hair follicles, sebaceous glands, and other appendigeal structures, is identified (Fig. 13-84). Occasional cases have a minor component of other teratomatous elements, including cysts lined by ciliated or intestinal-type epithelium, intestinal-type mucosa with accompanying muscularis mucosa, gastric pyloric-type epithelium, thyroid, pancreas, salivary gland, cartilage, smooth muscle, adipose tissue and bone.[300,551–553,584,585] Several have had a prominent lipogranulomatous reaction in the parenchyma adjacent to the cyst (Fig. 13-85), presumably caused by leakage of cyst contents.[553] The presence of IGCNU, as well as cytological atypia, is an indication for classification as teratoma. Documented metastasis from a pure dermoid cyst of the testis has not been reported,[300,551–553,585] and the distinction from teratoma is therefore important. Its pathogenesis, like that of prepubertal teratoma, is probably similar to that of the more common ovarian lesion.

### Epidermoid cyst

It is not entirely clear whether epidermoid cyst is teratomatous in origin, although it seems the likeliest explanation;[549,586] another alternative is from metaplasia of a mesothelial inclusion. If the origin is teratomatous, it must be similar to that of dermoid cyst because it is not associated with IGCNU,[57,554] and it is uniformly benign. It characteristically occurs in patients in the second to fourth decades of life.[549] Grossly, epidermoid cyst usually is 2–3 cm in diameter,[587] typically located at the periphery of the testis close to the tunica albuginea, and filled with white to yellow, friable, often pungent, keratinous material (Fig. 13-86). Microscopically, there is a single cyst lined by squamous epithelium with a granular cell layer and a fibrous wall of variable thickness (Fig. 13-87). The lining is often compressed to just a few flattened layers of cells. Unlike dermoid cyst, there are no adnexal structures in the wall of the cyst. It is important to examine the surrounding testis for teratomatous or other germ cell tumor elements and IGCNU in the seminiferous tubules; any of these findings would lead to reclassification of the lesion as teratoma. Epidermoid cyst requires no additional therapy after orchiectomy.[549,550] In rare cases where testicular preservation is considered essential, it may be justifiable to locally excise the cyst and a rim of surrounding testis, with frozen section examination to determine the presence of IGCNU or other forms of germ cell tumor.[585,588] Follow-up in conservatively managed patients has been uneventful,[554] but it is important to sample enough of the testicular parenchyma to confidently exclude IGCNU.

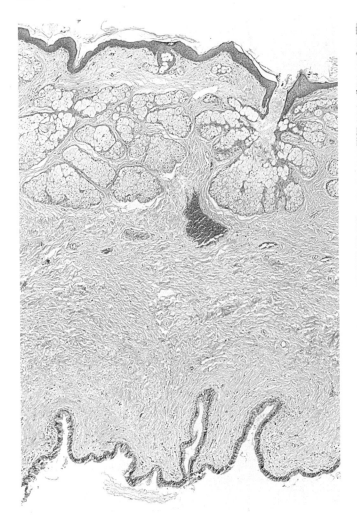

**Fig. 13-84** Dermoid cyst. Note the skin-like arrangement of adnexal structures and the additional glandular cyst (bottom).

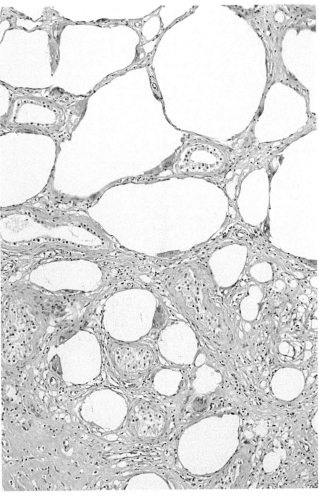

**Fig. 13-85** Lipogranulomatous reaction adjacent to a dermoid cyst.

# Choriocarcinoma and other trophoblastic neoplasms

## Clinical features

Choriocarcinoma is an uncommon component of mixed germ cell tumors (present in 15% of cases[490]), and pure choriocarcinoma is quite rare, representing only 0.3% of testicular tumors in a registry of 6000 cases.[300] Most patients with choriocarcinoma present with symptoms secondary to metastases, unlike other testicular tumors, in which a palpable mass is the usual presenting complaint. Often the testicular tumor remains occult even after the diagnosis of metastatic choriocarcinoma. Typically, metastases are in a hematogenous distribution, often affecting the lungs, brain, and gastrointestinal tract, although retroperitoneal lymph node involvement may occur. In rare instances patients may present with cutaneous[589] or pancreatic metastases.[590] Most patients are in the second and third decades, and choriocarcinoma has not been reported prior to puberty.[274] Serum levels of hCG may be highly elevated, resulting in secondary hormonal manifestations such as

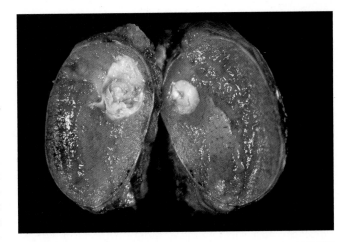

**Fig. 13-86** Epidermoid cyst containing friable, yellow-white keratinous material. Note proximity to tunica albuginea.

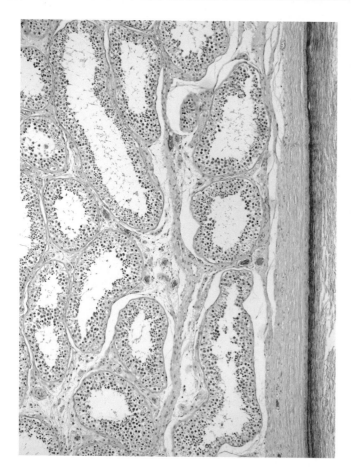

**Fig. 13-87** Epidermoid cyst showing a thin, compressed layer of stratified squamous epithelium (right) lining a space filled with keratin. The surrounding seminiferous tubules show intact spermatogenesis with no evidence of IGCNU.

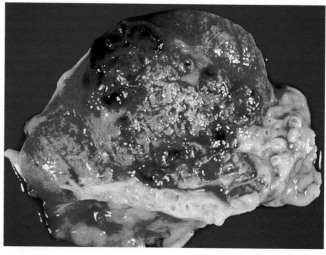

**Fig. 13-88** Choriocarcinoma of the testis. Note hemorrhagic, granular lesion.

gynecomastia and thyrotoxicosis, owing to cross-reactivity of hCG with gonadotropins and thyroid-stimulating hormone, respectively.[390,499,591]

## Pathologic features

Grossly, the testis may be externally normal; the cut surface usually shows a hemorrhagic and necrotic nodule (Fig. 13-88), although in some instances regression of the primary lesion has occurred, with residual scar as the only evidence of prior neoplasm. Classically, choriocarcinoma consists of a random mixture of mononucleated trophoblast cells with clear to lightly staining cytoplasm (cytotrophoblasts and intermediate trophoblasts) and multinucleated syncytiotrophoblast cells, often with smudged or degenerate-appearing nuclei and densely eosinophilic cytoplasm (Fig. 13-89). The syncytiotrophoblast cells may have intracytoplasmic lacunae containing an eosinophilic precipitate or erythrocytes. The area surrounding a choriocarcinoma is almost always hemorrhagic, and the central portions of the neoplasm are typically hemorrhagic and necrotic. Extensive sampling of such tumors may therefore be necessary to demonstrate the diagnostic cell types, usually at the periphery (Fig. 13-90). In the best-organized examples of choriocarcinoma the syncytiotrophoblast cells appear to surround or

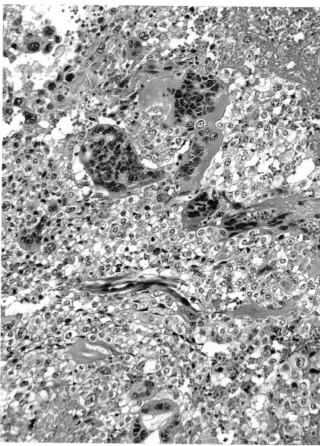

**Fig. 13-89** Characteristic mixture of syncytiotrophoblast cells and mononucleated trophoblast cells in choriocarcinoma. The background is hemorrhagic.

'cap' masses of mononucleated trophoblast cells, similar to the arrangement in immature placental villi (Fig. 13-91). However, in some cases the syncytiotrophoblast cells are inconspicuous, having relatively scant cytoplasm and a

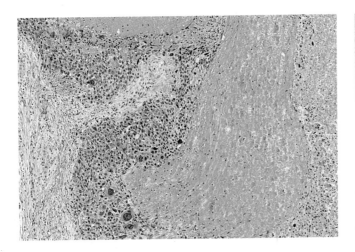

**Fig. 13-90** Viable choriocarcinoma forms a rim around pools of blood and fibrin.

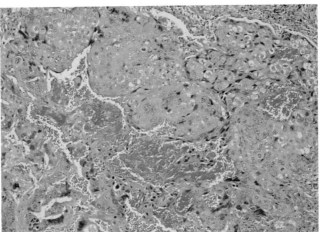

**Fig. 13-92** Choriocarcinoma in which the syncytiotrophoblast cells are inconspicuous, appearing as intermingled, smudged cells. Note the hemorrhage and typical syncytiotrophoblast cells at the bottom.

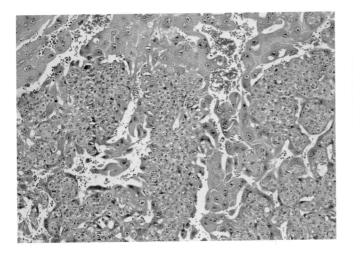

**Fig. 13-91** Choriocarcinoma with syncytiotrophoblast cells capping mononucleated trophoblast cells in a villus-like fashion.

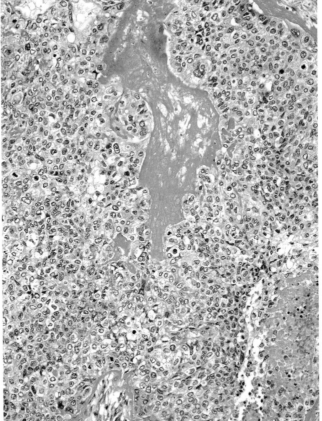

**Fig. 13-93** 'Monophasic' choriocarcinoma. There is a diffuse pattern of mostly mononucleated trophoblast cells in a hemorrhagic background.

degenerate appearance (Fig. 13-92). In other cases, descriptively characterized as 'monophasic choriocarcinoma,'[592] a biphasic pattern of intermingled syncytiotrophoblast and mononucleated trophoblast cells is absent; instead, there is a proliferation of atypical trophoblastic cells of varying size.[592] These are usually mononucleated and occasionally binucleated trophoblast cells, and the background typically remains hemorrhagic (Fig. 13-93). Angioinvasive foci are commonly identified in all variants.

There are other trophoblastic tumors in the testis apart from choriocarcinoma. One such is the placental site trophoblastic tumor[592] that resembles the uterine tumor of the same name (Fig. 13-94). This lesion consists of a nodular proliferation of 'intermediate' trophoblast cells that stain positively for human placental lactogen. There is a lack of the biphasic pattern of choriocarcinoma. In other non-choriocarcinomatous trophoblastic tumors there are cells that resemble cytotrophoblast cells and which line hemorrhagic cysts (Fig. 13-95). Occasionally, mononucleated, squamoid

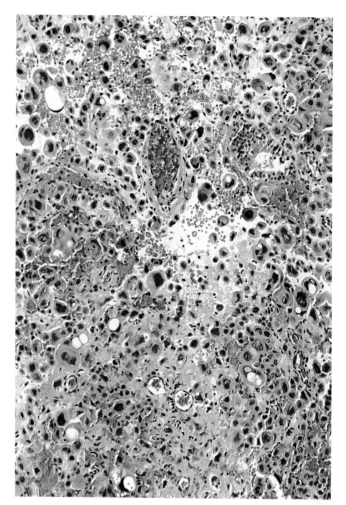

**Fig. 13-94** Placental site trophoblastic tumor. There is a sheet-like arrangement of intermediate trophoblast cells with densely eosinophilic cytoplasm in a hemorrhagic background. The tumor cells were strongly and diffusely reactive for human placental lactogen.

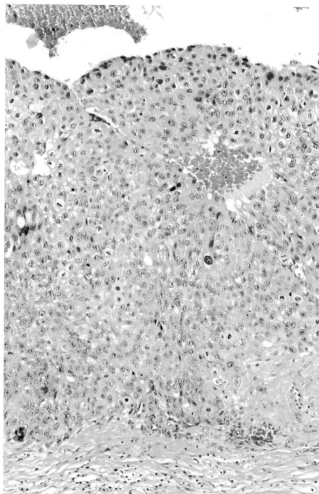

**Fig. 13-95** Trophoblastic proliferation in which mononucleated trophoblast cells line a hemorrhagic cyst.

trophoblastic cells with only rare mitotic figures may line cystic spaces (Fig. 13-96).

### Special studies

Immunostains for hCG are useful in establishing the diagnosis of a trophoblastic proliferation, including choriocarcinoma. Positivity for hCG is strongest in syncytiotrophoblast cells and in large mononucleated trophoblast cells that may represent transitional forms between cytotrophoblast cells and syncytiotrophoblast cells.[27,40,593] Cytotrophoblast cells generally have only weak or absent staining for hCG. Similarly, pregnancy-specific $\beta_1$-glycoprotein and human placental lactogen may be identified in syncytiotrophoblast cells and intermediate-sized trophoblast cells, but are not seen in the cytotrophoblast population.[593] Inhibin-$\alpha$ is positive in the syncytiotrophoblast cells.[511,594,595] About half of choriocarcinomas stain for PLAP,[27] and carcinoembryonic antigen (CEA) can be identified in both syncytiotrophoblast cells and cytotrophoblast cells in about 25% of cases.[27,596] Cytokeratin is readily identifiable in both the syncytiotrophoblastic and cytotrophoblastic components of choriocarcinoma,[27,301]

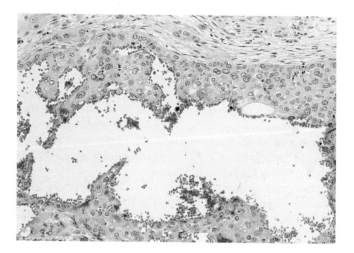

**Fig. 13-96** Squamoid, mononucleated trophoblastic cells line a hemorrhagic cyst.

including cytokeratins 7, 8, 18, and 19.[597] EMA positivity is noted in about half of choriocarcinomas, usually within syncytiotrophoblast cells,[27] whereas most other non-teratomatous germ cell tumors of the testis do not express EMA.

Ultrastructurally, the multinucleated syncytiotrophoblast cells have prominent cisternae of rough endoplasmic reticulum, which often contain electron-dense material, and show interdigitating microvilli on the cell surface.[41,598] Cytotrophoblast cells lack the prominent rough endoplasmic reticulum but have numerous free cytoplasmic ribosomes. Desmosomes are identified in all cell types.

### Differential diagnosis

Other types of germ cell tumor may contain trophoblast cells, but they are scattered as individual cells or small nests and lack the biphasic pattern of choriocarcinoma. For example, the syncytiotrophoblast cells that occur in many seminomas are randomly distributed as separate cells and small islands without accompanying mononucleated trophoblast cells. Nor is there a distinct nodule of trophoblast cells of varying sizes, as may be seen in some cases of choriocarcinoma. Embryonal carcinoma may show degenerate cells that mimic choriocarcinoma with a poorly defined syncytiotrophoblastic component. The lack of hemorrhage and hCG reactivity and the presence of OCT3/4 reactivity in such cases distinguish them from choriocarcinoma (see page 785). Rare cases of embryonal carcinoma may show transformation to choriocarcinoma;[599] if the background is hemorrhagic and the admixed multinucleated cells contain hCG, and OCT3/4 reactivity is lacking, choriocarcinoma should be diagnosed rather than embryonal carcinoma. 'Monophasic' variants of choriocarcinoma[592] should be distinguished from seminoma and solid pattern yolk sac tumor. Diffuse hCG reactivity is helpful in this regard, as is the absence of AFP and OCT3/4 staining and a greater degree of pleomorphism than in seminoma. The placental site trophoblastic tumor should be distinguished from choriocarcinoma based on its lack of a biphasic pattern and its strong and diffuse reactivity for human placental lactogen.

### Treatment and prognosis

Choriocarcinoma tends to metastasize prior to detection of the primary lesion, and most patients have advanced-stage tumor at the time of diagnosis. It often shows a less orderly pattern of metastasis than other germ cell tumors, frequently skipping the retroperitoneum and metastasizing in a hematogenous pattern to the lungs, liver, central nervous system, and other sites.[300,531] The prognosis is therefore worse than for other germ cell tumors. It is also likely that mixed germ cell tumors with a component of choriocarcinoma have a worse prognosis, but it remains unclear how much choriocarcinoma in such cases is required for deterioration in outcome. This concept is supported by several studies demonstrating a poorer prognosis in patients with non-seminomatous germ cell tumors who had elevated serum hCG levels,[390,600,601] and in those with choriocarcinoma in mixed germ cell tumors.[390,600,602,603] Patients with choriocarcinoma can achieve substantial tumor-free survival with chemotherapy.[390]

In the single reported example of the placental site trophoblastic tumor, the patient, a 16-month-old boy, had no evidence of disease at 8 years' follow-up after orchiectomy in the absence of any adjuvant therapy.[592]

## Mixed germ cell tumor

Mixed germ cell tumors are composed of more than one type of germ cell tumor element, including one or more non-seminomatous element, and are thus classified as non-seminomatous tumors, even if seminoma is the chief component. Mixed germ cell tumors are quite common, accounting for about one-third of germ cell tumors and 69% of all non-seminomatous germ cell tumors of the testis.[269] Virtually any combination of elements may be present. Common combinations include embryonal carcinoma and teratoma; embryonal carcinoma and seminoma; embryonal carcinoma, yolk sac tumor, and teratoma; embryonal carcinoma, teratoma, and choriocarcinoma; embryonal carcinoma, teratoma, and seminoma; and teratoma and seminoma.[269] Although seminoma with syncytiotrophoblast cells is histopathologically a mixed germ cell tumor, it is classified as a variant of seminoma rather than a mixed, non-seminomatous neoplasm because the natural history and treatment are similar to those of seminoma.

### Clinical features

Patients with mixed germ cell tumor have the same clinical features as those with non-seminomatous germ cell tumor, and most present with a testicular mass. Those with a predominance of embryonal carcinoma in mixed germ cell tumor average 28 years of age, whereas patients with a predominance of seminoma average 33 years.[604] AFP and hCG elevation occurs in about 60% and 55% of patients with mixed germ cell tumor, respectively.[284]

### Pathologic features

Grossly, mixed germ cell tumor is often variegated because of its different components (Fig. 13-97). Foci of hemorrhage and necrosis are common. The microscopic features are similar to those of the individual components described elsewhere in this chapter. It is common for foci of yolk sac tumor with microcystic or vacuolated patterns to be contiguous with areas of embryonal carcinoma, and such foci are easily overlooked (Fig. 13-98). A 'double-layered' pattern of embryonal carcinoma has been described in which ribbons of columnar embryonal carcinoma cells are accompanied by a parallel ribbon of flattened tumor cells (see page 781 and Fig. 13-41);[433,605] the intense AFP immunoreactivity of this flattened cell layer, together with its morphology, indicates yolk sac tumor differentiation, and this pattern should therefore be classified as a form of mixed germ cell tumor (embryonal carcinoma and yolk sac tumor). Some regard this pattern as 'diffuse embryoma' (see below).

## Polyembryoma and diffuse embryoma

Polyembryoma is a distinct form of mixed germ cell tumor that recapitulates small embryoid bodies. The embryoid body consists of a central core of cuboidal to columnar, sometimes stratified, embryonal carcinoma cells, a 'ventral'

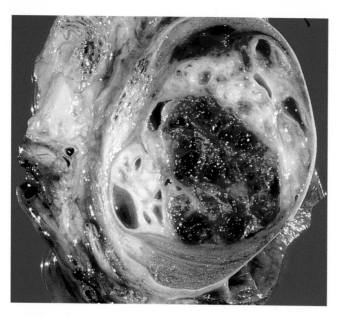

**Fig. 13-97** Variegated appearance of mixed germ cell tumor, with hemorrhagic, cystic, and fleshy areas.

yolk sac tumor component forming a yolk sac-like vesicle, and a 'dorsal' amniotic-like space (Fig. 13-99).[606,607] The embryoid body is surrounded by loose, myxomatous, richly vascular tissue, similar to extraembryonic mesenchyme, which is also commonly identified in yolk sac tumor (Fig. 13-99). Because of the yolk sac tumor component, patients with polyembryoma may have substantial AFP elevation.[606] In some cases intestinal and squamous differentiation of the 'amniotic' epithelium is present, as well as hepatic differentiation in the yolk sac-like zone.[606] Imperfectly formed embryoid bodies are occasionally seen in mixed germ cell tumors, consisting of small nodular collections of embryonal carcinoma admixed with yolk sac tumor, surrounded by a myxomatous to fibrous stroma (Fig. 13-100). Diffuse embryoma consists of a sheet-like admixture of embryonal carcinoma and yolk sac tumor in approximately equal proportions,[608] (Fig. 13-101) with the two components retaining their expected immunohistochemical reactivities.[609] The 'double-layered' tumor pattern (Fig. 13-41) may also be considered 'diffuse embryoma.' The behavior and treatment of polyembryoma and diffuse embryoma are similar to those of other mixed germ cell tumors with these components.

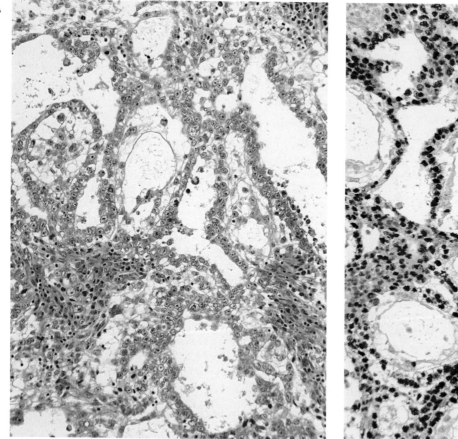

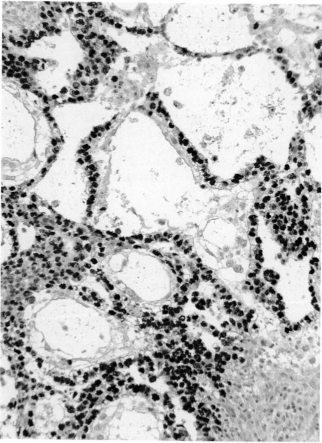

**Fig. 13-98** **(A)** There are luminal spaces lined by embryonal carcinoma cells with yolk sac tumor cells on the adluminal aspect. **(B)** OCT3/4 highlights the nuclei of the embryonal carcinoma but spares those of the yolk sac tumor.

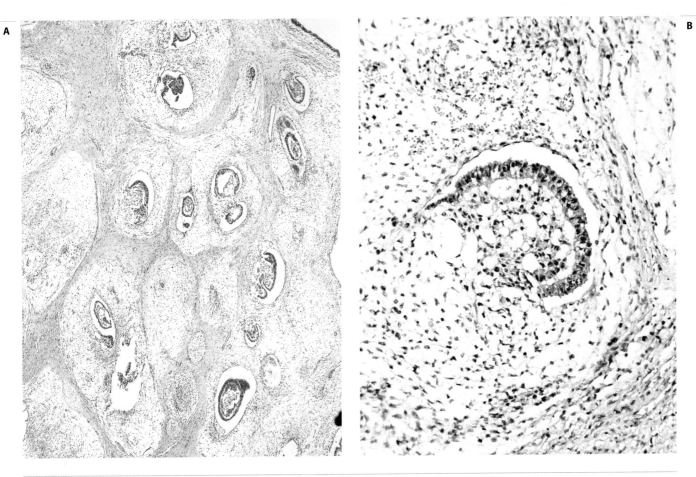

**Fig. 13-99** (**A**) Polyembryoma consists of embryoid bodies in a myxoid stroma. (**B**) Embryoid body composed of a central core of embryonal carcinoma, a 'ventral' yolk sac tumor component, and a 'dorsal' amnion.

## Treatment and prognosis

Patients with mixed germ cell tumors are managed like those with non-seminomatous tumors. Tumors consisting of embryonal carcinoma and teratoma are less likely to metastasize than tumors having the same volume of embryonal carcinoma but lacking a teratomatous component, suggesting that the ability of embryonal carcinoma to differentiate is associated with a decrease in metastatic potential.[610] A similar observation has been made for cases having a yolk sac tumor component, with a decrease in metastatic potential.[466]

## Regression of germ cell tumor ('burnt-out' germ cell tumor)

Some patients with extragonadal germ cell tumor lack clinical evidence of a primary testicular tumor.[611–614] Some have primary extragonadal germ cell tumor, especially those with tumor confined to the mediastinum or pineal region without retroperitoneal involvement. Accumulating evidence indicates that retroperitoneal tumor, frequently thought in the past to be a common site of primary extragonadal germ cell tumor, is often due to regression of a testicular primary.[263,614] Examination of the testis in such cases often demonstrates foci of testicular scarring and, less frequently, IGCNU.[263] This

phenomenon of primary testicular tumor regression in the presence of metastases is documented in autopsy studies, and almost 10% of patients who die of metastatic testicular germ cell tumor show 'burnt-out' primary tumors.[615] In our experience,[435] essentially all types of germ cell tumor are susceptible to regression and, not unexpectedly, regressed seminoma comprises the single greatest proportion of cases, given the large fraction of testicular germ cell tumors that it represents. It is also clear that many of the cases of 'pure' teratoma of the adult testis represent what were originally mixed germ cell tumors that had regression of the non-teratomatous components.[616]

Regression can be recognized from a constellation of findings (Fig. 13-102). All cases have scarred areas that may have either nodular or stellate configurations. These scars often contain a variably intense lymphoplasmacytic infiltrate and have prominent numbers of curvilinear blood vessels. They usually also have 'ghost' remnants of hyalinized seminiferous tubules, which therefore do not represent evidence for a non-neoplastic process causing scarring.[161,435] Coarse intratubular calcifications in the scar provide very good evidence for a regressed germ cell tumor that had an intratubular embryonal carcinoma component, as these commonly undergo comedonecrosis in the tubules with dystrophic calcification. Peripheral to the scar there is invariably tubular

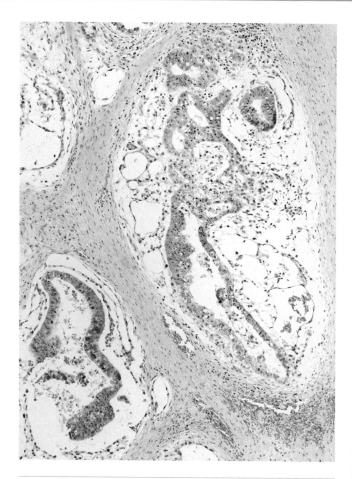

**Fig. 13-100** Complex embryoid body.

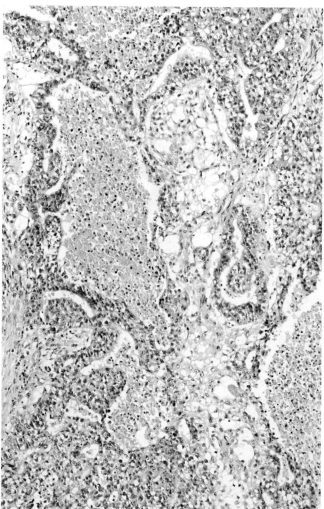

**Fig. 13-101** Diffuse embryoma consists of an approximately equal mixture of embryonal carcinoma and yolk sac tumor.

atrophy and impaired spermatogenesis, reflecting the usual testicular background upon which germ cell tumors develop. Additional findings include IGCNU in about half of cases, tubular microliths in about one-third, and prominent clusters of Leydig cells in about 40%.[435]

## Post-chemotherapy specimens

Chemotherapy in patients with metastatic testicular germ cell tumor often results in a marked decrease in tumor size, although large masses may persist. Persistent masses are often surgically excised, and the pathologic findings are of prime importance in determining the future treatment for these patients.[478,617]

Following chemotherapeutic cytoreduction, residual masses may consist of necrosis (often associated with a xanthomatous reaction), fibrosis, and viable-appearing germ cell tumor histologically similar to the original tumor or with an altered morphology. Additionally, malignant neoplasms resembling non-germ cell tumors (e.g., sarcoma, primitive neuroectodermal tumor and carcinoma) may occur.[478,563,566] Patients with necrosis, fibrosis, and mature (although often atypical-appearing) teratomatous lesions following chemotherapy are not usually treated with additional chemotherapy; conversely, those who have persistent embryonal carcinoma, yolk sac tumor, choriocarcinoma, or seminoma are candidates for second-line ('salvage') chemo-

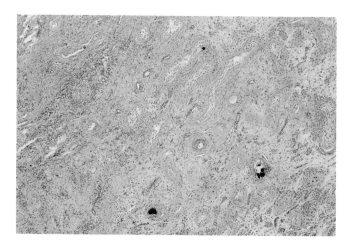

**Fig. 13-102** Regressed germ cell tumor consisting of scarring with lymphocytes, siderophages, and intratubular calcifications.

therapy, sometimes with bone marrow transplantation. The treatment of post-chemotherapy sarcoma, primitive neuroectodermal tumor and carcinoma is problematic and often ineffective, but is usually primarily by surgical resection.[560,565,566] In one study of 101 patients with advanced,

non-seminomatous germ cell tumor treated with cisplatin-based chemotherapy and resection of residual masses, 51% had necrosis or fibrosis, 37% had residual mature teratoma, and 12% had residual malignant, non-teratomatous germ cell tumor.[618]

Necrotic foci in post-chemotherapy resections often appear as tan, granular nodules surrounded by a thin yellow rim (Fig. 13-103). Microscopically, there is central, coagulative necrosis consisting of eosinophilic debris with ghost-like outlines of necrotic tumor cells, typically lacking prominent karyorrhectic debris. Macrophages with abundant, foamy cytoplasm surround the areas of necrosis (Fig. 13-104), accounting for the grossly visible yellow rim (Fig. 13-103). The nuclei of these cells may be mildly atypical which, in conjunction with the clear cytoplasm, can lead to misinterpretation as seminoma (Fig. 13-105).[478] The absence of significant atypia and inconspicuous mitotic activity are usually sufficient to permit separation without resorting to special stains for glycogen, placental alkaline phosphatase, OCT3/4, and macrophage markers. If immunohistochemical staining is necessary, OCT3/4 immunohistochemistry is a sensitive and specific marker for metastatic seminoma and embryonal carcinoma.[619] An active fibroblastic proliferation may be intermingled with the foamy macrophages, creating a fibroxanthomatous reaction.

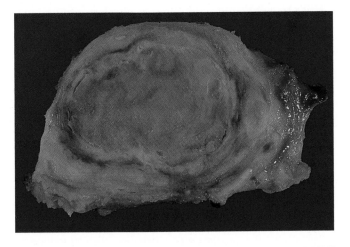

**Fig. 13-103** Tumor necrosis following chemotherapy. A tan, granular nodule is surrounded by a yellow rim with peripheral fibrosis.

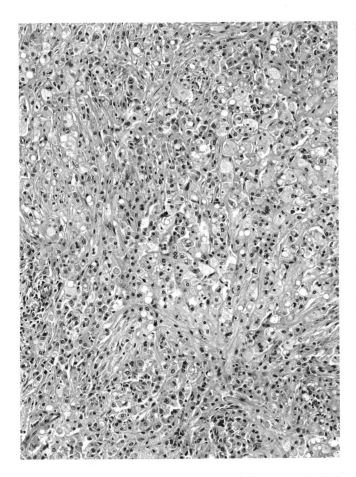

**Fig. 13-104** The fibroxanthomatous reaction that often surrounds foci of tumor necrosis induced by chemotherapy may be highly cellular.

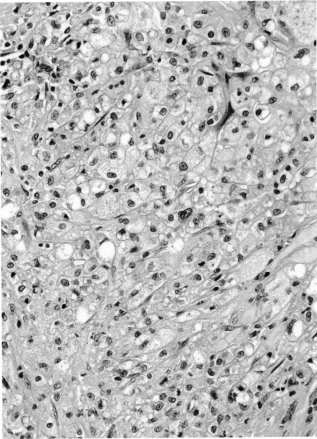

**Fig. 13-105** The histiocytes in the fibroxanthomatous reaction adjacent to necrotic tumor may show mild cytological atypia.

Grossly, fibrosis in post-chemotherapy resections is firm and white and, microscopically, consists of scattered spindle cells set in dense collagenous tissue. Some spindle cells may be enlarged and cytologically atypical but do not form fascicles and are scattered randomly, creating a hypocellular appearance (Fig. 13-106). Some of these fibrous lesions apparently represent post-chemotherapy persistence of the hypocellular, mesenchymal component of yolk sac tumor, based on the identification of this yolk sac tumor pattern in the orchiectomy specimen and the intense cytokeratin reactivity of the spindle cells.[501] It is probably best, however, to consider the hypocellular, collagenous lesions as 'fibrosis' rather than creating clinical confusion by characterizing it as persistence of a yolk sac tumor component.

Some spindle cell lesions observed after chemotherapy display increased cellularity and mitotic activity with a more myxomatous background; these are apparently derived from the mesenchymal component of yolk sac tumor (Fig. 13-107).[501] AFP positivity is usually absent in these lesions (AFP is also absent from the spindle cell component of the primary lesion),[501] although rare 'transitional' cases show persistent foci of an epithelioid, microcystic pattern of yolk sac tumor. Some of these sarcomatoid proliferations differentiate to embryonal rhabdomyosarcoma, often preceded by multiple recurrences having gradually increasing cellularity (Fig. 13-108). The prognosis of patients with high-grade spindle cell lesions in post-chemotherapy resections is guarded.[501]

Teratomatous lesions following chemotherapy are common and are readily diagnosed by those aware of the phenomenon of metastatic teratoma following orchiectomy for mixed germ cell tumor or pure, non-teratomatous germ cell tumor.[620] Metastatic teratoma appears as a multicystic mass with intervening fibrous tissue (Fig. 13-109); the cysts usually contain clear, serous fluid, but mucoid or hemorrhagic cyst contents may also be seen. Microscopically, there are often glands, squamous nests, islands of cartilage, smooth and striated muscle, and intervening fibrous stroma. Significant cytological atypia can be identified in these tumors.[621] Glandular epithelium, although confined to round, non-invasive glands, may be stratified with enlarged, hyperchromatic, and mitotically active nuclei, which raise concern for embryonal carcinoma (Fig. 13-110). However, the primitive, vesicular nuclei and macronucleoli of embryonal carcinoma are absent. These glands often have intestinal differentiation, with goblet cells and eosinophilic absorptive-type cells. Squamous nests and cartilage may also display cytological atypia. Stromal invasion by highly atypical elements indicates a diagnosis of carcinoma or sarcoma; the criteria for invasion are the same as in primary teratoma with a secondary malignant component (see page 800).

Metastatic teratoma may be life-threatening. Mature teratoma may undergo progressive enlargement, according to serial radiographic studies, and impinge on vital structures, especially in the mediastinum. This has been described as the 'growing teratoma syndrome'[622-625] and is one reason for complete excision of metastatic teratomatous tumor whenever feasible.[623] Although often diagnosed as mature teratoma, these tumors contain cells with a malignant genotype (as well as phenotype) based on karyotypic and ploidy studies.[472,543,626] Consequently, such lesions should be surgically excised before evolution to a more aggressive clone of cells results in overgrowth with a malignancy of teratoma-

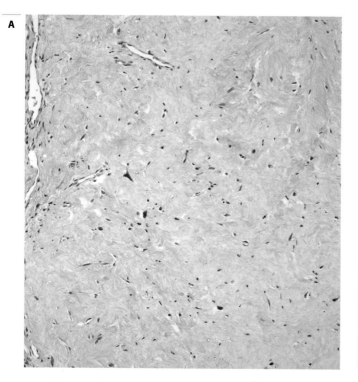

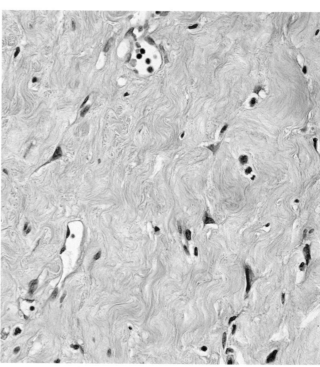

**Fig. 13-106** (**A**) Fibrous lesion following chemotherapy contains widely scattered spindle and stellate cells. (**B**) High power shows mild cytological atypia.

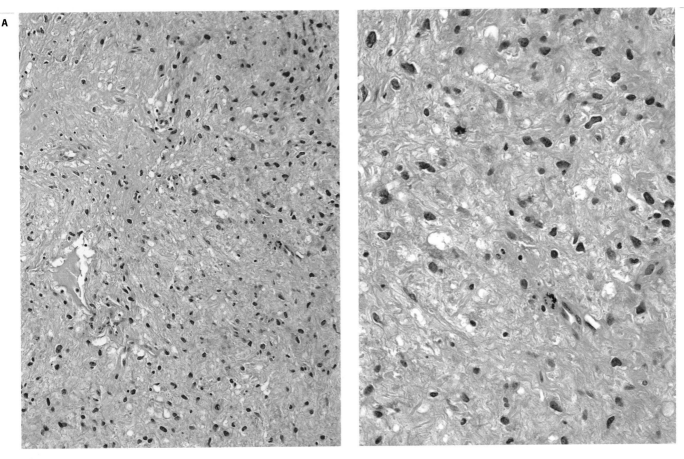

**Fig. 13-107** (**A**) Low grade fibromyxoid tumor after chemotherapy. The tumor cells in these lesions are usually cytokeratin reactive. (**B**) High power showing cytologic atypia and mitotic figures.

tous origin.[546,547,626] Despite the cytological atypia that occurs in metastatic teratomatous lesions following polychemotherapy, in the absence of evolution to an invasive malignant neoplasm such atypia does not appear to have prognostic significance.[621]

A variety of malignancies resembling tumors of non-germ cell origin may be identified in post-chemotherapy resections. These consist of fleshy or necrotic areas among fibrous tissue and cysts. Embryonal rhabdomyosarcoma and primitive neuroectodermal tumor are the most common tumors of this type; others include adenocarcinoma, undifferentiated carcinoma, and undifferentiated sarcoma.[563] The prognosis in such cases is guarded.[565]

The morphology of persistent, post-chemotherapy, non-teratomatous germ cell tumor is usually similar to that of primary testicular neoplasms. However, there are exceptions to this rule, particularly with trophoblastic proliferations. Unlike the biphasic proliferation of syncytiotrophoblast and cytotrophoblast cells in classic choriocarcinoma, the trophoblastic proliferations in post-chemotherapy resections often lack definite syncytiotrophoblast cells. Instead, mononucleated trophoblast cells may be identified in the absence of a syncytiotrophoblast component. Mazur[627] described this pattern in patients treated for gestational choriocarcinoma as 'atypical choriocarcinoma.' In some cases the trophoblast

cells are exclusively mononuclear and form the epithelial lining of cysts, closely mimicking teratomatous cysts composed of atypical squamous epithelium[628] (Fig. 13-111) but having focal hCG reactivity. The distinction between these cystic trophoblastic tumors and teratoma does not appear to be clinically important if there is no evidence of stromal invasion. We found no difference in outcome when such cystic trophoblastic lesions were identified with teratoma in post-chemotherapy resections compared to historical outcomes for teratoma alone in the same setting.[629] They may, however, be associated with minor elevation in serum hCG. Solid, monophasic proliferations of trophoblastic cells, on the other hand, merit additional chemotherapy, when feasible. Additionally, we have found that the appearance of yolk sac tumor may be different in post-chemotherapy resections, especially in the context of late recurrence. There tends to be a predominance of glandular, hepatoid and parietal patterns in this setting, often to the extent that the clinical history of late recurrence can be predicted from the morphology.[498]

The outcome of patients undergoing excision of persistent masses following chemotherapy for metastatic testicular germ cell tumor varies depending on the pathologic findings. Eighty-eight percent of patients with only necrosis in retroperitoneal lymph node dissections were well on follow-

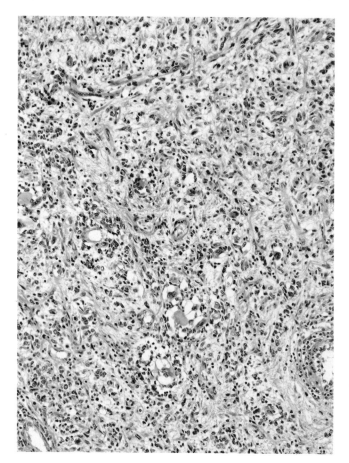

**Fig. 13-108** Embryonal rhabdomyosarcoma following chemotherapy.

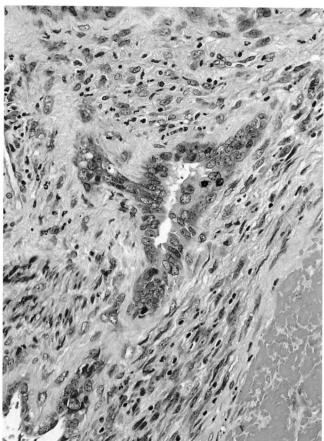

**Fig. 13-110** High-grade epithelial atypia in a teratomatous gland embedded in atypical stroma.

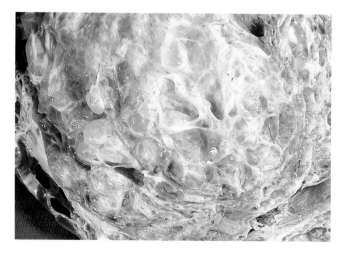

**Fig. 13-109** Metastatic teratoma following chemotherapy, showing the characteristic multicystic appearance.

reported a 5-year survival of 51%.[634] For patients with persistent, apparently viable germ cell tumor other than teratoma in post-chemotherapy resections, the prognosis is also guarded. Those who do well include patients who have complete surgical excision of persistent tumor, who have received only primary chemotherapy before resection, and who also receive post-resection chemotherapy; patients with retroperitoneal tumor who meet these criteria have a 70% disease-free survival.[635] Patients who have persistent retroperitoneal germ cell tumor other than teratoma after salvage therapy and who are completely resected have a 40% disease-free survival.[635] Inability to completely resect viable germ cell tumor other than teratoma after primary or salvage chemotherapy carries a poor prognosis, with only 9% remaining clinically tumor free.[635] Additionally, only about one-third of patients with late recurrence of non-teratomatous germ cell tumor remain disease free after resection.[498]

## Sex cord–stromal tumors

Sex cord–stromal tumors make up only about 4% of testicular neoplasms.[150,587] They include Leydig cell tumor, Sertoli cell tumor, granulosa cell tumor, and sex cord–stromal tumors of mixed and unclassified (indeterminate) types.

up.[630] Similarly, only one of 25 patients (4%) with fibrosis relapsed on follow-up.[631] Residual mature teratoma is also associated with a good prognosis: a combination of three series reported benign follow-up in 90% of 42 cumulative patients.[631-633] Conversely, 24 of 30 patients (80%) with malignant, somatic-type neoplasms developed recurrent tumor following resection,[566,621] and another series

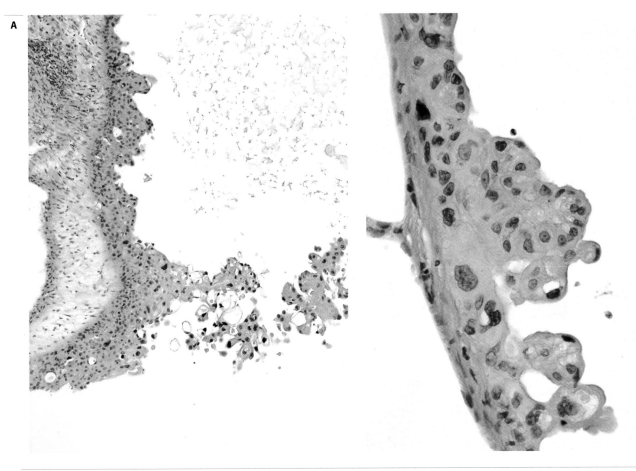

**Fig. 13-111** Cystic trophoblastic tumor showing (**A**) intracystic proliferation of stratified trophoblast cells, some of which have cytoplasmic lacunae. (**B**) High power view of the trophoblast cells lining the cyst.

Many authors also include within the sex cord–stromal tumor category those hyperplastic or hamartomatous lesions of the testis in patients with adrenogenital syndrome, Nelson's syndrome, and androgen insensitivity syndrome, which are derived from interstitial cells and Sertoli cells, although those occurring with the adrenogenital syndrome and Nelson's syndrome are almost always hyperplasias induced by high levels of adrenocorticotrophic hormone. These lesions are discussed with the neoplasm that they most closely resemble: Leydig cell tumor for the adrenogenital syndrome and Nelson's syndrome, and Sertoli cell tumor for the androgen insensitivity syndrome.

## Leydig cell tumor

### Clinical features

Leydig cell tumor accounts for about 3% of testicular neoplasms.[636] It has two age peaks, with about 20% of cases occurring in children[637] (most commonly between 5 and 10 years of age[638] and exceptionally rare in infants under 2 years[639,640]) and 80% occurring in adults (most commonly between 20 and 60 years[636]). Children usually present with significantly smaller tumors because of the early clinical detection of androgen production manifest by isosexual pseudoprecocity, the presenting feature in virtually all pedi-

atric cases.[636] Such patients may not have palpable tumors, and testicular ultrasound or differential testicular vein sampling for androgens may be required for clinical diagnosis. About 10% of children have gynecomastia superimposed upon virilization.[638] Adults, in whom neoplastic androgen production is much less readily detected than in children, most commonly present with a testicular mass, with about 30% of patients developing gynecomastia.[636] Bilateral involvement occurs in about 3% of cases.[636] Leydig cell tumor shares some of the epidemiological features of testicular germ cell tumors, occurring more commonly in patients with cryptorchidism, testicular atrophy, and infertility, and almost exclusively in white patients.[641] Familial occurrence is described,[642] and Leydig cell tumors may be seen, along with hereditary leiomyomatosis and renal cell carcinoma, in association with germline fumarate hydratase mutations.[643] Additionally, some Leydig cell tumors in children have been found to have acquired activating mutations in the luteinizing hormone receptor.[644–646]

### Pathologic features

Most Leydig cell tumors appear as yellow, brown, or tan, solid, sometimes lobulated, intratesticular nodules, infrequently with areas of necrosis or hemorrhage (Fig. 13-112).

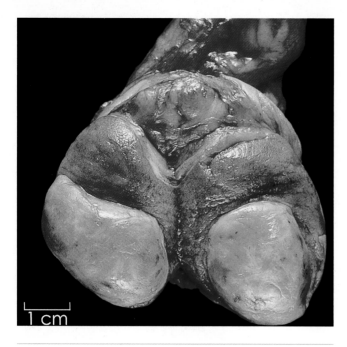

**Fig. 13-112** Leydig cell tumor with a solid, yellow-tan cut surface.

The majority are 2–5 cm in diameter, but some exceed 10 cm;[636] children more often have Leydig cell tumors less than 1 cm in diameter. Extratesticular extension occurs in about 10% of cases.[636] A variety of light microscopic patterns may be seen; the solid, sheet-like pattern is most common (Figs 13-113, 13-114), but pseudoglandular (Fig. 13-115), cord-like (trabecular), and compact nested patterns may also be present, often in the same neoplasm. Rare tumors may have a microcystic pattern, potentially causing confusion with yolk sac tumor (Fig. 13-116),[647] and also rare are those cases where the tumor cells are spindle shaped, either focally or as the predominant pattern (Fig. 13-117).[648] It is common for nodular aggregates of tumor cells to be separated by edematous or fibrous stroma (Fig. 13-118). The cells are polygonal, with abundant, eosinophilic cytoplasm, round, variably sized nuclei, and prominent, central nucleoli (Fig. 13-119). Finely granular lipofuscin pigment is present in the cytoplasm of tumors from postpubertal patients (Fig. 13-119) (usually giving a tan to brown gross appearance) and careful search allows the identification of rod-shaped, intra-cytoplasmic crystals of Reinke in up to 40% of cases (Fig. 13-114).[587] Cytoplasmic accumulation of lipid imparts a clear, finely vacuolated appearance resembling the zona fas-ciculata of the adrenal cortex in some cases and, in rare tumors, the cells may have optically clear cytoplasm (Fig.

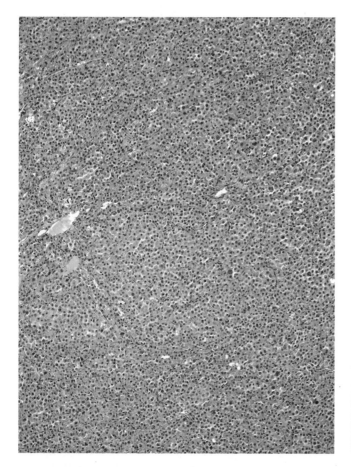

**Fig. 13-113** Sheets of eosinophilic cells in a Leydig cell tumor.

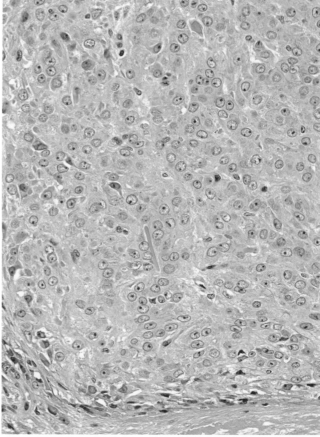

**Fig. 13-114** Prominent Reinke crystals in a Leydig cell tumor.

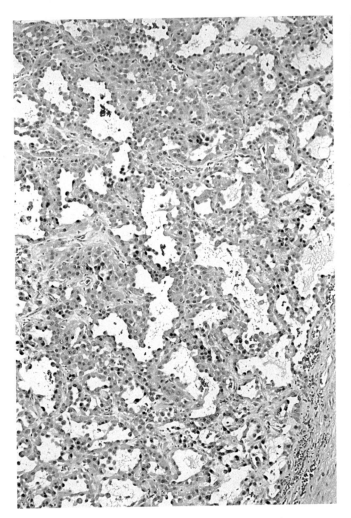

**Fig. 13-115** Pseudoglandular pattern in a Leydig cell tumor.

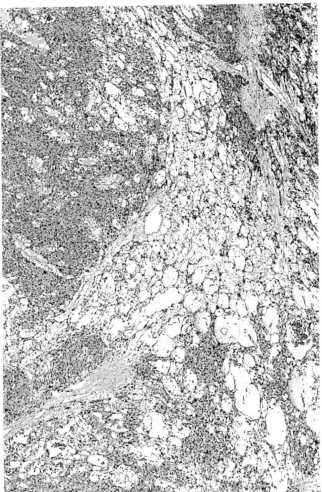

**Fig. 13-116** Microcystic change in a Leydig cell tumor. The more usual, solid pattern is also present.

13-120). Infrequently, fat cells are seen as a component of Leydig cell tumors (Fig. 13-121), deriving either from lipid accumulation within tumor cells or from differentiation of stromal cells.[648,649] Rarely, calcifications and ossification may be seen,[648,650,651] apparently more frequently in tumors with fatty metaplasia.[648] Mitotic figures are usually infrequent, and a rate of 3 or more per 10 high-power fields is a feature that suggests malignancy (see below).

Immunohistochemistry can assist with the diagnosis of Leydig cell tumor. Inhibin-α is positive in almost all Leydig cell tumors,[511,652,653] as are stains for MelanA (MART-1)[654] and calretinin.[655] CD99 is detected in about two-thirds of cases.[511] p53 is detected in some malignant cases and may be helpful in recognizing malignant examples.[656,657] Infrequently, Leydig cell tumors may stain for placental alkaline phosphatase.[511] Vimentin is the dominant cytoplasmic intermediate filament,[658] although cytokeratin reactivity may also be seen. One case with enkephalin immunoreactivity has been described.[659] Ultrastructurally, Leydig cell tumor has features of steroid hormone-synthesizing cells, including abundant lipid droplets, prominent cisternae of smooth endoplasmic reticulum, and mitochondria with tubular cristae.[660,661] Reinke crystals appear as sharply demarcated

geometric shapes, such as hexagons, rectangles and rhomboids, which have a lattice-like substructure.[662]

### Treatment and prognosis

About 10% of Leydig cell tumors are clinically malignant. Some clinical features correlate with the natural history of Leydig cell tumor, including that older patients are more likely to have malignant tumors,[663] that malignant behavior has not been reported before puberty,[636,637,664] and that gynecomastia is more common with benign cases.[636] Malignant behavior also correlates with a number of pathologic features (Fig. 13-122), including larger tumors (>5 cm), high mitotic rate (>3–5 mitotic figures per 10 high-power fields), atypical mitotic figures, vascular space invasion, significant nuclear atypia, necrosis, infiltrative borders, invasion of the rete testis or beyond, DNA aneuploidy, high proliferative activity (>5%) as assessed by staining with the MIB-1 antibody, and increased expression of p53 protein by the tumor cells.[636,656,657,665,666] None of these features, however, is pathognomonic of malignancy, and some non-metastasizing tumors may have a limited number of them, including

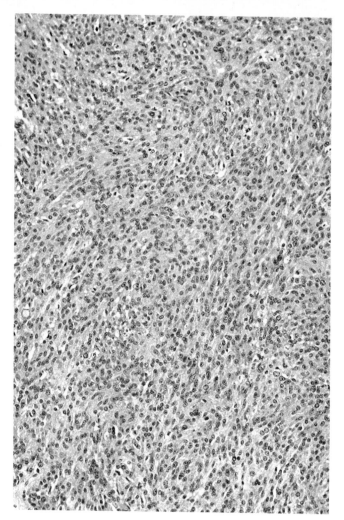

**Fig. 13-117** Leydig cell tumor with a vaguely fascicular arrangement of spindle cells.

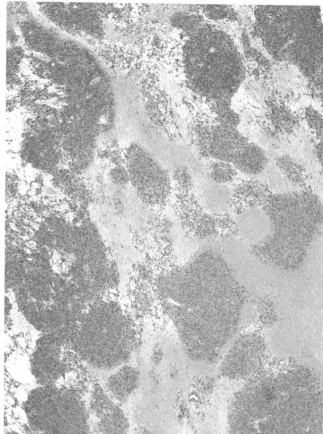

**Fig. 13-118** Nodular pattern in Leydig cell tumor.

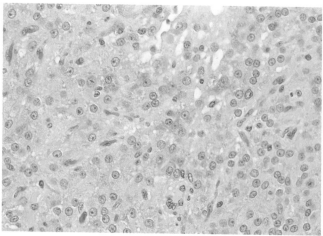

**Fig. 13-119** Leydig cell tumor with intracytoplasmic lipofuscin. Note the eosinophilic cytoplasm and round nuclei with moderate-sized nucleoli.

a single recent case reported in a 1-year-old boy.[640] Radiation and chemotherapy are not effective in the treatment of malignant Leydig cell tumor. Retroperitoneal lymphadenectomy may be performed in patients with testicular sex cord–stromal tumors with malignant features, but the therapeutic role of this intervention remains unclear.[667] Mean survival of patients with malignant Leydig cell tumor is about 4 years,[663] but some may develop metastases more than 10 years after orchiectomy.

### Differential diagnosis

Several entities should be considered in the differential diagnosis of Leydig cell tumor.[587] Leydig cell hyperplasia, although usually diffuse, may form nodules that mimic Leydig cell tumor. However, this is an interstitial, non-destructive process that preserves many seminiferous tubules.[668] It may be seen in patients with elevated gonadotropin levels, including those with elevated hCG levels. Apparent Leydig cell hyperplasia occurs in many cases of testicular atrophy because of a normal population of Leydig cells in a reduced testicular volume. It is seen in Klinefelter's

syndrome where other pathologic features of that disorder are present and help with the diagnosis (see Chapter 12). Patients who have the adrenogenital syndrome[669,670] or Nelson's syndrome[671] (Cushing's syndrome associated with occult pituitary adenoma that becomes clinically evident with high levels of adrenocorticotrophin after bilateral adre-

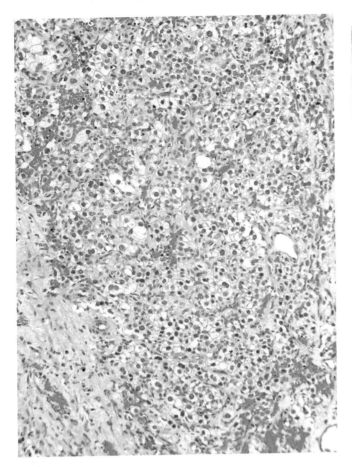

**Fig. 13-120** Leydig cell tumor with prominent clear cells, initially interpreted as seminoma.

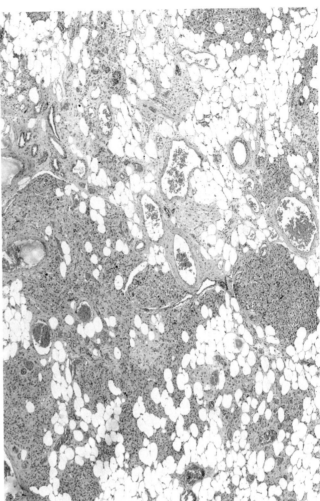

**Fig. 13-121** Leydig cell tumor with fatty metaplasia.

nalectomy) may develop testicular nodules that closely resemble Leydig cell tumor. These nodules appear to be hyperplastic and are usually distinguished from Leydig cell tumor by their multifocality, bilaterality, uniform absence of Reinke crystals, frequent fibrous bands and tendency for prominent lipofuscin deposits.[587] They often regress with treatment that causes the adrenocorticotrophin levels to decrease. Clinical history is of value in such cases. Large cell calcifying Sertoli cell tumor, an entity that is associated with Carney's syndrome (see page 824), may resemble Leydig cell tumor because the neoplastic cells are usually polygonal with abundant eosinophilic cytoplasm.[3,5,672,673] Unlike Leydig cell tumor, large cell calcifying Sertoli cell tumor may be bilateral and multifocal (when Carney's syndrome is associated), lacks Reinke crystals, is more consistently associated with calcifications (and sometimes ossification), may show intratubular growth, and tends to have a more myxoid stroma, often with a neutrophilic infiltrate.[5,587] There is significant overlap in the immunostaining patterns of these two neoplasms,[352] although it has been claimed that patchy (as opposed to diffuse) positivity for MelanA and CD10, as well as reactivity for S100 protein-β, favor large cell calcifying Sertoli cell tumor.[674] Young and Talerman[587] reported metastatic prostate carcinoma to the testis mimicking Leydig cell tumor, but immunostains against prostate specific antigen

and prostatic acid phosphatase were positive, resolving the differential diagnosis. Leydig cell tumor with prominent cytoplasmic clarity may be misinterpreted as seminoma, but the clarity is due to lipids, often yielding a finely vacuolated appearance, rather than glycogen, as in seminoma, which causes a 'water-clear' appearance. Additionally, there is no association with IGCNU, and the characteristic lymphoid infiltrate and granulomatous reaction of seminoma are absent. Malakoplakia may resemble Leydig cell tumor but has intratubular infiltrates of eosinophilic histiocytes and cytoplasmic calcifications that are not seen in Leydig cell tumor.

## Sertoli cell tumor

### Usual type ('Sertoli cell tumor, NOS')

#### Clinical features

Sertoli cell tumor is rare, accounting for about 1% of testicular neoplasms in both children[675] and adults. It can occur at virtually any age but is most common in middle age. Most patients present with a testicular mass,[638] but estrogen production by the tumor can cause gynecomastia or impotence,

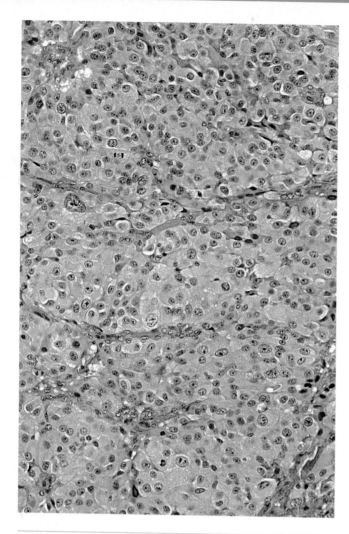

**Fig. 13-122** Malignant Leydig cell tumor. There is cellular pleomorphism and an elevated mitotic rate.

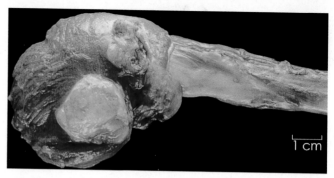

**Fig. 13-123** Sertoli cell tumor with a gray-white cut surface.

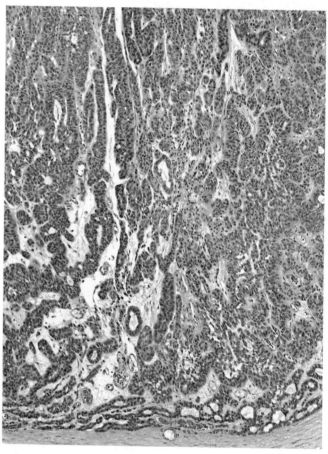

**Fig. 13-124** Sertoli cell tumor composed of mostly solid tubules.

which can be the presenting complaints.[676] Isolated gynecomastia may be the initial manifestation of Sertoli cell tumor in a child; children with Leydig cell tumor, in contrast, do not develop gynecomastia without virilization.[638] Patients with Peutz–Jeghers syndrome have been reported with testicular Sertoli cell tumor,[4] but most of these appear to represent intratubular proliferations of Sertoli cells[7] (see page 825).

## Pathologic features

Grossly, Sertoli cell tumor of the usual type (designated 'not otherwise specified' – NOS) is typically a solid, gray, white, tan or yellow nodule, usually under 4 cm in diameter; large tumors may occur but should raise a concern for malignancy (Fig. 13-123).[677] Occasional tumors have cystic change. On microscopic examination the hallmark is tubule formation.[377] These may be either hollow or solid, usually in a fibrous (often hyalinized) to myxoid stroma (Fig. 13-124). Sheet-like arrays of tumor cells, solid nests (Fig. 13-125), trabeculae and cords may also occur, but are not diagnostic alone. Rarely a retiform pattern may be seen (Fig. 13-126). The tumor cells typically have scant to moderate amounts of

pale to clear cytoplasm. Prominent cytoplasmic vacuolization may create a microcystic pattern (Fig. 13-127). The nuclei are round to oval, relatively uniform, and usually lack large nucleoli. The cytoplasmic clarity is due to abundant cellular lipid, which may be demonstrable on fresh tissue with special stains. One case of a Sertoli cell tumor with a heterologous sarcomatous component has been reported.[678]

On immunohistochemical study, 30–90% of Sertoli cell tumors are inhibin-α reactive,[511,652,679,680] 60–80% are positive for cytokeratin,[652,679,681] 90–100% are positive for

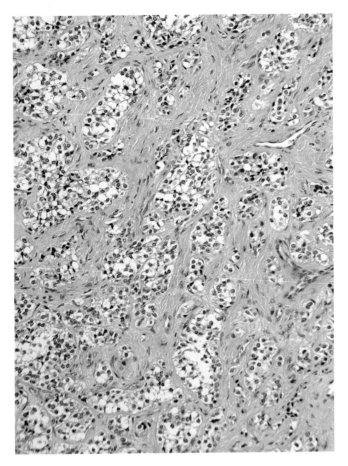

**Fig. 13-125** Solid nests and focal tubules in a Sertoli cell tumor.

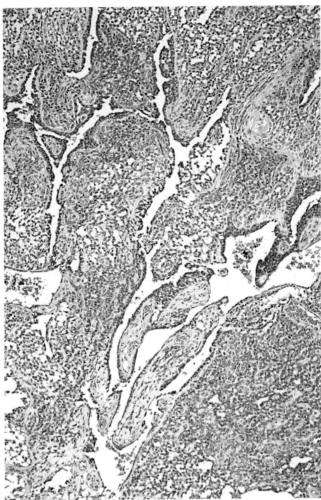

**Fig. 13-126** Retiform pattern in a Sertoli cell tumor.

vimentin,[679,681] 30–64% are positive for S100,[652,679] 0–82% are positive for chromogranin,[511,652] and 45% are reactive for synaptophysin[652] and usually negative for EMA,[679] although in our experience with malignant examples, EMA reactivity occurred in most.[378] In our experience about half of Sertoli cell tumors NOS stain for calretinin, although such positivity may be quite focal. NSE positivity has been described in several cases,[677] and very focal reactivity for anti-müllerian hormone has been reported.[682] Features of steroid synthesizing cells are identified ultrastructurally, including abundant cisternae of smooth endoplasmic reticulum and numerous intracytoplasmic lipid droplets. Adjacent cells are connected by desmosomes.[683] Charcot–Böttcher filaments (perinuclear arrays of filaments) are considered pathognomonic of Sertoli cell differentiation. They have been identified in ovarian Sertoli cell tumor[684] and in large cell calcifying Sertoli cell tumor,[673,685,686] but most reports of testicular Sertoli cell tumor NOS have not mentioned their presence.

About 10% of Sertoli cell tumors are malignant, and, in contrast to Leydig cell tumor, malignant cases may occur in children.[129,378,676,677,687] Gynecomastia appears to be more common with malignant tumors than with benign ones.[677] As in Leydig cell tumor, malignant behavior in Sertoli cell tumor NOS may be difficult to predict from pathologic features alone. Features that correlate with an increased likelihood of malignancy include a size of 5 cm or more, significant cytological atypia and pleomorphism, invasive borders, mitotic activity in excess of five mitotic figures per 10 high-power fields, vascular invasion and necrosis[677,688–691] (Fig. 13-128). In the study of Young and coworkers,[377] the malignant cases had at least two of these features (they did not include invasive borders as a criterion). MIB-1 proliferation index >30% correlates with malignant behavior,[680] and we noted malignant behavior in a group of Sertoli cell tumors with predominance of a diffuse growth pattern.[378]

### Differential diagnosis

Sertoli cell tumor must be distinguished from the rare seminoma with a tubular pattern,[305] a differential diagnosis discussed on page 775. Patients with the androgen insensitivity syndrome (AIS; also known as the testicular feminization syndrome) may develop multiple hamartomatous testicular nodules composed of closely spaced tubules lined by Sertoli cells but, in contrast to true Sertoli cell tumor, these lesions also have intervening Leydig cells within the interstitium

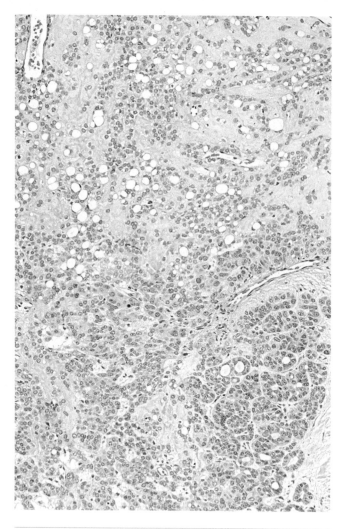

**Fig. 13-127** Sertoli cell tumor with cytoplasmic vacuolization.

(Fig. 13-129). [143,148] About 25% of patients with AIS also develop multifocal, bilateral Sertoli cell adenomas composed of pure proliferations of Sertoli cell-lined tubules (Fig. 13-130).[148] These lesions may be indistinguishable from well-differentiated Sertoli cell tumor, and it is uncertain whether they are neoplastic or hamartomatous. Some have a prominent component of globular basement membrane deposits. Malignant behavior in pure Sertoli cell proliferations in patients with AIS have not been reported; thus the term 'Sertoli cell adenoma' is appropriate even though it connotes a neoplastic process.[143,148] A unique case of a malignant sex cord–stromal tumor in a patient with AIS did not have the features of a typical 'Sertoli cell adenoma' and more closely resembled juvenile granulosa cell tumor, although ultrastructure supported Sertoli cell differentiation.[692]

Microscopic, non-encapsulated nodules composed of small tubules lined by immature-appearing Sertoli cells are common in orchiectomy specimens, and may be more common in cryptorchid testes (Fig. 13-131).[174,175,693] These 'Sertoli cell nodules' often contain central accumulations of basement membrane which can be seen in continuity with thickened peripheral basement membrane surrounding the tubules. In contrast to true Sertoli cell tumor, these are almost always[693] incidental microscopic findings. In patients with germ cell tumor they may be colonized by IGCNU, simulating gonadoblastoma (Fig. 13-132). Occasional Sertoli cell nodules may also contain spermatogenic cells, unlike Sertoli cell tumor.

Sertoli cell tumors may show large areas of sheet-like arrangement and, furthermore, have an associated lymphocytic infiltrate and prominence of clear or pale cytoplasm (Fig. 13-133). These features mimic seminoma and can be a source of serious diagnostic error.[378] Features of assistance include, in the Sertoli cell tumor, the absence of IGCNU, foci with typical tubules, less atypical appearing nuclei and lower mitotic rates. Immunohistochemistry is also helpful, with OCT3/4, PLAP, and inhibin showing opposite patterns of reactivity in Sertoli cell tumor and seminoma.[378]

The distinction of Sertoli cell tumor from Leydig cell tumor depends on the formation of tubules, at least focally, in the former. Leydig cell tumor may show Reinke crystalloids, unlike Sertoli cell tumor. Inhibin-α is less consistently expressed in Sertoli cell tumor than in Leydig cell tumor. Inhibin-α is positive in 30–80% of Sertoli cell tumors[511,680] but in virtually all Leydig cell tumors. CD99 is also more commonly expressed in Leydig cell tumors than in Sertoli cell tumors.[511]

### Treatment and prognosis

As for Leydig cell tumor, malignant Sertoli cell tumors do not usually respond to radiation and chemotherapy. Retroperitoneal lymphadenectomy therefore remains an important option if the tumor has not disseminated beyond the scope of the dissection.

### Sclerosing Sertoli cell tumor

Sclerosing Sertoli cell tumor is a variant of Sertoli cell tumor that occurs in patients with an average age of 35 years (range, 18–80 years).[694] All patients have presented with a testicular mass without associated hormonal symptoms, or the tumor has been found incidentally.[694-698] Grossly, sclerosing Sertoli cell tumor consists of solid, white to yellow-tan nodules. Microscopically it is composed of cords, solid or hollow tubules, and nests of Sertoli cells set in a densely collagenous stroma (Fig. 13-134). The nuclei vary from large and vesicular to small and hyperchromatic, and the cytoplasm is pale and sometimes vacuolated. Mitotic activity and cytological atypia were significant in only one of the reported cases, but, despite this finding all cases had a benign outcome.[694] The cord-like pattern may be misinterpreted as trabecular carcinoid tumor, but most primary carcinoids have an insular pattern and may be associated with teratomatous elements. The presence of a cord-like or tubular pattern with vacuolated cells may suggest adenomatoid tumor, but the primarily paratesticular location of adenomatoid tumor and immunohistochemical negativity for inhibin and strong reactivity for EMA are helpful differential features.

### Large cell calcifying Sertoli cell tumor

Large cell calcifying Sertoli cell tumor is another variant of Sertoli cell tumor that has some unique clinical associa-

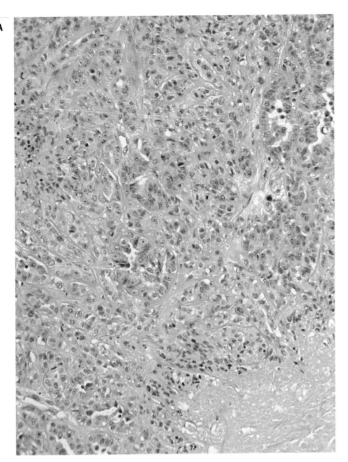 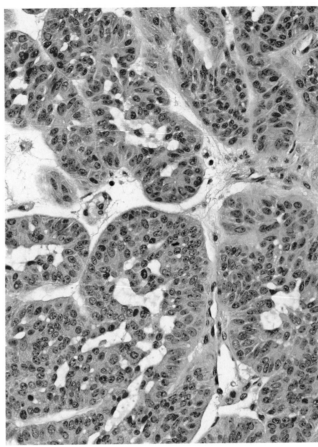

**Fig. 13-128** Metastasizing Sertoli cell tumor showing (**A**) foci of necrosis and (**B**) cytological atypia and mitotic figures.

tions.[3,699–701] It is now apparent that large cell calcifying Sertoli cell tumor is a component of Carney's syndrome, in which patients develop lentigines of the face; myxomas of the heart, skin, soft tissue, and elsewhere; myxoid fibroadenomas of the breast; blue nevi of the skin; pigmented nodules of the adrenal cortex associated with Cushing's syndrome; growth hormone-producing adenomas of the pituitary gland; and psammomatous melanotic schwannomas.[2,3,673,702–705] Because 40% or so of large cell calcifying Sertoli cell tumors are associated with Carney's syndrome, its diagnosis should prompt consideration of this association because of the potential life-threatening complications of cardiac myxomas. Typically, patients with Carney's syndrome-associated tumors have small, bilateral and multifocal tumors and present in childhood or adolescence, whereas those who have the tumor on a sporadic basis have solitary lesions and are older.[5,698] A testicular mass is the usual presenting complaint, but gynecomastia and isosexual pseudoprecocity may also occur,[685,706] especially in those that are syndrome associated. The hormones responsible for these manifestations may be produced by the neoplasm or by associated nodules of hyperplastic Leydig cells.

Grossly, large cell calcifying Sertoli cell tumor is usually tan or yellow with associated 'gritty' calcification, and may be multifocal, with a 40% frequency of bilaterality.[3,702] Microscopically, there are nests and cords of cells with abun-

dant, eosinophilic cytoplasm in a myxoid to collagenous stroma that is calcified or even ossified in about half of cases (Fig. 13-135). A neutrophilic stromal infiltrate is characteristic. Intratubular neoplasm and calcifications are common. Nuclei are usually round and may have prominent nucleoli, but mitotic figures are usually rare. Malignant cases do occur but are uncommon.[3,5,707] They usually occur on a sporadic basis in patients over 25 years of age rather than in association with Carney's syndrome;[698,707] hence malignant tumors are solitary and can be recognized as having metastatic potential on the basis of size >4 cm, extratesticular growth, tumor cell necrosis, high-grade atypia, vascular space invasion, or mitotic rate in excess of three mitotic figures per 10 high-power fields.[5] Immunohistochemical study has shown vimentin, inhibin, S100, NSE, desmin, EMA and focal cytokeratin reactivity.[5,653,700,708,709] Ultrastructural studies of large cell calcifying Sertoli cell tumor have demonstrated Charcot–Böttcher filaments and other features of Sertoli cells.[673,685] The main differential diagnostic problem is separation from Leydig cell tumor (see page 821).

### Sertoli cell tumors in Peutz–Jeghers syndrome

Patients with the Peutz–Jeghers syndrome develop multifocal, bilateral intratubular proliferations of Sertoli cells having abundant eosinophilic cytoplasm, similar to those seen in large cell calcifying Sertoli cell tumor.[6,7,710] Descriptively

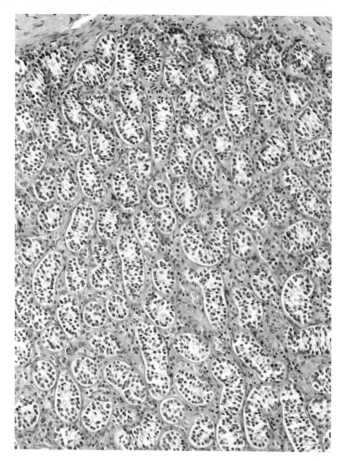

**Fig. 13-129** Nodule of seminiferous tubules lined by small, immature-appearing Sertoli cells with intertubular Leydig cells in a patient with the androgen insensitivity syndrome. Such lesions are considered hamartomas.

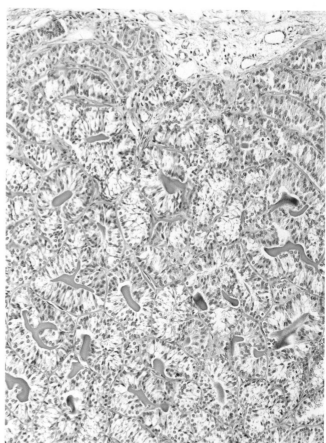

**Fig. 13-130** Sertoli cell adenoma in a patient with the androgen insensitivity syndrome. There is a circumscribed proliferation of closely packed tubules lined by immature Sertoli cells. Basement membrane deposits are prominent.

termed 'large cell hyalinizing Sertoli cell neoplasia,' these intratubular lesions occur in conjunction with a thickened, peritubular basement membrane that is internalized into the expanded tubules and infrequently calcified (Fig. 13-136).[7] These expanded tubules occur in lobular clusters throughout the parenchyma. Most patients present in childhood with gynecomastia or, less commonly, isosexual pseudoprecocity due to the production of estrogen or androgen, respectively, by the tumor. Occasional invasive tumors are seen in association with the intratubular tumor, and these may be very similar in appearance to the large cell calcifying Sertoli cell tumor, but they more commonly do not have calcifications or the prominent fibromyxoid stroma with neutrophils.[7] Conservative management of patients with no evidence of an invasive tumor (the majority), by ultrasonographic follow-up, permits testicular preservation in many patients, although the development of a distinct mass or hormonal complications may necessitate orchiectomy. Malignant behavior has not been reported.[6,7]

The differential diagnosis includes large cell calcifying Sertoli cell tumor, which, in contrast to the Peutz–Jeghers lesion, is dominated by invasive tumor. Furthermore, the intratubular component in these cases does not show as great a degree of tubular expansion or as prominent base-

ment membrane deposits, and often displays prominent calcifications. Sertoli cell nodules may also be confused with the Peutz–Jeghers lesion because of their clustered seminiferous tubules with basement membrane deposits, but they have small fetal-type Sertoli cells and may contain spermatogonia.

## Granulosa cell tumor

### Adult type

There are two major types of granulosa cell tumor of the testis: adult and juvenile. The adult type is rare,[711–717] occurring in patients from 16 to 76 years of age,[587] and is frequently associated with hyperestrogenism, often causing gynecomastia.[715] Grossly, the adult type may be solid, cystic, or both, and is typically yellow to gray.[587,713] Gross hemorrhage and necrosis may correlate with malignant behavior.[716] Microscopically, the patterns of the common granulosa cell tumor of the ovary may be identified, including microfollicular, macrofollicular, trabecular, gyriform, insular (Fig. 13-137), and diffuse patterns. Call–Exner bodies are characteristic of the microfollicular pattern. The cells have scant, lightly staining cytoplasm, and the nuclei are pale, round to oval, and frequently grooved. Mitotic figures are usually

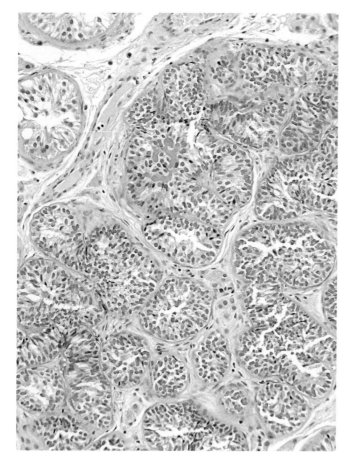

**Fig. 13-131** Sertoli cell nodule in a cryptorchid testis. The tubules are smaller than the surrounding seminiferous tubules, are lined only by fetal-type Sertoli cells, and have focal central accumulations of basement membrane.

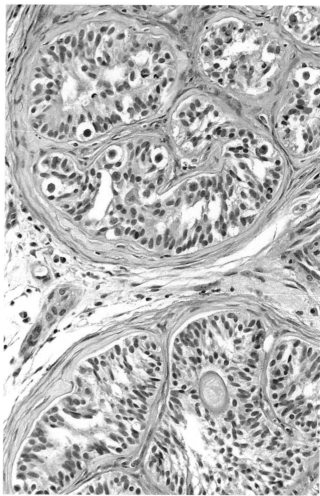

**Fig. 13-132** Sertoli cell nodule partially populated by IGCNU cells.

infrequent, but there may rarely be up to six per 10 high-power fields.[716] Positivity for inhibin, vimentin, cytokeratins 8 and 18, and CD99 has been reported,[711,714,717–719] although one study reported an absence of cytokeratin reactivity in five of five cases;[716] EMA is negative.[711,714,716,718] Ultrastructural studies have shown results similar to ovarian granulosa cell tumor.[712,714] Most reported cases have been benign, but malignant behavior is a possibility.[715,716] Large tumor size (>7 cm), vascular invasion, hemorrhage, and necrosis are considered useful in identifying cases with the greatest risk of malignant behavior.[716]

### Juvenile type

Juvenile granulosa cell tumor of the testis is similar in appearance to its ovarian counterpart but occurs in a more restricted age range, with most patients under 5 months of age.[519,720–723] There is one case report of this tumor presenting in a 4-year-old boy.[724] There are no well-established risk factors, although a disproportionate number occur in patients with either gonadal dysgenesis or anomalies of sex chromosomes, including patients with X/XY mosaicism.[209,725,726] A testicular mass is invariably the presenting feature. Grossly, it consists of a solid to cystic, gray to yellow

nodule (Fig. 13-138).[519] The cystic foci are filled with mucoid to watery fluid. Microscopically, juvenile granulosa cell tumor has solid, cellular zones admixed with follicle-like, cystic structures filled with watery, faintly mucicarminophilic fluid (Fig. 13-139). Often the follicles are lined by several layers of stratified tumor cells and surrounded by a spindle cell stroma (Fig. 13-139). The solid areas may display prominently hyalinized, collagenous stroma. There is often a lobular arrangement of follicular and solid areas. The neoplastic cells have abundant pale to eosinophilic cytoplasm with round, hyperchromatic nuclei and identifiable nucleoli.[519,587] Mitoses and cellular apoptosis may be prominent (Fig. 13-139), but malignant behavior has not been reported,[519,681,727,728] another feature that differs from ovarian juvenile granulosa cell tumor. Immunohistochemical studies reveal inhibin, vimentin, CD99 and focal cytokeratin, smooth muscle actin and desmin reactivity.[681,723,727,729] AFP is negative. The histogenesis of this tumor is controversial, with some favoring a Sertoli cell derivation rather than granulosa cell differentiation[729] (Talerman, personal communication 1993). Because of the exclusive occurrence in infants and young children, and the solid and cystic pattern, juve-

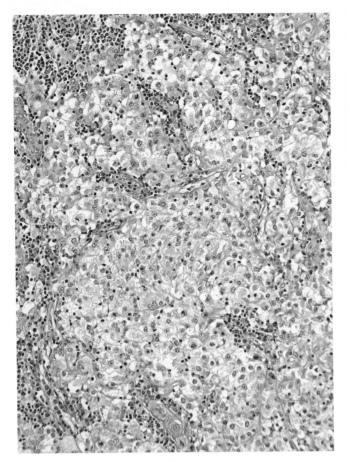

**Fig. 13-133** This malignant Sertoli cell tumor has a sheet-like pattern of pale cells and a prominent inflammatory reaction that mimic seminoma.

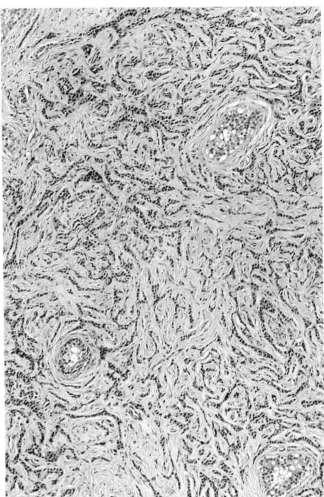

**Fig. 13-134** Cord-like growth in a sclerosing Sertoli cell tumor. Note densely collagenous stroma.

nile granulosa cell tumor may be confused with testicular yolk sac tumor. This differential diagnosis is discussed on page 795. Testis-sparing enucleation has been suggested for suspected juvenile granulosa cell tumors in infants with serum AFP in the normal range for age.[728]

## Tumors in the fibroma/thecoma group

Testicular tumors resembling ovarian fibroma or thecoma are exceptionally rare; some reported examples probably represent unclassified sex cord–stromal tumors with a predominance of spindle cells. Jones et al.[730] reported three intratesticular examples of usual or cellular fibromas in men 28–35 years old who presented with painless masses. These were circumscribed, solid, yellow-white tumors that lacked hemorrhage or necrosis. On microscopic examination there is moderate to dense cellularity and short fascicles of uniform spindle cells with focal storiform arrangements (Fig. 13-140). Acellular, hyaline plaques of collagen may be seen (Fig. 13-140). Mitotic activity is usually fewer than five mitotic figures per 10 high-power fields. Vimentin, actin, and desmin are identified on immunohistochemical study, but S100, CD34 and cytokeratin stains are negative.[730] Behavior is benign.

## Mixed and unclassified sex cord–stromal tumors

A sizable group of sex cord–stromal neoplasms of the testis show admixtures of various forms of differentiation or incomplete differentiation. Such cases are classified as mixed or unclassified sex cord–stromal tumors, respectively. An example of a mixed sex cord–stromal tumor is adult granulosa cell tumor with tubules lined by Sertoli cells. Unclassified sex cord–stromal tumors consist of proliferations of incompletely differentiated sex cord or stromal elements that cannot be further characterized at the light microscopic level. These neoplasms are heterogeneous and have been grouped into a 'wastebasket' category. Mixed and unclassified sex cord–stromal tumors occur at all ages, with 50% occurring in children.[731] They usually present as a testicular mass, and 15% of cases are associated with gynecomastia.[587] Most consist of gray, tan, or yellow solid nodules of variable size. Both epithelial (sex cord) and stromal differentiation may be apparent at the light-microscopic level (Fig. 13-141), and reticulum stains may enhance the different elements, surrounding groups of sex cord-like cells and individual stromal cells. In some tumors non-specific sex cord elements

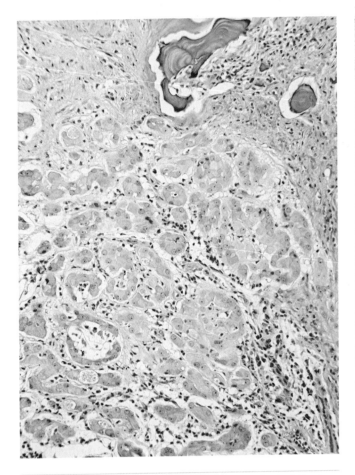

**Fig. 13-135** Large cell calcifying Sertoli cell tumor. Note focal calcification and neutrophilic infiltrate.

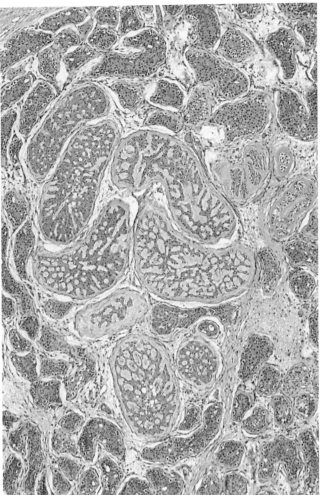

**Fig. 13-136** Cluster of expanded seminiferous tubules containing proliferations of large Sertoli cells with abundant, eosinophilic cytoplasm and prominent basement membrane deposits in a patient with Peutz–Jeghers syndrome.

may compose most of or the entire tumor. In other cases the stromal component may be dominant, consisting of a relatively pure spindle cell proliferation.[732,733] Many of those cases are small (1–2 cm), occur close to the rete testis, and have benign features.[734] Occasional cases are overtly sarcomatoid, sometimes having 'heterologous' mesenchymal differentiation.[735]

The demonstration of epithelial features by electron microscopy and immunohistochemistry suggests that some of these 'stromal' tumors are spindled forms of epithelial (sex cord) origin.[732,736] In other cases the presence of myofilaments in spindled stromal tumors suggests origin from myofibroblastic cells of the testicular interstitium, especially the peritubular myoid cells.[737–739] Such cases should be classified as pure mesenchymal tumors (see page 837) rather than unclassified sex cord–stromal tumors.

Both S100 and smooth muscle actin have been identified in the spindled examples,[734] with CD99 and inhibin reactivity occurring in the sex cord component of some.[732] Mixed and unclassified sex cord–stromal tumors have thus far behaved in a benign fashion in children under 10 years of age, but in 20% of older patients metastases develop.[727,731,740] The presence of cellular atypia and pleomorphism, a high mitotic rate, necrosis, vascular invasion, invasive margins, and large tumor size are features that identify patients at risk

for metastases. These tumors are usually managed by radical orchiectomy, with retroperitoneal lymph node dissection reserved for patients with clinical evidence of metastatic involvement or 'high risk' pathologic features.

# Mixed germ cell and sex cord–stromal tumors

## Gonadoblastoma

### Clinical features

Gonadoblastoma is composed of a mixture of seminoma-like cells and sex cord cells having features of Sertoli cells, with Charcot–Böttcher filaments in the cytoplasm.[741,742] Gonadoblastoma usually arises in abnormal, dysgenetic gonads of patients with an intersex syndrome; 80% are phenotypically female and 20% are phenotypically male, but ambiguous genitalia occur in many cases.[743] Phenotypically male patients present in childhood or early adolescence with

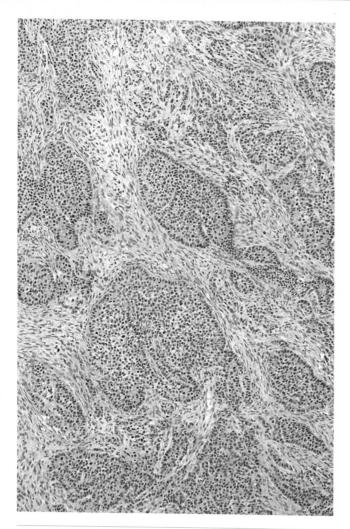

**Fig. 13-137** Testicular granulosa cell tumor of the adult type showing the characteristic solid nests with a peripheral palisade and cellular stroma.

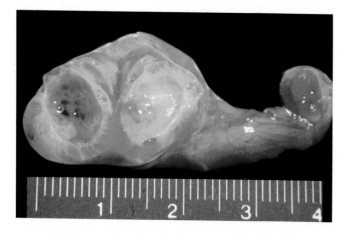

**Fig. 13-138** Juvenile granulosa cell tumor has a solid and cystic, yellow to tan cut surface. (Courtesy of Dr Carlos Galliani, Fort Worth, TX.)

cryptorchidism, hypospadias, or other anomalies of the external genitalia, and gynecomastia. Surgical exploration of the cryptorchid testes often demonstrates persistence of female-type internal genital structures stemming from failure of involution of the müllerian ductal system.[147] Bilateral involvement by gonadoblastoma occurs in about one-third of cases.[743] Karyotypic analysis of the patients, regardless of sexual phenotype, almost always reveals a Y chromosome, with 46XY and 45X/46XY occurring most commonly.[147]

## Pathologic features

Grossly, gonadoblastoma usually forms solid, yellow and tan nodules with gritty calcifications. Microscopically the nodules usually consist of well-defined, rounded nests of large, pale seminoma-like cells admixed with small, dark, angular, sex cord cells that may form a peripheral palisade around the cellular nests (Fig. 13-142). Foci of hyalinized basement membrane can be seen in the center of these nests and at the periphery. Calcifications appear initially on this basement membrane, and may become quite prominent. In some gonadoblastomas a trabecular growth pattern of seminoma-like cells and sex cord cells may occur in tandem. In the stroma adjacent to gonadoblastoma, collections of Leydig-like cells lacking Reinke crystals may be seen in about two-thirds of cases.[147,743]

## Special studies

The germ cell component of gonadoblastoma has the immunohistochemical reactivities seen in IGCNU.[231] The sex cord component stains for inhibin and the Wilms' tumor gene protein (WT1).[744] Fluorescence-in-situ hybridization in patients with gonadoblastoma and 45,X/46,XY mosaicism has demonstrated disproportionate representation of the Y chromosome in the gonadoblastoma cells, implicating it in tumor genesis.[745] Mapping studies have defined a susceptibility region on the Y chromosome[746,747] that encompasses five candidate genes.[748] Accumulation of OCT3/4-positive germ cells and loss of expression of testis-specific protein on the Y chromosome (TSPY) has been observed by immunohistochemistry in the progression from gonadoblastoma to invasive germ cell tumor.[749]

## Treatment and prognosis

Gonadoblastoma is a premalignant lesion from which invasive germ cell tumors can develop; most are seminomas, but any non-seminomatous germ cell tumor may occur.[743] Excision of a gonad with gonadoblastoma prior to the development of an invasive lesion is curative. Bilateral gonadectomy is indicated because of the dysgenetic nature of the gonads and the high frequency of bilaterality of gonadoblastoma.

## Differential diagnosis

Sertoli cell nodules colonized by IGCNU may be misinterpreted as gonadoblastoma (see page 824, Fig. 13-132). However, this lesion is almost always microscopic rather than macroscopic, and the associated gonad is not dysgenetic, nor does the patient have somatosexual ambiguity. In some cases the colonization by IGCNU is focal and the

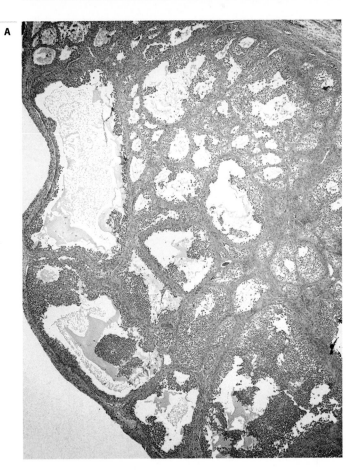
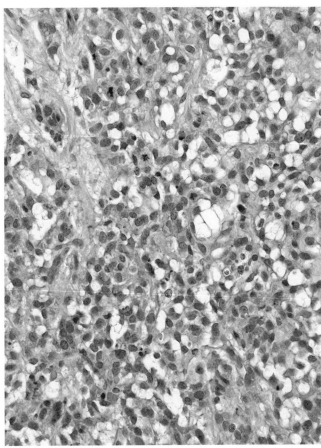

**Fig. 13-139** Juvenile granulosa cell tumor with (**A**) follicle-like structures mantled by multiple layers of tumor cells and containing watery to mucoid secretion and (**B**) solid foci with mitotic figures and apoptosis.

seminoma-like cells are not uniformly distributed throughout the Sertoli cell nodule, whereas gonadoblastoma contains seminoma-like cells that are an integral and diffusely distributed component. Additionally, we have shown that the constituent cells of these lesions contain both X and Y chromosomes by FISH methods, unlike gonadoblastoma.[750] This distinction is important because the diagnosis of gonadoblastoma implies an underlying dysgenetic gonad and a much higher risk of bilateral gonadal involvement by a premalignant lesion. In contrast, a patient with a Sertoli cell nodule with IGCNU probably has a risk of bilateral involvement similar to that of any patient with IGCNU in one testis – approximately 1–5% of cases.

## Other mixed germ cell–sex cord–stromal tumors

The legitimacy of this form of tumor is questionable (see below). If they do occur, they are quite rare.[751] Such tumors have been reported in adults between 27 and 69 years of age and present as asymptomatic testicular masses;[752,753] the features of gonadal dysgenesis or an intersex syndrome are absent.[751,753] Grossly, the reported tumors were usually fleshy, solid, and gray-white, although some had foci of cystic degeneration. Microscopically, there were sheets or nests of germ cells admixed with dark sex cord-like cells that

sometimes formed distinct areas similar to granulosa cell tumor and Sertoli cell tumor. Spindle stromal cells were variably prominent. The germ cell component in these cases was described as seminoma-like, but we believe that many of the putative cases of this entity actually represent sex cord–stromal tumors with entrapped, non-neoplastic spermatogonia having a uniform, fine chromatin and lacking the vesicular nuclei and large nucleoli of seminoma (Fig. 13-143).[752] Some reported cases have been PLAP negative, OCT3/4 negative, and negative for 12p amplification,[753] suggesting that the germ cells are entrapped non-neoplastic cells.[754] Tumors placed in the category would typically either represent Sertoli cell tumors or fall in the unclassified category. It is not clear whether all the examples of mixed germ cell–sex cord–stromal tumor can be attributed to a similar process of entrapment, or whether there are legitimate examples that contain a component of neoplastic germ cells. By way of differential diagnosis, the discrete, small nests typical of gonadoblastoma are not identified, and the surrounding testis does not have dysgenetic features. Furthermore, overgrowth of germ cell elements in the form of a typical germ cell tumor has not been reported, nor have metastases. Treatment consists of orchiectomy, with assessment of the sex cord–stromal tumor for the features associated with malignant behavior, as mentioned in earlier sections. If malignant

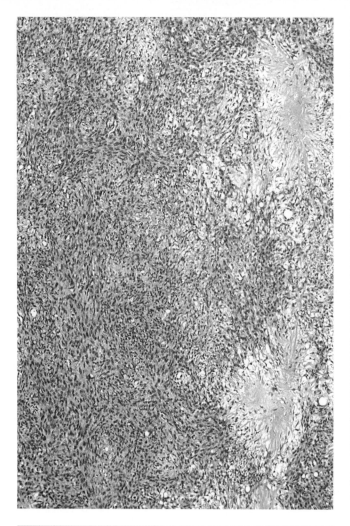

**Fig. 13-140** Cellular fibroma. Note the plaques of hyalinized collagen.

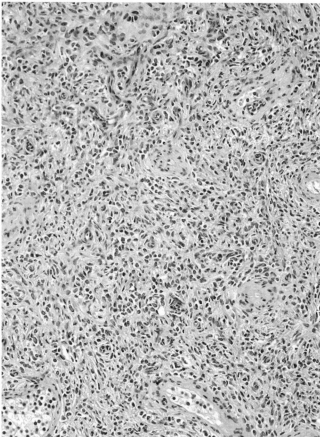

**Fig. 13-141** Unclassified sex cord stromal tumor has clusters of sex cord cells admixed with spindle cells.

features are present, consideration should be given to retroperitoneal lymph node dissection.

## Ovarian-type epithelial tumors

Tumors that resemble the surface epithelial tumors of the ovary may occur in and near the testis. More commonly they occur in the paratestis, involving the surface of the testis or structures such as the epididymis, and these are discussed in Chapter 14. Occasionally, however, they are found within the parenchyma and therefore merit a few comments here.

Borderline tumors of serous[755-757] or mucinous[758] types may occur in the testis, as may mucinous cystadenoma,[759,760] benign or malignant Brenner tumors,[761-763] serous carcinoma,[764] and endometrioid adenocarcinoma.[756] They occur over a wide age range and typically present as palpable masses. These are usually cystic lesions, in keeping with their frequently borderline nature. The histologic appearances are similar to those seen in the much more common ovarian examples. In the mucinous tumors, several of the cases we have seen were associated with extravasation of mucin into the parenchyma, with consequent fibrosis and dystrophic calcifications (Fig. 13-144). Some of the cases had marked cytological atypia in the absence of stromal invasion[758] – so-called intraepithelial carcinoma.

The distinctive appearance of the serous borderline tumors readily permits their diagnosis, although this diagnosis in the paratestis is complicated by the differential with papillary mesothelioma.[765-767] Mucinous tumors and Brenner tumors are potentially subject to confusion with teratoma. The absence of other teratomatous elements and of IGCNU assists with this differential, which may be facilitated by an older patient age, although there is overlap in the age range with patients having teratomas.[768] Orchiectomy appears to be curative for tumors lacking stromal invasion.

## Neoplasms and tumor-like lesions of the rete testis

### Adenocarcinoma

Adenocarcinoma of the rete testis is very rare, occurring in patients from 20 to 91 years old.[769-771] Most are over 60 years old.[770] Many present with symptoms of testicular pain and swelling. The initial clinical impression is often epididymitis

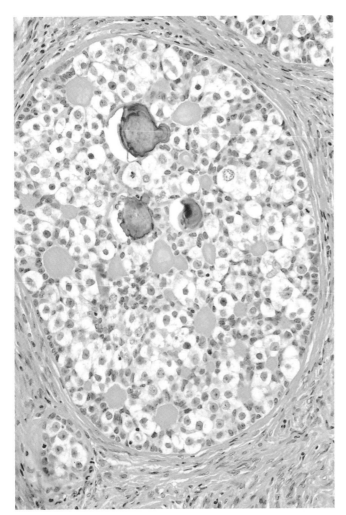

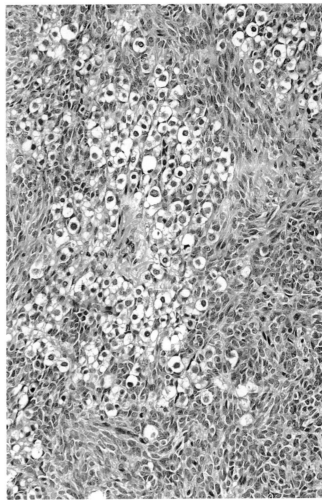

**Fig. 13-142** Gonadoblastoma composed of a nested arrangement of seminoma-like cells with clear cytoplasm and small, dark sex cord cells. The sex cord cells form palisades at the periphery of the nest and around eosinophilic matrix that is focally calcified.

**Fig. 13-143** Unclassified sex cord–stromal tumor with entrapped germ cells. Clusters of germ cells resembling spermatogonia are present amidst the tumor cells.

or hydrocele, and hydrocele is found associated with the tumor in 25% of cases.[769] Because of the posterior location of the tumor, a mass may be difficult to palpate. Some patients present with metastatic scrotal or perineal nodules. Grossly, there is a white to tan, yellow or brown ill-defined mass near the testicular hilum, often with extension into paratesticular structures. Some degree of cystic change may be present, but is usually not prominent. Microscopically the tumor displays solid, papillary, and glandular patterns. The tumor often has an intraluminal component, which distends the spaces of the rete, as well as a component that infiltrates the supporting stroma of the rete (Fig. 13-145). Ideally, a transition from benign to malignant epithelium is seen in the lining of the rete (Fig. 13-145).[769] The solid pattern is often punctuated by slit-like lumina, and a spindle cell pattern rarely occurs.[772] The papillae may have hyalinized fibrous cores and project into cysts. The tumor cells typically have round to oval nuclei, sometimes with grooves, and scant cytoplasm. Immunohistochemical studies typically yield positive reactions for cytokeratins and EMA and less

consistent reactivity for CEA. Lymphatic metastases occur most commonly and initially involve retroperitoneal lymph nodes; sometimes there is involvement of the skin of the scrotum or perineum.[773] The prognosis is poor, with only 36% of patients being tumor-free on follow-up.[769] The differential diagnosis includes carcinomas and low malignant potential tumors of ovarian epithelial type (see Chapter 14); these occur more commonly in the paratesticular area, probably from metaplasia of the mesothelium, but also rarely occur within the testis, perhaps from mesothelial inclusions. It is likely that some cases of papillary serous tumor of low malignant potential have been reported as adenocarcinoma of the rete testis,[769] thus leading to an overly optimistic prognosis for rete testis carcinoma. Psammoma bodies, squamous metaplasia, or mucinous cell type should raise the question of müllerian-type neoplasms. The differential is probably not of great importance except when it involves the distinction of a low malignant potential tumor from an invasive carcinoma. Mesothelioma, which in some cases is associated with a history of asbestos exposure,[774] should also

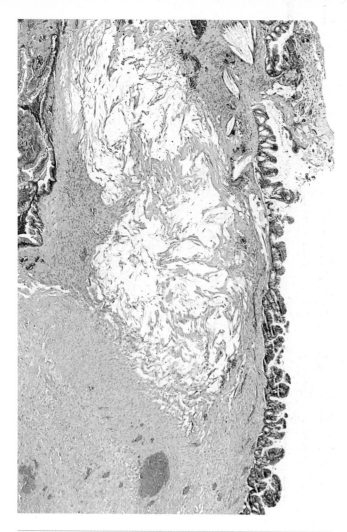

**Fig. 13-144** Borderline mucinous tumor with extravasated mucin. Note the characteristic filigree pattern of the lining epithelium.

be considered, and immunohistochemical studies to distinguish between adenocarcinoma and mesothelioma may help in difficult cases. Malignant mesothelioma of the tunica vaginalis consistently expresses calretinin and EMA, and thrombomodulin, cytokeratin 7, and cytokeratin 5/6 reactivity is also seen in most cases.[767] Prostatic carcinoma may involve the rete testis, but the clinical history and immunostains for prostate-specific antigen should allow identification.

## Adenoma

Adenoma of the rete testis is rare, consisting of papillary or glandular proliferations of cytologically bland cells.[775–777] Four adenomas were reported in patients from 21 to 79 years of age.[770] They ranged from 1.5 to 3.6 cm in diameter and were composed of cysts lined by bland, sometimes stratified or tufted epithelium, with prominent intervening fibrous stroma.

Four cases of 'Sertoliform cystadenoma' were reported in patients from 34 to 62 years old.[770] These cystic and solid lesions were centered in the testicular hilum and had an appearance similar to that of Sertoli cell tumor, though much of the proliferation occurred within the dilated channels of the rete testis (Fig. 13-146). One tumor was shown to be inhibin positive.

Cystadenomas,[770] adenofibromas,[778] and a complex multilocular cystic lesion of the rete testis with smooth muscle hyperplasia[779] are also reported.

## Adenomatous hyperplasia (see also Chapter 12)

Hartwick and co-workers[780] described nine cases of adenomatous hyperplasia of the rete testis in patients ranging from 30 to 74 years of age; in three cases the hyperplasia produced grossly evident, solid and cystic masses in the testicular hilum. Nistal et al.[781] reported 20 cases in patients ranging in age from 2 months to 74 years, 11 of which were associated with cryptorchidism and four with a germ cell tumor. Microscopically, these lesions are tubulopapillary proliferations of bland cells within distended rete testis. (This lesion is illustrated in Chapter 12). Whether these cases are distinct from adenoma is unclear: they do not appear to be similar to the hyperplastic reaction of the rete testis typically seen in cases of germ cell tumor (see page 796, Fig. 13-71).[521]

## Cystic dysplasia

Scattered case reports describe cystic dysplasia of the rete testis associated with absence or dysplasia of the ipsilateral kidney.[782,783] These lesions present mostly in children and young adults. There is often prominent dilatation of the rete, with compression of residual testicular parenchyma (see Chapter 12).

# Neoplasms of lymphoid and hematopoietic cells

## Lymphoma

Lymphoma in the testis usually represents secondary spread from lymph nodes,[371,373] although there are occasional cases that meet the criteria for primary testicular lymphoma.[371,376,784] These include principal involvement of the testis and absence of nodal involvement after careful staging.[371] However, these restrictions may be inadequate for recognizing lymphoma originating in the testis. The tendency for apparently primary testicular lymphoma to progress rapidly after excision, with high rates of recurrence, supports the belief that many originated elsewhere but spread to the testis and became clinically evident.[371,373,374,785,786] Consistent clonal rearrangements of the immunoglobulin light chain genes in synchronous, bilateral testicular lymphoma probably indicate occult dissemination of lymphoma with seeding of the testes,[787] and argue against primary bilateral testicular lymphoma. The poor survival of patients with bilateral lymphoma provides additional support for this view.[784] In many studies of testicular lymphoma it is not clear whether the tumor is primary extranodal lymphoma or lymphoma that originated elsewhere and subsequently spread to the testis, making interpretation of this literature difficult.

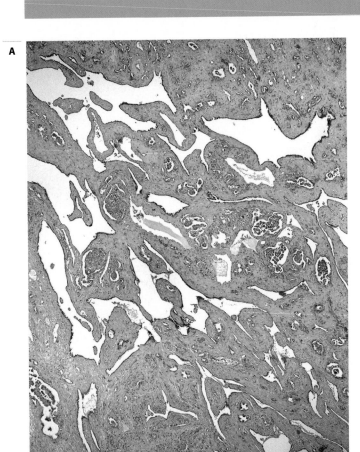

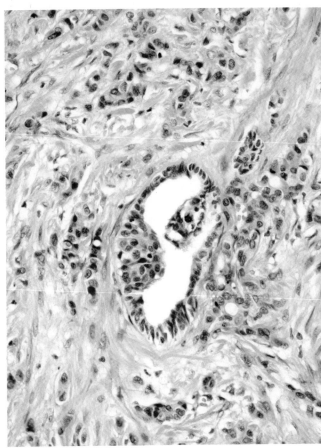

**Fig. 13-145** (**A**) Rete testis carcinoma grows as plugs of tumor in dilated channels of the rete and invades the stroma. (**B**) There is possible in-situ change in the rete epithelium, with adjacent invasive tumor.

## Clinical features

Patients with testicular lymphoma are usually older than those with germ cell tumors, with a mean age of about 60 years;[368–373,784] 50% of testicular neoplasms occurring in patients over 60 are lymphoma.[587] Although most patients present secondary to a testicular mass, systemic symptoms such as fever, sweats, and weight loss also occur.[371] Bilateral testicular involvement occurs in about 20% of cases[369,371–373,788] and is usually metachronous, but may also be synchronous.

## Pathologic features

Grossly, testicular lymphoma forms a fleshy, white-gray to pink mass which often diffusely replaces the testicular parenchyma (Fig. 13-147). Foci of necrosis may be conspicuous. It may be difficult to distinguish grossly from seminoma, although extension into the paratesticular structures suggests lymphoma rather than seminoma.[376,784] Microscopically, lymphoma often has an interstitial pattern, with neoplastic cells surrounding but not replacing seminiferous tubules deep within the tumor (Fig. 13-148). Transtubular migration of the neoplastic cells may occur, and there may rarely be conspicuous intratubular involvement[789] (Fig. 13-149). Despite interstitial growth, the

seminiferous tubules may eventually be destroyed and replaced by tumor, so the absence of an interstitial pattern does not exclude lymphoma. Most testicular lymphomas in adults are diffuse large cell type[312,368,370–372,784,786,790,791] with B-cell immunophenotype.[312,368,784,790,791] They are furthermore mostly of the non-germinal cell type of B-cell lymphoma,[792] a type associated with a more aggressive course. They are generally not associated with Epstein–Barr virus or human herpes virus 8.[790] Many express bcl-2 protein in the absence of a 14:18 chromosomal translocation.[793] In children, Burkitt's lymphoma is the most common lymphoma in the testis[788] and shows the characteristic features, including small, mitotically active cells with round nuclei having several small nucleoli intermixed with macrophages containing phagocytosed nuclear debris. Infrequent cases of pediatric testicular follicular lymphoma have been reported.[794,795] Rare cases of Burkitt's lymphoma of the testis have occurred in adults,[796] and Hodgkin's disease involving the testis is rare.[784,788,797] Several additional types have been described in the testis: anaplastic large cell lymphoma[789,798,799] (sometimes showing conspicuous intratubular involvement), nasal-type T/natural killer cell lymphoma,[800–802] follicular lymphoma,[795,803] low-grade T-helper cell lymphoma,[804] and histiocytic sarcoma.[805] A discussion of the features of these lymphomas is beyond the scope of this chapter.

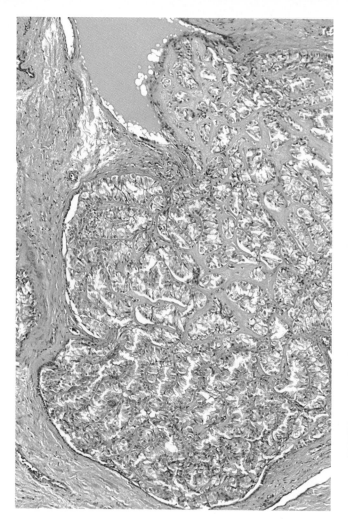

**Fig. 13-146** Sertoliform cystadenoma of the rete testis. A tubular proliferation of Sertoli-like cells is present in dilated channels of the rete testis.

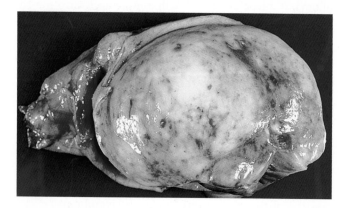

**Fig. 13-147** Lymphoma in the testis. Note fleshy, pink to cream-colored tumor.

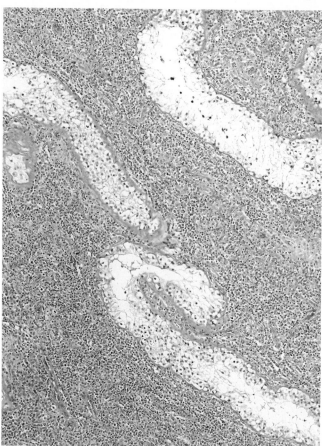

**Fig. 13-148** Typical interstitial pattern of lymphoma, with preservation of several seminiferous tubules.

## Prognosis

The stage of testicular lymphoma is the most important prognostic factor. In patients with stage I disease there is a 60% 5-year tumor-free survival, whereas those with more advanced stage disease have only a 17% 5-year tumor-free survival.[784] Histologic classification is also prognostically useful:[372] in a multivariate analysis, lymphoma with sclerosis had a significantly better outcome, and, for unclear reasons, so did right-sided testicular lymphoma.[784]

## Differential diagnosis

A major differential diagnostic consideration in testicular lymphoma is seminoma, which is addressed on page 775. Anaplastic large cell lymphoma with intratubular growth may be confused with embryonal carcinoma. Both are CD30 reactive and may show prominent comedo-type necrosis of the intratubular component, but the strong cytokeratin and OCT3/4 reactivity of embryonal carcinoma serves to assist in the distinction, as does the absence of IGCNU in lymphoma. Chronic orchitis may also be confused with lymphoma but contains a heterogeneous cell population, consisting of lymphocytes, plasma cells, and neutrophils without atypia. Reactive lymphoid hyperplasia within the testis is a rare condition and has been described as testicular

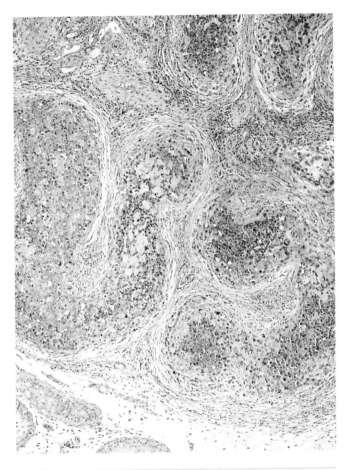

**Fig. 13-149** Unusual growth pattern of large cell lymphoma within seminiferous tubules. Note comedo-like tumor necrosis.

'pseudolymphoma;'[806] its distinction from lymphoma is based on the same criteria used at other sites.

## Plasmacytoma

Plasmacytoma of the testis is rare and usually occurs in older patients with an established or concurrent diagnosis of multiple myeloma.[807-811] Some of these patients may have bilateral involvement, either synchronous or asynchronous.[810,811] Even more rarely, however, testicular plasmacytoma may be an apparently isolated finding, and in such cases the patient must be carefully investigated and followed for multiple myeloma,[809,810,812] although some have not progressed.[812] Autopsy studies of patients with multiple myeloma demonstrate about a 2% frequency of testicular involvement, but the majority of such involvement remains clinically inapparent.[587] Grossly, plasmacytoma often appears as a soft, fleshy, gray-white and hemorrhagic intratesticular mass. Microscopically, sheets of variably differentiated neoplastic plasma cells are identified. Unlike with chronic orchitis, a polymorphic cell population is absent. In poorly differentiated examples misinterpretation as seminoma, lymphoma or metastatic melanoma is possible.[810] Immunostains for light chain restriction, CD138, CD79a, and with monoclonal antibody VS38 are often helpful in identifying plasmacytoma.

## Leukemia, including granulocytic sarcoma

Leukemic infiltrates occur commonly in the testis, with frequency rates at autopsy between 40% and 65% of patients with acute leukemia and 20–35% of patients with chronic leukemia.[797,813] Acute lymphoblastic leukemia is especially prone to testicular involvement, and the testis may be a 'sanctuary' site for leukemic cells, such that testicular biopsy may detect leukemic infiltrates during periods of otherwise complete remission. The detection of leukemia in the testis in such cases occurs in 5–10% of patients and is predictive of subsequent systemic relapse.[814-816] The probability of a second remission from non-B-cell childhood leukemia is higher for patients with isolated testicular relapse than for those with relapse at other sites.[817] The leukemic testis is usually not enlarged, and the diagnosis is established by biopsy of patients at risk. Occasionally, diffuse testicular enlargement or induration or a testicular mass may be observed.[816] Bilateral involvement is common. Exceptionally, leukemia may initially present as testicular enlargement.[587,818] Microscopically, leukemia usually shows an interstitial pattern of infiltration, similar to lymphoma. The neoplastic cells are characteristic of the particular type of leukemia. It may not be possible morphologically to distinguish between some types of lymphoma and leukemia, and clinical information regarding peripheral blood involvement and bone marrow studies are required. The distinction between neoplastic monocytic and myelocytic infiltrates and lymphoid neoplasia may require histochemical and immunohistochemical studies.

Rarely, granulocytic sarcoma occurs in the absence of leukemia;[819] typically, subsequent leukemia is found,[820,821] although one patient who was treated for lymphoma because of pathologic misinterpretation survived for 12 years without evidence of leukemia.[822] Granulocytic sarcoma, because of its frequent paratesticular involvement[821,822] and overlapping morphology, is prone to misinterpretation as lymphoma or plasmacytoma.[822] If eosinophilic myelocytes are present, the correct diagnosis is greatly facilitated. CD45 may be positive and therefore may not discriminate between granulocytic sarcoma and lymphoma.[822] More helpful are stains directed against myeloperoxidase and lysozyme, as well as chloroacetate esterase stains.[822]

# Miscellaneous lesions

## Soft tissue tumors

A variety of soft tissue tumors of the testis arise from interstitial stromal cells, endothelium, and probably peritubular myoid cells.[737,738] It may be difficult to separate some of these from unclassified sex cord–stromal tumor, but that distinction should be based on the absence of recognizable sex cord or epithelial differentiation, and possibly lack of inhibin reactivity. Thus, neurofibroma,[823] hemangioma[824-828] (including epithelioid hemangioma[829,830]), leiomyoma,[831-833] hemangioendothelioma,[834,835] osteosarcoma,[836,837] chondrosarcoma,[838] leiomyosarcoma,[839-841] fibrosarcoma,[837,842] rhabdomyosarcoma,[843-845] and unclassified sarcoma[840] of the testis have been reported. Some of these may represent overgrowth of teratomatous elements of a germ cell tumor; we have seen several cases of pure testicular embryonal rhabdomyosarcoma associated with IGCNU, and one other case has been reported in the literature,[846] suggesting that some testicular sarcomas are teratomatous in origin. As patients who have testicular sarcoma developing from germ cell tumor may have conventional germ cell tumor elements at metastatic sites (which would be amenable to chemotherapy), the distinction of primary sarcoma versus sarcoma of germ cell tumor origin is important. The occurrence of testicular sarcoma in younger adults is a suspicious finding for sarcoma in the context of germ cell tumor. Additionally, some sarcomas may occur as a 'dedifferentiation' phenomenon in Leydig cell tumors[648] and spermatocytic seminomas.[399,400]

## Metastatic tumors

Metastases to the testis are most commonly identified in patients with known malignancies, and the most common sites of origin (excluding leukemia and lymphoma) are the prostate,[847-849] stomach, lung,[850,851] skin (melanoma),[848,852] colon/rectum, kidney,[852-854] and elsewhere.[850,855-859] It is likely that the predominance of the prostate in this ranking represents a selection bias resulting from routine examination of orchiectomy specimens from patients with metastatic prostatic carcinoma.[860] In children there is a predominance of neuroblastoma and rhabdomyosarcoma.[850,861-864] Rarely metastases to the testis may present as apparent primary testicular tumors, including those originating in the prostate, lung, kidney, gastrointestinal tract (stomach and colon), skin (melanoma), pancreas, and liver, as well as carcinoid tumor.[587,852,855,858,865] Although bilateral involvement may be seen in some cases, often the tumors are unilateral and solitary,[850,852,858] complicating the distinction from primary tumors. A proclivity to involve the right testis has been identified in several studies.[850,852,858] Metastatic carcinoma or melanoma may be misinterpreted as embryonal carcinoma, Leydig cell tumor, or Sertoli cell tumor,[852,855,858] or metastatic carcinoid may be misinterpreted as primary testicular carcinoid.[569] We have seen several metastatic prostate carcinomas that had a prominent intratubular component (Fig. 13-150), potentially causing confusion with primary testicular neoplasms. The nested and tubular pattern of metastatic renal cell carcinoma of clear cell type is prone to misinterpretation as Sertoli cell tumor.[858] Some metastatic melanomas may show prominent foamy tumor cells, overlapping with an appearance that may be seen in Leydig cell tumor.[852] Additionally, melanomas may have relatively scant cytoplasm and display prominent intertubular growth, features that are readily confused with lymphoma (Fig. 13-151). The presence of an extensive interstitial pattern, prominent microvascular involvement, multifocality, and bilaterality are features that favor metastasis rather than primary testicular tumor (Fig. 13-150),[855,860] but they are not always present. The clinical history may also be of value, as patients with metastatic lesions to the testis are older (average age 57 years) than patients with a germ cell tumor such as embryonal carcinoma, (average age 30 years). However, patients with meta-

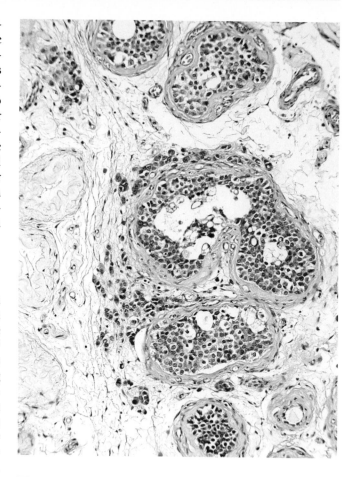

**Fig. 13-150** Metastatic prostate carcinoma to the testis with a prominent intratubular component.

static stomach and small intestinal cancer may fall within the usual age range of those with testicular germ cell tumor.[866] Serum AFP and hCG levels are much more likely to be elevated in patients with germ cell tumor. The absence of IGCNU in the surrounding seminiferous tubules increases the probability of a metastatic tumor over germ cell tumor, as do EMA positivity and PLAP and OCT3/4 negativity.[333] Other immunohistochemical studies may prove useful, including prostate-specific antigen, renal cell carcinoma and melanoma markers and inhibin stains.

## Diagnostic approach to testicular tumors

From the above it is apparent that several recurring morphologic patterns are observed in testicular tumors. The differential diagnostic considerations for tumors with certain patterns may include tumors of germ cell origin, tumors of sex cord–stromal origin, and secondary tumors. In most cases, careful attention to the morphologic features, along with the clinical history, will allow the correct diagnosis to be established. In some of these cases immunohistochemical staining provides crucial supportive evidence.

Some of the common patterns include solid tumors composed of cells with pale cytoplasm; tumors with a glandular

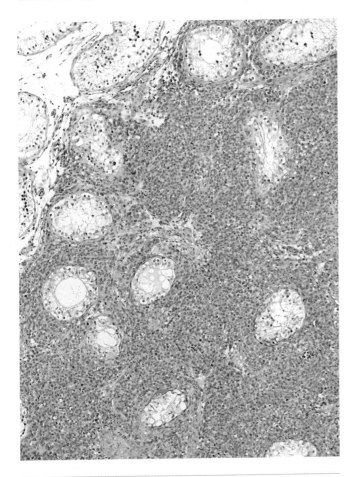

**Fig. 13-151** Metastatic melanoma. The tumor cells show prominent interstitial growth, mimicking the low-power appearance of lymphoma.

and/or tubular pattern; tumors with a microcystic pattern; oxyphilic tumors with a predominantly solid pattern; and tumors with spindle cell morphology.

Solid tumors composed of cells with pale cytoplasm include seminoma of usual type, spermatocytic seminoma, solid pattern embryonal carcinoma, solid pattern yolk sac tumor, metastatic adenocarcinoma, and lymphoma. A number of light-microscopic features and immunohistochemical reactions assist the separation of these entities (Fig. 13-152). These may be distinguished based on the presence of associated IGCNU, the presence of focal glandular architecture, the presence of a predominantly interstitial growth pattern, and the immunohistochemical staining pattern for OCT3/4, PLAP, CD30, AFP, LCA, and inhibin (Fig. 13-152).

Tumors with a glandular and/or tubular pattern include embryonal carcinoma, yolk sac tumor, tubular pattern seminoma, rete testis neoplasms, metastatic adenocarcinoma, and Sertoli cell tumor (Fig. 13-153). These may be distinguished based on the presence of associated IGCNU, nuclear features and the presence of elongated glandular spaces, the presence of hyaline globules and other patterns of yolk sac tumor, the presence of intertubular growth pattern or solid tubules, and OCT3/4, PLAP, CD30, AFP, keratin, and inhibin staining patterns (Fig. 13-153).

Tumors that may have a microcystic pattern include yolk sac tumor, seminoma, Sertoli cell tumor, Leydig cell tumor, and adenomatoid tumor (Fig. 13-154). Features helpful in distinguishing these tumors include the presence of IGCNU, nuclear features such as nuclear size variability and flattened cellular profiles within the cysts, the presence of cords of tumor cells and lipid-rich cells, and staining for keratin,

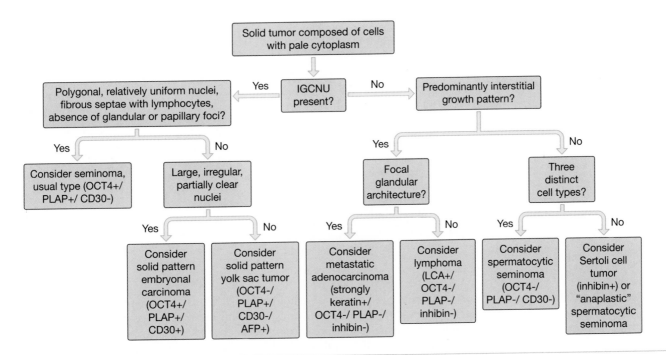

**Fig. 13-152** A general approach for the diagnosis of tumors with a diffuse arrangement of pale to clear cells. (Reproduced with permission from Emerson RE, Ulbright TM. Morphological approach to tumours of the testis and paratestis. J Clin Pathol 2007; 60: 866–880.)

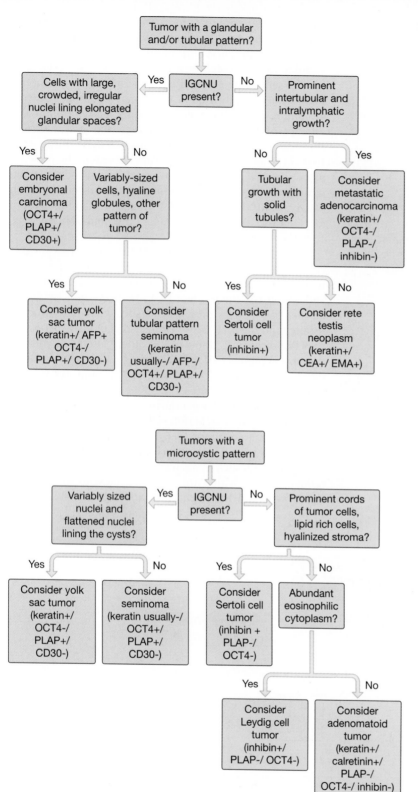

**Fig. 13-153** A general approach for the diagnosis of tumors with a glandular/tubular arrangement. (Reproduced with permission from Emerson RE, Ulbright TM. Morphological approach to tumors of the testis and paratestis. J Clin Pathol 2007; 60: 866–880.)

**Fig. 13-154** A general approach for the diagnosis of tumors with a microcystic pattern. (Reproduced with permission from Emerson RE, Ulbright TM. Morphological approach to tumors of the testis and paratestis. J Clin Pathol 2007; 60: 866–880.)

OCT3/4, PLAP, CD20, inhibin, and calretinin (Fig. 13-154).

Oxyphilic tumors with a predominantly solid pattern include Leydig cell tumor, large cell calcifying Sertoli cell tumor, hepatoid pattern yolk sac tumor, carcinoid tumor, metastatic adenocarcinoma, melanoma, plasmacytoma, and

adenomatoid tumor (Fig. 13-155). Cytoplasmic lipofuscin or Reinke crystals, the presence of associated fibromyxoid stroma, the presence of IGCNU, the presence of insular and trabecular patterns or teratomatous elements, the presence of overtly malignant nuclear features and intratubular growth, and staining patterns with keratin, inhibin,

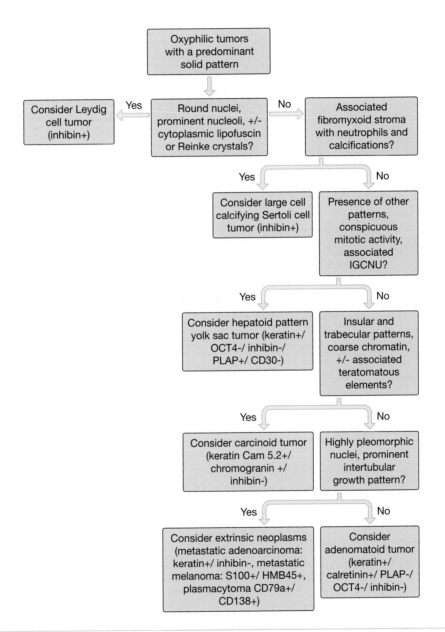

**Fig. 13-155** A general approach for the diagnosis of tumors composed mostly of oxyphilic cells. (Reproduced with permission from Emerson RE, Ulbright TM. Morphological approach to tumours of the testis and paratestis. J Clin Pathol 2007; 60: 866–880.)

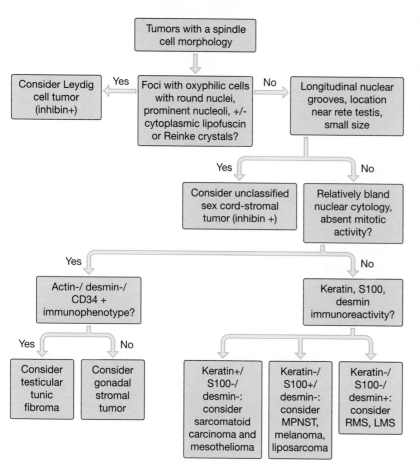

**Fig. 13-156** A general approach for the diagnosis of tumors composed mostly of spindle cells. LMS, leiomyosarcoma; MPNST, malignant peripheral nerve sheath tumor; RMS, rhabdomyosarcoma. (Reproduced with permission from Emerson RE, Ulbright TM. Morphological approach to tumours of the testis and paratestis. J Clin Pathol 2007; 60: 866–880.)

OCT3/4, PLAP, calretinin, and markers specific for extrinsic neoplasms can be useful in differentiating these tumors (Fig. 13-155).

Tumors with a largely or entirely spindle cell pattern include Leydig cell tumor, unclassified sex cord–stromal tumor, sarcomatoid carcinoma, mesothelioma, some benign lesions such as testicular tunic fibroma, and a variety of sarcomas (Fig. 13-156). These may be distinguished by the presence of foci of recognizable oxyphilic Leydig cells, nuclear cytology and mitotic activity, and immunohistochemical staining pattern for actin, desmin, CD34, keratin, and S100 protein (Fig. 13-156).

## REFERENCES

1. Giwercman A, Müller J, Skakkebaek NE. Prevalence of carcinoma in situ and other histopathological abnormalities in testes from 399 men who died suddenly and unexpectedly. J Urol 1991; 145: 77–80.
2. Buchino JJ, Uhlenhuth ER. Large-cell calcifying Sertoli cell tumor. J Urol 1989; 141: 953–954.
3. Proppe KH, Scully RE. Large-cell calcifying Sertoli cell tumor of the testis. Am J Clin Pathol 1980; 74: 607–619.
4. Wilson DM, Pitts WC, Hintz RL, et al. Testicular tumors with Peutz–Jeghers syndrome. Cancer 1986; 57: 2238–2240.
5. Kratzer SS, Ulbright TM, Talerman A, et al. Large cell calcifying Sertoli cell tumor of the testis. contrasting features of six malignant and six benign tumors and a review of the literature. Am J Surg Pathol 1997; 21: 1271–1280.
6. Venara M, Rey R, Bergada I, et al. Sertoli cell proliferations of the infantile testis. an intratubular form of Sertoli cell tumor? Am J Surg Pathol 2001; 25: 1237–1244.
7. Ulbright TM, Amin MB, Young RH. Intratubular large cell hyalinizing Sertoli cell neoplasia of the testis: a report of 8 cases of a distinctive lesion of the Peutz–Jeghers syndrome. Am J Surg Pathol 2007; 31: 827–835.
8. American Joint Committee on Cancer. Testis. In: Greene FL, Page DL, Fleming ID, et al., eds. AJCC cancer staging handbook. New York: Springer-Verlag, 2002; 347–354.
9. Morse MJ, Whitmore WF. Neoplasms of the testis. In: Walsh PC, Gittes RF, Perlmutter AD, et al., eds. Campbell's urology. Philadelphia: WB Saunders, 1986; 1535–1582.
10. Donohue JP. Metastatic pathways of nonseminomatous germ cell tumors. Semin Urol 1984; 2: 217–229.
11. Richie JP. Diagnosis and staging of testicular tumors. In: Skinner DG, Lieskovsky G, eds. Diagnosis and management of genitourinary cancer. Philadelphia: WB Saunders, 1988; 498–507.
12. Bredael JJ, Vugrin D, Whitmore WF, Jr. Autopsy findings in 154 patients with germ cell tumors of the testis. Cancer 1982; 50: 548–551.
13. Nazeer T, Ro JY, Kee KH, et al. Spermatic cord contamination in testicular cancer. Mod Pathol 1996; 9: 762–766.
14. Dry SM, Renshaw AA. Extratesticular extension of germ cell tumors preferentially occurs at the hilum. Am J Clin Pathol 1999; 111: 534–538.
15. Mostofi FK, Sesterhenn IA. Histological typing of testis tumours. Berlin: Springer-Verlag, 1998.

16. Pugh RCB. Testicular tumours – introduction. In: Pugh RCB, ed. Pathology of the testis. Oxford: Blackwell Scientific, 1976; 139–159.

17. Skakkebaek NE. Possible carcinoma-in-situ of the undescended testis. Lancet 1972; 2: 516–517.

18. Rorth M, Rajpert-De Meyts E, Andersson L, et al. Carcinoma in situ in the testis. Scand J Urol Nephrol 2000; 205: 166–186.

19. Scully RE. Intratubular germ cell neoplasia (carcinoma in situ): what it is and what should be done about it. World Urol Update Ser Lesson 1982; 17: 1–66.

20. Young RH, Scully RE. Testicular tumors. Chicago: ASCP Press, 1990.

21. Gondos B, Migliozzi JA. Intratubular germ cell neoplasia. Semin Diagn Pathol 1987; 4: 292–303.

22. Schulze C, Holstein AF. On the histology of human seminoma. development of the solid tumor from intratubular seminoma cells. Cancer 1977; 39: 1090–1100.

23. Giwercman A, Marks A, Bailey D, et al. M2A – a monoclonal antibody as a marker for carcinoma-in-situ germ cells of the human adult testis. Acta Pathol Microbiol Immunol Scand [A] 1988; 96: 667–670.

24. Giwercman A, Andrews PW, Jorgensen N, et al. Immunohistochemical expression of embryonal marker TRA-1–60 in carcinoma in situ and germ cell tumors of the testis. Cancer 1993; 72: 1308–1314.

25. Jacobsen GK, Norgaard-Pedersen B. Placental alkaline phosphatase in testicular germ cell tumours and carcinoma-in-situ of the testis: an immunohistochemical study. Acta Pathol Microbiol Immunol Scand [A] 1984; 92: 323–329.

26. Koide O, Iwai S, Baba K, et al. Identification of testicular atypical germ cells by an immunohistochemical technique for placental alkaline phosphatase. Cancer 1987; 60: 1325–1330.

27. Niehans GA, Manivel JC, Copland GT, et al. Immunohistochemistry of germ cell and trophoblastic neoplasms. Cancer 1988; 62: 1113–1123.

28. Klys HS, Whillis D, Howard G, et al. Glutathione S-transferase expression in the human testis and testicular germ cell neoplasia. Br J Cancer 1992; 66: 589–593.

29. Jones TD, Ulbright TM, Eble JN, et al. OCT4: A sensitive and specific biomarker for intratubular germ cell neoplasia of the testis. Clin Cancer Res 2004; 10: 8544–8547.

30. Willmore-Payne C, Holden JA, Chadwick BE, et al. Detection of c-kit exons 11- and 17-activating mutations in testicular seminomas by high-resolution melting amplicon analysis. Mod Pathol 2006; 19: 1164–1169.

31. Hoei-Hansen CE, Almstrup K, Nielsen JE, et al. Stem cell pluripotency factor NANOG is expressed in human fetal gonocytes, testicular carcinoma in situ and germ cell tumours. Histopathology 2005; 47: 48–56.

32. El-Naggar AK, Ro JY, McLemore D, et al. DNA ploidy in testicular germ cell neoplasms. histogenetic and clinical implications. Am J Surg Pathol 1992; 16: 611–618.

33. Delahunt B, Mostofi FK, Sesterhenn IA, et al. Nucleolar organizer regions in seminoma and intratubular malignant germ cells. Mod Pathol 1990; 3: 141–145.

34. Malmi R, Söderström KO. Lectin histochemistry of embryonal carcinoma. APMIS 1991; 99: 233–243.

35. Johnson DE, Appelt G, Samuels ML, et al. Metastases from testicular carcinoma. Study of 78 autopsied cases. Urology 1976; 8: 234–239.

36. Friedman NB, Moore RA. Tumors of the testis. a report on 922 cases. Military Surg 1946; 99: 573–593.

37. Czaja JT, Ulbright TM. Evidence for the transformation of seminoma to yolk sac tumor, with histogenetic considerations. Am J Clin Pathol 1992; 97: 468–477.

38. Mostofi FK, Sesterhenn IA. Pathology of germ cell tumors of testes. Prog Clin Biol Res 1985; 203: 1–34.

39. von Hochstetter AR, Sigg C, Saremaslani P, et al. The significance of giant cells in human testicular seminomas. A clinicopathological study. Virchows Arch [A] 1985; 407: 309–322.

40. Jacobsen GK, Jacobsen M. α-Fetoprotein (AFP) and human chorionic gonadotropin in testicular germ cell tumours. a prospective immunohistochemical study. Acta Pathol Microbiol Scand [A] 1983; 91: 165–176.

41. Srigley JR, Mackay B, Toth P, et al. The ultrastructure and histogenesis of male germ cell neoplasia with emphasis on seminoma with early carcinomatous features. Ultrastruct Pathol 1988; 12: 67–86.

42. de Jong B, Oosterhuis JW, Castedo SM, et al. Pathogenesis of adult testicular germ cell tumors. A cytogenetic model. Cancer Genet Cytogenet 1990; 48: 143–167.

43. Oosterhuis JW, Castedo SM, de Jong B, et al. Ploidy of primary germ cell tumors of the testis. Pathogenetic and clinical relevance. Lab Invest 1989; 60: 14–21.

44. Faulkner SW, Leigh DA, Oosterhuis JW, et al. Allelic losses in carcinoma in situ and testicular germ cell tumours of adolescents and adults: evidence suggestive of the linear progression model. Br J Cancer 2000; 83: 729–736.

45. Rajpert-De Meyts E, Bartkova J, Samson M, et al. The emerging phenotype of the testicular carcinoma in situ germ cell. APMIS 2003; 111: 267–278.

46. Rosenberg C, van Gurp RJ, Geelen E, et al. Overrepresentation of the short arm of chromosome 12 is related to invasive growth of human testicular seminomas and nonseminomas. Oncogene 2000; 19: 5858–5862.

47. Roelofs H, Mostert MC, Pompe K, et al. Restricted 12p amplification and RAS mutation in human germ cell tumors of the adult testis. Am J Pathol 2000; 157: 1155–1166.

48. Summersgill B, Osin P, Lu YJ, et al. Chromosomal imbalances associated with carcinoma in situ and associated testicular germ cell tumours of adolescents and adults. Br J Cancer 2001; 85: 213–220.

49. Datta MW, Macri E, Signoretti S, et al. Transition from in situ to invasive testicular germ cell neoplasia is associated with the loss of p21 and gain of mdm-2 expression. Mod Pathol 2001; 14: 437–442.

50. Bartkova J, Thullberg M, Rajpert-De Meyts E, et al. Cell cycle regulators in testicular cancer. loss of p18INK4C marks progression from carcinoma in situ to invasive germ cell tumours. Int J Cancer 2000; 85: 370–375.

51. Oosterhuis JW, Gillis AJ, van Putten WJ, et al. Interphase cytogenetics of carcinoma in situ of the testis. Numeric analysis of the chromosomes 1, 12 and 15. Eur Urol 1993; 23: 16–21.

52. Berney DM, Lee A, Randle SJ, et al. The frequency of intratubular embryonal carcinoma: implications for the pathogenesis of germ cell tumours. Histopathology 2004; 45: 155–161.

53. Visfeldt J, Jorgensen N, Muller J, et al. Testicular germ cell tumours of childhood in Denmark, 1943–1989: incidence and evaluation of histology using immunohistochemical techniques. J Pathol 1994; 174: 39–47.

54. Hawkins E, Heifetz SA, Giller R, et al. The prepubertal testis (prenatal and postnatal): its relationship to intratubular germ cell neoplasia. a combined Pediatric Oncology Group and Children's Cancer Study Group. Hum Pathol 1997; 28: 404–410.

55. Jorgensen N, Muller J, Giwercman A, et al. DNA content and expression of tumour markers in germ cells adjacent to germ cell tumours in childhood: probably a different origin for infantile and adolescent germ cell tumours. J Pathol 1995; 176: 269–278.

56. Manivel JC, Simonton S, Wold SE, et al. Absence of intratubular germ cell neoplasia in testicular yolk sac tumors in children. Arch Pathol Lab Med 1988; 112: 641–645.

57. Manivel JC, Reinberg Y, Niehans GA, et al. Intratubular germ cell neoplasia in testicular teratomas and epidermoid cysts. Correlation with prognosis and possible biologic significance. Cancer 1989; 64: 715–720.

58. Bussey KJ, Lawce HJ, Olson SB, et al. Chromosome abnormalities of eighty-one pediatric germ cell tumors: sex-, age-, site-, and histopathology-related differences. A Children's Cancer Group

study. Genes Chromosomes Cancer 1999; 25: 134–146.

59. Mostert M, Rosenberg C, Stoop H, et al. Comparative genomic and in situ hybridization of germ cell tumors of the infantile testis. Lab Invest 2000; 80: 1055–1064.

60. Perlman EJ, Hu J, Ho D, et al. Genetic analysis of childhood endodermal sinus tumors by comparative genomic hybridization. J Pediatr Hematol Oncol 2000; 22: 100–105.

61. Oosterhuis JW, Looijenga LH. Testicular germ-cell tumours in a broader perspective. Nature Rev Cancer 2005; 5: 210–222.

62. Forman D, Gallagher R, Moller H, et al. Aetiology and epidemiology of testicular cancer: report of consensus group. Prog Clin Biol Res 1990; 357: 245–253.

63. Pearce N, Sheppard RA, Howard JK, et al. Time trends and occupational differences in cancer of the testis in New Zealand. Cancer 1987; 59: 1677–1682.

64. Swerdlow AJ. The epidemiology of testicular cancer. Eur Urol 1993; 23: 35–38.

65. Muir C, Waterhouse J, Mack T, et al. Cancer incidence in five continents. Vol. V. Lyon, France: International Agency for Research on Cancer, 1987.

66. Schottenfeld D, Warshauer ME, Sherlock S, et al. The epidemiology of testicular cancer in young adults. Am J Epidemiol 1980; 112: 232–246.

67. Thompson IM, Optenberg S, Byers R, et al. Increased incidence of testicular cancer in active duty members of the Department of Defense. Urology 1999; 53: 806–807.

68. Moller H. Clues to the aetiology of testicular germ cell tumours from descriptive epidemiology. Eur Urol 1993; 23: 8–13.

69. Osterlind A. Diverging trends in incidence and mortality of testicular cancer in Denmark, 1943–1982. Br J Cancer 1986; 53: 501–505.

70. Adami HO, Bergstrom R, Mohner M, et al. Testicular cancer in nine northern European countries. Int J Cancer 1994; 59: 33–38.

71. Moller H. Trends in incidence of testicular cancer and prostate cancer in Denmark. Hum Reprod 2001; 16: 1007–1011.

72. Hoff Wanderas E, Tretli S, Fossa SD. Trends in incidence of testicular cancer in Norway 1955–1992. Eur J Cancer 1995; 31A: 2044–2048.

73. Pike MC, Chilvers CE, Bobrow LG. Classification of testicular cancer in incidence and mortality statistics. Br J Cancer 1987; 56: 83–85.

74. Forman D, Moller H. Testicular cancer. Cancer Surv 1994; 19–20: 323–341.

75. Power DA, Brown RS, Brock CS, et al. Trends in testicular carcinoma in England and Wales, 1971–99. BJU Int 2001; 87: 361–365.

76. Boyle P, Kaye SB, Robertson AG. Changes in testicular cancer in Scotland. Eur J Cancer Clin Oncol 1987; 23: 827–830.

77. Stone JM, Cruickshank DG, Sandeman TF, et al. Trebling of the incidence of testicular cancer in Victoria, Australia (1950–1985). Cancer 1991; 68: 211–219.

78. Weir HK, Marrett LD, Moravan V. Trends in the incidence of testicular germ cell cancer in Ontario by histologic subgroup, 1964–1996. CMAJ 1999; 160: 201–205.

79. Agnarsson BA, Gudbjartsson T, Einarsson GV, et al. Testicular germ cell tumours in Iceland: a nationwide clinicopathological study. APMIS 2006; 114: 779–783.

80. Swerdlow AJ, Skeet RG. Occupational associations of testicular cancer in south east England. Br J Indust Med 1988; 45: 225–230.

81. McDowall ME, Balarajan R. Testicular cancer mortality in England and Wales 1971–80: variations by occupation. J Epidemiol Commun Health 1986; 40: 26–29.

82. Ross RK, McCurtis JW, Henderson BE, et al. Descriptive epidemiology of testicular and prostatic cancer in Los Angeles. Br J Cancer 1979; 39: 284–292.

83. Graham S, Gibson R, West D, et al. Epidemiology of cancer of the testis in Upstate New York. J Natl Cancer Inst 1977; 58: 1255–1261.

84. Davies JM. Testicular cancer in England and Wales: some epidemiological aspects. Lancet 1981; 1: 928–932.

85. Akre O, Ekbom A, Hsieh CC, et al. Testicular nonseminoma and seminoma in relation to perinatal characteristics. J Natl Cancer Inst 1996; 88: 883–889.

86. Harding M, Hole D, Gillis C. The epidemiology of non-seminomatous germ cell tumours in the west of Scotland 1975–89. Br J Cancer 1995; 72: 1559–1562.

87. Haughey BP, Graham S, Brasure J, et al. The epidemiology of testicular cancer in upstate New York. Am J Epidemiol 1989; 130: 25–36.

88. Hardell L, Nasman A, Ohlson CG, et al. Case–control study on risk factors for testicular cancer. Int J Oncol 1998; 13: 1299–1303.

89. Marshall EG, Melius JM, London MA, et al. Investigation of a testicular cancer cluster using a case–control approach. Int J Epidemiol 1990; 19: 269–273.

90. Anonymous. Testicular cancer in leather workers – Fulton County, New York. MMWR 1989; 38: 105–106.

91. Fleming LE, Bean JA, Rudolph M, et al. Cancer incidence in a cohort of licensed pesticide applicators in Florida. J Occup Environ Med 1999; 41: 279–288.

92. Rhomberg W, Schmoll HJ, Schneider B. High frequency of metalworkers among patients with seminomatous tumors of the testis: a case–control study. Am J Indust Med 1995; 28: 79–87.

93. Davis RL, Mostofi FK. Cluster of testicular cancer in police officers exposed to hand-held radar. Am J Indust Med 1993; 24: 231–233.

94. Ducatman AM, Conwill DE, Crawl J. Germ cell tumors of the testicle among aircraft repairmen. J Urol 1986; 136: 834–836.

95. Foley S, Middleton S, Stitson D, et al. The incidence of testicular cancer in Royal Air Force personnel. Br J Urol 1995; 76: 495–496.

96. Gallagher RP, Huchcroft S, Phillips N, et al. Physical activity, medical history, and risk of testicular cancer (Alberta and British Columbia, Canada). Cancer Causes Control 1995; 6: 398–406.

97. Swerdlow AJ, Huttly SR, Smith PG. Prenatal and familial associations of testicular cancer. Br J Cancer 1987; 55: 571–577.

98. DePue RH, Pike MC, Henderson BE. Estrogen exposure during gestation and risk of testicular cancer. J Natl Cancer Inst 1983; 71: 1151–1155.

99. Strohsnitter WC, Noller KL, Hoover RN, et al. Cancer risk in men exposed in utero to diethylstilbestrol. J Natl Cancer Inst 2001; 93: 545–551.

100. Ekbom A. Growing evidence that several human cancers may originate in utero. Semin Cancer Biol 1998; 8: 237–244.

101. Crawford RD. The case for iron repletion as a promoter in testicular cancer. Med Hypoth 1998; 51: 129–132.

102. Anonymous. Social, behavioural and medical factors in the aetiology of testicular cancer: results from the UK study. UK Testicular Cancer Study Group. Br J Cancer 1994; 70: 513–520.

103. Majsky A, Abrahamova J, Korinkova P, et al. HLA system and testicular germinative tumours. Oncology 1979; 36: 228–231.

104. Carr BI, Bach FH. Possible association between HLA-Aw24 and metastatic germ-cell tumours. Lancet 1979; 1: 7156–7157.

105. Pollack MS, Vugrin D, Hennessy W, et al. HLA antigens in patients with germ cell cancers of the testis. Cancer Res 1982; 42: 2470–2473.

106. Dieckmann KP, von Keyserlingk HJ. HLA association of testicular seminoma. Klin Wschr 1988; 66: 337–339.

107. Kratzik C, Aiginger P, Kuzmits R, et al. HLA-antigen distribution in seminoma, HCG-positive seminoma and non-seminomatous tumours of the testis. Urol Res 1989; 17: 377–380.

108. Oliver RT. HLA phenotype and clinicopathological behaviour of germ cell tumours: possible evidence for clonal evolution from seminomas to nonseminomas. Int J Androl 1987; 10: 85–93.

109. DeWolf WC, Lange PH, Einarson ME, et al. HLA and testicular cancer. Nature 1979; 277: 216–217.

110. Dieckmann KP, Klan R, Bunte S. HLA antigens, Lewis antigens, and blood

groups in patients with testicular germ-cell tumors. Oncology (Basel) 1993; 50: 252–258.

111. Moss AR, Osmond D, Bacchetti P, et al. Hormonal risk factors in testicular cancer: a case–control study. Am J Epidemiol 1986; 124: 39–52.

112. Weir HK, Kreiger N, Marrett LD. Age at puberty and risk of testicular germ cell cancer (Ontario, Canada). Cancer Causes Control 1998; 9: 253–258.

113. Braun MM, Ahlbom A, Floderus B, et al. Effect of twinship on incidence of cancer of the testis, breast, and other sites (Sweden). Cancer Causes Control 1995; 6: 519–524.

114. Swerdlow AJ, De Stavola BL, Swanwick MA, et al. Risks of breast and testicular cancers in young adult twins in England and Wales: evidence on prenatal and genetic aetiology. Lancet 1997; 350: 1723–1728.

115. Lykkesfeldt G, Bennett P, Lykkesfeldt AE, et al. Testis cancer. Ichthyosis constitutes a significant risk factor. Cancer 1991; 67: 730–734.

116. Dexeus FH, Logothetis CJ, Chong C, et al. Genetic abnormalities in men with germ cell tumors. J Urol 1988; 140: 80–84.

117. Li FP, Fraumeni JF, Jr. Testicular cancers in children: epidemiologic characteristics. J Natl Cancer Inst 1972; 48: 1575–1582.

118. Sigg C, Pelloni F. Dysplastic nevi and germ cell tumors of the testis – a possible further tumor in the spectrum of associated malignancies in dysplastic nevus syndrome. Dermatologica 1988; 176: 109–110.

119. Harries LW, Stubbins MJ, Forman D, et al. Identification of genetic polymorphisms at the glutathione S-transferase Pi locus and association with susceptibility to bladder, testicular and prostate cancer. Carcinogenesis 1997; 18: 641–644.

120. Knight JA, Marrett LD. Parental occupational exposure and the risk of testicular cancer in Ontario. J Occup Environ Med 1997; 39: 333–338.

121. Bergstrom R, Adami HO, Mohner M, et al. Increase in testicular cancer incidence in six European countries: a birth cohort phenomenon. J Natl Cancer Inst 1996; 88: 727–733.

122. Ekbom A, Akre O. Increasing incidence of testicular cancer – birth cohort effects. APMIS 1998; 106: 225–229.

123. Nienhuis H, Goldacre M, Seagroatt V, et al. Incidence of disease after vasectomy: a record linkage retrospective cohort study. Br Med J 1992; 304: 743–746.

124. Hewitt G, Logan CJ, Curry RC. Does vasectomy cause testicular cancer? Br J Urol 1993; 71: 607–608.

125. Moller H, Knudsen LB, Lynge E. Risk of testicular cancer after vasectomy: cohort study of over 73,000 men. Br Med J 1994; 309: 295–299.

126. Rosenberg L, Palmer JR, Zauber AG, et al. The relation of vasectomy to the risk of cancer. Am J Epidemiol 1994; 140: 431–438.

127. Van den Eeden SK, Weiss NS, Strader CH, et al. Occupation and the occurrence of testicular cancer. Am J Indust Med 1991; 19: 327–337.

128. Halme A, Kellokumpu-Lehtinen P, Lehtonen T, et al. Morphology of testicular germ cell tumours in treated and untreated cryptorchidism. Br J Urol 1989; 64: 78–83.

129. Lanson Y. Epidemiology of testicular cancers. Prog Clin Biol Res 1985; 203: 155–159.

130. Javadpour N, Bergman S. Recent advances in testicular cancer. Curr Prob Surg 1978; 15: 1–64.

131. Henderson BE, Benton B, Jing J, et al. Risk factors for cancer of the testis in young men. Int J Cancer 1979; 23: 598–602.

132. Pottern LM, Brown LM, Hoover RN, et al. Testicular cancer risk among young men: role of cryptorchidism and inguinal hernia. J Natl Cancer Inst 1985; 74: 377–381.

133. Pike MC, Chilvers C, Peckham MJ. Effects of age at orchidopexy on risk of testicular cancer. Lancet 1986; 1: 1246–1248.

134. Giwercman A, Grindsted J, Hansen B, et al. Testicular cancer risk in boys with maldescended testis: a cohort study. J Urol 1987; 138: 1214–1216.

135. Giwercman A, Berthelsen JG, Muller J, et al. Screening for carcinoma-in-situ of the testis. Int J Androl 1987; 10: 173–180.

136. Dieckmann KP, Loy V. Prevalence of bilateral testicular germ cell tumors and early detection by testicular intraepithelial neoplasia. Eur Urol 1993; 23: 22–23.

137. Loy V, Dieckmann KP. Prevalence of contralateral testicular intraepithelial neoplasia (carcinoma in situ) in patients with testicular germ cell tumour. Results of the German multicentre study. Eur Urol 1993; 23: 120–122.

138. Dieckmann KP, Skakkebaek NE. Carcinoma in situ of the testis: review of biological and clinical features. Int J Cancer 1999; 83: 815–822.

139. Fuller DB, Plenk HP. Malignant testicular germ cell tumors in a father and two sons. Case report and literature review. Cancer 1986; 58: 955–958.

140. Tollerud DJ, Blattner WA, Fraser MC, et al. Familial testicular cancer and urogenital developmental anomalies. Cancer 1985; 55: 1849–1854.

141. Dieckmann KP, Pichlmeier U. The prevalence of familial testicular cancer. an analysis of two patient populations and a review of the literature. Cancer 1997; 80: 1954–1960.

142. Forman D, Oliver RT, Brett AR, et al. Familial testicular cancer. a report of the UK family register, estimation of risk and an HLA class 1 sib-pair analysis. Br J Cancer 1992; 65: 255–262.

143. Rutgers JL, Scully RE. Pathology of the testis in intersex syndromes. Semin Diagn Pathol 1987; 4: 275–291.

144. Hughesdon PE, Kumarasamy T. Mixed germ cell tumours (gonadoblastomas) in normal and dysgenetic gonads: case reports and review. Virchows Arch [A] 1970; 349: 258–280.

145. Manuel M, Katayama KP, Jones HW. The age of occurrence of gonadal tumors in intersex patients. Am J Obstet Gynecol 1976; 124: 293–306.

146. Morris JM. The syndrome of testicular feminization in male pseudohermaphrodites. Am J Obstet Gynecol 1953; 65: 1192–1211.

147. Rutgers JL. Advances in the pathology of intersex syndromes. Hum Pathol 1991; 22: 884–891.

148. Rutgers JL, Scully RE. The androgen insensitivity syndrome (testicular feminization): a clinicopathologic study of 43 cases. Int J Gynecol Pathol 1991; 10: 126–145.

149. Senturia YD. The epidemiology of testicular cancer. Br J Urol 1987; 60: 285–291.

150. Mostofi FK. Testicular tumors: epidemiologic, etiologic, and pathologic features. Cancer 1973; 32: 1186–1201.

151. Swerdlow AJ, Huttly SRA, Smith PG. Testicular cancer and antecedent disease. Br J Cancer 1987; 55: 97–103.

152. Brendler H. Cryptorchidism and cancer. Prog Clin Biol Res 1985; 203: 189–196.

153. Miller A, Seljelid R. Histopathologic classification and natural history of malignant testis tumors in Norway, 1959–1963. Cancer 1971; 28: 1054–1062.

154. Whitaker RH. Neoplasia in cryptorchid men. Semin Urol 1988; 6: 107–109.

155. Swerdlow AJ, Higgins CD, Pike MC. Risk of testicular cancer in cohort of boys with cryptorchidism. Br Med J 1997; 314: 1507–1511.

156. Gilbert JB, Hamilton JB. Studies in malignant testis tumors. III – incidence and nature of tumors in ectopic testes. Surg Gynecol Obstet 1940; 71: 731–743.

157. Johnson DE, Woodhead DM, Pohl DR, et al. Cryptorchidism and testicular tumorigenesis. Surgery 1968; 63: 919–922.

158. Prener A, Engholm G, Jensen OM. Genital anomalies and risk for testicular cancer in Danish men. Epidemiology 1996; 7: 14–19.

159. Batata MA, Chu FCH, Hilaris BS, et al. Testicular cancer in cryptorchids. Cancer 1982; 49: 1023–1030.

160. Bobba VS, Mittal BB, Hoover SV, et al. Classical and anaplastic seminoma: difference in survival. Radiology 1988; 167: 849–852.

161. Fram RJ, Garnick MB, Retik A. The spectrum of genitourinary abnormalities in patients with cryptorchidism, with emphasis on testicular carcinoma. Cancer 1982; 50: 2243–2245.

162. Cortes D, Thorup J, Frisch M, et al. Examination for intratubular germ cell neoplasia at operation for undescended testis in boys. J Urol 1994; 151: 722–725.

163. Cortes D, Thorup JM, Visfeldt J. Cryptorchidism: aspects of fertility and neoplasms. A study including data of 1,335 consecutive boys who underwent testicular biopsy simultaneously with surgery for cryptorchidism. Horm Res 2001; 55: 21–27.

164. Collins DH, Pugh RCB. Classification and frequency of testicular tumours. Br J Urol 1964; 36: 1–11.

165. Morrison AS. Cryptorchidism, hernia, and cancer of the testis. J Natl Cancer Inst 1976; 56: 731–733.

166. Giwercman A, Muller J, Skakkebaek NE. Carcinoma in situ of the undescended testis. Semin Urol 1988; 6: 110–119.

167. Pedersen KV, Bolesen P, Zetter-Lund CG. Experience of screening for carcinoma-in-situ of the testis among young men with surgically corrected maldescended testes. Int J Androl 1987; 10: 181–185.

168. Skakkebaek NE, Berthelsen JG, Giwercman A, et al. Carcinoma-in-situ of the testis: possible origin from gonocytes and precursor of all types of germ cell tumours except spermatocytoma. Int J Androl 1987; 10: 19–28.

169. Giwercman A, von der Maase H, Skakkebaek NE. Epidemiological and clinical aspects of carcinoma in situ of the testis. Eur Urol 1993; 23: 104–110.

170. Giwercman A, Bruun E, Frimodt-Moller C, et al. Prevalence of carcinoma-in-situ and other histopathologic abnormalities in testes of men with a history of cryptorchidism. J Urol 1989; 142: 998–1002.

171. Cappelen T, Fossa SD, Stenwig AE, et al. False-negative biopsy for testicular intraepithelial neoplasia and high-risk features for testicular cancer. Acta Oncol 2000; 39: 105–109.

172. Dieckmann KP, Souchon R, Hahn E, et al. False-negative biopsies for testicular intraepithelial neoplasia. J Urol 1999; 162: 364–368.

173. Nistal M, Codesal J, Paniagua R. Carcinoma in situ of the testis in infertile men. A histological, immunocytochemical, and cytophotometric study of DNA content. J Pathol 1989; 159: 205–210.

174. Stalker AL, Hendry WT. Hyperplasia and neoplasia of the Sertoli cell. J Pathol Bacteriol 1952; 64: 161–168.

175. Hedinger CE, Huber R, Weber E. Frequency of so-called hypoplastic or dysgenetic zones in scrotal and otherwise normal human testes. Virchows Arch A [Pathol Anat] 1967; 342: 165–168.

176. Scheiber K, Ackermann D, Studer UE. Bilateral testicular germ cell tumors. a report of 20 cases. J Urol 1987; 138: 73–76.

177. Dieckmann KP, Boeckmann W, Brosig W, et al. Bilateral testicular germ cell tumors. Report of nine cases and review of the literature. Cancer 1986; 57: 1254–1258.

178. Kristianslund S, Fossä SD, Kjellevold K. Bilateral malignant testicular germ cell cancer. Br J Urol 1986; 58: 60–63.

179. Osterlind A, Berthelsen JG, Abildgaard N, et al. Incidence of bilateral testicular germ cell cancer in Denmark, 1960–84: preliminary findings. Int J Androl 1987; 10: 203–208.

180. Bokemeyer C, Schmoll HJ, Schoffski P, et al. Bilateral testicular tumours: prevalence and clinical implications. Eur J Cancer 1993; 29A: 874–876.

181. Dieckmann KP, Loy P, Buttner P. Prevalence of bilateral testicular germ cell tumours and early detection based on contralateral testicular intra-epithelial neoplasia. Br J Urol 1993; 71: 340–345.

182. van Basten JP, Hoekstra HJ, van Driel MF, et al. Cisplatin-based chemotherapy changes the incidence of bilateral testicular cancer. Ann Surg Oncol 1997; 4: 342–348.

183. Tekin A, Aygun YC, Aki FT, et al. Bilateral germ cell cancer of the testis: a report of 11 patients with a long-term follow-up. BJU Int 2000; 85: 864–868.

184. van der Poel HG, Sedelaar JP, Debruyne FM, et al. Recurrence of germ cell tumor after orchiectomy. Urology 2000; 56: 467–473.

185. Pamenter B, de Bono JS, Brown IL, et al. Bilateral testicular cancer: a preventable problem? Experience from a large cancer centre. BJU Int 2003; 92: 43–46.

186. Che M, Tamboli P, Ro JY, et al. Bilateral testicular germ cell tumors: twenty-year experience at MD Anderson Cancer Center. Cancer 2002; 95: 1228–1233.

187. Dieckmann KP, Loy V. The value of the biopsy of the contralateral testis in patients with testicular germ cell cancer: the recent German experience. APMIS 1998; 106: 13–23.

188. Kliesch S, Thomaidis T, Schutte B, et al. Update on the diagnostic safety for detection of testicular intraepithelial neoplasia (TIN). APMIS 2003; 111: 70–74.

189. Harland SJ, Cook PA, Fossä SD, et al. Risk factors for carcinoma in situ of the contralateral testis in patients with testicular cancer. An interim report. Eur Urol 1993; 23: 115–118.

190. Harland SJ, Cook PA, Fossä SD, et al. Intratubular germ cell neoplasia of the contralateral testis in testicular cancer: defining a high risk group. J Urol 1998; 160: 1353–1357.

191. Zingg EJ, Zehntner C. Bilateral testicular germ cell tumors. Prog Clin Biol Res 1985; 203: 673–680.

192. Albers P, Goll A, Bierhoff E, et al. Clinical course and histopathologic risk factor assessment in patients with bilateral testicular germ cell tumors. Urology 1999; 54: 714–718.

193. Ware SM, Heyman J, Al-Askari S, et al. Bilateral testicular germ cell malignancy. Urology 1982; 19: 366–372.

194. Dieckmann KP, Becker T, Jonas D, et al. Inheritance and testicular cancer. Arguments based on a report of 3 cases and a review of the literature. Oncology 1987; 44: 367–377.

195. Hayakawa M, Mukai K, Nagakura K, et al. A case of simultaneous bilateral germ cell tumors arising from cryptorchid testes. J Urol 1986; 136: 470–472.

196. Dada R, Kumar R, Kucheria K. A 2-year-old baby with Down's syndrome, cryptorchidism and testicular tumour. Eur J Med Genet 2006; 49: 265–268.

197. Ryberg D, Heimdal K, Fossa SD, et al. Rare Ha-ras1 alleles and predisposition to testicular cancer. Int J Cancer 1993; 53: 938–940.

198. Nistal M, Gonzalez-Peramato P, Regadera J, et al. Primary testicular lesions are associated with testicular germ cell tumors of adult men. Am J Surg Pathol 2006; 30: 1260–1268.

199. Heimdal K, Olsson H, Tretli S, et al. Familial testicular cancer in Norway and southern Sweden. Br J Cancer 1996; 73: 964–969.

200. Hartley AL, Birch JM, Kelsey AM, et al. Are germ cell tumors part of the Li-Fraumeni cancer family syndrome? Cancer Genet Cytogenet 1989; 42: 221–226.

201. Heimdal K, Olsson H, Tretli S, et al. Risk of cancer in relatives of testicular cancer patients. Br J Cancer 1996; 73: 970–973.

202. Heimdal K, Lothe RA, Lystad S, et al. No germline TP53 mutations detected in familial and bilateral testicular cancer. Genes Chromosomes Cancer 1993; 6: 92–97.

203. Peng HQ, Hogg D, Malkin D, et al. Mutations of the p53 gene do not occur in testis cancer. Cancer Res 1993; 53: 3574–3578.

204. Bartkova J, Bartek J, Lukas J, et al. p53 protein alterations in human testicular cancer including pre-invasive intratubular germ-cell neoplasia. Int J Cancer 1991; 49: 196–202.

205. Ulbright TM, Orazi A, de Riese W, et al. The correlation of p53 protein expression with proliferative activity and occult metastases in clinical stage I non-seminomatous germ cell tumors of the testis. Mod Pathol 1994; 7: 64–68.

206. Heimdal K, Olsson H, Tretli S, et al. A segregation analysis of testicular cancer based on Norwegian and Swedish families. Br J Cancer 1997; 75: 1084–1087.

207. Rapley EA, Crockford GP, Teare D, et al. Localization to Xq27 of a susceptibility gene for testicular germ-cell tumours. Nature Genet 2000; 24: 197–200.

208. Crockford GP, Linger R, Hockley S, et al. Genome-wide linkage screen for testicular germ cell tumour

susceptibility loci. Hum Mol Genet 2006; 15: 443–451.

209. Gourlay WA, Johnson HW, Pantzar JT, et al. Gonadal tumors in disorders of sexual differentiation. Urology 1994; 43: 537–540.

210. Slowikowska-Hilczer J, Szarras-Czapnik M, Kula K. Testicular pathology in 46,XY dysgenetic male pseudohermaphroditism: an approach to pathogenesis of testis cancer. J Androl 2001; 22: 781–792.

211. Ramani P, Yeung CK, Habeebu SSM. Testicular intratubular germ cell neoplasia in children and adolescents with intersex. Am J Surg Pathol 1993; 17: 1124–1133.

212. Collins GM, Kim DU, Logrono R, et al. Pure seminoma arising in androgen insensitivity syndrome (testicular feminization syndrome): a case report and review of the literature. Mod Pathol 1993; 6: 89–93.

213. Chen CP, Chern SR, Wang TY, et al. Androgen receptor gene mutations in 46,XY females with germ cell tumours. Hum Reprod 1999; 14: 664–670.

214. Morris JM, Mahesh VB. Further observations on the syndrome, 'testicular feminization.' Am J Obstet Gynecol 1963; 87: 731–748.

215. Korsch E, Peter M, Hiort O, et al. Gonadal histology with testicular carcinoma in situ in a 15-year-old 46,XY female patient with a premature termination in the steroidogenic acute regulatory protein causing congenital lipoid adrenal hyperplasia. J Clin Endocrinol Metab 1999; 84: 1628–1632.

216. Cohen MB, Friend DS, Molnar JJ, et al. Gonadal endodermal sinus (yolk sac) tumor with pure intestinal differentiation: a new histologic type. Pathol Res Pract 1987; 182: 609–616.

217. Swerdlow AJ, Huttly SR, Smith PG. Testis cancer: post-natal hormonal factors, sexual behaviour and fertility. Int J Cancer 1989; 43: 549–553.

218. Giwercman A, Skakkebaek NE. Carcinoma-in-situ (gonocytoma-in-situ) of the testis. In: Burger H, de Kretser D, eds. The testis. New York: Raven Press, 1989; 475–491.

219. Perry A, Wiley EL, Albores-Saavedra J. Pagetoid spread of intratubular germ cell neoplasia into rete testis: a morphologic and histochemical study of 100 orchiectomy specimens with invasive germ cell tumors. Hum Pathol 1994; 25: 235–239.

220. Berney DM, Lee A, Shamash J, et al. The association between intratubular seminoma and invasive germ cell tumors. Hum Pathol 2006; 37: 458–461.

221. Coffin CM, Ewing S, Dehner LP. Frequency of intratubular germ cell neoplasia with invasive testicular germ cell tumors. Histologic and immunocytochemical features. Arch Pathol Lab Med 1985; 109: 555–559.

222. Manivel JC, Jessurun J, Wick MR, et al. Placental alkaline phosphatase immunoreactivity in testicular germ cell tumors. Am J Surg Pathol 1987; 11: 21–29.

223. Burke AP, Mostofi FK. Intratubular malignant germ cells in testicular biopsies. clinical course and identification by staining for placental alkaline phosphatase. Mod Pathol 1988; 1: 475–479.

224. Giwercman A, Cantell L, Marks A. Placental-like alkaline phosphatase as a marker of carcinoma-in-situ of the testis: comparison with monoclonal antibodies M2A and 43–9F. APMIS 1991; 99: 586–594.

225. Burke AP, Mostofi FK. Placental alkaline phosphatase immunohistochemistry of intratubular malignant germ cells and associated testicular germ cell tumors. Hum Pathol 1988; 19: 663–670.

226. de Jong J, Stoop H, Dohle GR, et al. Diagnostic value of OCT3/4 for pre-invasive and invasive testicular germ cell tumours. J Pathol 2005; 206: 242–249.

227. Marks A, Sutherland DR, Bailey D, et al. Characterization and distribution of an oncofetal antigen (M2A antigen) expressed on testicular germ cell tumours. Br J Cancer 1999; 80: 569–578.

228. Sonne SB, Herlihy AS, Hoei-Hansen CE, et al. Identity of M2A (D2–40) antigen and gp36 (Aggrus, T1A-2, podoplanin) in human developing testis, testicular carcinoma in situ and germ-cell tumours. Virchows Arch 2006; 449: 200–206.

229. Giwercman A, Lindenberg S, Kimber SJ, et al. Monoclonal antibody 43–9F as a sensitive immunohistochemical marker of carcinoma in situ of human testis. Cancer 1990; 65: 1135–1142.

230. Hiraoka N, Yamada T, Abe H, et al. Establishment of three monoclonal antibodies specific for prespermatogonia and intratubular malignant germ cells in humans. Lab Invest 1997; 76: 427–438.

231. Jorgensen N, Muller J, Jaubert F, et al. Heterogeneity of gonadoblastoma germ cells: similarities with immature germ cells, spermatogonia and testicular carcinoma in situ cells. Histopathology 1997; 30: 177–186.

232. Franke FE, Pauls K, Kerkman L, et al. Somatic isoform of angiotensin I-converting enzyme in the pathology of testicular germ cell tumors. Hum Pathol 2000; 31: 1466–1476.

233. Moore BE, Banner BF, Gokden M, et al. p53: a good diagnostic marker for intratubular germ cell neoplasia, unclassified. Appl Immunohistochem Mol Morphol 2001; 9: 203–206.

234. Lifschitz-Mercer B, Elliott DJ, Leider-Trejo L, et al. Absence of RBM expression as a marker of intratubular (in situ) germ cell neoplasia of the testis. Hum Pathol 2000; 31: 1116–1120.

235. Jorgensen N, Giwercman A, Muller J, et al. Immunohistochemical markers of carcinoma in situ of the testis also expressed in normal infantile germ cells. Histopathology 1993; 22: 373–378.

236. Sigg C, Hedinger C. Atypical germ cells of the testis. Comparative ultrastructural and immunohistochemical investigations. Virchows Arch [A] 1984; 402: 439–450.

237. Nielsen H, Nielsen M, Skakkebaek NE. The fine structure of possible carcinoma-in-situ in the seminiferous tubules in the testis of four infertile men. Acta Pathol Microbiol Scand [A] 1974; 82: 235–248.

238. Gondos B, Berthelsen JG, Skakkebaek NE. Intratubular germ cell neoplasia (carcinoma in situ): a preinvasive lesion of the testis. Ann Clin Lab Sci 1983; 13: 185–192.

239. Albrechtsen R, Nielsen MH, Skakkebaek NE, et al. Carcinoma in situ of the testis. Some ultrastructural characteristics of germ cells. Acta Pathol Microbiol Immunol Scand [A] 1982; 90: 301–303.

240. Holstein AF, Körner F. Light and electron microscopical analysis of cell types in human seminoma. Virchows Arch [A] 1974; 363: 97–112.

241. Hu LM, Phillipson J, Barsky SH. Intratubular germ cell neoplasia in infantile yolk sac tumor: verification by tandem repeat sequence in situ hybridization. Diagn Mol Pathol 1992; 1: 118–128.

242. Cortes D, Thorup J, Visfeldt J. Multinucleated spermatogonia in cryptorchid boys: a possible association with an increased risk of testicular malignancy later in life? APMIS 2003; 111: 25–30.

243. Skakkebaek NE, Berthelsen JG, Muller J. Carcinoma-in-situ of the undescended testis. Urol Clin North Am 1982; 9: 377–385.

244. Skakkebaek NE, Berthelsen JG, Visfeldt J. Clinical aspects of testicular carcinoma-in-situ. Int J Androl 1981; 4: 153–162.

245. Krabbe S, Skakkebaek NE, Berthelsen JG, et al. High incidence of undetected neoplasia in maldescended testes. Lancet 1979; 1: 999–1000.

246. von der Maase H, Rorth M, Walbom-Jorgensen S, et al. Carcinoma in situ of contralateral testis in patients with testicular germ cell cancer: study of 27 cases in 500 patients. Br Med J 1986; 293: 1398–1401.

247. Berthelsen JG, Skakkebaek NE, von der Maase H, et al. Screening for carcinoma in situ of the contralateral testis in patients with germinal testicular cancer. Br Med J 1982; 285: 1683–1686.

248. West AB, Butler MR, Fitzpatrick J, et al. Testicular tumors in subfertile men: report of 4 cases with implications for management of patients presenting with infertility. J Urol 1985; 133: 107–109.

249. Muller J, Skakkebaek NE, Ritzén M, et al. Carcinoma in situ of the testis in

children with 45,X/46,XY gonadal dysgenesis. J Pediatr 1985; 106: 431–436.

250. MacMahon RA, Cussen LJ. Detection of gonadal carcinoma in situ in childhood and implications for management. Aust NZ J Surg 1991; 61: 667–669.

251. Muller J, Skakkebaek NE. Testicular carcinoma in situ in children with the androgen insensitivity (testicular feminisation) syndrome. Br Med J 1984; 288: 1419–1420.

252. Skakkebaek NE. Carcinoma in situ of the testis in testicular feminization syndrome. Acta Pathol Microbiol Scand [A] 1979; 87: 87–89.

253. Skakkebaek NE. Carcinoma in situ of the testis: frequency and relationship to invasive germ cell tumours in infertile men. Histopathology 1978; 2: 157–170.

254. Pryor JP, Cameron KM, Chilton CP, et al. Carcinoma in situ in testicular biopsies in men presenting with infertility. Br J Urol 1983; 55: 780–784.

255. Jacobsen GK, Henriksen OB, von der Maase H. Carcinoma in situ of testicular tissue adjacent to malignant germ-cell tumors: a study of 105 cases. Cancer 1981; 47: 2660–2662.

256. Skakkebaek NE. Atypical germ cells in the adjacent 'normal' tissue of testicular tumours. Acta Pathol Microbiol Scand [A] 1975; 83: 127–130.

257. Muller J, Skakkebaek NE, Parkinson MC. The spermatocytic seminoma: views on pathogenesis. Int J Androl 1987; 10: 147–156.

258. Jorgensen N, Muller J, Visfeldt J, et al. Infantile germ cell tumors associated with carcinoma-in-situ of the testis. [Abstract] Onkologie 1991; 14: 8.

259. Stamp IM, Barlebo H, Rix M, et al. Intratubular germ cell neoplasia in an infantile testis with immature teratoma. Histopathology 1993; 22: 69–72.

260. Parkinson MC, Ramani P. Intratubular germ cell neoplasia in an infantile testis. Histopathology 1993; 23: 99–100.

261. Hawkins EP, Hicks MJ. Solid tumors and germ cell tumors induce nonneoplastic germ cell proliferations in testes of infants and young children. Hum Pathol 1998; 29: 1547–1548.

262. Berthelsen JG, Skakkebaek NE. Value of testicular biopsy in diagnosing carcinoma in situ testis. Scand J Urol Nephrol 1981; 15: 165–168.

263. Daugaard G, von der Maase H, Olsen J, et al. Carcinoma-in-situ testis in patients with assumed extragonadal germ-cell tumours. Lancet 1987; 2: 528–530.

264. Chen KT, Cheng AC. Retroperitoneal seminoma and intratubular germ cell neoplasia. Hum Pathol 1989; 20: 493–495.

265. von der Maase H, Giwercman A, Muller J, et al. Management of carcinoma-in-situ of the testis. Int J Androl 1987; 10: 209–220.

266. Bottomley D, Fisher C, Hendry WF, et al. Persistent carcinoma in situ of the testis after chemotherapy for advanced testicular germ cell tumours. Br J Urol 1990; 66: 420–424.

267. von der Maase H, Meinecke B, Skakkebaek NE. Residual carcinoma-in-situ of contralateral testis after chemotherapy. Lancet 1988; 1: 477–478.

268. Christensen TB, Daugaard G, Geertsen PF, et al. Effect of chemotherapy on carcinoma in situ of the testis. Ann Oncol 1998; 9: 657–660.

269. Jacobsen GK, Barlebo H, Olsen J, et al. Testicular germ cell tumours in Denmark 1976–1980. Pathology of 1058 consecutive cases. Acta Radiol Oncol 1984; 23: 239–247.

270. von Hochstetter AR, Hedinger CE. The differential diagnosis of testicular germ cell tumors in theory and practice: a critical analysis of two major systems of classification and review of 389 cases. Virchows Arch [A] 1982; 396: 247–277.

271. Fischer CG, Waechter W, Kraus S, et al. Urologic tumors in the Federal Republic of Germany: data on 56,013 cases from hospital cancer registries. Cancer 1998; 82: 775–783.

272. Moul JW, Schanne FJ, Thompson IM, et al. Testicular cancer in blacks. A multicenter experience. Cancer 1994; 73: 388–393.

273. Perry C, Servadio C. Seminoma in childhood. J Urol 1980; 124: 932–933.

274. Kay R. Prepubertal testicular tumor registry. J Urol 1993; 150: 671–674.

275. Thackray AC, Crane WAJ. Seminoma. In: Pugh RCB, ed. Pathology of the testis. Oxford: Blackwell Scientific, 1976; 164–198.

276. Duparc C, Boissiere-Veverka G, Lefebvre H, et al. An oestrogen-producing seminoma responsible for gynaecomastia. Horm Metab Res 2003; 35: 324–329.

277. Taylor JB, Solomon DH, Levine RE, et al. Exophthalmos in seminoma: regression with steroids and orchiectomy. JAMA 1978; 240: 860–861.

278. Mann AS. Bilateral exophthalmos in seminoma. J Clin Endocrinol Metab 1967; 27: 1500–1502.

279. da Silva MA, Edmondson JW, Eby C, et al. Humoral hypercalcemia in seminomas. Med Pediatr Oncol 1992; 20: 38–41.

280. Lundberg WB, Mitchell MS. Transient warm autoimmune hemolytic anemia and cryoglobulinemia associated with seminoma. Yale J Biol Med 1977; 50: 419–427.

281. Voltz R, Gultekin SH, Rosenfeld MR, et al. A serologic marker of paraneoplastic limbic and brain-stem encephalitis in patients with testicular cancer. N Engl J Med 1999; 340: 1788–1795.

282. Javadpour N. Management of seminoma based on tumor markers. Urol Clin North Am 1980; 7: 773–781.

283. Nazeer T, Ro JY, Amato RJ, et al. Histologically pure seminoma with elevated alpha-fetoprotein: a clinicopathologic study of ten cases. Oncol Rep 1998; 5: 1425–1429.

284. Rustin GJ, Vogelzang NJ, Sleijfer DT, et al. Consensus statement on circulating tumour markers and staging patients with germ cell tumours. Prog Clin Biol Res 1990; 357: 277–284.

285. Scheiber K, Mikuz G, Frommhold H, et al. Human chorionic gonadotropin positive seminoma: is this a special type of seminoma with a poor prognosis? Prog Clin Biol Res 1985; 203: 97–104.

286. Javadpour N. The role of biologic tumor markers in testicular cancer. Cancer 1980; 45: 1755–1761.

287. Mann K, Siddle K. Evidence for free beta-subunit secretion in so-called human chorionic gonadotropin-positive seminoma. Cancer 1988; 62: 2378–2382.

288. Dieckmann KP, Due W, Bauer HW. Seminoma testis with elevated serum beta-HCG – a category of germ cell cancer between seminoma and nonseminoma. Int Urol Nephrol 1989; 21: 175–184.

289. Javadpour N. Tumor markers in testicular cancer – an update. Prog Clin Biol Res 1985; 203: 141–154.

290. Chisolm GG. Tumour markers in testicular tumours. Prog Clin Biol Res 1985; 203: 81–91.

291. Schwartz BF, Auman R, Peretsman SJ, et al. Prognostic value of BHCG and local tumor invasion in stage I seminoma of the testis. J Surg Oncol 1996; 61: 131–133.

292. Mumperow E, Hartmann M. Spermatic cord beta-human chorionic gonadotropin levels in seminoma and their clinical implications. J Urol 1992; 147: 1041–1043.

293. Hartmann M, Pottek T, Bussar-Maatz R, et al. Elevated human chorionic gonadotropin concentrations in the testicular vein and in peripheral venous blood in seminoma patients. An analysis of various parameters. Eur Urol 1997; 31: 408–413.

294. Fossä A, Fossä SD. Serum lactate dehydrogenase and human chorionic gonadotropin in seminoma. Br J Urol 1989; 63: 408–415.

295. Suzuki K, Nakazato H, Kurokawa K, et al. Treatment of stage I seminoma: should beta-HCG positive seminoma be treated aggressively? Int J Urol Nephrol 1998; 30: 593–598.

296. Koshida K, Stigbrand T, Munck-Wikland E, et al. Analysis of serum placental alkaline phosphatase activity in testicular cancer and cigarette smokers. Urol Res 1990; 18: 169–173.

297. Kuzmits R, Schernthaner G, Krisch K. Serum neuron-specific enolase: a marker for response to therapy in seminoma. Cancer 1987; 60: 1017–1021.

298. Gross AJ, Dieckmann KP. Neuron-specific enolase: a serum tumor marker

in malignant germ-cell tumors? Eur Urol 1993; 24: 277–278.

299. Weissbach L, Bussar-Maatz R, Mann K. The value of tumor markers in testicular seminomas. Results of a prospective multicenter study. Eur Urol 1997; 32: 16–22.

300. Mostofi FK, Price EB Jr. Tumors of the male genital system. In: Armed Forces Institute of Pathology. Atlas of tumor pathology, 2nd Series, Fascicle 8. Washington DC: Armed Forces Institute of Pathology, 1973.

301. Jacobsen GK, Talerman A. Atlas of germ cell tumours. Copenhagen: Munksgaard, 1989.

302. Browne TJ, Richie JP, Gilligan TD, et al. Intertubular growth in pure seminomas. associations with poor prognostic parameters. Hum Pathol 2005; 36: 640–645.

303. Henley JD, Young RH, Wade CL, et al. Seminomas with exclusive intertubular growth. a report of 12 clinically and grossly inconspicuous tumors. Am J Surg Pathol 2004; 28: 1163–1168.

304. Kahn DG. Ossifying seminoma of the testis. Arch Pathol Lab Med 1993; 117: 321–322.

305. Young RH, Finlayson N, Scully RE. Tubular seminoma. Report of a case. Arch Pathol Lab Med 1989; 113: 414–416.

306. Zavala-Pompa A, Ro JY, El-Naggar AK, et al. Tubular seminoma. an immunohistochemical and DNA flow cytometric study of four cases. Am J Clin Pathol 1994; 102: 397–401.

307. Talerman A. Tubular seminoma. Arch Pathol Lab Med 1989; 113: 1204.

308. Takeshima Y, Sanda N, Yoneda K, et al. Tubular seminoma of the testis. Pathol Int 1999; 49: 676–679.

309. Ulbright TM, Young RH. Seminoma with tubular, microcystic, and related patterns: a study of 28 cases of unusual morphologic variants that often cause confusion with yolk sac tumor. Am J Surg Pathol 2005; 29: 500–505.

310. Bell DA, Flotte TJ, Bhan AK. Immunohistochemical characterization of seminoma and its inflammatory cell infiltrate. Hum Pathol 1987; 18: 511–520.

311. Strutton GM, Gemmell E, Seymour GJ, et al. An immunohistological examination of inflammatory cell infiltration in primary testicular seminomas. Aust NZ J Surg 1989; 59: 169–172.

312. Wilkins BS, Williamson JM, O'Brien CJ. Morphological and immunohistological study of testicular lymphomas. Histopathology 1989; 15: 147–156.

313. Bentley AJ, Parkinson MC, Harding BN, et al. A comparative morphological and immunohistochemical study of testicular seminomas and intracranial germinomas. Histopathology 1990; 17: 443–449.

314. Akaza H, Kobayashi K, Umeda T, et al. Surface markers of lymphocytes infiltrating seminoma tissue. J Urol 1980; 124: 827–828.

315. Wei YQ, Hang ZB, Liu KF. In situ observation of inflammatory cell-tumor cell interaction in human seminomas (germinomas): light, electron microscopic, and immunohistochemical study. Hum Pathol 1992; 23: 421–428.

316. Grobholz R, Verbeke CS, Schleger C, et al. Expression of MAGE antigens and analysis of the inflammatory T-cell infiltrate in human seminoma. Urol Res 2000; 28: 398–403.

317. Dixon FJ, Moore RA. Tumors of the male sex organs. In: Atlas of tumor pathology, 1st series, Fascicles 31b & 32. Washington, DC: Armed Forces Institute of Pathology, 1952.

318. von Hochstetter AR. Mitotic count in seminomas–an unreliable criterion for distinguishing between classical and anaplastic types. Virchows Arch [A] 1981; 390: 63–69.

319. Zuckman MH, Williams G, Levin HS. Mitosis counting in seminoma: an exercise of questionable significance. Hum Pathol 1988; 19: 329–335.

320. Suzuki T, Sasano H, Aoki H, et al. Immunohistochemical comparison between anaplastic seminoma and typical seminoma. Acta Pathol Jpn 1993; 43: 751–757.

321. Tickoo SK, Hutchinson B, Bacik J, et al. Testicular seminoma. A clinicopathologic and immunohistochemical study of 105 cases with special reference to seminomas with atypical features. Int J Surg Pathol 2002; 10: 23–32.

322. Hedinger C, von Hochstetter AR, Egloff B. Seminoma with syncytiotrophoblastic giant cells. A special form of seminoma. Virchows Arch [A] 1979; 383: 59–67.

323. Berney DM, Lee A, Shamash J, et al. The frequency and distribution of intratubular trophoblast in association with germ cell tumors of the testis. Am J Surg Pathol 2005; 29: 1300–1303.

324. Uchida T, Shimoda T, Miyata H, et al. Immunoperoxidase study of alkaline phosphatase in testicular tumor. Cancer 1981; 48: 1455–1462.

325. Hustin J, Collettee J, Franchimont P. Immunohistochemical demonstration of placental alkaline phosphatase in various states of testicular development and in germ cell tumours. Int J Androl 1987; 10: 29–35.

326. Strohmeyer T, Reese D, Press M, et al. Expression of the c-kit proto-oncogene and its ligand stem cell factor (SCF) in normal and malignant human testicular tissue. J Urol 1995; 153: 511–515.

327. Kraggerud SM, Berner A, Bryne M, et al. Spermatocytic seminoma as compared to classical seminoma. an immunohistochemical and DNA flow cytometric study. APMIS 1999; 107: 297–302.

328. Jones TD, Ulbright TM, Eble JN, et al. OCT4 staining in testicular tumors: a sensitive and specific marker for seminoma and embryonal carcinoma. Am J Surg Pathol 2004; 28: 935–940.

329. Looijenga LH, Stoop H, de Leeuw HP, et al. POU5F1 (OCT3/4) identifies cells with pluripotent potential in human germ cell tumors. Cancer Res 2003; 63: 2244–2250.

330. Hart AH, Hartley L, Parker K, et al. The pluripotency homeobox gene NANOG is expressed in human germ cell tumors. Cancer 2005; 104: 2092–2098.

331. Fogel M, Lifschitz-Mercer B, Moll R, et al. Heterogeneity of intermediate filament expression in human testicular seminomas. Differentiation 1990; 45: 242–249.

332. Cheville JC, Rao S, Iczkowski KA, et al. Cytokeratin expression in seminoma of the human testis. Am J Clin Pathol 2000; 113: 583–588.

333. Wick MR, Swanson PE, Manivel JC. Placental-like alkaline phosphatase reactivity in human tumors: an immunohistochemical study of 520 cases. Hum Pathol 1987; 18: 946–954.

334. Murakami SS, Said JW. Immunohistochemical localization of lactate dehydrogenase isoenzyme 1 in germ cell tumors of the testis. Am J Clin Pathol 1984; 81: 293–296.

335. Denk H, Moll R, Weybora W, et al. Intermediate filaments and desmosomal plaque proteins in testicular seminomas and non-seminomatous germ cell tumours as revealed by immunohistochemistry. Virchows Arch [A] 1987; 410: 295–307.

336. Boseman FT, Giard RWM, Kruseman ACN, et al. Human chorionic gonadotropin and alpha-fetoprotein in testicular germ cell tumors: a retrospective immunohistochemical study. Histopathology 1980; 4: 673–684.

337. Berney DM, Shamash J, Pieroni K, et al. Loss of CD30 expression in metastatic embryonal carcinoma: the effects of chemotherapy? Histopathology 2001; 39: 382–385.

338. Janssen M, Johnston WH. Anaplastic seminoma of the testis: ultrastructural analysis of three cases. Cancer 1978; 41: 538–544.

339. Min KW, Scheithauer BW. Pineal germinomas and testicular seminoma: a comparative ultrastructural study with special references to early carcinomatous transformation. Ultrastruct Pathol 1990; 14: 483–496.

340. Damjanov I. Is seminoma a relative or a precursor of embryonal carcinoma? Lab Invest 1989; 60: 1–3.

341. Baretton G, Diebold J, DePascale T, et al. Deoxyribonucleic acid ploidy in seminomas with and without syncytiotrophoblastic cells. J Urol 1994; 151: 67–71.

342. Rukstalis DB, DeWolf WC. Molecular biological concepts in the etiology of testicular and other urologic malignancies. Semin Urol 1988; 6: 161–170.

343. Castedo SM, de Jong B, Oosterhuis JW, et al. Cytogenetic analysis of ten human seminomas. Cancer Res 1989; 49: 439–443.

344. Delozier-Blanchet CD, Walt H, Engel E, et al. Cytogenetic studies of human testicular germ cell tumours. Int J Androl 1987; 10: 69–77.

345. van Echten J, Oosterhuis JW, Looijenga LH, et al. No recurrent structural abnormalities apart from i(12p) in primary germ cell tumors of the adult testis. Genes Chromosomes Cancer 1995; 14: 133–144.

346. Looijenga LH, Oosterhuis JW. Pathogenesis of testicular germ cell tumours. Rev Reprod 1999; 4: 90–100.

347. Looijenga LH, Rosenberg C, van Gurp RJ, et al. Comparative genomic hybridization of microdissected samples from different stages in the development of a seminoma and a non-seminoma. J Pathol 2000; 191: 187–192.

348. Kersemaekers AM, van Weeren PC, Oosterhuis JW, et al. Involvement of the Fas/FasL pathway in the pathogenesis of germ cell tumours of the adult testis. J Pathol 2002; 196: 423–429.

349. Houldsworth J, Reuter V, Bosl GJ, et al. Aberrant expression of cyclin D2 is an early event in human male germ cell tumorigenesis. Cell Growth Differ 1997; 8: 293–299.

350. Chaubert P, Guillou L, Kurt AM, et al. Frequent p16INK4 (MTS1) gene inactivation in testicular germ cell tumors. Am J Pathol 1997; 151: 859–865.

351. Sakuma Y, Sakurai S, Oguni S, et al. Alterations of the c-kit gene in testicular germ cell tumors. Cancer Sci 2003; 94: 486–491.

352. Bennett AK, Ulbright TM, Ramnani DM, et al. Immunohistochemical expression of calretinin, CD99, and alpha-inhibin in Sertoli and Leydig cells and their lesions, emphasizing large cell calcifying Sertoli cell tumor. Mod Pathol 2005; 18: 128A.

353. Hayashi T, Yamada T, Kageyama Y, et al. Expression failure of the notch signaling system is associated with the pathogenesis of testicular germ cell tumor. Tumour Biol 2004; 25: 99–105.

354. Eyzaguirre E, Gatalica Z. Loss of Fhit expression in testicular germ cell tumors and intratubular germ cell neoplasia. Mod Pathol 2002; 15: 1068–1072.

355. Jacobsen R, Moller H, Thoresen SO, et al. Trends in testicular cancer incidence in the Nordic countries, focusing on the recent decrease in Denmark. Int J Androl 2006; 29: 199–204.

356. Mulder MP, Keijzer W, Verkerk A, et al. Activated ras genes in human seminoma: evidence for tumor heterogeneity. Oncogene 1989; 4: 1345–1351.

357. Lifschitz-Mercer B, Elliott DJ, Issakov J, et al. Localization of a specific germ cell marker, DAZL1, in testicular germ cell neoplasias. Virchows Arch 2002; 440: 387–391.

358. Strohmeyer T, Peter S, Hartmann M, et al. Expression of the hst-1 and c-kit protooncogenes in human testicular germ cell tumors. Cancer Res 1991; 51: 1811–1816.

359. Yoshida T, Tsutsumi M, Sakamoto H. Expression of the HST1 oncogene in human germ cell tumors. Biochem Biophys Res Commun 1988; 155: 1324–1329.

360. Misaki H, Shuin T, Yao M, et al. Expression of myc family oncogenes in primary human testicular cancer. Nippon Hinyokika Gakkai Zasshi 1989; 80: 1509–1513.

361. Saksela K, Mäkelä TP, Alitalo K. Oncogene expression in small-cell lung cancer cell lines and a testicular germ-cell tumor: activation of the N-myc gene and decreased RB mRNA. Int J Cancer 1989; 44: 182–185.

362. Shuin T, Misaki H, Kubota Y, et al. Differential expression of protooncogenes in human germ cell tumors of the testis. Cancer 1994; 73: 1721–1727.

363. Hara I, Hara S, Miyake H, et al. Expression of MAGE genes in testicular germ cell tumors. Urology 1999; 53: 843–847.

364. Leroy X, Augusto D, Leteurtre E, et al. CD30 and CD117 (c-kit) used in combination are useful for distinguishing embryonal carcinoma from seminoma. J Histochem Cytochem 2002; 50: 283–285.

365. Visfeldt J, Giwercman A, Skakkebaek NE. Monoclonal antibody 43–9F: an immunohistochemical marker of embryonal carcinoma of the testis. APMIS 1992; 100: 63–70.

366. Badve S, Morimiya A, Agarwal B, et al. Podoplanin: a histological marker for seminoma. Mod Pathol 2006; 19: 129A.

367. Ulbright TM, Roth LM, Brodhecker CA. Yolk sac differentiation in germ cell tumors: a morphologic study of 50 cases with emphasis on hepatic, enteric and parietal yolk sac features. Am J Surg Pathol 1986; 10: 151–164.

368. Nonomura N, Aozasa K, Ueda T, et al. Malignant lymphoma of the testis: histological and immunohistological study of 28 cases. J Urol 1989; 141: 1368–1371.

369. Hamlin JA, Kagan AR, Friedman NB. Lymphomas of the testicle. Cancer 1972; 29: 1352–1356.

370. Hayes MM, Sacks MI, King HS. Testicular lymphoma. A retrospective review of 17 cases. S Afr Med J 1983; 64: 1014–1016.

371. Paladugu RR, Bearman RM, Rappaport H. Malignant lymphoma with primary manifestation in the gonad: a clinicopathologic study of 38 patients. Cancer 1980; 45: 561–571.

372. Turner RR, Colby TV, MacKintosh FR. Testicular lymphomas: a clinicopathologic study of 35 cases. Cancer 1981; 48: 2095–2102.

373. Sussman EB, Hajdu SI, Lieberman PH, et al. Malignant lymphoma of the testis: a clinicopathologic study of 37 cases. J Urol 1977; 118: 1004–1007.

374. Fonseca R, Habermann TM, Colgan JP, et al. Testicular lymphoma is associated with a high incidence of extranodal recurrence. Cancer 2000; 88: 154–161.

375. Duncan PR, Checa F, Gowing NF, et al. Extranodal non-Hodgkin's lymphoma presenting in the testicle: a clinical and pathologic study of 24 cases. Cancer 1980; 45: 1578–1584.

376. Talerman A. Primary malignant lymphoma of the testis. J Urol 1977; 118: 783–786.

377. Young RH, Koelliker DD, Scully RE. Sertoli cell tumors of the testis, not otherwise specified: a clinicopathologic analysis of 60 cases. Am J Surg Pathol 1998; 22: 709–721.

378. Henley JD, Young RH, Ulbright TM. Malignant Sertoli cell tumors of the testis: a study of 13 examples of a neoplasm frequently misinterpreted as seminoma. Am J Surg Pathol 2002; 26: 541–550.

379. Hunter M, Peschel RE. Testicular seminoma. Results of the Yale University experience, 1964–1984. Cancer 1989; 64: 1608–1611.

380. Babaian RJ, Zagars GK. Testicular seminoma: the M.D. Anderson experience. An analysis of pathological and patient characteristics, and treatment recommendations. J Urol 1988; 139: 311–314.

381. Fossä SD, Aass N, Kaalhus O. Radiotherapy for testicular seminoma Stage I: treatment results and long-term post irradiation morbidity in 365 patients. Int J Rad Oncol Biol Phys 1989; 16: 383–388.

382. Brunt AM, Scoble JE. Para-aortic nodal irradiation for early stage testicular seminoma. Clin Oncol 1992; 4: 165–170.

383. Fossä SD, Horwich A, Russell JM, et al. Optimal planning target volume for stage I testicular seminoma. A Medical Research Council randomized trial. Medical Research Council Testicular Tumor Working Group. J Clin Oncol 1999; 17: 1146.

384. Bauman GS, Venkatesan VM, Ago CT, et al. Postoperative radiotherapy for Stage I/II seminoma: results for 212 patients. Int J Radiat Oncol Biol Phys 1998; 42: 313–317.

385. Vallis KA, Howard GC, Duncan W, et al. Radiotherapy for stages I and II testicular seminoma: results and morbidity in 238 patients. Br J Radiol 1995; 68: 400–405.

386. Horwich A, Dearnaley DP. Treatment of seminoma. Semin Oncol 1992; 19: 171–180.

387. Milosevic MF, Gospodarowicz M, Warde P. Management of testicular seminoma. Semin Surg Oncol 1999; 17: 240–249.

388. Fossä SD, Oliver RT, Stenning SP, et al. Prognostic factors for patients with advanced seminoma treated with

platinum-based chemotherapy. Eur J Cancer 1997; 33: 1380–1387.

389. Evensen JF, Fosså SD, Kjellevold K, et al. Testicular seminoma: histological findings and their prognostic significance for stage II disease. J Surg Oncol 1987; 36: 166–169.

390. Logothetis CJ, Samuels ML, Selig DE, et al. Cyclic chemotherapy with cyclophosphamide, doxorubicin, and cisplatin plus vinblastine and bleomycin in advanced germ cell tumors: results with 100 patients. Am J Med 1986; 81: 219–228.

391. Motzer RJ, Bosl GJ, Geller NL, et al. Advanced seminoma: the role of chemotherapy and adjuvant surgery. Ann Intern Med 1988; 108: 513–518.

392. Javadpour N. Human chorionic gonadotropin in seminoma. J Urol 1984; 131: 407.

393. Eble JN. Spermatocytic seminoma. Hum Pathol 1994; 25: 1035–1042.

394. Masson P. Étude sur le seminome. Rev Can Biol 1946; 5: 361–387.

395. Talerman A. Spermatocytic seminoma. clinicopathological study of 22 cases. Cancer 1980; 45: 2169–2176.

396. Cummings OW, Ulbright TM, Eble JN, et al. Spermatocytic seminoma: an immunohistochemical study. Hum Pathol 1994; 25: 54–59.

397. Burke AP, Mostofi FK. Spermatocytic seminoma: a clinicopathologic study of 79 cases. J Urol Pathol 1993; 1: 21–32.

398. Rosai J, Silber I, Khodadoust K. Spermatocytic seminoma. I. Clinicopathologic study of six cases and review of the literature. Cancer 1969; 24: 92–102.

399. True LD, Otis CN, Delprado W, et al. Spermatocytic seminoma of testis with sarcomatous transformation. A report of five cases. Am J Surg Pathol 1988; 12: 75–82.

400. Floyd C, Ayala AG, Logothetis CJ, et al. Spermatocytic seminoma with associated sarcoma of the testis. Cancer 1988; 61: 409–414.

401. Matoska J, Talerman A. Spermatocytic seminoma associated with rhabdomyosarcoma. Am J Clin Pathol 1990; 94: 89–95.

402. Batata MA, Chu FC, Hilaris BS, et al. TNM staging of testis cancer. Int J Radiat Oncol Biol Phys 1980; 6: 291–295.

403. Chung PW, Bayley AJ, Sweet J, et al. Spermatocytic seminoma: a review. Eur Urol 2004; 45: 495–498.

404. Scully RE. Spermatocytic seminoma of the testis: a report of 3 cases and review of the literature. Cancer 1961; 14: 788–794.

405. Albores-Saavedra J, Huffman H, Alvarado-Cabrero I, et al. Anaplastic variant of spermatocytic seminoma. Hum Pathol 1996; 27: 650–655.

406. Dekker I, Rozeboom T, Delemarre J, et al. Placental-like alkaline phosphatase and DNA flow cytometry in spermatocytic seminoma. Cancer 1992; 69: 993–996.

407. Stoop H, van Gurp R, de Krijger R, et al. Reactivity of germ cell maturation stage-specific markers in spermatocytic seminoma: diagnostic and etiological implications. Lab Invest 2001; 81: 919–928.

408. Rosai J, Khodadoust K, Silber I. Spermatocytic seminoma. II. Ultrastructural study. Cancer 1969; 24: 103–116.

409. Romanenko AM, Persidsky YV, Mostofi FK. Ultrastructure and histogenesis of spermatocytic seminoma. J Urol Pathol 1993; 1: 387–395.

410. Talerman A, Fu YS, Okagaki T. Spermatocytic seminoma. Ultrastructural and microspectrophotometric observations. Lab Invest 1984; 51: 343–349.

411. Takahashi H. Cytometric analysis of testicular seminoma and spermatocytic seminoma. Acta Pathol Jpn 1993; 43: 121–129.

412. Takahashi H, Aizawa S, Konishi E, et al. Cytofluorometric analysis of spermatocytic seminoma. Cancer 1993; 72: 549–552.

413. Walsh TJ, Grady RW, Porter MP, et al. Incidence of testicular germ cell cancers in US children. SEER program experience 1973 to 2000. Urology 2006; 68: 402–405.

414. Matoska J, Ondrus D, Hornák M. Metastatic spermatocytic seminoma. A case report with light microscopic, ultrastructural, and immunohistochemical findings. Cancer 1988; 62: 1197–1201.

415. Steiner H, Gozzi C, Verdorfer I, et al. Metastatic spermatocytic seminoma – an extremely rare disease. Eur Urol 2006; 49: 183–186.

416. Hittmair A, Rogatsch H, Hobisch A, et al. CD30 expression in seminoma. Hum Pathol 1996; 27: 1166–1171.

417. Damjanov I. Tumors of the testis and epididymis. In: Murphy WM, ed. Urological pathology. Philadelphia: WB Saunders, 1989; 314–379.

418. Mostofi FK, Sesterhenn IA, Davis CJ, Jr. Developments in histopathology of testicular germ cell tumors. Semin Urol 1988; 6: 171–188.

419. Damjanov I, Andrews PW. Ultrastructural differentiation of a clonal human embryonal carcinoma cell line in vitro. Cancer Res 1983; 43: 2190–2198.

420. Damjanov I, Clark RK, Andrews PW. Cytoskeleton of human embryonal carcinoma cells. Cell Differ 1984; 15: 133–139.

421. Motoyama T, Watanabe H, Yamamoto T, et al. Human testicular germ cell tumors in vitro and in athymic nude mice. Acta Pathol Jpn 1987; 37: 431–448.

422. Pera MF, Blasco Lafita MJ, Mills J. Cultured stem-cells from human testicular teratomas: the nature of human embryonal carcinoma, and its comparison with two types of yolk-sac carcinoma. Int J Cancer 1987; 40: 334–343.

423. Pera MF, Mills J, Parrington JM. Isolation and characterization of a multipotent clone of human embryonal carcinoma cells. Differentiation 1989; 42: 10–23.

424. Damjanov I, Fox N, Knowles BB, et al. Immunohistochemical localization of stage-specific embryonic antigens in human testicular germ cell tumors. Am J Pathol 1982; 108: 225–230.

425. Mostofi FK. Pathology of germ cell tumors of testis: a progress report. Cancer 1980; 45: 1735–1754.

426. Hawkins EP, Finegold MJ, Hawkins HK, et al. Nongerminomatous malignant germ cell tumors in children: a review of 89 cases from the Pediatric Oncology Group, 1971–1984. Cancer 1986; 58: 2579–2584.

427. Kusumakumary P, Mathew BS, Hariharan S, et al. Testicular germ cell tumors in prepubertal children. Pediatr Hematol Oncol 2000; 17: 105–111.

428. Rodriguez PN, Hafez GR, Messing EM. Nonseminomatous germ cell tumor of the testicle: does extensive staging of the primary tumor predict the likelihood of metastatic disease? J Urol 1986; 136: 604–608.

429. Saukko P, Lignitz E. Sudden death caused by malignant testicular tumors [German]. Zeitschr Rechtsmed 1990; 103: 529–536.

430. Aronsohn RS, Nishiyama RH. Embryonal carcinoma. An unexpected cause of sudden death in a young adult. JAMA 1974; 229: 1093–1094.

431. Bosl GJ, Lange PH, Nochomovitz LE, et al. Tumor markers in advanced non-seminomatous testicular cancer. Cancer 1981; 47: 572–576.

432. Tsuruta T, Ogawa A, Ishii K, et al. CA19-9: a possible serum marker for embryonal carcinoma. Urol Int 1997; 58: 20–24.

433. Jacobsen GK. Histogenetic considerations concerning germ cell tumours. Morphological and immunohistochemical comparative investigation of the human embryo and testicular germ cell tumours. Virchows Arch [A] 1986; 408: 509–525.

434. Azzopardi JG, Mostofi FK, Theiss EA. Lesions of testes observed in certain patients with widespread choriocarcinoma and related tumors. Am J Pathol 1961; 38: 207–225.

435. Balzer BL, Ulbright TM. Spontaneous regression of testicular germ cell tumors: an analysis of 42 cases. Am J Surg Pathol 2006; 30: 858–865.

436. Mostofi FK, Sesterhenn IA, Davis CJ, Jr. Immunopathology of germ cell tumors of the testis. Semin Diagn Pathol 1987; 4: 320–341.

437. Wittekind C, Wichmann T, Von Kleist S. Immunohistological localization of AFP and HCG in uniformly classified testis tumors. Anticancer Res 1983; 3: 327–330.

438. Lamm DL, Wepsic HT, Feldman P, et al. Importance of alpha-fetoprotein

in patients with seminoma. Urology 1977; 10: 233–235.

439. Lifschitz-Mercer B, Fogel M, Moll R, et al. Intermediate filament protein profiles of human testicular non-seminomatous germ cell tumors: correlation of cytokeratin synthesis to cell differentiation. Differentiation 1991; 48: 191–198.

440. Battifora H, Sheibani K, Tubbs RR, et al. Antikeratin antibodies in tumor diagnosis: distinction between seminoma and embryonal carcinoma. Cancer 1984; 54: 843–848.

441. Ferreiro JA. Ber-H2 expression in testicular germ cell tumors. Hum Pathol 1994; 25: 522–524.

442. Pallesen G, Hamilton-Dutoit SJ. Ki-1 (CD30) antigen is regularly expressed in tumor cells of embryonal carcinoma. Am J Pathol 1988; 133: 446–450.

443. Jacobsen GK, Jacobsen M, Clausen PP. Distribution of tumor-associated antigens in the various histologic components of germ cell tumors of the testis. Am J Surg Pathol 1981; 5: 257–266.

444. Ulbright TM, Goheen MP, Roth LM, et al. The differentiation of carcinomas of teratomatous origin from embryonal carcinoma. A light and electron microscopic study. Cancer 1986; 57: 257–263.

445. Henegariu O, Vance GH, Heiber D, et al. Triple-color FISH analysis of 12p amplification in testicular germ-cell tumors using 12p band-specific painting probes. J Mol Med 1998; 76: 648–655.

446. Motzer RJ, Rodriguez E, Reuter VE, et al. Genetic analysis as an aid in diagnosis for patients with midline carcinomas of uncertain histologies. J Natl Cancer Inst 1991; 83: 341–346.

447. Rodriguez E, Mathew S, Mukherjee AB, et al. Analysis of chromosome 12 aneuploidy in interphase cells from human male germ cell tumors by fluorescence in situ hybridization. Genes Chromosomes Cancer 1992; 5: 21–29.

448. Blough RI, Smolarek TA, Ulbright TM, et al. Bicolor fluorescence in situ hybridization on nuclei from formalin-fixed, paraffin-embedded testicular germ cell tumors: comparison with standard metaphase analysis. Cancer Genet Cytogenet 1997; 94: 79–84.

449. Zynger DL, Dimov ND, Luan C, et al. Glypican 3: a novel marker in testicular germ cell tumors. Am J Surg Pathol 2006; 30: 1570–1575.

450. Ota S, Hishinuma M, Yamauchi N, et al. Oncofetal protein glypican-3 in testicular germ-cell tumor. Virchows Arch 2006; 449: 308–314.

451. de Bruin MJ, Oosterhof GO, Debruyne FM. Nerve-sparing retroperitoneal lymphadenectomy for low stage testicular cancer. Br J Urol 1993; 71: 336–339.

452. Rowland RG, Donohue JP. Scrotum and testis. In: Gillenwater JY, Grayhack JT, Howards SS, et al., eds. Adult and pediatric urology. St. Louis: Mosby Year Book, 1991; 1565–1598.

453. Hermans BP, Sweeney CJ, Foster RS, et al. Risk of systemic metastases in clinical stage I nonseminoma germ cell testis tumor managed by retroperitoneal lymph node dissection. J Urol 2000; 163: 1721–1724.

454. Sweeney CJ, Hermans BP, Heilman DK, et al. Results and outcome of retroperitoneal lymph node dissection for clinical stage I embryonal carcinoma-predominant testis cancer. J Clin Oncol 2000; 18: 358–362.

455. Albers P, Siener R, Kliesch S, et al. Risk factors for relapse in clinical stage I nonseminomatous testicular germ cell tumors: results of the German Testicular Cancer Study Group Trial. J Clin Oncol 2003; 21: 1505–1512.

456. Francis R, Bower M, Brunstrom G, et al. Surveillance for stage I testicular germ cell tumours: results and cost benefit analysis of management options. Eur J Cancer 2000; 36: 1925–1932.

457. Sogani PC, Fair WR. Surveillance alone in the treatment of clinical Stage I nonseminomatous germ cell tumor of the testis (NSGCT). Semin Urol 1988; 6: 53–56.

458. Moriyama N, Daly JJ, Keating MA, et al. Vascular invasion as a prognosticator of metastatic disease in nonseminomatous germ cell tumors of the testis. Importance in 'surveillance only' protocols. Cancer 1985; 56: 2492–2498.

459. Fung CY, Kalish LA, Brodsky GL, et al. Stage I nonseminomatous germ cell testicular tumor: prediction of metastatic potential by primary histopathology. J Clin Oncol 1988; 6: 1467–1473.

460. Dunphy CH, Ayala AG, Swanson DA, et al. Clinical stage I nonseminomatous and mixed germ cell tumors of the testis. A clinicopathologic study of 93 patients on a surveillance protocol after orchiectomy alone. Cancer 1988; 62: 1202–1206.

461. Jacobsen GK, Rorth M, Osterlind K, et al. Histopathological features in stage I non-seminomatous testicular germ cell tumours correlated to relapse. Danish Testicular Cancer Study Group. APMIS 1990; 98: 377–382.

462. Wishnow KI, Johnson DE, Swanson DA, et al. Identifying patients with low-risk clinical stage I nonseminomatous testicular tumors who should be treated by surveillance. Urology 1989; 34: 339–343.

463. Javadpour N, Canning DA, O'Connell KJ, et al. Predictors of recurrent clinical stage I nonseminomatous testicular cancer. A prospective clinicopathologic study. Urology 1986; 27: 508–511.

464. Costello AJ, Mortensen PH, Stillwell RG. Prognostic indicators for failure of surveillance management of stage I non-seminomatous germ cell tumours. Aust NZ J Surg 1989; 59: 119–122.

465. Fossä SD, Aass N, Kaalhus O. Testicular cancer in young Norwegians. J Surg Oncol 1988; 39: 43–63.

466. Freedman LS, Parkinson MC, Jones WG, et al. Histopathology in the prediction of relapse of patients with stage I testicular teratoma treated by orchidectomy alone. Lancet 1987; 2: 294–298.

467. Sturgeon JF, Jewett MA, Alison RE, et al. Surveillance after orchidectomy for patients with clinical stage I nonseminomatous testis tumors. J Clin Oncol 1992; 10: 564–568.

468. Moul JW, McCarthy WF, Fernandez EB, et al. Percentage of embryonal carcinoma and of vascular invasion predicts pathological stage in clinical stage I nonseminomatous testicular cancer. Cancer Res 1994; 54: 362–364.

469. Heidenreich A, Sesterhenn IA, Mostofi FK, et al. Prognostic risk factors that identify patients with clinical stage I nonseminomatous germ cell tumors at low risk and high risk for metastasis. Cancer 1998; 83: 1002–1011.

470. Moul JW, Foley JP, Hitchcock CL, et al. Flow cytometric and quantitative histological parameters to predict occult disease in clinical stage I nonseminomatous testicular germ cell tumors. J Urol 1993; 150: 879–883.

471. Albers P, Ulbright TM, Albers J, et al. Tumor proliferative activity is predictive of pathological stage in clinical stage A nonseminomatous testicular germ cell tumors. J Urol 1996; 155: 579–586.

472. Castedo SM, de Jong B, Oosterhuis JW, et al. Chromosomal changes in mature residual teratomas following polychemotherapy. Cancer Res 1989; 49: 672–676.

473. Albers P, Orazi A, Ulbright TM, et al. Prognostic significance of immunohistochemical proliferation markers (Ki-67/MIB-1 and proliferation-associated nuclear antigen), p53 protein accumulation, and neovascularization in clinical stage A nonseminomatous testicular germ cell tumors. Mod Pathol 1995; 8: 492–497.

474. Allhoff EP, Liedkes S, Wittekind C, et al. DNA content in NSGCT/CSI: a new prognosticator for biologic behaviour. [Abstract] J Cancer Res Clin Oncol 1990; 1: 592.

475. de Graaff WE, Sleijfer DT, de Jong B, et al. Significance of aneuploid stemlines in testicular nonseminomatous germ cell tumors. Cancer 1993; 72: 1300–1304.

476. Mazumdar M, Bacik J, Tickoo SK, et al. Cluster analysis of p53 and Ki67 expression, apoptosis, alpha-fetoprotein, and human chorionic gonadotrophin indicates a favorable prognostic subgroup within the embryonal carcinoma germ cell tumor. J Clin Oncol 2003; 21: 2679–2688.

477. Einhorn LH. Chemotherapy of disseminated testicular cancer. In:

Skinner DG, Lieskovsky G, eds. Diagnosis and management of genitourinary cancer. Philadelphia: WB Saunders, 1988; 526–531.

478. Ulbright TM, Roth LM. A pathologic analysis of lesions following modern chemotherapy for metastatic germ cell tumors. Pathol Annu 1990; 25: 313–340.

479. Mead GM, Stenning SP, Parkinson MC, et al. The Second Medical Research Council study of prognostic factors in nonseminomatous germ cell tumors. Medical Research Council Testicular Tumour Working Party. J Clin Oncol 1992; 10: 85–94.

480. Vogelzang NJ. Prognostic factors in metastatic testicular cancer. Int J Androl 1987; 10: 225–237.

481. Stoter G, Sylvester R, Sleijfer DT, et al. Multivariate analysis of prognostic variables in patients with disseminated non-seminomatous testicular cancer: results from an EORTC multi-institutional phase III study. Int J Androl 1987; 10: 239–246.

482. Sledge GW Jr, Eble JN, Roth BJ, et al. Relation of proliferative activity to survival in patients with advanced germ cell cancer. Cancer Res 1988; 48: 3864–3868.

483. Teilum G. Gonocytoma: homologous ovarian and testicular tumors I, with discussion of 'mesonephroma ovarii' (Schiller. Am J Cancer 1939). Acta Pathol Microbiol Scand 1946; 23: 242–251.

484. Teilum G. 'Mesonephroma ovarii' (Schiller) – an extra-embryonic mesoblastoma of germ cell origin in the ovary and the testis. Acta Pathol Microbiol Scand 1950; 27: 249–261.

485. Teilum G. Endodermal sinus tumors of the ovary and testis. comparative morphogenesis of the so-called mesonephroma ovarii (Schiller) and extraembryonic (yolk sac-allantoic) structures of the rat's placenta. Cancer 1959; 12: 1092–1105.

486. Pohl HG, Shukla AR, Metcalf PD, et al. Prepubertal testis tumors: actual prevalence rate of histological types. J Urol 2004; 172: 2370–2372.

487. Kaplan GW, Cromie WC, Kelalis PP, et al. Prepubertal yolk sac testicular tumors – report of the testicular tumor registry. J Urol 1988; 140: 1109–1112.

488. Brosman SA. Testicular tumors in prepubertal children. Urology 1979; 13: 581–588.

489. Pierce GB, Bullock WK, Huntington RW. Yolk sac tumors of the testis. Cancer 1970; 25: 644–658.

490. Talerman A. Endodermal sinus (yolk sac) tumor elements in testicular germ-cell tumors in adults: comparison of prospective and retrospective studies. Cancer 1980; 46: 1213–1217.

491. Brown LM, Pottern LM, Hoover RN, et al. Testicular cancer in the United States: trends in incidence and mortality. Int J Epidemiol 1986; 15: 164–170.

492. Kuo JY, Hsieh YL, Chin TW, et al. Testicular yolk sac tumors in children. Chin Med J 1999; 62: 92–97.

493. Talerman A, Haije WG, Baggerman L. Serum alphafetoprotein (AFP) in patients with germ cell tumors of the gonads and extragonadal sites: correlation between endodermal sinus (yolk sac) tumor and raised serum AFP. Cancer 1980; 46: 380–385.

494. Jacobsen GK. Alpha-fetoprotein (AFP) and human chorionic gonadotropin (HCG) in testicular germ cell tumours. Acta Pathol Microbiol Immunol Scand [A] 1983; 91: 183–190.

495. Talerman A. Germ cell tumors. In: Talerman A, Roth LM, eds. Pathology of the testis and its adnexa. New York: Churchill Livingstone, 1986; 29–65.

496. Martinazzi M, Crivelli F, Zampatti C. Immunohistochemical study of hepatic and enteric structures in testicular endodermal sinus tumors. Bas Appl Histochem 1988; 32: 239–245.

497. Clement PB, Young RH, Scully RE. Endometrioid-like variant of ovarian yolk sac tumor. A clinicopathological analysis of eight cases. Am J Surg Pathol 1987; 11: 767–778.

498. Michael H, Lucia J, Foster RS, et al. The pathology of late recurrence of testicular germ cell tumors. Am J Surg Pathol 2000; 24: 257–273.

499. Teilum G. Special tumors of ovary and testis and related extragonadal lesions. Philadelphia: JB Lippincott, 1976.

500. Michael H, Ulbright TM, Brodhecker CA. The pluripotential nature of the mesenchyme-like component of yolk sac tumor. Arch Pathol Lab Med 1989; 113: 1115–1119.

501. Ulbright TM, Michael H, Loehrer PJ, et al. Spindle cell tumors resected from male patients with germ cell tumors. a clinicopathologic study of 14 cases. Cancer 1990; 65: 148–156.

502. Moran CA, Suster S. Yolk sac tumors of the mediastinum with prominent spindle cell features: a clinicopathologic study of three cases. Am J Surg Pathol 1997; 21: 1173–1177.

503. Teilum G. Classification of endodermal sinus tumor (mesoblastoma vitellinum) and so-called 'embryonal carcinoma' of the ovary. Acta Pathol Microbiol Scand 1965; 64: 407–429.

504. Jacobsen GK, Jacobsen M. Possible liver cell differentiation in testicular germ cell tumours. Histopathology 1983; 7: 537–548.

505. Nakashima N, Fukatsu T, Nagasaka T, et al. The frequency and histology of hepatic tissue in germ cell tumors. Am J Surg Pathol 1987; 11: 682–692.

506. Horie Y, Kato M. Hepatoid variant of yolk sac tumor of the testis. Pathol Int 2000; 50: 754–758.

507. Prat J, Bhan AK, Dickersin GR, et al. Hepatoid yolk sac tumor of the ovary (endodermal sinus tumor with hepatoid differentiation): a light microscopic, ultrastructural, and immunohistochemical study of seven cases. Cancer 1982; 50: 2355–2368.

508. Damjanov I, Amenta PS, Zarghami F. Transformation of an AFP-positive yolk sac carcinoma into an AFP-negative neoplasm: evidence for in vivo cloning of the human parietal yolk sac carcinoma. Cancer 1984; 53: 1902–1907.

509. Eglen DE, Ulbright TM. The differential diagnosis of yolk sac tumor and seminoma: usefulness of cytokeratin, alpha-fetoprotein, and alpha-1-antitrypsin immunoperoxidase reactions. Am J Clin Pathol 1987; 88: 328–332.

510. Miettinen M, Virtanen I, Talerman A. Intermediate filament proteins in human testis and testicular germ-cell tumors. Am J Pathol 1985; 120: 402–410.

511. Kommoss F, Oliva E, Bittinger F, et al. Inhibin-alpha CD99, HEA125, PLAP, and chromogranin immunoreactivity in testicular neoplasms and the androgen insensitivity syndrome. Hum Pathol 2000; 31: 1055–1061.

512. Fan Z, van de RM, Montgomery K, et al. Hep par 1 antibody stain for the differential diagnosis of hepatocellular carcinoma: 676 tumors tested using tissue microarrays and conventional tissue sections. Mod Pathol 2003; 16: 137–144.

513. Fujimoto J, Hata J, Ishii E, et al. Differentiation antigens defined by mouse monoclonal antibodies against human germ cell tumors. Lab Invest 1987; 57: 350–358.

514. Gonzalez-Crussi F, Roth LM. The human yolk sac and yolk sac carcinoma: an ultrastructural study. Hum Pathol 1976; 7: 675–691.

515. Nogales-Fernandez F, Silverberg SG, Bloustein PA, et al. Yolk sac carcinoma (endodermal sinus tumor): ultrastructure and histogenesis of gonadal and extragonadal tumors in comparison with normal human yolk sac. Cancer 1977; 39: 1462–1474.

516. Roth LM, Gillespie JJ. Pathology and ultrastructure of germinal neoplasia of the testis. In: Einhorn LH, ed. Testicular tumors: management and treatment. New York: Masson, 1980; 1–28.

517. Oosterhuis JW, Castedo SM, de Jong B, et al. Karyotyping and DNA flow cytometry of an orchidoblastoma. Cancer Genet Cytogenet 1988; 36: 7–11.

518. Vogelzang NJ, Bronson D, Savino D, et al. A human embryonal–yolk sac carcinoma model system in athymic mice. Cancer 1985; 55: 2584–2593.

519. Lawrence WD, Young RH, Scully RE. Juvenile granulosa cell tumor of the infantile testis. A report of 14 cases. Am J Surg Pathol 1985; 9: 87–94.

520. Wu JT, Book L, Sudar K. Serum alpha fetoprotein (AFP) levels in normal infants. Pediatr Res 1981; 15: 50–52.

521. Ulbright TM, Gersell DJ. Rete testis hyperplasia with hyaline globule formation. A lesion simulating yolk sac tumor. Am J Surg Pathol 1991; 15: 66–74.

522. Loehrer PJ Sr, Williams SD, Einhorn LH. Testicular cancer. the quest continues. J Natl Cancer Inst 1988; 80: 1373–1382.

523. Logothetis CJ, Samuels ML, Trindade A, et al. The prognostic significance of endodermal sinus tumor histology among patients treated for stage III nonseminomatous germ cell tumors of the testes. Cancer 1984; 53: 122–128.

524. Grady RW, Ross JH, Kay R. Patterns of metastatic spread in prepubertal yolk sac tumor of the testis. J Urol 1995; 153: 1259–1261.

525. Carroll WL, Kempson RL, Govan DE, et al. Conservative management of testicular endodermal sinus tumor in childhood. J Urol 1985; 13: 1011–1014.

526. Kramer SA. Pediatric urologic oncology. Urol Clin North Am 1985; 12: 31–42.

527. Marshall S, Lyon RP, Scott MP. A conservative approach to testicular tumors in children: 12 cases and their management. J Urol 1983; 129: 350–351.

528. Kaplan WE, Firlit CF. Treatment of testicular yolk sac carcinoma in the young child. J Urol 1981; 126: 663–664.

529. Liu HC, Liang DC, Chen SH, et al. The stage I yolk sac tumor of testis in children younger than 2 years: chemotherapy or not? Pediatr Hematol Oncol 1998; 15: 223–228.

530. Nseyo UO, Englander LS, Wajsman Z, et al. Histological patterns of treatment failures in testicular germ cell neoplasms. J Urol 1985; 133: 219–220.

531. Barsky SH. Germ cell tumors of the testis. In: Javadpour N, Barsky SH, eds. Surgical pathology of urologic diseases. Baltimore: Williams & Wilkins, 1987; 224–246.

532. Pugh RCB, Cameron KM. Teratoma. In: Pugh RCB, ed. Pathology of the testis. Oxford: Blackwell Scientific, 1976; 199–244.

533. Kooijman CD. Immature teratomas in children. Histopathology 1988; 12: 491–502.

534. Grady RW, Ross JH, Kay R. Epidemiological features of testicular teratoma in a prepubertal population. J Urol 1997; 158: 1191–1192.

535. Hasegawa T, Maeda K, Kamata N, et al. A case of immature teratoma originating in intra-abdominal undescended testis in a 3-month-old infant. Pediatr Surg Int 2006; 22: 570–572.

536. Kusuda L, Leidich RB, Das S. Mature teratoma of the testis metastasizing as mature teratoma. J Urol 1986; 135: 1020–1022.

537. Kedia K, Fraley EE. Adult teratoma of the testis metastasizing as adult teratoma: case report and review of literature. J Urol 1975; 114: 636–639.

538. Cameron-Strange A, Horner J. Differentiated teratoma of testis metastasizing as differentiated teratoma in adult. Urology 1989; 33: 481–482.

539. Wogalter H, Scofield GF. Adult teratoma of the testicle metastasizing as adult teratoma. J Urol 1962; 87: 573–576.

540. Simmonds PD, Lee AH, Theaker JM, et al. Primary pure teratoma of the testis. J Urol 1996; 155: 939–942.

541. Leibovitch I, Foster RS, Ulbright TM, et al. Adult primary pure teratoma of the testis. The Indiana experience. Cancer 1995; 75: 2244–2250.

542. Ulbright TM. Gonadal teratomas: a review and speculation. Adv Anat Pathol 2004; 11: 10–23.

543. Sella A, el Naggar A, Ro JY, et al. Evidence of malignant features in histologically mature teratoma. J Urol 1991; 146: 1025–1028.

544. Eble JN, Sauter G, Epstein JI, Sesterhenn IA (eds) Pathology and genetics of tumours of the urinary system and male genital organs. Lyon, France: IARC Press, 2004.

545. Trojanowski JQ, Hickey WF. Human teratomas express differentiated neural antigens: an immunohistochemical study with anti-neurofilament, anti-glial filament, and anti-myelin basic protein monoclonal antibodies. Am J Pathol 1984; 115: 383–389.

546. Oosterhuis JW, de Jong B, Cornelisse CJ, et al. Karyotyping and DNA flow cytometry of mature residual teratoma after intensive chemotherapy of disseminated nonseminomatous germ cell tumor of the testis. a report of two cases. Cancer Genet Cytogenet 1986; 22: 149–157.

547. Molenaar WM, Oosterhuis JW, Meiring A, et al. Histology and DNA contents of a secondary malignancy arising in a mature residual lesion six years after chemotherapy for a disseminated nonseminomatous testicular tumor. Cancer 1986; 58: 264–268.

548. van Echten J, van der Vloedt WS, van de Pol M, et al. Comparison of the chromosomal pattern of primary testicular nonseminomas and residual mature teratomas after chemotherapy. Cancer Genet Cytogenet 1997; 99: 59–67.

549. Shah KH, Maxted WC, Chun B. Epidermoid cysts of the testis: a report of three cases and an analysis of 141 cases from the world literature. Cancer 1981; 47: 577–582.

550. Price EB, Jr. Epidermoid cysts of the testis: a clinical and pathologic analysis of 69 cases from the testicular tumor registry. J Urol 1969; 102: 708–713.

551. Burt AD, Cooper G, MacKay C, et al. Dermoid cyst of the testis. Scott Med J 1987; 32: 146–148.

552. Dockerty MB, Priestly JT. Dermoid cysts of the testis. J Urol 1942; 48: 392–400.

553. Ulbright TM, Srigley JR. Dermoid cyst of the testis: a study of five postpubertal cases, including a pilomatrixoma-like variant, with evidence supporting its separate classification from mature testicular teratoma. Am J Surg Pathol 2001; 25: 788–793.

554. Dieckmann KP, Loy V. Epidermoid cyst of the testis: a review of clinical and histogenetic considerations. Br J Urol 1994; 73: 436–441.

555. Gao F, Maiti S, Alam N, et al. The Wilms' tumor gene, Wt1, is required for Sox9 expression and maintenance of tubular architecture in the developing testis. Proc Natl Acad Sci USA 2006; 103: 11987–11992.

556. Shukla AR, Woodard C, Carr MC, et al. Experience with testis sparing surgery for testicular teratoma. J Urol 2004; 171: 161–163.

557. Johnson DE, Bracken RB, Blight EM. Prognosis for pathologic Stage I non-seminomatous germ cell tumors of the testis managed by retroperitoneal lymphadenectomy. J Urol 1976; 116: 63–68.

558. Dixon FJ, Moore RA. Testicular tumors: a clinicopathologic study. Cancer 1953; 6: 427–454.

559. Michael H, Hull MT, Ulbright TM, et al. Primitive neuroectodermal tumors arising in testicular germ cell neoplasms. Am J Surg Pathol 1997; 21: 896–904.

560. Ganjoo KN, Foster RS, Michael H, et al. Germ cell tumor associated primitive neuroectodermal tumors. J Urol 2001; 165: 1514–1516.

561. Emerson RE, Ulbright TM, Zhang S, et al. Nephroblastoma arising in a germ cell tumor of testicular origin. Am J Surg Pathol 2004; 28: 687–692.

562. Michael H, Hull MT, Foster RS, et al. Nephroblastoma-like tumors in patients with testicular germ cell tumors. Am J Surg Pathol 1998; 22: 1107–1114.

563. Ulbright TM, Loehrer PJ, Roth LM, et al. The development of non-germ cell malignancies within germ cell tumors. A clinicopathologic study of 11 cases. Cancer 1984; 54: 1824–1833.

564. Mostofi FK. Histological change ostensibly induced by therapy in the metastasis of germ cell tumors of testis. Prog Clin Biol Res 1985; 203: 47–60.

565. Motzer RJ, Amsterdam A, Prieto V, et al. Teratoma with malignant transformation: diverse malignant histologies arising in men with germ cell tumors. J Urol 1998; 159: 133–138.

566. Comiter CV, Kibel AS, Richie JP, et al. Prognostic features of teratomas with malignant transformation: a clinicopathological study of 21 cases. J Urol 1998; 159: 859–863.

567. Ahmed T, Bosl GJ, Hajdu SI. Teratoma with malignant transformation in germ cell tumors in men. Cancer 1985; 56: 860–863.

568. Talerman A, Gratama S, Miranda S, et al. Primary carcinoid tumor of the testis: case report, ultrastructure and review of the literature. Cancer 1978; 42: 2696–2706.

569. Berdjis CC, Mostofi FK. Carcinoid tumors of the testis. J Urol 1977; 118: 777–782.

570. Zavala-Pompa A, Ro JY, El-Naggar A, et al. Primary carcinoid tumor of the testis: immunohistochemical, ultrastructural, and DNA flow cytometric study of three cases with a review of the literature. Cancer 1993; 72: 1726–1732.

571. Sullivan JL, Packer JT, Bryant M. Primary malignant carcinoid of the testis. Arch Pathol Lab Med 1981; 105: 515–517.

572. Kim HJ, Cho MY, Park YN, et al. Primary carcinoid tumor of the testis: immunohistochemical, ultrastructural and DNA flow cytometric study of two cases. J Korean Med Sci 1999; 14: 57–62.

573. Ordonez NG, Ayala AG, Sneige N, et al. Immunohistochemical demonstration of multiple neurohormonal polypeptides in a case of pure testicular carcinoid. Am J Clin Pathol 1982; 78: 860–864.

574. Ogawa A, Sugihara S, Nakazawa Y. A case of primary carcinoid tumor of the testis. Gan No Rinsho 1988; 34: 1629–1634.

575. Reyes A, Moran CA, Suster S, et al. Neuroendocrine carcinomas (carcinoid tumor) of the testis. A clinicopathologic and immunohistochemical study of ten cases. Am J Clin Pathol 2003; 120: 182–187.

576. Lewin KJ, Ulich T, Yang K, et al. The endocrine cells of the gastrointestinal tract: Tumors, part II. Pathol Annu 1986; 21: 181–215.

577. Ulbright TM, Young RH. Carcinoid tumor of the testis. Am J Clin Pathol 2004; 121: 297.

578. Ulbright TM, Amin MB, Young RH. Tumors of the testis, adenexa, spermatic cord and scrotum. In: Atlas of tumor pathology, Third series. Washington, DC: Armed Forces Institute of Pathology, 1999.

579. Merino J, Zuluaga A, Gutierrez-Tejero F, et al. Pure testicular carcinoid associated with intratubular germ cell neoplasia. J Clin Pathol 2005; 58: 1331–1333.

580. Aguirre P, Scully RE. Primitive neuroectodermal tumor of the testis. Report of a case. Arch Pathol Lab Med 1983; 107: 643–645.

581. Nocks BN, Dann JA. Primitive neuroectodermal tumor (immature teratoma) of testis. Urology 1983; 22: 543–544.

582. Nistal M, Paniagua R. Primary neuroectodermal tumour of the testis. Histopathology 1985; 9: 1351–1359.

583. Assaf G, Mosbah A, Homsy Y, et al. Dermoid cyst of testis in five-year-old-child. Urology 1983; 22: 432–434.

584. Gupta AK, Gupta MK, Gupta K. Dermoid cyst of the testis (a case report). Indian J Cancer 1986; 23: 21–23.

585. Kressel K, Schnell D, Thon WF, et al. Benign testicular tumors: a case for testis preservation? Eur Urol 1988; 15: 200–204.

586. Younger C, Gu J, Ulbright TM, et al. Loss of heterozygosity in epidermoid cysts of the testis. Mod Pathol 2001; 14: 130A.

587. Young RH, Talerman A. Testicular tumors other than germ cell tumors. Semin Diagn Pathol 1987; 4: 342–360.

588. Goldstein AM, Mendez R, Vargas A, et al. Epidermoid cysts of testis. Urology 1980; 15: 186–189.

589. Chhieng DC, Jennings TA, Slominski A, et al. Choriocarcinoma presenting as a cutaneous metastasis. J Cutan Pathol 1995; 22: 374–377.

590. Wang L, Pitman MB, Castillo CF, et al. Choriocarcinoma involving the pancreas as first manifestation of a metastatic regressing mixed testicular germ cell tumor. Mod Pathol 2004; 17: 1573–1580.

591. Giralt S, Dexeus F, Amato R, et al. Hyperthyroidism in men with germ cell tumors and high levels of beta-human chorionic gonadotropin. Cancer 1992; 69: 1286–1290.

592. Ulbright TM, Young RH, Scully RE. Trophoblastic tumors of the testis other than classic choriocarcinoma. 'monophasic' choriocarcinoma and placental site trophoblastic tumor. A report of two cases. Am J Surg Pathol 1997; 21: 282–288.

593. Manivel JC, Niehans G, Wick MR, et al. Intermediate trophoblast in germ cell neoplasms. Am J Surg Pathol 1987; 11: 693–701.

594. McCluggage WG, Ashe P, McBride H, et al. Localization of the cellular expression of inhibin in trophoblastic tissue. Histopathology 1998; 32: 252–256.

595. Pelkey TJ, Frierson HF Jr, Mills SE, et al. Detection of the alpha-subunit of inhibin in trophoblastic neoplasia. Hum Pathol 1999; 30: 26–31.

596. Lind HM, Haghighi P. Carcinoembryonic antigen staining in choriocarcinoma. Am J Clin Pathol 1986; 86: 538–540.

597. Clark RK, Damjanov I. Intermediate filaments of human trophoblast and choriocarcinoma cell lines. Virchows Arch [A] 1985; 407: 203–208.

598. Pierce GB Jr, Midgley AR Jr. The origin and function of human syncytiotrophoblastic giant cells. Am J Pathol 1963; 43: 153–173.

599. Motoyama T, Sasano N, Yonezawa S, et al. Early stage of development in testicular choriocarcinomas. Acta Pathol Jpn 1993; 43: 320–326.

600. Vaeth M, Schultz HP, von der Maase H, et al. Prognostic factors in testicular germ cell tumours: experiences with 1058 consecutive cases. Acta Radiol Oncol, 1984; 23: 271–285.

601. Bosl GJ, Geller NL, Cirrincione C, et al. Multivariate analysis of prognostic variables in patients with metastatic testicular cancer. Cancer Res 1983; 43: 3403–3407.

602. Stoter G, Sylvester R, Sleijfer DT, et al. A multivariate analysis of prognostic factors in disseminated non-seminomatous testicular cancer. Prog Clin Biol Res 1988; 269: 381–393.

603. Seguchi T, Iwasaki A, Sugao H, et al. Clinical statistics of germinal testicular cancer. Nippon Hinyokika Gakkai Zasshi 1990; 81: 889–894.

604. Brawn PN. The origin of germ cell tumors of the testis. Cancer 1983; 51: 1610–1614.

605. Okamoto T. A human vitelline component in embryonal carcinoma of the testis. Acta Pathol Jpn 1986; 36: 41–48.

606. Nakashima N, Murakami S, Fukatsu T, et al. Characteristics of 'embryoid body' in human gonadal germ cell tumors. Hum Pathol 1988; 19: 1144–1154.

607. Evans RW. Developmental stages of embryo-like bodies in teratoma testis. J Clin Pathol 1957; 10: 31–39.

608. Cardoso de Almeida PC, Scully RE. Diffuse embryoma of the testis. A distinctive form of mixed germ cell tumor. Am J Surg Pathol 1983; 7: 633–642.

609. de Peralta-Venturina MN, Ro JY, Ordonez NG, et al. Diffuse embryoma of the testis. An immunohistochemical study of two cases. Am J Clin Pathol 1994; 102: 402–405.

610. Brawn PN. The characteristics of embryonal carcinoma cells in teratocarcinomas. Cancer 1987; 59: 2042–2046.

611. Burt ME, Javadpour N. Germ-cell tumors in patients with apparently normal testes. Cancer 1981; 47: 1911–1915.

612. Meares EM Jr, Briggs EM. Occult seminoma of the testis masquerading as primary extragonadal germinal neoplasm. Cancer 1972; 30: 300–306.

613. Asif S, Uehling DT. Microscopic tumor foci in testes. J Urol 1968; 99: 776–779.

614. Bohle A, Studer UE, Sonntag RW, et al. Primary or secondary extragonadal germ cell tumors. J Urol 1986; 135: 939–943.

615. Bär W, Hedinger C. Comparison of histologic types of primary testicular germ cell tumors with their metastases: consequences for the WHO and the British Nomenclatures? Virchows Arch [A] 1976; 370: 41–54.

616. Heidenreich A, Moul JW, McLeod DG, et al. The role of retroperitoneal lymphadenectomy in mature teratoma of the testis. J Urol 1997; 157: 160–163.

617. Ulbright TM. Testis risk and prognostic factors. The pathologist's perspective. Urol Clin North Am 1999; 26: 611–626.

618. Fossä SD, Aass N, Ous S, et al. Histology of tumor residuals following

chemotherapy in patients with advanced nonseminomatous testicular cancer. J Urol 1989; 142: 1239–1242.

619. Cheng L. Establishing a germ cell origin for metastatic tumors using OCT4 immunohistochemistry. Cancer 2004; 101: 2006–2010.

620. Moran CA, Travis WD, Carter D, et al. Metastatic mature teratoma in lung following testicular embryonal carcinoma and teratocarcinoma. Arch Pathol Lab Med 1993; 117: 641–644.

621. Davey DD, Ulbright TM, Loehrer PJ, et al. The significance of atypia within teratomatous metastases after chemotherapy for malignant germ cell tumors. Cancer 1987; 59: 533–539.

622. Jeffery GM, Theaker JM, Lee AH, et al. The growing teratoma syndrome. Br J Urol 1991; 67: 195–202.

623. Gelderman WA, Scraffordt Koops H, Sleijfer DT, et al. Late recurrence of mature teratoma in nonseminomatous testicular tumors after PVB chemotherapy and surgery. Urology 1989; 33: 10–14.

624. Logothetis CJ, Samuels ML, Trindade A. The growing teratoma syndrome. Cancer 1982; 50: 1629–1635.

625. Tongaonkar HB, Deshmane VH, Dalal AV, et al. Growing teratoma syndrome. J Surg Oncol 1994; 55: 56–60.

626. Looijenga LH, Oosterhuis JW, Ramaekers FC, et al. Dual parameter flow cytometry for deoxyribonucleic acid and intermediate filament proteins of residual mature teratoma. All tumor cells are aneuploid. Lab Invest 1991; 64: 113–117.

627. Mazur MT, Lurain JR, Brewer JI. Fatal gestational choriocarcinoma: clinicopathologic study of patients treated at a trophoblastic disease center. Cancer 1982; 50: 1833–1846.

628. Ulbright TM, Loehrer PJ. Choriocarcinoma-like lesions in patients with testicular germ cell tumors. Two histologic variants. Am J Surg Pathol 1988; 12: 531–541.

629. Ulbright TM, Henley JD, Cummings OW, et al. Cystic trophoblastic tumor: a nonaggressive lesion in postchemotherapy resections of patients with testicular germ cell tumors. Am J Surg Pathol 2004; 28: 1212–1216.

630. Donohue JP, Roth LM, Zachary JM, et al. Cytoreductive surgery for metastatic testis cancer: tissue analysis of retroperitoneal masses after chemotherapy. J Urol 1982; 127: 1111–1114.

631. Bracken RB, Johnson DE, Frazier OH, et al. The role of surgery following chemotherapy in Stage III germ cell neoplasms. J Urol 1983; 129: 39–43.

632. Einhorn LH, Williams SD, Mandelbaum I, et al. Surgical resection in disseminated testicular cancer following chemotherapeutic cytoreduction. Cancer 1981; 48: 904–908.

633. Vugrin D, Whitmore WF Jr, Sogani PC, et al. Combined chemotherapy and surgery in treatment of advanced germ-cell tumors. Cancer 1981; 47: 2228–2231.

634. Cagini L, Nicholson AG, Horwich A, et al. Thoracic metastasectomy for germ cell tumours. long term survival and prognostic factors. Ann Oncol 1998; 9: 1185–1191.

635. Fox EP, Weathers TD, Williams SD, et al. Outcome analysis for patients with persistent nonteratomatous germ cell tumor in postchemotherapy retroperitoneal lymph node dissections. J Clin Oncol 1993; 11: 1294–1299.

636. Kim I, Young RH, Scully RE. Leydig cell tumors of the testis. A clinicopathological analysis of 40 cases and review of the literature. Am J Surg Pathol 1985; 9: 177–192.

637. Kaplan GW, Cromie WJ, Kelalis PP, et al. Gonadal stromal tumors: a report of the Prepubertal Testicular Tumor Registry. J Urol 1986; 136: 300–302.

638. Dilworth JP, Farrow GM, Oesterling JE. Non-germ cell tumors of testis. Urology 1991; 37: 399–417.

639. Wheeler JE. Anatomy, embryology, and physiology of the testis and its ducts. In: Hill GS, ed. Uropathology. New York: Churchill-Livingstone, 1989; 935–954.

640. Drut R, Wludarski S, Segatelli V, et al. Leydig cell tumor of the testis with histological and immunohistochemical features of malignancy in a 1-year-old boy with isosexual pseudoprecocity. Int J Surg Pathol 2006; 14: 344–348.

641. Dieckmann KP, Loy V. Metachronous germ cell and Leydig cell tumors of the testis: do testicular germ cell tumors and Leydig cell tumors share common etiologic factors? Cancer 1993; 72: 1305–1307.

642. Bokemeyer C, Kuczyk M, Schoffski P, et al. Familial occurrence of Leydig cell tumors. a report of a case in a father and his adult son. J Urol 1993; 150: 1509–1510.

643. Carvajal-Carmona LG, Alam NA, Pollard PJ, et al. Adult Leydig cell tumors of the testis caused by germline fumarate hydratase mutations. J Clin Endocrinol Metab 2006; 91: 3071–3075.

644. Canto P, Soderlund D, Ramon G, et al. Mutational analysis of the luteinizing hormone receptor gene in two individuals with Leydig cell tumors. Am J Med Genet 2002; 108: 148–152.

645. Richter-Unruh A, Wessels HT, Menken U, et al. Male LH-independent sexual precocity in a 3.5-year-old boy caused by a somatic activating mutation of the LH receptor in a Leydig cell tumor. J Clin Endocrinol Metab 2002; 87: 1052–1056.

646. Liu G, Duranteau L, Carel JC, et al. Leydig-cell tumors caused by an activating mutation of the gene encoding the luteinizing hormone receptor. N Engl J Med 1999; 341: 1731–1736.

647. Billings SD, Roth LM, Ulbright TM. Microcystic Leydig cell tumors mimicking yolk sac tumor: a report of four cases. Am J Surg Pathol 1999; 23: 546–551.

648. Ulbright TM, Srigley JR, Hatzianastassiou DK, et al. Leydig cell tumors of the testis with unusual features. Adipose differentiation, calcification with ossification, and spindle-shaped tumor cells. Am J Surg Pathol 2002; 26: 1424–1433.

649. Santonja C, Varona C, Burgos FJ, et al. Leydig cell tumor of testis with adipose metaplasia. Appl Pathol 1989; 7: 201–204.

650. Minkowitz S, Soloway H, Soscia J. Ossifying interstitial cell tumor of the testes. J Urol 1965; 94: 592–595.

651. Balsitis M, Sokal M. Ossifying malignant Leydig (interstitial) cell tumour of the testis. Histopathology 1990; 16: 599–601.

652. Iczkowski KA, Bostwick DG, Roche PC, et al. Inhibin A is a sensitive and specific marker for testicular sex cord–stromal tumors. Mod Pathol 1998; 11: 774–779.

653. McCluggage WG, Shanks JH, Whiteside C, et al. Immunohistochemical study of testicular sex cord–stromal tumors, including staining with anti-inhibin antibody. Am J Surg Pathol 1998; 22: 615–619.

654. Busam KJ, Iversen K, Coplan KA, et al. Immunoreactivity for A103, an antibody to melan-A (Mart-1), in adrenal cortical and other steroid tumors. Am J Surg Pathol 1998; 22: 57–63.

655. Augusto D, Leteurtre E, De La TA, et al. Calretinin. a valuable marker of normal and neoplastic Leydig cells of the testis. Appl Immunohistochem Mol Morphol 2002; 10: 159–162.

656. McCluggage WG, Shanks JH, Arthur K, et al. Cellular proliferation and nuclear ploidy assessments augment established prognostic factors in predicting malignancy in testicular Leydig cell tumours. Histopathology 1998; 33: 361–368.

657. Hekimgil M, Altay B, Yakut BD, et al. Leydig cell tumor of the testis: comparison of histopathological and immunohistochemical features of three azoospermic cases and one malignant case. Pathol Int 2001; 51: 792–796.

658. Miettinen M, Wahlstrom T, Virtanen I, et al. Cellular differentiation in ovarian sex-cord–stromal and germ-cell tumors studied with antibodies to intermediate filament proteins. Am J Surg Pathol 1985; 9: 640–651.

659. Descheemaeker T, Fontaine P, Racadot A, et al. Enkephalin-like immunoreactivity in Leydig cell tumor. Ann Endocrinol (Paris) 1989; 50: 513–516.

660. Kay S, Fu Y-S, Koontz WW, et al. Interstitial-cell tumor of the testis: tissue culture and ultrastructural studies. Am J Clin Pathol 1975; 63: 366–376.

661. Sohval AR, Churg J, Suzuki Y, et al. Electron microscopy of a feminizing

Leydig cell tumor of the testis. Hum Pathol 1977; 8: 621–634.

662. Sohval AR, Churg J, Gabrilove JL, et al. Ultrastructure of feminizing testicular Leydig cell tumors. Ultrastruct Pathol 1982; 3: 335–345.

663. Grem JL, Robins HI, Wilson KS, et al. Metastatic Leydig cell tumor of the testis. Report of three cases and review of the literature. Cancer 1986; 58: 2116–2119.

664. Thomas JC, Ross JH, Kay R. Stromal testis tumors in children: a report from the prepubertal testis tumor registry. J Urol 2001; 166: 2338–2340.

665. Cheville JC, Sebo TJ, Lager DJ, et al. Leydig cell tumor of the testis: a clinicopathologic, DNA content, and MIB-1 comparison of nonmetastasizing and metastasizing tumors. Am J Surg Pathol 1998; 22: 1361–1367.

666. Bhatia-Gaur R, Donjacour AA, Sciavolino PJ, et al. Roles for Nkx3.1 in prostate development and cancer. Genes Dev 1999; 13: 966–977.

667. Mosharafa AA, Foster RS, Bihrle R, et al. Does retroperitoneal lymph node dissection have a curative role for patients with sex cord–stromal testicular tumors? Cancer 2003; 98: 753–757.

668. Naughton CK, Nadler RB, Basler JW, et al. Leydig cell hyperplasia. Br J Urol 1998; 81: 282–289.

669. Rutgers JL, Young RH, Scully RE. The testicular 'tumor' of the adrenogenital syndrome. A report of six cases and review of the literature on testicular masses in patients with adrenal cortical disorders. Am J Surg Pathol 1988; 12: 503–513.

670. Srikanth MS, West BR, Ishitani M, et al. Benign testicular tumors in children with congenital adrenal hyperplasia. J Pediatr Surg 1992; 27: 639–641.

671. Johnson RE, Scheithauer B. Massive hyperplasia of testicular adrenal rests in a patient with Nelson's syndrome. Am J Clin Pathol 1982; 77: 501–507.

672. Proppe KH, Dickersin GR. Large-cell calcifying Sertoli cell tumor of the testis: light microscopic and ultrastructural study. Hum Pathol 1982; 13: 1109–1114.

673. Tetu B, Ro JY, Ayala AG. Large cell calcifying Sertoli cell tumor of the testis: a clinicopathologic, immunohistochemical, and ultrastructural study of two cases. Am J Clin Pathol 1991; 96: 717–722.

674. Sato K, Ueda Y, Sakurai A, et al. Large cell calcifying Sertoli cell tumor of the testis: comparative immunohistochemical study with Leydig cell tumor. Pathol Int 2005; 55: 366–371.

675. Borer JG, Tan PE, Diamond DA. The spectrum of Sertoli cell tumors in children. Urol Clin North Am 2000; 27: 529–541.

676. Wheeler JE. Testicular tumors. In: Hill GS, ed. Uropathology. New York: Churchill Livingstone, 1989; 1047–1100.

677. Jacobsen GK. Malignant Sertoli cell tumors of the testis. J Urol Pathol 1993; 1: 233–255.

678. Gilcrease MZ, Delgado R, Albores-Saavedra J. Testicular Sertoli cell tumor with a heterologous sarcomatous component. immunohistochemical assessment of Sertoli cell differentiation. Arch Pathol Lab Med 1998; 122: 907–911.

679. Amin MB, Young RH, Scully RE. Immunohistochemical profile of Sertoli and Leydig cell tumors of the testis. [Abstract] Mod Pathol 1998; 11: 76A.

680. Comperat E, Tissier F, Boye K, et al. Non-Leydig sex-cord tumors of the testis. The place of immunohistochemistry in diagnosis and prognosis. A study of twenty cases. Virchows Arch 2004; 444: 567–571.

681. Harms D, Kock LR. Testicular juvenile granulosa cell and Sertoli cell tumours: a clinicopathological study of 29 cases from the Kiel Paediatric Tumour Registry. Virchows Arch 1997; 430: 301–309.

682. Rey R, Sabourin JC, Venara M, et al. Anti-mullerian hormone is a specific marker of sertoli- and granulosa-cell origin in gonadal tumors. Hum Pathol 2000; 31: 1202–1208.

683. Able ME, Lee JC. Ultrastructure of a Sertoli-cell adenoma of the testis. Cancer 1969; 23: 481–486.

684. Tavassoli FA, Norris HJ. Sertoli cell tumors of the ovary: a clinicopathologic study of 28 cases with ultrastructural observations. Cancer 1980; 46: 2281–2297.

685. Waxman M, Damjanov I, Khapra A, et al. Large cell calcifying Sertoli tumor of the testis. Light microscopic and ultrastructural study. Cancer 1984; 54: 1574–1581.

686. Horn T, Jao W, Keh PC. Large-cell calcifying Sertoli cell tumor of the testis: a case report with ultrastructural study. Ultrastruct Pathol 1983; 4: 359–364.

687. Kolon TF, Hochman HI. Malignant Sertoli cell tumor in a prepubescent boy. J Urol 1997; 158: 608–609.

688. Rosvoll R, Woodard JR. Malignant Sertoli cell tumor of the testis. Cancer 1968; 22: 8–13.

689. Talerman A. Malignant Sertoli cell tumor of the testis. Cancer 1971; 28: 446–454.

690. Morin LJ, Loening S. Malignant androblastoma (Sertoli cell tumor) of the testis: a case report with a review of the literature. J Urol 1975; 114: 476–480.

691. Koppikar DD, Sirsat MV. A malignant Sertoli cell tumor of the testis. Br J Urol 1973; 45: 213–217.

692. O'Dowd J, Gaffney EF, Young RH. Malignant sex cord stromal tumour in a patient with androgen insensitivity syndrome. Histopathology 1990; 16: 279–282.

693. Riemersma SA, Oudejans JJ, Vonk MJ, et al. High numbers of tumour-infiltrating activated cytotoxic T lymphocytes, and frequent loss of HLA class I and II expression, are features of aggressive B cell lymphomas of the brain and testis. J Pathol 2005; 206: 328–336.

694. Zukerberg LR, Young RH, Scully RE. Sclerosing Sertoli cell tumor of the testis: a report of 10 cases. Am J Surg Pathol 1991; 15: 829–834.

695. Anderson GA. Sclerosing Sertoli cell tumor of the testis: a distinct histological subtype. J Urol 1995; 154: 1756–1758.

696. Gravas S, Papadimitriou K, Kyriakidis A. Sclerosing sertoli cell tumor of the testis – a case report and review of the literature. Scand J Urol Nephrol 1999; 33: 197–199.

697. Abbas F, Bashir NW, Hussainy AS. Sclerosing Sertoli cell tumor of the testis. J Coll Phys Surg Pakistan 2005; 15: 437–438.

698. Giglio M, Medica M, De Rose AF, et al. Testicular sertoli cell tumours and relative subtypes. Analysis of clinical and prognostic features. Urol Int 2003; 70: 205–210.

699. Washecka R, Dresner MI, Honda SA. Testicular tumors in Carney's complex. J Urol 2002; 167: 1299–1302.

700. Plata C, Algaba F, Andujar M, et al. Large cell calcifying Sertoli cell tumour of the testis. Histopathology 1995; 26: 255–259.

701. Noszian IM, Balon R, Eitelberger FG, et al. Bilateral testicular large-cell calcifying sertoli cell tumor and recurrent cardiac myxoma in a patient with Carney's complex. Pediatr Radiol 1995; 25: S236–S237.

702. Blix GW, Levine LA, Goldberg R, et al. Large cell calcifying Sertoli cell tumor of the testis. Scand J Urol Nephrol 1992; 26: 73–75.

703. Carney JA, Gordon H, Carpenter PC, et al. The complex of myxomas, spotty pigmentation, and endocrine overactivity. Medicine 1985; 64: 270–283.

704. Carney JA. Psammomatous melanotic schwannoma: a distinctive, heritable tumor with special associations, including cardiac myxoma and the Cushing syndrome. Am J Surg Pathol 1990; 14: 206–222.

705. Carney JA, Toorkey BC. Myxoid fibroadenoma and allied conditions (myxomatosis) of the breast: a heritable disorder with special associations including cardiac and cutaneous myxomas. Am J Surg Pathol 1991; 15: 713–721.

706. Perez-Atayde AR, Nunez AE, Carroll WL, et al. Large-cell calcifying Sertoli cell tumor of the testis. An ultrastructural, immunocytochemical, and biochemical study. Cancer 1983; 51: 2287–2292.

707. De Raeve H, Schoonooghe P, Wibowo R, et al. Malignant large cell calcifying Sertoli cell tumor of the testis. Pathol Res Pract 2003; 199: 113–117.

708. Cano-Valdez AM, Chanona-Vilchis J, Dominguez-Malagon H. Large cell

calcifying Sertoli cell tumor of the testis: a clinicopathological, immunohistochemical, and ultrastructural study of two cases. Ultrastruct Pathol 1999; 23: 259–265.

709. Bufo P, Pennella A, Serio G, et al. Malignant large cell calcifying Sertoli cell tumor of the testis (LCCSCTT). Report of a case in an elderly man and review of the literature. Pathologica 1999; 91: 107–114.

710. Young S, Gooneratne S, Straus FH, et al. Feminizing Sertoli cell tumors in boys with Peutz-Jeghers syndrome. Am J Surg Pathol 1995; 19: 50–58.

711. Düe W, Dieckmann KP, Niedobitek G, et al. Testicular sex cord stromal tumour with granulosa cell differentiation: detection of steroid hormone receptors as a possible basis for tumour development and therapeutic management. J Clin Pathol 1990; 43: 732–737.

712. Gaylis FD, August C, Yeldandi A, et al. Granulosa cell tumor of the adult testis: ultrastructural and ultrasonographic characteristics. J Urol 1989; 141: 126–127.

713. Talerman A. Pure granulosa cell tumour of the testis. Report of a case and review of the literature. Appl Pathol 1985; 3: 117–122.

714. Nistal M, Läzaro R, Garcïa J, et al. Testicular granulosa cell tumor of the adult type. Arch Pathol Lab Med 1992; 116: 284–287.

715. Matoska J, Ondrus D, Talerman A. Malignant granulosa cell tumor of the testis associated with gynecomastia and long survival. Cancer 1992; 69: 1769–1772.

716. Jimenez-Quintero LP, Ro JY, Zavala-Pompa A, et al. Granulosa cell tumor of the adult testis: a clinicopathologic study of seven cases and a review of the literature. Hum Pathol 1993; 24: 1120–1126.

717. Al Bozom IA, El Faqih SR, Hassan SH, et al. Granulosa cell tumor of the adult type: a case report and review of the literature of a very rare testicular tumor. Arch Pathol Lab Med 2000; 124: 1525–1528.

718. Chadha S, van der Kwast TH. Immunohistochemistry of ovarian granulosa cell tumours: the value of tissue specific proteins and tumour markers. Virchows Arch [A] 1989; 414: 439–445.

719. Morgan DR, Brame KG. Granulosa cell tumour of the testis displaying immunoreactivity for inhibin. BJU Int 1999; 83: 731–732.

720. Nistal M, Redondo E, Paniagua R. Juvenile granulosa cell tumor of the testis. Arch Pathol Lab Med 1988; 112: 1129–1132.

721. Pinto MM. Juvenile granulosa cell tumor of the infant testis: case report with ultrastructural observations. Pediatr Pathol 1985; 4: 277–289.

722. Chan YF, Restall P, Kimble R. Juvenile granulosa cell tumor of the testis:

report of two cases in newborns. J Pediatr Surg 1997; 32: 752–753.

723. Perez-Atayde AR, Joste N, Mulhern H. Juvenile granulosa cell tumor of the infantile testis. Evidence of a dual epithelial–smooth muscle differentiation. Am J Surg Pathol 1996; 20: 72–79.

724. Fidda N, Weeks DA. Juvenile granulosa cell tumor of the testis: a case presenting as a small round cell tumor of childhood. Ultrastruct Pathol 2003; 27: 451–455.

725. Raju U, Fine G, Warrier R, et al. Congenital testicular juvenile granulosa cell tumor in a neonate with X/XY mosaicism. Am J Surg Pathol 1986; 10: 577–583.

726. Tanaka Y, Sasaki Y, Tachibana K, et al. Testicular juvenile granulosa cell tumor in an infant with X/XY mosaicism clinically diagnosed as true hermaphroditism. Am J Surg Pathol 1994; 18: 316–322.

727. Goswitz JJ, Pettinato G, Manivel JC. Testicular sex cord–stromal tumors in children: clinicopathologic study of sixteen children with review of the literature. Pediatr Pathol Lab Med 1996; 16: 451–470.

728. Shukla AR, Huff DS, Canning DA, et al. Juvenile granulosa cell tumor of the testis: contemporary clinical management and pathological diagnosis. J Urol 2004; 171: 1900–1902.

729. Groisman GM, Dische MR, Fine EM, et al. Juvenile granulosa cell tumor of the testis: a comparative immunohistochemical study with normal infantile gonads. Pediatr Pathol 1993; 13: 389–400.

730. Jones MA, Young RH, Scully RE. Benign fibromatous tumors of the testis and paratesticular region: a report of 9 cases with a proposed classification of fibromatous tumors and tumor-like lesions. Am J Surg Pathol 1997; 21: 296–305.

731. Lawrence WD, Young RH, Scully RE. Sex cord–stromal tumors. In: Talerman A, Roth LM, eds. Pathology of the testis and its adnexa. New York: Churchill Livingstone, 1986; 67–92.

732. de Pinieux G, Glaser C, Chatelain D, et al. Testicular fibroma of gonadal stromal origin with minor sex cord elements: clinicopathologic and immunohistochemical study of 2 cases. Arch Pathol Lab Med 1999; 123: 391–394.

733. Tarjan M, Sarkissov G, Tot T, et al. Unclassified sex cord/gonadal stromal testis tumor with predominance of spindle cells. APMIS 2006; 114: 465–469.

734. Renshaw AA, Gordon M, Corless CL. Immunohistochemistry of unclassified sex cord–stromal tumors of the testis with a predominance of spindle cells. Mod Pathol 1997; 10: 693–700.

735. Oosterhuis JW, Castedo SM, de Jong B, et al. A malignant mixed gonadal stromal tumor of the testis with

heterologous components and i(12p) in one of its metastases. Cancer Genet Cytogenet 1989; 41: 105–114.

736. Miettinen M, Salo J, Virtanen I. Testicular stromal tumor. Ultrastructural, immunohistochemical, and gel electrophoretic evidence of epithelial differentiation. Ultrastruct Pathol 1986; 10: 515–528.

737. Greco MA, Feiner HD, Theil KS, et al. Testicular stromal tumor with myofilaments: ultrastructural comparison with normal gonadal stroma. Hum Pathol 1984; 15: 238–243.

738. Evans HL. Unusual gonadal stromal tumor of the testis. Case report with ultrastructural observations. Arch Pathol Lab Med 1977; 101: 317–320.

739. Nistal M, Puras A, Perna C, et al. Fusocellular gonadal stromal tumour of the testis with epithelial and myoid differentiation. Histopathology 1996; 29: 259–264.

740. Eble JN, Hull MT, Warfel KA, et al. Malignant sex cord–stromal tumor of testis. J Urol 1984; 131: 546–550.

741. Ishida T, Tagatz GE, Okagaki T. Gonadoblastoma: ultrastructural evidence for testicular origin. Cancer 1976; 37: 1770–1781.

742. Roth LM, Eglen DE. Gonadoblastoma: immunohistochemical and ultrastructural observations. Int J Gynecol Pathol 1989; 8: 72–81.

743. Scully RE. Gonadoblastoma. A review of 74 cases. Cancer 1970; 25: 1340–1356.

744. Hussong J, Crussi FG, Chou PM. Gonadoblastoma: an immunohistochemical localization of mullerian-inhibiting substance, inhibin, WT-1 and p53. Mod Pathol 1997; 10: 1101–1105.

745. Iezzoni JC, von Kap-Herr C, Golden WL, et al. Gonadoblastomas in 45,X/46,XY mosaicism: analysis of chromosome distribution by fluorescence in situ hybridization. Am J Clin Pathol 1997; 108: 197–201.

746. Tsuchiya K, Reijo R, Page DC, et al. Gonadoblastoma: molecular definition of the susceptibility region on the Y chromosome. Am J Hum Genet 1995; 57: 1400–1407.

747. Salo P, Kaariainen H, Petrovic V, et al. Molecular mapping of the putative gonadoblastoma locus on the Y-chromosome. Genes Chromosomes Cancer 1995; 14: 210–214.

748. Lau Y, Chou P, Iezzoni J, et al. Expression of a candidate gene for the gonadoblastoma locus in gonadoblastoma and testicular seminoma. Cytogenet Cell Genet 2000; 91: 160–164.

749. Kersemaekers AM, Honecker F, Stoop H, et al. Identification of germ cells at risk for neoplastic transformation in gonadoblastoma. An immunohistochemical study for OCT3/4 and TSPY. Hum Pathol 2005; 36: 512–521.

750. Cummings OW, Henley JD, Vance G, et al. Gonadoblastoma in the scrotal testis of phenotypically normal males with germ cell tumors: fact or fantasy? Mod Pathol 2002; 15: 158A–159A.

751. Matoska J, Talerman A. Mixed germ cell-sex cord stroma tumor of the testis. A report with ultrastructural findings. Cancer 1989; 64: 2146–2153.

752. Ulbright TM, Srigley JR, Reuter VE, et al. Sex cord–stromal tumors of the testis with entrapped germ cells: a lesion mimicking unclassified mixed germ cell sex cord–stromal tumors. Am J Surg Pathol 2000; 24: 535–542.

753. Michal M, Vanecek T, Sima R, et al. Mixed germ cell sex cord–stromal tumors of the testis and ovary. Morphological, immunohistochemical, and molecular genetic study of seven cases. Virchows Arch 2006; 448: 612–622.

754. Ulbright TM, Young RH. Reply: mixed germ cell sex cord–stromal tumors of the testis and ovary. Virchows Arch. 450, 131–132. 2007.

755. Axiotis CA. Intratesticular serous papillary cystadenoma of low malignant potential: an ultrastructural and immunohistochemical study suggesting mullerian differentiation. Am J Surg Pathol 1988; 12: 56–63.

756. Young RH, Scully RE. Testicular and paratesticular tumors and tumor-like lesions of ovarian common epithelial and mullerian types. A report of four cases and review of the literature. Am J Clin Pathol 1986; 86: 146–152.

757. De Nictolis M, Tommasoni S, Fabris G, et al. Intratesticular serous cystadenoma of borderline malignancy. A pathological, histochemical and DNA content study of a case with long-term follow-up. Virchows Arch [A] 1993; 423: 221–225.

758. Ulbright TM, Young RH. Primary mucinous tumors of the testis and paratestis. Mod Pathol 2002; 15: 184A–185A.

759. Shimbo M, Araki K, Kaibuchi T, et al. Mucinous cystadenoma of the testis. J Urol 2004; 172: 146–147.

760. Teo CH, Chua WJ, Consigliere DT, et al. Primary intratesticular mucinous cystadenocarcinoma. Pathology 2005; 37: 92–94.

761. Brennan MK, Srigley JR. Brenner tumor of the testis: case report and review of other intrascrotal examples. J Urol Pathol 2002; 10: 219–228.

762. Caccamo D, Socias M, Truchet C. Malignant Brenner tumor of the testis and epididymis. Arch Pathol Lab Med 1991; 115: 524–527.

763. Goldman RL. A Brenner tumor of the testis. Cancer 1970; 26: 853–856.

764. Remmele W, Kaiserling E, Zerban U, et al. Serous papillary cystic tumor of borderline malignancy with focal carcinoma arising in testis: case report with immunohistochemical and ultrastructural observations. Hum Pathol 1992; 23: 75–79.

765. Cabay RJ, Siddiqui NH, Alam S. Paratesticular papillary mesothelioma: a case with borderline features. Arch Pathol Lab Med 2006; 130: 90–92.

766. Jones MA, Young RH, Scully RE. Malignant mesothelioma of the tunica vaginalis: a clinicopathologic analysis of 11 cases with review of the literature. Am J Surg Pathol 1995; 19: 815–825.

767. Winstanley AM, Landon G, Berney DM, et al. The immunocytochemical profile of malignant mesotheliomas of the tunica vaginalis: a study of 20 cases. Am J Surg Pathol 2006; 30: 1–6.

768. Ch TA, Tsampoulas C, Giannakopoulos X, et al. Solitary fibrous tumour of the epididymis. MRI features. Br J Radiol 2005; 78: 565–568.

769. Nochomovitz LE, Orenstein JM. Adenocarcinoma of the rete testis: review and regrouping of reported cases and a consideration of miscellaneous entities. J Urogenit Pathol 1991; 1: 11–40.

770. Jones EC, Murray SK, Young RH. Cysts and epithelial proliferations of the testicular collecting system (including rete testis). Semin Diagn Pathol 2000; 17: 270–293.

771. Perimenis P, Athanasopoulos A, Speakman M. Primary adenocarcinoma of the rete testis. Int Urol Nephrol 2003; 35: 373–374.

772. Visscher DW, Talerman A, Rivera LR, et al. Adenocarcinoma of the rete testis with a spindle cell component. A possible metaplastic carcinoma. Cancer 1989; 64: 770–775.

773. Nochomovitz LE, Orenstein JM. Adenocarcinoma of the rete testis. Case report, ultrastructural observations, and clinicopathologic correlates. Am J Surg Pathol 1984; 8: 625–634.

774. Gorini G, Pinelli M, Sforza V, et al. Mesothelioma of the tunica vaginalis testis: report of 2 cases with asbestos occupational exposure. Int J Surg Pathol 2005; 13: 211–214.

775. Altaffer LF III, Dufour DR, Castleberry GM, et al. Coexisting rete testis adenoma and gonadoblastoma. J Urol 1982; 127: 332–335.

776. Gupta RK. Benign papillary tumor of the rete testis. Indian J Cancer 1974; 11: 480–481.

777. Yadav SB, Patil PN, Karkhanis RB. Primary tumors of the spermatic cord, epididymis, and rete testis. J Postgrad Med 1969; 15: 49–52.

778. Janane A, Ghadouane M, Alami M, et al. Paratesticular adenofibroma. Scand J Urol Nephrol 2003; 37: 179–180.

779. Fridman E, Skarda J, Ofek-Moravsky E, et al. Complex multilocular cystic lesion of rete testis, accompanied by smooth muscle hyperplasia, mimicking intratesticular Leydig cell neoplasm. Virchows Arch 2005; 447: 768–771.

780. Hartwick RW, Ro JY, Srigley JR, et al. Adenomatous hyperplasia of the rete testis. A clinicopathologic study of nine cases. Am J Surg Pathol 1991; 15: 350–357.

781. Nistal M, Castillo MC, Regadera J, et al. Adenomatous hyperplasia of the rete testis. A review and report of new cases. Histol Histopathol 2003; 18: 741–752.

782. Nistal M, Regadera J, Paniagua R. Cystic dysplasia of the testis: light and electron microscopic study of three cases. Arch Pathol Lab Med 1984; 108: 579–583.

783. Camassei FD, Francalanci P, Ferro F, et al. Cystic dysplasia of the rete testis: report of two cases and review of the literature. Pediatr Dev Pathol 2002; 5: 206–210.

784. Ferry JA, Harris NL, Young RH, et al. Malignant lymphoma of the testis, epididymis, and spermatic cord. A clinicopathologic study of 69 cases with immunophenotypic analysis. Am J Surg Pathol 1994; 18: 376–390.

785. Martenson JA Jr, Buskirk SJ, Ilstrup DM, et al. Patterns of failure in primary testicular non-Hodgkin's lymphoma. J Clin Oncol 1988; 6: 297–302.

786. Baldetorp LA, Brunkvall J, Cavallin-Stähl E, et al. Malignant lymphoma of the testis. Br J Urol 1984; 56: 525–530.

787. Bentley RC, Devlin B, Kaufman RE, et al. Genotypic divergence precedes clinical dissemination in a case of synchronous bilateral B-cell malignant lymphoma of the testes. Hum Pathol 1993; 24: 675–678.

788. Doll DC, Weiss RB. Malignant lymphoma of the testis. Am J Med 1986; 81: 515–524.

789. Ferry JA, Ulbright TM, Young RH. Anaplastic large cell lymphoma presenting in the testis. J Urol Pathol 1997; 5: 139–147.

790. Hyland J, Lasota J, Jasinski M, et al. Molecular pathological analysis of testicular diffuse large cell lymphomas. Hum Pathol 1998; 29: 1231–1239.

791. Hasselblom S, Ridell B, Wedel H, et al. Testicular lymphoma – a retrospective, population-based, clinical and immunohistochemical study. Acta Oncol 2004; 43: 758–765.

792. Al-Abbadi MA, Hattab EM, Tarawneh MS, et al. Primary testicular diffuse large B-cell lymphoma belongs to the nongerminal center B-cell-like subgroup. A study of 18 cases. Mod Pathol 2006; 19: 1521–1527.

793. Lambrechts AC, Looijenga LH, van't Veer MB, et al. Lymphomas with testicular localisation show a consistent BCL-2 expression without a translocation (14; 18): a molecular and immunohistochemical study. Br J Cancer 1995; 71: 73–77.

794. Pileri SA, Sabattini E, Rosito P, et al. Primary follicular lymphoma of the testis in childhood: an entity with peculiar clinical and molecular characteristics. J Clin Pathol 2002; 55: 684–688.

795. Lu D, Medeiros J, Eskenazi AE, et al. Primary follicular large cell lymphoma of the testis in a child. Arch Pathol Lab Med 2001; 125: 551–554.

796. Root M, Wang TY, Hescock H, et al. Burkitt's lymphoma of the testicle: report of 2 cases occurring in elderly patients. J Urol 1990; 144: 1239–1241.

797. Givler RL. Testicular involvement in leukemia and lymphoma. Cancer 1969; 23: 1290–1295.

798. Akhtar M, Al-Dayel F, Siegrist K, et al. Neutrophil-rich Ki-1-positive anaplastic large cell lymphoma presenting as a testicular mass. Mod Pathol 1996; 9: 812–815.

799. Lee SN, Nam E, Cha JH, et al. Adult T-cell leukemia/lymphoma with features of CD30-positive anaplastic large cell lymphoma – a case report. J Korean Med Sci 1997; 12: 364–368.

800. Chan JK, Tsang WY, Lau WH, et al. Aggressive T/natural killer cell lymphoma presenting as testicular tumor. Cancer 1996; 77: 1198–1205.

801. Guler G, Altinok G, Uner AH, et al. CD56+ lymphoma presenting as a testicular tumor. Leuk Lymphoma 1999; 36: 207–211.

802. Kim YB, Chang SK, Yang WI, et al. Primary NK/T cell lymphoma of the testis. A case report and review of the literature. Acta Haematol 2003; 109: 95–100.

803. Finn LS, Viswanatha DS, Belasco JB, et al. Primary follicular lymphoma of the testis in childhood. Cancer 1999; 85: 1626–1635.

804. Hull DR, Alexander HD, Markey GM, et al. Histiocytic lymphoma presenting as a testicular tumour and terminating in acute monoblastic leukaemia. J Clin Pathol 2000; 53: 788–790.

805. Vos JA, Abbondanzo SL, Barekman CL, et al. Histiocytic sarcoma: a study of five cases including the histiocyte marker CD163. Mod Pathol 2005; 18: 693–704.

806. Algaba F, Santaularia JM, Garat JM, et al. Testicular pseudolymphoma. Eur Urol 1986; 12: 362–363.

807. Senzaki H, Okada H, Izuno Y, et al. An autopsy case of multiple myeloma accompanied by extensive nodular infiltration into the extraskeletal tissue. Gan No Rinsho 1990; 36: 2491–2495 (Japanese).

808. Avitable AM, Gansler TS, Tomaszewski JE, et al. Testicular plasmacytoma. Urology 1989; 34: 51–54.

809. Oppenheim PI, Cohen S, Anders KH. Testicular plasmacytoma. A case report with immunohistochemical studies and literature review. Arch Pathol Lab Med 1991; 115: 629–632.

810. Ferry JA, Young RH, Scully RE. Testicular and epididymal plasmacytoma: a report of 7 cases, including three that were the initial manifestation of plasma cell myeloma. Am J Surg Pathol 1997; 21: 590–598.

811. Castagna M, Gaeta P, Cecchi M, et al. Bilateral synchronous testicular involvement in multiple myeloma. Case report and review of the literature. Tumori 1997; 83: 768–771.

812. Kremer M, Ott G, Nathrath M, et al. Primary extramedullary plasmacytoma and multiple myeloma: phenotypic differences revealed by immunohistochemical analysis. J Pathol 2005; 205: 92–101.

813. Kuhajda FP, Haupt HM, Moore GW, et al. Gonadal morphology in patients receiving chemotherapy for leukemia: evidence for reproductive potential and against a testicular tumor sanctuary. Am J Med 1982; 72: 759–767.

814. Askin FB, Land VJ, Sullivan MP, et al. Occult testicular leukemi: testicular biopsy at three years continuous complete remission of childhood leukemia. A Southwest Oncology Group study. Cancer 1981; 47: 470–475.

815. Nesbit ME Jr, Robison LL, Ortega JA, et al. Testicular relapse in childhood acute lymphoblastic leukemia: association with pretreatment patient characteristics and treatment. A report for Children's Cancer Study Group. Cancer 1980; 45: 2009–2016.

816. Tiedemannn K, Chessells JM, Sandland RM. Isolated testicular relapse in boys with acute lymphoblastic leukaemia: treatment and outcome. Br Med J 1982; 285: 1614–1616.

817. Schroeder H, Garwicz S, Kristinsson J, et al. Outcome after first relapse in children with acute lymphoblastic leukemia: a population-based study of 315 patients from the Nordic Society of Pediatric Hematology and Oncology (NOPHO). Med Pediatr Oncol 1995; 25: 372–378.

818. McIlwain L, Sokol L, Moscinski LC, et al. Acute myeloid leukemia mimicking primary testicular neoplasm. Presentation of a case with review of literature. Eur J Haematol 2003; 70: 242–245.

819. Valbuena JR, Admirand JH, Lin P, et al. Myeloid sarcoma involving the testis. Am J Clin Pathol 2005; 124: 445–452.

820. Economopoulos T, Alexopoulos C, Anagnostou D, et al. Primary granulocytic sarcoma of the testis. Leukemia 1994; 8: 199–200.

821. Walker BR, Cartwright PC. Granulocytic sarcoma presenting as testicular and paratesticular masses in infancy. J Urol 2001; 165: 224.

822. Ferry JA, Srigley JR, Young RH. Granulocytic sarcoma of the testis: a report of two cases of a neoplasm prone to misinterpretation. Mod Pathol 1997; 10: 320–325.

823. LiVolsi VA, Schiff M. Myxoid neurofibroma of the testis. J Urol 1977; 118: 341–342.

824. Tada M, Takemura S, Takimoto Y, et al. A case of cavernous hemangioma of the testis. Hinyokika Kiyo 1989; 35: 1969–1971.

825. Nistal M, Paniagua R, Regadera J, et al. Testicular capillary haemangioma. Br J Urol 1982; 54: 433.

826. D'Esposito RF, Ferraro LR, Wogalter H. Hemangioma of the testis in an infant. J Urol 1976; 116: 677–678.

827. Mazal PR, Kratzik C, Kain R, et al. Capillary haemangioma of the testis. J Clin Pathol 2000; 53: 641–642.

828. Suriawinata A, Talerman A, Vapnek JM, et al. Hemangioma of the testis: report of unusual occurrences of cavernous hemangioma in a fetus and capillary hemangioma in an older man. Ann Diagn Pathol 2001; 5: 80–83.

829. Banks ER, Mills SE. Histiocytoid (epithelioid) hemangioma of the testis. The so-called vascular variant of 'adenomatoid tumor.' Am J Surg Pathol 1990; 14: 584–589.

830. Mazzella FM, Sieber SC, Lopez V. Histiocytoid hemangioma of the testis: a case report. J Urol 1995; 153: 743–744.

831. Honore LH, Sullivan LD. Intratesticular leiomyoma: a case report with discussion of differential diagnosis and histogenesis. J Urol 1975; 114: 631–635.

832. Gonzalez CM, Victor TA, Bourtsos E, et al. Monoclonal antibody confirmation of a primary leiomyoma of the testis. J Urol 1999; 161: 1908.

833. Mak CW, Tzeng WS, Chou CK, et al. Leiomyoma arising from the tunica albuginea of the testis: sonographic findings. J Clin Ultrasound 2004; 32: 309–311.

834. Cricco CF Jr, Buck AS. Hemangioendothelioma of the testis: second reported case. J Urol 1980; 123: 131–132.

835. Tsolos C, Polychronidis A, Sivridis E, et al. Epithelioid hemangioendothelioma of the testis. J Urol 2001; 166: 1834.

836. Mathew T, Prabhakaran K. Osteosarcoma of the testis. Arch Pathol Lab Med 1981; 105: 38–39.

837. Zukerberg LR, Young RH. Primary testicular sarcoma: a report of two cases. Hum Pathol 1990; 21: 932–935.

838. Washecka RM, Mariani AJ, Zuna RE, et al. Primary intratesticular sarcoma: immunohistochemical ultrastructural and DNA flow cytometric study of three cases with a review of the literature. Cancer 2002; 77: 1524–1528.

839. Yachia D, Auslaender L. Primary leiomyosarcoma of the testis. J Urol 1989; 141: 955–956.

840. Washecka RM, Mariani AJ, Zuna RE, et al. Primary intratesticular sarcoma. Immunohistochemical ultrastructural and DNA flow cytometric study of three cases with a review of the literature. Cancer 1996; 77: 1524–1528.

841. Singh R, Chandra A, O'Brien TS. Primary intratesticular leiomyosarcoma in a mixed race man: a case report. J Clin Pathol 2004; 57: 1319–1320.

842. Val-Bernal JF, Azcarretazabal T, Torio B, et al. Primary pure intratesticular fibrosarcoma. Pathol Int 1999; 49: 185–189.

843. Davis AE Jr. Rhabdomyosarcoma of the testicle. J Urol 1962; 87: 148–154.

844. Ravich L, Lerman PH, Drabkin JW, et al. Pure testicular rhabdomyosarcoma. J Urol 1965; 94: 596–599.

845. Alexander F. Pure testicular rhabdomyosarcoma. Br J Cancer 1968; 22: 498–501.

846. Nistal M, Fachal C, Paniagua R. Testicular carcinoma in situ associated with rhabdomyosarcoma of the spermatic cord. J Urol 1989; 142: 358–360.

847. Johansson JE, Lannes P. Metastases to the spermatic cord, epididymis and testicles from carcinoma of the prostate – five cases. Scand J Urol Nephrol 1983; 17: 249–251.

848. Tiltman AJ. Metastatic tumours in the testis. Histopathology 1979; 3: 31–37.

849. Tu SM, Reyes A, Maa A, et al. Prostate carcinoma with testicular or penile metastases. Clinical, pathologic, and immunohistochemical features. Cancer 2002; 94: 2610–2617.

850. Dutt N, Bates AW, Baithun SI. Secondary neoplasms of the male genital tract with different patterns of involvement in adults and children. Histopathology 2000; 37: 323–331.

851. Garcia-Gonzalez R, Pinto J, Val Bernal JF. Testicular metastases from solid tumors: an autopsy study. Ann Diagn Pathol 2000; 4: 59–64.

852. Datta MW, Young RH. Malignant melanoma metastatic to the testis: a report of three cases with clinically significant manifestations. Int J Surg Pathol 2000; 8: 49–57.

853. Dieckmann KP, Due W, Loy V. Intrascrotal metastasis of renal cell carcinoma. Case reports and review of the literature. Eur Urol 1988; 15: 297–301.

854. Lauro S, Lanzetta G, Bria E, et al. Contralateral solitary testis metastasis antedating renal cell carcinoma: a case-report and review. Anticancer Res 1998; 18: 4683–4684.

855. Haupt HM, Mann RB, Trump DL, et al. Metastatic carcinoma involving the testis: clinical and pathologic distinction from primary testicular neoplasms. Cancer 1984; 54: 709–714.

856. Rosser CJ, Gerrard E. Metastatic small cell carcinoma to the testis. South Med J 2000; 93: 72–73.

857. Han M, Kronz JD, Schoenberg MP. Testicular metastasis of transitional cell carcinoma of the prostate. J Urol 2000; 164: 2026.

858. Datta MW, Ulbright TM, Young RH. Renal cell carcinoma metastatic to the testis and its adnexa: a report of five cases including three that accounted for the initial clinical presentation. Int J Surg Pathol 2001; 9: 49–56.

859. Tozawa K, Akita H, Kusada S, et al. Testicular metastases from carcinoma of the bile duct. a case report. Int J Urol 1998; 5: 106–107.

860. Bhasin SD, Shrikhande SS. Secondary carcinoma of testis – a clinicopathologic study of 10 cases. Indian J Cancer 1990; 27: 83–90.

861. Backhaus BO, Kaefer M, Engum SA, et al. Contralateral testicular metastasis in paratesticular rhabdomyosarcoma. J Urol 2000; 164: 1709–1710.

862. Kumari PK, Surendran N, Chellam VG, et al. Neuroblastoma with testicular metastasis. Review of literature and report of a case. Indian J Cancer 1994; 31: 52–55.

863. Simon T, Hero B, Berthold F. Testicular and paratesticular involvement by metastatic neuroblastoma. Cancer 2000; 88: 2636–2641.

864. Gallagher BL, Vibhakar R, Kao S, et al. Bilateral testicular masses: an unusual presentation of neuroblastoma. Urology 2006; 68: 672–677.

865. Richardson PG, Millward MJ, Shrimankar JJ, et al. Metastatic melanoma to the testis simulating primary seminoma. Br J Urol 1992; 69: 663–665.

866. Pienkos EJ, Jablokow VR. Secondary testicular tumors. Cancer 1972; 30: 481–485.

867. Ulbright TM, Roth LM. Testicular and paratesticular neoplasms. In: Sternberg SS, ed. Diagnostic surgical pathology. New York: Raven Press, 1994; 1885–1947.

# CHAPTER 14

# Spermatic cord and testicular adnexae

David G. Bostwick

The paratesticular region includes the testicular tunics, efferent ductules, epididymis, spermatic cord, and vas deferens. Most studies of paratesticular region pathology include the rete testis despite its intratesticular location.[1] Numerous rare and interesting lesions arise in this region, including cysts, 'celes,' inflammatory diseases, embryonic remnants, neoplasms, and neoplasm-like proliferations (Table 14-1). In children, one of the common neoplasms is paratesticular rhabdomyosarcoma. In adults, the most common pathologic conditions in order of frequency, excluding 'celes,' are epididymitis, lipoma of the spermatic cord, adenomatoid tumor of the epididymis, and sarcoma of the spermatic cord.[2]

It is often difficult to diagnose paratesticular masses prior to or during surgery owing to their varied morphologic appearance and rarity. An inguinal surgical approach is usually indicated when there is a suspicion of malignancy. The pathologist should document the anatomic site of origin, histologic classification, and extent of spread of the lesion.

# Embryology and normal anatomy

The paratesticular region contains numerous anatomically complex epithelial and mesenchymal structures, often within embryonic remnants (Fig. 14-1). The rete testis of the mediastinum of the testis, the first element of the wolffian collecting system, connects the seminiferous tubules and efferent ductules.

The most common abnormalities of the paratesticular region are benign, including hydrocele, lipoma, and inflammatory conditions such as epididymitis, but a variety of cystic and proliferative lesions also occur and are diagnostically challenging.

## Embryology

The embryology of the testis and its adnexa is described in Chapter 12; herein is a brief summary of significant events in the development of paratesticular tissues. The testis and head of the epididymis arise from the genital ridge. The wolffian ducts, the male genital ducts, are paired tubes that are associated with the developing gonads and degenerating mesonephric tubules. The body and tail of the epididymis, the vas deferens, and the ejaculatory duct arise from the mesonephric tubules; other degenerating tubules often persist as embryonic remnants, including the appendix epididymis, paradidymis, and cranial and caudal aberrant ductules (Fig. 14-1). The paired vasa deferentia connect to the ejaculatory ducts within the prostate, which in turn have their outlets in the prostatic urethra adjacent to the müllerian tubercle. Blind diverticula of the distal vas deferens form the seminal vesicles. The müllerian duct, or paramesonephros, regresses in men, but may persist as embryonic remnants such as the appendix testis and prostatic utricle.

## Anatomy

### Scrotum and testicular tunics

The sac of the scrotum is divided by a partial median septum into two compartments, each of which contains a testis and epididymis and the lower portion of the spermatic cord. The scrotal wall consists of six layers, from the inside outward: the tunica vaginalis, the internal spermatic fascia, the cremasteric muscle, the external spermatic fascia, the dartos muscle, and the skin. The tunica vaginalis is a thin mesothelium-covered

**Table 14-1** Paratesticular tumors and cysts in the Canadian reference center for cancer pathology, 1949–1986

| | Number of Cases |
|---|---|
| **CYSTS** | |
| Mesothelial cyst | 4 |
| Epididymal cyst | 1 |
| **Benign Neoplasms and Pseudotumors** | |
| Adenomatoid tumor | 23 |
| Nodular and diffuse fibrous proliferation | 6 |
| Leiomyoma | 6 |
| Cystadenoma of epididymis | 3 |
| Hamartoma of rete testis | 1 |
| Adenomatous hyperplasia of epididymis | 1 |
| Adenomatous hyperplasia of rete testis | 1 |
| Mixed gonadal stromal tumor | 1 |
| Adrenal cortical heterotopia | 1 |
| Rhabdomyoma | 1 |
| Miscellaneous soft-tissue tumors | 8 |
| **Malignant Neoplasms** | |
| **Primary** | |
| Rhabdomyosarcoma | 14 |
| Liposarcoma | 9 |
| Leiomyosarcoma | 7 |
| Malignant mesothelioma | 7 |
| Malignant fibrous histiocytoma | 3 |
| Malignant mesenchymoma | 1 |
| Plasmacytoma | 1 |
| Papillary serous cystadenocarcinoma of low malignant potential | 1 |
| Sarcoma, not otherwise specified | 3 |
| **Secondary** | |
| Metastatic carcinoma | 4 |
| Metastatic carcinoid tumor | 2 |
| Metastatic non-Hodgkin's lymphoma | 2 |

From Srigley JR, Hartwick RWH: Tumors and cysts of the paratesticular region, Pathol Annu 25(Part2):51–108, 1990 (review); with permission.

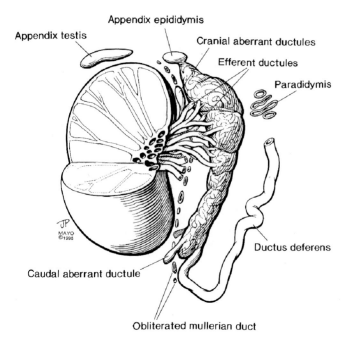

Appendix testis

Appendix epididymis

Cranial aberrant ductules

Efferent ductules

Paradidymis

Ductus deferens

Caudal aberrant ductule

Obliterated mullerian duct

**Fig. 14-1** Anatomy of the testis and paratesticular adnexae, including embryonic remnants.

layer of the parietal peritoneum that also covers the white fibrous tunica albuginea of the testis and epididymis; it is initially in contact with the peritoneal cavity from which it arises, but becomes isolated with regression of the processus vaginalis. It is likely that a common stimulus such as androgens are required for obliteration of the processus vaginalis and development of the epididymis, a hypothesis supported by the common coexistence of epididymal anomalies and patency of the processus vaginalis.[3]

The internal spermatic fascia is a continuation of the transversalis fascia, and the external fascia is a continuation of the external oblique aponeurosis. The cremasteric muscle consists of incomplete slips of muscle, usually in the upper part of the scrotal wall. The dartos muscle consists of smooth muscle embedded in loose areolar tissue. The scrotum is supplied by the external and internal pudendal, cremasteric, and testicular arteries. Lymphatics drain to the superficial inguinal lymph nodes.

### Rete testis

The rete testis is formed by the convergence of the seminiferous tubules (see Chapter 12). The tubules follow a cranial and dorsal course through the fibrous connective tissue of the mediastinum testis, eventually merging into 12–20 ducts (the efferent ductules, or ductuli efferentes) that perforate the tunica vaginalis and form the head of the epididymis at the upper pole of the testis. After puberty, elastic fibers are present in the muscular coat of the ductules, epididymis, and vas deferens.

### Epididymis

The epididymis is a highly convoluted tubule attached to the dorsomedial portion of the testis, connecting the efferent

ductules of the rete testis with the vas deferens. It is about 6 m long. The head consists of a series of conical masses, the lobules, each of which contains a single duct measuring 15–20 cm; it is lined by tall columnar epithelium and invested with a thick layer of smooth muscle (Fig. 14-2). The body of the epididymis is a single, highly convoluted tube that increases in diameter distally to form the tail. The tail distally merges with the vas deferens.

Development of the efferent ducts and ductus epididymidis follows a biphasic pattern. Progressive development occurs from the fetal period to infants 2–4 months of age, but this development is transient and regresses during infancy. Definitive development is initiated in childhood and completed at puberty. These changes are probably related to the androgen dependence of the epididymis, the different stages of testicular maturation, and the steroidogenic activity of Leydig cells.[4] The epididymis plays a critical role in maturation and viability of spermatozoa.[5]

A variety of morphologic variations occur in the epididymal columnar cells and vas deferens, including cribriform hyperplasia (42% of patients),[6–9] patchy or diffuse eosinophilic granular cell change (Paneth cell-like metaplasia) (8.3%),[10] intranuclear eosinophilic inclusions,[11] nuclear atypia with 'monstrous' cells (14%),[12] adenomatous hyperplasia, prostate-type glands,[13] epithelial luminal pitting,[14] multiple diverticula in the cauda epididymis in the elderly,[15] and accumulation of lipofuscin pigment.[16,17]

### Vas deferens (ductus deferens) and spermatic cord

The vas deferens is about 46 cm long, traversing the spermatic cord and inguinal canal to connect the tail of the epididymis with the ejaculatory ducts. In the spermatic cord, it is invested with a thick muscular coat that includes the internal spermatic, cremasteric, and external spermatic fasciae; other structures of the spermatic cord include the pampiniform plexus, the testicular artery, lymphatics, and nerves. Upon exiting the spermatic cord, the vas deferens passes extraperitoneally upward and laterally in the pelvis, passes medial to the distal ureter and the posterior wall of the bladder, and terminates at an acute angle in a dilated ampulla which, together with the duct of the seminal vesicle, forms the ejaculatory duct. The vas deferens is supplied by its own artery, the artery of the vas deferens, which is usually a branch of the internal iliac or umbilical artery.

The vas deferens is lined by low folds of columnar epithelium, with morphologic variations similar to those in the epididymis (see above). The wall of the vas deferens consists of three layers of smooth muscle: the inner longitudinal, middle circular, and outer longitudinal layers. Elastic fibers appear in the muscular wall after puberty.

## Congenital anomalies

Abnormal development of the paratesticular region may result in a variety of anomalies, including embryonic rem-

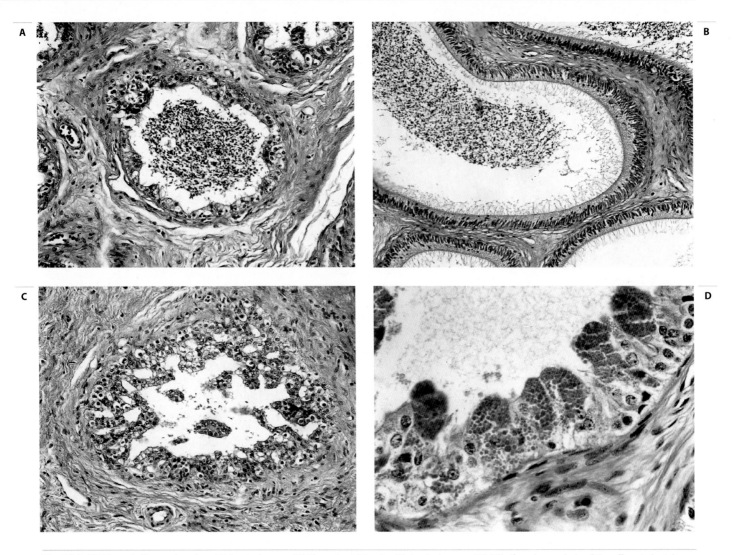

**Fig. 14-2 (A)** Normal efferent ductules with luminal sperm. **(B)** Normal epididymis with luminal sperm. **(C)** Cribriform hyperplasia of the efferent ductules. **(D)** Coarse granular cytoplasmic change of the vas deferens.

nants, agenesis, atresia, ectopia, and cysts. There is an increased frequency of anomalies in boys with cryptorchidism and congenital rubella. Bilateral anomalies result in sterility.

Agenesis and atresia of the testis, epididymis, and vas deferens result from failure of development of the genital ridge, often with anomalies of other wolffian derivatives and renal ectopia, agenesis, or dysplasia. Congenital absence of the vas deferens may be autosomal recessive, partial or complete, unilateral or bilateral, and is often associated with cystic fibrosis (see below). Testicular biopsies in patients with congenital absence of the vas deferens reveal normal spermatogenesis or hypospermatogenesis in up to 45% of cases, and clinical investigation should include semen analysis, renal ultrasound, and genetic cystic fibrosis screening.[18,19] Congenital unilateral absence of the vas deferens is more commonly associated with renal agenesis than bilateral absence (74% vs 12%, respectively).[18]

Duplications may involve any structure of the adnexae, but are rare. Ectopic insertion of the ureteric bud in the epididymis, vas deferens, or seminal vesicles may also occur.

Congenital or developmental cysts of the epididymis are extremely rare, and may be associated with intrauterine exposure to diethylstilbesterol.[20] The cysts are usually solitary, but may be multiple and bilateral. Ectopic epididymis may be found anterior to the testis, in the retroperitoneum, and within the kidney.

Epididymal abnormalities are commonly associated with ectopic or cryptorchid testes (72% of cases), ranging from simple elongation of the epididymis (33%) to more complex changes such as complete disruption (39%).[21]

## Splenogonadal fusion

Splenogonadal fusion is a rare congenital anomaly in which there is fusion of the splenic and gonadal anlagen.[22] About 100 cases have been reported, usually on the left side (98%) in men (95%). Patients may present with a non-tender scrotal mass or intestinal obstruction, but most cases are discovered incidentally at autopsy or surgery for cryptorchidism or inguinal hernia. About 57% are associated with other congenital anomalies, including peromelia, micrognathia, and cardiac anomalies.

There are two types of splenogonadal fusion. The continuous type is characterized by connection of the spleen and the splenogonad by a fibrous cord. The cord usually arises in the upper pole of the spleen, and may be retroperitoneal or anterior to the small bowel or colon. Splenic tissue may be present at both ends of the cord or stud the cord throughout its length. The discontinuous type of splenogonadal fusion has no connection between the spleen and splenogonad. The splenic tissue appears within the tunica albuginea or scrotum or along the vascular pedicle.

Splenogonadal fusion probably results from early fusion of the spleen and gonad during embryonic development, perhaps as a result of inflammation or adhesions. The spleen develops during the fourth and fifth weeks of gestation, and rotates into proximity with the urogenital fold and developing gonadal mesoderm. During the eighth to 10th weeks the gonads migrate caudally, probably accompanied by a portion of the spleen in cases of splenogonadal fusion. The limb buds and mandible are developing at the same time, accounting for the close association of splenogonadal fusion with peromelia and micrognathia.

Preoperative diagnosis of splenogonadal fusion by splenic scan may avoid unnecessary orchiectomy. Splenogonadal fusion and accessory spleen are important to consider when splenic ablation is needed.

## Adrenal heterotopia and renal ectopia

Adrenal cortical tissue may be present anywhere along the route of descent of the testis from the abdomen to the scrotum (Fig. 14-3).[23] It is usually an incidental finding at inguinal herniorrhaphy or epididymo-orchiectomy, present in 1–3% of children undergoing such operations.[24–26] Adrenal cortical tissue has been identified in inguinal hernia sac, spermatic cord (Fig. 14-3), epididymis, and rete testis. It may present as a palpable tumor, and appears as small, round to oval 1–5 mm diameter yellow-orange nodules, usually near the inguinal ring. The lesions almost always consist of adrenal cortical tissue resembling zona glomerulosa and fasciculata. Rarely, they contain medullary tissue. Involution during childhood is the rule, but exceptional cases persist and become functional, rarely harboring neoplasms or developing into 'tumors' in adrenogenital syndrome and Nelson's syndrome. Removal of functional rests may result in adrenal insufficiency.

Ectopic renal tissue has rarely been observed in the scrotum, and consists of tubules and immature glomeruli.

## Wolffian and müllerian remnants

Numerous embryonic remnants are found in the paratesticular area, including the appendix testis (hydatid of Morgagni), appendix epididymis, paradidymis, and vasa aberrantia. Precise classification of cystic remnants may be challenging.[27,28]

### Appendix testis (hydatid of morgagni)

The appendix testis is present on more than 90% of testes at autopsy; ultrasound examination found an incidence of 44%.[29] This structure is located at the superior pole of the testis adjacent to the epididymis. Grossly, it varies from 2 to 4 mm, appearing as a polypoid or sessile nodular excrescence. Microscopically, it contains a fibrovascular core of loose connective tissue covered by simple cuboidal or low columnar müllerian-type epithelium that is in continuity with the tunica vaginalis at the base. The fibrovascular core may contain tubular inclusions lined by similar cuboidal epithelium. Torsion of the appendix testis may be painful and mimic testicular torsion, and is the most common cause of acute scrotum in children.[30]

### Appendix epididymis (vestigial caudal mesonephric collecting tubule)

The appendix epididymis is present on about 35% of testicles examined at autopsy; ultrasound examination found an incidence of 18%.[29] Grossly, it is a pedunculated spherical cystic or elongated structure arising from the anterosuperior pole of the head of the epididymis. Microscopically, it is lined by cuboidal to low columnar epithelium that may be ciliated and show secretory activity. The wall consists of loose connective tissue, and is covered on its outer surface by flattened mesothelial cells that are continuous with the visceral tunica vaginalis. The appendix epididymis may become dilated by serous fluid, and, when enlarged, may mimic a tumor. Torsion may occur, sometimes in cryptorchidism.

### Paradidymis (organ of Giraldes)

This wolffian duct embryonic remnant consists of clusters of tubules lined by cuboidal to low columnar epithelium within the connective tissue of the spermatic cord, superior to the head of the epididymis.[31]

### Vasa aberrantia (organ of Haller)

These wolffian duct remnants appear as clusters of tubules that are histologically similar to the paradidymis. They arise within the groove between the testis and epididymis. Torsion of the vas aberrans is rare.[32]

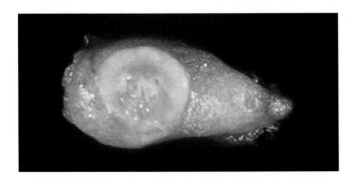

**Fig. 14-3** Heterotopic adrenal cortical tissue in the left spermatic cord forming a discrete yellow-orange nodule.

## Other lesions associated with the epididymis

Other rare epididymal lesions have been described, including cysts (Fig. 14-4), duplication, and ectopic epididymal tissue associated with inguinal hernia. Cysts and duplication may arise from the caudal vasa aberrantia.

### Walthard's rest

This remnant, probably of müllerian origin, consists of solid and cystic nests of uniform epithelial cells with oval nuclei and characteristic longitudinal grooves.

## Hernia sac specimens: glandular inclusions versus vas deferens or epididymis

Herniorrhaphy in children is surgically challenging, particularly in the commonly strangulated hernia sac, accounting for the vulnerability of the epididymis and vas deferens that may be inadvertently transected during the procedure. This problem is compounded by the diagnostic difficulty of classifying glandular inclusions in hernia sacs, and especially challenging in young children owing to the ambiguity of distinguishing features among the structures and embryonic remnants prior to puberty. Benign glandular inclusions in

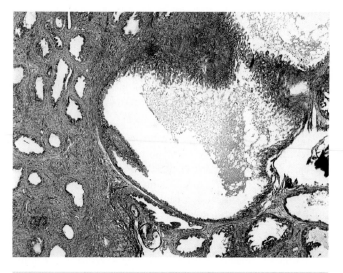

**Fig. 14-4** Small epididymal cyst that formed a palpable paratesticular mass.

inguinal herniorrhaphy specimens may represent müllerian remnants, wolffian remnants, transected vas deferens, or transected epididymis. It is critical to make this distinction owing to the potential impact on reproductive function and medicolegal issues.[33–36] Disruption of one vas deferens may generate antisperm antibodies.

Classification of glandular inclusions is often subjective, even with experienced pathologists; in one study, interobserver agreement was only 44–52% of cases.[34] The epididymis typically has a well-formed concentric muscular coat, whereas embryonic remnants lack a muscular coat but have a mantle of fibrous tissue. Some have advocated use of Masson's trichrome stain and muscle-specific actin to make this distinction, but this has been refuted by others as inconclusive.[34] Comparative analysis reveals that the combination of glandular diameter (with special attention to patient age, recognizing possible changes with advancing development) and histochemical and immunohistochemical stains (trichrome, muscle-specific actin, and CD10) should allow distinction in most cases (Table 14-2). Reliance on light microscopic features alone may be misleading.[33]

Should inguinal hernia repair specimens be submitted routinely for histopathologic examination? One study of 456 specimens from 371 patients under the age of 20 revealed four unexpected cases with epididymal tissue (1%), leading the authors to conclude that pathologic study was an unnecessary expense.[37] In a study of almost 1500 inguinal herniorrhaphies, the authors found vas deferens in 0.13% of cases (Table 14-2).[38] Another report of more than 7000 consecutive pediatric herniorrhaphies found 0.23% vas deferens, 0.3% epididymis, and 0.41% embryonal rests.[34]

Inguinal hernias characteristically show cremasteric muscle fiber hypertrophy, which accounts for the palpable thickening of the spermatic cord (see Hamartoma, below).[39]

## Cystic fibrosis

Cystic fibrosis is a genetic abnormality that often affects the testicular adnexae, resulting in infertility due to agenesis or atresia of mesonephric structures or anomalies of the testes (see Chapter 12). Patients with congenital bilateral absence of the vas deferens often have cystic fibrosis, although this finding may occur in patients without cystic fibrosis.

**Table 14-2** Glandular inclusions in herniorrhaphies: comparative features

| | Incidence in herniorrhaphies (%) | Mean diameter (mm) | Immunophenotype |
|---|---|---|---|
| Embryonic remnants | 1.5[35]<br>2.6[222]<br>2.9[34]<br>6.0[36] | 0.17[35]<br>0.20[222] | Muscle-specific actin negative; CD10 negative[33] |
| Vas deferens | 0.16[35]<br>0.23[34] | 0.6[33]<br>1.2–1.4 (age 4 months)[35] | Muscle-specific actin positive in wall; CD10 positive[33] |
| Epididymis | 0.16[35]<br>0.30[34]<br>0.88[37] | 0.20[222] | Muscle-specific actin positive in wall; CD10 positive in epithelium[33] |

# Non-neoplastic diseases of the spermatic cord and testicular adnexae

## 'Celes' and cysts

### Hydrocele

This mesothelial-lined cyst results from the accumulation of serous fluid between the parietal and the visceral tunica vaginalis of the testis (Fig. 14-5). Congenital hydrocele occurs when a patent processus vaginalis within the spermatic cord communicates with the peritoneal cavity. The prevalence of congenital hydrocele is about 6% at birth and 1% in adulthood. Most cases of hydrocele are idiopathic, but may be associated with inguinal hernia, scrotal trauma, epididymo-orchitis, or tumors of the testis or paratesticular region. Possible causes of idiopathic hydrocele include excessive secretion within the testicular tunics by parietal mesothelial cells, decreased reabsorption, and congenital absence of efferent lymphatics.

Hydrocele is lined by a single layer of cuboidal or flattened mesothelial cells, sometimes with prominent atypia, with underlying connective tissue stroma. The luminal fluid is usually clear and serous unless complicated by infection or hemorrhage. The surface is often covered by fibrinous adhesions and inflammation, and subepithelial chronic inflammation and fibrosis may be present. In some cases, progressive fibrosis narrows or obliterates the cyst lumen, creating adhesions and multiple cysts. Spermatocele may rupture into the hydrocele sac.

### Hematocele (hematoma)

Hematocele refers to the accumulation of blood in the space between the parietal and visceral tunica vaginalis, often in association with hydrocele (Fig. 14-5). Long-standing hematocele becomes calcified and fibrotic, with numerous hemosiderin-laden macrophages. The causes of hematocele are similar to those of hydrocele.

Idiopathic hematoma arising in the spermatic cord or epididymis may be mistaken for neoplasm.[40]

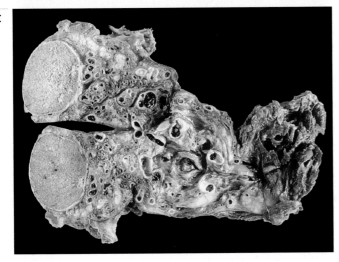
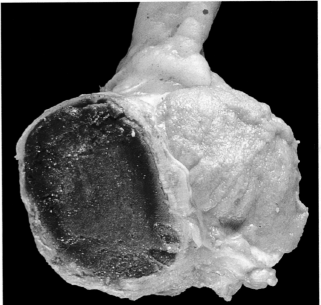
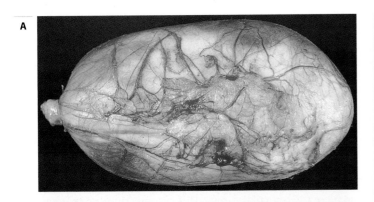
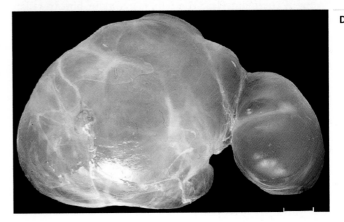

**Fig. 14-5 (A)** Hydrocele. **(B)** Encapsulated hematocele. **(C)** Varicocele. **(D)** Spermatocele.

## Varicocele

Varicocele is a mass of dilated tortuous veins of the pampiniform venous plexus of the spermatic cord that occurs posterior and superior to the testis, sometimes extending into the inguinal ring (Fig. 14-5). The venous plexus normally empties into the internal spermatic vein near the internal inguinal ring; poor drainage and progressive dilatation and elongation result from incompetent valves of the left internal spermatic vein that empties into the renal vein. The right internal spermatic vein is less likely to be involved with varicocele because it drains directly into the inferior vena cava, and is less likely to have incompetent valves. Microscopic changes in the pampiniform plexus with varicocele include variable vascular wall thickening, segmental obliteration, medial hypertrophy of longitudinal smooth muscle fibers, fragmentation of the internal elastic lamina, and occasional occlusive thrombi.[41,42]

Varicocele results from a number of conditions, but most cases are idiopathic. Unilateral varicocele in older men may indicate the presence of a renal tumor that has invaded the renal vein and occluded the drainage of the spermatic vein. Varicocele is associated with maternal exposure to diethylstilbestrol. Patients with varicocele sometimes present with testicular pain associated with sexual activity.

Long-standing varicocele causes testicular atrophy and infertility in the affected testis. Treatment consists of ligation of the internal spermatic vein at the level of the internal inguinal ring, and does not usually yield a pathologic specimen for analysis.

## Spermatocele (acquired epididymal cyst)

Spermatocele is a dilatation of an efferent ductule in the region of the rete testis or caput epididymis.[43] The inner lining consists of a single layer of cuboidal to flattened epithelial cells that are often ciliated. The wall is composed of fibromuscular soft tissue, often with chronic inflammation, and the cyst may be unilocular or multilocular (Fig. 14-5).[44] Spermatocele is distinguished from hydrocele by the presence of spermatozoa in the cyst fluid, a distinction that can be made by aspiration cytology. Torsion is a rare complication of spermatocele.[45,46]

Benign papilloma may arise within the epithelial lining of spermatoceles. The papillae contain fibrovascular cores lined by a single layer of columnar epithelium with vacuolated cytoplasm. The epithelium appears cytologically benign, and there is no evidence of subepithelial invasion.

## Mesothelial cyst

Mesothelial cyst arises within the tunica vaginalis, tunica albuginea, or, less commonly, the epididymis and spermatic cord. The cyst may be single or multiple, measuring up to 2.5 cm in diameter, and is lined by a single layer of uniform cuboidal to flattened attenuated mesothelial cells.

Mesothelial cyst of the tunica vaginalis arises from the connective tissue of the tunica. There may be nodular or diffuse proliferation of mesothelial cells, sometimes with squamous metaplasia. This cyst is probably an embryonic remnant or an inclusion of vaginalis mesothelium resulting from inflammation, trauma, or neoplasm, similar to mesothelial cyst of the tunica albuginea.

Mesothelial cyst of the tunica albuginea most often occurs in men over 40 years, but all ages are affected. It is usually located anterior and lateral to the testis, measuring up to 4 cm in diameter. The cyst is filled with clear or blood-tinged serous fluid, and the lining consists of typical mesothelial cells with a wall composed of hyalinized fibrous tissue.

Unilocular and multilocular mesothelial cyst of the spermatic cord is rare, and probably arises from embryonic mesothelial remnants such as the processus vaginalis.[47]

## Epidermoid cyst (epidermal cyst)

Epidermoid cyst is common in the testis, comprising about 1% of testicular tumors, but may also rarely arise in the paratesticular area and epididymis.[48] Epidermoid cyst consists of a lining of benign keratinizing squamous epithelium and a wall composed of fibrous connective tissue, often with inflammation. Diligent search is required to exclude the presence of adnexal structures or teratomatous elements. Paratesticular epidermoid cyst may arise from squamous metaplasia of wolffian duct structures, displacement of squamous epithelium from the scrotal skin to paratesticular structures during embryogenesis, squamous metaplasia of mesothelial cyst, or monomorphic epidermal development of a teratoma. Epidermoid cyst in the paratesticular area does not recur after surgical excision. Some consider this tumor to be a cholesteatoma when it arises in the epididymis.

## Dermoid cyst (mature teratoma)

Dermoid cyst most often involves the testis and paratesticular structures, but may occur in the spermatic cord and, very rarely, in the testicular tunics. This cyst measures up to 4 cm in diameter, and contains soft, cheesy yellow-white amorphous material with or without hair and calcifications. The cyst is lined by keratinized squamous epithelium, and the wall contains typical dermal adnexal structures such as pilosebaceous units, although these may be difficult to identify without thorough sectioning. Dermoid cyst does not recur or metastasize after excision.

## Simple cyst and cystic dysplasia of the rete testis

Simple cyst of the rete testis is rare, and is typically unilocular, up to 1 cm in diameter, lined by normal rete testis tubular epithelium, and bulges into the testis proper. When multilocular, it is often associated with epididymal cysts.[49]

Cystic dysplasia of the rete testis is a benign congenital lesion of newborns and young boys that is frequently associated with ipsilateral renal agenesis and dysplasia.[50] Clinically it mimics testicular cancer. Long-term follow-up for possible recurrence is recommended.

Cystic transformation of the rete testis and epididymis is common in men undergoing dialysis for chronic renal insufficiency. Histologic changes include columnar transformation of the epithelium, accumulation of calcium oxalate crystals, fibrosis, and giant cell reaction.[51-53] Other causes of cystic transformation include mechanical obstruction of the epididymis by tumor or trauma, ischemia, hormonal alterations such as those in hepatic cirrhosis, or cryptorchidism.[54]

Patients with cryptorchidism display changes in the rete testis referred to in one report as dysgenetic rete testis; changes included metaplastic epithelium with columnar or large cuboidal cells, rete testis hypoplasia, combined hypoplasia and cystic dysplasia, or adenomatous hyperplasia.[9,55] These findings may result from a primary abnormality of the rete testis or incomplete pubertal maturation.

A rare case was reported of a 35-year-old with a seminal vesicle cyst that extended through the inguinal canal.[56]

## Inflammatory and reactive diseases

### Epididymitis

Epididymitis may be acute or chronic, depending on the inciting agent and the duration of infection.[57] It usually occurs in association with orchitis or after trauma, but rarely is an isolated finding. Most cases result from retrograde spread by vesicoepididymal urinary reflux, but hematogenous and lymphatic spread account for some cases. Congenital anomalies such as ureteral ectopia may cause epididymitis in infants. The surgical pathologist rarely receives specimens of these diseases. Urethral and epididymal smears and cultures are useful in identifying the causative infectious agent.

#### Acute epididymitis

Patients with acute epididymitis usually present with unilateral painful enlargement of the epididymis, more commonly on the right side, often involving the testicle (50% of cases have epididymo-orchitis) and vas deferens (Fig. 14-6). The epididymis is thickened, congested, and edematous, with white fibrinopurulent exudate in the tubules and stroma. Microabscesses and fistulae may occur, but rupture is uncommon. The tubules may be damaged or destroyed by the inflammation, sometimes with squamous metaplasia and regenerative changes.

Acute epididymitis is commonly caused by bacteria. Coliforms account for most cases in children, whereas *Neisseria gonorrheae* and *Chlamydia trachomatis* are most frequent in young men, and *Escherichia coli* and *Pseudomonas* predominate in older men.[58] Other bacteria that may cause acute epididymitis include *Klebsiella, Staphylococcus, Streptococcus pneumoniae, Neisseria meningitidis, Aerobacter aerogenes*, and *Hemophilus influenzae*. The epididymis is a reservoir for *Neisseria gonorrheae*, and although infection may be asymptomatic, microabscesses and edema are common, usually without extensive necrosis. The round cytoplasmic inclusions of *C. trachomatis* are difficult to identify in routinely stained sections, and immunohistochemical stains, culture, or genotypic studies are usually required for diagnosis.

Clinical and histopathologic findings allow separation of some cases of chlamydial and bacterial epididymitis (Table 14-3).[59] *C. trachomatis*-positive cases are clinically indolent, with minimally destructive periductal and intraepithelial inflammation and epithelial regeneration.[60] Lymphoepithelial complexes and squamous metaplasia are sometimes present. *E. coli*-positive cases are characterized by scrotal pain, pyuria, leukocytosis, and highly destructive epididymitis with abscesses and xanthogranulomas.

Viral causes of acute epididymitis include mumps and cytomegalovirus, similar to those causing orchitis (see

**Table 14-3** Comparison of bacterial and chlamydial epididymitis*

| | Bacterial Epididymitis[†] | Chlamydial Epididymitis |
|---|---|---|
| **CLINICAL FEATURES** | | |
| Patient age (yr) | 59.8 (39–79) | 42.8 (22–74) |
| Pain | Yes | Infrequent |
| **LABORATORY FEATURES** | | |
| Pyuria | Frequent | Infrequent |
| Elevated ESR | Yes | No |
| Elevated C-Reactive Protein | Yes | No |
| **PATHOLOGIC FEATURES** | | |
| Tissue Destruction | Yes | Minimal |
| Xanthogranulomas | Yes | Minimal |
| Abscesses and Necrosis | Yes | Minimal |
| Cytoplasmic Location of Antigens | Histiocytes | Epithelial Cells |

*For details see Hori S, Tsutsumi Y: Histologic differentiation and bacterial epididymitis: nondestructive and proliferative versus destructive and abscess forming – immunohistochemical and clinicopathologic findings, Hum Pathol 26:402–407, 1995.
[†]Usually *E.coli*.
ESR, erythrocytic sedimentation rate.

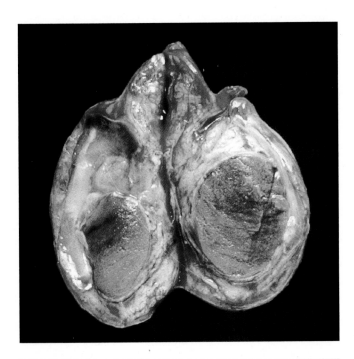

**Fig. 14-6** Acute epididymitis with associated testicular infarction.

Chapter 10). Mumps epididymitis, present in 85% of cases of mumps orchitis, occurs before testicular involvement, usually appearing as unilateral scrotal swelling following parotiditis. The epididymis shows vascular congestion, edema, and interstitial lymphocytic inflammation; neutrophils are usually not a prominent feature. Cytomegaloviral epididymitis may occur in patients with AIDS[61] or those receiving immunosuppression for transplantation.[62]

Parasitic infection by *Wuchereria bancrofti* preferentially involves intrascrotal juxtatesticular lymphatic vessels, with nests of microfilaria with a mean diameter of 0.3 cm² observable by ultrasonography.[63]

Traumatic acute epididymitis is characterized by vascular congestion, petechial hemorrhages, and hematocele. Drugs such as amiodarone may also cause epididymitis.[64]

### Chronic epididymitis

Although many cases of acute epididymitis resolve, some become chronic. The epididymis in chronic epididymitis is indurated and scarred, with cystically dilated tubules, marked fibrosis, chronic inflammation, and sperm granulomas; similar changes may account for the 'late vasectomy syndrome,' in which patients complain of pain many months or years after vasectomy.[65] The epithelium shows reactive or metaplastic changes, often with cytoplasmic vacuolization and luminal hyaline aggregates. Epididymitis nodosa, a proliferative lesion of the epididymis, may result from chronic inflammation or trauma, reminiscent of vasitis nodosa.[66] Coarse granular cytoplasmic changes appear in the epididymis in the setting of ductal obstruction. Calcification is common in chronic epididymitis, and there may be a foreign body giant cell reaction. Xanthogranulomatous epididymitis may also occur. Special stains for bacteria and fungi may be of value.

Specific causes of chronic epididymitis include tuberculosis, leprosy, malakoplakia, sarcoidosis, and sperm granuloma. The epididymis is the reservoir for tuberculous involvement in the male genital tract, with secondary testicular involvement and other local sites of involvement in about 80% of cases; for example, 40% of cases of renal tuberculosis are accompanied by epididymal infection. Patients usually present with painless scrotal swelling, but other signs and symptoms include unilateral or bilateral mass,[67] infertility, and scrotal fistula. Caseating granulomatous inflammation is prominent, with fibrous thickening and enlargement of the epididymis and adjacent structures (Fig. 14-7). Rarely, miliary tuberculosis causes small punctate white lesions. One case of bilateral tuberculous epididymo-orchitis followed intravesical Bacille Calmette–Guérin therapy for urothelial carcinoma of the bladder.[68] The auramine–rhodamine stain is preferred over the Ziehl–Neelsen stain because of its greater sensitivity (60% positive in aspiration smears).[69] Fine needle aspiration cytology was diagnostic in 27 of 40 patients with tubercular epididymitis or epididymo-orchitis, with epithelioid cell granulomas with caseation, but non-diagnostic in the rest.[69]

Lepromatous leprosy frequently involves the epididymis, usually following testicular involvement, but rarely spreads to the vas deferens. Patients complain of painful scrotal

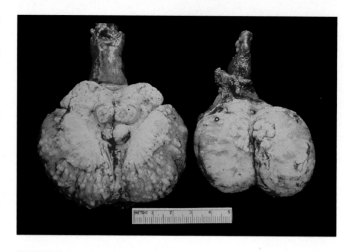

**Fig. 14-7** Tuberculosis of the epididymis and testis.

swelling, and the epididymis and testis are thickened and enlarged. The inflammation consists chiefly of perivascular and perineural lymphocytic infiltrates, often with sheets of macrophages containing acid-fast bacilli set in a dense sclerotic stroma. Sterility results from testicular azoospermia rather than epididymal blockage. The dartos muscle of the testicular tunics shows a predilection for lepromatous myositis.

Malakoplakia of the epididymis is uncommon, usually occurring with testicular involvement.[70] Patients are asymptomatic or present with painful scrotal swelling or hydrocele. The histologic findings are similar to those of malakoplakia at other sites.

Sarcoidosis involves the genital tract in about 5% of cases at autopsy, but is rarely symptomatic. The epididymis is the most common site of genital involvement.[71–73] Patients present with painful or painless scrotal swelling that is bilateral in about 33% of cases. Non-necrotizing granulomatous inflammation is typical, similar to involvement at other sites. The main differential diagnostic consideration is sperm granuloma, but extravasated sperm are absent in sarcoidosis.

Epididymitis may also result from other fungi, bacteria, parasites, and viruses. *Candida albicans* epididymo-orchitis with candiduria is rare, usually following instrumentation of the urinary tract.[74] *Histoplasma capsulatum* creates necrotizing inflammation and abscesses that mimic sperm granuloma; typical silver-stained 2–4 μm fungal spores are usually present.[75] *Coccidioides immitis* produces necrotizing and non-necrotizing granulomas of the epididymis and prostate; silver-stained fungal spherules measuring about 100 μm in diameter contain numerous endospores. Systemic *Blastomyces dermatidis* involves the epididymis in up to 30% of systemic cases, producing microabscesses that contain silver-stained budding fungal spores up to 15 μm in diameter, with thick refractile capsules.[76] Other causes of epididymitis include *Paracoccidioides brasiliensis*, *Actinomyces*, *Sporothrix schenckii*, *Schistosoma hematobium*, *Treponema pallidum*, typhoid, brucellosis, rickettsia, and hydatid cyst. The degenerating worms of *Wuchereria bancrofti* filariasis produce granulomas, often with prominent tissue and blood eosinophilia; scrotal and penile elephantiasis results from lymphatic obstruction.[77] Human papillomavirus was identified by polymerase chain reaction in dysplastic squamous metaplastic epithelium of the epididymis in a 39-year-old man.[78]

Young's syndrome is characterized by the association of sinobronchial disease and azoospermia resulting from bilateral epididymitis-associated obstruction in the distal ductuli efferentes.[79,80]

Idiopathic granulomatous epididymitis is a rare but significant finding at autopsy or during surgery (less than 1% incidence), arising in the caput epididymis.[81] This lesion contains zonal necrosis of efferent ducts with epithelial damage and regeneration. Macrophages are plentiful, as well as cholesterol crystals, foreign body-type giant cells, and spermatozoa.

### Sperm granuloma

Sperm granuloma is an exuberant foreign body giant cell reaction to extravasated sperm, and occurs in up to 42% of patients after vasectomy[82] and 2.5% of routine autopsies. Patients may have no symptoms, but often present with a history of pain and swelling of the upper pole of the epididymis, spermatic cord, and, rarely, the testis. Others have a history of trauma, epididymiditis, and orchitis. In some cases, sperm granuloma mimics testicular or spermatic cord tumor.

Sperm granuloma appears as a solitary yellow nodule or multiple small indurated nodules measuring up to 3 cm in diameter. Foreign body-type granulomas are present, with necrosis in the early stages and progressive fibrosis in late stages (Fig. 14-8). Extravasated sperm are often present in large numbers, but are quickly engulfed by macrophages (referred to as spermiophages) and eventually disappear. Yellow-brown ceroid pigment, a lipid degradation product of sperm, may persist. Vasitis nodosa occurs in about one-third of cases of sperm granuloma.

Disruption of the tubules and extravasation of sperm results in sperm granuloma, but isolated sperm may be present in the interstitium without significant inflammation. Ligation vasectomy accounts for most cases of sperm granuloma, whereas cauterization vasectomy rarely results in granuloma. Secondary oxalosis with crystal deposition from chronic renal failure may be accompanied by sperm granuloma.[52] Experimental injection of ceroid pigment produces granulomatous inflammation, suggesting that destruction of sperm initiates the process. An autoimmune process has been proposed but is not favored.

### Vasitis and vasitis nodosa

Inflammation of the vas deferens (vasitis, or deferentitis), usually occurs in association with epididymitis or posterior urethritis.[83] Vasitis nodosa is a benign ductular proliferation that produces nodular and fusiform enlargement of the vas deferens, often following vasectomy. It resembles salpingitis isthmica nodosa and clinically mimics sperm granuloma.

In vasitis nodosa, the vas deferens may be more than 1 cm in diameter, with diffuse enlargement or rounded indurated masses punctuated by small lumina. The ductular proliferation is prominent, and may be mistaken for metastatic prostatic adenocarcinoma (Fig. 14-9). Chronic inflammation and fibrosis are always observed, albeit in variable amounts, and are sometimes accompanied by muscular hyperplasia of the wall. The ductules vary from discrete round acinar structures to plexiform masses of irregular acini. The cells are cuboidal or low columnar, with a moderate amount of pale granular cytoplasm, central large nuclei with uniform chromatin, and single enlarged nucleoli. Cilia may be present. Perineural invasion is common and often extensive, and may be mistaken for malignancy; benign vascular invasion may also occur. Sperm granulomas are present in about 50% of cases, and sperm are often present in the acinar lumina of vasitis nodosa. As the number of sperm granulomas declines, the amount of ceroid pigment increases, resulting from lipid breakdown products of spermatozoa. A histologically similar process may occur in the epididymis (epididymitis nodosa).

Vasitis nodosa is a benign reactive process. Trauma or surgery results in epithelial rupture with the release of sperm into the soft tissues of the vas deferens, invariably invoking a prominent fibroinflammatory response. However, some cases have no history of trauma and are idiopathic.

### Funiculitis (inflammation of the spermatic cord)

Inflammation of the spermatic cord, or funiculitis, often accompanies vasitis, usually as the result of direct extension from the vas deferens, but isolated involvement may occur by hematogenous spread from other sites of inflammation.[84] Funiculitis appears as painful enlargement of the spermatic cord. Tuberculous funiculitis is rare, presenting as multiple large discrete masses or diffuse thickening with typical necrotizing granulomatous inflammation.[85] Perforation of an incarcerated hernia may cause extravasation of fecal contents and vegetable fibers, resulting in an exuberant foreign body giant cell reaction in the cord. Sclerosing endophlebitis and thrombosis of the pampiniform plexus may accompany funiculitis, resulting in necrosis and gangrene. Recent reports described diabetes-associated

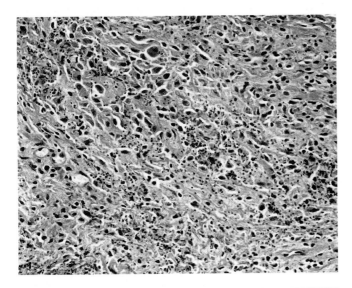

**Fig. 14-8** Sperm granuloma.

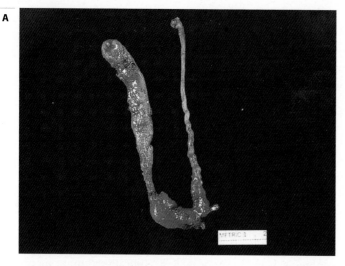

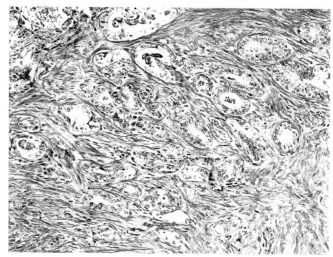

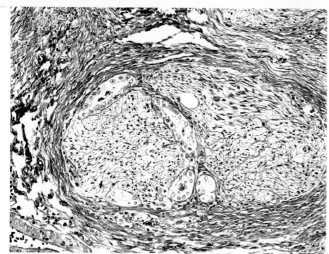

**Fig. 14-9** Vasitis nodosa. **(A)** Grossly apparent nodularity in the midportion (bottom) of the vas deferens. **(B)** Proliferation of small tubules mimicking prostatic adenocarcinoma. **(C)** Perineural invasion by vasitis nodosa.

*Actinomyces*-infected xanthogranulomatous funiculitis[58] and *Dirofilaria repens*-induced chronic funiculitis and epididymitis.[86] *Schistosoma hematobium*-induced funiculitis can be diagnosed by semen analysis in infected men.[87]

### Meconium-induced inflammation

Prenatal or antenatal perforation of the colon may cause meconium leakage through the patent processus vaginalis into the scrotum, resulting in foreign body giant cell reaction, chronic inflammation, and scarring; this is referred to as meconium periorchitis, meconium granuloma, or meconium vaginalisitis.[88] Fewer than 30 cases are reported, rarely in association with cystic fibrosis. Grossly, the tunica vaginalis contains a single mass or is studded with numerous orange or green nodules composed of chronically inflamed myxoid stroma, sometimes containing bile, cholesterol, or lanugo hairs within histiocytes. Hydrocele is often present.

### Vasculitis

Systemic vasculitides may affect the epididymal and testicular vessels, sometimes resulting in hydrocele or swelling of the affected structures.[89,90] Polyarteritis nodosa is observed in these vessels at autopsy in 80% of affected patients, although clinical involvement is rare.[91,92] Isolated epididymal or spermatic cord vasculitis is rare.[93,94] There are no apparent histopathologic differences between systemic vasculitis and most forms of isolated necrotizing vasculitis of testicular and epididymal tissue.

## Other non-neoplastic diseases

### Torsion of the spermatic cord and embryonic remnants

Torsion of the spermatic cord results in hemorrhagic infarction of the testis (see Chapter 12), as well as thrombosed veins surrounded by fat necrosis with cystic cavities bounded by wavy hyaline membranes.[95,96] Torsion of embryonic remnants is a much rarer event that may clinically mimic torsion of the cord. Torsion of a hernia sac is very rare, presenting as acute scrotum in children.[97]

Torsion is a common abnormality of the appendix testis. Patients complain of acute scrotal pain, often following vigorous exercise. About 90% of patients are boys between 10 and 12 years of age, accounting for the most common cause of acute scrotum in children, but men of all ages are affected. Typical histologic features of torsion are present, including

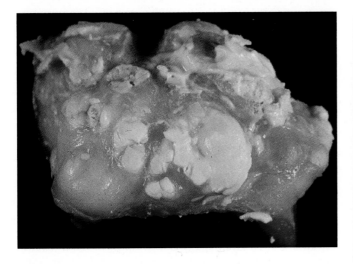

**Fig. 14-10** Idiopathic scrotal and epididymal calcinosis in an otherwise healthy 37-year-old man forming a multinodular mass measuring 3 cm in greatest dimension.

severe congestion, edema, and hemorrhagic infarction. Severe acute inflammation is associated with longer duration of symptoms.[98] Bilateral involvement is rare.[99]

Torsion of the appendix epididymis is much less common than that of the appendix testis, and the histologic findings are similar. Torsion of the vasa aberrantia is extremely rare, with fewer than 10 reported cases.

### Calculi and calcification

Acute and chronic epididymitis and vasitis predispose to calculus formation, usually in the epididymis, vas deferens, and scrotum (Fig. 14-10). The calculi are brown and composed of phosphates and carbonates, measuring up to 1 cm in diameter. Their occurrence in varicose veins has been referred to as 'varicolithiasis.'[100]

Idiopathic mural calcification of the vas deferens occurs in up to 15% of diabetics. These deposits in the smooth muscle are focal and variable in appearance, rarely with osseous metaplasia. Inflammation-induced calcifications are scattered throughout the smooth muscle, usually associated with chronic inflammation and fibrosis.

Myositis ossificans has also been reported forming a spermatic cord tumor,[101] as has heterotopic ossification.[102] Osseous metaplasia of the epididymis occurs sporadically in association with fibrous pseudotumor, sometimes forming a mass that may be mistaken for a neoplasm. Microscopically, it consists of trabecular bone set in connective tissue stroma.

## Neoplasms

### Benign neoplasms and pseudotumors

A variety of unusual tumors and tumor-like proliferations arise in the paratesticular region, often of uncertain histogenesis. Because of the rarity of many of these benign tumors, they may be erroneously considered malignant.

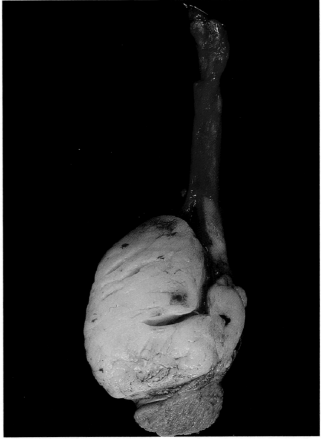

**Fig. 14-11** Lipoma of the cord dwarfing the testis.

### Lipoma

Lipoma is the most common paratesticular tumor, accounting for up to 90% of spermatic cord tumors (Fig. 14-11).[103] It usually occurs in adults, but may be seen at all ages. Grossly, it is a circumscribed unencapsulated mass of lobulated yellow adipose tissue up to 30 cm in diameter and weighing as much as 3.2 kg.[104] The microscopic appearance is similar to that of lipoma at other sites, consisting of mature adipose tissue. Variants include angiolipoma, hibernoma, fibrolipoma, fibromyxolipoma, myxolipoma, and myxoid myolipoma.

Lipoma was identified in 23% of 217 consecutive hernia repairs; of these, 51% were associated with indirect hernia, 17% with direct hernia, 1% with pantaloon and femoral hernia, and 31% without hernia.[105] Autopsy study with careful inguinal dissection revealed 75% with discrete masses of adipose tissue within the inguinal canal, and the majority of lipomas measured more than 4 cm, with pedunculation and a bulbous distal tip.[106]

### Adenomatous hyperplasia

Adenomatous hyperplasia of the rete testis and epididymis consists of a poorly circumscribed tubular or tubulopapillary proliferation of uniform benign cuboidal to low columnar epithelial cells with back-to-back crowding; there is no stromal invasion or other features of malignancy. This lesion is a frequent finding in the undescended testis, and is considered benign.[107]

## Adenomatoid tumor (benign non-papillary mesothelioma)

Adenomatoid tumor is the most common tumor of the epididymis and cord and second in frequency only to lipoma in the paratesticular area; it accounts for about one-third of non-lipoma paratesticular tumors.[108,109] It also arises in the tunica vaginalis or tunica albuginea, and may be present in association with hydrocele.

Adenomatoid tumor is usually seen in men between 20 and 50 years of age, but has been reported in men as old as 79. Patients often present with a painless scrotal mass, but some lesions are found incidentally at epididymo-orchiectomy or autopsy. Adenomatoid tumor consists of a firm, circumscribed solid mass measuring up to 2 cm in greatest dimension, usually arising in the head of the epididymis or rarely in the lower pole of the epididymis, testicular tunics, or spermatic cord. The cut surface is homogeneous and white-gray (Fig. 14-12). The characteristic microscopic finding is irregular tubules, cell nests, and solid trabeculae of cuboidal to flattened epithelioid or endothelioid cells (Fig. 14-12).[110] The tumor cells are eosinophilic, with variably sized cytoplasmic vacuoles. In some cases, excessive vacuolization creates thin strands of cytoplasm spanning lumina; alternatively, it creates a signet ring-cell pattern. Nuclei are small and vesicular with inconspicuous nucleoli. The stroma contains fibroblasts, blood vessels, and smooth muscle. Focal stromal hyalinization may be present, and the tumor may infiltrate the testis. Adenomatoid leiomyoma consists of adenomatoid tumor in association with prominent smooth muscle.

A mesothelial origin is likely for adenomatoid tumor because of the anatomic continuity between the surface mesothelium of the tunica vaginalis and tumor cells in some cases, as well as the identification of rare adenomatoid tumor in the abdominal peritoneum.

Tumor cell cytoplasm contains hyaluronidase-sensitive acid mucopolysaccharides, similar to mesothelioma. Immunohistochemistry reveals cytoplasmic staining for cytokeratin in most cases, focal luminal surface staining for epithelial membrane antigen in some cases, and negative staining for carcinoembryonic antigen, vimentin, Factor VIII-related antigen, and *Ulex europaeus* agglutinin 1, although focal staining for Factor VIII has occasionally been reported. Proliferative activity by MIB-1 staining is less than 1%, and the tumor is diploid.[111] Ultrastructural studies reveal mesothelial differentiation, including slender microvilli, intermediate filaments adjacent to the nuclei, intracellular canaliculi, desmosomes, basal lamina, and transition forms with features of both typical mesothelial cells and stromal spindle cells. The mesothelial theory of histogenesis has displaced earlier theories, including endothelial origin, mesonephric origin, and müllerian origin.

Despite the potential for local invasion, adenomatoid tumor is benign, with no metastatic potential. Intraoperative frozen section diagnosis allows local resection with preservation of the epididymis and testis. This tumor may recur if incompletely excised, but does not recur after complete excision.

## Hamartoma (smooth muscle hyperplasia)

Separation of smooth muscle hamartoma (tumor-like overgrowth of normal tissue) and hyperplasia may be difficult and perhaps arbitrary, according to a recent study of 16 cases in which there was predominantly concentric periductal, perivascular, or interstitial proliferation of muscle fascicles.[112] Hamartoma of the spermatic cord may be composed chiefly of smooth muscle (Fig. 14-13) or fibrous connective tissue. One case of hamartoma of the rete testis arose as a testicular

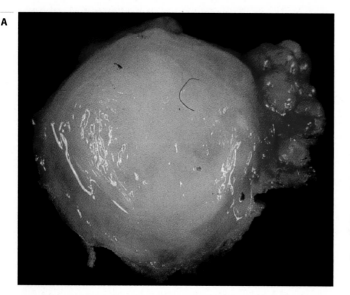

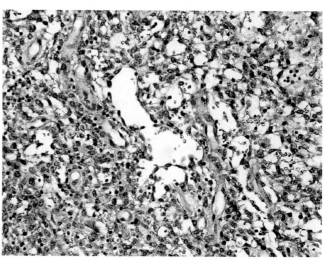

**Fig. 14-12** Adenomatoid tumor of the epididymis. **(A)** Grossly, the tumor was a firm white-gray mass. **(B)** Anastomosing tubules lined by cells with small nuclei and punctuated by thin-walled vessels.

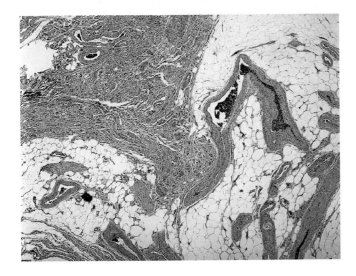

**Fig. 14-13** Smooth muscle hamartoma of the epididymis.

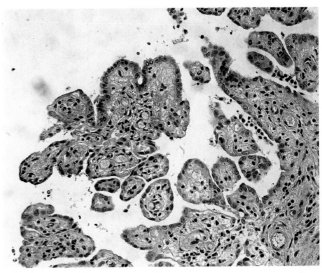

**Fig. 14-14** Benign papillary mesothelioma of the tunica vaginalis.

mass in a 2-year-old. The tumor consisted of a disorganized cluster of tubules embedded in a loose connective tissue stroma. The tubules were lined by cells that were cytologically similar to normal rete testis. Another case of smooth muscle hyperplasia of the rete testis arose in association with multilocular cyst and myxoid stroma with scattered Leydig cells mimicking Leydig cell tumor.[113]

### Reactive mesothelial hyperplasia

Reactive mesothelial hyperplasia appears as a small solid nodule of mesothelial cells that is usually microscopic and clinically asymptomatic. It probably arises as a result of mechanical irritation or inflammation. Reactive mesothelial hyperplasia has also been described in association with hydrocele, hematocele, inguinal hernia sac, and fibrous pseudotumor. Reactive hyperplasia consists of solid nests, tubules, simple papillae, or small cysts of cytologically benign mesothelium set in a fibrous stroma, often appearing beneath the surface mesothelium. Mild cytologic atypia may be present, and squamous metaplasia is rarely seen. Histologic mimics include benign papillary mesothelioma, malignant mesothelioma, and metastatic adenocarcinoma. Benign papillary mesothelioma has a more complex papillary architecture. Malignant mesothelioma is also architecturally complex, often with nuclear atypia, increased mitotic activity, and stromal infiltration. Metastatic adenocarcinoma usually shows severe nuclear abnormalities that stand in contrast to the adjacent surface mesothelium; stains for neutral or hyaluronidase-resistant mucin may also be of value, with negative staining suggesting adenocarcinoma rather than mesothelioma.

### Benign papillary mesothelioma

This rare tumor of the tunica vaginalis usually appears in young men.[114,115] Grossly, it consists of a hydrocele sac with papillary or adenomatous excrescences and cystic or solid areas. Microscopically, there are complex papillae covered by cuboidal, columnar, or flattened mesothelial cells with large vesicular nuclei and glassy eosinophilic cytoplasm (Fig.

14-14). There is no significant nuclear atypia. Psammoma bodies are often present. A careful search should be made to determine whether the papillary lining of the tumor is in continuity with the mesothelium of the adjacent tunica vaginalis. The tumor contains hyaluronidase-sensitive mucin, and ultrastructural study reveals mesothelial differentiation.

Multicystic mesothelioma rarely arises in the spermatic cord.[116]

### Papillary cystadenoma of the epididymis

Papillary cystadenoma of the epididymis is a benign tumor that accounts for about one-third of all primary epididymal tumors; one case was located in the spermatic cord.[117] It occurs in men between 16 and 81 years of age, with a mean of 36 years. More than 50 cases have been reported.[118] About 40% of cases of papillary cystadenoma of the epididymis are bilateral, and these appear as cystic masses in the head of the epididymis that measure up to 6 cm in diameter. The cut surface is gray-brown with yellow foci, and often contains cyst fluid that varies from clear and colorless to yellow, green, or blood-tinged (Fig. 14-15).

Microscopically, papillary cystadenoma consists of dilated ducts lined by papillae with a single or double layer of cuboidal to low columnar epithelium (Fig. 14-15).[119] The cells have characteristic clear glycogen-filled cytoplasm with secretory droplets and cilia at the surface. The papillary cores and cyst walls consist of fibrous connective tissue that may be hyalinized or inflamed. This appearance may be mistaken for metastatic renal cell carcinoma.[120] The cells stain with soybean agglutinin lectin,[121] and are immunoreactive for low and intermediate weight cytokeratins Cam 5.2 and AE1/AE3, epithelial membrane antigen, $\alpha_1$-antitrypsin, $\alpha_1$-antichymotrypsin, and vimentin.[120]

About two-thirds of cases of papillary cystadenoma of the epididymis occur in patients with von Hippel–Lindau syndrome, and are more frequently bilateral in this syndrome.[122] Other manifestations of von Hippel–Lindau syndrome

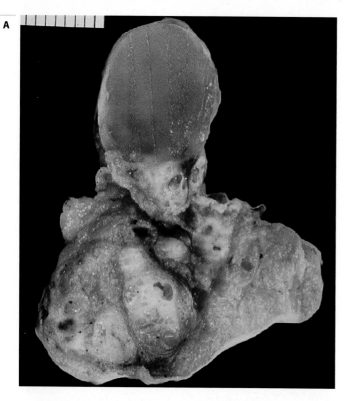

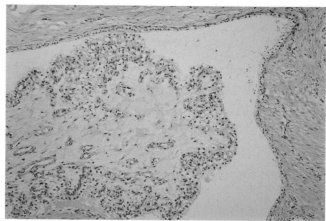

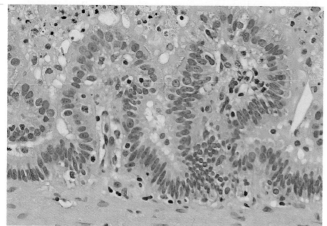

**Fig. 14-15** Papillary cystadenoma of the epididymis. **(A)** Grossly, the tumor consisted of a papillary mass. **(B)** Cystic space containing well-formed papillae. This 35-year-old man had a history of von Hippel–Lindau syndrome, including bilateral renal cell carcinoma and cerebellar and retinal hemangioblastomas. **(C)** Another case of papillary cystadenoma from a patient without a history of von Hippel–Lindau syndrome (A and B courtesy of Dr Bernd Scheithauer, Rochester, MN).

include hemangioblastoma of the cerebellum, cerebrum, spinal cord, retina, pancreas, and urinary bladder; meningioma; syringomyelia; paraganglioma; renal cell carcinoma; pheochromocytoma; islet cell tumor; adrenal cortical adenoma; and a variety of cysts of the liver, kidney, adrenal, and pancreas. Somatic VHL mutations are present in some cases.[120]

### Fibrous pseudotumor (nodular and diffuse fibrous proliferation)

Fibrous pseudotumor encompasses a wide variety of fibroproliferative lesions of the testicular tunics, epididymis, and spermatic cord.[123,124] This lesion has been referred to as chronic periorchitis, proliferative funiculitis,[125,126] fibrous proliferation of the tunics, fibroma, non-specific paratesticular fibrosis, nodular fibrous periorchitis, nodular fibropseudotumor, inflammatory pseudotumor, reactive periorchitis, and pseudofibromatous periorchitis. Early cases of spermatic cord and epididymal fibroma were probably fibrous pseudotumor. This non-neoplastic fibroinflammatory reactive lesion clinically mimics testicular and paratesticular neoplasms, especially when it encases the testis and manifests grossly as an indurated testis. Patients are usually in the third decade of life, but range in age from 7 to 95 years. The lesion usually involves the tunics, and may be associated with hydrocele, hematocele, or both. Less commonly, the epididymis or spermatic cord are involved. A history of epididymo-orchitis, trauma,[127] or inflamed hydrocele is often elicited.

Fibrous pseudotumor is a nodular or diffuse thickening of firm white tissue up to 9.5 cm in diameter, often with focal yellow calcifications (Fig. 14-16). Histologically, it consists of granulation tissue with chronic inflammation, but long-standing tumors contain only paucicellular hyalinized

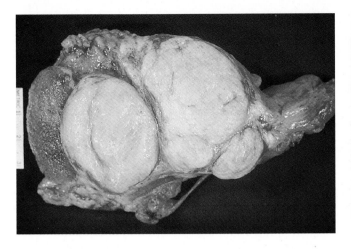

**Fig. 14-16** Fibrous pseudotumor of the testicular tunics.

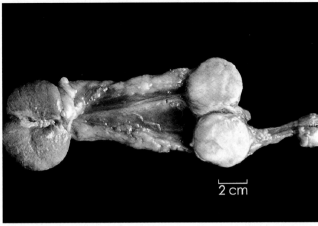

**Fig. 14-18** Leiomyoma of the vas deferens.

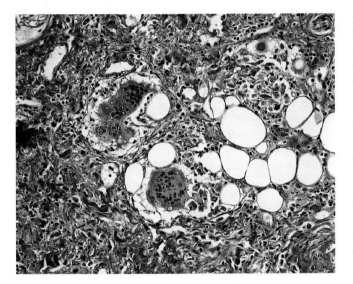

**Fig. 14-17** Sclerosing lipogranuloma of the spermatic cord.

fibrous connective tissue with calcification and ossification. Sclerosing lipogranuloma-like changes may be present (Fig. 14-17).

The condition is considered reactive. Resection of the tumor, perhaps with the tunica vaginalis, is curative, but it is frequently difficult to confirm the benign nature of the process preoperatively, and orchiectomy is often employed.[127] One case was associated with lipoma and diffuse mast cell infiltration of unknown significance.[128]

The differential diagnosis includes solitary fibrous tumor, idiopathic fibromatosis, neurofibroma, and leiomyoma.

### Leiomyoma

Reports of the relative frequencies of leiomyoma to adenomatoid tumor of the epididymis vary from 1:9 to almost 1:1.[129,130] Men with genital leiomyoma range in age from 25 to 81 years, with a mean of 48 years. A hydrocele or hernia sac is identified in up to 21% of cases, and up to 39% are bilateral.[131] Leiomyoma appears as a round, firm, gray-white mass measuring up to 8 cm in diameter; the cut surface is homogeneous and whorled, and bulges from the adjacent soft tissues (Fig. 14-18). It has typical microscopic features of leiomyoma, including interlacing fascicles of spindled smooth muscle cells with few or no mitotic figures. Tumor cells are immunoreactive for vimentin, desmin, and smooth muscle actin.[132] Rare cases of leiomyoma with bizarre nuclei have been described.[133] Angioleiomyoma has also been reported.[134] Surgical excision of epididymal leiomyoma is curative.

Differential diagnostic considerations include smooth muscle hyperplasia, low-grade leiomyosarcoma, and solitary fibrous tumor. The number of mitotic figures is the most reliable criterion for making this separation, but quantitative reporting in smooth muscle tumor of the epididymis and spermatic cord has not been validated.

Leiomyoma is less common in the spermatic cord than the epididymis, with fewer than 20 reported cases. Patient age is similar.

### Melanotic neuroectodermal tumor of infancy (progonoma; retinal anlage tumor)

Rare cases of melanotic neuroectodermal tumor of infancy have arisen in the head of the epididymis and para-testis.[135-138] Patients range in age from newborn to 24 months, with a mean of about 7 months. The tumor is a solitary circumscribed solid blue-brown or black mass measuring up to 3 cm in diameter. Microscopically, it consists of cells with uniform round nuclei and abundant melanin granules lining small cystic spaces of variable size. Smaller round cells with hyperchromatic nuclei, prominent nucleoli, and minimal cytoplasm are observed within luminal spaces and the stroma. Tumor cells resemble neuroblasts and may form glomeruloid bodies, sometimes surrounded by a fibrous matrix set in a collagenous stroma.

Melanotic neuroectodermal tumor of infancy may replace the epididymis, but there are no reports of testicular or spermatic cord invasion. No recurrences of metastases have been identified at this site, but the number of cases is small and the duration of follow-up limited; some speculate that this tumor has the potential for local recurrence and lymph node involvement.

### Brenner tumor

Brenner tumor of the testicular tunics is rare, occurring in men between 37 and 61 years of age. The tumors are small, usually less than 3 cm in diameter, and appear as solid masses with smooth external surfaces and typical histologic features of Brenner tumor elsewhere. Brenner tumor may share a common histogenesis with adenomatoid tumor or Walthard's cell rest.

### Gonadal stromal tumor

Gonadal stromal tumor accounts for up to 3% of testicular tumors, and rare extratesticular examples have been reported.

Embryogenesis of the testis can account for extratesticular nests of germ cells and stromal cells. Microscopic foci of gonadal interstitial cells are occasionally observed in extratesticular sites, such as the spermatic cord and epididymis in orchiectomy specimens removed for other reasons, and these may account for gonadal stromal tumor at such sites.

### Other benign tumors

Other rare benign paratesticular tumors and tumor-like conditions include mucinous adenoid tumor, desmoid,[139] neurofibroma,[140,141] pheochromocytoma/paraganglioma,[142,143] blue nevus,[144] and hemangioma of the testicular tunics.[145] Lymphangiectasia,[146] lymphangioma,[147] hemangioma,[148] angiomyolipoma,[149] angiomyofibroblastoma,[150] angiomyofibroblastoma-like tumor (cellular angiofibroma),[151] and neurofibroma may arise in the spermatic cord or epididymis. There have been rare case reports of granular cell tumor, paratesticular myxoma, carcinoid,[152] solitary fibrous tumor,[153,154] extratesticular Leydig cell tumor,[155] and rhabdomyoma of the spermatic cord.[156–159] Aggressive angiomyxoma of the spermatic cord was reported in two 13-year-old boys, appearing as a benign myxoid tumor immunoreactive for vimentin and smooth muscle actin.[160] Another case arose in an 82-year-old that was also positive for vimentin but negative for actin, desmin, and CD34.[161] A recent report of four cases of aggressive angiomyoma found estrogen and progesterone immunoreactivity in the majority, similar to cases in women.[162] Fibrous hamartoma of infancy occasionally arises in the scrotum or spermatic cord.[163]

## Malignant neoplasms

### Liposarcoma

The most common sarcoma of the paratesticular region in adults is spermatic cord liposarcoma.[164,165] Mean patient age is about 63 years,[166] with a range from 16 to 90 years. Grossly, liposarcoma is a lobulated mass of yellow tissue ranging from 3 to 30 cm (mean, 12 cm) that often resembles lipoma.[166] Microscopically, the most common pattern is well-differentiated liposarcoma (lipoma-like liposarcoma), often with prominent sclerosis.[167] Myxoid/round cell liposarcoma[168,169] and dedifferentiated/pleomorphic liposarcoma may also occur.[166,170,171]

Paratesticular liposarcoma is treated by radical orchiectomy with high ligation of the spermatic cord. Hemiscrotectomy may be required in cases with inadequate surgical resection margins to avoid local recurrence. Lymphadenectomy is not usually indicated, especially with well-differentiated and myxoid liposarcoma. The role of radiation therapy and chemotherapy is uncertain, but both are commonly employed. The majority of patients with paratesticular liposarcoma treated by resection with negative surgical margins are clinically free of tumor, and those with well-differentiated liposarcoma have a prolonged course, sometimes with late recurrences[166]; however, 23% of all patients with liposarcoma develop local recurrence, and less than 10% develop metastases, invariably in those with dedifferentiated or high-grade liposarcoma.

The differential diagnosis of well-differentiated liposarcoma includes sclerosing lipogranuloma and lipoma. Myxoid liposarcoma should be distinguished from rhabdomyosarcoma and myxoid malignant fibrous histiocytoma. Pleomorphic liposarcoma may be difficult to distinguish from other types of high-grade sarcoma.

### Rhabdomyosarcoma

Paratesticular rhabdomyosarcoma may arise in the testicular tunics, epididymis, or spermatic cord. When the tumor is large or locally invasive, the exact site of origin cannot be determined. Rhabdomyosarcoma is the most common sarcoma of the paratesticular area in children, with a peak incidence at about 9 years, although it may occur at any age.[172–175]

Grossly, rhabdomyosarcoma is an encapsulated white-gray mass with focal hemorrhage and cystic degeneration that measures up to 20 cm in diameter. Most are embryonal, consisting of small round cells with dark nuclei, scant cytoplasm, and variable numbers of cells showing myoblastic differentiation. The connective tissue stroma may be myxoid. Alveolar, botryoid, and pleomorphic patterns have rarely been observed at this site.[173]

Rhabdomyosarcoma usually spreads to retroperitoneal lymph nodes, and patients without distant metastases are treated by radical inguinal orchiectomy with high ligation of the spermatic cord and ipsilateral or bilateral retroperitoneal or pelvic lymphadenectomy. Retroperitoneal lymphadenectomy can be avoided after radical inguinal orchiectomy when radiologic studies such as computerized tomography (CT) are negative. The extent of lymphadenectomy determines the likelihood of postoperative fertility. Locally invasive rhabdomyosarcoma that involves the skin or arises with clinically suspicious inguinal lymph nodes is treated by orchiectomy, scrotectomy, and inguinal lymphadenectomy. Long-term survival rates of more than 80% are observed in patients receiving adjuvant radiation therapy and combination chemotherapy.

### Leiomyosarcoma

Leiomyosarcoma is more common in the spermatic cord than in the epididymis, with more than 100 reported cases.[176,177] It arises in patients of all ages, with a peak in the sixth and seventh decades; more than 80% of patients are over 40 years of age.[166,178]

Grossly, leiomyosarcoma is a solid gray-tan mass, 2–9 cm in diameter, involving the intrascrotal portion of the spermatic cord, scrotal subcutis and dartos muscle, epididymis, or testicular tunics (Fig. 14-19).[179] It consists of a spindle cell proliferation with typical features of leiomyosarcoma at other sites. Features that definitely separate low-grade leiomyosarcoma and leiomyoma are lacking, although the presence of necrosis, large numbers of mitotic figures, nuclear pleomorphism, and marked cellularity suggest malignancy. Most cases are high grade at diagnosis, although this has been refuted.[179]

Paratesticular leiomyosarcoma is treated by radical inguinal orchiectomy. The role of retroperitoneal lymphadenectomy is uncertain, and is usually not recommended owing to the propensity of leiomyosarcoma for hematogenous rather than lymphatic spread. Adjuvant radiation therapy and chemotherapy are considered palliative. Leiomyosarcoma may recur locally and metastasize, and about one-third of patients die of metastases. Survival rates after treatment are 75% and 50% at 5 and 10 years, respectively.[180] Enucleation was undertaken in one patient, with good long-term results.[181]

## Malignant mesothelioma

Paratesticular malignant mesothelioma is rare, with fewer than 70 reported cases. Most occur in the tunica vaginalis,[182,183] with very few in the spermatic cord and epididymis. Mean patient age is about 55 years, ranging from 12 to 84 years. Primary peritoneal malignant mesothelioma may present as a mass in an inguinal hernia. Malignant mesothelioma of the tunica vaginalis may appear in pipe-fitters with asbestos exposure, raising the possibility of asbestos as a contributory factor, similar to pleural and peritoneal mesothelioma. Bilateral mesothelioma of the tunica vaginalis occurs rarely.

Grossly, malignant mesothelioma appears as multiple friable cystic and solid masses and small nodules studding the lining of a hydrocele sac, hernia sac, or the peritoneum (Fig. 14-20). Continuity between the tumor and adjacent mesothelium of the tunica vaginalis may be apparent, and there may be invasion of adjacent structures.

Histologically, paratesticular malignant mesothelioma is similar to mesothelioma at other sites, and may be epithelial, spindle cell, or biphasic, with a wide morphologic spectrum (Fig. 14-20). The epithelial pattern is most common, accounting for about 75% of cases, and may be mixed with papillary, tubular, and solid areas. Spindle cells predominate in the sarcomatous pattern, and may merge perceptively with solid epithelioid nests. Tumor cells are cuboidal or flattened, with variable amounts of eosinophilic cytoplasm and atypical vesicular nuclei, often with prominent nucleoli. Mitotic figures are usually present. The combination of calretinin, cytokeratins 5/6, and thrombomodulin appears to be useful in separating epithelioid mesothelioma from metastatic carcinoma; these markers are also positive in benign and reactive mesothelium.[184]

Malignant mesothelioma is aggressive, with a potential for late recurrence or metastasis. It recurs locally along the vas deferens or in the pelvis, and usually spreads by lymphatic routes to pelvic, retroperitoneal, or distant lymph nodes. Radical inguinal orchiectomy is recommended, with high ligation of the spermatic cord at the internal inguinal ring. Hemiscrotectomy or hemiscrotal irradiation may be useful to avoid local recurrence when a transscrotal incision is made. Primary retroperitoneal lymphadenectomy is often employed in patients with clinical or radiologic evidence of lymphatic metastases or in those without distant metastases. The utility of adjuvant chemotherapy is uncertain. About half of patients remain free of tumor for up to 18 years after treatment.

The predominance of the epithelial or spindle cell component determines the differential diagnostic considerations. Epithelial malignant mesothelioma may be mistaken for reactive mesothelial hyperplasia, adenomatoid tumor, benign papillary mesothelioma, adenocarcinoma of the epididymis, paratesticular müllerian serous tumor, and metastatic adenocarcinoma. Paratesticular mesothelioma should

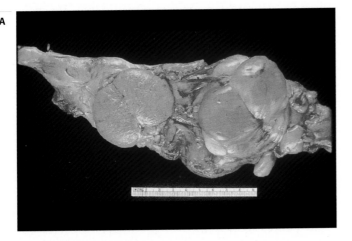

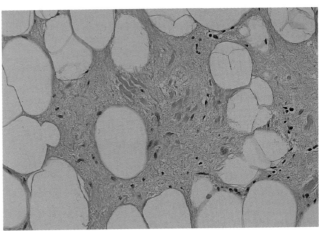

**Fig. 14-19** Liposarcoma of the spermatic cord. **(A)** Grossly, the tumor consisted of a multinodular mass of firm tan tissue. **(B)** Delicate fibrosis and increased cellularity was observed within adipose tissue.

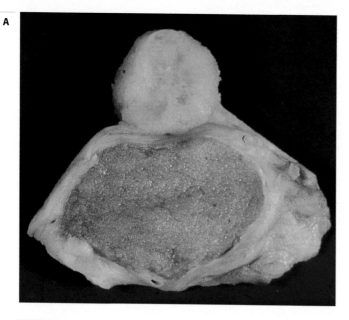

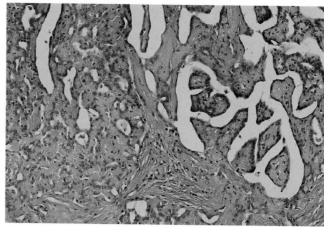

**Fig. 14-20** Malignant mesothelioma of the tunica vaginalis. **(A)** Grossly, the tumor consisted of a large exophytic papillary mass. **(B)** Micropapillations are lined by flattened to cuboidal tumor cells. (Courtesy of Dr Jan Kennedy, Atlanta, Georgia.)

be suspected in cases with in situ mesothelioma in the adjacent tunics, typical tubulopapillary architecture, and a lack of extrascrotal involvement. Spindle cell malignant mesothelioma should be distinguished from the variety of soft tissue sarcomas that arise at this site. Biphasic mesothelioma may be confused with stromal fibrosis, synovial sarcoma, and carcinosarcoma.

### Papillary serous tumor of müllerian epithelium (benign and malignant)

Rarely, müllerian epithelial tumors (also referred to as ovarian-type epithelial tumors, or OTET) arise in the testis and paratesticular structures, perhaps from embryonic remnants such as the appendix testis.[135,185] One case arose in the torsed appendix testis of a young boy.[186] Some early reports of adenocarcinoma of the testicular appendages apparently represent papillary serous tumor of müllerian epithelium or malignant mesothelioma.

Papillary serous tumor of low malignant potential may occur in the tunica vaginalis, testis, spermatic cord, and epididymis, and is grossly, microscopically, and immunohistochemically identical to its ovarian counterpart.[111,187] Patients range in age from 6 to 77 years (mean, 56 years), and present with an apparent testicular tumor. Proliferative activity by MIB-1 staining ranges from 1% to 10% (mean, 5.5%), and most are diploid. Radical orchiectomy is the treatment of choice, and the tumor does not recur or metastasize after complete resection.[111]

Papillary serous carcinoma typically consists of invasive papillae lined by serous cuboidal or columnar cells with eosinophilic cytoplasm, frank nuclear anaplasia, and abundant psammoma bodies.[188] Cancer cells display immunoreactivity for broad-spectrum keratin AE1/3, S100 protein, epithelial membrane antigen, and Ber-EP4; variable positive staining is seen with Leu M1, B72.3, CEA, PLAP, and vimen-

tin. Serum concentration of CA-125 is elevated in some patients. Cancer tends to recur within 5–7 years.

The differential diagnosis of serous tumor of müllerian epithelium includes papillary cystadenoma of the epididymis, benign papillary mesothelioma, malignant mesothelioma, adenocarcinoma of the rete testis or epididymis, and metastatic adenocarcinoma.

### Adenocarcinoma of the epididymis

Fewer than 30 cases of epididymal adenocarcinoma have been reported.[7,189–192] Mean patient age is 44 years, with a range from 5 to 78 years. The tumors measure up to 9 cm in diameter, and may be multicystic or solid. About half are associated with hydrocele.

Microscopically, there are typical features of adenocarcinoma, including papillary, glandular, mucinous,[193] and solid undifferentiated patterns; clear cells often predominate. Squamous cell carcinoma may also be admixed. The main differential diagnostic consideration is metastatic renal cell carcinoma.[194]

Nearly half of reported patients develop metastases. Treatment is uncertain, but surgery and chemotherapy are most often used; palliative radiation therapy has no apparent durable effect on cancer progression.[195]

### Malignant fibrous histiocytoma

Fewer than 40 cases of malignant fibrous histiocytoma (MFH) involving the spermatic cord and paratesticular area have been reported.[196–199] Most occurred in patients over 50 years of age. Grossly, the tumor is solid gray or yellow-white, has a whorled cut surface, and measures up to 10 cm in diameter. Histologic patterns include myxoid, inflammatory, and pleomorphic malignant fibrous histiocytoma; the storiform–pleomorphic pattern accounted for more than 80% of reported cases.[197]

About one-third of patients with MFH develop local recurrence or distant metastases. The treatment of choice is radical inguinal orchiectomy with high ligation of the spermatic cord. The value of adjuvant therapy is unknown, although one patient was cancer-free 6 years after adjuvant radiation therapy.[200] Tumor size did not predict outcome.[197]

## Other sarcomas and malignancies

More than 60 cases of spermatic cord and epididymal fibrosarcoma have been described, but some of these probably represent other forms of sarcoma.[201] Most occur in adults, but all ages may be affected. The gross and microscopic appearances of fibrosarcoma of the paratesticular area are similar to those of other sites. More than half of patients die of locally recurrent or metastatic tumor.

Most types of sarcoma have been described in the paratesticular area, including primary neuroblastoma,[202] neurofibrosarcoma, angiosarcoma, chondrosarcoma, myxofibrosarcoma,[203] and undifferentiated sarcoma. Peripheral neuroectodermal tumor (extraskeletal Ewing's sarcoma) has also been reported (Fig. 14-21).[204]

## Germ cell tumor

A variety of germ cell tumors have been described in the paratesticular area, including seminoma, embryonal carcinoma, and teratoma; rare cases may be burned out and pose a diagnostic challenge.[205] The epididymis is more commonly involved than the spermatic cord, but germ cell tumor at either site is rare. The demographic and pathologic features of paratesticular germ cell tumor are similar to those of the testis. These tumors probably arise from misplaced germinal elements. Contiguous subepithelial spread of seminoma along the vas deferens was reported in a 56-year-old man.[206]

## Malignant lymphoma and hematopoietic neoplasms

Malignant lymphoma is the most common tumor of the testis in men over 50, yet paratesticular lymphoma is uncommon.[207] Rare cases of primary epididymal or spermatic cord lymphoma have been described.[208–210] Secondary lymphoma has been described in all sites of the paratesticular area, invariably in association with testicular involvement. Occlusion of spermatic cord vessels by lymphoma may result in testicular ischemia.[211] Plasmacytoma of the epididymis and spermatic cord has also been reported.[212]

## Metastases

Metastases to the paratesticular area are rare, and usually arise from the prostate,[213] kidney,[214] lung,[215] and stomach.[216]

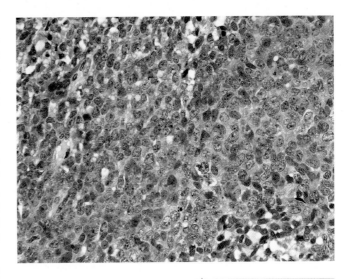

**Fig. 14-21** Peripheral neuroectodermal tumor (extraskeletal Ewing's tumor) of the spermatic cord. Tumor cells displayed MIC-2 immunoreactivity.

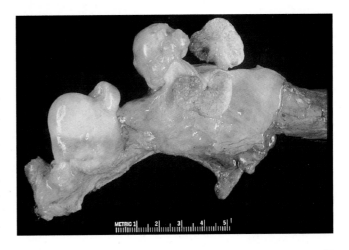

**Fig. 14-22** Hernia sac containing multiple nodules of metastatic colonic adenocarcinoma.

A renal primary should always be considered in clear cell carcinoma at this site; misdiagnoses include Sertoli cell tumor, Sertoli–Leydig cell tumor, and clear cell cystadenoma of the epididymis.[217] Rare cases have originated from colonic adenocarcinoma[218,219] (Fig. 14-22), pancreatic adenocarcinoma, prostatic adenocarcinoma,[220] urothelial carcinoma,[221] ileal carcinoid, and malignant melanoma. Patients with paratesticular metastases usually have a poor outcome.

## REFERENCES

1. Srigley JR. The paratesticular region: histoanatomic and general considerations. Semin Diagn Pathol 2000; 17: 258–269.

2. Lioe TF, Biggart JD. Tumours of the spermatic cord and paratesticular tissue. A clinicopathological study. Br J Urol 1993; 71: 600–606.

3. Han CH, Kang SH. Epididymal anomalies associated with patent processus vaginalis in hydrocele and cryptorchidism. J Korean Med Sci 2002; 17: 660–662.

4. De Miguel MP, Marino JM, Martinez-Garcia F, et al. Pre- and post-natal growth of the human ductus epididymidis. A morphometric study. Reprod Fertil Dev 1998; 10: 271–277.

5. Bedford JM. The status and the state of the human epididymis. Hum Reprod 1994; 9: 2187–2199.

6. Oliva E, Young RH. Paratesticular tumor-like lesions. Semin Diagn Pathol 2000; 17: 340–358.

7. Jones EC, Murray SK, Young RH. Cysts and epithelial proliferations of the testicular collecting system (including rete testis). Semin Diagn Pathol 2000; 17: 270–293.

8. Sharp SC, Batt MA, Lennington WJ. Epididymal cribriform hyperplasia. A variant of normal epididymal histology. Arch Pathol Lab Med 1994; 118: 1020–1022.

9. Butterworth DM, Bisset DL. Cribriform intra-tubular epididymal change and adenomatous hyperplasia of the rete testis – a consequence of testicular atrophy? Histopathology 1992; 21: 435–438.

10. Coyne JD. Eosinophilic granular cell change of Sertoli cells and of epididymal columnar cells. Histopathology 2004; 44: 86–87.

11. Oshima S, Okayasu I, Uchima H, Hatakeyama S. Histopathological and morphometrical study of the human epididymis and testis. Acta Pathol Jpn 1984; 34: 1327–1342.

12. Kuo T, Gomez LG. Monstrous epithelial cells in human epididymis and seminal vesicles. A pseudomalignant change. Am J Surg Pathol 1981; 5: 483–490.

13. Bromberg WD, Kozlowski JM, Oyasu R. Prostate-type gland in the epididymis. J Urol 1991; 145: 1273–1274.

14. Nistal M, Iniguez L, Paniagua R. Pitted pattern in the human epididymis. J Reprod Fertil 1990; 89: 655–661.

15. Nistal M, Iniguez L, Paniagua R, Regadera J. Diverticula of the ductus epididymis in men. J Urol 1986; 136: 1224–1227.

16. Shah VI, Ro JY, Amin MB, et al. Histologic variations in the epididymis: findings in 167 orchiectomy specimens. Am J Surg Pathol 1998; 22: 990–996.

17. Jayaram N, Ramaprasad AV, Chethan M, Sujay RP. Tumours and tumour-like conditions of the para-testicular region – a study of morphological features. Indian J Pathol Microbiol 1998; 41: 287–295.

18. Weiske WH, Salzler N, Schroeder-Printzen I, Weidner W. Clinical findings in congenital absence of the vasa deferentia. Andrologia 2000; 32: 13–18.

19. Wagenknecht LV, Lotzin CF, Sommer HJ, Schirren C. Vas deferens aplasia: clinical and anatomical features of 90 cases. Andrologia 1983; 15: 605–613.

20. Conley GR, Sant GR, Ucci AA, Mitcheson HD. Seminoma and epididymal cysts in a young man with known diethylstilbestrol exposure in utero. JAMA 1983; 249: 1325–1326.

21. Koff WJ, Scaletscky R. Malformations of the epididymis in undescended testis. J Urol 1990; 143: 340–343.

22. Pendse AK, Mathur PN, Sharma MM, Gupta OP. Splenic-gonadal fusion. Br J Surg 1975; 62: 624–628.

23. Habuchi T, Mizutani Y, Miyakawa M. Ectopic aberrant adrenals with epididymal abnormality. Urology 1992; 39: 251–253.

24. Oguzkurt P, Oz S, Kayaselcuk F. Ectopic adrenal tissue: an incidental finding during inguinoscrotal operations in children. Hernia 2002; 6: 62–63.

25. Savas C, Candir O, Bezir M, Cakmak M. Ectopic adrenal cortical nodules along the spermatic cord of children. Int Urol Nephrol 2001; 32: 681–685.

26. Vaos G, Zavras N, Boukouvalea I. Ectopic adrenal cortical tissue along the inguinoscrotal path of children. Int Surg 2006; 91: 125–128.

27. Schned AR, Seremetis GM, Rous SN. Paratesticular multicystic mass of Wolffian, probably paradidymal, origin. Am J Clin Pathol 1994; 101: 543–546.

28. Nistal M, Iniguez L, Paniagua R, et al. Tubular embryonal remnants in the human spermatic cord. Urol Int 1987; 42: 260–264.

29. Kantarci F, Ozer H, Adaletli I, Mihmanli I. Cystic appendix epididymis: a sonomorphologic study. Surg Radiol Anat 2005; 27: 557–561.

30. Skorpil M, Silseth C, Berne M. Torsion of the hydatid of Morgagni – a hereditary disease? The most common cause of acute scrotum in children. Lakartidningen 1999; 96: 1320–1322.

31. Wollin M, Marshall FF, Fink MP, Malhotra R, Diamond DA. Aberrant epididymal tissue: a significant clinical entity. J Urol 1987; 138: 1247–1250.

32. Virdi JS, Conway W, Kelly DG. Torsion of the vas aberrans. Br J Urol 1990; 66: 435.

33. Cerilli LA, Sotelo-Avila C, Mills SE. Glandular inclusions in inguinal hernia sacs: morphologic and immunohistochemical distinction from epididymis and vas deferens. Am J Surg Pathol 2003; 27: 469–476.

34. Steigman CK, Sotelo-Avila C, Weber TR. The incidence of spermatic cord structures in inguinal hernia sacs from male children. Am J Surg Pathol 1999; 23: 880–885.

35. Popek EJ. Embryonal remnants in inguinal hernia sacs. Hum Pathol 1990; 21: 339–349.

36. Walker AN, Mills SE. Glandular inclusions in inguinal hernial sacs and spermatic cords. Mullerian-like remnants confused with functional reproductive structures. Am J Clin Pathol 1984; 82: 85–89.

37. Miller GG, McDonald SE, Milbrandt K, Chibbar R. Routine pathological evaluation of tissue from inguinal hernias in children is unnecessary. Can J Surg 2003; 46: 117–119.

38. Partrick DA, Bensard DD, Karrer FM, Ruyle SZ. Is routine pathological evaluation of pediatric hernia sacs justified? J Pediatr Surg 1998; 33: 1090–1092; discussion 3–4.

39. Brisson P, Patel H, Feins N. Cremasteric muscle hypertrophy accompanies inguinal hernias in children. J Pediatr Surg 1999; 34: 1320–1321.

40. Nistal M, Martin L, Paniagua R. Idiopathic hematoma of the epididymis: presentation of three cases. Eur Urol 1990; 17: 178–180.

41. Gioffre L. Structure of the venous wall of the pampiniform plexus in idiopathic varicocele. G Chir 2001; 22: 213–216.

42. Tanji N, Fujiwara T, Kaji H, et al. Histologic evaluation of spermatic veins in patients with varicocele. Int J Urol 1999; 6: 355–360.

43. Mavrov K, Takov R, Tsvetkov D. Clinico-morphological studies of epididymal cysts. Khirurgiia (Sofiia) 1990; 43: 56–61.

44. Yagi H, Igawa M, Shiina H, et al. Multilocular spermatocele: a case report. Int Urol Nephrol 2001; 32: 413–416.

45. Takimoto K, Okamoto K, Wakabayashi Y, Okada Y. Torsion of spermatocele: a rare manifestation. Urol Int 2002; 69: 164–165.

46. Jassie MP, Mahmood P. Torsion of spermatocele: a newly described entity with 2 case reports. J Urol 1985; 133: 683–684.

47. Nistal M, Iniguez L, Paniagua R. Histological classification of spermatic cord cysts in relation to their histogenesis. Eur Urol 1987; 13: 327–330.

48. Katergiannakis V, Lagoudianakis EE, Markogiannakis H, Manouras A. Huge epidermoid cyst of the spermatic cord in an adult patient. Int J Urol 2006; 13: 95–97.

49. Brown DL, Benson CB, Doherty FJ, et al. Cystic testicular mass caused by dilated rete testis: sonographic findings in 31 cases. AJR Am J Roentgenol 1992; 158: 1257–1259.

50. Wojcik LJ, Hansen K, Diamond DA, et al. Cystic dysplasia of the rete testis: a benign congenital lesion associated with ipsilateral urological anomalies. J Urol 1997; 158: 600–604.

51. Nistal M, Jimenez-Heffernan JA, Garcia-Viera M, Paniagua R. Cystic transformation and calcium oxalate deposits in rete testis and efferent ducts in dialysis patients. Hum Pathol 1996; 27: 336–341.

52. Coyne J, al-Nakib L, Goldsmith D, O'Flynn K. Secondary oxalosis and sperm granuloma of the epididymis. J Clin Pathol 1994; 47: 470–471.

53. Nistal M, Santamaria L, Paniagua R. Acquired cystic transformation of the rete testis secondary to renal failure. Hum Pathol 1989; 20: 1065–1070.

54. Nistal M, Mate A, Paniagua R. Cystic transformation of the rete testis. Am J Surg Pathol 1996; 20: 1231–1239.

55. Nistal M, Jimenez-Heffernan JA. Rete testis dysgenesis. A characteristic lesion of undescended testes. Arch Pathol Lab Med 1997; 121: 1259–1264.

56. Inoue K, Higaki Y, Yoshida H. Inguinal hernia of seminal vesicle cyst. Int J Urol 2004; 11: 1039–1040.

57. Mikuz G, Damjanov I. Inflammation of the testis, epididymis, peritesticular membranes, and scrotum. Pathol Annu 1982; 17: 101–128.

58. Nistal M, Gonzalez-Peramato P, Serrano A, Regadera J. Xanthogranulomatous funiculitis and orchiepididymitis: report of 2 cases with immunohistochemical study and literature review. Arch Pathol Lab Med 2004; 128: 911–914.

59. Doble A, Taylor-Robinson D, Thomas BJ, et al. Acute epididymitis: a microbiological and ultrasonographic study. Br J Urol 1989; 63: 90–94.

60. Ostaszewska I, Zdrodowska-Stefanow B, Darewicz B, et al. Role of Chlamydia trachomatis in epididymitis. Part II: Clinical diagnosis. Med Sci Monit 2000; 6: 1119–1121.

61. Dalton AD, Harcourt-Webster JN. The histopathology of the testis and epididymis in AIDS – a post-mortem study. J Pathol 1991; 163: 47–52.

62. McCarthy JM, McLoughlin MG, Shackleton CR, et al. Cytomegalovirus epididymitis following renal transplantation. J Urol 1991; 146: 417–419.

63. Reddy GS, Das LK, Pani SP. The preferential site of adult Wuchereria bancrofti: an ultrasound study of male asymptomatic microfilaria carriers in Pondicherry, India. Natl Med J India 2004; 17: 195–196.

64. Gasparich JP, Mason JT, Greene HL, et al. Amiodarone-associated epididymitis: drug-related epididymitis in the absence of infection. J Urol 1985; 133: 971–972.

65. Chen TF, Ball RY. Epididymectomy for post-vasectomy pain: histological review. Br J Urol 1991; 68: 407–413.

66. Schned AR, Selikowitz SM. Epididymitis nodosa. An epididymal lesion analogous to vasitis nodosa. Arch Pathol Lab Med 1986; 110: 61–64.

67. Segawa N, Abe H, Nishida T, Katsuoka Y. Spermatic cord tuberculosis: a case report. Hinyokika Kiyo 2005; 51: 347–349.

68. Muttarak M, Lojanapiwat B, Chaiwun B, Wudhikarn S. Preoperative diagnosis of bilateral tuberculous epididymo-orchitis following intravesical Bacillus Calmette–Guérin therapy for superficial bladder carcinoma. Australas Radiol 2002; 46: 183–185.

69. Sah SP, Bhadani PP, Regmi R, et al. Fine needle aspiration cytology of tubercular epididymitis and epididymo-orchitis. Acta Cytol 2006; 50: 243–249.

70. Dieckmann KP, Henke RP, Zimmer-Krolzig G. Malacoplakia of the epididymis. Report of a case and review of the literature. Urol Int 1995; 55: 222–225.

71. Esser R, Rothenberger KH. Sarcoidosis of the spermatic cord and epididymus. Aktuelle Urol 2003; 34: 354–355.

72. Gazaigne J, Mozziconacci JG, Mornet M, Provendier B. Epididymal and renal sarcoidosis. Br J Urol 1995; 75: 413–414.

73. Ryan DM, Lesser BA, Crumley LA, et al. Epididymal sarcoidosis. J Urol 1993; 149: 134–136.

74. Jenkin GA, Choo M, Hosking P, Johnson PD. Candidal epididymo-orchitis: case report and review. Clin Infect Dis 1998; 26: 942–945.

75. Kauffman CA, Slama TG, Wheat LJ. Histoplasma capsulatum epididymitis. J Urol 1981; 125: 434–435.

76. Seo R, Oyasu R, Schaeffer A. Blastomycosis of the epididymis and prostate. Urology 1997; 50: 980–982.

77. Jungmann P, Figueredo-Silva J, Dreyer G. Bancroftian lymphangitis in northeastern Brazil: a histopathological study of 17 cases. J Trop Med Hyg 1992; 95: 114–118.

78. Svec A, Urban M, Mikyskova I, Tachezy R. Human papillomavirus in squamous metaplastic epithelium with dysplasia of the epididymis detected by PCR method. Am J Surg Pathol 1999; 23: 1437–1438.

79. Matsuda T, Horii Y, Nishimura K, et al. Young's syndrome: report of two Japanese cases. Urol Int 1991; 47: 53–56.

80. Handelsman DJ, Conway AJ, Boylan LM, Turtle JR. Young's syndrome. Obstructive azoospermia and chronic sinopulmonary infections. N Engl J Med 1984; 310: 3–9.

81. Nistal M, Mate A, Paniagua R. Granulomatous epididymal lesion of possible ischemic origin. Am J Surg Pathol 1997; 21: 951–956.

82. McDonald SW. Cellular responses to vasectomy. Int Rev Cytol 2000; 199: 295–339.

83. Warner JJ, Kirchner FK Jr, Wong SW, Dao AH. Vasitis nodosa presenting as a mass of the spermatic cord. J Urol 1983; 129: 380–381.

84. Tsurusaki T, Maruta N, Iwasaki S, et al. Idiopathic bilateral panniculitis of the spermatic cord in an elderly male patient. J Urol 2000; 164: 1657–1658.

85. Tanaka M, Tsumatani K, Mibu H, Saka T. Genital tuberculosis occurring in the spermatic cord: a case report. Hinyokika Kiyo 2002; 48: 753–755.

86. Pampiglione S, Rivasi F, Angeli G, et al. Dirofilariasis due to Dirofilaria repens in Italy, an emergent zoonosis: report of 60 new cases. Histopathology 2001; 38: 344–354.

87. Durand F, Brion JP, Terrier N, et al. Funiculitis due to Schistosoma haematobium: uncommon diagnosis using parasitologic analysis of semen. Am J Trop Med Hyg 2004; 70: 46–47.

88. Heydenrych JJ, Marcus PB. Meconium granulomas of the tunica vaginalis. J Urol 1976; 115: 596–598.

89. Al-Arfaj A. Limited Wegener's granulomatosis of the epididymis. Int J Urol 2001; 8: 333–335.

90. San Miguel P, Fernandez GC, Pesqueira Santiago D, et al. Spermatic cord mass as a manifestation of systemic vasculitis: a case report and review of the literature. Actas Urol Esp 2005; 29: 777–781.

91. Hashiguchi Y, Matsuo Y, Torii Y, et al. Polyarteritis nodosa of the epididymis. Abdom Imag 2001; 26: 102–104.

92. Kameyama K, Kuramochi S, Kamio N, et al. Isolated periarteritis nodosa of the spermatic cord presenting as a scrotal mass: report of a case. Heart Vessels 1998; 13: 152–154.

93. Kessel A, Toubi E, Golan TD, et al. Isolated epididymal vasculitis. Israel Med Assoc J 2001; 3: 65–66.

94. Karnauchow PN, Steele AA. Isolated necrotizing granulomatous vasculitis of the spermatic cords. J Urol 1989; 141: 379–381.

95. Nistal M, Gonzalez-Peramato P, Paniagua R. Lipomembranous fat necrosis in three cases of testicular torsion. Histopathology 2001; 38: 443–447.

96. Sirvent JJ, Bernat R, Navarro MA, et al. Spermatic cord torsion: morphologic and functional study, with special reference to the Leydig cells. Actas Urol Esp 1988; 12: 443–448.

97. Matsumoto A, Nagatomi Y, Sakai M, Oshi M. Torsion of the hernia sac within a hydrocele of the scrotum in a child. Int J Urol 2004; 11: 789–791.

98. Rakha E, Puls F, Saidul I, Furness P. Torsion of the testicular appendix: importance of associated acute inflammation. J Clin Pathol 2006; 59: 831–834.

99. Mumtaz FH, Khan MA, Morgan RJ. Synchronous bilateral torsion of the appendix testis. Urol Int 1998; 60: 128–129.

100. Kilciler M, Saglam M, Sumer F, et al. Lithiasis in varicocele veins: 'varicolithiasis.' J Urol 2002; 168: 630.

101. Ozgur A, Tarcan T, Simsek F, Ahiskali R. An unusual tumor of the spermatic cord: myositis ossificans. Arch Esp Urol 2003; 56: 1072–1074.

102. Demirci D, Ekmekcioglu O, Inci M, Akgun H. Heterotopic ossification of the spermatic cord. Int Urol Nephrol 2003; 35: 513–514.

103. Montgomery E, Buras R. Incidental liposarcomas identified during hernia repair operations. J Surg Oncol 1999; 71: 50–53.

104. Greeley DJ Jr, Sullivan JG, Wolfe GR. Massive primary lipoma of the scrotum. Am Surg 1995; 61: 954–955.

105. Lilly MC, Arregui ME. Lipomas of the cord and round ligament. Ann Surg 2002; 235: 586–590.

106. Heller CA, Marucci DD, Dunn T, et al. Inguinal canal 'lipoma.' Clin Anat 2002; 15: 280–285.

107. Cooper K, Govender D. Adenomatous hyperplasia of the rete testis in the undescended testis. J Pathol 1990; 162: 333–334.

108. Racioppi M, D'Addessi A, Di Pinto A, et al. Three consecutive cases of adenomatoid tumour of the epididymis: histological considerations and therapeutical implications. Review of the literature. Arch Ital Urol Androl 1996; 68: 115–119.

109. Tammela TL, Karttunen TJ, Makarainen HP, et al. Intrascrotal adenomatoid tumors. J Urol 1991; 146: 61–65.

110. Perez-Campos A, Jimenez-Heffernan JA, Perez F, Vicandi B. Cytologic features of paratesticular adenomatoid tumor. Acta Cytol 2004; 48: 457–458.

111. McClure RF, Keeney GL, Sebo TJ, Cheville JC. Serous borderline tumor of the paratestis: a report of seven cases. Am J Surg Pathol 2001; 25: 373–378.

112. Barton JH, Davis CJ Jr, Sesterhenn IA, Mostofi FK. Smooth muscle hyperplasia of the testicular adnexa clinically mimicking neoplasia: clinicopathologic study of sixteen cases. Am J Surg Pathol 1999; 23: 903–909.

113. Fridman E, Skarda J, Ofek-Moravsky E, Cordoba M. Complex multilocular cystic lesion of rete testis, accompanied by smooth muscle hyperplasia, mimicking intratesticular Leydig cell neoplasm. Virchows Arch 2005; 447: 768–771.

114. Rosales Leal JL, Tallada Bunuel M, Espejo Maldonado E, et al. Multicystic mesothelioma of the testicular tunica vaginalis. Arch Esp Urol 2003; 56: 1154–1157.

115. Xiao SY, Rizzo P, Carbone M. Benign papillary mesothelioma of the tunica vaginalis testis. Arch Pathol Lab Med 2000; 124: 143–147.

116. Tobioka H, Manabe K, Matsuoka S, et al. Multicystic mesothelioma of the spermatic cord. Histopathology 1995; 27: 479–481.

117. Geenen RW, Bevers RF, Gielis C, Boon TA. Papillary cystadenoma located in the spermatic cord. J Urol 1997; 158: 546.

118. Raimoldi A, Berti GL, Canclini L, et al. Papillary cystadenoma of the epididymis. 2 case reports. Arch Ital Urol Androl 1997; 69: 309–311.

119. Calder CJ, Gregory J. Papillary cystadenoma of the epididymis: a report of two cases with an immunohistochemical study. Histopathology 1993; 23: 89–91.

120. Gilcrease MZ, Schmidt L, Zbar B, et al. Somatic von Hippel–Lindau mutation in clear cell papillary cystadenoma of the epididymis. Hum Pathol 1995; 26: 1341–1346.

121. Kragel PJ, Pestaner J, Travis WD, et al. Papillary cystadenoma of the epididymis. A report of three cases with lectin histochemistry. Arch Pathol Lab Med 1990; 114: 672–675.

122. Handra-Luca A, Toublanc M, Richard S, et al. Papillary cystadenoma of the epididymis revealing von Hippel–Lindau disease. Ann Pathol 2001; 21: 102–103.

123. Polsky EG, Ray C, Dubilier LD. Diffuse fibrous pseudotumor of the tunica vaginalis testis, epididymis and spermatic cord. J Urol 2004; 171: 1625–1626.

124. Yamashina M, Honma T, Uchijima Y. Myofibroblastic pseudotumor mimicking epididymal sarcoma. A clinicopathologic study of three cases. Pathol Res Pract 1992; 188: 1054–1059.

125. Milanezi MF, Schmitt F. Pseudosarcomatous myofibroblastic proliferation of the spermatic cord (proliferative funiculitis). Histopathology 1997; 31: 387–388.

126. Hollowood K, Fletcher CD. Pseudosarcomatous myofibroblastic proliferations of the spermatic cord ('proliferative funiculitis'). Histologic and immunohistochemical analysis of a distinctive entity. Am J Surg Pathol 1992; 16: 448–454.

127. Tobias-Machado M, Correa Lopes Neto A, Heloisa Simardi L, et al. Fibrous pseudotumor of tunica vaginalis and epididymis. Urology 2000; 56: 670–672.

128. Shintaku M, Ukikusa M. Proliferative funiculitis with a prominent infiltration of mast cells. Pathol Int 2003; 53: 897–900.

129. Yusim IE, Neulander EZ, Eidelberg I, et al. Leiomyoma of the genitourinary tract. Scand J Urol Nephrol 2001; 35: 295–299.

130. Elmer EB, Levine R, Nolan J. Leiomyoma of spermatic cord with unusual features. Urology 1989; 33: 236–237.

131. Bruno S, Leone V, Mincione GP. Bilateral leiomyoma of the epididymis. Pathologica 1993; 85: 129–133.

132. Kato Y, Hori J, Taniguchi N, et al. Solitary genital leiomyoma of the tunica dartos: a case report and review of the literature in Japan. Hinyokika Kiyo 2005; 51: 699–701.

133. Borri A, Nesi G, Bencini L, Pernice LM. Bizarre leiomyoma of the epididymis. A case report. Minerva Urol Nefrol 2000; 52: 29–31.

134. Ghei M, Arun B, Maraj BH, et al. Case report: angioleiomyoma of the spermatic cord: a rare scrotal mass. Int Urol Nephrol 2005; 37: 731–732.

135. Henley JD, Ferry J, Ulbright TM. Miscellaneous rare paratesticular tumors. Semin Diagn Pathol 2000; 17: 319–339.

136. Toda T, Sadi AM, Kiyuna M, et al. Pigmented neuroectodermal tumor of infancy in the epididymis. A case

report. Acta Cytol 1998; 42: 775–780.

137. Kobayashi T, Kunimi K, Imao T, et al. Melanotic neuroectodermal tumor of infancy in the epididymis. Case report and literature review. Urol Int 1996; 57: 262–265.

138. Calabrese F, Danieli D, Valente M. Melanotic neuroectodermal tumor of the epididymis in infancy: case report and review of the literature. Urology 1995; 46: 415–418.

139. Lai FM, Allen PW, Chan LW, et al. Aggressive fibromatosis of the spermatic cord. A typical lesion in a 'new' location. Am J Clin Pathol 1995; 104: 403–407.

140. Milathianakis KN, Karamanolakis DK, Mpogdanos IM, Trihia-Spyrou EI. Solitary neurofibroma of the spermatic cord. Urol Int 2004; 72: 271–274.

141. Jiang R, Chen JH, Chen M, Li QM. Male genital schwannoma, review of 5 cases. Asian J Androl 2003; 5: 251–254.

142. Young IE, Nawroz IM, Aitken RJ. Phaeochromocytoma of the spermatic cord. J Clin Pathol 1999; 52: 305–306.

143. Bacchi CE, Schmidt RA, Brandao M, et al. Paraganglioma of the spermatic cord. Report of a case with immunohistochemical and ultrastructural studies. Arch Pathol Lab Med 1990; 114: 899–901.

144. Gonzalez-Campora R, Galera-Davidson H, Vazquez-Ramirez FJ, Diaz-Cano S. Blue nevus: classical types and new related entities. A differential diagnostic review. Pathol Res Pract 1994; 190: 627–635.

145. Liokumovich P, Herbert M, Sandbank J, et al. Cavernous hemangioma of spermatic cord: report of a case with immunohistochemical study. Arch Pathol Lab Med 2002; 126: 357–358.

146. Kaido M, Iwai S, Ide Y, Koide O. Epididymal lymphangiectasis. J Urol 1993; 150: 1251–1252.

147. Postius J, Manzano C, Concepcion T, et al. Epididymal lymphangioma. J Urol 2000; 163: 550–551.

148. Chetty R. Epididymal cavernous haemangiomas. Histopathology 1993; 22: 396–398.

149. Castillenti TA, Bertin AP. Angiomyolipoma of the spermatic cord: case report and literature review. J Urol 1989; 142: 1308–1309.

150. Siddiqui MT, Kovarik P, Chejfec G. Angiomyofibroblastoma of the spermatic cord. Br J Urol 1997; 79: 475–476.

151. Canales BK, Weiland D, Hoffman N, et al. Angiomyofibroblastoma-like tumors (cellular angiofibroma). Int J Urol 2006; 13: 177–179.

152. Zeng L, Xia T, Kong X, et al. Primary carcinoid tumor of the epididymis. Chin Med J [Engl] 2001; 114: 544–545.

153. Xambre L, Lages R, Cerqueira M, et al. Solitary fibrous tumor. Two additional

cases with urologic implications. Actas Urol Esp 2003; 27: 832–838.

154. Fisher C, Bisceglia M. Solitary fibrous tumour of the spermatic cord. Br J Urol 1994; 74: 798–799.

155. Lanzafame S, Leonardi R, Torrisi A. Extratesticular Leydig cell tumor of the spermatic cord. J Urol 2004; 171: 1238–1239.

156. Kurzrock EA, Busby JE, Gandour-Edwards R. Paratesticular rhabdomyoma. J Pediatr Surg 2003; 38: 1546–1547.

157. Wehner MS, Humphreys JL, Sharkey FE. Epididymal rhabdomyoma: report of a case, including histologic and immunohistochemical findings. Arch Pathol Lab Med 2000; 124: 1518–1519.

158. Matsunaga GS, Shepherd DL, Troyer DA, Thompson IM. Epididymal rhabdomyoma. J Urol 2000; 163: 1876.

159. Maheshkumar P, Berney DM. Spermatic cord rhabdomyoma. Urology 2000; 56: 331.

160. Carlinfante G, De Marco L, Mori M, et al. Aggressive angiomyxoma of the spermatic cord. Two unusual cases occurring in childhood. Pathol Res Pract 2001; 197: 139–144.

161. Madrigal B, Veiga M, Vara A, et al. An aggressive inguinal (parafunicular) angiomyxoma in a male patient. Arch Esp Urol 1999; 52: 785–788.

162. Idrees MT, Hoch BL, Wang BY, Unger PD. Aggressive angiomyxoma of male genital region. Report of 4 cases with immunohistochemical evaluation including hormone receptor status. Ann Diagn Pathol 2006; 10: 197–204.

163. Popek EJ, Montgomery EA, Fourcroy JL. Fibrous hamartoma of infancy in the genital region: findings in 15 cases. J Urol 1994; 152: 990–993.

164. Merimsky O, Terrier P, Bonvalot S, et al. Spermatic cord sarcoma in adults. Acta Oncol 1999; 38: 635–638.

165. Schwartz SL, Swierzewski SJ 3rd, Sondak VK, Grossman HB. Liposarcoma of the spermatic cord: report of 6 cases and review of the literature. J Urol 1995; 153: 154–157.

166. Montgomery E, Fisher C. Paratesticular liposarcoma: a clinicopathologic study. Am J Surg Pathol 2003; 27: 40–47.

167. Dundar M, Erol H, Kocak I, Kacar F. Liposarcoma of the spermatic cord. Urol Int 2001; 67: 102–103.

168. Panagis A, Karydas G, Vasilakakis J, et al. Myxoid liposarcoma of the spermatic cord: a case report and review of the literature. Int Urol Nephrol 2003; 35: 369–372.

169. Ikinger U, Westrich M, Pietz B, et al. Combined myxoid liposarcoma and angiolipoma of the spermatic cord. Urology 1997; 49: 635–637.

170. Hornick JL, Bosenberg MW, Mentzel T, et al. Pleomorphic liposarcoma: clinicopathologic analysis of 57 cases. Am J Surg Pathol 2004; 28: 1257–1267.

171. Henricks WH, Chu YC, Goldblum JR, Weiss SW. Dedifferentiated liposarcoma: a clinicopathological analysis of 155 cases with a proposal for an expanded definition of dedifferentiation. Am J Surg Pathol 1997; 21: 271–281.

172. Kizer WS, Dykes TE, Brent EL, et al. Paratesticular spindle cell rhabdomyosarcoma in an adult. J Urol 2001; 166: 606–607.

173. Furlong MA, Mentzel T, Fanburg-Smith JC. Pleomorphic rhabdomyosarcoma in adults: a clinicopathologic study of 38 cases with emphasis on morphologic variants and recent skeletal muscle-specific markers. Mod Pathol 2001; 14: 595–603.

174. Perez Herms S, Castellanos Acosta R, Cortadellas Angel R, et al. Paratesticular rhabdomyosarcoma. Report of 2 cases. Actas Urol Esp 1991; 15: 491–494.

175. Rodriguez Garcia N, Llanes Gonzalez L, Pascual Mateo C, Berenguer Sanchez A. Spermatic cord rhabdomyosarcoma in an adult. Arch Esp Urol 2005 Nov; 58: 956–9.

176. Watanabe J, Soma T, Kawa G, Hida S, Koisi M. Leiomyosarcoma of the spermatic cord. Int J Urol 1999; 6: 536–538.

177. Stein A, Kaplun A, Sova Y, et al. Leiomyosarcoma of the spermatic cord: report of two cases and review of the literature. World J Urol 1996; 14: 59–61.

178. Varzaneh FE, Verghese M, Shmookler BM. Paratesticular leiomyosarcoma in an elderly man. Urology 2002; 60: 1112.

179. Fisher C, Goldblum JR, Epstein JI, Montgomery E. Leiomyosarcoma of the paratesticular region: a clinicopathologic study. Am J Surg Pathol 2001; 25: 1143–1149.

180. Llarena Ibarguren R, Azurmendi Sastre V, Martin Bazaco J, et al. Paratesticular leiomyosarcoma. Review and update. Arch Esp Urol 2004; 57: 525–530.

181. Lopes RI, Leite KR, Lopes RN. Paratesticular leiomyosarcoma treated by enucleation. Int Braz J Urol 2006; 32: 66–67.

182. Reynard JM, Hasan N, Baithun SI, et al. Malignant mesothelioma of the tunica vaginalis testis. Br J Urol 1994; 74: 389–390.

183. Kamiya M, Eimoto T. Malignant mesothelioma of the tunica vaginalis. Pathol Res Pract 1990; 186: 680–684; discussion 5–6.

184. Cury PM, Butcher DN, Fisher C, et al. Value of the mesothelium-associated antibodies thrombomodulin, cytokeratin 5/6, calretinin, and CD44H in distinguishing epithelioid pleural mesothelioma from adenocarcinoma metastatic to the pleura. Mod Pathol 2000; 13: 107–112.

185. Kurian RR, Prema NS, Belthazar A. Paratesticular papillary serous cystadenocarcinoma – a case report. Indian J Pathol Microbiol 2006; 49: 36–37.

186. Johnson DB, Sarda R, Uehling DT. Mullerian-type epithelial tumor arising within a torsed appendix testis. Urology 1999; 54: 561.

187. McCluggage WG, Shah V, Nott C, et al. Cystadenoma of spermatic cord resembling ovarian serous epithelial tumour of low malignant potential: immunohistochemical study suggesting müllerian differentiation. Histopathology 1996; 28: 77–80.

188. Jones MA, Young RH, Srigley JR, Scully RE. Paratesticular serous papillary carcinoma. A report of six cases. Am J Surg Pathol 1995; 19: 1359–1365.

189. Arocena Garcia Tapia J, Sanz Perez G, Diez-Caballero Alonso F, et al. Epididymal carcinoma. Bibliographic review in reference to a case. Arch Esp Urol 2000; 53: 273–275.

190. Ganem JP, Jhaveri FM, Marroum MC. Primary adenocarcinoma of the epididymis: case report and review of the literature. Urology 1998; 52: 904–908.

191. Jones MA, Young RH, Scully RE. Adenocarcinoma of the epididymis: a report of four cases and review of the literature. Am J Surg Pathol 1997; 21: 1474–1480.

192. Yu CC, Huang JK, Chiang H, et al. Papillary cystadenocarcinoma of the epididymis: a case report and review of the literature. J Urol 1992; 147: 162–165.

193. Nistal M, Revestido R, Paniagua R. Bilateral mucinous cystadenocarcinoma of the testis and epididymis. Arch Pathol Lab Med 1992; 116: 1360–1363.

194. Kurihara K, Oka A, Mannami M, Iwata Y. Papillary adenocarcinoma of the epididymis. Acta Pathol Jpn 1993; 43: 440–443.

195. Chauhan RD, Gingrich JR, Eltorky M, Steiner MS. The natural progression of adenocarcinoma of the epididymis. J Urol 2001; 166: 608–610.

196. Sethi S, Ashok S. Malignant fibrous histiocytoma of the spermatic cord. J Indian Med Assoc 2003; 101: 599–600.

197. Lin BT, Harvey DA, Medeiros LJ. Malignant fibrous histiocytoma of the spermatic cord: report of two cases and review of the literature. Mod Pathol 2002; 15: 59–65.

198. Bosch-Princep R, Martinez-Gonzalez S, Alvaro-Naranjo T, et al. Fine needle aspiration and touch imprint cytology of a malignant fibrous histiocytoma of the spermatic cord. Case report. Acta Cytol 2000; 44: 423–428.

199. Glazier DB, Vates TS, Cummings KB, Pickens RL. Malignant fibrous histiocytoma of the spermatic cord. J Urol 1996; 155: 955–957.

200. Ikinger U, Westrich M, Bersch W, Bottinger K. Malignant fibrous histiocytoma of the epididymis. Case report and review of the literature. Urol Int 1999; 62: 106–109.

201. Folpe AL, Weiss SW. Paratesticular soft tissue neoplasms. Semin Diagn Pathol 2000; 17: 307–318.

202. Calonge WM, Heitor F, Castro LP, et al. Neonatal paratesticular neuroblastoma misdiagnosed as in utero torsion of testis. J Pediatr Hematol Oncol 2004; 26: 693–695.

203. Ozkan B, Ozguroglu M, Ozkara H, et al. Adult paratesticular myxofibrosarcoma: report of a rare entity and review of the literature. Int Urol Nephrol 2006; 38: 5–7.

204. Matsumoto H, Inoue R, Tsuchida M, et al. Primitive neuroectodermal tumor of the spermatic cord. J Urol 2002; 167: 1791–1792.

205. Rzeszutko M, Rzeszutko W, Nienartowicz E, Jelen M. Paratesticular localization of burned out non-seminomatous germ cell tumor – NSGCT: a case report. Pol J Pathol 2006; 57: 55–57.

206. Lockett CJ, Nandwani GM, Stubington SR. Testicular seminoma – unusual histology and staging with sub epithelial spread of seminoma along the vas deferens. BMC Urol 2006; 6: 5.

207. Ferry JA, Harris NL, Young RH, et al. Malignant lymphoma of the testis, epididymis, and spermatic cord. A clinicopathologic study of 69 cases with immunophenotypic analysis. Am J Surg Pathol 1994; 18: 376–390.

208. Vega F, Medeiros LJ, Abruzzo LV. Primary paratesticular lymphoma: a report of 2 cases and review of literature. Arch Pathol Lab Med 2001; 125: 428–432.

209. Novella G, Porcaro AB, Righetti R, et al. Primary lymphoma of the epididymis: case report and review of the literature. Urol Int 2001; 67: 97–99.

210. Suzuki K, Sai S, Kato K, Murase T. A case of malignant lymphoma of the epididymis. Hinyokika Kiyo 2000; 46: 291–293.

211. Tranchida P, Bayerl M, Voelpel MJ, Palutke M. Testicular ischemia due to intravascular large B-cell lymphoma: a novel presentation in an immunosuppressed individual. Int J Surg Pathol 2003; 11: 319–324.

212. Ferry JA, Young RH, Scully RE. Testicular and epididymal plasmacytoma: a report of 7 cases, including three that were the initial manifestation of plasma cell myeloma. Am J Surg Pathol 1997; 21: 590–598.

213. Wiebe B, Warnoe H, Klarlund M, Jacobsen AK. Epididymal metastasis from prostatic carcinoma. Scand J Urol Nephrol 1993; 27: 553–555.

214. Mabjeesh NJ, Bar-Yosef Y, Schreiber-Bramante L, et al. Spermatic vein tumor thrombus in renal cell carcinoma. Sci World J 2004; 4: 192–194.

215. Kaya C, Tanrikulu H, Yilmaz G, et al. Spermatic cord metastasis as an initial manifestation of non-small cell carcinoma of the lung. Int J Urol 2006; 13: 846–848.

216. Dutt N, Bates AW, Baithun SI. Secondary neoplasms of the male genital tract with different patterns of involvement in adults and children. Histopathology 2000; 37: 323–331.

217. Datta MW, Ulbright TM, Young RH. Renal cell carcinoma metastatic to the testis and its adnexa: a report of five cases including three that accounted for the initial clinical presentation. Int J Surg Pathol 2001; 9: 49–56.

218. Salesi N, Fabi A, Di Cocco B, et al. Testis metastasis as an initial manifestation of an occult gastrointestinal cancer. Anticancer Res 2004; 24: 1093–1096.

219. Kanno K, Ohwada S, Nakamura S, et al. Epididymis metastasis from colon carcinoma: a case report and a review of the Japanese literature. Jpn J Clin Oncol 1994; 24: 340–344.

220. Mishra VC, Tindall SF. Case report – Prostatic carcinoma presenting as an epididymal nodule. Int Urol Nephrol 2001; 33: 511.

221. Issa MM, Kabalin JN, Dietrick DD, et al. Spermatic cord metastasis from transitional cell carcinoma of the bladder. Urology 1994; 43: 561–563.

222. Gomez-Roman JJ, Mayorga M, Mira C, et al. Glandular inclusions in inguinal hernia sacs: a clinicopath-ological study of six cases. Pediatr Pathol 1994; 14: 1043–1049.

# CHAPTER 15

# Penis and scrotum

Jae Y. Ro, Kyu-Rae Kim, Mahul B. Amin, Alberto G. Ayala

# PENIS

## Normal anatomy and histology

The penis consists of three portions: the root, the body, and the glans. The root lies in the superficial perineal pouch and provides fixation and stability. The body constitutes the major part of the penis and is composed of three cylinders of spongy erectile tissue: the paired corpora cavernosa and the single corpus spongiosum. The two cavernous bodies lie on the dorsum of the penis and are surrounded by a double layer of dense fibrous connective tissue called Buck's fascia and tunica albuginea. The corpus spongiosum lies in the ventral aspect of the penis and surrounds the urethra in its center. The glans is the distal expansion of the corpus spongiosum; it is conical and normally ensheathed by the loose skin of the prepuce. In the uncircumcised male, five to six layers of stratified non-keratinizing squamous epithelium line the mucosal surface of the glans; after circumcision these become keratinized.

The foreskin or prepuce of the penis is remarkably thin, dark, and loosely connected to the tunica albuginea. It has features of true skin but is devoid of subcutaneous adipose tissue. Sebaceous glands without associated hair follicles and sweat glands are present in the superficial dermis.

Histologically, the foreskin comprises five layers: epidermis, dermis, dartos muscle, lamina propria, and squamous mucosa. The squamous mucosa of the foreskin is a prolongation of that of the glans and the balanopreputial sulcus. Langerhans' cells are present in the mucosal epithelium of the foreskin, and are more numerous than those occurring in the female cervical tissue.[1] The foreskin is highly vascular. Most of its blood supply arises from the internal pudendal artery, which has three main branches: the deep artery, the bulbar artery, and the urethral artery. The venous return is through three channels: the cavernous veins, the deep veins, and the superficial dorsal veins. The lymphatic drainage is through the superficial and deep inguinal lymph nodes that drain to the external and common iliac nodes.

The glans is composed of epithelium, lamina propria, corpus spongiosum, tunica albuginea, and corpora cavernosa. The epithelium of the glans is keratinized or non-keratinized depending on the status of circumcision. The lamina propria is 1–3 mm thick and consists of a layer of loose connective tissue containing small vessels, lymphatics, nerves and occasional Vater–Pacini corpuscles.

The corpus spongiosum is the main structure of the glans; it is 8–10 mm thick and consists of highly vascularized erectile tissue with variably sized vessels, smooth muscle fibers, and peripheral nerves. The transition between the lamina propria and corpus spongiosum is usually not well delineated and often difficult to determine (Fig. 15-1). The corpora cavernosa are present in the glans to a variable degree from man to man. The corpus spongiosum is separated from the corpora cavernosa by a dense white fibroelastic membrane, the tunica albuginea (Fig. 15-2). This is 1–2 mm thick in the flaccid state, but becomes thinner during erection, and serves

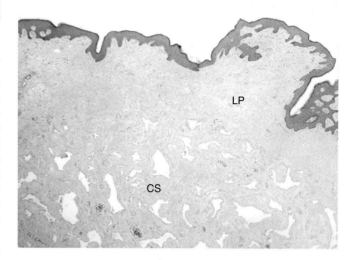

**Fig. 15-1** Glans penis with lamina propria (LP) corpus spongiosum (CS).

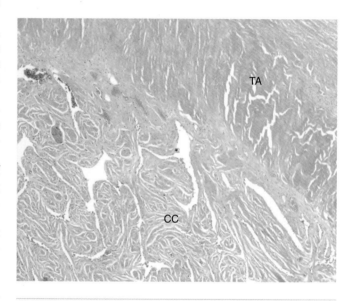

**Fig. 15-2** Tunica albuginea (TA) and corpus cavernosum (CC).

as an important barrier to the spread of cancer to the corpora cavernosa.

The coronal sulcus between the glans and the shaft is a narrow and circumferential 'cul de sac' located just below the corona of the penis. The sulcus is composed of squamous mucosa, lamina propria, dartos muscle, and Buck's fascia, and is a common site for recurrence of carcinoma or a positive margin in cases of primary foreskin carcinoma.[2]

The body or shaft of the penis is composed of a thin, wrinkled, pigmented epidermis with few adnexal structures; dermis; dartos muscle; adipose tissue; Buck's fascia with numerous vessels and nerves; tunica albuginea; and erectile tissue of corpora cavernosa and corpus spongiosum, the latter encasing the urethra (Fig. 15-3). Histogenetically, the penis has two separate origins for its three erectile bodies. Genital tubercles are responsible for the corpora cavernosa,

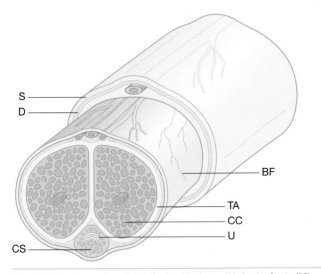

**Fig. 15-3** Anatomy of penile shaft: skin (S), dartos (D), Buck's fascia (BF), tunica albuginea (TA), corpora cavernosa (CC), corpus spongiosum (CS), and urethra (U).

whereas the urethra and corpus spongiosum are formed from the urogenital sinus and the urogenital folds.

The spectrum of penile diseases is listed in Table 15-1.

## Congenital abnormalities

Congenital absence of the upper wall of the urethra is known as epispadias. In this anomaly, the urethral opening appears on the dorsum of the penis as a groove or cleft. The incidence of epispadias is 1 in 117 000 male births.[3,4] According to location, there are three types of epispadias: penopubic, penile, and glanular, the first being most frequent.[3] Urinary incontinence is frequently observed with penopubic epispadias and occasionally with penile type, but is not associated with glanular epispadias.[4] Associated congenital anomalies include diastasis of the pubic symphysis, bladder exstrophy, renal agenesis, and ectopic pelvic kidney.[4–10]

Hypospadias is a developmental anomaly in which the urethra opens on the underside of the penile shaft or on the perineum (Fig. 15-4A, B).[11,12] Hypospadias is frequently associated with chordee (Fig. 15-5), but can occur in isolation. Hypospadias is classified based on the location of the

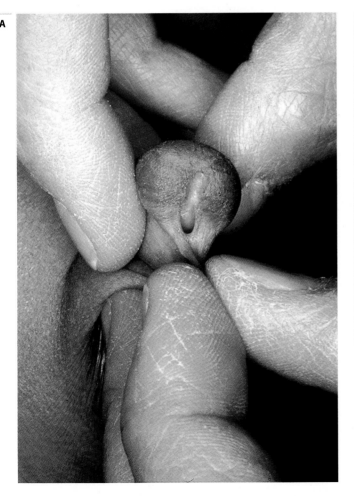

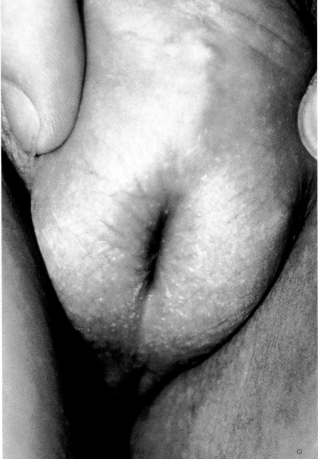

**Fig. 15-4** (**A**) Distal hypospadias with the urethral meatus at the junction of the glans and penile shaft. (**B**) Proximal hypospadias with the urethral meatus at the base of scrotum. (Courtesy of Dr Hyum Yul Rhew, Kosin University, Busan, Korea.)

**Table 15-1** Diseases of the penis

| | |
|---|---|
| **Congenital Abnormalities** | Glomus tumor |
| **Non-neoplastic Diseases Inflammation** | Fibrous histiocytoma |
| Phimosis and paraphimosis | Granular cell tumor |
| Fibroepithelial polyp | Myointioma |
| Balanoposthitis | Nevi and other benign melanocytic proliferations |
| Plasma cell balanitis (Zoon's balanitis) | *Premalignant lesions* |
| Balanitis xerotica obliterans (lichen sclerosus et atrophicus) | Erythroplasia of Queyrat |
| Reiter's syndrome | Bowen's disease |
| Peyronie's disease | Bowenoid papulosis |
| Os penis | *Maliguant neoplasms* *Malignant epithelial tumors* |
| Penile prosthesis | Squamous cell carcinoma |
| Priapism | Usual type |
| **Infections** | Variants |
| Gonorrhea | Basaloid |
| Syphilis | Warty (condylomatous) |
| Herpes simplex | Verrucous |
| Lymphogranuloma venereum | Papillary, not otherwise specified |
| Granuloma inguinale | Pseudohyperplastic non-verruciform carcinoma |
| Chancroid (soft chancre) | Sarcomatoid (spindle cell) carcinoma* |
| Candidiasis | Mixed (hybrid) carcinomas |
| Scabies | Adenosquamous carcinoma |
| Pediculosis pubis | Clear cell carcinoma |
| Molluscum contagiosum | Basal cell carcinoma |
| Erythrasma | Paget's disease (See in the scrotum) |
| Penile lesions in AIDS | *Melanocytic tumors* |
| **Tumor-Like Conditions** | Malignant melanoma |
| Condyloma | *Malignant mesenchymal tumors (Sarcoma)* |
| Pearly penile papules | Kaposi's sarcoma |
| Penile cysts | Angiosarcoma |
| Pseudoepitheliomatous keratotic and micaceous balanitis | Leiomyosarcoma |
| Verruciform xanthoma | Rhabdomyosarcoma |
| **Neoplastic Diseases** | Epithelioid sarcoma |
| *Benign neoplasms* | Others |
| Papilloma | *Hematopoietic tumors* |
| Hemangioma | Malignant lymphoma |
| Neurofibroma, schwannoma | **Secondary (Metastatic) Tumors** |
| Leiomyoma | |

*For the purposes of this work carcinosarcoma is included with sarcomatoid carcinoma. These tumors are also designated metaplastic carcinoma by some authors.

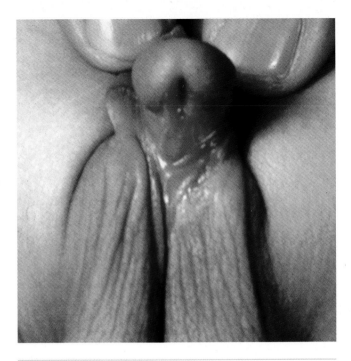

Fig. 15-5 Hypospadias with chordee. (Courtesy of Dr Hyun Yun Rhew, Kosin University, Busan Korea.)

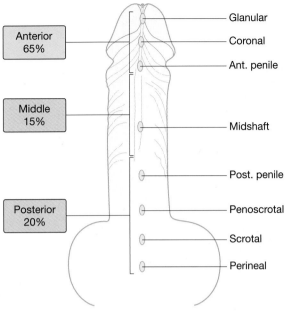

Fig. 15-6 Location of hypospadias. (From Mr Subhendu Chakraborty, Methodist Hospital, Houston, Tx.)

meatus (glanular, subcoronal, distal penile, midshaft, proximal penile, penoscrotal, scrotal, scrotal and perineal) (Fig. 15-6). The glanular and subcoronal types constitute anterior hypospadias (Fig. 15-4A), which accounts for 50% of all cases. Distal penile, midshaft, and proximal types make up middle hypospadias, accounting for 30% of cases. The remaining 20% are posterior hypospadias and include penoscrotal, scrotal (Fig. 15-4B), and perineal types.[11,12] The incidence of hypospadias is 1 per 300 live male births.[12,13] Associated anomalies include cryptorchidism and inguinal hernia. Association with anomalies of the upper urinary tract is uncommon unless other anomalies are present in other organ systems.[12–14]

A micropenis is a normally formed penis with a size 2 or more standard deviation below the mean. The ratio of the length of the penile shaft to its circumference is normal (Fig. 15-7). The corpora cavernosa may be severely hypoplastic. The scrotum is generally fused but often diminutive, and the testes are usually small and frequently cryptorchid. A webbed or concealed penis often resembles a micropenis, but the penile shaft is of normal length. The three most common causes of micropenis are hypogonadotropic hypogonadism, hypergonadotropic hypogonadism (primary testicular failure), and idiopathic.[15,16]

A concealed penis is a normally developed penis that becomes buried in a suprapubic fat pad (Fig. 15-8). This anomaly may be congenital or idiopathic following circumcision. A concealed penis may be visualized by retracting skin lateral to the penile shaft.[17]

Aphallia (penile agenesis) results from failure of the genital tubercle to develop. The incidence is 1 in 10 000 000 live male births; only 70 cases have been reported.[18,19] The usual appearance is that of a well-developed scrotum with descended testes but no penile shaft. In most cases the urethra opens at the anal verge adjacent to a small skin tag

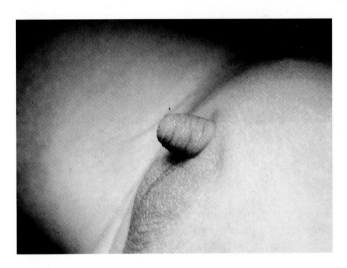

Fig. 15-7 Micropenis. (Courtesy of Dr Hyun Yun Rhew, Kosin University, Busan, Korea.)

or, in other cases, into the rectum. Associated malformations include cryptorchidism, vesicoureteral reflux, horseshoe kidney, renal agenesis, imperforate anus, and musculoskeletal and cardiopulmonary abnormalities.[18,19]

Diphallus, or duplication of the penis, is a rare anomaly that ranges from a small accessory penis to complete duplication (Fig. 15-9).[20] Associated anomalies include hypospadias, bifid scrotum, duplication of the bladder, renal agenesis or ectopia, and diastasis of the pubic symphysis. Anal and cardiac anomalies are also common.[20,21]

Chordee, a congenital or acquired bend of the penis, is caused by reduced elasticity in one or more of the fascial layers of the penis, leading to shortness of one corpus cavernosum when erection occurs. The bend may be ventral,

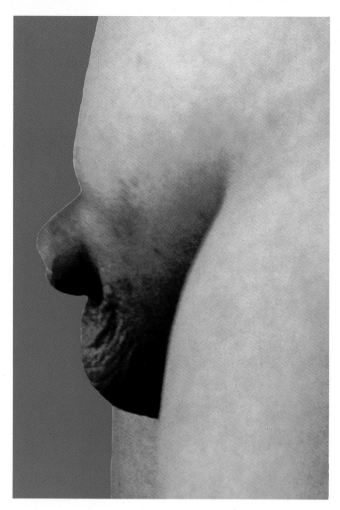

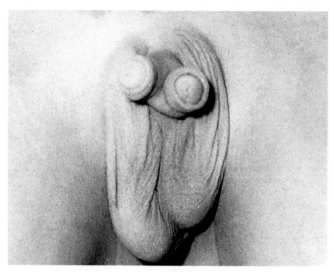

**Fig. 15-9** Diphallus. (Courtesy of Dr Hyun Yun Rhew, Kosin University, Busan, Korea.)

**Fig. 15-8** Concealed penis. (Courtesy of Dr Hyun Yun Rhew, Kosin University, Busan, Korea.)

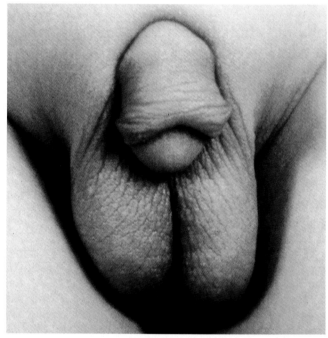

**Fig. 15-10** Scrotal engulfment. (Courtesy of Dr Hyun Yun Rhew, Kosin University, Busan, Korea.)

dorsal, lateral, or complex. Chordee is most frequently associated developmentally with hypospadias when the mesenchyme distal to the meatus ceases to differentiate, creating a fan-shaped band of dysgenetic fascia.[22] Acquired chordee may result from trauma or Peyronie's disease.[23]

Scrotal engulfment (penoscrotal transposition) results from incomplete migration of the inferomedial labioscrotal swelling (Fig. 15-10). This has been termed bifid scrotum, doughnut scrotum, prepenile scrotum, and shawl scrotum. Frequently it occurs in conjunction with perineal, scrotal, or penoscrotal hypospadias with chordee.[24]

Ectopic scrotum is rare and refers to the anomalous position of one hemiscrotum along the inguinal canal, most commonly the suprainguinal canal, although it may be within the infrainguinal canal or the perineum. Associated anomalies include cryptorchidism, inguinal hernia, exstrophy, popliteal pterygium syndrome, renal agenesis, renal dysplasia, and ectopic urethra.[25] A recent paper evaluated the utility of magnetic resonance imaging (MRI) in the evaluation of congenital anomalies of the external genitalia and concluded that this technique renders excellent anatomic interpretation of complex genital anomalies and associated

abnormal pelvic tissues, thereby assisting surgeons in conceptualizing the anomalous structures and contributing to management.[26] After surgical correction of anomalies, long-term follow-up studies have shown that adulthood satisfaction with respect to voiding and sexual function is achieved in about two-thirds of patients and some degree of dissatisfaction in one-third. Epispadias repair is a much more complicated procedure and long-term results are seldom reported. Nevertheless, good results are achieved with respect to continence (approximately 80% success) and sexual function.[27]

# Non-neoplastic diseases

## Inflammation

### Phimosis and paraphimosis

Phimosis is a condition in which the foreskin cannot be retracted behind the glans penis (Fig. 15-11). In adolescents and adults the foreskin can normally be retracted beyond the corona with relative ease, but it is important to note that in children less than 5 years old the foreskin is not retractable.[28] Phimosis may arise in uncircumcised men at any age.

Phimosis may be congenital or acquired. Congenital phimosis is much rarer and is secondary to a small preputial orifice or to an abnormally long foreskin. Secondary phimosis usually results from an accumulation of smegma, which is due to poor hygiene and can lead to chronic inflammation, edema, and fibrosis. Balanoposthitis (inflammation of the glans and prepuce) and balanitis xerotica obliterans may cause phimosis.[28,29]

Circumcision is the treatment for phimosis, regardless of etiology. Surgical specimens from men should be carefully examined for areas of induration which might indicate dysplastic or neoplastic lesions.[28] Microscopically, phimotic prepuces may be histologically normal or show varying degrees of inflammation, fibrosis, edema, and vascular congestion. Lymphocytes and plasma cells are the predominant inflammatory components.[30] Patients with phimosis often complain of irritation, but significant pain is uncommon unless there is ballooning of the foreskin due to urinary obstruction.

Paraphimosis is a condition in which the foreskin has been retracted behind the glans penis and cannot be advanced back over the glans.[28] Constriction of the glans causes pain as a result of vascular engorgement and edema. Paraphimosis is often iatrogenic, occurring after examina-tion of the penis or after urinary tract instrumentation. Rarer reported causes include *Plasmodium falciparum* malaria[31] and carcinoma metastatic to the penis.[32] Paraphimosis requires circumcision or emergency dorsal slit surgery.[28]

Phimosis often coexists with penile carcinoma and is a risk factor for it (see below).[33,34] Difficulty in foreskin retraction and phimosis are risk factors for penile carcinoma that may be related to the anatomically variable length of the foreskin. Recently Velazquez et al.[35] compared foreskin length and status in the general population and in patients with penile cancer, and found that 77% of men without cancer had a long foreskin and only 7% had phimosis. Cancer patients had a long foreskin in 78% of cases, and phimosis was significantly increased in frequency (52%; $P < 0.001$). Coexistence of a long foreskin and phimosis may explain the high incidence of penile cancer in some geographic regions. Because phimosis appears to be a major factor, the presence of a long foreskin may be a necessary but not a sufficient condition for cancer development. For these reasons Velazquez et al. supported preventive circumcision in patients with long and phimotic foreskins living in high-risk areas.[35]

### Fibroepithelial polyp

Fibroepithelial polyp is very rare in the penis and usually presents as a polypoid or cauliflower-like mass or masses involving the glans penis or prepuce.[36-38] It ranges in size from less than 1 cm to 7.5 cm in greatest dimension, and is strongly associated with long-term condom catheter use, or rarely may develop in association with phimosis. The age of the patients ranges from 4 to 58 years (median, 40 years) at the time of initial surgical resection, and the preoperative duration varies from 6 months to 10 years. The majority of fibroepithelial polyps affect the ventral surface of the glans near the urethral meatus.

Histologically, fibroepithelial polyp of the penis is similar to that in other sites, with a polypoid configuration and keratinizing squamous epithelial surface. The underlying stroma is notably edematous, with telangiectasia of pre-existing vessels, and in many instances there is a focal mild small vessel proliferation. The stroma exhibits mildly to moderately increased cellularity with mononucleated and multinucleated stromal cells. Mild inflammation is often present. Immunohistochemically, the stromal cells demonstrate limited immunoreactivity for muscle-specific actin, α-smooth muscle actin, and desmin, and show no reactivity for S100 protein or CD34. Surgical intervention consists of local excision. Although fibroepithelial polyp may recur, recurrences are also managed by local excision.[36]

### Balanoposthitis

Balanoposthitis (inflammation of the glans penis and prepuce) and balanitis (inflammation of the glans penis) occur most commonly in uncircumcised men.[39-41] The usual cause is poor hygiene. Failure to regularly retract and clean the foreskin leads to the accumulation of smegma (desquamated epithelial cells and debris), which incites an inflammatory response, and may subsequently result in phimosis.

Balanoposthitis can also result from specific dermatologic lesions or infectious agents (Table 15-2). In a series of 86

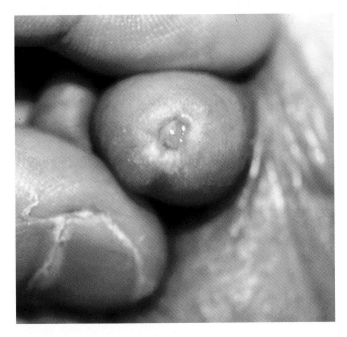

**Fig. 15-11** Phimosis. (Courtesy of Dr Hyun Yun Rhew, Kosin University, Busan, Korea.)

**Table 15-2** Balanoposthitis: inflammation of glans penis and prepuce

| |
|---|
| Balanoposthitis NOS |
| Candidal balanitis |
| Plasma cell balanitis (Zoon's balanitis) |
| Balanitis xerotica obliterans (lichen sclerosus et atrophicus) |
| Papulosquamous diseases |
| Lichen planus |
| Psoriasis |
| Balanitis circinata of Reiter's syndrome |
| Contact dermatitis |
| Allergic |
| Irritant |
| Vesiculobullous diseases—may simulate balanitis clinically |
| Cicatricial pemphigoid |
| Fixed drug eruption |

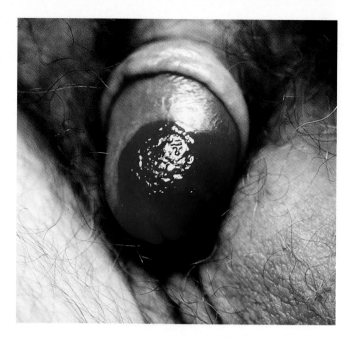

**Fig. 15-12** Zoon's balanitis. (Courtesy of Dr. Hans Stricker, Henry Ford Hospital, Detroit, MI.)

patients with balanoposthitis and balanitis, 41% had no attributable etiologic factor; *Candida* species accounted for 30%, and β-hemolytic streptococci were responsible for 11% of cases.[42] Candidal balanoposthitis is discussed below in the section on infectious diseases of the penis. Discussion of papulosquamous and vesiculobullous diseases is beyond the scope of this text.

### Plasma cell balanitis (Zoon's balanitis)

Plasma cell balanitis (Zoon's balanitis, or balanitis circumscripta plasmacellularis) is a disorder that was first described in 1952 by Zoon.[44] The disease is not rare, and is important because it clinically resembles squamous cell carcinoma in situ of the glans penis.[45,46] Plasma cell balanitis is a benign disorder of unknown etiology that is thought to represent a reaction to a multitude of diverse stimuli. Recently, Houser et al.[47] reported a case of Zoon's balanitis in an African-American man with human immunodeficiency virus (HIV). Plasma cell balanitis affects only uncircumcised males.[48] It is similar clinically and histologically to its vulvar counterpart, vulvitis circumscripta plasmacellularis. It usually presents as a single large (2 cm or greater) bright red, moist patch on the glans or inner prepuce (Fig. 15-12). Rarely, multiple patches may be present, and in severe cases it may consist of extensive visibly eroded lesions. The clinical appearance of the lesion overlaps with that of candidal balanitis and squamous cell carcinoma in situ, so biopsy is mandatory.

Histologically, the hallmark of plasma cell balanitis is a distinct upper dermal band-like infiltrate containing numerous plasma cells (Fig. 15-13A, B).[48–50] In some cases the number of plasma cells may be scant or moderate, and the histologic findings must be correlated with the clinical observations. The dermis also contains numerous dilated capillaries adjacent to extravasated erythrocytes or hemosiderin deposits. The overlying epidermis is thin and may occasionally be absent or partially separated from the dermis. The most distinctive feature within the epidermis is the presence of flattened or diamond- or rhomboid-shaped keratinocytes that are separated from one another by uniform intercellular edema.

Mucinous metaplasia of the penis is an uncommon lesion that occurs usually in elderly men and appears to be a metaplastic change associated with severe chronic inflammation, especially with Zoon's balanitis. Mucinous metaplasia may affect the glans penis as well as the mucosal surface of the foreskin.[51,52] Currently, the treatment of choice is circumcision,[45,46,50] but laser surgery[48,53] and topical application of retin-A preparations or steroids have been employed with variable success.

### Balanitis xerotica obliterans (penile lichen sclerosus)

Lichen sclerosus is a chronic and atrophic mucocutaneous condition affecting epidermis and dermal connective tissue that most commonly involves the genital and perianal skin of both males and females.[54] Extragenital lesions may accompany genital lesions, although they may also occur alone.[54] Balanitis xerotica obliterans is a term used as a synonym for lichen sclerosus of the glans penis and prepuce.[55] This lesion has been found to be associated with penile carcinoma, and it has been postulated to be a preneoplastic condition for at least some types of penile cancers, particularly in non-human papilloma virus variants of squamous cell carcinoma.[56–68]

Balanitis xerotica obliterans is commonly encountered in preputial resectates for phimosis in older men. In contrast, the prepubertal incidence in a series of 117 cases was only 4%.[69] The idiopathic form of balanitis xerotica obliterans is not associated with phimosis and presents with classic clinical and pathologic features. The cause of this classic form is unknown, but an autoimmune mechanism has been suggested.[55,70–72] Patients with lichen sclerosus may have increased organ-specific antibodies (thyroid microsomal and parietal cell antibodies in women, and smooth muscle and parietal cell antibodies in men).[70–72] Association with autoimmune diseases, including vitiligo and alopecia areata,

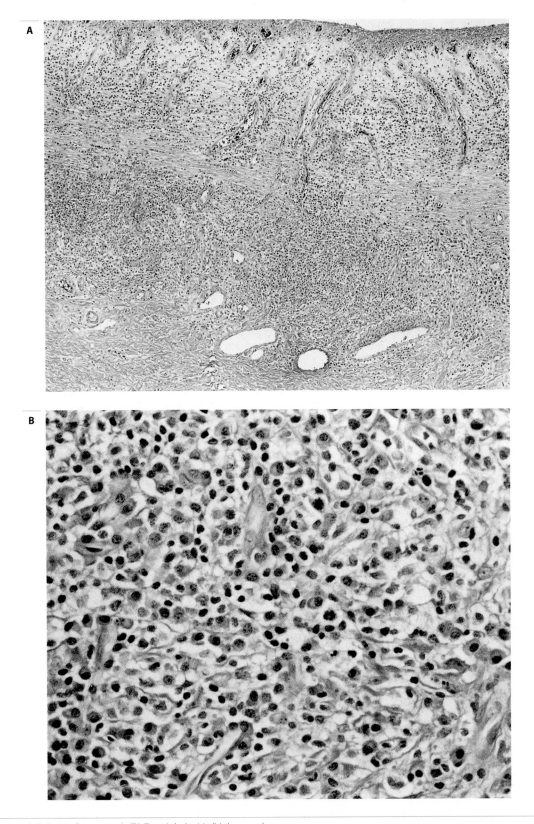

**Fig. 15-13** (**A**) Zoon's balanitis (low power). (**B**) Zoon's balanitis (high power).

further supports the premise that autoimmune pathogenetic mechanisms may play an important role in this disease.

Clinically, balanitis xerotica obliterans presents as a well-defined and marginated white patch on the glans penis or prepuce that envelops or involves the urethral meatus (Fig. 15-14). It may also present as a lichenoid scale with a roughened surface. In long-standing cases the lesion is firm due to underlying fibrosis, which may cause phimosis in uncircumcised men. Most lesions occur on the glans penis or prepuce, but occasionally the shaft is involved. Urethral involvement may cause stricture.[73] Pruritus, pain, and dyspareunia are common in vulvar lichen sclerosus et atrophicus, but balanitis xerotica obliterans is usually asymptomatic.

Histologically, active lesions of balanitis xerotica obliterans show pronounced orthokeratotic hyperkeratosis accompanied by striking atrophy of the epidermis, a distinctive combination of features. Basal cell vacuolation and clefting of the dermoepidermal junction may also occur; in rare instances there may be bullae. Orthokeratotic plugging of cutaneous follicles, a feature of lichen sclerosus et atrophicus, is not seen in balanitis xerotica obliterans because of the absence of follicles in this area.[59,60] The upper dermis is markedly edematous and the collagen forms a homogenized band, beneath which there may be a lymphoplasmacytic infiltrate (Fig. 15-15).

Over time, four principal changes occur: the basal layer of the epidermis becomes mature; the upper dermis is gradually replaced by sclerotic collagen; the inflammation in the mid-dermis becomes patchy or absent and inflammation is seen in the superficial dermis; and areas of epithelial hyperplasia may alternate with atrophy. In rare cases, frank atypia may be evident. Small capillaries in the upper dermis and papillary dermis may be widely patent owing to retraction by the sclerotic collagen. The chief differential diagnostic considerations are lupus erythematosus, morphea, and lichen planus.

The treatment of balanitis xerotica obliterans is often difficult. Circumcision, laser therapy, and topical administration of steroids, antifungal agents, and retinoids have been used, with variable results.

Balanitis xerotica obliterans may precede, coexist with, or arise subsequent to the development of carcinoma. Whether lichen sclerosus precedes penile keratinizing squamous carcinoma is a matter of debate. Lichen sclerosus is preferentially associated with non-human papilloma virus variants of squamous cell carcinoma. When lichen sclerosus is associated with malignancy it often shows, in addition to hyperplastic epithelium, low-grade squamous intraepithelial lesion. These findings suggest that lichen sclerosus may represent a preneoplastic condition for at least some types of penile cancer, in particular those not related to human papilloma virus (HPV).[74]

## Reiter's syndrome

In 1916, Reiter described a patient who developed systemic illness with polyarthritis, conjunctivitis, and nongonococcal urethritis after an episode of bloody diarrhea.[75] Although this was not the first reported case, the syndrome characterized by the triad of arthritis, urethritis, and conjunctivitis is now commonly referred to as Reiter's syndrome. More than two-thirds of patients have associated mucocutaneous lesions, supporting the argument that Reiter's syndrome is better defined by a tetrad of symptoms that includes mucocutaneous lesions.[75] More than 90% of patients are male, with onset of symptoms in the third and fourth decades.[76] Epidemic (enteric) and endemic (urogenital) modes of presentation have been described, the latter being much more common.[76–78] Patients frequently report a history of recent sexual contact with a new partner that is followed by the development of urethritis. The less common epidemic form is secondary to enteric infection and also occurs in children. Urethritis occurs in 90% of the postdysenteric or enteric forms of the disease, so it should not be assumed that urethritis and Reiter's syndrome are always sexually transmitted.

*Chlamydia trachomatis* is probably the most common cause of the sexually acquired form of Reiter's syndrome, although *Ureaplasma urealyticum*, *Shigella flexneri*, *Salmonella* species, *Campylobacter* species, *Yersinia enterocolitica*, and *Neisseria gonorrhoeae* have also been implicated.[75–80] Genetic susceptibility also plays an important role: 60–80% of patients are HLA-B27 positive. It is postulated that HLA-B27, either owing to molecular mimicry or by virtue of its relation to antigens linked to genes controlling immune responses to certain infectious agents, produces an exaggerated or

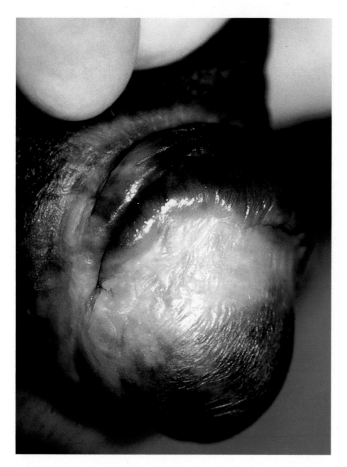

**Fig. 15-14** Balanitis xerotica obliterans.

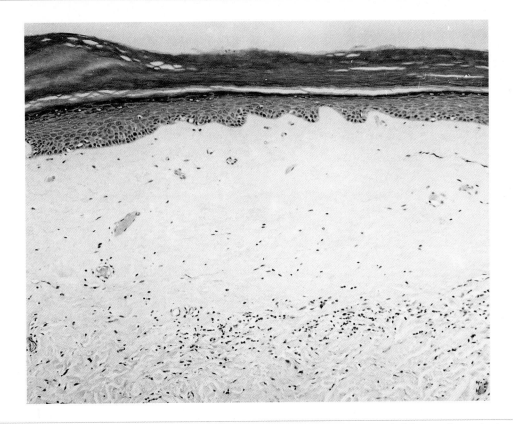

**Fig. 15-15** Balanitis xerotica obliterans showing homogeneous collagen in the upper dermis with a thin band of chronic inflammation just below.

abnormal immune response to specific microbiologic agents that culminates in the inflammatory manifestations of the disease.[81]

Genital involvement occurs as part of the mucocutaneous manifestations of Reiter's syndrome and is common in the sexually acquired form of the disease. The lesions take two forms, known as balanitis circinata and keratoderma blenorrhagica. Balanitis circinata is the more common form and occurs in up to 85% of men with the sexually acquired form of the syndrome.[82-84] It consists of a painless lesion which begins as small red papules that enlarge centrifugally to form a circular or ring-like configuration. In circumcised men the lesion is hyperkeratotic and resembles the second lesion, keratoderma blenorrhagica. Keratoderma blenorrhagica is predominantly a cutaneous lesion, most commonly affecting the palms and soles. It begins as erythematous macules that enlarge to form hyperkeratotic papules with red haloes. This form is clinically and histologically similar to psoriasis, and some cases of Reiter's syndrome progress to become indistinguishable from psoriatic arthritis.[84]

Histologically, the early lesions are indistinguishable from psoriasis vulgaris or pustular psoriasis, and demonstrate psoriasiform hyperplasia, hyperkeratosis, parakeratosis, and neutrophilic exocytosis within the stratum corneum together with the formation of spongiform pustules.[85] The spongiform pustules seen in the upper epidermis are the most characteristic histologic feature of Reiter's syndrome. The papillary dermis is thickened due to edema and may contain a neutrophilic perivascular infiltrate. In later stages the pustules are absent and the epidermis shows non-specific findings, including acanthosis, hyperkeratosis, and focal parakeratosis. Reliable distinction of Reiter's syndrome from pustular psoriasis and psoriasis vulgaris may be difficult and requires clinicopathologic correlation.

## Peyronie's disease

Peyronie's disease (also called plastic induration, fibrous sclerosis, and fibrous cavernositis) presents with painful erection accompanied by distortion, bending, or constriction of the erect penis.[86-89] Observations resembling Peyronie's disease were made in 1561 by the Italian anatomist Fallopius, but the first detailed description was by de la Peyronie, in a series of patients with deformities of the erect penis.

Peyronie's disease affects men between the ages of 20 and 80 years (median, 53 years) but is uncommon in men less than 40 years old. The prevalence of patients presenting under the age of 40 is 1.5%.[90,91] Peyronie's disease is more prevalent in patients with diabetes and urolithiasis.[92] More than 66% of patients complain of painful erection. In contrast, in patients without pain the presenting symptom is penile bending (Fig. 15-16), which varies in duration from an 'overnight' appearance to a few months or, in some instances, a few years. Patients concerned about the presence of tumor may also seek attention after feeling a plaque. These lesions are often palpable as firm nodules or plaques on the dorsal surface of the erect penis. Examination of the flaccid penis may be unremarkable. Rarely, there may be multiple plaques. Some have suggested that Peyronie's disease may be related to fibromatosis because of its associa-

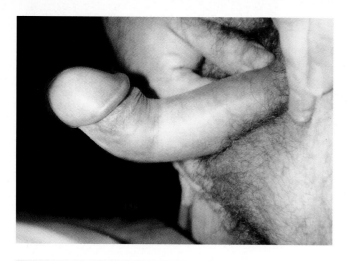

**Fig. 15-16** Peyronie's disease.

tion with Dupuytren's contractures or palmar or plantar fibromatosis, seen in 10–20% of patients.[93] Others have suggested that it may be an inflammatory fibrotic reaction secondary to urethritis. Peyronie's disease also appears to be related to coital trauma and urethral instrumentation, and has been associated with the use of β-blockers, hypertension, diabetes, and immune reactions.[94–98] Hauck et al.[100] recently found an increased frequency of the homozygous genotype of the single nucleotide polymorphism G915C in patients with Peyronie's disease compared to healthy controls (89.2% vs 79%, P = 0.04). However, there were no significant differences in allelic frequencies of the single nucleotide polymorphism T869C. These results indicate that the homozygous wild type of the G915C single nucleotide polymorphism in the coding region of the TGF-β1 gene, which was recently associated with elevated TGF-β1 production and pulmonary fibrosis, may influence the predisposition to Peyronie's disease. However, it does not represent a major genetic risk factor.[100] The expression levels of TGF-β1 and pro- and anti-fibrotic gene products, as well as the nitric oxide/reactive oxygen species (NO/ROS) ratio in the tunica albuginea, appear to be essential for the formation and progression of the Peyronie's disease plaque and affect the expression of multiple genes. This can be assessed with recently developed DNA-based chip arrays, and results with the Peyronie's disease plaque have been encouraging. OSF-1 (osteoblast recruitment), MCP-1 (macrophage recruitment), procollagenase IV (collagenase degradation), and other fibrotic genes have been identified as possible candidate regulatory genes. Gene-based therapy for the treatment of Peyronie's disease is being investigated and may eventually reduce the need for surgical intervention.[101]

Although some earlier studies suggested a relationship between specific human leukocyte antigen (HLA) types and Peyronie's disease, further studies failed to corroborate this association.[99,102] In addition, Hauck et al.[103] failed to demonstrate the occurrence of 16S rDNA in Peyronie's disease which is a highly sensitive marker for the presence of bacteria in inflammatory processes. The results of this study argue against an association between Peyronie's disease and bacterial infection. Bivens et al.[104] reported six patients with Peyronie's disease and carcinoid syndrome, and suggested a causal role for elevated serum serotonin levels. Guerneri et al.[105] found chromosomal aberrations in nine of 14 cases.

Although the chief pathologic finding in Peyronie's disease is fibrosis of the tunica albuginea, it does not affect the erectile tissue of the corpora cavernosa. Calcification and ossification may occur in the fibrous plaques. Histologically, Peyronie's disease begins with perivascular inflammation in the loose connective tissue between the tunica albuginea and the sinusoids of the corpora cavernosa. Deposition of fibrin in the tunica albuginea may be the primary event, followed by inflammation, fibrosis, and collagenization. In surgical specimens the histologic features are less dramatic than the clinical presentation, often consisting only of a cellular proliferation resembling fibromatosis or merely fibrosis (Fig. 15-17A, B). Studies have shown excessive amounts of type III collagen in the plaques.[106]

The clinical course is variable. The disease resolves spontaneously in less than one-third of patients, progresses in up to 40%, and remains stable in the rest.[107] Treatment has included surgical excision of the plaques, intracavernosal plaque excision, radiotherapy, intralesional injections of interferon, steroid injections, and extracorporeal shock-wave therapy.[99–112] The combination of colchicine and vitamin E (which has anti-fibrotic, anti-mitotic and anti-inflammatory effects) in modifying the early stages of Peyronie's disease has been utilized in one study and was an effective and well-tolerated way to stabilize the disease, but more extensive study is needed, comparing these results with other oral therapies.[113] Prostheses may be required to restore potency.[114]

Heterotopic penile bone (os penis) is occasionally found in the plaques of Peyronie's disease, particularly in elderly men.[115] In children, the presence of os penis is considered a congenital anomaly related to the normal occurrence of penile bone in numerous carnivorous animals, a feature lost in humans.[116] The bone is usually deposited just beneath the tunica albuginea.

## Penile prosthesis

Penile prostheses are surgically implanted devices that aid in erection by providing penile rigidity.[117] Since their introduction in the early 1970s the technology has advanced greatly, chiefly because of better understanding of erectile physiology and pathophysiology. These developments have resulted in widespread patient and physician acceptance of these devices, as well as a substantial reduction in complications.

The indication for prosthetic implantation is impotence, both organic and psychogenic. Organic causes include diabetes, paraplegia, quadriplegia, and Peyronie's disease. Therapeutic advances in vascular surgery and pharmacotherapy are leading to reduced use of penile prostheses in patients with organic causes because other modalities offer better results.[117]

There are two general categories of penile prosthesis: malleable devices and inflatable devices. These differ from one

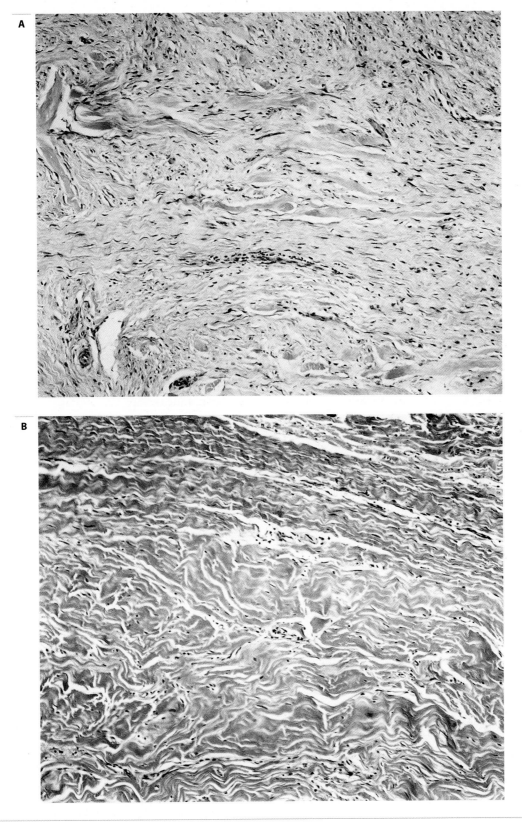

**Fig. 15-17** (**A**) Peyronie's disease, cellular region. (**B**) Peyronie's disease, densely collagenous region.

another in their construction and operation.[117-119] Malleable devices provide simplicity of implantation and have no mechanical parts that may fail. They require very little manual dexterity as they need merely to be bent upward before use. They are disadvantageous because neither the size nor the rigidity of the penis changes. Inflatable devices are based on hydraulic principles that allow inflation for sexual intercourse and deflation in the detumescent phase. These devices are more difficult to implant and have a limited lifespan owing to eventual mechanical failure.

Complications of penile prostheses may occur during surgery (usually crural or corporal perforation), postoperatively (mainly infection or component failure), or later owing to device erosion. Although more than 90% of patients report satisfaction, the reoperation rate is as high as 44%. Slightly lower rates have been reported recently and are expected to improve further with new designs and surgical advances.[120-122]

## Priapism

Priapism is defined as prolonged painful erection unrelated to sexual desire. Typically, pain and tenderness result after 6–8 hours and are related to ensuing ischemia. Priapism is a relatively uncommon condition that may present as a medical emergency associated with significant pain and anxiety in the veno-occlusive or low-flow variant.[123]

Priapism may be primary, secondary, or idiopathic. Secondary causes include genital trauma, thromboembolism, hemostasis and leukostasis (fat embolism, sickle cell anemia, leukemia), neurologic defects (anesthetic agents, spinal cord injury, and autonomic dysfunction), infiltration by cancer, pharmacologic effects (alcohol, drugs acting on central nervous system, total parenteral nutrition), and intracavernosal injections for diagnostic procedures (papaverine hydrochloride, prostaglandin E, and phentolamine).[123,124] Pohl et al.[125] reviewed 230 cases from the literature: more than 33% were idiopathic; 21% were reactions to drugs and alcoholism, 12% were caused by trauma; 11% were caused by sickle cell anemia (an important cause of priapism in children), and less than 1% were due to neoplasms. Priapism can be caused by hematologic malignancy with hypercoagulation, or metastatic disease involving the corpora cavernosa with thrombosis of the venous outflow from the penis.[125,126]

Data on pathologic findings in priapism are extremely limited. The corporeal tissue may be edematous, indurated, and ultimately sclerotic. Ultrastructural examination reveals interstitial edema within 12 hours, destruction of sinusoidal endothelium and exposure of basement membrane with adherence of platelets by the end of 24 hours, and, finally, vascular thrombi associated with ischemic necrosis of smooth muscle tissue at 48 hours.[127]

Besides control of the precipitating factors, treatment includes conservative therapy with analgesics, sedatives, and fluids; control of pain with penile block; aspiration and injection of anesthetic agent, injection of α-adrenergic receptor agonists, intracavernosal injection of thrombolytic medications, and surgery for cavernosal shunt.[128,129]

## Infections

### Gonorrhea

Gonorrhea is caused by *Neisseria gonorrhoeae*, a Gram-negative, non-motile, non-spore-forming, biscuit-shaped diplococcus. The term gonorrhea was coined by Galen in the second century and means 'flow of semen,' referring to the exudate of gonorrheal urethritis. The disease was recorded before the common era in descriptions by Hippocrates and Celcus. The latter treated gonorrheal strictures by catheterization.[130]

In men, gonorrhea typically produces urethritis with urethral discharge, which may be profuse, purulent, or scant (gleet), and burning micturition.[130,131] The disease is sexually acquired, and the risk of infection increases as the number of sexual partners increases. The penis is involved only as a complication of the disease, with cutaneous lesions, infection of the median raphe, penile abscess, and gonococcal tysonitis (inflammation of the preputial glands).[132,133] The chief complication is urethral stricture. Laboratory tests are essential as the disease is frequently mimicked by, and coexists with, chlamydial infection.[134] Standard diagnostic procedures include Gram stain, culture, and microbial susceptibility testing.[130,131] The Center for Disease Control and Prevention has given guidelines for its treatment, which consist primarily of antibiotic therapy.[135]

### Syphilis

*Know syphilis in all its manifestations and relations, and all other things will be added unto you.*

Sir William Osler (1897)

Syphilis is one of the most fascinating diseases affecting humans and has been investigated and described by clinical scholars, playwrights, and poets, including Fracastoro,[136] who in 1530 wrote in his poem about the suffering shepherd Syphilis. Although the disease was thought to be declining in incidence, it seems to have made a comeback in recent years.[137-140] Syphilis is produced by *Treponema pallidum*, a microaerophilic Gram-negative spirochete, after a 9–90-day incubation period. In its classic form, untreated syphilis occurs in three stages: primary, secondary, and tertiary.

In the primary stage, penile involvement commences as a tiny papule, usually at the site of genital trauma on the glans penis, coronal sulcus, prepuce, frenulum, or shaft. In homosexual men the lesion may occur in the anal canal or rectum. The lesion progresses through the papular phase into an ulcerated chancre. The classic chancre is a single round painless ulcer with sharp margins and a clean, indurated base (Fig. 15-18). Lymphadenopathy develops within a week, and the nodes are typically painless, rubbery, and non-suppurative. With or without therapy, the primary ulcer heals within 6–8 weeks.[136,137]

Dark-field microscopy is the mainstay of diagnosis during this phase of the disease, because the antibody response lags.[137] Biopsy is usually not necessary, but may be performed if the diagnosis of syphilis is not suspected. Histopathologic features include epidermal ulceration with

specific, because in up to 25% of cases the plasma cell infiltrate and capillary endothelial proliferation typical of syphilis are absent.[143] The lesions lacking plasma cells and endothelial proliferation may mimic other cutaneous diseases, such as lichen planus or psoriasis. A pronounced lymphocytic response may also be mistaken for mycosis fungoides.[144] The epidermal changes include parakeratotic scales, acanthosis, ulceration, spongiosis, exocytosis, dyskeratosis, and basal vacuolation. Condyoma latum shows prominent epithelial hyperplasia that may become 'pseudoepitheliomatous,' with ulceration and exocytosis with neutrophils.[145]

The third stage (tertiary syphilis) is characterized by granulomas referred to as gummata. These lesions may be nodular or gummatous, that is, accompanied by central necrosis. Nodular lesions lack tissue necrosis and are composed of 'hard' granulomas accompanied by endothelial proliferation and perivascular inflammation. Central caseous necrosis heralds the gummatous phase, which has an intense inflammatory infiltrate in addition to the granulomas.

Until recently syphilis was considered a major cause of penile cancer, but the possible role of syphilis was discarded without much debate with the acceptance of certain human papilloma viruses as etiologic agents. A recent study showed that patients with penile cancer did not have a syphilis history significantly more often than control colon and stomach cancer patients, and the authors concluded that syphilis should be removed from the list of risk factors for penile cancer.[146]

Therapy is stage dependent, consists predominantly of antimicrobial drugs, and is successful if it is timely. The Centers for Disease Control and Prevention recommends counseling all patients for risks and testing for HIV infection, which also reactivates syphilis.

## Herpes simplex

Herpes (from the Greek 'to creep') simplex virus infection involving the genital system is an important sexually transmitted disease that may have a causal role in cervical carcinoma and has high morbidity and mortality in infants. The virus is a double-stranded DNA virus that has two subtypes. Herpes simplex virus type 1 produces oral lesions, whereas herpes simplex virus type 2 predominantly affects the genitalia; only 10–25% of herpes simplex virus type 2 infections produce oral lesions.[147,148] Herpes genitalis and infections caused by HPV are increasingly common, particularly in young, sexually active people. However, herpes simplex virus infection remains the most common infectious cause of genital ulceration, with evidence that many infections are asymptomatic.[148,149]

Clinical manifestations are more severe and fulminant in the first episode than in recurrent disease.[150,151] First episodes often have systemic symptoms (fever, malaise, and headache) and affect multiple extragenital and genital sites. Pain, itching, urethral discharge, dysuria, and tender lymphadenopathy are the most common local symptoms. The genital lesions appear as multiple vesicles with erythematous bases that may coalesce, rupture, form pustules, and eventually become encrusted (Fig. 15-20A). Asymptomatic viral shedding may occur for a prolonged period.[152] The clinical diag-

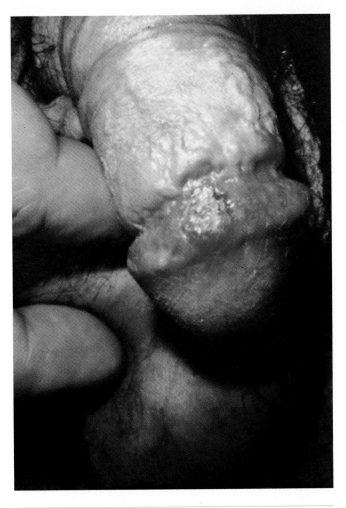

**Fig. 15-18** Syphilitic chancre.

acanthosis at the margins. The submucosa or dermis contains an inflammatory infiltrate of lymphocytes and plasma cells that is mostly diffuse but which may be concentrated perivascularly and associated with pronounced proliferation of endothelial cells (Fig. 15-19).[136,141] Warthin–Starry or Levaditi staining reveals spirochetes in the epidermis or in the dermis around capillaries. The organisms typically have eight to 12 convolutions, but reticulin fibers may mimic them and interpretation must be cautious.[141] The lymph nodes exhibit follicular hyperplasia with many plasma cells and endothelial proliferation. Special stains may also show numerous spirochetes in lymph nodes.

In secondary syphilis, penile involvement is usually part of the systemic mucocutaneous manifestations of this stage. The T. pallidum organisms circulate in the blood and lymphatic systems for 6 weeks to 6 months after the primary stage, producing symmetric skin lesions and generalized lymphadenopathy. The skin lesions are maculopapular, annular, and usually hyperpigmented. Secondary syphilis may present with nodular lesions.[142] Condyloma latum and mucous patches are included in the constellation of mucocutaneous lesions. Smears from these lesions should be examined by dark-field microscopy for organisms. A biopsy may yield variable histological features and by itself is non-

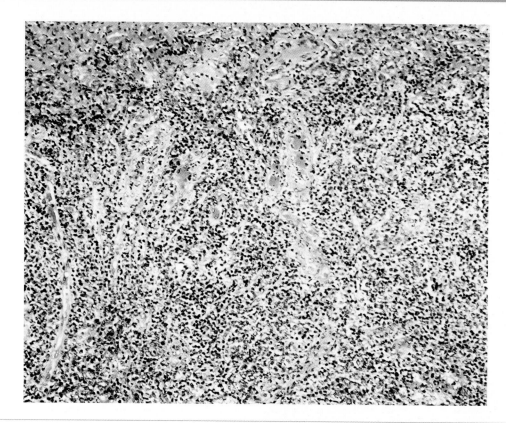

**Fig. 15-19** Syphilis: dense chronic inflammatory infiltrate with endothelial hyperplasia.

nosis may be confirmed by scraping the lesion and obtaining a Tzank smear (stained with Wright–Giemsa, toluidine blue, or Papanicolaou procedures), which reveals large multinucleated giant cells with ballooning degeneration and characteristic intranuclear inclusions. However, this method cannot differentiate between herpes simplex virus and varicella-zoster infection. For this distinction, other techniques such as immunofluorescent antigen detection, virus isolation by culture, and serology are necessary.[153]

Histologically, herpes simplex and varicella-zoster lesions are identical, characterized by unilocular or multilocular intraepidermal vesicles produced by profound acantholysis (Fig. 15-20B).[154] The vesicles contain proteinaceous material and are surrounded by epidermal cells with reticular and ballooning degeneration – features that are hallmarks of herpes infection but absent in other vesiculobullous diseases – that may enter into the differential diagnosis. Cytopathic changes may be evident in adnexal and pilosebaceous structures, endothelial cells, and fibroblasts, but are typically seen in the epidermal cells, which exhibit chromatin margination and inclusion bodies (ranging from small demarcated acidophilic bodies to large, homogeneous, ground-glass acidophilic to basophilic bodies) surrounded by haloes. Classic 3M (multinucleation, margination of chromatin and molding of nuclei) are commonly seen.

Complications of herpes include neonatal complications; nervous system abnormalities (aseptic meningitis, encephalitis, radiculopathies);[155] extragenital lesions on the buttocks, groin, thighs, or other sites; disseminated infection resulting in arthritis, hepatitis, or hematologic disorders; superinfec-

tions; intractable non-healing ulcers in patients with acquired immunodeficiency syndrome (AIDS); and possibly cervical cancer in women. Treatment options are limited. Aciclovir and phosphonoformate trisodium are effective in reducing the intensity and duration of both primary and recurrent episodes, but are not curative.

## Lymphogranuloma venereum

Lymphogranuloma venereum is a sexually transmitted disease caused by *Chlamydia trachomatis* subtypes L1, L2, and L3. It was established as a clinicopathologic entity separate from other venereal diseases in 1913 by Durand, Nicolas, and Favre.[156] Lymphogranuloma venereum is sporadic in the United States and most European countries, but is highly prevalent in Africa, Asia, and South America. Rarely, it is associated with HIV infection.

Like syphilis, lymphogranuloma venereum has three stages: primary genital stage; secondary inguinal stage characterized by acute lymphadenitis with bubo formation; and a rare chronic tertiary stage with genital ulcers, fistulas, elephantiasis, and rectal strictures.[157,158] After an incubation period of 3 days to 6 weeks, the lesion begins as a papule which transforms into a pustule and heals without treatment; therefore in 50% of patients the penile lesion is not clinically examined. The pathognomonic clinical sign is inguinal lymphadenopathy, commonly known as bubo. It is painful, usually unilateral (66%), and may enlarge to form an abscess and rupture (33%).[157–159]

The histologic features are non-specific and non-diagnostic. The ulcer is coated with exudate and neutrophils; the base is composed of granulation tissue, with a mixed

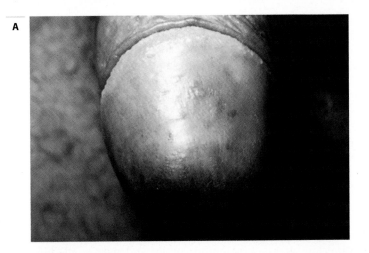

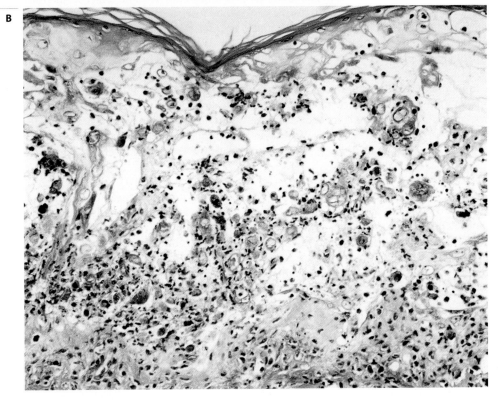

**Fig. 15-20** (**A**) Herpes simplex. (**B**) Herpes simplex vesicle.

inflammatory infiltrate containing large mononuclear cells with occasional granulomas.[160] Giemsa stains may demonstrate purple chlamydial inclusions in the macrophages, but this procedure lacks specificity and sensitivity. The lymph nodes show follicular hyperplasia and elongated stellate abscesses similar to those of cat-scratch disease, tularemia, and fungal and atypical mycobacterial infections.

Culture of the organisms by aspirating the lymph nodes is a useful method of detection, but is technically difficult and costly. Frei's test is no longer used, but serologic tests have gained wide acceptance for diagnosis of lymphogranuloma venereum.[161] Genetic testing is now widely available and is rapid and specific. Antibiotics are effective if the diagnosis is achieved in a timely fashion.

## Granuloma inguinale (donovanosis)

Granuloma inguinale is a chronic, progressive, sexually transmitted disease caused by *Calymmatobacterium granulomatis*, a non-motile, Gram-negative, pleomorphic intracellular bacillus of uncertain classification. Although rare in the United States, it is more prevalent in areas of Australia, India, the Caribbean, and Africa.[162,163]

Granuloma inguinale is only mildly contagious and affects the penis, anal region, and vulva. The incubation period varies from 8 to 80 days. The lesion starts as single or multiple small papules which subsequently form ulcers that bleed readily and have abundant beefy-red granulation tissue at their bases.[162–165] Ulcers are the hallmark of the disease and are typically non-tender, indurated, and firm. A verrucous form occurs in the perianal region and may simulate carcinoma.[166-168] Severe ulcerative genital diseases can cause destruction of the prepuce, glans, or sometimes the entire penis (phagedena). Partial destruction of the prepuce from donovanosis has been reported.[168]

Histologically, granuloma inguinale consists of a central ulcer bordered by acanthotic epidermis with features of pseudoepitheliomatous hyperplasia.[166,167] The dermis below the ulcer contains granulation tissue with vascular ectasia and endothelial proliferation, microabscesses with neutrophils, and large histiocytes (25-90 μm). These histiocytes have cytoplasmic vacuoles that contain dark particulate inclusions (Donovan bodies), seen best with Giemsa or Warthin–Starry stains.[169] Donovan bodies are often easier to see in smears than in histologic sections. Mimicking granuloma inguinale, organisms may be evident within histiocytes in rhinoscleroma, histoplasmosis, coccidioidomycosis, and leishmaniasis; but the small size (1–2 μm) of C. granulomatis is an important distinguishing feature for granuloma inguinale.[170] The diagnosis must be established by microscopy because the bacilli are not readily cultured.[171] Serologic testing using indirect immunofluorescence is available in some laboratories.[172] Antibiotic therapy is usually curative, although relapses may occur when drugs are withdrawn early.

## Chancroid (soft chancre)

Chancroid is a sexually transmitted disease caused by the Gram-negative facultatively anaerobic, biochemically relatively inert bacteria Haemophilus ducreyi. It is characterized by necrotizing genital ulceration that may be accompanied by inguinal lymphadenitis or bubo formation in 50% of cases. First described by Ricord in France in 1838, chancroid is a major cause of genital ulceration in Africa, which recently increased in prevalence in the United States.[173,174,180]

The ulcer develops following a 4–7-day incubation period, beginning as a tender erythematous papule which erodes, ulcerates, and becomes pustular. The ulcer is not indurated, but has undermined edges and is covered by grayish-yellow exudate. The lymphadenitis is unilateral, and the lymph nodes may enlarge and rupture spontaneously.[174]

Histologically, the cutaneous findings are relatively distinctive, forming three zones: a surface zone containing exudate, fibrin, neutrophils, and debris at the base of the ulcer; a wide intermediate zone in which there is prominent vascular proliferation and ectasia with focal thrombosis; and a deep zone containing a dense infiltrate of lymphocytes and plasma cells.[175] The adjacent epidermis may show acanthosis, spongiosis, and a neutrophilic infiltrate. The presumptive diagnosis based on the recognition of these typical zonal histologic features may be confirmed by demonstrating the bacteria by Giemsa, Gram, or methylene blue stains. The bacteria are more easily seen in smears than in histologic sections.[175] In smears, the organisms have a 'railroad track' or 'school of fish' pattern of alignment of short rods.[176] The organisms may be cultured on a selective agar medium[177] and directly detected by polymerase chain reaction.[178]

There is evidence that chancroid is a risk factor for heterosexual spread of HIV.[179-181] Cell-mediated immunity in the host response to Hemophilus ducreyi infection may play a more critical role in the transmission of HIV than humoral immunity.[182] Antibiotic therapy is usually curative, although cases associated with HIV infection do not respond as well.

## Candidiasis

Candidiasis of the penis mimics balanitis or balanoposthitis, visible clinically as bright red patches, numerous minute pustules and erosions. It is common in uncircumcised men, in whom heat and retained moisture within the preputial sac create a favorable environment.[28,183,184] Diabetes mellitus, lengthy antibiotic treatment, and immunosuppression are other predisposing factors.[185] Candida albicans is the most common species and may be identified in the curd-white exudate that often overlies the lesions. Microscopy of a wet-mount preparation with potassium hydroxide is sufficient for diagnosis. Conversely, positive culture alone is not diagnostic because fungi may colonize other forms of balanitis. Therapy consists of eliminating environmental factors predisposing to the infection, improving local hygiene, and application of topical antifungal agents. If local treatment fails, circumcision may be necessary. Patients may have concurrent candidal intertrigo. Severe life-threatening infections with the formation of emphysematous lesions are rare.[186]

## Scabies

Believed to be the first human disease with a known causative agent, scabies was discovered in 1687 to be due to the bite of the human itch mite (Sarcoptes scabiei).[187] Prolonged personal contact is required for transmission, and several members of a family or sexual partners are likely to be infected.[188,189] Scabies may also be an undetected contributor to recurrent staphylococcal or streptococcal infections. A recent report described an AIDS patient with Norwegian scabies who presented with a single, crusted plaque localized to the glans penis.

Scabies is clinically characterized by severe pruritus that is more pronounced at night and may be severe enough to provoke profound excoriation. In addition to the genitalia, the palms, wrists, feet, and elbows may be involved. Burrowing by female mites produces scaly red patches that may be papular, nodular, or excoriated. Vesicles may be visible at the ends of burrows.[188,149]

The diagnosis may be made by teasing the mite out from the burrow with a needle, or by scraping the skin with a sharp scalpel and examining the fragments with a microscope (Fig. 15-21A). Definitive histopathologic diagnosis requires the demonstration of the mite or its products. The burrow is housed within the horny layer where the female mite, approximately 400 μm long, resides (Fig. 15-21B).[190-193] In the absence of the mite, eggs containing larvae or egg shells (chitin walls with marked eosinophilia and periodic acid–Schiff positivity) are diagnostic of scabies. Epidermal spongiosis and dermal eosinophilia are clues aiding recognition. Treatment consists of antipruritic agents and antiscabietic drugs, which should also be administered to family members and sexual partners.[194]

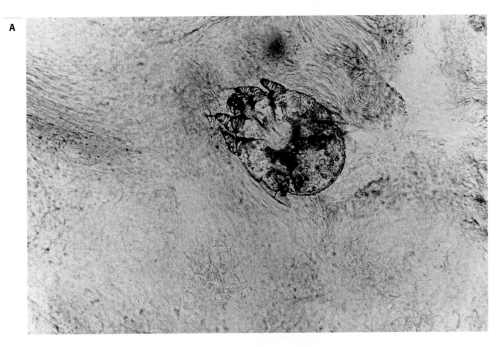

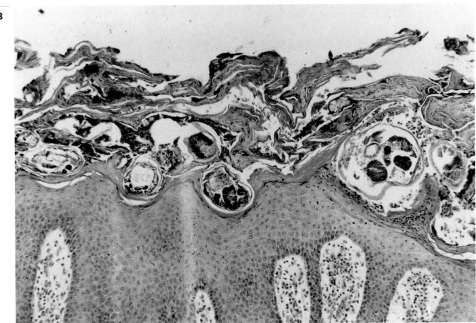

**Fig. 15-21 (A)** Scabies mite. **(B)** Scabies burrow in the epidermis.

## Pediculosis pubis

Pediculosis pubis or pthiriasis is caused by infection with *Pthirus pubis*, the crab louse, which, along with the head louse, accounts for nearly 3 million cases annually in the United States. History and physical examination and a high index of suspicion are necessary to make the correct diagnosis.[149,195] Pediculosis should be suspected when there is itching of hair-bearing regions of the groin, scrotum, and thighs. Penile lesions may be evident as 'blue spots.' Transmission occurs through physical contact and contamination of clothing.[196,197] The lice and mites may be seen in the pubic hair with a magnifying lens. Treatment – essential for the patient, sexual partners, and close family members – consists of mechanical measures, such as combing, topical insecticide in cream or shampoo form, and, if necessary, antibiotics for secondary infection.[198,199]

## Molluscum contagiosum

Molluscum contagiosum is a fairly common viral mucocutaneous disorder caused by a large brick-shaped DNA pox virus.[200] The lesion was named in 1817 by Bateman for its pedunculated gross appearance and contagious nature.

Lymphangioma circumscriptum of the penis may clinically mimic molluscum contagiosum.[201]

The incubation period is 2–7 weeks, and the lesions appear as multiple, discrete, dome-shaped, 3–6 mm papules (Fig. 15-22) with small central umbilications through which milky-white contents may be extruded under pressure.[202] Molluscum contagiosum occurs in children, adolescents, young adults, and in immunocompromised patients (including those with AIDS). In immunocompromised patients there may be hundreds of lesions which fail to involute.

Histologically, the characteristic low-power picture is of a cup-shaped invagination of acanthotic epidermis into the

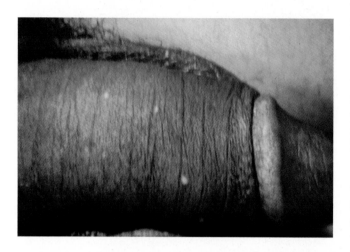

**Fig. 15-22** Molluscum contagiosum.

dermis (Fig. 15-23).[203,204] The basal layer is uninvolved, but the cells of the stratum malpighii acquire cytoplasmic inclusions that progressively enlarge as they reach the surface. The inclusions, known as molluscum bodies (Henderson–Patterson bodies), contain viral particles. The inclusions initially are eosinophilic, but gradually acquire basophilia and granularity as they enlarge and displace the nuclei. The stratum corneum ultimately ruptures, releasing the molluscum bodies through a central crater. The underlying dermis usually lacks significant inflammation unless the molluscum bodies and epidermal contents rupture into it.[205]

Most lesions regress spontaneously within 6–12 months, but treatment is necessary to prevent autoinoculation and transmission to others. Treatment consists of curettage with application of podophyllin or silver nitrate, or laser vaporization.

### Erythrasma

Erythrasma is a superficial, asymptomatic, non-inflammatory disease caused by the diphtheroid organism *Corynebacterium minutissimum*.[206] The lesions are often overlooked, appearing as sharply delineated, round to oval patches or plaques with fine scales in intertriginous areas (the genitocrural form). Examination with a Wood's light (ultraviolet light in the ultraviolet A range) reveals characteristic coral-red fluorescence. The histologic abnormalities are limited to the stratum corneum, where hyperkeratosis and small Gram-positive bacilli are seen.[207,208] The basal epidermis and dermis lack specific histologic changes. The disease is more common in tropical and subtropical climates. Treatment with antibiotics is effective.

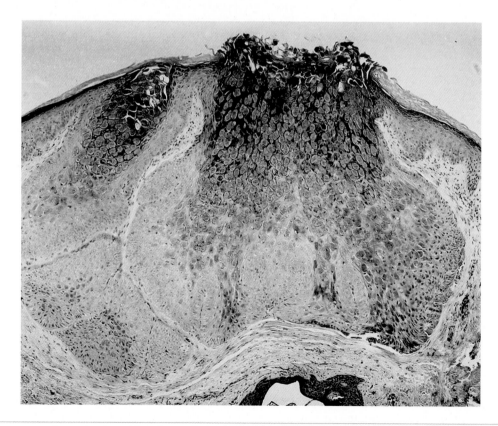

**Fig. 15-23** Molluscum contagiosum showing epidermal crater filled with molluscum bodies.

## Penile lesions in AIDS

Almost all sexually transmitted diseases are common in AIDS patients. These include gonorrhea, syphilis, herpes, candidiasis, chancroid, molluscum contagiosum, HPV, scabies, Reiter's syndrome, and others.[209-213] In patients with AIDS these diseases are generally more severe, of longer duration, and less responsive to therapy than in other patients.

Kaposi's sarcoma, multiple squamous carcinomas, and multifocal carcinoma in situ are malignancies of the penile skin associated with AIDS.[214-217] Condyloma acuminata and squamous cell carcinoma in situ also arise in the perianal region of homosexual males. Foscarnet (trisodium phosphonoformate hexahydrate), an agent used therapeutically for herpes and cytomegalovirus infections in AIDS patients, may induce penile ulcers, mimicking an infectious disease.[218,219]

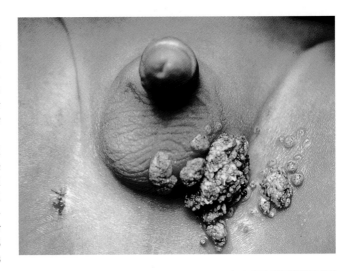

**Fig. 15-24** Condyloma acuminatum. (Courtesy of Dr Julian Wan, State University of New York, Buffalo.)

# Tumor-like conditions

## Condyloma acuminata

The most common tumor-like lesion of the penis is condyloma acuminata, an infection caused by HPV. Condyloma acuminata, typically a disease of young adults, has reached epidemic proportions during the last decade.[220-222]

The incidence of condyloma is reported to be around 5% among adults aged 20–40 years.[223,224] The great majority are sexually transmitted. Men whose sexual partners have HPV-related cervical lesions have an increased (50–85%) incidence of penile condyloma.[225] When genital condyloma occurs in children, sexual abuse should be suspected.[226] After the initial infection, autoinfection is common. The incubation period for penile condyloma varies from several weeks to months or even years.[227] Condyloma is most often located on the corona of the glans, the penile meatus, or the fossa navicularis urethrae, but also occurs on the scrotal skin and perineum (Fig. 15-24).[227] Condyloma is flat, delicately papillary, or warty and cauliflower-like. Histologically, it consists of a proliferation of squamous epithelium with an acanthotic and papillomatous architecture, showing orderly epithelial maturation (Fig. 15-25A). Hyperkeratosis, parakeratosis, and koilocytic atypia are common (Fig. 15-25B).[228] Although cytologic atypia is usually minimal in penile condyloma and mitotic figures are confined to the basal layer, treatment with podophyllin or lasers may cause bizarre cytologic changes that mimic malignancy.[229] To avoid an erroneous diagnosis of carcinoma, information about treatment should be obtained. Human papilloma virus can be demonstrated in condyloma by in-situ hybridization or immunohistochemistry.[230-232] Human papilloma viruses 6 and 11 are common in typical condyloma without dysplasia, whereas 16, 18, 31, and 33 are common in dysplastic condyloma.[230,231] Although condyloma may regress spontaneously, it persists in approximately 50% of cases. The lesion is usually treated with topical podophyllin or laser, and in

the great majority of cases responds to treatment.[232] The relationship of HPV infection to carcinogenesis is discussed later in the chapter.

## Pearly penile papules

Pearly penile papules, also called hirsutoid papillomas, are common penile lesions without clinical significance that are present in approximately 10–20% of males.[233] They are thought to be embryologic remnants of an organ that is well developed in other mammals. They must also be distinguished from the preputial glands (Tyson's glands). Pearly penile papules are typically 1–3 mm in diameter, appearing as yellow-white papules on the corona or, rarely, on the frenulum of the penis.[234] The individual lesions are dome-like, resembling hair, and are usually arranged in a row. Histologically, they show epithelial thickening covering a central fibrovascular core resembling angiofibroma, and lack glandular elements.[235] Pearly penile papules are associated with no known infectious agent and have no potential for malignant transformation; they require no treatment.

## Penile cysts

Epidermal cyst is the most common cystic lesion of the penis and usually occurs on the penile shaft. It varies in size from 0.1 to 1 cm in diameter.[236] Mucoid cyst of the penis arises from ectopic urethral mucosa.[237] It is lined by stratified columnar epithelium with mucous cells and is filled with mucoid material. Usually located on the prepuce or the glans, most are unilocular and range from 0.2 to 2 cm in diameter. Median raphe cyst arises during embryogenesis as a result of incomplete closure of the genital fold. This cyst is lined by pseudostratified columnar epithelium and may be unilocular or multilocular.[236,238-240]

## Pseudoepitheliomatous keratotic and micaceous balanitis

This is a rare lesion that appears as hyperkeratotic, micaceous growths on the glans penis.[241] It was first described by

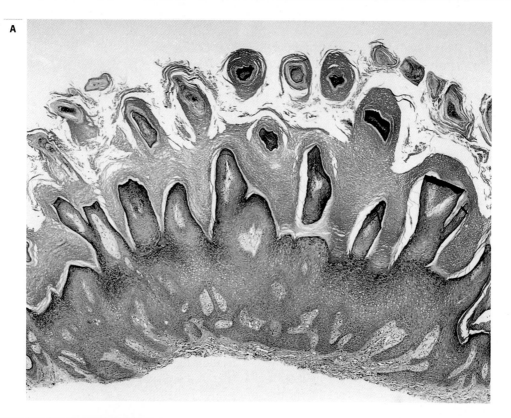

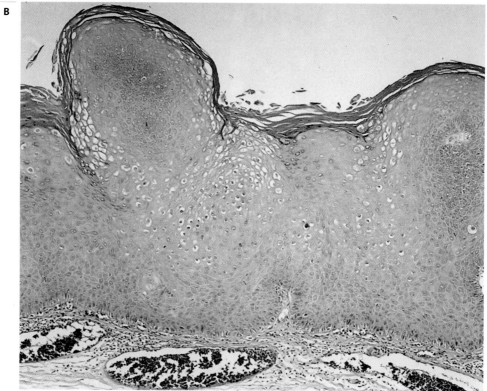

**Fig. 15-25** (**A**) Condyloma acuminatum with marked papillomatosis and hyperkeratosis. (**B**) Condyloma acuminatum with koilocytic atypia.

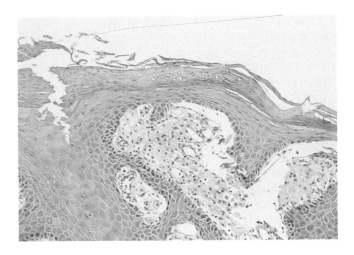

**Fig. 15-26** Verruciform xanthoma with infiltrate of foamy histiocytes.

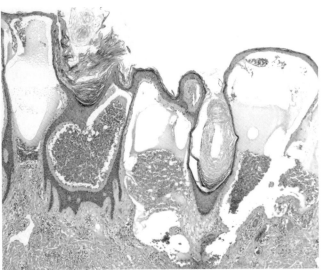

**Fig. 15-27** Angiokeratoma with dilated vascular channels.

Lortat-Jacob and Civatte[242] as a rare scaling, raised lesion of the glans characterized by acanthosis, hyperkeratosis, and pseudoepitheliomatous hyperplasia. Pseudoepitheliomatous keratotic and micaceous balanitis often recurs and may be a precursor of verrucous carcinoma.

### Verruciform xanthoma

Verruciform xanthoma is a warty lesion characterized by acanthosis, hyperkeratosis, and parakeratosis, with long rete ridges associated with a neutrophilic infiltrate. A variable (often prominent) xanthomatous infiltrate occupies the dermis between the rete ridges (Fig. 15-26). This lesion is usually solitary and arises in the oral cavity, and only a few genital lesions have been described (scrotal, penile, and vulvar areas). Despite the architectural resemblance of verruciform xanthoma to other verruciform mucocutaneous lesions of the penis related to HPV infection, this lesion is most likely not an HPV-associated penile lesion.[243] The xanthoma cells have been reported to be weakly and focally positive for cytokeratin, KP1, Mac 387, and Factor XIIIa, but negative for S100 protein and HPV immunostains. Mohsin et al.[244] postulated that the xanthoma (foam) cells, a histologic hallmark of the lesion, are possibly derived from dermal dendritic cells.

## Neoplastic diseases

### Benign neoplasms

Benign tumors of epithelial origin are rare, but squamous papilloma has been described.[245] Among the benign soft tissue tumors of the glans penis, tumors of vascular origin, including capillary or cavernous hemangioma, epithelioid hemangioma, and lymphangioma, are the most common,[246] followed by neurofibroma, schwannoma, leiomyoma, glomus tumor, fibrous histiocytoma, and granular cell tumor.[246–249] Epithelioid hemangioma can be exuberant and often confused with epithelioid hemangioendothelioma and epithelioid angiosarcoma.[250] Benign soft tissue tumors are more often located on the distal part, and malignant

lesions are more common on the proximal shaft. Angiokeratoma is a distinctive benign vascular lesion, but is not considered to be a true neoplasm. This lesion characteristically involves the scrotum, but may involve the penis. Morphologically, this lesion reveals superficial vascular ectasia with overlying warty epidermal changes (Fig. 15-27). There are four clinical types: angiokeratoma corporis diffusum in association with Fabry's disease, in which multiple angiokeratomas appear late in childhood; angiokeratoma of Mibelli, in which bilateral angiokeratomas are found on the dorsum of fingers and toes; angiokeratoma of Fordyce, in which angiokeratoma characteristically occurs on the scrotum; and solitary angiokeratoma.

Another recently described lesion, 'myointioma (myointimal proliferation),' involves the corpus spongiosum of the glans penis.[251] Patients range in age from 2 to 61 years (mean, 29 years) and present with a mass that varies in size from 0.5 to 1.9 cm in greatest dimension. The lesion is present from 4 days to more than 6 months before surgical intervention. Microscopically there is a prominent, often occlusive, fibrointimal proliferation with plexiform architecture involving the vasculature of the corpus spongiosum. The proliferation consists of stellate and spindled cells embedded in abundant fibromyxoid matrix. Occasional lesional cells have well-developed myoid characteristics with moderately abundant eosinophilic cytoplasm, blunt-ended nuclei, and juxtanuclear vacuoles. Foci with degenerative changes, including ghost cell morphology, are also present. The myointimal process is extensively immunoreactive for smooth muscle actin, muscle-specific actin (HHF-35), and calponin, but minimally reactive for desmin. The myointimal cells are non-reactive for S100 protein, and keratin. Factor VIIIrAg, CD31, and CD34 highlight intact endothelial cells lining suboccluded vessels, scattered capillaries that penetrate the proliferation, and the normal uninvolved vasculature. Follow-up data demonstrated that the lesions were benign without evidence of metastasis. Myofibroma, late-stage intravascular (nodular) fasciitis, vascular leiomyoma, and plexiform fibrohistiocytic tumor are potential differential diagnoses.

Benign melanocytic lesions such as melanocytic nevi, melanosis, and lentiginous melanosis also occur on the penis. These lesions pre-exist or coexist with penile melanoma.

## Premalignant lesions

One of the major areas of confusion in the nomenclature of penile lesions is the terminology of premalignant epithelial proliferations. The terms erythroplasia of Queyrat, Bowen's disease, and bowenoid papulosis have been used to describe lesions that are histologically similar but which may have different clinical presentations and biologic behaviors (Table 15-3).[73,252,253] Whether erythroplasia of Queyrat and Bowen's disease are the same lesion or different clinicopathologic entities remains controversial. Some have recommended that these two names be replaced by terms such as intraepithelial neoplasia or carcinoma in situ.[254–258] Squamous hyperplasia and squamous intraepithelial lesions of low and high grade are probably precursors of invasive squamous cell carcinoma.[258] Recently Cubilla et al.[257] reported that the presence of two groups of lesions in the precancerous and invasive carcinomas (typical squamous carcinoma and the warty basaloid carcinoma) is consistent with the bimodal hypothesis of the existence of non-HPV (the typical squamous) and HPV-related (warty or basaloid) tumors.

### Erythroplasia of Queyrat

Although originally described by Tarnovsky in 1891, it was in 1911 that Queyrat[259] applied the term erythroplasia to bright red, well-defined, minimally raised, glistening, velvety, and persistent plaques on the glans penis and the prepuce.[259] Erythroplasia of Queyrat has been reported in patients of all ages but usually occurs in men in the fifth and sixth decades of life. In the 100 cases studied by Graham and Helwig[260] the median age was 51 years. Circumcision protects against the development of erythroplasia of Queyrat, as it does against invasive squamous carcinoma (see the discussion on squamous cell carcinoma later in the chapter).

Clinically, erythroplasia of Queyrat appears as a shiny, elevated, red, velvety, oozing, erythematous plaque located on the glans penis or prepuce.[260,261] It may also involve the urethral meatus, frenulum, or neck of the penis. In more than 50% of patients erythroplasia of Queyrat is solitary.[260] Histologically, it consists of full-thickness alteration of the squamous epithelium with loss of polarity, large hyperchromatic nuclei, dyskeratosis, multinucleated cells, and numerous typical and atypical mitotic figures (Fig. 15-28). The underlying stroma contains a band of chronic inflammation and vascular proliferation. About 10% of patients progress to invasive squamous cell carcinoma, and 2% develop distant metastases.[260] The cause of erythroplasia of Queyrat is largely unknown. HPV type 16 DNA has previously been detected only in very few distinctly characterized patients. Recently Wieland et al.[261] reported that HPV DNA was detected in all eight patients with erythroplasia of Queyrat and in none of the controls with inflammatory penile lesions. HPV types 8, 16, 39 and 51 were detected in erythroplasia of Queyrat patients. However, HPV type 8 was not detected in cervical or vulvar precancerous and cancerous lesions and in Bowen's disease lesions that carried genital HPV types. The data suggested that in contrast to other genital neoplasias, in erythroplasia of Queyrat a co-infection with HPV type 8 and carcinogenic genital HPV types occurs. The presence or absence of HPV type 8 might help to distinguish between penile erythroplasia of Queyrat and Bowen's diseases.

A number of different diseases may produce penile lesions that are clinically similar to erythroplasia of Queyrat, including Zoon's balanitis, other inflammatory processes, and penile manifestations of benign dermatoses such as drug eruption, psoriasis, and lichen planus.[262]

### Bowen's disease

Bowen's disease was first described by Bowen in 1912, and the term has been used to designate squamous cell carcinoma in situ of both sun-exposed and sun-protected skin. The term is used to denote a lesion histologically similar to erythroplasia of Queyrat when it involves the shaft of the penis, or when the lesion does not have the red clinical

**Table 15-3** Distinguishing features of three different preneoplastic conditions of the penis

| Features | Erythroplasia of Queyrat | Bowen's disease | Bowenoid papulosis |
|---|---|---|---|
| Site | Glans, prepuce | Shaft | Shaft |
| Age | 5th and 6th decade | 4th and 5th decade | 3rd and 4th decade |
| Lesion | Erythematous plaque | Scaly plaque | Papules |
| Hyperkeratosis | – | + | + |
| Maturation | – | – | + |
| Sweat gland involvement | – | – | + |
| Pilosebaceous involvement | – | + | – |
| Progression to carcinoma | 10% | 5–10% | – |
| Association with internal cancer | – | + | – |
| Spontaneous regression | – | – | + |

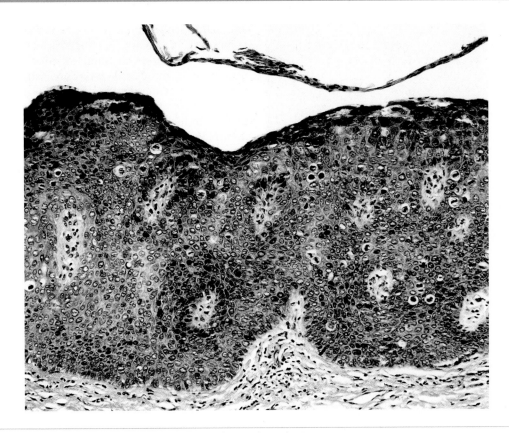

**Fig. 15-28** Erythroplasia of Queyrat showing severe nuclear abnormalities and acanthosis.

appearance of erythroplasia of Queyrat.[73,254,263] Bowen's disease occurs most often in men in the fourth and fifth decades of life, a decade earlier than erythroplasia of Queyrat.[263] Typically, it is a crusted, sharply demarcated scaly plaque (Fig. 15-29). Rarely, Bowen's disease is papillomatous.[264] Histologically, it shows features indistinguishable from those of erythroplasia of Queyrat (Fig. 15-30). Some authors have pointed to minor histologic differences, but these are mainly the result of differing anatomic locations.[251] Bowen's disease is hyperkeratotic and commonly involves pilosebaceous units, features not seen in erythroplasia of Queyrat that occurs in the mucocutaneous epithelium (Table 15-3).[254,260,265]

The incidence of progression to invasive squamous cell carcinoma is similar (approximately 5–10%) for both erythroplasia of Queyrat and Bowen's disease. They are considered separate entities because of differences in their natural histories. It has been believed that up to 33% of patients with Bowen's disease develop visceral cancer (often respiratory, gastrointestinal, or urogenital).[260] In contrast, erythroplasia of Queyrat has no such association.[260,266,267] The distinction has become less clear because recent studies of Bowen's disease have cast doubt on its association with visceral cancer.[254]

### Bowenoid papulosis

The term bowenoid papulosis was first used by Wade et al.[268] in 1978 to describe lesions on the penile shaft or perineum in young men. Histologically, bowenoid papulosis closely resembles squamous cell carcinoma in situ. However, it is multicentric and has an indolent clinical course.[265,269] In all reported cases the lesions either responded to conservative treatment (local excision, topical or laser treatment) or regressed spontaneously.[265,270] Bowenoid papulosis is considered the male counterpart of multifocal vulvovaginal dysplasia in young women.[271]

Bowenoid papulosis usually occurs in young men, with a mean age of 29.5 years.[271] The lesions occur most commonly on the penile shaft and are usually multicentric papules ranging in size from 2 to 10 mm.[271] The papules sometimes coalesce to form plaques resembling condyloma acuminata.

Bowenoid papulosis is characterized by varying degrees of hyperkeratosis, parakeratosis, irregular acanthosis, and papillomatosis (Fig. 15-31).[265] Although scattered atypical keratinocytes and mitotic figures may be seen even in the superficial layers of the epithelium, there is usually more maturation of keratinocytes in bowenoid papulosis than in Bowen's disease or erythroplasia of Queyrat. Patterson et al.[265] pointed out that the atypical keratinocytes in bowenoid papulosis involve the upper parts of sweat glands, usually sparing pilosebaceous units (see Table 15-3); this pattern is reversed in Bowen's disease.[265] A recent paper described a significant difference in the morphometric evaluation between Bowen's disease and bowenoid papulosis. The nuclei were larger, more oval, with more irregular margins in Bowen's disease than in bowenoid papulosis.[272] However, the minor histologic differences between bowenoid papulosis and Bowen's disease and erythroplasia of Queyrat do not allow for an accurate diagnosis on the basis of histo-

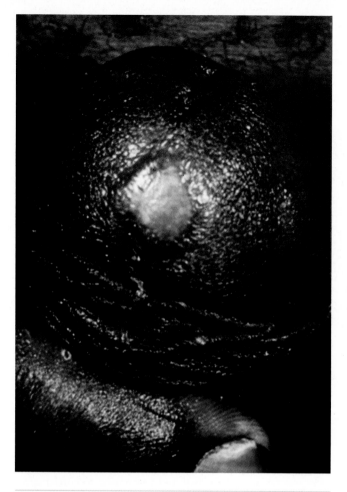

**Fig. 15-29** Bowen's disease.

logic findings alone. Bowenoid papulosis should be suspected when a young man has multiple skin lesions that range histologically from dysplasia to squamous carcinoma in situ on the penile shaft.

The etiology of bowenoid papulosis is unknown, but viral, immunologic, and chemical causes have been suggested.[265] HPV DNA has been demonstrated in several cases of bowenoid papulosis.[273–275]

The clinical behavior of bowenoid papulosis differs significantly from that of Bowen's disease or erythroplasia of Queyrat. Spontaneous regression has been reported in a number of cases. Neither progression to invasive carcinoma nor association with visceral cancer has been observed.[276] Recent reports, however, stated that bowenoid papulosis with high-risk human papilloma viruses may develop to invasive squamous cell carcinoma.[277,278]

## Malignant neoplasms

Cancer of the penis is uncommon, affecting approximately 1 in 100 000 men and accounting for less than 0.5% of all neoplasms in men in North America and Europe.[256,279] According to the American Cancer Society, a total of 1280 cases were diagnosed in 2007, with 290 deaths.[280] In some countries, such as Paraguay, Uganda, Brazil, Jamaica, Mexico,

and Haiti, penile cancer is more common than in the US, comprising as many as 10–12% of malignancies in men.[279,281,282] Worldwide, more than 95% of cases of penile cancer are squamous cell carcinoma, with sarcoma accounting for most of the remaining 4–5%. Rarely, other cancers such as melanoma and basal cell carcinoma arise in the penis. Urothelial carcinoma usually arises in the penile urethra (see Chapter 9).

### Squamous cell carcinoma

Risk factors for squamous cell carcinoma of the penis include lack of circumcision, poor hygiene, phimosis, smoking, viruses, and the presence of underlying lichen sclerosus.[56,57,66–68,279–284] Squamous cell carcinoma is extremely unusual among individuals who were circumcised in infancy; for example, it is rare among Jews, who practice circumcision shortly after birth.[285] Circumcision in late childhood or adolescence seems to confer partial protection;[286–288] a higher incidence of penile squamous cell carcinoma has been reported in Muslims, who are circumcised later in childhood.[288] In India, more than 95% of cases occur in Hindus, who do not customarily undergo circumcision.[286] Although the data indicate that circumcision at birth provides excellent protection, it appears that equally low incidence rates can be achieved in uncircumcised males who practice good hygiene. The very low rate of penile carcinoma in Northern European countries, where males are not circumcised but where good hygiene is practiced, supports this conclusion.[289] Almost 50% of patients with penile carcinoma also have phimosis.[290] Experimental evidence suggests that smegma plays an important role in penile carcinogenesis.[279] Retention of smegma or its derivatives is thought to have an irritating effect on penile epithelium, and in phimosis this effect may be exacerbated.[279] *Mycobacterium smegmatis* may be a factor in carcinogenesis, either directly or by converting smegma sterols into carcinogenic sterols.

A viral etiology has also been suggested for penile carcinoma. Human papilloma viruses 16 and 18 are present in approximately 50% of cases.[291–296] There is an increase in the incidence of cervical cancer in the spouses or ex-spouses of men with penile carcinoma, supporting the hypothesis that a sexually transmitted agent plays a causative role.[297] There are significant differences in HPV prevalence in different histological cancer subtypes, higher in basaloid and warty subtypes than in keratinizing squamous cell carcinoma and verrucous carcinoma.[298,299] Although an early report demonstrated the presence of HPV6,[300] HPV16 is more frequently implicated[301] and has been found in bowenoid papulosis[302] and in an early penile carcinoma associated with a cutaneous horn.[303] Nucleic acid analysis by in-situ hybridization for HPV16 or 18 has demonstrated this virus in both primary and metastatic penile cancer.[294,304] Human papilloma viruses 11 and 30 have also been associated with penile carcinoma.

Ultraviolet radiation also may contribute to squamous cell carcinoma of the penis and scrotum, according to studies of patients with psoriasis who have been treated with oral 8-methoxy-psoralen and ultraviolet A phototherapy or ultraviolet B.[305] Two different pathways of penile carcinogenesis seem to exist, similar to vulvar cancer. In contrast to basaloid and

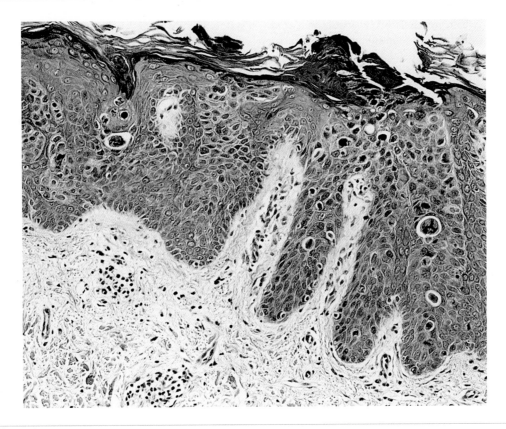

**Fig. 15-30** Bowen's disease with marked nuclear pleomorphism and abnormal mitotic figures.

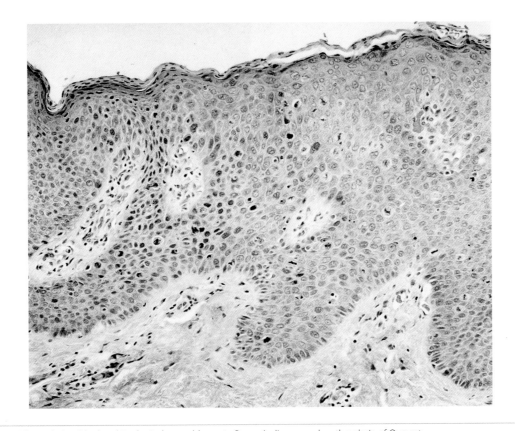

**Fig. 15-31** Bowenoid papulosis with close histological resemblance to Bowen's disease and erythroplasia of Queyrat.

warty penile cancer, which are regularly HPV associated (about 80–100%), only a minority of keratinizing and verrucous penile carcinomas appear to be related to HPV (33–35%).

Penile intraepithelial neoplasia, including Bowen's disease, erythroplasia of Queyrat, and bowenoid papulosis, is a precursor of basaloid and warty carcinoma. Precursors of keratinizing carcinoma and verrucous carcinoma are not established. Recently Cubilla et al.[258] suggested that squamous hyperplasia is a precursor despite its benign appearance, owing to the high frequency and preferential association of these cancers as well as the subtle morphologic differences. Whether lichen sclerosus is a precancerous lesion is uncertain.

Penile carcinoma usually occurs in older men.[298,306–309] Patient age at diagnosis ranges from 20 to 90 years, but patients are rarely younger than 40.[309,310] This may be changing, however. In a 1992 study from the United States, 22% of the patients were under 40 and 7% were younger than 30.[309]

Patients usually have an exophytic or ulcerated mass. Penile pain, discharge, difficulty in voiding, and lymphadenopathy are presenting symptoms.[279] The majority arise in the glans or the prepuce,[279,309] and rarely primarily involve the penile shaft and urethral meatus (Table 15-4).[307–310]

There are two main types of penile carcinoma: fungating/exophytic, and ulcerating/infiltrating (Fig. 15-32, 15-33). There is no unique grading system for penile squamous cell carcinoma; instead, the grading system for cutaneous squamous cell carcinoma is used. In the modified Broders' grading system (Table 15-5)[311] the degree of keratinization is the most important feature. Most squamous cell carcinomas are low grade at the time of biopsy. Well-differentiated squamous cell carcinoma consists of finger-like downward projections of atypical squamous cells that originate from a thickened, hyperkeratotic, papillomatous epidermis (Fig. 15-34). These projections often resemble nests of cells within the dermis. Concentrically arranged masses of cells often surround accumulations of anucleate keratin known as keratin pearls (Fig. 15-35A). These represent a disorganized attempt by the malignant cells to undergo differentiation. Intercellular bridges often are prominent (Fig. 15-35B). Well-differentiated (grade 1) cancer has limited atypia, consisting of nuclear enlargement and pleomorphism and the presence of one or more large nucleoli. Mitotic figures can usually be found, but are rare. Individual cells may be dyskeratotic with deeply eosinophilic cytoplasm. The dermis along the tumor margin usually contains a dense lymphocytic or mixed inflammatory infiltrate. Poorly differentiated squamous cell carcinoma (grade 3) forms few or no keratin pearls (Fig. 15-36), but it has marked nuclear pleomorphism and hyperchromasia and may have areas of necrosis and superinfection. Mitotic figures are usually numerous, and the cancer is deeply invasive (Fig. 15-37). Moderately

**Table 15-4** Primary sites of squamous carcinoma of the penis

| Site(s) | Frequency (%) |
| --- | --- |
| Glans | 48 |
| Prepuce | 21 |
| Glans, prepuce, and shaft | 14 |
| Glans and prepuce | 9 |
| Coronal sulcus | 6 |
| Shaft | 2 |

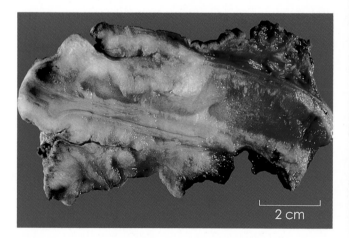

**Fig. 15-32** Squamous cell carcinoma of penis. The glans and prepuce are eroded and replaced by a fungating mass, which invades the corpus cavernosum (sagittal section in plane of urethra).

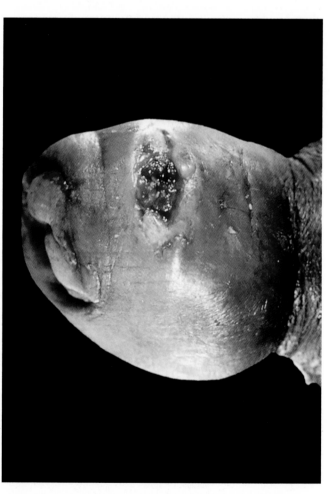

**Fig. 15-33** Squamous cell carcinoma of penis has eroded through the foreskin of this uncircumcised penis.

differentiated carcinoma (grade 2) shows histologic differentiation intermediate between grades 1 and 3, with moderate nuclear atypia, and more mitotic activity and fewer keratin pearls than grade 1.

Maiche et al.[312] proposed a scoring system for grading squamous cell carcinoma of the penis on the basis of four criteria: the degree of keratinization, the number of mitotic figures per high-power field (×400), the degree of nuclear atypia, and the presence of inflammatory cells (Table 15-6). They reported that this grading system was practical and showed a correlation between histologic grade and stage.[312] In their series, stages I and II cancers were grades 1 and 2 more frequently than were stages III and IV. The highest proportion of poorly differentiated grade 4

cancer was found in patients with stage IV disease. These authors also found that histologic grade was a valuable prognostic factor. The 5- and 10-year relative survival rates are highest for patients with grade 1 tumors and lowest for those with grade 4 cancer. There is no significant difference in the survival rates between patients with grades 2 and 3 cancer.[312]

A prognostic index was described for penile cancer based on histologic grade and location. Cancer was categorized as low prognostic index (score 1–3), intermediate (score 4) and high prognostic index (scores 5 and 6) (Table 15-7).[263]

Penile cancer spreads superficially through the epithelial mucosal compartment, following the penile fascia, following spaces formed by feeding vessels in the tunica albuginea, by direct vertical invasion, or along the urethral epithelium.[313,314]

The urethra and periurethral tissues, including the penile fascia, are common sites of involvement, followed by the corpus spongiosum and corpora cavernosa (Fig. 15-38),[314] and fistulas may be created. Despite the rich vascularity of the corpus cavernosum, hematogenous spread is uncommon. Infrequent involvement of the corpora cavernosa probably reflects the barrier function of the tunica albuginea.[314] Distant metastasis usually occurs through lymphatics, and the inguinal lymph nodes are generally the first involved. The lymphatics of the penis consist of richly anastomosing channels that cross the midline along the shaft and at the penile base. Therefore, metastasis may be to either side or both sides. The number of lymph nodes containing metastases correlates with prognosis.[315]

Infection of the primary tumor can cause inguinal lymph node enlargement without metastases; therefore, sentinel

**Table 15-5** Grading of squamous carcinoma (modified Broders' system)

| Grade | | Histologic features |
|---|---|---|
| 1 | Well | Prominent intercellular bridges<br>Prominent keratin pearl formation<br>Minimal cytologic atypia<br>Rare mitotic figures |
| 2/3 | Moderately | Occasional intercellular bridges<br>Fewer keratin pearls<br>Increased mitotic activity<br>Moderate nuclear atypia |
| 4 | Poorly | Marked nuclear pleomorphism<br>Numerous mitotic figures<br>Necrosis<br>No keratin pearls |

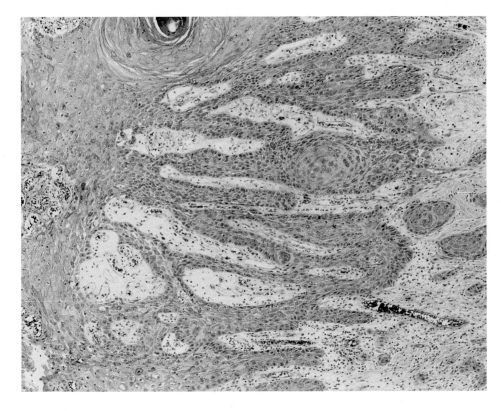

**Fig. 15-34** Fingerlike projections of well-differentiated squamous cell carcinoma extend into the dermis.

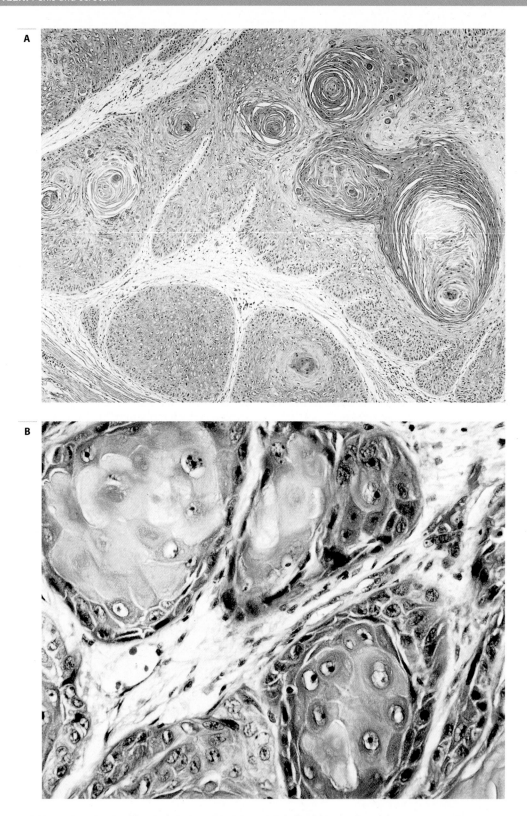

**Fig. 15-35** (**A**) Squamous cell carcinoma forming keratin pearls. (**B**) Squamous cell carcinoma of penis at higher magnification showing glassy cytoplasm of keratinizing cells with intercellular bridges.

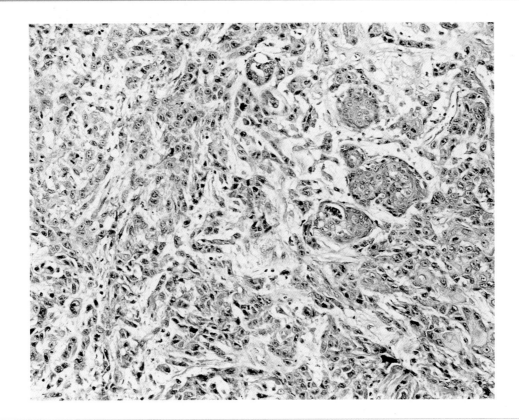

**Fig. 15-36** Squamous cell carcinoma infiltrating the penis as small nests of cells.

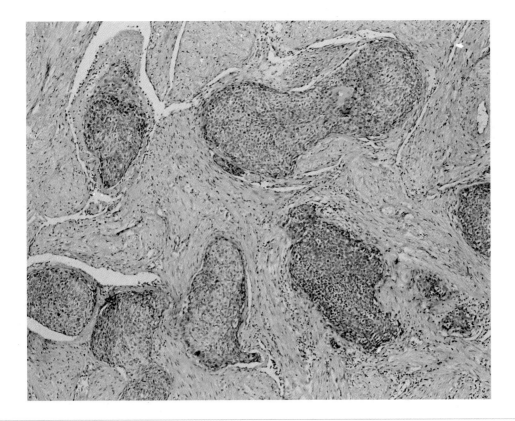

**Fig. 15-37** Deeply invasive poorly differentiated squamous cell carcinoma.

**Table 15-6** Histologic scoring system for squamous cell carcinoma of the penis

| Degree of keratinization | |
| --- | --- |
| Points | |
| 0: | No keratin pearls. Keratin in <25% of cells |
| 1: | No keratin pearls. Keratin in 25–50% of cells |
| 2: | Keratin pearls incomplete or keratin in 50–75% of cells |
| 3: | Keratin pearls complete or keratin in >75% of cells |
| **Mitotic activity** | |
| Points | |
| 0: | 10 or more mitotic cells/field |
| 1: | 6–9 mitotic cells/field |
| 2: | 3–5 mitotic cells/field |
| 3: | 0–2 mitotic cells/field |
| **Cellular atypia** | |
| Points | |
| 0: | All cells atypical |
| 1: | Many atypical cells/field |
| 2: | Moderate number of atypical cells/field |
| 3: | Few atypical cells/field |
| **Inflammatory cells** | |
| Points | |
| 0: | No inflammatory cells present |
| 1: | Inflammatory cells (lymphocytes) present |
| Grade 1: | 8–10 points |
| Grade 2: | 5–7 points |
| Grade 3: | 3–4 points |
| Grade 4: | 0–2 points |

From Maiche AG, Pyrhonen S, Karkinen M. Histological grading of squamous cell carcinoma of the penis. A grading system. Br J Urol 1991; 67:522–526.

**Table 15-7** Prognostic index for squamous carcinoma of the penis

**Numerical Values of Histologic Grade**

| Grade | Value |
| --- | --- |
| I | 1 |
| II | 2 |
| III | 3 |

**Numerical Values of Anatomic Levels of Invasion**

| Site | Level | Value |
| --- | --- | --- |
| Glans | Epithelium | 0 |
| | Lamina propria | 1 |
| | Corpus spongiosum | 2 |
| | Corpora cavernosa | 3 |
| Foreskin | Epithelium | 0 |
| | Lamina propria | 1 |
| | Dartos | 2 |
| | Skin | 3 |
| Coronal sulcus | Epithelium | 0 |
| | Lamina propria | 1 |
| | Dartos | 2 |
| | Buck's fascia | 3 |

node biopsy is commonly performed to stage the tumor accurately. Although most patients present with clinical stage I or II, controversy exists about the role of prophylactic bilateral inguinal node dissection.[316–322] Palpation of the inguinal lymph nodes is 70–85% sensitive and 50% specific for the detection of metastases. If clinical evaluation of the groin lymph nodes is delayed several weeks after excision of the primary tumor, the false-positive rate drops to around 15%. Bilateral inguinal lymph node dissection carries a significant risk of morbidity and mortality, so many surgeons have advocated that inguinal dissection be performed only for patients with palpable lymph nodes several weeks after primary surgery to allow the inflammatory reaction in the nodes to subside. Alternately, biopsy of sentinel lymph nodes may detect inguinal metastasis, and can be followed by inguinal dissection in patients with metastasis.[317–323]

Cubilla et al.[324] classified penile carcinoma as superficially spreading squamous cell carcinoma, vertical growth squamous cell carcinoma, verruciform carcinoma (including warty or condylomatous carcinoma), verrucous carcinoma, papillary carcinoma, not otherwise specified, and multicentric carcinoma. Superficially spreading carcinoma occurred most frequently. Inguinal lymph node metastases were found in 82% of patients with vertical growth carcinoma, 42% with superficially spreading carcinoma, and 33% with multicentric carcinoma. Superficial spreading carcinoma usually involves more than one compartment (glans, foreskin, or coronal sulcus), but occasionally is confined to either the glans or the foreskin. When vertical growth occurs, there may be invasion of the corpora or skin of the prepuce.

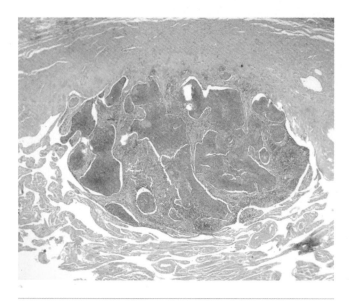

**Fig. 15-38** Tumor emboli in corpus cavernosum.

Approximately 20% of cases of penile carcinoma display vertical growth, characterized by a large, fungating, often ulcerated, whitish-gray or hemorrhagic mass.

Exophytic penile carcinoma forms a large polypoid mass. Histologically, most are well-differentiated squamous cell carcinomas, with extensive keratinization and finger-like projections invading the stroma. Ulcerating carcinoma tends to originate on the glans penis, grows invasively, and is usually moderately to poorly differentiated, with a higher incidence of lymph node metastases than the exophytic type.

The extent of penile shaft involvement of squamous cell carcinoma, the growth pattern, mean depth of invasion, and vascular invasion[325] correlate with the frequency of lymph node metastases. Patients with tumors of the shaft and those with ulcerating growth have a greater likelihood of metastases. Inguinal lymph node metastases are frequent in cases with vertical growth and skin involvement.[314] The size of the primary tumor, the grade, and the length of the delay in diagnosis do not correlate with the incidence of lymph node metastases.[309,315,325] There are limitations in interpretation of biopsies in patients with penile squamous cell carcinoma. Therefore, important pathologic prognostic factors cannot depend on biopsy information alone, as this may be insufficient to make a decision whether to perform a groin dissection or to predict those patients in whom other treatment modalities should be considered.[326]

Palpable inguinal lymphadenopathy is present at diagnosis in 58% of patients.[279] Of these, fewer than 50% have metastases; the others have inflammatory lymphadenopathy resulting from infection of the primary tumor. About 20% of patients with non-palpable lymph nodes have metastases.[279] In patients with squamous carcinoma of the penis the presence and extent of metastases involving the inguinal nodes are the most important predictors of survival. Favorable prognostic indicators of survival in surgically treated patients in whom metastases develop include minimal nodal disease; unilateral involvement; no evidence of extranodal extension of cancer; and absence of pelvic nodal metastases. Therefore, prophylactic lymphadenectomy in selected patients at high risk for metastases seems reasonable.[327] Dynamic sentinel node biopsy is now recommended for patients with clinically node-negative penile cancer to reduce the morbidity of radical inguinal lymphadenectomy.[328-330] Perdona et al.[328] reported that this procedure is minimally invasive and easy to perform, with similar results to those of radical inguinal lymphadenectomy, and has lower morbidity. Kroon et al.[331] compared the clinical outcome of early and delayed excision of lymph node metastases in patients with penile squamous cell carcinoma, and found that the cancer-specific 3-year survival of patients with positive lymph nodes detected during surveillance was 35%, whereas those who underwent early resection of occult inguinal metastases detected on dynamic sentinel biopsy had 85% survival (P = 0.0017). However, Izawa et al.[332] reported that dynamic sentinel node biopsy utilizing intraoperative lymphatic mapping is a promising technique, but requires further testing in high-volume centers for penile cancer. Contemporary superficial and modified inguinal dissection techniques with intraop-erative frozen section remain the 'gold standard' for identifying microscopic metastases. Tabatabaei et al.[333] evaluated lymphotrophic nanoparticle-enhanced magnetic resonance imaging (LNMRI) with ferumoxtran-10 to determine the presence of regional lymph node metastases in patients with penile cancer. They found that LNMRI had sensitivity, specificity, and positive and negative predictive values of 100%, 97%, 81.2%, and 100%, respectively. Venous and/or lymphatic embolization predicted lymph node involvement, and could be used to determine which patients with clinically negative lymph nodes should undergo immediate lymphadenectomy.[334] Among the pathologically node-positive patients, factors adversely influencing survival in multivariate analysis were bilateral nodal metastases, number of positive inguinal nodes, pelvic nodal metastases, and extranodal extension.[335] Presentation with distant metastases is rare in the absence of regional lymph node metastasis. Hematogenous dissemination is rare: less than 2% of patients with penile carcinoma have distant visceral metastases at the time of diagnosis. However, hepatic, pulmonary, and osseous metastases can occur in untreated cases.[336,337] The presence of HPV does not influence the prognosis.[338]

The most widely used clinical staging systems for penile cancer are Jackson's system (Table 15-8)[339] and the American Joint Committee on Cancer system (Table 15-9).[340] Grade and stage are the most reliable prognostic factors for penile carcinoma, although stage is dominant. Survival is shortened when there is spread to inguinal or iliac lymph nodes, or distant metastases. Histologic grade correlates well with the clinical stage. Patients with low-grade cancer have a favorable prognosis, and more than 80% are long-term survivors. Patients with high-grade cancer tend to have advanced stage at presentation and a poor prognosis. About 50% of cancers appearing on the shaft are high-grade, compared to only 10% arising in the prepuce.[341]

DNA flow cytometric analysis may also be a useful prognostic factor in penile cancer.[342-345] Yu et al.[342] reported that patients with diploid cancer had longer survival than those with aneuploid cancer, and low S-phase fraction was associated with favorable outcome. The incidence of aneuploidy rises with increasing stage. Yu et al.[342] also reported that all patients who appeared cured had diploid tumors, whereas 80% of patients dying of cancer had aneuploid tumors. Gustafson et al.[343] reported similar results: they found that low-grade cancer was predominantly diploid, whereas high-grade cancer was not. Only one of 14 patients with diploid cancer

**Table 15-8** Jackson's staging system for squamous cell carcinoma of the penis (From Jackson SM. The treatment of carcinoma of the penis. Br J Surg 1966; 53: 33–35)

| Stage | Description |
| --- | --- |
| I | Confined to glans, prepuce, or both |
| II | Extending onto penile shaft or corpora |
| III | Operable inguinal lymph node metastases |
| IV | Inoperable inguinal lymph node metastases, adjacent structure involvement and/or distant metastases |

died from cancer, but four of 12 patients with non-diploid cancer did so.[343]

The treatment of choice for penile cancer is surgical resection with inguinal lymphadenectomy; there have been few therapeutic advances in the last two decades. Major progress includes methods for less disfiguring treatment of the primary lesion for some patients; improved survival by altering the timing of groin dissection for those at risk for metastases; and multimodal therapy (radiotherapy and chemotherapy)

**Table 15-9** TNM: The staging system of the American Joint Committee on Cancer (From Greene FL, Page DL, Fleming ID, et al. American Joint Committee on Cancer: Cancer staging manual, 6th edn. New York: Springer Verlag, 2002)

| Primary Tumor (T) | |
| --- | --- |
| TX | Primary tumor cannot be assessed. |
| T0 | No evidence of primary tumor |
| Tis | Carcinoma in situ |
| Ta | Noninvasive verrucous carcinoma |
| T1 | Tumor invades subepithelial connective tissue |
| T2 | Tumor invades the corpus spongiosum or cavernosum |
| T3 | Tumor invades the urethra or prostate |
| T4 | Tumor invades other adjacent structures |

| Regional Lymph Nodes (N) | |
| --- | --- |
| NX | Regional lymph node cannot be assessed |
| N0 | No regional lymph node metastasis |
| N1 | Metastasis in a single superficial inguinal lymph node |
| N2 | Metastasis in multiple or bilateral superficial inguinal lymph node |
| N3 | Metastasis in deep inguinal or pelvic lymph node(s), unilateral or bilateral |

| Distant Metastasis (M) | |
| --- | --- |
| MX | Presence of distant metastasis cannot be assessed |
| M0 | No distant metastasis |
| M1 | Distant metastasis |

for treating metastases.[346,347] Assessment of penile cancer on the basis of clinical findings alone often results in inaccurate staging and suboptimal treatment. Imaging of primary site and metastases optimizes treatment planning. Both $T_1$- and $T_2$-weighted MRI scans are the most accurate imaging modality in the assessment of primary penile cancer.[348] Resection margin control is critical for cancer control, but the traditional 2-cm free resection margin is unnecessary. Minhas et al.[349] reported that excision margins of only a few millimeters offered excellent control. The role of sentinel lymph node biopsy, lymphatic mapping, prophylactic lymphadenectomy, and the template for lymph node dissection will be better defined in the future.[350]

## Variants of squamous cell carcinoma (Table 15-10)

### Basaloid carcinoma

Basaloid carcinoma is an unusual but distinctive variant of squamous cell carcinoma, that is frequently associated with HPV,[298] deeper invasion and a higher mortality rate than typical squamous cell carcinoma. It is similar to basaloid cancer occurring at other sites such as the vulva,[351] and it may coexist with other types of squamous cell carcinoma, such as typical squamous carcinoma, warty, pseudoglandular, anaplastic, and spindle types. The tumor usually appears as a mass in the glans and perimeatus, but may extend to the coronal sulcus, skin of the penile shaft and urethra, and infiltrate deeply into the corpus cavernosum, corpus spongiosum, Buck's fascia, dartos muscle, skin, and the urethra. Grossly, it presents with a white-gray, flat or elevated, irregular, firm mass with necrotic foci. Microscopically, there is often downward proliferation of closely packed solid nests, with focal central comedonecrosis. The cells have basaloid features with uniform, small, basophilic nuclei having inconspicuous nucleoli and numerous mitotic figures (Fig. 15-39). Individual cell necrosis occasionally forms a 'starry sky' appearance. The differential diagnosis includes typical squamous cell carcinoma, urothelial carcinoma, basal cell carcinoma, small cell (neuroendocrine) carcinoma, and metastatic carcinoma.

**Table 15-10** Variants of squamous cell carcinoma

| | Basaloid | Warty | Verrucous | P Ca NOS | Sarcomatoid |
| --- | --- | --- | --- | --- | --- |
| HPV | + | + | – | – | – |
| Age (mean) | 55 | 61 | 50 | 60 | 60 |
| Incidence | 10% | 6% | 5–16% | 10% | 1.4–4% |
| Size | >4 cm | 4 cm | 3 cm | upto 14 cm | 5–7 cm |
| Koilocytosis | Absent | Prominent | Absent | Absent | Absent |
| Fibrovascular core | Rare | Present | Rare | Present | Absent |
| Base | Irregular and infiltrative | Rounded or irregular | Regular, pushing | Irregular, jagged | Irregular, jagged |
| Metastasis | Yes | Rare | No | Yes | Yes |
| Prognosis | Poor | Good | Excellent | Fair | Poor |

P Ca NOS, papillary carcinoma, not otherwise specified.

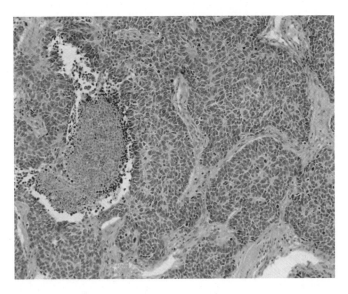

**Fig. 15-39** Basaloid carcinoma.

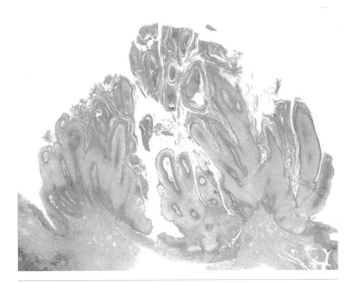

**Fig. 15-40** Warty (verrucous) carcinoma.

## Warty (condylomatous carcinoma)

Warty carcinoma is a morphologically distinct verruciform neoplasm that is similar to its counterpart in the vulva. The cancer may involve single or multiple anatomic sites, such as the glans, coronal sulcus and foreskin.[352]

Grossly, warty cancer forms exophytic, cauliflower-like, firm white/gray masses that are mainly papillomatous, with acanthosis, hyperkeratosis, and horny cysts (Fig. 15-40). The papillae contain prominent fibrovascular cores, and the epithelium has large, wrinkled, hyperchromatic, often binucleated nuclei and clear cytoplasm. The epithelial–stromal border is infiltrative, pushing, or mixed.[298] HPV DNA is present in up to 45% of cases – more than with typical squamous cell carcinoma.[292,298] The differential diagnosis includes other verruciform neoplasms, such as verrucous carcinoma, giant condyloma, and papillary squamous carcinoma not otherwise specified.

It is difficult to identify the early cases of warty carcinoma in the literature because of the diverse nomenclature used in the past for the verruciform lesions, including giant condyloma, Buschke–Löwenstein tumor, verrucous carcinoma, and papillary squamous cell carcinoma. A useful feature is its preferential association with HPV compared to other types of penile cancer, and it may be a malignant counterpart of giant condyloma.[292,298] The tumor has a definite risk of regional lymph node metastasis, although this is less frequent than with typical squamous cell carcinoma.[292,298] Therefore, it is important to distinguish this tumor from verrucous carcinoma and other verruciform tumors.[298,299,353]

## Verrucous carcinoma

Since its first description in the oral cavity, verrucous carcinoma has been identified in numerous organs, including the larynx, vulva, vagina, anus, and penis. Verrucous carcinoma of the penis accounts for 5–16% of penile malignancies.[354] It is commonly seen in middle-aged men.[354–360] Typically, it appears as a large, fungating, frequently ulcerated warty lesion that burrows through the normal tissues (Fig. 15-41A, B). Most arise on the coronal sulcus and spread to the glans and preputial skin. Microscopically, verrucous carcinoma is a very well-differentiated squamous cell carcinoma with exophytic and endophytic papillary growth (Fig. 15-42). Central fibrovascular cores are not prominent. Characteristically, the tumor shows a broad-based 'pushing' pattern of infiltration. Cytologic atypia is minimal, and mitotic figures are very rare and usually confined to the deeper aspect of the tumor (Fig. 15-43). There is no cytoplasmic clearing and/or koilocytotic nuclear atypia seen in HPV-related tumors (Table 15-11).[359]

Verrucous carcinoma tends to grow locally and does not metastasize. If it is treated inadequately, multiple recurrences may appear. The differential diagnoses include condyloma acuminatum, warty carcinoma, and the usual type of keratinizing squamous cell carcinoma. When the lesion is large, giant condyloma of Buschke–Löwenstein enters into the differential diagnosis. Whether verrucous carcinoma and giant condyloma of Buschke–Löwenstein are the same or different entities remains controversial. The consistent absence of human papilloma viruses 6, 11, 16, 18, and 31 in verrucous carcinoma suggests a fundamental difference between verrucous carcinoma and giant condyloma.[359] Masih et al.[359] reported the uniform absence of the common genital human papilloma viruses in their cases of verrucous carcinoma, and concluded that verrucous carcinoma is a distinct clinicopathologic entity that does not have a place in the morphologic spectrum of condyloma acuminatum and giant condyloma (penile giant condyloma of Buschke–Löwenstein has the same human HPV subtypes as condyloma acuminatum, with similar frequency).[361,362] Conversely, some authors found human papilloma viruses 6 and 11 as well as pre-existing condyloma acuminatum in some cases of verrucous carcinoma, suggesting a viral etiology.[358,360] The lack of cytologic atypia, mitotic figures, and infiltrative growth pattern are helpful features in differentiating verrucous carcinoma from the usual type of squamous cell carcinoma. According to Saeed et al.,[363] the mean Bcl-2/Bax ratio

A

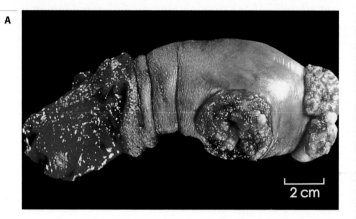

B

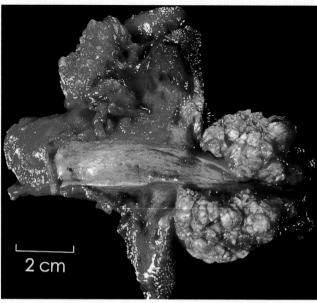

**Fig. 15-41** (**A**) Verrucous carcinoma has grown out of the preputial orifice and eroded through the prepuce. (**B**) Dissection reveals that verrucous carcinoma has grown extensively in the glans and prepuce, obliterating the preputial space. (From Fletcher CDM. Diagnostic histopathology of tumors, Edinburgh: Churchill Livingstone, 1995.)

**Table 15-11** Histopathologic features of verrucous carcinoma

| Morphologic features | Frequency |
| --- | --- |
| Club-shaped, hyperplastic rete ridges | +++ |
| Pushing deep margins | +++ |
| Well-differentiated squamous epithelium | +++ |
| Polygonal squamous cells with glassy cytoplasm | +++ |
| Intercellular bridges | +++ |
| Centrally located vesicular nuclei | +++ |
| Central single nucleolus | +++ |
| Well-formed intercellular edema | +++ |
| Individual cell necrosis | +++ |
| Hyperkeratosis | +++ |
| Parakeratosis | +++ |
| Keratin-filled clefts | +++ |
| Cystic degeneration of rete ridges | +++ |
| Heavy subepithelial inflammatory cell infiltrates | ++ |
| Intact basement membrane | ++ |
| Crust formation | ++ |
| Epithelial abscesses | ++ |
| Koilocyte-like cells | ++ |
| Superficial fibrovascular cores | ++ |
| Keratohyaline granules | + |
| Dermal abscesses | + |
| Anaplastic foci (hybrid verrucous and regular) | + |
| True koilocytes | − |
| True fibrovascular cores | − |

was significantly lower in verrucous carcinoma than in typical squamous cell carcinoma. Bax expression was comparable in verrucous carcinoma and low-grade squamous cell carcinoma, but Bcl-2 expression was significantly higher in higher grades of squamous cell carcinoma. These findings indicate that penile verrucous carcinoma and typical squamous cell carcinoma are immunophenotypically distinct.

Clinical outcome for patients with verrucous carcinoma varies according to the type of treatment. Partial or radical penectomy reduces the recurrence rate to 33%, compared to 80% in patients treated with local excision.[354,359,360] Therefore, partial or total penectomy is recommended. Radiation therapy is contraindicated as it induces dedifferentiation of verrucous carcinoma.[354,359,360,364]

### Papillary carcinoma, not otherwise specified

This is an exophytic squamous cell carcinoma lined by atypical cells without HPV-related features and with infiltrative borders. This variant occurs commonly in the fifth and sixth decades. Microscopically it is a well-differentiated, hyperkeratotic carcinoma with irregular, complex papillae, with or without fibrovascular cores. Unlike verrucous carcinoma, the interface with the underlying stroma is infiltrative and irregular. Although papillary carcinoma NOS can invade the corpus spongiosum or cavernosum, regional lymph node metastases are exceptional and therefore the prognosis is excellent.

### Pseudohyperplastic non-verruciform squamous cell carcinoma

This variant of penile carcinoma was recently described by Cubilla et al.[74] as well-differentiated squamous cell carcinoma with pseudohyperplastic features. The majority of low-grade penile cancers are verruciform, either verrucous or papillary carcinoma NOS subtypes. The median age at pre-

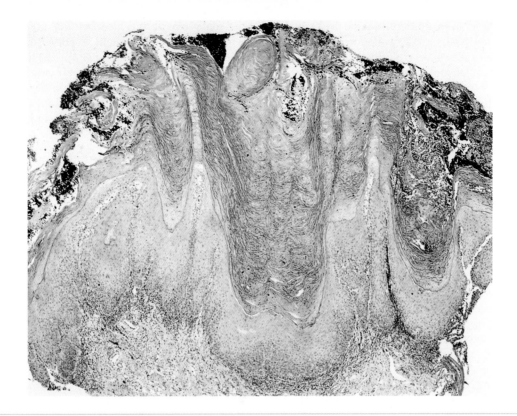

**Fig. 15-42** Verrucous carcinoma with marked hyperkeratosis and regular border with the dermis.

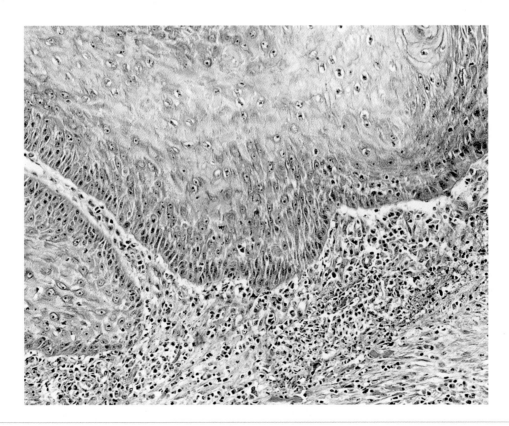

**Fig. 15-43** Deep margin of verrucous carcinoma showing lack of infiltration. Note the lack of nuclear atypia.

sentation is 69 years. Most are multicentric, and preferentially involve the inner mucosal surface of the foreskin. Grossly, pseudohyperplastic carcinoma is typically flat or slightly elevated, white and granular, and measures approximately 2 cm in diameter. Characteristic histologic features include downgrowth pattern with pseudoepitheliomatous hyperplasia and keratinizing nests of squamous cells with minimal atypia surrounded by a reactive fibrous stroma. In biopsies or select foci of resected specimens separation from pseudoepitheliomatous hyperplasia is very difficult, but samples of sufficient size contain obvious evidence of infiltration. The adjacent squamous epithelium typically shows changes often associated with squamous cell carcinoma, including squamous hyperplasia and low-grade/high-grade squamous intraepithelial neoplasia. Well-developed lichen sclerosus is invariably present. Patients are treated by circumcision or partial penectomy, and with rare exceptions are cured.

### Spindle-cell (sarcomatoid) squamous cell carcinoma

Although spindle-cell squamous cell carcinoma is common in the oral cavity, upper respiratory tract, and esophagus, only a few cases have been reported in the penis.[365,366] Two recent series reported that the incidence of the spindle-cell carcinoma is 1.4–4%.[367,368] The cancer tends to form polypoid masses on the glans penis and deeply invades corpora cavernosa. Histologically, it is composed predominantly of spindle cells with focal squamous differentiation (Fig. 15-44). Marked nuclear pleomorphism and numerous mitotic figures are common in the spindle-cell component. Sarcomatous differentiation may include osteoid (osteosarcomatous component), myxoid, pseudoangiomatous, malignant fibrous histiocytoma, fibrosarcoma, or leiomyosarcomatous component.[367] HPV is negative, and high molecular weight cytokeratin (34βE12) and p63 appear to be the more specific and sensitive markers to confirm epithelial derivation.[367] Most cases are very aggressive, with early lymph node metastasis and distant metastases, including to lung, skin, bone, pericardium, and pleura.[365,367,368]

### Mixed carcinoma

About 25% of cases of penile verrucous carcinoma contain microscopic foci of cellular anaplasia, higher mitotic activity, and ruptured basement membranes.[354,359] These tumors are referred to as hybrid squamous–verrucous carcinoma, similar to their counterpart in the oral cavity.[369] Hybrid squamous–verrucous carcinoma and verrucous carcinoma have multiple similarities, including patient age, location, and outcome after treatment, although the data on hybrid squamous–verrucous carcinoma are limited.[354,359] DNA ploidy and cell-cycle studies by Masih et al.[359] showed that both verrucous carcinoma and hybrid squamous–verrucous carcinoma are diploid and have similar proliferative indices. Other mixed carcinomas include warty–basaloid carcinoma, adenocarcinoma–basaloid carcinoma (adenobasaloid carcinoma), and squamous–neuroendocrine carcinoma.

### Adenosquamous carcinoma

Adenosquamous carcinoma of the penis is a rare, biphasic malignant tumor with squamous cell carcinoma and adenocarcinoma components. Several cases report that the squamous component is warty and the usual types of squamous carcinoma and adenocarcinoma are mucin secreting. For the

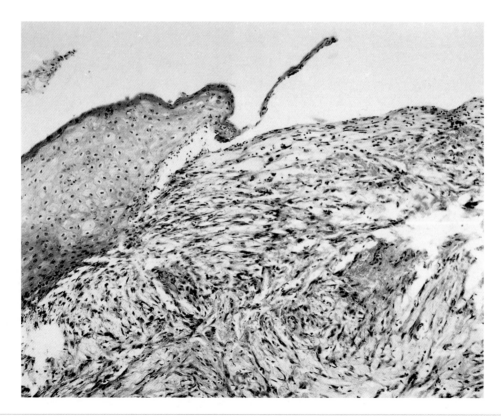

**Fig. 15-44** Spindle cell squamous cell carcinoma.

diagnosis of adenosquamous carcinoma, we recommend that the adenocarcinoma component be truly glandular with either definite gland formation or mucin production. Acantholysis of the squamous component (acantholytic squamous carcinoma, adenoid squamous carcinoma) with pseudogland formation should not be included as adenosquamous carcinoma. Rarely, adenosquamous carcinoma follows a relatively indolent course. A case of mucoepidermoid carcinoma arising in the glans penis was reported with a more aggressive course than those previously reported.[370]

### Clear cell carcinoma

Leigl and Regauer[371] recently described five cases of penile clear cell carcinoma presenting on the inner side of the foreskin in middle-aged men. The cancer was large, exophytic, partly ulcerated, and widely invasive, with sharp demarcation from the adjacent benign skin and mucosa. Histologically, clear cell carcinoma was composed of large clear cells with intracytoplasmic diastase-resistant PAS-positive material and extensive lymphatic and blood vessel invasion. Intense cytoplasmic immunoreactivity for Muc-1, EMA, and CEA was typical. All carcinomas contained HPV16, although only one displayed HPV-related cytologic changes. All patients had extensive, partly cystic inguinal lymph node metastases with striking clear cell differentiation and focal dense sclerotic basement membrane material either at diagnosis or within several months. Two patients were alive after 7 and 10 years; one patient died after 9 months with widespread cancer; and two other patients were alive at 7 and 17 months with widespread lymphatic and hematogenous metastases despite adjuvant chemotherapy and radiation therapy. In contrast to squamous cell carcinoma, penile clear cell carcinoma showed extensive vascular and lymphatic invasion and early metastases to regional lymph nodes. Therefore, clear cell carcinoma appears to represent a distinct group of penile cancers that have a different clinical behavior from typical squamous cell carcinoma. However, more cases are required to confirm these observations.

### Basal cell carcinoma

Basal cell carcinoma is the most common malignant skin tumor elsewhere in the body, but is rare in penile or scrotal skin.[372-375] It may involve any portion of the penis, but most often involves the shaft (56%), the glans (30%), and the prepuce (14%).[374,375] Rarely, it may arise from the inner surface of the foreskin.[376] Patients range in age from 37 to 79 years.[374,375] Most patients are white, although one Japanese patient was reported.[375] Grossly, basal cell carcinoma presents as a small, irregular, ulcerated mass. Histologically, it contains nests of small, uniform basaloid cells with peripheral palisading (Fig. 15-45). The cells tend to form nests with bulbous finger-like invaginations from the epidermis. The cells lack intercellular bridges, and the nuclei display little variation in size, shape, or intensity of staining; there are no abnormal mitotic figures. The stroma adjacent to the tumor often shows a proliferation of 'young' fibroblasts; alternatively, it may appear mucinous. Frequently, the stroma retracts about the islands of basal cell carcinoma, resulting in peritumoral lacunae or cleft-like spaces. The clinical course tends to be indolent, and local excision is usually curative.

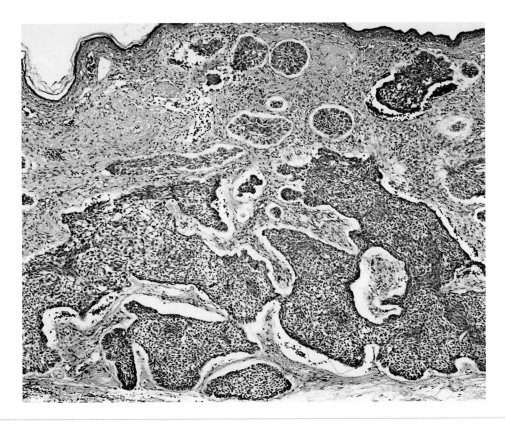

**Fig. 15-45** Basal cell carcinoma.

## Malignant melanoma

There are about 100 reported cases of malignant melanoma of the penis, including melanoma in situ, accounting for less than 1% of all penile cancers.[377-384] Most occur in white men in their fifth and sixth decades of life, a decade older than is typical for most cutaneous melanomas.[385] In contrast to squamous cell carcinoma, penile malignant melanoma is rare in men of African ancestry. In the majority of cases it arises on the glans (Fig. 15-46).[64,383]

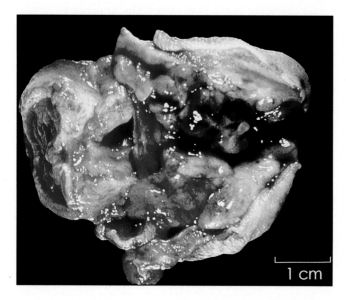

**Fig. 15-46** Malignant melanoma arising in the glans penis.

Patients present with a black, brown, or blue variegated papule or ulcerated plaque. The histologic findings are identical to those in other mucosal or cutaneous sites (Fig. 15-47).[64] Variants of penile malignant melanoma include nodular, superficial spreading, and acral lentiginous types.[381-386]

Stage I melanoma is confined to the penis; stage II melanoma is metastatic to regional lymph nodes; and stage III has distant metastases. The prognosis depends on the depth of invasion and the stage. Penile melanoma with a thickness of 0.75 mm or less has an excellent prognosis, whereas a depth of invasion of 1.5 mm or more carries an extremely poor prognosis because of the high frequency of metastases.[64,383] Overall, 50% of patients have lymph node metastases at the time of diagnosis.[64] Prophylactic superficial lymph node dissection is recommended as an adjunct to penectomy for stage I penile malignant melanoma more than 1.5 mm thick. Bilateral inguinal lymph node dissection is standard treatment for stage II melanoma.[383]

Malignant melanoma of soft parts (clear cell sarcoma) is an uncommon neoplasm that occurs most frequently in the tendons and aponeuroses of the extremities, and rarely arises in the penis.[387]

## Sarcoma

Sarcoma is the second most common type of penile cancer, accounting for less than 5% of penile malignancies. Sarcoma arises in men of all ages, with a typical peak occurrence in the fifth and sixth decades of life; exceptions include rhabdomyosarcoma (young children) and epithelioid sarcoma (young adults).[388,389] With the exception of Kaposi's sarcoma, which most commonly arises on the glans penis, sarcoma is most frequently located on the shaft.[389]

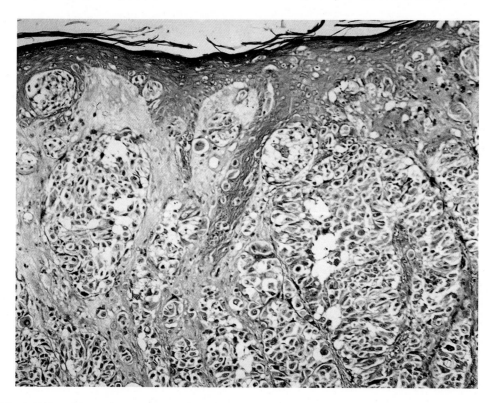

**Fig. 15-47** Nests of malignant melanoma cells undermine the epidermis.

Vascular sarcomas, including Kaposi's sarcoma, epithelioid hemangioendothelioma, and angiosarcoma, are the most common type of penile sarcoma. Sarcoma of myogenic, neurogenic, and fibrous origin also occurs.[390] The histologic features of these lesions are similar to those of their counterparts arising at other locations.

AIDS-related Kaposi's sarcoma of the penis is increasing in frequency.[391-393] Approximately 20% of male AIDS patients with Kaposi's sarcoma have lesions on the penis, and as many as 3% initially present with penile Kaposi's sarcoma (Fig. 15-48). The penis is rarely the first site of involvement of Kaposi's sarcoma, and in its occurrence there is usually associated with systemic lesions.[394] The tumor usually involves the skin of the shaft or the glans. When it involves the glans or corpus spongiosum, Kaposi's sarcoma may cause urethral obstruction. Spindle-shaped tumor cells stain for Factor VIII and CD34 (Fig. 15-49A, B). Human herpes virus 8 is detected in tumor tissue and in peripheral blood mononuclear cells. Kaposi's sarcoma may arise in HIV-negative patients.[395-397] Local excision is effective for small localized lesions, as is radiation therapy.[398,399]

Rarely, vascular sarcoma arises in the corpora cavernosa; about 35 cases have been reported.[400] The majority are hemangioendotheliomas and tend to be indolent. Epithelioid hemangioendothelioma is composed of anastomosing networks of irregularly shaped vascular spaces lined by plump, often piled-up, endothelial cells with low-grade morphology.[401-403] High-grade tumors with solid masses of anaplastic tumor cells, hemorrhage, and necrosis have also been reported. These may metastasize to lymph nodes or hematogenously to distant sites such as lung, liver, and bone.

Leiomyosarcoma of the penis is very rare, with fewer than 30 reported cases. It usually occurs in the fifth to seventh decades of life and involves the prepuce, distal shaft, circumcision scar line, or base of the penis.[404-406] Superficial leiomyosarcoma is thought to arise from the smooth muscle of the glans, frenulum, or the dermis of the shaft, and usually forms subcutaneous nodules.[407] Patients with superficial leiomyosarcoma tend to do well with local excision, but the tumor may recur locally. Deep leiomyosarcoma (Fig. 15-50) is less common, arising from the smooth muscle of the corpora cavernosa and tending to invade the urethra and metastasize early. Tumor depth and size are currently the best predictors of outcome for primary leiomyosarcoma. Small (<2 cm diameter) superficial tumors are best managed by wide local excision, but large (>5 cm), deep-seated sarcomas have a poor prognosis because of their tendency for widespread metastases despite aggressive surgical inter-

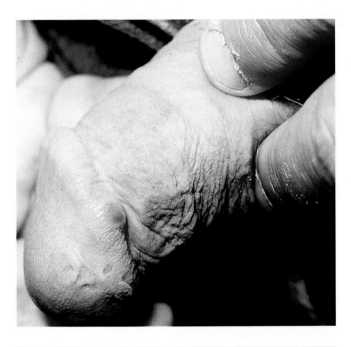

**Fig. 15-48** Kaposi's sarcoma presenting as a small purple nodule on the corona of the glans penis. (Courtesy of Dr A Hood, Indiana University, Indianapolis, IN.)

A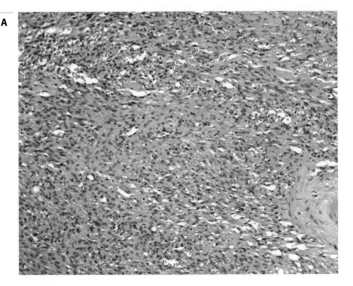

B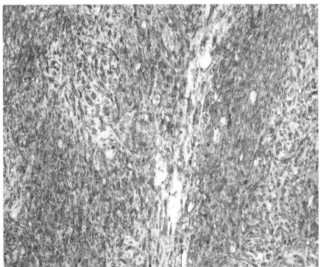

**Fig. 15-49** (**A**) Kaposi's sarcoma showing monomorphic spindle cells arranged in ill-defined fascicles with slit-like vessels and extravasated red blood cells. (**B**) CD34 immunostaining demonstrated immunoreactivity of spindle cells.

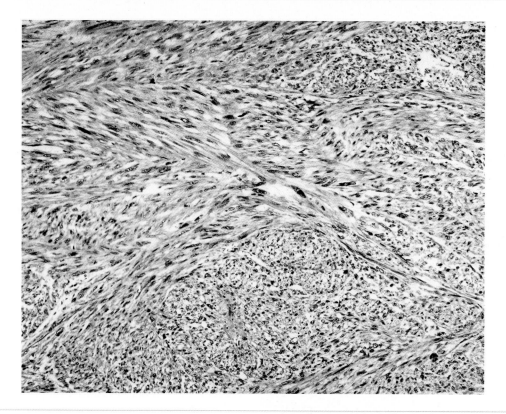

**Fig. 15-50** Leiomyosarcoma.

vention.[404,408] Adjuvant radiation and chemotherapy are unproven as primary treatment of penile leiomyosarcoma.

Fibrosarcoma can be superficial or deep, and usually presents as a slow-growing, firm, non-tender mass on the dorsum of the shaft or glans. It shares many clinical and gross features with leiomyosarcoma.[409,410] Immunohistochemical stains (cytokeratin, smooth muscle actin, desmin, and vimentin) and the absence of overlying in situ carcinoma are useful to confirm soft tissue derivation and rule out spindle-cell squamous cell carcinoma.

Malignant fibrous histiocytoma is rare in the penis, with only two cases reported in the literature, including one case of inflammatory malignant fibrous histiocytoma.[411,412]

Rhabdomyosarcoma in the penis arises on the shaft near the root. Most reported cases appeared in children, and were embryonal rhabdomyosarcoma.[413,414]

Fewer than 20 cases of epithelioid sarcoma of the penis have been reported.[415-418] Patients ranged in age from 23 to 43 years (mean, 32). The sarcoma presented as single or multiple, firm, slow-growing, painless subcutaneous nodules. The masses may produce surface ulceration, resulting in erectile pain or dysuria. Therefore, epithelioid sarcoma may mimic Peyronie's disease, urethral stricture, or ulcerating squamous carcinoma. Radical excision is the preferred method of treatment, although local excision combined with radiation therapy has been used with success. Epithelioid sarcoma is a slow-growing but aggressive tumor in the penis, as elsewhere in the body. Regardless of therapy, up to 80% recur locally. Metastases to the lung have been reported in two cases, but most reports lack long-term follow-up. So-called proximal type of epithelioid sarcoma has been reported in the penis.[418]

Other soft tissue sarcomas, including hemangiopericytoma, malignant schwannoma, and extraskeletal osteosarcoma with malignant fibrous histiocytoma-like component may arise in the penis.[419]

## Lymphoma

Primary lymphoma of the penis is extremely rare, with fewer than two dozen reported cases. Most are high-grade diffuse large B-cell lymphoma, but other subtypes, including T-cell lymphomas, MALT lymphoma, and Hodgkin's disease, have been reported.[420-422] Penile lymphoma at presentation may simulate Peyronie's disease, appearing as a bulky scrotal mass with priapism and inflammatory ulcers. Patients commonly describe painless, progressive swelling or ulceration of the shaft or glans penis. Wedge biopsy is essential to achieve the correct diagnosis, and histological analysis must include immunohistochemical tests in order to differentiate lymphoma from undifferentiated sarcoma or carcinoma, as well as to distinguish between B- and T-cell lymphoma. The absence of lymphoid tissue in the penis suggests that penile lymphoma is a manifestation of occult nodal disease or part of a systemic process; this is the rationale for combined treatment modalities (chemotherapy, radiation therapy, or surgery). Primary lymphoma appears to have a good prognosis, and treatment is the same as for diffuse lymphoma. Chemotherapy with radiotherapy may be considered the treatment of choice to obtain complete remission and optimize quality of life.[420,421]

### Metastases to the penis

Although the penis has a rich and complex vascular circulation interconnected to the pelvic organs, metastases are rare and usually represent a late manifestation of systemic metastasis.[423,424] In all reported series the most common primary site was the prostate, followed by the bladder, the rectosigmoid, and the kidney.[423-431] Less common primary sites include the testes, ureters, and non-pelvic organs such as the lung, pancreas, nasopharynx, larynx, thyroid, and bone.[124,423-439] Tu et al.[423] found that ductal–endometrioid carcinoma of the prostate was most prone to develop penile metastasis.

The most common site for metastatic deposits is the corpus cavernosum.[426] Clinically, metastases usually present as multiple, palpable, painless nodules that involve the skin and ulcerate, mimicking syphilitic chancre. In 50% of patients diffuse involvement of the corpus cavernosum causes priapism.[426] Hematuria and dysuria may also occur. In the great majority of cases penile metastases occur in the terminal stage of known cancer and pose no diagnostic difficulty, although rarely they may be the primary presentation of an occult cancer.[435,436] Metastases to the penis should be suspected in any patient with known cancer who has an onset of priapism or an unusual penile lesion.

The prognosis is poor for patients with metastases to the penis: Paquin and Roland[437] reported that 95% of patients died within weeks to months of diagnosis. Similarly, Mukamel et al.[438] reported that 71% of patients died within 6 months of diagnosis, and they have suggested that total penectomy may be indicated for relief of pain or severe urinary symptoms if metastases are confined to the penis without extension to the pelvis or pelvic diaphragm.

## SCROTUM

## Normal anatomy and histology

The scrotum consists of skin, the dartos muscle, and external spermatic, cremasteric, and internal spermatic fasciae. The internal fascia is loosely attached to the parietal layer of the tunica vaginalis. The epidermis covers the dermis, and the deepest layer of the dermis merges with the smooth muscle bundles of the dartos tunic. Although scattered fat cells are present, there is no subcutaneous adipose tissue layer. The dermis contains hair follicles and apocrine, eccrine, and sebaceous glands.

The scrotum contains the testes and the lower parts of the spermatic cords. The surface of the scrotum is divided into right and left halves by a cutaneous raphe which continues ventrally to the inferior penile surface and dorsally along the midline of the perineum to the anus. The left side of the scrotum is usually lower because of the greater length of the left spermatic cord.

Embryologically, the scrotum originates from the genital swellings that meet ventral to the anus and unite to form the two scrotal sacs. A median raphe of fibrovascular connective tissue separates the two halves. The scrotum derives its blood supply from the external and internal pudendal arteries, and additional blood comes to it from the cremasteric and testicular arteries that traverse the spermatic cords. Lymphatic drainage of the scrotum is to the superficial inguinal nodes.

## Non-neoplastic diseases

### Fournier's gangrene

Fournier's gangrene is an idiopathic form of necrotizing fasciitis of the subcutaneous tissue and skeletal muscle of the genitals and perineum, particularly that of the scrotum.[440,441] It begins as reddish plaques with necrosis (Fig. 15-51) and is accompanied by severe systemic symptoms, including pain and fever. The lesions progress to develop localized edema, become insensitive, and form blisters that overlie an area of cellulitis. Most cases have accompanying scrotal emphysema. Without prompt diagnosis and aggressive treatment, ulceration and gangrene ensue.

Fournier's gangrene probably results from infection by staphylococcal or streptococcal species, which may be pure or, more commonly, are mixed with other Gram-negative bacilli and anaerobic bacteria. Diabetes, alcoholism, immunosuppression, recent surgical intervention, trauma, and morbid obesity are predisposing factors, but are not necessary for the development of Fournier's gangrene.[441] Fournier's gangrene is a serious, life-threatening condition that requires vigorous and prompt therapy.[440,442] Clinically, the infection resembles clostridial gas gangrene, and in the past frozen sections were performed to detect gas bubbles. Today,

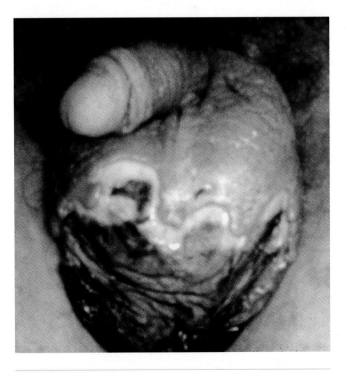

**Fig. 15-51** Fournier's gangrene. (Courtesy of Dr Hans Stricker, Henry Ford Hospital, Detroit, MI.)

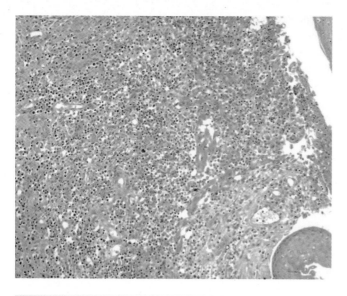

**Fig. 15-52** Acute necrotizing gangrenous inflammation.

most believe that this does not yield clinically significant information and is unnecessary. Definitive treatment includes wide debridement, intravenous broad-spectrum antibiotics, and skin grafting.[442] Squamous cell carcinoma may develop in the scar of Fournier's gangrene after a long delay, which differentiates it from other scar carcinomas or Marjolin's ulcer.[443]

A necrotizing inflammatory process that is clinically similar to Fournier's gangrene but which involves the glans penis is called Corbus' disease or gangrenous balanitis.[444–446] This condition is caused by anaerobic bacteria and can cause total necrosis of the glans penis (Fig. 15-52). Gangrene of the penis may also be caused by constricting bands from external urinary drainage devices[447] and other constricting injuries.[448]

## Hidradenitis suppurativa

Hidradenitis suppurativa is a chronic, suppurative inflammatory disease that is part of the follicular occlusion triad of: hidradenitis suppurativa, acne conglobata, and perifollicular capitis.[449] First described by Verneuil in 1854,[450] hidradenitis suppurativa is included with other lesions of the triad because of their histologic and pathogenetic similarities.

The term hidradenitis suppurativa is a misnomer, as it is an inflammatory process of apocrine and eccrine glands that are obstructed by follicular hyperkeratosis. Thus, follicular hyperkeratosis is the main cause of the rupture of dilated pilosebaceous structures, which extrudes keratin and apocrine and eccrine products and commensal bacteria into the dermis, inciting the acute necrotizing and granulomatous reaction with abscess formation that extends into the deep connective tissue and upward onto the epidermis as sinus tracts in the lesions typically seen by surgical pathologists.

The cause of the obstructing follicular hyperkeratosis is not fully understood, but may include genetic, hormonal,

mechanical, and environmental factors.[451,452] Women with androgenic disturbances, obese patients, and those with intertrigo are especially predisposed to hidradenitis suppurativa. Puberty also is a risk factor. Cultures are often negative, but superinfection is usually due to staphylococci, streptococci, or a mixture of bacteria, including anaerobes and *Actinomyces* species.[453]

Clinically, hidradenitis suppurativa begins as tender erythematous papules and progresses to form fluctuant nodules that may have draining sinuses. Coalescence of adjacent involved follicles forms large plaques. The axilla is the most common site, but it also occurs in the skin of the groin, perianal, areolar, and periumbilical regions. Treatment is difficult, and antibiotics and intralesional steroid injections may be ineffective. Incision and drainage or localized excision is frequently necessary.[454]

## Idiopathic scrotal calcinosis

Scrotal calcinosis occurs in two settings: calcification of pre-existing epidermal or pilar cysts, and calcification of dermal connective tissue in the absence of cysts (idiopathic scrotal calcinosis).[455,456] The hypothesis for the latter form favors origin from eccrine duct milia because of immunoreactivity for carcinoembryonic antigen, a marker for eccrine sweat glands.[457] A recent study indicated that the idiopathic form may be related to trauma.[458]

Approximately 123 cases of scrotal calcinosis have been described.[459] Saladi et al.[460] classified scrotal calcinosis according to the proposed causal mechanisms: calcific degeneration of epidermoid cysts (34 cases); dystrophic calcification of dartos muscle (three cases); calcification of eccrine sweat ducts (four cases); and idiopathic/undetermined (82 cases).

Patients are usually young men, but children and older men have also been affected. They usually have multiple (up to 50) long-standing, firm to hard nodules varying in size from a few millimeters up to 3 cm. The overlying skin is usually intact but may ulcerate, releasing cheesy material. Occasionally, a single hard nodule may be present.[461]

Histologically, scrotal calcinosis lies within the dermis and contains granules and globules of hematoxylinophilic calcific material. It may or may not be accompanied by giant cell granulomatous inflammation and recognizable cyst wall fragments (Fig. 15-53). It is plausible that idiopathic scrotal calcinosis represents an end-stage phenomenon of numerous 'old' epidermal cysts that over time have lost their cyst walls.[462–464] Treatment may be unnecessary for asymptomatic lesions, but surgery is indicated for infected, recurrent, or extensive lesions.

## Lipogranuloma

Lipogranuloma (also known as paraffinoma, sclerosing lipogranuloma, and Tancho's nodules) may involve the penile or scrotal skin. Penile lipogranuloma is usually due to hypodermic injection of substances such as paraffin, silicone, oil, or wax into the penis for penile enlargement or sexual gratification.[465–468] In the scrotum, trauma, cold weather, and topical application of ointment (suggesting percutaneous

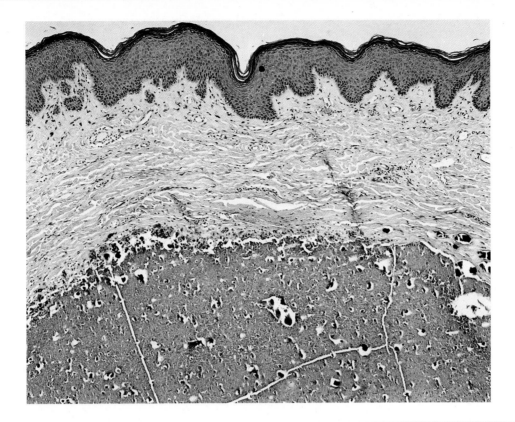

**Fig. 15-53** Scrotal calcinosis.

absorption) have also been implicated.[465,469] Most lipogranulomas arise in men younger than 40 years, who complain of a localized plaque or mass that may be tender and indurated and as large as several centimeters in diameter. Biopsy is necessary, especially in the absence of a clinical history of injection of exogenous material. The importance of lipogranuloma lies in differentiating it from malignancy to avoid extensive surgery. It is normally treated with total or partial excision. However, a recent report stated that surgery should be reserved for recurrent or refractory cases when steroids have failed as first-line treatment.[470]

Microscopically, lipogranuloma consists of lipid vacuoles embedded in a sclerotic stroma, usually accompanied by a histiocytic or foreign-body granulomatous infiltrate with or without eosinophils (Fig. 15-54).[469] The differential diagnosis includes signet ring cell carcinoma and malakoplakia. The diagnosis of lipogranuloma may be confirmed by histochemical stains for lipid, but light microscopy is usually sufficient.

## Epidermal cyst

Epidermal cyst (keratinous cyst) is common in the scrotum.[64,471–473] It presents as single or multiple rubbery-firm subdermal or intradermal nodules. Typically, it contains gray-white cheesy material[471] resulting from exfoliation of the keratinizing squamous epithelium. Homayoon et al.[472] reported epidermal cysts in children, and none had a history of exposures to diethylstilbestrol, cryptorchidism, cystic fibrosis, or von Hippel–Lindau disease. Only one

patient required surgical excision owing to persistent pain, and the epidermal cysts resolved in other patients who completed follow-up.

## Fat necrosis

Fat necrosis of the scrotum usually occurs in children and adolescents,[474] appearing as firm nodules in the lower portion of the scrotal wall. Two-thirds of patients have bilateral nodules.[474] The lesion may develop when scrotal fat crystallizes following exposure to cold.

## Neoplastic diseases

A hamartomatous lesion with angioleiomyomatous features (angioleiomyomatous hyperplasia) rarely occurs in the scrotum and may simulate malignancy. This lesion is probably underrecognized and has been poorly described in the literature, labeled variously as hamartoma, muscular hyperplasia, leiomyoma or vascular leiomyoma.[475–477] Van Kooten et al.[476] reported that chronic scrotal lymphedema may induce hyperplasia of the dartos muscle, resulting in the histological appearance of scrotal hamartoma.

Benign and malignant neoplasms of the scrotum are rare and most arise from the skin and adnexal structures.[64,478–481] Melanoma of the scrotum is uncommon, and a series[383] of six cases has been reported as well as a single case report.[482] Hemangioma, lymphangioma, leiomyoma, angiomyofibro-

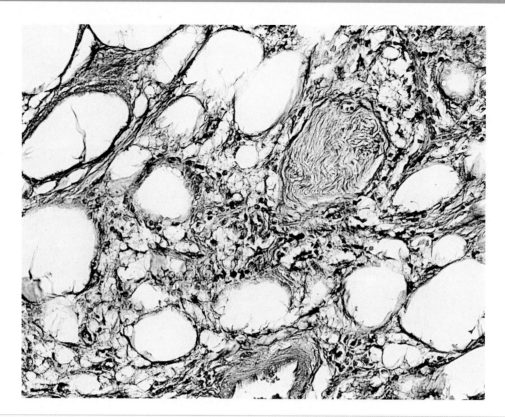

**Fig. 15-54** Scrotal lipogranuloma.

blastoma, neurofibroma, fibrous hamartoma, and angiokeratoma are the most common benign scrotal neoplasms.[64,483–491] Atypical fibrous histiocytoma,[492] lipoblastoma,[493] ganglioneuroma,[494] and granular cell tumor[495] also have been reported. Squamous cell carcinoma is the most common scrotal cancer.[496–498] Merkel cell carcinoma and basal cell carcinoma also arise in the scrotum.[499,500] Cases of metastatic carcinoma to the scrotum have been also reported.[501] Recently, cases of aggressive angiomyxoma and angiomyofibroblastoma were reported at this site.[502–506]

## Squamous cell carcinoma

Scrotal squamous cell carcinoma was the first cancer linked to occupational exposure to a carcinogen. In the 18th century, men exposed to soot and dust (for example chimney sweeps and cotton factory workers) had an increased incidence of scrotal squamous cell carcinoma. Pott[507] described this association, and the tumor was subsequently referred to as Pott's cancer or chimney sweep's cancer. Squamous cell carcinoma of the scrotum also occurs in men with other occupations, including tar workers, paraffin and shale oil workers, machine operators in the engineering industry, petroleum wax pressmen, workers in the screw-making industry, and automatic lathe operators.[497] Later, 3'4'-benzpyrene was discovered to be the causative agent.[508] Other risk factors include psoriasis treated with coal tar, arsenic or UV therapy, condyloma acuminatum, HPV, and multiple cutaneous epitheliomas.[497,508–510]

The incidence of squamous cell carcinoma of the scrotum is much lower than that of penile carcinoma.[496–498] To date,

more than 100 cases have been reported. It usually presents as a solitary slow-growing pimple, wart, or nodule, usually on the anterolateral aspect of the scrotum. It later ulcerates and forms raised, rolled edges with variable amounts of seropurulent discharge. Invasion of the scrotal contents or the penis may occur in patients with advanced cancer. Some authors have suggested that scrotal cancer is uncommon among black men; however, the relatively small number of cases in each reported series limits current understanding of the racial distribution.[488,498]

Squamous cell carcinoma of the scrotum occurs primarily in the sixth and seventh decades of life.[497,498] The left scrotum is more frequently affected than the right,[497,498] and this predominance seems to reflect the site of exposure to carcinogens. When occupational exposure is excluded, the sides are equally frequently affected. Ipsilateral inguinal lymphadenopathy is observed at the time of initial presentation in 50% of patients.[497]

Microscopically, squamous cell carcinoma of the scrotum is similar to that of the penis. It is usually well or moderately differentiated, and keratinization is common. The adjacent epidermis shows hyperkeratosis, acanthosis, and dyskeratosis. There is a strong correlation between stage and survival, but grade does not appear to add prognostic information, although most studies are limited by small sample size.

Pigmented squamous cell carcinoma has also been reported in the scrotum in a 70-year-old man, similar to its counterpart in the oral cavity and conjunctiva. Microscopically, the tumor had typical features, including keratinization, intercellular bridges, and colonization by plump dendritic melanocytes with marked pigmentation. The tumor

**Table 15-12** Staging system for scrotal carcinoma (From Lowe FC. Squamous cell carcinoma of the scrotum. J Urol 1983; 130: 423–427.)

| Stage | Description |
|---|---|
| A1 | Localized to scrotal wall |
| A2 | Locally extensive tumor invading adjacent structure (testis, spermatic cord, penis, pubis, perineum) |
| B | Metastatic disease involving inguinal lymph nodes |
| C | Metastatic disease involving pelvic lymph nodes without evidence of distant spread |
| D | Metastatic disease beyond the pelvic lymph nodes involving distant organs |

cells were positive for high molecular weight cytokeratin and the colonizing melanocytes for HMB-45. Because the tumor was associated with a lentiginous lesion, melanocytes entrapped from the lentigo may therefore have been activated during cancer enlargement, resulting in melanocytic colonization.[511]

The differential diagnosis of scrotal squamous cell carcinoma includes a wide variety of lesions, including nevus, epidermal cyst, eczema, psoriasis, folliculitis, syphilis, tuberculous epididymitis, periurethral abscess, as well as benign and malignant neoplasms such as hemangioma, lymphangioma, basal cell carcinoma, malignant melanoma, Paget's disease, and sarcoma.[512]

The staging system for scrotal cancer was proposed by Lowe (Table 15-12).[513] The prognosis is poor for those with squamous cell carcinoma, the 5-year survival rate being 30–52%. Ray and Whitmore[514] reported a 5-year survival rate of 70% for patients with stage A carcinoma and 44% for patients with stage B. Patients with stage C or stage D cancer have little chance of long-term survival.[512]

## Basal cell carcinoma

Basal cell carcinoma of the scrotum is rare, accounting for less than 10% of scrotal malignancies.[496,515–519] Mean patient age is 65 years (range, 42–82).[517] Clinically, it presents as painless plaques or ulcerated nodules. Non-ulcerative basal cell carcinoma may also occur, clinically mimicking angiokeratoma or seborrheic keratosis.[520] There is a predilection for the left side of the scrotum.[516] Unlike squamous cell carcinoma, there is no known occupational risk factor or carcinogen. HPV infection does not appear to play a role.[521] A case of basal cell carcinoma associated with Langerhans' cell histiocytosis was reported in a patient with occupational exposure to coal tar and dust.[522] Basal cell carcinoma of the scrotum is more likely to metastasize than basal cell carcinoma arising at other sites.[517,523–525]

## Paget's disease

Extramammary Paget's disease rarely involves the penile or scrotal skin.[526–530] The great majority of cases arise in apocrine gland-bearing skin, most commonly the vulva followed by the perianal region, although other sites have been reported less commonly, including the male genitalia. Unlike mammary Paget's disease, most cases of extramammary Paget's disease

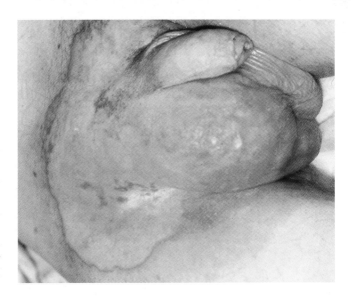

**Fig. 15-55** Extramammary Paget's disease.

do not arise in association with an underlying malignancy, but occasional cases are associated with an underlying carcinoma (either adnexal or visceral), including cancers of the urinary bladder, prostate, rectum, and urethra.[530–532] Penile and scrotal Paget's disease most often occurs during the sixth and seventh decades of life, usually presenting as a scaly, eczematous lesion (Fig. 15-55). Microscopically, extramammary Paget's disease consists of an intraepithelial proliferation of atypical cells with vacuolated cytoplasm and large vesicular nuclei (Fig. 15-56). The atypical cells tend to cluster at the tips of the rete ridges. Hyperkeratosis, parakeratosis, and papillomatosis are common. The intraepithelial neoplastic cells contain intracytoplasmic neutral and acidic mucopolysaccharides that can be demonstrated by periodic acid–Schiff, mucicarmine, Alcian blue, and aldehyde fuscin stains. Primary scrotal involvement may rarely coexist with Bowen's disease alone[530] or HPV 31-positive Bowen's disease and condyloma acuminatum.[535]

The differential diagnosis of extramammary Paget's disease includes squamous cell carcinoma in situ and malignant melanoma. Intracytoplasmic mucin is not a feature of melanoma or squamous carcinoma in situ, so mucin stain is helpful in establishing the diagnosis. Immunohistochemical stains for carcinoembryonic antigen, S100 protein, and HMB-45 also may be helpful because the cells of Paget's disease often contain carcinoembryonic antigen, whereas melanoma cells are negative; and melanoma cells are usually positive for either S100 protein or HMB-45, whereas the cells of Paget's disease are negative for these markers.[533] Paget's cells in cases of extramammary disease express a uniform phenotype of mucin (MUC1+MUC2–MUC5AC+) which is different from that of mammary Paget's disease (MUC1+MUC2–MUC5AC–).[534] The differential diagnosis of pagetoid Bowen's disease includes primarily Paget's disease, malignant melanoma in situ, and other less common entities.[535] Williamson et al.[536] reported two cases of pagetoid Bowen's disease, one in a 65-year-old man with a thigh lesion and the other in a 25-year-old man with a lesion in the penile/

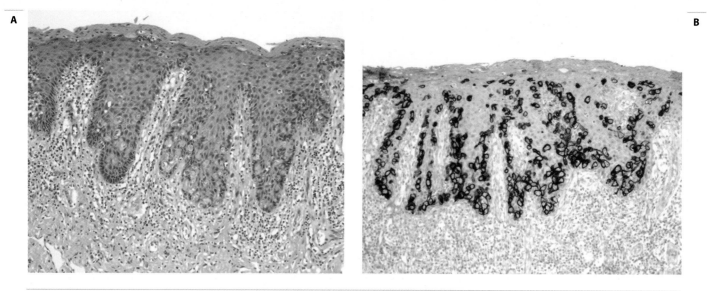

**Fig. 15-56** Extramammary Paget's disease. (**A**) Large atypical cells with vacuolated cytoplasm, mainly located at the basal layer of the epidermis. (**B**) CK7 immunoreactivity demonstrates immunoreactivity of tumor cells.

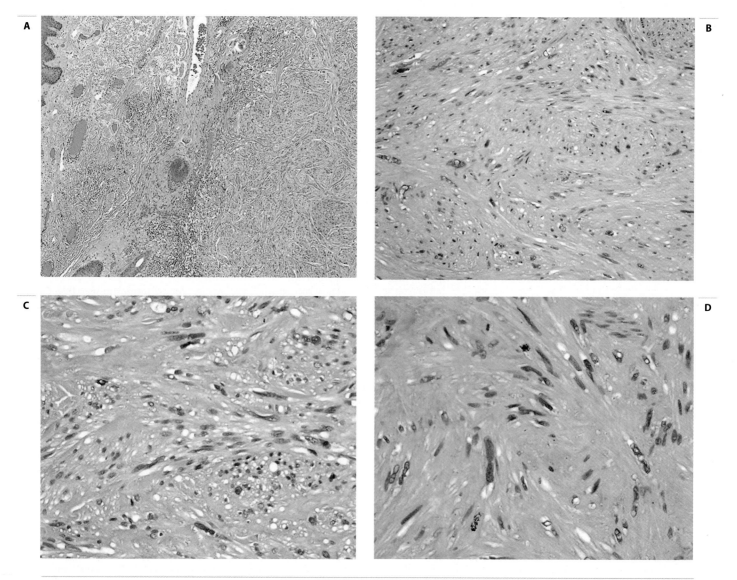

**Fig. 15-57** Leimyosarcoma of the scrotum. Leiomyosarcoma arising from dartos muscle showing fascicular growth patterns with focal cytologic atypia and mitotic figures.

scrotal region. Neither had clinical evidence of an internal malignant neoplasm. In both cases, the neoplastic cells were positive for cytokeratin 7 and 19 and were negative for CK 18, CK 20, carcinoembryonic antigen, GCDFP-15, c-erbB2, S100 protein, and HMB-45. Others have shown that CK 7 is an almost invariable marker of Paget's disease. These two cases illustrated that CK 7 can be expressed by pagetoid Bowen's disease and should not be a cause of confusion in the differential diagnosis.[536]

Choi et al.[537] found that the best predictors of late recurrence for extramammary Paget's disease were lymphovascular invasion and surgical margin involvement. Yang et al.[538] reported that patients with positive surgical margins developed local recurrence at a median of 8 months, and therefore recommended local excision with intraoperative frozen biopsy analysis.

## Sarcoma

Sarcoma of the scrotum, excluding extension of sarcoma from the spermatic cord, is extremely rare.[539] The most common type is leiomyosarcoma, which arises from the dartos muscle; fewer than 20 cases have been reported.[540-545] The age at presentation ranges from 35 to 89 years. A case of radiation-induced leiomyosarcoma was reported in the scrotum.[540] Only five patients have long-term follow-up, and four of these developed distant metastases.[539] Scrotal leiomyosarcoma appears to behave similarly to subcutaneous leiomyosarcoma (Fig. 15-57). Lymphatic metastases are rare, but long-term follow-up is necessary because of the possibility of late visceral metastases or recurrence. Recently, a case with combined features of liposarcoma and leiomyosarcoma was reported in the scrotum.[546] Cases of liposarcoma, malignant fibrous histiocytoma, epithelioid sarcoma, and synovial sarcoma arising from the scrotal wall have also been reported.[547-551] Other malignant tumors are extremely rare and include malignant lymphoma, and melanoma. Froehner et al.[552] reported a case of gastrointestinal stromal tumor (GIST) extending through the right inguinal canal that presented as a scrotal mass. Scrotal post-traumatic spindle-cell nodule may mimic sarcoma.[553] To avoid misdiagnosis, clinicopathologic evaluation is required.

## REFERENCES

1. Patterson BK, Landay A, Siegel JN, et al. Susceptibility to human immunodeficiency virus-1 infection of human foreskin and cervical tissue grown in explant culture. Am J Pathol 2002; 161: 867–873.
2. Bissada NK, Yakout HH, Fahmy WE, et al. Multi-institutional long-term experience with conservative surgery for invasive penile carcinoma. J Urol 2003; 169: 500–502.
3. Dees JE. Congenital epispadias with incontinence. J Urol 1949; 62: 513–522.
4. Kramer SA, Kelalis PP. Assessment of urinary continence in epispadias: review of 94 patients, J Urol 1982; 128: 290–293.
5. Campbell M. Epispadias: a report of 15 cases. J Urol 1952; 67: 988–999.
6. Arap S, Nahas WC, Giron AM, et al. Incontinent epispadias. surgical treatment of 38 cases. J Urol 1988; 140: 577–581.
7. Hynes PJ, Fraher JP. The development of the male Genitourinary system. I. The origin of the urorectal septum and the formation of the perineum. Br J Plast Surg 2004; 57: 27–36.
8. Hammouda HM. Results of complete penile disassembly for epispadias repair in 42 patients. J Urol 2003; 170: 1963–1965.
9. Grady RW, Mitchell ME. Management of epispadias. Urol Clin North Am 2002; 29: 349–360.
10. Mollard P, Basset T, Mure PY. Male epispadias: experience with 45 cases. J Urol 1998; 160: 55–59.
11. Duckett JW. Hypospadias. In: Walsh PC, Retik AB, Stamey TA, et al., eds. Campbell's urology, 6th edn. Philadelphia: WB Saunders, 1992, 1893–1919.
12. Juskiewenski S, Vaysse P, Guitard J, et al. Traitement des hypospadias anterieurs: place de la balanoplastie. J Urol (Paris) 1983; 89: 153–156.
13. Sweet RA, Schrott HG, Kurland R, et al. Study of the incidence of hypospadias in Rochester, Minnesota, 1940–1970, and a case–control comparison of possible etiologic factors. Mayo Clin Proc 1974; 49: 52–59.
14. Sheldon TB, Noe HN. The role of excretory urography in patients with hypospadias. J Urol 1985; 135: 97–100.
15. Gonzales JR. Micropenis. AUA Update Series 1983; 2: 1.
16. Lee PA, Mazur T, Danish R, et al. Micropenis. I. Criteria, etiologies and classification. Johns Hopkins Med J 1980; 146: 156–163.
17. Marizels M, Zaontz M, Donovan J, et al. Surgical correction of the buried penis: description of a classification system and technique to correct the diagnosis. J Urol 1986; 136: 268–271.
18. Skoog SJ, Belman AB. Aphallia: its classification and management. J Urol 1989; 141: 589–592.
19. Gilbert J, Clark RD, Koyle MA. Penile agenesis: a fatal variation of an uncommon lesion. J Urol 1990; 143: 338–339.
20. Hollowell JG, Witherington R, Ballagas AJ, et al. Embryologic considerations of diphallus and associated anomalies. J Urol 1977; 117: 728–732.
21. Kapoor R, Saha MM. Complete duplication of the bladder, urethra and external genitalia in a neonate: a case report. J Urol 1987; 137: 1243–1244.
22. Kaplan GW, Brock WA. The etiology of chordee. Urol Clin North Am 1981; 8: 383–387.
23. Gelbard MK, Dorey F, James K. The natural history of Peyronie's disease. J Urol 1990; 144: 1376–1379.
24. Cohen-Addad N, Zarafu IW, Hanna MK. Complete penoscrotal transposition. Urology 1985; 26: 149–152.
25. Elder JS, Jeffs RD. Suprainguinal ectopic scrotum and associated anomalies. J Urol 1982; 127: 336–338.
26. Lapointe SP, Wei DC, Hricak H, et al. Magnetic resonance imaging in the evaluation of congenital anomalies of the external genitalia. Urology 2001; 58: 452–456.
27. Ringert RH, Hermanns M, Zoeller G. Outcome after repair of congenital penile malformations. Andrologia 1999; 31: 21–6.
28. Lynch DF, Schellhammer PF. Tumors of the penis. In: Walsh PC, Retik AB, Stamey TA, et al., eds. Campbell's urology, 7th edn. Philadelphia: WB Saunders, 1998.
29. Robson WL, Leung AK. The circumcision question. Postgrad Med J 1992; 91: 237–242.
30. Clemmensen OJ, Krogh J, Petri M. The histologic spectrum of prepuces from patients with phimosis. Am J Dermatopathol 1988; 10: 104–108.
31. Gozal D. Paraphimosis apparently associated with Plasmodium falciparum infection. Trans Roy Soc Trop Med Hyg 1991; 85: 443.
32. Romero-Perez P, Amat-Cecilia M, Amdrada-Becerra E. Metastasis in the glans of prostatic adenocarcinoma.

Apropos of a case. Actas Urol Esp 1991; 15: 284–287.

33. Reddy CRRM, Devendranath V, Pratap S. Carcinoma of penis – role of phimosis. Urology 1984; 24: 85–88.

34. Brinton LA, Li JY, Rong SD, et al. Risk factors for penile cancer: results from a case–control study in China. Int J Cancer 1991; 47: 504–509.

35. Velazquez EF, Bock A, Soskin A, et al. Preputial variability and preferential association of long phimotic foreskins with penile cancer. An anatomic comparative study of types of foreskin in a general population and cancer patients. Am J Surg Pathol 2003; 27: 994–998.

36. Fetsch JF, Davis CJ Jr, Hallman JR, et al. Lymphedematous fibroepithelial polyps of the glans penis and prepuce: a clinicopathologic study of 7 cases demonstrating a strong association with chronic condom catheter use. Hum Pathol 2004; 35: 190–195.

37. Yildirim I, Irkilata C, Sumer F, et al. Fibroepithelial polyp originating from the glans penis in a child. Int J Urol 2004; 11: 187–188.

38. Turgut M, Yenilmez A, Can C, et al. Fibroepithelial polyp of glans penis. Urology 2005; 65: 593.

39. Escala JM, Rickwood AM. Balanitis. Br J Urol 1989; 63: 196–197.

40. Vohra S, Badlani G. Balanitis and balanoposthitis. Urol Clin North Am 1992; 19: 143–147.

41. Waugh MA. Balanitis. Dermatol Clin 1998; 16: 757–762.

42. Margolis DJ. Cutaneous diseases of the male external genitalia. In: Walsh PC, Retik AB, Vaughan ED, et al., eds. Campbell's urology, 7th edn. Philadelphia: WB Saunders, 1998, 717–732.

43. Abdullah AN, Drake SM, Wade AA, et al. Balanitis (balanoposthitis) in patients attending a department of Genitourinary medicine. Int J STD AIDS 1992; 3: 128–129.

44. Zoon JJ. Balanophosthite chronique circonscrite benigne plasmocytes. Dermatologica 1952; 105: 1–7.

45. Jolly BB, Krishnamurty S, Vaidyanathan S. Zoon's balanitis. Urol Int 1993; 50: 182–184.

46. Arango-Toro O, Rosales-Bordes A, Vese-Llanes J, et al. Plasmacellular balanoposthitis of Zoon. Arch Esp Urol 1990; 43: 337–339.

47. Houser ER, Gaston KE, Funkhouser WK, et al. Plasma cell (Zoon's) balanitis with concomitant HIV infection. Urology 66: 657, 2005.

48. Retamar RA, Kien MC, Chouela EN. Zoon's balanitis: presentation of 15 patients, five treated with a carbon dioxide laser. Int J Dermatol 2003; 42: 305–307.

49. Brodin M. Balanitis circumscripta plasmacellularis. J Am Acad Dermatol 1980; 2: 33–35.

50. Pastar Z, Rados J, Lipozencic J, et al. Zoon plasma cell balanitis: an overview and role of histopathology. Acta Dermatovenerol Croatia 2004; 12: 268–273.

51. Fang AW, Whittaker MA, Theaker JM. Mucinous metaplasia of the penis. Histopathology 2002; 40: 177–179.

52. Val-Bernal JF, Hernandez-Nieto E. Benign mucinous metaplasia of the penis. A lesion resembling extramammary Paget's disease. J Cutan Pathol 2000; 27: 76–79.

53. Baldwin HE, Geronemus RG. The treatment of Zoon's balanitis with the carbon dioxide laser. J Dermatol Surg Oncol 1989; 15: 491–494.

54. Rowell NR. Lupus erythematosus, scleroderma and dermatomyositis. The 'collagen' or 'connective-tissue' diseases. In: Rook A, Wilkinson DS, Ebling FJG, et al., eds. Textbook of dermatology, 4th edn. Oxford: Blackwell Scientific, 1986; 1281–1392.

55. Datta C, Dutta SK, Chaudhuri A. Histopathological and immunological studies in a cohort of balanitis xerotica obliterans. J Indian Med Assoc 1993; 91: 146–148.

56. Velazquez EF, Cubilla AL. Lichen sclerosus in 68 patients with squamous cell carcinoma of the penis: frequent atypias and correlation with special carcinoma variants suggests a precancerous role, Am J Surg Pathol 2003; 27: 1448–1453.

57. Powell J, Robson A, Cranston D, et al. High incidence of lichen sclerosus in patients with squamous cell carcinoma of the penis. Br J Dermatol 2001; 145: 85–89.

58. Powell J, Robson A, Cranston D, et al. High incidence of lichen sclerosus in patients with squamous cell carcinoma of the penis. Br J Dermatol 2003; 148: 1083–1084.

59. Post B, Janner M. Lichen sclerosus et atrophicus penis. Zeitschr Hautkr 1975; 50: 675–681.

60. Yesudian PD, Sugunendran H, Bates CM, O'Mahony C. Lichen sclerosus. Int J STD AIDS 2005; 16: 465–73.

61. Harrington CI, Dunsmore IR. An investigation into the incidence of autoimmune disorders in patients with lichen sclerosus et atrophicus. Br J Dermatol 1981; 104; 563–566.

62. Thomas RHM, Ridley CM, Black MM. The association of lichen sclerosus et atrophicus related disease in males. Br J Dermatol 1983; 109: 661–664.

63. Harrington CI, Gelsthorpe K. The association between lichen sclerosus et atrophicus and HLA-B40. Br J Dermatol 1981; 104: 561–562.

64. Hewan-Lowe K, Moreland A, Finnerty DP. Penis and scrotum, tumors and related disorders. In: Someren A, ed. Urologic pathology with clinical and radiologic correlations. New York: Macmillan, 1989; 611–659.

65. Dore B, Grange P, Irani J, et al. Atrophicus sclerosis lichen and cancer of the glans. J Urol (Paris) 1989; 95: 415–418.

66. Barbagli G, Palminteri E, Mirri F, et al. Penile carcinoma in patients with genital lichen sclerosus: a multicenter survey. J Urol 2006; 175: 1359–1363.

67. Goolamali SI, Pakianathan M. Penile carcinoma arising in balanitis xerotica obliterans. Int J STD AIDS 2006; 17: 135–136.

68. Aquilina C, Viraben R. Rapid onset of acute carcinoma of the glans penis arising three years after a lichen sclerosus. Eur J Dermatol 2005; 15: 497–499.

69. Campus GV, Alia F, Bosincu L. Squamous cell carcinoma and lichen sclerosus et atrophicus of the prepuce. Plast Reconstr Surg 1992; 89: 692–694.

70. Pride HB, Miller OF, Tyler WB. Penile squamous cell carcinoma arising from balanitis xerotica obliterans. J Am Acad Dermatol 1993; 29: 469–473.

71. Bouyssou-Gauthier ML, Boulinguez S, Dumas JP, et al. Penile lichen sclerosus: follow-up study. Ann Dermatol Venereol 1999; 126: 804–807.

72. Nasca MR, Innocenzi D, Micali G. Penile cancer among patients with genital lichen sclerosus. J Am Acad Dermatol 1999; 41: 911–914.

73. Kumaran MS, Kanwar AJ. Squamous cell carcinoma in untreated lichen sclerosus of the penis: a rare complication. J Dermatol 2004; 31: 239–241.

74. Cubilla AL, Velazquez EF, Young RH. Pseudohyperplastic squamous cell carcinoma of the penis associated with lichen sclerosus. An extremely well-differentiated, nonverruciform neoplasm that preferentially affects the foreskin and is frequently misdiagnosed. A report of 10 cases of a distinctive clinicopathologic entity. Am J Surg Pathol 2004; 28: 895–900.

75. Perry HO, Mayne JG. Psoriasis and Reiter's syndrome. Arch Dermatol 1965; 92: 129–136.

76. Keat A. Reiter's syndrome and reactive arthritis in perspective. N Engl J Med 1983; 309: 1606–1615.

77. Calin A. Reiter's syndrome. In: Kelly WN, Harris ED Jr, Ruddy S, et al., eds. Textbook of rheumatology, 3rd edn. Philadelphia: WB Saunders, 1989.

78. Keat A, Rowe I. Reiter's syndrome and associated arthritides. Rheum Dis Clin North Am 1991; 17: 25–42.

79. Cuttica RJ, Scheines EJ, Garay SM, et al. Juvenile onset Reiter's syndrome. A retrospective study of 26 patients. Clin Exp Rheumatol 1992; 10: 285–288.

80. Rehman MU, Cantwell R, Johnson CC, et al. Inapparent genital infection with Chlamydia trachomatis and its potential role in the genesis of Reiter's syndrome. DNA Cell Biol 1992; 11: 215–219.

81. Tuncer T, Arman MI, Akyokus A, et al. HLA B27 and clinical features in Reiter's syndrome. Clin Rheumatol 1992; 11: 239–242.

82. Hansfield HH, Pollock PS. Arthritis associated sexually transmitted

diseases. In: Holmes KK, Mardh P, Sparling PF, et al., eds. Sexually transmitted diseases, 2nd edn. New York: McGraw-Hill, 1990.

83. Schneider JM, Matthews JH, Graham BS. Reiter's syndrome. Cutis 2003; 71: 198–200.

84. Edirisinghe DN, Sankar KN, Pattman RS. Reiter's syndrome and keratoderma blennorrhagica on glans penis – is this unusual? Int J STD AIDS 2002; 13: 133–134.

85. Toussaint S, Kamino H. Noninfectious erythematous papular and squamous diseases of the skin. In: Elder D, Elenitsas R, Jaworsky C, Johnson B, eds. Histopathology of the skin, 8th edn. Philadelphia: Lippincott-Raven, 1997.

86. Wilson SK, Delk JR. A new treatment for Peyronie's disease: modeling the penis over an inflatable penile prosthesis. J Urol 1994; 152: 1121–1123.

87. Maan Z, Arya M, Shergill I, Joseph JV, Patel HR. Peyronie's disease: an update of the medical management. Expert Opin Pharmacother 2004; 5: 799–805.

88. Hellstrom WJ. History, epidemiology, and clinical presentation of Peyronie's disease. Int J Impotence Res 2003; 15: s91–92.

89. Briganti A, Salonia A, Deho F, et al. Peyronie's disease: a review. Curr Opin Urol 2003; 13: 417–422.

90. Levine LA, Estrada CR, Storm DW, Matkov TG. Peyronie disease in younger men: characteristics and treatment results. J Androl 2003; 24: 27–32.

91. Mulhall JP, Schiff J, Guhring P. An analysis of the natural history of Peyronie's disease. J Urol 2006; 175: 2115–2118.

92. Sommer F, Schwarzer U, Wassmer G, et al. Epidemiology of Peyronie's disease. Int J Impotence Res 2002; 14: 379–383.

93. Enzinger FM, Weiss SW. Fibromatoses. In: Weiss SW, Goldblum JR eds. Soft tissue tumors, 4th edn. St. Louis: Mosby, 2001; 309–346.

94. Neyberg LM, Bias WB, Hochberg MC, et al. Identification of an inherited form of Peyronie's disease with autosomal dominant inheritance and association with Dupuytren's contracture and histocompatibility B7 cross reacting antigens. J Urol 1982; 128: 48–51.

95. Vande Berg JS, Devine CJ, Horton CE, et al. Peyronie's disease: an electron microscopic study. J Urol 1981; 126: 333–336.

96. Hinman F Jr. Etiologic factors in Peyronie disease. Urol Int 1980; 35: 407–413.

97. Kaufman JJ. Peyronie's: its cause. Scand J Urol Nephrol 1991; 138: 219.

98. Bjekic MD, Vlajinac HD, Sipetic SB, Marinkovic JM. Risk factors for Peyronie's disease: a case-control study. BJU Int 2006; 97: 570–574.

99. Hauck EW, Hauptmann A, Weidner W, et al. Prospective analysis of HLA classes I and II antigen frequency in patients with Peyronie's disease. J Urol 2003; 170: 1443–1446.

100. Hauck EW, Hauptmann A, Schmelz HU, et al. Prospective analysis of single nucleotide polymorphisms of the transforming growth factor beta-1 gene in Peyronie's disease. J Urol 2003; 169: 369–372.

101. Gonzalez-Cadavid NF, Magee TR, Ferrini M, et al. Gene expression in Peyronie's disease. Int J Impotence Res 2002; 14: 361–374.

102. Rompel R, Weidner W, Mueller-Eckhardt G. HLA association of idiopathic Peyronie's disease: an indication of autoimmune phenomena in etiopathogenesis? Tissue Antigens 1991; 38: 104–106.

103. Hauck EW, Domann E, Hauptmann A, et al. Prospective analysis of 16S rDNA as a highly sensitive marker for bacterial presence in Peyronie's disease plaques. J Urol 2003; 170: 2053–2056.

104. Bivens CH, Maracek RL, Feldman JM. Peyronie's disease – a presenting complaint of the carcinoid syndrome. N Engl J Med 1973; 289: 844–846.

105. Guerneri S, Stioui S, Mantovani F, et al. Multiple clonal chromosome abnormalities in Peyronie's disease. Cancer Genet Cytogenet 1991; 52: 181–185.

106. Chiang PH, Chiang CP, Shen MR, et al. Study of the changes in collagen of the tunica albuginea in venogenic impotence and Peyronie's disease. Eur Urol 1992; 21: 48–51.

107. McRoberts JW. Peyronie's disease. Surg Gynecol Obstet 1969; 129: 1291–1294.

108. Dang G, Matern R, Bivalacqua TJ, et al. Intralesional interferon-alpha-2B injections for the treatment of Peyronie's disease. South Med J 2004; 97: 42–46.

109. Hauck EW, Mueller UO, Bschleipfer T, et al. Extracorporeal shock wave therapy for Peyronie's disease: exploratory meta-analysis of clinical trials. J Urol 2004; 171: 740–745.

110. Ralph DJ, Minhas S. The management of Peyronie's disease. BJU Int 2004; 93: 208–215.

111. Darewicz JS, Darewicz BA, Galek LM, et al. Surgical treatment of Peyronie's disease by the intracavernosal plaque excision method: a new surgical technique. Eur Urol 2004; 45: 77–81.

112. Hauck EW, Diemer T, Schmelz HU, Weidner W. A critical analysis of nonsurgical treatment of Peyronie's disease. Eur Urol 2006; 49: 987–997.

113. Prieto Castro RM, Leva Vallejo ME, Regueiro Lopez JC, et al. Combined treatment with vitamin E and colchicine in the early stages of Peyronie's disease. BJU Int 2003; 91: 522–524.

114. Montorsi F, Guazzoni G, Bergamaschi F, et al. Patient-partner satisfaction with semirigid penile prostheses for Peyronie's disease: a 5-year followup study. J Urol 1993; 150: 1819–1821.

115. Gelbrad MK. Dystrophic penile calcification in Peyronie's disease. J Urol 1988; 139: 738–740.

116. Hoeg OM. Human penile ossification. A case report. Scand J Urol Nephrol 1986; 20: 231–232.

117. Goldstein I, Krane RJ. Diagnosis and therapy of erectile dysfunction. In: Walsh PC, Retik AB, Stamey TA, et al., eds. Campbell's urology, 6th edn. Philadelphia: WB Saunders, 1992; 3033–3072.

118. Petrou AP, Barrett DM. The use of penile prosthesis in erectile dysfunction. Semin Urol 1990; 8: 138–152.

119. Kessler R. Surgical experience with the inflatable penile prosthesis. J Urol 1980; 124: 611–613.

120. Kasebayashi Y, Hayashi Y, Hirao K, et al. A case of penile cavernitis following a penile prosthesis implantation. Hinyokika Kiyo 1991; 37: 1555–1557.

121. Fulow WL, Goldwasser B, Gundian JC. Implantation of model AMS 700 penile prosthesis: long-term results. J Urol 1988; 139: 741–742.

122. Rahman NU, Carrion RE, Bochinski D, Lue TF. Combined penile plication surgery and insertion of penile prosthesis for severe penile curvature and erectile dysfunction. J Urol 2004; 171: 2346–2349.

123. Sadeghi-Nejad H, Dogra V, Seftel AD, Mohamed MA. Priapism. Radiol Clin North Am 2004; 42: 427–443.

124. Inamoto T, Azuma H, Iwamoto Y, et al. A rare case of penile metastasis of testicular cancer presented with priapism. Hinyokika Kiyo 2005; 51: 639–642.

125. Pohl J, Pott B, Kleinhans G. Priapism: a three-phase concept of management according to aetiology and prognosis. Br J Urol 1986; 8: 113–118.

126. Russo P. Urologic emergencies in the cancer patient. Semin Oncol 2000; 27: 284–298.

127. Spycher MA, Hauri D. The ultrastructure of the erectile tissue in priapism. J Urol 1986; 135: 142–150.

128. Winter CC, McDowell G. Experience with 105 patients with priapism: update review of all aspects. J Urol 1988; 140: 980–983.

129. Vilke GM, Harrigan RA, Ufberg JW, Chan TC. Emergency evaluation and treatment of priapism. Emerg Med 2004; 26: 325–329.

130. Judson FN. Gonorrhea. Med Clin North Am 1990; 74: 1353–1366.

131. Hawley HB. Gonorrhea. Finding and treating a moving target. Postgrad Med 1993; 94: 105–111.

132. Ramon QD, Betlloch MI, Jimenez MR. Gonococcal infection of the penile median raphe. Int J Dermatol 1987; 26: 242–243.

133. Gaffoor PM, Bayyari KH. Gonococcal tysonitis: an unusual penile infection. Indian J Dermatol 1989; 34: 90–91.

134. Nsuami M, Cammarata CL, Brooks BN, et al. Chlamydia and gonorrhea co-occurrence in a high school population. Sex Transm Dis 2004; 31: 424–427.

135. Levenson D. Increasing cases of drug-resistant gonorrhea prompt new CDC treatment recommendations for gay and bisexual men. Rep Med Guide Outcomes Res 2004; 15: 8–9.

136. Sparling PF. Natural history of syphilis. In: Holmes KK, Mardh P, Sparling PF, eds. Sexually transmitted diseases. New York: McGraw-Hill, 1990.

137. Hutchinson CM, Hook EW III. Syphilis in adults. Med Clin North Am 1990; 74: 1389–1416.

138. Tramont EC. Syphilis in HIV-infected persons. AIDS Clin Rev 1993–1994; 61–72.

139. Mencus A, Antal GM. The endemic treponematoses: not yet eradicated. World Health Stat Q 1992; 45: 228–237.

140. Pariser H. Syphilis. Prim Care 1989; 16: 603–619.

141. Jeerapaet P, Ackerman AB. Histologic patterns of secondary syphilis. Arch Dermatol 1973; 107: 373–377.

142. Dave S, Gopinath DV, Thappa DM. Nodular secondary syphilis, Dermatol Online J 2003; 9: 9.

143. Abell E, Marks R, Wilson-Jones E. Secondary syphilis: a clinicopathological review. Br J Dermatol 1975; 93: 53–61.

144. Cochran RIE, Thomson J, Fleming KA, et al. Histology simulating reticulosis in secondary syphilis. Br J Dermatol 1976; 95: 251–254.

145. Poulsen A, Kobayasi T, Secher L, et al. Treponema pallidum in macular and papular secondary syphilis skin eruptions. Acta Dermatol Venereol 1986; 66: 251–258.

146. Frisch M, Jorgensen BB, Friis S, Melbye M. Syphilis and the risk of penis cancer. Sex Transm Dis 1996; 23: 471–474.

147. Nahmias AJ, Roizman D. Infection with herpes simplex virus 1 and 2. N Engl J Med 1973; 29: 667–719.

148. Rudlinger R, Norval M. Herpes simplex virus infections: new concepts in an old disease. Dermatologica 1989; 178: 1–5.

149. Buechner SA. Common skin disorders of the penis. BJU Int 2002; 90: 498–506.

150. Corey L. Herpes simplex virus infections during the decade since the licensure of acyclovir. J Med Virol 1993; 1: 7–12.

151. Arbesfeld DM, Thomas I. Cutaneous herpes simples virus infections. Am Fam Phys 1991; 43: 1655–1664.

152. Stenzel-Poore MP, Hallick LM, Fendrick JL, et al. Herpes simplex virus shedding in genital secretions. Sex Transm Dis 1987; 14: 17–22.

153. Ashley RL. Laboratory techniques in the diagnosis of herpes simplex infection. Genitourinary Med1993; 69: 174–183.

154. McSorley J, Shapiro L, Brownstein MH, et al. Simplex and varicella-zoster: comparative cases. Int J Dermatol 1974; 13: 69–75.

155. Whitley RJ. Neonatal herpes simplex virus infections. J Med Virol 1993; 1: 13–21.

156. Favre M, Hellerstrom S. The epidemiology, aetiology and prophylaxis of lymphogranuloma inguinale. Acta Dermatol Venereol 1954; 34: 1–9.

157. Burgoyne RA. Lymphogranuloma venereum. Prim Care 1990; 17: 153–157.

158. Aggarwal K, Jain VK, Gupta S. Bilateral groove sign with penoscrotal elephantiasis. Sex Transm Infect 2002; 78: 458.

159. Heaton ND, Yates-Bell A. Thirty-year follow-up of lymphogranuloma venereum. Br J Urol 1992; 70: 693–694.

160. Sheldon WH, Heyman A. Lymphogranuloma venereum. Am J Pathol 1947; 23: 653–664.

161. Schubiner HH, LeBar WD, Joseph S, et al. Evaluation of two rapid tests for the diagnosis of Chlamydia trachomatis genital infections. Eur J Clin Microbiol Infect Dis 1992; 11: 553–556.

162. Bassa AG, Hoosen AA, Moodley J, et al. Granuloma inguinale (donovanosis) in women. An analysis of 61 cases from Durban, South Africa. Sex Transm Dis 1993; 20: 164–167.

163. Richens J. The diagnosis and treatment of donovanosis (granuloma inguinale). Genitourinary Med1991; 67: 441–452.

164. Sayal SK, Kar PK, Anand LC. A study of 255 cases of granuloma inguinale. Indian J Dermatol 1987; 32: 91–97.

165. Sehgal VN, Sharma HK. Donovanosis. J Dermatol 1992; 19: 932–946.

166. Beerman H, Sonck CE. The epithelial changes in granuloma inguinale. Am J Syph 1952; 36: 501–510.

167. Fritz GS, Hubler WR, Dodson RF, et al. Mutilating granuloma inguinale. Arch Dermatol 1975; 111: 1464–1465.

168. Gupta S, Kumar B. Dorsal perforation of prepuce: a common end point of severe ulcerative genital diseases? Sex Transm Infect 2000; 76: 210–212.

169. Davis CM, Collins C. Granuloma inguinale: an ultrastructural study of Calymmatobacterium granulomatis. J Invest Dermatol 1969; 53: 315–321.

170. Barnes R, Masood S, Lammert N, et al. Extragenital granuloma inguinale mimicking a soft-tissue neoplasm: a case report and review of the literature. Hum Pathol 1990; 21: 559–561.

171. Van-Dyck E, Piot P. Laboratory techniques in the investigation of chancroid, lymphogranuloma venereum and donovanosis. Genitourinary Med 1992; 68: 130–133.

172. Freinkel AL, Dangor Y, Koornhof HJ, et al. A serological test for granuloma inguinale. Genitourinary Med 1992; 68: 269–272.

173. Steen R. Eradicating chancroid. Bull WHO 2001; 79: 818–826.

174. Schmid GP, Sanders LL Jr, Blount JH, et al. Chancroid in the United States: reestablishment of an old disease. JAMA 1987; 258: 3265–3268.

175. Freinkel AL. Histological aspects of sexually transmitted genital lesions. Histopathology 1987; 11: 819–831.

176. Gaisin A, Heaton CL. Chancroid: alias the soft chancre. Int J Dermatol 1975; 14: 188–197.

177. Jones CC, Rosen T. Cultural diagnosis of chancroid. Arch Dermatol 1991; 127: 1823–1827.

178. Chui L, Albritton W, Paster B, et al. Development of the polymerase chain reaction for diagnosis of chancroid. J Clin Microbiol 1993; 31: 659–664.

179. Jessamine PG, Plummer FA, Ndinya-Achola JO, et al. Human immunodeficiency virus, genital ulcers and the male foreskin: synergism in HIV-1 transmission. Scand J Infect Dis 1990; 69: 181–186.

180. Simonsen JN, Cameron DW, Yakinya MN, et al. Human immunodeficiency virus infection in men with sexually transmitted diseases. N Engl J Med 1988; 319: 274–278.

181. Lewis DA. Chancroid: clinical manifestations, diagnosis, and management. Sex Transm Infect 2003; 79: 68–71.

182. Magro CM, Crowson AN, Alfa M, et al. A morphological study of penile chancroid lesions in human immunodeficiency virus (HIV)-positive and -negative African men with a hypothesis concerning the role of chancroid in HIV transmission. Hum Pathol 1996; 27: 1066–1070.

183. Mayser P. Mycotic infections of the penis. Andrologia 1999; 31: 13–16.

184. David LM, Walzman M, Rajamanoharan S. Genital colonisation and infection with candida in heterosexual and homosexual males. Genitourinary Med 1997; 73: 394–396.

185. Burchard KW. Fungal sepsis. Infect Dis Clin North Am 1992; 6: 677–692.

186. Humayun H, Maliwan N. Emphysematous genital infection caused by Candida albicans. J Urol 1982; 128: 1049–1054.

187. Heilesen B. Studies on Ascaris scabiei and scabies. Acta Dermatol Venereol 1946; 26: 1–370.

188. Barrett NG, Morse DL. The resurgence of scabies. Commun Dis Rep CDR Rev 1993; 3: 32–34.

189. Perna AG, Bell K, Rosen T. Localised genital Norwegian scabies in an AIDS patient. Sex Transm Infect 2004; 80: 72–73.

190. Fernandez N, Torres A, Ackerman AB. Pathological finding in human scabies. Arch Dermatol 1977; 113: 320–324.

191. Hejazi N, Mehregan AH. Scabies. Histological study of inflammatory lesions. Arch Dermatol 1975; 111: 37–39.

192. Orkin M, Maibach HI. This scabies pandemic. N Engl J Med 1978; 289: 496–498.

193. Yang SA, Lu CF, Kuo MC, et al. Clinical and scanning electron microscopic studies on Norwegian scabies infection. Kao Hsiung I Hsueh Ko Hsueh Tsa Chih 1992; 8: 569–575.

194. Estes SA, Estes J. Therapy of scabies: nursing homes, hospitals, and the homeless. Semin Dermatol 1993; 12: 26–33.

195. Billstein SA, Mattaliano VJ Jr. The nuisance sexually transmitted diseases: molluscum contagiosum, scabies, and crab lice. Med Clin North Am 1990; 74: 1487–1505.

196. Levine GI. Sexually transmitted parasitic diseases. Prim Care 1991; 18: 101–128.

197. Wendel K, Rompalo A. Scabies and pediculosis pubis: an update of treatment regimens and general review. Clin Infect Dis 2002; 35: S146–S151.

198. Ko CJ, Elston DM. Pediculosis. J Am Acad Dermatol 2004; 50: 1–12.

199. Hutchinson DB, Farquhar JA. Trimethoprim-sulfamethoxazole in the treatment of malaria, toxoplasmosis, and pediculosis. Rev Infect Dis 1982; 4: 419–425.

200. Porter CD, Blake NW, Cream JJ, et al. Molluscum contagiosum virus. Mol Cell Biol Hum Dis Ser 1992; 1: 233–257.

201. Gupta S, Radotra BD, Javaheri SM, Kumar B. Lymphangioma circumscriptum of the penis mimicking venereal lesions. J Eur Acad Dermatol Venereol 2003; 17: 598–600.

202. Epstein WL. Molluscum contagiosum. Semin Dermatol 1992; 11: 184–189.

203. Lutzner MA. Molluscum contagiosum, verruca and zoster viruses. Arch Dermatol 1963; 23: 436–444.

204. Mescon H, Gray M, Moretti G. Molluscum contagiosum. J Invest Dermatol 1954; 23: 293–308.

205. Henao M, Freeman RG. Inflammatory molluscum contagiosum. Arch Dermatol 1964; 90: 479–482.

206. Golledge CL, Phillips G. *Corynebacterium minutissimum* infection. J Infect 1991; 23: 73–76.

207. Sarkany I, Taplin D, Blank H. Incidence and bacteriology of erythrasma. Arch Dermatol 1962; ;85: 578–582.

208. Montes LF, Black SH, McBride ME. Bacterial invasion of the stratum corneum in erythrasma. Ultrastructural evidence for a keratolytic action exerted by *Corynebacterium minutissimum*. J Invest Dermatol 1967; 49: 474–485.

209. Saffrin S. Treatment of acyclovir-resistant herpes simplex virus infections in patients with AIDS. J AIDS 1992; l5: S29–S32.

210. Coleman DC, Bennett DE, Sullivan DJ, et al. Oral candida in HIV infection and AIDS: new perspectives/new approaches. Crit Rev Microbiol 1993; 19: 61–82.

211. Schwartz JJ, Myskowski PL. Molluscum contagiosum in patients with human immunodeficiency virus infection. A review of twenty-seven patients. J Am Acad Dermatol 1992; 27: 583–588.

212. Orkin M. Scabies in AIDS. Semin Dermatol 1993; 12: 9–14.

213. Brancato L, Itescu S, Skovron ML, et al. Aspects of the spectrum, prevalence and disease susceptibility determinants of Reiter's syndrome and related disorders associated with HIV infection. Rheumatol Int 1989; 9: 137–141.

214. Demopoulos BP, Vamvakas E, Ehrlich JE, Demopoulos R. Non-acquired immunodeficiency syndrome-defining malignancies in patients infected with human immunodeficiency virus. Arch Pathol Lab Med 2003; 127: 589–592.

215. Kaplan MH, Sodick N, McNutt NS, et al. Dermatologic findings and manifestations of acquired immunodeficiency syndrome (AIDS). J Am Acad Dermatol 1987; 16: 485–506.

216. Milburn PB, Brandsma JL, Goldsman CI, et al. Disseminated warts and evolving squamous cell carcinoma in a patient with AIDS. J Am Acad Dermatol 1988; 19: 401–405.

217. Croxson T, Chabow AB, Rorat E, et al. Intraepithelial carcinoma of the anus in homosexual men. Dis Colon Rectum 1984; 27: 325–330.

218. Gelquin J, Weiss L, Kazatchkine MD. Genital and oral erosions induced by foscarnet. Lancet 1990; 335: 287.

219. Fegueux S, Salmon D, Picard C, et al. Penile ulceration with foscarnet. Lancet 1990; 335: 547.

220. Rosenberg SK, Reid R. Sexually transmitted papilloma viral infections in the male. I. Anatomic distribution and clinical features. Urology 1987; 29: 488–492.

221. Chuang T-Y. Condyloma acuminata (genital warts). An epidemiologic view. J Am Acad Dermatol 1987; 16: 376–384.

222. Buechner SA. Common skin disorders of the penis. BJU Int 2002; 90: 498–506.

223. Chuang T-Y, Perry HO, Kurland LT, et al. Condyloma acuminatum in Rochester, Minn, 1950–1978. I. Epidemiology and clinical features. Arch Dermatol 1984; 120: 469–475.

224. Syrjanen K, Syrjanen S. Epidemiology of human papilloma virus infections and genital neoplasia. Scand J Infect Dis 1990; 69: 7–17.

225. Bleeker MC, Hogewoning CJ, Van Den Brule AJ, et al. Penile lesions and human papilloma virus in male sexual partners of women with cervical intraepithelial neoplasia. J Am Acad Dermatol 2002; 47: 351–357.

226. Schackner L, Hankin DE. Assessing child abuse in childhood condyloma acuminatum. J Am Acad Dermatol 1985; 123: 157–160.

227. Oriel JD. Natural history of genital warts. Br J Venereal Dis 1971; 47: 1–13.

228. Margolis S. Genital warts and molluscum contagiosum. Urol Clin North Am 1984; 11: 163–170.

229. Goette DK. Review of erythroplasia of Queyrat and its treatment. Urology 1976; 8: 311–315.

230. O'Brien WM, Jenson AB, Lancaster WD, et al. Human papilloma virus typing of penile condyloma. J Urol 1989; 141: 863–865.

231. Nuovo GJ, Hochman HA, Eliezri HA, et al. Detection of human papilloma virus DNA in penile lesions histologically negative for condylomata. Analysis by in-situ hybridization and the polymerase chain reaction. Am J Surg Pathol 1990; 14: 829–836.

232. Weaver MG, Abdul-Karim FM, Dale G, et al. Detection and localization of human papilloma virus in penile condylomas and squamous cell carcinomas using in-situ hybridization with biotinylated DNA viral probes. Mod Pathol 1989; 2: 94–100.

233. Glicksman JM, Freeman RG. Pearly penile papules. A statistical study of incidence. Arch Dermatol 1966; 93: 56–59.

234. Johnson BL, Baxter DL. Pearly penile papules. Arch Dermatol 1964; 90: 166–167.

235. Tannenbaum MH, Becker SW. Papillae of the corona of the glans penis. J Urol 1965; 93: 391–395.

236. Elder D, Elenitsas R, Ragsdale BD. Tumors of the epidermal appendages. In: Elder D, Elenitsas R, Jaworsky C, Johnson B, eds. Histopathology of the skin. Philadelphia: Lippincott-Raven, 1997; 747–804.

237. Cole LA, Helwig EB. Mucoid cysts of the penile skin. J Urol 1976; 115; 397–400.

238. Golitz LE, Robin M. Median raphe canals of the penis. Cutis 1981; 27: 170–172.

239. Asarch RG, Golitz LE, Sausker WF, et al. Median raphe cysts of the penis. Arch Dermatol 1979; 115: 1084–1086.

240. Cardoso R, Freitas JD, Reis JP, Tellechea O. Median raphe cyst of the penis. Dermatol Online J 2005; 11: 37.

241. Gray MR, Ansell ID. Pseudo-epitheliomatous hyperkeratotic and micaceous balanitis: evidence for regarding it as pre-malignant. Br J Urol 1990; 66: 103–104.

242. Lortat-Jacob E, Civatte J. Balanite pseudoépithéliomateuse kératosique et micacée. Bull Soc Franc Dermatol Syph 1961; 68: 164–167.

243. Ersahin C, Szpaderska AM, Foreman K, Yong S. Verucciform xanthoma of the penis not associated with human papilloma virus infection. Arch Pathol Lab Med 2005; 129: e62–64.

244. Mohsin SK, Lee MW, Amin MB, et al. Cutaneous verruciform xanthoma. A report of five cases investigating the etiology and nature of xanthoma cells. Am J Surg Pathol 1998; 22: 479–487.

245. Lam KY, Chan KW. Molecular pathology and clinicopathologic features of penile tumors. With special reference to analyses of p21 and p53 expression and unusual histologic features. Arch Pathol Lab Med 1999; 123; 895–904.

246. Dehner LP, Smith BH. Soft tissue tumors of the penis. A clinicopathologic study of 46 cases. Cancer 1970; 25: 1431–1447.

247. Laskin WB, Fetsch JF, Davis CJ Jr, Sesterhenn IA. Granular cell tumor of the penis. clinicopathologic evaluation of 9 cases. Hum Pathol 2005; 36: 291–298.

248. Bulstrode NW, Sandison A, Martin DL. Granular cell tumor of the glans penis. Br J Plast Surg 2004; 57: 83–5.

249. Park DS, Cho TW, Kang H. Glomus tumor of the glans penis. Urology 2004; 64: 1031.

250. Fetsch JF, Sesterhenn IA, Miettinen M, Davis CJ. Epithelioid hemangioma of the penis. A clinicopathologic and immunohistochemical analysis of 19 cases, with special reference to exuberant examples often confused with epithelioid hemangioendothelioma and epithelioid angiosarcoma. Am J Surg Pathol 2004; 28: 523–533.

251. Fetsch JF, Brinsko RW, Davis CJ Jr, et al. A distinctive myointimal proliferation ('myointimoma') involving the corpus spongiosum of the glans penis: a clinicopathologic and immunohistochemical analysis of 10 cases, Am J Surg Pathol 2000; 24: 1524–1530.

252. Porter WM, Francis N, Hawkins D, et al. Penile intraepithelial neoplasia. clinical spectrum and treatment of 35 cases. Br J Dermatol 2002; 147: 1159–1165.

253. Von Krogh G, Horenblas S. Diagnosis and clinical presentation of premalignant lesions of the penis. Scand J Urol Nephrol 2000; 205: 201–214.

254. Kaye V, Zhang G, Dehner LP, et al. Carcinoma in situ of penis: is distinction between erythroplasia of Queyrat and Bowen's disease relevant? Urology 1990; 36: 479–482.

255. Aynaud O, Ionesco M, Barrasso R. Penile intraepithelial neoplasia: specific clinical features correlate with histologic and virologic findings. Cancer 1994; 74: 1762–1767.

256. Gerber GS. Carcinoma in situ of the penis. J Urol 1994; 151: 829–833.

257. Cubilla AL, Meijer CJ, Young RH. Morphological features of epithelial abnormalities and precancerous lesions of the penis. Scand J Urol Nephrol 2000; 205: 215–219.

258. Cubilla AL, Velazquez EF, Young RH. Epithelial lesions associated with invasive penile squamous cell carcinoma: a pathologic study of 288 cases. Int J Surg Pathol 2004; 12: 351–364.

259. Queyrat L. Erythroplasie du gland. Bull Soc Franc Dermatol Syph 1911; 22: 378–382.

260. Graham JH, Helwig EB. Erythroplasia of Queyrat: a clinicopathologic and histochemical study. Cancer 1973; 32: 1396–1414.

261. Wieland U, Jurk S, Weissenborn S, et al. Erythroplasia of Queyrat: coinfection with cutaneous carcinogenic human papilloma virus type 8 and genital papilloma viruses in a carcinoma in situ. J Invest Dermatol 2000; 115: 396–401.

262. Davis-Daneshfar A, Trueb RM. Bowen's disease of the glans penis (erythroplasia of Queyrat) in plasma cell balanitis. Cutis 2000; 65: 395–398.

263. Young RH, Srigley JR, Amin MB, et al. The penis and scrotum. In: Young RH, Srigley JR, Amin MB, et al., eds. Tumors of the prostate gland, seminal vesicles, male urethra, and penis. Atlas of tumor pathology. Washington, DC: Armed Forces Institute of Pathology, 2000; 403–488.

264. Haneke E. Skin diseases and tumors of the penis. Urol Int 1982; 37: 172–182.

265. Patterson JW, Kao GF, Graham JH, et al. Bowenoid papulosis: a clinicopathologic study with ultrastructural observations. Cancer 1986; 57: 823–836.

266. Chuang TY, Tse J, Reizner GT. Bowen's disease (squamous cell carcinoma in-situ) as a skin marker for internal malignancy: a case–control study. Am J Prev Med 1990; 6: 238–243.

267. Callen JP, Headington JT. Bowen's and non-Bowen's squamous intraepithelial neoplasia of the skin: relationship to internal malignancy. Arch Dermatol 1980; 116: 422–426.

268. Wade TR, Kopf AW, Ackerman AB. Bowenoid papulosis of the penis. Cancer 1978; 42: 1890–1903.

269. Taylor DR Jr, South DA. Bowenoid papulosis: a review. Cutis 1981; 27: 92–98.

270. Eisen RF, Bhawan J, Cahn TH. Spontaneous regression of bowenoid papulosis of the penis. Cutis 1983; 32: 269–272.

271. Chesney TM, Murphy WM. Diseases of the penis and scrotum. In: Murphy WM, ed. Urological pathology. Philadelphia: WB Saunders, 1989; 401–429.

272. Yu DS, Kim G, Song HJ, Oh CH. Morphometric assessment of nuclei in Bowen's disease and bowenoid papulosis. Skin Res Technol 2004; 10: 67–70.

273. Endo M, Yamashita T, Jin HY, et al. Detection of human papilloma virus type 16 in bowenoid papulosis and nonbowenoid tissues. Int J Dermatol 2003; 42: 474–476.

274. Pala S, Poleva I, Vocatura A. The presence of HPV types 6/11, 16/18, 31/33/51 in Bowenoid papulosis demonstrated by DNA in situ hybridization. Int J STD AIDS 2000; 11: 823–824.

275. Castren K, Vahakangas K, Heikkinen E, Ranki A. Absence of p53 mutations in benign and pre-malignant male genital lesions with over-expressed p53 protein. Int J Cancer 1998; 77: 674–678.

276. Barnes RD, Sarembock LA, Abratt RP, et al. Carcinoma of penis. J Roy Coll Surg Edin 1989; 34: 44–46.

277. Yoneta A, Yamashita T, Jin HY, Iwasawa A, et al. Development of squamous cell carcinoma by two high-risk human papilloma viruses (HPVs), a novel HPV-67 and HPV-31 from bowenoid papulosis. Br J Dermatol 2000; 143: 604–608.

278. Park KC, Kim KH, Youn SW, et al. Heterogeneity of human papilloma virus DNA in a patient with Bowenoid papulosis that progressed to squamous cell carcinoma. Br J Dermatol 1998; 139: 1087–1091.

279. Sufrin G, Huben R. Benign and malignant lesions of the penis. In: Gillenwater JY, Grayhack JT, Howards SS, et al., eds. Adult and pediatric urology, 4th edn. St Louis: Mosby-Year Book, 2002; 1975–2010.

280. Jemal A, Siegel R, Mard E, et al. Cancer statistics 2007. CA Cancer J Clin 2006; 57: 43–66.

281. Dodge OG, Linsell CA. Carcinoma of the penis in Uganda and Kenya Africans. Cancer 1963; 16: 1255–1263.

282. Riveros M, Lebron R. Geographic pathology of cancer of penis. Cancer 1963; 16: 798–811.

283. Brinton LA, Li JY, Rong SD, et al. Risk factors for penile cancer: results from a case–control study in China. Int J Cancer 1991; 47: 504–509.

284. Daling JR, Madeleine MM, Johnson LG, et al. Penile cancer: importance of circumcision, human papilloma virus and smoking in in situ and invasive disease. Int J Cancer 2005; 116: 606–616.

285. Bissada NK, Morcos RR, El-Senoussi M. Post-circumcision carcinoma of the penis: clinical aspects. J Urol 1986; 135: 283–285.

286. Leiter E, Lefkovits AM. Circumcision and penile cancer. NY State J Med 1975; 75: 1520–1525.

287. Dagher R, Selzer ML, Lapides J. Carcinoma of the penis and the anti-circumcision crusade. J Urol 1980; 110: 79–80.

288. Apt A. Circumcision and prostatic cancer. Acta Med Scand 1965; 178: 493–504.

289. Jensen MS. Cancer of the penis in Denmark 1942 to 1962 (511 cases). Dan Med Bull 1977; 24: 66–72.

290. Tsen HF, Morgenstern H, Mack T, et al. Risk factors for penile cancer: results of a population-based case–control study in Los Angeles County (United States). Cancer Causes Control 2001; 12: 267–277.

291. Gross G, Pfister H. Role of human papilloma virus in penile cancer, penile intraepithelial squamous cell

neoplasias and in genital warts. Med Microbiol Immunol (Berl) 2004; 193: 35–44.

292. Ferreux E, Lont AP, Horenblas S, et al. Evidence for at least three alternative mechanisms targeting the p16$^{ink4A}$/cyclin D/Rb pathway in penile carcinoma, one of which is mediated by high-risk human papilloma virus. J Pathol 2003; 201; 109–118.

293. Masih AS, Stoler MH, Farrow GM, et al. Human papilloma virus in penile squamous cell lesions: a comparison of an isotopic RNA and two commercial nonisotopic DNA in situ hybridization methods. Arch Pathol Lab Med 1993; 117: 302–307.

294. Scinicariello F, Rady P, Saltzstein D, et al. Human papilloma virus 16 exhibits a similar integration pattern in primary squamous cell carcinoma of the penis and in its metastasis. Cancer 1992; 70: 2143–2148.

295. Starkar FH, Miles BJ, Plieth DM, et al. Detection of human papilloma virus in squamous neoplasm of the penis. J Urol 1992; 147: 389–392.

296. Wiener JS, Effert PJ, Humphrey PA, et al. Prevalence of human papilloma virus types 16 and 18 in squamous cell carcinoma of the penis: a retrospective analysis of primary and metastatic lesions by differential polymerase chain reaction. Int J Cancer 1992; 50: 694–701.

297. Maiche AG, Pyrhonen S. Risk of cervical cancer among wives of men with carcinoma of the penis. Acta Oncol 1990; 29: 569–571.

298. Bezerra AL, Lopes A, Landman G, et al. Clinicopathologic features and human papilloma virus DNA prevalence of warty and squamous cell carcinoma of the penis. Am J Surg Pathol 2001; 25; 673–678.

299. Rubin MA, Kleter B, Zhou M, et al. Detection and typing of human papilloma virus DNA in penile carcinoma: evidence for multiple independent pathways of penile carcinogenesis. Am J Pathol 2001; 159: 1211–1218.

300. Villa LL, Lopes A. Human papilloma virus DNA sequences in penile carcinomas in Brazil. Int J Cancer 1986; 37: 853–855.

301. Zur Hausen H. Papilloma viruses in human cancers. Mol Carcinog 1988; 1: 147–150.

302. Obalek S, Jablonska S, Beaudenon S, et al. Bowenoid papulosis of the male and female genitalia: risk of cervical neoplasia. J Am Acad Dermatol 1986; 14: 433–444.

303. Solivan GA, Smith KJ, James WD. Cutaneous horn of the penis: its association with squamous cell carcinoma and HPV-16 infection. J Am Acad Dermatol 1990; 23: 969–972.

304. Rosemberg SK, Herman G, Elfont E. Sexually transmitted papillomaviral infection in males. VII. Is cancer of penis sexually transmitted? Urology 1991; 37: 437–440.

305. Stern RS, and Members of the Photochemotherapy Follow-up Study. Genital tumors among men with psoriasis exposed to psoralens and ultraviolet A radiation (PUVA) and ultraviolet B radiation. N Engl J Med 1990; 332: 1093–1097.

306. Droller MJ. Carcinoma of penis: an overview. Urol Clin North Am 1980; 7: 783–784.

307. Jones WG, Hamers H, Van Den Bogaert W. Penis cancer. A review by the joint radiotherapy committee of the European Organization for Research and Treatment of Cancer (EORTC) Genitourinary and Radiotherapy Groups. J Surg Oncol 1989; 40: 227–231.

308. Fossa SD, Hall KS, Johannessen NB, et al. Cancer of the penis. Eur Urol 1987; 13: 372–377.

309. Burgers JK, Badalament RA, Drago JR. Penile cancer: clinical presentation, diagnosis, and staging. Urol Clin North Am 1992; 19: 247–256.

310. Derrick FC Jr, Lynch KM Jr, Kretkowski RC, et al. Epidermoid carcinoma of the penis: computer analysis of 87 cases. J Urol 1973; 110: 303–305.

311. Lucia MS, Miller GJ. Histopathology of malignant lesions of the penis. Urol Clin North Am 1992; 19: 227–246.

312. Maiche AG, Pyrhonen S, Karkinen M. Histological grading of squamous cell carcinoma of the penis. A new grading system. Br J Urol 1991; 67: 522–526.

313. Bissada NK, Yakout HH, Fahmy WE, et al. Multi-institutional long-term experience with conservative surgery for invasive penile carcinoma. J Urol 2003; 169: 500–502.

314. Velazquez EF, Soskin A, Bock A, et al. Positive resection margins in partial penectomies. Site of involvement and proposal of local routes of spread of penile squamous cell carcinoma. Am J Surg Pathol 2004; 28; 384–389.

315. Pow-Sang JE, Benavente V, Pow-Sang JM, et al. Bilateral inguinal lymph node dissection in the management of cancer of the penis. Semin Surg Oncol 1990; 6: 241–242.

316. Ornellas AA, Seixas ALC, de Moraes JR. Analysis of 200 lymphadenectomies in patients with penile carcinoma. J Urol 1991; 146: 330–332.

317. Srinivas V, Joshi A, Agarwal B, et al. Penile cancer – the sentinel lymph node controversy. Urol Int 1991; 47: 108–109.

318. Horenblas S, van Tinteren H, Delemarre JFM, et al. Squamous cell carcinoma of the penis. III. Treatment of regional lymph nodes. J Urol 1993; 149: 492–497.

319. Young MJ, Reda DJ, Waters WB. Penile carcinoma: a twenty-five-year experience. Urology 1991; 38: 529–532.

320. Maiche AG, Pyrhonen S. Clinical staging of cancer of the penis: by size? by localization? or by depth of infiltration ? Eur Urol 1990; 18: 16–22.

321. Fraley EE, Zhang G, Manivel C, et al. The role of ilioinguinal lymphadenectomy and significance of histological differentiation in treatment of carcinoma of the penis. J Urol 1989; 142: 1478–1482.

322. Ayyappan K, Ananthakrishnan N, Sankaran V. Can regional lymph node involvement be predicted in patients with carcinoma of the penis? Br J Urol 1994; 73: 549–553.

323. Horenblas S, van Tinteren H. Squamous cell carcinoma of the penis. IV. Prognostic factors of survival: analysis of tumor, nodes and metastasis classification system. J Urol 1994; 151: 1239–1243.

324. Cubilla AL, Barreto J, Caballero C, et al. Pathologic features of epidermoid carcinoma of the penis: a prospective study of 66 cases. Am J Surg Pathol 1993; 17: 753–763.

325. Emerson RE, Ulbright TM, Eble JN, et al. Predicting cancer progression in patients with penile squamous cell carcinoma. The importance of depth of invasion more than 6mm and vascular invasion. Mod Pathol 2001; 14: 963–968.

326. Velazquez EF, Barreto JE, Rodriquez I, et al. Limitations in the interpretation of biopsies in patients with penile squamous cell carcinoma. Int J Surg Pathol 2004; 12: 139–146.

327. Sanchez-Ortiz RF, Pettaway CA. The role of lymphadenectomy in penile cancer. Urol Oncol 2004; 22: 236–244.

328. Perdona S, Autorino R, De Sio M, et al. Dynamic sentinel node biopsy in clinically node-negative penile cancer versus radical inguinal lymphadenectomy: a comparative study. Urology 2005; 66: 1282–6.

329. Perdona S, Autorino R, Gallo L, et al. Role of dynamic sentinel node biopsy in penile cancer. Our experience. J Surg Oncol 2006; 93: 181–185.

330. Kroon BK, Lont AP, Valdes Olmos RA, et al. Morbidity of dynamic sentinel node biopsy in penile carcinoma. J Urol 2005; 173: 813–815.

331. Kroon BK, Horenblas S, Lont AP, et al. Patients with penile carcinoma benefit from immediate resection of clinically occult lymph node metastases. J Urol 2005; 173: 816–819.

332. Izawa J, Kedar D, Wong F, Pattaway CA. Sentinel lymph node biopsy in penile cancer: evolution and insights. Can J Urol 2005; 12: 24–29.

333. Tabatabaei S, Harisinghani M, McDougal WS. Regional lymph node staging using lymphotropic nanoparticle enhanced magnetic resonance imaging with ferumoxtran-10 in patients with penile cancer. J Urol 2005; 174: 923–927.

334. Ficarra V, Zattoni F, Cunico SC, et al. Lymphatic and vascular embolization are independent predictive variables of inguinal lymph node involvement in patients with squamous cell carcinoma of the penis. Gruppo Uro-Oncologico del Nord Est (Northeast Uro-

Oncological Group) Penile Cancer Data Base data. Cancer 2005; 103: 2507–2516.

335. Pandey D, Mahajan V, Kannan RR. Prognostic factors in node-positive carcinoma of the penis. J Surg Oncol 2006; 93: 133–138.

336. Lynch D, Schellhammer PF. Tumors of the penis. In: Walsh PC, Retik AB, Vaughan ED, et al., eds. Campbell's urology, 7th edn. Philadelphia: WB Saunders, 1998.

337. Johnson DE, Fuerst DE, Ayala AG. Cancer of the penis: experience with 153 cases. Urology 1973; 1: 404–408.

338. Bezerra ALR, Lopes A, Santiago GH, et al. Human papilloma virus as a prognostic factor in carcinoma of the penis. Analysis of 82 patients treated with amputation and bilateral lymphadenectomy. Cancer 2001; 91: 2315–2321.

339. Jackson SM. The treatment of carcinoma of the penis. Br J Surg 1966; 53: 33–35.

340. Greene FL, Page DL, Fleming ID, et al. American Joint Committee on Cancer. Cancer staging manual, 6th edn. Philadelphia: Springer Verlag, 2002.

341. Nitti VW, Macchia RJ. Neoplasms of the penis. In: Hashmat AI, Das S, eds. The penis. Philadelphia: Lea and Febiger, 1993.

342. Yu DS, Chang SY, Ma CP. DNA ploidy, S-phase fraction and cytomorphometry in relation to survival of human penile cancer. Urol Int 1992; 48: 265–269.

343. Gustafsson O, Tribukait B, Nyman CR, et al. DNA pattern and histopathology of penis. A prospective study. Scand J Urol Nephrol 1988; 110: 219–222.

344. Hoofnagle RF, Mahin EJ, Lamm DL, et al. Deoxyribonucleic acid flow cytometry of squamous cell carcinoma of the penis. J Urol 1990; 143: 352A.

345. Pettaway CA, Stewart D, Vuitch F, et al. Penile squamous carcinoma. DNA flow cytometry versus histopathology for prognosis. J Urol 1991; 145: 367A.

346. Busby JE, Pettaway CA. What's new in the management of penile cancer? Curr Opin Urol 2005; 15: 350–357.

347. McDougal WS. Advances in the treatment of carcinoma of the penis. Urology 2005; 66: 114–117.

348. Singh AK, Saokar A, Hahn PF, Harisinghani MG. Imaging of penile neoplasms. Radiographics 2005; 25: 1629–1638.

349. Minhas S, Kayes O, Hegarty P, et al. What surgical resection margins are required to achieve oncological control in men with primary penile cancer? BJU Int 2005; 96: 1040–1043.

350. Siow WY, Cheng C. Penile cancer: current challenges. Can J Urol 2005; 12: 18–23.

351. Cubilla AL, Reuter VE, Gregoire L, et al. Basaloid squamous cell carcinoma. A distinctive human papilloma virus-related penile neoplasm. A report of 20 cases. Am J Surg Pathol 1998; 22; 755–761.

352. Cubilla AL, Velazques EF, Reuter VE, et al. Warty (condylomatous) squamous cell carcinoma of the penis. Am J Surg Pathol 2000; 24: 505–512.

353. Davis SW. Giant condyloma acuminata: incidence among cases diagnosed as carcinoma of the penis. J Clin Pathol 1965; 18: 142–149.

354. Johnson DE, Lo RK, Srigley J, et al. Verrucous carcinoma of the penis. J Urol 1985; 133: 216–218.

355. McKee PH, Lowe D, Haigh RJ. Penile verrucous carcinoma. Histopathology 1983; 7: 897–906.

356. Kraus FT, Perez-Mesa C. Verrucous carcinoma. Clinical and pathologic study of 105 cases involving oral cavity, larynx, and genitalia. Cancer 1966; 19: 26–38.

357. Yeager JK, Findlay RF, McAleer IM. Penile verrucous carcinoma. Arch Dermatol 1990; 126: 1208–1210.

358. Blessing K, McLaren K, Lessells A. Viral etiology for verrucous carcinoma. Histopathology 1986; 10: 1101–1102.

359. Masih AS, Stoler MH, Farrow GM, et al. Penile verrucous carcinoma: a clinicopathologic, human papilloma virus typing and flow cytometric analysis. Mod Pathol 1992; 5: 48–55.

360. Noel JC, Vandenbossche M, Peny MO, et al. Verrucous carcinoma of the penis: importance of human papilloma virus typing for diagnosis and therapeutic decision. Eur Urol 1992; 22: 83–85.

361. de Villiers EM, Schneider A, Gross G, et al. Analysis of benign and malignant urogenital tumors for human papilloma virus infection by labelling cellular DNA. Med Microbiol Immunol 1986; 174: 281–286.

362. Gissmann L, de Villiers EM, zur Hausen H. Analysis of human genital warts (condylomata acuminata) and other genital tumors for human papilloma virus type 6 DNA. Int J Cancer 1982; 29: 143–146.

363. Saeed S, Keehn CA, Khalil FK, Morgan MB. Immunohistochemical expression of Bax and Bcl-2 in penile carcinoma. Ann Clin Lab Sci 2005; 35: 91–96.

364. Fukunaga M, Yokoi K, Miyazawa Y, et al. Penile verrucous carcinoma with anaplastic transformation following radiotherapy. Am J Surg Pathol 1994; 18: 501–505.

365. Manglani KS, Manaligod JR, Biswamay R. Spindle cell carcinoma of the glans penis: a light and electron microscopic study. Cancer 1980; 46: 2266–2272.

366. Wood EW, Gardner WA Jr, Brown FM. Spindle cell squamous carcinoma of the penis. J Urol 1972; 107: 990–991.

367. Velazquez EF, Melamed J, Barreto JE, et al. Sarcomatoid carcinoma of the penis: a clinicopathologic study of 15 cases. Am J Surg Pathol 2005; 29: 1152–1158.

368. Lont AP, Gallee MP, Snijders P, Horenblas S. Sarcomatoid squamous cell carcinoma of the penis: a clinical and pathological study of 5 cases. J Urol 2004; 172: 932–935.

369. Medina JE, Dichtel W, Luna MA. Verrucous–squamous carcinomas of the oral cavity: a clinicopathologic study of 104 cases. Arch Otolaryngol Head Neck Surg 1984; 110: 437–440.

370. Layfield LJ, Liu K. Mucoepidermoid carcinoma arising in the glans penis. Arch Pathol Lab Med 2000; 124: 148–151.

371. Liegl B, Regauer S. Penile clear cell carcinoma: a report of 5 cases of a distinct entity. Am J Surg Pathol 2004; 28: 1513–1517.

372. Rahbari H, Mehregan AH. Basal cell epitheliomas in usual and unusual sites. J Cutan Pathol 1979; 6: 425–431.

373. Hall TC, Britt DB, Woodhead DM. Basal cell carcinoma of the penis. J Urol 1968; 99: 314–315.

374. McGregor DH, Tanimura A, Weigel JW. Basal cell carcinoma of penis. Urology 1982; 20: 320–323.

375. Goldminz D, Scott G, Klaus S. Penile basal cell carcinoma. Report of a case and review of the literature. J Am Acad Dermatol 1989; 20: 1094–1097.

376. Manavi K, Kemmett D. A case of penile superficial basal cell carcinoma involving the inner surface of foreskin. Int J STD AIDS 2005; 16: 766–767.

377. Stillwell TJ, Zincke H, Gaffey TA, et al. Malignant melanoma of the penis. J Urol 1988; 140: 72–75.

378. Oldbring J, Mikulowski P. Malignant melanoma of the penis and male urethra. Report of nine cases and review of the literature. Cancer 1987; 59: 581–587.

379. Begun FP, Grossman HB, Diokno AC, et al. Malignant melanoma of the penis and male urethra. J Urol 1984; 132: 123–125.

380. Manivel JC, Fraley EE. Malignant melanoma of the penis and male urethra: 4 case reports and literature review. J Urol 1988; 139: 813–816.

381. Johnson DE, Ayala AG. Primary melanoma of the penis. Urology 1973; 2: 174–177.

382. Rashid AMH, Williams RM, Horton LWL. Malignant melanoma of penis and male urethra: is it a difficult tumor to diagnose? Urology 1993; 41: 470–471.

383. Sanchez-Ortiz R, Huang SF, Tamboli P, et al. Melanoma of the penis, scrotum and male urethra: a 40-year single institution experience. J Urol 2005; 173: 1958–1965.

384. Betti R, Menni S, Crosti C. Melanoma of the glans penis. Eur J Dermatol 2005; 15: 113–115.

385. Konigsberg HA, Gray GF. Benign melanosis and malignant melanoma of penis and male urethra. Urology 1976; 7: 323–326.

386. Jaeger N, Wirtler H, Tschubel K. Acral lentiginous melanoma of penis. Eur Urol 1982; 8: 182–184.

387. Saw D, Tse CH, Chan J, et al. Clear cell sarcoma of the penis. Hum Pathol 1986; 17: 423–425.

388. Ormsby AH, Liou LS, Oriba HA, et al. Epithelioid sarcoma of the penis:

report of an unusual case and review of the literature. Ann Diagn Pathol 2000; 4: 88–94.

389. Corsi A, Perugia G, De Matteis A. Epithelioid sarcoma of the penis. Clinicopathologic study of a tumor with myogenic features and review of the literature concerning this unusual location. Pathol Res Pract 1999; 195: 441–448;.

390. Dehner LP, Smith BH. Soft tissue tumors of the penis. A clinicopathologic study of 46 cases. Cancer 1970; 25: 1431–1447.

391. Casado M, Jimenez F, Borbujo J, et al. Spontaneous healing of Kaposi's angiosarcoma of the penis. J Urol 1988; 139: 1313–1315.

392. Lowe FC, Lattimer G, Metroka CE. Kaposi's sarcoma of the penis in patients with acquired immunodeficiency syndrome. J Urol 1989; 142: 1475–1477.

393. Bayne P, Wise G. Kaposi sarcoma of penis and genitalia. a disease of our times, Urology 31: 22–25, 1988.

394. Saftel AD, Sadick NS, Waldbaum RS. Kaposi's sarcoma of the penis in a patient with the acquired immunodeficiency syndrome. J Urol 1986; 136: 673–675.

395. Pacifico A, Piccolo D, Fargnoli MC, Peris K. Kaposi's sarcoma of the glans penis in an immunocompetent patient. Eur J Dermatol 2003; 13: 182–583.

396. Micali G, Nasca MR, De Pasquale R, Innocenzi D. Primary classic Kaposi's sarcoma of the penis: report of a case and review. J Eur Acad Dermatol Venereol 2003; 17: 320–323.

397. Morelli L, Pusiol T, Piscioli F, et al. Herpesvirus 8-associated penile Kaposi's sarcoma in an HIV-negative patient: first report of a solitary lesion. Am J Dermatopathol 2003; 25: 28–31.

398. Vapnek JM, Quivey JM, Carroll PR. Acquired immunodeficiency syndrome-related Kaposi's sarcoma of the male genitalia: management with radiation therapy. J Urol 1991; 146: 333–336.

399. Lands RH, Ange D, Hartman DL. Radiation therapy for classic Kaposi's sarcoma presenting only on the glans penis. J Urol 1992; 147: 468–470.

400. Rasbridge SA, Parry JRW. Angiosarcoma of the penis. Br J Urol 1989; 63: 440–441.

401. Weiss SW, Enzinger FM. Epithelioid hemangioendothelioma: a vascular tumor often mistaken for a carcinoma. Cancer 1982; 50: 970–981.

402. Deutsch M, Lee RLS, Mercado R. Hemangioendothelioma of the penis with late appearing metastases: report of a case with review of the literature. J Surg Oncol 1973; 5: 27–34.

403. Calonje E, Fletcher CDM, Wilson-Jones E, et al. Retiform hemangioendothelioma: a distinctive form of low-grade angiosarcoma delineated in a series of 15 cases. Am J Surg Pathol 1994; 18: 115–125.

404. Fetsch JF, Davis CJ, Miettinen M, Sesterhenn IA. Leiomyosarcoma of the penis. A clinicopathologic study of 14 cases with review of the literature and discussion of the differential diagnosis. Am J Surg Pathol 2004; 28; 115–125.

405. Dominici A, Delle Rose A, Stomaci N, et al. A rare case of leiomyosarcoma of the penis with a reappraisal of the literature. Int J Urol 2004; 11: 440–444.

406. Antunes AA, Nesrallah LJ, Goncalves PD, et al. Deep-seated sarcomas of the penis. Int Braz J Urol 2005; 31: 245–250.

407. Mendis D, Bott SR, Davies JH. Subcutaneous leiomyosarcoma of the frenulum. Sci World J 2005; 5: 571–575.

408. Pow-sang MR, Orihuela E. Leiomyosarcoma of the penis. J Urol 1994; 151: 1643–1645.

409. Wilson LS, Lockhart JL, Bergman H, et al. Fibrosarcoma of the penis. Case report and review of the literature. J Urol 1983; 129: 606–607.

410. Pandit GA, Kudrimoti JK, Kokandakar HR, Bhople KS. Fibrosarcoma of penis – a case report. Indian J Pathol Microbiol 2004; 47: 389–390.

411. Parsons MA, Fox M. Malignant fibrous histiocytoma of the penis. Eur Urol 1988; 14: 75–76.

412. Fletcher CDM, Lowe D. Inflammatory fibrous histiocytoma. Histopathology 1984; 8: 1079–1084.

413. Dalkin B, Zaontz MR. Rhabdomyosarcoma of the penis in children. J Urol 1989; 141: 908–909.

414. Pak K, Sakaguchi N, Takayama H, et al. Rhabdomyosarcoma of the penis. J Urol 1986; 136: 438–439.

415. Huang DJ, Stanisic TH, Hansen KK. Epithelioid sarcoma of the penis. J Urol 1992; 147: 1370–1372.

416. Gower RL, Pambakian H, Fletcher CDM. Epithelioid sarcoma of the penis: a rare tumour to be distinguished from squamous carcinoma. Br J Urol 1987; 59: 592–593.

417. Guillo L, Wadden C, Coindre JM, et al. 'Proximal-type' epithelioid sarcoma: a distinctive aggressive neoplasm showing rhabdoid features. Clinicopathologic, immunohistochemical, and ultrastructural study of a series. Am J Surg Pathol 1997; 21: 130–146.

418. Corsi A, Perugia G, de Matteis A. Epithelioid sarcoma of the penis. Clinicopathologic study with myogenic features and review of the literature concerning this unusual location. Pathol Res Pract 1999; 195: 441–448.

419. Bacetic D, Knezevic M, Stojsic Z, et al. Primary extraskeletal osteosarcoma of the penis with a malignant fibrous histiocytoma-like component. Histopathology 1988; 33: 185–186.

420. Arena F, di Stefano C, Peracchia G, et al. Primary lymphoma of the penis. Diagnosis and treatment. Eur Urol 2001; 39: 232–235;.

421. Thorns C, Urban H, Remmler K, et al. Primary cutaneous T-cell lymphoma of the penis. Histopathology 2003; 42: 513–514.

422. Haque S, Noble J, Wotherspoon A, et al. MALT lymphoma of the foreskin. Leuk Lymphoma 2004; 45: 1699–701.

423. Tu SM, Reyes A, Maa A, et al. Prostate carcinoma with testicular or penile metastases. Clinical, pathologic, and immunohistochemical features. Cancer 2002; 94: 2610–2617.

424. Dutt N, Bates AW, Baithun SI. Secondary neoplasms of the male genital tract with different patterns of involvement in adults and children. Histopathology 2000; 37: 323–331.

425. Perez-Mesa C, Oxenhandler R. Metastatic tumors of the penis. J Surg Oncol 1989; 42: 11–15.

426. Haddad FS. Penile metastases secondary to bladder cancer. Review of the literature. Urol Int 1984; 39: 125–142.

427. Robey EL, Schellhammer PF. Four cases of metastases to the penis and review of the literature. J Urol 1984; 132: 992–994.

428. Khubchandani M. Metachronous metastasis to the penis from carcinoma of the rectum. Report of a case. Dis Colon Rectum 1986; 29: 52–54.

429. 429. Pomara G, Pastina I, Simone M, et al. Penile metastasis from primary transitional cell carcinoma of the renal pelvis: first manifestation of systemic spread. BMC Cancer 2004; 4: 90.

430. Bordeau KP, Lynch DF. Transitional cell carcinoma of the bladder metastatic to the penis. Urology 2004; 63: 981–983.

431. Vilmaz E, Batislam E, Altinok G, et al. Isolated late penile metastasis of an adenocarcinoma of the rectum. Urol Int 2004; 72: 261–263.

432. Hashimoto H, Saga Y, Watabe Y, et al. Case report: secondary penile carcinoma. Urol Int 989; 44: 56–57.

433. Ordonez NG, Ayala AG, Bracken RB. Renal cell carcinoma metastatic to penis. Urology 1982; 19: 417–419.

434. Perez LM, Shumway RA, Carson CC, et al. Penile metastasis secondary to supraglottic squamous cell carcinoma: review of the literature. J Urol 1992; 147: 157–160.

435. Adjiman S, Flam TA, Zerbib M, et al. Delayed nonurothelial metastatic lesions to the penis. A report of two cases. Eur Urol 1989; 16: 391–392.

436. Powell FC, Venencie PY, Winkelmann RK. Metastatic prostate carcinoma manifesting as penile nodules. Arch Dermatol 1984; 20: 1604–1606.

437. Paquin AJ, Roland SI. Secondary carcinoma of the penis: a review of the literature and a report of nine new cases. Cancer 1956; 9: 626–632.

438. Mukamel E, Farrer J, Smith RB, et al. Metastatic carcinoma to penis: when is total penectomy indicated? Urology 1987; 29: 15–18.

439. Grimm MO, Spiegelhalder P, Heep H, et al. Penile metastasis secondary to follicular thyroid carcinoma. Scand J Urol Nephrol 2004; 38: 253–255.

440. Paty R, Smith AD. Gangrene and Fournier's gangrene. Urol Clin North Am 1992; 19: 149–162.

441. Ecker KW, Derouet H, Omlor G, et al. Fournier's gangrene. Chirurgie 1993; 64: 58–62.

442. de Roos WK, van Lanschot JJ, Bruining HA. Fournier's gangrene: the need for early recognition and radical surgical debridement. Neth J Surg 1991; 43: 184–188.

443. Chintamani, Shankar M, Singhal V, et al. Squamous cell carcinoma developing in the scar of Fournier's gangrene – case report. BMC Cancer 2004; 4: 16.

444. Corbus BC, Harris FG. Erosive and gangrenous balanitis. The fourth venereal disease. JAMA 1909; 52: 1474–1477.

445. Barile MF, Blumberg JM, Kraul CW, et al. Penile lesions among US Armed Forces personnel in Japan. The prevalence of herpes simplex and the role of pleuropneumonia-like organisms. Arch Dermatol 1962; 86: 273–281.

446. Schneider PR, Russell RC, Zook EG. Fournier's gangrene of the penis: a report of two cases. Ann Plast Surg 1986; 17: 87–90.

447. Jayachandran S, Mooppan UMM, Kim H. Complications from external (condom) urinary drainage devices. Urology 1985; 25: 31–34.

448. Sheinfeld J, Cos LR, Etruck E, et al. Penile tourniquet injury due to a coil of hair. J Urol 1985; 133: 1042–1043.

449. Lane JE. Hidrosadenitis axillaris of Verneuil. Arch Dermatol Syphilol 1933; 28: 609–614.

450. Brunsting HA. Hidradenitis and other variants of acne. Arch Dermatol Syphilol 1952; 65: 303–315.

451. Shelly WB, Cahn MM. The pathogenesis of hidradenitis suppurativa in man. Arch Dermatol 1955; 72: 562–565.

452. Curry SS, Gaither DH, King LE Jr. Squamous cell carcinoma arising in dissecting perifolliculitis of the scalp. J Am Acad Dermatol 1981; 4: 673–678.

453. Moyer DG, Williams RM. Perifolliculitis capitis abscedens et suffodiens. Arch Dermatol 1962; 85: 378–384.

454. Banerjee AK. Surgical treatment of hidradenitis suppurativa. Br J Surg 1992; 79: 863–866.

455. Shapiro L, Platt N, Torres-Rodriguez VM. Idiopathic calcinosis of the scrotum. Arch 1970; 102: 199–204.

456. Swinehart JM, Golitz LE. Scrotal calcinosis. Dystrophic calcification of epidermoid cysts. Arch Dermatol 1982; 118: 985–988.

457. Dare AJ, Axelsen RA. Scrotal calcinosis: origin from dystrophic calcification of eccrine duct milia. J Cutan Pathol 1988; 15: 142–149.

458. Turksoy O, Ozcan N, Tokgoz H. Extratesticular scrotal calcifications. their relationship. J Ultrasound Med 2006; 25: 141–142.

459. Tosun Z, Karaçor Z, Özkan A, Toy H, Savac N. Two scrotal calcinosis cases with different causal mechanisms. Plast Reconstr Surg 2005; 116: 1834–1835.

460. Saladi RN, Persaud AN, Phelps RG, Cohen SR. Scrotal calcinosis. Is the cause still unknown? J Am Acad Dermatol 2004; 51: 97.

461. Kaskas M, Dabrowski A, Sabbah M, et al. Idiopathic calcinosis of the scrotum. Apropos of a case. Review of the literature. J Urol (Paris) 1991; 97: 287–290.

462. Song DH, Lee KH, Kang WH. Idiopathic calcinosis of the scrotum: histopathologic observations of fifty-one nodules. J Am Acad Dermatol 1988; 19: 1095–1101.

463. Akosa AB, Gilliland EA, Ali MH, et al. Idiopathic scrotal calcinosis: a possible aetiology reaffirmed. Br J Plast Surg 1989; 42: 324–327.

464. Fetsch JF, Montgomery EA, Meis JM. Calcifying fibrous pseudotumor. Am J Surg Pathol 1993; 17: 502–508.

465. Matsuchima M, Tajima M, Maki A, et al. Primary lipogranuloma of the male genitalia. Urology 1988; 31: 75–77.

466. Steward RC, Beason ES, Hayes CW. Granulomas of the penis from self-injection with oils. Plast Reconstr Surg 1979; 64: 108–111.

467. Matsuda T, Shichiri Y, Hida S, et al. Eosinophilic sclerosing lipogranuloma of the male genitalia not caused by exogenous lipids. J Urol 1988; 140: 1021–1024.

468. Gilmore JAI, Weingad DA, Burgdorf WHC. Penile nodules in Southeast Asian men. Arch Dermatol 1983; 119: 446–447.

469. Takihara H, Takahashi M, Ueno T, et al. Sclerosing lipogranuloma of the male genitalia: analysis of the lipid constituents and histological study. Br J Urol 1993; 71: 58–62.

470. Lawrentschuk N, Angus D, Bolton DM. Sclerosing lipogranuloma of the genitalia treated with corticosteroids. Int Urol Nephrol 2006; 38: 97–9.

471. Yamamoto S, Maekawa T, Kumata N, et al. Giant epidermoid cyst of the scrotum. Hinyokikakiyo 1992; 38: 1273–1276.

472. Homayoon K, Suhre CD, Steinhardt GF. Epidermal cysts in children: natural history. J Urol 2004; 171: 1274–6.

473. Yang WT, Whitman GJ, Tse GM. Extratesticular epidermal cyst of the scrotum. AJR Am J Roentgenol 2004; 183: 1084.

474. Hollander JB, Begun FP, Lee RD. Scrotal fat necrosis. J Urol 1985; 134: 150–151.

475. Nuciforo PG, Roncalli M. Pathologic quiz case: a scrotal sac mass incidentally discovered during autopsy. Paratesticular hamartoma with angioleiomyomatous features (angioleiomyomatous hyperplasia).

476. van Kooten EO, Hage JJ, Meinhardt W, et al. Acquired smooth-muscle hamartoma of the scrotum: a histological simulator. J Cutan Pathol 2004; 31: 388–392.

477. Oiso N, Fukai K, Ishii M, et al. A case of acquired smooth muscle hamartoma of the scrotum. Clin Exp Dermatol 2005; 30: 523–524.

478. Evans J, Datta MW, Goolsby M, Langenstroer P. Eccrine porocarcinoma of the scrotum. Can J Urol 2005; 12: 2722–2723.

479. Bechara FG, Altmeyer P, Jansen T. Unilateral angiokeratoma scroti: a rare manifestation of a vascular tumor. J Dermatol 2004; 31: 39–41.

480. Kawaguchi H, Tatewaki S, Takeuchi M. A case of polypoid clear cell acanthoma on the scrotum. J Dermatol 2004; 31: 236–238.

481. Lin TP, Pan CC, Huang WJ, Murphy GF. Primary sweat gland carcinosarcoma of the scrotal skin. J Cutan Pathol 2004; 31: 678–682.

482. Damala K, Tsanou E, Pappa L, et al. A rare case of primary malignant melanoma of the scrotum diagnosed by fine-needle aspiration. Diagn Cytopathol 2004; 31: 413–416.

483. Popek EJ, Montgomery EA, Fourcroy JL. Fibrous hamartoma of infancy in the genital region: findings of 15 cases. J Urol 1994; 152: 990–993.

484. Gioglio L, Porta C, Moroni M, et al. Scrotal angiokeratoma (Fordyce): histopathological and ultrastructural findings. Histol Histopathol 1992; 7: 47–55.

485. Slone S, O'Connor D. Scrotal leiomyomas with bizarre nuclei: a report of three cases. Mod Pathol 1998; 11: 282–287.

486. Fadare O, Wang S, Mariappan MR. Pathologic quiz case: a 69-year-old asymptomatic man with a scrotal mass. Atypical (symplastic or bizarre) leiomyoma of the scrotum. Arch Pathol Lab Med 2004; 128: e37–38.

487. Kingsly KA, Sant GR. Images in clinical urology. Scrotal lymphangioma in an adult. Urology 1999; 53: 820–821.

488. Yoshimura K, Maeda O, Saiki S, et al. Solitary neurofibroma. J Urol 1990; 143: 823.

489. Yagmurlu A, Gokcora IH, Duran E, Gollu G. A children's disease of rarity: 'scrotal lymphangioma circumscriptum.' Int Urol Nephrol 2004; 36: 229–233.

490. Celia A, Bruschi M, De Stefani S, et al. Bizarre leiomyoma of scrotum. Arch Ital Urol Androl 2005; 77: 113–114.

491. Turkyilmaz Z, Sonmez K, Karabulut R, et al. A childhood case of intrascrotal neurofibroma with a brief review of the literature. J Pediatr Surg 2004; 39: 1261–1263.

492. Huan Y, Vapnek J, Unger PD. Atypical fibrous histiocytoma of the scrotum. Ann Diagn Pathol 2003; 7: 370–373.

Arch Pathol Lab Med 2003; 127: 239–240.

493. Somers GR, Teshima I, Nasr A, et al. Intrascrotal lipoblastoma with a complex karyotype: a case report and review of the literature. Arch Pathol Med 2004; 128: 797–800.

494. Hanna SJ, Muneer A, Coghill SB, Miller MA. Ganglioneuromas in the adult scrotum. J Roy Coll Med 2005; 98: 63–64.

495. Craig E, Rodriguez R, Ruben B. Granular cell tumor of the scrotum. Dermatol Online J 2005; 11: 25.

496. Parys BT, Hutton JL. Fifteen-year experience of carcinoma of the scrotum. Br J Urol 1991; 68: 414–417.

497. Andrews PE, Farrow GM, Oesterling JE. Squamous cell carcinoma of the scrotum: long-term followup of 14 patients. J Urol 1991; 146: 1299–1304.

498. Gross DJ, Schosser RH. Squamous cell carcinoma of the scrotum. Cutis 1991; 47: 402–404.

499. Best TJ, Metcalfe JB, Moore RB, Nguyen GK. Merkel cell carcinoma of the scrotum. Ann Plast Surg 1994; 33: 83–85.

500. Ribuffo D, Alfano C, Ferrazzoli PS, Scuderi N. Basal cell carcinoma of the penis and scrotum with cutaneous metastases. Scand J Plast Reconstr Surg Hand Surg 2002; 36: 180–182.

501. Aridogan IA, Satar N, Doran E, Tansug MZ. Scrotal skin metastases of renal cell carcinoma: a case report. Acta Chir Belg 2004; 104: 599–600.

502. Laskin WB, Fetsch JF, Mostofi FK. Angiomyofibroblastoma-like tumor of the male genital tract: analysis of 11 cases with comparison to female angiomyofibroblastoma and spindle cell lipoma. Am J Surg Pathol 1998; 1: 6–16.

503. Kim HS, Park SH, Chi JG. Aggressive angiomyxoma of childhood: two unusual cases developed in the scrotum. Pediatr Dev Pathol 2003; 6: 187–191.

504. Tsang WY, Chan JK, Lee KC, et al. Aggressive angiomyxoma occurring in men. Am J Surg Pathol 1992; 16: 1059–1065.

505. Chihara Y, Fujimoto K, Takada S, et al. Aggressive angiomyxoma in the scrotum expressing androgen and progesterone receptors. Int J Urol 2003; 10: 672–675.

506. Dursun H, Bayazit AK, Buyukcelik M, et al. Aggressive angiomyxoma in a child with chronic renal failure. Pediatr Surg Int 2005; 21: 563–565.

507. Pott P. Cancer scroti. In: Hawes L, Clarke W, Collins R, eds. Chirurgical works. London: Longman, 1775.

508. Waldron HA. On the history of scrotal cancer. Ann Roy Coll Surg Engl 1983; 65: 420–422.

509. Taniguchi S, Furukawa M, Kutsuna H, Sowa J, Ishii M. Squamous cell carcinoma of the scrotum. Dermatology 1996; 193: 253–254.

510. Orihuela E, Tyring SK, Pow-Sang M, et al. Development of human papilloma virus type 16 associated squamous cell carcinoma of the scrotum in a patient with Darier's disease treated with systemic isotretinoin. J Urol 1995; 153: 1940–1943.

511. Matsumoto M, Sonobe H, Takeuchi T, et al. Pigmented squamous cell carcinoma of the scrotum associated with a lentigo. Br J Dermatol 2000; 142: 184.

512. Lowe FC. Squamous cell carcinoma of the scrotum. Urol Clin North Am 1992; 19: 397–405.

513. Lowe FC. Squamous cell carcinoma of the scrotum. J Urol 1983; 130: 423–427.

514. Ray B, Whitmore WF. Experience with carcinoma of the scrotum. J Urol 1977; 117: 741–745.

515. Grossman HB, Sogani PC. Basal cell carcinoma of scrotum. Urology 1981; 17: 241–242.

516. Greider HE, Vernon SD. Basal cell carcinoma of the scrotum. A case report and literature review. J Urol 1982; 127: 145–146.

517. Nahass GT, Blauvelt A, Leonardi CL, et al. Basal cell carcinoma of the scrotum. J Am Acad Dermatol 1992; 26: 574–578.

518. Parys BT. Basal cell carcinoma of the scrotum. A rare clinical entity. Br J Urol 1991; 68: 434–435.

519. Handa Y, Kato Y, Ishikawa H, Tomita Y. Giant superficial basal cell carcinoma of the scrotum. Eur J Dermatol 2005; 15: 186–188.

520. Takahashi H. Non-ulcerative basal cell carcinoma arising on the genitalia. J Dermatol 2000; 27: 798–801.

521. Gibson GE, Ahmed I. Perianal and genital basal cell carcinoma. A clinicopathologic review of 51 cases. J Am Acad Dermatol 2001; 45: 68–71.

522. Izikson L, Vanderpool J, Brodsky G, et al. Combined basal cell carcinoma and Langerhans' cell histiocytosis of the scrotum in a patient with occupational exposure to coal tar and dust. Int J Dermatol 2004; 43: 678–680.

523. Ribuffo D, Alfano C, Ferrazzoli PS, Scuderi N. Basal cell carcinoma of the penis and scrotum with cutaneous metastases. Scand J Plast Reconstr Surg Hand Surg 2002; 36: 180–182.

524. Nahass GT, Blauvelt A, Penneys NS. Metastases from basal cell carcinoma of the scrotum. J Am Acad Dermatol 1992; 26: 509–510.

525. Kinoshita R, Yamamoto O, Yasuda H, Tokura Y. Basal cell carcinoma of the scrotum with lymph node metastasis: report of a case and review of the literature. Int J Dermatol 2005; 44: 54–56.

526. Hoch WH. Adenocarcinoma of the scrotum (extramammary Paget's disease). A case report and review of the literature. J Urol 1984; 132: 137–139.

527. Mitsudo S, Nakanishi I, Koss L. Paget's disease of the penis and adjacent skin. Its association with fatal sweat gland carcinoma. Arch Pathol Lab Med 1981; 105: 518–520.

528. Perez MA, Larossa DD, Tomaszewski JE. Paget's disease primarily involving the scrotum. 1989; 63: 970–975.

529. Takahashi Y, Komeda H, Horie M, et al. Paget's disease of the scrotum. Hinyokikakiyo 1988; 34: 1069–1072.

530. Quinn AM, Sienko A, Basrawala Z, Campbell SC. Extramammary Paget disease of the scrotum with features of Bowen disease. Arch Pathol Lab Med 2004; 128: 84–86.

531. Salamanca J, Benito A, Garcia-Penalver C, et al. Paget's disease of the glans penis secondary to transitional cell carcinoma of the bladder: a report of two cases and review of the literature. J Cutan Pathol 2004; 31: 341–345.

532. Kim KJ, Lee DP, Lee MW, et al. Penoscrotal extramammary Paget's disease in a patient with rectal cancer: double primary adenocarcinomas differentiated by immunoperoxidase staining. Am J Dermatopathol 2005; 27: 171–172.

533. Ordonez NG, Awalt H, Mackay B. Mammary and extramammary Paget's disease: an immunohistochemical and ultrastructural study. Cancer 1987; 59: 1173–1183.

534. Kuan SF, Montag AG, Hart J, et al. Differential expression of mucin genes in mammary and extramammary Paget's disease. Am J Surg Pathol 2001; 25: 1469–1477.

535. Egawa K, Honda Y. Simultaneous human papilloma virus 6 (HHP 6)-positive condyloma acuminatum, HPV 31-positive Bowen's disease, and non HPV-associated extramammary Paget's disease coexisting within an area presenting clinically as condyloma acuminatum. Am J Dermatopathol 2005; 27: 439–442.

536. Williamson JD, Maria I, Colome MI, et al. Pagetoid Bowen disease: a report of 2 cases that express cytokeratin 7. Arch Pathol Lab Med 2000; 124: 427–430.

537. Choi YD, Cho NH, Park YS, et al. Lymphovascular and marginal invasion as useful prognostic indicators and the role of c-erbB-2 in patients with male extramammary Paget's disease: a study of 31 patients. J Urol 2005; 174: 561–565.

538. Yang WJ, Kim DS, Im YJ, et al. Extramammary Paget's disease of penis and scrotum. Urology 2005; 65: 972–975.

539. Moon TD, Sarma DP, Rodriguez FH. Leiomyosarcoma of the scrotum. J Am Acad Dermatol 1989; 20: 290–292.

540. Dalton DP, Rushovich AM, Victor TA, Larson R. Leiomyosarcoma of the scrotum in a man who had received scrotal irradiation as a child. J Urol 1988; 139: 136–138.

541. Washecka RM, Sidhu G, Surya B. Leiomyosarcoma of scrotum. Urology 1989; 34: 144–146.

542. Naito S, Kaji S, Kumazawa J. Leiomyosarcoma of the scrotum. Case report and review of literature. Urol Int 1988; 43: 242–244.

543. Desai SR, Angarkar NN. Leiomyosarcoma of the scrotum. Indian J Pathol Microbiol 2003; 46: 212–213.

544. John T, Portenier D, Auster B, et al. Leiomyosarcoma of scrotum – a case report and review of literature. Urology 2006; 67: 424,e213; 424,e15.

545. Persichetti P, Di Lella F, Marangi GF, et al. Leiomyosarcoma of the scrotum arising from the dartos muscle: a rare clinicopathological entity. Vivi 2004; 18: 553–554.

546. Suster S, Wong TY, Moran CA. Sarcomas with combined features of liposarcoma and eiomyosarcoma. Study of two cases of an unusual soft-tissue tumor showing dual lineage differentiation. Am J Surg Pathol 1993; 17: 905–911.

547. Watanabe K, Ogawa A, Komatsu H, et al. Malignant fibrous histiocytoma of the scrotal wall: a case report. J Urol 1988; 140: 151–152.

548. Chan JA, McMenamin ME, Fletcher CD. Synovial sarcoma in older patients: clinicopathological analysis of 32 cases with emphasis on unusual histological features. Histopathology 2003; 43: 72–83.

549. Bajaj P, Aiyer H, Sinha BK, et al. Pitfalls in the diagnosis of epithelioid sarcoma presenting in an unusual site: a case report. Diagn Cytopathol 2001; 24: 36–38.

550. Kochman A, Jablecki J, Rabczynski J. Recurrent primary well-differentiated intrascrotal liposarcoma: case report and review of the literature. Tumori 1999; 85: 135–136.

551. Thanakit V, Nelson SD, Udomsawaengsup S. Round cell liposarcoma of scrotum with indolent course in young adult. J Med Assoc Thai 2005; 88: 1302–1307.

552. Froehner M, Ockert D, Aust DE, et al. Gastrointestinal stromal tumor presenting as a scrotal mass. Int J Urol 2004; 11: 445–447.

553. Papadimitriou JC, Drachenberg CB. Posttraumatic spindle cell nodules. Immunohistochemical and ultrastructural study of two scrotal lesions. Arch Pathol Lab Med 1994; 118: 709–711.

THE LIBRARY
THE LEARNING AND DEVELOPMENT CENTRE
THE CALDERDALE ROYAL HOSPITAL
HALIFAX HX3 0PW

# CHAPTER 16

# The adrenal glands

Ernest E. Lack, Jacqueline A. Wieneke

# Embryology and normal gross anatomy

## Adrenal cortex

The primordium of the adrenal cortex becomes evident at Carnegie stage 14 (approximately 5–7 mm and 32 days) just lateral to the base of the dorsal mesentery near the cranial end of the mesonephros.[1,2] The adrenal cortical primordia are of mesodermal origin, and during development in the late embryo and fetus the portion of the developing cortex that occupies the greatest volume is referred to as the fetal or provisional cortex. This layer of cortex comprises about 80% of the newborn adrenal gland and undergoes marked regression in the first weeks of life; this is shown graphically in Figure 16-1, in which the combined weight of the adrenal glands decreases by almost 50% by the ninth to the 14th week after birth.[3] The adult or definitive cortex forms a much thinner outer zone beneath the adrenal capsule and ultimately becomes the trilayered adrenal cortex of the adult. There is convincing evidence for centripetal migration or displacement of adrenal cortical cells in experimental animals, thus supporting the original cell migration theory of Gottschau,[3] which proposed that migrating adrenal cortical cells were capable of producing all of the major adrenal cortical steroids.

On gross examination the late fetal or neonatal adrenal gland is relatively soft, and in transverse sections there may be rather dark coloration of the fetal zone, which at this stage is quite broad. This dark appearance, shown in Figure 16-2, may be misinterpreted as adrenal hemorrhage or apoplexy. The adrenal glands in newborns have smoother external surfaces than in adults. In the adult, the right adrenal gland is roughly pyramidal and the left is more elongated (Fig. 16-3). Inspection of the intact capsular surface of the gland following removal of periadrenal connective tissue and fat may reveal small capsular extrusions of cortex; some of these are directly connected with the underlying cortex, but others seem to lie free on the capsular surface or unattached in periadrenal fat. Transverse sections of adrenal gland in the adult reveal a bright yellow, relatively uniform cortex with a gray-white medulla that is concentrated in the head and body of the gland (Fig. 16-4). A cuff of cortical cells may be noted partially or entirely surrounding larger tributaries of the adrenal vein. The dorsal surface of the adrenal gland has a longitudinal ridge or crista flanked by medial and lateral extensions or alae (wings). The anterior (or ventral) surface of the adrenal gland is relatively smooth, and it is from this surface of the gland that the adrenal veins exit and drain into the inferior vena cava on the right side and the renal vein on the left. The orientation of the adrenal gland in vivo differs from that depicted in gross photographs of specimens in surgical or autopsy material. As seen in Figure 16-5, the glands are oriented in a more vertical axis with the ridge (or crista) projecting posteriorly and flanked by medial and lateral alae. The thickness of the adult cortex is 2 mm or more throughout

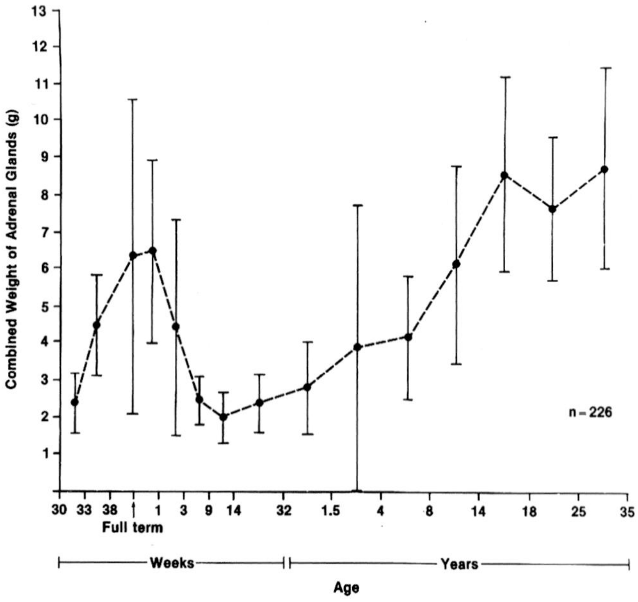

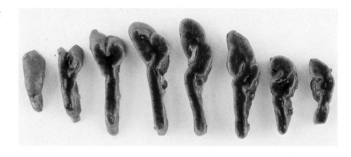

**Fig. 16-2** Adrenal gland from a newborn infant. Note the dark congested fetal (provisional) cortex and thin rim of pale adult (definitive) cortex. Cortical extrusion is also present centrally.

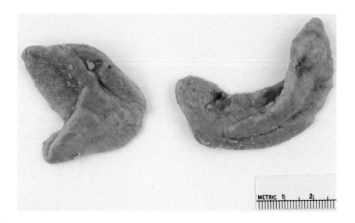

**Fig. 16-3** Normal adrenal glands from an adult. The right is roughly pyramidal (left side of photo), whereas the left is elongated (right side of photo). The longitudinal ridge (crista) is flanked by lateral extensions (alae).

**Fig. 16-1** Average combined weight of the adrenal glands from 226 autopsies by age. Note the marked reduction in combined weight in the first few weeks of life caused by regression of the fetal (provisional) cortex. (From Lack EE, Kozakewich HPW. Embryology, developmental anatomy, and selected aspects of non-neoplastic pathology. In: Lack EE, ed. Pathology of the adrenal glands. New York: Churchill Livingstone, 1990; 1–74.)

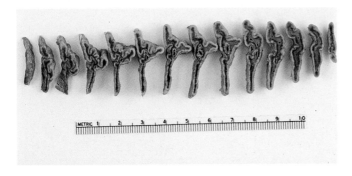

**Fig. 16-4** Normal adrenal from an adult. An incomplete cuff of cortical cells is present around a central adrenal vein in the medulla. The adrenal vein is present on the ventral surface toward the head of the gland. The dorsal ridge (crista) is flanked by lateral and medial extensions (alae). Medullary tissue is concentrated in the body and head and appears gray-white, in contrast to the bright yellow cortex.

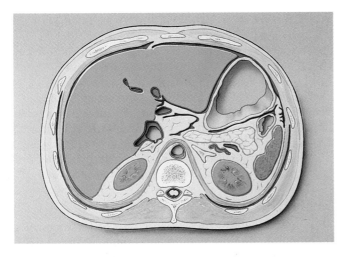

**Fig. 16-5** Diagram of transverse cut of abdomen in an adult showing orientation of the adrenal glands and relation with kidneys. Ventral aspect of both glands is relatively flat while dorsal surface has longitudinal ridge (crista). Lateral extensions (alae) are often referred to as medial and lateral limbs on CT scans.

most of the gland, although there may be some variability from area to area, and cortical nodularity may complicate the morphology.[3]

## Adrenal medulla

Chromaffin tissue of the adrenal medulla in the fetal and newborn adrenal gland is inconspicuous on gross examination of transverse sections of the gland. In the adult, however, chromaffin tissue is concentrated in the body and head of the gland, with the latter regions being directed inferomedially in vivo.[3,4] As seen in Figure 16-6, the ratio of area occupied by cortex relative to that of medulla decreases considerably from the tail to the body and head of the gland. The normal overall ratio of cortex to medulla is about 10:1. The distribution and amount of chromaffin tissue within the gland, as well as other factors such as adrenal weight, may be important in determining whether there is adrenal medullary hyperplasia.[4] Another consideration is morphologic abnormalities of the adrenal cortex, such as adrenal cortical atrophy, which can affect the overall ratio. The adrenal medulla is composed of chromaffin cells derived from primitive sympathicoblasts of neural crest origin that migrate into the dorsomedial aspect of the adrenal primordium and become apparent at Carnegie stages 16 and 17 (approximately 11–14 mm and 41 days).[1,2] Most of the developing chromaffin tissue in fetal life is extra-adrenal, with the largest collections of cells in the para-aortic region, near the origin of the superior mesenteric and renal arteries down to the aortic bifurcation; these chromaffin structures were first characterized in the human fetus by Zuckerkandl[5] in 1901, who referred to them as the aortic bodies.

## Microscopic anatomy

At birth, the thin rim of adult (definitive) cortex blends imperceptibly into cells of the fetal (provisional) cortex. The definitive cortex apparently begins to grow soon after birth,[6] with zonation into the zona glomerulosa and zona fasciculata first appearing at 2–4 weeks. According to some investigators, the zona reticularis appears at about 4 years,[6] but others contend that it appears before 1 year.[7] The zona glomerulosa contains cells with dark round nuclei and rela-

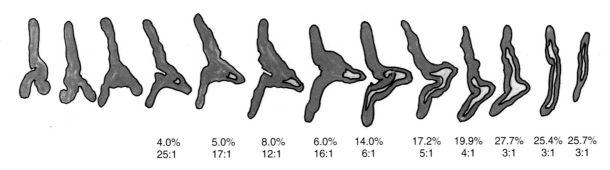

| 4.0% | 5.0% | 8.0% | 6.0% | 14.0% | 17.2% | 19.9% | 27.7% | 25.4% | 25.7% |
| 25:1 | 17:1 | 12:1 | 16:1 | 6:1 | 5:1 | 4:1 | 3:1 | 3:1 | 3:1 |

**Fig. 16-6** Schematic drawing of transverse sections of adrenal gland from an adult. Chromaffin tissue is concentrated in the body and head. Figures indicate the percentage of cross-sectional area occupied by medulla (top row) and ratio of areas of cortex to medulla (bottom row).

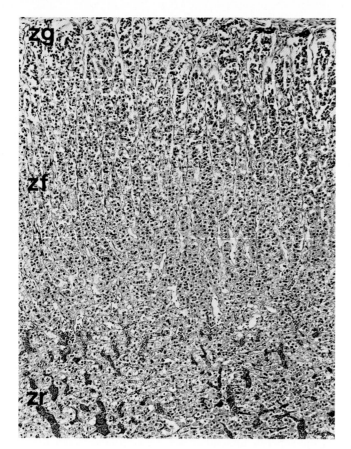

**Fig. 16-7** Normal adult adrenal cortex. Zona glomerulosa (zg) is at top of field beneath the adrenal capsule and forms a thin, discontinuous layer of cells. Most of cortex is occupied by radial interconnecting cords of zona fasciculata (zf), which contain cells with pale-staining, lipid-rich cytoplasm. The zona reticularis (zr) has interconnecting short cords of cells with compact, eosinophilic cytoplasm and congested microvasculature.

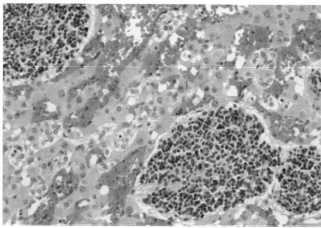

**Fig. 16-8** Neuroblastic nodules in the provisional zone of a 16-week fetal adrenal gland.

tively scant cytoplasm arranged in interlacing cords and spherules; this zone is normally thin, ill-defined, and may appear discontinuous in the normal adult gland (Fig. 16-7). This layer blends imperceptibly into the zona fasciculata, which constitutes most of the adult cortex, and consists of long columns of larger cells with pale finely vacuolated cytoplasm in the unstressed gland. The transition between the innermost zona fasciculata and the zona reticularis contains cells with more compact eosinophilic cytoplasm separated by thin-walled sinusoids and irregular short cords of cells. Reticularis cells may contain prominent granular pigment representing lipofuscin. Chromaffin cells of the adrenal medulla are polyhedral and arranged in short anastomosing cords or nests with a prominent vascular network, or there may be a more solid or diffuse arrangement of cells. Adrenal chromaffin cells secrete predominantly epinephrine, with lesser amounts of norepinephrine.[4] In the fetal and neonatal adrenal, one may encounter small nests of primitive neuroblastic cells (Fig. 16-8), which may be a part of normal developmental anatomy[3,4] (see discussion under In situ neuroblastoma, later in this chapter).

The zona glomerulosa is the site of aldosterone production and is responsive to stimulation by angiotensin as well

as adrenocorticotrophic hormone (ACTH). The zona fasciculata produces corticosteroids such as cortisol, whereas the zona reticularis is responsible for sex steroid production. Longitudinal pillars of smooth muscle are found predominantly in the head of the adrenal gland around tributaries of the adrenal vein, and are thought to act as 'sluice gates' that retard the flow of blood from the medullary venous sinuses and plexus reticularis during muscle contraction.[8] The muscular bundles may help to regulate medullary blood flow and may influence the degree of congestion in the zona reticularis and zona fasciculata of the adjacent cortex.

## Examination of the adrenal glands

Examination of the intact adrenal gland is best accomplished by careful removal of as much investing connective tissue and fat as possible in order to obtain an accurate weight. The weight of the cleanly dissected gland may provide valuable information regarding adrenal cortical or medullary pathology. In the study by Stoner et al.,[6] the average combined weight of the adrenal glands at birth was 10 g (range, 2–17 g), whereas the average weight was 6 g at 7 days of age and 5 g at 2 weeks of age. Quinan and Berger[9] studied the adult adrenal, concentrating on ostensibly healthy subjects who had died suddenly, and found that the average weight of each gland was 4.15 g with no significant difference between the right and left sides. Studzinski et al.[10] examined surgically removed adrenal glands from women with breast cancer and reported an average weight of 4 g, with little variation (standard deviation, 0.8 g). Adrenal glands obtained at autopsy from individuals who had not died suddenly or unexpectedly tended to be heavier, with an average individual weight of 6 g; this difference was attributed to the stress of illness and the trophic influence of endogenous ACTH.[10] Using these data, each normal adrenal gland should weigh less than 6 g, provided excess periadrenal fat and connective tissue are carefully removed.

# Congenital abnormalities

## Adrenal aplasia and hypoplasia

Complete bilateral adrenal aplasia is rare and may occur in a familial setting.[11] There are four forms of congenital adrenal hypoplasia: a sporadic form associated with hypopituitarism; an autosomal recessive form; an X-linked cytomegalic form associated with hypogonadotropic hypogonadism; and a form associated with glycerol kinase deficiency.[12,13] The hereditary form is divided into a miniature type, which affects both sexes and causes extremely small adrenal glands with normal architecture, and the more common cytomegalic type, which has an X-linked pattern of inheritance.[3] In the cytomegalic type, affected males have small adrenal glands that are architecturally abnormal and contain scattered cytomegalic cells that are sometimes vacuolated and may contain intranuclear pseudoinclusions. The onset of adrenal cortical insufficiency is variable and depends chiefly on the endocrine reserve of the existing adrenal cortex. Affected infants may present in the newborn period with weight loss, vomiting, dehydration, and a tendency towards severe salt loss. Prompt recognition of this rare adrenoprival condition results in improved survival. Males with the X-linked cytomegalic form of adrenal hypoplasia typically have hypogonadotropic hypogonadism in adolescence. A recently discovered mutation in the DAX-1 gene gives rise to X-linked adrenal hypoplasia congenita and is also believed to play a role in hypogonadotropic hypogonadism.[14-18] Adrenal insufficiency has also been reported in several other conditions, including familial glucocorticoid deficiency, glycerol kinase deficiency, and selective hypoaldosteronism.[3]

## Adrenal heterotopia

During embryologic development the adrenal primordium is in close proximity to the urogenital ridge, accounting for the accessory and heterotopic adrenal tissue that may occur in sites in the upper abdomen and along lines of descent of the gonads.[3] Heterotopic adrenal tissue has been described in up to 32% of patients in the region of the celiac axis, and at this site about half of the lesions contained both cortex and medulla.[19] Accessory adrenal tissue in sites further removed from the upper abdomen usually consists of cortical tissue alone, without the distinctive zones of the normal adult adrenal gland. Other sites of heterotopia include the broad ligament near the ovary (23%),[20] kidney (6%, usually subcapsular),[21] along the spermatic cord (3.8–9.3%; higher incidence observed for males undergoing surgery for an undescended testis),[22,23] the testicular adnexa (7.5%),[24] and other rarely described sites that defy ready embryologic explanation, such as the placenta,[25] lung,[26,27] and an intracranial intradural location.[28] Only rarely have intratesticular[29] or intraovarian[30] cortical rests occurred within the substance of the gonads. There have been reports of hyperplastic cortical nodules arising from accessory adrenal tissue along the spermatic cord and the broad ligament,[31] and adenomas have rarely been reported in hepatic parenchyma[32] and the spinal canal.[33]

## Union and adhesion

Union or adhesion of the adrenal gland to kidney or liver has also been reported, the distinction being whether or not a continuous connective tissue capsule separates the two organs.[34] Adrenal fusion is a rare anomaly in which the adrenal glands are fused in the midline, and may be associated with other congenital midline defects such as spinal dysraphism or indeterminate visceral situs.[3] Abnormal adrenal shape has also been reported in some cases of renal agenesis, where the glands may be ovoid with smoother contours.[3]

## Adrenal cytomegaly

Congenital adrenal cytomegaly is usually an incidental finding in an adrenal gland that otherwise appears grossly normal. It has been reported in about 3% of newborn autopsies and 6.5% of premature stillborns.[35] The cytomegaly affects cells of the fetal (provisional) cortex, and may be bilateral or unilateral, focal or diffuse. The cytomegalic cell has an enlarged hyperchromatic nucleus and increased volume of cytoplasm. Nuclei may be markedly pleomorphic and occasionally contain intranuclear 'pseudoinclusions,' which are indentations of the nucleus with invagination of cytoplasm; despite the marked nuclear abnormalities, mitotic figures are characteristically absent.

Adrenal cytomegaly is a characteristic component of the Beckwith–Wiedemann syndrome (Fig. 16-9),[36-38] sometimes called the EMG syndrome, which refers to a major triad of findings: exomphalos, macroglossia, and gigantism.[3] The estimated frequency of this disorder is 1 in 13 000 births; most reported cases are sporadic, although some seem to have a mendelian pattern of inheritance.[3] The disorder is caused by dysregulation of growth regulatory genes within the 11p15 region, resulting in loss of normal growth control and increased incidence of certain cancers.[39,40] The adrenal glands in this disorder are enlarged, with combined weights as high as 16 g. The adrenal cytomegaly is usually marked and is typically bilateral and diffuse. Curiously, adrenal chromaffin tissue may be hyperplastic or inappropriately mature.[4,38] There may be visceromegaly affecting the kidneys and pancreas, and some infants develop severe neonatal hypoglycemia, which may prove fatal. There is also an increased incidence of malignant tumors in this disorder, usually Wilms' tumor or adrenal cortical carcinoma, but other neoplasms have also been reported, including neuroblastoma, pancreatoblastoma, and hepatoblastoma.[3,41-44] The presence of hemihypertrophy in children predicts a greater risk for the development of a malignant neoplasm.

## Adrenoleukodystrophy

Adrenoleukodystrophy occurs in multiple forms. The neonatal form usually has an autosomal recessive inheritance, and the childhood form is an X-linked disorder; an adult variant of adrenoleukodystrophy known as adrenomyeloneuropathy is recognized in which there is progressive spastic paraparesis and distal polyneuropathy, with onset usually in the second or third decade of life.[3] Adrenoleukodystrophy or adrenomyeloneuropathy should be considered in the

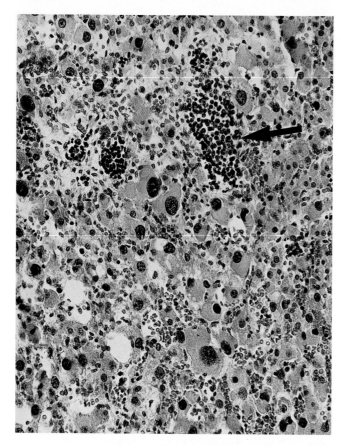

**Fig. 16-9** Adrenal in Beckwith–Wiedemann syndrome. Provisional zone of the fetal adrenal gland shows prominent cytomegaly with cells having greatly enlarged hyperchromatic nuclei. Small nests of neuroblastic cells are also evident (arrow).

differential diagnosis of boys or young men who present with unexplained adrenal cortical insufficiency because neurologic symptoms may not be evident at the time of presentation. Adrenoleukodystrophy is a peroxisomal disorder resulting from diminished capacity to oxidize branched or very long-chain fatty acids of 24–30 carbon atoms. Most work has been done on the X-linked form, the gene responsible for this disorder having been identified as the X-ADL gene (X-linked adrenoleukodystrophy gene).[45,46] The lipid material accumulates in tissue as cholesterol esters that may exert a toxic effect on cells, with crystallization of lamellae and disruption of cell membranes.[3] This mechanism may account for the pathogenesis of adrenal cortical insufficiency and degeneration of white matter, particularly involving the posterior cerebrum, cerebellum, and descending corticospinal tracts.

The adrenal glands in adrenoleukodystrophy are often quite small. There is thinning of the adrenal cortex, with characteristic enlargement of cortical cells having abundant 'ground glass' or 'waxy' cytoplasm;[47] these cells have been called balloon cells, and may have a fibrillar or striated appearance caused by lipid material being extracted during routine processing. On ultrastructural examination bilamellar and lamellar lipid inclusions can be seen, which are virtually

pathognomonic for the disorder. The adrenal cortical insufficiency in this disorder is primary and not caused by pituitary or hypothalamic dysfunction. The recent molecular advances regarding the X-linked form of this disease have major implications for the possibility of gene-based therapy.[45,48]

## Congenital adrenal hyperplasia

Congenital adrenal hyperplasia (adrenogenital syndrome) is a rare autosomal recessive disorder caused by a deficiency of one of five different enzymes in the steroid biosynthetic pathway of the adrenal cortex (Fig. 16-10).[3,49] The first unmistakable and thorough description of congenital adrenal hyperplasia was in 1865 by the Italian anatomist de Crecchio,[50] who dissected the cadaver of an apparent male of about 40 years of age who had bilateral cryptorchidism and partial hypospadias; however, further examination revealed a vagina, uterus, fallopian tubes, ovaries, and very large adrenal glands. The subject was also said to have had frequent diarrhea and vomiting, and in his final days had extreme weakness and exhaustion, which almost certainly represented an addisonian crisis.

The most common cause of congenital adrenal hyperplasia is 21-hydroxylase deficiency, which accounts for about 90–95% of cases.[51,52] This deficiency has been divided into a classic form, with an incidence of 1:5000 to 1:15000 live births in most white populations; a non-classic form, which is among the most frequent of autosomal recessive disorders in the white population; and a cryptic form in which patients are asymptomatic despite having the same biochemical abnormality.[51] Mutations in the encoding gene have been confirmed as the basis of endocrine disease in all adrenal steroidogenic enzymes required for the synthesis of cortisol, except for cholesterol desmolase.[52] In 21-hydroxylase deficiency there is insufficient production of cortisol, resulting in a lack of negative feedback at the hypothalamopituitary level and secondary trophic stimulation of the adrenal glands by increased ACTH levels. In about two-thirds of cases of the classic disorder biosynthesis of aldosterone is also affected, leading to 'salt wasting'; if unrecognized or severe enough, this may result in death in the first few weeks of life.[3] The remaining one-third of cases have 'simple virilizing disease' without significant impairment of aldosterone biosynthesis. Because of the enzymatic block, precursor steroids accumulate and are diverted into the sex steroid pathway with increased androgen production. The development of external genitalia is under the control of androgens in utero, and because of this affected females usually have ambiguous genitalia with clitoromegaly and fusion of the labioscrotal folds, although the internal female organs develop normally. In females the ambiguous genitalia may be so extreme that the child is incorrectly assumed to be male. Affected males usually appear normal at birth. For this reason, males with the disorder may not be diagnosed until they present with more severe symptoms, often related to a potentially fatal 'salt-wasting' crisis. The identification of mutations in the CYP21 gene which encodes the 21-hydroxylase enzyme has led to advances in DNA diagnosis, including prenatal and newborn screening programs.[53–55]

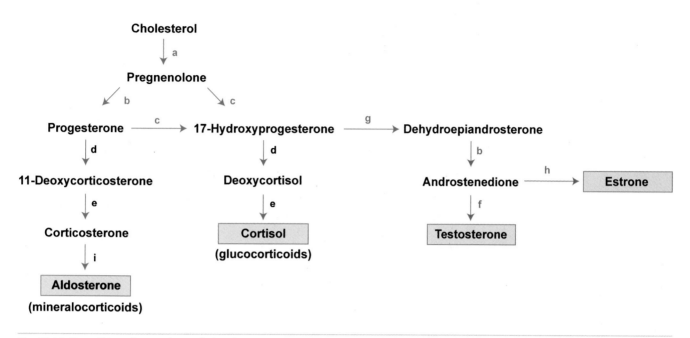

**Fig. 16-10** Normal biosynthetic pathway of adrenal cortical steroid synthesis. a = 20,22 hydroxylase and 20,22 desmolase; b = 3β-hydroxysteroid dehydrogenase; c= 17-hydroxylase; d = 21-hydroxylase; e = 11β- hydroxylase; f = 17-ketosteroid reductase; g = 17, 20 desmolase; h = P450 aromatase; i = 18-hydroxylase and 18-aldehyde synthetase.

About 5–8% of cases of congenital adrenal hyperplasia are caused by the classic form of 11β-hydroxylase deficiency[51] owing to mutations of the CYP11B1 gene.[56,57] Other enzymatic defects causing congenital adrenal hyperplasia include deficiency of 3β-hydroxysteroid dehydrogenase, 17α-hydroxylase, and the rare deficiency of cholesterol desmolase, the enzyme involved in early steroidogenesis.

## Pathology of adrenal glands in congenital adrenal hyperplasia

Nowadays it is very uncommon to examine the adrenal glands of patients who died of unrecognized or untreated congenital adrenal hyperplasia. Grossly, the adrenal glands are enlarged, often with a convoluted or cerebriform surface with excess cortical plications and folding. The glands frequently have a light brown color reminiscent of the zona reticularis, resulting from the sustained trophic effect of ACTH and the conversion of lipid-rich, pale-staining cells to cortical cells which have lipid-depleted compact eosinophilic cytoplasm (Fig. 16-11). In children, the weight of each adrenal gland may be 10–15 g, whereas in older individuals each gland may weigh 30–35 g.[3] Cholesterol desmolase (cytochrome P450scc [side chain cleavage]) deficiency is also called congenital lipoid hyperplasia because there is accumulation of cholesterol and cholesterol esters, which gives the gland a bright-yellow or white appearance on cross-section.

### Testicular tumors in congenital adrenal hyperplasia

Occasionally, male patients with congenital adrenal hyperplasia – particularly the salt-losing form of 21-hydroxylase deficiency – develop one or more testicular tumors in adolescence or young adulthood. The tumors are often bilateral (83%) and may cause testicular pain and tenderness.[58] Several reports in the literature clearly document that the tumors are ACTH dependent, as evidenced by reduction in testicular size and associated symptoms with suppressive doses of dexamethasone, and recrudescence of testicular enlargement with ACTH stimulation. Laboratory testing has also demonstrated ACTH-dependent steroidogenesis by the tumors.[59]

The tumors may be 2–10 cm in diameter in older patients. Most of the smaller tumors appear to be located in the hilum of the testis, but with larger tumors the precise site of origin is difficult to determine.[58] On cross-section the tumors often have a lobulated appearance with bulging, tan to dark brown nodules; the histologic appearance resembles that of a Leydig cell tumor, although Reinke crystalloids are absent. Nuclei

**A**

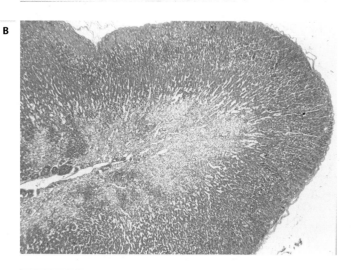

**B**

Fig. 16-11  Adrenal gland in congenital adrenal hyperplasia. **(A)** Note the convoluted or cerebriform surface of the gland in this whole-mount section. **(B)** Microscopically, the adrenal cortical cells have a compact eosinophilic cytoplasm with depletion of the normal lipid content.

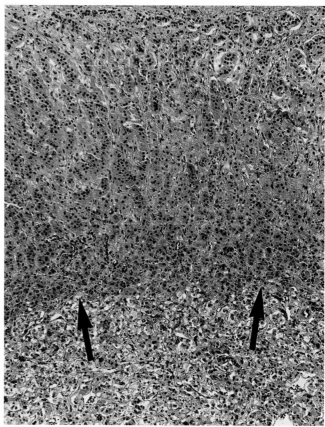

Fig. 16-12  Adrenal gland of an adult who died of AIDS. The cortex showed severe lipid depletion, characterized by numerous cells with compact eosinophilic cytoplasm. The corticomedullary junction is indicated by arrows.

are usually round to oval with a single prominent nucleolus, which may be central or somewhat eccentric. Cells have granular, pink cytoplasm with relatively distinct cell borders. The cells are usually arranged in sheets or small nests with intersecting fibrous bands, and reticulum stain often demonstrates an intimate pattern of isolation of individual and small clusters of cells.

Virtually identical testicular tumors of this type have been reported in males with Nelson's syndrome;[60] rarely, a female with Nelson's syndrome may develop similar adrenal rest tumors in the region of the ovaries where heterotopic adrenal cortical tissue occasionally is found.[31] The histogenesis of these interesting testicular tumors is not clear; possibilities include origin from Leydig cells, adrenal cortical rests, or multipotent testicular stromal cells capable of differentiation into either Leydig or adrenal cortical cells, depending on the hormonal milieu. It is unclear whether these tumors are true neoplasms or hyperplastic nodules. In favor of hyperplasia are their ACTH dependence, bilaterality, and the fact that malignant progression has never occurred. Recently, a case of a histologically similar tumor arising in the ovary of a 36-year-old woman with congenital adrenal hyperplasia due

to 21-hydroxylase deficiency was reported[61] and may represent the first case of this so-called 'testicular tumor' to arise in the ovary.

### Other tumors associated with congenital adrenal hyperplasia

Rare cases of adrenal cortical adenoma and carcinoma have been reported in patients with congenital adrenal hyperplasia.[3,62] It has been suggested that persistent ACTH stimulation may result in neoplastic transformation of some adrenal cortical cells, but this is unproven. Other tumors have been reported in association with congenital adrenal hyperplasia, including osteosarcoma and Ewing's sarcoma,[63] but their relationship with congenital adrenal hyperplasia and the underlying biochemical abnormality is unclear.

### Stress-related changes of the adrenal gland

One of the most common histologic changes observed in the adrenal gland of patients under stress is the conversion of lipid-rich, pale-staining cortical cells of the zona fasciculata to cells with compact, lipid-depleted eosinophilic cytoplasm. This is particularly common in acquired immunodeficiency syndrome (AIDS) (Fig. 16-12). Another abnormality reported in stress-related conditions is degeneration of the outer zona fasciculata, initially described as 'tubular degeneration;' this abnormality appears with scattered necrosis of cortical cells, shedding of vacuolated cytoplasm, and exudation of fluid into cords of cortical cells in the outer zona fasciculata.[64] A peculiar vacuolization of the fetal adrenal cortex has been described in infants with erythroblastosis fetalis, and nearly identical changes have been observed in thalassemia major.[3] A relationship with intrauterine stress and hypoxia has been suggested. A pattern of focal lipid depletion has also been reported as lipid reversion, which suggests recovery from stress and replenishment of lipid in cells of the inner zona fasciculata. In areas of lipid reversion the outer aspect of the adrenal cortex contains little or no lipid, although lipid is prominent in the inner zona fasciculata.[7]

## Other abnormalities

There may be conspicuous iron accumulation in the form of hemosiderin in cells of the outer cortex, particularly the zona glomerulosa, in conditions such as primary hemochromatosis and transfusion hemosiderosis.[3] In some cases there may be associated hypothalamopituitary dysfunction caused by excess iron deposition, which may result in endocrine insufficiency of the gonads, thyroid, and adrenal glands. A variety of drugs and cytotoxic agents also have direct anti-adrenal activity; examples include dichlorodiphenyltrichloroethane (DDT) and its derivative o,p'DDD, which has been used for palliative treatment of patients with adrenal cortical carcinoma because of its adrenolytic effect on normal and neoplastic cortical cells. Another agent with anti-adrenal activity is ketoconazole, a broad-spectrum antifungal drug that blocks adrenal steroid synthesis.[3] Linear hyaline fibrosis has also been reported in the zona reticularis following radiation, probably because of structural damage of the vascular plexus in this zone.[65]

Anencephaly is a severe developmental defect of anterior neural tube structures with agenesis of much of the brain and cranial vault. The pituitary gland is difficult to find grossly but is often identified in histologic sections, albeit reduced in amount. The adrenal glands are often extremely small in this disorder, with an average combined weight in one study of 1.8 g, but a significant number weighed less than 1 g.[66] The fetal cortex is often normal in size and structure until approximately 20 weeks of gestation, after which it progressively involutes, similar to changes that normally occur following birth; chromaffin tissue may appear relatively prominent.

## Non-neoplastic diseases

## Chronic adrenal cortical insufficiency (Addison's disease)

### Idiopathic or autoimmune Addison's disease

The most common type of Addison's disease is idiopathic or autoimmune, and is regarded as an organ-specific autoimmune form of adrenalitis. One proposed mechanism is aberrant expression of class II major histocompatibility antigens by target cells and the presentation of adrenal-specific autoantigen to T-helper lymphocytes, which in turn initiate an autoimmune response.[3] It is uncertain whether class II antigen expression is a primary event or mediated by lymphokines, which are related to the inflammatory infiltrate. Recently, it has been shown that the presence of 21-hydroxylase autoantibodies is a sensitive and specific diagnostic marker for autoimmune Addison's disease and may be helpful in predicting the risk of developing the disease.[67-69]

The adrenal gland in this disorder may be greatly reduced in size and volume, making gross identification difficult at autopsy unless numerous tissue blocks from the suprarenal bed are examined. The adrenal cortex has a large endocrine reserve, and it is estimated that up to 90% or more of the cortex must be ablated before functional impairment is apparent.[3] In some cases intercurrent illness, infection, or surgery may precipitate an addisonian crisis. The residual cortex is often thin and discontinuous, with scattered islands of cortical cells (Fig. 16-13) admixed with lymphocytes, plasma cells, and occasional lymphoid follicles, sometimes with reactive germinal centers. Cortical cells may be enlarged, with ample compact, eosinophilic cytoplasm and occasional nuclear alteration, including 'pseudoinclusions.' On

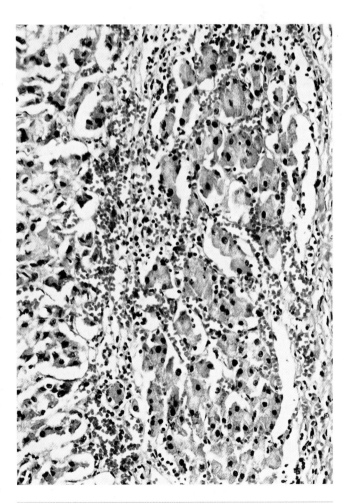

**Fig. 16-13** Primary idiopathic or autoimmune form of Addison's disease. Atrophic adrenal cortex (right side) contains cells with compact, eosinophilic cytoplasm. The medulla is present on the left.

occasion, residual cortex may be difficult to identify and there may be little or no inflammation.

Autoimmune polyendocrinopathy–candidiasis–ectodermal dystrophy (APECED) is an autosomal recessive disorder with endocrine insufficiency involving various organs, including the adrenal cortex. Numerous mutations in the gene responsible for the disease, AIRE (autoimmune regulator), have been identified. The gene is located on chromosome 21 and encodes a protein involved in transcriptional regulation.[70–73] This disorder has also been called autoimmune polyglandular disease type I, and has a variety of manifestations.[74] The combination of non-tuberculous Addison's disease and thyroid insufficiency is called Schmidt's syndrome.[75]

## Adrenal tuberculosis

Adrenal tuberculosis once was the leading cause of Addison's disease.[76] According to the review by Guttman[77] of cases between 1900 and 1929, 70% resulted from tuberculosis and 19% were caused by primary or idiopathic atrophy. The endemic nature of bovine tuberculosis in the early decades of the 20th century is reflected in the comment by Dunlop,[78] who characterized cream on top of the milk in those days as often being composed of 'tuberculous pus.' The tuberculous adrenal is often enlarged, with extensive areas of caseous necrosis. A classic granulomatous reaction with numerous epithelioid histiocytes is present typically in extra-adrenal sites but not the adrenal, suggesting that the locally high levels of adrenal corticosteroids dampen the host inflammatory response.[3]

## Histoplasmosis and other fungal infections

Disseminated histoplasmosis is a recognized cause of Addison's disease and typically involves the glands bilaterally. In a study of almost 100 cases, 7% of patients had chronic adrenal cortical insufficiency.[79] Similar to tuberculosis, extensive caseous necrosis is a common finding, although a granulomatous response is the exception rather than the rule. Perivasculitis involving extracapsular adrenal vessels may lead to extensive infarction and caseous necrosis, resulting in loss of adrenal parenchyma and development of Addison's disease. Other mycotic infections causing Addison's disease are less frequent, including North American blastomycosis, South American blastomycosis, and coccidioidomycosis.[3] On microscopic examination the organisms are often found clustered within the cytoplasm of macrophages (Fig. 16-14). They are spherical to oval in shape and typically have single buds attached by a relatively narrow base.

## Amyloidosis

The adrenal may be involved in primary and secondary (AA) forms of amyloidosis. In primary amyloidosis there tends to be involvement of arterioles, whereas in the secondary form there is usually extensive involvement of the cortex by the characteristic homogeneous eosinophilic material, resulting in severe atrophy and distortion of cells in the zona fasciculata and zona reticularis (Fig. 16-15).

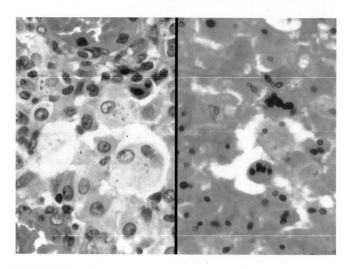

**Fig. 16-14** *Histoplasma capsulatum* infection of the adrenal gland (left). Fungal organisms present within macrophages are highlighted by Gomori's methenamine silver (GMS) stain (right).

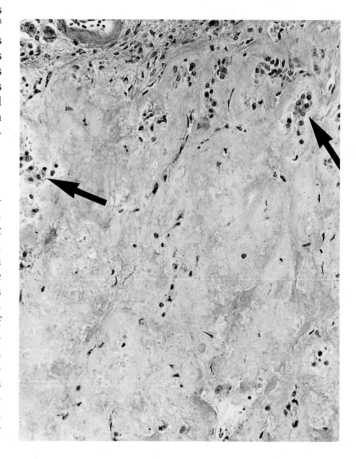

**Fig. 16-15** Amyloidosis of the adrenal cortex. Only small nests of cortical cells remain (arrows).

## Acute adrenal cortical insufficiency

Acute adrenal cortical insufficiency can occur in the setting of systemic infection with Waterhouse–Friderichsen syndrome, but is seldom documented by laboratory or biochemical studies. Waterhouse–Friderichsen syndrome is seen classically in meningococcemia, but occasionally other bacteria, such as *Streptococcus pneumoniae*, are causative. The course of the disease is usually fulminant, with a fatal outcome within 48 hours of onset, accompanied by muco-cutaneous petechial hemorrhages and vascular collapse. The adrenal is usually intensely hemorrhagic, with confluent areas of coagulative necrosis, often associated with small fibrin deposits within sinusoids; occasionally there is more extensive hemorrhage, with expansion of the gland and peri-adrenal hemorrhage (Fig. 16-16).

## Inflammation and other infections

### Non-specific adrenalitis

Focal chronic adrenalitis is common and has been found in up to 48% of autopsies, appearing as small aggregates of lymphocytes admixed with plasma cells adjacent to veins or venules in the corticomedullary junction.[80] Focal chronic adrenalitis of this type is not considered to be a primary adrenal disorder, but represents a non-specific inflammatory reaction, possibly related to inflammation in neighboring organs such as chronic pyelonephritis. Autoantibodies may be directed against adrenal medullary or chromaffin cells in type 1 (insulin-dependent) diabetes mellitus, and this organ-specific autoimmunity might be related to diabetic auto-nomic neuropathy.[4]

### Herpetic adrenalitis

Members of the herpes virus group may infect the adrenal gland, including herpes simplex, cytomegalovirus, and vari-cella zoster virus. A characteristic pattern of herpetic adrenal-itis occurs with disseminated herpes simplex infection in newborns, referred to as neonatal hepatoadrenal necrosis and first described by Haas in 1935.[81] The foci of herpes simplex or varicella zoster infections tend to be small, circumscribed, 'punched-out' areas of coagulative necrosis, with scant inflammation. The necrosis within the cortex may become widespread and confluent.[3] Eosinophilic Cowdry type A intranuclear inclusions are the diagnostic hallmark, usually occurring in cells bordering the zones of necrosis (Fig. 16-17 A). It may not be possible to distinguish varicella zoster infec-tion from herpes simplex by routine light microscopy.

Disseminated cytomegalovirus (CMV) infection in the newborn involves a wide variety of organs and tissues, including the adrenal gland. Some infants may have multi-ple mobile blue-gray subcutaneous nodules caused by dermal erythropoiesis. The appearance of the pigmented nodules may be striking, giving the infant an appearance described as 'blueberry muffin.'[3] The viral cytopathic effect in CMV adrenalitis is virtually pathognomonic, with sharply defined large amphophilic intranuclear inclusions having characteristic haloes and small, basophilic granules within the cytoplasm (Fig. 16-17B). CMV adrenalitis is relatively common in patients with AIDS; death is attributed in part in some cases to adrenal cortical insufficiency. In one study about 50% of patients with AIDS had evidence of CMV infection at autopsy, and the adrenal glands were most com-monly involved (75%) with cortical or medullary necrosis.[82] Necrosis of the medulla caused by CMV infection may be

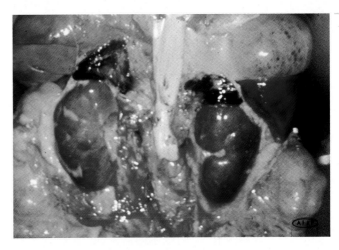
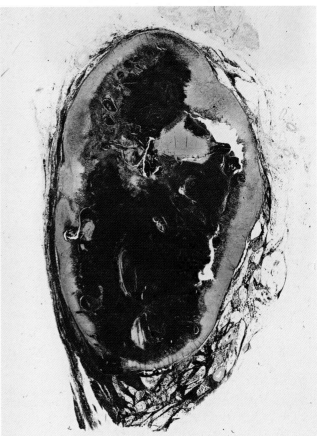

**Fig. 16-16** Adrenal glands in Waterhouse–Friderichsen syndrome. **(A)** In situ photograph showing bilateral hemorrhagic adrenal glands in a suprarenal location (autopsy specimen, from files of Armed Forces Institute of Pathology). **(B)** Extensive necrosis and hemorrhage are seen in this adrenal gland and extend into periadrenal connective tissue. (From Lack EE, Kozakewich HPW. Pathology. In: Javadpour N, ed. Principles and management of adrenal cancer. Berlin: Springer-Verlag, 1987; 19–55).

greater than that of the cortex, and it is useful to note that there is no deficiency syndrome caused by destruction of the adrenal medulla. CMV infection of the adrenal in AIDS may result in latent or overt adrenal cortical insufficiency, requir-ing prophylactic treatment with corticosteroids.[83]

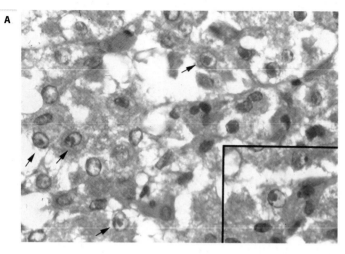

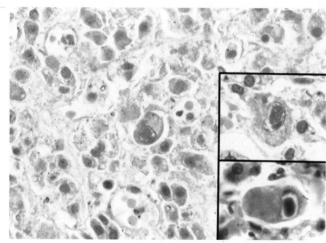

**Fig. 16-17** Herpetic adrenalitis. **(A)** Herpes simplex virus (HSV) infection. Note multiple intranuclear eosinophilic 'Cowdry type A' inclusions (arrows) with peripheral displacement of nuclear chromatin (inset). **(B)** Cytomegalovirus (CMV) infection. The adrenal cortical cells infected by the virus show the characteristic cytomegalic changes. Insets highlight the large, amphophilic intranuclear inclusions with peripheral halo.

### Rare infections

Rarely the adrenal is involved by other infectious agents, such as *Pneumocystis carinii* (Fig. 16-18), usually in patients with AIDS.[84] Malakoplakia of the adrenal gland has also been reported.[85,86] Echinococcal cyst of the adrenal gland is usually an incidental autopsy finding.[87]

## Adrenal cortical hyperplasia

### Nodular adrenal gland

Cortical nodularity in the adrenal can pose significant diagnostic problems for the pathologist at the autopsy table and in surgical material. Nodularity usually occurs in individuals without biochemical or clinical signs or symptoms of adrenal cortical hyperfunction. By definition, hyperplasia refers to an increase in the number of cells in tissue or in an organ, which in the adrenal cortex results in diffuse, symmetric thickening with or without cortical nodules (Fig. 16-19). The spectrum of diffuse and nodular adrenal cortical hyperplasia is broad.

The incidence of cortical nodularity with eucorticalism can be analyzed from material obtained at autopsy or in patients who are discovered to have cortical nodules in vivo.

### Nodular adrenal gland at autopsy

Early studies of adrenal cortical nodularity at autopsy considered any solitary adrenal cortical nodule greater than 3–5 mm in diameter to be a non-functional adenoma.[3] Several studies have shown that the incidence of cortical nodularity increases with age,[88] and may be associated with hypertension[88] and diabetes mellitus.[89] The early study by Spain and Weinsaft[90] identified solitary adrenal cortical adenomas in 29% of elderly women. Another autopsy study reported a cortical adenoma 1.5 cm or larger in up to 20% of hypertensive individuals, compared to only 1.8% of normotensive patients.[91] In two of the largest studies of adrenal cortical adenomas detected at autopsy the frequency was 1.5–2.9% of cases in a study population of over 16 000.[92,93] The study by Dobbie[88] showed that incidental adrenal cortical nodules may be present in virtually every region of the cortex, with the degree of nodularity varying widely from gland to gland. Adrenal nodularity was almost always bilateral, and in some cases there was significant disparity in the weights of the glands from an individual patient. Some nodules are as large as 3 cm in diameter and may display lipomatous or myelolipomatous metaplasia. Occasionally degenerative features such as fibrosis or microcystic change are noted. Although there are no specific size criteria for distinguishing between nodules versus adenomas, most cortical nodules are less than 1 cm in diameter. In Dobbie's study[88] some nodules were related to capsular arteriopathy, which in turn was related to aging. For many of these cortical nodules it seems inappropriate to use the term adenoma, which implies a true neoplasm. Cortical hyperplasia implies some degree of cortical hyperfunction in addition to the increase in cortical tissue volume. However, this is not always the case and the designation non-hyperfunctional may be appropriate.

The pathogenesis of nonhyperfunctional cortical nodules is uncertain. There is a significant correlation between adrenal capsular arteriopathy and cortical nodularity;[88] hyalinization and intimal proliferation with luminal obstruction may be an important etiologic factor, resulting in localized cortical ischemia with secondary regenerative change and hyperplasia and the subsequent formation of one or more cortical nodules. Based on this hypothesis, most cortical nodules can be regarded as secondary to hypertension rather than a cause of it. Other investigators have logically questioned the validity of this theory.

### Incidental pigmented cortical nodule

Incidental pigmented nodules of adrenal cortex vary from 0.1 cm to 1.5 cm in diameter and are usually located in the zona reticularis, often with expansion and distortion of the adjacent cortex or medulla (Fig. 16-20). The frequency of grossly identifiable pigmented nodules at autopsy varies according to the method of adrenal sectioning, the number of sections examined, and the level of interest of the pathologist searching for the lesions. Retrospective studies of autopsy material show pigmented adrenal cortical nodules

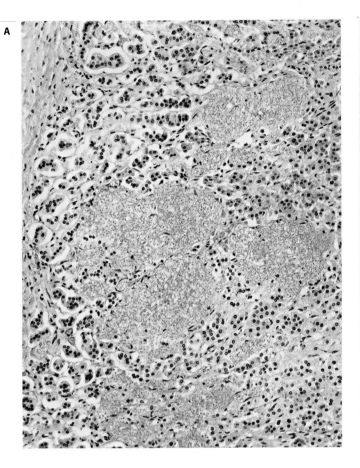

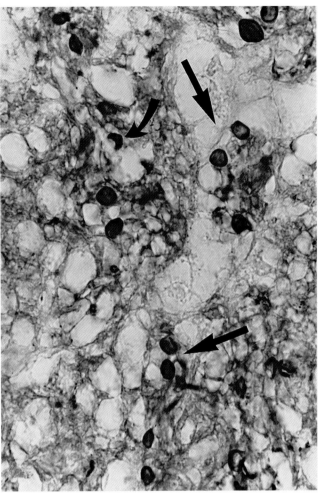

**Fig. 16-18 (A)** Adrenal gland extensively involved by *Pneumocystis carinii* infection in a patient with AIDS. Note the characteristic 'foamy' exudate in the cortex. The adrenal capsule is on the left side. **(B)** Gomori methenamine silver stain shows several *Pneumocystis carinii* organisms (straight arrows), some with cup-shaped indentations when viewed in profile (curved arrow).

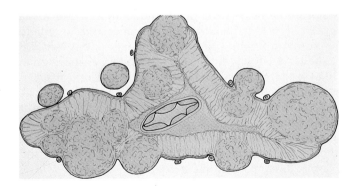

**Fig. 16-19** Schematic view of nodular adrenal gland in transverse section. Accessory nodules of cortical cells may be seen lying free within periadrenal fat, on the capsular surface, or attached to underlying cortex (capsular extrusion). A dominant macronodule within the cortex can simulate a neoplasm. Multiple small capsular arterioles are present on the surface of the gland. The central adrenal vein in the medullary compartment has discontinuous bundles of smooth muscle, allowing close contact of chromaffin cells or cortical cells with vascular lumina. Occasionally one may see a mushroom-like intravascular protrusion by cortical or medullary cells.

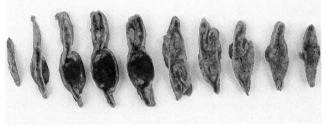

**Fig. 16-20** Incidental pigmented adrenal cortical nodule. The adjacent cortex contained numerous small pale-yellow nodules.

in 2.2–10.4% of cases.[94,95] When the glands were thinly sectioned in a prospective study, pigmented nodules were detected in 37% of cases.[94] Pigmented nodules are usually solitary but may be multiple, and in 11% of cases are bilateral. Histologically, the cells have compact eosinophilic cytoplasm with variable amounts of intracellular granular

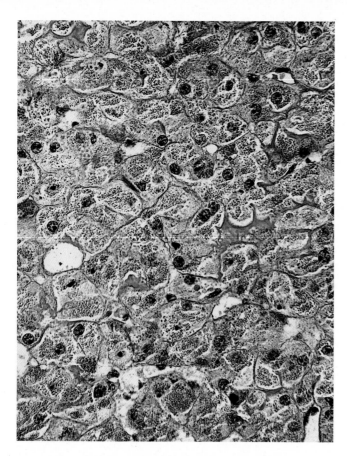

**Fig. 16-21** Incidental pigmented adrenal cortical nodule. Cells contain abundant granular lipofuscin pigment. Nuclei are uniform and many contain a small central to eccentric nucleolus.

brown pigment, which has staining characteristics similar to those of lipofuscin (Fig. 16-21). One study suggested the presence of neuromelanin.[95]

## Incidental cortical nodules discovered in vivo: incidentalomas

The increasing use of sensitive imaging studies such as computed tomography (CT) has identified many adrenal masses in asymptomatic patients. The prevalence of these asymptomatic masses (incidentalomas) varied from 0.6% to 1.3% in three combined series in which CT scans were performed on over 5000 patients.[96-98] The average size of the incidental adrenal nodules in one study was 2.8 cm, but some reached 5 cm in diameter. Another study looked at 342 cases of incidentally discovered adrenal masses. Fifty-two of these patients underwent surgical resection, of which five turned out to be malignant, four were adrenal cortical carcinomas, and one a metastatic carcinoma of undetermined primary site. Interestingly, the minimum size of the malignant tumors was 5 cm, and of the benign, incidentally discovered lesions only 6% were 5 cm or larger.[99]

Magnetic resonance imaging (MRI) may provide some information on tissue characterization of adrenal masses; $T_2$-weighted pulse sequences provide some specificity in separating non-hyperfunctioning cortical adenomas, which have low signal intensity, from metastases with intermediate signal intensity and pheochromocytomas, which tend to have high signal intensity.[100] MRI does not allow distinction between functional and non-functional (or non-hyperfunctional) cortical adenomas, or small adrenal cortical carcinomas that lack necrosis and other secondary changes. Adrenal cortical scintigraphy with a radioiodinated cholesterol precursor often shows tracer uptake, indicating cortical steroid synthesis.[101-104] Various enzymes in cortical steroid synthesis are present, according to immunohistochemical staining, indicating that the nodules have the capacity for corticosteroidogenesis, although not in sufficient amounts to elicit signs or symptoms of endocrine hyperfunction or abnormal biochemical findings to alter the hypothalamopituitary–adrenal axis.[105] Many incidental cortical nodules (or adenomas) are therefore considered non-hyperfunctional rather than non-functional, without excess production of adrenal cortical steroids. Cortical nodularity in this setting has been compared with nodular euthyroid (non-toxic) goiter.

### Approach to the nodular adrenal discovered in vivo

In general, all functional, incidentally discovered masses should be surgically resected. The incidentally discovered, non-hyperfunctioning adrenal mass is a diagnostic challenge in a patient without a known malignancy. Fine needle aspiration under CT or ultrasound guidance may provide valuable information,[106] particularly when it is not possible to reliably distinguish a metastasis from an adrenal cortical nodule or neoplasm (Fig. 16-22). Further classification between adrenal cortical adenoma and carcinoma is not always reliable by FNA. Occasionally, aspiration yields cells with bare nuclei stripped of cytoplasm, which might be confused with a small cell malignancy. Correlation of cytologic findings with imaging results, clinical findings, and endocrinologic data is essential. Adrenal cortical carcinoma should be considered in the differential diagnosis. If one assumes that the prevalence of biochemically silent adrenal cortical carcinoma is 1 : 250 000 of the population, it is estimated that over 60 operations would have to be performed on patients with an adrenal mass 6 cm in diameter to remove one adrenal cortical carcinoma.[107] The size of the adrenal mass alone assumes importance as a distinguishing feature in decision making, although the reported threshold for size varies from 3 to 5 cm or more.[99,108-111] A National Institutes of Health (NIH) consensus panel was convened in 2002 to address questions concerning the 'clinically inapparent adrenal mass'[112,113] with the following conclusions: all patients with adrenal incidentaloma should undergo a 1-mg dexamethasone suppression test and measurement of plasma-free metanephrines; patients with hypertension should undergo measurement of serum potassium and plasma aldosterone concentration–plasma renin activity ratio; patients with biochemical evidence of pheochromocytoma, tumors larger than 6 cm and patients with tumors larger than 4 cm who meet other criteria should undergo surgical resection of the mass; and patients with tumors smaller than 4 cm and no other suspicious features are generally monitored (Table 16-1).[113] It is estimated that up to 20% of patients with adrenal incidentalomas have abnormal cortisol production and could be classified as having subclinical Cushing's syndrome.[114]

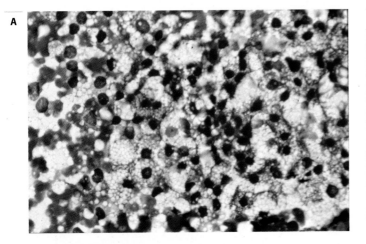

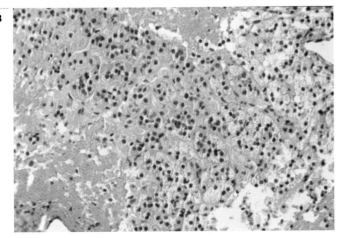

**Fig. 16-22** Adrenal 'incidentaloma.' **(A)** Fine needle aspiration (Diff Quik stain) of adrenal cortical adenoma showing clusters of adrenal cortical cells with microvesiculated cytoplasm and eccentrically placed, round to oval nuclei. **(B)** The corresponding cell block preparation (hematoxylin and eosin stain) shows a proliferation of adrenal cortical cells, some with microvesiculated, lipid-filled cytoplasm (right) interspersed by cells with a more compact eosinophilic cytoplasm (left).

**Table 16-1** NIH Consensus Conference on Adrenal Incidentalomas[112, 113]

| |
| --- |
| All patients with an incidentaloma should have a 1-mg dexamethasone suppression test and measurement of plasma free metanephrines. |
| Patients with hypertension should also undergo measurement of serum potassium and plasma aldosterone concentration–plasma renin activity ratio. |
| A homogenous mass with a low attenuation value (<10 HU) on computed tomography is probably a benign adenoma. |
| Surgery should be considered in all patients with functional adrenal cortical tumors that are clinically apparent. |
| All patients with biochemical evidence of pheochromocytoma should undergo surgery. |
| Data are insufficient to indicate the superiority of a surgical or non-surgical approach to manage patients with subclinical hyperfunctioning adrenal cortical adenomas. |
| Recommendations for surgery based on tumor size are derived from studies not standardized for inclusion criteria, length of follow-up, or methods of estimating the risk for carcinoma. Nevertheless, patients with tumors >6 cm usually are treated surgically, while those with tumors <4 cm are generally monitored. In patients with tumors between 4 and 6 cm, criteria in addition to size should be considered in the decision to monitor or proceed to adrenalectomy. |
| The literature on adrenal incidentaloma has proliferated in the last several years. Unfortunately, the lack of controlled studies makes formulating diagnostic and treatment strategies difficult. Because of the complexity of the problem, the management of patients with adrenal incidentalomas will be optimized by a multidisciplinary team approach involving physicians with expertise in endocrinology, radiology, surgery and pathology. The paucity of evidence-based data highlights the need for well-designed prospective studies. |
| Open or laparoscopic adrenalectomy is an acceptable procedure for resection of an adrenal mass. The procedure choice will depend on the likelihood of an invasive adrenal cortical carcinoma, technical issues, and the experience of the surgical team. |
| In patients with tumors that remain stable on two imaging studies done at least 6 months apart and do not exhibit hormonal hypersecretion over 4 years, further follow-up may not be warranted. |

## Adrenal cortical hyperplasia with hypercortisolism

There are several basic non-iatrogenic causes of Cushing's syndrome (Fig. 16-23). The three most common causes are pituitary-dependent ACTH overproduction, commonly referred to as Cushing's disease, which accounts for about 60–70% of cases in adults; adrenal cortical neoplasm with autonomous overproduction of cortisol, which accounts for 17–25% of cases in adults; and ectopic production of ACTH (15–16% of cases), or rarely ectopic production of corticotrophin-releasing factor.[115-120] In childhood, Cushing's syndrome is most often caused by a cortisol-producing cortical neoplasm, particularly in the very young,[121] whereas older children are more likely to have a pituitary-dependent form of hypercortisolism (Cushing's disease). Most patients with a pituitary-dependent form caused by ACTH overproduction have a pituitary microadenoma or macroadenoma.[122-124] In some cases no pituitary tumor is detected, and the disease may result from hyperplasia of ACTH-producing cells or abnormal hypothalamic regulation with secondary ACTH hypersecretion.

## Pituitary-dependent hypercortisolism (Cushing's disease)

### Diffuse and micronodular adrenal cortical hyperplasia

With the high success rate of trans-sphenoidal adenomectomy for ACTH-producing pituitary neoplasms,[117,125] the pathologist rarely has the opportunity to examine adrenal glands in this disorder. Bilateral adrenalectomy is usually done only after failed resection of a pituitary adenoma or when the primary ACTH-secreting neoplasm cannot be removed. Bilateral laparoscopic adrenalectomy has gained an increasing role as a safe and effective therapeutic option.[126,127] The pathologic alterations in the adrenal may be so subtle that the gland might be regarded as 'normal' if the alterations are not correlated with clinical and biochemical data.[3,62] The size and weight of the mildly stimulated gland may be only slightly increased – usually between 6 and 12 g; the average weight in the study by Smals et al. was 8.2 g.[128]

On transverse sectioning the adrenal gland may have a somewhat rounded contour, and the larger glands may demonstrate a mild degree of nodularity (Fig. 16-24) with nodules up to 3 mm in diameter randomly distributed throughout the cortex. Capsular extrusions may appear accentuated, as well as the cuff of cortical cells around tributaries of the central adrenal vein. The microscopic hallmark of ACTH stimulation in Cushing's disease is conversion of lipid-rich, pale-staining cortical cells in the inner one-third to one-half of the cortex into cells with compact eosinophilic cytoplasm, similar to those in the zona reticularis (Fig. 16-25). The net effect is what appears to be a greatly expanded zona reticularis except for the absence of lipochrome pigment in the outer part, which actually is zona fasciculata.[3,62] The extent to which vacuolated, lipid-rich cells are converted into compact, lipid-depleted cells is variable and may be influenced by a variety of physiologic factors.[3] The zona glomerulosa may be even more difficult to identify because of expansion of the zona fasciculata. Some cortical cells may extend irregularly into periadrenal adipose tissue or intermingle in irregular nests with chromaffin cells. Some of these changes may be subtle, particularly in mildly stimulated glands, and correlation with clinical and biochemical data is crucial.[3,62]

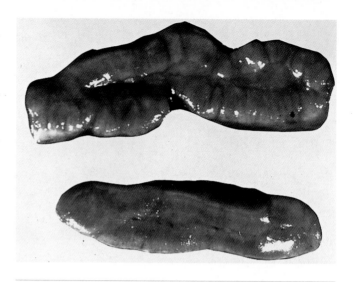

**Fig. 16-24** Transverse sections of a 3.5 g adrenal gland with mild nodularity surgically resected from an 8-year-old boy with Cushing's disease. Patient underwent several attempts at trans-sphenoidal pituitary resection. The patient was also treated with radiation (4800 cGy), but the tumor recurred on several occasions. Nelson's syndrome subsequently developed, with radiologically detectable changes in the sella.

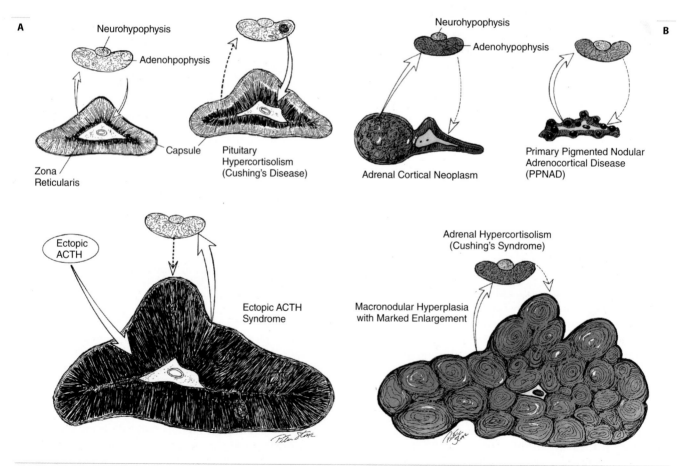

**Fig. 16-23 (A)** Normal hypothalamopituitary–adrenal axis (upper left). Pituitary (or adrenocorticotrophic hormone)-dependent hypercortisolism (upper right) is characteristic of Cushing's disease. Ectopic adrenocorticotrophic hormone syndrome (lower half) with enlarged, dark adrenal gland caused by trophic influence of adrenocorticotrophic hormone with predominance of cells with compact, lipid-depleted cytoplasm. **(B)** Non-iatrogenic causes of Cushing's syndrome. Cortisol-secreting cortical neoplasm (upper left) with autonomous hyperfunction and feedback inhibition of adrenocorticotrophic hormone release from adenohypophysis. Rare examples of Cushing's syndrome are caused by primary pigmented nodular adrenal cortical disease (upper right) and macronodular hyperplasia with marked adrenal enlargement (lower half).

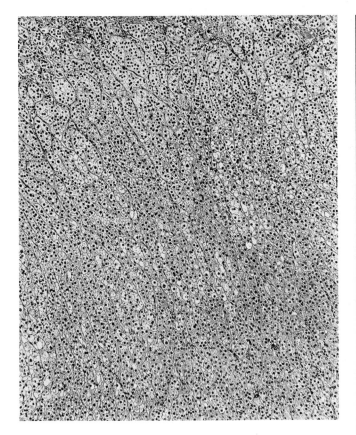

**Fig. 16-25** Adrenal in Cushing's disease caused by an adrenocorticotrophic hormone-producing pituitary adenoma. The cortex is hyperplastic, with conversion of many cells throughout the zona fasciculata into reticularis-type cells with compact, eosinophilic cytoplasm caused by lipid depletion.

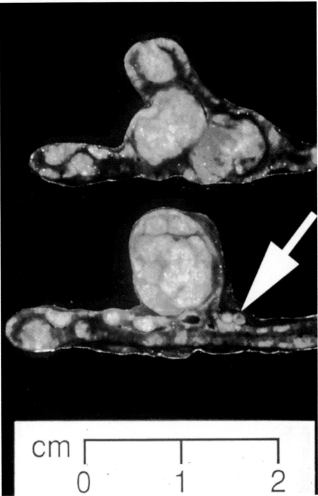

**Fig. 16-26** Macronodular adrenal cortical hyperplasia in a patient with MEN I who developed Cushing's syndrome caused by a presumed adrenocorticotrophic hormone-producing pituitary adenoma. Multiple pale cortical nodules range up to 1.5 cm in diameter, including small capsular extrusions (arrow). (Modified from Lack EE, Travis WD, Oertel JE. Adrenal cortical nodules, hyperplasia, and hyperfunction. In: Lack EE, ed. Pathology of the adrenal glands. New York: Churchill Livingstone, 1990; 75–113.)

## Macronodular hyperplasia

Macronodular hyperplasia is present in about 20% of cases of hyperplasia with Cushing's disease,[3] but this is variable.[128,129] The morphology may be more confusing than that of diffuse or micronodular hyperplasia. Nodules up to 2 cm in diameter or larger (Fig. 16-26) protrude from one or more sides of the gland; they may also be situated deep within the adrenal, identifiable only when the gland is sectioned in the transverse plane. Smals et al.[128] used the designation macronodular hyperplasia for grossly visible nodules 0.5 cm or more in diameter, with some nodules up to 5 cm in diameter. Separation of micronodular and macronodular hyperplasia is difficult, and there is a morphologic continuum between the two processes, making this distinction arbitrary.

Macronodular hyperplasia is characterized by disparity in size and weight between the adrenals. In the study by Smals et al.[128] the female:male ratio for macronodular hyperplasia was 5:1, identical to that for diffuse and micronodular hyperplasia. However, there are several important differences between micronodular and macronodular hyperplasia. The average age of patients with macronodular hyperplasia (44 years) is considerably older than those with diffuse and micronodular hyperplasia (31 years), and disease duration is longer with macronodular hyperplasia (8 years vs 2 years). The average adrenal in macronodular hyperplasia weighs 16 g, nearly twice the observed weight in diffuse and micronodular hyperplasia.[128] As noted by Cohen et al.,[130] the medullary compartment may be compressed by the prominent cortical nodules, and in many sections it may be difficult to recognize (Fig. 16-27). There may be foci of lipomatous or myelolipomatous metaplasia.

### Ectopic ACTH syndrome with secondary hypercortisolism

About 15–20% of cases of Cushing's syndrome in adults result from ectopic production of ACTH[131,132] by bronchial carcinoid tumor, bronchogenic small cell carcinoma, pancreatic endocrine neoplasm, medullary thyroid carcinoma, pheochromocytoma, or other rare neoplasms. Ectopic production of corticotrophin-releasing factor may rarely occur, and be accompanied by orthotopic ACTH secretion by the pituitary.[3,62] Nearly all normal tissues are capable of producing small amounts of the inactive precursor of ACTH, probably pro-opiomelanocortin, and cancers may overproduce this substance, although few convert it into ACTH; in this regard ectopic ACTH production may not be 'ectopic.'[133]

Correct identification of the source of ACTH secretion is essential in order to avoid unnecessary pituitary surgery.[134,135] In ectopic ACTH syndrome serum levels of ACTH are usually quite elevated, sometimes over 250 pg/mL, whereas in Cushing's disease ACTH levels are rarely over 200 pg/mL and are commonly in the upper range of normal or only slightly elevated.[62] Inferior petrosal sinus sampling can identify a pituitary source of ACTH via central (petrosal sinus) to peripheral blood concentration gradient with an estimated 94–100% accurracy.[119,132,136] Some patients with aggressive fast-growing tumors such as bronchogenic small cell carcinoma lack signs and symptoms of Cushing's syndrome, with the clinical findings dominated by electrolyte disturbances and cachexia. Some slowly growing neoplasms such as bronchial carcinoid tumor may be associated with marked changes of Cushing's syndrome, although the primary tumor remains occult, sometimes for years.[137]

On gross examination the adrenal glands are often symmetrically enlarged with rounded contours, and frequently weigh 10–15 g each; occasionally the individual adrenal may weigh more than 20 g, or rarely 30 g.[3,62] In this setting the adrenal glands are under intense and persistent trophic stimulation by ACTH, and on transverse sectioning may be tan to brown because of the conversion of lipid-rich, pale-staining cortical cells to cells with more compact eosinophilic cytoplasm (Fig. 16-28). The cortex is hyperplastic, being 0.3–0.4 cm thick, but in some cases may be even thicker. There is typically diffuse cortical hyperplasia, but sometimes there may be vague nodularity (Fig. 16-29).

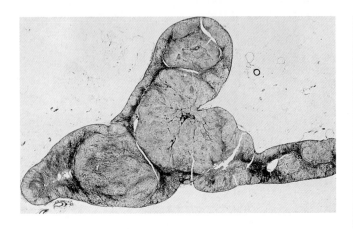

**Fig. 16-27** Pituitary-dependent macronodular adrenal cortical hyperplasia (same as in Fig. 16-26). Irregular expansile cortical nodules blend with adjacent hyperplastic cortex. The adrenal medulla was difficult to identify in random transverse sections of the gland. (From Lack EE, Travis WD, Oertel JE. Adrenal cortical nodules, hyperplasia, and hyperfunction. In: Lack EE, ed. Pathology of the adrenal glands. New York: Churchill Livingstone, 1990; 75–113.)

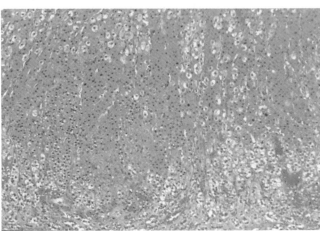

**Fig. 16-29** Ectopic adrenocorticotrophic hormone syndrome. The adrenal cortex is markedly hyperplastic, with columns and cords of lipid-depleted cells. Faint nodularity was evident in some areas.

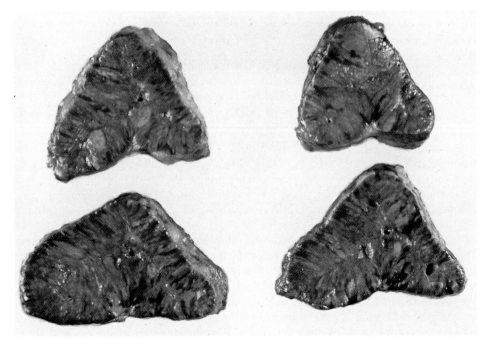

**Fig. 16-28** Ectopic adrenocorticotrophic hormone syndrome caused by a bronchial carcinoid tumor that was occult for several years. The right adrenal gland weighed 12 g and the left 11 g. The dark appearance on cross-section is caused by intense stimulation by adrenocorticotrophic hormone with conversion of lipid-rich cortical cells to lipid-depleted cells with compact, eosinophilic cytoplasm. (From Lack EE, Travis WD, Oertel JE. Adrenal cortical nodules, hyperplasia, and hyperfunction. In: Lack EE, ed. Pathology of the adrenal glands. New York: Churchill Livingstone, 1990; 75–113.)

### Primary pigmented nodular adrenal cortical disease

Primary pigmented nodular adrenal cortical disease (PPNAD) is a rare form of pituitary or ACTH-independent hypercortisolism typically seen in young individuals, with a predilection for females. It is a benign, bilateral adrenal cortical hyperplasia that can be seen as an isolated process but which may be found in association with Carney's complex (see below).[138-141] The associated Cushing's syndrome may be severe, with bone pain and pathologic fractures.[138] A variety of endocrinologic studies, including dynamic endocrine testing, indicate a primary adrenal source for the hypercortisolism.[142] Imaging studies of the sella and pituitary fossa reveal no abnormalities, and selective venous sinus sampling of the inferior petrosal sinus excludes a pituitary origin for PPNAD.

The adrenal glands in PPNAD are usually normal on CT scans, but unilateral or bilateral nodularity may be present, including macronodules >1 cm in diameter.[62] The weight of each gland varies from 0.9 to 13.4 g, with an average combined weight of 9.6 g; the gland is usually normal in size.[142] Small pigmented micronodules, 1–3 mm in diameter, may be seen through the intact capsular surface of the gland, but transverse sections usually reveal the pigmented nodules to better advantage (Fig. 16-30). Complete removal of the investing connective tissue and fat may be impeded by these small nodules when they protrude through the capsule or extend into the periadrenal fat. The pigmented nodules are light gray, gray-brown, dark brown, or jet black. The term micronodular is somewhat arbitrary because many of the intensely pigmented nodules are grossly apparent, even when they are less than 1 mm in diameter.

The gross pathology of the pigmented nodules are much more striking than the histologic features (Fig. 16-31). The pigmented nodules are usually round to oval and are present within the zona reticularis or interface with the adjacent medulla. Their configuration varies from hourglass and strings of beads to links of sausages. The pigmented nodules

are typically unencapsulated, but have expansile borders and may cause distortion or compression of adjacent uninvolved cells (Fig. 16-32). Occasionally there is intraluminal projection of a small pigmented nodule into tributaries of the central adrenal vein at sites with interrupted bundles of smooth muscle. In most nodules the cells contain compact eosinophilic cytoplasm with variable amounts of coarse granular pigment, which usually has the staining characteristics of lipofuscin. Some nodules contain cells with pale-staining lipid-rich cytoplasm, and, occasionally, cells may be large with a ballooned appearance. Sparse lymphocytic infiltrates have rarely been noted around vessels or actually within the nodules, and occasionally one may see a lipomatous or even myelolipomatous metaplastic component.[62]

The etiology and pathogenesis of primary pigmented nodular adrenal cortical disease are unknown, but several theories have been proposed,[142] such as hamartomatous malformation or dysplasia of the cortex; primary abnormality of the zona reticularis; occult adrenocorticotrophic hormone-producing pituitary adenoma with adrenal cortical

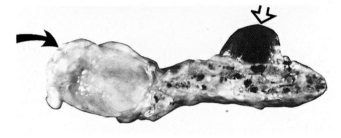

**Fig. 16-30** Primary pigmented nodular adrenal cortical disease. Transverse section of the adrenal gland shows numerous dark pigmented nodules, one nearly 1 cm in diameter (open arrow). Another nodule (curved arrow) is pale-yellow and has small foci of necrosis. The patient was a member of a family with the complex of myxomas, spotty pigmentation, and endocrine overactivity.

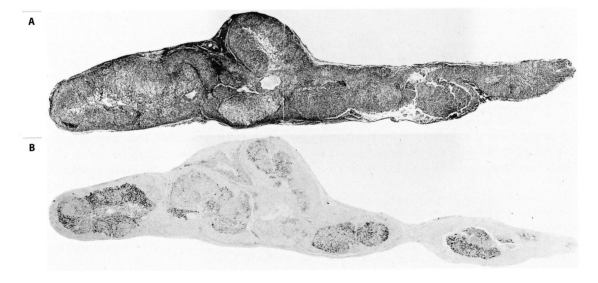

**Fig. 16-31 (A)** Primary pigmented nodular adrenal cortical disease. Numerous pigmented nodules were apparent in a transverse section of the gland, but were much more clearly delineated on gross examination. **(B)** Pigmented nodules contain cells that are argentaffin positive, causing them to stand out in contrast to the remaining gland. Some areas show marked atrophy of the internodular cortex.

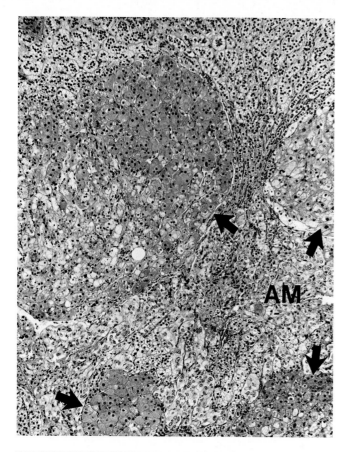

**Fig. 16-32** Several pigmented micronodules in primary pigmented nodular adrenal cortical disease (arrows) are located in the inner aspect of the cortex and impinge on the medulla (AM).

nodules becoming functionally autonomous; embryonic developmental error in the cortex at the adrenarche; block in evolution of zona fasciculata cells into cells of the zona reticularis, with accumulation of autonomous cells at the interface; and organ-specific autoimmune hypercortisolism (Cushing's syndrome).

The autoimmune theory of hypercortisolism is based on reports of circulating adrenal stimulating immunoglobulin in this disorder;[143] the adrenal-stimulating immunoglobulin is presumably directed against ACTH receptors or receptor-binding sites. Further study should determine whether PPNAD is an autoimmune disorder or one in which the circulating adrenal stimulating immunoglobulin is merely an epiphenomenon. An immunohistochemical study of PPNAD revealed the nodules to be strongly reactive for synaptophysin, whereas the extra- or internodular cortex was nonreactive.[144] This immunohistochemical differential may be helpful in the detection of small nodules in apparently unaffected cortex, as well as suggesting a possible neuroendocrine role for the genes involved. A previous report revealed intense immunoreactivity for all enzymes involved in steroidogenesis in cells of the cortical nodules, particularly those with abundant eosinophilic cytoplasm, unlike cells of the internodular cortex.[145]

The treatment of choice for PPNAD is bilateral adrenalectomy,[146] with the removal of both adrenal glands even if they appear normal or small. In some cases subtotal resection

may be possible, although about one-third of patients initially treated by unilateral or subtotal adrenalectomy require completion or total adrenalectomy because of persistence or recurrence of Cushing's syndrome.[142] It is important to note that Nelson's syndrome has not been reported following bilateral adrenalectomy in patients with PPNAD.

## Complex of myxomas, spotty pigmentation, and endocrine overactivity: Carney's complex

This is a complex array of diverse abnormalities which, in the review by Carney et al.,[147] included cardiac myxoma (72%), spotty mucocutaneous pigmentation (65%), testicular tumors, particularly large cell calcifying Sertoli cell tumor (56% of males), PPNAD (45%), cutaneous myxoma (45%), mammary myxoid fibroadenoma (30% of females), and other abnormalities such as growth hormone-secreting pituitary tumor and psammomatous melanotic schwannoma.[3,62,147] Recently, Carney et al.[148] reported four cases of unusual congenital bone tumors associated with Carney's complex which they have provisionally named 'osteochondromyxoma of bone.' Carney's complex has an autosomal dominant inheritance. Two chromosomal loci, 17q22-24 and 2p16, have been identified which are believed to harbor the genes for PPNAD and/or Carney's complex.[140,141] Germline inactivating mutations (PRKAR1A) have been observed in both Carney's complex and PPNAD.[149,150] Cardiac myxomas have a significant risk of morbidity and mortality, especially in the setting of Cushing's syndrome. Therefore, if a patient has two or more elements of this complex, particularly PPNAD, bilateral large cell calcifying Sertoli cell tumor of the testis, or mucocutaneous pigmentation, investigation for cardiac myxoma (which may be multiple) is recommended for early detection and treatment.

## Macronodular hyperplasia with marked adrenal enlargement

Macronodular hyperplasia with marked adrenal enlargement (MHMAE) is a rare primary autonomous form of adrenal hypercortisolism that is ACTH and pituitary independent.[3,62] It is a heterogenous disorder in which cortisol secretion can be mediated by hormones other than ACTH following the aberrant or ectopic expression of various hormone receptors. Ectopic receptors for gastric inhibitory polypeptide, β-adrenergic receptor agonists, vasopression, 5-hydroxytryptamine, and probably angiotensin II have been identified.[62] Careful endocrinologic investigation, including dynamic endocrine testing, usually reveals elevated plasma cortisol levels, undetectable ACTH levels, and loss of diurnal rhythmicity, suggesting a primary adrenal cortical neoplasm. Paradoxically, radiographic imaging reveals bilateral adrenal gland enlargement and there is no detectable abnormality of the sella or pituitary fossa, including one patient who was reinvestigated almost 26 years later.[151] An unusual case of ACTH-independent MHMAE occurred in a male patient who presented with feminization and Cushing's syndrome; the combined adrenal glands weighed 86 g.[62] Another reported case describes massive adrenal gland enlargement, with the left gland weighing 199 g and the right gland weighing 93 g.[152] The average patient age is about 50 years, with a slight male preponderance (although one series reports a 3:1 female preponderance[153]), and the duration of Cushing's syndrome ranged from about 1 to 10 years in one study.[151]

The adrenal glands in MHMAE are significantly enlarged and can simulate an adrenal neoplasm.[62] Typically, the combined weight ranges from 60 g to 180 g, with an extraordinary degree of nodular cortical hyperplasia; the nodules in one study ranged in size from 0.2 to 3.8 cm (Fig. 16-33).[151] The nodules are yellow or golden-yellow, typically unencapsulated, and blend imperceptibly with the hyperplastic cortex. The medullary compartment may be distorted and difficult to recognize in random sections of the gland, similar to macronodular hyperplasia. Cortical cells have a variable amount of finely vacuolated, lipid-rich pale-staining cytoplasm (Fig. 16-34). There may be scattered cells with compact eosinophilic cytoplasm. Rarely cells with large ballooned vacuolated cytoplasm are present, and occasionally one may see lipomatous or myelolipomatous metaplasia. There is weak immunoreactivity in MHMAE for 3β-hydroxysteroid dehydrogenase and other enzymes involved in steroidogenesis, whereas strong staining is noted in adrenal cortical adenoma[154] and PPNAD.[145] In situ hybridization study of P-450c17 has also been used to localize the site of steroido-genesis, and results suggest that the degree of corticosteroidogenesis by individual cortical cells is low and that a significant increase in cell numbers is necessary before excessive cortisol production causes Cushing's syndrome.[155] As indicated in Figure 16-35, a possible relationship between MHMAE and macronodular hyperplasia of Cushing's disease cannot be definitively established in most cases. The treatment proposed for this rare disorder is bilateral adrenalectomy. As in macronodular hyperplasia in Cushing's disease, the clinical and biochemical features may be misleading and suggest an underlying adrenal cortical neoplasm.

## Multiple endocrine neoplasia type 1

Multiple endocrine neoplasia (MEN) type 1 (Wermer's syndrome)[156] occurs as an autosomal dominant trait with somewhat variable expression or affects family members in whom manifestations are detectable only after close scrutiny. The genetic defect is located on chromosome 11q13.[157] In a review by Ballard et al.,[158] adrenal findings at autopsy included cortical adenoma, 'miliary' adenoma, hyperplasia, multiple adenomas, and nodular hyperplasia, but only one of 31 patients had clinical hypercortisolism. Cushing's disease may occur in MEN 1, but is rare (see Figs 16-26 and 16-27).[159] A recent study reports 12 malignant endocrine neoplasms in 42 cases of MEN 1, two of which were adrenal cortical carcinomas; thus, although malignancies tend to play a lesser role in MEN 1 than in the other MEN syndromes, patients still need to be examined and followed with this possibility in mind.[160]

## Other rare causes of Cushing's syndrome

There are several other rare causes of Cushing's syndrome that are reviewed elsewhere.[62] These include McCune–Albright syndrome (triad of café au lait spots, polyostotic fibrous dysplasia, and sexual precocity) with hyperfunction of various endocrine glands, including adrenal hypercorti-

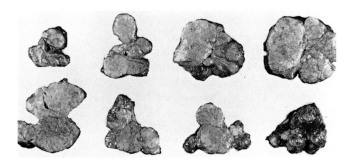

**Fig. 16-33** Macronodular adrenal cortical hyperplasia with marked adrenal enlargement. Transverse sections of one adrenal gland are displayed. The combined weight of both glands was about 90 g.

**Fig. 16-34** Macronodular adrenal cortical hyperplasia with marked adrenal enlargement. Note multiple irregular nodules of hyperplastic adrenal cortex as well as small area of metaplastic fat. Most hyperplastic cells had lipid-rich, pale-staining cytoplasm.

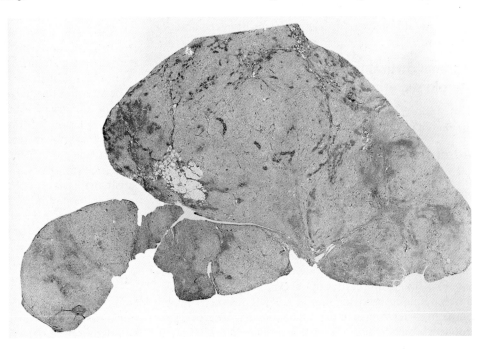

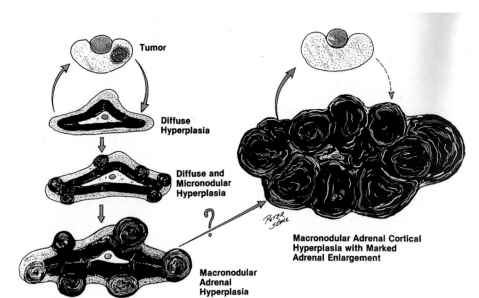

**Fig. 16-35** Schematic diagram of progression of pituitary (or adrenocorticotrophic hormone)-dependent Cushing's disease into micronodular and macronodular adrenal cortical hyperplasia. Macronodular adrenal cortical hyperplasia with marked adrenal enlargement appears to be a primary form of adrenal hypercortisolism (Cushing's syndrome) by sensitive imaging and biochemical studies. The relationship with macronodular adrenal hyperplasia (lower left) is uncertain.

solism due to a somatic mutation with activation of a signal transduction pathway generating cAMP,[161,162] and food-dependent Cushing's syndrome caused by abnormal responsiveness of the adrenal glands to physiologic postprandial secretion of gastric inhibitory polypeptide.[163,164]

## Adrenal cortical hyperplasia with hyperaldosteronism

Up to 35% of cases of primary hyperaldosteronism are idiopathic, with bilateral hyperplasia of the zona glomerulosa,[165] but a higher incidence is noted in milder forms of the disorder.[166] Patients are usually managed medically; adrenalectomy is reserved for patients with an aldosterone-producing adenoma because of a more predictable response in terms of amelioration or normalization of systemic hypertension.[62,167] The cause of this disorder is uncertain, but may be due to an aldosterone-stimulating factor from the anterior pituitary.[168,169]

## Adrenal cortical hyperplasia with excess sex steroid secretion

This disorder is essentially limited to cases of congenital adrenal hyperplasia.

## Adrenal medullary hyperplasia

Adrenal medullary hyperplasia is either inherited or occurs sporadically. The inherited form usually arises in the setting of MEN types 2a and 2b, may be diffuse or nodular, and is often multicentric and bilateral.[170,171] Sporadic adrenal medullary hyperplasia is now accepted as an entity, occurring in patients with symptoms of pheochromocytoma, including paroxysmal or sustained hypertension, headaches, palpitations, and diaphoresis; surgical exploration fails to reveal a catecholamine-secreting tumor. Adrenal medullary hyperplasia in this setting is in the differential diagnosis of 'pseudopheochromocytoma.' Adrenal medullary hyperplasia has

also been reported in patients with cystic fibrosis and the Beckwith–Wiedemann syndrome.[4,38,62]

In MEN types 2a and 2b, one of the earliest manifestations of adrenal medullary hyperfunction is an elevated ratio of epinephrine to norepinephrine in the urine.[170] One suggested treatment for such patients is bilateral total adrenalectomy. Others suggest good long-term results with conservative unilateral adrenalectomy, with removal of the larger gland.[171,172] Involvement of the adrenal glands by adrenal medullary hyperplasia may be symmetric or asymmetric. The distinction between adrenal medullary hyperplasia and pheochromocytoma in MEN 2 is arbitrary. Carney et al.[173] adopted a cut-off point of 1 cm in diameter to separate adrenal medullary hyperplasia and pheochromocytoma. Nodules larger than 1 cm are considered pheochromocytoma. This size was chosen because it was the lower limit of size range of pheochromocytomas reported in the first series fascicle from the Armed Forces Institute of Pathology (AFIP)[173a] dealing with tumors of the adrenal gland. Histologically, adrenal medullary hyperplasia consists of expansile nodular growth of the medulla with distortion of the adjacent cortex or adjacent normal-appearing medulla. There may be numerous extensively vacuolated cells, as well as intracytoplasmic hyaline globules, some of which appear to be present in the extracellular space. Mitotic figures may be present but are usually not numerous, and there may be some nuclear pleomorphism. In a study of adrenal medullary hyperplasia and pheochromocytoma, DNA content was found to be diploid or euploid in normal and hyperplastic glands, whereas 87% of clinically benign pheochromocytomas (33 of 38 cases) and all five malignant pheochromocytomas had non-diploid or aneuploid DNA histograms.[174]

## Adrenal cyst

Non-neoplastic adrenal cysts are uncommon, usually occurring in the fifth and sixth decades, although cases have been reported from birth to 76 years.[175] There is a predilection for

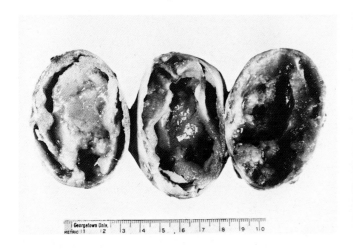

**Fig. 16-36** Adrenal pseudocyst on cross-section contains grumous, soft, pale-tan debris. Dystrophic calcification was present in the cyst wall.

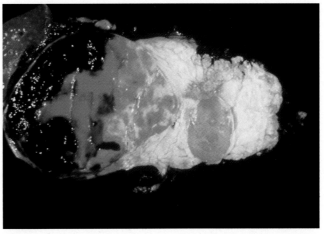

**Fig. 16-37** Adrenal myelolipoma. The tumor is well circumscribed with a thin fibrous capsule. On cross-section it is red-brown because of abundant hematopoietic elements with a focal area of hemorrhage. The lesion appears quite large and is enveloped by abundant adipose tissue.

women, with a female:male ratio of about 3:1.[176] Adrenal cysts are usually small and discovered incidentally at autopsy. Rarely they may be extremely large, containing several liters of fluid and compressing the abdominal contents. Adrenal cysts have been classified as parasitic[177] (7% of cases, usually echinococcal), epithelial (9%), endothelial (45%), and pseudocyst (39%).[175] Epithelial cysts are subdivided into three categories: true glandular or retention cysts; embryonal cysts lined by cylindrical epithelium derived from displaced urogenital tissue that has undergone cystic transformation; and cystic change within an adrenal adenoma, carcinoma, or pheochromocytoma.[178] It has also been proposed that an epithelial-lined adrenal cyst rarely may develop from entrapped mesothelium.[179,180]

Adrenal pseudocysts are the most common type of adrenal cyst seen at surgery and often appear as a large unilocular cyst with an irregular lining, containing red-brown bloody fluid (Fig. 16-36). Some adrenal pseudocysts probably arise by hemorrhage into normal or pathologic adrenals; a small number result from hemorrhage into an underlying tumor.[175,178,181] Immunohistochemical studies show a vascular endothelial lining in some adrenal pseudocysts.[181–184] Some hemorrhagic cysts may also arise when hemorrhage occurs in an existing vascular malformation.[183] There may be entrapment of nests of cortical cells by extravasated blood, and this hemorrhagic cyst should be distinguished from a necrotic adrenal cortical neoplasm.[183] Breast carcinoma has initially presented as metastasis to an adrenal cyst, and mature adipose tissue and myelolipomatous metaplasia have also been described within adrenal pseudocysts.[185]

Microscopic cysts are a frequent histologic finding in the permanent cortex of fetal and premature adrenal glands, being reported in up to 62% of stillbirths under 35 weeks' gestational age.[186] A significant correlation with short gestation and short survival after birth has been reported.[187] Three possible pathogenetic mechanisms have been proposed: an intrinsic developmental process, infection, and a generalized reaction to stress.

## Myelolipoma

Adrenal myelolipoma is a benign tumefactive lesion consisting of mature adipose tissue admixed with a variable amount of hematopoietic elements. This lesion occurs most frequently in the adrenal gland, although it also occurs in extra-adrenal sites,[188] including the stomach, liver,[189] mediastinum,[190,191] pleura,[192] spleen,[193] and the presacral region.[178,194] The pathogenesis is unknown, although some data suggest that it arises under hormonal influence by metaplasia of adrenal cortical or stromal cells.[178] Intra-adrenal fat and hematopoietic tissue have been induced experimentally by injecting crude pituitary ACTH extract into adrenal glands,[195] and myelolipomatous foci may be seen in patients with excess cortical activity, such as hyperfunctioning adrenal cortical adenoma or adrenal cortical hyperplasia. Others have suggested that myelolipoma derives from emboli from the bone marrow or from embryonic rests of hematopoietic tissue.[178] A recent study suggests a clonal origin for myelolipoma, as supported by non-random X-chromosome inactivation.[196]

The incidence of adrenal myelolipoma at autopsy is 0.01–0.2%, and it is most common in persons over 40 years of age, with a roughly equal gender predilection.[197] Most patients are asymptomatic, and most cases are discovered incidentally. When patients are symptomatic it is usually because of the large size of the myelolipoma, resulting in abdominal or flank pain, dysuria, hematuria, or rarely, catastrophic spontaneous retroperitoneal hemorrhage.[198–200] It may occur in patients with concurrent endocrinologic disorders, such as Cushing's disease,[201,202] Cushing's syndrome,[203] Conn's syndrome,[204] Addison's disease, and congenital adrenal hyperplasia.[62] A case of subclinical Cushing's syndrome due to adrenal myelolipoma has been reported.[205]

Grossly, myelolipoma forms a soft, well-circumscribed mass that is variegated yellow to red-brown (Fig. 16-37). It ranges in size from a few millimeters up to 34 cm. Microscopically, there is hematopoietic tissue comprising various combinations of the three cell lines, with an admixture of mature adipose tissue (Fig. 16-38). Bony trabeculae, hemor-

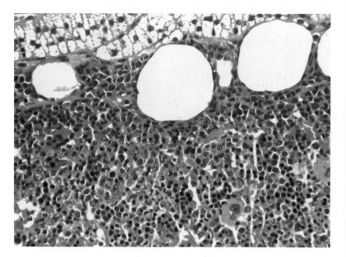

**Fig. 16-38** Myelolipoma consists of fat mixed with hematopoietic elements, including megakaryocytes. Note the rim of compressed adrenal cortical tissue (top).

rhage, and fibrosis are occasionally seen. Myelolipoma is detected more frequently with the advent of CT and MRI scanning; fine needle aspiration biopsy has proved useful in preoperative diagnosis.[206] Treatment varies from radiographic surveillance for small lesions in asymptomatic patients to surgical excision of large or symptomatic lesions.

## Adrenal hemorrhage

Adrenal hemorrhage can complicate cardiac disease, thromboembolic disease, sepsis, postoperative or postpartum state, or coagulopathy (e.g., heparin administration).[3] Patients may become symptomatic with abdominal or lower chest pain and fever. Newborn infants may also present with manifestations of adrenal hemorrhage or hematoma formation.[3,178] Occasionally, adrenal hemorrhage is bilateral and massive.[207] Unfortunately, the diagnosis is made only infrequently during life. A high index of suspicion is required owing to the non-specific clinical presentation and the frequent comorbidity of other factors. Imaging techniques are useful in establishing a timely diagnosis so that appropriate intervention can prevent the overall poor outcome.[208]

## Adrenal neoplasms

### Adrenal cortical neoplasms

#### Adrenal cortical adenoma with Cushing's syndrome

Adrenal cortical adenoma (ACA) is usually small, weighing less than 50 g. In one series[209] the tumors had an average weight of 36 g (range, 12.5–126 g). On transverse section it usually appears as a sharply circumscribed or encapsulated mass.[62,210] Almost all tumors are unilateral and solitary, although there are rare exceptions.[211,212] Adenomas may be yellow or golden-yellow throughout, or have irregular mottling or diffuse dark brown areas (Fig. 16-39). The color of the tumor depends on a number of factors, including the presence of congestion or hemorrhage and the content of neutral lipid and lipofuscin.[62,210,213]

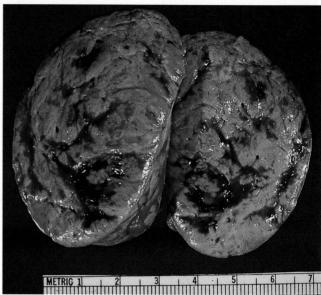

**Fig. 16-39** Adrenal cortical adenoma in Cushing's syndrome.

Although many tumors appear grossly encapsulated, histologic study may reveal a relatively smooth expansile border, in some cases with formation of a pseudocapsule. Compression of adjacent adrenal parenchyma and connective tissue, including the expanded adrenal capsule itself, contributes to the encapsulation of the ACA. Adenomas usually consist of cells with relatively abundant pale, lipid-rich cytoplasm resembling the zona fasciculata, but there may be cells with more compact eosinophilic cytoplasm. Architecturally, the cells are arranged in short trabeculae, blunt cords, or a nesting or alveolar pattern (Fig. 16-40). Nuclei are usually vesicular, with a single, small nucleolus. There may be nuclear enlargement and pleomorphism, but it is usually focal and mild to moderate in degree (Fig. 16-41). Also, there may be foci of lipomatous or myelolipomatous metaplasia. Endocrinologic data and clinical information are often essential to distinguish an adrenal cortical neoplasm associated with Cushing's syndrome from an incidental nonhyperfunctioning adenoma or one associated with a different endocrine syndrome.[62,210] An important clue to the presence of Cushing's syndrome is cortical atrophy in the attached adrenal or the contralateral gland. In most cases ultrastructural study reveals abundant intracytoplasmic lipid (Fig. 16-42). Mitochondria may have tubulovesicular cristae, similar to normal cells of zona fasciculata, or lamellar cristae characteristic of the zona reticularis. Smooth endoplasmic reticulum is usually abundant.

### Adrenal cortical adenoma with primary hyperaldosteronism (Conn's syndrome)

It has been estimated that 65–85% of cases of primary hyperaldosteronism are caused by an aldosterone-secreting ACA, but recent data indicate that idiopathic bilateral hyperplasia may be a more frequent cause, particularly if mild examples are included. The aldosterone-secreting ACA is an important surgical lesion because it may be a curable form of systemic hypertension. The prevalence of an aldosterone-

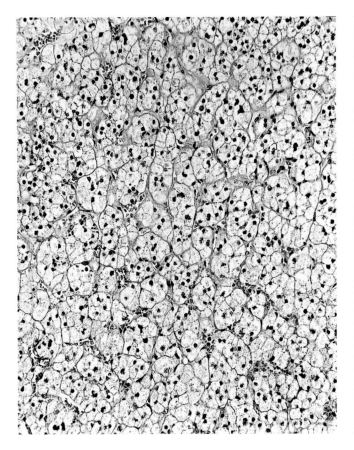

**Fig. 16-40** Adrenal cortical adenoma in Cushing's syndrome. Cells are arranged in alveoli or short cords.

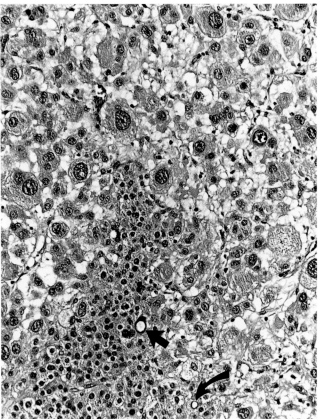

**Fig. 16-41** Adrenal cortical adenoma in Cushing's syndrome. Note focally marked variability in nuclear size and hyperchromasia. Many cells in this field have compact, eosinophilic cytoplasm and several have nuclear 'pseudoinclusions' (arrows).

secreting adenoma in the hypertensive population ranges from 0.5% to 8%,[210] although Conn[214] suggested that primary hyperaldosteronism may be the cause of up to 20% of all cases of essential hypertension based on the incidence of a solitary 'adenoma' 1.5 cm or more in diameter reported in hypertensive individuals at autopsy (20%).[91] However, incidental cortical nodules are relatively common in patients 50–80 years of age, as well as in those with hypertension.[88] It is uncertain whether hypertension results from the incidental nodule or adenoma or is a cause of it, perhaps in some cases related to capsular arteriopathy. This controversy can forever be rekindled, however, because one can postulate that over time there may be conversion of glomerulosa-type cells within these incidental nodules to cells having different functional characteristics; when the incidental 'adenoma' is discovered the patient may already have established systemic hypertension without the expected biochemical profile of an aldosterone-secreting adenoma.[210]

Aldosterone-secreting ACA (aldosteronoma) is usually solitary, small, and measures only a few centimeters in diameter; many are smaller than 2 cm,[210] although most are large enough to be visible on abdominal CT scan. Grossly, the tumor may project from one portion of the gland, although it may be difficult to appreciate in the intact gland without transverse sectioning. It is often homogeneous and diffusely bright yellow-orange, and may be sharply demarcated from the adjacent cortex, simulating encapsulation (Fig. 16-43).

Architectural patterns include alveolar or nesting arrangement, short cords or trabeculae of cells (Fig. 16-44).

Four types of cells have been described by light microscopy, often with multiple types in the same tumor.[7] The most common cell type is large, with pale-staining lipid-rich cytoplasm resembling cells of the zona fasciculata. A second cell type appears as clusters of smaller cells resembling those of the zona glomerulosa, with a high nuclear to cytoplasmic ratio and a small amount of vacuolated cytoplasm. The third type consists of scattered cells with compact eosinophilic cytoplasm similar to cells of the zona reticularis. The fourth cell type, 'hybrid' cells, has morphologic features intermediate between zona glomerulosa-type and zona fasciculata-type cells. The attached or contralateral adrenal may show hyperplasia of the zona glomerulosa with a broad focal or discontinuous zone beneath the capsule (Fig. 16-45), sometimes with small tongues of glomerulosa-type cells extending inward from the capsule. The term 'hybrid' refers to the capacity of the cell to synthesize cortical steroids, which are normally produced by the zona glomerulosa (aldosterone) or the zona fasciculata (cortisol). Aldosterone-secreting adenomas may originate from hybrid cells or zona fasciculata-type cells. This would account for the functional behavior of tumor cells in vivo, as evidenced by modulation of aldosterone secretion by ACTH, lack of responsiveness to angioten-

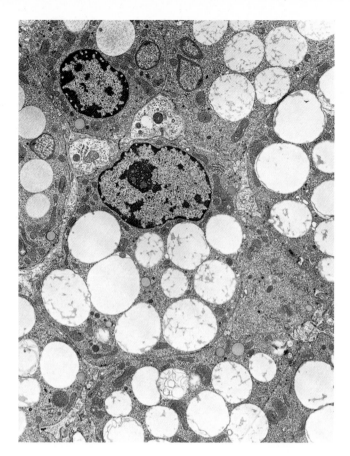

**Fig. 16-42** Adrenal cortical adenoma in Cushing's syndrome. Cells contain large lipid globules and prominent smooth endoplasmic reticulum. (×3500) (From Lack EE, Travis WD, Oertel JE. Adrenal cortical neoplasms. In: Lack EE, ed. Pathology of the adrenal glands. New York: Churchill Livingstone, 1990; 115–171.)

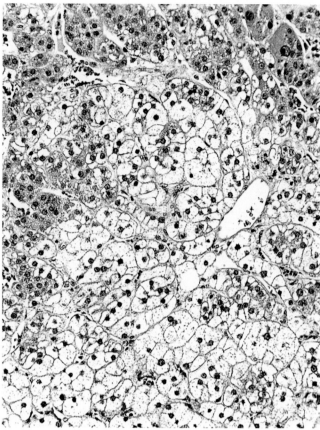

**Fig. 16-44** Aldosterone-producing adrenal cortical adenoma. Most cells have lipid-rich, finely vacuolated cytoplasm.

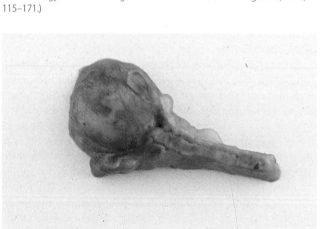

**Fig. 16-43** Aldosterone-secreting adrenal cortical adenoma. The tumor was 1 cm in diameter and yellow-orange on cross-section.

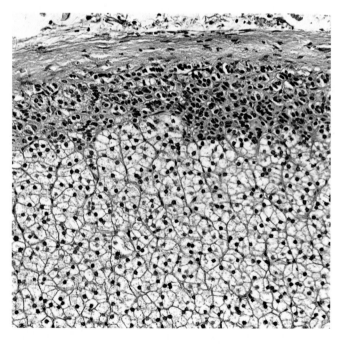

**Fig. 16-45** Hyperplasia of the zona glomerulosa is apparent as a continuous band of cells beneath the capsule. Numerous foci such as this may be present in the cortex adjacent to aldosterone-secreting adenomas.

sin II (the dominant secretagogue and trophic hormone for the glomerulosa-type cells under normal conditions), secretion of the hybrid steroids in large quantities, and the ability of the cells to produce cortisol in vitro and sometimes in large quantities in vivo.[215] Ultrastructurally, these cells show morphologic heterogeneity,[62,216] including round to elongated mitochondria with cristae that are short and tubular, vesicular, or lamellar, typical of zona glomerulosa-type cells.

Spironolactone bodies are lightly eosinophilic, scroll-like intracytoplasmic inclusions which have been described in the zona glomerulosa of the non-neoplastic cortex or occasionally within the tumor cells; these occur in patients treated with the aldosterone antagonist spironolactone (Aldactone) (Fig. 16-46).[62,210,217] Ultrastructural study suggests origin from tightly packed tubules of endoplasmic reticulum.[218] The spironolactone bodies typically range in size from 2 to 12 μm, but most are equal in size or slightly larger than the adjacent nucleus. These structures may be highlighted with Luxol fast blue stain because of their rich

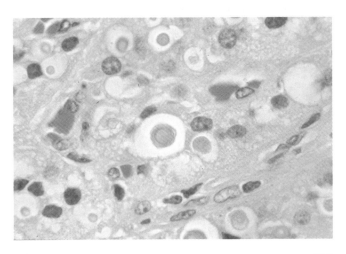

**Fig. 16-46** Spironolactone bodies appear as single scroll-like, eosinophilic inclusions within zona glomerulosa cells. Many are surrounded by a clear space.

phospholipid content.[62,210] Although the specificity of these inclusions has been questioned, they are generally regarded as rather specific markers for spironolactone administration. In one study, the number of spironolactone bodies within cells of the aldosterone-secreting adenoma correlated positively with the proportion of glomerulosa-type cells.[219]

### Functional pigmented (black) ACA

Pigmented (black) ACA is characterized by diffuse black pigmentation on cross-section (Fig. 16-47), although there may be some areas that are dark-brown or yellow-brown.[220] Pigmented ACA is usually diagnosed in the third to the fifth decades of life, with a distinct predilection for females.[210] This tumor is most often associated with Cushing's syndrome, although it has also been reported with primary hyperaldosteronism.[62,210] Microscopically, the architectural patterns are similar to those of other adenomas. The histologic hallmark is the conspicuous brown or golden-brown granular pigment in the cytoplasm (Fig. 16-48), which has the staining characteristics of lipofuscin. One study, however, suggested that some of the pigment may be neuromelanin.[95] As with other adenomas, there may be areas of lipomatous or myelolipomatous metaplasia.[62] Ultrastructurally, the cells contain relatively few lipid globules, but have a variable number of electron-dense granules that are often associated with small lipid vacuoles (Fig. 16-49) characteristic of lipfuscin.[62,210] There are no melanosomes or premelanosomes.

### Adrenal cortical neoplasms with virilization or feminization

Adrenal cortical neoplasms associated with virilization or feminization are clinically important because of the potential for malignant behavior. Many have unfavorable gross or microscopic findings, such as large size and areas of necrosis. A review of women with virilizing adrenal cortical tumors found that at least 17% were clinically malignant;[221] an even greater proportion of feminizing adrenal cortical neoplasms were malignant.[222] Histologically, there is often a predominance of cells with compact eosinophilic cytoplasm,

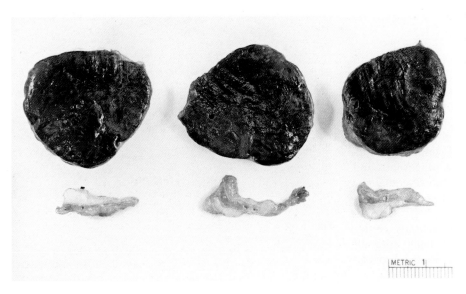

**Fig. 16-47** Pigmented (black) adrenal cortical adenoma with Cushing's syndrome. The tumor is 3. 5 cm in diameter. Sectioned surface s of tumor are diffusely black, with vague lobulation. Residual adrenal gland (lower row) shows marked cortical atrophy.

METRIC 1

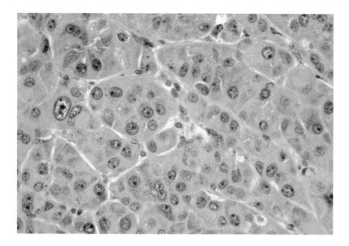

**Fig. 16-48** Pigmented (black) adenoma causing Cushing's syndrome. Tumor cells form nests and short cords and have abundant intracytoplasmic granular lipofuscin pigment.

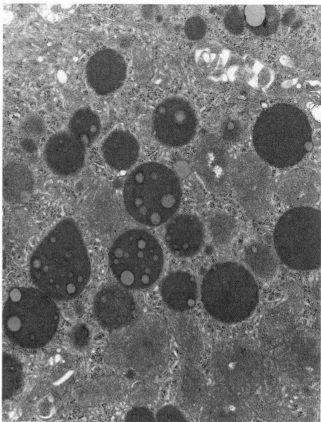

**Fig. 16-49** Black adenoma of adrenal gland from a patient with Cushing's syndrome. Note numerous electron-dense structures, some containing small lipid droplets. (×17 000).

but this histologic pattern is not specific. Virilization has also been reported with tumors classified as Leydig cell adenoma of the adrenal gland, which contain Reinke crystalloids, a pathognomonic feature of Leydig (or hilus) cells.[223] Rarely, Leydig cells are present in the adrenal cortex, probably because of the close embryologic relation between developing adrenal primordia and gonads.[224]

## Oncocytic adrenal cortical neoplasms (adrenal oncocytoma)

Rarely adrenal cortical neoplasms are composed of cells with abundant, finely granular, eosinophilic cytoplasm typical of oncocytoma (Fig. 16-50).[225–228] The vast majority of these tumors are clinically non-functional, but some may exhibit low levels of enzyme activity in cortical steroidogenesis.[226] Although most adrenal cortical oncocytic neoplasms are benign, cases of malignant oncocytic carcinomas have been reported.[229–232]

## Adrenal cortical carcinoma

Adrenal cortical carcinomas (ACC) are rare, occurring annually in about two persons per million population in the United States.[233] A number of large series of ACC have been reported in the last few decades, mainly in adults. There is a slight female preponderance, and the peak incidence is in the fifth to seventh decades of life, although there is a second peak in childhood.[234] Presenting signs and symptoms include abdominal pain, a palpable mass, fatigue, weight loss, and, in 10–20% of patients, intermittent low-grade fever that may be caused by tumor necrosis.[62,210] Regional or distant metastases occur in 25% or more of patients.[62,210,235,236] Because ACCs are usually inefficient producers of steroids, clinical evidence of excess hormone secretion usually does not become apparent until the tumor is large. Some tumors are

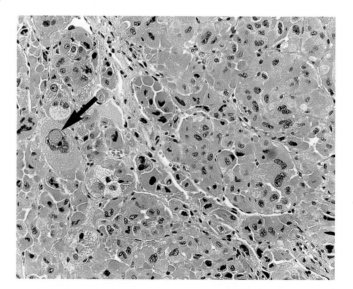

**Fig. 16-50** Incidental non-hyperfunctional adrenal cortical adenoma is composed of cells with abundant, granular eosinophilic cytoplasm (oncocytoma). Nuclei are moderately pleomorphic and hyperchromatic, with occasional nuclear 'pseudoinclusions' (arrow). The tumor weighed less than 15 g.

therefore classified clinically as functionally inactive. When adrenal cortical neoplasms are functional they most commonly produce cortisol, but in some cases the patient may present with a mixed endocrine syndrome, e. g. Cushing's syndrome and virilization. Purely virilizing ACC is uncommon in adults, and feminizing ACC is rare. Primary hyperaldosteronism caused by ACC is also relatively uncommon.[62,210] A study reported five adrenal cortical neoplasms clinically mimicking pheochromocytoma with biochemical evidence of elevated catecholamine secretion in serum or urine;[237] two were ACC, three were ACA.

ACC is usually large, and careful gross examination may often suggest malignancy with areas of necrosis, hemorrhage and cystic change.[62,210] On cross-section the tumors are usually yellow, yellow-orange, or tan-brown. Larger tumors are often coarsely lobulated with intersecting fibrous bands (Fig. 16-51). The average recorded weight in several series ranged from 705 to 1210 g.[62] Tang and Gray[238] reported that all adrenal cortical tumors over 95 g were malignant, whereas those weighing less than 50 g were benign. However, weight alone is not entirely reliable as a distinguishing characteristic, because some small ACCs have metastasized, including tumors weighing 40 g or less.[62,210,239] Also, some adrenal cortical neoplasms weighing more than 1000 g may prove to be clinically benign after prolonged follow-up. Size has been reported to be an important indicator of malignancy. Copeland[107] reported that 92% of the ACCs they reviewed were greater than 6 cm in diameter; subsequently, there have been a number of reports of small ACCs measuring less than 5 cm.[240] The reverse is also true. Adrenal cortical adenomas may be quite large – more than 5 cm – usually due to central degeneration, hemorrhage, and/or calcification and fibrosis.[241] Most recently, however, a study of the SEER database[242] indicated that for adrenal cortical neoplasms 4 cm or larger the likelihood of malignancy essentially doubles to approximately 10%, and increases more than ninefold in tumors 8 cm or larger.[242]

ACC has a variety of architectural patterns, including trabecular, alveolar (nesting), and solid (diffuse). The most characteristic pattern is a trabecular arrangement of cells with broad anastomosing columns separated by delicate elongated vascular spaces (Fig. 16-52). Some of the trabeculae, when cut in cross-section or oblique planes, appear as free-floating islands of tumor cells. Rarely, a pseudoglandular arrangement of cells may be seen, or the tumor may have a myxoid appearance.[62,210] Most tumor cells in ACC have compact, eosinophilic cytoplasm that is lipid poor. Foci of vascular invasion usually appear as unattached plugs of tumor within vascular spaces. Nuclear pleomorphism and hyperchromasia can be spectacular in ACC, but nuclear atypia alone is not a reliable indicator of malignancy and can also be seen in ACA (Fig. 16-53).[62,210] Mitotic figures may be numerous in ACC, and are rare in adenoma and adrenal hyperplasia (Fig. 16-54). In the study by Weiss,[243] only two non-metastasizing adrenal cortical tumors contained fewer

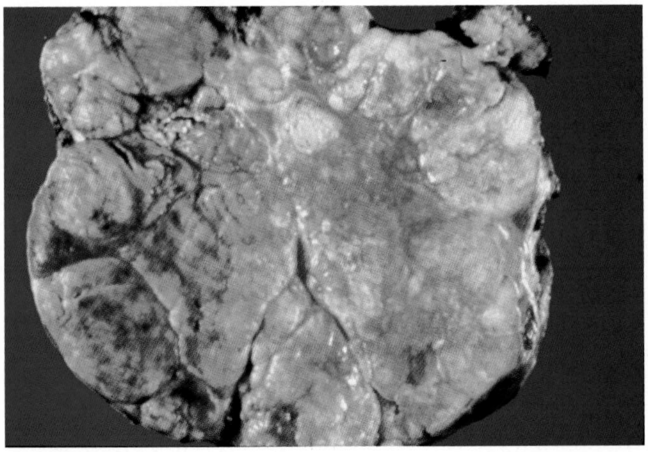

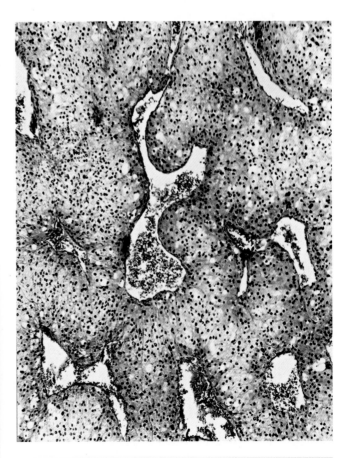

**Fig. 16-52** Adrenal cortical carcinoma. The tumor has broad anastomosing trabeculae and gaping sinusoids with delicate endothelium. Tumor cells have compact, eosinophilic cytoplasm and small, uniform nuclei. The patient died of metastases within a year of diagnosis, and at autopsy had massive invasion of the inferior vena cava.

**Fig. 16-51** Adrenal cortical carcinoma. Note the coarsely nodular cut surface.

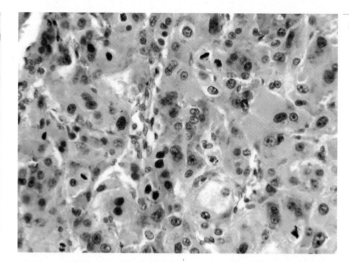

**Fig. 16-53** Adrenal cortical adenoma. Tumor cells have marked nuclear pleomorphism and hyperchromasia. The tumor was found incidentally on CT and weighed 99 g. The patient was alive and well 11 yrs. later.

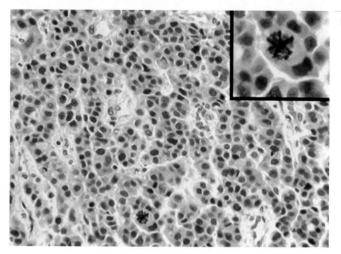

**Fig. 16-54 (A)** Adrenal cortical carcinoma with several mitotic figures seen in this single, high-power field. **(B)** Another case of adrenal cortical carcinoma composed of cells with dense, compact eosinophilic cytoplasm arranged in a trabecular growth pattern; an atypical mitotic figure is highlighted (inset).

than three mitotic figures per 50 high-power fields (hpf), whereas 78% of ACCs contained more than five mitotic figures per hpf, and 17% had more than 50 per 50 hpf. In addition to mitotic activity, tumor necrosis is more frequent in ACC than in adrenal cortical adenoma;[236,244–247] one investigation of 56 cases reports no necrosis in eight of the adrenal cortical adenomas reviewed, whereas 45 of the 48 ACCs displayed variable amounts of necrosis.[236]

An unusual feature of ACC (and some adenomas) is the presence of intracytoplasmic hyaline globules, similar to those commonly seen in pheochromocytomas (Fig. 16-55).[62] An ACC with an alveolar growth pattern and cells with compact, eosinophilic cytoplasm along with intracytoplasmic globules may be mistaken for a pheochromocytoma. Another pitfall in the diagnosis of adrenal cortical neoplasms is immunoreactivity for synaptophysin and/or neuron-specific enolase (NSE), markers that are used for documenting neuroendocrine differentiation.[248,249] Ultrastructurally, intracytoplasmic lipid vacuoles are often sparse or absent, and cellular organelles may be moderate or few in number.[250] There may be flattened cisternae of rough endoplasmic reticulum in stacks or short parallel lamellae. Smooth endoplasmic reticulum may form an intricate anastomosing network.

A number of studies have proposed histologic criteria to predict malignant behavior. Hough et al.[244] reported that the strongest predictors were broad fibrous bands, a diffuse growth pattern, and vascular invasion. Weiss et al[246] analyzed the predictive value of nine histologic parameters and found that recurrence or metastasis occurred only in tumors with a mitotic rate greater than five per 50 hpf, atypical mitotic figures, and invasion of venous structures. Van Slooten et al.[245] used a histologic index based on seven histologic parameters to predict outcome. Despite these findings, it is clear that a small but significant number of adrenal cortical neoplasms have unpredictable biologic behavior, and long-term follow-up in some of these troublesome cases is the final arbiter in diagnosis.[210] Mitotic rate has been used to

separate low- and high-grade ACC; the median survival for patients with low-grade ACC (≤20 mitotic figures per 50 hpf) was 58 months, compared to 14 months for high-grade tumors (>20 mitotic figures per 50 hpf).[246] DNA ploidy analysis has also been used to predict outcome, but the results have been controversial.[62,251–254] According to some investigators, the greatest value of DNA ploidy analysis in predicting outcome is in patients undergoing potentially curative surgical resection.[255] More recently, molecular studies have revealed multiple chromosomal aberrations that may be related to ACC. Some chromosomal loci correlate with abnormal familial syndromes, including Li–Fraumeni syndrome (p53, 17p13), MEN 1 (11q13), Beckwith–Wiedemann syndrome (11p15. 5 associated with IGFII over-expression), and Carney's complex (2p16).[240,256] Additionally, loss of heterozygosity (LOH) on chromosomes 11p, 13q and 17p has been reported in ACCs, whereas these chromosomal changes have not been seen in adrenal cortical adenomas or hyperplasia.[257,258] Numerous other studies on chromosomal

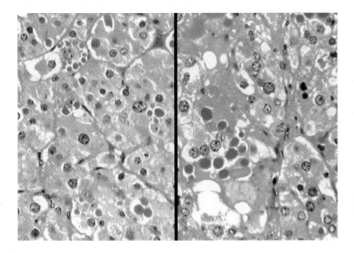

**Fig. 16-55** Adrenal cortical adenoma with intracytoplasmic globules, similar to what is more commonly encountered in pheochromocytoma. Right side: high power image of globules.

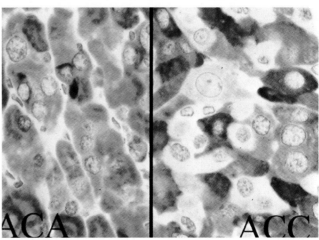

**Fig. 16-56** Adrenal cortical adenoma (ACA) and adrenal cortical carcinoma (ACC), both showing strong cytoplasmic staining with antibodies to the α subunit of inhibin.

associations with malignancy in adrenal cortical tumors have been reported in recent years, the results of which are beyond the scope of this chapter.[259–267] Suffice it to say that as our understanding of the molecular pathogenesis of these neoplasms progresses, improved diagnostic and treatment strategies may become available.

The pattern of metastasis of ACC reflects both lymphatic and hematogenous dissemination. The sites of metastases in patients dying of ACC include liver (92%), lung (78%), retroperitoneum (48%), intra-abdominal lymph nodes (32%), intrathoracic lymph nodes (26%), and other sites such as bone.[210,247]

Percutaneous fine needle aspiration may be helpful in the preoperative diagnosis of ACC, but extreme caution must be exercised in trying to differentiate ACC from a benign adrenal cortical neoplasm on cytologic features alone.[62,210] A major drawback to the cytologic differentiation of adrenal cortical carcinoma versus adenoma is sampling error. If one obtains a good specimen with obvious cytologic features of carcinoma the diagnosis can be made with a fair amount of certainty.[62] However, if the specimen has only minor cytologic abnormalities that could be seen in adrenal cortical adenoma, to definitively rule out the possibility of carcinoma on an FNA specimen would not be prudent. Careful correlation with clinical and endocrinologic data is needed, combined with a knowledge of other features such as tumor size and imaging characteristics.[62] The same can be said for core needle biopsy specimens.

The differential diagnosis of ACC may be aided by special studies, including immunohistochemistry. Adrenal cortical neoplasms in general do not have a pathognomonic immunohistochemical profile. Typically, adrenal cortical neoplasms are positive for vimentin and negative for epithelial markers such as cytokeratin, CAM 5.2 and EMA; however, occasionally adrenal cortical neoplasms may express keratin reactivity. Antibodies to the α subunit of inhibin have been found to be expressed by adrenal cortical tissue, both normal and abnor-

mal or neoplastic (Fig. 16-56). Thus, it is quite useful in differentiating adrenal cortical neoplasms from other neoplasms that arise in the adrenal gland, such as adrenal medullary tumors, i.e. pheochromocytomas, and metastatic tumors, especially renal cell carcinoma.[268,269] Other studies suggest the utility of MelanA (MART-1) immunoreactivity and nuclear expression of D-11 in adrenal cortical neoplasms.[270–272]

Disease-free and overall survival rates have been strongly correlated with ACC stage. Most patients have relatively advanced disease at the time of diagnosis, only about 30% of patients having tumor confined to the adrenal gland (Table 16-2).[62,273]

Adrenal cortical neoplasms in children remain somewhat of an enigma for pathologists. Their clinical and biologic behavior can be quite distinct from that of histologically similar counterparts in adults. Attempts to identify pathologic criteria of malignancy have been made, with some success, but further studies will be required for a better understanding of adrenal cortical neoplasms in children.[274,275] A big factor in the difficulty of assessing these lesions is the rarity with which adrenal cortical carcinoma occurs in this population.

### Other adrenal cortical neoplasms

Several examples of adrenal carcinosarcoma have been reported in adults, consisting of mixtures of sarcomatous elements and ACC.[276–278] An example of virilizing adrenal cortical blastoma was reported in an infant who had an elevated serum level of α-fetoprotein.[279]

### Pheochromocytoma

Pheochromocytoma is a catecholamine-secreting tumor arising from neural crest-derived chromaffin cells of the sympathoadrenal system. It is relatively uncommon in surgical pathology practice, with an estimated average annual incidence of eight per million person-years (excluding familial

**Table 16-2** Staging of adrenal cortical carcinoma (From Lack EE. Tumors of the adrenal glands and extra-adrenal paraganglia. 3rd series. Atlas of Tumor Pathology, 19. Washington, DC: Armed Forces Institute of Pathology, 1997)

| % | Stage | TNM | | Staging criteria |
|---|---|---|---|---|
| 2.8 | I | $T_1N_0M_0$ | $T_1$ | Tumor less than or equal to 5 cm, no invasion |
| 29 | II | $T_2N_0M_0$ | $T_2$ | Tumor greater than 5 cm, no invasion |
| 19.3 | III | $T_1N_1M_0$ | $T_3$ | Tumor of any size, locally invasive but not involving adjacent organs |
| | | $T_2N_1M_0$ | | |
| | | $T_3N_0M_0$ | $T_4$ | Tumor of any size, with invasion of adjacent organs |
| 48.9 | IV | Any T, any N, $M_1$ | $N_0$ | Negative regional lymph nodes |
| | | $T_3, N_1$ | $N_1$ | Positive regional lymph nodes |
| | | $T_4$ | $M_0$ | No distant metastases |
| | | | $M_1$ | Distant metastases |

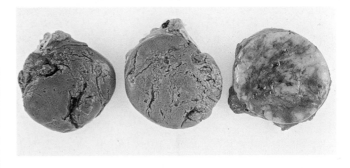

**Fig. 16-57** Pheochromocytoma. Cross-section of a 3.5 cm tumor on the right is fleshy, pale tan with mottled areas of congestion. Two other portions of the same tumor had been fixed in Zenker's solution and show a positive chromaffin reaction with a mahogany brown color.

cases).[280] It has been suggested that for every pheochromocytoma diagnosed during life, there are two that remain undiscovered, but recent data show more of them diagnosed during life, probably reflecting increased clinical awareness, heightened diagnostic acumen, and more sensitive laboratory testing. Pheochromocytoma has been referred to as the '10% tumor' –10% bilateral, 10% extra-adrenal, 10% malignant, and 10% occurring in childhood – but this is only an approximation that must be correlated with other factors, such as tumor location, patient age, and familial predisposition.[4,281] About 95% of cases of sporadic pheochromocytoma in adults are solitary, 5% are bilateral, and 5–10% are extra-adrenal in location. Interestingly, a recent study found that almost 25% of patients with apparently sporadic pheochromocytoma may be carriers of mutations, including RET, VHL, SDHD and SDHB (succinate dehydrogenase subunit D and subunit B).[282,283] Additionally, mutations in the SDHB gene appear to correlate with extra-adrenal location of pheochromocytomas.[284] Over 50% of cases of familial pheochromocytoma are bilateral, and the tumor may be multicentric within the adrenal gland.[4,281] In childhood there is an increased incidence of bilateral pheochromocytomas, as well as multicentric and extra-adrenal tumors. A higher incidence of malignant pheochromocytoma/paraganglioma has recently been reported in the pediatric population.[285] The peak incidence is in the fifth decade of life, but pheochromocytoma can occur at virtually any age. Most clinical series report a roughly equal gender incidence.

Sporadic pheochromocytoma usually forms a unicentric spherical or oval mass that is often sharply circumscribed and may appear encapsulated. Histologic sections taken at the periphery of the tumor often show a fibrous pseudocapsule or, at times, no capsule at all. Most pheochromocytomas are 3–5 cm in diameter, with an average weight in several large series ranging from 73 to 156.5 g.[4,281] The average weight of clinically malignant tumors tends to be greater than that of benign tumors. Pheochromocytoma is usually resiliently firm, with a glistening gray-white surface (Fig. 16-57), which may be altered by degenerative change such as congestion, hemorrhage, or necrosis, and some tumors undergo cystic change that may be marked. Rarely, pheochromocytoma grows into the inferior vena cava, and may extend into the right atrium, mimicking renal cell carcinoma.[4,281]

Pheochromocytoma usually has an anastomosing cell cord pattern (Fig. 16-58), or sometimes an alveolar or 'zell-ballen' architectural growth pattern in which the neoplastic cells form rounded to oval nests that are surrounded by a delicate fibrovascular network of supporting cells, the most characteristic supporting cell being the sustentacular cell (Fig. 16-58). Sustentacular cells are typically not apparent on routine stained sections. Occasionally, tumor cells are arranged in a predominantly solid or diffuse pattern (Fig. 16-59). There may be a compressed fibrous pseudocapsule between the pheochromocytoma and the adjacent cortex, but sometimes there is no intervening fibrous connective tissue (Fig. 16-60). There may even be intermingling with non-neoplastic cortical cells at the periphery. Alterations in the supporting stroma, including sclerosis, edema, and changes in the vasculature, which could create diagnostic confusion, may also be present. One study reported amyloid in 14 of 20 pheochromocytomas (70%), but no electron microscopic illustrations were provided.[286] Another study identified amyloid deposition in only two of 22 cases (9.1%) examined with supporting special stains, immunohistochemical stains, and electron microscopy.[287]

The pheochromocytoma cells or 'pheochromocytes' are typically polygonal in shape with a finely granular cytoplasm that is basophilic to lightly eosinophilic. Nuclear 'pseudoinclusions' have been reported in about one-third of pheochromocytomas,[4,281] and typically appear as sharply defined

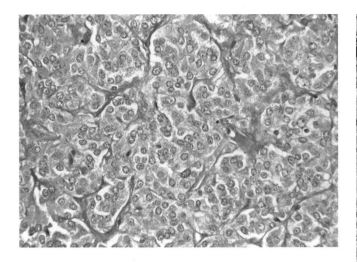

**Fig. 16-58** Pheochromocytoma with an anastomosing cell cord pattern. The cells have a finely granular, basophilic cytoplasm with round to oval, eccentrically placed nuclei.

round to oval structures that contain cytoplasm having the same staining intensity as the remainder of the cell, although they sometimes appear pale or empty (Fig. 16-61). Some tumors contain cells with prominent nuclear hyperchromasia and pleomorphism, but these features alone are not useful in predicting biologic behavior. Cytoplasmic hyaline globules can be found in some pheochromocytomas and are characteristically PAS positive and resistant to diastase predigestion. The globules are slightly refractile and identical to those that may be found in the normal medullary chromaffin cells. These globules are detected in almost 50% of cases of sympathoadrenal paraganglioma,[288] and are possibly related to secretory activity. Rarely, in some tumors the cytoplasm is deeply eosinophilic and copious, reminiscent of oncocytic changes.[289,290] Lipid degeneration gives the cytoplasm a clear vacuolated appearance that can mimic an adrenal cortical neoplasm.[291,292] Some pheochromocytomas contain scattered cells resembling neuronal or ganglion cells with tapering cytoplasmic processes and peripheral aggregation of basophilic material resembling Nissl substance. Periadrenal brown fat may be associated with pheochromocytoma,[293] but its incidence and functional importance are uncertain.[294] Pigmented pheochromocytoma and extra-adrenal paraganglioma are extremely rare.[62,295,296] These tumors may have a jet-black gross appearance caused by an abundance of intracytoplasmic granules of lipofuscin (Fig. 16-62). The differential diagnosis of pigmented (black) adrenal neoplasms includes cortical adenoma, pheochromocytoma, and malignant melanoma (primary or secondary).

## Pheochromocytoma in MEN

Multiple endocrine neoplasia syndrome type 2a (Sipple's syndrome) is an autosomal dominant disorder with a high degree of penetrance, including various combinations of pheochromocytoma, medullary thyroid carcinoma, and parathyroid hyperplasia.[297,298] MEN 2b also has an autosomal dominant mode of inheritance, but some patients

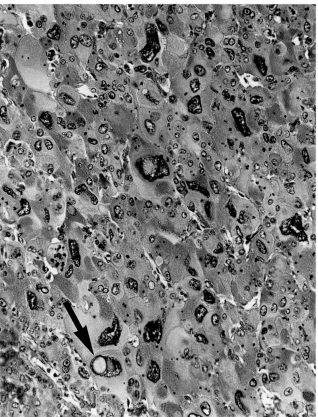

**Fig. 16-59** Pheochromocytoma with solid or diffuse growth pattern. Cells have abundant amphophilic cytoplasm. Note marked nuclear pleomorphism and hyperchromasia as well as nuclear 'pseudoinclusion' (arrow).

appear to have the isolated or sporadic form of the disorder. It is possible that clinically aggressive medullary thyroid carcinoma that occurs in this setting causes death at an early age without the patient being able to pass the syndrome on to a future generation.[4] Some cases may be truly sporadic as a result of gene mutations. The pheochromocytomas in MEN types 2a and 2b are frequently multicentric (Fig. 16-63) and bilateral (Fig. 16-64), and in some cases where residual chromaffin tissue is recognizable there may be extratumoral adrenal medullary hyperplasia.[299] Gross morphologic features may be sufficiently distinctive that the surgical pathologist may be alerted to the possibility of the associated syndrome.[4]

The phenotypic expression of MEN type 2b is very distinctive. Medullary thyroid carcinoma in this syndrome is usually aggressive, and recurrence and metastasis are its most pernicious components.[4] Pheochromocytoma is often preceded by adrenal medullary hyperplasia.[170,173] There is a low incidence of clinical and biochemical hyperfunction of the parathyroid glands, in contrast to MEN 2a.[4] There is very characteristic mucosal neuromatous proliferation involving the lips, tongue (Fig. 16-65), oral mucosa, and conjunctivae; ganglioneuromatosis may involve the upper aerodigestive and lower gastrointestinal tracts. This may lead to a variety

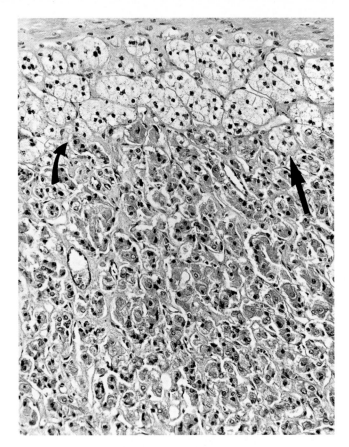

**Fig. 16-60** Pheochromocytoma with an alveolar or nesting pattern. Section taken through the periphery of the tumor shows junction with the residual cortex (arrows) and lack of encapsulation.

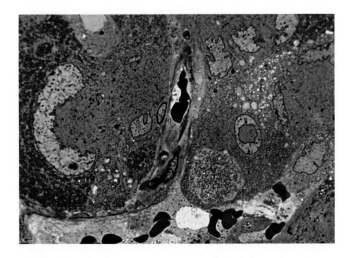

**Fig. 16-61** Pheochromocytoma. A nuclear 'pseudoinclusion' is present in the right side of field viewed en face. Nucleus of tumor cell on left side shows a deep indentation with a jagged border that represents a 'pseudoinclusion' viewed in profile. (Toluidine blue stain ×1000.)

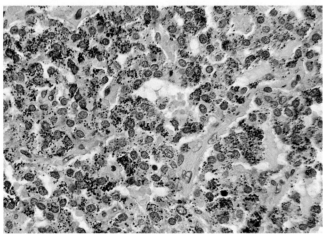

**Fig. 16-62** Pigmented pheochromocytoma with abundant granular pigment that is consistent with lipofuscin. Ultrastructural study revealed no melanosomes or premelanosomes. A heavily pigmented tumor such as this may be mistaken for a pigmented black adenoma or malignant melanoma.

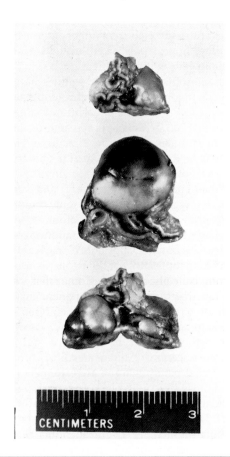

**Fig. 16-63** Multifocal nodular hyperplasia of adrenal medulla with early pheochromocytomas in MEN 2a (Sipple's syndrome). The adrenal glands had similar gross appearances. Transverse sections of the left adrenal gland show multiple nodules expanding the medullary compartment, with the largest nodule 1.5 cm in diameter. (From Lack EE. Pathology of adrenal and extra-adrenal paraganglia. In: Major problems in pathology, Vol 29. Philadelphia: WB Saunders, 1994; 220–272.)

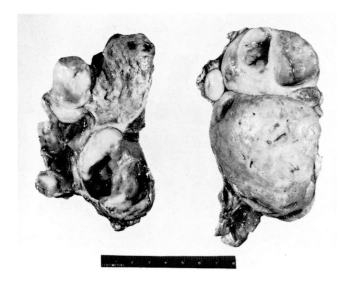

**Fig. 16-64** Bilateral pheochromocytomas in MEN 2a. The tumors weighed 168 and 220 g.

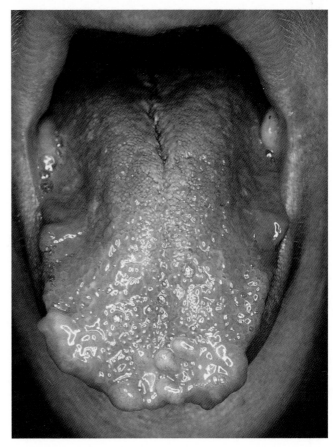

**Fig. 16-65** Patient with MEN 2b. The tongue is studded with neuromas, particularly along the lateral borders and the tip. (From Lack EE. Adrenal medullary hyperplasia and pheochromocytoma. In: Lack EE ed. Pathology of the adrenal glands. New York: Churchill Livingstone, 1990; 173–235.)

of intestinal manifestations, including motility disorders and megacolon mimicking Hirschsprung's disease.[4] Other findings include ocular abnormalities such as thickened corneal nerves, conjunctival and eyelid neuromas, and rarely failing vision. Various neuromuscular abnormalities have been described, such as marfanoid habitus, elongated facies, dolichocephaly, laxity of joints, lordosis, kyphosis, pes cavus, and coxa valga. The gastrointestinal manifestations in MEN 2b are very important to recognize because they may form a prominent component of the syndrome, often antedating the endocrine neoplasms.[300]

### Composite pheochromocytoma

The term composite pheochromocytoma refers to pheochromocytomas in which there is a component that resembles neuroblastoma, ganglioneuroblastoma (Fig. 16-66), ganglioneuroma, or malignant peripheral nerve sheath tumor (malignant schwannoma).[4,301] A few have secreted vasoactive intestinal peptide (VIP), causing the watery diarrhea syndrome. The capacity for synthesis and secretion of VIP has been associated with a neuronal or ganglionic phenotype. Neoplastic chromaffin cells in vitro may exhibit intense neuritic outgrowth of cell processes, indicative of one of several neuronal characteristics. The existence of composite pheochromocytoma with neural and endocrine features in vivo is ample testimony to the close morphologic and functional kinship of the nervous system and the endocrine system.[4] Not uncommonly, these composite tumors occur in association with neurocutaneous phakomatosis, most commonly neurofibromatosis. Recently, an example of composite pheochromocytoma/ganglioneuroma of the adrenal gland was described in a patient with MEN 2a, which appears to be the first reported case.[302]

### Pseudopheochromocytoma

The term pseudopheochromocytoma refers to the unusual circumstance in which a patient has signs and/or symptoms of a pheochromocytoma, but on surgical exploration no neoplasm is found. Examples include adrenal medullary hyperplasia, adrenal myelolipoma, renal cyst, coarctation of abdominal aorta, and astrocytoma.[4] Rarely, patients may develop signs and symptoms suggesting pheochromocytoma following surreptitious administration of epinephrine or other agents that produce provocative clinical manifestations.[4]

### Immunohistochemistry and other features

The catecholamine-synthesizing enzymes tyrosine hydroxylase, dopamine β-hydroxylase, and phenylethanolamine *N*-methyltransferase have been identified in pheochromocytoma, and correlate with the functional capacity of this tumor to produce norepinephrine and epinephrine.[4] The ratio of epinephrine to norepinephrine in the normal adrenal medulla is about 4 : 1, whereas in pheochromocytomas norepinephrine predominates.[4] The immunohistochemical profile of pheochromocytoma is quite broad:[303] it typically expresses neuron-specific enolase and other neuroendocrine

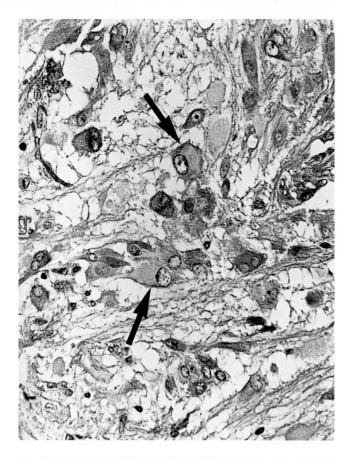

**Fig. 16-66** Composite pheochromocytoma. Cells (arrows) have neuronal or ganglionic features with eccentric, prominent nuclei, abundant cytoplasm with distinct borders and tapering extensions, and some have peripheral granular cytoplasmic basophilia consistent with Nissl substance. Note the prominent fibrillar matrix resembling neuropil. Other areas have the typical morphology of a pheochromocytoma.

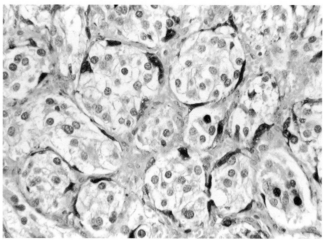

**Fig. 16-67** Pheochromocytoma. Sustentacular cells are demonstrated by immunostaining for S100 protein, which highlights nuclei and slender cytoplasmic extensions. These cells are located at the periphery of nests and cords of pheochromocytoma cells.

markers, such as chromogranin A and synaptophysin. Pheochromocytoma can also express a broad array of other regulatory peptides and hormones, including enkephalins, somatostatin, VIP, substance P, ACTH, and calcitonin.[303] Rare cases are associated with a paraneoplastic syndrome caused by the secretion of one of the neuropeptides such as VIP with watery diarrhea syndrome and ACTH with Cushing's syndrome.[4] Sustentacular cells are the supporting cells in pheochromocytoma, appearing as S100 protein immunoreactive cells at the periphery of cords and clusters of neoplastic chromaffin cells (Fig. 16-67). Recently, there have been some reports of cytokeratin reactivity in pheochromocytoma.[289,290] However, another report fails to support this keratin reactivity, which was noted in only extra-adrenal paragangliomas.[304] It is possible that the keratin reactivity that can be seen in pheochromocytomas represents nonspecific staining of the cytoplasmic granules rather than true staining of intermediate filaments.

The ultrastructural hallmark of pheochromocytoma is the presence of dense-core neurosecretory-type granules, which have variable distribution and density within neoplastic cells.[305] Sparse numbers of these granuless in some cells may help to explain a low to absent intensity of immunostaining for neuroendocrine markers such as chromogranin A in some cases. Tannenbaum[306] found that granule morphology correlated with catecholamine content as determined biochemically. Two distinct types of granules were recognized. Those associated with norepinephrine storage had a distinctly prominent, eccentric halo or electron-lucent space adjacent to the dense core, and those associated with epinephrine storage were more uniform (Fig. 16-68). Given the wide array of neuropeptides and hormones that may be detected in pheochromocytomas, the distinction based solely on granule morphology is no longer tenable.[4,281] Some granules, in fact, may be quite pleomorphic and may contain more than one peptide.

Fine needle aspiration of pheochromocytoma may create problems in cytologic interpretation, and malignant diagnoses rendered solely on the basis of cytologic and nuclear atypia may be erroneous.[4] Occasional complications have also been reported, including catecholamine crisis with a marked alteration in blood pressure, and sometimes with uncontrollable intra-abdominal hemorrhage.[4] In smear and imprint preparations of pheochromocytoma, nuclei may appear suspended in a syncytium of ill-defined cytoplasm and there may be considerable variation in nuclear size and shape (Fig. 16-69). Other cytologic features include intranuclear 'pseudoinclusions' and enlarged hyperchromatic nuclei, sometimes stripped of cell cytoplasm.[4]

The incidence of clinically malignant adrenal pheochromocytoma is relatively low, and it is important to consider these separately from extra-adrenal paragangliomas, which have a significantly higher incidence of malignant behavior.[4] Early reviews cite a frequency of malignant behavior in

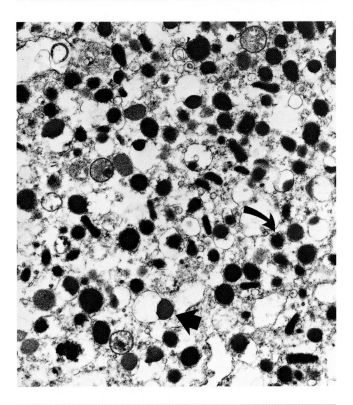

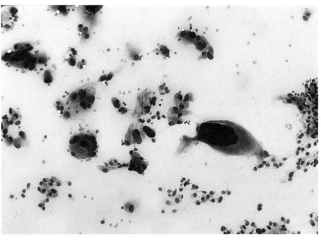

**Fig. 16-69** Pheochromocytoma. Touch imprint smear of resected tumor shows marked variation in nuclear size, which might lead to a presumptive diagnosis of malignancy. (Diff Quik stain.)

**Fig. 16-68** Pheochromocytoma. Electron micrograph shows numerous dense-core neurosecretory granules; some have an investing membrane with a uniform thin halo (curved arrow), whereas others have an eccentric dense core with a wide asymmetric halo (straight arrow). Other neurosecretory granules are pleomorphic. (×15 000.)

adrenal pheochromocytoma of 2.4–2.8% in adults,[307–309] whereas in children 2.4% were malignant.[308] A recent study from 2006 reports a relatively high incidence (47%) of malignancy in 30 children with pheochromocytoma/paraganglioma.[285] In this study, however, 18 of the children had extra-adrenal paraganglioma and only 12 had pheochromocytoma (defined as tumors arising from the adrenal medulla), which may account for the higher incidence. Overall, recent studies show an incidence of malignancy ranging from 7% to 14%.[4] It is notoriously difficult on gross and histologic evaluation to predict which tumors will prove to be malignant. The histology of benign and malignant pheochromocytoma overlaps to such an extent that the most important criterion acceptable for malignancy is the presence of metastases in sites where non-neoplastic chromaffin tissue is not normally found.[310] However, some histologic features have been noted to be more frequently associated with malignant behavior.[311] These include loss of the small alveolar/nesting pattern, to be replaced by larger cell nests lacking the well-formed fibrovascular supporting network; a diffuse growth pattern; tumor cell spindling; confluent tumor necrosis; increased mitotic rate (>3/10 hpf); and the presence of atypical mitotic figures.[312] Subsequent studies have attempted to validate these findings in both pheochromocytomas and

extra-adrenal pheochromocytomas with some success,[313,314] but additional studies are required. In some studies DNA quantification has suggested that ploidy may be an independent prognostic factor, as none of the patients with diploid tumors died of pheochromocytoma.[315,316] Aneuploid histograms have been reported in pheochromocytomas, which are clinically benign or cured by surgery. A low proportion (or absence) of S100 protein immunoreactive cells has also been correlated with malignant behavior of paraganglioma,[317,318] but may not be a reliable discriminator in the evaluation of individual cases.[319] Other markers recently investigated as possible predictors of malignant behavior in pheochromocytomas include MIB-1 labeling >3%, and expression of telomerase activity.[320,321]

Surgical resection has been the mainstay of treatment for pheochromocytoma. With the recent development of laparoscopic adrenalectomy, such surgical resection has become less invasive for patients. Although there are reports of success with laparoscopic adrenalectomy for pheochromocytoma,[322,323] others have reported recurrence due to local spillage of tumor during laparoscopic manipulation.[324]

## Neuroblastic tumors: neuroblastoma, ganglioneuroblastoma, and ganglioneuroma

Neuroblastic tumors (NT) are defined as embryonal tumors of the sympathetic nervous system derived from the neural crest and arise in the adrenal medulla, paravertebral sympathetic ganglia, and sympathetic ganglia.[325] They include a spectrum of lesions ranging from neuroblastoma and ganglioneuroblastoma to ganglioneuroma.

An understanding of the development and biologic behavior of these tumors is essential. During embryologic development, primitive cells of neural crest origin migrate and give rise to cells that eventually develop into the adrenal medulla, neuronal cells of the autonomic nervous system, Schwann cells, melanocytes, various neuroendocrine cells, and some mesenchymal-type cells of the head and neck region.[325] These tumors demonstrate unique biologic behaviors: involution/spontaneous regression, maturation, or aggressive proliferation.[325]

Neuroblastoma ranks fourth in frequency of malignant tumors in patients under 15 years of age, exceeded only by leukemia, brain tumors, and malignant lymphoma.[326] The incidence of neuroblastoma/ganglioneuroblastoma is estimated at 9.1 per million. Age is a strong factor bearing on incidence, with neuroblastoma predominating in children under 5 years of age and the vast majority of those arising during infancy.[326] There is a slight increased incidence of neuroblastoma in males (9.8 per million) compared to females (9.2 per million). In a series of 118 patients from Boston Children's Hospital, 88% were 5 years of age or younger at diagnosis, with a median age of 21 months.[327] Neuroblastoma and ganglioneuroblastoma are rare in the second decade of life, and exceedingly rare in adults.[328] When these tumors do arise in adolescents or adults they appear to have different biologic characteristics from their pediatric counterparts, and have a poor prognosis regardless of stage.[328] Occasionally, neuroblastoma appears in several members of a family, and some data suggest an autosomal dominant pattern of inheritance, but there are obvious difficulties in determining the incidence and penetrance of an inherited susceptibility because of the capacity for regression or spontaneous maturation, as well as early death and long-term treatment complications that prevent reproduction and the evaluation of multiple pedigrees.[329,330] Neuroblastoma and ganglioneuroblastoma may have some unusual associations: watery diarrhea syndrome due to VIP production, Cushing's syndrome, opsoclonus/myoclonus, and alopecia. Heterochromia iridis has also been reported with mediastinal and cervical neuroblastoma and ganglioneuroma.[4,331]

The first screening for neuroblastoma began in Japan in 1974, and others have followed.[4,332–337] Screening in Japan has resulted in an increased annual detection rate for these tumors (93 per million) compared to the baseline rate of 13.3 per million. Children are screened at 6 months of age with a qualitative vanillylmandelic acid spot test. The prognosis for children with neuroblastoma detected by screening is favorable because of low clinical stage and early age at diagnosis, both independent prognostic factors.[4] Most infants are considered to be in a low-risk subgroup with potential for spontaneous regression, and although screening programs do increase the number of newly diagnosed cases[338] they do not appear to reduce population-based mortality in infants, nor do they result in a decreased incidence of advanced-stage disease in older children.[339–341]

The distribution of neuroblastoma and ganglioneuroblastoma parallels that of the sympathetic nervous system, with tumors arising anywhere from the neck to the pelvis. The anatomic distribution of primary tumors in a report of 118 patients was as follows: intra-abdominal (67.8%), with most arising in the adrenal glands (38.1%) and 29.7% being non-adrenal; intrathoracic (20.3%); cervical (3.4%); pelvic (3.4%); and in 5.1% the precise anatomic origin was undetermined.[327] Patients with neuroblastoma and ganglioneuroblastoma may have spinal cord compression caused by an extradural intraspinal ('dumb-bell') configuration of the tumor; similar spinal cord compression may occasionally be seen with ganglioneuroma.[4]

Neuroblastoma and ganglioneuroblastoma usually present as a solitary unicentric mass or a confluent mass of nodules. Rarely, the tumors grow into the inferior vena cava and occasionally tumors are quite large, measuring up to 10 cm or more.[4,331] On cross-section they are variable in appearance and consistency depending on the amount of immature neuroblastic tissue present. Usually, the tumors have coarse lobulations with areas of hemorrhage and necrosis (Fig. 16-70). Viable tumors may appear pale gray and have a soft encephaloid consistency.

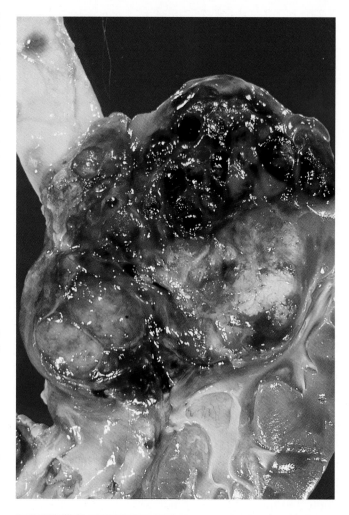

**Fig. 16-70** At autopsy neuroblastoma virtually replaces the entire adrenal gland and compresses the adjacent kidney. The cut surface of the tumor has coarse lobulations and is hemorrhagic.

Neuroblastoma and ganglioneuroblastoma often have a lobular growth pattern with delicate, incomplete fibrovascular septa, but some cases have a diffuse or solid pattern. There is a continuum in the morphologic appearance of neuroblastoma and ganglioneuroblastoma.[4,342] Within this morphologic spectrum there may be patterns merging imperceptibly with ganglioneuroblastoma, which are well differentiated (Shimada stroma predominant, well-differentiated category) and simulate mature ganglioneuroma; at the other end of the spectrum the tumor pattern is that of undifferentiated neuroblastoma.[4,331,343] Typical Homer Wright rosettes can be found in some tumors[344] (Fig. 16-71) and there may be broad, matted tangles of neuritic processes. The degree of ganglion cell differentiation varies from tumor to tumor, and also within different areas of the same tumor. The nuclei of neuroblastoma often have a stippled or dispersed 'salt and pepper' pattern of nuclear chromatin (Fig. 16-72). Anaplastic neuroblastoma has marked cellular and nuclear pleomorphism,[345] but this finding has no apparent impact on survival after controlling for disease stage.[346]

Morphologic evidence of ganglion cell differentiation includes nuclear enlargement, increased amount of eosinophilic cytoplasm, distinct cell borders, prominent nucleolus, and peripheral granular material within the cytoplasm that represents Nissl substance (Fig. 16-73). A variety of stromal alterations may be seen in neuroblastoma and ganglioneuroblastoma, including hemorrhage, necrosis, dystrophic calcification, and marked cystic degeneration.[4,331] Cystic neuroblastoma may simulate an adrenal cyst or hematoma. Immunostaining for S100 protein highlights slender dendritic cells near fibrovascular septa, which represent satellite cells or indicate differentiation into Schwann cells. Large numbers of S100 protein immunoreactive cells in undifferentiated neuroblastoma are associated with a good prognosis;[347] conversely, large numbers of ferritin-positive cells have been associated with a poor prognosis.[4]

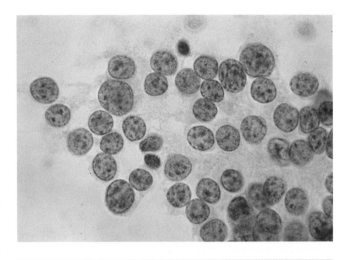

**Fig. 16-72** Touch imprint of neuroblastoma (stroma-poor in the Shimada classification). Nuclei have dispersed chromatin ('salt and pepper' nuclei), and are separated by pale pink cytoplasm with indistinct borders.

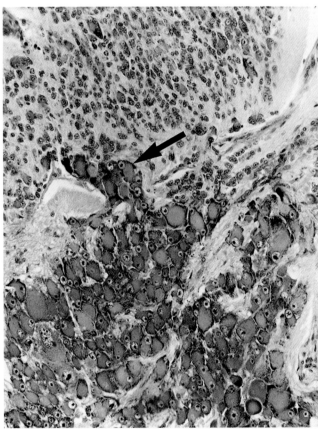

**Fig. 16-73** Ganglioneuroblastoma with well-developed ganglion cells (arrow).

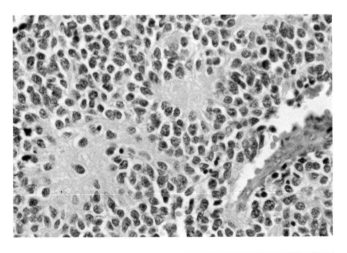

**Fig. 16-71** Neuroblastoma (stroma-poor in the Shimada classification). The cells are closely packed, with indistinct cellular borders. Note the Homer Wright rosettes.

Ultrastructural characteristics of neuroblastoma and ganglio-neuroblastoma include neuritic extensions with neurofilaments, neurotubules, and dense-core neurosecretory granules, which are usually few in number (Fig. 16-74).[305]

A variety of grading systems have been proposed for childhood neuroblastoma and ganglioneuroblastoma. Beckwith and Martin[348] recognized four grades of differentiation: grade I had the highest level of ganglion cell differentiation with good survival, and grade IV was undifferentiated with poor survival. Other grading systems employed three levels of differentiation.[4,349] In 1984, Shimada et al.[350] introduced an age-linked grading of neuroblastoma, based on the patient's age at diagnosis, degree of maturation or percentage of differentiating elements, and the mitosis–karyorrhexis index (MKI). The stroma-rich catgory shows extensive growth of schwannian and other supporting elements, with three groups (Fig. 16-75): the well-differentiated and intermixed groups had a favorable prognosis (92–100% 5-year survival), and the nodular group had an unfavorable prognosis (18% survival). The stroma-poor category had two groups (Fig. 16-76): the favorable group had a 5-year survival of 84%, and the unfavorable group a 5-year survival of 4.5%. Several studies have supported the utility of the Shimada grading system.[351,352]

A histologic grading system was subsequently proposed by Joshi et al.[353] in which the grade of the neoplasm was based on the mitotic rate or presence of calcification. Two risk groups were defined: the low-risk group consisted of patients in both age groups (<1 year and >1 year) with grade 1 tumors (i.e., low mitotic rate (<10 per 10 hpf), calcifications present) and patients less than 1 year of age with grade 2 tumors (low mitotic rate or calcification present); and the high-risk group consisted of patients over 1 year of age with grade 2 tumors and patients in both age groups with grade 3 tumors (high mitotic rate (>10 per 10 hpf), no calcification). A high degree of concordance was seen between the low-risk and high-risk groups (84%) and the favorable and unfavorable histology groups in the Shimada classification. The survival curves are therefore very similar.[353]

The International Neuroblastoma Pathology Committee is an international collaborative effort that was convened with the aim of establishing a prognostically significant and

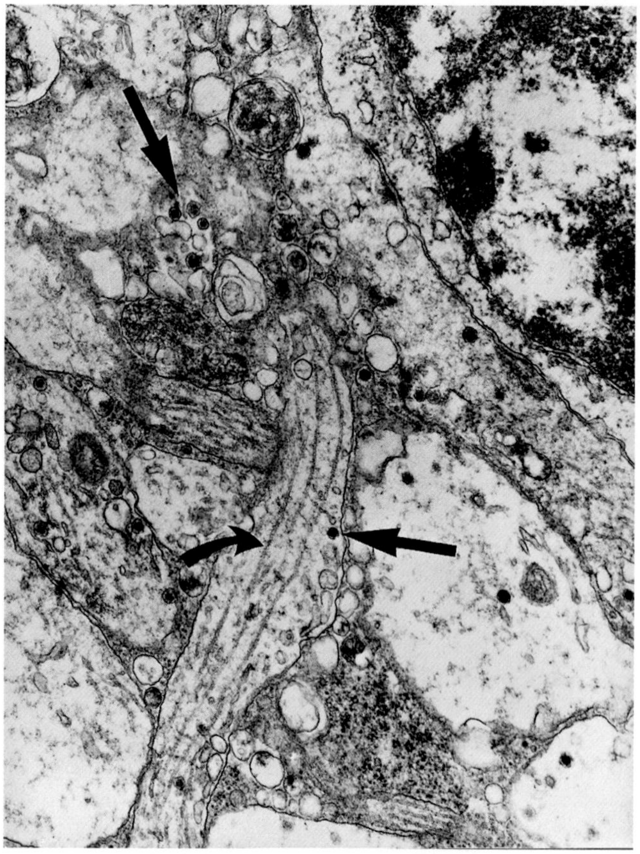

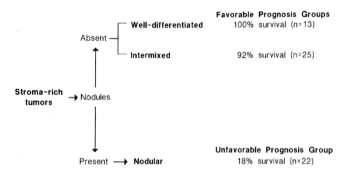

**Fig. 16-75** Stroma-rich neuroblastoma according to the Shimada age-linked classification. Survival data are indicated for the favorable and unfavorable groups. (From Lack EE, ed. Pathology of adrenal and extra-adrenal paraganglia. In: Major problems in pathology, Vol 29. Philadelphia: WB Saunders, 1994; 315–370.)

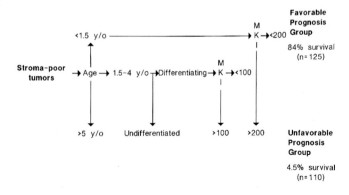

**Fig. 16-76** Stroma-poor neuroblastoma according to the Shimada age-linked classification. Favorable and unfavorable prognosis groups are indicated along with survival data. MKI, mitosis–karyorrhexis index. (From Lack EE, ed. Pathology of adrenal and extra-adrenal paraganglia. In: Major problems in pathology, Vol 29. Philadelphia: WB Saunders, 1994; 315–370.)

**Fig. 16-74** Neuroblastoma. Neuritic processes contain microtubules (curved arrow) and sparse numbers of dense-core neurosecretory granules (straight arrows). (×27 000.)

biologically relevant classification scheme for the diagnosis of neuroblastic tumors. The system, referred to as the International Neuroblastoma Pathology Classification (INPC), is based on a framework of the Shimada classification with minor modifications.[325,350,354] It is a an age-linked system dependent on histologic differentiation, the schwannian stromal component, and the cellular turnover index (Table 16-3).[354] Its prognostic significance has since been confirmed.[355,356]

Based on this INPC classification scheme,[354] neuroblastic tumors can show a wide range of differentiation between tumors from different patients, and often within the same tumor. Neuroblastomas are NTs that are schwannian stroma-poor and are either undifferentiated or poorly differentiated. The undifferentiated tumors typically are composed of small to medium-sized cells with a minimal amount of cytoplasm and vaguely defined cytoplasmic borders. The nuclei are round to oval and may show the characteristic stippled chromatin pattern of neuroendocrine tumors. Identifiable neuropil is absent. Usually, ancillary studies such as immunohistochemistry, electron microscopy and/or cytogenetics are necessary to confirm the diagnosis. The poorly differentiated subtype is composed of undifferentiated neuroblastic cells with an identifiable background of neuropil. The extent of neuropil will often vary, but for the purpose of subtyping the presence of definitive identifiable neuropil is sufficient to place it in the poorly differentiated category. The importance of distinguishing between undifferentiated and poorly differentiated tumors is of practical importance because of the poor prognosis associated with the undifferentiated subtype.

The differentiating subtype usually has abundant neuropil, with 5% or more of the tumor cells showing differentiation toward ganglion cells. A cell in the transitional stage of ganglionic maturation should show evidence of differentiation of the nucleus with a vesicular chromatin pattern and single prominent nucleolus, as well as differentiation of the cytoplasm showing a conspicuous eosinophilic or amphophilic appearance. The amount of neuropil is not a discriminating feature between poorly differentiated and differentiating subtypes.

There appears to be a histologic continuum in the morphologic appearance of neuroblastoma and ganglioneuroblastoma. Ganglioneuroblastoma, referred to in the original Shimada system as 'stroma-rich, intermixed,' consists of an NT of transitional appearance with evidence of maturation toward fully differentiated mature ganglion cells but which is not totally complete. There still remain scattered foci of neuroblastic cells. In order to fit into this category the ganglioneuromatous component should exceed 50% relative to the neuroblastomatous component. These microscopic nests of neuroblastic cells are randomly intermixed within the ganglioneuromatous component. Abundant neuropil is typically present.

Table 16-3 Prognostic Evaluation of Neuroblastic Tumors According to the International Neuroblastoma Pathology Classification (From Shimada H, et al. The International Neuroblastoma Pathology Classification (the Shimada System). Cancer 1999; 86: 364–372)

| International Neuroblastoma Pathology Classification | | Original Shimada classification | Prognostic group |
|---|---|---|---|
| Neuroblastoma | Schwannian stroma-poor | Stroma-poor | |
| Favorable | Favorable | Favorable | |
| <1.5 yrs | Poorly differentiated or differentiating & low or intermediate MKI tumor | | |
| 1.5–5 yrs | Differentiating & low MKI tumor | | |
| Unfavorable | Unfavorable | Unfavorable | |
| <1.5 yrs | a) undifferentiated tumor | | |
| | b) high MKI tumor | | |
| 1.5-5 yrs | a) undifferentiated or poorly-differentiated tumor | | |
| | b) intermediate or high MKI tumor | | |
| >5 yrs | All tumors | | |
| Ganglioneuroblastoma, intermixed | Schwannian stroma-rich | Stroma-rich Intermixed (favorable) | Favorable* |
| Ganglioneuroma Maturing Mature | Schwannian stroma-dominant | Well-differentiated (favorable) Ganglioneuroma | Favorable* |
| Ganglioneuroblastoma, nodular composite | Schwannian stroma-rich stroma-dominant and stroma-poor | Stroma-rich nodular (unfavorable) | Unfavorable* |

*Prognostic grouping for these tumor categories is not related to age.
MKI, mitosis–karyorrhexis index.

The ganglioneuroblastoma, nodular (GNBn) category (composite schwannian stroma-rich/stroma-dominant and stroma poor) is made up of NTs with the principal feature of macroscopic, usually hemorrhagic, neuroblastic nodules admixed with ganglioneuroblastoma, intermixed component or ganglioneuroma (stroma-dominant component). The proportion of the stroma-rich or stroma-dominant component to the neuroblastic component is not critical to the diagnosis. Rarely, the neuroblastic nodules may become so large that the stroma-rich/stroma-dominant areas cannot be identified. In such cases, examination of the periphery of the tumor or the fibrous septa may be helpful in locating the ganglioneuroblastoma or ganglioneuroma component. In the original INPC, all GNBns were classified into an unfavorable histology group.[354] Subsequently, it has been reported that GNBn can be subdivided into two prognostic groups: favorable subset (FS) and unfavorable subset (US), based on age-linked criteria and previously established morphologic characteristics of the nodular component.[357,358]

The mitosis–karyorrhexis index (MKI) was introduced by Shimada in his original classification scheme[350] and has subsequently been incorporated into the new INPC. It is used as a prognostic indicator and is defined as the number of mitotic figures and karyorrhectic cells per 5000 neuroblastic cells.[325] One of three MKI scores is reported: low: <2% (<100/5000); intermediate: 2–4% (100–200/5000); and high: >4% (>200/5000). The MKI should reflect an average of all tumor sections available. For optimal results the sections should be thin, preferably 3 μm, evenly stained, and contain at least 5000 viable tumor cells from multiple microscopic fields. A reproducible correlation between a high MKI and adverse clinical and biologic outcome has been noted.[359] Myc-N amplification in NTs produces an excess of Myc-N protein. Myc-N protein prevents cellular differentiation and promotes cellular proliferation and apoptosis. Thus, tumors with Myc-N amplification are usually undifferentiated or poorly differentiated subtypes with increased mitotic rate and karyorrhectic cells, i.e. high MKI.[325,360]

The staging classification proposed by Evans et al. has been popular for decades and continues to provide valuable prognostic information.[4,361–363] An interim working staging system has also been proposed, and incidence as well as survival data are shown in Table 16-4, based on stage at diagnosis.[364] Sixty to 70% of patients with neuroblastoma and ganglioneuroblastoma have metastases at the time of presentation (i.e., stages IV and IV-S), and 30–40% have localized disease (stages I, II, and III).[4] Children with a tumor primary in the cervical, intrathoracic, or pelvic areas have a better prognosis stage for stage than do patients with intra-abdominal primaries, but a disproportionate number may have low-stage tumor or be under 2 years of age and frequently less than 1 year of age at diagnosis.[4] Other staging classifications for neuroblastoma and ganglioneuroblastoma have been proposed. Revisions of the International Neuroblastoma Staging System (INSS) were reported in 1993 and vary slightly from those in Table 16-4 (see Table 16-5).[365]

The term 'in situ neuroblastoma' refers to a small nodule of primitive neuroblastic cells within the adrenal that is histologically indistinguishable from childhood neuroblastoma, without evidence of tumor elsewhere in the body.[366]

**Table 16-4** Staging system proposed by the International Staging System Working Party with incidence and survival according to stage of tumor and diagnosis (From Philip T. Overview of current treatment of neuroblastoma. Am J Pediatr Hematol/Oncol 1992; 14: 97–102)

| | Staging criteria | Incidence (%) | Survival at 5 years (%) |
|---|---|---|---|
| Stage I | Localized tumor confined to the area of origin, complete gross excision, with or without microscopic residual disease; identifiable ipsilateral and contralateral lymph nodes negative microscopically | 5 | 90 or greater |
| Stage IIa | Unilateral tumor with incomplete gross excision; identifiable ipsilateral and contralateral lymph nodes negative microscopically | 10 | 70–80 |
| Stage IIb | Unilateral tumor with complete or incomplete gross excision; with positive ipsilateral regional lymph nodes; identifiable contralateral lymph nodes negative microscopically | | |
| Stage III | Tumor infiltrating across the midline with or without regional lymph node involvement; or, midline tumor with bilateral regional lymph node involvement | 25 | 40–70 (depending on completeness of surgical resection) |
| Stage IV | Dissemination of the tumor to distant lymph nodes, bone, bone marrow, liver and/or other organs (except as defined in stage IV-S) | 60 | More than 60 if age at diagnosis is younger than 1 year; 20 if age at diagnosis is older than 1 year and under 2 years; 10 if age at diagnosis is over 2 years |
| Stage IVS | Localized primary tumor as defined for stage I or II with dissemination limited to liver, skin, and/or bone marrow | 5 | More than 80 |

**Table 16-5** International neuroblastoma staging system (From Brodeur GM, et al. Revisions of the international criteria for neuroblastoma diagnosis, staging and response to treatment. J Clin Oncol 1993; 11: 1466–1477)

| Stage | Definition |
|---|---|
| 1 | Localized tumor with complete gross excision, with or without microscopic residual disease; representative ipsilateral lymph nodes negative for tumor microscopically (nodes attached to and removed with the primary tumor may be positive) |
| 2A | Localized tumor with incomplete gross excision; representative ipsilateral non-adherent lymph nodes negative for tumor microscopically |
| 2B | Localized tumor with or without complete gross excision, with ipsilateral non-adherent lymph nodes positive for tumor. Enlarged contralateral lymph nodes must be negative microscopically |
| 3 | Unresectable unilateral tumor infiltrating across midline,* with or without regional lymph node involvement; or localized unilateral tumor with contralateral regional lymph node involvement; or midline tumor with bilateral extension by infiltration (unresectable) or by lymph node involvement |
| 4 | Any primary tumor with dissemination to distant lymph nodes, bone, bone marrow, liver, skin and/or other organs (except as defined for stage 4S) |
| 4S | Localized primary tumor (as defined for stage 1, 2A, or 2B), with dissemination limited to skin, liver, and/or bone marrow+ (limited to infants <1 year of age) |

*Midline is defined as the vertebral column. Tumors originating on one side and crossing the midline must infiltrate to or beyond the opposite side of the vertebral column.
+Marrow involvement in stage 4S should be minimal, i.e. <10% of total nucleated cells identified as malignant on bone marrow biopsy or on marrow aspirate. More extensive involvement would be considered to be stage 4. MIBG scan (if performed) should be negative in the marrow.

In the series by Beckwith and Perrin,[366] the nodules ranged in size from 0.7 to 9.5 mm in diameter. The incidence is estimated to be one per 224 infants. In situ neuroblastoma is about 45 times more common than clinical neuroblastoma. The obvious conclusion, if these lesions are indeed neoplastic, is that many undergo spontaneous involution or maturation, or remain clinically occult. It may be difficult to distinguish nodules of neuroblastic cells that are a normal part of the embryologic development of the adrenal gland (see Fig. 16-8) from in situ neuroblastoma.[4,331,367]

Stage IV-S (S = special) neuroblastoma refers to a distinctive group of patients with disseminated neuroblastoma involving liver, skin, or bone marrow without radiologic or other evidence of bone metastases[4,331,361] and limited to less than 1 year of age[365] (median, about 3 months). These children usually have a small adrenal primary, but in a minority of cases no primary can be identified.[368] Overall the prognosis is good, with survival rates of 80% or more, and many of the tumors undergo spontaneous regression. There is, however, a poor prognostic group of stage IV-S that may be predicted histologically (Shimada system) and/or biologically (Myc-N amplification).[369] In addition, there is a small subset of children with stage IV-S neuroblastoma, usually in the first 6 weeks of life, where there is marked abdominal distension due to massive liver involvement by tumor. The outlook for these patients is less favorable because massive hepatomegaly may cause secondary complications such as compromise in cardiorespiratory function.[370] Some authors speculate that stage IV-S neuroblastoma is a mass of hyperplastic nodules of mutated cells that lack the genetic events for transformation into an overtly malignant tumor.[371]

A fascinating aspect of neuroblastoma and ganglioneuroblastoma is occasional spontaneous regression or maturation into fully mature ganglioneuroma.[4,372] The concept of Collins' law[373] has been applied to children with neuroblastoma, and gives a rough approximation of the doubling time of a tumor measured as a period of risk that is equal to the patient's age at diagnosis plus 9 months. According to this concept, a child with neuroblastoma who has not been cured of the tumor will relapse within this timespan; theoretically, older children must therefore be followed for a much longer time because of the expanded period of risk. Two syndromes of metastatic neuroblastoma can be found in the early literature: the Pepper syndrome with prominent hepatic metastases, and the Hutchison syndrome with skull metastases presenting at a somewhat later age.[374] The cases described as Pepper in 1901 probably correspond to stage IV-S neuroblastoma.[4] Because there is no correlation between the laterality of the adrenal tumor and the pattern of metastases, the concept of these syndromes is obsolete. Metastatic spread of neuroblastoma and ganglioneuroblastoma occurs by both hematogenous and lymphatic routes, with involvement of sites such as bone and lymph nodes. Cranial involvement by metastatic neuroblastoma is usually confined to calvarial bone, leptomeninges, and dura, with intrinsic involvement of brain parenchyma being very rare.[4]

## Ganglioneuroma

Ganglioneuroma consists of mature or mildly dysmorphic ganglion cells set in an abundant mixture of mature Schwann cells.[4] This benign tumor is usually located in the posterior mediastinum; it may also be seen in the retroperitoneum; it is relatively uncommon in the adrenal gland.[4] Ganglioneuroma typically presents as a circumscribed tumor that is firm, rubbery, and gray-white to tan-yellow (Fig. 16-77). Grossly, ganglioneuroma may have a trabecular or whorled appearance reminiscent of leiomyoma. Larger tumors may have degenerative features such as hemorrhage and cystic change. Histologically, there is often considerable variation in the distribution and density of ganglion cells; areas with a paucity or absence of ganglion cells may be mistaken for a neurofibroma. Ganglion cells may be exceedingly well differentiated, with Nissl substance and a complete or partial collarette of cells resembling satellite cells, and some ganglion cells may contain granular tan to brown pigment (Fig. 16-78).

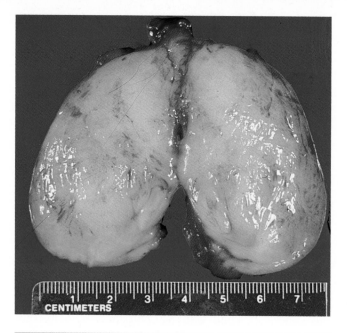

**Fig. 16-77** Ganglioneuroma is homogeneous pale tan on cross-section. The tumor measured 7 × 5 × 4 cm.

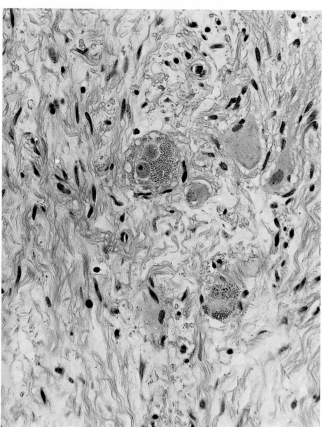

**Fig. 16-78** Ganglioneuroma. Ganglion cells mingle with Schwann cells. Some ganglion cells contain granular pigment.

Whether ganglioneuroma arises de novo or by maturation (differentiation) of a pre-existing neuroblastoma or ganglio-neuroblastoma remains controversial. Transformation of ganglioneuroma to malignant peripheral nerve sheath tumor (malignant schwannoma) has been rarely observed.[4,62] In some cases, malignant schwannoma has arisen de novo without any history of chemotherapy, radiation treatment, or von Recklinghausen's disease, but other cases have developed following radiation therapy. There have also been a few examples of adrenal ganglioneuroma with hilus or Leydig cells containing typical crystalloids of Reinke;[375] the tumor reported by Aguirre and Scully[376] was associated with masculinization.

The 'well-differentiated' neuroblastic tumor in the original Shimada system may resemble a ganglioneuroma because of the predominant schwannian stroma, but these tumors, despite having fully mature ganglion cells, also have scattered microscopic foci of differentiating neuroblasts. Ganglioneuromas are referred to in the recent INPC classification as 'ganglioneuroma, mature subtype' (Table 16-3).[354] By definition, a neuroblastomatous component, even microscopic, is absent.

## Other adrenal tumors

### Adenomatoid tumor

Although rare, adenomatoid tumors have been described in extragenital sites, including the adrenal gland,[377–381] mesentery of the small intestine,[382] retroperitoneum,[383] and omentum.[384]

Adenomatoid tumors of the adrenal gland[385,386] are benign tumors believed to be of mesothelial origin, with the characteristic histomorphology of adenomatoid tumors more commonly seen in or near the genital tract. The tumor may have an infiltrative border and typically has a sieve-like appearance. It is composed of epithelioid cells with uniform nuclei and intracytoplasmic vacuoles forming tubular or gland-like spaces (Fig. 16-79). Immunohistochemical evaluation shows strong immunoreactivity for cytokeratin and vimentin, weak reactivity for epithelial membrane antigen (EMA), and negative immunoreactivity for carcinoembryonic antigen (CEA), Factor VIII-related antigen, and CD34.[378–381] Strong staining for calretinin is also seen[385–386] (Fig. 16-80). Electron microscopy reveals desmosomes, tonofilaments, and long 'bushy' cytoplasmic microvilli typical of mesothelial cells.

### Malignant lymphoma

Malignant lymphoma secondarily involving the adrenal gland usually occurs in the setting of widespread or advanced-stage tumor, with an incidence of fatal cases of 18–25%.[4,178] Bilateral adrenal involvement has been reported in 9% of cases of Hodgkin's disease and 18% of non-Hodgkin's malignant lymphoma.[178] Malignant lymphoma rarely presents

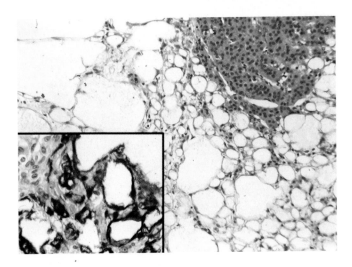

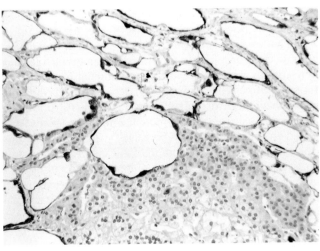

**Fig. 16-79** Adenomatoid tumor. Note the uninvolved adrenal cortical tissue (upper right) intimately adjacent to the tumor cells, forming cystic, tubular and gland-like spaces. The inset demonstrates strong staining of the tumor cells with antibodies to cytokeratin (AE1/AE3, CK1).

**Fig. 16-80** Adenomatoid tumor. Immunohistochemical stain showing the tumor cells immunoreactive for calretinin.

primarily in the adrenal without detectable extra-adrenal involvement, although recently there have been several reported cases.[387–389] Addison's disease may rarely result from massive involvement of the adrenal glands by malignant lymphoma, and the adrenal cortical insufficiency may resolve after treatment with combination chemotherapy.[62,178,390] Adrenal cortical insufficiency has also been reported with a form of malignant lymphoma having prominent vascular involvement, intravascular lymphomatosis, previously referred to as malignant angioendotheliomatosis. Plasmacytoma presenting primarily in the adrenal gland is extremely unusual[391] and may represent an early stage of malignant lymphoma with plasmacytoid features.[178] A study suggesting a possible association between Epstein–Barr virus (EBV) infection and the development of adrenal lymphoma has been reported.[392]

## Mesenchymal tumors

Primary angioformative neoplasms of the adrenal glands are extremely unusual. Adrenal hemangioma may be found incidentally at autopsy, but several cases have been detected during life as a surgical lesion. Visceral hemangioma may also occur in the setting of hereditary hemorrhagic telangiectasia (Rendu–Osler–Weber syndrome), but adrenal involvement is very rare.[178] Adrenal hemangioma is usually of the cavernous type, although capillary hemangioma has also been reported. Adrenal angiosarcoma has been rarely reported and may have epithelioid features[393–395] that include the presence of epithelial-specific immunohistochemical markers such as cytokeratin.[394,395]

Both leiomyoma and leiomyosarcoma occur rarely in the adrenal, with histologic features similar to those of smooth muscle neoplasms occurring in other sites.[62,396–398]

Neurilemmoma and neurofibroma arising in the adrenal gland are extremely unusual.[62] Malignant peripheral nerve sheath tumor (malignant schwannoma) has also been reported,[399] and in one case was part of a composite pheochromocytoma.[400]

## Malignant melanoma

Primary melanoma of the adrenal gland is extremely rare and highly malignant, usually occurring in middle-aged individuals.[62,401–403] Origin of a malignant melanoma within the adrenal is reasonable given the common embryogenesis of adrenal chromaffin cells and melanocytes from the neural crest. Melanin pigment is typically present in varying amounts, but the tumor may be amelanotic. There may be a nesting pattern or a biphasic growth pattern consisting of epithelioid and spindle cells. Rarely, a meningothelial-like growth pattern may be seen. Immunohistochemical studies are important in confirming the diagnosis. The neoplastic cells of an adrenal melanoma, like those of other melanomas, typically show strong reactivity with S100, HMB-45 and tyrosinase. MelanA (MART-1) is a recently developed immunomarker that stains for melanoma, but this marker should be used with caution in making a diagnosis of melanoma in the adrenal gland, as there are reports of positive reactivity to MelanA in adrenal cortical neoplasms.[271] It may be very difficult to exclude the possibility of primary mucocutaneous malignant melanoma that has metastasized to the adrenal.

## Other unusual tumors and tumor-like lesions

Ovarian thecal metaplasia is an incidental microscopic lesion composed of bland spindle cells. It is typically wedge-shaped and attached to the adrenal capsule, and may contain small nests of cortical cells.[3,62] Foci measure up to 2 mm and may be multiple.[404] Most cases occur in females, but rare cases have been seen in males. Rarely, such lesions may arise in association with ectopic adrenal tissue.[62] Macroscopic tumefactive spindle cell lesions of the adrenal glands have been described in two individuals, one male and one female, and S100 protein immunoreactivity suggested an origin from Schwann cells.[405] An incidentally discovered solitary fibrous tumor of the adrenal gland was reported in a woman during abdominopelvic ultrasonographic examination,[406] as well as a case associated with pregnacy.[407] A case of granulosa cell tumor of the adrenal gland has also been reported.[408] Leydig cells have been described in the adrenal gland as an incidental finding, a component of adrenal ganglioneuroma, or rarely a pure adrenal Leydig cell adenoma.

## Tumors metastatic to the adrenal glands

The adrenal gland is the fourth most common site of metastatic cancer, following lung, liver, and bone; per unit weight, it is more frequently involved than the other sites (Fig. 16-81),[62,178] probably because the adrenal vascular supply has a high flow volume and a sinusoidal vascular pattern. Metastases to the adrenal most commonly originate in the lung (Fig. 16-82) and breast, but other primary sites include the kidney, stomach, pancreas, and skin (malignant melanoma). Rarely, metastases to the adrenal are massive, resulting in adrenal cortical insufficiency (Addison's disease).[62,178] CT- or ultrasound-guided fine needle aspiration biopsy may be useful in documenting the presence of adrenal metastases. Metastases to the adrenal can simulate poorly differentiated adrenal cortical carcinoma.

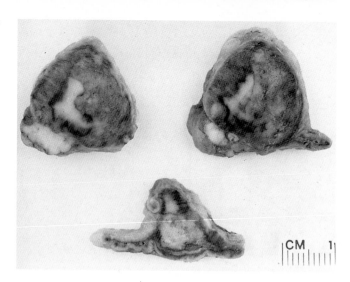

**Fig. 16-81** Bronchial carcinoma metastatic to the adrenal gland has a variegated color with geographic zones of necrosis having hyperemic borders.

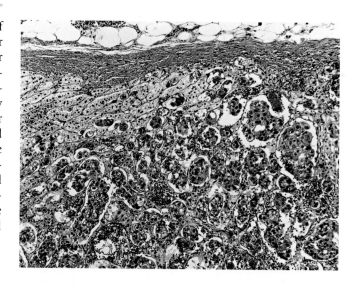

**Fig. 16-82** Bronchogenic adenocarcinoma metastatic to the adrenal gland.

## REFERENCES

1. Crowder R. The development of the adrenal gland in man, with special reference to origin and ultimate location of cell types and evidence in favor of the 'cell migration' theory. Contrib Embryol Carneg Inst 1957; 36: 193–210.

2. O'Rahilly R. The timing and sequence of events in the development of the human endocrine system during the embryonic period proper. Anat Embryol 1983; 166: 439–451.

3. Lack EE, Kozakewich HPW. Embryology, developmental anatomy and selected aspects of non-neoplastic pathology. In: Lack EE, ed. Pathology of the adrenal glands. New York: Churchill Livingstone, 1990.

4. Lack EE. Pathology of adrenal and extra-adrenal paraganglia. In: Major problems in pathology. Vol 29. Philadelphia: WB Saunders, 1994; 186–219.

5. Zuckerkandl E. Ueber Nebenorgane des sympathicus im Retroperitonaealraum des Menschen. Verh Dtsch Anat Ges 1901; 15: 95–107.

6. Stoner HB, Whiteley HJ, Emery JL. The effect of systemic disease on the adrenal cortex of the child. J Pathol Bacteriol 1953; 66: 171–183.

7. Symington T. Functional pathology of the human adrenal gland. Baltimore: Williams & Wilkins, 1969.

8. Dobbie JW, Symington T. The human adrenal gland with special reference to the vasculature. J Endocrinol 1966; 34: 479–489.

9. Quinan C, Berger AA. Observations on human adrenals with special reference to the relative weight of the normal medulla. Ann Intern Med 1933; 6: 1180–1192.

10. Studzinski GP, Hay DCF, Symington T. Observations on the weight of the human adrenal gland and the effect of preparations of corticotropin of different purity on the weight and morphology of the human adrenal gland. J Clin Endocrinol Metab 1963; 23: 248–254.

11. Pakravan P, Kenny FM, Depp R et al. Familial congenital absence of adrenal glands: evaluation of glucocorticoid, mineralocorticoid, and estrogen metabolism in the perinatal period. J Pediatr 1974; 4: 74–78.

12. Wise JE, Metalon R, Morgan AM, et al. Phenotypic features of patients with congenital adrenal hypoplasia and glycerol kinase deficiency. Am J Dis Child 1987; 141: 744–747.

13. Clark RA, Howard N, O'Sullivan WJ, et al. Glycerol kinase deficiency and adrenal hypoplasia congenita. J Inherit Metab Dis 1997; 20: 609.

14. Zanaria E, Muscatelli F, Baradoni B, et al. An unusual member of the nuclear hormone receptor superfamily responsible for X-linked adrenal hypoplasia congenita. Nature 1994; 372: 635–641.

15. Muscatelli F, Strom TM, Walker AP, et al. Mutations in the DAX-1 gene give rise to both X-linked adrenal hypoplasia congenita and hypogonadotropic hypogonadism. Nature 1994; 372: 672–676.

16. Guo W, Mason JS, Stone CG, et al. Diagnosis of X-linked adrenal hypoplasia congenita by mutation analysis of the DAX-1 gene. JAMA 1995; 274: 324–330.

17. Reutens AT, Achermann JC, Ito M, et al. Clinical and functional effects of mutations in the DAX-1 gene in patients with adrenal hypoplasia congenita. J Clin Endocrinol Metab 1999; 84: 504–511.

18. Fujieda K, Tajima T. Molecular basis of adrenal insufficiency. Pediatr Res 2005; 57: 62R–69R.

19. Graham LS. Celiac accessory adrenal glands. Cancer 1953; 6: 149–152.

20. Falls JL. Accessory adrenal cortex in the broad ligament: incidence and functional significance. Cancer 1955; 8: 143–150.

21. Apitz K. Die geschwülste und gewebsmissbildungen der Nierenrinde. I. Die intrarenalen Nebenniereninseln. Virchows Arch [Pathol Anat] 1944; 311: 285–305.

22. Mares AJ, Shkolni, A, Sacks M, et al. Aberrant (ectopic) adrenal cortical tissue along the spermatic cord. J Pediatr Surg 1980; 15: 289–292.

23. Habuchi T, Mizutani Y, Miyakawa M. Ectopic aberrant adrenals with epididymal abnormality. Urology 1992; 39: 251–253.

24. Dahl EV, Bahn RC. Aberrant adrenal cortical tissue near the testis in human infants. Am J Pathol 1962; 40: 587–598.

25. Labarrere CA, Caccamo D, Telenta M, et al. A nodule of adrenal cortical tissue within a human placenta: light microscopic and immunocytochemical findings. Placenta 1984; 5: 139–144.

26. Bozic C. Ectopic fetal adrenal cortex in the lung of a newborn. Virchows Arch A [Pathol Anat Histol] 1974; 363: 371–374.

27. Armin A, Castelli M. Congenital adrenal tissue in the lung with adrenal cytomegaly. Am J Clin Pathol 1984; 82: 225–228.

28. Weiner MF, Dallgard SA. Intracranial adrenal gland. Arch Pathol 1959; 67: 228–233.

29. Roosen-Runge EC, Lund J. Abnormal sex cord formation and an intratesticular adrenal cortical nodule in a human fetus. Anat Rec 1972; 173: 57–68.

30. Symonds DA, Driscoll SG. An adrenal cortical rest within the fetal ovary: report of a case. Am J Clin Pathol 1973; 60: 562–564.

31. Verdonk C, Guerin C, Lufkin E, et al. Activation of virilizing adrenal rest tissues by excessive ACTH production. An unusual presentation of Nelson's syndrome. Am J Med 1982; 73: 455–459.

32. Contreras P, Altieri E, Liberman C, et al. Adrenal rest tumor of the liver causing Cushing's syndrome: treatment with ketoconazole preceding an apparent surgical cure. J Clin Endocrinol Metab 1985; 60: 21–28.

33. Kepes JJ, O'Boynick P, Jones S, et al. Adrenal cortical adenoma in the spinal canal of an 8-year-old girl. Am J Surg Pathol 1990; 14: 481–484.

34. Dolan MF, Janovski NA. Adreno-hepatic fusion. Arch Pathol 1968; 86: 22–24.

35. Craig JM, Landing BH. Anaplastic cells of fetal adrenal cortex. Am J Clin Pathol 1951; 21: 940–949.

36. Beckwith JB. Extreme cytomegaly of the adrenal fetal cortex, omphalocele, hyperplasia of kidneys and pancreas, and Leydig cell hyperplasia: another syndrome? Presented at Annual Meeting of Western Society for Pediatric Research, Los Angeles, 11 November 1963.

37. Wiedemann HR. Complexe malformatif familial avec hernie umbilicale et macroglossia: un 'syndrome nouveau?' J Genet Hum 1964; 13: 223–232.

38. Beckwith JB. Macroglossia, omphalocele, adrenal cytomegaly, gigantism and hyperplastic visceromegaly. Birth Defects, Original Article Series 1969; 5: 188–196.

39. Li M, Squire JA, Weksberg R. Molecular genetics of Wiedemann–Beckwith syndrome. Am J Med Genet 1998; 79: 253–259.

40. Weksberg R, Shuman C, Smith AC. Beckwith–Wiedemann syndrome. Am J Med Genet C Semin Med Genet 2005; 137: 12–23.

41. Martelli C, Blandamura S, Massaro S, et al. A case study of Beckwith–Wiedemann syndrome associated with hepatoblastoma. Clin Exp Obstet Gynecol 1993; 20: 82–87.

42. Worth LL, Slopis JM, Herzog CE. Congenital hepatoblastoma and schizencephaly in an infant with Beckwith–Wiedemann syndrome. Med Pediatr Oncol 1999; 33: 591–593.

43. Porteus MH, Narkool P, Neuberg D, et al. Characteristics and outcome of children with Beckwith–Wiedemann syndrome and Wilms' tumor: a report from the National Wilms Tumor Study Group. J Clin Oncol 2000; 18: 2026–2031.

44. McNeil De, Brown M, Ching A, et al. Screening for Wilms' tumor and hepatoblastoma in children with Beckwith–Wiedemann syndrome. A cost effective model. Med Pediatr Oncol 2001; 37: 349–356.

45. Unterrainer G, Molzer B, Forss-Petter, et al. Co-expression of mutated and normal adrenoleukodystrophy protein reduces protein function: implications for gene therapy of X-linked adrenoleukodystrophy. Hum Mol Genet 2000; 9: 2609–2616.

46. Berger J, Gartner J. X-linked adrenoleukodystrophy. Clinical, biochemical and pathogenetic aspects. Biochim Biophys Acta 2006; 26 (Epub).

47. Powers JM, Schaumberg HH. The adrenal cortex in adrenoleukodystrophy. Arch Pathol 1973; 96: 305–310.

48. Alger S, Green A, Kohler W, et al. Proceedings of the 4th international workshop of the Adrenoleukodystrophy International Research Group (ALD-IRG), University of York, 3 September 1998. J Inherit Metab Dis 2000; 23: 449–452.

49. New MI. An update on congenital adrenal hyperplasia. Ann NY Acad Sci 2004; 1038: 14–43.

50. de Crecchio L. Sopra un caso di apparenzi virili in una donna. Morgagni 1865; 7: 154–188.

51. White PC, New MI, Dupont B. Congenital adrenal hyperplasia. N Engl J Med 1987; 316: 1519–1524 (part I), 316: 1580–1586, (part II).

52. Kalaitzoglou G, New MI. Congenital adrenal hyperplasia. Molecular insights learned from patients. Receptor 1993; 3: 211–222.

53. Mercado AB, Wilson RC, Cheng KC, et al. Prenatal treatment and diagnosis of congenital adrenal hyperplasia owing to steroid 21-hydroxylase deficiency. J Clin Endocrinol Metab 1995; 80: 2014–2020.

54. Pang S. Congenital adrenal hyperplasia. Endocrinol Metab Clin North Am 1997; 26: 853–891.

55. Lee HH, Kuo JM, Chao HT, et al. Carrier analysis and prenatal diagnosis of congenital adrenal hyperplasia caused by 21-hydroxylase deficiency in Chinese. J Clin Endocrinol Metab 2000; 85: 597–600.

56. Geley S, Kapelari K, Hohrer K, et al. CYP11B1 mutations causing congenital adrenal hyperplasia due to 11 beta-hydroxylase deficiency. J Clin Endocrinol Metab 1996; 81: 2896–2901.

57. Krone N, Grischuk Y, Muller M, et al. Analyzing the functional and structural consequences of two point mutations (P94L and A368D) in the CYP11B1 gene causing congenital adrenal hyperplasia resulting from 11-hydroxylase deficiency. J Clin Endocrinol Metab 2006; 91: 2682–2688.

58. Rutgers JL, Young RL, Scully RE. The testicular 'tumor' of the adrenogenital syndrome. A report of six cases and review of the literature on testicular masses in patients with adrenal cortical disorders. Am J Surg Pathol 1988; 12: 503–513.

59. Radfar N, Bartter FC, Easley R, et al. Evidence for endogenous LH suppression in a man with bilateral testicular tumors and congenital adrenal hyperplasia. J Clin Endocrinol Metab 1977; 45: 1194–1204.

60. Johnson RE, Scheithauer B. Massive hyperplasia of testicular adrenal rests in a patient with Nelson's syndrome. Am J Clin Pathol 1982; 77: 501–507.

61. Al-Ahmadie HA, Stanek J, Liu J, et al. Ovarian 'tumor' of the adrenogenital syndrome: the first reported case. Am J Surg Pathol 2001; 25: 1443–1450.

62. Lack EE. Tumors of the adrenal gland and extra-adrenal paraganglia. In: Atlas of tumor pathology, Series 4. Washington, DC: Armed Forces Institute of Pathology, 2007.

63. Duck SC. Malignancy associated with congenital adrenal hyperplasia. J Pediatr 1981; 99: 423–424.

64. Rich AR. A peculiar type of adrenal cortical damage associated with acute infection, and its possible relation to circulatory collapse. Bull Johns Hopkins Hosp 1944; 74: 1–15.

65. Sommers SC, Carter ME. Adrenal cortical postirradiation fibrosis. Arch Pathol 1975; 99: 421–423.

66. Benirschke K. Adrenals in anencephaly and hydrocephaly. Obstet Gynecol 1956; 8: 412–425.

67. Soderbergh A, Winqvist O, Norheim I, et al. Adrenal autoantibodies and organ-specific autoimmunity in patients with Addison's disease. Clin Endocrinol 1996; 45: 453–460.

68. Falorni A, Laureti S, Nikoshkov A, et al. 21-hydroxylase autoantibodies in adult patients with endocrine autoimmune disease are highly specific for Addison's disease. Clin Exp Immunol 1997; 107: 341–346.

69. Gambelunghe G, Falorni A, Ghaderi M, et al. Microsatellite polymorphism of the MHC class I chain-related (MIC-A and MIC-B) genes marks the risk for autoimmune Addison's disease. J Clin Endocrinol Metab 1999; 84: 3701–3707.

70. Nagamine K, Peterson P, Scott HS, et al. Positional cloning of the APECED gene. Nature Genet 1997; 17: 393–398.

71. The Finnish-German APECED Consortium. An autoimmune disease, APECED, caused by mutation in a novel gene featuring two PHD-type zinc-finger domains. Nature Genet 1997; 17: 399–403.

72. Scott HS, Heino M, Peterson P, et al. Common mutations in autoimmune polyendocrinopathy–candidiasis–ectodermal dystrophy patients of different origins. Mol Endocrinol 1998; 12: 1112–1119, 1998.

73. Betterle C, Zanchetta. Update on autoimmune polyendocrine syndromes (APS). Acta Biomed Ateneo Parmense 2003; 74: 9–33.

74. Ahonen P, Myllärniemi S, Sipilä I, et al. Clinical variation of autoimmune polyendocrinopathy-candidiasis–ectodermal dystrophy (APECED) in a series of 68 patients. N Engl J Med 1990; 322: 1829–1836.

75. Schmidt MB. Eine biglanduläre Erkrankung (Nebennieren und Schilddrüse) bei morbus Addisonii. Verh Dtsch Ges Pathol 1926; 21: 212–221.

76. Alevritis EM, Sarubbi FA, Jordan RM, et al. Infectious causes of adrenal insufficiency. South Med J 2003; 96: 888–890.

77. Guttman PH. Addison's disease. A statistical analysis of five hundred and sixty-six cases and a study of the pathology. Arch Pathol 1930; 10: 742–785.

78. Dunlop D. Eighty-six cases of Addison's disease. Br Med J 1963; 12: 887–891.

79. Goodwin RA Jr, Shapiro JL, Thurman GH, et al. Disseminated histoplasmosis: clinical and pathologic correlations. Medicine 1980; 59: 1–33.

80. Griffel B. Focal adrenalitis. Its frequency and correlation with similar lesions in the thyroid and kidney. Virchows Arch A [Pathol Anat Histol] 1974; 364: 191–198.

81. Hass GM. Hepato-adrenal necrosis with intranuclear inclusion bodies: report of a case. Am J Pathol 1935; 11: 127–142.

82. Klatt EC, Shibata D. Cytomegalovirus infection in the acquired immunodeficiency syndrome. Clinical and autopsy findings. Arch Pathol Lab Med 1988; 112: 540–544.

83. Donovan DS Jr, Dluhy RG. AIDS and its effect on the adrenal gland. Endocrinologist 1991; 1: 227–232.

84. Cote RJ, Rosenblum M, Telzak EE. Disseminated Pneumocystis carinii infection causing extrapulmonary organ failure: clinical, pathologic, and immunohistochemical analysis. Mod Pathol 1990; 3: 25–30.

85. Sinclair-Smith C, Kahn LB, Sidney C. Malacoplakia in childhood. Arch Pathol 1975; 99: 198–203.

86. Benjamin E, Fox H. Malakoplakia of the adrenal gland. J Clin Pathol 1981; 34: 606–611.

87. Bartsch G, Bodner E, Buchsteiner R, et al. Echinococcal cyst of the adrenal gland. Eur Urol 1975; 1: 240–242.

88. Dobbie JW. Adrenal cortical nodular hyperplasia: the aging adrenal. J Pathol 1969; 99: 1–18.

89. Hedeland H, Östberg G, Hökfelt B. On the prevalence of adrenal cortical adenomas in an autopsy material in relation to hypertension and diabetes. Acta Med Scand 1968; 184: 211–214.

90. Spain DM, Weinsaft P. Solitary adrenal cortical adenoma in elderly female. Frequency. Arch Pathol 1964; 78: 231–233.

91. Shamma AH, Goddard JW, Sommers SC. A study of the adrenal status in hypertension. J Chronic Dis 1958; 8: 587–595.

92. Russi S, Blumenthal HT, Gray SH. Small adenomas of the adrenal cortex in hypertension and diabetes. Arch Intern Med 1945; 76: 284–291.

93. Commons RR, Callaway CP. Adenomas of the adrenal cortex. Arch Intern Med 1948; 81: 37–41.

94. Robinson MJ, Pardo V, Rywlin AM. Pigmented nodules (black adenomas) of the adrenal. An autopsy study of incidence, morphology and function. Hum Pathol 1972; 3: 317–325.

95. Damron TA, Schelper RL, Sorensen L. Cytochemical demonstration of neuromelanin in black pigmented adrenal nodules. Am J Clin Pathol 1987; 87: 334–341.

96. Glazer HS, Weyman PJ, Sagel SS, et al. Non-functioning adrenal masses: incidental discovery on computed tomography. AJR Am J Roentgenol 1982; 139: 81–85.

97. Prinz RA, Brooks MH, Churchill R, et al. Incidental asymptomatic adrenal masses detected by computed tomographic scanning. JAMA 1982; 248: 701–704.

98. Abecassis M, McLoughlin MJ, Longer B, et al. Serendipitous adrenal masses: prevalence, significance and management. Am J Surg 1985; 149: 783–788.

99. Herrera MF, Grant CS, van Heerden JA, et al. Incidentally discovered adrenal tumors: an institutional perspective. Surgery 1991; 110: 1014–1021.

100. Keiser HR, Doppman JL, Robertson CN, et al. Diagnosis, localization, and management of pheochromocytoma. In: Lack EE, ed. Pathology of the adrenal glands. New York: Churchill Livingstone, 1990.

101. Beierwaltes WH, Sturman MF, Ryo U, et al. Imaging functional nodules of the adrenal glands with I 131–19 iodocholesterol. J Nucl Med 1974; 15: 246–251.

102. Rizza RA, Wahner HW, Spelsberg TC, et al. Visualization of nonfunctional adrenal adenomas with iodocholesterol: possible relationship to subcellular distribution of tracer. J Nucl Med 1978; 19: 458–463.

103. Gross MD, Valk TW, Freitas JE, et al. The relationship of adrenal iodomethylnorcholesterol (NP-59) uptake to indices of adrenal cortical function in Cushing's syndrome. J Clin Endocrinol Metab 1981; 52: 1062–1066.

104. Gross MD, Wilton GP, Shapiro B, et al. Functional and scintigraphic evaluation of the silent adrenal mass. J Nucl Med 1987; 28: 1401–1407.

105. Suzuki T, Sasano H, Sawai T, et al. Small adrenal cortical tumors without apparent clinical endocrine abnormalities. Immunolocalization of steroidogenic enzymes. Pathol Res Pract 1992; 188: 883–889.

106. Krestin GP, Friedmann G, Fishbach R, et al. Evaluation of adrenal masses in oncology patients: dynamic contrast-enhanced MR vs CT. J Comput Assist Tomogr 1991; 15: 104–110.

107. Copeland PM. The incidentally discovered adrenal mass. Ann Intern Med 1983; 98: 940–945.

108. Ross NS, Aron DC. Hormonal evaluation of the patient with an incidentally discovered adrenal mass. N Engl J Med 1990; 323: 1401–1405.

109. Nadler JL, Rabin R. Evaluation and management of the incidentally discovered adrenal mass. Endocrinologist 1991; 1: 5–9.

110. Roubidoux M, Dunnick NR. Adrenal cortical tumors. Bull NY Acad Med 1991; 67: 119–130.

111. Case Records of the Massachusetts General Hospital. Case 6–1991. N Engl J Med 1991; 324: 400–408.

112. Anon. NIH state-of-the-science statement on management of the clinically inapparent adrenal mass ('incidentaloma'). NIH Consensus State Sci Statements 2002; 19: 1–25.

113. Grumbach MM, Biller BMK, Braunstein GD, et al. Management of the clinically inapparent adrenal mass ('incidentaloma'). Ann Intern Med 2003; 138: 424–429.

114. Sippel RS, Chen H. Subclinical Cushing's syndrome in adrenal incidentalomas. Surg Clin North Am 2004; 84: 875–885.

115. Orth DN, Liddle GW. Results of treatment in 108 patients with Cushing's syndrome. N Engl J Med 1971; 285: 243–247.

116. Liddle GW. Cushing's syndrome. Ann NY Acad Sci 1977; 297: 594–602.

117. Carpenter PC. Cushing's syndrome: update of diagnosis and management. Mayo Clin Proc 1986; 61: 49–58.

118. Invitti C, Giraldi F, De Martin M, et al. Diagnosis and management of Cushing's syndrome: results of an Italian multicentre study. J Clin Endocrinol Metab 1999; 84: 440–448.

119. Newell-Price J, Grossman AB. The differential diagnosis of Cushing's syndrome. Ann Endocrinol 2001; 62: 173–179.

120. Boscaro M, Barzon L, Fallo F, et al. Cushing's syndrome. Lancet 2001; 357: 783–791.

121. Mandel S. Cushing's syndrome in infancy. Endocrinologist 1994; 4: 28–32.

122. Mampalan TJ, Tyrell JB, Wilson CB. Transsphenoidal microsurgery for Cushing's disease: a report of 216 cases. Ann Intern Med 1988; 109: 487–493.

123. Klibanski A, Zervas NT. Diagnosis and management of hormone-secreting pituitary adenomas. N Engl J Med 1991; 324: 822–831.

124. Miller J, Crapo L. The biochemical diagnosis of hypercortisolism. Endocrinologist 1994; 4: 7–16.

125. Hammer GD, Tyrell JB, Lamborn KR, et al. Transsphenoidal microsurgery fro Cushing's disease: initial outcome and long-term results. J Clin Endocrinol Metab 2004; 80: 6348–6357.

126. Vella A, Thompson GB, Grant CS, et al. Laparoscopic adrenalectomy for adrenocorticotropin-dependent Cushing's syndrome. J Clin Endocrinol Metab 2001; 86: 1596–1599.

127. Young WF Jr, Thompson GB. Laparoscopic adrenalectomy for patients who have Cushing's syndrome. Endocrinol Metab Clin North Am 2005; 34: 489–499.

128. Smals AGH, Pieters GFFM, van Haelst UJG, et al. Macronodular, adrenal cortical hyperplasia in longstanding Cushing's disease. J Clin Endocrinol Metab 1984; 58: 25–31.

129. Doppman JL, Miller DL, Dwyer AJ, et al. Macronodular adrenal hyperplasia in Cushing's disease. Radiology 1988; 166: 347–352.

130. Cohen RB, Chapman WB, Castleman B. Hyperadrenocorticism (Cushing's disease): a study of surgically resected adrenal glands. Cancer 1959; 35: 537–561.

131. Grua JR, Nelson DH. ACTH-producing tumors. Endocrinol Metab Clin N Am 1991; 20: 319–362.

132. Nieman LK. The evaluation of ACTH-dependent Cushing's syndrome. Endocrinologist 1999; 9: 93–98.

133. Odell WD. Ectopic ACTH secretion. A misnomer. Endocrinol Metab Clin North Am 1991; 20: 371–379.

134. Doppman JL. The search for occult ectopic ACTH-producing tumors. Endocrinologist 1992; 2: 41–46.

135. Aniszewski JP, Young WF, Thompson GB, et al. Cushing syndrome due to adrenocorticotropic hormone secretion. World J Surg 2001; 25: 934–940.

136. Ilias I, Torpy DJ, Pacak K, et al. Cushing's syndrome due to ectopic corticotropin secretion: twenty years' experience at the National Institutes of Health. J Clin Endocrinol Metab 2005; 90: 4955–4962.

137. Leinung MC, Young WF Jr, Whitaker MD, et al. Diagnosis of corticotropin-producing bronchial carcinoid tumors causing Cushing's syndrome. Mayo Clin Proc 1990; 65: 1314–1321.

138. Shenoy BV, Carpentar PC, Carney JA. Bilateral primary pigmented nodular adrenal cortical disease. Rare cause of Cushing's syndrome. Am J Surg Pathol 1984; 8: 335–344.

139. Stratakis CA, Sarlis N, Kirschner LS, et al. Paradoxical response to dexamethasone in the diagnosis of primary pigmented nodular adrenal cortical disease. Ann Intern Med 1999; 131: 585–591.

140. Stratakis CA, Kirschner LS, Carney JA. Clinical and molecular features of the Carney complex: diagnostic criteria and recommendations for patient evaluation. J Clin Endocrinol Metab 2001; 86: 4041–4046.

141. Stratakis CA. Genetics of adrenal cortical tumors. Carney complex. Ann Endocrinol 2001; 62: 180–184.

142. Carney JA, Young WF Jr. Primary pigmented nodular adrenal cortical disease and its associated conditions. Endocrinologist 1992; 2: 6–21.

143. Wulffra-at NM, Drexhagge HA, Wiersinga WM, et al. Immunoglobulins of patients with Cushing's syndrome due to pigmented adrenal cortical micronodular dysplasia stimulate in vitro steroidogenesis. J Clin Endocrinol Metab 1988; 66: 301–307.

144. Stratakis CA, Carney JA, Kirschner LS, et al. Synaptophysin immunoreactivity in primary pigmented nodular adrenal cortical disease: neuroendocrine properties of tumors associated with Carney complex. J Clin Endocrinol Metab 1999; 84: 1122–1128.

145. Sasano H, Miyazaki S, Sawai T, et al. Primary pigmented nodular adrenal cortical disease (PPNAD): immunohistochemical and in situ

hybridization analysis of steroidogenic enzymes in eight cases. Modern Pathol 1992 5: 23–29.

146. Grant CS, Carney JA, Carpenter PC, et al. Primary pigmented nodular adrenal cortical disease: diagnosis and treatment. Surgery 1986; 100: 1178–1184.

147. Carney JA, Gordon H, Carpenter PC, et al. The complex of myxomas, spotty pigmentation, and endocrine overactivity. Medicine 1985; 64: 270–283.

148. Carney JA, Boccon-Gibod L, Jarka DE, et al. Osteochondromyxoma of bone. A congenital tumor associated with lentigines and other unusual disorders. Am J Surg Pathol 2001; 25: 164–176.

149. Bertherat J, Gimenez-Roqueplo AP. New insights in the genetics of adrenal cortical tumors, pheochromocytomas and paragangliomas. Horm Metab Res 2005; 37: 384–390.

150. Groussin L, Horvath A, Jullian E, et al. A PRKAR1A mutation associated with primary pigmented nodular adrenal cortical disease in 12 kindreds. J Clin Endocrinol Metab 2006; 91: 1943–1949.

151. Doppman JL, Nieman LK, Travis WD, et al. CT and MR imaging of massive macronodular adrenal cortical disease: a rare cause of autonomous primary adrenal hypercortisolism. J Comput Assist Tomogr 1991; 15: 773–779.

152. Lieberman SA, Eccleshall TR, Feldman D. ACTH-independent massive bilateral adrenal disease (AIMBAD): a subtype of Cushing's syndrome with major diagnosis and therapeutic implications. Eur J Endocrinol 1994; 131: 67–73.

153. Doppman JL, Chrousos GP, Papanicolaou DA, et al. Adrenocorticotropin-independent macronodular adrenal hyperplasia: an uncommon cause of primary adrenal hypercortisolism. Radiology 2000; 216: 797–802.

154. Aiba M, Hirayama A, Iri H, et al. Adrenocorticotropic hormone-independent bilateral adrenal cortical macronodular hyperplasia as a distinct subtype of Cushing's syndrome. Enzyme histochemical and ultrastructural study of four cases with a review of the literature. Am J Clin Pathol 1991; 96: 334–340.

155. Sasano H, Suzuki T, Nagura H. ACTH-independent macronodular adrenal cortical hyperplasia: immunohistochemical and in situ hybridization studies of steroidogenic enzymes. Mod Pathol 1994; 7: 215–219.

156. Wermer P. Genetic aspects of adenomatosis of endocrine glands, Am J Med 16: 363–371, 1954.

157. Skogseid B, Larsson C, Lindgren P-G, et al. Clinical and genetic features of adrenal cortical lesions in multiple endocrine neoplasia type 1.

158. Ballard HS, Frame B, Hartsock RJ. Familial multiple endocrine adenoma–peptic ulcer complex. Medicine 1964; 43: 481–516.

159. Miyagawa K, Ishibashi M, Kasuga M, et al. Multiple endocrine neoplasia type I with Cushing's disease primary hyperparathyroidism and insulin-glucagonoma. Cancer 1988; 61: 1232–1236.

160. Dotzenrath C, Goretzki PE, Cupisti K, et al. Malignant endocrine tumors in patients with MEN I disease. Surgery 2001; 129: 91–95.

161. Weinstein LS, Shenker A, Gejman PV, et al. Activating mutations of the stimulatory G protein in McCune–Albright syndrome. N Engl J Med 1991; 325: 1688–1695.

162. Bertagna X. New causes of Cushing's syndrome. N Engl J Med 1992; 327: 1024–1025.

163. Reznik Y, Allali-Zerah V, Chayvialle JA, et al. Food-dependent Cushing's syndrome mediated by aberrant adrenal sensitivity to gastric inhibitory polypeptide. N Engl J Med 1992; 327: 981–986.

164. Lacroix A, Bolté E, Tremblay J, et al. Gastric inhibitory polypeptide-dependent cortisol hypersecretion – a new cause of Cushing's syndrome. N Engl J Med 1992; 327: 974–980.

165. Neville AM, O'Hare MJ. Histopathology of the human adrenal cortex. Clin Endocrinol Metab 1985; 14: 791–820.

166. Young WF Jr, Hogan MJ, Klee GG, et al. Primary aldosteronism: diagnosis and treatment. Mayo Clin Proc 1990; 65: 96–110.

167. Puccino M, Iacconi P, Bernini G, et al. Conn syndrome: 14 years' experience from two European centres. Eur J Surg 1998; 164: 811–817.

168. Carey RM, Sen S, Doland LM, et al. Idiopathic hyperaldosteronism: a possible role for aldosterone-stimulating factor. N Engl J Med 1984; 311: 94–100.

169. Gill JR Jr. Hyperaldosteronism. In: Becker KL, ed. Principles and practice of endocrinology and metabolism. Philadelphia: JB Lippincott, 1990.

170. DeLellis RA, Wolfe HJ, Gagel RT, et al. Adrenal medullary hyperplasia. A morphometric analysis in patients with familial medullary thyroid carcinoma. Am J Pathol 1976; 83: 177–190.

171. Dralle H, Schroder S, Gratz KF, et al. Sporadic unilateral adrenomedullary hyperplasia with hypertension cured by adrenalectomy. World J Surg 1990; 14: 308–315.

172. Jansson S, Khorram-Manesh A, Nilsson O, et al. Treatment of bilateral pheochromocytoma and adrenal medullary hyperplasia. Ann NY Acad Sci 2006; 1073: 429–435.

173. Carney JA, Sizemore GW, Sheps SG. Adrenal medullary disease in multiple endocrine neoplasia, type 2. Pheochromocytoma and its precursors. Am J Clin Pathol 1976; 66: 279–290.

173a. Karsner HT. Tumor of the adrenal. In: Atlas of Tumor Pathology. Fasc 29, sec VIII. WASH., D. C., AFIP, 1950.

174. Padberg B-C, Garbe E, Achilles E, et al. Adrenomedullary hyperplasia and phaeochromocytoma. DNA photometric findings in 47 cases. Virchows Arch A [Pathol Anat] 1990; 416: 443–446.

175. Foster DG. Adrenal cysts. Review of the literature and report of case. Arch Surg 1966; 92: 131–143.

176. Abeshouse GA, Goldstein RB, Abeshouse BS. Adrenal cysts: review of the literature and report of three cases. J Urol 1959; 81: 711–719.

177. Akcay MN, Akcay G, Balik AA, et al. Hydatid cysts of the adrenal gland: review of nine patients. World J Surg 2004; 28: 97–99.

178. Travis WD, Oertel JE, Lack EE. Miscellaneous tumors and tumefactive lesions of the adrenal gland. In: Lack EE, ed. Pathology of the adrenal glands. New York: Churchill Livingstone, 1990, 351–378.

179. Medeiros LJ, Weiss LM, Vickery AL. Epithelial-lined (true) cyst of the adrenal gland: a case report. Hum Pathol 1989; 20: 491–492.

180. Fukushima N, Oonishi T, Yamaguchi K, et al. Mesothelial cyst of the adrenal gland. Pathol Int 1995; 45: 156–159.

181. Erickson LA, Lloyd RV, Hartman R, et al. Cystic adrenal neoplasms. Cancer 2004; 101: 1537–1544.

182. Groben PA, Roberson JB, Anger SR, et al. Immunohistochemical evidence for the vascular origin of primary adrenal pseudocysts. Arch Pathol Lab Med 1986; 110: 121–123.

183. Gaffey MJ, Mills SE, Fechner RE, et al. Vascular adrenal cysts. A clinicopathologic and immunohistochemical study of endothelial and hemorrhagic (pseudocystic) variants. Am J Surg Pathol 1989; 13: 740–747.

184. Torres C, Ro JY, Batt MA, et al. Vascular adrenal cysts: a clinicopathologic and immunohistochemical study of six cases and a review of the literature. Mod Pathol 1997; 10: 530–536.

185. Gaffey MJ, Mills SE, Medeiros LJ, et al. Unusual variants of adrenal pseudocysts with intracystic fat, myelolipomatous metaplasia, and metastatic carcinoma. Am J Clin Pathol 1990; 94: 706–713.

186. Oppenheimer EH. Cyst formation in the outer adrenal cortex: studies in the human fetus and newborn. Arch Pathol 1969; 87: 653–659.

187. Rodin AE, Hsu FL, Whorton EB. Microcysts of the permanent adrenal

cortex in perinates and infants. Arch Pathol Lab Med 1976; 100: 499–502.

188. Hunter SB, Schemankewitz EH, Patterson C, et al. Extra-adrenal myelolipoma. A report of two cases. Am J Clin Pathol 1992; 97: 402–404.

189. Nishizaki T, Kanematsu T, Matsumata T, et al. Myelolipoma of the liver. A case report. Cancer 1989; 63: 930–934.

190. Minamiya Y, Abo S, Kitamura M, et al. Mediastinal extra-adrenal myelolipoma: report of a case. Surg Today 1997; 27: 971–972.

191. Kawanami, S, Watanabe H, Aoki T, et al. Mediastinal myelolipoma. CT and MRI appearances. Eur Radiol 2000; 10: 691–693.

192. Spanta R, Saleh HA, Khatib G. Fine needle aspiration diagnosis of extra-adrenal myelolipoma presenting as a pleural mass: a case report. Acta Cytol 1999; 43: 295–298.

193. Cina SJ, Gordon BM, Curry NS. Ectopic adrenal myelolipoma presenting as a splenic mass. Arch Pathol Lab Med 1995; 119: 561–563.

194. Giuliani A, Tocchi A, Caporale A, et al. Presacral myelolipoma in a patient with colon carcinoma. J Exp Clin Cancer Res 2001; 20: 451–454.

195. Seyle S, Stone H. Hormonally induced transformation of adrenal into myeloid tissue. Am J Pathol 1950; 26: 211–233.

196. Bishop E, Eble JN, Cheng L, et al. Adrenal myelolipomas show nonrandom X-chromosome inactivation in hematopoietic elements and fat: support for a clonal origin of myelolipomas. Am J Surg Pathol 2006; 30: 838–843.

197. Plaut A. Myelolipoma in the adrenal cortex (myeloadipose structures). Am J Pathol 1958; 34: 487–515.

198. Del Gaudio A, Solidaro G. Myelolipoma of the adrenal gland: report of two cases with a review of the literature. Surgery 1986; 99: 293–301.

199. Hoeffel C, Chelle C, Clement A, et al. Spontaneous retroperitoneal hemorrhage from a giant adrenal myelolipoma. J Urol 1996; 155: 639.

200. Amano T, Takemae K, Niikura S, et al. Retroperitoneal hemorrhage due to spontaneous rupture of adrenal myelolipoma. Int J Urol 1999; 6: 585–588.

201. Bennett BD, McKenna T, Hough AJ, et al. Adrenal myelolipoma associated with Cushing's disease. Am J Clin Pathol 1980; 73: 443–447.

202. Yoshioka M, Fujimori K Wakasugi M, et al. Cushing's disease associated with adrenal myelolipoma, adrenal calcification and thyroid cancer. Endocr J 1994; 41: 461–466.

203. Vyberg M, Sestoft L. Combined adrenal myelolipoma and adenoma associated with Cushing's syndrome. Am J Clin Pathol 1986; 86: 541–545.

204. Whaley D, Becker S, Presbrey T, et al. Adrenal myelolipoma associated with Conn's syndrome. CT evaluation. J Comput Assist Tomogr 1985; 9: 959–960.

205. Boronat M, Moreno A, Ramon y Cajal S, et al. Subclinical Cushing's syndrome due to adrenal myelolipoma. Arch Pathol Lab Med 1997; 121: 735–737.

206. DeBlois GG, DeMay RM. Adrenal myelolipoma diagnosed by computed tomography-guided fine needle aspiration. Cancer 1985; 55: 848–850.

207. Rao RH, Vagnucci AH, Amico JA. Bilateral massive adrenal hemorrhage: early recognition and treatment. Ann Intern Med 1989; 110: 227–235.

208. Vella A, Nippoldt TB, Morris JC. Adrenal hemorrhage: a 25 year experience at the Mayo Clinic. Mayo Clin Proc 2001; 76: 161–168.

209. Bertagna C, Orth DN. Clinical and laboratory findings and results of therapy in 58 patients with adrenal cortical tumors admitted to a single medical center (1951–1978). Am J Med 1981; 71: 855–875.

210. Lack EE, Travis WD, Oertel JE. Adrenal cortical neoplasms. In: Lack EE, ed. Pathology of the adrenal glands. New York: Churchill Livingstone, 1990, 115–171.

211. Aiba M, Kawakami M, Ito Y, et al. Bilateral adrenal cortical adenomas causing Cushing's syndrome. Report of two cases with enzyme histochemical and ultrastructural studies and a review of the literature. Arch Pathol Lab Med 1992; 116: 146–150.

212. Kato S, Masunaga R, Kawabe T, et al. Cushing's syndrome induced by hypersecretion of cortisol from only one of bilateral adrenal cortical tumors. Metabolism 1992; 41: 260–263.

213. O'Leary TJ, Liotta LA, Gill JR. Pigmented adrenal nodules in Cushing's syndrome. Arch Pathol Lab Med 1982; 106: 257.

214. Conn JW. Plasma renin activity in primary aldosteronism. Importance in differential diagnosis and in research of essential hypertension. JAMA 1964; 190: 222–225.

215. Ganguly A. Cellular origin of aldosteronomas. Clin Invest 1992; 70: 392–395.

216. Eto T, Kumamoto K, Kawasaki T, et al. Ultrastructural types of cells in adrenal cortical adenoma with primary aldosteronism. J Pathol 1979; 128: 1–6.

217. Janigan DT. Cytoplasmic bodies in the adrenal cortex of patients treated with spironolactone. Lancet 1963; 1: 850–852.

218. Jenis EH, Hertzog RW. Effect of spironolactone on the zona glomerulosa of the adrenal cortex:

light and electron microscopy. Arch Pathol 1969; 88: 530–539.

219. Cohn D, Jackson RV, Gordon RD. Factors affecting the frequency of occurrence of spironolactone bodies in aldosteronomas and non-tumorous cortex. Pathology 1983; 15: 273–277.

220. Komiya I, Takasu N, Aizawa T, et al. Black (or brown) adrenal cortical adenoma: its characteristic features on computed tomography and endocrine data. J Clin Endocrinol Metab 1985; 61: 711–717.

221. Mattox JH, Phelan S. The evaluation of adult females with testosterone producing neoplasms of the adrenal cortex. Surg Gynecol Obstet 1987; 164: 98–101.

222. Gabrilove JL, Sharma DC, Wotiz HH, et al. Feminizing adrenal cortical tumors in the male. A review of 52 cases including a case report. Medicine 1965; 44: 37–79.

223. Pollock WJ, McConnell CF, Hilton C, et al. Virilizing Leydig cell adenoma of adrenal gland. Am J Surg Pathol 1986; 10: 816–822.

224. Lack EE, Nauta RJ. Intracortical Leydig cells in a patient with an aldosterone-secreting adrenal cortical adenoma. J Urol Pathol 1993; 1: 411–418.

225. Erlandson RA, Reuter VE. Oncocytic adrenal cortical adenoma. Ultrastr Pathol 1991; 15: 539–547.

226. Sasano H, Suzuki T, Sano T, et al. Adrenal cortical oncocytoma. A true nonfunctioning adrenal cortical tumor. Am J Surg Pathol 1991; 15: 949–956.

227. Nguyen G-K, Vriend R, Ronaghan D, et al. Heterotopic adrenal cortical oncocytoma. A case report with light and electron microscopic studies. Cancer 1992; 70: 2681–2684.

228. Kitching PA, Patel V, Harach HR. Adrenal cortical oncocytoma. J Clin Pathol 1999; 52: 151–153.

229. Lin BT, Bonsib SM, Mierau GW, et al. Oncocytic adrenal cortical neoplasms: a report of seven cases and review of the literature. Am J Surg Pathol 1998; 22: 603–614.

230. Hoang MP, Ayala AG, Albores-Saavedra J. Oncocytic adrenal cortical carcinoma: a morphologic, immunohistochemical and ultrastructural study of four cases. Mod Pathol 2002; 15: 973–978.

231. Bisceglia M, Ludovico O, DiMattia A, et al. Adrenal cortical oncocytic tumors: report of 10 cases and review of the literature. Int J Surg Pathol 2004; 12: 231–243.

232. Song SY, Park S, Kim SR, et al. Oncocytic adrenal cortical carcinomas. A pathological and immunohistochemical study of four cases in comparison with conventional adrenal cortical carcinomas. Pathol Int 2004; 54: 603–610.

233. Third National Cancer Survey: incidence data. DHEW Publ. No.

(NIH) 75–787. NCI monograph. Bethesda: National Cancer Institute, 1975; 41.

234. Wooten MD, King DK. Adrenal cortical carcinoma. Epidemiology and treatment with mitotane and a review of the literature. Cancer 1993; 72: 3145–3155.

235. King DR, Lack EE. Adrenal cortical carcinoma. A clinical and pathologic study of 49 cases. Cancer 1979; 44: 239–244.

236. Evans HL, Vassilopoulou-Sellin R. Adrenal cortical neoplasms, a study of 56 cases. Am J Clin Pathol 1996; 105: 76–86.

237. Alsabeh R, Mazoujian G, Goates J, et al. Adrenal cortical tumors clinically mimicking pheochromocytoma. Am J Clin Pathol 1995; 104: 382–390.

238. Tang CK, Gray GF. Adrenal cortical neoplasms. Prognosis and morphology. Urology 1975; 5: 691–695.

239. Gandour MJ, Grizzle WE. A small adrenal cortical carcinoma with aggressive behavior. An evaluation of criteria for malignancy. Arch Pathol Lab Med 1986; 110: 1076–1079.

240. Dackiw APB, Lee JE, Gagel RF, et al. Adrenal cortical carcinoma. World J Surg 2001; 25: 914–926.

241. Newhouse JH, Heffess CS, Wagner BJ, et al. Large degenerated adrenal adenomas. Radiologic–pathologic correlation. Radiology 1999; 210: 385–391.

242. Sturgeon C, Shen WT, Clark OH, et al. Risk assessment in 457 adrenal cortical carcinomas: how much does tumor size predict the likelihood of malignancy? J Am Coll Surg 2006; 202: 423–30.

243. Weiss LM. Comparative histologic study of 43 metastasizing and nonmetastasizing adrenal cortical tumors. Am J Surg Pathol 1984; 8: 163–169.

244. Hough AJ, Hollifield JW, Page DL, et al. Prognostic factors in adrenal cortical tumors. A mathematical analysis of clinical and morphologic data. Am J Clin Pathol 1979; 72: 390–399.

245. Van Slooten H, Schaberg A, Smeenk D, et al. Morphologic characteristics of benign and malignant adrenal cortical tumors. Cancer 1985; 55: 766–773.

246. Weiss LM, Medeiros LJ, Vickery AL Jr. Pathologic features of prognostic significance in adrenal cortical carcinoma. Am J Surg Pathol 1989; 13: 202–206.

247. Lack EE, Mulvihill JJ, Travis WD, et al. Adrenal cortical neoplasms in the pediatric and adolescent age group. Clinicopathologic study of 30 cases with emphasis on epidemiological and prognostic factors. Pathol Annu 1992; 27: 1–53.

248. Miettinen M. Neuroendocrine differentiation in adrenal cortical carcinoma. New immunohistochemical findings supported by electron microscopy. Lab Invest 1992; 66: 169–174.

249. Schröder S, Padberg B-C, Achilles E, et al. Immunocytochemistry in adrenal cortical tumors: a clinicopathological study of 72 neoplasms. Virchows Arch A [Pathol Anat] 1992; 420: 65–70.

250. Mackay B, El-Naggar A, Ordonez NG. Ultrastructure of adrenal cortical carcinoma. Ultrastruct Pathol 1994; 18: 181–190.

251. Cibas ES, Medeiros LJ, Weinberg DS, et al. Cellular DNA profiles of benign and malignant adrenal cortical tumors. Am J Surg Pathol 1990; 14: 948–955.

252. Camuto P, Citrin D, Schinella R, et al. Adrenal cortical carcinoma: flow cytometric study of 22 cases on ECOG study. Urology 1991; 37: 380–384.

253. Zerbini C, Kozakewich HPW, Weinberg DS, et al. Adrenal cortical neoplasms in childhood and adolescence: analysis of prognostic factors including DNA content. Endocrinol Pathol 1992; 3: 116–128.

254. Bugg MF, Ribeiro RC, Roberson PK, et al. Correlation of pathologic features with clinical outcome in pediatric adrenal cortical neoplasia: a study of a Brazilian population. Am J Clin Pathol 1994; 101: 625–629.

255. Hosaka Y, Rainwater LM, Grant CS, et al. Adrenal cortical carcinoma: nuclear deoxyribonucleic acid ploidy studies by flow cytometry. Surgery 1987; 102: 1027–1034.

256. Reincke M. Mutations in adrenal cortical tumors. Horm Metab Res 1998; 30: 447–455.

257. Yano T, Linehan M, Anglard P, et al. Genetic changes in human adrenal cortical carcinomas. J Natl Cancer Inst 1989; 81: 518–523.

258. Fogt F, Vargas MP, Zhuang Z, et al. Utilization of molecular genetics in the differentiation between adrenal cortical adenomas and carcinomas. Hum Pathol 1998; 29: 518–521.

259. Ivesmake V, Kahri AI, Miettien PJ, et al. Insulin-like growth factors (IGFs) and their receptors in adrenal tumors: high IGF-II expression in functional adrenal cortical carcinomas. J Clin Endocrinol Metab 1993; 77: 852–858.

260. Reincke M, Karl M, Travis WH, et al. p53 mutation in human adrenal cortical neoplasms: immunohistochemical and molecular studies. J Clin Endocrinol Metab 1994; 78: 790–794.

261. Wagner J, Portwine C, Rabin K, et al. High frequency of germline p53 mutations in childhood adrenal cortical cancer. J Natl Cancer Inst 1994; 86: 1707–1710.

262. Backlin C, Rastad J, Skogseid B, et al. Immunohistochemical expression of insulin-like growth factor 1 and its receptor in normal and neoplastic human adrenal cortex. Anticancer Res 1995; 15: 2453–2459.

263. Gicquel C, Raffin Sanson ML, Gaston V, et al. Structural and functional abnormalities at 11p15 are associated with the malignant phenotype in sporadic adrenal cortical tumors: study on a series of 82 tumors. J Clin Endocrinol Metab 1997; 82: 2559–2565.

264. McNicol Am, Nolan CE, Struthers AJ, et al. Expression of p53 in adrenal cortical tumors: clinicopathologic correlations. J Pathol 1997; 181: 146–152.

265. Reincke M, Mora P, Beuschlein F, et al. Deletion of the adrenocorticotropin receptor gene in human adrenal cortical tumors: implications for tumorigenesis. J Clin Endocrinol Metab 1997; 82: 3054–3058.

266. Weber MM, Auernhammer CJ, Engelhardt D. Insulin-like growth factor receptors in normal and tumorous adult human adrenal cortical glands. Eur J Endocrinol 1997; 136: 296–303.

267. Boulle N, Logie A, Gicquel C, et al. Increased levels of insulin-like growth factor II (IGF-II) and IGF-binding protein-2 are associated with malignancy in sporadic adrenal cortical tumors. J Clin Endocrinol Metab 1998; 83: 1713–1720.

268. Nishi Y, Haji M, Takayanagi R, et al. In vivo and in vitro evidence for the production of inhibin-like immunoreactivity in human adrenal cortical adenomas and normal adrenal glands: relatively high secretion from adenomas manifesting Cushing's syndrome. Eur J Endocrinol 1995; 132: 292–299.

269. Pelkey TJ, Frierson HF, Mills SE, et al. The alpha subunit of inhibin in adrenal cortical neoplasia. Mod Pathol 1998; 11: 516–524.

270. Tartour E, Caillou B, Tenebaum F, et al. Immunohistochemical study of adrenal cortical carcinoma. Predictive value of the D11 monoclonal antibody. Cancer 1993 2: 3296–3303.

271. Busam KJ, Iversen K, Coplan KA, et al. Immunoreactivity for A103, an antibody to Melan-A (MART-1), in adrenal cortical and other steroid tumors. Am J Surg Pathol 1998; 22: 57–63.

272. Pan CC, Chen PC, Tsay SH, et al. Differential immunoprofiles of hepatocellular carcinoma, renal cell carcinoma and adrenal cortical carcinoma: a systemic immunohistochemical survey using tissue array technique. Appl Immunohistochem Mol Morphol 2005; 13: 347–351.

273. Kebebew E, Reiff E, Duh Qy, et al. Extent of disease at presentation and outcome for adrenal

cortical carcinoma: have we made progress? World J Surg 2006; 30: 872–878.

274. Wieneke JA, Thompson LDR, Heffess CS. Adrenal cortical neoplasms in the pediatric population. Am J Surg Pathol 2003; 27: 867–881.

275. Sbragia L, Oliveira-Filho Ag, Vassallo J, et al. Adrenal cortical tumors in Brazilian children: immunohistochemical markers and prognostic factors. Arch Pathol Lab Med 2005; 129: 1127–1131.

276. Decorato JW, Gruber H, Petti M, et al. Adrenal carcinosarcoma. J Surg Oncol 1990; 45: 134–136.

277. Fischler DF, Nunez C, Levin HS, et al. Adrenal carcinosarcoma presenting in a woman with clinical signs of virilization. A case report with immunohistochemical and ultrastructural findings. Am J Surg Pathol 1992; 16: 626–631.

278. Barksdale SK, Marincola FM. Carcinosarcoma of the adrenal cortex presenting with mineralocorticoid excess. Am J Surg Pathol 1993; 17: 941–945.

279. Molberg K, Vuitch F, Stewart D, et al. Adrenal cortical blastoma. Hum Pathol 1992; 23: 1187–1190.

280. Beard CM, Sheps SG, Kurland LT, et al. Occurrence of pheochromocytoma in Rochester, Minnesota, 1950 through 1979. Mayo Clin Proc 1983; 58: 802–804.

281. Lack EE. Adrenal medullary hyperplasia and pheochromocytoma. In: Lack EE, ed. Pathology of the adrenal glands. New York: Churchill Livingstone, 1990, 173–235.

282. Abbott MA, Nathanson KL, Nightingale S, et al. The early von Hippel–Lindau (VHL) germline mutation V84L manifests as early-onset bilateral pheochromocytoma. Am J Med Genet A 2006; 140: 685–690.

283. Neumann HPH, Bausch B, McWhinney SR, et al. Germ line mutations in nonsyndromic pheochromocytoma. N Engl J Med 2002; 346: 1459–1466.

284. Van Nederveen FH, Dinjens WN, Korpershoek E, et al. The occurrence of SDHB gene mutations in pheochromocytoma. Ann NY Acad Sci 2006; 1073: 177–182.

285. Pham TH, Moir C, Thompson GB, et al. Pheochromocytoma and paraganglioma in children: review of medical and surgical management at a tertiary care center. Pediatrics 2006; 118: 1109–1117.

286. Steinhoff MM, Wells SA Jr, DeSchryver-Kecskemeti K. Stromal amyloid in pheochromocytomas. Hum Pathol 1992; 23: 33–36.

287. Miranda RN, Wu D, Nayak RN, et al. Amyloid in adrenal gland pheochromocytomas. Arch Pathol Lab Med 1995; 119: 827–830.

288. Linnoila RI, Keiser HR, Steinberg SM, et al. Histopathology of benign versus malignant sympathoadrenal paragangliomas. Clinicopathologic study of 120 cases including unusual histologic features. Hum Pathol 1990; 21: 1168–1180.

289. Wang BY, Gabrilove L, Pertsemlidis D, et al. Oncocytic pheochromocytoma with cytokeratin reactivity (case report). Int J Surg Pathol 5: 61–68, 1997.

290. Li M, Wenig BM. Adrenal oncocytic pheochromocytoma (case report). Am J Surg Pathol 2000; 24: 1552–1557.

291. Ramsay JA, Asa SL, van Nostrand AWP, et al. Lipid degeneration in pheochromocytomas mimicking adrenal cortical tumors. Am J Surg Pathol 1987; 11: 480–486.

292. Unger PD, Cohen JM, Thung SN, et al. Lipid degeneration in a pheochromocytoma histologically mimicking an adrenal cortical tumor. Arch Pathol Lab Med 1990; 114: 892–894.

293. Melicow MM. Hibernating fat and pheochromocytoma. Arch Pathol 1957; 63: 367–372.

294. Medeiros LJ, Katsas GG, Balogh K. Brown fat and adrenal pheochromocytoma. Association or coincidence? Hum Pathol 1985; 16: 970–972.

295. Lack EE, Kim H, Reed K. Pigmented ('black') extra-adrenal paraganglioma. Am J Surg Pathol 1998; 22: 265–269.

296. Handa U, Khullar U, Mohan H. Pigmented pheochromocytoma. A report of a case with diagnosis by fine needle aspiration. Acta Cytol 2005; 49: 421–423.

297. Gertner ME, Kebebew E. Multiple endocrine neoplasia type 2. Curr Treat Options Oncol 2004; 5: 315–325.

298. Carney JA. Familial multiple endocrine neoplasia: the first 100 years. Am J Surg Pathol 2005; 29: 254–274.

299. Webb TA, Sheps SG, Carney JA. Differences between sporadic pheochromocytoma and pheochromocytoma in multiple endocrine neoplasia, type 2. Am J Surg Pathol 1980; 4: 121–126.

300. Carney JA, Go VLW, Sizemore GW, et al. Alimentary-tract ganglioneuromatosis. A major component of the syndrome of multiple endocrine neoplasia, type 2b. N Engl J Med 1976; 295: 1287–1291.

301. Lam KY, Lo CY. Composite pheochromocytoma-ganglioneuroma of the adrenal gland: an uncommon entity with distinctive clinicopathologic features. Endocrinol Pathol 1999; 10: 343–352.

302. Brady S, Lechan RM, Schwaitzberg SD, et al. Composite pheochromocytoma/ganglioneuroma of the adrenal gland associated with multiple endocrine neoplasia 2A. Am J Surg Pathol 1997; 21: 102–108.

303. Linnoila RI, Lack EE, Steinberg SM, et al. Decreased expression of neuropeptides in malignant paragangliomas: an immunohistochemical study. Hum Pathol 1988; 19: 41–50.

304. Chetty R, Pilla-ay P, Jaichand V. Cytokeratin expression in adrenal phaeochromocytomas and extra-adrenal paragangliomas. J Clin Pathol 1998; 51: 477–478.

305. Erlandson RA. Diagnostic transmission electron microscopy of tumors. New York: Raven Press, 1994.

306. Tannenbaum M. Ultrastructural pathology of adrenal medullary tumors. Pathol Annu 1970; 5: 145–171.

307. Symington T, Goodall AL. Studies in pheochromocytoma. I. Pathological aspects. Glas Med J 1953; 34: 75–96.

308. Hume DM. Pheochromocytoma in the adult and in the child. Am J Surg 1960; 99: 458–496.

309. Melicow MM. One hundred cases of pheochromocytoma (107 tumors) at the Columbia-Presbyterian Medical Center 1926–1976. A clinicopathological analysis. Cancer 1977; 40: 1987–2004.

310. Neville AM. The adrenal medulla. In: Symington T, ed. Functional pathology of the human adrenal gland. Baltimore: Williams & Wilkins, 1969; 219–324.

311. Wenig BM, Heffess CS, Adair CF. Neoplasms of the adrenal gland. In: Wenig BM, Heffess CS, Adair CF, eds. Atlas of endocrine pathology. Philadelphia: WB Saunders, 1997; 288–329.

312. Thompson LDR. Pheochromocytoma of the adrenal gland scaled score (PASS) to separate benign from malignant neoplasms: a clinicopathologic and immunophenotypic study of 100 cases. Am J Surg Pathol 2002; 26: 551–566.

313. Kimura N, Watanabe T, Noshiro T, et al. Histologic grading of adrenal and extra-adrenal pheochromocytomas and relationship to prognosis: a clinicopathological analysis of 116 adrenal pheochromocytomas and 30 extra-adrenal sympathetic paragangliomas including 38 malignant tumors. Endocrinol Pathol 2005; 16: 23–32.

314. Gao B, Meng F, Bian W, et al. Development and validation of pheochromocytoma of the adrenal gland scaled score for predicting malignant pheochromocytomas. Urology 2006; 68: 282–286.

315. Hosaka Y, Rainwater LM, Grant CS, et al. Pheochromocytoma: nuclear deoxyribonucleic acid patterns studied by flow cytometry. Surgery 1986; 100: 1003–1010.

316. Nativ O, Grant CS, Sheps SG, et al. The clinical significance of nuclear DNA ploidy pattern in 184 patients

with pheochromocytoma. Cancer 1992; 69: 2683–2687.

317. Kliewer KE, Wen D-R, Cancilla PA, et al. Paragangliomas: assessment of prognosis by histologic, immunohistochemical, and ultrastructural techniques. Hum Pathol 1989; 20: 29–39.

318. Kliewer KE, Cochran AJ. A review of the histology, ultrastructure, immunohistology, and molecular biology of extra-adrenal paragangliomas. Arch Pathol Lab Med 1989; 113: 1209–1218.

319. Linnoila RI, Becker RL Jr, Steinberg SM, et al. The role of S-100 protein containing cells in the prognosis of sympathoadrenal paragangliomas. Mod Pathol 1993; 6: 39A.

320. Clarke MR, Weyant RJ, Watson CG, et al. Prognostic markers in pheochromocytoma. Hum Pathol 1998; 29: 522–526.

321. Kubota Y, Nakada T, Sasagawa I, et al. Elevated levels of telomerase activity in malignant pheochromocytoma. Cancer 1998; 82: 176–179.

322. Easter DW, Katz M. Laparoscopic adrenalectomy for pheochromocytoma – a new standard? Curr Surg 2002; 59: 450–454.

323. Guerrieri M, Baldarelli M, Scarpelli M, et al. Laparoscopic adrenalectomy in pheochromocytoma. J Endocrinol Invest 2005; 28: 523–527.

324. Li ML, Fitzgerald PA, Price DC, et al. Iatrogenic pheochromocytomatosis: a previously unreported result of laparoscopic adrenalectomy. Surgery 2001; 130: 1072–1077.

325. Shimada J, Ambros IM, Dehner LP, et al. Terminology and morphologic criteria of neuroblastic tumors. Cancer 1999; 86: 349–363.

326. Ries LA, Smith MA, Gurney JG, et al. (eds) Cancer incidence and survival among children and adolescents; United States SEER Program 1975–1995. Bethesda, MD: National Cancer Institute, SEER Program, 1999. NIH Pub. No. 99-4649.

327. Rosen EM, Cassady JR, Frantz CN, et al. Neuroblastoma: the Joint Center for Radiation Therapy/Dana-Farber Cancer Institute/Children's Hospital experience. J Clin Oncol 1984; 2: 719–732.

328. Franks LM, Bollen A, Seeger RC, et al. Neuroblastoma in adults and adolescents. Cancer 1997; 79: 2028–2035.

329. Kushner BH, Gilbert F, Helson L. Familial neuroblastoma: case reports, literature review and etiologic considerations. Cancer 1986; 57: 1887–1893.

330. Brodeur GM. Molecular biology and genetics of human neuroblastoma. In: Pochedly C, ed. Neuroblastoma: tumor biology and therapy. Boca Raton: CRC Press, 1990, 31–50.

331. Lack EE, Kozakewich HPW. Adrenal neuroblastoma, ganglioneuroblastoma, and related tumors. In: Lack EE, ed. Pathology of the adrenal glands. New York: Churchill Livingstone, 1990; 277–309.

332. Sawada T. Past and future of neuroblastoma screening in Japan. Am J Ped Hematol Oncol 1992; 14: 320–326.

333. Seviour JA, McGill AC, Craft AW, et al. Screening for neuroblastoma in the northern region of England. Laboratory aspects. Am J Pediatr Hematol Oncol 1992; 14: 332–336.

334. Treuner J, Shilling FH. Neuroblastoma mass screening: the arguments for and against. Eur J Cancer 1995; 31A: 565–568.

335. Kerble R, Urban CE, Ambros PF, et al. Screening for neuroblastoma in late infancy by the EIA method: 115,000 screened infants in Austria. Eur J Cancer 1996; 32A. 2298–2305.

336. Nishi M, Miyake H, Takeda T, et al. Mass screening for neuroblastoma targeting children age 14 months in Sapporo City. Cancer 1998; 82: 1973–1977.

337. Ater JL, Gardner KL, Foxhall LE, et al. Neuroblastoma screening in the United States. Results of the Texas outreach program for neuroblastoma screening. Cancer 1998; 82: 1593–1602.

338. Hachitanda Y, Ishimoto K, Naito M, et al. 100 neuroblastomas detected through mass screening system in Japan. Mod Pathol 1993; 6: 4.

339. Woods WG, Tuchman M, Robison LL, et al. A population-based study of the usefulness of screening for neuroblastoma. Lancet 1996; 348: 1682–1697.

340. Woods WG, Gao RN, Shuster JJ, et al. Screening of infants and mortality due to neuroblastoma. N Engl J Med 2002; 346: 1041–1046.

341. Schilling F, Spiz C, Berthold F, et al. Neuroblastoma screening at one year of age. N Engl J Med 2002; 346: 1047–53.

342. Adam A, Hochholzer L. Ganglioneuroblastoma of the posterior mediastinum. Cancer 1981; 47: 373–381.

343. Triche TJ. Differential diagnosis of neuroblastoma and related tumors. In: Lack EE, ed. Pathology of the adrenal glands. New York: Churchill Livingstone, 1990; 323–350.

344. Wright JH. Neurocytoma or neuroblastoma, a kind of tumor not generally recognized. J Exp Med 1910; 12: 556–561.

345. Cozzutto C, Carbone A. Pleomorphic (anaplastic) neuroblastoma. Arch Pathol Lab Med 1988; 112: 621–625.

346. Chatten J. Anaplastic neuroblastoma. Arch Pathol Lab Med 1989; 113: 9–10.

347. Shimada H, Aoyama C, Chiba T, et al. Prognostic subgroups for undifferentiated neuroblastoma: immunohistochemical study with anti-S-100 protein antibody. Hum Pathol 1985; 16: 471–476.

348. Beckwith JB, Martin RF. Observations on the histopathology of neuroblastomas. J Pediatr Surg 1986; 3: 106–110.

349. Hughes M, Marsden HB, Palmer MK. Histologic patterns of neuroblastoma related to prognosis and clinical staging. Cancer 1974; 34: 1706–1711.

350. Shimada H, Chatten J, Newton WA Jr, et al. Histopathologic prognostic factors in neuroblastic tumors: definition of subtypes of ganglioneuroblastoma and an age-linked classification of neuroblastomas. J Natl Cancer Inst 1984; 73: 405–416.

351. Chatten J, Shimada H, Sather HN, et al. Prognostic value of histopathology in advanced neuroblastoma: a report from the Children's Cancer Study Group. Hum Pathol 1988; 19: 1187–1198.

352. Joshi VV, Chatten J, Sather HN, et al. Evaluation of the Shimada classification in advanced neuroblastoma with a special reference to the mitosis–karyorrhexis index: a report from the Children's Cancer Study Group. Mod Pathol 1991; 4: 139–147.

353. Joshi VV, Cantor AB, Altschuler G, et al. Age-linked prognostic categorization based on a new histologic grading system of neuroblastomas: a clinicopathologic study of 211 cases from the Pediatric Oncology Group. Cancer 1992; 69: 2197–2211.

354. Shimada H, Ambros I, Dehner L, et al. The International Neuroblastoma Pathology Classification (the Shimada System). Cancer 1999; 86: 364–372.

355. Shimada H, Umehara S, Monobe Y, et al. International neuroblastoma pathology classification for prognostic evaluation of patients with peripheral neuroblastic tumors. A report from the Children's Cancer Group. Cancer 2001; 92: 2451–2461.

356. Sano H, Bonadio J, Gerbing RB, et al. International neuroblastoma pathology classification adds independent prognostic information beyond the prognostic contribution of age. Eur J Cancer 2006; 42: 1113–1119.

357. Umeharar S, Nakagawa A, Matthay KK, et al. Histopathology defines prognostic subsets of ganglioneuroblastoma, nodular. Cancer 2000; 89: 1150–1161.

358. Peuchmaur M, d'Amore ESG, Joshi VV, et al. Revision of the international neuroblastoma pathology classification. Confirmation of favorable and unfavorable prognostic subsets in ganglioneuroblastoma, nodular. Cancer 2003; 98: 2274–2281.

359. Shimada H, Stram DO, Chatten J, et al. Identification of subsets of neuroblastomas by combined histopathologic and N-myc analysis. J Natl Cancer Inst 1995; 87: 1470–1476.

360. Goto S, Umehara S, Gerbing RB, et al. Histopathology (international neuroblastoma pathology classification) and myc-N status in patients with peripheral neuroblastic tumors. Cancer 2001; 92: 2699–2708.

361. Evans AE, D'Angio GJ, Randolph J. A proposed staging for children with neuroblastoma. Children's Cancer Study Group A. Cancer 1971; 27: 374–378.

362. Evans AE, D'Angio GJ, Sather HN, et al. A comparison of four staging systems for localized and regional neuroblastoma: a report from the Children's Cancer Study Group. J Clin Oncol 1990; 8: 678–688.

363. Bowman LC, Santana VM, Green AA, et al. Staging systems in neuroblastoma: which is best? J Clin Oncol 1991; 9: 189–193.

364. Philip T. Overview of current treatment of neuroblastoma. Am J Pediatr Hematol Oncol 1992; 14: 97–102.

365. Brodeur GM, Pritchard J, Berthold F, et al. Revisions of the international criteria for neuroblastoma diagnosis, staging, and response to treatment. J Clin Oncol 1993; 11: 1466–1477.

366. Beckwith JB, Perrin EV. In situ neuroblastomas: a contribution to the natural history of neural crest tumors. Am J Pathol 1963; 43: 1089–1104.

367. Turkel SB, Itabashi HH. The natural history of neuroblastic cells in the fetal adrenal gland. Am J Pathol 1974; 76: 225–236.

368. Evans AE, Baum E, Chard R. Do infants with stage IV-S neuroblastoma need treatment? Arch Dis Child 1981; 56: 271–274.

369. Hachitanda Y, Hata J. Stage IVS Neuroblastoma. A clinical, histological and biological analysis of 45 cases. Hum Pathol 1996; 27: 1135–1138.

370. Stephenson SR, Cook BA, Mease AD, et al. The prognostic significance of age and pattern of metastases in stage IV-S neuroblastoma. Cancer 1986; 58: 372–375.

371. Knudson AG Jr, Meadows AT. Regression of neuroblastoma IV-S: a genetic hypothesis. N Engl J Med 1980; 302: 1254–1256.

372. Cushing H, Wolbach SB. The transformation of a malignant paravertebral sympathicoblastoma into a benign ganglioneuroma. Am J Pathol 1927; 3: 203–216.

373. Collins VP. Wilms' tumor: its behavior and prognosis. J La State Med Soc 1955; 107: 474–480.

374. Willis RA. The spread of tumors in the human body, 3rd edn. London: Butterworths, 1973, 102–105.

375. Scully RE, Cohen RB. Ganglioneuroma of adrenal medulla containing cells morphologically identical to hilus cells (extraparenchymal Leydig cells). Cancer 1961; 14: 421–425.

376. Aguirre P, Scully RE. Testosterone-secreting adrenal ganglioneuroma containing Leydig cells. Am J Surg Pathol 1983; 7: 699–705.

377. Evans CP, Vaccaro JA, Storrs BG, et al. Suprarenal occurrence of an adenomatoid tumor. J Urol 1988; 139: 348.

378. Simpson PR. Adenomatoid tumor of the adrenal gland. Arch Pathol Lab Med 1990; 114: 725–727.

379. Travis WD, Lack EE, Azumi N, et al. Adenomatoid tumor of the adrenal gland with ultrastructural and immunohistochemical demonstration of a mesothelial origin. Arch Pathol Lab Med 1990; 114: 722–724.

380. Ra-af HN, Grant LD, Santoscoy C, et al. Adenomatoid tumor of the adrenal gland: a report of four new cases and a review of the literature. Mod Pathol 1996; 9: 1046–1051.

381. Angeles-Angeles A, Reyes E, Munoz-Fernandez L, et al. Adenomatoid tumor of the right adrenal gland in a patient with AIDS. Endocrinol Pathol 1997; 8: 59–63.

382. Craig JR, Hart WR. Extragenital adenomatoid tumor: evidence for mesothelial theory of origin. Cancer 1979; 43: 1678.

383. Benisch BM. A retroperitoneal mesonephric cystadenoma with features of the adenomatoid tumor of the genital tract. J Urol 1973; 110: 44.

384. Hanrahan JB. A combined papillary mesothelioma and adenomatoid tumor of the omentum: report of a case. Cancer 1963; 16: 1497–1500.

385. Isotalo PA, Keeney GL, Sebo TJ, et al. Adenomatoid tumor of the adrenal gland: a clinicopathologic study of five cases and review of the literature. Am J Surg Pathol 2003; 27: 969–977.

386. Garg K, Lee P, Ro JY, et al. Adenomatoid tumor of the adrenal gland: a clinicopathologic study of 3 cases. Ann Diagn Pathol 2005; 9: 11–15.

387. Airaghi L, Greco I, Carrabba M, et al. Unusual presentation of large B cell lymphoma: a case report and review of literature. Clin Lab Haematol 2006; 28: 338–342.

388. Li Y, Sun H, Gao S, et al. Primary bilateral adrenal lymphoma: 2 case reports. J Comput Assist Tomogr 2006; 30: 791–793.

389. Thompson MA, Habra MA, Routbort MJ, et al. Primary adrenal natural killer/T-cell nasal type lymphoma: first case report in adults. Am J Hematol 2006 [Epub].

390. Diamanti-Kandarakis E, Chatzismalis P, Economou F, et al. Primary adrenal lymphoma presented with adrenal insufficiency. Hormones 2004; 3: 68–72.

391. Page DL, DeLellis RA, Hough AJ. Tumors of the adrenal. In: Atlas of tumor pathology, AFIP 2nd series, fascicle 23. Washington, DC: Armed Forces Institute of Pathology, 1986, 162–173.

392. Ohsawa M, Tomita Y, Hashimoto M, et al. Malignant lymphoma of the adrenal gland. Its possible correlation with the Epstein–Barr virus. Mod Pathol 1996; 9: 534–543.

393. Livaditou A, Alexiou G, Floros D, et al. Epithelioid angiosarcoma of the adrenal gland associated with chronic arsenical intoxication? Pathol Res Pract 1991; 187: 284–289.

394. Ben-Izhak O, Auslander L, Rabinson S, et al. Epithelioid angiosarcoma of the adrenal gland with cytokeratin expression. Report of a case with accompanying mesenteric fibromatosis. Cancer 1992; 69: 1808–1812.

395. Wenig BM, Abbondanzo SL, Heffess CS. Epithelioid angiosarcoma of the adrenal glands. A clinicopathologic study of nine cases with a discussion of the implications of finding 'epithelial-specific' markers. Am J Surg Pathol 1994; 18: 62–73.

396. Lin J, Wasco MJ, Korokbin M, et al. Leiomyoma of the adrenal gland presenting as a non-functioning adrenal incidentaloma: case report and review of the literature. Endocr Pathol (in press).

397. Lack EE, Graham CW, Azumi N, et al. Primary leiomyosarcoma of adrenal gland. Case report with immunohistochemical and ultrastructural study. Am J Surg Pathol 1991; 15: 899–905.

398. Zetler PJ, Filipenko D, Bilbey JH, et al. Primary adrenal leiomyosarcoma in a man with acquired immunodeficiency syndrome. Arch Pathol Lab Med 1995; 119: 1164–1167.

399. Ayala GE, Ettinghausen SE, Epstein AH, et al. Primary malignant peripheral nerve sheath tumor of the adrenal gland. Case report and literature review. J Urol Pathol 1994; 2: 265–272.

400. Min KW, Clemens A, Bell J, Kick H. Malignant peripheral nerve sheath tumor and pheochromocytoma. A composite tumor of the adrenal. Arch Pathol Lab Med 1988; 112: 266–270.

401. Dao AH, Page DL, Reynolds VH, et al. Primary malignant melanoma of the adrenal gland. A report of two cases and review of the literature. Am Surg 1990; 56: 199–203.

402. Granero LE, Al-Lawati T, Bobin UY. Primary melanoma of the adrenal gland, a continuous dilemma. Report of a case. Surg Today 2004; 34: 554–556.

403. Bastide C, Arroua F, Carcenas A, et al. Primary malignant melanoma of the adrenal gland. Int J Urol 2006; 13: 608–610.

404. Fidler WJ. Ovarian thecal metaplasia in adrenal glands. Am J Clin Pathol 1977; 67: 318–323.

405. Carney JA. Unusual tumefactive spindle cell lesions in the adrenal glands. Hum Pathol 1987; 18: 980–985.

406. Prevot S, Penna C, Imbert, JC, et al. Solitary fibrous tumor of the adrenal gland. Mod Pathol 1996; 9: 1170–1174.

407. Bongiovanni M, Viberti L, Giraudo G, et al. Solitary fibrous tumour of the adrenal gland associated with pregnancy. Virchows Arch 2000; 437: 445–449.

408. Orselli RC, Bassler TJ. Theca granulosa tumor arising in the adrenal. Cancer 1973; 31: 474–477.

Page numbers in **bold** represent tables, those in *italics* represent figures

**THE LIBRARY**
THE LEARNING AND DEVELOPMENT CENTRE
THE CALDERDALE ROYAL HOSPITAL
HALIFAX HX3 0RW

THE LIBRARY
THE ............ NG AND DEVELOPMENT CENTRE
THE CALDERDALE ......... HOSPITAL
HALIFAX HX3 0PW